### Want to Know





### Clinical Pathways

# Foundations of Maternal-Newborn Nursing

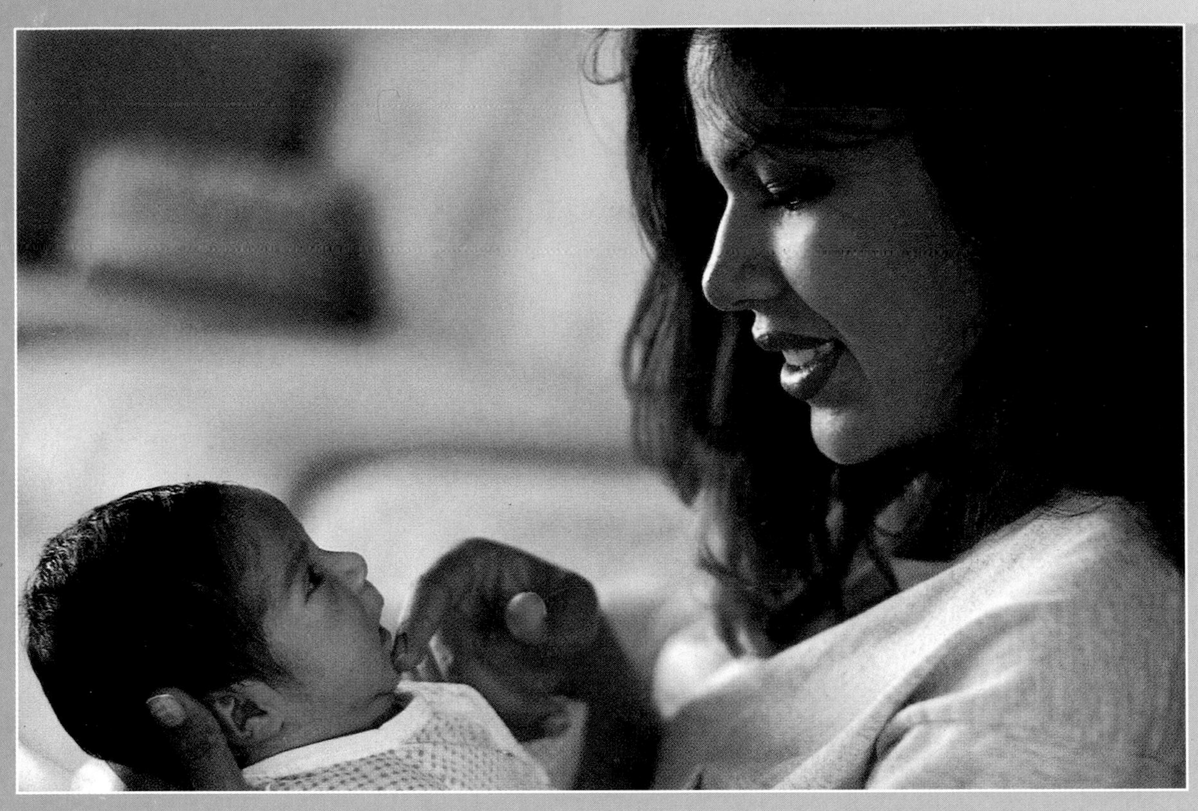

W.B. SAUNDERS COMPANY
*A Division of Harcourt Brace & Company*

Philadelphia London Toronto Montreal Sydney Tokyo

Trula Myers Gorrie, M.N., R.N.,C.
Professor Emeritus
Golden West College
Huntington Beach, California

Emily Slone McKinney, M.S.N., R.N.,C.
Formerly Faculty of Grayson County College
Sherman-Denison, Texas and
Tarrant County Junior College
Fort Worth, Texas

Sharon Smith Murray, M.S.N., R.N.,C.
Professor, Health Professions
Golden West College
Huntington Beach, California

# *Foundations of* Maternal-Newborn Nursing

second edition

**W.B. SAUNDERS COMPANY**
*A Division of Harcourt Brace & Company*

The Curtis Center
Independence Square West
Philadelphia, Pennsylvania 19106

**NOTICE**

Nursing is an ever-changing field. Standard safety precautions must be followed, but as new research and clinical experience broaden our knowledge, changes in treatment and drug therapy become necessary or appropriate. Readers are advised to check the product information currently provided by the manufacturer of each drug to be administered to verify the recommended dose, the method and duration of administration, and contraindications. It is the responsibility of the treating physician relying on experience and knowledge of the patient to determine dosages and the best treatment for the patient. Neither the Publisher nor the editor assumes any responsibility for any injury and/or damage to persons or property.

THE PUBLISHER

**Library of Congress Cataloging-in-Publication Data**

Gorrie, Trula.

Foundations of maternal-newborn nursing / Trula Myers Gorrie, Emily Slone McKinney, Sharon Smith Murray.—2nd ed.

p. cm.

Includes bibliographical references and index.

ISBN 0–7216–8652–4

1. Maternity nursing. I. McKinney, Emily Slone. II. Murray, Sharon Smith. III. Title.
[DNLM: 1. Maternal-Child Nursing. 2. Family Health. WY 157.3 G673f 1998]

RG951.G668 1998 610.73′678—dc21

DNLM/DLC 97–18556

Foundations of Maternal-Newborn Nursing ISBN 0–7216–8652–4



Printed in the United States of America

Last digit is the print number: 9 8 7 6 5 4 3 2 1

*To Clayton, my support and comfort through this and all other projects. And to the next generation — Macy, Brian, Michele, and Jacie — with love and thanksgiving.*
T.M.G.

*To Michael. I am so glad God gave you to me.*
E.S.M.

*To Skip for his love and encouragement. To Vicki, Holly, and Shannon for their understanding and support. To my mother, Clare, my role model throughout life, and to Marina and Nicholas for bringing great joy to us all.*
S.S.M.

## Reviewers

Katherine G. Bowman, M.S.N., R.N.
Instructor of Clinical Nursing, University of Missouri, Columbia, Missouri

Linda L. Reeder Breidigam, M.S.N., R.N., C.C.E.
School of Nursing, Alvernia College, Reading, Pennsylvania

Sandra Godman Brown, D.S.N., R.N.
College of Nursing, Medical University of South Carolina, Charleston, South Carolina

Janis M. Byers, M.S.N., R.N.
School of Nursing, Sewickley Valley Hospital, Sewickley, Pennsylvania

Donna F. Cheatham, M.S., R.N.
School of Nursing, Kettering College of Medical Arts, Kettering, Ohio

Patricia A. Creehan, M.S.N., R.N.,C.
Palos Community Hospital, Palos Heights, Illinois

Francine de Montigny, M.S.N., R.N.
Professor, Department of Nursing, University of Quebec in Hull, Hull, Quebec, Canada

Velora Elthea Ferris, M.N., R.N.
School of Nursing, Mt. San Antonio College, Walnut, California

Linda S. Foley, M.S.N., R.N.
Associate Professor of Nursing, Nebraska Methodist College, Omaha, Nebraska

Kathleen K. Furniss, M.S.N., R.N.,C.
School of Nursing, University of Medicine and Dentistry of New Jersey, Newark; and Associates in Women's Health Care, Wayne, New Jersey

Debra A. Gilhooly, B.S.N., R.N.
Cochran School of Nursing, St. John's Riverside Hospital, Yonkers, New York

Janice G. Harris, M.S.N., R.N.,C.
Associate Professor of Nursing, Columbus State University, Columbus, Georgia

Mary Katherine Bourgeois Harris, M.S.N., C.F.N.P.
Certified Lactation Consultant, ASPO/Lamaze Instructor, Kaiser Permanente Hospital, Huntingon Beach, California

Linda C. Hildenbrand, M.S., R.N.
School of Nursing, Hagerstown Junior College, Hagerstown, Maryland

Patricia L. Hiser, M.S., R.N.
Associate Professor of Nursing, Clinton Community College, Plattsburgh, New York

Carolyn May Kaple, M.S., R.N.
Associate Professor of Nursing, North Central Technical College, Mansfield, Ohio

Cynthia Kirbie, C.R.N.A., A.N.P.
John Peter Smith Hospital, and Adjunct Faculty, Texas Wesleyan University, Fort Worth, Texas

Catherine Gannon Kocur, M.B.A., M.S., R.N.,C.
Cochran School of Nursing, St. John's Riverside Hospital, Yonkers, New York

Linda Koehl, M.S., R.N.,C.
Mt. Sinai Hospital Medical Center, Chicago, Illinois

Nancy A. Markin, M.S.N., M.S., R.N.
School of Nursing, Oakton Community College, Des Plaines, Illinois

Cheryl M. Martin, M.S.N., O.G.N.P., R.N.,C.
School of Nursing, Bethel College, Mishawaka, Indiana

Gloria Mondor Matsuura, M.S., R.N., C.N.M., A.C.C.E.
School of Nursing, University of Minnesota, Minneapolis, Minnesota

Alison Benzies Miklos, M.S.N., R.N.,C.
Christ Hospital and Medical Center, Oak Lawn, Illinois

Karen Sanders Moore, M.S.N., R.N.,C., I.B.C.L.C.
St. John's Mercy Medical Center, St. Louis, Missouri

Joyce J. Morris, M.S., R.N., A.R.N.P., C.N.M.
Family Health Center of Southwest Florida, Inc., Ft. Myers, Florida

Alyce Rochelle Patterson, M.S.N., R.N.
School of Nursing, Southern West Virginia Community and Technical College, Logan, West Virginia

Kathleen Ann Russell, M.S.N., R.N.,C.
School of Nursing, Front Range Community College, Westminster, Colorado

Barbara A. Schell, M.M.Ed., R.N.
School of Nursing, Western Pennsylvania Hospital, Pittsburgh, Pennsylvania

Elizabeth S. Sergio, M.S.N., R.N.,C.
School of Nursing, Massachusetts Bay Community College, Wellesley, Massachusetts

LuAnn R. Smith, B.S.N., R.N., I.B.C.L.C.
York Health System, York, Pennsylvania

Mary Ellen Burke Sosa, M.S., R.N.,C.
Women and Infants Hospital of Rhode Island and Brown University School of Medicine, Providence, Rhode Island

Sheila Hughes Stewart, M.S.N., C.R.N.P.
School of Nursing, Alvernia College, Reading, Pennsylvania

Jean Tillman, M.S.N., R.N.
School of Nursing, Holyoke Community College, Holyoke, Massachusetts

Paula A. Viau, Ph.D., R.N.
College of Nursing, University of Rhode Island, Kingston, Rhode Island

Catherine L. Witt, M.S., N.N.P.
Women's and Children's Services, P/SL Medical Center, Denver, Colorado

Linda Sue Wood, M.S.N., R.N.
School of Nursing, DePaul Medical Center, Norfolk, Virginia

Marian Yavorka, M.S., M.S.N., R.N.
School of Nursing, Mercy Hospital, Pittsburgh, Pennsylvania

# Preface

The challenge of nursing education is to keep pace with rapid changes in technology and in health care delivery and, at the same time, to prepare students to participate in care during their brief clinical rotations. Although health care delivery has changed dramatically, with more emphasis on outcomes management and clinical pathways to decrease the length of stay in the birth facility, there has been no lessening of the family's need for education and support during the childbearing period. Nurses have responded to families' needs by expanding alternatives. Clinical experience is no longer confined to the birth facility but may now take place in the home and in a variety of community clinics.

We recognize that nursing students differ in learning abilities and experience. Therefore, an effective textbook must present comprehensive content that can be read with ease. Major objectives of the second edition of *Foundations of Maternal-Newborn Nursing* are to present complex material as simply and clearly as possible and to provide step-by-step instruction in assessments and interventions so students can function quickly in the clinical area at a beginning level. To this end, proven learning aids, such as summaries, illustrations, tables, and highlights, are used generously throughout the book.

## Content

Maternity nurses must be flexible to accommodate families with different languages and different health beliefs. Nurses must be prepared to use critical thinking skills to devise culture-specific care that includes providing necessary education and support. The six elements we consider most important are a scientific base of information, nursing process, communication, client teaching, critical thinking, and cultural diversity.

### SCIENTIFIC BASE

Effective nursing care depends on a sound understanding of the physiologic bases for medical treatments and nursing actions. Although anatomy and physiology courses are part of every curriculum, students often need a review, particularly of the specific content related to childbearing. Because of this, we have incorporated sound principles of physiology and pathophysiology throughout the book. We have presented these scientific concepts in a clear and understandable manner so the reader can comprehend the forces that underlie both health and dysfunction.

Chapters 4, 5, and 6 provide basic information about reproductive physiology, genetics, and the process of conception and fetal development. Chapters 7, 12, 17, and 19 explain physiologic adaptation during pregnancy, birth, and the postpartum period, and in the newborn. Part V, Families at Risk During the Childbearing Period, describes the pathophysiologic, psychological, and social bases of complications in the mother and in the newborn.

### NURSING PROCESS

Nursing process is the accepted framework for client assessment and analysis of client needs. It is used to plan and provide nursing care and to evaluate the client's response to care. Client needs are often a mixture of those for which nurses have the primary accountability and those for which another discipline provides definitive therapy yet for which nurses have some responsibility. Thus, when analyzing client needs we have chosen either a *nursing diagnosis* or a *collaborative problem* depending on whether nurses are primarily responsible for helping the client meet those needs. All nursing diagnoses are drawn from the most recent list of those approved by the North American Nursing Diagnosis Association (NANDA).

Both narrative text and nursing care plans are used to show the student how nursing process can be applied to maternity care. In each method we lead the reader through the five steps of the nursing process. In the narrative text, basic knowledge is presented and nursing care follows, organized by the steps of nursing process and supported by rationales. Because nursing students often have difficulty transferring knowledge to the care of a specific client, we have also created nursing care plans based on scenarios of client situations frequently encountered in maternity nursing.

### COMMUNICATION

Although they are seldom included as core content in maternal-newborn nursing texts, communication skills are essential to provide adequate care for a childbearing family. We reinforce the student's previous learning and give practical examples of how to use communication skills in the maternity setting.

Guidelines and examples of effective communication and potential blocks are reviewed in Chapter 2. Color-highlighted *communication cues* in the text give tips on how to interact with families. Tips include ways to avoid potentially embarrassing situations, role modeling of effective communication styles, and reading nonverbal signals. Communication cues are listed in the index for easy access.

In addition, dialogues throughout the text present realistic possible nurse-client interactions. As the interaction develops, we identify communication techniques and explain the rationale. Because no one is perfect, we occasionally insert communication blocks, identify them, and suggest alternate responses.

#### CLIENT TEACHING

Childbearing families expect, and are entitled to, comprehensive information about how to achieve the best pregnancy outcome. Nurses are the primary instructors in most areas of maternal-newborn nursing, and to be effective they must be well prepared and well organized. We present client teaching in three ways:

- Teaching-learning principles are reviewed in Chapter 2.
- Chapters are organized to highlight key content so that the student can gather information and translate it into client teaching. For example, Chapter 22, Infant Feeding, lays a foundation of basic information, discusses some of the common problems, identifies relevant assessments, and presents nursing interventions devoted to teaching parents how to feed their infant successfully.
- Client teaching guidelines are highlighted in *Want to Know* features, which give practical instructions on how to answer the most common client questions. These features have been constructed to show students how to present information in everyday language so the family will better understand the teaching. Many boxed features relate to home care. For instance, the feature "When to Go to the Hospital or Birth Center" addresses the learning needs of a woman who is concerned that she may not recognize the signs of true labor.

#### CRITICAL THINKING

Nurses must learn critical thinking skills to overcome habits or impulses that can lead to poor clinical decisions. Chapter 3 discusses steps in critical thinking and describes how critical thinking is used in each step of the nursing process. In addition, critical thinking exercises are presented in two ways. First, there are exercises throughout the text that are based on common clinical scenarios with questions to stimulate critical thinking. Answers to the questions follow each exercise to provide positive reinforcement for student learning. Second, specific nursing care plans, described earlier, contain critical thinking exercises that require participation by the student. This makes the care plans interactive and reinforces the concept of critical thinking in clinical practice.

#### CULTURAL DIVERSITY

Cultural values are among the most significant factors that influence a woman's perception of childbirth, and effective nursing care must be culture specific. This requires nurses to consider their own cultural values and to examine how these values may create conflict with those whose values are different.

Chapter 1 offers an overview of Western cultural values and identifies some areas, such as communication and health beliefs, that may be a source of conflict. Because there are many different cultural groups in the United States and Canada, emphasis is placed on how to do a cultural assessment. Plans for care can then show respect for cultural differences and traditional healing practices.

Additional information is integrated throughout the book in specific areas, such as nutrition, birth, the postpartum period, and care of the newborn.

## Organization

The second edition of *Foundations of Maternal-Newborn Nursing* is divided into six parts. Part I presents an overview of contemporary maternity care, including ethical, social, and legal aspects. A review of reproductive anatomy and physiology and the hereditary and environmental factors that affect care are also presented. This material is especially important for students who have not recently completed a full anatomy and physiology course.

**Part II, The Family Before Birth,** begins with conception and fetal development. The chapters also cover the physiologic and psychosocial adaptations to pregnancy and include a thorough explanation of recommended nutrition during pregnancy and after childbirth.

**Part III, The Family During Birth,** addresses the physiologic processes of birth and nursing care during labor and birth. These chapters include intrapartum fetal monitoring, pain management, and obstetric procedures, such as cesarean birth.

**Part IV, The Family Following Birth,** describes care of the new mother and infant. Alternative methods for continuing care, such as nurse-managed postpartum clinics and home care, are also covered. Separate chapters address infant nutrition and home care of the infant.

**Part V, Families at Risk During the Childbearing Period,** includes a chapter on the family with special needs, such as age-related concerns, childbearing in a substance-abusing or violent environment, birth of an infant with congenital anomalies, and responses to fetal and neonatal death. Additional chapters describe the most common complications of pregnancy, childbirth, and the postpartum and neonatal periods.

**Part VI, Other Reproductive Issues,** focuses on family planning, care of the infertile couple, and women's health care.

## Features

- *Visual Appeal.* The book is visually appealing with numerous full color illustrations and photographs that are used to clarify concepts and reinforce learning. Beautiful color pictures also illustrate a childbirth story and cesarean birth.
- *Objectives and Definitions.* Each chapter begins with a list of objectives that spells out the purposes of the chapter. A list of key terms with their definitions follows the objectives. A glossary at the back of the book summarizes key terms from all chapters.
- *Check Your Reading Questions.* At intervals throughout each chapter we have included questions that help students monitor their understanding of the material presented. Answers to questions are presented in Appendix E so students can have immediate feedback.
- *Critical Thinking Exercises.* Clinical situations are boxed and set apart to stimulate critical thinking. We believe strongly that immediate feedback is a powerful learning tool, so answers to critical thinking exercises in the text and in the specific nursing care plans are also included.
- *Critical to Remember.* The most important points of information are boxed and set apart to alert students that these are critical facts.
- *Want to Know.* These include answers to the most common questions that women or parents ask. They can be used by students who must begin teaching very early in their clinical rotation.
- *Procedures and Drug Guides.* Illustrated procedures that are specific to maternity nursing, such as assessment of the uterine fundus, are presented in a step-by-step format with rationales for each step. Drug guides for drugs commonly administered in maternity nursing and women's health care are also available in appropriate chapters.
- *Summary Concepts.* A concise review of content is provided at the end of each chapter. In addition, tables and flow charts are frequently used to summarize complex material.
- *Keys to Clinical Practice.* A description of how to prepare for clinical experience is presented in Appendix D. This feature provides care guides for assessments and interventions for the woman in labor, the woman following childbirth, and the infant. It also provides teaching on key topics, for example, assisting the inexperienced mother to breastfeed. This feature is designed to help students through their first clinical experiences.

## Teaching and Learning Support

- The *Instructor's Manual* was written by Carrie Pierce and Elizabeth Tipping, experienced educators in maternity nursing. The *Manual* contains suggested outlines for lectures, extra credit activities, critical thinking exercises, and suggestions for teaching-learning activities.
- *Transparencies* include 70 illustrations that we believe will be most useful in classroom teaching.
- A *Test Bank,* prepared by Patricia Montpas, Ed.D., R.N., provides 500 items that address the content of each chapter and relate to the chapter's objectives. Each item is assigned a cognitive level of knowledge, comprehension, or application. The test bank is also available in a computerized version, EXAM*aster*+, which offers the instructor numerous options in test construction.
- The *Study Guide,* new with this edition, presents a variety of additional activities designed to help students master content and to become more proficient in the clinical area. Numerous review questions, at various levels of difficulty, are included.
- A *Clinical Practice Manual* that provides a concise guide to maternal-newborn nursing is also available. The manual complements *Foundations of Maternal-Newborn Nursing* but can be used alone by nurses who need only a review. Its handy size makes it a portable reference book for the novice nurse or nursing student. It provides essential background information as well as an outline of assessments and interventions for the childbearing family.

## Acknowledgments

The second edition of *Foundations of Maternal-Newborn Nursing* would not have been possible without the contributions of many people. We were very fortunate to work with a group of reviewers who read the manuscript, shared their insights, and encouraged us by their comments. Their names are listed on a separate page. In addition, we want to thank Fountain Valley Regional Hospital and Medical Center, Saddleback Memorial Medical Center, and University of California, Irvine, Medical Center for helping us meet our needs for photographs as well as the many nurses, nursing students, and new parents who were so gracious in posing for them.

We owe a special debt of gratitude to Eric Woodward for the beautiful pictures that capture in color the concepts that are so difficult to put into words.

Every project has a key person, and for us that person was Marie Thomas, Editorial Assistant at W.B. Saunders Company, who was present throughout the entire project. She kept manuscript moving, patiently answered numerous questions, and calmly smoothed ruffled feathers.

We give special thanks to developmental editors Sharon Cloud Hogan and Debra Osnowitz. They gave necessary criticism in a most constructive manner and helped refine and organize this complex project. We are grateful to Lee Ann Draud, Copy Editor at Saunders, whose careful attention to detail smoothed our writing and helped create a seamless text. Laurie Sander, Production Manager, efficiently guided our project while patiently reassuring us that we were going to finish on time.

Sandra Sevigny, medical illustrator, worked with us to create illustrations that add so much to the text. Pat Morrison, Director of Art and Design, provided invaluable assistance with illustrations throughout the long process. We thank Karen O'Keefe, Designer, for the cover that conveys our commitment to mothers and infants and for the clear and attractive page layouts.

We thank Ilze Rader, former Editor, for bringing the three of us together and initiating the text. We also want to thank Maura Connor, Senior Editor at Saunders, and Victoria Legnini, Editorial Assistant, for helping us put the finishing touches on the text and for assistance with all the ancillaries.

TRULA MYERS GORRIE
EMILY SLONE MCKINNEY
SHARON SMITH MURRAY

# Brief Contents



Test II - 1, 2, 6, 7, 8, 9, 10, 11, 25, 26

# Detailed Contents

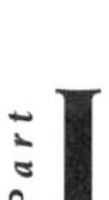 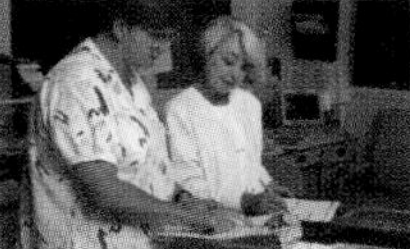

## Foundations for Nursing Care of Childbearing Families 1



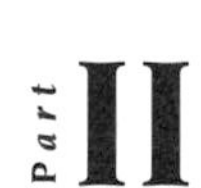 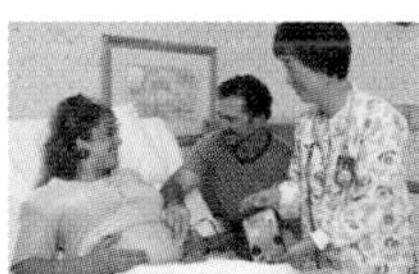

## The Family Before Birth 95

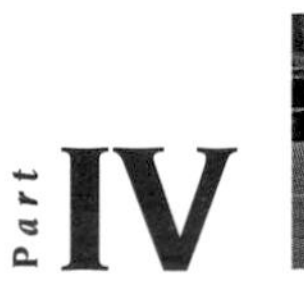
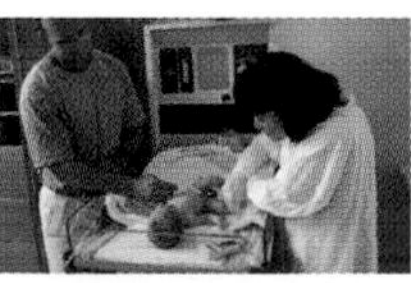

## Part IV The Family Following Birth 425

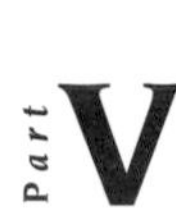
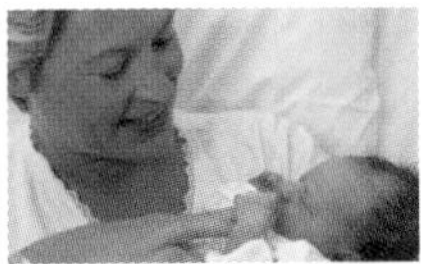

# Part V Families at Risk During the Childbearing Period 635

# Part I

# Foundations for Nursing Care of Childbearing Families

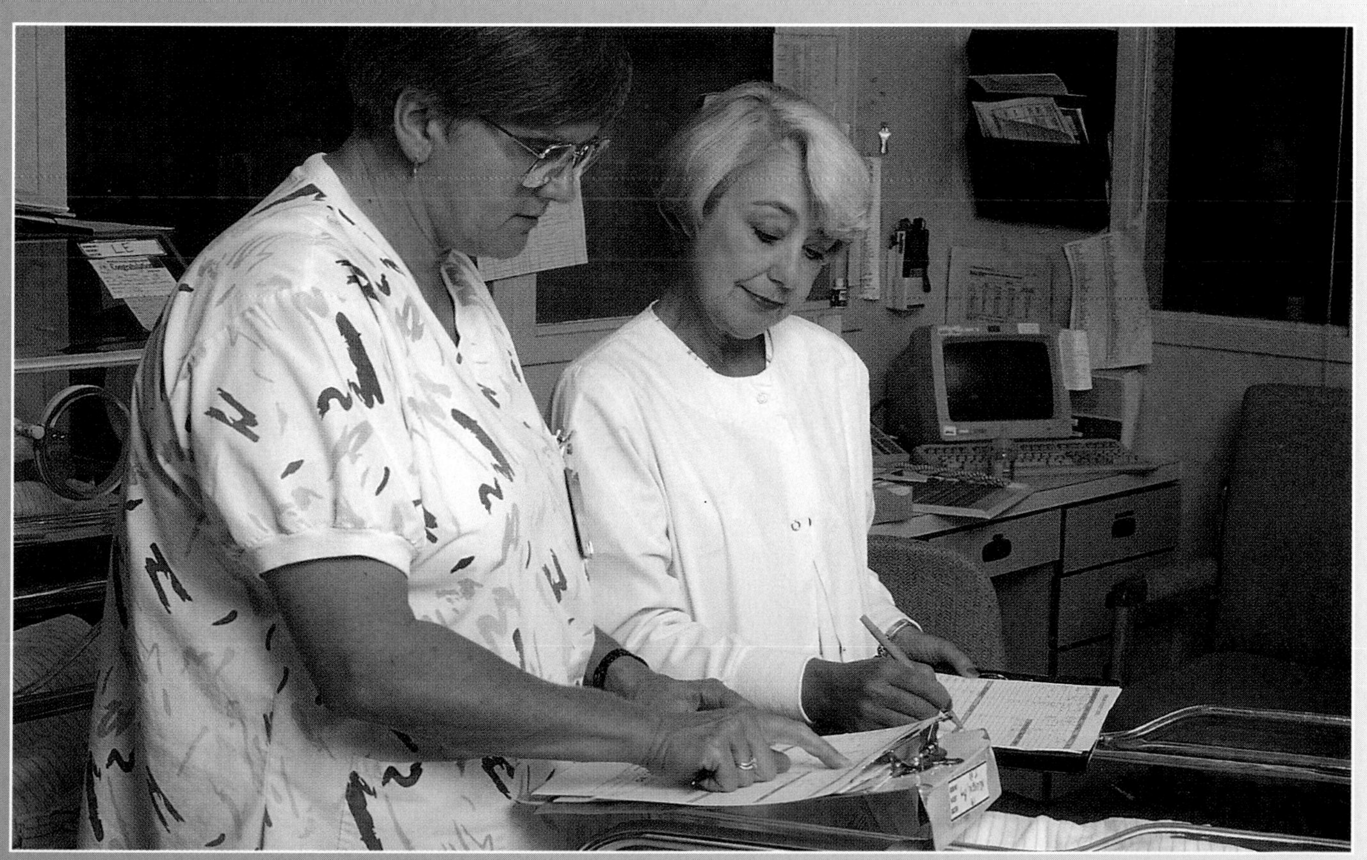

# 1

# Maternity Care Today

## OBJECTIVES

1. Describe changes in maternity care from home birth with lay midwives to the emergence of medical management.
2. Compare current settings for childbirth both within and outside the hospital setting.
3. Identify trends that led to the development of family-centered maternity care.
4. Describe current trends that affect perinatal nursing, including cost containment, outcomes management, home care, and advances in technology.
5. Explain changes in family structure and their impact on family functioning.
6. Compare Western cultural values with those of differing cultural groups.
7. Describe the effect of cultural diversity on nursing practice.
8. Discuss the downward trends in infant and maternal mortality rates, and compare current infant mortality rates for specific ethnic groups and nations.

## DEFINITIONS

**antepartum** *Term describing the pregnant woman before the onset of labor.*

**culture** *Sum of values, beliefs, and practices of a group of people that are transmitted from one generation to the next.*

**ethnic** *Pertaining to religious, racial, national, or cultural group characteristics, especially speech patterns, social customs, and physical characteristics.*

**ethnicity** *Condition of belonging to a particular ethnic group; also refers to ethnic pride.*

**ethnocentrism** *Opinion that the beliefs and customs of one's own ethnic group are superior.*

**infant mortality rate** *Number of deaths per 1000 live births that occurs within the first 12 months of life.*

**intrapartum** *Term describing the time of labor and childbirth.*

**lactation** *Secretion of milk from the breasts; also describes the time when a child is breastfed.*

**maternal mortality rate** *Number of maternal deaths from births and complications of pregnancy, childbirth, and puerperium (the first 42 days after termination of the pregnancy) per 100,000 live births.*

**neonatal mortality rate** *Number of deaths per 1000 live births occurring at birth or within the first 28 days of life.*

**postpartum** *Term describing the first 6 weeks following childbirth.*

Major changes in maternity care took place in the first half of the 20th century as childbirth moved from the home to a hospital setting. Rapid change continues as health care reform attempts to control the increasing cost of care while advances in technology accelerate. Despite changes, health care professionals attempt to maintain the quality of care. Alterations in family structure and function, as well as differing cultural beliefs and customs, also affect nursing care. Although improvements in health care have resulted in a significant decline in maternal and infant mortality in the United States, statistics show a wide disparity between whites and nonwhites.

## Historical Perspectives on Childbearing

### "Granny" Midwives

Before the 20th century, childbirth occurred most often in the home with the assistance of a "granny" midwife whose training was obtained through an apprenticeship with a more experienced granny midwife. Physicians were involved in childbirth only if there were serious problems.

Although many women and infants fared well when a lay midwife assisted with birth in the home, maternal and infant death rates resulting from childbearing were high. The primary causes of maternal death were postpartum hemorrhage; postpartum infection, also known as puerperal sepsis (or "childbed fever"); and toxemia, now known as pregnancy-induced hypertension. The primary causes of infant death were prematurity, dehydration from diarrhea, and contagious diseases.

### Emergence of Medical Management

In the late 19th century, technologic developments which were available to physicians but not to midwives, led to a decline in home births and an increase in physician-assisted hospital births. Significant discoveries that set the stage for a change in maternity care included the following:

- The discovery by Semmelweis that puerperal infection could be prevented by hygienic practices
- The development of forceps to facilitate birth
- The discovery of chloroform, which was used to control pain during childbirth
- The use of drugs to start labor (induction) or to increase uterine contractions (augmentation of labor)
- Advances in operative procedures, such as cesarean birth

With good intentions—to prevent infections—hospitals hurried to develop policies and procedures to meet the needs of physicians and to take advantage of technology (Wertz & Wertz, 1992).

Maternity care became highly regimented. All antepartum, intrapartum, and postpartum care was managed by physicians. Lay midwifery became illegal in many areas, and nurse-midwifery was not well established. The woman's role in childbirth was seen as passive, as the physician "delivered" the infant. Nurses' primary functions were to assist the physician and to follow prescribed medical orders following childbirth. Teaching and counseling were not valued nursing functions at that time.

Unlike home births, hospital births hindered bonding between parents and infant. During labor, the woman received medication, such as "twilight sleep"—a combination of a narcotic and scopolamine—that provided pain relief but left her disoriented, confused, and heavily sedated. Because of this practice and because little was known of the importance of early contact between parents and child, many mothers did not see the infant for several hours after the delivery. The father was relegated to a waiting area and was not allowed to see the mother until some time after the birth of the infant. By 1960, 90 percent of all births in the United States occurred in hospitals.

Despite the technologic advances and the move from home to hospital, maternal and infant mortality have declined slowly. The slow decline was primarily due to problems that could have been prevented, such as poor nutrition, infectious diseases, and inadequate prenatal care. These stubborn problems remained because of inequalities in health care delivery. Whereas affluent families could afford comprehensive medical care that began early in the pregnancy, poor families had very limited access to care or to information about childbearing. Two concurrent trends, federal involvement and consumer demands, led to additional changes in maternity care.

### Government Involvement in Maternal-Infant Care

The high rates of maternal and infant mortality among indigent women provided the impetus for federal involvement in maternity care. The Sheppard-Towner Act of 1921, the first federally sponsored program, provided funds for state-managed programs for mothers and children. Although this act was later repealed, it set the scene for future allocation of federal funds. Today, the federal government supports several programs to improve the health of mothers, infants, and young children (Table 1–1). Although government funds partially solved the problem of maternal and infant mortality, the *distribu-*

**TABLE 1–1 FEDERAL PROJECTS FOR MATERNAL-CHILD CARE**

| Program | Purpose |
|---|---|
| Title V of Social Security Act | Provides funds for maternal-child health programs |
| National Institute of Health and Human Development | Supports research and education of personnel needed for maternal and child health programs |
| Title V Amendment of Public Health Service Act | Established the Maternal and Infant Care (MIC) projects to provide comprehensive prenatal and infant care in public clinics |
| Title XIX of Medicaid Program | Provides funds to facilitate access to care by pregnant women and young children |
| Head Start | Provides educational opportunities for low-income children of preschool age |
| National Center for Family Planning | A clearinghouse for contraceptive information |
| Women, Infants, and Children (WIC) | Provides supplemental food and nutrition information |

*tion* of health care remained inequitable. Most physicians practiced in urban or suburban areas where the affluent could afford to pay for medical services, but women in rural or inner city areas had difficulty obtaining care. Distribution of health care is a problem that persists today.

The ongoing problem of providing health care for poor women and children left the door open for nurses to expand their roles, and advanced programs of education prepared nurses as nurse-midwives, nurse practitioners, and clinical specialists. Chapter 2 provides a more complete description of the nurse's role in current maternal-infant care.

### Impact of Consumer Demands on Health Care

In the early 1950s, consumers began to insist on their right to be involved in the health care they received. Pregnant women were no longer willing to accept only what was offered. They wanted information about planning and spacing their children, and they wanted to know what to expect during pregnancy. Moreover, the father, siblings, and grandparents wanted to be part of the extraordinary events of pregnancy and childbirth. Parents also wanted more say in how the birth was accomplished.

Early in the 1950s, Dr. Grantly Dick-Read proposed a method of childbirth that allowed the mother to control her fear and thus to control her pain during labor so that birth without pharmacologic intervention was possible. Additional methods, such as Lamaze and Bradley, quickly gained favor (see Chapter 11). Moreover, a growing consensus among child psychologists and nurse researchers indicated that the benefits of early, extended parent-newborn contact far outweighed the risks of infection. As a result, knowledgeable parents began to insist that the infant remain with them at all times. The practice of separating the infant from the family was abandoned, and family-centered maternity care gradually evolved.

### Development of Family-Centered Maternity Care

*Family-centered maternity care* is the term used to describe safe, quality care that recognizes and adapts to both the physical and psychosocial needs of the family, including those of the newborn. The emphasis is on fostering family unity while maintaining physical safety.

The basic principles of family-centered care are as follows:

- Childbirth is usually a normal, healthy event in the life of a family.
- Childbirth affects the entire family, and restructuring of family relationships is required.
- Families are capable of making decisions about care, provided that they are given adequate information and professional support.

Family-centered care greatly increased the responsibilities of nurses. It is no longer enough for nurses to provide only physical care and to assist physicians. Nurses now assume a major role in teaching, counseling, and supporting families in their decisions. (See Chapter 2 for additional information about the nurse's role in maternity care.)

## Current Settings for Childbirth

### Traditional Hospital Setting

In traditional hospitals of the past, labor often took place in a functional hospital room. When birth was imminent, the mother was moved to a delivery area similar to an operating room. Following childbirth, the mother was transferred to a recovery area for 1 to 2 hours of observation and then taken to the postpartum unit, which resembled a standard hospital room. The infant was usually moved to the newborn nursery when the mother was transferred to the recovery area. Mother and infant were reunited when the mother was settled in the postpartum unit. Beginning in the 1970s, the father or another significant support person could usually remain with the mother throughout labor, birth, and recovery.

Although birth in a traditional hospital setting was safe, the setting was impersonal and uncomfortable. Having to move so many times was a major disadvantage. The move from the labor room to the delivery room just before the birth of the baby was particularly difficult for the mother. Furthermore, each move disrupted the family's time together and often separated the parents from the infant. Because of these disadvantages, hospitals began to devise settings that were more comfortable and that facilitated family participation.

### Labor, Delivery, and Recovery Rooms

Today, most hospitals offer alternative settings in some form. The most common is the labor, delivery, and recovery (LDR) room. In an LDR room, normal labor, childbirth, and recovery from childbirth take place in one setting. Some LDR rooms are quite luxurious, with hardwood floors, paintings, refrigerators, televisions, and video players; in some facilities, whirlpool baths are available. The furniture can, however, quickly be transformed into a well-equipped delivery room. Paintings slide to the side, revealing suction and oxygen apparatus; ceiling spotlights are activated; and wood chests open to reveal fetal monitors and all equipment desired for the birth. A typical LDR room is illustrated in Figure 1–1.

During labor, the woman's significant others are allowed to remain with her. These people may include a number of relatives, friends, and even her other children, depending on the policies of the agency and the mother's desires. Once she has given birth, the mother typically remains in the LDR room for 1 to 2 hours, after which she is transferred to the postpartum unit. The infant may remain with the mother throughout her stay in the LDR room. When she is transferred to the postpartum unit, the infant may be transferred to the nursery for assessments or may remain with the mother.

The major advantages of LDR rooms are that the setting is more comfortable and home-like and that the family can remain with the mother throughout. Disadvantages for the family include the amount of technology used, such as electronic fetal monitoring; the administration of intravenous fluids; and the continuous epidural anesthesia. These measures can be frightening unless families are prepared in advance.

### Labor, Delivery, Recovery, and Postpartum Rooms

Some hospitals offer rooms that are similar to LDR rooms in layout and in function, but the mother is not transferred to a postpartum unit. She and the infant remain in the labor, delivery, recovery, and postpartum (LDRP) room until discharge. Fathers are encouraged to stay with the mother and infant, and many facilities provide beds so they can stay through the night.

### Birth Centers

Free-standing birth centers are designed to provide maternity care to low-risk women outside the hospital setting. In addition to care during childbirth, birth centers also provide antepartum and postpartum care. The mother usually attends classes there to prepare her for childbirth, breastfeeding, and infant care. Both the mother and infant continue to receive follow-up care during the first 6 weeks. This may include help with breastfeeding problems, a postpartum examination at 4 to 6 weeks, family planning

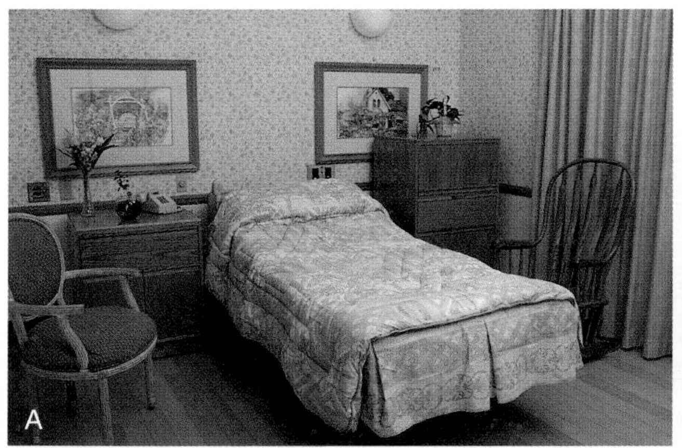


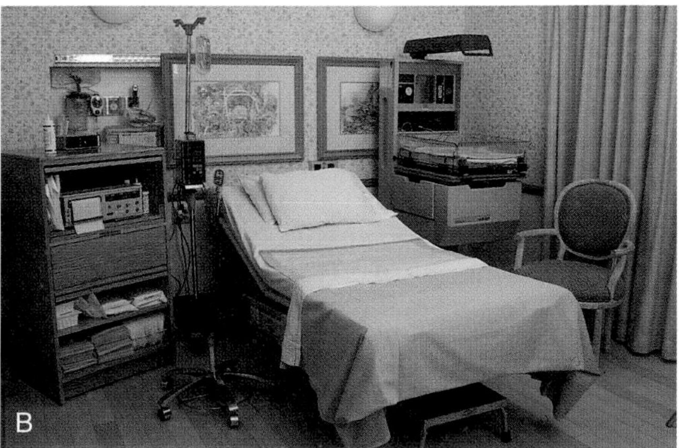


**FIGURE 1–1**

A typical labor, delivery, and recovery room. Home-like furnishings (A) can be adapted quickly to reveal needed technical equipment (B).

information, and examination of the newborn. Birth is often assisted by certified nurse-midwives who have provided care for the woman throughout her pregnancy and will continue to provide primary care for both the mother and the infant.

Birth centers generally charge less than traditional hospitals, which provide advanced technology that may be unnecessary for low-risk clients. Moreover, women who want a safe, home-like birth in a familiar setting with staff they have known throughout their pregnancies express a very high rate of satisfaction.

The major disadvantage is that most free-standing birth centers are not equipped for obstetric emergencies. Should unforeseen difficulties develop during labor, the woman must be transferred by ambulance to a nearby hospital to the care of a back-up physician who has agreed to perform this role. Although procedures have been worked out to deal with problems, a sudden transfer is frightening for the family.

### Home Births

In the United States, only a small number of women have their babies at home. Because malpractice insurance for midwives attending home births is expensive and difficult to obtain, the number of midwives who offer this service has decreased greatly. Many have moved their practices to hospitals or birth centers. Mothers who once sought home births have found that they can have many of the advantages of family-centered care in the safe environment of a hospital LDR room or a birth center while avoiding the disadvantages and potential dangers of home birth.

Home birth provides the advantages of keeping the family together in their own familiar environment throughout the childbirth experience. When all goes well, birth at home can be a growth-enhancing experience for every family member. Young siblings are not separated from their mothers and are able to establish positive relationships with the new baby immediately after birth. Bonding with the infant is unimpeded by hospital routines, and breastfeeding is highly encouraged and supported. Women who have their babies at home maintain a feeling of control because they actively plan and prepare for each detail of the birth.

Disadvantages of home births must also be noted. Women who plan a home birth must be screened carefully to make sure that they have a very low risk for complications. Opponents of home birth cite the need for immediate highly technologic care of the woman or fetus if complications develop. Even when transfer is to a nearby hospital, the time needed may be too long. Other problems of home birth include the need for the parents to provide a setting and adequate supplies for the birth. Moreover, the mother must take care of herself and the infant without the professional help she would have in a hospital setting.

**✓ CHECK YOUR READING**

1. What two trends created change in maternity care in the last 4 decades?
2. How does family-centered maternity care differ from previous maternity care?
3. How do LDR and LDRP rooms differ from birth centers and home births in their advantages and disadvantages?

## Current Trends in Maternity Care

In the last few years there has been a concerted effort by the government, insurance companies, hospitals, and health care providers to reform health care delivery in the United States. One goal of the reform is to control the ever-increasing cost of health care. This trend has involved a change in where and how money is spent. In the past most of the health care budget was spent in acute-care settings, where the facility charged for services after they were provided. Because they were paid for whatever services they provided, hospitals had no incentive to be efficient or cost conscious.

### Cost Containment

One way in which the payers of health care have attempted to control costs of health care is by shifting to a *prospective* form of payment—that is, they will no longer pay whatever charges the hospital decides on for service provided. Instead, a fixed amount of money is agreed in advance for necessary services for specifically diagnosed conditions. One example of this approach is *diagnosis-related groups* (DRGs).

#### DIAGNOSIS-RELATED GROUPS

Diagnosis-related grouping is a method of classifying related medical diagnoses based on the amount of resources that are generally required by the client. This method became a standard in 1987, when the federal government set the amount of money that would be paid by Medicare for each DRG. If the hospital delivers more services than what is paid for by that DRG, the hospital must absorb the costs. Conversely, if the hospital delivers the care at less cost than the payment for that DRG, the hospital keeps the remaining money. Hospitals obviously benefit financially if they can reduce the client's length of stay (LOS) in the facility and thereby reduce the costs for service. Although the DRG system originally applied only to Medicare clients, most states have adopted the system for Medicaid payments, and many insurance companies use a similar system. Diagnosis-related groups are being developed for outpatient and ambulatory care as well. Table 1–2 lists the most common DRGs in perinatal care.

#### MANAGED CARE

Health insurance companies also examined the cost of health care and instituted an alternative health care delivery system that has been labeled *managed care*. Examples of managed care organizations are *health maintenance organizations* (HMOs) and *preferred provider organizations* (PPOs). In return for a set fee or premium, HMOs are responsible for providing relatively comprehensive health services for persons enrolled in the organization. Similarly, PPOs are groups of health care providers who agree to provide health services to a specific group of clients on a discounted basis. When the client requires medical treatment, managed care includes strategies such as payment arrangements and preadmission authorization to control costs.

### Effects of Cost Containment on Maternity Care

Prospective payment plans have had major effects on maternity care. First, the LOS of mothers and infants in the birth facility has been reduced by about 40 percent. Mothers who have a normal vaginal birth may leave the birth facility within 24 to 48 hours, and mothers who give birth by cesarean may go home within 72 hours. This policy of early discharge has received intense criticism because problems have developed with mothers or infants who have needed readmittance to the birth facility. As a result, legislation has been passed that mandates a 48-hour LOS for vaginal deliveries and 4 days for women who have had cesarean births.

Reduced LOS has also affected caregivers, particularly nurses. Within the last 5 years nurses have become increasingly concerned with meeting the needs of families who leave the hospital a short time after the birth of an infant. Nurses find it especially difficult to provide adequate information about self-care and infant care within the first 24 hours, when the mother is still recovering from childbirth.

#### OUTCOMES MANAGEMENT

The determination to lower health care costs while maintaining the quality of care has led to a clinical practice model called *outcomes management*. This is a systematic method to identify client outcomes and to focus care on interventions that will accomplish the stated outcomes for specific case types, such as the woman who has just given birth or the normal newborn. The planning tools used by the health care team to identify and meet stated outcomes are *clinical pathways*.

#### CLINICAL PATHWAYS

Clinical pathways—also called critical paths, care paths, or care MAPS (multidisciplinary action plans)—are guidelines developed by each facility in a collaborative process that includes physicians, nurses, and other key professionals. In general, clinical pathways define expected client outcomes, appropriate LOS, and specific interventions by the health care team that will help accomplish the stated outcomes. Most clinical pathways also set the time and sequence of interventions of nurses, physicians, and other health care providers for a particular case type.

Many facilities differ in how they use clinical pathways. For instance, they may be used for change-of-shift reports to indicate information about LOS, individual needs, and priorities of the shift for each client. They may also be used as an adjunct to, or instead of, nursing care plans and to document the client's progress in meeting the outcomes. Many are particularly helpful in identifying families that require follow-up care.

**Variances.** Clinical pathways are guidelines that are meant for clients who are expected to progress along the timeline to meet the expected outcomes. Deviations, often called *variances*, may occur, either in the timeline or in the expected outcomes. A variance is the difference between what was expected and what actually happened. A variance may be positive or negative. A positive variance occurs when a client progresses more rapidly than expected and is discharged earlier than planned. A negative variance occurs when progress is slower than expected, outcomes are not met within the designated time frame, and LOS is prolonged. Any variance must be analyzed, and the treatment plan must be adjusted to meet individual or family needs.

**TABLE 1–2 COMMON DIAGNOSIS-RELATED GROUPS (DRGs) IN PERINATAL CARE**

| DRG | Description |
|---|---|
| 370 | Cesarean section with complications |
| 371 | Cesarean section without complications |
| 372 | Vaginal delivery with complications |
| 373 | Vaginal delivery without complications |
| 375 | Vaginal delivery with operative procedures |
| 379 | Therapeutic abortion |
| 382 | False labor |
| 386 | Prematurity with respiratory distress syndrome |
| 387 | Prematurity without other complications |
| 388 | Prematurity with other complications |
| 389 | Full-term neonate with complications |

Text continued on page 12

**YORK HOSPITAL**
YORK, PENNSYLVANIA
**CLINICAL PATHWAY**
**VAGINAL DELIVERY**

| CLINICAL PATH DAY | EXPECTED PATIENT/ FAMILY OUTCOMES | MULTIDISCIPLINARY ASSESSMENT | TESTS | CONSULT |
|---|---|---|---|---|
| Pre-natal<br>Date | ☐ Prenatal test results available [4]<br>☐ 8 or more prenatal visits complete [4]<br>☐ Attended baby care and post-partum classes [3]<br>☐ Risk assessment complete and referral(s) to appropriate agency made as needed [6]<br>☐ Low risk pregnancy or monitored high risk pregnancy [4]<br>☐☐☐ ______ | Each visit—maternal weight; BP; urine dipstick-sugar, protein ketones; FHT<br>S/S of pregnancy complication<br>Perinatal risk assessment<br>Social support<br>Knowledge of self and newborn care<br>Knowledge of warning signs of complications<br>Knowledge of signs of labor<br>☐ RECORDED ON PRENATAL RECORD AND/OR MOTHER CHILD CLINIC PRENATAL CARE PATH WAY | Type & Rh<br>Antibody Screen<br>H & H<br>Sickle cell<br>Rubella<br>RPR<br>HBSAG<br>Trutol or 3h GTT<br>GC, Chlamydia<br>Triple Screen<br>Group B Step<br>☐ RECORDED ON PRENATAL RECORD AND/OR MOTHER CHILD CLINIC PRENATAL CARE PATH WAY | ☐ ______<br>______ |
| Admission<br>Date | ☐ Demonstrates use of breathing and relaxation technique [1,2,3]<br>☐ Support person present [2]<br>☐ Referral made for identified risk factors<br>☐ Admission procedures completed [4]<br>☐ ______ | ☐ Admission assessment<br>☐ Knowledge of breathing and relaxation techniques<br>☐ Support system<br>☐ ______ | ☐ WCBC<br>☐ Type & Rh<br>☐ Tube to hold<br>☐ US scan prn<br>☐ ______ | ☐ ______<br>______ |
| Labor First Stage | N D E<br>☐☐☐ Demonstrates use of breathing and relaxation technique [1,2,3]<br>☐☐☐ Support person present [2]<br>☐☐☐ Referral made for identified maternal/fetal risk during labor<br>☐☐☐ Mother demonstrates normal physiologic parameters [4]<br>☐☐☐ Fetus demonstrates normal physiologic parameters [4]<br>☐☐☐ ______ | N D E<br>☐☐☐ FHR q 30 min<br>☐☐☐ UC q 30-60 min<br>☐☐☐ P, R, BP q 2h<br>☐☐☐ T q 4° (q 2 if ROM)<br>☐☐☐ Support system<br>☐☐☐ Progress of labor<br>☐☐☐ Comfort status<br>☐☐☐ ______ | N D E<br>☐☐☐<br>______ | N D E<br>☐☐☐<br>______<br>☐☐☐<br>______ |
| Labor 2nd Stage | ☐☐☐ Pushing effectively [4]<br>☐☐☐ Support person present [2]<br>☐☐☐ Referral made for identified maternal/fetal risk during labor<br>☐☐☐ Mother demonstrates normal physiologic parameters [4]<br>☐☐☐ Fetus demonstrates normal physiologic parameters [4] | ☐☐☐ FHR q 5 min<br>☐☐☐ BP q 30 min<br>☐☐☐ Vaginal exam prn<br>☐☐☐ ______ | ☐☐☐<br>______<br>______ | ☐☐☐<br>______<br>______ |

| NAME | INITIALS | NAME | INITIALS |
|---|---|---|---|
| | | | |
| | | | |

8030 (4/96)

**FIGURE 1–2**

Clinical pathway for vaginal delivery. (Courtesy of Women and Children Services of the York Health System, York, Pennsylvania.)

**DOCUMENTATION CODES**
Initial = Meets Standard
* = Exception on pathway identified
C = Chronic problems
N = Not applicable

**PATIENT/FAMILY PROBLEMS**
1. Pain r/t childbirth
2. Anxiety r/t childbirth and/or parenting
3. Knowledge deficit r/t childbirth and/or parenting
4. Potential alteration maternal/fetal homeostasis
5. Bonding
6. Potential for alteration in parenting r/t inadequate support systems
7. ______
8. ______

| TREATMENTS | MEDS | NUTRITION | EDUC & DC PLANNING |
|---|---|---|---|
| ☐ ______<br>______ | Perinatal vitamin, $FeSO_4$ as per order<br>☐ ______<br>______<br>☐ RECORDED ON PRENATAL RECORD AND/OR MOTHER CHILD CLINIC PRENATAL CARE PATHWAY | Regular diet<br>☐ RECORDED ON PRENATAL RECORD AND/OR MOTHER CHILD CLINIC PRENATAL CARE PATHWAY | Childbirth preparation class<br>Baby care class<br>Breastfeeding class when appropriate<br>Prenatal education<br>☐ RECORDED ON PRENATAL RECORD AND/OR MOTHER CHILD CLINIC PRENATAL CARE PATHWAY |
| ☐ Bedrest with fetal monitor x 30 minutes<br>☐ ______ | ☐ IV/mini cath<br>☐ ______ | ☐ NPO with ice chips<br>☐ ______ | ☐ Orient pt/SO/family to L & D area<br>☐ Reinforce breathing and relaxation techniques<br>☐ ______ |
| N D E<br>☐☐☐ Insertion of scalp electrode and IUPC as appropriate<br>☐☐☐ Warm/cold compress, massage, position change, ambulates and warm showers prn<br>☐☐☐ Encourage to void q 1-2°<br>☐☐☐ EFM as ordered<br>☐☐☐ Vaginal exam prn<br>☐☐☐ Catheterize prn | N D E<br>☐☐☐ IV as ordered<br>☐☐☐ Analgesia prn as ordered<br>☐☐☐ Epidural as ordered<br>☐☐☐ Induction/augmentation of labor as ordered<br>☐☐☐ ______ | N D E<br>☐☐☐ NPO with ice chips | N D E<br>☐☐☐ Reinforce breathing and relaxation technique<br>☐☐☐ Encourage support person involvement<br>☐☐☐ Provide explanation of labor progress prn |
| ☐☐☐ Position for comfort<br>☐☐☐ Catheterize prn<br>☐☐☐ Warm/cold compress, massage, position change and void prn<br>☐☐☐ ______ | ☐☐☐ IV as ordered<br>☐☐☐ Continue epidural as ordered<br>☐☐☐ Augmentation of labor as ordered<br>☐☐☐ ______ | ☐☐☐ NPO with ice chips | ☐☐☐ Assist with pushing<br>☐☐☐ Encourage support person involvement<br>☐☐☐ ______ |

| NAME | INITIALS | NAME | INITIALS |
|---|---|---|---|
| | | | |
| | | | |

*Illustration continued on following page*

| CLINICAL PATH DAY | EXPECTED PATIENT/ FAMILY OUTCOMES | MULTIDISCIPLINARY ASSESSMENT | TESTS | CONSULT |
|---|---|---|---|---|
| **Delivery** Date<br>Time | ☐ Deliver live newborn vaginally [4]<br>☐ Support person present [2]<br>☐ ________ | ☐ Fundus, bleeding<br>☐ ________ | ☐ Cord blood<br>☐ Rh studies when indicated<br>☐ Placenta to pathology as ordered | ☐ ________<br>________ |
| **Early Recovery** Date | ☐ Postpartum parameters stable [4]<br>☐ Pain relief [1]<br>☐ ________ | ☐ Temp X 1<br>☐ P, R, BP, fundus, lochia, bladder, episiotomy q 15 min x 4, & q 30 min x 2<br>☐ ________ | ☐ ________<br>________ | ☐ ________<br>________ |
| **Postpartum <12°** Date | ☐ Pain relief [1]<br>☐ Demonstrates self-care ADL [3]<br>☐ Postpartum parameters stable<br>☐ Voiding qs [4]<br>☐ **Adequate home support system identified [6]**<br>☐ ________ | ☐ T, P, R, BP, breasts, fundus, lochia, bladder, episiotomy q 4h<br>☐ Knowledge of self and newborn care<br>☐ Home Support System<br>☐ ________ | ☐ ________ | ☐ ________ |
| **Postpartum 12°-24°** Date | ☐ Pain relief [1]<br>☐ V.S. and postpartum physiological parameters stable [4]<br>☐ **Referral made for identified problems r/t home support system**<br>☐ Voiding qs [4]<br>☐ ________ | ☐ T, P, R, BP, q 4h<br>☐ Breasts, fundus, lochia, bladder, episiotomy q shift WA<br>☐ ________ | ☐ WCBC | ☐ ________ |
| **Discharge** Date | ☐☐☐ Pain relief [1]<br>☐☐☐ V.S. & postpartum physiological parameters within D/C guidelines [4]<br>☐☐☐ Voiding qs [4]<br>☐ **Patient/SO/family verbalization of D/C Instructions [3].**<br>☐ **Postpartum home visit scheduled [4,6]**<br>☐ **Discharge within 2 days after delivery**<br>☐☐☐ ________ | ☐☐☐ T, P, R, BP bid shift<br>☐☐☐ Breasts, fundus, lochia, bladder, episiotomy bid shift WA<br>☐☐☐ Pt/SO/family knowledge of postpartum care<br>☐☐☐ ________ | ☐ ________ | ☐ ________ |

| NAME | INITIALS | NAME | INITIALS |
|---|---|---|---|
| | | | |
| | | | |
| | | | |

NOTE: EACH PATIENT REQUIRES AN INDIVIDUAL ASSESSMENT & TREATMENT PLAN. THIS CLINICAL PATH IS A RECOMMENDATION FOR THE AVERAGE PATIENT WHICH REQUIRES MODIFICATION WHEN NECESSARY BY THE PROFESSIONAL STAFF.

| TREATMENTS | MEDS | NUTRITION | EDUC & DC PLANNING |
|---|---|---|---|
| ☐ Catheterize prn<br>☐ Continue IV<br>☐ Continue epidural or local anesthetic<br>☐ ______ | ☐ Oxytocin after placenta delivered as ordered<br>☐ ______ | ☐ NPO | ☐ Support parent/infant bonding<br>☐ ______ |
| ☐ OOB with assist first time<br>☐ Perineal ice pack q 30 min prn<br>☐ Cath prn<br>☐ Shower<br>☐ ______ | ☐ Analgesia prn<br>☐ Continue epidural if PPTL<br>☐ Continue IV oxytocin as ordered<br>☐ D/C IV<br>☐ ______ | ☐ Reg diet as tolerated | ☐ Support parent/infant bonding<br>☐ Teach pericare<br>☐ ______ |
| ☐ OOB with assist first time, then OOB ad lib<br>☐ Catheterize per protocol<br>☐ Epifoam, Tucks prn<br>☐ Ice pack prn<br>☐ ______ | ☐ Analgesia prn<br>☐ ______ | ☐ Advance to regular diet as tolerated | ☐ Initiate materal/newborn education record, D/C instructions<br>☐ ______ |
| ☐ OOB ad lib<br>☐ Epifoam, Tucks prn<br>☐ Sitz bath 12° after delivery & prn<br>☐ Ice pack prn<br>☐ ______ | ☐ Analgesia prn<br>☐ ______ | ☐ Regular diet | ☐ Continue maternal newborn education record |
| ☐☐☐ OOB ad lib<br>☐☐☐ Epifoam, Tucks prn<br>☐☐☐ Sitz bath prn<br>☐☐☐ ______ | ☐☐☐ Analgesia prn<br>☐ **Rhogam, when indicated**<br>☐ **Rubella, when indicated**<br>☐ ______ | ☐☐☐ Regular diet | ☐ Completion of maternal newborn education record<br>☐ Physican discharge instructions<br>☐ Support services in community:<br>☐ Breastfeeding Support Services<br>☐ Perinatal Coaching<br>☐ City/State Health<br>☐ Other |

| NAME | INITIALS | NAME | INITIALS |
|---|---|---|---|
| | | | |
| | | | |
| | | | |

**Students Using Clinical Pathways.** Clinical pathways are guidelines for care. Assessments, tests, treatments, consultations, and client education are listed in a specific time sequence to accomplish identified outcomes. Figure 1–2 is an example of a clinical pathway that could be used when vaginal births occur in an LDRP room. Outcomes statements have been developed for the prenatal period as well as for labor, childbirth, and the postpartal period.

Although this pathway provides insight into the scheduling of assessments and care, it is not meant to teach nursing skills and procedures. For example, outcomes in the first stage of labor state that the woman demonstrates use of breathing and relaxation techniques and the fetus demonstrates normal physiologic parameters. Before they can assess these outcome statements, students must learn breathing and relaxation techniques that are used during labor, and they must know the normal fetal heart rate and its reaction to uterine contractions.

One purpose of this book is to provide ample information so students can *use* clinical pathways in a clinical setting. This involves teaching *why and how to perform* assessments and interpreting the significance of the data obtained. The text also provides detailed information about normal values and expected behaviors for recognizing when family members are progressing toward the stated outcome and when they are not. Moreover, the book emphasizes ways of providing information, care, and comfort for childbearing families as they progress along a clinical pathway.

## Home Care

Perinatal home care has experienced dramatic growth since 1990. The expansion of services is due to recognition of cost benefits; increased reimbursement by the federal government, which pays for approximately 30 percent of health care; and increased reimbursement by state governments, which pay for about 10 percent of all health care costs (Finkler & Kovner, 1993). Advances in portable technology, such as state-of-the-art electronic fetal monitors or infusion pumps for the administration of intravenous nutrition or subcutaneous medications, allow nurses to perform complicated procedures in the home. In addition, consumers often prefer home care because of decreased stress on the family when a woman or newborn is able to remain at home rather than be separated from the family support system because of the need for hospitalization. As in acute-care facilities, clinical pathways are sometimes used to define client outcomes and to direct the time and sequencing of interventions to meet these outcomes in the home. (See Chapter 17 for an example of a postpartum and newborn clinical pathway.)

### STANDARDS FOR PERINATAL HOME CARE

Home care is a unique practice setting governed by standards that nurses who practice in home health should know. Standards are guidelines or models for practice established by agencies or organizations.

**Agency Standards.** Each home care agency is required to have policies, procedures, and protocols to define and guide all elements of care. These standards, which must comply with established national standards, must be kept current and accessible to the nursing staff.

**Organizational Standards.** In addition to agency standards, nurses who provide home care must also be aware of organizational standards. For perinatal services, the Association of Women's Health, Obstetric, and Neonatal Nurses (AWHONN) is recognized as the national professional organization. AWHONN publishes competency statements, position papers, and practice guidelines. *Didactic Content and Clinical Skills Verification for Professional Nurse Providers of Perinatal Home Care* (1994) provides written statements regarding the scope of services, policies, procedures, and protocols for perinatal home care. Standards set by other professional organizations, such as the American College of Obstetricians and Gynecologists, the National Association of Home Care, and the American Academy of Pediatrics, may also influence standards for perinatal nurses.

**Legal Standards.** Professionals practicing in any health care delivery system, including home care, must be knowledgeable about the definition of nursing practice and the rules and regulations that govern that practice. For instance, in most states, home health care agencies, as well as registered nurses, must be licensed to provide care. Nurses must also be aware of their scope of practice, which is defined by nurse practice acts. (Chapter 3 gives additional information on legal aspects of nursing.)

Other regulatory bodies, such as Occupational Safety and Health Administration (OSHA), Food and Drug Administration (FDA), and Centers for Disease Control and Prevention (CDC), also provide guidelines for practice. Accrediting agencies, such as Joint Commission on Accreditation of Healthcare Organizations (JCAHO) and Community Health Accreditation Program (CHAP), give their approval after visiting facilities and observing whether standards are being met in practice.

### PERINATAL HOME CARE NURSING

The emerging specialty of perinatal home health encompasses antepartum, postpartum, and neonatal care. Because care is given in an environment that is physically separated from an acute-care institution, nurses must be able to function independently and must be confident of their clinical skills. They should be proficient at interviewing, counseling, and teaching. They often assume a leadership role in coordinating all the services a family may require, and they frequently supervise the work of other care providers.

**Antepartum Home Care.** Most preconceptional and low-risk antepartum care takes place in private offices or public clinics. High-risk clients who once would have been routinely hospitalized are frequently cared for in the home today because home care is both less expensive and more agreeable to most women. High-risk clients are defined as those who have known conditions that will, or can, have a strong potential to compromise the health of the pregnant woman, her fetus, or both (AWHONN, 1994). The goal of care is to monitor the effects of identified risk factors and to prevent complications. Some of the most common conditions are preterm labor, hyperemesis gravidarum (intractable vomiting during pregnancy), bleeding problems, premature rupture of membranes (bag of waters), hypertension, and diabetes during pregnancy. Because home care is a growing part of maternity care, throughout the text home care nursing is discussed for specific conditions.

**Postpartum and Neonatal Home Care.** Shorter hospital stays have increased the need for postpartum home care, particularly during the first weeks when many physical and emotional adaptations take place. The American Academy of Pediatrics and the American College of Obstetricians and Gynecologists guidelines (1992) recommend that all infants leaving the hospital within 24 hours of birth be seen for evaluation and support within 48 hours of discharge. AWHONN takes the position that nurse-managed postpartum follow-up care should be available to all childbearing families (AWHONN, 1994).

The most common problems encountered by new mothers are discomfort—such as perineal, incisional, or nipple pain—and uterine cramping. Additional problems include fatigue, constipation, breastfeeding difficulties, and problems with self-care or infant care (Williams & Cooper, 1993).

Infants who leave the hospital within the first 24 hours following birth are at risk for a variety of problems that may be prevented or alleviated by nursing management. These conditions include jaundice, feeding difficulties, significant weight loss or inadequate weight gain, rashes, and conjunctivitis (Keppler, 1995).

A variety of services are offered for home care. These include telephone calls, home visits, information lines, and lactation consultations. In addition, nurse-managed outpatient clinics provide care for mothers and infants in some areas. (See Chapters 18 and 23 for additional information about home care for mothers and infants.)

**Home Care for High-Risk Neonates.** Perinatal nurses must also be prepared to provide care for infants who are discharged from the acute-care facility with serious medical conditions. Parents of preterm or low-birth-weight infants require a great deal of information and support. Infants with congenital anomalies, such as cleft palate, may require care that is adapted to their condition. Moreover, increasing numbers of technology-dependent infants are now cared for at home. The numbers include infants requiring ventilator assistance, total parenteral nutrition, intravenous medications, apnea monitoring, and other device-associated nursing care.

Coordinating care for the high-risk newborn is a major challenge for home care nurses. The involvement of multiple specialty providers—physicians, nurses, respiratory therapists, equipment vendors, and others—may result in duplication or fragmentation of services. Duplication of services results in unnecessary costs, and fragmentation of services can result in dangerous gaps in care. (See Chapters 29 and 30 for home care for high risk infants.)

## Community-Based Perinatal Care

Ample evidence shows that the health care system of the future will be community oriented, with greater numbers of clients cared for in the home and through community agencies. Public health agencies have existed for many years, and many women obtain all antepartum, postpartum, and neonatal care in these clinics. The number of free-standing birth centers is increasing as hospitals become highly specialized centers of critical care. Other community facilities, such as neighborhood health centers, shelters for women and children, school-aged mothers programs, and nurse-managed postpartum centers, also provide care to a variety of families.

Nurses need a broad array of skills to function effectively in community-based care. They need an understanding of the communities within which they practice and the diverse nature of those communities. Nurses need to develop skills in working with a multidisciplinary team. They are often responsible for assisting clients through high-technology choices and thus need to be proficient in communicating and teaching.

## Advances in Technology

Perinatal care must change constantly to keep pace with technologic advances. Procedures that were new a short time ago, such as amniocentesis, ultrasonography, and electronic fetal monitoring, are now used extensively. Newer technology includes sophisticated genetic testing and manipulation, fetal surgery, assisted-reproduction techniques, and mechanical systems, sometimes called artificial wombs, that facilitate ongoing maturation of preterm infants. Biomedical research in areas of pregnancy prevention may reduce the number of unplanned or unwanted pregnancies. In some areas, health care professionals can already use computer technology to compute and document medications, feedings, and intravenous solutions.

Nowhere is technology developing faster than in the fields of information and communication. At this time, health care professionals can instantly access on-line information from a variety of data bases. In the near future, so-called expert systems that mimic the decision-making processes of experts in the field will be used to generate client outcomes and to direct client care. Video and digital imaging technology will preserve and recall crisp images that allow image overlay and computerized comparison. Personal computer systems will be linked to share information about staffing, scheduling, and communication.

All nurses in practice today need to learn to use computers and find out how they can help to organize and facilitate the practice of nursing. They need to know basic word processing to enter data and how to move between computer screen fields. Learning about networks and electronic mail opens the windows to global connections with other systems. In the future, nurses will be active in designing clinical practice systems that will directly affect their responsibilities.

**CHECK YOUR READING**

4. How do cost-containment strategies affect maternal-newborn nursing?
5. What are the functions of clinical pathways?
6. How do standards guide home care?

## The Family

Families are sometimes categorized into three groups: traditional, nontraditional, and high-risk. In theory, traditional families require care that differs from that needed by nontraditional or high-risk families. See Table 1–3 for definitions of general family types.

### Traditional Families

Traditional families (also called nuclear families) are headed by a couple that views parenting as the major priority in their lives and whose energies are not depleted by stressful conditions, such as poverty, illness, or substance abuse. Generally, traditional families are motivated to learn all they can about pregnancy, childbirth, and parenting. These families are best served by providing information as the need arises. Traditional families can be single-income or dual-income.

**TABLE 1–3 GENERAL FAMILY TYPES**

| Family Type | Definition |
|---|---|
| **Traditional (nuclear)** | |
| | Mother, father, and subadult children (either natural or adopted) living in same household; may depend on single or dual income |
| **Nontraditional** | |
| Single-parent | Never-married, divorced, or widowed adult and his or her natural or adopted children |
| Blended | A parent, stepparent, children, and stepchildren living in the same household |
| Extended | Nuclear family plus relatives of either or both spouses living in the same household |
| Communal | Several households of adults and their children living in a common geographic area and working together in a common way to achieve the group's goals |
| Foster | Care provided by family other than biologic or adoptive parents |
| **High-Risk** | |
| | At increased risk for problems (those below poverty level, headed by single teenaged parent, with unanticipated stress, uncertain lifestyle) |

#### SINGLE-INCOME FAMILIES

In the 1950s and 1960s, the idealized single-income American family was epitomized in several long-running television series, such as "Leave It to Beaver." This family was composed of a father who was the sole provider, a mother who was homemaker and caregiver, and two children. Today, this family structure represents only a small minority of the nation's families.

#### DUAL-INCOME FAMILIES

Most two-parent families are now dependent on two incomes. This economic reality has created a great deal of stress on parents, subjecting them to many of the same problems that single-parent families face. For instance, reliable, competent child care has become a major issue and has increased the stress on traditional families.

## Nontraditional Families

Nontraditional families are defined by their unique structure and may be single-parent, blended, or extended. As with traditional families, nontraditional families require information. They often benefit from referral to meet specific needs, for instance, single-parenting classes, classes for mothers with twins, or group classes for adoptive families.

### SINGLE-PARENT FAMILIES

Millions of families are now headed by a single parent, most often the mother, who not only must function as homemaker and caregiver but also is often the major provider for the family's financial needs. Divorce is the most common cause of single-parent families, although childbirth among unmarried women is also a major factor.

Single-parent families are more likely to live below the poverty level and are vulnerable to a variety of problems. Parents may feel overwhelmed by the prospect of assuming all childrearing responsibilities and may be less prepared for illness or loss of a job than two-parent families.

Nurses can support and encourage single-parent families by listening to the unique problems of each family. Nurses are often the primary source of information about health care for many of these families and are often instrumental in initiating the necessary referrals.

### BLENDED FAMILIES

Blended families are formed when divorced or widowed parents remarry and bring children from a previous marriage into the new relationship. Many times the couple desires children with each other, creating a contemporary family structure commonly described as "yours, mine, and ours." These families may have difficulty forming a cohesive family unit unless they can overcome differences in parenting styles and values. Differing expectations of children's behavior and development as well as differing beliefs about discipline often cause family conflict.

### EXTENDED FAMILIES

The extended family includes members from three generations living under one roof. This family structure is becoming increasingly common in the United States and has given rise to the term *boomerang* families. This expression refers to adult children who return to the parents' homes, either because they are unable to support themselves or because they want the additional support that the grandparents provide for the grandchildren. Extended families are vulnerable to generational conflicts and may require education and referral to prevent disintegration of the family unit.

### HOMOSEXUAL FAMILIES

Although homosexual families are proportionately uncommon, they are recognized increasingly in the United States. Children in homosexual families may be offspring of previous heterosexual unions, or they may be adopted children or children conceived by artificial insemination of one or both members of a lesbian couple. This couple may face a great many challenges from a community that is unaccustomed to alternative lifestyles.

### ADOPTIVE FAMILIES

Persons who adopt a child may have problems that biologic parents do not face. Biologic parents have the long period of gestation and the gradual changes of pregnancy to help them adjust emotionally and socially to the birth of a child. The needs of adoptive parents may be overlooked after the adoption process is over. Adoptive parents as well as biologic parents need information, support, and guidance to prepare them to care for the infant and to maintain their own relationship.

## High-Risk Families

High-risk families include those below the poverty level, those headed by a single teenaged parent, and those with unanticipated stress, such as an infant who is preterm, ill, or handicapped. In addition, families with lifestyle problems such as alcoholism, use of illicit drugs, or family violence are considered at high risk for problems in providing adequate care for the infant.

Many high-risk families require specialized services. In such cases, the major responsibility of staff nurses is to refer families in need to agencies that can provide comprehensive care. Some of the most common referrals are to social service agencies for financial assistance, crisis intervention, home visits, or drug rehabilitation programs. (Chapter 24 provides additional information about substance abuse, teenaged parenting, and the effect of poverty on family structure and function.)

## Characteristics of a Healthy Family

In general, healthy families are able to adapt to changes that occur in the family unit. Pregnancy and childbirth create some of the most powerful changes that a family experiences. The relationship between adults must change to include the care of a helpless infant. Children must learn to share the attention of parents with a new sibling. The healthy, viable family is able to adapt to these changes without undue stress, but the family that is unprepared for change may suffer conflict.

Healthy families exhibit some common characteristics that provide a framework for assessing how all families function:

- Members of healthy families communicate openly with one another to express the concerns and needs of each family member.
- Healthy families remain flexible in role assignment so that if one person is unable to complete the assigned tasks, another member offers assistance.
- Adults in healthy families agree on the basic principles of parenting so that there is minimal discord about such things as discipline and sleep schedules.
- Healthy families are adaptable and are not overwhelmed by changes that occur in the home and in relationships as a result of childbirth. For instance, adaptable families can tolerate less-than-perfect housekeeping, an irregular schedule of meals, and interrupted sleep, which are common when an infant is added to the family structure.
- Members of healthy families volunteer assistance without waiting to be asked. Some young parents feel guilty if they must ask for help with the tasks of parenting but are relieved when assistance is offered.

### Factors That Interfere with Family Functioning

Nurses need to recognize factors that interfere with the family's ability to provide for the individual needs of family members. These factors include lack of financial resources, absence of adequate family support, birth of an infant who requires specialized care, unhealthy habits such as smoking or abuse of other substances, and inability to make mature decisions that are necessary to provide care for an infant.

**CHECK YOUR READING**

7. How do structures of traditional and nontraditional families differ?
8. What are four reasons why families might be identified as high risk?
9. What are the characteristics of a healthy family?
10. What factors interfere with family functioning?

## Cultural Perspectives in Childbearing

*Culture* is the sum of the beliefs and values that are learned, shared, and transmitted from generation to generation by a particular group. Cultural values guide the thinking, decisions, and actions of the group, particularly in pivotal events such as childbearing. *Ethnicity* is the condition of belonging to a particular group that shares race, language and dialect, religious faiths, traditions, values, and symbols, as well as food preferences, literature, and folklore. Cultural beliefs and values vary among different groups, and nurses must be aware that individuals often believe their cultural values and patterns of behavior are superior. This belief, termed *ethnocentrism*, forms the basis for many conflicts that occur when persons from different cultural groups have frequent contact.

Nurses must be aware that culture is composed of visible and invisible layers that could be said to resemble an iceberg (Fig. 1–3). The behaviors that one observes can be compared with the visible part—the tip of the iceberg. The history, beliefs, values, and religion are not observed, but they are the hidden foundation on which behaviors are based and can be likened to the large submerged part of the iceberg. To fully comprehend cultural behavior, one must seek knowledge of the hidden beliefs that behaviors express.

### Implications of Cultural Diversity for Perinatal Nurses

Many immigrants and refugees are of childbearing age, which means that perinatal nurses in most localities will provide care for culturally diverse families. To provide effective care, nurses must be aware that culture is among the most significant factors that influence a woman's perception of childbirth.

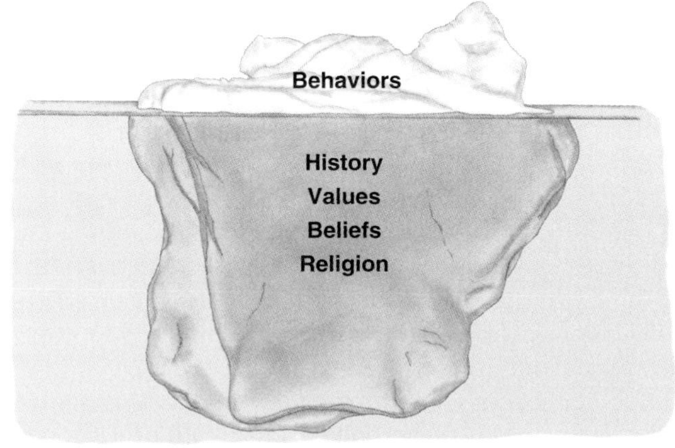


**FIGURE 1–3**

Visible and hidden layers of culture are like the visible and submerged parts of an iceberg. Many cultural differences are hidden below the surface.

#### WESTERN CULTURAL BELIEFS

Nursing practice in the United States is based largely on Western beliefs. It is imperative that nurses recognize that these beliefs may differ significantly from those of other societies and that the differences may cause a great deal of conflict.

Leininger (1978) identified seven dominant Western cultural values. These values greatly influence the thinking and action of nurses in the United States but may not be shared by their clients.

1. *Democracy* is a cultural value not shared by families who believe that decisions are made by elders or other higher authorities in the group. Fatalism, or a belief that events and results are predestined, may also affect health care decisions.
2. *Individualism* conflicts with the values of many cultural groups in which individual goals are subordinated to the greater good of the group.
3. *Cleanliness* is an American "obsession" viewed with amazement by many.
4. *Preoccupation with time,* which is measured by health care professionals in minutes and hours, is a major source of conflict with those who mark time by different standards, such as seasons or body needs.
5. *Reliance on machines and equipment* may intimidate families who have not reached even minimal comfort with technology.
6. *The belief that optimal health is a right* is in direct conflict with beliefs in many cultures in the world in which health is not a major emphasis or even an expectation.
7. *Admiration of self-sufficiency and financial success* may conflict with beliefs of other societies that place less value on wealth and more value on less tangible things, such as spirituality.

#### COMMUNICATION

Communication may also be a source of conflict between "dominant culture" health care professionals and those from other cultures. This is particularly true for Southeast Asians, Latinos, African-Americans, and Middle-Eastern immigrants.

**Southeast Asians.** Language is the greatest barrier to health care for those from Southeast Asia (Mattson, 1995). Besides the national languages of Vietnam, Cambodia, and Laos, numerous tribal languages are spoken in each country. Moreover, people from Southeast Asia speak softly and avoid prolonged eye contact, which they consider rude, in contrast to the Western belief that eye contact denotes honesty and forthrightness. They invariably show respect to the elderly, to priests, and to physicians. When medication or therapy is recommended, they seldom say no. They may accept the prescription or medication sample but not take the medicine or may agree to undergo a procedure but not keep the appointment.

**Latinos.** Latinos include those whose origin is Mexico, Central and South America, and Puerto Rico. Latinos tend to be polite and gracious in conversation. Preliminary social interaction is particularly important, and Latinos may be insulted if a problem is addressed directly without taking time for "small talk." This is counter to the Western value of "getting to the point" and may cause frustration for the client as well as for the health care worker.

**African-Americans.** African-Americans sometimes use a communication style that may cause conflict when they seek health care. They may use idioms, colloquial expressions, or speech patterns that are unfamiliar to many health care workers. Nurses must often clarify what is being said so that misunderstandings can be avoided and teaching can be effective.

**Middle Easterners.** Middle-Eastern immigrants come from a variety of countries that include Lebanon, Syria, Arabia, Egypt, Turkey, Iran, and Palestine. Communication in these countries is an elaborate system, but obtaining information may be difficult because Islam (the primary religion) dictates that family affairs should be kept within the family. Personal information is shared only with personal friends, and health assessment must be done gradually. When interpreters are used, they should be of the same country and religion, if possible, because of regional differences and hostilities. Because Muslim society tends to be paternalistic, it is wise to ask the man's permission or opinion when family members require health care.

## Cross-Cultural Health Beliefs

There are more than 100 different ethnocultural groups in the United States, and numerous traditional health beliefs are observed among these groups. For example, there are often culturally based definitions of health. Women of Asian origin may view health as the balance of "yin and yang." Those of African or Haitian origin may define health as "harmony with nature." Those from Mexico, Central and South America, and Puerto Rico often see health as a balance of "hot and cold."

#### TRADITIONAL METHODS OF PREVENTING ILLNESS

The traditional methods of preventing illness rest in the woman's ability to understand the cause of a given illness in her culture. These causes may include the following:

- Agents such as hexes, spells, or the evil eye, which may strike a person (often a child) and cause injury, illness, or misfortune.

- Phenomena such as soul loss or accidentally provoking envy, jealousy, or hate of a friend or acquaintance.
- Environmental factors such as bad air and natural events such as solar eclipses.

Practices to prevent illness developed from beliefs about the cause of illness. Obviously, one must avoid those known to transmit hexes and spells. Elaborate methods are used to prevent inciting envy or jealousy of others and to avoid the evil eye. Protective or religious objects, such as amulets with magic powers, or consecrated religious objects (talismans) are frequently worn or carried to prevent illness. There are also numerous food taboos and traditional combinations that are prescribed in traditional belief systems to prevent illness. For instance, people from many ethnic backgrounds eat raw garlic to prevent illness. Those of African origin may consume nonfood substances such as starch to make labor easier.

#### TRADITIONAL PRACTICES TO MAINTAIN HEALTH

A variety of traditional practices are used to maintain health. For instance, wearing proper clothing, such as a scarf, may prevent drafts and thus maintain the health of a woman who is pregnant and believes she must avoid cool air. Another example is eating the proper diet. For instance, women of Asian origin eat rice daily. Mental and spiritual health is maintained by activities such as silence, meditation, and prayer. Many people view illness as punishment for breaking a religious code and adhere strictly to religious morals and practices to maintain health.

#### TRADITIONAL PRACTICES TO RESTORE HEALTH

Traditional practices to restore health often conflict with Western medical practice. Some of the most common practices include the use of natural substances, such as herbs and plants, to treat illness. Religious charms, holy words, or traditional healers may be tried before seeking a medical opinion. Illness may also be treated by wearing religious medals, carrying prayer cards, or performing sacrifices.

A variety of substances may be ingested for the treatment of illnesses. An effort should be made to identify what the woman is taking and to determine whether the active ingredient may alter the effects of prescribed medication.

Dermabrasion, the rubbing or irritation of the skin to relieve discomfort, is a common health care practice. The most popular form is *coining* in which an area is covered with an ointment and the edge of a coin is rubbed over the area. All dermabrasion methods leave marks resembling bruises or burns on the skin and may be mistaken for signs of physical abuse (Mattson, 1995).

### Cultural Assessment

All health care professionals must develop skill in performing a cultural assessment so they can understand the meaning of childbirth in different cultural groups. The following questions might be considered in making such an assessment:

- Is childbearing viewed as a normal process, a time of vulnerability, or a state of illness?
- What are the prescribed practices, customs, or rituals related to diet, activity, or behavior during pregnancy and childbirth?
- What maternal restrictions or precautions are necessary during pregnancy and childbirth?
- Who provides support during pregnancy, childbirth, and beyond?
- What are the prescribed practices and restrictions related to care of the newborn?
- Who in the family hierarchy makes health care decisions?
- How is time marked—by minutes and hours or by seasons and body needs?
- What are the views of life and death, including predestination and fatalism?
- How can health care professionals be most helpful?

After such an assessment, plans for care should show respect for cultural differences and traditional healing practices. Additional information is presented throughout this book relating to specific areas such as nutrition, pregnancy, birth, and the postpartum period.

**CHECK YOUR READING**

11. Why is it important for nurses to examine their own cultural values and beliefs?
12. How might communication be a source of conflict?
13. Why is culture compared to an iceberg?

## Statistics on Maternal and Infant Health

Statistics is the science of collecting and interpreting numeric data. In health and medical science, the data often focus on mortality rates within a given population. Mortality rates indicate the number of deaths that occur each year by different categories. They are important sources of information about the health of groups of people within a country. They may also be an indication of the value a society places on health care and the kind of health care available to the people.

## Maternal and Infant Mortality

Throughout history, the number of deaths of women and infants has been high, especially around the time of childbirth. In 1910, six of every 1000 women having a baby in the United States died of causes related to pregnancy and childbirth. In that same year, 130 of every 1000 children died before reaching their first birthday (Simkin, 1989).

Infant and maternal mortality rates began to fall when the health of the general population improved, basic principles of sanitation were applied, and medical knowledge increased. By 1940, major improvements in care reduced the infant mortality rate to half that of 1910. A further large decrease over the next 10 years was a result of the widespread availability of antibiotics, improvement in public health, and increased prenatal care. Today, mothers seldom die in childbirth and infant mortality rates continue downward. The downward trend in maternal and infant mortality rates, however, is greater for whites than for nonwhite groups.

### MATERNAL MORTALITY

Because few women today die in childbirth, the maternal mortality rate is determined by the number of deaths per 100,000 live births instead of per 1000 live births. In 1995, the rate was 7.1 for all women in the United States. African-American women are more likely to die from birth-related causes than white women. The maternal mortality rate for African-American women is 22.1, whereas that for white women is 4.2 (National Center for Health Statistics, 1997).

### INFANT MORTALITY

Improvements in infant mortality rates have been slower than those in maternal mortality. Unlike maternal rates, those for infants are calculated by the number of deaths under 1 year of age per 1000 live births. Between 1950 and 1990 infant mortality dropped from 29.2 to 9.8 deaths per 1000 live births. In 1995 the infant mortality rate (death before the age of 1 year) was 7.6 per 1000 live births, 6 percent lower than 1994, and the lowest ever recorded in the United States (National Center for Health Statistics, 1997). Moreover, the neonatal mortality rate (death before 28 days of life) dropped to 5.0 deaths per 1000 live births, or 8 percent less than the rate of 5.4 for 1993 (Singh et al., 1995).

Although infant mortality rates in the United States have declined overall, the decline for whites has remained significantly greater than that for African-Americans. In 1995 the mortality rate for white infants was 6.3. For black infants the rate was 15.1 (National Center for Health Statistics, 1997). Figure 1–4 compares the rates of infant mortality among whites and African-Americans for the last 53 years.

## Disparity Across Minority Groups

The disparity in maternal and infant mortality rates is most obvious between whites and African-Americans, who constitute the largest minority group. The discrepancy is primarily due to increases in the rate of low-birth-weight infants (below 2500 g). African-American infants are at twice the risk for low birth weight than other newborns, and they are twice as likely to die before their first birthday.

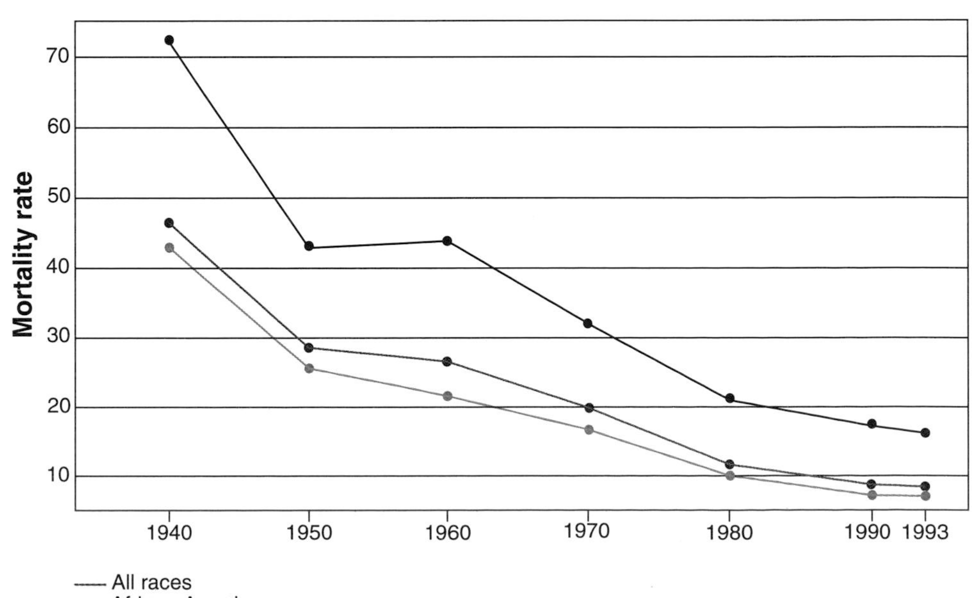


**FIGURE 1–4**

Infant mortality rates from 1940 to 1993 based on advance report on final mortality statistics. (National Center for Health Statistics. U.S. Department of Health and Human Services, Public Health Service, Centers for Disease Control and Prevention, 1994. *Monthly vital statistics report* 43[2], supplement.)

Poverty, not race, is the important factor. The rate of poverty is higher for nonwhites in the United States. People who live below the poverty level are unlikely to be in good health or to get the health care they need. Obtaining care becomes vital during pregnancy and infancy, and lack of care is reflected in the high mortality rates in all categories.

Two national health objectives for the year 2000 are (1) to reduce the overall infant mortality rate to no more than seven per 1000 and (2) to reduce the rate among black infants to no more than 11 per 1000 (U.S. Department of Health and Human Services, 1995).

### Infant Mortality Across Nations

One would expect that a country such as the United States, which has one of the highest gross national products in the world, would have one of the lowest infant mortality rates. Yet in 1994 (the most recent year for which comparative data are available) the mortality rate in the United States was worse than that of 20 other countries (Table 1–4).

The major reasons for this poor showing are (1) unequal access to health care for women of all socioeconomic levels and (2) the high rate of adolescent pregnancy, which is associated with the low birth weight and prematurity that contribute to infant mortality. Congenital anomalies and sudden infant death syndrome are also leading causes of infant mortality.

**TABLE 1–4 INFANT MORTALITY RATES FOR SELECTED COUNTRIES**

| Country | Infant Mortality (Per 1000 Live Births) |
|---|---|
| Japan | 4.2 |
| Singapore | 4.3 |
| Sweden | 4.4 |
| Finland | 4.7 |
| Hong Kong | 4.8 |
| Norway | 5.2 |
| Switzerland | 5.5 |
| Netherlands | 5.9 |
| Ireland | 5.9 |
| Australia | 6.1* |
| Austria | 6.1 |
| France | 6.1 |
| Canada | 6.2 |
| Germany | 6.2* |
| United Kingdom | 6.2 |
| Denmark | 6.5† |
| Italy | 6.7 |
| New Zealand | 7.2* |
| Spain | 7.2 |
| Belgium | 7.6 |
| United States | 7.6 |

* 1992 data.
† 1993 data.
Adapted from Guyer, B., Strobino, D.M., Ventura, S.J., MacDorman, M., & Martin, J.A. (1996). Annual summary of vital statistics—1995. *Pediatrics*, 98(6), 1007–1020.

**✓ CHECK YOUR READING**

14. Why is the infant mortality rate so much lower today than at the beginning of the twentieth century?
15. Why are African-American women and infants more likely to die than Caucasian women and children?
16. How does the infant mortality rate in the United States compare with the rates in other countries?

## SUMMARY CONCEPTS

- Changes in maternity care in the United States came about as a result of technologic advances, increased knowledge, government involvement, and consumer demands.
- Alternative settings for childbirth are now available within hospitals and in free-standing birth centers; home births are less frequently selected as an alternative.
- Family-centered maternity care, based on the principle that families can make decisions about health care if they have adequate information, has greatly increased the role of nurses.
- Outcomes management, which came about as a result of cost-containment strategies, has resulted in new tools to reduce the length of stay for mothers and infants in the birth facility.
- Clinical pathways are interdisciplinary guidelines for assessments and interventions that will accomplish the identified outcomes in the shortest time.
- Students must learn why and how to perform assessments and interventions so they can use clinical pathways to determine whether clients are achieving identified outcomes.
- Social trends such as poverty, early unplanned pregnancy, and increased rate of divorce have altered family structure and function and have increased the need for information and support provided by nurses.
- To provide care for culturally diverse clients, nurses must examine their own beliefs and become familiar with different cultural values and customs.
- Infant and maternal mortality rates have declined dramatically in the last 50 years; however, the United States continues to rank well below other industrialized nations, and there is still wide variation in mortality rates across ethnic groups.

### References

American Academy of Pediatrics & American College of Obstetricians and Gynecologists (1992). *Guidelines for perinatal care*, 3rd ed. p. 108.

AWHONN (1994). Shortened maternity and newborn hospital stays (position statement). Washington, D.C.: Author.

AWHONN (1994). Didactic content and clinical skills verification for professional nurse providers of perinatal home care. Washington, D.C.: Author.

Bailey, C. (1994). Education for home-care providers. *Journal of Obstetric, Gynecologic, and Neonatal Nursing*, 23(8), 714–719.

Brent, N.J. (1994). Risk management and legal issues in home care: The utilization of nursing staff. *Journal of Obstetric, Gynecologic, and Neonatal Nursing*, 23(8), 659–666.

Callister, L.C. (1995). Cultural meanings of childbirth. *Journal of Obstetric, Gynecologic, and Neonatal Nursing*, 24(4), 327–334.

Cassey, M.Z., & Savalle-Dunn, J. (1994). Sketching the future: Trends influencing nursing informatics. *Journal of Obstetric, Gynecologic, and Neonatal Nursing*, 23(2), 175–182.

Cohen, E.L., & Cesta, T.G. (1993). *Nursing case management: From concept to evaluation*. St. Louis: Mosby–Year Book.

DeWoody, S., and Price, J. (1994). A systems approach to multidimensional critical paths. *Nursing Management*, 25(11), 47–51.

Evans, C.J. (1995). Postpartum home care in the United States. *Journal of Obstetric, Gynecologic, and Neonatal Nursing*, 24(2), 180–186.

Finkler, S., & Kovner, C. (1993). *Financial management for nurse managers and executives*. Philadelphia: W.B. Saunders.

Fleschler, R.G., & King, B.P. (1995). Perinatal outcomes management: balancing quality with cost. *Journal of Perinatal-Neonatal Nursing*, 9(2), 21–28.

Goodwin, L. (1994). Essential program components for perinatal home care. *Journal of Obstetric, Gynecologic, and Neonatal Nursing*, 23(8), 667–673.

Grohar, J. (1994). Nursing protocols for antepartum home care. *Journal of Obstetric, Gynecologic, and Neonatal Nursing*, 23(8), 687–695.

Gupton, A. (1995). The Canadian perspective on postpartum home care. *Journal of Obstetric, Gynecologic, and Neonatal Nursing*, 24(2), 173–179.

Guyer, B., Strobino, D.M., Ventura, S.J., MacDorman, M., & Martin, J.A. (1996). Annual summary of vital statistics—1995. *Pediatrics*, 98(6), 1007–1020.

Hutchinson, M.K., & Baqi-Aziz, M. (1994). Nursing care of the childbearing Muslim family. *Journal of Obstetric, Gynecologic, and Neonatal Nursing*, 23(9), 767–772.

Ignatavicius, D.D., & Hausman, K.A. (1995). *Clinical pathways for collaborative practice*. Philadelphia: W.B. Saunders.

Keatley, M.A. (1994, September). Managing care through outcomes analysis. *Inside Case Management*, p. 7.

Keppler, A.B. (1995). Postpartum care center: Follow-up care in a hospital-based clinic. *Journal of Obstetric, Gynecologic, and Neonatal Nursing*, 24(1), 17–21.

Lamb, G.S., & Stempel, J.E. (1994). Nurse case management from the client's view: Growing as insider-expert. *Nursing Outlook*, 42(1), 7–12.

Leininger, M. (1978). *Transcultural nursing: Concepts, theories, practices*. New York: John Wiley & Sons.

Mattson, S. (1995). Culturally sensitive perinatal care for Southeast Asians. *Journal of Obstetric, Gynecologic, and Neonatal Nursing*, 24(4), 335–342.

Miller, M. (1995). Culture, spirituality, and women's health. *Journal of Obstetric, Gynecologic, and Neonatal Nursing*, 24(3), 257–263.

Nance, T.A. (1995). Intercultural communication: Finding common ground. *Journal of Obstetric, Gynecologic, and Neonatal Nursing*, 24(3), 249–255.

National Center for Health Statistics. (1996, November). *Healthy people 2000 review*, 1995–96. Hyattsville, Md.: Public Health Service.

National Center for Health Statistics. (1997). *Health, United States*, 1996–97 *and injury chartbook*. Hyattsville, Md.: Public Health Service.

Simkin, P. (1989). Childbearing in social context. *Women and Health*, 15(3), 5–21.

Singh, G.K., Mathews, T.J., Clarke, S.C., Yannicos, K., & Smith, B.L. (1995). A summary of births, marriages, divorces, and deaths, 1994. *Monthly Statistics Report*, Hyattsville, Md.: National Center for Health Statistics; September 21, 1995; 43(13).

U.S. Bureau of Census. (1995). *Statistical abstract of the United States* (115th ed.). Washington, D.C.: Author, pp. 87–90.

U.S. Department of Health and Human Services. (1995). *Healthy people* 2000 *review*, 1995–96. Washington, D.C.: Author.

Wertz, R., & Wertz, D. (1992). *Lying-in: A history of childbirth in America* (2nd ed.). New Haven, Conn.: Yale University Press.

Williams, L.R., & Cooper, M.K. (1993). Nurse-managed postpartum home care. *Journal of Obstetric, Gynecologic, and Neonatal Nursing*, 22(1), 25–32.

# 2

# The Nurse's Role in Maternity Care

## OBJECTIVES

1. Explain the roles of nurses with advanced preparation in maternal-newborn nursing. Include the roles of nurse-midwives, nurse practitioners, and clinical specialists.
2. Discuss the roles for nurses in maternity care. Include those of teacher, communicator, and manager.
3. Explain the importance of critical thinking, and describe how it may be learned.
4. Describe the steps of the nursing process and relate them to maternal-newborn nursing.
5. Explain how nursing process relates to critical thinking.
6. Discuss the importance of nursing research in clinical practice.

## DEFINITIONS

**ambiguity (ambiguous)** *Lack of clarity or certainty; having more than one meaning.*

**assumptions** *Beliefs taken for granted without examination.*

**baseline data** *Information that describes the status of the client before treatment begins.*

**bias** *A prejudice that sways the mind.*

**cesarean birth** *Surgical birth of the fetus through an incision in the abdominal wall and uterus.*

**delegated nursing interventions** *Physician-prescribed nursing actions that require nursing judgment because nurses are accountable for correct implementation. See also independent nursing interventions.*

**fetus** *The developing baby from 9 weeks after conception until birth. In everyday practice, the term is often used to describe a developing baby during pregnancy, regardless of age.*

**independent nursing interventions** *Nurse-prescribed actions used in both nursing diagnoses and collaborative problems. See also delegated nursing interventions.*

**inference** *The act of drawing a conclusion or making a deduction.*

**judgment** *An opinion.*

**reflection** *Meditation, attentive consideration.*

**skepticism** *Doubt in the absence of conclusive evidence.*

**suspend** *To delay or to bring to a stop temporarily.*

**validate** *To make certain that the information collected during assessment is accurate.*

As maternity care changed from regimented care of the mother and newborn to a family-centered approach, maternity nursing evolved to a new era of autonomy and independence. Nurses who work with childbearing families must be able to communicate and teach effectively. They must be able to think critically and to use nursing process to develop a plan of care that meets the unique needs of each family. They will be expected to use current research to problem solve and to collaborate with other health care providers. Moreover, many nurses complete advanced programs of education that allow them to provide primary care throughout pregnancy and the childbearing experience.

## Advanced Preparation for Maternal-Newborn Nurses

The gradual change to family-centered maternity care and the persistent challenge of providing health care for indigent women have led to an expanded role for nurses. Many nurses have completed advanced programs of education and are prepared as certified nurse-midwives, nurse practitioners, and clinical specialists.

### Certified Nurse-Midwives

Certified nurse-midwives are registered nurses who have completed an extensive program of study and clinical experience. They must pass a certification test administered by the American College of Nurse-Midwives. Certified nurse-midwives are qualified to take complete health histories and to perform physical examinations. They can provide complete care during pregnancy, childbirth, and the postpartum period. They attend both the mother and the infant as long as the mother's progress is normal. They are committed to providing information about preventive measures and preparation for normal pregnancy and childbirth. They spend a great deal of time counseling and supporting the childbearing family. The certified nurse-midwife also provides gynecologic services as well as family-planning information and counseling.

The effectiveness of care provided by nurse-midwives has a long history. In the 1930s, the Maternity Center Association, founded to provide care for indigent women, began to educate public health nurses in midwifery. At almost the same time, Mary Breckinridge, a nurse-midwife from England, founded the Frontier Nursing Service to provide primary care (including midwifery services) for destitute families in the remote mountains of Kentucky.

Despite the proven effectiveness of care, physicians opposed the widespread use of nurse-midwives. For many years restrictions were placed on the scope and location of their practice. In 1970, however, many of the restrictions were alleviated when the American College of Obstetricians and Gynecologists, together with the Nurses Association of the American College of Obstetricians and Gynecologists (NAACOG)—now known as the Association of Women's Health, Obstetric, and Neonatal Nurses (AWHONN)—issued a joint statement, which admitted nurse-midwives as part of the health care team. In 1981, Congress authorized Medicaid payments for the services of certified nurse-midwives. This measure has greatly increased use of nurse-midwives, particularly in health maintenance organizations (HMOs), in birth centers, and in some hospitals.

### Nurse Practitioners

Nurse practitioners are registered nurses with advanced preparation that allows them to provide primary care for specific groups of clients. They can take a complete health history, perform physical examinatons, order and interpret laboratory and other diagnostic studies, and provide primary care for health maintenance and health promotion. All nurse practitioners collaborate with physicians for treatments and medications that are beyond their scope of practice.

The responsibilities of nurse practitioners continue to expand despite restrictions against direct third-party payment to them. Nurse practitioners now specialize in many areas of practice, including maternal-child care.

The *maternity nurse practitioner,* or women's health practitioner, can assess the pregnant woman at prenatal appointments and evaluate the progress of the pregnancy. Although they do not assist with childbirth, nurse practitioners provide information and care during the postpartum period.

*Family nurse practitioners* are prepared to provide care for all family members. They care for women during uncomplicated pregnancies as well as provide follow-up care for the mother and infant after childbirth. Unlike certified nurse-midwives, they do not assist with childbirth.

*Pediatric nurse practitioners* provide health maintenance care for infants and children who do not require the services of physicians.

*Family planning nurse practitioners* often work in family planning clinics or with physicians in private practice. Major responsibilities include performing pelvic examinations and screening procedures for sexually transmitted diseases and providing family planning services.

### Clinical Nurse Specialists

Maternity clinical specialists are registered nurses who, through study and supervised practice at the graduate level (master's or doctorate), have become expert in the care of childbearing families. Four major subroles have been identified for clinical nurse specialists: expert practitioner, educator, researcher, and consultant. These professionals often function as clinical leaders, role models, client advocates, and change agents. They have been particularly active in the development of outcomes management systems described in Chapter 1. They also act as consultants to assist other nurses in planning care for difficult problems encountered in the maternity unit. Unlike nurse practitioners, clinical nurse specialists are not prepared to provide primary care.

## Implications of Changing Roles for Nurses

As maternity care has changed, so have the roles of maternal-newborn nurses. Nurses now work in a variety of highly specialized areas, such as fetal diagnostic centers, infertility clinics, and genetic counseling. Although they previously worked almost exclusively in the hospital setting, many are now involved in home care and in community-based clinics. Moreover, nurses have assumed primary responsibility for independent functions such as teaching, counseling, and intervening for a wide variety of nonmedical problems that trouble the childbearing family.

The added responsibilities of teaching and counseling make it necessary for all nurses to develop and maintain additional intrapersonal skills. These skills include communication, effective teaching, critical thinking, and the use of nursing process to identify and intervene for a variety of problems.

### Therapeutic Communication

Therapeutic communication, unlike social communication, is purposeful, goal directed, and focused. Although it may seem simple, therapeutic communication requires conscious effort and considerable practice. Therapeutic communication is a vital part of all nursing, and techniques are taught early in all curricula. Communication is emphasized throughout this book for three reasons: (1) to review the process, (2) to emphasize the importance of communication in maternal-newborn nursing, and (3) to provide examples for using therapeutic communication with childbearing families.

#### GUIDELINES FOR THERAPEUTIC COMMUNICATION

Therapeutic communication requires great flexibility and cannot depend on a particular set of learned techniques. Certain guidelines may prove helpful, however.

1. A calm setting that provides privacy, reduces distractions, and minimizes interruptions is essential.
2. Interactions should begin with introductions and clarification of the nurse's role: "My name is Claudia Lyall; I am here to complete the discharge teaching that was started yesterday." This introduction acknowledges the nurse's purpose and sets the scene to discuss concerns about what happens when the family is discharged from the hospital.
3. Therapeutic communication should be focused because it is directed toward meeting the needs expressed by the family. Beginning the interaction with an open-ended question is one method of focusing the interaction: "How do you feel about going home today?" It may also be necessary to redirect the conversation: "Thanks for showing me the beautiful pictures of the baby; I understand you are having a bit of trouble getting him to nurse."
4. Nonverbal behaviors may communicate more powerful messages than the spoken word. For example, facial expressions and eye movements can confirm or contradict what the woman says. Repetitive hand gestures, such as finger tapping or twirling a lock of hair, may indicate frustration, irritation, or boredom. Body posture, stance, and gait can convey energy, depression, or discomfort. Voice tone, pitch, rate, and volume may indicate joy, anger, or fear. Grooming also conveys messages about how the woman feels about herself. If she is tired or depressed, she may neglect grooming, although some may not verbalize a problem.
5. Active listening requires that the nurse "attend" to what is being said as well as to the nonverbal clues. Attending behaviors that convey the nurse's interest and a sincere desire to understand include the following:
   - Eye contact, which signals a readiness to interact
   - Relaxed posture, with the upper portion of the body inclined toward the client
   - Encouraging cues, such as nodding, leaning closer, and smiling; verbal cues include "Uh huh, go on," "Tell me about that," or "Can you give me an example?"
   - Touch, which can be a powerful response

when words would break a mood or fail to convey the depth of feeling experienced between the woman and the nurse.

6. Cultural differences influence communication. In some cultures (Chinese, Southeast Asian), prolonged eye contact is confrontational and initiates a great deal of concern. Some people from other cultures (Middle Eastern, Native American) are sometimes uncomfortable with touch and would be disturbed by unsolicited touching.
7. Clarifying communication involves a unique process of the listener receiving the message as the sender intended. It may be necessary for the nurse to ask questions if the meaning of a statement is unclear. For instance, the nurse might say, "I'm not sure I understand." "So you are undecided about breastfeeding?"
8. Emotions are part of communication, and nurses must often reflect feelings that are expressed verbally or nonverbally: "You looked forward to delivery in a birth center and are disappointed that you needed a cesarean birth?"

#### THERAPEUTIC COMMUNICATION TECHNIQUES

Therapeutic communication involves responding as well as listening, and nurses must learn to use responses that facilitate rather than block communication. These facilitative responses, often called communication techniques, focus on both the content of the message and the feeling that accompanies the message. Communication techniques include clarifying, reflecting, silence, questioning, and directing. A brief review of these and other communication techniques can be found in Table 2–1. In addition to being aware of effective communication techniques, nurses must be aware of blocks to communication. These are listed with examples and alternatives in Table 2–2.

#### ✓ CHECK YOUR READING

1. How does therapeutic communication differ from social communication?
2. What are the major communication techniques?
3. What are the major blocks to communication?

## The Nurse's Role in Teaching and Learning

Nurses can be the most significant teachers on the health care team because of the relationship between nurses and clients. Clients often perceive nurses as being less threatening than physicians and expect nurses to have time to respond to concerns that the physician may find trivial. Nurses teach in a variety of settings: in one-to-one interactions, in formal classes, and in group discussions (Fig. 2–1). To teach effectively, nurses must be familiar with the basic principles of teaching and learning.

#### PRINCIPLES OF TEACHING AND LEARNING

Application of the following principles will help nurses become effective teachers in the childbearing setting.

- Real learning depends on the readiness of the family to learn and the relevance of the content. Fortunately, childbearing families are highly motivated to learn. The parents want to be effective, and any content that is relevant to the health of either mother or child is eagerly sought.
- Active participation increases learning. Whenever possible, the learner should be involved in the educational process and not act as a passive listener or viewer. Therefore, learning is enhanced when goals are mutually developed by the family and the nurse and when ample time is allowed for

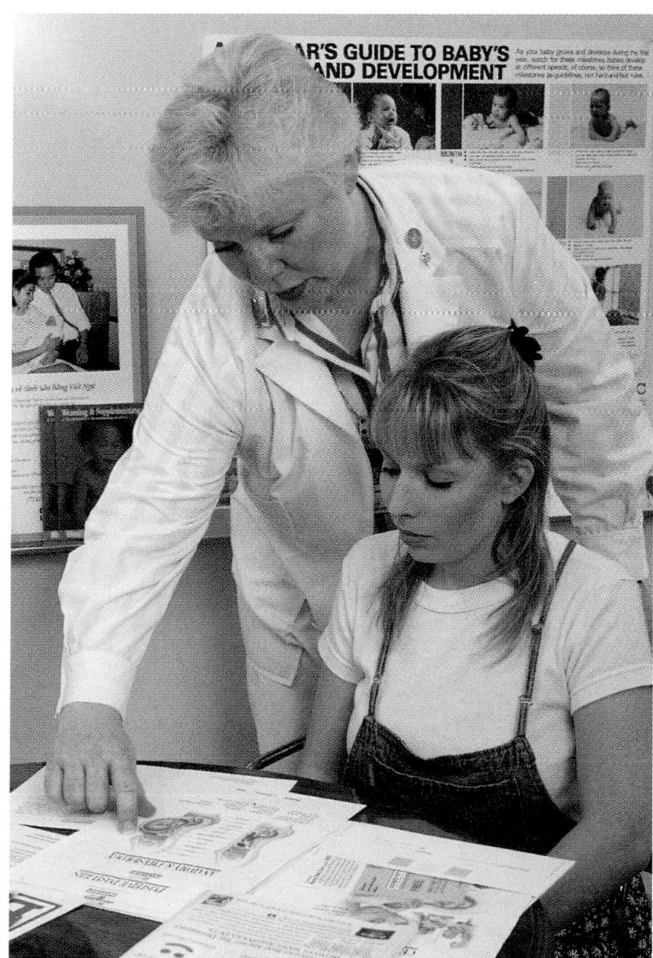


**FIGURE 2–1**

In the prenatal clinic, the nurse teaches a woman one-on-one.

## TABLE 2–1 COMMUNICATION TECHNIQUES

| Definition | Examples |
|---|---|
| **Clarifying** | |
| Clearing up or following up to understand both content and feelings expressed; to check the accuracy of how the nurse perceives the message. | "I'm confused about your plans; could you explain?" "Tell me what you mean when you say you don't feel like yourself."<br>"Are you saying that ______?"<br>"Can you tell me more about ______?" |
| **Paraphrasing** | |
| Restating in words other than those used by the client what the client seems to express; this is a form of clarification. | Example No. 1. Client: "My boyfriend won't even come into the room for the birth. I am furious with him."<br>Nurse: "You want him with you and you are angry because he won't be here?"<br>Example No. 2. Client: "I watch my diet, but I am gaining too much weight anyway."<br>Nurse: "You want to control your weight, but your diet isn't working?" |
| **Reflecting** | |
| Verbalizing comprehension of what the client said and what she seems to be feeling. It is important to link content and feeling and to reflect the client as a mirror reflects a person. The opinion, values, and personality of the nurse should not be in the reflected image. | Example No. 1. Client: "I don't know what to do. My husband doesn't think a cesarean is needed, but the doctor says the baby is showing some stress."<br>Nurse: "You're confused and frightened because they don't agree?"<br>Example No. 2. Woman in early labor: "It was my husband's idea for me to become pregnant. I wasn't too excited about it at first."<br>Nurse: "I'll bet the dad will be a pushover as a father." This reflects the nurse's opinion and fails to acknowledge the mother's statement. A better response might be: "Your husband was more excited early in the pregnancy than you?" |
| **Silence** | |
| Waiting and allowing time for the client to continue; verbal communication need not be constant. | The nurse waits quietly for the client to continue. |
| **Structuring** | |
| Creating guidelines or setting priorities. | "You said you don't know how to take care of the baby and also that you are afraid of getting pregnant again. What should we talk about first?" |
| **Pinpointing** | |
| Calling attention to differences or inconsistencies in statements. | "You say you feel wonderful, but I see some tears." |
| **Questioning** | |
| Eliciting information directly; using open-ended questions to avoid yes or no answers and to prevent controlling the answers. | "How do you feel about being pregnant?" instead of "Are you happy to be pregnant?" |
| **Directing** | |
| Using nonverbal responses or succinct comments to encourage the client to continue. | Nodding. "Um mm." "You were saying ______." "Please go on." |
| **Summarizing** | |
| Reviewing the main themes or issues that were discussed. | "You had two major concerns today ______." "We have talked about breastfeeding and how to bathe the baby today." |

**TABLE 2-2 BEHAVIORS THAT BLOCK COMMUNICATION**

| Behavior | Example | Alternative |
|---|---|---|
| Conveying lack of interest | Looking away, fidgeting | Attending behaviors such as eye contact, nodding. |
| Conveying sense of haste | Checking the time, standing near the door | Sitting at bedside |
| Closed posture | Arms crossed over chest, holding clip board in front of body | Arms relaxed, leaning forward. |
| Interrupting, finishing sentences | Woman: "I'm not sure how ______." Nurse: "We will have a bath demonstration later." | "Go on ______." "You were saying ______." |
| Providing false reassurance | "You're going to be okay." | "I sense you are concerned about how to care for the baby. I will help you give the bath today." |
| Inappropriate self-disclosure | To woman in labor: "I was in labor 12 hours, then had a cesarean." | "What concerns you most about labor?" |
| Giving advice | "You should ______." "If I were you, I would ______." | "How do you feel about that?" "What do you think is most important?" |
| Failure to acknowledge comments or feelings | Woman: "I'm sick of being pregnant; I feel like an incubator." Nurse: "You will soon have a beautiful baby." | "You're ready for this to be over?" |

questions and explanations. Moreover, a discussion format, in which all can participate, stimulates more learning than a straight lecture.

- Repetition of a skill increases retention as well as a feeling of competence. For example, parents experience real learning when they are allowed to bathe, feed, and diaper the infant more than once. This learning often begins during infant care classes that are presented in the prenatal period. It may continue during home visits made by the nurse soon after the mother and infant leave the birth facility.
- Praise and positive feedback are powerful motivators for learning. They are particularly important when the family is trying to master a frustrating task, such as breastfeeding an unresponsive infant.
- Role modeling is an effective method for demonstrating behavior. Parents benefit greatly from watching a competent nurse respond to the infant. Nurses must be aware that their behavior is scrutinized carefully at all times and that it may be copied later.
- Conflicts and frustration impede learning, and they should be recognized and resolved for learning to progress. For instance, couples sometimes do not agree about how the infant should be fed (breastfeeding versus formula feeding). This issue and the feelings it generates must be acknowledged before teaching about breastfeeding can be effective.
- Learning is enhanced when teaching is structured to present simple tasks before more complex material. For instance, the nurse teaches umbilical cord care, which is simple, before teaching how to bathe and shampoo the infant, which is more difficult.
- A variety of teaching methods are necessary to maintain interest and to illustrate concepts. Posters, videos, and printed materials supplement lectures and discussion. Models may be especially useful for teaching family planning or the processes of labor.
- Retention is greater when material is presented in small segments over a period of time. Abbreviated hospital stays are not supportive of this practice, making follow-up care particularly important.

### FACTORS THAT INFLUENCE LEARNING

A variety of factors influence learning. Some of the most important are the developmental level of the family, their primary language, their cultural orientation, and their previous experiences.

**Developmental Level.** It is not surprising that teenaged parents have concerns that are different from those of older couples. To be effective, the nurse must acknowledge this difference and structure teaching-learning sessions to meet the family's primary concerns. For example, very young parents often do not benefit from printed material to the same degree as older parents. However, teenagers often learn well from videos and group discussions with those who share similar problems.

**Language.** The ability to understand the language in which teaching takes place determines how much the family learns. Although many newly arrived immigrants speak English fairly well, they do not understand the idioms, nuances, medical words, or slang terms that are frequently used. It is critical to create a climate in which families feel free to ask questions when they do not understand.

It is sometimes helpful to ask those who speak a different language to describe what they have learned and how they will use the information. The nurse may also want to determine whether the information conflicts with what these parents have learned previously.

**Culture.** Background and culture influence learning. People tend to forget content with which they disagree. For instance, if the family is from a culture that believes certain foods should be eaten by the mother after childbirth, family members may not remember different foods the nurse recommends. Also, if there are conflicts between what elders in the family recommend and what nurses or physicians teach, many young parents follow the advice of the elders. Therefore, it is wise for the nurse to determine the cultural beliefs and attempt to reach an understanding about what information will be useful before beginning to teach.

**Previous Experiences.** Parents who already have children have unique concerns. These families may not need instruction in how to care for a newborn. They may, however, be very concerned about how older children will accept a new infant.

**Physical Environment.** Learning is also influenced by the physical environment. The hospital room is generally suitable for individual teaching. If group instruction is planned, it is helpful to arrange comfortable chairs in a circle, so that all persons can hear and participate in face-to-face communication.

**Organization and Skill of the Instructor.** The instructor must determine the objectives of the class, develop a plan for meeting the objectives, and gather all material before beginning the teaching session. If the objective is that all parents present will observe a bath demonstration, the nurse must decide how to demonstrate the bath, when care of the umbilical cord and circumcision will be presented, and which major principles should be addressed.

It is also very helpful to summarize the major principles discussed. For example, after a bath demonstration, the nurse might conclude by saying, "The important points to remember are to prevent the baby from becoming chilled; to be sure the infant doesn't fall; to start at the face, which is the cleanest area; and to bathe the bottom last."

#### EFFECTS OF EARLY DISCHARGE

Although the principles of teaching and learning should be used whenever possible, early discharge of the mother and infant makes this difficult (Fig. 2–2). Many mothers now leave the hospital within 24 hours after childbirth, and a great deal of teaching must be compressed into a few hours. As a result, there is not enough time for repetition and return demonstrations of infant care. Many families leave the hospital before they have attained any degree of comfort with infant care.

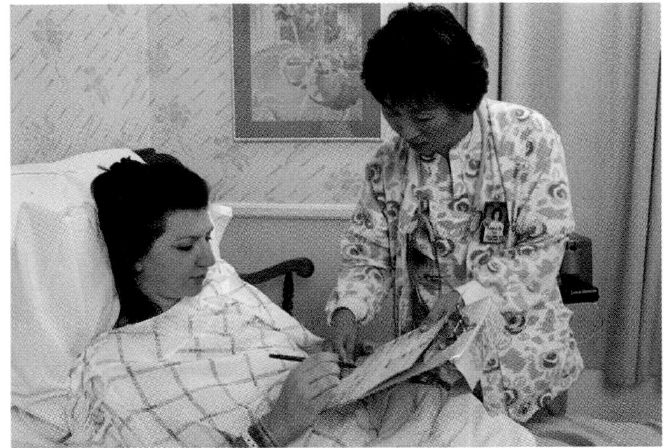

**FIGURE 2–2**

Often, the nurse must condense teaching by using a "check-off" sheet because mothers and infants leave the birth facility within 24 hours of childbirth.

Innovative methods have been developed to meet the needs of families who leave the birth facility feeling insecure. These include follow-up telephone calls, home visits, information lines, and mother-infant outpatient clinics. Moreover, there is greater emphasis on teaching self-care and infant care during the prenatal period. Of course, this information must be reviewed before mother and infant leave the birth facility, but review generally takes less time than providing information the first time.

## The Nurse's Role as Manager

As a result of the decreased length of stay (LOS) in the birth facility, the role of nurses has changed dramatically. Nurses are not often able to provide direct patient care. Instead, they delegate concrete tasks, such as giving a bath or taking vital signs, to others. As a result, nurses spend more time teaching and supervising nonlicensed personnel, planning and coordinating care, and collaborating with other professionals and agencies. Moreover, nurses are expected to understand the financial squeeze resulting from cost-containment strategies and to contribute to their institutions' economic viability. At the same time they must continue to act as patient advocates and to maintain a standard of care. (See Chapter 3 for information about the legal implications of delegating and supervising personnel.)

**CHECK YOUR READING**

4. What are the major principles of teaching and learning?
5. What factors affect learning?

## Critical Thinking

In recent years critical thinking has received widespread attention in nursing. In 1992 it became one of the National League for Nursing's mandatory criteria for accreditation. Clearly, nurses must be concerned with the development of critical thinking skills that are needed not only to pass the National Council Licensure Examination (NCLEX) but also to function in the clinical area.

### Definitions

Unlike undirected thinking, during which the mind wanders freely, critical thinking is controlled and directed toward finding solutions or forming opinions. To do this effectively, all involved must gain insight into their own unique thought processes. This process means analyzing one's own thinking by taking it apart to examine and criticize it. It includes recognizing and acknowledging specific habits and responses that can interfere with productive thinking.

Critical thinking is based on reason rather than on preference or prejudice. Moreover, critical thinking seeks to examine feelings so that one can understand how emotions affect thinking. Last, but certainly not least, critical thinking requires that one suspend judgment until there is adequate evidence to support inferences or conclusions.

### Purpose of Critical Thinking

The purpose of critical thinking is to identify and then to overcome habits or impulses that can result in poor decisions or inappropriate actions. Although it may not be recognized as such, critical thinking is used in many situations. For example, when buying a car, one might be tempted by a particular color or model, but after considering other factors, such as cost and gas mileage, a different, more suitable car might be selected.

The primary purpose of critical thinking in nursing is to help nurses make the best clinical judgments. The process begins when nurses realize that it is not enough to accumulate a fund of knowledge from texts and lectures. They must also be able to *apply* the knowledge to specific clinical situations and thus to reach conclusions that provide the most effective care in each situation.

In addition to acquiring knowledge and learning to apply that knowledge, nurses must also honestly examine their own thought processes for flaws that can lead to inaccurate conclusions or poor judgments. Although this examination requires a great deal of self-analysis, a series of steps makes the process easier. Critical thinking exercises are presented throughout the book to help students develop skill in critical thinking and applying knowledge.

### Steps in Critical Thinking

A series of steps may help clarify how critical thinking is learned. These steps may be called the ABCDEs of critical thinking. They include a recognition of *assumptions*, an examination of personal *biases*, an analysis of how much pressure one has for *closure*, an examination of how one collects and analyzes *data*, and an evaluation of how *emotions* may interfere with one's ability to think critically.

#### RECOGNIZING ASSUMPTIONS

*Assumptions* are ideas, beliefs, or values that are taken for granted without any basis in fact or reason. These unconscious assumptions lead to unexamined thoughts or unsound actions. For instance, what might be the consequences of the following assumptions: "Anyone who wants a job can get one." "Teenagers don't listen." "Every woman wants a baby." "Children should be seen but not heard."

When attempting to identify assumptions, it may be helpful to make a list of everything known about a specific situation. Then each item on the list should be analyzed to determine which is true, which could be true, and which is either untrue or lacks enough evidence to determine whether it is true or not.

#### ANALYZING BIASES

*Biases* are prejudices that sway the mind toward a particular conclusion or course of action on the basis of personal theories or stereotypes. Biases are based on unexamined beliefs, and many are widespread. For instance, "Fat people are lazy." "Women are bad drivers." "Men are insensitive."

People are often biased toward those of different races, religions, or lifestyles. When faced with a predisposition to judge a person or a group of persons, it may be wise to ask oneself (or a co-worker) a series of questions: "Why do you think that?" "What if this were a different client?" "What if there were different circumstances?" "What might someone who disagrees say?" "What is influencing my thinking?"

#### EXAMINING THE NEED FOR CLOSURE

Many persons look for immediate answers and experience a great deal of anxiety until a solution is found for any problem. In other words, they have very little tolerance for doubt or uncertainty, sometimes called ambiguity. As a result, they feel pressure to come to a decision or to reach *closure* as early as possible. This is one of the most important aspects of critical thinking because those who feel pressure to come to an early decision, or to find a quick solution, often do so with insufficient data.

To overcome the pressure to reach an early conclusion, a conscious effort must be made to suspend judgment. This is sometimes called *reflective skepticism*. The first step is to acknowledge the anxiety that postponing decisions creates. The next step involves deliberately waiting to make a decision. One could follow the example of judges who take information "under advisement" and announce they will "render a decision" at a later date.

Persons who jump to conclusions often stop with one answer. To overcome this tendency, they should always look for a second right answer. They could also imagine the problem from the perspective of someone else. They might also ask a series of questions: "What alternatives do we have?" "What else might work?" "What information supports this?" "What effect would that have?" "Is there good evidence to support that decision?" "Is there reason to doubt that evidence?"

Unlike those who feel pressure for closure, some persons can tolerate a great deal of doubt and uncertainty. They are comfortable with data collection and analysis but feel uncomfortable making decisions. They may procrastinate or put off coming to a decision for as long as possible. This course of action may be of little consequence. For instance, collecting information to decide whether to get a pet may go on for considerable time, and the decision may be of slight importance.

On the other hand, failure to make a decision in the clinical area may have serious consequences for clients and their families. Several questions may help overcome the tendency to put off coming to a decision. "What signs indicate something is wrong?" "Do I need to do something about it?" "How much time do I have?" "What happens if I don't do something about this?" "What could happen if I do?" "What should I do first?" "What resources can help me?" This step might also be called *priority setting*; it is one of the most important aspects of critical thinking.

### BECOMING EXPERT IN MANAGING DATA

Expertise in collecting, organizing, and analyzing data involves developing an attitude of *inquiry* and learning to live with questions. "Why?" "What if?" "What else?" "Is this relevant?" "How does it relate to that?" "How can I organize the data?" "Does it form patterns?" "What can I infer from those patterns?"

**Collecting Data.** To obtain complete data, one must develop skill in verbal communication. Asking open-ended questions elicits more information than asking questions that require only a one-word answer. Follow-up questions are often needed to clarify information or to pursue a particular train of thought.

**Validating Data.** Information that is unclear or incomplete should be validated. This process may involve rechecking physical signs, collecting additional information, or determining whether a perception is accurate. For instance, the comment "You seem uncomfortable" may result in the client's denying or acknowledging discomfort.

**Organizing and Analyzing Data.** Data is more useful when organized into patterns or clusters. The first step is to separate data that are relevant from data that may be interesting but that are not related to the current situation. For example, the fact that a neighbor is pregnant with twins has little bearing on how a new mother breastfeeds her infant.

The next step is to compare one's data with expected norms to determine what is within the expected range (normal) and what is not within expected levels (abnormal). Abnormal results provide cues that can be grouped or clustered so that conclusions can be made. For example, grouping all data that may indicate excessive bleeding, such as pulse rate, blood pressure, amount of vaginal bleeding, and skin color, may make the information more meaningful. Organizing data into clusters often reveals that additional data are needed before a decision can be reached.

### ACKNOWLEDGING OTHER FACTORS

A variety of *emotions* and *environmental factors* can influence critical thinking. For instance, the clinical area is often a noisy, fast-paced, and hectic environment with time limitations and distractions that make calm reflection and reasoning difficult. Moreover, nurses working 10- to 12-hour shifts are aware that fatigue may reduce their ability to concentrate. Inexperienced nurses and students may lack confidence in their knowledge and experience. As a result, they often feel anxious, which can reduce their ability to think critically.

Many nurses, both experienced and inexperienced, have a strong need to protect their self-image. As a result, they become very defensive when they have said or done something wrong. This response is a serious barrier to critical thinking and requires that all health care professionals learn to acknowledge mistakes and to feel comfortable with constructive criticism.

Extreme emotions, such as anger or frustration, impede critical thinking by narrowing the focus only to data that support the intense feeling. For example, persons who are extremely frustrated may repeat the perceived cause of their frustration over and over and may be unable to move on to other information so the problem can be addressed.

The first step in dealing with factors or emotions that impede thinking is to recognize and acknowledge them. For example, it may be necessary to say, "I feel flustered by all the activity and need to find a quiet spot for a few minutes of concentration." To develop critical thinking skills, one must learn to admit mistakes and become comfortable saying, "I was wrong." Asking for assistance, verification, or validation is wise when fatigue is a problem or when lack of confidence creates anxiety.

It is essential for the person who experiences intense frustration or anger to recognize the emotions and their impact on rational thought. It may be helpful to ask a trusted colleague to point out when signs of these emotions, such as repetitive vehement comments, occur. Some persons use other methods of control, such as visualizations; a series of breathing exercises; or, when possible, a brief, self-imposed "time-out" from the precipitating situation.

**CHECK YOUR READING**

6. What is the purpose of critical thinking?
7. What steps may be helpful in learning critical thinking?
8. What is meant by reflective skepticism?

## Application of Nursing Process: Maternal-Newborn Nursing

Nursing process forms the basis for maternal-newborn nursing, as it does for all of nursing. Nursing process consists of five distinct steps: (1) assessment, (2) analysis, (3) planning, (4) implementation, and (5) evaluation. In maternal-newborn nursing, nursing process must be adapted to a population that is generally healthy and that is experiencing a life event that holds the potential for growth as well as for problems. Much maternal-newborn nursing activity is devoted to assessing and diagnosing client strengths and healthy functioning. Interventions often focus on promoting and enhancing these strengths to help families achieve the highest level of wellness. This focus differs somewhat from providing care for clients who are ill and presents some difficulty for maternal-newborn nurses when they use the list of largely problem-oriented nursing diagnoses provided by the North American Nursing Diagnosis Association (NANDA).

### Assessment

Nursing assessment is accomplished in a systematic, deliberate manner and includes not only physiologic data but also information related to other life processes that involve psychological, social, and cultural considerations. Thus, although the mother or the infant may be the primary client, nurses must assess the belief systems, available support, perceptions, and plans of other family members in an effort to provide the best nursing care. Two levels of nursing assessment are used to collect comprehensive data: (1) data base assessment and (2) focus assessments.

#### DATA BASE ASSESSMENT

The data base assessment is usually performed at the initial contact with the woman. Its purpose is to gather information about all aspects of her health. This information, called *baseline data*, describes the client's health status before interventions begin. It forms the basis for identifying both strengths and problems.

A variety of methods may be used to organize the assessment. For example, information may be grouped according to body systems. Also assessment can be organized around nursing models that are based on nursing theory, such as Roy's adaptation to stress theory or Orem's self-care deficit theory.

#### FOCUS ASSESSMENT

A focus assessment is used to gather information that is specifically related to an actual health problem or a problem that the client or family is at risk for acquiring. A focus assessment is often performed at the beginning of a shift and centers on areas relevant to childbearing. For instance, in maternal-newborn nursing, one should assess the breasts and nipples because the mother is at risk for problems if she does not have adequate information about breastfeeding or care of the nipples.

### Analysis

The data gathered during assessment must be analyzed so that problems or potential problems and their causes can be identified. Data are validated and grouped in a process of critical thinking so that cues and inferences can be determined. Health problems that nurses can treat independently and for which they are legally accountable are termed *nursing diagnoses*. At this time more than 100 nursing diagnoses have been identified by NANDA.

### Nursing Diagnosis

Each health problem identified by NANDA as a nursing diagnosis consists of three components:

- The *title* offers a concise description of the health problem.
- *Defining characteristics* refer to a cluster of signs and symptoms that are often seen with that particular diagnosis.
- *Etiologic and related factors* are factors that can cause or contribute to the problem. The etiology may be pathophysiologic, situational, or maturational.

Nursing diagnoses may be *actual* or *risk*. Actual nursing diagnoses indicate the problem exists at the time and can be validated by the presence of defining characteristics. Risk nursing diagnoses are appropriate when the problem does not exist but the individual or family is at risk for it to develop later. Table 2–3 provides examples of actual and risk diagnoses.

Any nursing diagnosis may be appropriate for maternal-newborn nursing. Some nursing diagnostic categories, however, are particularly common (Table 2–4).

## Planning

The third step in nursing process involves planning care for problems that were identified during assessment and that are reflected in the nursing diagnoses. During this step, nurses set priorities, develop goals or outcomes that state what is to be accomplished by a certain time, and plan interventions that help to accomplish them.

**TABLE 2–3 EXAMPLES OF ACTUAL AND RISK NURSING DIAGNOSES**

**Actual Nursing Diagnoses**

| Problem | Etiology | Signs and Symptoms |
|---|---|---|
| Alteration in Nutrition: Less Than Body Requirement | Knowledge deficit of nutritional needs during lactation | Weight loss of 5 kg and daily caloric intake <1500 calories |
| Ineffective Breastfeeding | Nipple trauma | Cracked nipples and reports of discomfort during nursing |

**Risk Nursing Diagnoses**

| Problem | Risk Factors |
|---|---|
| Risk for Ineffective Breastfeeding | Lack of knowledge of correct positioning of infant and appropriate breast care |
| Risk for Alteration in Nutrition: Less Than Body Requirements | Knowledge deficit of nutritional needs during lactation |

**TABLE 2–4 COMMON NURSING DIAGNOSES IN MATERNAL-NEWBORN NURSING**

Anxiety
Body Image Disturbance
Breastfeeding, Effective
Breastfeeding, Ineffective
Breastfeeding, Interrupted
Communication, Impaired Verbal
Constipation
Decisional Conflict
Family Coping: Potential for Growth
Family Processes, Altered
Fatigue
Fluid Volume Deficit, Risk for
Health Maintenance, Altered
Health Seeking Behaviors
Infection, Risk for
Knowledge Deficit
Nutrition: Less Than Body Requirements, Altered
Nutrition: More Than Body Requirements, Altered
Organized Infant Behavior, Potential for Enhanced
Pain
Parent/Infant/Child Attachment, Risk for Altered
Parental Role Conflict
Parenting, Altered
Role Performance, Altered
Self-Esteem, Situational Low
Sexuality Patterns, Altered
Sleep Pattern Disturbance
Thermoregulation, Ineffective
Urinary Elimination, Altered
Urinary Retention

### SETTING PRIORITIES

Setting priorities includes (1) determining what problems need immediate attention (i.e., life-threatening problems) and taking immediate action; (2) determining whether there are potential problems that call for a physician's orders for diagnosis, monitoring, or treatment; and (3) identifying actual nursing diagnoses that take precedence over at-risk diagnoses.

### ESTABLISHING GOALS AND EXPECTED OUTCOMES

Although the terms *goals* and *outcomes* are sometimes used interchangeably, they are different. Generally, broad goals do not state the specific outcome criteria and are less measurable than outcome statements. If broad goals are developed, they should be linked with more specific and measurable outcome criteria. For example, if the goal is that the parents will demonstrate effective parenting by discharge, *outcome criteria* that serve as evidence might be prompt, consistent responses to infant signals and competence in bathing, feeding, and comforting the infant.

Certain rules should be followed when writing outcomes:

- Outcomes should be stated in client terms. This wording identifies who is expected to achieve the goal.
- Measurable verbs must be used. For example, "identify," "demonstrate," "express," "walk," "relate," and "list" are verbs that are observable and measurable. Examples of verbs that are difficult to measure are "understand," "appreciate," "feel," "accept," "know," and "experience." For instance, "Ms. Brown will experience less anxiety about assuming care of her infant" poses a problem because it is difficult to determine whether she experiences less anxiety. This outcome can be reworded "Ms. Brown will express less anxiety about assuming care of her infant and will participate in infant care (umbilical cord, circumcision, bathing) before discharge."
- A time frame is necessary. When is the person expected to perform the action? By the first postpartum day? By discharge? Within the second trimester?
- Goals and outcomes must be realistic and attainable. For instance, if a nursing diagnosis of "pain related to uterine contractions and lack of knowledge of the processes of labor" is formulated, a realistic goal or outcome might be "will use learned relaxation and breathing techniques during contractions to manage discomfort." Other goals, such as "will remain free of pain throughout labor" are not attainable by nursing interventions only.
- Goals and outcomes are worked out in collaboration with the client and family to ensure their participation in the plan of care.

#### DEVELOPING NURSING INTERVENTIONS

Once the goals and outcomes are developed, it is necessary to write nursing interventions that will help the client meet the established outcomes.

**Planning Interventions for Actual Nursing Diagnoses.** Nursing interventions for actual nursing diagnoses are aimed at reducing or eliminating the causes or related factors. For instance, suppose the nursing diagnosis is "Altered Parenting related to interruption of bonding process secondary to illness of infant as manifested by absences of attachment behaviors (eye contact, holding)." The desired outcome might be that the parents will demonstrate progressive attachment behaviors, such as touching, palming, eye contact, and participation in infant care within 1 week. Nursing interventions would focus on increasing contact between parents and infant and on facilitating attachment behaviors.

A second example may help to clarify the process. Suppose the nursing diagnosis is "Constipation related to insufficient fluid and fiber intake and inadequate exercise as manifested by painful defecation of small, hard stools." The desired outcome is that the patient will establish a pattern of soft, painless stools occurring more than three times per week. Appropriate nursing interventions seek to bring about increased fluid and fiber intake and to initiate a realistic exercise regimen.

**Planning Interventions for At-Risk Nursing Diagnoses.** Interventions are aimed at (1) monitoring for onset of the problem, (2) reducing or eliminating risk factors, and (3) preventing the problem. For example, suppose the nursing diagnosis for an infant is "Risk for Impaired Skin Integrity related to frequent, loose stools." The planned outcome is that the skin will remain intact, with nursing interventions to include monitoring the condition of the skin at prescribed times for signs and symptoms of skin impairment and initiating measures to keep the skin clean and dry.

### Implementing Interventions

A major problem with implementing nursing interventions occurs because written interventions are often not specific and do not spell out clearly exactly what should be done. Nursing interventions should be as specific as physician's orders. When a physician orders "morphine sulfate, 10 mg IM every 3 hours prn for pain," the order specifies what is to be given, how much is to be given, how it is to be administered, at what time, and why it is necessary. A well-written nursing intervention is equally specific: "Provide 200 ml of fluid (water or juice of choice) q2h while the woman is awake."

Conversely, poorly written interventions, such as "assist with breastfeeding" provide generalizations rather than specific steps to follow. Spelling out exactly how the nurse should assist the mother to breastfeed is more effective: "Demonstrate correct positioning in cradle and football hold at first attempt to breastfeed. Teach mother to elicit rooting reflex by stroking infant's lips with nipple. Demonstrate how to latch infant to nipple, and request a return demonstration before mother is discharged."

### Evaluation

The evaluation determines how well the plan worked or how well the goals or outcomes were met. To evaluate, the nurse must assess the status of the client and compare the current status with the goals or outcome criteria that were developed during the planning step. The nurse then judges how well the client is progressing toward goal achievement and makes a decision. Should the plan be continued? Modified? Abandoned? Are the problems resolved or the causes diminished? Is another nursing diagnosis more relevant?

Nursing process is dynamic, and evaluation frequently results in expanded assessment and additional or modified nursing diagnoses and interventions. Nurses are cautioned not to view lack of goal achievement as a failure. Instead, it is simply time to reassess and to begin the process anew.

## Individualized Nursing Care Plans

Nurses are responsible for documenting nursing diagnoses, expected outcomes, and interventions for each problem. This information is often communicated to colleagues through a written plan of care. Many institutions have *standards of care* for groups of clients, such as those who have had normal spontaneous vaginal births. Individual nursing care plans may be necessary, however, on the basis of needs or problems identified during the assessment step of nursing process. When an individualized plan of care is written, nurses implement the plan through interventions that direct the care. Table 2–5 summarizes the procedure for creating a nursing care plan.

**TABLE 2-5 DEVELOPING INDIVIDUALIZED NURSING CARE THROUGH THE NURSING PROCESS**

Although nursing process is the foundation for maternal-newborn nursing, initially it is a challenging process to apply in the clinical area. It requires proficiency in focus assessments of the new mother and infant as well as the ability to analyze data and plan nursing care for individual clients and families. It may be helpful to pose questions at each step of the nursing process.

**Assessment**

1. Were there data that were not within normal limits or expected parameters? For example, the client states that she feels "dizzy" when she tries to ambulate.
2. If so, what else should be assessed? (What else should I look for? What might be related to this symptom?) For instance, what are the blood pressure, pulse, skin color, temperature, and amount of lochia if the client feels "dizzy"?
3. Did the assessment identify the cause of the abnormal data? What are the hemoglobin count, hematocrit value, and estimated blood loss during childbirth?
4. Are there other factors? What medication is the client taking? How long since she has eaten? Is the environment a related factor (crowded, warm, unfamiliar)? Is she reluctant to ask for assistance?

**Analysis**

1. Are adequate data available to reach a conclusion? What else is needed? (What do you wish you had assessed? What would you look for next time?)
2. What is the major concern? (On the basis of the data, what are you worried about?) The client who is "dizzy" may fall as she ambulates to the bathroom.
3. What might happen if no action is taken? (What might happen to the client if you do nothing?) She may suffer an injury or a complication.
4. Is there a NANDA-approved diagnostic category that reflects your major concern? How is it defined? Suppose during analysis you decide the major concern is that the patient will faint and suffer an injury. What diagnostic category most closely reflects this concern? High Risk for Injury? Definition: The state in which an individual is at risk for harm because of a perceptual or physiologic deficit, a lack of awareness of hazards, or maturational age.
5. Do this category and definition "fit" this client? Is she at greater risk for a problem than others in a similar situation? Why? What are the additional risk factors?
6. Is this a problem that nurses can manage independently? Are medical interventions also necessary?
7. If the problem can be managed by nurses, is it an actual problem (defining characteristics are present), at-risk (risk factors are present), or possible (you have a "hunch" and some data but not enough)?

**Planning**

1. What outcomes are desired? That the client will remain free of injury during hospital stay? That she will demonstrate position changes that reduce the episodes of vertigo?
2. Would the outcomes be clear, specific, and measurable to anyone reading them?
3. What nursing interventions should be initiated and carried out to accomplish these goals or outcomes?
4. Are your written interventions specific and clear? Are action verbs used ("assess," "teach," "assist")? After you have written the interventions, look them over. Do they define exactly what is to be done (when, what, how far, how often)? Will they prevent the client from suffering an injury?
5. Are the interventions based on sound rationale? For instance, dehydration that may occur during labor causes weakness that may result in falls; loss of blood during delivery often exceeds 500 ml, which results in hypotension that is aggravated when the client stands suddenly.

**Implementing Nursing Interventions**

1. What are the expected effects of the prescribed intervention? Are there potential adverse effects? What are they?
2. Are the interventions acceptable to the client and family?
3. Are the interventions clearly written so that they can be carefully followed?

**Evaluation**

1. What is the status of the client right now?
2. What were the goals and outcomes? Are they specific? Can they be measured?
3. Compare the current status of the client with the stated goals and outcomes.
4. What should be done now?

*Abbreviation*: NANDA, North American Nursing Diagnosis Association.

### Nursing Process Related to Critical Thinking

Although nursing process and critical thinking are similar and overlap in many respects, there are major differences. The five steps of nursing process provide a logical method for problem solving. Problem solving begins with a specific problem and ends with a solution. Conversely, critical thinking is open-ended; it goes before and beyond problem solving. Figure 2–3 illustrates the relationship between critical thinking and nursing process. Critical thinking may be triggered not only by a problem but also by a positive event or an opportunity to improve. It focuses on appraisal of how one thinks and emphasizes reflective skepticism. Critical thinking is used throughout each step of the nursing process (Table 2–6).

**CHECK YOUR READING**

9. How does data base assessment differ from focus assessment?
10. How do actual nursing diagnoses differ from high-risk nursing diagnoses?
11. How should goals and outcomes be stated?
12. Why are interventions sometimes difficult to implement? How can this difficulty be corrected?

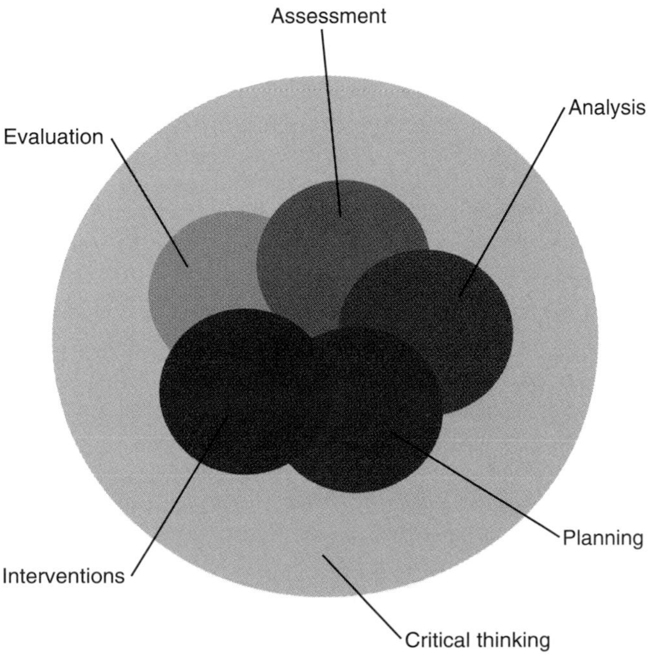

**FIGURE 2–3**

Relationship between the nursing process and critical thinking.

**TABLE 2–6 HOW CRITICAL THINKING IS USED IN NURSING PROCESS**

| Nursing Process | Critical Thinking Skills |
|---|---|
| Assessment | Collecting complete data, validating data<br>Clustering data (normal versus abnormal, important versus unimportant, relevant versus irrelevant)<br>Identifying emotions |
| Analysis | Identifying cues and making inferences<br>Reflecting and suspending judgment<br>Examining thought processes for biases and assumptions<br>Identifying alternatives<br>Determining priorities |
| Planning | Examining need for closure<br>Searching for alternative solutions<br>Validating plan with client, co-worker<br>Communicating plan<br>Acknowledging defensive behavior |
| Implementation | Applying knowledge<br>Testing plan<br>Carrying out plan |
| Evaluation | Examining insights gained<br>Recognizing new ways of thinking, acting<br>Examining options and criteria for action<br>Appraising self and others in the situation |

## Collaborative Problems

In addition to nursing diagnoses, which describe problems that respond to independent nursing functions, nurses must also deal with problems that are beyond the scope of independent nursing practice. These are sometimes termed *collaborative problems*—physiologic complications that usually occur in association with a specific pathologic condition or treatment. They are unlike medical diagnoses, in that they represent situations that are the primary responsibility of nurses.

Nurses monitor to detect the onset of the complication and collaborate with physicians to manage changes in client status. Both physician-prescribed and nursing-prescribed interventions are necessary to minimize complications (Carpenito, 1995). Examples of collaborative problems in maternal-newborn nursing include excessive bleeding following childbirth or labor that begins before the fetus is fully developed.

### Planning

It is inappropriate to identify client-centered goals for a collaborative problem because the goals cannot be achieved by independent nursing action. Client-centered goals for collaborative problems incorrectly imply accountability for problems that nurses cannot manage independently (Carpenito, 1995).

Collaborative problems should reflect the nurse's responsibility in situations requiring physician-prescribed interventions. The responsibility includes the following:

- Monitoring for signs of complications
- Consulting standing orders, protocols, and physicians if signs of complications are observed
- Performing specific actions to minimize the severity of an event or situation (Carpenito, 1995)

### Interventions

Nursing interventions for collaborative problems include (1) performing frequent assessments to monitor the status of the client and detect signs and symptoms of complications, (2) communicating with the physician when signs and symptoms of complications are noted, (3) performing physician-prescribed interventions to prevent or correct the complication, and (4) performing nursing interventions described in the standards of care or policy and procedure manuals.

### Evaluation

Although client-centered goals or outcomes are not developed for collaborative problems, the nurse collects and compares data with established norms and judges whether the data are within normal limits. If data are not within normal limits, the nurse communicates with the physician for additional direction and implements physician-prescribed interventions as well as nursing interventions.

**✓ CHECK YOUR READING**

13. How do nursing diagnoses differ from collaborative problems?
14. Why are client-centered goals inappropriate for collaborative problems?

## Nursing Research

As maternal-newborn nursing and the health care system change, nurses will be challenged to demonstrate that what they do improves client outcomes and is cost effective. To meet this challenge, nurses must participate in research and encourage the utilization of research. With the establishment of the National Institute of Nursing Research as a full-fledged member of the National Institutes of Health, nurses now have an infrastructure in place to ensure that nursing research is supported and that a group of well-prepared nurse researchers will be educated.

The amount of clinically based nursing research conducted is increasing rapidly as nurse researchers strive to develop an independent body of knowledge that demonstrates the value of nursing interventions. Although knowledge is being generated, there is a gap between knowledge acquired by the research team and application of that knowledge to care of the client in the clinical area.

Although students and inexperienced nurses may not participate in research projects, they must take advantage of the knowledge obtained by the research team. Professional journals—such as *Lifelines*; *Journal of Obstetric, Gynecologic, and Neonatal Nursing* (JOGNN); *Nursing Research*; and *Comprehensive Neonatal Nursing*—are the best sources of new information that can help nurses provide improved care and demonstrate that what they do makes a difference in client outcomes.

## SUMMARY CONCEPTS

- Registered nurses with advanced education are prepared to provide primary care for women and children as certified nurse-midwives and nurse practitioners.
- Clinical nurse specialists function as educators, researchers, and consultants to provide in-depth interventions for many problems encountered in maternity care.
- As maternity care has changed, so has the role of nurses, who must be adept at communication techniques and blocks to communication to meet their responsibilities as educators and counselors.
- A primary responsibility of nurses is to provide information to childbearing families; nurses must know the principles of teaching and learning to fulfill the role of educator.
- Nurses must learn to think critically by examining their own thought processes for flaws that can lead to inaccurate conclusions or poor clinical judgments.
- Nursing process begins with assessment and includes analysis of data that may result in nursing diagnoses. These are problems that nurses are legally accountable for identifying and managing independently.
- Collaborative problems are usually physiologic complications that require both physician-prescribed and nurse-prescribed interventions.
- Professional journals are the best sources for information about research projects that demonstrate the effectiveness of nursing interventions.

### References and Readings


Alfaro-LeFevre, R. (1995). *Critical thinking in nursing: A practical approach*, Philadelphia: W.B. Saunders.

Arnold, E., & Boggs, K. (1995). *Interpersonal relationships: Professional communication skills for nurses* (2nd ed.). Philadelphia: W.B. Saunders.

Bowers, B. (1993). Developing analytic thinking skills in early undergraduate education. *Journal of Nursing Education*, 32(3), 107–114.

Brown, H., & Sorrell, J. (1993). Use of clinical journals to enhance critical thinking. *Nurse Educator*, 18(5), 16–18.

Carpenito, L.J. (1995). *Nursing diagnosis: Application to clinical practice* (6th ed.). Philadelphia: J.B. Lippincott.

Case, B. (1994). Walking around the elephant: A critical-thinking strategy for decision making. *Journal of Continuing Education in Nursing*, 25(3), 101–109.

Hendrikson, M., Wall, G., Lethbridge, D., & McClurg, V. (1992). Nursing diagnosis and obstetric, gynecologic, and neonatal nursing: Breastfeeding as an example. *Journal of Obstetric, Gynecologic, and Neonatal Nursing*, 21(6), 446–456.

Kramer, M.K. (1993). Concept clarification and critical thinking: Integrated processes. *Journal of Nursing Education*, 32(9), 406–414.

National League for Nursing (1992a). *Criteria for the evaluation of associate degree programs in nursing*. New York, NY.

National League for Nursing (1992b). *Criteria for the evaluation of baccalaureate and higher degree programs in nursing*. New York, NY.

North American Nursing Diagnosis Association. *Nursing diagnoses: Definitions & classification* (1997–1998). Philadelphia.

Pless, B., & Clayton, G. (1993). Clarifying the concept of critical thinking in nursing. *Journal of Nursing Education*, 32(9), 425–428.

Rubenfeld, M.G., & Scheffer, B.K. (1995). *Critical thinking in nursing: An interactive approach*. Philadelphia: J.B. Lippincott.

Tucker, D.A., & Flannery, J. (1996). The student process for success: The nursing care plan. *Nurse Educator*, 21(1), 47–50.

Wilkinson, J.M. (1992). *Nursing process in action: A critical thinking approach*. Redwood City, Calif: Addison-Wesley Nursing.

# 3

# Ethical, Social, and Legal Issues

## OBJECTIVES

1. Apply theories and principles of ethics to ethical dilemmas.
2. Describe how the steps of the nursing process can be applied to ethical decision making.
3. Discuss ethical conflicts related to reproductive issues such as elective abortion, forced contraception, and infertility.
4. Relate how major social issues, such as poverty and access to health care, affect maternal-newborn nursing.
5. Describe the legal basis for nursing practice.
6. Identify measures to prevent malpractice claims.
7. Identify current trends in health care and their implications for nursing.

## DEFINITIONS

**bioethics** *Rules or principles that govern right conduct, specifically those that relate to health care.*

**deontologic theory** *Ethical theory holding that the right course of action is the one dictated by ethical principles and moral rules.*

**ethical dilemma** *A situation in which no solution seems completely satisfactory.*

**ethics** *Rules or principles that govern right conduct and distinctions between right and wrong.*

**malpractice** *Negligence by a professional person.*

**negligence** *Failure to act in the way a reasonable, prudent person of similar background would act in similar circumstances.*

**nurse practice acts** *Laws that determine the scope of nursing practice in each state.*

**standard of care** *Level of care that can be expected of a professional. This level is determined by laws, professional organizations, and health care agencies.*

**standardized procedures** *Procedures determined by nurses, physicians, and administrators that allow nurses to perform duties usually part of the medical practice.*

**utilitarian theory** *Ethical theory stating that the right course of action is the one that produces the greatest good.*

Maternal-newborn nurses often grapple with ethical and social dilemmas that affect childbearing families. Nurses must know how to approach these issues in a knowledgeable and systematic way. Some ethical and social issues result in the passage of laws that regulate reproductive practice. It is important for nurses to understand the legal basis for their scope of practice to decrease the risk of involvement in malpractice claims.

## Ethics and Bioethics

Ethics involves determining the best course of action in a certain situation. Ethical reasoning is the analysis of what is morally right and reasonable. Bioethics is the application of ethics to health care. Ethical behavior for nurses is discussed in various codes, such as the American Nurses' Association Code for Nurses. Ethical issues have become more complex as developing technology has allowed more options in health care. These issues are controversial because there is lack of agreement over what is right or best and because moral support is possible for more than one course of action.

### Ethical Dilemmas

An ethical dilemma is a situation in which no solution seems completely satisfactory. Opposing courses of action may seem equally desirable, or all possible solutions may seem undesirable. Ethical dilemmas are among the most difficult situations in nursing practice. Finding solutions involves applying ethical theories and principles and determining the burdens and benefits of any course of action.

#### ETHICAL THEORIES

Two major theories guide ethical decision making. Few people use one theory exclusively. Instead, they make decisions by examining both theories and trying to determine which one is most appropriate for the circumstances.

##### DEONTOLOGIC THEORY

The deontologic approach determines what is right by applying ethical principles and moral rules. It does not vary the solution according to individual situations. One example is the rule "life must be maintained at all costs and in all circumstances." Strictly used, the deontologic approach would not consider the quality of life or weigh the use of scarce resources against the likelihood that the life maintained would be near normal.

##### UTILITARIAN THEORY

The utilitarian theory approaches ethical dilemmas by analyzing the benefits and burdens of any course of action to find one that will result in the greatest amount of good. With this theory, the appropriate actions may vary according to the situation. It is a pragmatic approach concerned with the consequences of actions more than the actual actions themselves. In its simplest form, this is an "end justifies the means" approach. If the outcome is positive, the method of arriving at that outcome is less important.

#### ETHICAL PRINCIPLES

Ethical principles are also important in solving ethical dilemmas. Four of the most important principles are beneficence, nonmaleficence, autonomy, and justice (Table 3–1). Although principles guide decision making, in some situations it may be impossible to apply one without conflicting with another. In such cases, one principle may outweigh another in importance.

For example, treatments designed to do good may also cause some harm. A cesarean birth may prevent permanent harm to a fetus in distress. However, the surgery that saves the fetus also harms the mother, causing pain, temporary disability, and possible financial hardship. Both mother and health care providers may decide that the principle of beneficence outweighs the principle of nonmaleficence. A third possibility is that if the mother does not want surgery, the principles of autonomy and justice must also be considered. Is the mother's right to determine what happens to her body more or less important than the right of the fetus to fair and equal treatment?

#### APPLICATION OF ETHICAL THEORIES AND PRINCIPLES

Nurses are often involved in supporting parents when tragedy strikes at birth. They must be knowledgeable, not only of the disease process and the nursing care that is appropriate in these situations but also of the support families need when ethical dilemmas arise. An example is the birth of an infant with anencephaly (congenital absence of brain tissue). A newborn with anencephaly has no chance of survival. Ethical theories and principles can be ap-

**TABLE 3–1 ETHICAL PRINCIPLES**

*Beneficence*: One is required to do or promote good for others.
*Nonmaleficence*: One must avoid risking or causing harm to others.
*Autonomy*: People have the right to self-determination. This includes the right to respect, privacy, and information necessary to make decisions.
*Justice*: All people should be treated equally and fairly regardless of disease or social or economic status.

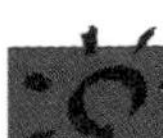

## CRITICAL THINKING EXERCISE

The parents of an infant with anencephaly state that they would like to donate the organs from their dying infant to another infant who might live as a result. They feel that in this way their own infant will live on as a part of another baby. Although these transplants have been performed in the past, they are not currently practiced because of the ethical concerns.

**Q:**

1. What is the deontologic view of this decision?
2. How would the utilitarian view differ?
3. What ethical principles are involved? If such transplants became routine, what potential problems might arise?

**A:**

1. The deontologic view is that it is wrong to take organs necessary for life from one human being to give to another, even when the donor cannot survive. This view disapproves of aggressive treatment necessary to maintain perfusion to the organs until a recipient is located because treatment does not help the dying infant and may increase suffering. This concern invokes the principle of nonmaleficence.
2. The utilitarian view is that anencephalic infants cannot survive but that their organs could provide great benefit to other infants (beneficence). Because this family feels strongly that helping other infants allows good to come from their own tragedy, the greatest good would be for an organ transplant.
3. Potential problems include the possibility that transplants might someday be required, even against the parents' will (and might deny them autonomy). A woman might be forced to carry a pregnancy to term so that the organs could be harvested, even if the parents would rather terminate the pregnancy. If anencephalic infants are used for organ donation, perhaps people with profound mental retardation or persistent vegetative states might be placed in the same situation. Choosing infants to benefit would also be a concern, involving principles of justice. An overriding concern would be determining who would make the decisions necessary.

plied to determine whether it is acceptable to use the organs from an anencephalic infant to save the lives of other infants.

### SOLVING ETHICAL DILEMMAS

There are many approaches to solving ethical dilemmas. Although an approach does not guarantee a right decision, it provides a logical, systematic method for going through the steps of decision making. Because the nursing process is also a method of problem solving, a similar approach can be used for solving ethical dilemmas (Table 3–2).

Decision making in ethical dilemmas may seem straightforward, but it may not result in answers agreeable to everyone. Many agencies, therefore, have bioethics committees to formulate policies for ethical situations, provide education, and help make decisions in specific cases. The committees include a variety of professionals such as nurses, physicians, social workers, ethicists, and clergy members. The woman and family also participate, if possible. A satisfactory solution to ethical dilemmas is more likely to occur when a variety of people work together.

Ethical dilemmas may also have legal ramifications. For example, although the American Medical Association has stated that anencephalic organ donation is ethically permissible, it may be illegal. In many states, the legal criteria for death include both cardiopulmonary and brain death. Anencephalic infants do not meet those criteria, so that donation of their organs would be illegal, even if it were ethical (Rhodes, 1996a).

## ✓ CHECK YOUR READING

1. What is the difference between ethics and bioethics?
2. How does the deontologic theory differ from the utilitarian theory?
3. When might two ethical principles conflict?
4. How do the steps of the nursing process relate to ethical decision making?

## Ethical Issues in Reproduction

Reproductive issues often involve conflicts in which a woman behaves in a way that may cause harm to her

### TABLE 3–2 APPLYING NURSING PROCESS TO SOLVE ETHICAL DILEMMAS

*Assessment*: Gather data to clearly identify the problem and the decisions necessary. Obtain viewpoints of all who will be affected by the decision as well as legal, agency policy, and common practice standards that may apply.

*Analysis*: Decide whether an ethical dilemma exists. Analyze the situation using ethical theories and principles. Determine whether and how these conflict.

*Planning*: Identify as many options as possible, their advantages and disadvantages, and which are most realistic. Predict what is likely to happen if each option is followed. Include the option of doing nothing. Choose the solution.

*Implementation*: Carry out the solution. Determine who will implement the solution and how. Identify all interventions necessary and what support is needed.

*Evaluation*: Analyze the results. Determine whether further interventions are necessary.

fetus or that is disapproved of by some or most members of society. Conflicts between a mother and fetus occur when the mother's needs, behavior, or wishes may injure the fetus. The most obvious instances are those involving abortion, substance abuse, or a mother's refusal to follow the advice of caregivers. Health care workers and society in general may respond to such a woman with anger rather than support. The rights of both mother and fetus must be examined, however.

### ELECTIVE ABORTION

Abortion was a volatile legal, social, and political issue even before the *Roe v. Wade* decision by the U.S. Supreme Court in 1973. Before that time, states could prohibit abortion, making the procedure illegal. In *Roe v. Wade* the Supreme Court stated that abortion was legal anywhere in the United States and that existing state laws prohibiting abortion were unconstitutional because they interfered with the mother's constitutional right to privacy. The Supreme Court decision stipulated that (1) a woman could obtain an abortion at any time during the first trimester, (2) the state could regulate abortions during the second trimester only to protect the woman's health, and (3) the state could regulate or prohibit abortion during the third trimester, except when the mother's life might be jeopardized by continuing the pregnancy.

For many, the woman's constitutional right to privacy conflicts with the fetus' right to life. The Supreme Court did not rule, however, on when life begins. This omission provokes debate between those who believe life begins at conception and those who believe life begins when the fetus is viable, or capable of living outside the uterus. Those who believe life begins at conception may be opposed to abortion at any time during pregnancy. Those who believe life begins when the fetus is viable (20 to 26 weeks of gestation) may oppose abortion after that time. Nurses need to be knowledgeable about past Supreme Court decisions related to abortion and about the conflicting beliefs that divide society on this issue.

**Conflicting Beliefs About Abortion.** Perhaps no issue creates greater division or incites more powerful emotions among Americans than that of elective abortion. Some people believe abortion should be illegal at any time because it deprives the fetus of life. In contrast, others believe that women have the right to control their reproductive function and that political discussion of reproductive rights is an invasion of the most private decisions of women.

***Belief That Abortion Is a Private Choice.*** At the heart of political action to keep abortion legal is the conviction that women have the right to make decisions about their reproductive function on the basis of their own ethical and moral beliefs and that the government has no place in these decisions. Many women who support this view state that they would not choose abortion for themselves. Still, they support the right of each woman to make her own decision and view government action as interference in a very private part of women's lives. Many people who support legal abortions prefer to call themselves "pro-choice" rather than "pro-abortion," as they believe that the word "choice" expresses their philosophical and political position more accurately.

Each year there are more than 1.2 million legal abortions in the United States. In 1994, the rate was 21 abortions for every 1000 women aged 15 to 44 years. Many abortions are obtained by minors (Department of Health and Human Services, 1997). Advocates of the legal right to abortion point out that abortion, either legal or illegal, has always been a reality of life and will continue regardless of legislation or judicial rulings. Advocates express concern about the unsafe conditions that accompany illegal abortion, citing the deaths that occurred as a result of illegal abortions performed before the *Roe v. Wade* decision.

***Belief That Abortion Is Taking a Life.*** Many people believe that legalized abortion condones taking a life and feel morally bound to protect the lives of fetuses. This position is called "pro-life." The term has become emotionally charged, and some feel it polarizes opinion and implies that those who do not agree with the anti-abortion position are not concerned about life or are "anti-life."

Persons opposed to abortion have demonstrated their commitment by organizing to become a potent political force. They have willingly been arrested for civil disobedience when they attempted to prevent admissions to clinics that perform abortions.

**Legal Aspects of *Roe v. Wade*.** Abortion has been a complex legal issue since 1973, and the U.S. Supreme Court has made major decisions that affect abortion law since that time. Some decisions have strengthened the original *Roe v. Wade* ruling, and others have weakened it. Because nurses should know about the legal history of abortion, some of these decisions are enumerated in Table 3–3. Legislation introduced in 1995 banning late-term abortions received a presidential veto because it did not provide an exception when the mother's health is at risk. Other versions of this bill will probably be introduced in the future and, if passed, may come before the Supreme Court.

**Political Aspects of Abortion.** The abortion question is one of the primary issues confronting political candidates, who are often asked to explain their stand on abortion. Abortion-rights advocates are emphasizing that their message is to keep government out of the daily lives of citizens and that it is uncon-

**TABLE 3-3 SUPREME COURT DECISIONS ON ABORTION SINCE *ROE v. WADE***

1976: States cannot give a husband veto power over his spouse's decision to have an abortion.
1977: States do not have an obligation to pay for abortions as part of government-funded health care programs (considered by abortion rights advocates to be unfair discrimination against poor women who are unable to pay for an abortion).
1979: Physicians have broad discretion in determining fetal viability, and states have leeway to restrict abortions of viable fetuses.
1979: States may require parental consent for minors seeking abortions as long as an alternative, such as the minor getting a judge's aproval, is also available.
1989: Upheld a Missouri law barring abortions performed in public hospitals and clinics or performed by public employees. Also required physicians to conduct tests for fetal viability at 20 weeks of gestation.
1990: States may require notification of both parents before a person under the age of 18 years has an abortion. A judge can authorize the abortion without parental consent.
1992: Validated Pennsylvania law imposing restrictions on abortions. The restrictions upheld include the following:
- A woman must be told about fetal development and alternatives to abortion.
- She must wait at least 24 hours after this explanation before having an abortion.
- Unmarried women under the age of 18 must obtain consent from their parents or a judge.
- Physicians must keep detailed records of each abortion, subject to public disclosure.

Struck down only one requirement of the Pennsylvania law: that a married woman must inform her husband before having an abortion.
1993: Rescinded the so-called gag rule, which restricted counseling that health care professionals (with the exception of physicians) could provide at federally funded family planning clinics.
1995: Upheld a ruling that states cannot withhold state funds for abortions in case of pregnancies resulting from rape or incest or when the mother's life is in danger.

stitutional to abridge women's right to abortion. Anti-abortion leaders will probably continue a confrontational strategy to bring attention to their point of view. In addition, they will continue to try to pass legislation that would hinder abortion.

**Implications for Nurses.** As health care professionals, nurses are involved in the conflict between differing beliefs about abortion. Nurses have several responsibilities that cannot be ignored. First, they must be informed about the complexity of the abortion issue from a legal and ethical standpoint and know the exact regulations and laws in their state. Second, they must realize that, for many, abortion is an ethical dilemma that results in confusion, ambivalence, and personal distress. Next, they must also recognize that the issue is not a dilemma for many but is a fundamental violation of the personal or religious views that give meaning to their lives. Finally, it is absolutely essential that nurses acknowledge the sincere convictions and the strong emotions of all sides of the issue.

***Personal Values.*** Nurses respond to abortion in ways that illustrate the complexity of the issue and the ambivalence that it often produces. For instance, some nurses have no objection to participating in abortions. Others do not assist with abortions but may care for women after the procedure. Some nurses assist with a first-trimester abortion but may object to later abortions. Many nurses are comfortable assisting in abortion if the fetus has severe anomalies but are uncomfortable in other circumstances. Some nurses feel that they could not provide care before, during, or after an abortion but that they are bound by conscience to try to dissuade a woman from the decision to abort.

***Professional Obligations.*** Nurses have no obligation to support a position with which they disagree. Many states have laws that allow nurses to refuse to assist with the procedure if abortions violate ethical, moral, or religious beliefs. Nurses are obligated, however, to disclose this information before they are employed in an institution that performs abortions. It would be unethical for a nurse to withhold this information until assigned to care for a woman having an abortion and then refuse to provide care. As always, nurses must respect the decisions of women who look to nurses for care. If nurses feel that they are not able to provide compassionate care because of personal convictions, they must inform a supervisor so that appropriate care can be arranged.

**✓ CHECK YOUR READING**

5. How did the *Roe v. Wade* ruling affect state laws related to abortion in the United States?
6. What are the major conflicting beliefs about abortion?
7. What are some Supreme Court decisions that have modified the *Roe v. Wade* ruling?
8. What are nurses' responsibilities if they are morally opposed to abortion?

### MANDATED CONTRACEPTION

The availability of long-term contraceptive devices that are injected or implanted under the skin has led to speculation about whether certain women should be forced to use them. In fact, the procedure has already been used as a condition of probation, allowing women accused of child abuse to avoid jail terms. Legislative efforts have been made to require women who receive Aid to Families with Dependent Children (AFDC) to use the implants.

Some feel that forced contraception is a way to prevent additional births to women considered unsuitable parents and a way to decrease government expenses for dependent children. This punitive approach to social and ethical problems, however, does not provide long-term solutions. In addition, coercing the poor to use birth control to limit the money spent supporting them is questionable both legally and ethically.

Such a practice would interfere with a woman's constitutional rights to privacy, to reproduction, to refusal of medical treatment, and to freedom from cruel and unusual punishment. In addition, the implants may pose health risks to the woman. Other methods of limiting unwanted pregnancies, such as access to free or low-cost information on family planning, would be more appropriate.

### FETAL INJURY

If a mother's actions cause injury to her fetus, the question of whether she should be restrained or prosecuted has both legal and ethical implications. In some instances, courts have issued jail sentences to women who have caused or who may cause injury to the fetus. This response punishes the woman and places her in a situation in which she cannot further harm the fetus. In other cases, women have been forced to undergo cesarean births against their will when physicians have testified that such a procedure was necessary to prevent injury to the fetus.

The state has an interest in protecting children, and the Supreme Court has ruled that a child has the right to begin life with a sound mind and body. Many states have laws requiring reporting evidence of prenatal drug exposure, which is considered child abuse. Women have been charged with negligence, involuntary manslaughter, delivering drugs to a minor, and child endangerment.

Yet forcing a woman to behave in a certain way because she is pregnant violates the principles of autonomy, self-determination of competent adults, bodily integrity, and personal freedom. Because of fear of prosecution, this practice could impede health care during pregnancy instead of advancing it. Women are unlikely to seek prenatal care or treatment for substance abuse unless they feel safe. The American Nurses' Association is one of many professional groups opposing criminalization of substance abuse in pregnancy, considering it to be counterproductive ("Opposition," 1992).

The punitive approach to fetal injury also raises the question of how much control the government seeking to protect the fetus should have over a pregnant woman. Laws could be passed mandating fetal testing, use of tocolytics for preterm labor, intrauterine surgery, or even the foods the woman eats during pregnancy. It could be hard to decide just how much control should be allowed in the interests of fetal safety.

### FETAL THERAPY

Fetal therapy is in its early phases but may become more widespread as techniques improve. Although intrauterine blood transfusions are relatively standard practice in some areas, most fetal surgery is still at the research stage.

The risks and benefits of surgery for major fetal anomalies must be considered in every case. Even when surgery is successful, the fetus may not survive, may have other serious problems, or may be born preterm. The mother may need weeks of bedrest and a cesarean birth. Yet in spite of the risks, successful surgery may result in birth of an infant who could not otherwise have survived.

Parents need help in balancing the potential risks to the mother with the best interests of the fetus. There is a danger that they might feel pressured to have surgery or other fetal treatment they do not understand. As with any situation involving informed consent, women need adequate information before making a decision. They should understand whether procedures are still experimental, what are the chances of success, and what alternatives are available.

### ISSUES IN INFERTILITY

**Infertility Treatment.** Perinatal technology has found ways for some infertile couples to bear children (see Chapter 32). There are many happy results from such practices when infertile couples are finally able to give birth, but there have been some ethical concerns as well.

Concerns include the high cost and overall low success of various treatments. Because the costs are usually not covered by insurance, their use is limited to the affluent. The high price of research on techniques that will benefit only a few has also been questioned. Some think that the money should be spent on research that will help a greater number of people. Even with highly technologic infertility treatment, many couples will never give birth. Success rates for these procedures are still low. Also, when treatment is successful, there is a high risk of multiple births and premature infants, leading to extensive complications and expensive care associated with preterm birth.

Other ethical concerns focus on the fate of unused embryos. Should they be frozen for later use by the woman or someone else, or could they be used in genetic research? Who should make these decisions? In multiple pregnancies with more fetuses than can be expected to survive intact, reduction surgery may be used to destroy one or more fetuses for the benefit of those remaining. The ethical and long-term psychological implications of this procedure are also controversial.

Assisted reproductive techniques now allow postmenopausal women to become mothers. What are the ethical implications of giving birth to children who may very well be orphaned at an early age? Should the age and health of the parents be a factor in determining whether this treatment is offered? Should the risk these women face for developing complications that might result in low-birth-weight infants be considered?

**Surrogate Parenting.** In surrogate parenting, a woman agrees to bear an infant for another woman. Conception may take place outside the body using ova and sperm from the couple who wish to become parents. These "test-tube babies" are then implanted into the surrogate mother, or the surrogate may be inseminated artificially with sperm from the intended father.

Cases in which the surrogate mother has wanted to keep the child have been controversial. There are no standard regulations governing these cases, which are decided on an individual basis. Ethical concerns involve who should be a surrogate mother, what her role should be after birth, and who should make these decisions. Screening of parents as well as surrogates may be necessary to determine whether they are suitable for their roles. But who should do the screening? Should it be left to the private interests of those involved, or should the government become involved? There are no definite answers to these questions at this time.

**✓ CHECK YOUR READING**

9. What dangers are involved in punitive approaches to ethical and social problems?
10. What problems are involved in the use of advanced reproductive techniques?

## Social Issues

Nurses are exposed to many social issues that influence health care and often have ethical implications. Some of the issues that affect maternity care include poverty, homelessness, access to care, and allocation of funds.

### Poverty

Poverty is an underlying factor in problems such as inadequate access to health care and homelessness. One of every four children in the United States is born to a family in poverty (March of Dimes, 1993). Minority children and families headed by females with children under 18 have higher poverty rates. In 1991, 40 percent of white and 60 percent of black or Latino families headed by a female had resources falling below the poverty level (Horton, 1995). Because of adverse living conditions and poor health care, infants born to low-income women are more likely to have health problems such as low birth weight. Poverty affects the health of women and children throughout their lives because health care is less available to the poor.

Poverty tends to breed poverty. In poor families, children may leave the educational system early, making them less likely to learn skills necessary to obtain good jobs. Childbearing at an early age is common and interferes with education and the ability to work. The cycle of poverty may continue from one generation to another as a result of hopelessness and apathy (Fig. 3–1).

Even people with incomes above the poverty level may not be able to pay for health care. The working poor have jobs but receive wages that barely meet their day-to-day needs. They have little opportunity to save for emergencies such as serious illness. In 1995, 16.5 percent of the population younger than 65 years in the United States had no health insurance (National Center for Health Statistics, 1997). Millions of others have only limited insurance and would not be able to survive financially should serious illness occur. People without insurance seek care only when absolutely necessary. Health maintenance and illness prevention may seem costly and unnecessary to them. Some receive no health care during pregnancy until they arrive at the hospital for birth.

Various government programs help the poor. One is AFDC, which provides money for basic living costs of poor children and their families. Eligibility requirements, however, vary among the states, and many families, although poor, have incomes too high to meet the requirements.

### Homelessness

Families, many of which are composed of single women and their children, are the fastest-growing group of homeless people. Their health problems are immense. Some of the women are substance abusers. Both women and children are poorly nourished and are exposed to tuberculosis, human immunodeficiency virus (HIV) infection, and sexually transmitted diseases, to name a few. Rape and assault are problems, with a high rate of pregnancy among homeless girls. Infants born to homeless women are subject to a lower birth weight and a greater likelihood of neonatal mortality (Beal & Redlener, 1995).

Pregnancy and birth, especially as a teenager, are important contributing causes for becoming homeless. Pregnancy interferes with a woman's ability to work and may decrease her income to the point at which she loses her housing. Without child care or a home address, she may have less chance of obtain-

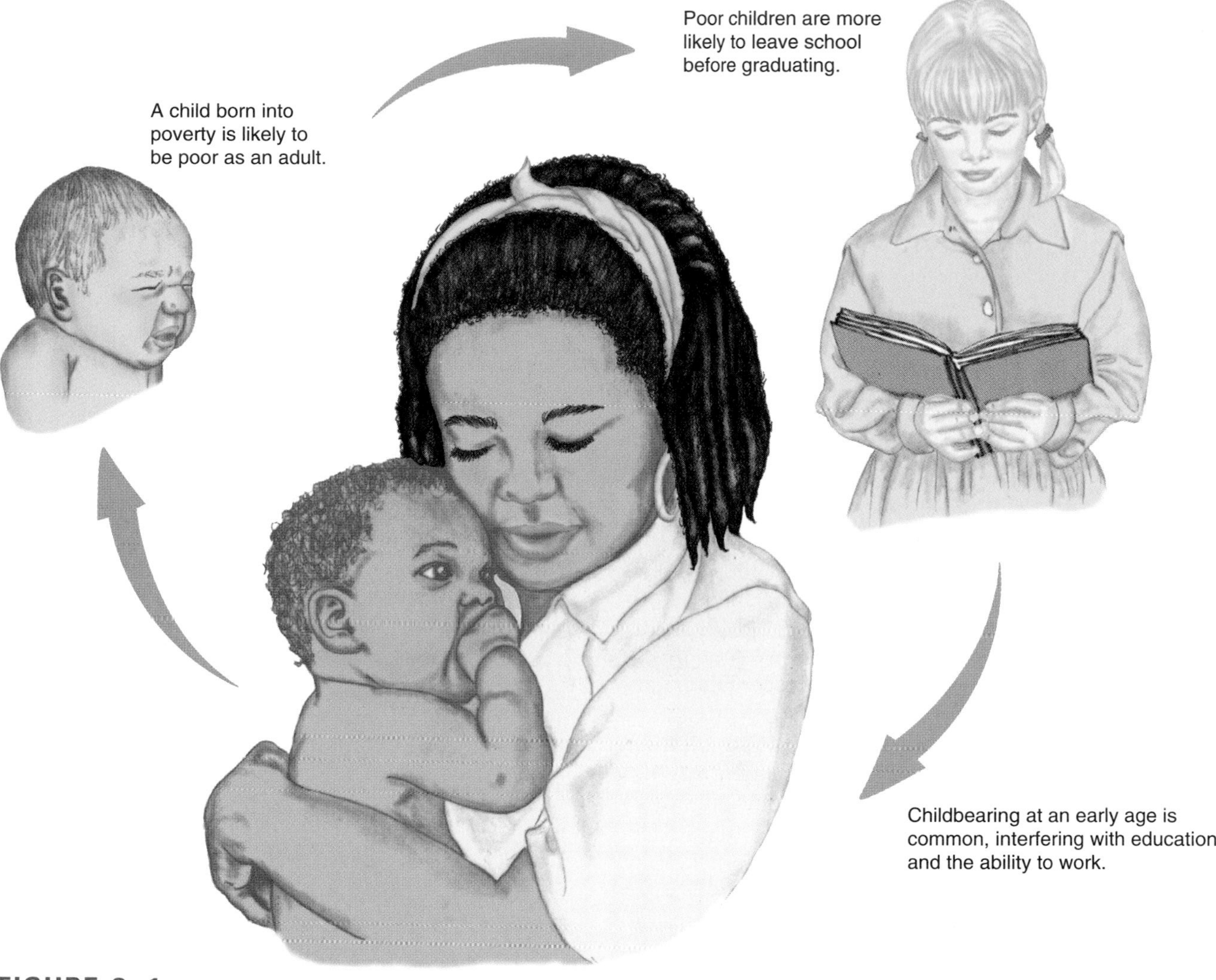

A child born into poverty is likely to be poor as an adult.
Poor children are more likely to leave school before graduating.
Childbearing at an early age is common, interfering with education and the ability to work.


**FIGURE 3–1**

The cycle of poverty.

ing and keeping employment. In addition, her children are more likely to be sick because of inadequate food and shelter. Without money to pay for insurance or early health care, there is an increased chance that children will need hospitalization.

## Access to Health Care

As Chapter 1 explained, the United States ranks 21st in infant mortality compared with other countries. Data for 1995 show that for every 1000 live births each year in the United States, 7.6 infants die before they reach their first birthday. This is approximately 80 infants each day (National Center for Health Statistics, 1997). Many of these deaths are related to low birth weight and other prenatal factors.

### PRENATAL CARE IN THE UNITED STATES

Prenatal care is widely accepted as an important element in improving pregnancy outcome. In 1994 in the United States, approximately 475 infants were born each day to mothers who began prenatal care in the third trimester or had no prenatal care at all (Guyer et al., 1996). Inadequate prenatal care refers to care begun after the fourth month of pregnancy or less than half the 13 prenatal visits recommended by the American College of Obstetricians and Gynecologists. Poor prenatal care often occurs because care is not easily available.

Lack of access to care is a major reason for the high infant mortality rate and the large number of low-birth-weight infants born each year in the United States. Because preterm infants form the largest category of those needing intensive care, millions of dollars could be saved each year by ensuring adequate prenatal care. Even a small improvement in an infant's birth weight decreases complications and hospital time.

Some factors that interfere with access to care are summarized in Table 3–4. Many of them overlap. For example, poverty is often associated with the other characteristics listed. In the United States, minority women are more likely to be poor, less likely to

**TABLE 3-4 FACTORS RELATED TO LACK OF ACCESS TO HEALTH CARE**

| |
|---|
| Poverty |
| Unemployment |
| Lack of medical insurance |
| Adolescence |
| Minority group membership |
| Inner city residence |
| Rural residence |
| Unmarried mother status |
| Less than high school education |
| Inability to speak English |

obtain adequate prenatal care, and more likely to die in childbirth when compared with white women.

In the United States, adolescent pregnancy rates are high, with approximately 1465 teens giving birth daily (March of Dimes, 1995). Although the rate has decreased from 62.1 per 1000 women 15 to 19 years old in 1991 to 56.9 in 1995, the number of teenagers is increasing (Guyer et al., 1996). This change in the population will further increase adolescent pregnancies.

In some situations, women can obtain prenatal care but choose not to do so. These women may not understand the importance of the care or may deny they are pregnant. Some have had such unsatisfactory past experiences with the health care system that they avoid it as long as possible. Others want to hide substance use or other habits from disapproving health care workers. When women have overwhelming problems, prenatal care is not a priority. Language and cultural differences also play a part in whether a woman seeks prenatal care. Although these are not access issues as such, they must be addressed to improve health care.

#### GOVERNMENT PROGRAMS FOR HEALTH CARE

**Medicaid.** More than 44 percent of all money spent on health care in 1995 was publicly funded (National Center for Health Statistics, 1997). One government program that increases access to health care is Medicaid, which has existed since 1965. Medicaid provides health care for the poor, aged, and disabled, with pregnant women and young children especially targeted. Medicaid is funded by both the federal and the state governments. The states administer the program and determine which services are offered. Although there is variation among the states in just how poor one must be to qualify for assistance, all women under 133 percent of the current federal poverty level for income are eligible for perinatal care.

Medicaid has a number of problems. It often takes weeks for a client to go through the process to become eligible. The woman must fill out lengthy, complicated forms, provide documentation of income, then wait for determination of eligibility. If a woman is not already enrolled at the beginning of her pregnancy, she is unlikely to finish the process in time to receive early prenatal care.

Some physicians are unwilling to care for Medicaid patients who are likely to be at high risk. Many are especially unwilling when the reimbursement rate for physicians and hospitals may be slow and less than that paid by other insurers. With their continual concern about malpractice suits, physicians may be less inclined to accept high-risk, lower-paying clients.

Medicaid patients may receive care in clinics rather than from private physicians. Clinics, however, are often understaffed and attended by large numbers of clients. Clinics may be located in areas not easily accessible to pregnant women who have transportation problems. Long waits for appointments may necessitate taking time off from work. A mother may not have anyone to care for other children while she visits the clinic. These problems decrease the chance that women who do not understand the importance of prenatal care will be willing to go through the difficulties involved in obtaining care.

**Shelters and Health Care for the Homeless.** Federal funding has provided assistance with shelter and health care for homeless people. The homeless, however, have the same difficulties in obtaining health care as other poor people with lack of transportation, inconvenient hours, and lack of continuity of care.

Quality as well as quantity of care in clinics may be poor because of inadequate funding. Nurses have been instrumental in opening shelters, clinics, and outreach services, with nurse practitioners often playing a major role. Nurses also help inform the public and legislatures about the needs of the homeless.

**Innovative Programs.** Innovative programs to see that all women receive good prenatal care are necessary. Many different programs are available in various areas of the country, but there are not enough to meet the need. Some include outreach programs designed to improve health in women who traditionally do not seek prenatal care. Bilingual health care workers and bilingual educational classes are part of some programs. Many programs employ nurse practitioners and are located in schools, shopping centers, workplaces, or neighborhoods so that clients have easy access. More such programs will be necessary if adequate health care for women and children is to become a reality.

## Allocation of Health Care Resources

In 1995, the United States spent $988.5 billion on health care. This amount is $3621 per person (National Center for Health Statistics, 1997). Expenditures continue to climb every year. Methods of reforming health care financing have drawn increasing attention in recent times, and many changes are occurring. How to provide care for the poor, the uninsured or underinsured, and those with long-term care needs are areas that must be addressed. The distribution of the limited funds available for health care among all these areas is a major concern.

#### CARE VERSUS CURE

One problem to be addressed is whether the focus of health care should be on preventive and caring measures or on cure of disease. Medicine has traditionally centered more on treatment and cure than on prevention and care. Yet prevention not only avoids suffering but is also less expensive than treating diseases once they are diagnosed.

The focus on cure has resulted in great technologic advances that have enabled some people to live longer, healthier lives. Financial resources are limited, however, and the costs of expensive technology must be balanced against the benefits obtained. Indeed, the cost of one organ transplant would pay for prenatal care for many low-income mothers.

Although low-birth-weight infants make up a small percentage of all infants born, they require a large percentage of total hospital expenditures. The expenses of one preterm infant for a single day in an intensive care nursery are more than enough to pay for care of the mother throughout her pregnancy and birth. Yet, if the mother had received prenatal care, the infant might not have needed intensive care.

In addition, "quality of life" issues are important in regard to technology. Neonatal nurseries are able to keep very-low-birth-weight babies alive because of advances in knowledge. Some of these infants go on to lead normal or near-normal lives. Others gain time but not quality of life. Families and health care professionals face difficult decisions about when to treat, when to terminate treatment, and when suffering outweighs the benefits.

#### HEALTH CARE RATIONING

Modern technology has had a great impact on health care rationing. Some might argue that such rationing does not exist, but it occurs when some people have no access to care and there is not enough money for all people to share equally in the technology available. Advanced medical care often benefits only a small number of people but at great cost. Health care is also rationed when it is more freely given to those who have money to pay for it than to those who do not.

Many questions will need answers as the costs of health care increase faster than the funds available. Is health care a fundamental right? Should a certain level of care be guaranteed to all citizens? What should that care entail? Should the cost of treatment and its effectiveness be considered when one is deciding how much government or third-party payers will cover? Nurses will be instrumental in finding solutions to these vital questions.

**✓ CHECK YOUR READING**

11. How do poverty and inadequate prenatal care affect infant mortality and morbidity?
12. How does a decision to spend money on technology sometimes conflict with issues of disease prevention?

## Legal Issues

The legal foundation for the practice of nursing provides safeguards for health care and sets standards by which nurses can be evaluated. Nurses need to understand how the law applies specifically to them. When nurses do not meet the standards expected, they may be held legally accountable.

### Safeguards for Health Care

Three categories of safeguards determine how the law views nursing practice: (1) nurse practice acts, (2) standards of care set by professional organizations, and (3) rules and policies set by the institution employing the nurse.

#### NURSE PRACTICE ACTS

Every state has a nurse practice act that determines the scope of practice of registered nurses in that state. Nurse practice acts define what the nurse is and is not allowed to do in caring for clients. Some parts of the law may be very specific. Others are stated broadly enough to allow interpretation of the law that permits flexibility in the role of nurses. Nurse practice acts vary from state to state, and nurses must be knowledgeable about these laws wherever they practice. Nurses should have a copy of the nurse practice act for their state and should refer to it when there are questions about their scope of practice.

Laws relating to nursing practice also delineate methods, called *standardized procedures,* by which nurses may assume certain duties commonly considered part of medical practice. The procedures are written by committees of nurses, physicians, and administrators. They specify the nursing qualifications required for practicing the procedures, define the appropriate situations, and list the education required. Standardized procedures allow for changing the role of the nurse to meet the needs of the community and of expanding knowledge.

#### STANDARDS OF CARE

Although courts do not have the force of laws, they have generally held that nurses must practice according to established standards and health agency policies. Standards of care are set by professional associations and describe the level of care that can be expected from practitioners. For example, perinatal nurses are held to the standards published by the Association of Women's Health, Obstetric, and Neonatal Nurses (AWHONN, formerly NAACOG), a widely respected organization for nurses in this field. AWHONN publishes national standards for nursing care as well as specific practice resources when a consistent minimum standard of care is desirable. These standards are based on research and the agreement of experts.

AWHONN also publishes practice resources, position statements, and other guidelines for nurses. It is essential that nurses be familiar with the latest standards of care that cover their own practice.

#### AGENCY POLICIES

Each health care agency sets specific policies, procedures, and protocols that govern nursing care. All nurses should be familiar with those that apply in the agencies in which they work. Nurses are frequently involved in writing nursing policies and procedures and in revising them when necessary.

### Malpractice

*Negligence* is the failure to perform the way a reasonable, prudent person of similar background would act in a similar situation. Negligence may consist of doing something that should not be done or failing to do something that should be done.

*Malpractice* is negligence by professionals, such as nurses or physicians, in the performance of their duties. Nurses may be accused of malpractice if they do not perform according to established standards of care and in the manner of a reasonable, prudent nurse with similar education and experience. Four elements must be present to prove negligence. They include duty, breach of duty, damage, and proximate cause.

> **Critical to Remember**
>
> **ELEMENTS OF NEGLIGENCE**
>
> **Duty.** The nurse must have a duty to act or give care to the client. It must be part of the nurse's responsibility.
> **Breach of duty.** A violation of that duty must occur. The nurse fails to conform to established standards in performing that duty.
> **Damage.** There must be actual injury or harm to the client as a result of the nurse's breach of duty.
> **Proximate cause.** The nurse's breach of duty must be proved to be the cause of harm to the client.

### Prevention of Malpractice Claims

Malpractice claims have escalated in recent years. As a result of awards from such claims, the cost of malpractice insurance has risen for all health care workers. In addition, more health care workers practice defensively, accumulating evidence that they are acting in the patient's best interest. For example, nurses must be careful to include detailed data when they chart. This responsibility is especially important in perinatal nursing, because this is the area in which most suits occur.

There are many reasons for perinatal malpractice claims. Complications are usually unexpected because parents view pregnancy and birth as normal. The birth of a child with a problem is a tragic surprise, and they may look for someone to blame. Although very small preterm infants now survive, some have long-term disabilities that require expensive care. Statutes of limitations vary in different states, but plaintiffs often have more than 20 years for lawsuits that involve a newborn. Therefore, there is a longer period during which a malpractice suit may be filed.

Health care agencies and individual nurses must work together to prevent malpractice claims. Hospitals have paid millions of dollars for lawsuits claiming malpractice. Although nurses are not often sued, there has been an increase in the number of nurses named in lawsuits. Nurses are responsible and accountable for their own actions. Therefore, they must be aware of the limits of their knowledge and scope of practice, and they must practice within those limits.

Prevention of claims is sometimes referred to as "risk management" or "quality assurance." Although it may not be possible to prevent all malpractice claims, nurses can help prevent malpractice judgments against themselves by following guidelines for informed consent, refusal of care, and documentation; acting as a client advocate; and maintaining their level of expertise.

#### INFORMED CONSENT

When clients receive adequate information, they are less likely to file malpractice suits. Informed consent is an ethical concept that has been enacted into law. Clients have the right to decide whether to accept or reject treatment options as part of their right to function autonomously. To make wise decisions, they need full information about treatments offered.

### Critical to Remember

**REQUIREMENTS OF INFORMED CONSENT**

Client's competence to consent
Full disclosure of information needed
Client's understanding of information
Client's voluntary consent

**Competence.** Certain requirements must be met before consent can be considered "informed." The first is that the client be competent, or able to think through a situation and make rational decisions. A client who is comatose or severely mentally retarded or an infant or child is incapable of making such decisions. A client who has received drugs that impair ability to think is temporarily incompetent. In these cases, another person would be appointed to make decisions for the client.

**Full Disclosure.** The second requirement is that of full disclosure of information, including what the treatment entails and the expected results. The risks, side effects, and benefits as well as other treatment options must be explained to clients. The client must also be informed as to what would happen if no treatment were chosen.

**Understanding of Information.** The client must comprehend information about proposed treatment. Health professionals must explain the facts in terms the person can understand. If a client does not speak English, an interpreter may be necessary. Nurses must be client advocates when they find a client does not fully understand a treatment or has questions about it. If it is a minor point, the nurse may be able to explain it. Otherwise, the nurse must inform the physician so that the client's misconceptions can be clarified.

**Voluntary Consent.** Clients must be allowed to make choices voluntarily without undue influence or coercion from others. Although others can give information, the client alone makes the decision. Clients should not feel pressured to choose in a certain way or that their future care depends on their decision.

#### REFUSAL OF CARE

Sometimes clients decline treatment offered by health care workers. Clients refuse treatment when they believe that the benefits of treatment are insufficient to balance the burdens of the treatment or the life they will have after that treatment. Clients do have the right to refuse care, and they can withdraw agreement to treatment at any time. When a person makes this decision, a number of steps should be taken.

First, it should be established by the physician or nurse that the client understands the treatment and the results of refusal. The physician, if unaware of the client's decision, should be notified by the nurse. The nurse documents the refusal, explanations given the client, and notification of the physician on the chart. If the treatment is considered vital to the client's well-being, the physician discusses the need with the client and documents the results. Opinions by other physicians may be offered to the client as well.

Clients may be asked to sign a form indicating that they understand the possible results of rejecting treatment. This measure is to prevent a later lawsuit in which a client claims lack of knowledge of the possible results of a decision. If there is no ethical dilemma, the client's decision stands.

In cases of an ethical dilemma, a referral may be made to the hospital ethics committee. In rare situations, the physician may seek a court ruling to force treatment. One example is a woman's refusal of a cesarean birth, even though her decision is likely to cause grave harm to the fetus. This situation is the only legal instance in which a person is forced to undergo surgery for the health of another. Women who are poor or of minority status are more likely to have a court-ordered cesarean birth (Lindgren, 1996). Court action is avoided if possible, however, because it places the woman and her caregiver in adversarial positions. In addition, it invades the woman's privacy and interferes with her autonomy and right to informed consent. If legally mandated surgery became widespread and women avoided health care during pregnancy, the resulting harm would affect more women and infants than the surgery would protect.

Coercion is illegal (as well as unethical) in obtaining consent. Even though the nurse may strongly believe that the client should receive the treatment, the client should not feel forced to submit to unwanted procedures. Nurses must be sure that personal feelings do not adversely affect the care they give. Clients have the right to good nursing care, regardless of their decision to accept or reject treatment.

#### DOCUMENTATION

Documentation is especially important when there is a question of liability because it is the best evidence that a standard of care has been maintained. All information recorded about a client should reflect that standard of care. This information includes nurses' notes, fetal monitoring strips, flow sheets, and any other data recorded in the chart. In many instances, notations on hospital records are the only proof that care has been given. Unfortunately, accurate and thorough documentation is the most common area missing (Simpson & Chez, 1996). When documentation is not present, juries tend to assume that care was not given.

It is especially important that documentation be specific and complete in perinatal nursing. This careful step is needed because of the long statute of limitations when a newborn is involved. Nurses are unlikely to be able to remember situations that happened years in the past and, if sued, must rely on their documentation to explain their care. Documentation must show that the client was assessed appropriately, that continuing monitoring of problems was provided, that problems were identified and correct interventions were instituted, and that changes in the client's condition were reported to the primary care provider.

**Documenting Fetal Monitoring.** Fetal monitor strips are important sources of information about the mother and fetus during labor and birth. Nurses record a great deal of information about nursing care on the monitor strip. Sometimes the client requires the nurse's full attention, and completion of other charting must be delayed temporarily. In this situation, the nurse's notes on the monitor strip provide the basis for later charting.

Although monitor strips are a legal part of the chart, they may become lost. This risk makes it particularly important that all information from the strip be recorded in the nurse's notes. Complete, detailed charting ensures that the nurse's actions will be clear many years later in a court of law even without the monitor strip.

**Documenting Discharge Teaching.** With length of stay becoming shorter, discharge teaching becomes increasingly important to ensure clients know how to take care of themselves and their infants. To prevent lawsuits, nurses must document the teaching they perform as well as the client's understanding of that teaching. Various documentation forms are used to show that parents received teaching about important topics. It is important to include information about the parents' degree of understanding of teaching. The nurse should also note the need for reinforcement and how that reinforcement was provided. If follow-up home care is planned for the mother and infant, teaching can be continued at home and documented on forms by the home care nurse.

**Documenting Incidents.** Another form of documentation used in risk management is the incident report, sometimes called a "quality assurance report" or a "variance report." The nurse completes a report when something occurs that might result in legal action, such as in injury to a client. The report warns the agency legal department that there may be a problem. It also identifies situations that might endanger clients in the future. Incident reports are not a part of the client's chart and should not be referred to on the chart. When an incident occurs, documentation on the chart should include the same type of factual information on the client's condition that would be recorded in any other situation.

### THE NURSE AS CLIENT ADVOCATE

Malpractice suits may be brought if nurses fail in their role of client advocate. Nurses are ethically and legally bound to act as the client's advocate. This means that the nurse must act in the client's best interests at all times. When nurses feel that the client's best interests are not being served, they are obligated to seek help for the patient from appropriate sources. This usually involves taking the problem through the normal chain of command. The nurse consults a supervisor and the client's physician. If the results are not satisfactory, the nurse continues through administrative channels to the director of nurses, hospital administrator, and chief of the medical staff, if necessary. All nurses should know the chain of command process for their workplaces.

In seeking help for clients, nurses must document their efforts. For example, when postpartum patients are experiencing excessive bleeding, nurses document what they have done to control the bleeding. They also document each time they call the physician, what information was given the physician, and the response received. When nurses cannot contact the physician or do not receive adequate instructions, they should document their efforts to seek instruction from others, such as the supervisor. They should also complete an incident report. It is essential that they continue in their efforts until the patient receives the care needed.

### MAINTAINING EXPERTISE

Maintaining expertise is another way for the nurse to prevent malpractice liability. To ensure that nurses maintain their expertise to provide safe care, most states require proof of continuing education for renewal of nursing licenses. Nursing knowledge grows and changes rapidly, and it is essential that all nurses keep current. Incorporating new information learned by attending classes or conferences and reading nursing journals can help nurses perform the way a reasonably prudent peer would perform. Journals provide information about nursing research that may be important in updating nursing practice. It is important for all nurses to analyze research articles to determine whether changes in client care are indicated.

Employers often provide continuing education classes for their nurses. Many workshops and seminars are available on a wide variety of nursing subjects. Membership in professional organizations, such as state branches of the American Nurses' Association or specialty organizations like AWHONN, gives nurses access to new information through publications as well as nursing conferences and other educational offerings.

Maintaining expertise may be a concern when nurses are "floated" or required to work with clients who have needs different from those of their usual clients. A nurse may be floated from one maternal-newborn setting to another or to a nonmaternity setting. In these situations, nurses may need cross-training: orientation and education to perform care safely in new areas. The employer must provide cross-training for nurses who float, when appropriate. Nurses who work outside their usual expertise must assess their own skills and avoid performing tasks or taking responsibilities in areas in which they are not competent. Many nurses learn to provide care in two or three different areas and are floated only to those areas. This system meets the need for flexible staffing while providing safe client care.

**CHECK YOUR READING**

13. How do standards of care and agency policies, which are not laws, influence judgments about malpractice?
14. What is the difference between negligence and malpractice?
15. How can nurses help to prevent malpractice claims?

# Current Trends and Their Legal and Ethical Implications

Recent health care changes have affected the way nurses give care and may have legal and ethical implications as well. These changes result from efforts to lower health care costs. Two of special concern are the use of unlicensed assistive personnel and early discharge.

## Use of Unlicensed Assistive Personnel

In an effort to reduce health care costs, many agencies have increased the use of unlicensed assistive personnel to perform direct client care, and have decreased the number of nurses who supervise them. An unlicensed person may be trained to do everything from housekeeping tasks to drawing blood and performing other diagnostic testing to giving medications, all in the same day. This practice raises grave concerns about the quality of care clients receive when the nurse becomes responsible for the care of more clients but must rely on unlicensed persons to perform much of the care formerly provided by professionals.

Nurses must be aware of their legal responsibilities in these situations. They must know that the nurse is always responsible for client assessments and must make the critical judgments that are necessary to ensure client safety. Nurses must know what each unlicensed person caring for clients is able to do and must supervise them closely enough to ensure that they perform delegated tasks competently. The American Nurses Association and state boards of nursing have issued statements to help nurses understand their role in working with unlicensed assistive personnel (American Nurses Association, 1994).

## Early—and Earlier—Discharge

The time from hospital admission to discharge continues to decrease. When discharge within 24 hours of birth was mandated by many third-party payers, health care professionals were apprehensive about client safety. In some areas, the time limit began when the woman entered the birth facility in labor instead of when she gave birth. In others, the woman may go home 6 to 12 hours after birth. Discharge after cesarean birth has been as early as the second morning after surgery. In addition, women and newborns with complications may be discharged from the hospital as soon as they are stable but before they are well.

There have been attempts to reverse the trend toward early discharge after birth. In 1996 federal legislation was passed to require insurance companies to allow the option of a 48-hour hospital stay after vaginal birth and a 4-day stay after cesarean birth. Discharge may be sooner if deemed appropriate after discussion between the physician and the client. Although the federal law did not require follow-up, many states mandate prompt follow-up in the client's home, an office, or a clinic when early discharge occurs.

### CONCERNS ABOUT EARLY DISCHARGE

Health care professionals are concerned about women's ability to take over complete care of themselves and their infants so soon after birth. Women may be exhausted from a long labor or illness and unable to take in all the information that nurses attempt to teach before discharge. Once home, many women must care for other children as well, often without family members or friends to help them. The lack of support for the important role changes that take place after a birth may have long-term effects on the family. The woman with complications may have inadequate resources to care for herself and her family while on bedrest.

During the time mothers remain in the birth facility, nurses are able to detect indications of maternal or infant complications that may not be apparent to parents. Mothers at home may not recognize developing signs of serious maternal or neonatal infection or of jaundice, and care may be delayed until the illness is severe. There may be legal implications if a mother or infant develops a complication after early discharge. The ethics of sending a mother home before she is ready to care for herself and her newborn adequately is also a concern. More research must be performed to determine the long-term effects of this practice on the family.

#### METHODS OF DEALING WITH THE PROBLEM

Nurses must establish ways of helping clients who go home soon after birth. New teaching tactics may be necessary, with more teaching taking place during pregnancy when the mother's physical needs do not interfere with her ability to comprehend the new knowledge. Careful documentation and notification of the primary care provider is essential when abnormal findings develop so that clients are not discharged inappropriately. Methods of follow-up such as home visits, phone calls, or return visits by the families to the birth facility for nursing assessments in the first 24 to 48 hours after birth have become increasingly important. In addition, home care nurses must be knowledgeable about caring for high-risk pregnancies and newborns and all the technology that now can be used at home.

### Increase in Home Health Nursing

As hospital stays continue to shorten, home health nursing has increased as a cost-effective alternative to hospitalization. Clients are cared for by nurses as well as a number of other caregivers, many of whom are unlicensed. This may increase ethical and legal concerns. Correlating a client's needs for extensive home visits with the push to keep costs low is an ethical concern. Supervision of unlicensed personnel when the nurse makes only occasional visits may lead to legal questions. Nurses involved in home care must be certain they have the education necessary to care for clients in an out-of-the-hospital setting. Standards for nursing care include the education levels recommended to work in home health settings. These are available from professional groups such as AWHONN and other regulatory groups (AWHONN, 1994).

Home care agencies often provide telephone access to a nurse for clients who have questions or concerns after discharge. When giving advice by telephone, nurses must have specialized training and use protocols developed by a multidisciplinary team to ensure that all clients receive adequate advice and to avoid liability. All calls must be documented carefully.

#### ✓ CHECK YOUR READING

16. What concerns do nurses have about unlicensed personnel?
17. Why is early discharge a concern for nurses?

## SUMMARY CONCEPTS

- Ethical dilemmas are a difficult area and are best solved by applying ethical theories and principles as well as the steps of the nursing process.
- When ethical principles of beneficence, nonmaleficence, autonomy, and justice result in ethical dilemmas, nursing process may be used to guide ethical decision making.
- Elective abortion is a controversial issue that generates strong feelings in two opposing factions in the United States. Decisions by the Supreme Court have limited or upheld the right of states to impose restrictions on abortion.
- Nurses must examine their beliefs and come to a personal decision about abortion before they are faced with the situation in their own practice.
- Punitive approaches to ethical and social problems may prevent women from seeking adequate prenatal care.
- Issues in fetal therapy include weighing the risks and benefits for the mother versus those for the fetus and determining whose rights should prevail.
- Issues in infertility concern the high cost and low success rate of some treatments, the fate of unused embryos and multiple fetuses, and the rights of surrogate parents.
- Poverty is a major social issue that leads to questions about allocation of health care resources, access to prenatal care, government programs to increase health care to indigent women and children, and health care rationing.
- Nurses are expected to perform in accordance with nurse practice acts, standards of care, and agency policies to provide expected care and to avoid malpractice claims.
- Nurses can help to prevent malpractice claims by following guidelines for informed consent, refusal of care, and documentation and by maintaining their level of expertise.
- To give informed consent, the client must be competent, receive full information, understand that information, and consent voluntarily.
- Documentation is the best evidence of the standard of care received by a client. Therefore, nurses must ensure that their documentation accurately reflects the care given.
- New trends include early discharge, use of unlicensed assistive personnel, and increase in home health nursing.

#### *References and Readings*

American Medical Association Board of Trustees. (1992). Requirements or incentives by government for the use

of long-acting contraceptives. *Journal of the American Medical Association*, 267(13), 1818–1821.
American Nurses Association. (1994). *Registered professional nurses and unlicensed assistive personnel*. Washington, D.C.: Author.
Association of Women's Health, Obstetric, and Neonatal Nurses (AWHONN). (1994). *Didactic content and clinical skills verification for professional nurse providers of perinatal home care*. Washington, D.C.: Author.
AWHONN. (1995a). *The role of the nurse in clinical ethical decision making*. Washington, D.C.: Author.
AWHONN. (1995b). Shortened maternity, newborn stay issue gaining momentum. AWHONN *Voice*, 3(9), 13, 20.
Beal, A.C., & Redlener, I. (1995). Enhancing perinatal outcome in homeless women: The challenge of providing comprehensive health care. *Seminars in Perinatology*, 19(4), 307–313.
Brent, N.J. (1994). Risk management and legal issues in home care: The utilization of nursing staff. *Journal of Obstetric, Gynecologic, and Neonatal Nursing*, 23(8), 659–665.
Collins, J.E. (1994). Fetal surgery: Changing the outcome before birth. *Journal of Obstetric, Gynecologic, and Neonatal Nursing*, 23(2), 166–169.
Department of Health and Human Services. (1997). *Morbidity and Mortality Weekly Report*, 46(SS-4).
Doblin, B.H., Gelberg, L., & Freeman, H.E. (1992). Patient care and professional staffing patterns in McKinney Act clinics providing primary care to the homeless. *Journal of the American Medical Association*, 267(5), 698–701.
Driscoll, K.M. (1993). Legal aspects of perinatal care. In C. Kenner, A. Brueggemeyer, & L.P. Gunderson (Eds.), *Comprehensive neonatal nursing, a physiologic perspective*. Philadelphia: W.B. Saunders.
Ferguson, S.L., & Engelhard, C.L. (1997). Short stay: The art of legislating quality and economy. AWHONN's *Lifelines*, 1(1), 17–23.
Fiesta, J. (1994). Incident reports—confidential or not? *Nursing Management*, 25(10), 17–18.
Freda, M.C. (1994). Childbearing, reproductive control, aging women, and health care: The projected ethical debates. *Journal of Obstetric, Gynecologic, and Neonatal Nursing*, 23(2), 144–152.
Gardner, S.L., & Hagedorn, M.E. (1997). Holding nurses accountable. AWHONN's *Lifelines*, 1(1), 55–56.
Guyer, B., Strobino, D.M., Ventura, S.J., MacDorman, M., & Martin, J.A. (1996). Annual summary of vital statistics—1995. *Pediatrics*, 98(6), 1007–1019.
Horton, J.A. (Ed.). (1995). Demographic classification. *The women's health data book* (2nd ed.). Washington, D.C.: Jacobs Institute of Women's Health.
Johnson, S.A. (1992). Ethical dilemma: A patient refuses a life-saving cesarean. MCN: *The American Journal of Maternal/Child Nursing*, 17(3), 121–125.
Jones, S.L. (1994). Genetic-based and assisted reproductive technology of the 21st century. *Journal of Obstetric, Gynecologic, and Neonatal Nursing*, 23(2), 160–165.
Kachoyeanos, M.K. (1995). Maintaining an ethical stand without jeopardizing your job. MCN: *The American Journal of Maternal/Child Nursing*, 20(5), 243–248.
Kjervik, D.K. (1996). Legal and ethical issues. In J. Cookfair, *Nursing care in the community*. St. Louis: C.V. Mosby.
Klerman, L.V. (1994). Perinatal health care policy: How it will affect the family in the 21st century. *Journal of Obstetric, Gynecologic, and Neonatal Nursing*, 23(2), 124–128.
Kotelchuck, M. (1994). The adequacy of prenatal care utilization index: Its U.S. distribution and association with low birthweight. *American Journal of Public Health*, 84(9), 1486–1490.
Ladebauche, P. (1995). Limiting liability to avoid malpractice litigation. MCN: *The American Journal of Maternal/Child Nursing*, 20(6), 339.
Lescale, K.B., Inglis, S.R., Eddleman, K.A., Peeper, E.Q., Chervenak, F.A., & McCullough, L.B. (1996). Conflicts between physicians and patients in non-elective cesarean delivery: Incidence and the adequacy of informed consent. *American Journal of Perinatology*, 13(3), 171–176.
Lindgren, K. (1996). Maternal-fetal conflict: Court-ordered cesarean section. *Journal of Obstetric, Gynecologic, and Neonatal Nursing*, 25(8), 653–656.
Locher, A.W. (1996). Ethics, women with HIV, and procreation: Implications for nursing practice. *Journal of Obstetric, Gynecologic, and Neonatal Nursing*, 25(6), 564–469.
March of Dimes Birth Defects Foundation. (1993). *Toward improving the outcome of pregnancy: The 90's and beyond*. White Plains, N.Y.: March of Dimes.
March of Dimes Birth Defects Foundation. (1995). *March of Dimes birth defects foundation mission*. White Plains, N.Y.: March of Dimes.
National Center for Health Statistics. (1997). *Health, United States, 1996–97 and injury chartbook*. Hyattsville, Md.: Author.
Opposition to the criminal prosecution. (1992). *Birth*, 19(1), 43.
Penticuff, J. (1994). Ethical issues in genetic therapy. *Journal of Obstetric, Gynecologic, and Neonatal Nursing*, 23(6), 498–501.
Penticuff, J. (1996). Ethical dimensions in genetic screening: A look into the future. *Journal of Obstetric, Gynecologic, and Neonatal Nursing*, 25(9), 785–789.
Piotrowski, K. (1996). Caring for the maternal-infant client. In J. Cookfair, *Nursing care in the community*. St. Louis: C.V. Mosby.
Rhodes, A.M. (1996a). Anencephalic organ donation. MCN: *The American Journal of Maternal/Child Nursing*, 21(1), 15.
Rhodes, A.M. (1996b). Drug use during pregnancy. MCN: *The American Journal of Maternal/Child Nursing*, 21(3), 127.
Rhodes, A.M. (1996c). Testing the standards of death. MCN: *The American Journal of Maternal/Child Nursing*, 21(2), 109.
Rhodes, A.M. (1997). Viable fetus vs. drug-abusing mother. MCN: *The American Journal of Maternal/Child Nursing*, 22(3), 127.
Simpson, K.R., & Chez, B.F. (1996). Professional and legal issues. In K.R. Simpson & P.A. Creehan (Eds.), *AWHONN's perinatal nursing*. Philadelphia: J.B. Lippincott.
Sorich, M.P., & Letizia, M. (1994). Nursing malpractice litigation: A personal journey. MCN: *The American Journal of Maternal/Child Nursing*, 19(5), 249–254.
Southwell, S.M., & Archer-Duste, H. (1993). Ethical aspects of perinatal care. In C. Kenner, A. Brueggemeyer, & L.P. Gunderson (Eds.), *Comprehensive neonatal nursing: A physiologic perspective*. Philadelphia: W.B. Saunders.
Taylor, D.L., & Woods, N.F. (1996). Changing women's health, changing nursing practice. *Journal of Obstetric, Gynecologic, and Neonatal Nursing*, 25(9), 791–802.
Wegman, M.E. (1996). Infant mortality: Some international comparisons. *Pediatrics*, 98(6), 1020–1027.
York, R., Grant, C., Gibeau, A., Beecham, J., & Kessler, J. (1996). A review of problems of universal access to prenatal care. *Nursing Clinics of North America*, 31(2), 279–292.

# 4

# Reproductive Anatomy and Physiology

**OBJECTIVES**

1. Explain female and male sexual development from prenatal life through sexual maturity.
2. Describe normal anatomy of the female and male reproductive systems.
3. Explain normal function of the female and male reproductive systems.
4. Explain normal structure and function of the female breast.

**DEFINITIONS**

**amenorrhea** *Absence of menstruation. Primary amenorrhea is a delay of the first menstruation. Secondary amenorrhea is cessation of menstruation after its initiation.*

**cilia** *Hair-like processes on the surface of a cell. Cilia beat rhythmically to move the cell or to move fluid or other substances over the cell surface.*

**climacteric** *Endocrine, body, and psychic changes occurring at the end of a woman's reproductive period. Also informally called menopause.*

**coitus** *Sexual union between a male and a female.*

**fornix (pl. fornices)** *An arch or pouch-like structure at the upper end of the vagina. Also called a cul-de-sac.*

**gamete** *Reproductive cell; in the female an ovum; and in the male a spermatozoon.*

**genetic sex** *Sex determined at conception by union of two X chromosomes (female) or an X and a Y chromosome (male). Also called chromosomal sex.*

**gonad** *Reproductive (sex) gland that produces gametes and sex hormones. The female gonads are ovaries; the male gonads are testes.*

**gonadotropic hormones** *Secretions of the anterior pituitary gland that stimulate the gonads, specifically follicle-stimulating hormone and luteinizing hormone. Chorionic gonadotropin is secreted by the placenta during pregnancy.*

**graafian follicle** *A small sac within the ovary that contains the maturing ovum.*

**menarche** *Onset of menstruation; average age is 13 years.*

**menopause** *Permanent cessation of menstruation during the climacteric.*

**puberty** *Period of sexual maturation accompanied by the development of secondary sex characteristics and the capacity to reproduce.*

**ruga (pl. rugae)** *Ridge or fold of tissue, as on the male's scrotum and in the female's vagina.*

**secondary sex characteristics** *Physical differences between mature males and females that are not directly related to reproduction.*

**somatic sex** *Gender assignment as male or female on the basis of form and structure of the external genitalia.*

**spermatogenesis** *Formation of male gametes (sperm) in the testes.*

**spinnbarkeit** *Clear, slippery, stretchy quality of cervical mucus during ovulation.*

To care for women during and after their reproductive years, the nurse must understand the structure and function of the reproductive organs. This chapter reviews basic prenatal development, sexual maturation, and structure and function of both female and male reproductive systems. Because of its emphasis in this book, the female reproductive system is discussed more extensively.

## Sexual Development

Sexual development begins at conception when the genetic sex is determined by union of an ovum and a sperm. During childhood, the sex organs are quiet. They become active during puberty as the person begins sexual maturation.

### Prenatal Development

The mother's ovum carries a single X chromosome. Each of the father's spermatozoa carries either an X chromosome or a Y chromosome. If an X-bearing spermatozoon fertilizes the ovum, the offspring's genetic sex is female. If a Y-bearing spermatozoon fertilizes the ovum, a male offspring results.

Although genetic sex is determined at conception, the reproductive system of both males and females is similar, or sexually undifferentiated, for the first 6 weeks of prenatal life. During the seventh week, differences between males and females appear in the internal structures. The external genitalia look similar until the ninth week, when these outer structures begin to change. Differentiation of the external sexual organs is complete at about 12 weeks.

The basic trend for prenatal sexual development is to have female structures. Presence of only a small part of the Y chromosome (the short arm) changes this trend and directs the early (primitive) sex cells to become testes. Absence of the critical part of a Y chromosome allows the primitive sex cells to continue on their course of becoming ovaries. Prenatal development of the reproductive organs is detailed in Chapter 6.

During fetal life, both ovaries and testes secrete their primary hormones, estrogen and testosterone, respectively. Testosterone causes development of male sex organs and external genitalia, and its absence results in development of female sex characteristics. Although estrogen is secreted by the fetal ovary, this hormone is not required to initiate development of female sex structures.

### Childhood

The sex glands of both girls and boys are inactive during infancy and childhood. At sexual maturity, the hypothalamus stimulates the anterior pituitary gland to produce hormones that, in turn, stimulate sex hormone production by the gonads.

### Sexual Maturation

Puberty refers to the time during which the reproductive organs become fully functional. It is not a single event but a series of changes occurring over several years during late childhood and early adolescence. Primary sex characteristics develop as the organs directly responsible for reproduction mature. Examples of primary sex characteristics are maturation of ova in the ovaries and production of sperm in the testes. Secondary sex characteristics are changes in other systems that differentiate females and males but that do not directly relate to reproduction. Table 4–1 cites examples of female and male secondary sex characteristics.

#### INITIATION OF SEXUAL MATURATION

All factors that initiate sexual maturation are not known. Secretions of the hypothalamus, the anterior pituitary, and the gonads all play a part. The hypothalamus is capable of secreting gonadotropin-releasing hormone (GnRH) to initiate puberty during infancy and early childhood, but it does not do so in significant amounts until late childhood. Production of even tiny quantities of sex hormones by the young child's ovaries or testes inhibits secretions of the hypothalamus, avoiding premature onset of puberty. Maturation of another brain area, as yet unknown, probably triggers the hypothalamus to initiate puberty (Guyton, 1996).

**TABLE 4–1 COMPARISON OF SECONDARY SEX CHARACTERISTICS IN FEMALES AND MALES**

| Females | Males |
|---|---|
| Development of glandular and ductal systems in the breast; deposition of fat selectively in the breast, buttocks, and thighs, resulting in a rounded figure | Muscle mass 50% greater |
| Wide, round pelvis | Narrow, upright, and heavier pelvis |
| Pubic and axillary hair | Pubic and axillary hair; facial and chest hair; increased amount of hair on upper back in some males; male pattern baldness, beginning on top of head |
| Soft, smooth skin texture | Coarser skin |
| Higher-pitched voice | Deeper voice |

**TABLE 4–2 MAJOR HORMONES IN REPRODUCTION**

| Produced by | Target Organs | Action in Female | Action in Male |
|---|---|---|---|
| **Gonadotropin-Releasing Hormone (GnRH)** | | | |
| Hypothalamus | Anterior pituitary | Stimulates release of FSH and LH, initiating puberty and sustaining female reproductive cycles; release is pulsatile | Stimulates release of FSH and LH, initiating puberty; release is pulsatile |
| **Follicle-Stimulating Hormone (FSH)** | | | |
| Anterior pituitary | Ovaries (female)<br>Testes (male) | 1. Stimulates production of estrogens, progesterone<br>2. Stimulates growth and maturation of graafian follicles before ovulation | Stimulates sperm formation in Sertoli cells of testes |
| **Luteinizing Hormone (LH)** | | | |
| Anterior pituitary | Ovaries (female)<br>Testes (male) | 1. Stimulates final maturation of follicle<br>2. Surge of LH about 14 days before next expected menstrual period causes ovulation<br>3. Stimulates transformation of graafian follicle into corpus luteum, which continues secretion of estrogens and progesterone for about 12 days if ovum is not fertilized. If fertilization occurs, placenta gradually assumes this function | Stimulates Leydig cells of testes to secrete testosterone |
| **Estrogens** | | | |
| 1. Ovaries and corpus luteum (female)<br>2. Placenta (pregnancy)<br>3. Formed in small quantities from testosterone in Sertoli cells of testes (male); other tissues, especially the liver, produce estrogen in the male | Female; internal and external reproductive organs; breasts<br>Male: testes | 1. Reproductive organs<br>a. Maturation at puberty<br>b. Stimulation of endometrium before ovulation<br>2. Breasts: induce growth of glandular and ductal tissue; initiate deposition of fat at puberty<br>3. Stimulate growth of long bones but cause closure of epiphyses, limiting mature height<br>4. Pregnancy: stimulate growth of uterus, breast tissue; inhibit active milk production; relax pelvic ligaments | Necessary for normal sperm formation |

The maturing child's hypothalamus gradually increases production of GnRH beginning about 8 years of age. The level of GnRH increases slowly until reaching a level adequate to stimulate the anterior pituitary to increase its production of follicle-stimulating hormone (FSH) and luteinizing hormone (LH). The ovaries and testes increase production of sex hormones and begin maturing gametes in response

**TABLE 4–2 MAJOR HORMONES IN REPRODUCTION** *Continued*

| Produced by | Target Organs | Action in Female | Action in Male |
|---|---|---|---|
| **Progesterone** | | | |
| Ovary, corpus luteum, placenta | Uterus, breasts | 1. Stimulates secretion of endometrial glands; causes endometrial vessels to become highly dilated and tortuous in preparation for possible embryo implantation<br>2. Pregnancy: induces growth of cells of fallopian tubes and uterine lining to nourish embryo; decreases contractions of uterus; prepares breasts for lactation but inhibits prolactin secretion | Not applicable |
| **Prolactin** | | | |
| Anterior pituitary | Female breasts | Stimulates secretion of milk (lactogenesis); estrogen and progesterone from placenta have an inhibiting effect on milk production until after placenta is expelled at birth; sucking of newborn stimulates prolactin secretion to maintain milk production | Not applicable |
| **Oxytocin** | | | |
| Posterior pituitary | Uterus, female breast | 1. Uterus; stimulates contractions during birth and stimulates postpartum contractions to compress uterine vessels and control bleeding<br>2. Stimulates let-down, or milk-ejection reflex during breast feeding | Not applicable |
| **Testosterone** | | | |
| Testes (male)<br>Adrenal glands (female)<br>Ovaries (female) | Sexual organs (male)<br>Male body conformation after puberty | Small quantities of androgenic (masculinizing) hormones from adrenal glands cause growth of pubic and axillary hair at puberty<br>Most androgens, such as testosterone, are converted to estrogen | 1. Induces development of male sex organs in fetus<br>2. Induces growth and division of the cells that mature sperm<br>3. Induces development of male secondary sex characteristics |

to higher levels of FSH and LH. The sex hormones also induce development of secondary sex characteristics. Table 4–2 presents the major hormones that play a role in reproduction.

There is individual variation in the age at which changes of puberty begin and in the time required to complete these changes. Nutritional state can influence the start of puberty, with the well-nourished child having an earlier onset. Girls are about 6 months to 1 year younger than boys when hormonal changes of puberty begin, although the girl's growth spurt earlier in puberty makes it seem that she begins puberty about 2 years before boys of the same age. Changes of puberty occur in an orderly sequence in both sexes. Growth in height and weight are dramatic during puberty but slow after puberty until the mature height and weight are attained.

### FEMALE PUBERTY CHANGES

The anterior pituitary gland secretes increasing amounts of FSH and LH in response to the hypothalamic secretion of GnRH as the girl matures. These two pituitary secretions stimulate secretion of estrogens and progesterone by the ovary, resulting in maturation of the reproductive organs and breasts and in development of secondary sex characteristics. The first noticeable changes of puberty begin at about 10 to 11 years in girls, with the development of breast buds. The first menstrual period (menarche) occurs 2 to 2½ years later, when the girl is about 12 to 13 years old.

**Breast Changes.** The earliest outward changes of puberty occur in the breasts. First, the nipple enlarges and protrudes. The areola surrounding the nipple enlarges and becomes somewhat protuberant, although less so than the nipple. These changes are followed by growth of the glandular and ductal tissue. Fat is deposited in the breasts to give them the characteristic rounded female appearance. During puberty, a girl's breasts often develop at different rates, resulting in a lopsided appearance until one catches up with the other.

**Body Contours.** The pelvis widens and assumes a rounded, basin-like shape that is favorable for passage of the fetus during childbirth. Fat is deposited selectively in the hips, giving them a rounder appearance than that of the male.

**Body Hair.** Pubic hair appears, downy at first, but becoming thicker as puberty progresses. Axillary hair appears near the time of menarche. The texture and quantity of pubic and axillary hair vary among women and in different ethnic groups. Women of African descent usually have body hair that is coarser and curlier than that of white women. Asian women often have sparser body hair than women of other racial groups.

**Skeletal Growth.** The girl grows taller for several years during early puberty in response to estrogen stimulation. The growth spurt begins about 1 year after initial breast development. Estrogen's other powerful effect on the skeleton is to cause the epiphyses (growth areas of the bone) to unite with the shaft of the bones; this eventually stops growth in height.

**Reproductive Organs.** The girl's external genitalia enlarge as fat is deposited in the mons pubis, labia majora, and labia minora. The vagina, uterus, fallopian tubes, and ovaries grow larger. In addition, the vaginal mucosa changes, becoming more resistant to trauma and infection in preparation for sexual activity. Cyclic changes in the reproductive organs occur during each female reproductive cycle.

**Menarche.** Two to 2½ years after a girl's breasts begin developing, she experiences her first menstrual period. Early menstrual periods are often irregular and scant. These early menstrual cycles are not usually fertile because ovulation occurs inconsistently. Fertile reproductive cycles require preparation of the uterine lining precisely timed with ovulation. However, ovulation may occur during any female reproductive cycle, including the first. The sexually active girl can conceive even before her first menstrual period.

Delayed onset of menstruation is called *primary amenorrhea* if the girl's periods have not begun by the age of 16 years. It may also be considered if the girl is more than 1 year older than her mother or sisters were when their menarche occurred. *Secondary amenorrhea* describes absence of menstruation for at least three cycles after regular cycles have been established. Both primary and secondary amenorrhea are more common in females who are thin. Girls and women who are competitive athletes or ballet dancers or who suffer from eating disorders (such as anorexia nervosa or bulimia) may have too little fat to produce enough sex hormones to stimulate ovulation and menstruation. Pregnancy is a common cause of secondary amenorrhea as well.

### MALE PUBERTY CHANGES

Secretion of GnRH by the hypothalamus begins rising about the age of 10 to 13 years, stimulating secretion of LH and FSH from the anterior pituitary. LH and FSH then stimulate secretion of testosterone and eventually spermatogenesis. Testosterone stimulates development of a boy's reproductive organs and secondary sex characteristics. The outward changes of puberty begin at about 13 to 16 years of age.

**Growth of the Testes and Penis.** The first outward evidence of male sexual maturation is growth of the testes. Growth in circumference and lengthening of the penis follow about a year after testicular growth begins. The skin of the scrotum thins and darkens.

**Nocturnal Emissions.** Often called "wet dreams," nocturnal emissions commonly occur during the teenage years. The boy experiences a spontaneous ejaculation of seminal fluid during sleep, often accompanied by dreams with sexual content. It is important to prepare boys for this normal occurrence so that they do not feel abnormal or ashamed.

**Body Hair.** Pubic hair growth begins at the base of the penis. Gradually, the hair coarsens, and growth spreads upward and in the midline of the abdomen. About 2 years later, axillary hair appears. Facial hair begins as a fine, downy mustache and progresses to the characteristic beard of the adult male. In most boys, chest hair develops, and some boys have hair on their upper backs. The amount and character of body hair vary among men of different racial groups, with Asian and Native American men often having less than White or African men. There is variation in the quantity and character of body hair among men of the same racial group as well.

**Body Composition.** Under the influence of testosterone, the male develops a greater average muscle mass than the female. At maturity, the man's muscle mass exceeds the woman's by 50 percent; this explains why a man has a biologic advantage over a woman in tasks that require muscle strength.

**Skeletal Growth.** Testosterone causes boys to undergo a rapid growth spurt, especially in height. A boy's linear growth begins about a year later than a girl's and lasts for a longer time. Testosterone eventually causes union of the epiphysis with the shaft of long bones, as estrogen does in girls. However, the height-limiting effect of testosterone is not as strong as that of estrogen in females, so boys grow in stature for several years longer than girls. The male's greater average height at maturity is the combined result of beginning the growth spurt at a later age and continuing it for a longer time.

A boy's shoulders broaden as his height increases. His pelvis assumes a more upright shape, with narrower diameters and heavier composition than the female's. A man's pelvis is structurally suited for tasks requiring load bearing.

**Voice Changes.** Hypertrophy of the laryngeal mucosa and enlargement of the larynx cause the male's voice to deepen. Before reaching its bass tones at maturity, many boys experience an embarrassing "cracking" or "squeaking" of their voice when they speak.

### Decline in Fertility

A woman's ability to reproduce decreases over a period of years called the climacteric. In most women, the climacteric occurs between the ages of 45 and 50. At this time, maturation of ova and production of ovarian hormones gradually decline. The external and internal reproductive organs atrophy somewhat as well. Menopause is the term used to describe the final menstrual period. However, *menopause* and *climacteric* are often used interchangeably to describe the entire gradual process of change. *Perimenopause* is the time from onset of symptoms associated with the climacteric until at least 1 year after the last menstrual period. See Chapter 33 for more information about the woman's needs during this phase of her life.

Males do not experience a distinct marker event like menopause. Their production of testosterone and sperm gradually declines, but men in their 50s, 60s, and beyond may still be able to father children.

**✓ CHECK YOUR READING**

1. What are the first noticeable changes of puberty in girls and in boys?
2. What are common differences in body hair characteristics among adult males of different races?
3. What are basic differences between the mature male and female pelves?
4. Why do males generally attain greater mature height than females?
5. What are common male and female secondary sex characteristics?

## Female Reproductive Anatomy

The nurse needs a basic knowledge of the structure and function of the external and internal reproductive organs to understand their role in pregnancy and childbirth. The functions of the female reproductive and accessory organs are summarized in Table 4–3.

### External Female Reproductive Organs

Collectively, the external female reproductive organs are called the *vulva*. These structures include the mons pubis, labia majora and minora, clitoris, structures of the vestibule, and perineum (Fig. 4–1).

#### MONS PUBIS

The mons pubis is the rounded, fleshy prominence over the symphysis pubis that forms the anterior border of the external reproductive organs. It is covered with varying amounts of pubic hair.

#### LABIA MAJORA AND LABIA MINORA

The labia majora are two rounded, fleshy folds of tissue that extend from the mons pubis to the perineum. They have slightly deeper pigmentation than surrounding skin and are covered with pubic hair. The labia majora protect the more fragile tissues of the external genitalia.

The labia minora run parallel to and within the labia majora. The labia minora extend from the clito-

**TABLE 4-3 FUNCTIONS OF FEMALE REPRODUCTIVE AND ACCESSORY ORGANS**

| Organ | Function |
|---|---|
| Vagina | 1. Passageway for the menstrual flow.<br>2. Female organ for coitus: receives male penis.<br>3. Passageway for the fetus during birth. |
| Uterus | Houses and nourishes fetus until sufficiently mature to function outside the mother's body; uterine muscle propels fetus to outside. |
| Fallopian tube | 1. Provides passageway for ovum as it travels from ovary to uterus.<br>2. Site of fertilization. |
| Ovaries | 1. Endocrine glands that secrete estrogens and progesterone.<br>2. Contain ova within follicles for maturation during the woman's reproductive life. |
| Breasts | |
| Alveoli | Acinar cells within alveoli secrete milk after childbirth. |
| Lactiferous ducts and sinuses | Collect milk from alveoli and conduct it to the outside. |

ris anteriorly and merge posteriorly to form the fourchette, or posterior rim of the vaginal introitus, or opening. The labia minora do not have pubic hair. They are highly vascular and respond to stimulation by becoming engorged with blood.

#### CLITORIS

The clitoris is a small projection at the anterior junction of the two labia minora. This structure is composed of highly sensitive erectile tissue that is similar to that of the penis. The labia majora merge to form a prepuce over the clitoris.

#### VESTIBULE

The vestibule refers to structures enclosed by the labia minora. The urinary meatus, vaginal introitus, and ducts of Skene's and Bartholin's glands lie within the vestibule. Skene's, or periurethral, glands provide lubrication for the urethra. Bartholin's glands provide lubrication for the vaginal introitus, particularly during sexual arousal.

The vaginal introitus is surrounded by erectile tissue. During sexual stimulation, blood flows into the erectile tissue, allowing the introitus to tighten around the penis. This adds a massaging feeling that heightens the male's sexual sensations, encouraging release of semen.

The hymen is a thin fold of mucosa partially separating the vagina from the vestibule. The intactness, or lack thereof, of the hymen is not a criterion of virginity. The hymen may be broken with injury, with

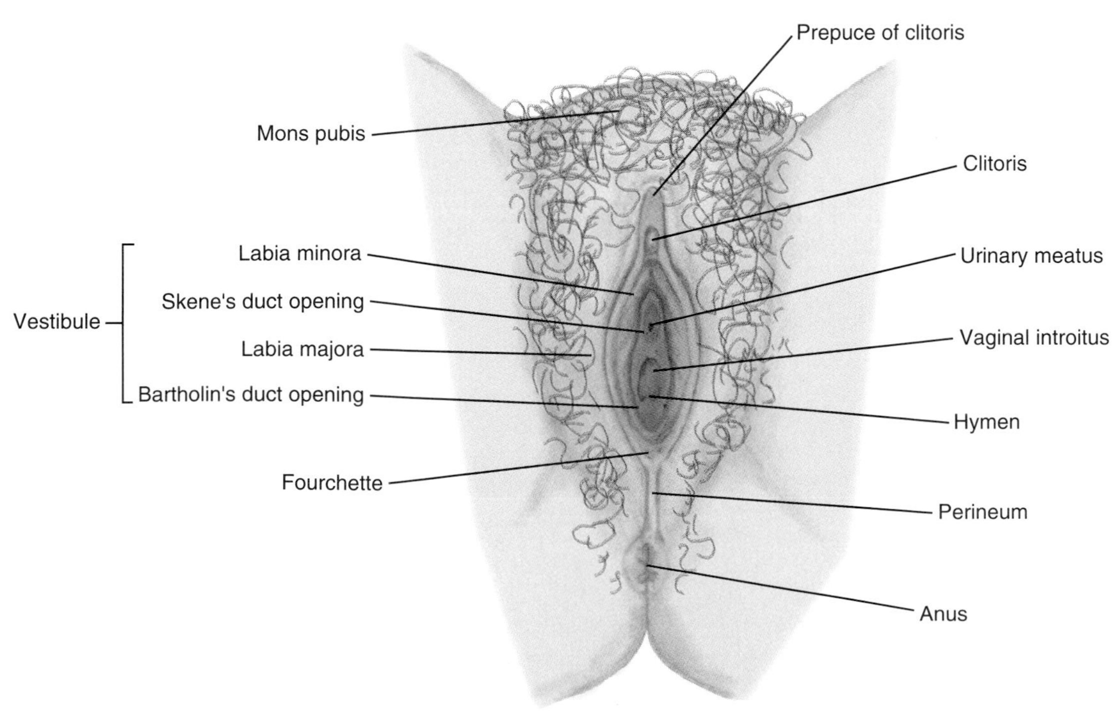


**FIGURE 4-1**
External female reproductive structures.

the use of tampons, during intercourse, or during childbirth.

### PERINEUM

The perineum is the most posterior part of the external female reproductive organs. The perineum extends from the fourchette anteriorly to the anus posteriorly. It is composed of fibrous and muscular tissues that provide support for pelvic structures. The perineum may be lacerated during childbirth, or it may be incised to enlarge the vaginal opening in a procedure called an *episiotomy*.

## Internal Female Reproductive Organs

The internal reproductive structures are the vagina, uterus, fallopian tubes, and ovaries (Figs. 4–2 and 4–3). These organs are supported and contained within the bony pelvis.

### VAGINA

The vagina is a tube of muscular and membranous tissue about 8 to 10 cm long, lying between the bladder anteriorly and the rectum posteriorly. The vagina connects the uterus above with the vestibule below. The vaginal lining has multiple folds, or rugae, and a muscular layer that are capable of marked distention during childbirth. The vagina is lubricated by secretions of the cervix, the lowermost part of the uterus, and by the Bartholin's glands.

The vagina does not end abruptly at the uterine opening but arches to form a pouch-like structure, the vaginal fornix. Each fornix is described by its location: anterior, posterior, or lateral.

The vagina has three major functions: (1) it allows discharge of the menstrual flow; (2) it is the female organ of coitus; and (3) during childbirth, it allows passage of the fetus from the uterus to the outside.

### UTERUS

The uterus is a hollow, thick-walled, muscular organ that is shaped like a flattened upside-down pear. The uterus houses and nourishes the fetus until birth, then contracts rhythmically during labor to expel the fetus. Each month, the uterus is prepared for a pregnancy, whether or not conception occurs.

The uterus measures about 7.5 × 5 × 2.5 cm and is larger in a woman who has borne children than in one who has not. It is suspended above the bladder and is anterior to the rectum. Its normal position is anteverted (rotated forward) and slightly anteflexed (flexed forward).

#### DIVISIONS OF THE UTERUS

The uterus has three divisions.

**Corpus.** The upper division is the corpus, or body, of the uterus. The uppermost part of the uterine corpus, above the area where the fallopian tubes enter the uterus, is the *fundus* of the uterus.

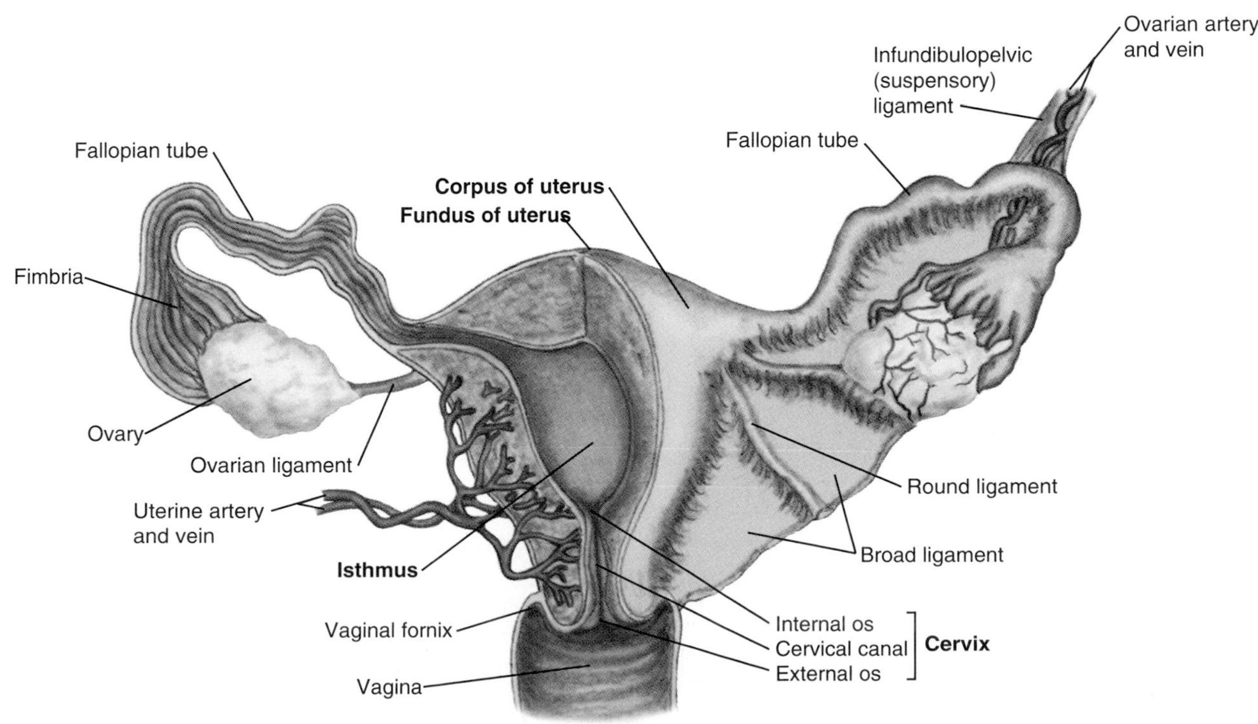


**FIGURE 4–2**
Internal female reproductive structures, anterior view.

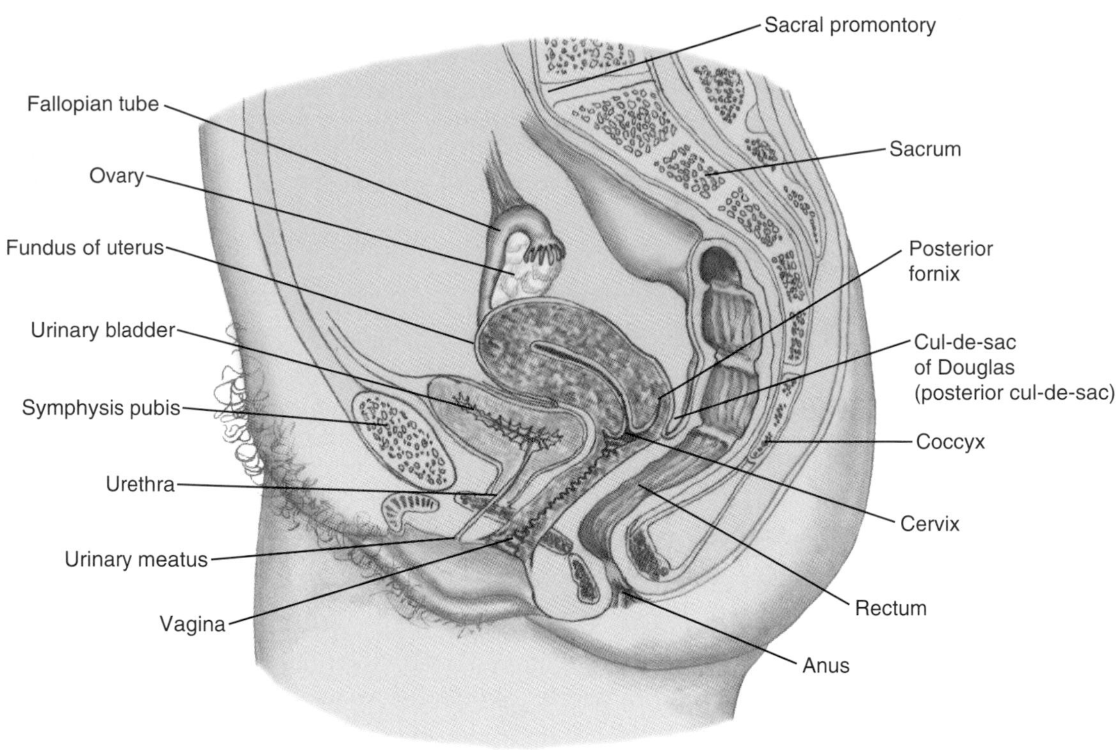


**FIGURE 4–3**

Internal female reproductive structures, midsagittal view.

**Isthmus.** A narrower transition zone, the isthmus, is between the corpus of the uterus and the cervix. During late pregnancy, the isthmus elongates and is known as the lower uterine segment.

**Cervix.** The cervix is the tubular "neck" of the lower uterus and is about 2 to 3 cm long. During labor, the cervix effaces (thins) and dilates (opens) to allow passage of the fetus. The os is the opening in the cervix that runs between the uterus and the vagina. The upper part of the cervix is marked by the internal os, and the lower cervix is marked by the external os. The external os of a childless woman is round and smooth. After vaginal birth, the external os has an irregular, slit-like shape and may have tags of scar tissue.

LAYERS OF THE UTERUS

The uterus has three layers.

**Perimetrium.** The perimetrium is the outer peritoneal layer of serous membrane that covers most of the uterus. Laterally, the perimetrium is continuous with the broad ligaments on either side of the uterus.

**Myometrium.** The myometrium is the middle layer of thick muscle. Most of the muscle fibers are concentrated in the upper uterus, and their number diminishes progressively toward the cervix. The myometrium contains three types of smooth muscle fiber, each suited to specific functions in childbearing (Fig. 4–4).

1. *Longitudinal fibers* are found mostly in the fundus and are designed to expel the fetus efficiently toward the pelvic outlet during birth.
2. *Interlacing figure-8 fibers* make up the middle layer. These fibers contract after birth to compress blood vessels that pass between them to limit blood loss.
3. *Circular fibers* form constrictions where the fallopian tubes enter the uterus and surround the internal cervical os. Circular fibers prevent reflux of menstrual blood and tissue into the fallopian tubes, promote normal implantation of the fertilized ovum by controlling its entry into the uterus, and retain the fetus until the appropriate time of birth.

**Endometrium.** The endometrium is the inner layer of the uterus. It is responsive to the cyclic variations of estrogen and progesterone during the female reproductive cycle (see p. 65). The endometrium has two layers:

1. The *basal layer*, the area nearest the myometrium that regenerates the functional layer of the en-

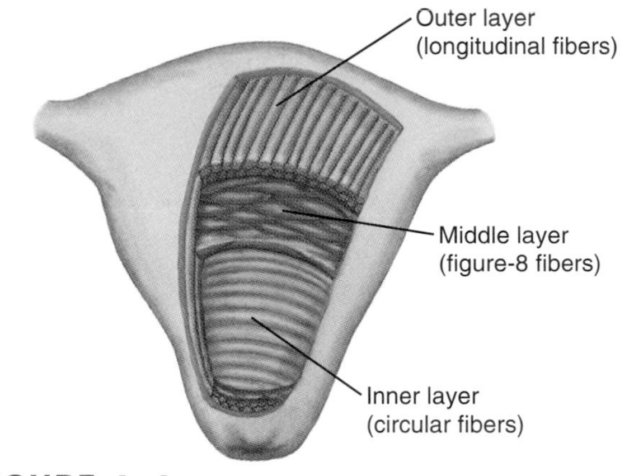


**FIGURE 4–4**

Layers of the myometrium, showing the three types of smooth muscle fiber.

dometrium after each menstrual period and after childbirth.

2. The *functional layer*, which lies above the basal layer and contains the endometrial arteries, veins, and glands; this layer is shed during each menstrual period and after childbirth in the *lochia*.

#### FALLOPIAN TUBES

The fallopian tubes, also called *oviducts*, are 8 to 14 cm long and quite narrow (2 to 3 mm at their narrowest and 5 to 8 mm at their widest). They are a pathway for the ovum between the ovary and the uterus. Fertilization occurs in the fallopian tubes. Each fallopian tube enters the upper uterus at the *cornu*, or horn, of the uterus.

The fallopian tubes are lined with folded epithelium containing cilia that beat rhythmically toward the uterine cavity to propel the ovum through the tube. The rough, folded surface of the lining combined with the small diameter makes the fallopian tube vulnerable to blockage from infection or scar tissue. Tubal blockage may result in sterility or a tubal pregnancy because the fertilized ovum cannot enter the uterus for proper implantation.

The tubes have four divisions:

1. The *interstitial* portion, which runs into the uterine cavity and lies within the uterine wall.
2. The *isthmus*, the narrow part adjacent to the uterus.
3. The *ampulla*, the wider area of the tube lateral to the isthmus, where fertilization occurs.
4. The *infundibulum*, the wide, funnel-shaped terminal end of the tube. *Fimbria* are finger-like processes surrounding the infundibulum.

The fallopian tubes are not directly connected to the ovary. At ovulation, the ovum is expelled into the abdominal cavity. Wave-like motions of the fimbria draw the ovum into the tube. The tubal isthmus, however, remains contracted until 3 days after conception to allow the fertilized ovum to develop within the tube. Initial growth of the fertilized ovum within the fallopian tube promotes its normal implantation in the fundal portion of the uterine corpus.

#### OVARIES

The ovaries are the female gonads, or sex glands. They have two functions: (1) sex hormone production and (2) maturation of an ovum during each reproductive cycle.

The ovaries secrete estrogen and progesterone in varying amounts during a woman's reproductive cycle to prepare the uterine lining for pregnancy. Ovarian hormone secretion gradually declines to very low levels during the climacteric.

At birth, the ovary contains all the ova that it will ever have. About one million immature ova are present at birth. Many of these degenerate until puberty, when 200,000 to 400,000 remain. Many ova begin the maturation process during each reproductive cycle, but most never reach maturity. During the course of a woman's reproductive life, only about 400 of the ova ever mature enough to be released and fertilized. By the time a woman reaches the climacteric, almost all of her ova have been released during ovulation or have regressed. The few remaining ova are unresponsive to stimulating hormones and do not mature.

#### CHECK YOUR READING

6. What is the vulva? Describe the location of each of these external female organs: Labia majora and minora; clitoris; urinary meatus; vaginal introitus; hymen; perineum.
7. What are the three divisions of the uterus? Where is the fundus located?
8. Describe the three myometrial layers of the uterus. What is the function of each layer?
9. How do the fallopian tubes conduct the ovum from the ovary to the uterus? Why does the fertilized ovum grow within the fallopian tube at first?
10. What are the two functions of the ovaries?

## Support Structures

The bony pelvis supports and protects the lower abdominal and internal reproductive organs. Muscles and ligaments provide added support for the internal organs of the pelvis against the downward force of gravity and the increases in intra-abdominal pressure.

## PELVIS

The bony pelvis is a basin-shaped structure at the lower end of the spine. Its posterior wall is formed by the sacrum. The side and anterior pelvic walls are composed of three fused bones: *ilium*, *ischium*, and *pubis*. Figure 4–5 illustrates important anatomic landmarks on the pelvis.

The linea terminalis, also called the pelvic brim or ileopectineal line, is an imaginary line that divides the upper, or false, pelvis from the lower, or true, pelvis. The false pelvis provides support for the internal organs and the upper part of the body. The true pelvis is most important during childbirth, and its divisions and measurements are discussed in Chapter 12.

## MUSCLES

Paired muscles enclose the lower pelvis and provide support for internal reproductive, urinary, and bowel structures (Fig. 4–6). In addition, a fibromuscular sheet, the *pelvic fascia*, provides support for the pelvic organs. Vaginal and urethral openings are in the pelvic fascia.

The *levator ani* is a collection of three pairs of muscles: the *pubococcygeus*, which is also called the *pubovaginal muscle* in the female; the *puborectal*; and the *iliococcygeus*. These muscles support internal pelvic structures and resist increases in the intra-abdominal pressure.

The *ischiocavernosus muscle* extends from the clitoris to the ischial tuberosities on each side of the lower bony pelvis. The two *transverse perineal muscles* extend from fibrous tissue of the perineum to the two ischial tuberosities, stabilizing the center of the perineum.

## LIGAMENTS

Seven pairs of ligaments maintain the internal reproductive organs, with their nerve and blood supplies, in their proper positions within the pelvis (see Fig. 4–2).

**Lateral Support.** Paired ligaments stabilize the uterus and ovaries laterally and keep them in the midline of the pelvis. The *broad ligament* is a sheet of tissue extending from each side of the uterus to the lateral pelvic wall. The *round ligament* and fallopian tube mark the upper border of the broad ligament, and the lower edge is bounded by the uterine blood vessels. Within the two broad ligaments are the ovarian ligaments, blood vessels, and lymphatics.

The right and left *cardinal ligaments* provide support to the lower uterus and vagina. They extend from the lateral walls of the cervix and vagina to the side walls of the pelvis.

The two *ovarian ligaments* connect the ovaries to the lateral uterine walls. The *infundibulopelvic (suspensory) ligaments* connect the lateral ovary and distal fallopian tubes to the pelvic side walls. The infundibulopelvic ligament also carries the blood vessel and nerve supply for the ovary.

**Anterior Support.** Two pairs of ligaments provide anterior support for the internal reproductive organs. The *round ligaments* connect the upper uterus to the connective tissue of the labia majora. These ligaments maintain the uterus in its normal anteflexed position and help direct the fetal presenting part against the cervix during labor.

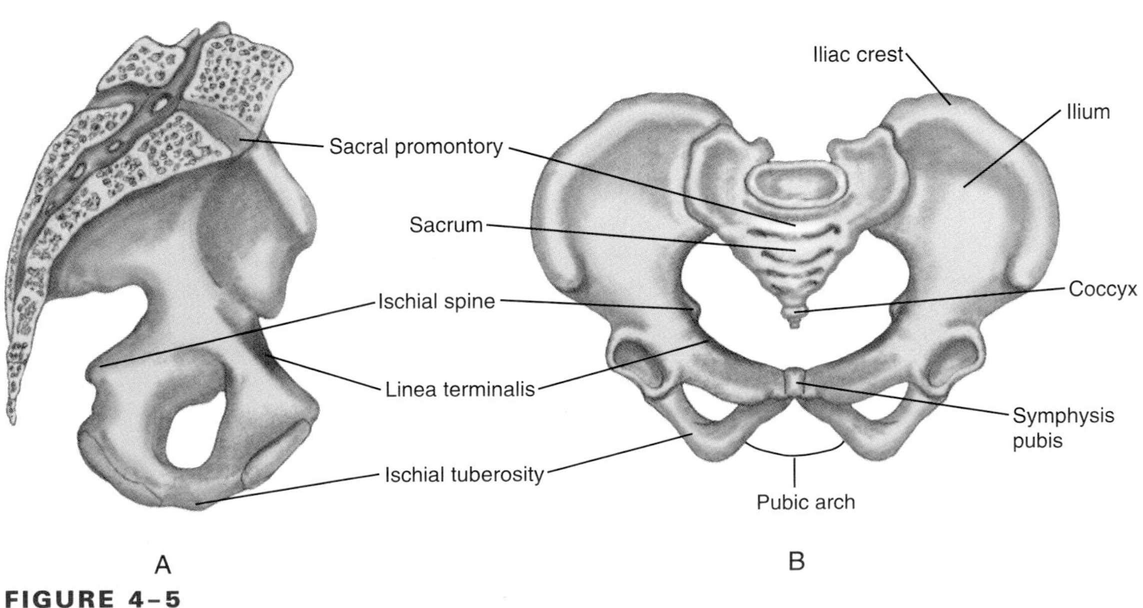


**FIGURE 4–5**

Structures of the bony pelvis, shown in lateral (A) and anterior (B) views.

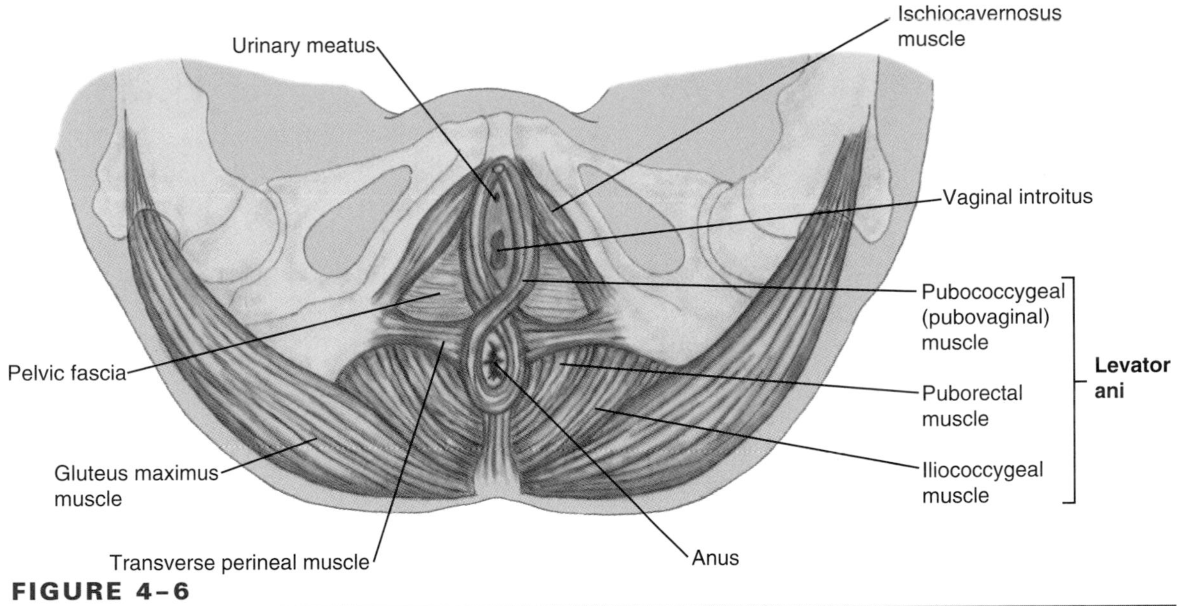


**FIGURE 4–6**

Muscles of the female pelvic floor.

The *pubocervical ligaments* support the cervix anteriorly. They connect the cervix to the interior surface of the symphysis pubis.

**Posterior Support.** The *uterosacral ligaments* provide posterior support, extending from the lower posterior uterus to the sacrum. These ligaments also contain sympathetic and parasympathetic nerves of the autonomic nervous system.

### BLOOD SUPPLY

The uterine blood supply is carried by the *uterine arteries*, which are branches of the internal iliac artery. These vessels enter the uterus at the lower border of the broad ligament, near the isthmus of the uterus. The vessels branch downward to supply the cervix and vagina and upward to supply the uterus. The upper branch also supplies the ovaries and fallopian tubes. The vessels are coiled to allow for elongation as the uterus enlarges and rises out of the pelvis during pregnancy. Blood drains into the *uterine veins* and from there into the internal iliac veins.

Additional ovarian and tubal blood supply is carried by the *ovarian artery*, which arises from the abdominal aorta. The ovarian blood supply drains into the two *ovarian veins*. The left ovarian vein drains into the left renal vein, but the right ovarian vein drains directly into the inferior vena cava.

### NERVE SUPPLY

Most functions of the reproductive system are under involuntary, or unconscious, control. Nerves of the autonomic nervous system from the uterovaginal plexus and inferior hypogastric plexus control automatic functions of the reproductive system.

Sensory and motor nerves that innervate the reproductive organs enter the spinal cord at the T12 through L2 levels. These nerves are important during childbearing in terms of pain management (see Chapter 15).

**✓ CHECK YOUR READING**

11. Where is the true pelvis located?
12. What are the purposes of the muscles of the pelvis? The purposes of the ligaments?

## Female Reproductive Cycle

The female reproductive cycle describes the regular and recurrent changes in the anterior pituitary secretions, ovaries, and uterine endometrium that are designed to prepare the body for pregnancy. Associated changes in the cervical mucus promote fertilization during each cycle. The female reproductive cycle is often called the *menstrual cycle* because menstruation provides a marker for each cycle's beginning and end if pregnancy does not occur. Figure 4–7 illustrates these interrelated changes during the cycle.

The female reproductive cycle is driven by a *feedback loop* between the anterior pituitary and the ovaries. A feedback loop is a change in the level of one secretion in response to a change in the level of

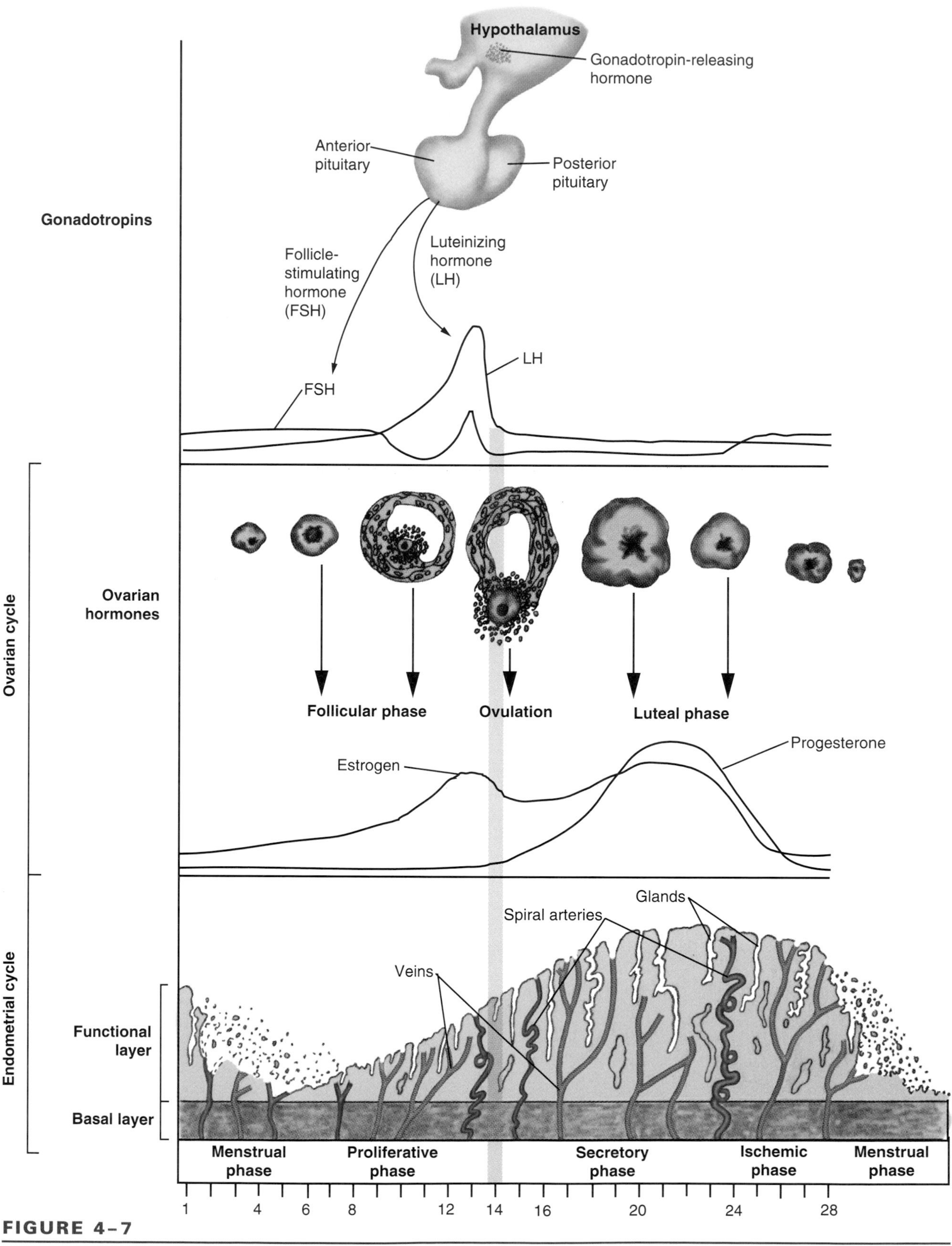


**FIGURE 4–7**

The female reproductive cycle, showing the changes in hormone secretion from the anterior pituitary and interrelated changes in the ovary and uterine endometrium.

another secretion. The feedback loop may be positive, in which rising levels of one secretion cause another to rise. The feedback loop may also be negative, in which rising levels of one secretion cause another to fall.

The duration of the cycle is about 28 days, although it may range from 20 to 45 days (Guyton, 1996). Significant deviations from the 28-day cycle are associated with reduced fertility. The first day of the menstrual period is counted as day 1 of the woman's cycle. The female reproductive cycle is further divided into two cycles that reflect changes in the ovaries and uterine endometrium.

## Ovarian Cycle

In response to GnRH from the woman's hypothalamus, the anterior pituitary secretes FSH and LH. The FSH and LH stimulate the ovaries to mature an ovum, release it, and to secrete other hormones that will prepare the endometrium for implantation of a fertilized ovum. The ovarian cycle consists of three phases: the follicular, ovulatory, and luteal phases.

### FOLLICULAR PHASE

The follicular phase is the period during which an ovum matures. It begins with the first day of menstruation and ends about 14 days later in a 28-day cycle. The length of this phase varies more among different women than do the lengths of the other two phases. The fall in estrogen and progesterone secretion by the ovary just before menstruation stimulates secretion of FSH and LH by the anterior pituitary. As the FSH and LH levels rise slightly, six to 12 graafian follicles, each containing an immature ovum, begin growing. Each follicle secretes fluid containing high levels of estrogen, which accelerates maturation by making the follicle more sensitive to the effects of FSH. Eventually, one follicle outgrows the others to reach maturity. The mature follicle secretes large amounts of estrogen, which depresses FSH secretion. The dip in FSH secretion just before ovulation blocks further maturation of the less-developed follicles. Occasionally, more than one follicle matures and releases its ovum, which can lead to a multifetal pregnancy.

### OVULATORY PHASE

Near the middle of a 28-day reproductive cycle, about 2 days before ovulation, LH secretion rises markedly. Secretion of FSH also rises but to a lesser extent than that of LH. These surges in LH and FSH cause a slight fall in follicular estrogen production and a rise in progesterone secretion, stimulating final maturation of a single follicle and release of its ovum. Ovulation marks the beginning of the luteal phase of the female reproductive cycle and occurs about 14 days before the next menstrual period.

The mature follicle is a mass of cells with a fluid-filled chamber. A smaller mass of cells houses the ovum within this chamber. At ovulation, a blister-like projection forms on the wall of the follicle (a *stigma*), the follicle ruptures, and the ovum with its surrounding cells is released from the surface of the ovary, where it is picked up by the fimbriated end of the fallopian tube for transport to the uterus.

### LUTEAL PHASE

After ovulation and under the influence of LH, the remaining cells of the old follicle persist for about 12 days as a *corpus luteum*. The corpus luteum secretes estrogen and large amounts of progesterone to prepare the endometrium for a fertilized ovum. Levels of FSH and LH decrease during this phase in response to higher levels of estrogen and progesterone. If the ovum is fertilized, it secretes a hormone (chorionic gonadotropin) that causes persistence of the corpus luteum to maintain an early pregnancy. If the ovum is not fertilized, FSH and LH fall to low levels, and the corpus luteum regresses. Decline of estrogen and progesterone with corpus luteum regression results in menstruation as the uterine lining breaks down.

The loss of estrogen and progesterone from the corpus luteum at the end of one cycle stimulates the anterior pituitary to again secrete more FSH and LH, initiating a new female reproductive cycle. The old corpus luteum is replaced by fibrous tissue called the *corpus albicans*.

## Endometrial Cycle

The uterine endometrium responds to ovarian hormone stimulation with cyclic changes. Three phases mark the changes in the endometrium: the proliferative phase, the secretory phase, and the menstrual phase.

### PROLIFERATIVE PHASE

The proliferative phase takes place as the ovum matures and is released during the first half of the ovarian cycle. After completion of a menstrual period, the endometrium is very thin. The basal layer of endometrial cells remains after menstruation. These cells multiply to form new endometrial epithelium and endometrial glands under the stimulation of estrogen secreted by the maturing ovarian follicles. Endometrial spiral arteries and endometrial veins elongate to accompany thickening of the functional endometrial layer and to nourish the proliferating cells. As ovulation time approaches, the endometrial glands secrete a thin, stringy mucus that aids entry of sperm into the uterus.

#### SECRETORY PHASE

The secretory phase occurs during the last half of the ovarian cycle as the uterus is prepared to receive a fertilized ovum. The endometrium continues to thicken under the influence of estrogen and progesterone from the corpus luteum, reaching its maximum thickness of 5 to 6 mm. The blood vessels and endometrial glands become twisted and dilated.

Progesterone from the corpus luteum causes the thick endometrium to secrete substances to nourish a fertilized ovum. Large quantities of glycogen, proteins, lipids, and minerals are stored within the endometrium, awaiting arrival of the ovum.

#### MENSTRUAL PHASE

If fertilization does not occur, the corpus luteum regresses and its production of estrogen and progesterone falls. About 2 days before the onset of the menses, vasospasm of the endometrial blood vessels causes the endometrium to become ischemic and necrotic. The necrotic areas of endometrium separate from the basal layers, resulting in the menstrual flow. The duration of the menstrual phase is about 5 days.

During a menstrual period, women lose about 40 ml of blood. Because of the recurrent loss of blood, many women are mildly anemic during their reproductive years, especially if their diets are low in iron.

### Changes in Cervical Mucus

During most of the female reproductive cycle, the mucus of the cervix is scant, thick, and sticky. Just before ovulation, cervical mucus becomes thin, clear, and elastic to promote passage of sperm into the uterus and fallopian tube, where they can fertilize the ovum. *Spinnbarkeit* refers to the elasticity of cervical mucus. A woman may assess the elasticity of her cervical mucus either to avoid conception or to promote conception.

**✓ CHECK YOUR READING**

13. Which ovarian structures secrete estrogen and progesterone during the female reproductive cycle?
14. What three ovarian phases occur during each female reproductive cycle?
15. How does the uterine endometrium change during a woman's reproductive cycle?
16. Why is it important for the cervical mucus to become thin, clear, and elastic around the time of ovulation?

## The Female Breast

### Structure

The breasts, or mammary glands, are not directly functional in reproduction, but they secrete milk after childbirth to nourish the infant. The small, raised nipple is at the center of each breast (Fig. 4–8). The nipple is composed of sensitive erectile tissue and may respond to sexual stimulation. Surrounding the nipple is a larger circular areola. Both the nipple and areola are darker than surrounding skin. Montgomery's tubercles are sebaceous glands in the areola. They are inactive and not obvious except during pregnancy and lactation, when they enlarge and secrete a substance that keeps the nipple soft.

Within each breast are lobes of glandular tissue that secrete milk. These lobes are arranged like spokes of a wheel around the hub. Fifteen to 20 of these lobes are arranged around and behind the nipple and areola. Fibrous tissue and fat in the breast support the glandular tissue, blood vessels, lymphatics, and nerves.

Alveoli are small sacs that contain acinar cells to secrete milk. The acinar cells extract substances needed from the mammary blood supply to manufacture milk when the breasts are properly stimulated by the anterior pituitary gland. Myoepithelial cells surround the alveoli to contract and eject the milk into the ductal system when signaled by secretion of the hormone oxytocin from the posterior pituitary gland.

The alveoli drain into lactiferous ducts, which connect to drain milk from all areas of the breast. The lactiferous ducts become wider under the areola and are called *lactiferous sinuses* in this area. The lactiferous sinuses narrow again as they open to the outside in the nipple.

### Function

The breasts are inactive until puberty, when rising estrogen levels stimulate growth of the glandular tissue. In addition, fat is deposited in the breasts, resulting in the mature female contour. The amount of fat is the major determinant of breast size; the amount of glandular tissue is similar for all mature women. Thus, breast size is unrelated to the amount of milk a woman can produce during lactation.

During pregnancy, high levels of estrogen and progesterone, produced by the placenta, stimulate growth of the alveoli and ductal system to prepare them for lactation. Prolactin secretion by the anterior pituitary gland stimulates milk production during pregnancy, but this effect is inhibited by estrogen and progesterone produced by the placenta. Inhibiting effects of estrogen and progesterone stop when the placenta is expelled after birth, and active milk production occurs in response to the infant's nursing.

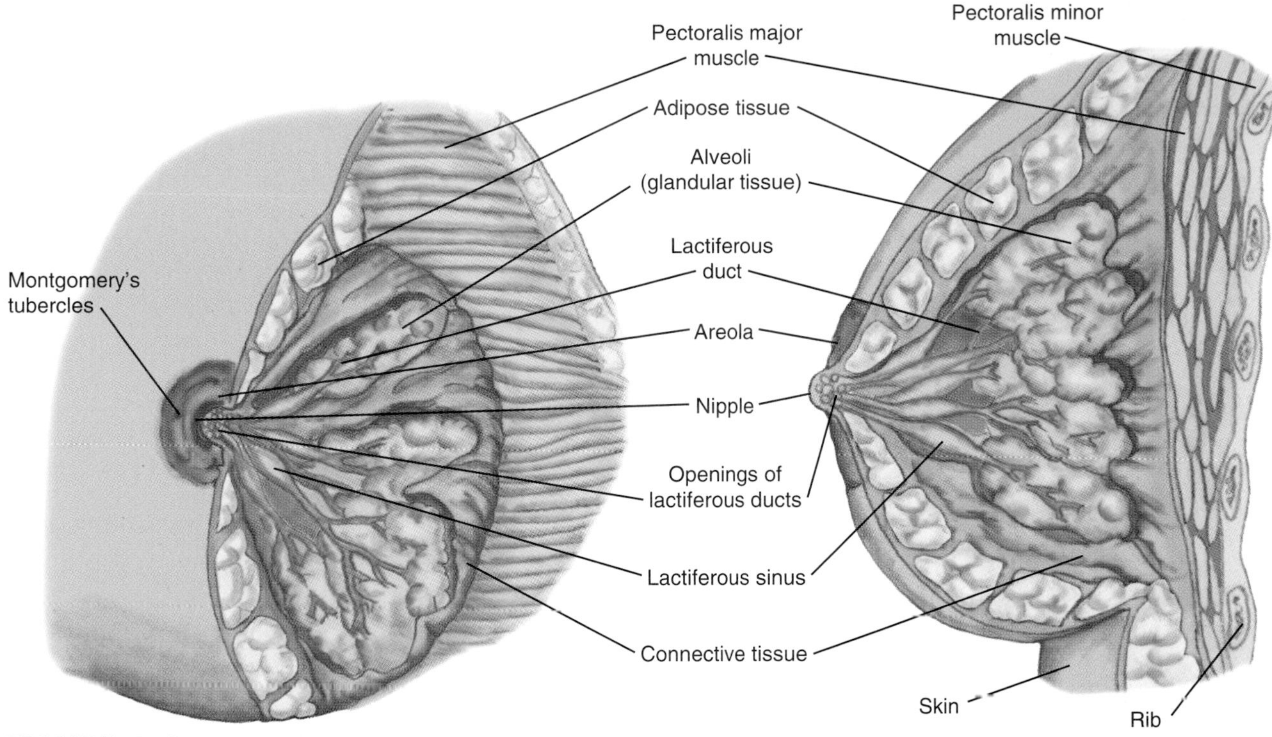


**FIGURE 4–8**

Structures of the female breast.

**CHECK YOUR READING**

17. What is the function of Montgomery's tubercles?
18. How is a woman's breast size related to the amount of milk she can produce?
19. Why is milk not actively secreted during pregnancy?

# Male Reproductive Anatomy and Physiology

## External Male Reproductive Organs

The male has two external organs of reproduction, the penis and the scrotum (Fig. 4–9).

### PENIS

The penis has two functions. As part of the urinary tract, it carries urine from the bladder to the exterior during urination. As a reproductive organ, the penis deposits semen into the female vagina during coitus.

The penis is composed mostly of erectile tissue, spongy tissues with many small spaces inside. There are three areas of erectile tissue: the corpus spongiosum, which surrounds the urethra, and two columns of the corpus cavernosum on each side of the penis.

The penis is flaccid most of the time because the small spaces within the erectile tissue are collapsed. During sexual stimulation, arteries within the penis dilate and veins are partly occluded, trapping blood in the spongy tissue. Entrapment of blood within the penis causes erection and enables the man to penetrate the vagina during sexual intercourse.

The glans is the distal end of the penis. The urinary meatus is centered in the end of the glans. Covering the glans is the loose skin of the prepuce, or foreskin. The prepuce may be removed during *circumcision*, a surgical procedure usually performed during the newborn period, although it may be performed later. The glans is very sensitive to tactile stimulation, adding to a man's sensation during coitus.

### SCROTUM

The scrotum is a pouch of thin skin and muscle that is suspended behind the penis. The skin of the scrotum is somewhat darker than the surrounding skin and is covered with small ridges called rugae. The scrotum is divided internally by a septum. One of the male gonads (testicle) is contained within each pocket of the scrotum.

The scrotum's main purpose is to keep the testes cooler than the core body temperature. Formation of normal male sperm requires that the testes not be too warm. A cremaster muscle is attached to each testicle to draw them closer to the body and warm them, or to relax, allowing the testes to fall away from the body and become cooler.

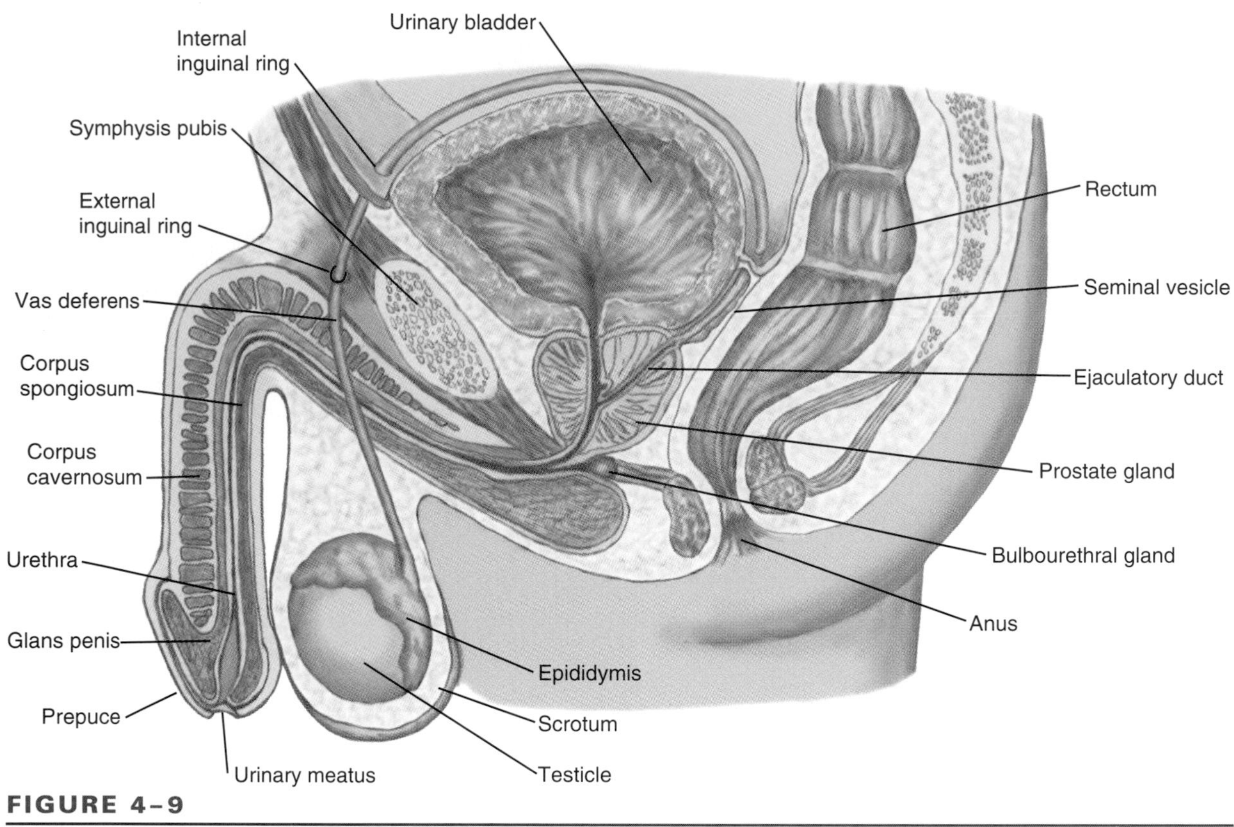


**FIGURE 4–9**

Structures of the male reproductive system, midsagittal view.

## Internal Male Reproductive Organs

The functions of the male external and internal organs are summarized in Table 4–4.

### TESTES

The male gonads, or testes, have two functions: (1) they serve as endocrine glands, and (2) they produce male gametes, or sperm, also called spermatozoa. Androgens (male sex hormones) are the primary endocrine secretions of the testes. Androgens are produced by Leydig cells of the testes. The primary androgen produced by the testes is testosterone.

Unlike the female, who experiences a cyclic pattern of hormone secretion, the male secretes testosterone in a relatively even pattern. A feedback loop

**TABLE 4–4 FUNCTIONS OF MALE REPRODUCTIVE AND ACCESSORY ORGANS**

| Organ | Function |
|---|---|
| Penis | 1. Conduit for urine from bladder.<br>2. Male organ of sexual intercourse. |
| Scrotum | Houses testes and maintains their temperature at a level cooler than the trunk of the body, thus promoting normal sperm formation. |
| Testes | 1. Endocrine glands that secrete the primary male hormone, testosterone.<br>2. Sperm formation. |
| Seminiferous tubules | Location of spermatogenesis within the testes. |
| Epididymis | 1. Storage of some sperm.<br>2. Final sperm maturation.<br>3. Where sperm develop ability to be motile. |
| Vas deferens | 1. Storage of sperm.<br>2. Conduction of sperm from epididymis to urethra. |
| Seminal vesicles, prostate, bulbourethral glands | Secretion of seminal fluids that carry sperm and provide for:<br>1. Nourishment of sperm.<br>2. Protection of sperm from hostile acidic environment of vagina.<br>3. Enhancement of motility of sperm.<br>4. Washing of all sperm from urethra. |

with the hypothalamus and anterior pituitary keeps testosterone levels stable. A small amount of testosterone is converted to estrogen in the male and is necessary for sperm formation.

Spermatogenesis occurs within tiny coiled tubes, the seminiferous tubules, of the testes (Fig. 4–10). Leydig cells are interstitial cells that support the seminiferous tubules and secrete testosterone, a hormone that is necessary for forming new cells that will mature into sperm. Sertoli cells within the seminiferous tubules respond to FSH secretion by nourishing and supporting sperm as they mature. Unlike the female, who has a lifetime supply of ova in her gonads at birth, the male does not begin producing sperm until puberty. The normal male produces new sperm throughout life, although production declines with age.

At ejaculation, about 400 million sperm are deposited in the vagina. This large number is needed for normal fertility, although a single sperm fertilizes the ovum. Only a few sperm ever reach the fallopian tube, where an ovum may be available for fertilization. When the first sperm penetrates the ovum, changes within the ovum prevent others from also fertilizing it. (See Chapter 6 for further discussion of sperm formation and conception.)

### ACCESSORY DUCTS AND GLANDS

From the seminiferous tubules, sperm pass into the epididymis within the scrotum for storage and final maturation. In the epididymis, sperm develop the ability to be motile, although secretions within the epididymis inhibit actual motility until ejaculation occurs.

The epididymis empties into the vas deferens,

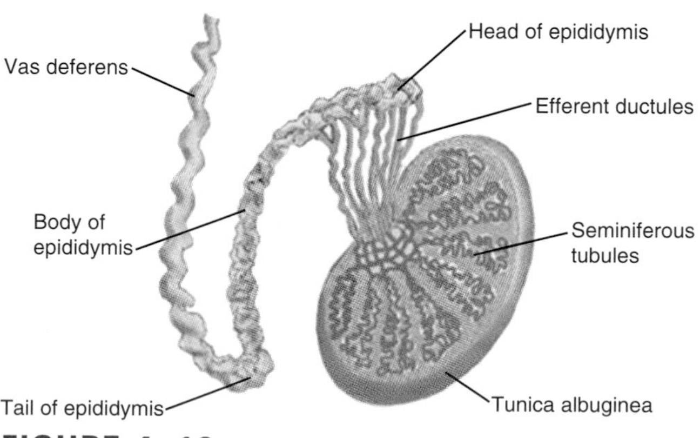


**FIGURE 4–10**

Internal structures of the testis. Initial production of sperm begins within the tiny, coiled seminiferous tubules. Immature sperm pass from the seminiferous tubules to the epididymis, and then to the vas deferens. During their passage through these structures, the sperm mature and acquire the ability to propel themselves.

where larger numbers of sperm are stored. The vas deferens then leads upward into the pelvis, then back down toward the penis through the internal and external inguinal rings. Within the pelvis, the vas deferens joins the ejaculatory duct before connecting to the urethra.

Three glands—the *seminal vesicles*, the *prostate*, and the *bulbourethral glands*—secrete seminal fluids that carry sperm into the vagina during intercourse. The seminal fluid (1) nourishes the sperm, (2) protects the sperm from the hostile pH (acidic) environment of the vagina, (3) enhances the motility of the sperm, and (4) washes the sperm out of the urethra so that the maximum number are deposited in the vagina.

**✓ CHECK YOUR READING**

20. What are the two functions of the penis?
21. What two types of erectile tissue are in the penis? What is their function?
22. Why is it important for the testes to be contained within the scrotum?
23. What are the two functions of the testes?

## SUMMARY CONCEPTS

- Initial prenatal development of the reproductive organs is similar for both males and females. If a critical part of the Y chromosome is not present at conception, female reproductive structures will develop.
- Puberty is the time when the reproductive organs become fully functional and secondary sex characteristics develop.
- Puberty begins about 6 months to 1 year earlier in girls than in boys, although the girl's early growth spurt makes it seem that she begins puberty much earlier than the boy.
- Females are generally shorter than males because they begin their growth spurt at an earlier age and complete it more quickly than boys.
- The onset of menstruation (menarche) is an obvious marker of puberty in girls.
- Girls often do not ovulate in early menstrual cycles, although they can ovulate even before the first one. Therefore, a girl can become pregnant before her first menstrual period if she is sexually active.
- The onset of puberty is more subtle in boys than in girls, beginning with growth of the testes and penis.
- Boys may have nocturnal emissions of seminal fluid; this may be distressing unless they are educated that these events are normal and expected.
- At birth, a woman has all the ova she will ever have. New ova are not formed after birth; almost all are depleted when she reaches the climacteric.

- The female reproductive cycle is often called the menstrual cycle. It includes changes in the anterior pituitary gland, ovaries, and uterine endometrium to prepare for a fertilized ovum. The character of cervical mucus also changes to encourage fertilization.
- Breast size is unrelated to glandular tissue or to the quantity or quality of milk a woman can produce for her infant after childbirth. Breast size is primarily related to the amount of fat present.
- For normal sperm formation, a man's testes must be cooler than his core body temperature.
- Seminal fluids secreted by the seminal vesicles, prostate, and bulbourethral glands nourish and protect the sperm, enhance their motility, and ensure that most sperm are deposited in the vagina during sexual intercourse.

### References and Readings

Applegate, E.J. (1995). *The anatomy and physiology learning system: Textbook.* Philadelphia: W.B. Saunders.

Blackburn, S.T., & Loper, D.L. (1992). *Maternal, fetal, and neonatal physiology.* Philadelphia: W.B. Saunders.

Cunningham, F.G., MacDonald, P.C., Gant, N.F., Leveno, K.J., Gilstrap, L.C., Hankins, G.D.V., et al. (1997). *Williams obstetrics* (20th ed.). Norwalk, Conn.: Appleton & Lange.

DiGeorge, A.M., & Garibaldi, L. (1996). Physiology of puberty. In W.E. Nelson, R.E. Behrman, R.M. Kliegman, & A.M. Arvin (Eds.), *Nelson textbook of pediatrics* (15th ed., pp. 1579–1580). Philadelphia: W.B. Saunders.

Georges, J.M. (1995). Structure and function of the female reproductive system. In L.C. Copstead (Ed.), *Perspectives on pathophysiology* (pp. 648–666). Philadelphia: W.B. Saunders.

Ginsburg, K.A., & Moghissi, K.S. (1994). Secondary amenorrhea. In F.P. Zuspan & E.J. Quilligan (Eds.), *Current therapy in obstetrics and gynecology* 4 (pp. 112–116). Philadelphia: W.B. Saunders.

Guyton, A.C. (1996). *Textbook of medical physiology* (9th ed.). Philadelphia: W.B. Saunders.

Mikkelsen, D. (1995). Structure and function of the male genitourinary system. In L.C. Copstead (Ed.), *Perspectives on pathophysiology* (pp. 612–633). Philadelphia: W.B. Saunders.

Moore, K.L., & Persaud, T.V.N. (1993). *Before we are born* (4th ed.). Philadelphia: W.B. Saunders.

Riddick, D.H. (1994). Primary amenorrhea. In F.P. Zuspan & E.J. Quilligan (Eds.), *Current therapy in obstetrics and gynecology* 4 (pp. 109–111). Philadelphia: W.B. Saunders.

# 5

# Hereditary and Environmental Influences on Childbearing

**OBJECTIVES**

1. Describe the structure and function of normal human genes and chromosomes.
2. Give examples of ways genes and chromosomes are studied.
3. Describe the transmission of single gene traits from parent to child.
4. Relate chromosomal abnormalities to spontaneous abortion and to birth defects in the infant.
5. Explain characteristics of multifactorial birth defects.
6. Identify environmental factors that can interfere with prenatal development and how their effects can be avoided or reduced.
7. Describe the process of genetic counseling.
8. Explain the role of the nurse in caring for individuals or families with concerns about birth defects.

**DEFINITIONS**

**allele** *An alternate form of a gene.*

**autosome** *Any of the 22 pairs of chromosomes other than the sex chromosomes.*

**birth defect** *An abnormality of structure, function, or body metabolism that often results in a physical or mental handicap, shortens life, or is fatal (according to the March of Dimes Birth Defects Foundation).*

**congenital** *Present at birth.*

**diploid** *Having a pair of chromosomes (46 in humans) that represents one copy of every chromosome from each parent; the number of chromosomes normally present in body cells other than gametes.*

**familial** *Presence of a trait or condition in a family more often than would be expected by chance alone.*

**gamete** *Reproductive cell; in the female an ovum and in the male a spermatozoon.*

**genetic** *Pertaining to the genes or the chromosomes.*

**genotype** *Genetic makeup of an individual.*

**haploid** *Having one copy of a chromosome from each pair (23 in humans, or half the diploid number). Gametes normally have a haploid number of chromosomes.*

**heterozygous** *Having two different alleles for a genetic trait.*

**homozygous** *Having two identical alleles for a genetic trait.*

**karyotype** *A photomicrograph of a cell's chromosomes, arranged from largest to smallest pairs.*

**monosomy** *Presence of only one of a chromosome pair in every body cell.*

**mutation** *Variation in a gene that affects its function.*

**pedigree** *A graphic representation of a family's medical and hereditary history and the relationships among the family members. May be called a genogram.*

**phenotype** *The outward expression of one's genetic makeup.*
**polymorphism** *Common variation in a gene that does not affect its function or the individual's health negatively.*
**polyploidy** *Having additional full sets of chromosomes.*
**sex chromosome** *The X or Y chromosome. Females have two X chromosomes; males have one X and one Y chromosome.*
**somatic cells** *Body cells other than the gametes, or germ cells.*
**teratogen** *An agent that can cause defects in a developing baby during pregnancy.*
**translocation** *Attachment of all or part of a chromosome to another chromosome.*
**trisomy** *Presence of three copies of a chromosome in each body cell.*

Hereditary and environmental forces influence one's development from before conception until death. The nurse needs a basic knowledge of these forces to better understand disorders evident at birth and those that develop later in life. This chapter reviews the basics of hereditary influences on development and the impact of environmental factors in causing birth defects. The nursing role in relation to genetic knowledge is also discussed.

## Hereditary Influences

Hereditary influences on development result from the directions for cellular functions provided by genes that make up the 46 chromosomes in every somatic cell. Disease or disorders can result if too much or too little genetic material is present in the cells, or if one or more genes are abnormal and provide incorrect directions.

### Structure of Genes and Chromosomes

A review of the structure of genes and chromosomes aids in understanding how disorders occur. Chromosomes are composed of genes that in turn are composed of DNA (Fig. 5–1).

#### DNA

DNA (deoxyribonucleic acid) is the basic building block of genes and chromosomes. It has three units: (1) a sugar (deoxyribose), (2) a phosphate group, and (3) one of four nitrogen bases (adenine, thymine, guanine, and cytosine).

DNA resembles a spiral ladder, with a sugar and a phosphate group forming each side of the ladder and a pair of nitrogen bases forming each rung. The four bases of the DNA molecule pair to one another in a fixed way, allowing the DNA to be accurately duplicated during each cell division.

- Adenine pairs with thymine.
- Guanine pairs with cytosine.

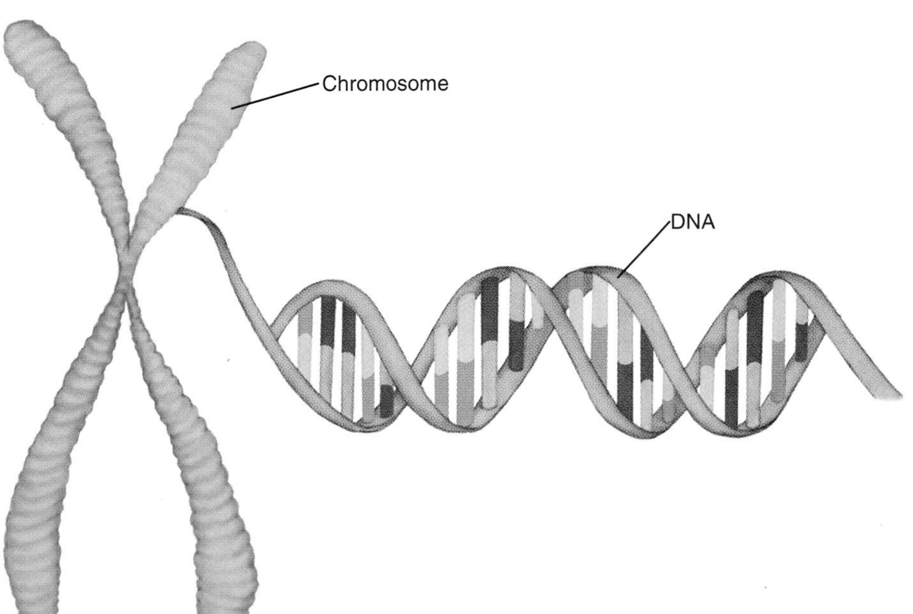


**FIGURE 5–1**
Diagrammatic representation of the DNA helix, which is the building block of genes and chromosomes.

The sequence of base pairs within the DNA determines which amino acids will be assembled to form a protein and the order in which they will be assembled. Some of these proteins form the structure of body cells, whereas others are enzymes that control metabolic processes within the cell. If the sequence of nitrogen bases in the DNA is incorrect or if some bases are missing or added, a defect in body structure or function may result.

### GENES

A gene is a segment of DNA that directs the production of a specific product needed for body structure or function. Humans may have as many as 100,000 genes, but not all genes function at the same time. Some are active only during prenatal life; others become functional at various times after birth.

Genes that code for the same trait often have two or more alternate forms (alleles). Many alleles are normal, such as those that code for a person's blood type. Normal alleles, or polymorphisms, provide genetic variation and sometimes a biologic advantage. However, abnormal alleles (mutations) may harm function, such as those that cause the production of abnormal hemoglobin in sickle cell disease.

Genes are too small to be seen under a microscope, but many can be studied by tissue analysis in several ways:

- By measuring the products that they direct cells to produce, such as an enzyme or other substance
- By direct study of the gene's DNA if its exact location is known
- By analyzing its close association (linkage) with another gene that can be studied in one of the previous two ways

The tissue used for study of a gene depends on where the gene product is present in the body and on the available technology. These tissues may include blood, skin cells, hair follicles, and fetal cells from the amniotic fluid or chorionic villi.

Genes that can be identified by direct analysis of DNA can be studied in any cells containing a nucleus, even if the gene product is not present in that tissue. Although not widely available, DNA analysis of the blastomere (eight-cell stage of prenatal development) has been used to select embryos to be implanted in the uterus following in vitro fertilization. Blastomere analysis may eventually be possible for embryos conceived through intercourse as well.

The Human Genome Project is a massive international effort begun in 1990 to identify all genes contained in the 46 human chromosomes. Approximately 2000 of the up to 100,000 genes have been identified, including around 900 that contribute to disease (Scanlon & Fibison, 1995). The potential impact of this project is enormous.

- Identification of the genetic alteration for a disorder may lead to a genetic test to determine the risk for, or presence of, that disorder in an individual.
- Direct testing for the gene can be done for anyone, not just for one having a family history of a genetic problem.
- Decisions about reproduction can be more specific because the information obtained will have greater accuracy.
- Identification of genetic susceptibility for a disorder allows lifestyle changes or other interventions, such as more frequent diagnostic tests.
- Gene therapy—modifying the defective gene itself rather than just compensating for an abnormal gene product—might be possible for some disorders.

Today's nurse must expect development of genetic prediction, diagnosis, and therapy for disorders never before thought to have a genetic basis. At the same time, the explosion of knowledge about the genetic basis for disease raises many legal and ethical issues for which we do not yet have answers. As our knowledge base grows, new issues are likely to emerge.

- Genetic information has implications for others in the person's family, raising privacy issues.
- Identification of genetic problems could lead to poor self-esteem, guilt, excessive caution, or, conversely, a reckless lifestyle.
- Presymptomatic identification of genetically influenced illness would be a source of long-term anxiety.
- Genetic knowledge could affect one's choice of a partner.
- Discrimination is a real possibility, such as the imposition of high insurance rates or the denial of coverage or the decision not to hire a qualified (but genetically compromised) person. One might be discriminated against for conditions that *might* occur, not for conditions that already have occurred.

### CHROMOSOMES

Genes are organized into 46 paired chromosomes in the nucleus of most somatic cells. A gene can be described as a single bead; a chromosome is like a string of beads. Each chromosome is composed of varying numbers of genes. Twenty-two chromosome pairs are autosomes, and the 23rd pair makes up the sex chromosomes. Added or missing chromosomes or structurally abnormal chromosomes are usually harmful.

Mature gametes have half the chromosomes (23) of other body cells. One chromosome from each pair is distributed randomly in the gametes, allowing variation of genetic traits among people. When the ovum and sperm unite at conception, the total is restored to 46 paired chromosomes.

Cells for chromosomal analysis must have a nucleus and must be living. Chromosomes can be studied using any of several types of cells: white blood cells, skin fibroblasts, bone marrow cells, and fetal cells from the chorionic villi (future placenta) or those suspended in amniotic fluid.

Unlike genes, chromosomes can be seen under the microscope but only during division of live cells. Specimens must be obtained and preserved carefully to provide enough living cells for chromosomal analysis. Temperature extremes, clotting of blood, or addition of improper preservatives can kill the cells and render them useless for analysis.

Chromosomes look jumbled when viewed under a microscope (Fig. 5–2). Photographing the chromosomes and then arranging the chromosomes in that picture into a karyotype (Fig. 5–3) allows systematic study. In a karyotype, autosomal pairs are arranged from largest to smallest. Letters describe groups that are of similar size and appearance. Sex chromosomes are arranged in a separate group.

A person's karyotype is abbreviated by a combination of numbers and letters. A number describes the total number of chromosomes, followed by either an XX to indicate that sex chromosomes are female or XY to indicate they are male. Thus, the chromosome complement of a normal female is abbreviated 46,XX and a normal male 46,XY. If the chromosome number is abnormal, such as that in Down syndrome, which has an extra 21 chromosome, an added abbreviation indicates the abnormality: 47 (total number of chromosomes), XY (male), +21 (the number that describes the added chromosome). Other abbreviations describe karyotypes having missing or structurally altered chromosomes.

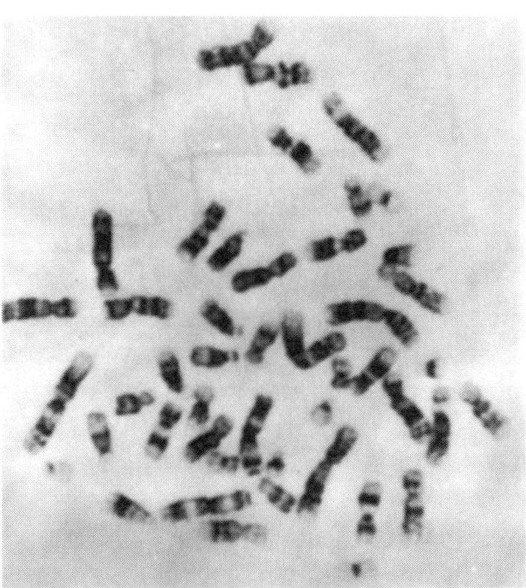

**FIGURE 5–2**

When viewed under a microscope, chromosomes appear jumbled. (From Thompson, M.W., McInnes, R.R., & Willard, H.F. [1991]. *Thompson and Thompson genetics in medicine* [5th ed., p. 16]. Philadelphia: W.B. Saunders. Courtesy of R.G. Worton, The Hospital for Sick Children, Toronto.)

A new way to analyze chromosomes makes use of fluorescent-labeled DNA probes that attach to specific chromosomes. This technique is called fluorescent in situ hybridization (FISH) and permits identification of abnormal numbers of chromosomes. Probes are being developed to identify chromosomal abnormalities that are too small to be seen under the microscope and for DNA sequences that code for single gene traits.

**✓ CHECK YOUR READING**

1. What is the relationship between DNA, genes, and chromosomes?
2. Can genes be studied by examining them under a microscope? What are the methods used to study them?
3. Why is it important to keep cell specimens for chromosomal analysis alive?
4. What do each of these abbreviations mean? 46,XY? 46,XX?

## Transmission of Traits by Single Genes

Inherited characteristics are passed from parent to child by the genes in each chromosome. These traits are classified according to whether they are dominant (strong) or recessive (weak) and whether the gene is located on one of the autosome pairs or on the sex chromosomes. Both normal and abnormal hereditary characteristics are transmitted by these mechanisms.

### ALLELES

Because humans have a pair of matched chromosomes (except the sex chromosomes in the male), they have one allele for a gene at the same location on each member of the chromosome pair. The paired alleles may be identical (homozygous) or different (heterozygous).

Some alleles, both normal and abnormal, occur more frequently in certain groups than they do in the population as a whole. For example, the gene that causes Tay-Sachs disease is carried by about one of every 27 Ashkenazi Jews, whose families have their roots in eastern Europe. However, only one of every 150 people outside this group carries the gene. Because the abnormal gene occurs more frequently in this group, their incidence of Tay-Sachs disease is also higher. Other disorders that are prevalent in certain ethnic groups are cystic fibrosis (primarily whites of northern European descent) and sickle cell disease (primarily people of African descent).

A new trait (harmful, neutral, or sometimes beneficial) may emerge because of a change in the gene

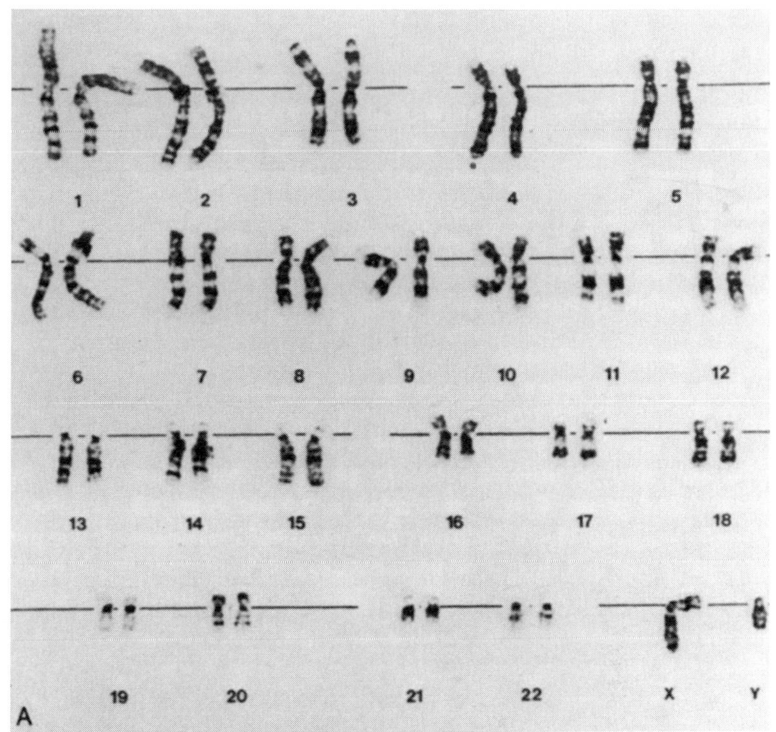


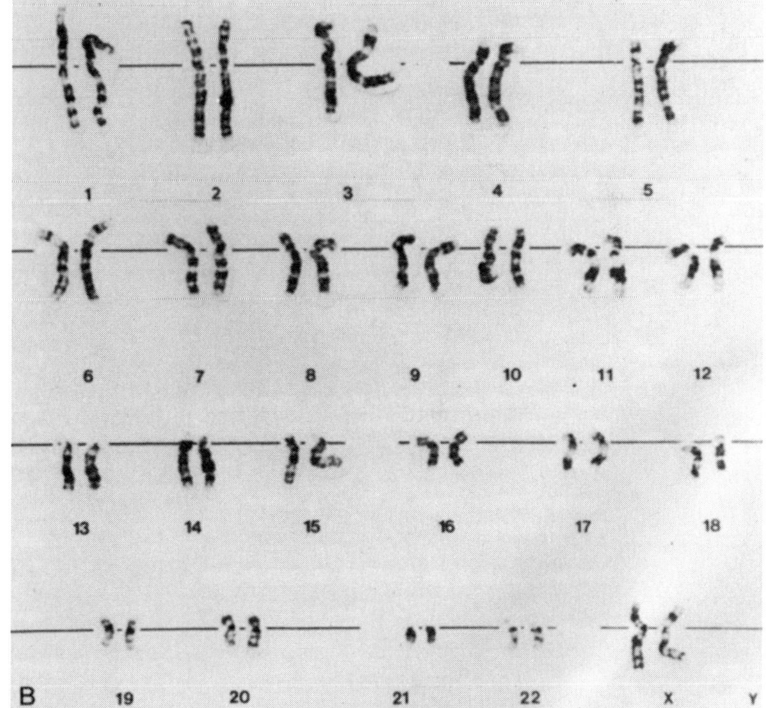


**FIGURE 5-3**

Chromosomes arranged in karyotypes. A, Normal male karyotype: 46,XY. B, Normal female karyotype: 46,XX. (From Knuppel, R.A., & Drukker, J.E. [1993]. *High-risk pregnancy: A team approach* [p. 666]. Philadelphia: W.B. Saunders. Courtesy of The Children's Hospital, Denver.)

within the gamete. The DNA in the gamete is then different from that in the person's somatic cells. The offspring who receives the new version of the gene will have it in all somatic cells and can transmit it to future generations.

### DOMINANCE

Dominance describes how one's genetic composition is translated into the phenotype, or observable characteristics. In the case of a dominant gene, one copy is enough to cause the trait to be expressed. For example, in the ABO blood system, genes for type A and type B are dominant. Therefore, a single copy of either of these genes is enough to be expressed in the person's blood type.

Two identical copies of a recessive gene are required for the trait to be expressed. The gene for blood group O is recessive. Only if a person receives a gene for blood group O from both parents will laboratory testing identify his or her blood group as O. If the person receives a gene for group O from one parent and group A from the other parent, group A will be expressed in laboratory blood typing.

On the basis of dominant and recessive forms of a gene, a person with group A blood can have one of two possible combinations of gene alleles:

- Two group A alleles
- One group A allele and one group O allele

Other alleles are equally dominant. The person who receives a gene for blood group A from one parent and group B from the other will have type AB blood because both alleles are equally dominant and both are expressed in blood typing.

Dominance and recessiveness are not absolute for all genes. Some people having a single copy of an abnormal recessive gene (carriers) may have a lower than normal level of the gene product (such as an enzyme) that can be detected by laboratory methods. These people usually do not have disease because the normal copy of the gene produces enough of the required product to allow normal or near-normal function.

#### CHROMOSOME LOCATION

Genes located on autosomes are either autosomal dominant or autosomal recessive, depending on the number of identical copies of the gene needed to produce the trait. However, genes located on the X chromosome are paired only in females because males have one X and one Y chromosome.

A female with an abnormal recessive gene on one of her X chromosomes usually has a normal gene on the other X chromosome that compensates and maintains relatively normal function. However, the male is at a disadvantage if his only X chromosome has an abnormal gene. The male has no compensating normal gene because his other sex chromosome is a Y. The abnormal gene will be expressed in the male because it is unopposed by a normal gene.

### TABLE 5-1 SINGLE GENE TRAITS

#### Pedigree Symbols

A pedigree is a way to symbolically represent a family's medical history and the relationships of its members to one another. It can help identify patterns of inheritance that may help distinguish one type of disorder from another.

Male

Female

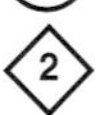
Sex not specified (number indicates the number of persons represented by the symbol)

Affected

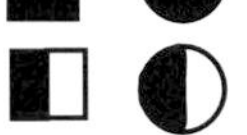
Carriers (heterozygous) for an autosomal recessive trait

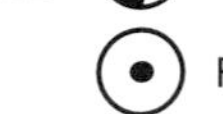
Female carrier of an X-linked recessive trait

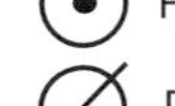
Deceased

Mating/marriage

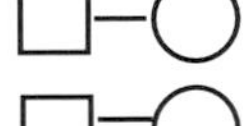
Consanguineous mating/marriage

I Roman numerals indicate generations

#### Autosomal Dominant

**Characteristics**

A single copy of the gene is enough to produce the trait.
Males and females are equally likely to have the trait.
Often appears in every generation of a family, although family members having the trait may have widely varying manifestations of it.
May have multiple and seemingly unrelated effects on body structure and function.

**Transmission of Trait from Parent to Child**

A parent with the trait has a 50% (1 in 2) chance of passing the trait to the child.
The trait may arise as a new mutation from an unaffected parent. The child who receives the mutated gene can then transmit it to future generations.

**Examples**

Normal traits: Blood groups A and B; Rh-positive blood factor.
Abnormal traits: Huntington's disease; neurofibromatosis.

**Pedigree**

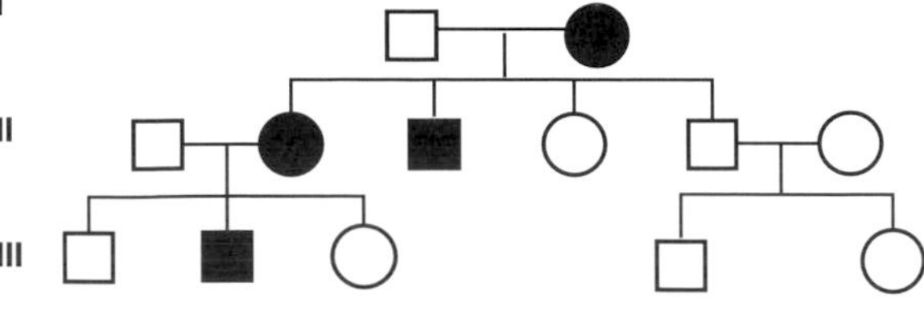

## Patterns of Single Gene Inheritance

Three important patterns of single gene inheritance are (1) autosomal dominant, (2) autosomal recessive, and (3) X-linked. Each pattern of inheritance has characteristics that distinguish it from the other two. Table 5–1 summarizes characteristics and transmission of each pattern. The inheritance patterns are graphically illustrated with a pedigree to represent a family's history and the relationships among family members.

**Be cautious when referring to the illustration of a family's genetic history as a pedigree. Some people may be offended because they associate that word with animals. Although the word *pedigree* is widely used among genetic professionals, the nurse may need to interpret it for the client. For example, when taking a genetic family history, the nurse might say, "I'm going to use several symbols to depict your family tree and its members' health histories. This diagram is usually called a pedigree."**

### TABLE 5–1 SINGLE GENE TRAITS *Continued*

#### Autosomal Recessive

**Characteristics**

Two autosomal recessive genes are required to produce the trait.
Males and females are equally likely to have the trait.
There is often no prior family history of the disorder before the first affected child.
If more than one family member is affected, they are usually full siblings.
Consanguinity (blood relationship) of the parents increases the risk for the disorder.
Disorders are more likely to occur in groups isolated by geography, culture, religion, or other factors.
Some autosomal recessive disorders are more common in specific ethnic groups.

**Transmission of Trait from Parent to Child**

Unaffected parents are carriers of the abnormal autosomal recessive trait.
Children of carriers have a 25% (1 in 4) chance for receiving both copies of the defective gene and thus having the disorder.
Children of carriers have a 50% (1 in 2) chance of receiving one copy of the gene and being carriers like the parents.
Children of carriers have a 25% (1 in 4) chance of receiving both copies of the normal gene. They are neither carriers nor affected.

**Examples**

Normal traits: Blood group O; Rh-negative blood factor.
Abnormal traits: Tay-Sachs disease; sickle cell disease; cystic fibrosis.

**Pedigree**

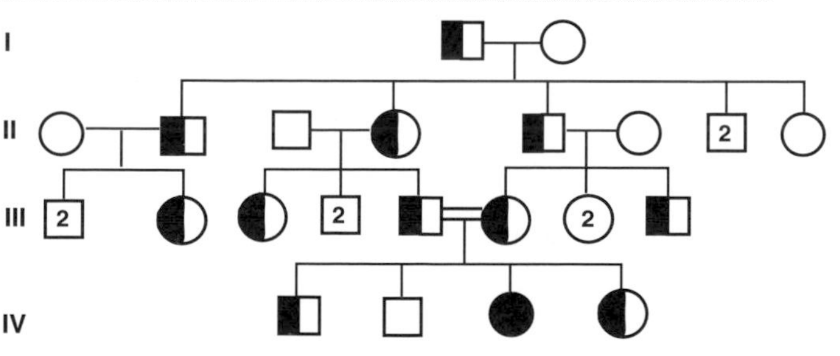


#### X-Linked Recessive

**Characteristics**

Although recessive, only one copy of the gene is needed to cause the disorder in the male, who does not have a compensating X without the trait.
Males are affected, with rare exceptions.
Females are carriers of the trait, but not usually adversely affected.
Affected males are related to one another through carrier females.
Affected males do not transmit the trait to their sons.

**Transmission of Trait from Parent to Child**

Males who have the disorder transmit the gene to
100% of their daughters.
None of their sons.
Sons of carrier females have a 50% (1 in 2) chance of being affected. They also have a 50% chance of being unaffected.
Daughters of carrier females have a 50% (1 in 2) chance of being carriers like their mothers. They also have a 50% chance of being neither affected nor carriers.
An abnormal X-linked recessive gene also may arise by mutation.

**Examples**

Colorblindness; Duchenne's muscular dystrophy; hemophilia A

**Pedigree**

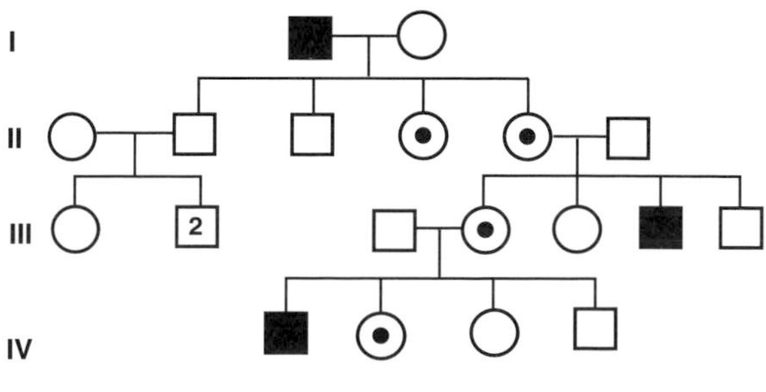

Single gene traits have mathematically predictable and fixed rates of occurrence. For example, if a couple has a child with an autosomal recessive disorder, the risk that future children will have the same disorder is one in four (25 percent) at every conception. It is not important how many of their children are affected; the *risk* is the same at every conception.

#### AUTOSOMAL DOMINANT TRAITS

An autosomal dominant trait is produced by a dominant gene on a nonsex chromosome. The expression of abnormal autosomal dominant genes may result in multiple and seemingly unrelated effects in the person. The gene's effects also may vary substantially in severity, leading a family to believe incorrectly that a trait skips a generation. A careful physical examination may reveal subtle evidence of the trait in each generation. Or, some people may carry the dominant gene but may have no apparent expression of it in their physical makeup.

In some autosomal dominant disorders, such as Huntington's disease, the person having the gene will always have the disease if he or she lives long enough. In other disorders, only a portion of those carrying the gene will ever exhibit the disease.

New mutations account for the introduction of abnormal autosomal dominant traits into a family that has no prior history. In this case, parents of the child will be normal because their body cells do not have the altered gene. Men who father children in their fifth decade or later are more likely to have offspring with a new autosomal dominant mutation.

The person who is affected with an autosomal dominant disorder is usually heterozygous for the gene. That is, the person has a normal gene on one chromosome and an abnormal gene on the other chromosome of the pair. However, the abnormal gene overrides the influence of the normal gene. Occasionally, a person receives two copies of the same abnormal autosomal dominant gene. Such an individual is usually much more severely affected than someone with only one copy.

#### AUTOSOMAL RECESSIVE TRAITS

An autosomal recessive trait occurs if a person receives two copies of a recessive gene carried on an autosome. Everyone carries two to six abnormal autosomal recessive genes without manifesting the disorder because they have a compensating normal gene. Because the probability that two unrelated people will share even one of the same abnormal genes is low, the incidence of autosomal recessive diseases is relatively low in the general population.

Situations that increase the likelihood of two parents sharing the same abnormal autosomal recessive gene are the following:

- Consanguinity (blood relationship of the parents).
- Groups that are isolated by culture, geography, religion, or other factors. The isolation allows abnormal genes to become concentrated over the years and occur at a greater frequency than they do in more diverse groups.

Many autosomal recessive disorders are severe, and affected persons may not live long enough to reproduce. Two exceptions are phenylketonuria and cystic fibrosis. Improved care of people with these disorders has allowed them to live into the reproductive years. If one member of the couple has the autosomal recessive disorder, all of their children will be carriers. Their risk for having similarly affected children is higher as well, depending on the prevalence of the abnormal gene in the general population.

#### X-LINKED TRAITS

X-linked recessive traits are more common than X-linked dominant ones, and they are the only X-linked pattern discussed here. Sex differences in the occurrence of X-linked recessive traits and the relationship of affected males to one another are important factors that distinguish these disorders from autosomal dominant or recessive disorders. In general, males are the only ones who show full effects of an X-linked recessive disorder because their only X chromosome has the abnormal gene on it. Females can show the full disorder in two uncommon circumstances:

- If a female has a single X chromosome (Turner's syndrome, p. 81)
- If a female child is born to an affected father and a carrier mother

X-linked recessive disorders can be relatively mild, such as colorblindness, or they may be severe,

### Critical to Remember

#### SINGLE GENE ABNORMALITIES

- A person affected with an autosomal dominant disorder has a 50 percent chance of transmitting the disorder to each of his or her children.
- Two healthy parents who carry the same abnormal autosomal recessive gene have a 25 percent chance of having a child affected with the disorder caused by this gene.
- Parental consanguinity increases the risk for having a child with an autosomal recessive disorder.
- One copy of an abnormal X-linked recessive gene is enough to produce the disorder in a male.
- Abnormal genes can arise as new mutations that are then transmitted to future generations.

such as hemophilia. In addition, those having the disorder may be affected with varying degrees of severity.

**CHECK YOUR READING**

5. If a parent has an autosomal dominant disorder, what is the chance that the child will have the same disorder?
6. Why are parents who are related by blood more likely to have a child with an autosomal recessive disorder?
7. If each member of a couple carries a gene for an autosomal recessive disorder, what is the chance that the children will have the disorder? What is the chance that the children will be carriers? What is the chance that the children will not receive the abnormal gene from either parent?
8. Why are males more often affected with X-linked recessive disorders? If a female carries an X-linked recessive disorder such as hemophilia, what are the chances that her sons will have the disorder? What is the chance that her daughters will be carriers?

## Chromosomal Abnormalities

Chromosomal abnormalities can be numerical or structural. They are quite common (50 percent or more) in the embryo or fetus that is spontaneously aborted. Chromosomal abnormalities often cause major defects because they involve many added or missing genes.

### NUMERICAL ABNORMALITIES

Numerical chromosomal abnormalities are those involving added or missing single chromosomes or those with multiple sets of chromosomes. Trisomy and monosomy are numerical abnormalities of single chromosomes. Polyploidy describes abnormalities involving whole sets of chromosomes.

**Critical to Remember**

**CHROMOSOME ABNORMALITIES**

Chromosome abnormalities are either numerical or structural.

| Numerical | Structural |
|---|---|
| Entire single chromosome added (trisomy) | Part of a chromosome missing or added |
| Entire single chromosome missing (monosomy) | Rearrangements of material within chromosome(s) |
| One or more added sets of chromosomes | Two chromosomes that adhere to each other |
| | Fragility of a specific site on the X chromosome |

**Trisomy.** A trisomy exists when each body cell contains an extra copy of one chromosome, bringing the total number to 47 (Fig. 5–4). Each chromosome is normal, but there are too many in every cell. The most common trisomy is *Down syndrome*, or trisomy 21. In Down syndrome, each cell has three copies of chromosome 21. Trisomies of chromosomes 13 and 18 are less common and have more severe effects. The incidence of trisomies increases with maternal age, so that most women who are 35 years old or older are offered prenatal diagnosis to determine whether the fetus has Down syndrome or another trisomy.

Infants with Down syndrome have characteristic features that are usually noticed shortly after birth (Fig. 5–5). Chromosomal analysis is done during the neonatal period to confirm the diagnosis and to determine whether Down syndromc is caused by trisomy 21 or a rarer chromosomal anomaly that involves a structural rather than a numerical abnormality.

Children with Down syndrome reach developmental milestones more slowly than normal children. They are mentally retarded, although the severity varies, just as intelligence varies in the general population. Early intervention programs and regular medical care help these children to reach their full ability and manage physical problems associated with Down syndrome.

**Monosomy.** A monosomy exists when each body cell has a missing chromosome, with a total number of 45. The only monosomy that is compatible with postnatal life is *Turner's syndrome*, or monosomy X (Fig. 5–6). People with Turner's syndrome have a single X chromosome and are always female. Turner's syndrome, like other chromosomal abnormalities, is very common in fetuses lost to spontaneous abortion.

Live-born infants have excess skin around the neck and edema that is most noticeable in the hands and feet. If Turner's syndrome is not identified and treated during infancy or childhood, an affected girl will remain very short and will not have menstrual periods or develop secondary sex characteristics. Children with Turner's syndrome usually have normal intelligence, although they may have difficulty with spatial relationships or solving visual problems, such as reading a map. Figure 5–7 shows an infant with Turner's syndrome and describes additional characteristics that may be present at birth or later in life.

**Polyploidy.** Polyploidy may occur when gametes do not halve their chromosome number during meiosis and retain both members of the pair or when two sperm fertilize an ovum simultaneously. The result is an embryo with one or more extra sets of chromosomes. The total number of chromosomes is a multiple of the haploid number of 23 (69 or 92 total

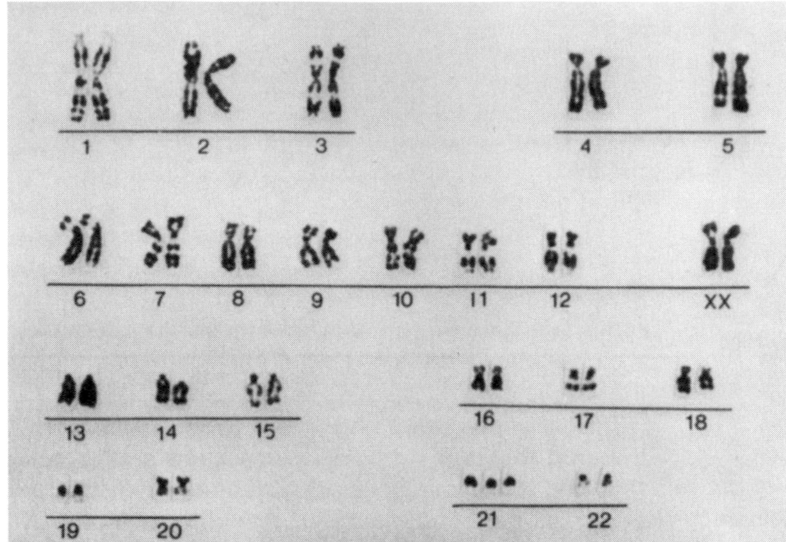


**FIGURE 5–4**

Karyotype of a female with trisomy 21 (Down syndrome: 47,XX, +21). (From Hacker, N., & Moore, J.G. [1992]. *Essentials of obstetrics and gynecology* [2nd ed., p. 95]. Philadelphia: W.B. Saunders.)

chromosomes). Polyploidy usually results in an early spontaneous abortion but may occasionally be seen in a live-born infant. This abnormality may be found in chorionic villus sampling (see p. 230) and may reflect an abnormality of the chorionic villi rather than the fetus.

### STRUCTURAL ABNORMALITIES

Chromosomal abnormalities may involve the structure of one or more chromosomes. Part of a chromosome may be missing or added, or DNA within the chromosome may be rearranged. Some of these rearrangements are common harmless variations. However, others are harmful because important genetic material is lost or duplicated in the structural abnormality, or the position of the genes in relation to other genes is altered so that normal function is not possible.

Another structural abnormality occurs when all or part of a chromosome is attached to another (trans-

Poor muscle tone at birth
Short, wide head with a flat occiput and a flat face
Upslanting eyes
Speckled iris (Brushfield's spots)
Epicanthal folds near the bridge of the nose
Short flat nose with a flat nasal bridge
Prominent or protruding tongue
Low-set ears
Wide, short fingers, often incurving toward the radius
Simian crease (single transverse palmar crease)
Wide space between the first two toes, with a prominent plantar crease
Cardiac defects
Gastrointestinal defects (duodenal atresia)
Prone to infections
Mental retardation (Intelligence Quotient [IQ] 25–70)

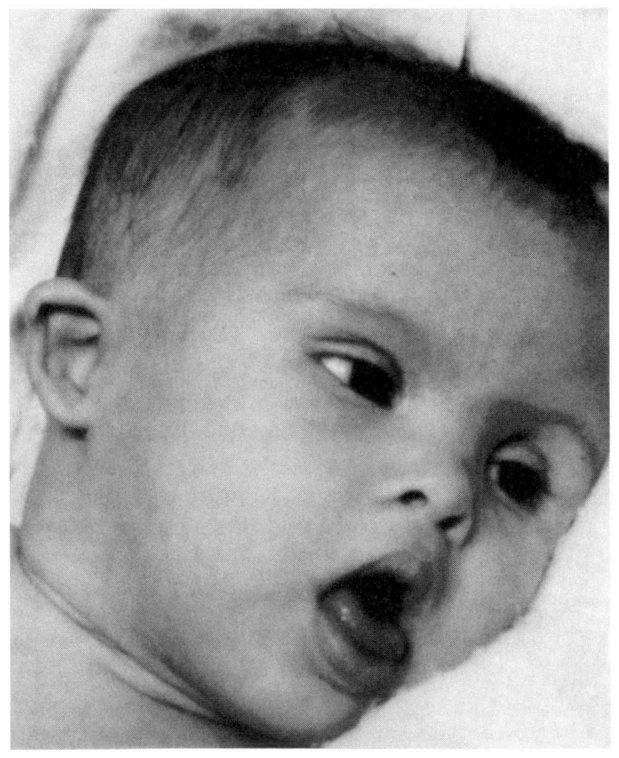

**FIGURE 5–5**

Infant with characteristic features of Down syndrome. (From Simpson, J.L., & Golbus, M.S. [1992]. *Genetics in obstetrics and gynecology* [2nd ed., p. 62]. Philadelphia: W.B. Saunders.)

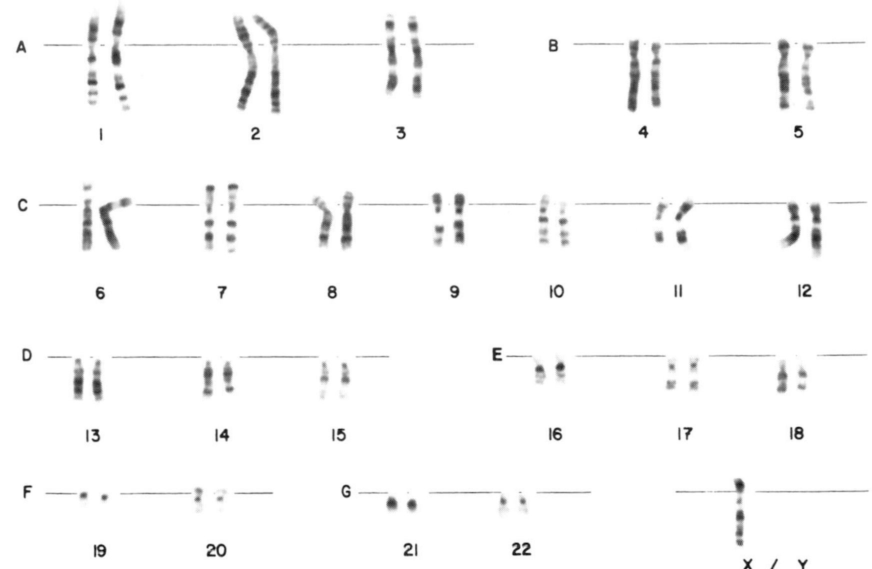


**FIGURE 5-6**

Karyotype of a female with monosomy X (Turner's syndrome: 45,X). (Courtesy of Dr. Mary Jo Harrod, University of Texas Southwestern Medical Center.)

location). Many people with a translocation chromosomal abnormality are clinically normal because the total of their genetic material is normal, or balanced (Fig. 5–8). If a parent has a balanced translocation, the offspring may have completely normal chromosomes or may have a balanced translocation like the parent. However, the offspring may receive too much or too little chromosomal material and may

Decreased birth weight
Edema at birth, noticeable on hands and feet
Short broad neck, with excess webbed skin
Low posterior hairline
Broad shield-shaped chest with widely spaced nipples
Cardiac anomalies (coarctation of the aorta)
Renal anomalies (horseshoe kidneys)
Permanently sexually immature with infantile appearance
Short adult height
Intelligence Quotient (IQ) normal, but difficulty with spatial relationships a possibility

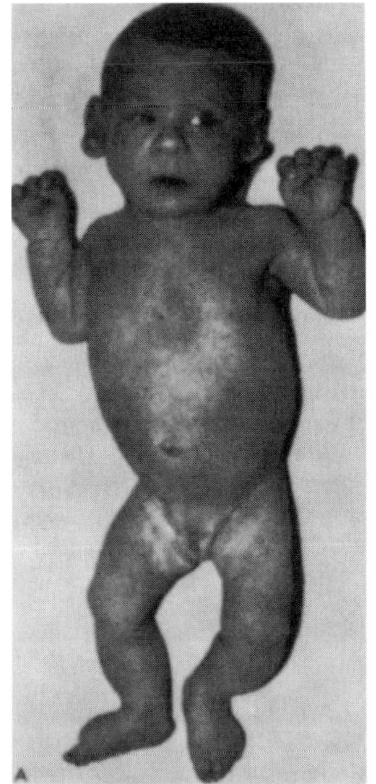


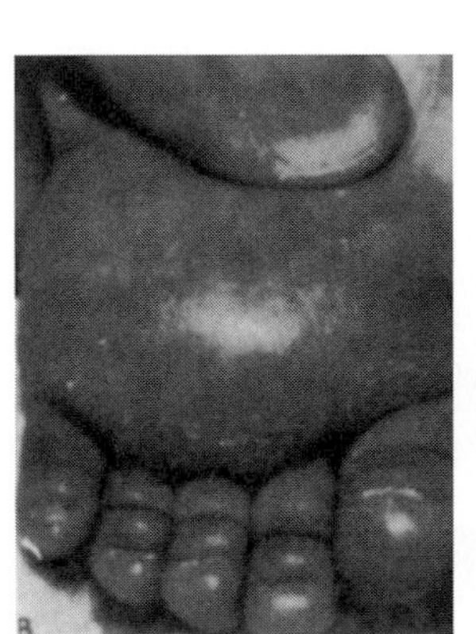


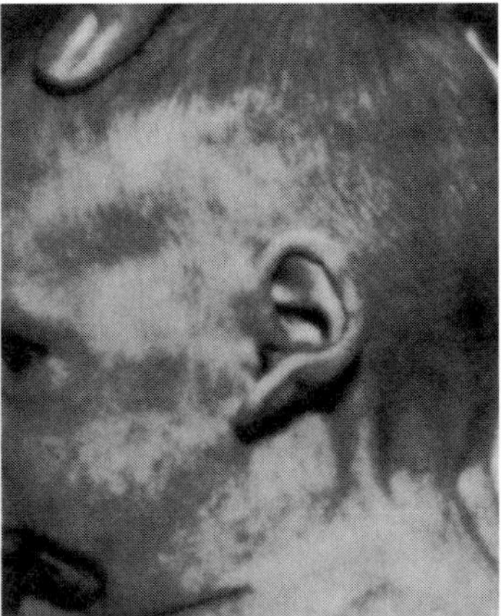

**FIGURE 5-7**

Infant with characteristic features of Turner's syndrome (monosomy X). (From Lemli, L., & Smith, D.W. [1963]. The XO syndrome: A study of the differentiated phenotype in 25 patients. *Journal of Pediatrics*, 63, 577.)

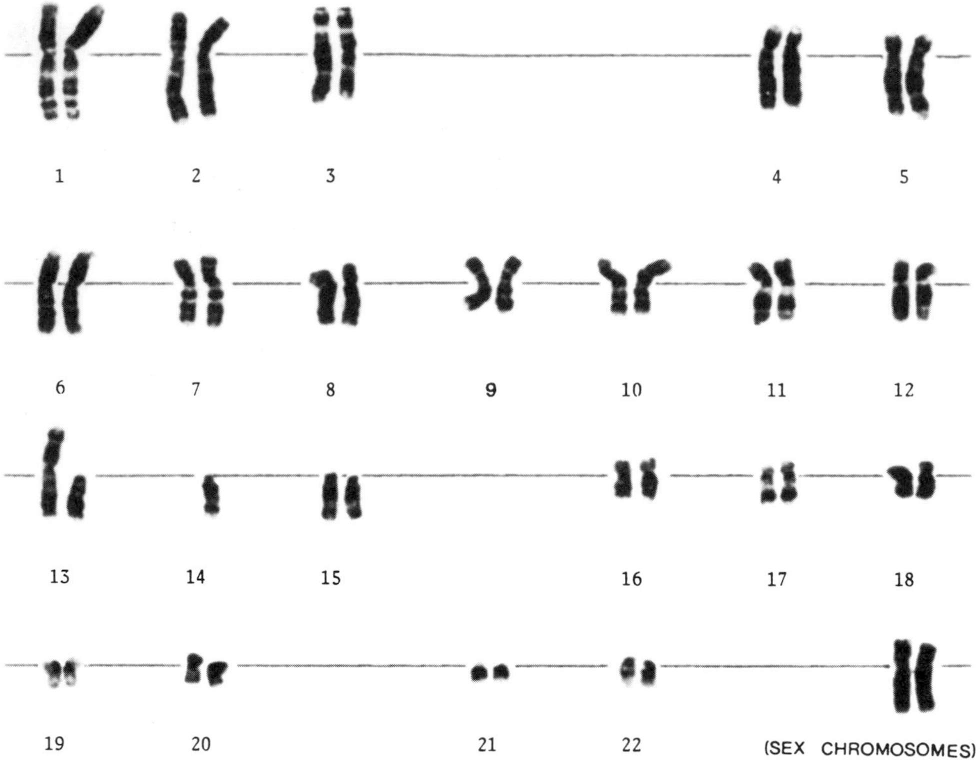


**FIGURE 5-8**

Karyotype of a balanced chromosome translocation. One of the 14th chromosome pair is attached to one of the 13th pair. (From Creasy, R.K., & Resnik, R. [1989]. *Maternal-fetal medicine: Principles and practice* [2nd ed., p. 37]. Philadelphia: W.B. Saunders.)

be spontaneously aborted or may have birth defects.

Balanced translocations are usually discovered when a pregnant woman undergoes amniocentesis and a translocation in the fetus is revealed, or they may be found during infertility evaluations if there is a history of recurrent spontaneous abortions. Either balanced or unbalanced chromosomal translocations may occur spontaneously in the offspring of parents who have no translocation.

X-linked mental retardation (fragile X syndrome) is a special type of chromosomal abnormality that exists on the X chromosome. A site on part of the X chromosome is more fragile than normal. As in X-linked recessive traits, males are more significantly affected than are females, who have a compensating X chromosome that is usually normal. Fragile X syndrome is the most common form of male mental retardation (Hall, 1996a).

**CHECK YOUR READING**

9. What is a chromosomal trisomy? Name a common trisomy.
10. What is a chromosomal monosomy? Which monosomy is compatible with life?
11. Why are structural chromosomal abnormalities often harmful?
12. What are the possible outcomes of the offspring of a parent who has a balanced chromosomal translocation?

## Multifactorial Disorders

Multifactorial disorders are those resulting from an interaction of genetic and environmental factors. The genetic tendency toward the disorder is modified by the environment. These interactions may influence prenatal and postnatal development either positively or negatively. For example, two embryos may have an equal genetic susceptibility for the development of a disorder such as spina bifida (open spine). However, the disorder will not occur unless an environment that favors its development, such as deficient maternal intake of folic acid, also exists.

### Characteristics

Multifactorial disorders have two characteristics that distinguish them from other types of birth defects. They are typically (1) present and detectable at birth and (2) isolated defects rather than ones that occur with other unrelated abnormalities.

A multifactorial defect may *cause* a secondary defect, however. For example, infants with spina bifida often have hydrocephalus (abnormal collection of spinal fluid within the brain) as well. The hydrocephalus is not a separate defect but one that occurs because abnormal development of the spine and spinal cord disrupts spinal fluid circulation, allowing it to build up within the brain's ventricular system.

The infant who has spina bifida plus defects other than those associated with disrupted central nervous

## Critical to Remember

### MULTIFACTORIAL BIRTH DEFECTS

- Multifactorial defects are some of the most common birth defects encountered in maternity and pediatric nursing practice.
- They are a result of interaction between one's genetic susceptibility and environmental factors during prenatal development.
- These are usually single, isolated defects, although the primary defect may cause secondary defects.
- Some occur more often in certain geographic areas.
- A greater risk of occurrence exists if
  - Several close relatives have the defect, whether mild or severe.
  - One close relative has a severe form of the defect.
  - The defect occurs in a child of the less frequently affected sex.
- Infants who have several major or minor defects, or both, that are not directly related probably *do not* have a multifactorial defect but have another syndrome, such as a chromosomal abnormality.

system development probably does *not* have a multifactorial disorder. In this case, the spina bifida is more likely to be part of a syndrome that may pose a much different risk for recurrence in a future child.

Multifactorial disorders represent some of the most common birth defects that a maternal-child nurse encounters. Examples include the following:

- Many heart defects
- Neural tube defects such as anencephaly (absence of most of the brain and skull) and spina bifida
- Cleft lip and cleft palate
- Pyloric stenosis

### Risk for Occurrence

Unlike single gene traits, multifactorial disorders are not associated with a fixed risk of occurrence or recurrence in a family. The risks are an average rather than a constant percentage. Factors that may affect the risk are as follows.

1. *Number of affected close relatives.* Risk increases as the number of affected close relatives (parent, full sibling, or child) increases.
2. *Severity of the disorder in affected family members.* For example, bilateral cleft lip is associated with a higher risk for recurrence in a close relative than is a unilateral cleft lip.
3. *Sex of affected person(s).* For example, pyloric stenosis occurs five times as often in males as in females. The couple who has a daughter with pyloric stenosis faces a higher risk for recurrence with subsequent children because there is a greater genetic influence for development of the defect if a female develops it.
4. *Geographic location.* The risk for some disorders, such as neural tube defects, is higher in some locations than in others. Neural tube disorders have shown greater prevalence in some areas, such as the Rio Grande Valley area in Texas.
5. *Seasonal variations.* With some multifactorial disorders seasonal variations are noted.

If multifactorial disorders had no environmental component, the risk for occurrence and recurrence would be a precise percentage rather than a range. However, if there were no genetic component (that is, if the disorder were totally related to environment), there would be little ability to predict the risk for occurrence or recurrence.

## Environmental Influences

Environment may influence prenatal development positively, such as good nutrition that supplies all necessary raw materials for fetal growth. However, some environmental influences are harmful, such as teratogens or mechanical forces that disrupt development.

Environmental influences on childbearing are those that do not now have an identified genetic component. At one time, the placenta was thought to be a shield against harmful agents within a pregnant woman's body. Now we recognize that most agents can cross the placenta and affect the developing fetus.

### Teratogens

Teratogens are agents in the fetal environment that either cause or increase the likelihood that a birth defect will occur. People often ask whether a certain drug or other substance will harm the baby. Some drugs have been definitely established as safe or harmful. For most agents, however, their potential for harming the fetus is not clear. Several factors make it difficult to establish the teratogenic potential of an agent.

1. *Retrospective study.* Investigators must rely on the mother's memory about substances she ingested or was exposed to during pregnancy. Only when many cases are collected in which the exposure history is similar and the birth defects are also similar is it possible to conclude that a specific agent is harmful and to identify the nature of that harm.

2. *Timing of exposure.* Agents may be harmful at one stage of prenatal development but not at another.
3. *Different susceptibility of organ systems.* Some agents affect only one fetal organ system, or they affect one system at one stage of development and another at a different stage of development.
4. *Noncontrolled fetal exposure.* Exposures cannot be controlled to eliminate extraneous agents or to ensure a consistent dose. Interactions with other agents may reduce or compound the fetal effects. An agent that is toxic at one dose may have no apparent effects at another.
5. *Placental transfer.* Agents vary in their ability to cross the placenta.
6. *Individual variations.* Fetuses show varying susceptibility to harmful agents.
7. *Nontransferability of animal studies.* Results of animal studies cannot always be applied to humans. Agents that do not harm animal fetuses may damage the human embryo or fetus.

Teratogens typically cause more than one defect, which distinguishes teratogenic defects from multifactorial disorders. However, children affected by single gene and chromosome defects are also likely to have multiple defects. Therefore, clinicians consider single gene disorders, chromosomal abnormalities, and effects of teratogenic agents when trying to diagnose an infant born with multiple anomalies.

Hundreds of individual agents are either known or suspected teratogens. Types of teratogens include the following:

- Maternal infectious agents (viruses or bacteria) that cross the placenta and damage the embryo or fetus
- Drugs and other substances used by the woman (therapeutic agents, illicit drugs, tobacco, alcohol)
- Pollutants, chemicals, or other substances to which the mother is exposed in her daily life
- Ionizing radiation
- Maternal hyperthermia
- Effects of maternal disorders, such as diabetes mellitus or phenylketonuria

Table 5–2 lists several common known or suspected teratogens.

It is theoretically possible to eliminate all or some of the risk to the developing fetus by avoiding exposure to the agent or changing the fetal environment in some way.

**TABLE 5-2 ENVIRONMENTAL SUBSTANCES KNOWN OR THOUGHT TO HARM THE FETUS**

Alcohol
Aminoglycosides
Antineoplastic agents
Antithyroid drugs
Cocaine
Diethylstilbestrol
Diphenylhydantoin (phenytoin)
Folic acid antagonists
Infections
  Cytomegalovirus
  Herpes simplex virus
  Human immunodeficiency virus
  Rubella
  Syphilis
  Toxoplasmosis
  Varicella
Lithium
Mercury
Retinoic acid
Tetracycline
Tobacco
Trimethadione
Valproic acid
Warfarin

### AVOIDING FETAL EXPOSURE

Ideally, avoiding exposure to harmful influences begins before conception because all major organ systems develop early in pregnancy, often before a woman realizes that she is pregnant. To avoid some agents, such as alcohol or illicit drugs, pregnant women must be committed to make substantial lifestyle changes.

**Infections.** Rubella immunization at least 3 months before pregnancy virtually eliminates the risk that the mother will contract this infection, which can damage the fetus severely. For infections that cannot be prevented by immunization, the nurse can counsel the woman to avoid situations in which acquiring the disease is more likely. (See Chapters 26 and 30 for other infections that may harm the fetus.)

**Drugs and Other Substances.** The U.S. Food and Drug Administration has established pregnancy categories for therapeutic drugs based on their potential to harm the fetus. The categories range from A through D, and X. Class A drugs have no demonstrated fetal risk in well-controlled studies. At the opposite end, pregnancy category X drugs are well established as being harmful. For about 80 percent of therapeutic drugs, it is unknown whether they are definitely safe or definitely unsafe. (See Appendix C for a list of common drugs and other substances that may affect the fetus adversely.) In addition, the physician must often balance the woman's need for the drug's therapeutic effects against the fetal need to avoid exposure to it.

It is especially difficult to establish whether an illicit drug can cause prenatal damage, because women who use illegal drugs often have other problems that complicate analysis of fetal effects. For example, these women may use multiple drugs and often have poor nutrition, untreated sexually transmissible diseases, inadequate prenatal care, and a stressful life. In addition, the purity of illicit drugs is unlikely, and substances used to dilute them may themselves be harmful.

The best action is for the woman to eliminate use of nontherapeutic drugs and substances such as alcohol. If she takes therapeutic drugs, the physician may be able to prescribe an alternative drug with a lower risk to the fetus or may eliminate therapeutic drugs that are not essential, such as acne medications.

The pregnant woman who abuses drugs presents a complicated picture because maintenance of her drug habit usually takes priority over other needs. Also, she often has late or no prenatal care, increasing the likelihood that fetal damage occurred long before she encountered health care professionals.

**Ionizing Radiation.** Nonurgent radiologic procedures may be done during the first 2 weeks after the menstrual period begins. This is usually before ovulation and thus before conception is possible. For urgent procedures, the lower abdomen should be shielded with a lead apron, if possible. The radiation dose is kept as low as possible to reduce fetal exposure.

**Maternal Hyperthermia.** An important teratogen is maternal hyperthermia. The mother's temperature may rise unavoidably during illness. However, pregnant women should be cautioned to avoid or limit exposure to heat such as saunas or hot tubs. Temperatures vary widely among public hot tubs, so it is difficult to give a specific guideline for duration of exposure. In addition, the important factor is how high the woman's body temperature rises and for how long, not just the sauna or hot tub temperature.

#### MANIPULATING THE FETAL ENVIRONMENT

Appropriate medical therapy can help a woman avoid fetal damage that could result from her illness. For example, a woman who has diabetes should try to keep her blood glucose levels normal and stable before and during pregnancy for the best possible fetal outcomes. A woman with phenylketonuria should return to her special low-phenylalanine diet before conception to avoid buildup of toxic metabolic products in her body that may damage the fetus.

Occasionally, a pregnant woman is given a drug to medicate her fetus, for example, digitalis for fetal cardiac arrhythmias. In these cases, it is the fetus who has the disorder, not the mother. The mother is the conduit for medicating the fetus to allow normal development and function.

### Mechanical Disruptions to Fetal Development

Mechanical forces that interfere with normal prenatal development include oligohydramnios and fibrous amniotic bands.

*Oligohydramnios*, an abnormally small volume of amniotic fluid, reduces the cushion surrounding the fetus and may result in deformations such as clubfoot. Prolonged oligohydramnios can interfere with fetal lung development because it does not allow normal development of the alveoli. Oligohydramnios may not be the primary fetal problem but rather may be related to other fetal anomalies.

*Fibrous amniotic bands* may result from tears in the inner sac (amnion) of the fetal membranes and can result in fetal deformations or intrauterine limb amputation. Fibrous bands are usually sporadic and unlikely to recur. Because these bands can cause multiple defects, they may be confused with birth defects from other causes such as chromosome or single gene abnormalities.

**✓ CHECK YOUR READING**

13. What are the usual characteristics of multifactorial disorders?
14. What are some factors that can vary the likelihood that a multifactorial disorder will occur or recur?
15. How can a woman avoid exposing her fetus to teratogens?
16. Why should a woman with phenylketonuria adhere to a low-phenylalanine diet before and during pregnancy?

## Genetic Counseling

Genetic counseling provides services to help people understand the disorder about which they are concerned and the risk that it will occur in their family. Those concerned about multifactorial or environmental hazards can receive up-to-date information at most centers, as can families having concerns about purely genetic disorders.

### Availability

Genetic counseling is often available through university medical centers. State departments of mental health and mental retardation or rehabilitation services also may provide counseling services. Local chapters of the March of Dimes are an important source of information about birth defects and counseling sites. Also, organizations that focus on specific birth defects provide valuable support and assistance in obtaining needed services for individuals and families affected by that disorder.

## Focus on the Family

Genetic counseling focuses on the family rather than on an individual. One family member may have a birth defect, but study of the entire family is often needed for accurate counseling. This may involve obtaining medical records or performing physical examinations or laboratory studies on numerous family members. Counseling is impaired if family members are unwilling to provide their medical records or agree to examinations or laboratory studies. Moreover, those who seek counseling may be unwilling to request cooperation from other family members or to share with them genetic information they acquire.

## Process of Genetic Counseling

Genetic counseling is often a slow process that is not always straightforward. Several visits spread over months may be needed. In addition, some tests may be performed at only one or a few laboratories in the world, and several weeks may be needed to complete them. Despite a comprehensive evaluation, a diagnosis may never be established. An accurate diagnosis is crucial for providing families with the best information about the risks for a specific birth defect, the prognosis for one affected, and options available to avoid or manage the disorder. Advances in knowledge about birth defects may allow a definite diagnosis later, and families are encouraged to contact the center for updates. Table 5–3 lists examples of procedures that may be used before conception, prenatally, and after birth to establish an accurate diagnosis related to birth defects.

Individuals or families may request genetic counseling before or during pregnancy or after a child has been born with a defect. A genetic evaluation may include many factors, such as the following:

- A complete medical history, including prenatal and perinatal history
- The medical history of other family members
- Laboratory, imaging, or other studies
- Physical assessment of a child with the birth defect and other family members as needed
- Examination of photographs, particularly for family members who are deceased or unavailable
- Construction of a pedigree to identify relationships among family members and their relevant medical history

If a diagnosis is established, genetic counseling educates the family about the following:

- What is known about the cause of the disorder
- The natural course of the disorder
- Options for care of an affected person
- The likelihood that the disorder will occur or recur
- Availability of prenatal diagnosis for the disorder
- How a couple may be able to avoid having an affected child
- Availability of treatment and services for the person with the disorder

Genetic counseling is nondirective; that is, the counselor does not tell the individual or parents what decision to make but educates them about options for dealing with the disorder. However, families often interpret the counseling subjectively. Some parents may regard a 50 percent risk of occurrence or recurrence as low, whereas others may think that a 1 percent risk is unacceptably high. Also, the family's values and beliefs influence whether they seek counseling and what they do with the information that is provided.

**TABLE 5–3 DIAGNOSTIC METHODS THAT MAY BE USED IN GENETIC COUNSELING**

**Pre-conception Screening**

- Family history to identify hereditary patterns of disease or birth defects
- Examination of family photographs
- Physical examination for obvious or subtle signs of birth defects
- Carrier testing
  - Persons from ethnic groups with a higher incidence of some disorders
  - Persons with a family history suggesting that they may carry a gene for a specific disorder
- Chromosomal analysis
- DNA analysis

**Prenatal Diagnosis for Fetal Abnormalities**

- Chorionic villus sampling
- Amniocentesis
- Ultrasonography
- Percutaneous umbilical blood sampling

**Postnatal Diagnosis for an Infant with a Birth Defect**

- Physical examination and measurements
- Imaging procedures (ultrasonography, radiography, echocardiography)
- Chromosomal analysis
- DNA analysis
- Tests for metabolic disorders (phenylketonuria, cystic fibrosis)
- Hemoglobin analysis for disorders such as sickle cell disease
- Immunologic testing for infections
- Autopsy

## Supplemental Services

Comprehensive genetic counseling includes services of professionals from many disciplines, such as biology, medicine, nursing, social work, and education.

These professionals provide added support for families and may offer referral to parent support groups, grief counseling, and intervention for problems that accompany the birth of a child with a birth defect, such as socioeconomic or family dysfunction.

## Nursing Care of Families Concerned About Birth Defects

Nurses have an important role in helping families that are concerned about birth defects. Some nurses work directly with family members who are undergoing genetic counseling. Many more nurses are generalists who bring their knowledge about birth defects and their prevention to those they encounter in everyday practice.

### Nurses as Part of a Genetic Counseling Team

Many genetic counseling teams include nurses. Genetic nursing may include the following:

- Providing counseling (after having additional education in this area)
- Guiding a woman or couple through prenatal diagnosis
- Supporting parents as they make decisions after receiving abnormal prenatal diagnostic results
- Helping the family deal with the emotional impact of a birth defect
- Assisting parents who have had a child with a birth defect to locate needed services and support
- Coordinating services of other professionals, such as social workers, physical and occupational therapists, psychologists, and dietitians
- Helping families find appropriate support groups to help them cope with the daily stresses associated with a child who has a birth defect

**Parents Want to Know**

**About Birth Defects**

*How can this birth defect be genetic? No one else in our family has ever had anything like it.*

Autosomal recessive disorders are carried by parents who themselves are unaffected. The abnormal gene may have been passed down through many generations, but there is no risk for an affected child until *two* carrier parents mate.

*Isn't there only a one-in-a-million chance that this birth defect will happen to another of our children?*

Autosomal recessive disorders have a 25 percent (1 in 4) chance of recurring in children of the same parents. Autosomal dominant disorders may pose a 50 percent risk for recurrence unless they resulted from a new mutation in the parental germ cells.

*Isn't this birth defect very likely to recur? We'd better not have any more children.*

Some birth defects are associated with a relatively high risk of recurrence; others have a relatively low risk. Prenatal diagnosis may offer parents a way to avoid having an affected child, or some disorders may be treated before birth.

*Since we've already had a child with this birth defect [an autosomal recessive one], will the next three be normal?*

If both parents are carriers for an autosomal recessive disorder, there is a 25 percent (1 in 4) risk that is constant with *each* conception. There is an equal chance that their children will be neither affected nor carriers.

*If I have an amniocentesis or other prenatal diagnostic test, can the test detect all birth defects?*

Although many disorders can be prenatally diagnosed, not all can be diagnosed in the same fetus. Testing is offered for one or more specific disorders after a careful family history is taken to determine appropriate tests.

*If the prenatal test is normal, will my baby be normal?*

Normal results from prenatal testing exclude those disorders that were specifically tested for. Every healthy couple has about a 5 percent risk of having a child with a birth defect, some of which are not obvious at birth. This baseline risk remains, even if all prenatal test results are normal.

*Will I have to have an abortion if my prenatal tests show that my baby is abnormal?*

Abortion may be an option for parents whose fetus is affected with a birth defect, but most parents are reassured by normal test results. If results are abnormal, some parents appreciate the time to prepare for a child with special needs. Better medical management can be planned for a newborn who is expected to have problems. Prenatal diagnosis gives many parents the confidence to have children despite their increased risk for having a child with a birth defect.

### Nurses in General Practice

Nurses who work in women's health care and those who work in antepartum, intrapartum, newborn, or pediatric settings often encounter families who are concerned about birth defects. These families may include a member who has a birth defect. Other families may believe that they have an increased risk for having a child with a birth defect. Generalist nurses provide care and support that complements those of nurses who work on a genetic counseling team.

#### WOMEN'S HEALTH NURSES

The nurse who provides care in women's health may encounter families who should be referred for genetic counseling. The ideal time to provide counseling is before conception so the childbearing couple has more options if problems are identified.

As in antepartum care, the primary nursing role is to identify families who might benefit from counsel-

**TABLE 5-4 REASONS FOR REFERRAL TO A GENETIC COUNSELOR**

Pregnant women who will be 35 years of age or older when the infant is born
Men who father children after age 40
Members of a group with an increased incidence of a specific disorder
Carriers of autosomal recessive disorders
Women who are carriers of X-linked disorders
Couples related by blood (consanguineous relationship)
Family history of birth defect or mental retardation
Family history of unexplained stillbirth
Women who experience multiple spontaneous abortions
Pregnant women exposed to known or suspected teratogens or other harmful agents, either before or during pregnancy
Pregnant women with abnormal prenatal screening results, such as alpha-fetoprotein, triple screen, or suspicious ultrasound findings

ing before conception. Personal and family histories are commonly taken at primary health care visits, and the nurse may identify a history that could affect a future child that the couple might conceive. For example, the nurse may identify a woman who belongs to a group in which the sickle cell gene is more frequent and arrange for testing to determine her carrier status. If testing reveals that she is a carrier for the gene, the woman can be advised that she could conceive a child with sickle cell disease if her partner is also a carrier. If her partner has not been tested, the nurse can arrange for the testing.

### ANTEPARTUM NURSES

During the initial antepartum interview, the nurse may identify the pregnant woman or family who may benefit from genetic counseling. The antepartum nurse also assists families with decision making, teaching, and emotional support.

**Identifying Families for Referral.** Nurses in antepartum settings often identify a woman or family who is appropriately referred for genetic counseling. The personal and family history of the woman and her partner may reveal factors that increase their risks for having a child with a birth defect. In addition to the usual medical history about disorders such as hypertension or diabetes, the woman should be questioned about a family history of birth defects, diseases that seem to "run in the family," mental retardation, or developmental delay. Table 5–4 lists common reasons for referral to a genetic counselor.

**Some people are reluctant to disclose that they have a family member with mental retardation or a birth defect. The nurse can gently probe for sensitive information by asking questions about whether there are family members who have learning problems or who are "slow." Using words that are lay oriented often elicits more information than using clinical terms that may seem harsh.**

**Helping the Family Decide About Genetic Counseling.** If genetic counseling is appropriate, the physician usually discusses it with the woman and offers to refer her and her partner to an appropriate center. However, the final decision rests with the couple. The nurse can help the family decide whether they want genetic counseling at all and weigh issues that are important to them.

Genetic counseling can raise issues that are uncomfortable, such as whether to undergo prenatal diagnosis, what to do if a condition cannot be prenatally diagnosed, and what options are acceptable if prenatal diagnosis shows abnormal results. Counseling may open family conflicts if information from other family members is needed or if family values differ on issues such as abortion of an abnormal fetus. In addition, the tests can show unexpected results (Table 5–5). The nurse must be careful not to allow personal values to influence the family's decision. It is the family members who must live with the decision they make.

**Teaching About Lifestyle.** Nurses can teach a pregnant woman about harmful factors in her lifestyle that can be modified to reduce the risk of defects to offspring. The nurse can support the woman in making lifestyle changes that may be difficult, such as stopping alcohol consumption, reducing or eliminating smoking, or improving her diet. Using liberal praise can motivate a woman to continue her efforts to promote an optimal outcome. However, a negative

**TABLE 5-5 PROBLEMS ENCOUNTERED IN GENETIC COUNSELING AND PRENATAL DIAGNOSIS**

Inadequate medical records
- Family members' refusal to share information
- Records that are incomplete, vague, or uninformative

Inconclusive testing
- Too few family members available when family studies are needed
- Inadequate number of live fetal cells obtained during amniocentesis
- Failure of fetal cells to grow in culture
- Ambiguous prenatal test results that are neither clearly normal nor clearly abnormal

Unexpected results from prenatal diagnosis
- Finding an abnormality other than the one tested for
- Non-paternity revealed

Inability to determine the severity of a prenatally diagnosed disorder
Inability to rule out all birth defects

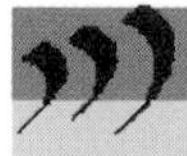

## THERAPEUTIC COMMUNICATION

### Assisting a Woman Who May Benefit from Genetic Counseling

Paula Crandall is a 41-year-old white woman who is 8 weeks pregnant with her first child after more than 10 years of infertility. Barbara Glenn is a nurse who works with Paula's obstetrician.

**Paula:** I know all about the risks at my age. I'm not so much worried about my own health, but the baby's.

**Barbara:** You're concerned that the baby might not be all right?

*Clarifying*

**Paula:** Sure, what woman wouldn't be? I know the baby is more likely to have Down syndrome and be mentally retarded if the mother is older . . . and I certainly qualify as older!

**Barbara:** Yes, you're right. The risks of having an infant with a chromosomal abnormality increase after the mother is 35 years old. Have you considered having prenatal diagnosis to see if the fetus has this kind of problem?

*Paraphrasing and giving information. Barbara also uses a closed-end question that tends to block communication because it can be answered with a simple "yes" or "no."*

**Paula:** Oh, yes. I know all about what's available. When I became 35 and wasn't yet pregnant, I just assumed that if I ever did get pregnant, I'd automatically have amniocentesis or whatever tests were recommended. I just don't know . . .

**Barbara:** You're reconsidering prenatal testing?

*Reflecting*

**Paula:** Well, not exactly reconsidering. It's just that I've waited so long for a baby, and this is probably the only one I'll ever have.

**Barbara:** [Waiting quietly, but attentively as Paula seems to be thinking.]

*Using silence*

**Paula:** I'm just worried about testing. I know amniocentesis has a low risk, but what if it causes me to lose a normal baby? It took me so long to finally get pregnant, and I'm running out of time. I don't think I'll get another chance.

**Barbara:** It must be a very difficult decision.

*Reflecting*

**Paula:** It is. Even if I have testing and the baby has Down syndrome, I'm not so sure I'd have an abortion. The outlook for people with Down syndrome is much better than it used to be. On the other hand, I worry about who would care for a handicapped child when I am no longer able to. Why even have prenatal testing if I wouldn't do anything about an abnormal baby?

**Barbara:** You certainly have some valid concerns. How does your husband feel about testing?

*Questioning using an open-ended question*

**Paula:** Oh, Bill is all for it. He keeps reminding me that the baby is probably normal and that I probably won't have a miscarriage if I have amniocentesis. But his cousin had a child with Down syndrome, and Bill doesn't think we should knowingly bring a child with a serious birth defect into the world. What would you do if you were in my place?

**Barbara:** I can't answer that question because I'm not in your place and I don't have to live with the decision. Let's review some of the issues so you can make the best decision for yourself and your family. First, you know you have an increased risk for having a baby with a chromosomal defect such as Down syndrome because of your age. Second, the odds that the baby will be normal are much higher than the risk that the baby will be abnormal. Third, amniocentesis poses a small but real risk of causing a miscarriage. Fourth, you are undecided about whether you would terminate a pregnancy if the fetus were abnormal. Another issue that you haven't specifically mentioned is time. If you choose prenatal diagnosis, amniocentesis is done between 16 and 17 weeks' gestation and chorionic villus sampling must be done within the next 2 to 4 weeks.

*Summarizing*

**Paula:** I know. I'm running out of time in more ways than one.

**Barbara:** If you like, I can set up an appointment with a genetic counselor. The counselor can provide you with the most accurate assessment of your risk for having a child with a birth defect and also the risks of any indicated prenatal diagnosis procedure. Then you can decide whether or not to have testing.

**Paula:** I think I'd like that, as long as I don't have to be committed to a particular decision before I go.

---

attitude from nurses or other professionals may make her feel like a failure, and she may abandon her efforts to create a healthier lifestyle.

**Providing Emotional Support.** The time between prenatal testing and results sometimes spans several difficult weeks. In the meantime, the pregnancy is becoming more obvious and the woman may begin to feel fetal movement. Many women delay telling friends or family about their pregnancy until they know that prenatal test results are normal. They often delay investing emotionally in their pregnancy because it seems so tentative until test results are known. When results are abnormal, women face more difficult decisions about whether to terminate or continue the pregnancy.

**Helping the Family Deal with Abnormal Results.** Because prenatal diagnostic tests are performed to detect disorders involving serious physical and often mental effects, the woman or couple whose test results are abnormal must confront painful decisions. For many of these disorders, no effective prenatal or postnatal treatment exists. In many cases, there are only two choices: continue the pregnancy or terminate it. In addition, the decision to terminate a pregnancy must be made in a short time. Arriving at "no decision" is effectively a decision to continue the pregnancy. Although the physician or genetic counselor is the one who discusses abnormal results and available options, the nurse reinforces the information given to these anxious families.

When test results are abnormal, nurses can expect the couple to grieve. Even if a pregnancy was unplanned, the woman who reaches the time of prenatal diagnosis has already made the initial decision to continue the pregnancy. If results are abnormal, she must decide all over again about terminating the pregnancy. Women who continue their pregnancies grieve over the expected normal infant.

### INTRAPARTUM AND NEONATAL NURSES

Nurses working in intrapartum and neonatal settings encounter families who have given birth to an infant with a birth defect that was often unexpected. Stillborn infants sometimes have birth defects that contributed to their intrauterine death. Besides the loss of their baby, these parents face added pain because of the associated abnormality. An autopsy may be performed to document all anomalies and to establish the most accurate diagnosis of the birth defect for future counseling. Nursing care for families experiencing a perinatal loss, whether a result of the infant's death or the loss of the expected normal infant, is addressed in Chapter 24.

Nurses who care for these families in the intrapartum and neonatal settings will find the parents anxious, depressed, and sometimes hostile because of the unexpected event. The family's usual coping mechanisms may be inadequate for the situation, yet they have not developed new ones. Various diagnostic studies are often recommended soon after the birth of an abnormal infant to establish a diagnosis and to give parents accurate information about the disorder and their options. However, a high anxiety level reduces their ability to understand the often massive amount of information received. The nurse is in the best position to evaluate the family's perception of the problem, help them understand the diagnostic tests, reinforce correct information, and correct misunderstandings. Moreover, the nurse is often most therapeutic by just being an available, active listener, helping to ease the family's pain over the event.

Nurses should encourage families to contact lay support groups. These groups are a significant source of support because they understand fully the daily problems encountered when caring for a child with a birth defect. They can help the parents deal with the stress and chronic grief associated with prolonged care of these children. Support groups can also help the parents see the positive aspects and victories when caring for their special-needs child.

### PEDIATRIC NURSES

Children with birth defects typically have numerous recurrent medical problems. They usually are hospitalized more often and for longer periods than children without birth defects. They may have to travel to specialized hospitals for care, adding to the family's stress. Their families often have large expenses for medical care and equipment that are not covered by insurance or public assistance programs. There may be lost income because one parent, usually the mother, stops working to care for the child.

Family dysfunction is common, and the strain of having a child with a serious birth defect may lead to divorce. Siblings of the child often feel left out of their parents' attention because the needs of the sick child demand so much of their time.

The pediatric nurse can reduce the family's stress by helping them locate appropriate support services. The nurse can contact social services departments to help the family find financial and other resources needed to care for the child. If parents have not connected with a lay support group, the pediatric nurse can encourage them to do so.

## SUMMARY CONCEPTS

- The 46 human chromosomes are long strands of DNA, each containing up to several thousand individual genes.
- With the exception of those genes located on the X and Y chromosomes in males, genes are inherited in pairs that may be identical or different. Some genes are dominant, and some are recessive.
- Many genes can be analyzed by the products they produce, their DNA, or their close association with another gene that is more easily analyzed.
- Cells for chromosome analysis must be living. Specimens must be handled carefully to preserve their viability.
- Chromosome abnormalities are either numerical, with the addition or deletion of an entire chromosome or chromosomes, or structural, with deletion, addition, rearrangement, or fragility of the chromosome material.

- Single gene disorders are associated with a fixed risk of occurrence or recurrence. The type of single gene abnormality (autosomal dominant, autosomal recessive, or X-linked) determines the risk.
- Multifactorial disorders occur because of a genetic predisposition combined with environmental factors.
- The risk for occurrence or recurrence of multifactorial disorders is not fixed but varies according to the number of close relatives that are affected, the severity of the defect in affected persons, the sex of the affected person, and the geographic locale. Seasonal variations may affect the risk for some disorders.
- Relatively few agents that can enter the fetal environment are known to be definitely teratogenic or definitely safe.
- The risk for fetal damage from environmental agents can be decreased by reducing exposure to the agent or manipulating the fetal environment.
- The purpose of genetic counseling is to educate individuals or families with accurate information so they can make informed decisions about reproduction and appropriate care for affected members.
- The nurse cares for people with concerns about birth defects by identifying those needing referral, by teaching, by coordinating services, and by offering emotional support.

### *References and Readings*


American Academy of Pediatrics and American College of Obstetricians and Gynecologists. (1992). *Guidelines for perinatal care* (3rd ed., pp. 56–62). Elk Grove Village, Ill., and Washington, D.C.: Author.

Collins, J.E. (1994). Fetal surgery: Changing the outcome before birth. *Journal of Obstetric, Gynecologic, and Neonatal Nursing, 23*(2), 166–169.

Conover, E. (1994). Hazardous exposures during pregnancy. *Journal of Obstetric, Gynecologic, and Neonatal Nursing, 23*(6), 524–531.

Forsman, I. (1994). Evolution of the nursing role in genetics. *Journal of Obstetric, Gynecologic, and Neonatal Nursing, 23*(6), 481–486.

Grabowski, G.A., & Whitsett, J.A. (1996). Gene therapy. In W.E. Nelson, R.E. Behrman, R.M. Kliegman, & A.M. Arvin (Eds.), *Nelson textbook of pediatrics* (15th ed., pp. 321–326). Philadelphia: W.B. Saunders.

Guyton, A.C., & Hall, J.E. (1996). *Textbook of medical physiology* (9th ed.). Philadelphia: W.B. Saunders.

Hall, J.G. (1996a). Chromosomal clinical abnormalities. In W.E. Nelson, R.E. Behrman, R.M. Kliegman, & A.M. Arvin (Eds.), *Nelson textbook of pediatrics* (15th ed., pp. 312–321). Philadelphia: W.B. Saunders.

Hall, J.G. (1996b). Genetic counseling. In W.E. Nelson, R.E. Behrman, R.M. Kliegman, & A.M. Arvin (Eds.), *Nelson textbook of pediatrics* (15th ed., p. 327). Philadelphia: W.B. Saunders.

James, D. (1994). Genetic counseling. In D.K. James, P.J. Steer, C.P. Weiner, & B. Gonik (Eds.), *High risk pregnancy: Management options* (pp. 9–20). London: W.B. Saunders.

Jones, K.L. (1994). Effects of therapeutic, diagnostic, and environmental agents. In R.K. Creasy & R. Resnik (Eds.), *Maternal-fetal medicine: Principles and practice* (3rd ed., pp. 171–180). Philadelphia: W.B. Saunders.

Jones, O.W., & Cahill, T.C. (1994). Basic genetics and patterns of inheritance. In R.K. Creasy & R. Resnik (Eds.), *Maternal-fetal medicine: Principles and practice* (3rd ed., pp. 3–60). Philadelphia: W.B. Saunders.

Jones, S.L. (1994). Assisted reproductive technologies: Genetic and nursing implications. *Journal of Obstetric, Gynecologic, and Neonatal Nursing, 23*(6), 492–497.

Jones, S.L. (1996). Genetics: Changing health care in the 21st century. *Journal of Obstetric, Gynecologic, and Neonatal Nursing, 25*(9), 777–783.

Mackta, J., & Weiss, J.O. (1994). The role of genetic support groups. *Journal of Obstetric, Gynecologic, and Neonatal Nursing, 23*(6), 519–523.

Moore, K.L. (1993). *Before we are born: Essentials of embryology and birth defects* (4th ed.). Philadelphia: W.B. Saunders.

Munro, C.L., & Pickler, R.H. (1994). The technology and use of blastomere analysis. *Journal of Obstetric, Gynecologic, and Neonatal Nursing, 23*(3), 229–234.

Penticuff, J.H. (1996). Ethical dimensions in genetic screening: A look into the future. *Journal of Obstetric, Gynecologic, and Neonatal Nursing, 25*(9), 785–789.

Pickler, R.H., & Munro, C.L. (1994). Blastomere analysis: Issues for discussion. *Journal of Obstetric, Gynecologic, and Neonatal Nursing, 23*(5), 379–382.

Raff, B.S., & Carroll, D. (1994). The genome project. *Journal of Obstetric, Gynecologic, and Neonatal Nursing, 23*(6), 488–491.

Rhodes, A.M. (1995). Liability for failure to offer prenatal AFP testing. *MCN: American Journal of Maternal-Child Nursing, 20*(3), 169.

Rogers, J., & Davis, B.A. (1995). How risky are hot tubs and saunas for pregnant women? *MCN: American Journal of Maternal-Child Nursing, 20*(3), 137.

Romanczuk, A.N., & Brown, J.P. (1994). Folic acid will reduce risk of neural tube defects. *MCN: American Journal of Maternal-Child Nursing, 19*(6), 331–334.

Scanlon, C., & Fibison, W. (1995). *Managing genetic information: Implications for nursing practice.* Washington, D.C.: American Nurses Association.

Shapiro, L.J. (1996a). Inheritance patterns. In W.E. Nelson, R.E. Behrman, R.M. Kliegman, & A.M. Arvin (Eds.), *Nelson textbook of pediatrics* (15th ed., pp. 308–312). Philadelphia: W.B. Saunders.

Shapiro, L.J. (1996b). The molecular basis of genetic disorders. In W.E. Nelson, R.E. Behrman, R.M. Kliegman, & A.M. Arvin (Eds.), *Nelson textbook of pediatrics* (15th ed., pp. 299–305). Philadelphia: W.B. Saunders.

Shapiro, L.J. (1996c). Molecular diagnosis. In W.E. Nelson, R.E. Behrman, R.M. Kliegman, & A.M. Arvin (Eds.), *Nelson textbook of pediatrics* (15th ed., pp. 305–308). Philadelphia: W.B. Saunders.

Simpson, J.L., & Elias, S. (1994). Prenatal diagnosis of genetic disorders. In R.K. Creasy & R. Resnik (Eds.), *Maternal-fetal medicine: Principles and practice* (3rd ed., pp. 61–88). Philadelphia: W.B. Saunders.

Simpson, J.L., & Golbus, M.S. (1992). *Genetics in obstetrics and gynecology* (2nd ed.). Philadelphia: W.B. Saunders.

Slaughter, L. (1997). Ensuring protection from genetic discrimination in health insurance. *Lifelines, 1*(3), 23.

Thompson, M.W., McInnes, R.R., & Willard, H.F. (1991). *Thompson and Thompson genetics in medicine* (5th Ed.). Philadelphia: W.B. Saunders.

Williams, J.K., & Lea, D.H. (1995). Applying new genetic technologies: Assessment and ethical considerations. *Nurse Practitioner, 20*(7), 16–26.

Wright, L. (1994). Prenatal diagnosis in the 1990s. *Journal of Obstetric, Gynecologic, and Neonatal Nursing, 23*(6), 506–515.

# Part II

# The Family Before Birth

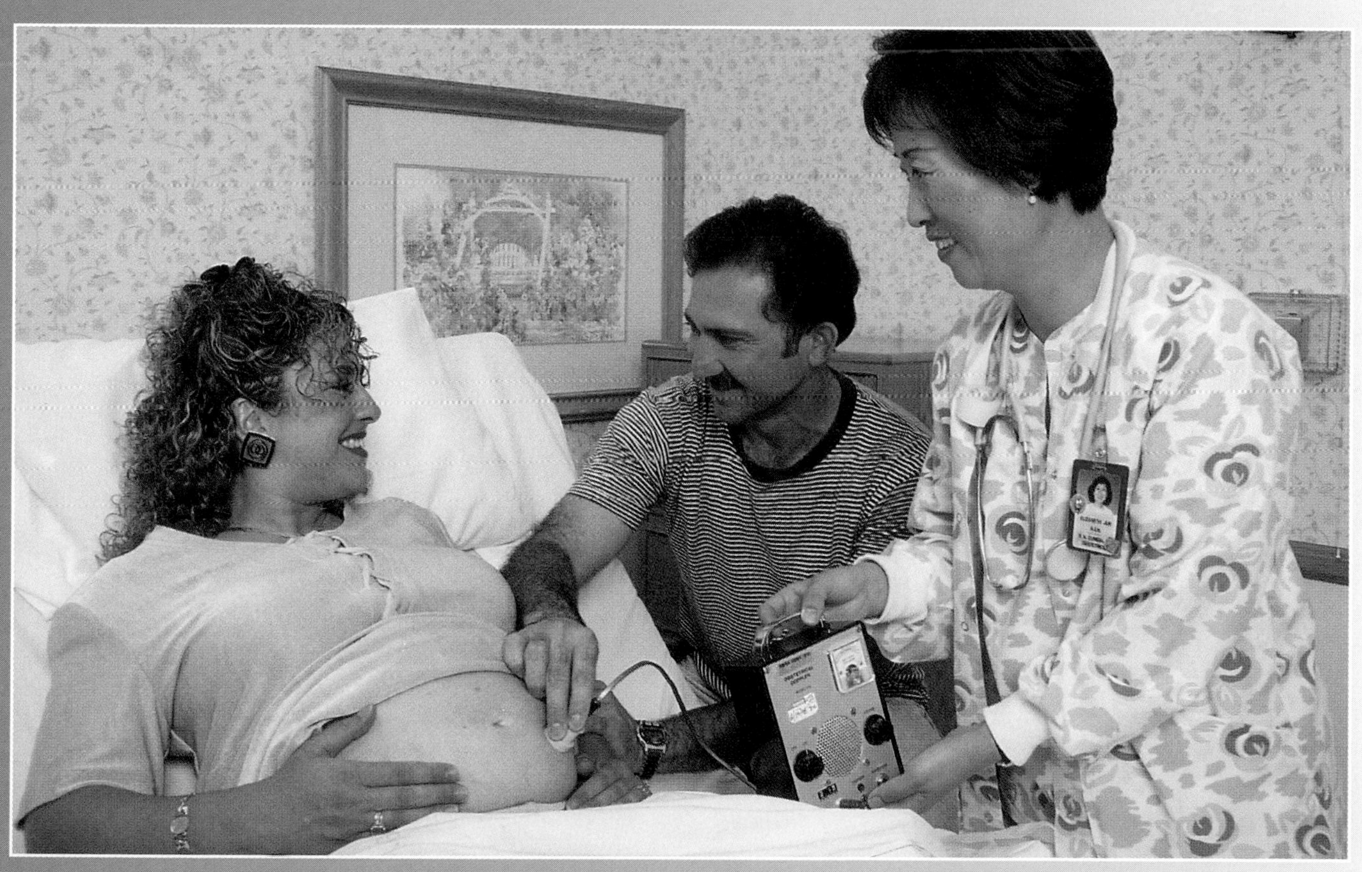

# 6

# Conception and Prenatal Development

## OBJECTIVES

1. Describe formation of the female and male gametes.
2. Relate ovulation and ejaculation to the process of human conception.
3. Explain implantation and nourishment of the embryo before development of the placenta.
4. Describe normal prenatal development from conception through birth.
5. Explain structure and function of the placenta, umbilical cord, and fetal membranes.
6. Describe how common deviations from usual conception and prenatal development occur.
7. Describe prenatal circulation and the circulatory changes after birth.
8. Explain how multifetal pregnancies can occur.

## DEFINITIONS

**autosome** *Any of the 22 pairs of chromosomes other than the sex chromosomes.*

**conceptus** *Cells and membranes resulting from fertilization of the ovum at any stage of prenatal development.*

**corpus luteum** *Graafian follicle cells remaining after ovulation that produce estrogen and progesterone.*

**diploid** *Having a pair of chromosomes (46 in humans) that represents one copy of every chromosome from each parent; the number of chromosomes normally present in body cells other than gametes.*

**ejaculation** *Expulsion of semen from the penis.*

**embryo** *The developing baby from the beginning of the third week through the eighth week after conception.*

**endometrium** *Lining of the uterus.*

**fertilization age** *Prenatal age of the developing baby calculated from the date of conception. Also called post-conceptional age.*

**fetus** *The developing baby from 9 weeks after conception until birth. In everyday practice, this term is often used to describe a developing baby during pregnancy, regardless of age.*

**gamete** *Reproductive cell; in the female an ovum, and in the male a spermatozoon.*

**gestational age** *Prenatal age of the developing baby (measured in weeks) calculated from the first day of the woman's last menstrual period. Also called menstrual age. About 2 weeks longer than the fertilization age.*

**graafian follicle** *A small sac within the ovary that contains the maturing ovum.*

**haploid** *Having one copy of a chromosome from each pair (23 in humans, or half the diploid number). Gametes normally have a haploid number of chromosomes.*

**meiosis** *Reduction cell division in gametes that halves the number of chromosomes in each cell.*

**mitosis** *Cell division in body cells other than the gametes.*

**nidation** *Implantation of the fertilized ovum (zygote) in the uterine endometrium.*
**oogenesis** *Formation of gametes (ova) in the female.*
**ovulation** *Release of the mature ovum from the ovary.*
**placenta** *Fetal structure that provides nourishment and removes wastes from the developing baby and secretes hormones necessary for the pregnancy to continue.*
**sex chromosome** *The X or Y chromosomes. Females have two X chromosomes; males have one X and one Y chromosome.*
**somatic cells** *Body cells other than the gametes, or germ cells.*
**spermatogenesis** *Formation of male gametes (sperm) in the testes.*
**teratogen** *An agent that can cause defects in a developing baby during pregnancy.*
**zygote** *The developing baby from conception through the first week of prenatal life.*

A basic understanding of conception and prenatal development helps the nurse to provide care to parents during normal childbearing and to better understand problems such as infertility and birth defects. This chapter addresses formation of the gametes, the process of conception, prenatal development, and important auxiliary structures that support normal prenatal development. A short discussion of how multifetal pregnancy, such as twinning, occurs is also included.

## Gametogenesis

Gametogenesis is the development of ova in the woman and sperm in the man. Production of gametes requires a different process than formation of somatic cells. Somatic cells reproduce by a process called mitosis. Each somatic cell has 46 paired chromosomes: 22 pairs of autosomes and one pair of sex chromosomes. During mitosis the cell divides into two new cells, each having 46 chromosomes, like the parent cell.

Gametogenesis requires a special reduction division called meiosis. Unlike mitosis, in which the diploid number of chromosomes is retained in the new cells, meiosis halves the number of chromosomes (haploid number). Only one of each chromosome pair is directed to the gamete, 22 autosomes and one sex chromosome. Also, each chromosome (other than the X and Y chromosomes in the male) exchanges some material with its mate so that the new chromosome in the gamete contains some material from the mother and some from the father. This process (crossing over) allows variation in genetic material while keeping the total amount of chromosome material constant from generation to generation.

When the sperm and ovum unite at conception,

**TABLE 6–1 COMPARISON OF FEMALE AND MALE GAMETOGENESIS**

| | Oogenesis | Spermatogenesis |
|---|---|---|
| *Time during which primary germ cells are produced* | Fetal life. No others develop after about 30 weeks of gestation. | Continuously after puberty |
| *Hormones controlling process* | GnRH<br>FSH<br>LH<br>Estrogen | GnRH<br>FSH<br>LH<br>Testosterone<br>Estrogen (small amounts converted from testosterone)<br>Growth hormone |
| *Number of mature germ cells that develop from each primary cell* | One | Four |
| *Quantity* | One during each reproductive cycle of about 28 days. | 200–600 million are released with each ejaculation. |
| *Size* | Large. Visible to naked eye. Abundant cytoplasm to nourish embryo until implantation. | Tiny compared to ovum. Little cytoplasm. Head is almost all nuclear material (chromosomes). |
| *Motility* | Relatively non-motile. Carried along by action of cilia and currents within fallopian tubes. | Independently motile by means of whip-like tail. Mitochondria in middle piece provide energy for motility. |
| *Chromosome complement* | 23 total: 22 autosomes plus one X sex chromosome. | 23 total: 22 autosomes, plus either an X or a Y sex chromosome. |

*Abbreviations:* GnRH, gonadotropin-releasing hormone; FSH, follicle-stimulating hormone; LH, luteinizing hormone.

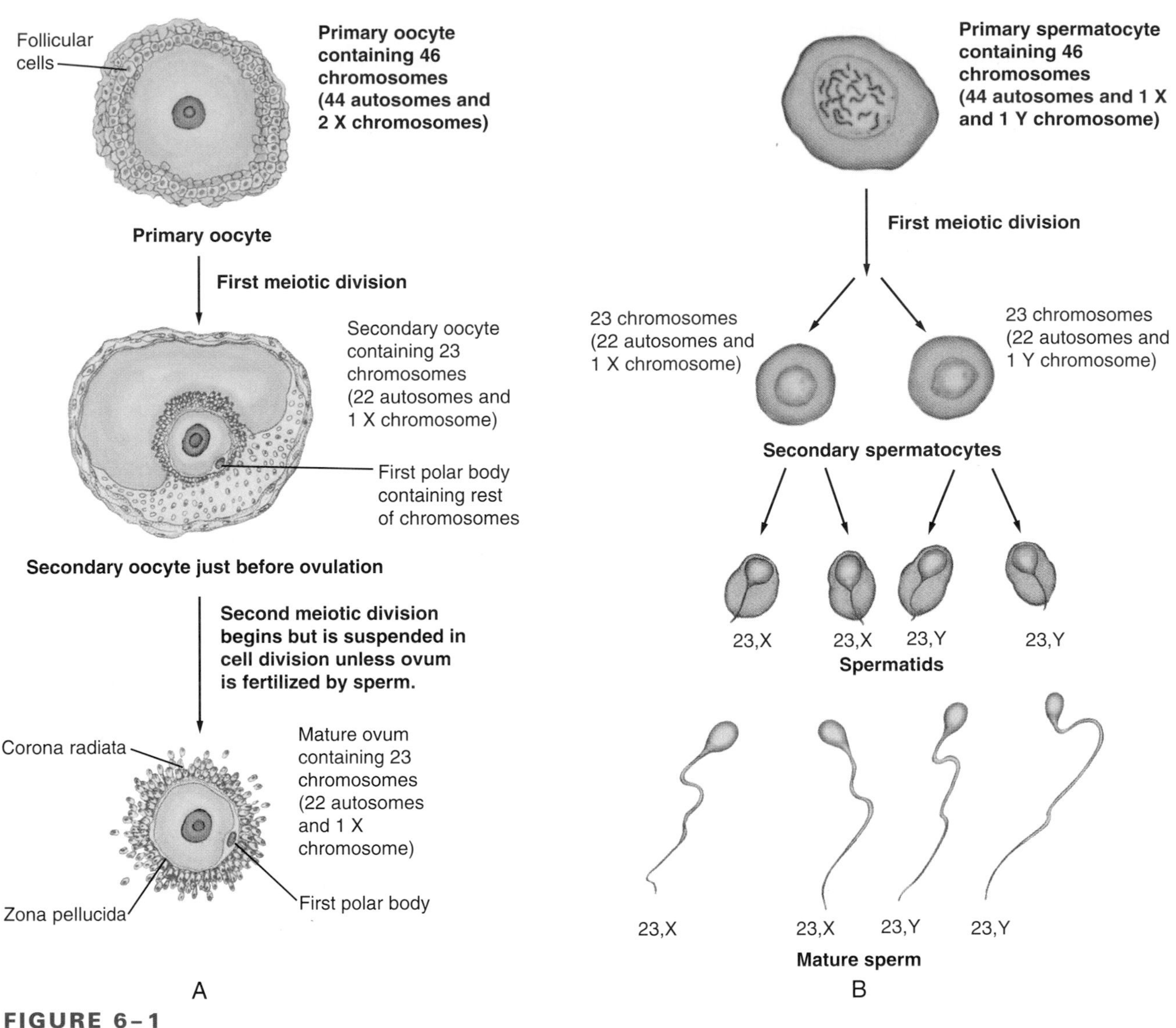


**FIGURE 6–1**

Gametogenesis. A, Formation of the mature ovum. B, Formation of mature sperm.

the "halves" form a new cell and restore the chromosome number to 46. Table 6–1 summarizes human gametogenesis and differences between males and females.

## Oogenesis

Oogenesis is the formation of female gametes (Fig. 6–1A) within the ovary. Oogenesis begins during prenatal life when primitive ova (oogonia) multiply by mitosis, like all other cells. Each oogonium contains 46 chromosomes (22 pairs of autosomes and a pair of X chromosomes), as do other body cells. Before birth, these oogonia enlarge to form primary oocytes with a layer of follicular cells surrounding each one. These are called *primary follicles.* The primary oogonium begins its first meiotic division during fetal life but does not complete the process until puberty. The primary follicle and its oogonium (still containing 46 chromosomes) remain dormant throughout childhood.

The female fetus has all the ova she will ever have by the 30th week of gestation. Many of these ova regress during childhood. When a girl's reproductive cycles begin at puberty, some of the primary follicles present at birth begin maturing. The process of gamete maturation continues throughout her reproductive years until the climacteric ("change of life").

When the oocyte matures, two meiotic divisions reduce the chromosome number from 46 paired to 23 unpaired chromosomes: 22 autosomes and an X. Shortly before ovulation, the primary oocyte completes its first meiotic division, which was begun during fetal life. A secondary oocyte, now containing 23 unpaired chromosomes, results. The primary cell's cytoplasm is divided unequally with this division, with most being retained by the secondary oocyte. The remainder of cytoplasm, plus the other half of the chromosomes, goes into a tiny, nonfunctional polar body that soon degenerates.

At ovulation, the secondary oocyte begins dividing again (second meiotic division) to form a mature ovum. The second meiotic division is prolonged, and the mature ovum remains suspended in metaphase, the middle part of cell division. If fertilization occurs, the second meiotic division is completed, resulting in a mature ovum containing 23 chromosomes and a second tiny polar body that degenerates. If the ovum is not fertilized, it does not complete the second meiotic division and degenerates. In oogenesis, one primary oocyte results in a single mature ovum.

When released from the ovary, the mature ovum is surrounded by two layers, the zona pellucida and the cells of the corona radiata. These layers protect the ovum and prevent fertilization by more than one sperm. For fertilization to occur, the sperm must penetrate these two layers to reach the ovum's cell nucleus.

### Spermatogenesis

Spermatogenesis (see Fig. 6–1B) begins during puberty in the male. Primitive sperm cells (*spermatogonia*) develop during the prenatal period and begin multiplying by mitosis during puberty. Unlike the female, the male continues throughout his lifetime to produce new spermatogonia that can mature into sperm. Although male fertility gradually declines with age, men can father children in their 50s, 60s, and beyond.

Each spermatogonium contains 46 paired chromosomes, like other body cells. In the mature male, a spermatogonium enlarges to become a primary spermatocyte, still containing all 46 chromosomes. The first meiotic division forms two secondary spermatocytes and reduces the number to 23 unpaired chromosomes: 22 autosomes and one sex chromosome, either an X or a Y. Each secondary spermatocyte divides again in the second meiotic division to form two spermatids. Therefore, half of the four spermatids that result from the two meiotic divisions of the spermatogonium carry an X chromosome and half carry a Y. The spermatids gradually evolve into mature sperm.

The gamete from a male determines the sex of the new baby. Each mature sperm contains 23 chromosomes: 22 autosomes and either an X or a Y. If an X-bearing spermatozoon fertilizes the ovum, the baby is a girl. If a Y-bearing spermatozoon fertilizes the ovum, the baby is a boy.

The mature sperm has three major sections: a head, a middle portion, and a tail (Fig. 6–2). The head is almost entirely a cell nucleus. The head contains the male chromosomes that join the chromosomes of the ovum. The middle portion supplies energy for the tail's whip-like action. The movement of the tail propels the sperm toward the ovum.

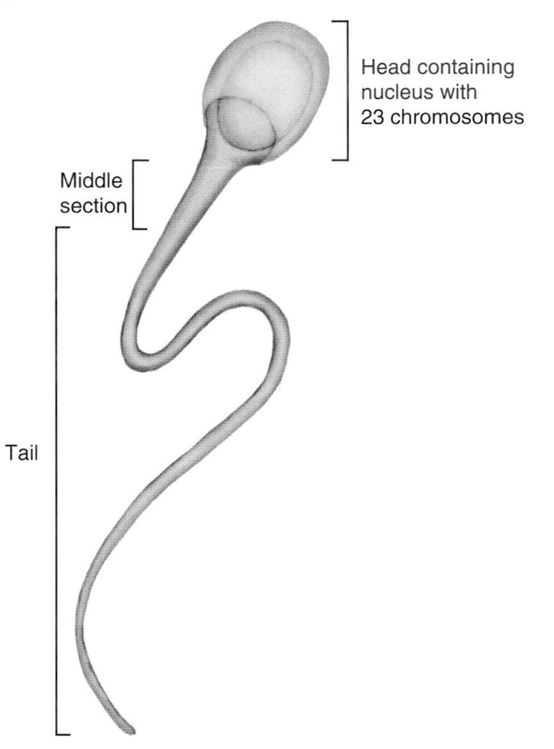


**FIGURE 6–2**

Mature sperm.

**CHECK YOUR READING**

1. What is the purpose of meiosis in the gametes?
2. How many mature ova can be produced by each oogonium? When does meiosis occur in the female?
3. How many mature spermatozoa can be produced by each spermatogonium? When does meiosis occur in the male?

## Conception

Conception requires correct timing between release of a mature ovum at ovulation and ejaculation of enough healthy, mature, motile sperm into the vagina. Although exact viability is unknown, the ovum may survive no longer than 24 hours after its release at ovulation. Most sperm survive no more than 24 hours in the female reproductive tract, although some remain fertile up to 72 hours.

### Preparation for Conception in the Female

Before ovulation, several oocytes begin to mature under the influence of follicle-stimulating hormone (FSH) and luteinizing hormone (LH) from the woman's anterior pituitary gland. The maturing oocytes are contained within a sac called the graafian follicle, which produces estrogen and progesterone to prepare the endometrium for a possible pregnancy. Eventually, one follicle outgrows the others. The less mature oocytes permanently regress.

#### RELEASE OF THE OVUM

Ovulation occurs about 14 days before a woman's next menstrual period would begin. The follicle develops a weak spot on the surface of the ovary and ruptures, releasing the mature ovum with its surrounding cells on the surface of the ovary. The collapsed follicle is transformed into the corpus luteum, which maintains high estrogen and progesterone secretion necessary to make final preparation of the uterine lining for a fertilized ovum.

#### OVUM TRANSPORT

The mature ovum is released on the surface of the ovary, where it is picked up by the fimbriated (fringed) ends of the fallopian tube as they sweep back and forth across the ovary. The ovum is transported through the tube by muscular action of the tube and movement of cilia within the tube. Fertilization normally occurs in the distal third of the fallopian tube, near the ovary. The ovum, fertilized or not, enters the uterus about 3 days after its release from the ovary.

### Preparation for Conception in the Male

The male preparation for fertilizing the ovum consists of ejaculation, movement of the sperm in the female reproductive tract, and preparation of the sperm for actual fertilization.

#### EJACULATION

When a male ejaculates during sexual intercourse, 200 to 600 million sperm are deposited in the upper vagina and over the cervix. The sperm are suspended in seminal fluid, which nourishes and protects the sperm from the acidic environment of the vagina. The seminal fluid coagulates slightly after ejaculation to hold the semen deeply in the vagina. The sperm are relatively immobile for about 15 to 30 minutes until other seminal enzymes dissolve the coagulated fluid and allow the sperm to begin moving upward through the cervix.

#### TRANSPORT OF SPERM IN THE FEMALE REPRODUCTIVE TRACT

Whip-like movement of the tails of spermatozoa propels them through the cervix, uterus, and fallopian tubes. Uterine contractions induced by prostaglandins in the seminal fluid enhance movement of the sperm toward the ovum. Only sperm cells enter the cervix. The seminal fluid remains in the vagina.

Many sperm are lost along the way. Some are digested by vaginal enzymes and phagocytes in the female reproductive tract, whereas others simply lose their way, moving into the wrong tube or past the ovum and out into the peritoneal cavity. Only a few hundred reach the fallopian tube where the ovum is located.

#### PREPARATION OF SPERM FOR FERTILIZATION

Sperm are not immediately ready to fertilize the ovum when they are ejaculated. While making the trip to the ovum, the sperm undergo changes that enable one of them to penetrate the protective layers surrounding the ovum (*capacitation*). During capacitation a glycoprotein coat and seminal proteins are removed from the acrosome (tip of the sperm head). After capacitation, the sperm look the same but are more active and can better penetrate the corona radiata and zona pellucida that surround the ovum.

The sperm that reach the ovum release an enzyme (hyaluronidase) to digest a pathway through the corona radiata and zona pellucida. Their tails beat harder to propel them toward the center of the ovum. Eventually, one spermatozoon penetrates the ovum.

### Fertilization

Fertilization occurs when one spermatozoon enters the ovum and the two nuclei containing the parents' chromosomes merge (Fig. 6–3).

#### ENTRY OF ONE SPERMATOZOON INTO THE OVUM

Entry of a spermatozoon into the ovum has two results. First, changes in the zona pellucida surrounding the ovum prevent other sperm from entering. Second, the ovum, which has been suspended in the middle of its second meiotic division since just before ovulation, completes meiosis. This results in a nucleus with 23 chromosomes and expulsion of a second nonfunctional polar body. The mature ovum now contains 23 unpaired chromosomes, 22 autosomes and one X chromosome, in its nucleus.

#### FUSION OF THE NUCLEI OF SPERM AND OVUM

Once a spermatozoon has penetrated the ovum, fusion of their nuclei begins. The sperm head enlarges, and the tail degenerates. The nuclei of the gametes move toward the center of the ovum, where the membranes surrounding their nuclei touch and dissolve. The 23 chromosomes from the sperm mingle with the 23 from the ovum, restoring the diploid number to 46, as in all other body cells. Fertilization is complete, and cell division can begin when the nuclei of the sperm and ovum unite.

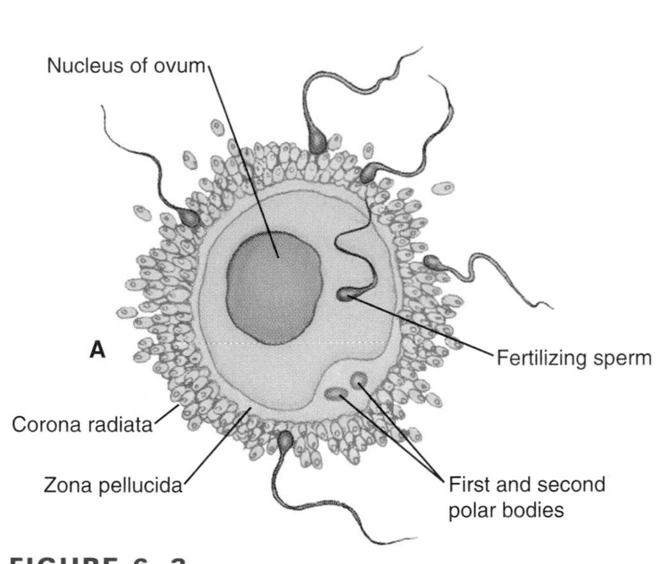


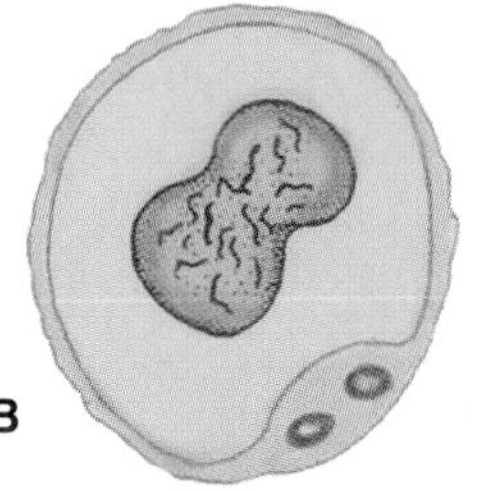


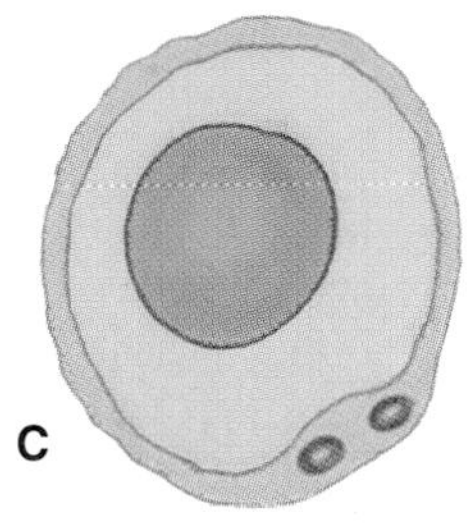


**FIGURE 6–3**

Process of fertilization. A, A sperm enters the ovum. B, The 23 chromosomes from the sperm mingle with the 23 chromosomes from the ovum, restoring the diploid number to 46. C, The fertilized ovum is now called a zygote and is ready for the first mitotic cell division.

**CHECK YOUR READING**

4. Where does fertilization usually occur?
5. What are the purposes of the seminal fluid?
6. What occurs when a spermatozoon penetrates the ovum?
7. When is fertilization complete and a new human conceived?

## Pre-embryonic Period

The pre-embryonic period is the first 2 weeks after conception. Prenatal development begins in the fallopian tube for the first 2 days after fertilization. On about the third day the zygote enters the uterus. Figure 6–4 illustrates the period from fertilization through implantation.

### Initiation of Cell Division

The zygote divides into two cells, then four, then eight cells. Up to the 16-cell stage, the cells become smaller with each division, so they occupy about the same amount of space as the original ovum. When the conceptus is a solid ball of 12 to 16 cells, it is called a *morula* because it resembles a mulberry.

The outer cells of the morula secrete fluid, forming a sac of cells with an inner cell mass placed off-center within the sac (*blastocyst*). The inner cell mass develops into the fetus. Part of the outer layer of cells develops into the placenta and fetal membranes.

### Entry of the Zygote into the Uterus

The conceptus enters the uterus about 3 days after conception, when it contains about 100 cells. It lingers in the uterus another 2 to 4 days before beginning implantation. The endometrium, now called the decidua, is in the secretory phase of the reproductive cycle, 1½ weeks before the woman would otherwise begin her menstrual period. The endometrial glands are secreting at their maximum, providing rich fluids to nourish the conceptus before placental circulation is established. The endometrial spiral arteries are well developed in the secretory phase, providing easy access for developing the placental blood supply.

### Implantation in the Decidua

The conceptus carries a small supply of nutrients for early cell division. However, implantation at the proper time and location in the uterus is crucial for continued development. Implantation (*nidation*) is not sudden but is a gradual process beginning 6 days after conception. Implantation is complete by the 10th day. During the relatively long process of implantation, embryonic structures also are developing.

### Maintaining the Decidua

Implantation and survival of the conceptus are critically dependent on a continuing supply of estrogen and progesterone to maintain the decidua in the

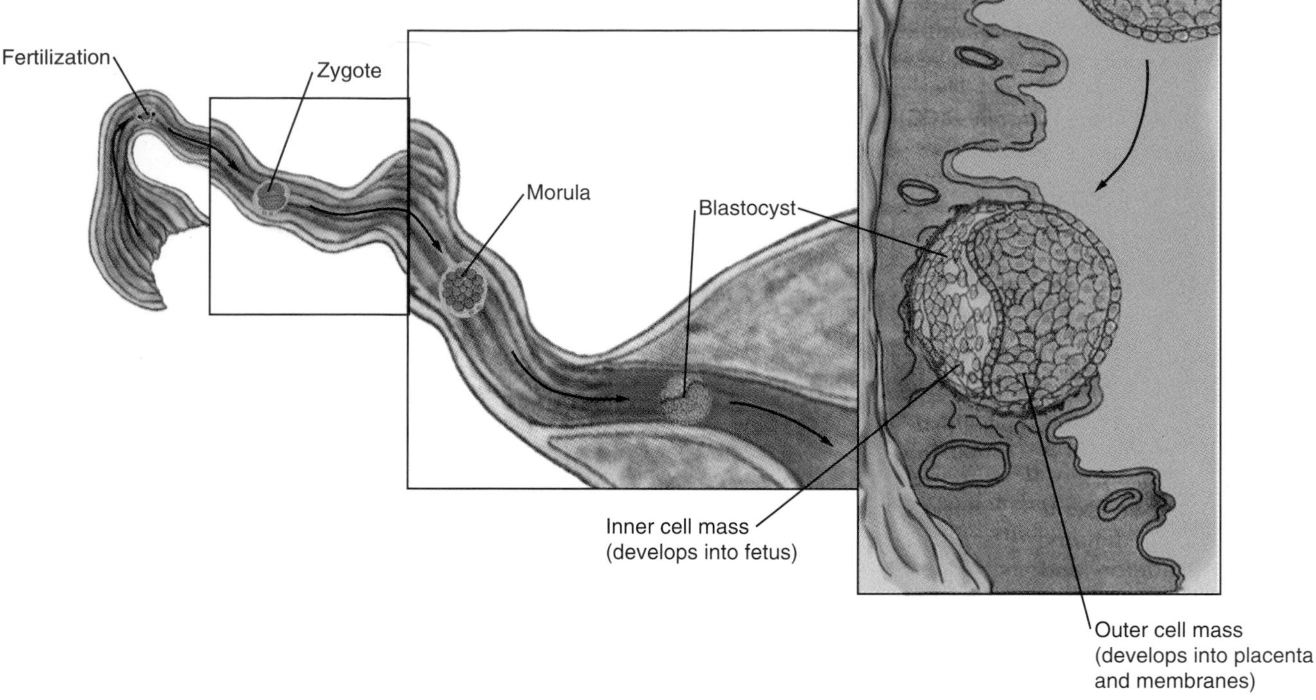


**FIGURE 6–4**

Prenatal development from fertilization through implantation of the blastocyst. Implantation gradually occurs from the sixth through the 10th day. Implantation is complete on the 10th day.

secretory phase. The zygote secretes human chorionic gonadotropin (hCG) to signal the woman's body that a pregnancy has begun. With continued hCG production by the conceptus, the corpus luteum persists and continues secreting estrogen and progesterone.

## Location of Implantation

The conceptus must be in the right place at the right time for normal implantation to occur. The site of implantation is important because that is where the placenta develops. Normal implantation occurs in the upper uterus (fundus). The fundus is the best area for implantation and placental development for three reasons:

- The fundus is richly supplied with blood for optimal fetal gas exchange and nutrition.
- The uterine lining is thick in the fundus, preventing the placenta from attaching so deeply that it cannot be easily expelled after birth.
- Fundal implantation limits blood loss after birth because strong interlacing muscle fibers in this area compress open vessels after the placenta detaches.

## Mechanism of Implantation

Enzymes produced by the conceptus erode the decidua, tapping maternal sources of nutrition. Primary chorionic villi are tiny projections on the surface of the conceptus that extend into the decidua basalis that lies between the conceptus and the wall of the uterus. The chorionic villi eventually form the fetal side of the placenta; the decidua basalis forms the maternal side of the placenta (see p. 111).

At this early stage, nutritive fluid passes to the embryo by *diffusion* (passive movement across a cell membrane from an area of higher concentration to one of lower concentration) because no circulatory system is yet established. The conceptus is fully embedded within the mother's uterine decidua by 10 days, and the site of implantation is almost invisible.

As the conceptus implants, usually near the time of the next expected menstrual period, a small amount of bleeding ("spotting") may occur at the site. Implantation bleeding may be confused with a normal menstrual period, particularly if the woman's menstrual periods are normally light. Implantation bleeding may cause inaccurate calculation of a pregnancy's duration if it is counted as a normal menstrual period.

**✓ CHECK YOUR READING**

8. When does implantation occur?
9. What are the advantages of implantation in the uterine fundus?
10. How is the embryo nourished before the placenta develops?

## TABLE 6–2 TIMETABLE OF PRENATAL DEVELOPMENT BASED ON FERTILIZATION AGE*

| Nervous/Sensory System | Cardiorespiratory System | Digestive System | Genitourinary System | Musculoskeletal System | Integumentary System |
|---|---|---|---|---|---|
| | | **3 WEEKS: 1.5 mm CRL** | | | |
| Flat neural plate begins closing to form neural tube. Neural tube still open at each end. | Heart consists of 2 parallel tubes that fuse into a single tube. Contractions of heart tube begin. Chorionic villi of early placenta connect with heart. | Endoderm (inner germ layer) will become digestive tract. | | Paired, cube-shaped swellings (somites) appear and will form most of the head and trunk skeleton. Muscle, bone, and cartilage develop from mesoderm. | Epidermis (outer skin layer) will develop from ectoderm (outer germ layer). Dermis (deep skin layer) and connective tissue will develop from mesoderm (middle germ layer). |
| | | **4 WEEKS: 4.0 mm CRL** | | | |
| Neural tube closed at each end. Cranial end of neural tube will form brain, caudal end will form spinal cord. Eye development begins as an outgrowth of forebrain. Nose development begins as two pits. Inner ear begins developing from hind brain. | Heart begins partitioning into 4 chambers and begins beating. Blood circulating through embryonic vessels and chorionic villi. Tracheal development begins as a bud on the upper gut and branches into two bronchial buds. | Development of primitive gut as embryo folds laterally. Stomach begins as a widening of the tube-shaped primitive gut. Liver, gallbladder, and biliary ducts begin as a bud from primitive gut. | Primordial germ (reproductive) cells are present on embryonic yolk sac. | Upper limb buds are present and look like flippers. Lower limb buds appear. | Mammary ridges that will develop into mammary glands appear. |
| | | **6 WEEKS: 13 mm CRL** | | | |
| Development of pituitary gland and cranial nerves. Head sharply flexed because of rapid brain growth. Eyelid development beginning. External ear development begins in neck region as six swellings. | Blood formation primarily in liver. Three right and two left lung lobes develop as outgrowths of the right and left bronchi. | Most intestines are contained within the umbilical cord because the liver and kidneys occupy most of the abdominal cavity. Stomach nearing final form. Development of upper and lower jaws. | Kidneys are near bladder in the pelvis. Kidneys occupy much of the abdominal cavity. Primordial germ cells incorporated into developing gonads. Male and female gonads are identical in appearance. | Arms paddle-shaped, fingers webbed. Feet and toes develop similarly, but a few days later than arms and hands. Bones cartilaginous, but ossification of skull begins. | Mammary glands begin development. Tooth buds for primary (deciduous) teeth begin developing. |
| | | **8 WEEKS: 30 mm CRL** | | | |
| Spinal cord stops at end of vertebral column. Taste buds begin developing. Eyelids fuse. Ears have final form but are low-set. | Heart partitioned into 4 chambers. Heart beat detectable with ultrasound. Additional branching of bronchi. | Stomach has reached final form. Lips are fused. Intestines remain in umbilical cord. | Testes begin developing under influence of Y chromosome. Ovaries will develop if a Y chromosome is not present. External genitalia begin to differentiate but still appear quite similar. | Fingers and toes still webbed, but distinct by end of eighth week. Bones begin to ossify. Joints resemble those of adults. | |
| | | **10 WEEKS: 61 mm CRL WEIGHT 14 g** | | | |
| Head flexion still present, but straighter. Eyelids closed and fused. Top of external ear is slightly below eye level. | May be possible to detect heart beat with Doppler transducer. Blood produced in spleen and lymphatic tissue. | Intestines contained within abdominal cavity as growth of this cavity catches up with digestive system development. Digestive tract patent from mouth to anus. | Kidneys are in their adult position. Male and female external genitalia have different appearance but are still easily confused. | Toes distinct, soles face each other. | Fingernails begin developing. Tooth buds for permanent teeth begin developing below those for primary teeth. |

*Table continued on following page*

**TABLE 6-2 TIMETABLE OF PRENATAL DEVELOPMENT BASED ON FERTILIZATION AGE*** *Continued*

| Nervous/Sensory System | Cardiorespiratory System | Digestive System | Genitourinary System | Musculoskeletal System | Integumentary System |
|---|---|---|---|---|---|
| **12 WEEKS: 87 mm CRL WEIGHT 45 g** | | | | | |
| Surface of brain is smooth, without sulci (grooves) or gyri (convolutions). Nasal septum and palate complete development. | Heart beat should be detected with Doppler transducer. | Sucking reflex present. Bile formed by liver. | Kidneys begin producing urine. Male and female external genitalia can be distinguished by appearance. | Limbs are long and thin. Involuntary muscles of viscera develop. | Downy lanugo begins developing at end of this week. |
| **16 WEEKS: 140 mm CRL WEIGHT 200 g** | | | | | |
| | Pulmonary vascular system developing rapidly. | Fetus swallows amniotic fluid and produces meconium (bowel contents). | Urine excreted into amniotic fluid. | Lower limbs reach final relative length, longer than upper limbs. A woman who has been pregnant before may begin to feel fetal movements. | External ears have enough cartilage to stand away from head somewhat. Blood vessels easily visible through the delicate skin. Fingerprints developing. |
| **20 WEEKS: 160 mm CRL WEIGHT 460 g** | | | | | |
| Myelination of nerves begins, and continues through first year of postnatal life. | Heartbeat should be detectable with regular fetoscope. | Peristalsis well developed. | Over 40% of nephrons are mature and functioning. Testes contained in abdomen, but begin descent toward scrotum. Primordial follicles of ovary develop. | Fetal movements felt by mother and may be palpable by an experienced examiner. | Skin is thin and covered with vernix caseosa. Brown fat production complete. Nipples begin development. |
| **24 WEEKS: 230 mm CRL WEIGHT 820 g** | | | | | |
| Spinal cord ends at level of first sacral vertebra because of more rapid growth of vertebral canal. | Primitive thin-walled alveoli (air sacs) have developed and are surrounded by capillary network. Surfactant production begins in lungs to reduce surface tension within alveoli. Respiration possible, but most fetuses die if born at this time. | | | Fetus is active. Fetal movements become progressively more noticeable to both mother and examiner. | Body appearance lean. Skin wrinkled and red. Fingerprints and footprints developed. Fingernails present. Eyebrows and lashes present. |
| **28 WEEKS: 270 mm CRL WEIGHT 1300 g** | | | | | |
| Major sulci and gyri are present. Eyelids no longer fused after 26 weeks. Responds to bitter substances on tongue. | Erythrocyte formation shifts completely to bone marrow. Sufficient alveoli, surfactant, and capillary network to allow respiratory function, although respiratory distress syndrome is common. Many infants born at this time survive with intensive care. | | Testes begin descent into scrotum. | | Skin slightly wrinkled, but smoothing out as subcutaneous fat is deposited under it. |

**TABLE 6–2 TIMETABLE OF PRENATAL DEVELOPMENT BASED ON FERTILIZATION AGE* *Continued***

| Nervous/Sensory System | Cardiorespiratory System | Digestive System | Genitourinary System | Musculoskeletal System | Integumentary System |
|---|---|---|---|---|---|
| | | **32 WEEKS: 300 mm CRL WEIGHT 2100 g** | | | |
| | | | Testes enter scrotum. | | Skin smooth and pigmented. Large vessels visible beneath skin. Fingernails reach fingertips. Lanugo disappearing. |
| | | **38 WEEKS: 360 mm CRL WEIGHT 3400 g** | | | |
| Sulci and gyri developed. Visual acuity about 20/600 at birth. | Newborn infant has about one-eighth to one-sixth the number of alveoli of an adult. Well-developed ability to exchange gas. | | Both testes usually palpable in scrotum at birth. The newborn girl's ovaries contain about 1 million follicles. No new ones are formed after birth. | | Fetus plump and skin smooth. Vernix caseosa present in major body creases. Lanugo present on shoulders and upper back only. Fingernails extend beyond the fingertips. Ear cartilage firm. |

*Fertilization age is about 2 weeks less than gestational age.
*Abbreviation*: CRL, crown-rump length.

## Embryonic Period

The embryonic period of development extends from the beginning of the third week through the eighth week after conception. Basic structures of all major body organs are completed during the embryonic period. Table 6–2 presents major developments in body systems during prenatal life. Figure 6–5 illustrates the external appearance of the embryo from the third through the eighth week after conception.

### Differentiation of Cells

The embryo progresses from having cells with essentially identical functions (undifferentiated) to differentiated, or specialized, body cells. By the end of the eighth week, all major organ systems are in place and many are functioning, although in a simple way.

Development of the specialized structures is controlled by three factors: (1) the genetic information in the chromosomes received from the parents, (2) interaction between adjacent tissues, and (3) timing. Although basic instructions are carried within the chromosomes, one tissue may induce change toward greater specialization in another, but only if a signal between the two tissues occurs at a specific time during development. In this way, structures develop with appropriate size and relationships to each other.

During the embryonic period, structures are vulnerable to damage from teratogens because they are developing rapidly; normal development of one structure often requires normal and properly timed development of another. Unfortunately, a woman may not even realize that she is pregnant at this sensitive time. For this reason, the possibility of pregnancy should be explored with her before drugs or diagnostic procedures, such as radiography, are prescribed. Some agents may be damaging at one time during pregnancy but not at another. Others may be damaging at any time during pregnancy. Appendix C contains information about substances that may cause prenatal damage.

### Weekly Developments

Development occurs simultaneously in all of the embryonic organ systems. Changes beginning the second week after conception are described next. Development of the embryo and fetus proceeds in a cephalocaudal (head-to-toe) and a central-to-peripheral direction. This developmental pattern continues after birth.

#### SECOND WEEK

Implantation is complete by the end of the second week. The most growth occurs in the outer cells (*trophoblast*), which eventually become the fetal part of the placenta. The inner cell mass that will develop

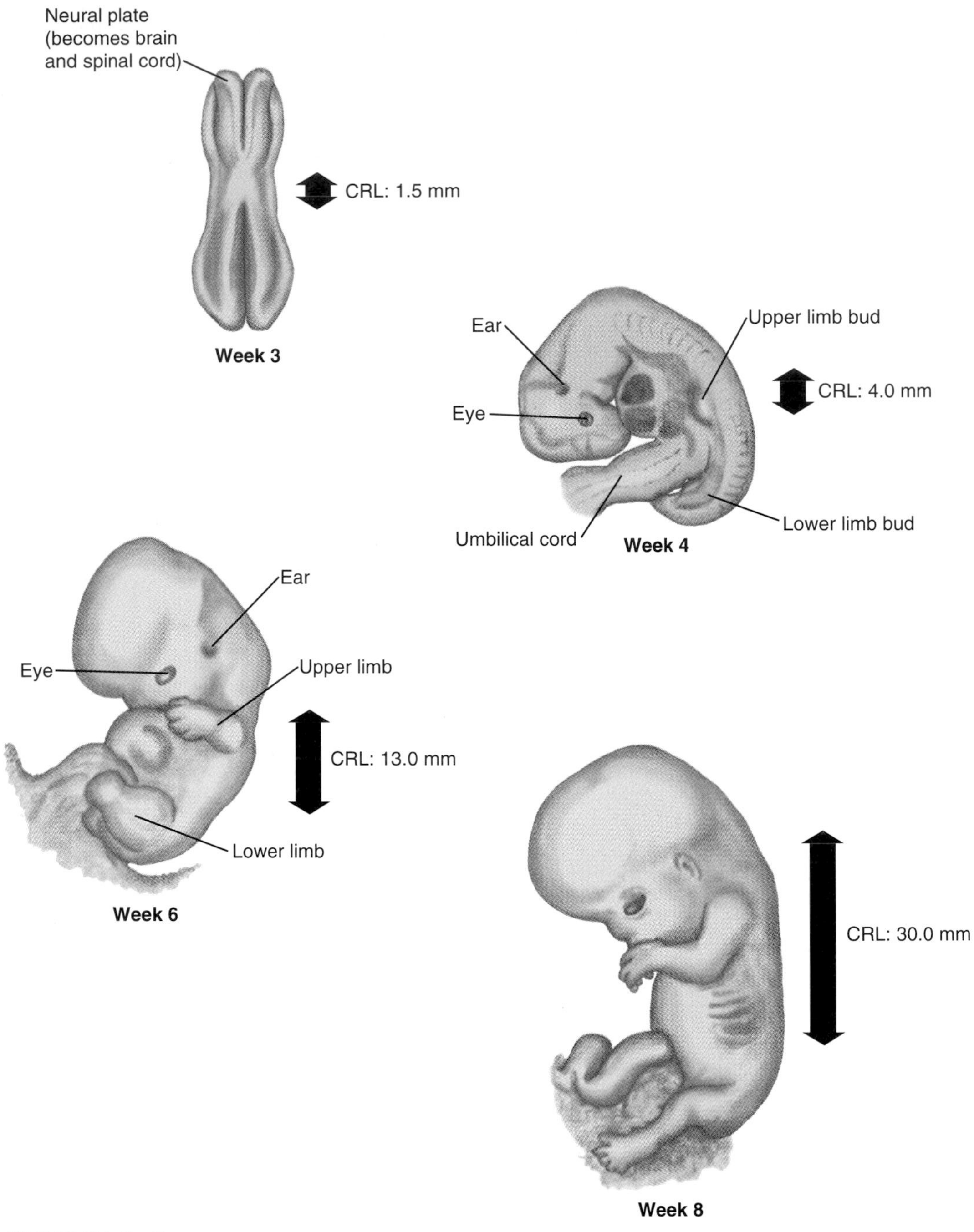


**FIGURE 6–5**

Embryonic development from 3 weeks through the eighth week after fertilization. CRL, crown-to-rump length.

into the baby becomes flattened into the *embryonic disk*. Cells that eventually form part of the fetal membranes develop.

### THIRD WEEK

Many women miss their first menstrual period during the third week of pregnancy. The embryonic disk develops three layers (*germ layers*) that, in turn, give rise to major organ systems of the body. The three germ layers are the ectoderm, the mesoderm, and the endoderm. Table 6–3 lists structures that develop from each germ layer.

The central nervous system begins developing during the third week. A thickened flat neural plate appears, extending toward the end of the embryonic disk that will become the head. The neural plate develops a longitudinal groove that folds to form the neural tube. At the end of the third week, the neural tube is fused in the middle but is still open at each end.

**TABLE 6–3 DERIVATIVES OF THE THREE GERM LAYERS**

| Ectoderm | Mesoderm | Endoderm |
|---|---|---|
| Brain and spinal cord | Cartilage | Lining of gastrointestinal and respiratory tracts |
| Peripheral nervous system | Bone | Tonsils |
| Pituitary gland | Connective tissue | Thyroid |
| Sensory epithelium of the eye, ear, and nose | Muscle tissue | Parathyroid |
| Epidermis | Heart | Thymus |
| Hair | Blood vessels | Liver |
| Nails | Blood cells | Pancreas |
| Subcutaneous glands | Lymphatic system | Lining of urinary bladder and urethra |
| Mammary glands | Spleen | Lining of ear canal |
| Tooth enamel | Kidneys | |
| | Adrenal cortex | |
| | Ovaries | |
| | Testes | |
| | Reproductive system | |
| | Lining membranes (pericardial, pleural, peritoneal) | |

Early heart development consists of a pair of parallel heart tubes that run longitudinally and join. The primitive heart begins beating at 21 to 22 days. Vessels developing in the chorionic villi and membranes join the heart tube. Primitive blood cells arise from the endoderm lining the distal blood vessels.

#### FOURTH WEEK

The shape of the embryo changes. It folds at the head and tail end and laterally. The embryo resembles a C-shaped cylinder by the end of the fourth week. A "tail" is apparent during the embryonic period because the brain and spinal cord develop more rapidly than other systems. The tail becomes less prominent and finally disappears as the rest of the body catches up with growth of the central nervous system.

The neural tube completes closure during the fourth week. If the neural tube does not close, defects such as anencephaly and spina bifida result.

Formation of the face and upper respiratory tract begins. Beginnings of the internal ear and the eye are apparent. The upper extremities appear as buds on the lateral body walls.

Because the embryo is sharply flexed anteriorly, the heart is near the embryo's mouth. Partitioning of the heart into four chambers begins during the fourth week and is completed by the end of the sixth week.

The lower respiratory tract begins growth as a branch off the upper digestive tract, which is tubular at this time. Gradually, the esophagus and trachea separate completely. The trachea branches to form the right and left bronchi. These bronchi in turn branch to form the three lobes of the right lung and two lobes of the left lung. Continued branching of the bronchi eventually forms the terminal air sacs (*alveoli*). The alveoli proliferate and become surrounded by a rich capillary network that enables oxygen and carbon dioxide exchange at birth.

#### FIFTH WEEK

The head is very large because the brain grows rapidly during the fifth week. The heart is beating and developing four chambers. Upper limb buds are paddle shaped with obvious notches between the fingers. Lower limbs form slightly later than upper ones. Lower limbs are also paddle shaped, but the area between the toes is not as well defined as the division between the fingers.

#### SIXTH WEEK

The head is prominent because of rapid development and is bent over the chest. The heart reaches its final four-chambered form. Upper and lower extremities continue to become more defined.

The eye continues to develop, and the beginning of the external ear is apparent as six small bumps near each side of the neck. Facial development begins with eyes, ears, and nasal pits widely separated, aligned with the body walls. Gradually, the embryo grows so that the face comes together in the midline.

#### SEVENTH WEEK

General growth and refinement of all systems occur. The face becomes more human looking. The eyelids begin to grow, and the extremities become longer and better defined. The trunk elongates and straightens, although a C-shaped spinal curve is still present in the newborn at birth.

The intestines have been growing faster than the abdominal cavity during the embryonic period. The relatively large liver and kidneys also occupy much of the abdominal cavity. Therefore, most of the intestines are contained within the umbilical cord while the abdominal cavity grows to accommodate them. The abdomen is large enough to contain all its normal contents by 10 weeks.

#### EIGHTH WEEK

The embryo has a definite human form, and refinements to all systems continue. The ears are low set but are approaching their final location. The eyes are pigmented but not yet fully covered by eyelids. Fingers and toes are stubby but well defined. The external genitalia begin to differentiate, but male and female characteristics are not distinct until after the 10th week.

**CHECK YOUR READING**

11. Why is the embryo particularly susceptible to damage from teratogens?
12. How does the lower respiratory tract develop?
13. Why are the intestines mostly contained within the umbilical cord until the 10th week?

## Fetal Period

The fetal period represents the longest part of prenatal development. It begins 9 weeks after conception and ends with birth. All major systems are present in their basic form. Dramatic growth and refinement in the structure and function of all organ systems occur during the fetal period. Teratogens may damage already formed structures but are less likely to cause major structural alterations. The central nervous system is vulnerable to damaging agents through the entire pregnancy. Figure 6–6 illustrates growth and development during the fetal period.

### Weeks 9 Through 12

At the beginning of this period, the head is large, about half the total length of the fetus. The body begins growing faster than the head. The extremities approach their final relative lengths, although the legs remain proportionally shorter than the arms. The first fetal movements begin but are too slight for the mother to detect.

The face is broad, with a wide nose and widely spaced eyes. The eyes close at 9 weeks and reopen about 26 weeks. The ears appear low set because the mandible is still small.

The intestinal contents that were partly contained within the umbilical cord enter the abdomen as the capacity of the abdominal cavity catches up with them in size. Blood formation occurs primarily in the liver during the ninth week but shifts to the spleen by the end of the 12th week. The fetus begins producing urine during this period, excreting it into the amniotic fluid.

Internal differences in males and females begin to be apparent in the seventh week. External genitalia look similar until the end of the ninth week. By the end of the 12th week, the fetal sex can be determined by the appearance of the external genitalia.

### Weeks 13 Through 16

The fetus grows rapidly in length, so the head becomes smaller in proportion to the total length. Movements strengthen, and some women, particularly those who have been pregnant before, are able to detect them (*quickening*).

The face looks human because the eyes face fully forward. The ears near their final position, in line with the eyes.

### Weeks 17 Through 20

Fetal movements feel like fluttering or "butterflies." Some women may not recognize these subtle sensations for what they are.

Changes in the skin and hair are evident. *Vernix caseosa*, a fatty cheese-like secretion of the fetal sebaceous glands, covers the skin to protect it from constant exposure to amniotic fluid. *Lanugo* is fine, downy hair that covers the fetal body. Lanugo helps the vernix adhere to the skin. Both vernix and lanugo diminish as the fetus reaches term. Eyebrows and head hair appear.

*Brown fat* is a special heat-producing fat that is deposited during this period. It is located on the back of the neck, behind the sternum, and around the kidneys. Brown fat helps the neonate maintain temperature stability after birth.

### Weeks 21 Through 24

The fetus continues growing and gaining weight, although he or she is thin and has little subcutaneous fat. The skin is translucent and looks red because the capillaries are close to its fragile surface.

The lungs begin to produce *surfactant*, a surface-active lipid substance that makes it easier for the baby to breathe after birth. Surfactant reduces surface tension in the lung alveoli and keeps them from collapsing with each breath. A ratio of two substances in the amniotic fluid is used to estimate the amount of surfactant and the maturity of the fetal lungs: lecithin (L) and sphingomyelin (S). These substances are initially present in equal amounts. During the middle of the third trimester, the level of lecithin increases while the sphingomyelin level remains constant. At about 35 weeks of gestation, the concentration of lecithin is about twice that of sphin-

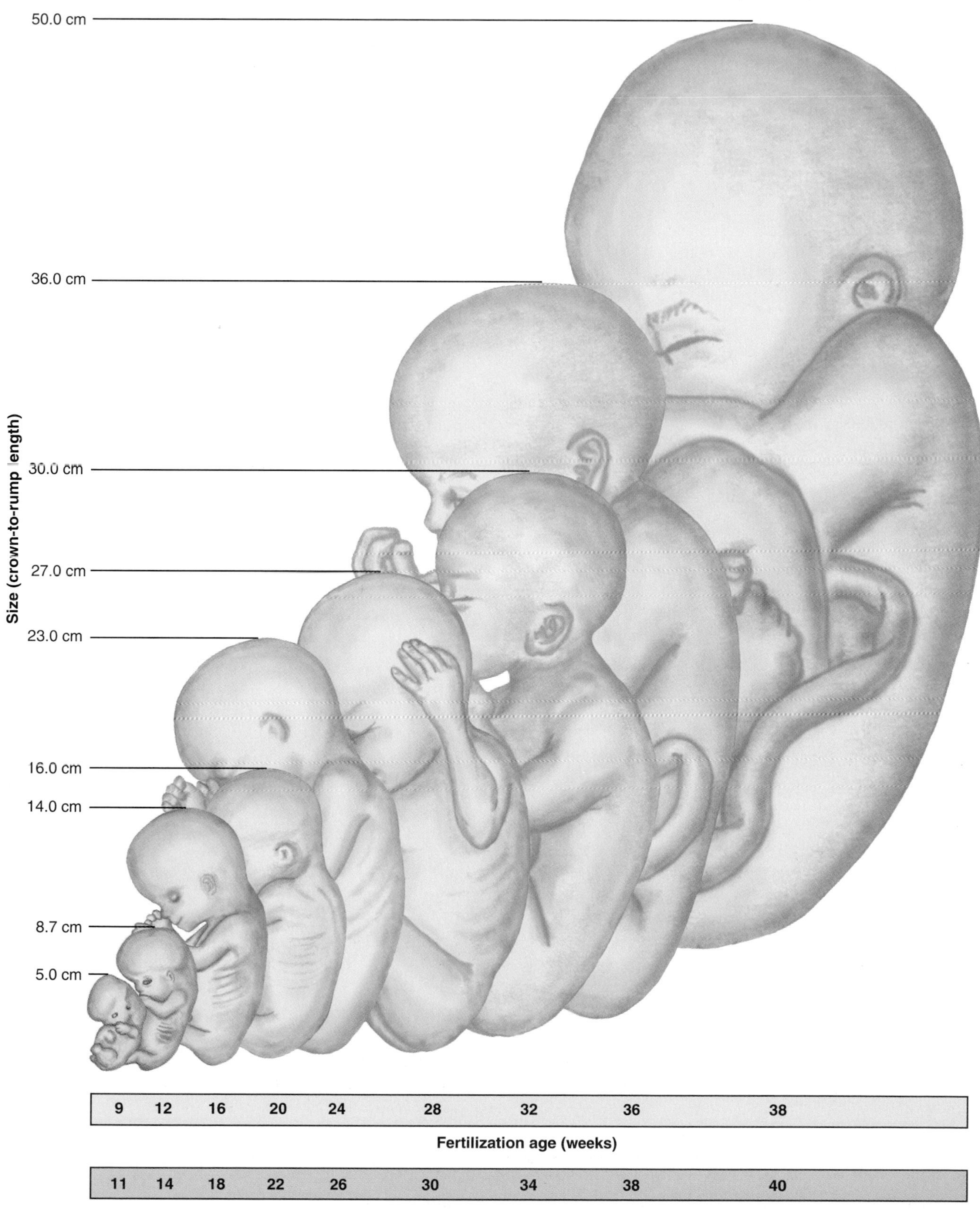


**FIGURE 6–6**

Fetal development from 9 weeks of fertilization age through 38 weeks of fertilization age. The gestational age, measured from the first day of the last menstrual period, is about 2 weeks longer than the fertilization age.

gomyelin (L/S ratio 2:1), which indicates lung maturity.

The capillary network surrounding the alveoli is increasing but is still very immature, although some gas exchange is possible. A fetus born at this time is unlikely to survive because adequate gas exchange is not possible. Other systems are extremely immature as well.

### Weeks 25 Through 28

The fetus may survive if born during this period because of maturation of the lungs, pulmonary capillaries, and central nervous system. The fetus becomes plumper and smoother skinned as subcutaneous fat is deposited under the skin. The skin gradually becomes less red. The eyes, closed since 9 weeks, reopen. Head hair is abundant. Blood formation shifts from the spleen to the bone marrow.

During early pregnancy, the fetus floats freely within the amniotic sac. However, the fetus usually assumes a head-down position during this time for two reasons:

- The uterus is shaped like an inverted egg. The overall shape of the fetus in flexion is similar, with the head being the small pole of the egg shape and the buttocks, flexed legs, and feet being the larger pole.
- The fetal head is heavier than the feet, and gravity causes the head to drift downward in the pool of amniotic fluid.

The head-down position is most favorable for normal birth as well.

### Weeks 29 Through 32

The skin is pigmented according to race and is smooth. Larger vessels are visible over the abdomen, but small capillaries cannot be seen. Toenails are present, and fingernails extend to the fingertips. The fetus has more subcutaneous fat, rounding the body contours. If the fetus is born during this period, chances of survival are good.

### Weeks 33 Through 38

Growth of all body systems continues until birth, but the rate of growth slows as full term approaches. The fetus is mainly gaining weight. The pulmonary system matures to enable efficient and unlabored breathing after birth.

The well-nourished term fetus is rotund, with abundant subcutaneous fat. At birth, boys are slightly heavier than girls. The skin is pink to brownish pink, depending on race. Lanugo may be present over the forehead, upper back, and upper arms. Vernix often remains in major creases, such as the groin and axillae.

The testes are in the scrotum. Breasts of both male and female infants are enlarged, and breast tissue is palpable beneath the areola and nipple.

Full term ranges from 36 to 40 weeks of fertilization age, or 38 to 42 weeks of gestational age. *Because conception occurs about 2 weeks after the first day of the last menstrual period, the fertilization age, used in this chapter, is about 2 weeks shorter than the gestational age. However, gestational age is most commonly used in practice because the last menstrual period provides a known marker, whereas most women do not know exactly when they conceived.*

**✓CHECK YOUR READING**

14. What is the purpose of each of these fetal structures or substances: Vernix caseosa? Lanugo? Brown fat? Surfactant?
15. Why does the fetus usually assume a head-down position in the uterus?
16. What is the difference between fertilization age and gestational age? Which term is more commonly used and why?

## Auxiliary Structures

Three auxiliary structures sustain the pregnancy and permit normal prenatal development: the placenta, the umbilical cord, and the fetal membranes. These structures develop simultaneously with the baby's development. Their structure and function are discussed, as is the route of fetal circulation.

### Placenta

The placenta is a thick, disk-shaped organ. The placenta has two components, maternal and fetal (Fig. 6–7). Its major functions are (1) metabolic, (2) transfer of substances between mother and fetus, and (3) endocrine. The fetal side is smooth, with branching vessels covering the membrane-covered surface. The maternal side is rough where it attaches to the uterus (see Fig. 12–14).

The umbilical cord is normally inserted on the fetal side of the placenta, near the center. However, it may insert off-center or even out on the fetal membranes. Figure 6–8 illustrates the normal insertion and variations from normal.

During early pregnancy, the placenta is larger than the embryo or fetus. However, the fetus grows faster than the placenta, so that the placenta is about one sixth the weight of the fetus at the end of a term pregnancy.

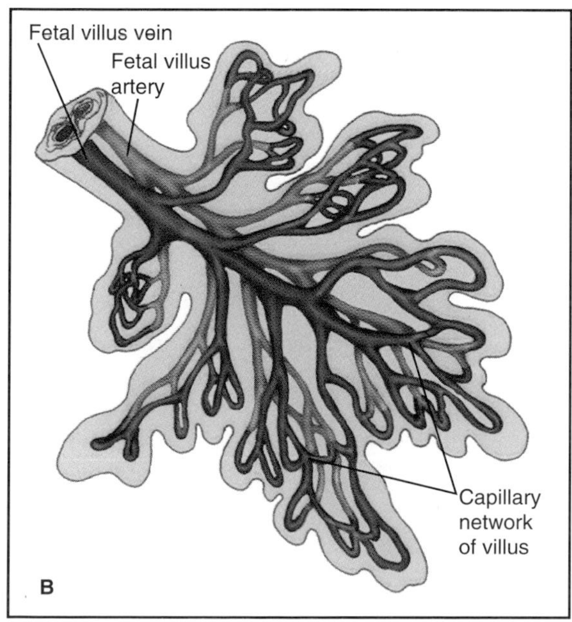


**FIGURE 6–7**

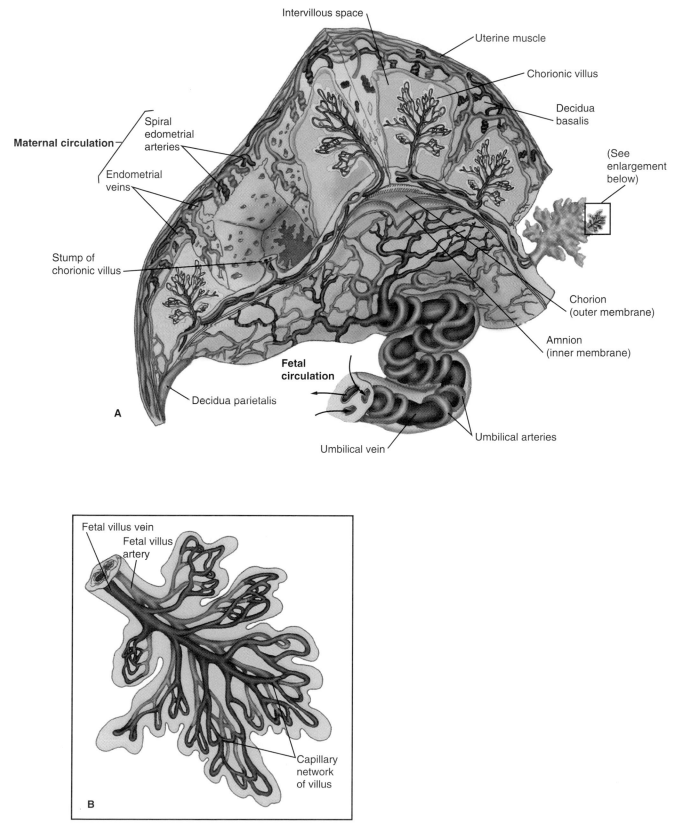

A, Placental structure, showing relationship of placenta, fetal membranes, and uterus. Arrows indicate the direction of blood flow between the fetus and placenta through the umbilical arteries and vein. Blood from the woman bathes the fetal chorionic villi within the intervillous spaces to allow exchange of oxygen, nutrients, and waste products without gross mixing of maternal and fetal blood. B, Structure of a chorionic villus, showing its fetal capillary network.

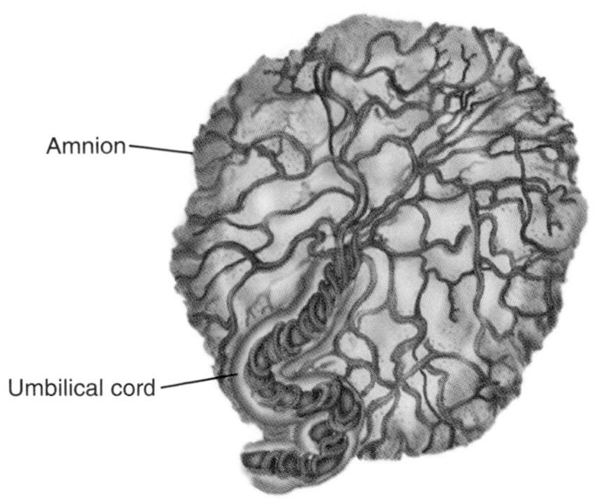


Normal placenta, with insertion of umbilical cord near center and branching of fetal umbilical vessels over the surface

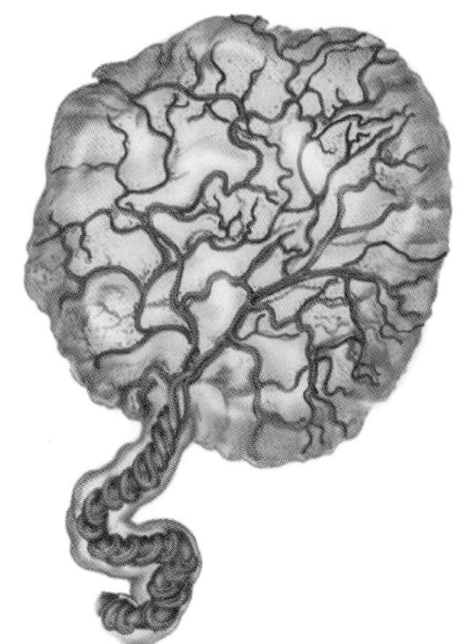

Placenta with cord inserted near margin of placenta

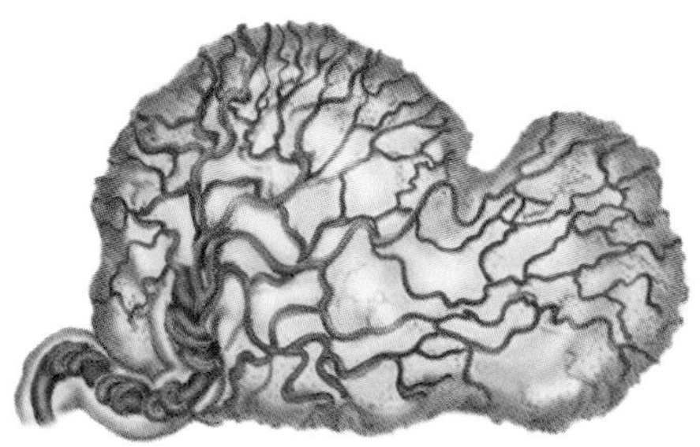

Placenta with a small accessory lobe

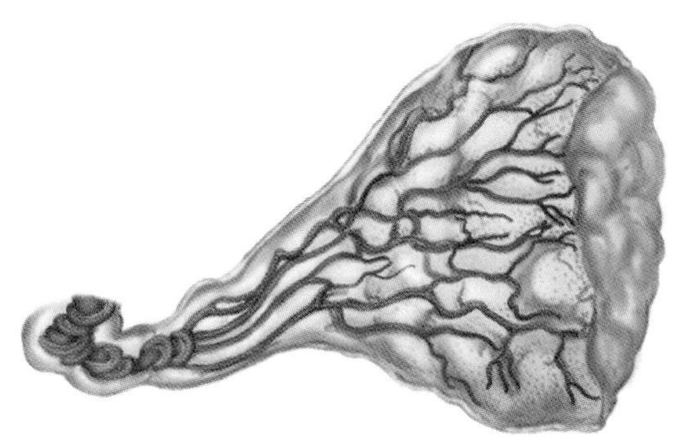

Velamentous insertion of umbilical cord. Cord vessels branch far out on membranes. When membranes rupture, fetal umbilical vessels may be torn and the fetus can hemorrhage.

**FIGURE 6–8**

Placental variations.

### MATERNAL COMPONENT

**Development.** When conception occurs, cells of the decidua undergo changes that promote early nutrition of the embryo and enable most of the uterine lining to be shed after birth. These changes convert endometrial cells into the *decidua*. In addition to providing nourishment for the embryo, the decidua may protect the mother from uncontrolled invasion of fetal placental tissue into the uterine wall.

There are three decidual layers:

- The *decidua basalis* underlies the developing embryo and forms the maternal side of the placenta.
- The *decidua capsularis* overlies the embryo and bulges into the uterine cavity as the embryo and fetus grow.
- The *decidua parietalis* lines the rest of the uterine cavity. By about 22 weeks of gestation, the decidua capsularis fuses with the decidua parietalis, filling the uterine cavity.

**Circulation in the Maternal Side.** Maternal and fetal blood do not mix in the placenta, although they flow very close to each other. Exchange of substances between mother and fetus occurs within the *intervillous spaces* of the placenta. While in the intervillous space, maternal blood is briefly outside her circulatory system. About 150 ml of maternal blood is contained within the intervillous space, and it is changed about three to four times per minute.

Maternal blood spurts into the intervillous spaces through 80 to 100 spiral arteries in the decidua. After the oxygenated and nutrient-bearing maternal blood washes over the chorionic villi containing the fetal vessels, it returns to the maternal circulation through the endometrial veins for elimination of fetal waste products.

### FETAL COMPONENT

**Development.** The fetal side of the placenta develops from the outer cell layer (trophoblast) of the blastocyst at the same time that the inner cell mass develops into the embryo and fetus. The primary chorionic villi are the initial structures that eventually form the fetal side of the placenta.

**Circulation in the Fetal Side.** The umbilical cord contains the umbilical arteries and vein to transport blood between the fetus and placenta. Tiny finger-like projections (*chorionic villi*) are bathed by oxygen-rich and nutrient-rich maternal blood in the maternal intervillous spaces. Each chorionic villus is supplied by a tiny fetal artery carrying deoxygenated blood and waste products from the fetus. The vein of the chorionic villus returns oxygenated blood and nutrients to the embryo and fetus.

Capillaries in the chorionic villi are separated from actual contact with the mother's blood by the membranes of each villus. This arrangement allows contact close enough for exchange and avoids mixing of maternal and fetal blood. The closed fetal circulation is important because the blood types of mother and fetus may not be compatible.

The placental arteries and veins converge in the blood vessels of the umbilical cord. Two umbilical arteries and one umbilical vein transport blood between the fetus and the fetal side of the placenta. Blood is circulated to and from the fetal side of the placenta by the fetal heart.

### METABOLIC FUNCTIONS

The placenta produces some nutrients needed by the embryo and for its own functions. Substances synthesized include glycogen, cholesterol, and fatty acids (Moore, 1993).

### TRANSFER FUNCTIONS

Exchange of oxygen, nutrients, and waste products across the chorionic villi occurs by several methods. Table 6–4 presents examples of how substances are transferred between the mother and the developing fetus.

Placental transfer of harmful substances also may occur. Most substances that enter the mother's blood stream can enter the fetal circulation, and many agents enter it almost immediately.

**Gas Exchange.** A key function of the placenta is respiration. Oxygen and carbon dioxide pass through the placental membrane by simple diffusion. The average oxygen partial pressure ($Po_2$) of maternal blood in the intervillous space is 50 mmHg. The average blood $Po_2$ in the umbilical vein (after oxygenation) is about 30 mmHg (Guyton, 1996).

The fetus can thrive in this low-oxygen environment for three reasons:

- Fetal hemoglobin can carry 20 to 50 percent more oxygen than adult hemoglobin.
- The fetus has a higher oxygen-carrying capacity because of a higher average hemoglobin (14.5 to 22.5 g/dl) and hematocrit value (about 48 to 69 percent).
- Hemoglobin can carry more oxygen at low carbon dioxide partial pressure ($Pco_2$) levels than it can at high ones (Bohr effect). Blood entering the placenta from the fetus has a high $Pco_2$, but carbon dioxide diffuses quickly to the mother's blood, where the $Pco_2$ is lower, reversing the levels of carbon dioxide in maternal and fetal bloods. Therefore, the fetal blood becomes more alkaline and the maternal blood becomes more acidic. This

**TABLE 6–4 MECHANISMS OF PLACENTAL TRANSFER**

| Mechanism | Description | Examples of Substances Transferred |
|---|---|---|
| Simple diffusion | Passive movement of substances across a cell membrane from an area of higher concentration to one of lower concentration | Oxygen and carbon dioxide<br>Carbon monoxide<br>Water<br>Urea and uric acid<br>Most drugs and their metabolites |
| Facilitated diffusion | Passage of substances across a cell membrane by binding with carrier proteins that assist transfer | Glucose |
| Active transport | Transfer of substances across a cell membrane against a pressure or electrical gradient, or from an area of lower concentration to one of higher concentration | Amino acids<br>Water-soluble vitamins<br>Minerals: Calcium, iron, iodine |
| Pinocytosis | Movement of large molecules by ingestion within cells | Maternal IgG class antibodies<br>Some passage of maternal IgA antibodies |

allows the mother's blood to give up oxygen and the fetal blood to combine with oxygen readily.

Fetal $P_{CO_2}$ is only about 2 to 3 mmHg higher than that of maternal blood. However, carbon dioxide is very soluble, allowing it to pass across the placental membrane into maternal blood at this low pressure gradient.

**Nutrient Transfer.** The growing fetus requires a constant supply of nutrients from the pregnant woman. Glucose, fatty acids, vitamins, and electrolytes pass readily across the placenta. Glucose is the major energy source for fetal growth and metabolic activities.

**Waste Removal.** In addition to carbon dioxide, urea, uric acid, and bilirubin are readily transferred from the fetus to the mother for disposal. Because the normal placenta removes wastes for the fetus, metabolic defects such as phenylketonuria are usually not evident until after birth.

**Antibody Transfer.** Many of the immunoglobulin G (IgG) class of antibodies are passed from mother to fetus through the placenta. This confers passive (temporary) immunity to the fetus against diseases such as measles if the mother is immune to them. Passage of antibodies against disease is beneficial because the newborn does not produce antibodies for several months after birth. The preterm infant has little protection from maternal antibodies because they are transferred during late pregnancy.

Passage of antibodies from expectant mother to fetus is not always beneficial. If maternal and fetal blood types are not compatible, the mother either may already have or may produce antibodies against fetal erythrocytes. The mother's antibodies may then destroy the fetal erythrocytes, causing fetal anemia or even fetal death. This situation may occur if the mother is Rh-negative and the fetus is Rh-positive.

**Transfer of Maternal Hormones.** Most maternal protein hormones do not reach the fetus in significant amounts. The female fetus exposed to androgenic hormones may have masculinization of her genitalia, and her true gender may be difficult to determine at birth.

One instance of adverse effects from fetal exposure to hormones is that of "DES daughters." In the late 1940s through the early 1960s, diethylstilbestrol (DES) was prescribed to prevent spontaneous abortion. The drug was ineffective for this purpose, and its use was abandoned. However, as the females who were prenatally exposed to DES reached their teens and early 20s, researchers noted an association between exposure to the DES and reproductive system problems. Vaginal carcinoma was noted in a few adolescent and young adult females. DES daughters have a higher incidence of infertility, spontaneous abortion, and preterm labor than do unexposed women. Although the effects on males have been less publicized than the effects on females, some sons of women who took DES also showed reproductive abnormalities.

#### ENDOCRINE FUNCTIONS

The placenta produces several hormones necessary for normal pregnancy. Human chorionic gonadotropin (hCG) causes the corpus luteum to persist and secrete estrogens and progesterone. As the placenta develops further, it produces estrogens and progesterone, and the corpus luteum gradually regresses after 20 weeks. When a Y chromosome is present in the male fetus, hCG also causes the fetal testes to secrete testosterone necessary for normal development of male reproductive structures.

Human placental lactogen, also called human chorionic somatomammotropin, is a placental hormone that promotes normal nutrition and growth of the fetus and maternal breast development for lactation. The hormone decreases maternal insulin sensitivity and utilization of glucose, making more glucose available for fetal nutrition.

Steroid hormones secreted by the placenta include estrogens and progesterone. Estrogens cause enlargement of the woman's uterus, enlargement of the breasts, growth of the ductal system of the breasts, and enlargement of the external genitalia.

Progesterone is essential for normal continuation of the pregnancy. Progesterone causes the endometrium to change into the decidua, providing nourishment for the early conceptus. Progesterone also reduces the contractions of the uterus to prevent spontaneous abortion. Progesterone acts with estrogens and other hormones to cause growth of the breasts, budding of the alveoli that will secrete milk, and development of secretory characteristics in the alveolar cells.

Other hormones produced by the placenta include human chorionic thyrotropin and human chorionic adrenocorticotropin.

#### CHECK YOUR READING

17. Which structure takes over functions of the corpus luteum?
18. What is the purpose of the intervillous spaces of the placenta?
19. Why is it important that fetal and maternal blood do not actually mix?
20. What factors enable the fetus to thrive in a low-oxygen environment?
21. What are the purposes of these placental hormones: Human chorionic gonadotropin? Human placental lactogen? Estrogen? Progesterone?

### Fetal Membranes and Amniotic Fluid

The two fetal membranes are the *amnion* (inner membrane) and the *chorion* (outer membrane). The two membranes are so close as to be one (the "bag of waters"), but they can be separated. If the membranes rupture in labor, amnion and chorion usually rupture together, releasing the amniotic fluid within the sac.

The amnion is continuous with the surface of the umbilical cord, joining the epithelium of the fetus' abdominal skin. Chorionic villi proliferate over the entire surface of the gestational sac for the first 8 weeks after conception. A conceptus observed at this time looks like a shaggy sphere with the embryo suspended inside. As the embryo grows, it bulges into the uterine cavity. The villi on the outer surface gradually atrophy and form the smooth-surfaced chorion. The remaining villi continue to branch and enlarge to form the fetal side of the placenta.

Amniotic fluid protects the growing fetus and promotes normal prenatal development. Amniotic fluid protects the fetus by

- Cushioning against impacts to the maternal abdomen
- Providing a stable temperature

Amniotic fluid promotes normal prenatal development by

- Allowing symmetric development as the major body surfaces fold toward the midline
- Keeping the membranes from adhering to developing fetal parts
- Allowing room and buoyancy for fetal movement

Amniotic fluid is derived from two sources: (1) fetal urine, and (2) fluid transported from the maternal blood across the amnion. Cast-off fetal epithelial cells and vernix are suspended in the amniotic fluid. The water of the amniotic fluid changes by absorption across the amnion, returning to the mother. The fetus also swallows amniotic fluid and absorbs it in the digestive tract; waste products are returned to the placenta via the umbilical arteries.

The volume of amniotic fluid increases during pregnancy, until it is about 500 to 1500 ml at term (Guyton, 1996; Blackburn & Loper, 1992). An abnormally small quantity of fluid (less than 50 percent of the amount expected for gestation, or under 500 ml at term) is called *oligohydramnios* and may be associated with poor fetal lung development and malformations that result from compression of fetal parts. Oligohydramnios may occur because the kidneys fail to develop, urine excretion is blocked, or placental blood flow is inadequate. *Hydramnios* (also called *polyhydramnios*) is the opposite situation, in which the quantity may exceed 2000 ml. Hydramnios may occur when the fetus has a severe malformation of the central nervous system or gastrointestinal tract that prevents normal ingestion of amniotic fluid.

## Fetal Circulation

The course of fetal blood circulation is from the fetal heart, to the placenta for exchange of oxygen and waste products, and back to the fetus for delivery to fetal tissues (Fig. 6–9A).

### Umbilical Cord

The fetal umbilical cord is the lifeline between the fetus and placenta. It has two arteries that carry deoxygenated blood and waste products away from the fetus to the placenta, where these substances are transferred to the mother's circulation. The umbilical vein carries freshly oxygenated and nutrient-laden blood from the placenta back to the fetus. The umbilical arteries and vein are coiled within the cord to allow them to stretch and prevent obstruction of blood flow through them. The entire cord is cushioned by a soft substance called *Wharton's jelly* to prevent obstruction due to pressure.

### Fetal Circulatory Circuit

Because the fetus does not breathe air, several alterations of the postbirth circulatory route are needed prenatally (see Fig. 6–9A). Three shunts in the fetal circulatory system divert most circulating blood away from the lungs: the ductus venosus, the foramen ovale, and the ductus arteriosus. At birth, the infant's lungs begin oxygenating the blood, so the need to bypass the lungs no longer exists. Shortly after birth, all three shunts are converted to functions unrelated to circulating the blood.

Oxygenated blood from the placenta enters the fetal body through the umbilical vein. About half the blood goes through the liver, and the rest bypasses the liver and enters the inferior vena cava through the first shunt, the *ductus venosus*. The blood then enters the right atrium. Most of the blood passes directly into the left atrium through the second shunt, the *foramen ovale*, where it mixes with the small amount of blood returning from the lungs. Blood is pumped from the left ventricle into the aorta to nourish the body. A small amount of blood from the right ventricle is circulated to the lungs to nourish the lung tissue. The rest of the blood from the right ventricle joins oxygenated blood in the aorta through the third shunt, the *ductus arteriosus*. The head and upper body receive the greatest amount of oxygenated blood.

The muscle wall of the right side of the fetal heart is thicker than that of the left because resistance to

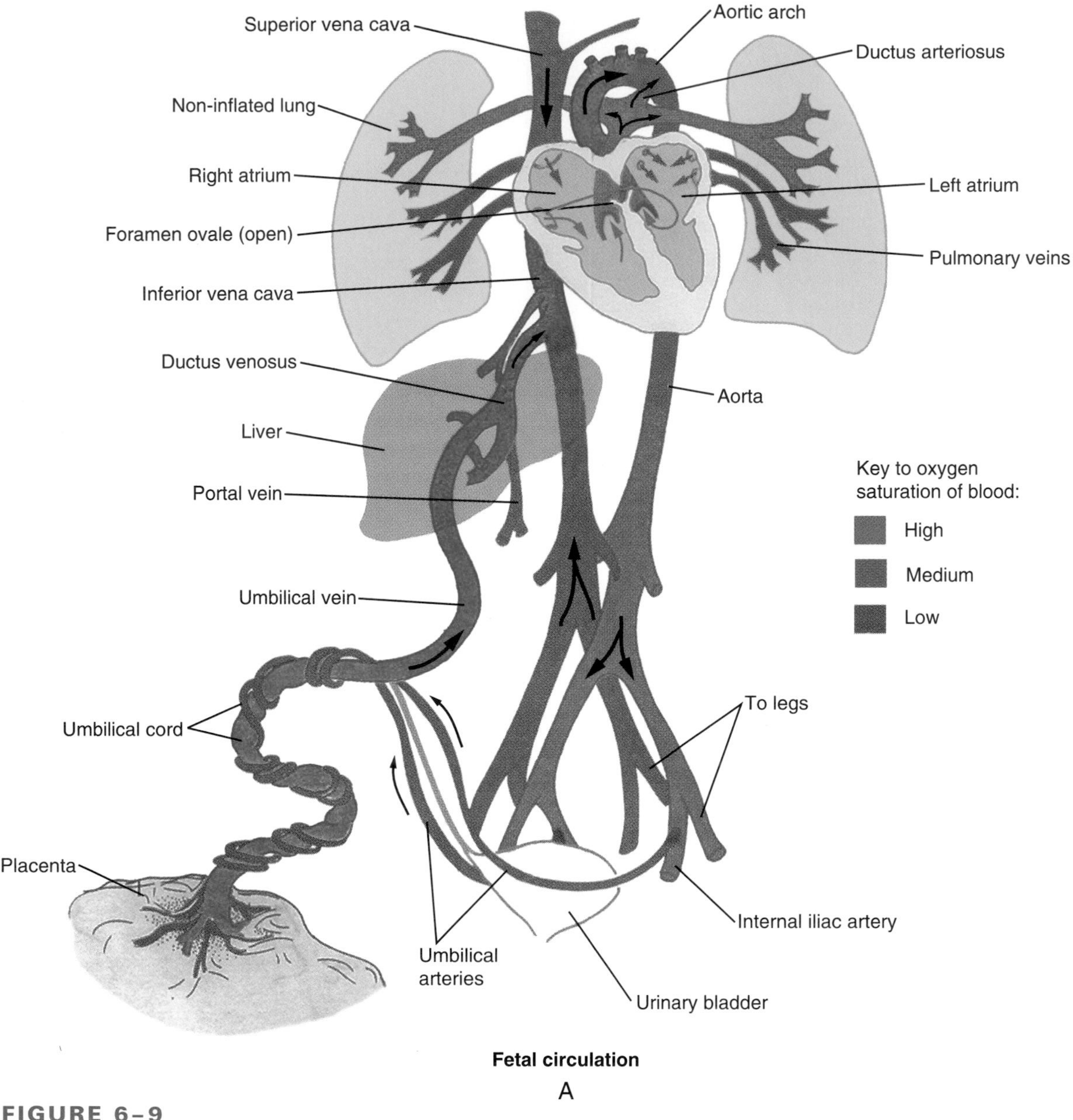


**FIGURE 6–9**

A, Fetal circulation. Three shunts exist to allow most blood from the placenta to bypass the fetal lungs and liver, the ductus venosus, the ductus arteriosus, and the foramen ovale.

blood flow through the uninflated lungs is high, similar to the resistance in other parts of the fetal body. When the infant begins breathing after birth, resistance to pulmonary blood flow falls dramatically and the right side of the heart does not need to be so thick. During infancy, the thickness of the right heart gradually decreases because its workload decreases.

## Changes in Blood Circulation After Birth

Fetal circulatory shunts are not needed after birth because the infant oxygenates blood in the lungs and is not circulating blood to the placenta (see Fig. 6–9B). As the infant breathes, blood flow to the lungs increases, pressure in the right heart falls, and the foramen ovale closes. The ductus arteriosus constricts as the arterial oxygen level rises. The ductus venosus constricts when flow of blood from the umbilical cord stops.

Transition to the postnatal circulatory pattern is gradual. Functional closure occurs when the infant breathes. The foramen ovale and ductus venosus are permanently closed as tissue proliferates in these structures. The ductus venosus becomes a ligament, as do the umbilical vein and arteries. Table 19–1 (see p. 490) lists the changes from fetal to neonatal circulation.

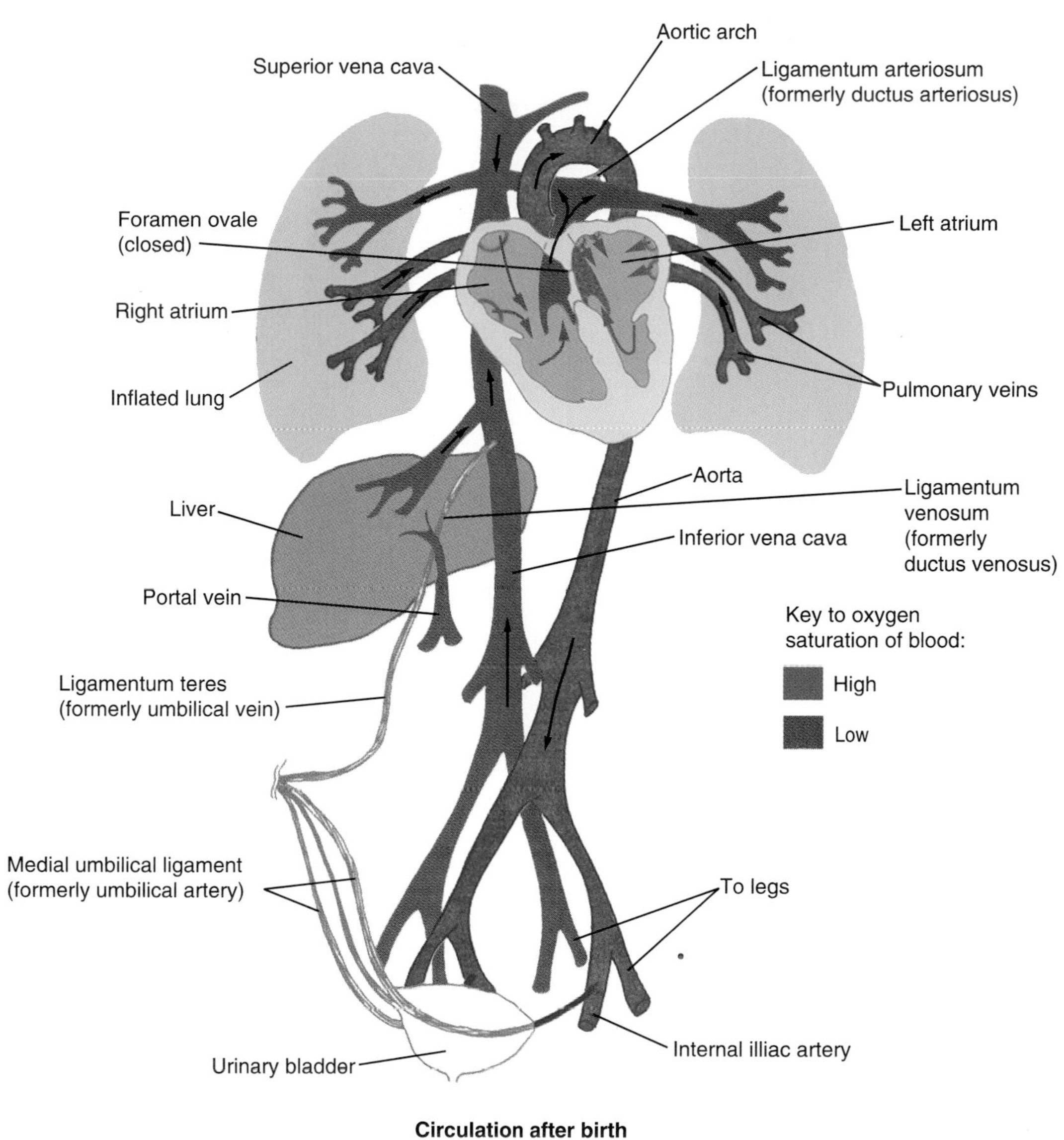


**FIGURE 6–9** *Continued*

B, Circulation after birth. Note that the fetal shunts have closed. The umbilical vessels, the ductus venosus and ductus arteriosus, have been converted to ligaments.

**CHECK YOUR READING**

22. What are the purposes of the fetal membranes and amniotic fluid?
23. Trace the path of fetal circulation from the placenta through the fetal body and back to the placenta.

## Multifetal Pregnancy

Multifetal pregnancy (multiple gestation) is a deviation from the usual course of gestation. Twins occur spontaneously about once in 90 pregnancies, triplets about once in 8100 pregnancies, quadruplets once in 729,000 pregnancies, and quintuplets only once in more than 65 million pregnancies (Moore, 1993).

Twinning is the most common form of multifetal pregnancy. The same processes that occur in twin pregnancies also may occur in other multiple gestations. Twins are often called "identical" or "fraternal" by lay people. They are more accurately described by their genetic origin, or the number of ova and sperm involved. The two types of twins are monozygotic and dizygotic. Figure 6–10 illustrates these two mechanisms of twinning.

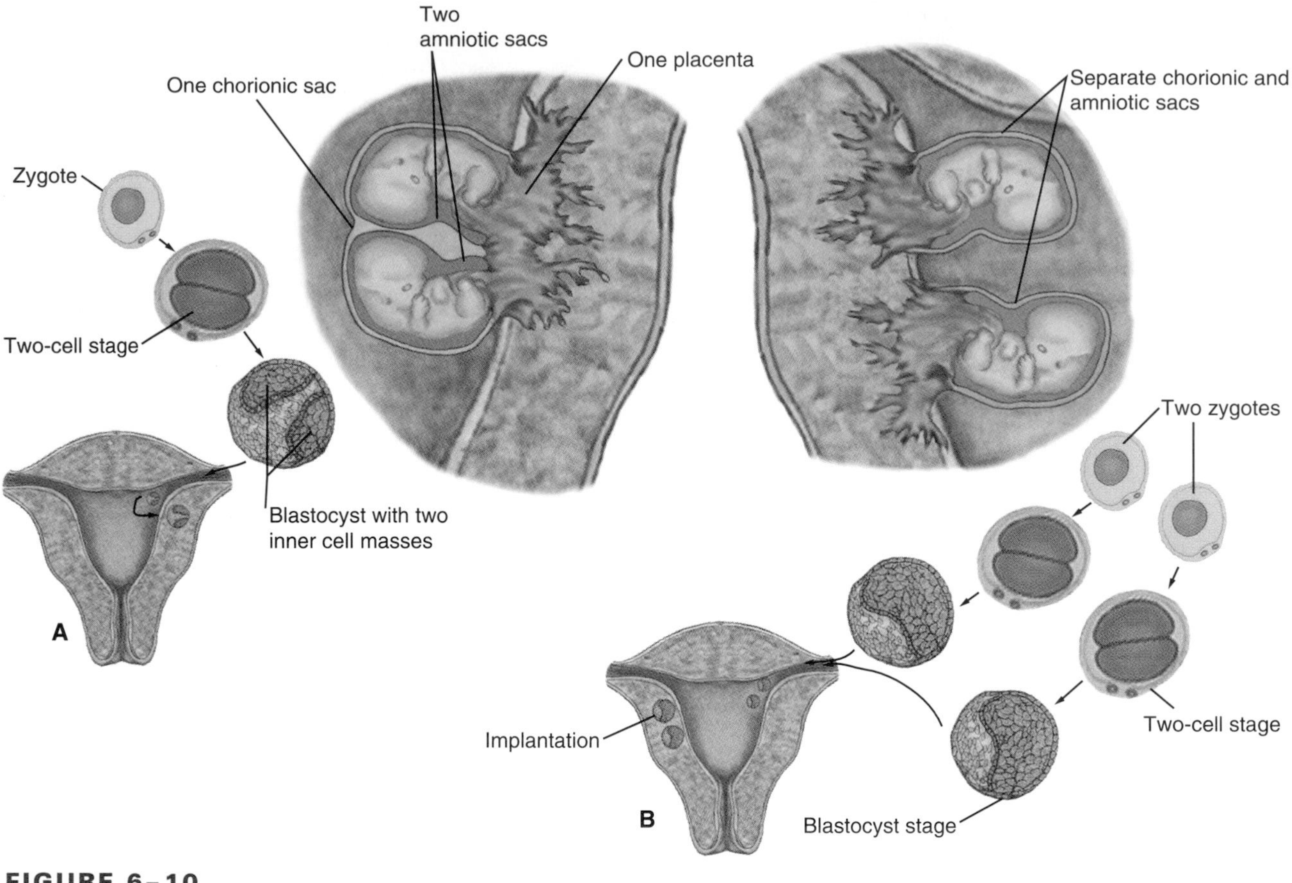


**FIGURE 6–10**

A, Monozygotic twinning. The single inner cell mass divides into two inner cell masses during the blastocyst stage. These twins have a single placenta and chorion, but each twin develops in its own amnion. B, Dizygotic twinning. Two ova are released during ovulation, and each is fertilized by a separate spermatozoon. The ova may implant near each other in the uterus, or they may be far apart.

## Monozygotic Twinning

Monozygotic twins are conceived by the union of a single ovum and spermatozoon, with later division of the conceptus into two. Monozygotic twins have identical genetic complements and are of the same sex. They may not always look identical at birth, however, because one twin may have grown much larger than the other, or one may have a birth defect, such as a cleft lip. Monozygotic twinning occurs essentially at random (1 in 250 births), and there is not a well-established hereditary component (Simpson & Golbus, 1992).

Monozygotic twinning occurs when a single conceptus divides early in gestation. In most cases of monozygotic twins (70 percent), when the *blastocyst* is formed, it has two inner cell masses instead of one. If this occurs, the fetuses have two amnions (inner membranes) but a single chorion (outer membrane).

If the conceptus divides earlier, two separate but identical morulas (and then blastocysts) develop and implant separately. These monozygotic twins have two amnions and two chorions. Although their placentas develop separately, they may fuse and appear as one at birth. Their chorions also may fuse during prenatal development. Therefore, examining the placenta and membranes after birth cannot always establish whether twins are monozygotic or dizygotic.

Late separation of the inner cell mass may result in twins having a single amnion and a single chorion. These twins often die because their umbilical cords become entangled. Incomplete separation of the inner cell mass may result in conjoined (formerly called "Siamese") twins.

## Dizygotic Twinning

Dizygotic twins arise from two ova that are fertilized by different sperm. Dizygotic twins may be the same or different sex, and they may or may not have similar physical traits.

Dizygotic twining may be hereditary in some families, presumably because of an inherited tendency of the females to release more than one ovum per cycle. Women of some races are more likely to have dizygotic twins as well:

- African: 1 in 20 births
- Asian: 1 in 150 births
- United States White: 1 in 80 births

There is an increased incidence of dizygotic twin births in women who conceive after age 40. Fertility treatments that induce ovulation also lead to an increased incidence of dizygotic multifetal gestations because multiple ova are released.

Because dizygotic twins arise from two separate zygotes, their membranes and placentas are separate. The membranes, placentas, or both may fuse during development if they implant closely. Dizygotic twins are not conjoined because they do not involve division of a single cell mass into two, but arise from two separate conceptions.

### Other Multifetal Gestations

Pregnancies resulting in more offspring than twins may arise from a single zygote or a combination of a single and multiple zygotes, or each may arise from a separate zygote. These pregnancies pose much greater hazards to both expectant mother and fetuses. The incidence of long-term handicaps is higher as the number of fetuses increases.

**✓ CHECK YOUR READING**

24. How do monozygotic twins occur?
25. Why can examination of the placenta and membranes in a multifetal pregnancy not always establish whether they are monozygotic or dizygotic?
26. Why are dizygotic twins often of different sex?

## SUMMARY CONCEPTS

- The purpose of gametogenesis is to produce ova and sperm that have half the full number of chromosomes, or 23 unpaired chromosomes. When an ovum and sperm unite at conception, the number is restored to 46 paired chromosomes.
- The female has all the ova she will ever have at 30 weeks of prenatal gestation. No other ova are formed after this time.
- One primary oocyte can mature into one mature ovum that contains 23 unpaired chromosomes (22 autosomes and an X chromosome).
- A male can continuously produce new sperm from puberty through the rest of his life, although fertility declines somewhat after age 40.
- One primary spermatocyte can result in production of four mature sperm. Two of the mature sperm have 22 autosomes and an X sex chromosome. Two have 22 autosomes and a Y sex chromosome.
- The male determines the baby's sex because only sperm carry either an X or Y sex chromosome. The female can contribute only an X chromosome to the baby.
- The basic structure of all organ systems is established during the first 8 weeks of pregnancy. Teratogens during this period may cause major structural and functional damage to the developing organs.
- The fetal period is one of growth and refinement of already established organ systems. Teratogens can still damage the fetus but are less likely to cause major structural damage. They may still cause major functional damage.
- The placenta is an embryonic or fetal organ with metabolic, respiratory, and endocrine functions.
- Transfer of substances between mother and embryo or fetus occurs by four mechanisms: simple diffusion, facilitated diffusion, active transport, and pinocytosis.
- Most substances in the maternal blood can be transferred to the fetus.
- The fetal membranes contain the amniotic fluid, which cushions the fetus, allows normal prenatal development, and maintains a stable temperature.
- The umbilical cord is the lifeline between the fetus and the placenta. Two umbilical arteries carry deoxygenated blood and waste products to the placenta for transfer to the mother's blood. One umbilical vein carries oxygenated and nutrient-rich blood to the fetus. Coiling of the vessels and enclosure in Wharton's jelly reduce the risk of obstruction of the umbilical vessels.
- Three fetal circulatory shunts are needed to partially bypass the fetal liver and lungs: the ductus venosus, the foramen ovale, and the ductus arteriosus. These structures close functionally after birth but are not closed permanently until several weeks or months later.
- Multifetal pregnancy may be monozygotic or dizygotic. Twins are the most common form of multifetal pregnancy.
- Examination of the placenta and membranes alone cannot conclusively establish whether multiple fetuses are monozygotic or dizygotic.
- Dizygotic twins are more likely to occur in certain families and racial groups, and especially in mothers older than 40 years and in women who take fertility treatments to induce ovulation.

#### References and Readings

Benirschke, K. (1994). Multiple gestation: Incidence, etiology and inheritance. In R.K. Creasy & R. Resnik (Eds.), *Maternal-fetal medicine: Principles and practice* (pp. 575–588). Philadelphia: W.B. Saunders.

Benirschke, K. (1994). Normal development. In R.K. Creasy & R. Resnik (Eds.), *Maternal-fetal medicine: Principles and practice* (pp. 96–105). Philadelphia: W.B. Saunders.

Blackburn, S.T., & Loper, D.L. (1992). *Maternal, fetal, and neonatal physiology: A clinical perspective.* Philadelphia: W.B. Saunders.

Brace, R.A. (1994). Amniotic fluid dynamics. In R.K. Creasy

& R. Resnik (Eds.), *Maternal-fetal medicine: Principles and practice* (pp. 106–114). Philadelphia: W.B. Saunders.

Glass, R.H. (1994). Gamete transport, fertilization, and implantation. In R.K. Creasy & R. Resnik (Eds.), *Maternal-fetal medicine: Principles and practice* (pp. 89–95). Philadelphia: W.B. Saunders.

Guyton, A.C. (1996). *Textbook of medical physiology* (9th ed.). Philadelphia: W.B. Saunders.

Moore, K.L. (1993). *Before we are born: Essentials of embryology and birth defects* (4th ed.). Philadelphia: W.B. Saunders.

Moore, K.L., Persaud, T.V.N., & Shiota, K. (1994). *Color atlas of clinical embryology*. Philadelphia: W.B. Saunders.

Simpson, J.L., & Golbus, M.S. (1992). *Genetics in obstetrics and gynecology* (2nd ed.). Philadelphia, W.B. Saunders.

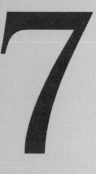

# Physiologic Adaptations to Pregnancy

## OBJECTIVES

1. Describe the physiologic changes that occur during pregnancy.
2. Differentiate presumptive, probable, and positive signs of pregnancy.
3. Compute gravida, para, and estimated date of delivery (birth).
4. Describe initial antepartum assessments in terms of history, physical examination, and risk assessment.
5. Identify subsequent antepartum assessments.
6. Discuss maternal adaptation to multifetal pregnancy.
7. Describe the common discomforts of pregnancy in terms of causes and measures that prevent or relieve them.
8. Explain cultural assessment and negotiation.
9. Discuss nursing process and critical thinking skills needed to develop nursing care plans for the most common problems and discomforts of pregnancy.

## DEFINITIONS

**amenorrhea** *Absence of menstruation. Primary amenorrhea is a delay of the first menstruation. Secondary amenorrhea is cessation of menstruation after its initiation.*

**Braxton Hicks contractions** *Irregular, mild uterine contractions that occur throughout pregnancy; they become stronger in the last trimester.*

**Chadwick's sign** *Bluish discoloration of the cervix, vagina, and labia during pregnancy as a result of increased vascular congestion.*

**chloasma** *Brownish pigmentation of the face during pregnancy; also called "mask of pregnancy."*

**colostrum** *Breast fluid secreted during pregnancy and the first 2 to 3 days following childbirth.*

**diastasis recti** *Separation of the longitudinal muscles of the abdomen (rectus abdominis) during pregnancy.*

**Goodell's sign** *Softening of the cervix, uterus, and vagina during pregnancy.*

**Hyperemia** *Excess of blood in a part of the body.*

**Physiologic anemia of pregnancy** *Decrease in hematocrit values caused by dilution of erythrocytes by expanded plasma volume rather than by an actual decrease in erythrocytes or hemoglobin.*

**Striae gravidarum** *Irregular reddish streaks resulting from tears in connective tissue; during pregnancy, these streaks generally appear on the woman's abdomen, breasts, or thighs.*

From the moment of conception, important changes occur in the pregnant woman's body that are necessary to support and nourish the fetus, to prepare the woman for childbirth and lactation, and to maintain her health. Pregnant women are often puzzled by the physical changes and unprepared for the discomforts that sometimes accompany them. Many pregnant women rely on nurses to provide accurate information and compassionate guidance throughout their pregnancies. To respond effectively, nurses must understand not only the physiologic changes but also the ways these changes affect the daily lives of expectant mothers.

## Changes in Body Systems

Although pregnancy challenges each body system to adapt to increasing demands of the fetus, the most obvious changes are in the reproductive system.

### Reproductive System

#### UTERUS

**Growth.** Perhaps the most dramatic change during pregnancy occurs in the uterus, which, before conception, is a small, pear-shaped organ entirely contained in the pelvic cavity. Before pregnancy, the uterus weighs approximately 60 g (2 ounces) and has a capacity of about 10 ml (one third of an ounce). At the end of pregnancy, the uterus extends to the level of the xiphoid process, weighs approximately 1000 g (2.2 pounds), and has sufficient capacity for the fetus, placenta, and amniotic fluid, a total of about 5000 ml.

Uterine growth occurs as the result of both hyperplasia and hypertrophy. During the first trimester, growth is due mainly to hyperplasia and the formation of new cells that result from stimulation of the myometrium by estrogen (Resnik, 1994). During the second and third trimesters, uterine growth is due to hypertrophy as the muscle fibers stretch in all directions to accommodate the growing fetus. In addition to muscle growth, fibrous tissue accumulates in the outer muscle layer of the uterus, and the amount of elastic tissue increases. These changes greatly increase the strength of the muscle wall.

Muscle fibers in the myometrium increase in both length and width. As a result, by the third trimester the uterine muscles are thin, and the fetus can be easily palpated through the abdominal wall. As the uterus expands into the abdominal cavity, it gradually displaces the intestine upward and laterally as it rotates to the right. The rotation is probably due to pressure of the rectosigmoid colon on the left side of the pelvis.

**Pattern of Uterine Growth.** The uterus grows in a predictable pattern that provides information about fetal growth and helps to confirm the expected date of delivery (EDD), sometimes called the expected date of birth (EDB) (Fig. 7–1). For instance, by 12 weeks of gestation, the uterus extends out of the maternal pelvis and can be palpated above the symphysis pubis; at 16 weeks, the fundus reaches midway between the symphysis pubis and the umbilicus; and at 20 weeks, the fundus is located at the umbilicus. By 36 weeks, the fundus reaches its highest level at the xiphoid process; it pushes against the diaphragm, and the expectant mother may experience shortness of breath, even during rest. By 40 weeks, the fetal head descends into the pelvic cavity, and the uterus sinks to a lower level. This descent of the fetal head is called *lightening* because it reduces pressure on the diaphragm and makes breathing easier.

**Contractility.** Throughout pregnancy, the uterus undergoes irregular, painless contractions that are called *Braxton Hicks contractions*. During the contraction, the uterus temporarily tightens and becomes firm. It then returns to its original relaxed state. During the first two trimesters, the contractions are infrequent. During the third trimester, the contractions occur more frequently and they may cause some discomfort at this time. They are termed

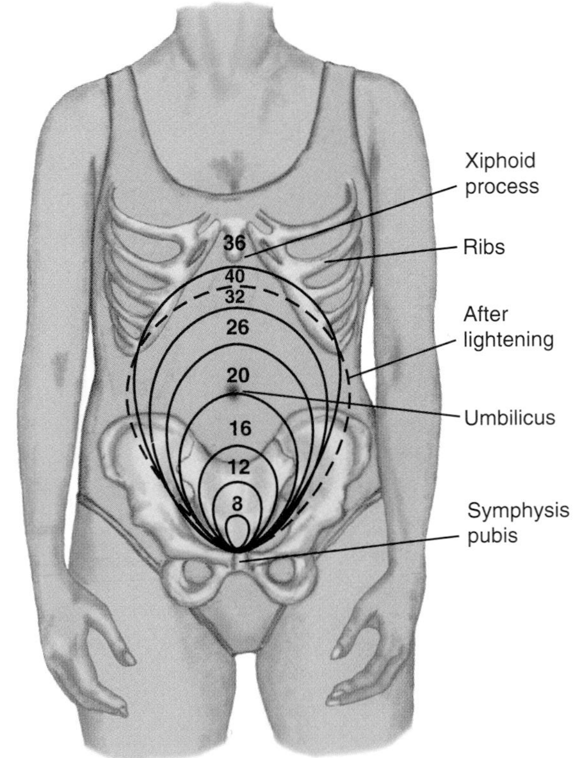


**FIGURE 7–1**

Uterine growth pattern during pregnancy.

"false" labor when they are mistaken for the onset of early labor.

**Uterine Blood Flow.** As the uterus increases in size, blood flow increases dramatically. In early pregnancy, when the uterus and placenta are relatively small, most of the blood flow is to the myometrium and endometrium. As pregnancy progresses, the delivery of most substances needed for fetal growth, as well as removal of metabolic wastes, depends on adequate perfusion of the placental intervillous spaces. Maternal blood, carried by the myometrial arteries, enters the intervillous spaces, where oxygen and nutrients are transferred to the chorionic villi and hence to the fetus. Metabolic wastes from the fetus diffuse into venous structures of the mother. (See Chapter 6 for additional information about placental and fetal circulation.)

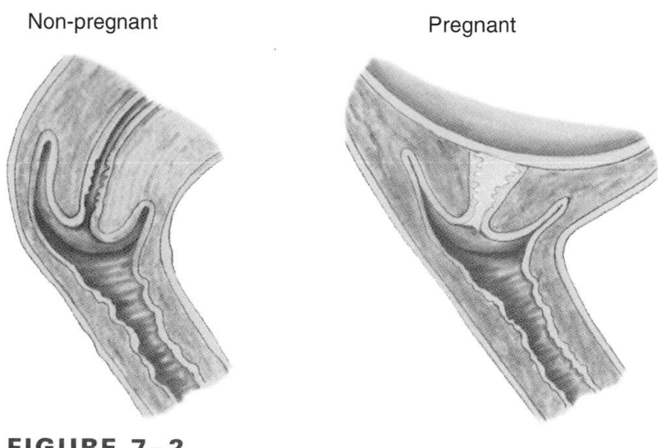


**FIGURE 7-2**

Cervical changes that occur during pregnancy. Note enlargement of spaces in cervical mucosa, which are filled with a thick mucus plug.

### CERVIX

The cervix also undergoes significant changes following conception. The most obvious changes occur in color and consistency. In response to the increasing levels of estrogen, the cervix becomes congested with blood (i.e., hyperemic), resulting in the characteristic bluish color that extends to include the vagina and labia. This discoloration, referred to as *Chadwick's sign*, is one of the earliest signs of pregnancy.

The cervix is largely composed of connective tissue that softens when the collagen fibers become swollen and loosely connected as a result of increased vascularity. Before pregnancy, the cervix has a consistency similar to that of the tip of the nose. After conception, the cervix feels more like the lobe of the ear. The cervical softening is referred to as *Goodell's sign*.

A less obvious change occurs as the cervical glands proliferate during pregnancy and the glandular walls become thin and widely separated. As a result, the endocervical tissue resembles a honeycomb that fills with mucus secreted by the cervical glands. The mucus forms a plug in the cervical canal; the plug is important because it blocks the ascent of bacteria from the vagina into the uterus during pregnancy and thus protects the membranes and fetus from infection (Fig. 7–2). The mucus plug remains in place until the onset of labor, when the cervix begins to thin and dilate, allowing the mucus plug to be expelled. One of the earliest signs of labor may be "bloody show," which consists of the mucus plug plus a small amount of blood produced by disruption of the cervical capillaries as the mucus plug is dislodged.

### VAGINA AND VULVA

Changes of the vagina are due to increased vascularity and are similar in some ways to those of the cervix. There is softening of the abundant connective tissue, which allows the vagina to distend during childbirth. Because of hyperemia, the vaginal walls, as well as the cervix, appear bluish. The vaginal mucosa thickens, and vaginal rugae (folds) become very prominent.

Vaginal cells contain increasing amounts of glycogen, which causes rapid sloughing and increased vaginal discharge. The pH of the vaginal discharge is acidic because of the increased production of lactic acid that results from the action of *Lactobacillus acidophilus* on glycogen in the vaginal epithelium (Cunningham et al., 1997). The acidic condition works to prevent growth of harmful bacteria found in the vagina. The glycogen-rich environment, however, favors the growth of *Candida albicans*, so that persistent yeast infections (candidiasis) are common during pregnancy.

Increased vascularity, edema, and connective tissue changes make the tissues of the vulva and perineum more pliable. Pelvic congestion during pregnancy can lead to heightened sexual interest and increased orgasmic experiences.

### OVARIES

Once conception occurs, the major function of the ovaries is to secrete progesterone for the first 6 to 7 weeks of the pregnancy. Progesterone (from Latin, *pro*, "for"; *gestare*, "bearing" or "reproduction") is called the *hormone of pregnancy*, and if the pregnancy is to be maintained, adequate progesterone must be available from the earliest stages. The corpus luteum secretes progesterone until the placenta is developed. Once developed, the placenta secretes progesterone throughout pregnancy, and the corpus luteum regresses because it is no longer needed.

Ovulation ceases during pregnancy because the circulating levels of estrogen and progesterone are

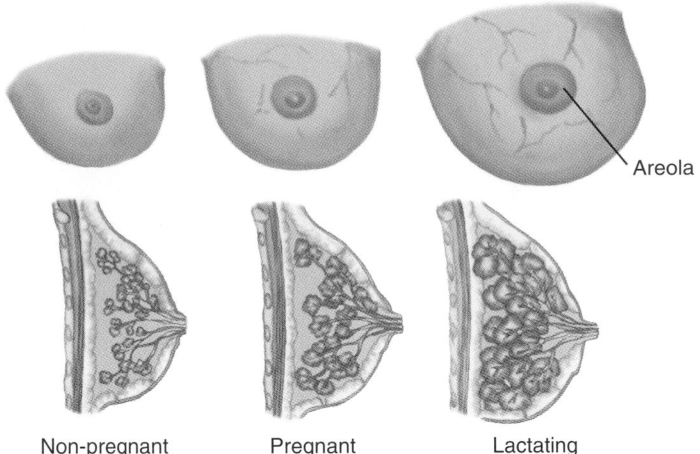


**FIGURE 7–3**

Breast changes that occur during pregnancy. The breasts increase in size and become more vascular, the areolae become darker, and the nipples become more erect.

high, inhibiting the release of follicle-stimulating hormone (FSH) and luteinizing hormone (LH), which are necessary for ovulation.

#### BREASTS

During pregnancy, the breasts change in both size and appearance (Fig. 7–3). The increase in size is due to the effects of estrogen and progesterone. Estrogen stimulates the growth of mammary ductal tissue; progesterone promotes the growth of lobes, lobules, and alveoli. The breasts become highly vascular, and a delicate network of veins is often visible just beneath the surface of the skin. If the increase in breast size is extensive, striations ("stretch marks") similar to those that occur on the abdomen may develop.

Characteristic changes in the nipples and areolae occur during pregnancy. The nipples increase in size and become more erect, and the areolae become larger and more pigmented. The degree of pigmentation varies with the complexion of the expectant mother. Women with very light complexions exhibit less change in pigmentation than those who have darker skin. Sebaceous glands, called *tubercles of Montgomery*, become more prominent during pregnancy and secrete a substance that lubricates the nipples. In addition, a thin yellowish breast fluid (*colostrum*) is present in greater or lesser amounts throughout pregnancy and can readily be expressed by the third trimester.

#### ✓ CHECK YOUR READING

1. What is the expected uterine growth at 20 weeks compared with that at 36 weeks?
2. How does uterine blood flow change during pregnancy?
3. What is the major purpose of progesterone?
4. What is the purpose of the cervical mucus plug?
5. How do the breasts change during pregnancy in size and appearance?

### Cardiovascular System

During pregnancy, alterations occur in heart size and position as well as in blood volume, blood flow, and blood components.

#### HEART

**Heart Size and Position.** Cardiac changes are slight, and they reverse soon after childbirth. The muscles of the heart (myocardium) enlarge slightly due to increased workload during pregnancy. The heart is pushed upward and toward the left as the uterus elevates the diaphragm during the third trimester. As a result of the change in position, the locations for auscultating (listening to) heart sounds may be shifted upward and laterally in late pregnancy.

**Heart Sounds.** During pregnancy some heart sounds may be altered to the extent that they would be considered abnormal in a non-pregnant state. The changes are first heard between 12 and 20 weeks and continue for 2 to 4 weeks after childbirth. The most common variations in heart sounds include splitting of the first heart sound and a systolic murmur that is found in 90 percent of pregnant women (Cunningham et al., 1997). In the non-pregnant state diastolic murmurs are evidence of heart disease, but during pregnancy these murmurs occur in 20 percent of pregnant women and are thought to be due to increased blood flow through the tricuspid or mitral valve or to physiologic dilation of the pulmonary artery (Blackburn & Loper, 1992).

#### BLOOD VOLUME

**Plasma Volume.** Total blood volume is a combination of plasma and solutes, such as red blood cells, white blood cells, and platelets. Plasma volume increases progressively from 6 to 8 weeks' gestation to approximately 5000 ml at 32 weeks. This is an increase of 45 percent (1200 to 1600 ml) above non-pregnant values (Monga & Creasy, 1994). The exact reason for plasma volume increase is unclear, but it may be related to estrogen stimulation of the renin-angiotensin-aldosterone system, which stimulates sodium and water retention.

Although the cause of plasma volume expansion is poorly understood, the increased volume is clearly needed for two reasons: (1) to transport nutrients and oxygen to the placenta, where they become available for the growing fetus, and (2) to meet the demands of the expanded maternal tissue in the uterus and breasts. An additional benefit of hypervolemia is that it provides a reserve to protect the pregnant woman from the adverse effects of blood loss that occurs during childbirth.

**Red Blood Cell Volume.** Red blood cell mass increases by 250 to 450 ml, about 20 to 30 percent above pre-pregnancy values (Monga & Creasy, 1994). Although both red blood cell volume and plasma volume expand, the increase in plasma volume is more pronounced and occurs earlier. The resulting dilution of red blood cell mass causes a decline in maternal hematocrit. This condition is frequently called *physiologic anemia* or *pseudoanemia of pregnancy* because it reflects dilution of red blood cells in greatly expanded plasma volume and does not indicate true anemia.

Although not true anemia, physiologic anemia should not be dismissed as unimportant. Frequent laboratory examinations may be needed to distinguish physiologic anemia from true anemia. Generally, iron deficiency anemia does not exist unless the hemoglobin is 10.5 g/dl or lower (Duffy, 1995) or the hematocrit is less than 33 percent. Iron supplementation is necessary if hemoglobin or hematocrit falls below these levels. Iron supplementation is often associated with constipation. (See Women Want To Know: How to Overcome the Common Discomforts of Pregnancy, p. 155, for measures to alleviate constipation.)

Dilution of red blood cells by plasma may also have a protective function. By decreasing blood viscosity, dilution may counter the tendency to form clots (thrombi) that can obstruct blood vessels and cause serious complications (see Chapter 28).

### CARDIAC OUTPUT

A major consequence of expanded vascular volume during pregnancy is an increase in cardiac output. Cardiac output is the amount of blood discharged from the heart each minute. It is based on stroke volume (the amount of blood pumped from the heart with each contraction) and heart rate (the number of times the heart beats each minute). Cardiac output rises rapidly during the first trimester and remains elevated throughout pregnancy. During pregnancy, the increase in cardiac output is due primarily to a gain in stroke volume, but the heart rate also rises about 15 to 20 beats per minute (Blackburn & Loper, 1992).

### PERIPHERAL VASCULAR RESISTANCE

Peripheral vascular resistance falls during pregnancy. This change is likely due to (1) smooth muscle relaxation in vessel walls due to the effects of progesterone; (2) the addition of the uteroplacental unit, which provides a greater area for circulation; (3) fetal heat production, which may produce vasodilation; and (4) increased synthesis of *prostaglandins* that cause resistance to circulating vasoconstrictors, such as angiotensin II and norepinephrine.

### BLOOD PRESSURE

The effect of decreased peripheral vascular resistance is that, despite the increase in blood volume, blood pressure remains stable during pregnancy. Systolic pressure remains largely unchanged, although diastolic pressure may decrease (about 10 mmHg) during the first and second trimesters (Monga & Creasy, 1994). During the third trimester, blood pressure rises slightly. Blood pressure should, however, remain at or near the normal levels of early pregnancy.

**Effect of Position on Blood Pressure.** Arterial blood pressure is affected by position during pregnancy. Pressure is lowest when the pregnant woman is in a lateral recumbent position. Pressures are significantly higher when she is standing than when she is sitting. Moreover, an increase in both systolic and diastolic pressure occurs when the arm is held in a dependent position (Knuppel & Drukker, 1993).

Each agency needs to standardize how blood pressure is taken and to document the position as well as the pressure so that the site of evaluation remains consistent. Moreover, controversy continues about whether Korotkoff's fifth phase (disappearance of sound) correlates better with the true diastolic pressure than does the fourth (muffling) phase. Facilities should select which phase is to be used and remain consistent throughout the prenatal, intrapartum, and postpartum periods. Blood pressures of 140/90 require additional evaluations.

**Mean Arterial Pressure.** The mean arterial pressure (MAP) is the average pressure within an artery over a complete cycle of one heart beat. It is estimated by computing one third of the pulse pressure (systolic pressure minus diastolic pressure) and adding that figure to the diastolic pressure. For example:

Blood pressure: 108/72

Pulse pressure: (108 − 72) = 36

MAP: 36 divided by 3 = 12 + 72 = 84

According to some researchers, an elevated MAP (above 85 mmHg) is thought to be predictive of hypertension.

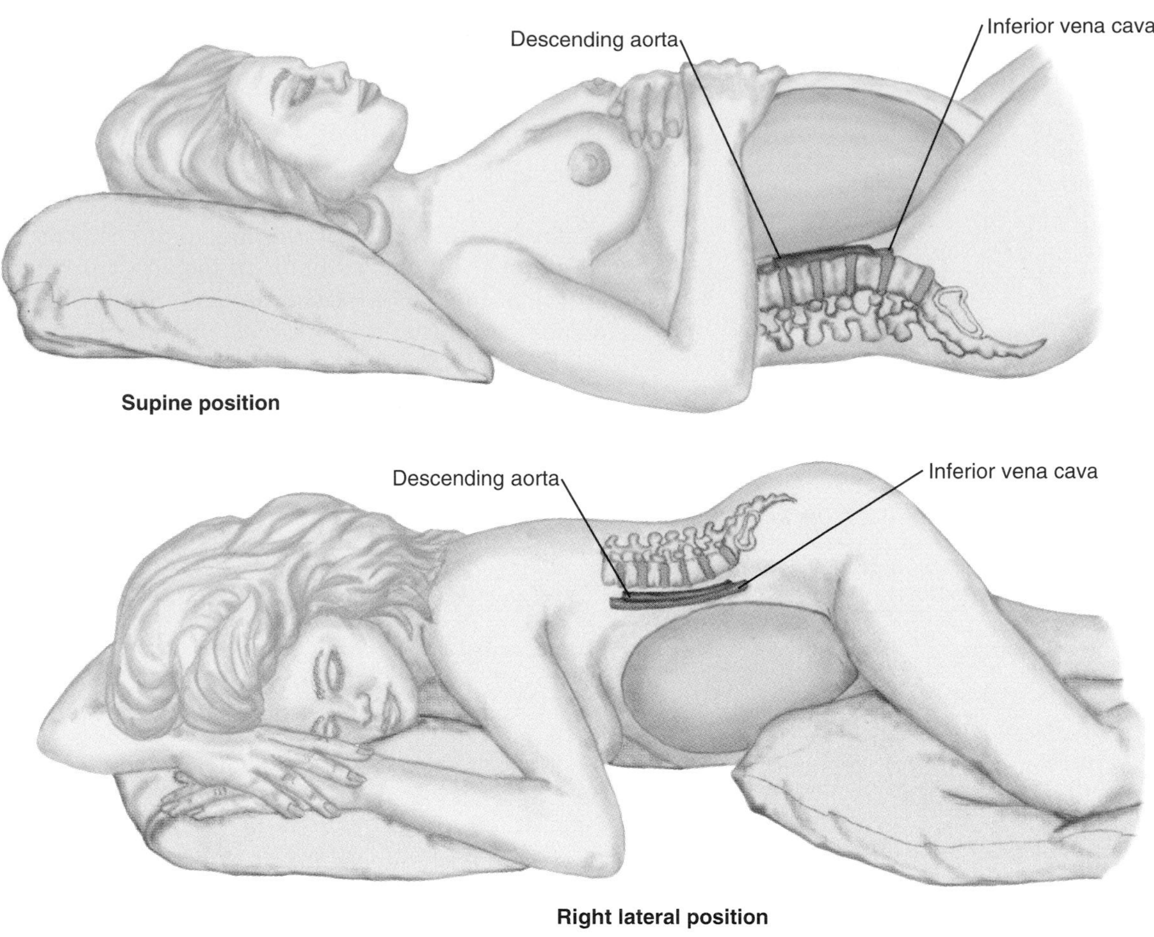


**FIGURE 7–4**

Vena caval syndrome, or supine hypotensive syndrome. When the woman is in the supine position, the weight of the gravid uterus partially occludes the vena cava and the descending aorta. Turning to a lateral recumbent position corrects supine hypotension.

**Supine Hypotension.** When the pregnant woman is in the supine position, particularly in the second and third trimesters, the weight of the *gravid* (*pregnant*) uterus partially occludes the vena cava and the descending aorta (Fig. 7–4). The occlusion impedes return of blood from the lower extremities and, as a consequence, reduces cardiac return, cardiac output, and blood pressure. This supine hypotensive syndrome is also called *vena caval syndrome*. Occlusion of the aorta, however, also causes decreased blood pressure in the lower extremities, and thus a more precise term is *supine hypotensive syndrome*. Symptoms include faintness, lightheadedness, dizziness, and agitation. Some may experience syncope, a brief lapse in consciousness. Blood flow through the placenta is also decreased if the woman remains in the supine position for a prolonged period of time, and this could result in fetal hypoxia.

Turning to a lateral recumbent position alleviates the pressure on the blood vessels and quickly corrects supine hypotension. Women should be advised to rest in a side-lying position to prevent supine hypotension from occurring as well as to correct it when it does occur. If they must assume a supine position for fetal surveillance testing, a wedge or pillow under the right hip may also be effective in decreasing supine hypotension.

### BLOOD FLOW

Four major changes in blood flow occur during pregnancy.

1. Blood flow is altered to include the uteroplacental unit; approximately 500 ml per minute is required to perfuse the placenta adequately.
2. Approximately 30 percent more blood must circulate through the maternal kidneys to remove the increased metabolic wastes that are generated by mother and fetus.
3. The woman's skin requires increased circulation to dissipate heat that is generated by increased metabolism during pregnancy.

4. The weight of the expanding uterus on the inferior vena cava and iliac veins partially obstructs blood return from veins in the legs, and blood pools in the deep and superficial veins of the legs. The resulting stasis of blood exerts pressure on the veins and may cause the veins to become distended. Prolonged engorgement of the veins of the lower legs may result in varicose veins of the legs, vulva, or rectum (hemorrhoids).

#### BLOOD COMPONENTS

During pregnancy, red blood cells (erythrocytes), white blood cells (leukocytes), and clotting factors increase. Erythrocytes increase by 20 to 30 percent. The rise reflects accelerated production of erythrocytes rather than prolonged red cell life. The gain in erythrocytes greatly increases the maternal demand for iron, which is necessary for hemoglobin formation.

Although iron absorption and iron-binding power are increased during pregnancy, sufficient iron is not always supplied by diet. Iron supplementation is necessary to promote hemoglobin synthesis and thus to ensure that erythrocyte production is sufficient to prevent the development of iron-deficiency anemia (which is described in Chapter 25).

Leukocytes increase from an average pre-pregnancy level of 5000 cells/$mm^3$ to an average of 10,000 cells/$mm^3$ (Baker, 1995). Leukocytes increase further during labor as a result of exertion and may reach 25,000 cells/$mm^3$ by the early postpartum period.

Several clotting factors are elevated during pregnancy, particularly plasma fibrinogen (factor I), which rises by about 50 percent. Elevated fibrinogen levels increase the ability to form clots, creating both a protective mechanism and an increased risk for the mother. It offers some protection from hemorrhage during childbirth, but it also increases the risk of clot formation (*thrombus*) in the legs and the development of thrombophlebitis. The risk is a particular concern if the woman must stand or sit for prolonged periods, with stasis of blood in the veins of the legs. (See Appendix C for additional changes in blood components.)

#### ✓ CHECK YOUR READING

6. How does the cause of physiologic anemia or pseudoanemia differ from iron deficiency anemia?
7. Why is circulation to the kidneys and skin increased during pregnancy?
8. Why do some pregnant women feel faint when they are in a supine position?
9. Why is it important to standardize techniques for taking blood pressure?

### Respiratory System

The major respiratory changes in pregnancy are due to three factors: increased oxygen consumption, hormonal factors, and physical effects of the enlarging uterus.

#### OXYGEN CONSUMPTION

Oxygen consumption increases by about 15 to 20 percent in pregnancy. Half the oxygen is used by the fetus, and the rest is consumed by the uterus, the breast tissue, and the increased respiratory and cardiac demands. To compensate for the increased need for oxygen, the woman breathes more deeply, although her respiratory rate remains unchanged. As a result, the tidal volume (the volume of gas moved into or out of the respiratory tract with each breath) as well as the respiratory minute volume (the volume of air inspired or expired in 1 minute) increase by about 40 percent. As a consequence of the elevated minute volume, the partial pressure of carbon dioxide ($Pco_2$) is lowered. The resulting respiratory alkalosis is partially compensated by renal excretion of bicarbonate. Decreased partial pressure of $Pco_2$ also promotes the transfer of carbon dioxide from fetal to maternal circulation.

#### HORMONAL FACTORS

**Progesterone.** Progesterone is believed to be a major factor in the respiratory changes of pregnancy. It plays a role in decreasing airway resistance by relaxing the smooth muscle in the respiratory tract. Progesterone is also believed to raise the sensitivity of the respiratory center (medulla oblongata) to carbon dioxide, thus stimulating the increase in minute ventilation and lowering the $Pco_2$. These two factors are responsible for the heightened awareness of the need to breathe (dyspnea) experienced by many women during pregnancy.

**Estrogen.** Estrogen causes increased vascularity of the mucous membranes of the upper respiratory tract. As the capillaries become engorged, edema and hyperemia develop within the nose, pharynx, larynx, and trachea. This congestion gives rise to several conditions commonly seen during pregnancy. These conditions include nasal and sinus stuffiness, epistaxis (nosebleeds), and changes in the voice. Increased vascularity also causes edema of the eardrum and eustachian tubes that may result in a sense of fullness in the ears or earaches.

#### PHYSICAL CHANGES

By the third trimester, the enlarging uterus lifts the diaphragm by about 4 cm (1.6 inches), which prevents the lungs from expanding as fully as they normally do. To compensate for the reduced space, the ribs flare; the substernal angle widens; and the circumference of the chest expands by about 6 cm (2.5 inches). Breathing becomes thoracic rather than abdominal, adding to the dyspnea many women experience.

## Gastrointestinal System

The gastrointestinal system undergoes changes that are clinically significant because they may cause discomfort for the expectant mother.

### MOUTH

Elevated levels of estrogen cause hyperemia of the tissues of the mouth and gums that may lead to gingivitis and bleeding gums. Some women develop severe vascular hypertrophy of the gums, which appear reddened and swollen and bleed easily. The condition regresses spontaneously after childbirth.

Some women experience *ptyalism*, or excessive salivation, that is unpleasant and embarrassing. The cause of ptyalism appears to be stimulation of the salivary glands by the ingestion of starch (Cunningham et al., 1997). Small, frequent meals, gum chewing, and oral lozenges offer limited relief for some women. The teeth are unaffected by pregnancy; contrary to common beliefs, they do not lose minerals to the fetus.

### ESOPHAGUS

The lower esophageal sphincter tone decreases during pregnancy, primarily because of the relaxant activity of progesterone on the smooth muscles. The reduced tone allows reflux of acidic stomach contents into the esophagus and produces heartburn (*pyrosis*).

### STOMACH AND SMALL INTESTINE

Elevated levels of progesterone relax all smooth muscle, leading to decreased tone and motility of the gastrointestinal tract. The stomach and small intestine take longer to empty, allowing additional time for nutrients to be absorbed. This slowed process benefits the growing fetus, but it may contribute to the nausea many expectant mothers experience.

### LARGE INTESTINE

Decreased motility in the large intestine allows time for more water to be absorbed, which tends to make the stool hard and may lead to constipation. Hemorrhoids may be caused or exacerbated by constipation if the expectant mother must strain to have bowel movements.

### LIVER AND GALLBLADDER

Although the size of the liver and gallbladder remains unchanged during pregnancy, functional changes occur, largely because of the effects of progesterone. The gallbladder becomes hypotonic, and emptying time is prolonged, resulting in thicker bile that can predispose to the development of gallstones. Reduced gallbladder tone also leads to a tendency to retain bile salts, which can lead to itching (pruritus).

The liver is pushed upward and backward by the enlarging uterus during the last trimester, and liver function is also altered. Serum alkaline phosphatase and serum cholesterol levels are almost doubled by the end of pregnancy, whereas levels of serum albumin fall gradually. These changes are due primarily to the effect of estrogen and to hemodilution.

## Urinary System

Changes in both the structure and the function of the urinary tract take place during pregnancy.

### BLADDER

During the first trimester, the uterus begins to expand within the pelvic cavity. Expansion applies pressure to the bladder, causing the woman to experience frequency and urgency of urination. During the second trimester, the uterus extends into the abdominal cavity, so that pressure on the bladder is relieved and the urge to void decreases. In addition, bladder capacity almost doubles as the bladder, like all smooth muscle, relaxes in response to increasing levels of progesterone.

Bladder mucosa also becomes congested with blood, and the bladder walls become hypertrophied as a result of stimulation from estrogen. Decreased drainage of blood from the base of the bladder results in edema of its tissues and renders the area susceptible to trauma and infection during childbirth.

Late in the third trimester, the fetus settles into the pelvis (through the process called lightening) and presses against the bladder. Once again, the woman experiences frequency, urgency, and nocturia. Although frequency and urgency are normal during early and late pregnancy, they are also signs of infection; if they are accompanied by burning sensations or pain, the woman should be assessed for urinary tract infection.

### KIDNEYS AND URETERS

**Changes in Size and Shape of the Kidneys.** During pregnancy, the kidneys change in both size and shape because dilation of the renal pelves, calyces, and ureters occurs above the pelvic brim. The dilation is caused by (1) the effect of progesterone, which relaxes the walls of the ureters and makes them more distensible, and (2) compression of the ureters between the enlarging uterus and the bony pelvic brim. As the flow of urine through the ureters is obstructed, particularly on the right side (the left ureter is cushioned by the sigmoid colon), the ureters dilate and apply hydrostatic pressure against the renal pelvis, which also dilates. The resulting stasis of urine is clinically significant because it allows time for bacteria to multiply and increases the risk of urinary tract infection during pregnancy.

**Functional Changes of the Kidneys.** Renal plasma flow, the total amount of plasma to flow through the kidneys, increases by 35 to 60 percent. The rise is due to increases in plasma volume and cardiac output. The glomerular filtration rate, the rate at which water and dissolved substances are filtered in the glomerulus, increases by as much as 50 percent. This increase is due to the rise in renal plasma flow and to decreased colloid osmotic pressure caused by a reduction in the concentration of plasma proteins.

The increases in renal plasma flow and glomerular filtration rate are necessary to excrete additional metabolic waste from the mother and fetus, but also affect the excretion of glucose. As glomerular filtration rate increases, the filtered load of glucose exceeds the ability of the renal tubules to reabsorb it, and glucose spills into the urine. Therefore, glycosuria is not uncommon during pregnancy, particularly after consumption of foods, such as candy or cookies, that are high in simple sugars. Furthermore, small quantities of amino acids and water-soluble vitamins are excreted. Bacteria thrive in urine that is rich in nutrients, so that glycosuria is one more reason why the incidence of urinary tract infections is increased during pregnancy.

Tests of renal function may be misleading during pregnancy. As a result of increased glomerular filtration rate, plasma concentrations of both creatinine and urea normally decline.

**CHECK YOUR READING**

10. How does the respiratory system compensate for the pressure exerted on the diaphragm by the enlarging uterus?
11. Why do some women experience dyspnea during pregnancy?
12. How does pregnancy affect the gastrointestinal system?
13. Why are pregnant women at increased risk for urinary tract infection?

## Integumentary System

### SKIN

Circulation to the skin increases during pregnancy, and encourages activity of the sweat and sebaceous glands. Pregnant women feel warmer and perspire more, particularly during the last trimester. Accelerated activity by the sebaceous glands fosters the development of facial blemishes, which are usually reduced by careful cleansing of the face several times each day. Additional changes include hyperpigmentation and vascular changes in the skin.

**Hyperpigmentation.** Increased pigmentation may begin as early as the second month, when levels of melanocyte-stimulating hormone (MSH) become elevated because of the effects of estrogen and progesterone. Brunettes and dark-skinned women exhibit more hyperpigmentation than women with very light skin. Areas of pigmentation include brownish patches, called *chloasma*, which usually involve the forehead, cheeks, and bridge of the nose. This sign is commonly called the *mask of pregnancy*. A dark line of pigmentation (*linea nigra*) may also extend from the umbilicus to the symphysis pubis. Preexisting moles become darker, and the areolae become darker as pregnancy progresses. Hyperpigmentation usually disappears following childbirth, when the levels of estrogen and progesterone decline.

**Cutaneous Vascular Changes.** Blood vessels dilate and proliferate during pregnancy. This change is thought to be due largely to the effect of estrogen. Changes in surface blood vessels are obvious during pregnancy, especially in white women. These include angiomas that appear as tiny red elevations that branch in all directions. Commonly called *vascular spiders* or telangiectasis, they appear most often on the face, neck, upper chest, and arms. Redness of the palms or soles of the feet, known as *palmar erythema*, also occurs in many white women and in some African-American women. Many times, vascular changes occur simultaneously, and although they may be emotionally distressing for the expectant mother, they are clinically insignificant and usually disappear shortly after childbirth.

### CONNECTIVE TISSUE

Linear tears may occur in the connective tissue, most often on the abdomen, breasts, and buttocks, appearing as slightly depressed, pink to purple streaks called *striae gravidarum*, or "stretch marks" (Fig. 7–5). Women are concerned about striae because, although the marks fade to silvery lines, they do not disappear after childbirth. Laser therapy is sometimes used after childbirth to reduce or eliminate severe striae. Many women insist that striae can be prevented by massage with oil or vitamin E, but the effectiveness of this treatment has not been documented. Antipruritic ointments may be effective in controlling the itching that accompanies severe striae.

### HAIR AND NAILS

Because fewer follicles are in the resting phase, hair grows more rapidly and less hair falls out during

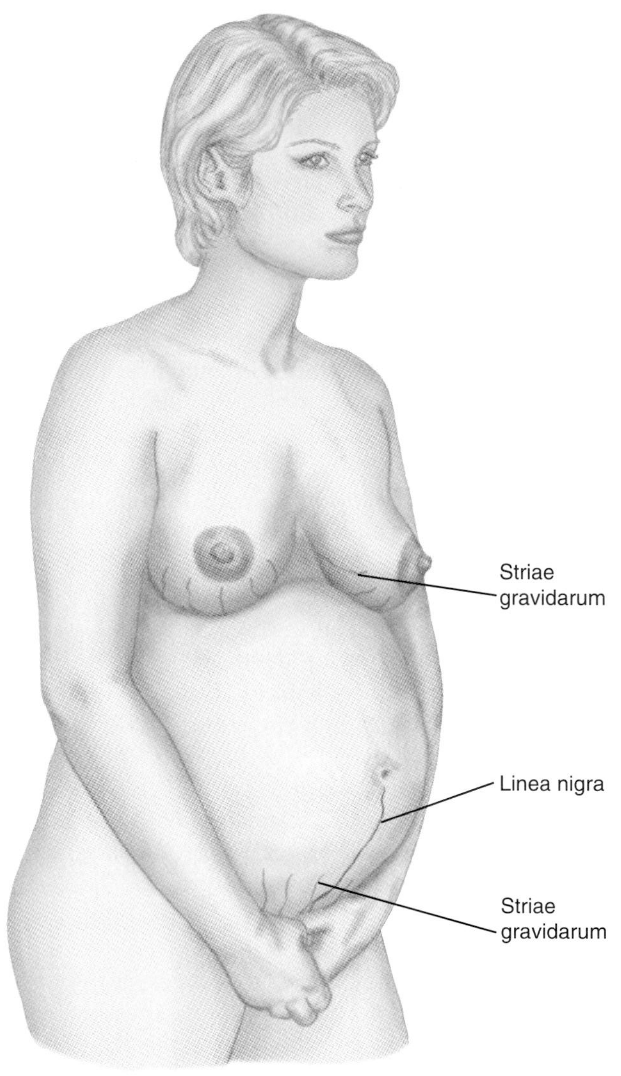


**FIGURE 7-5**

Striae gravidarum are linear tears that may occur in the connective tissue. Linea nigra, a dark line of pigmentation from the umbilicus to the symphysis pubis, may also appear.

pregnancy. After childbirth, hair follicles return to normal activity, and many women become concerned at the rate of hair loss. They need reassurance that more follicles have returned to the normal resting phase and that excessive hair loss will not continue.

Nail growth increases during pregnancy. Many women notice thinning and softening of the nails as pregnancy progresses, although reasons for this change are unclear.

## Musculoskeletal System

### POSTURAL CHANGES

Musculoskeletal changes are progressive. They begin in the second trimester, when maternal hormones (relaxin and progesterone) initiate gradual softening of the pelvic ligaments and joints to facilitate passage of the fetus through the pelvis at the time of birth. Relaxation of the pelvic joints creates pelvic instability, and the pregnant woman assumes a wide stance and the so-called waddling gait of pregnancy to compensate for a changing center of gravity.

During the third trimester, as the uterus increases in size, it becomes necessary for the expectant mother to lean backward to maintain her balance. This creates a progressive *lordosis*, or curvature of the lower spine (Fig. 7–6).

### ABDOMINAL WALL

Pregnancy also affects the abdominal muscles, which may be stretched beyond their capacity during the third trimester, causing the rectus abdominis muscles to separate (*diastasis recti*). The extent of the separation varies from slight, which is not clinically significant, to severe, when a large portion of the uterine wall is covered only by skin and fascia (see Chapter 17).

## Endocrine System

Numerous changes in hormones are related to pregnancy. See Table 7–1 for a summary.

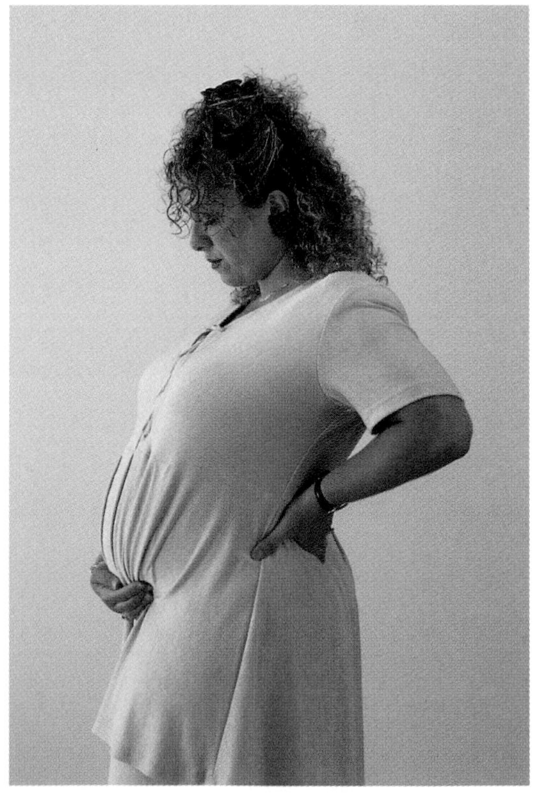

**FIGURE 7-6**

Lordosis increases by the third trimester as the uterus grows larger and the woman must lean backward to maintain her balance.

**TABLE 7-1 HORMONES RELATED TO PREGNANCY**

| Hormone | Source | Major Effects |
|---|---|---|
| Estrogen | Ovary, placenta | Stimulates uterine development to provide environment for fetus and stimulates breast to prepare for lactation |
| Progesterone | Ovary, placenta | Maintains uterine lining for implantation, relaxes all smooth muscle, including uterus; develops acini cells and lobes to prepare breasts for lactation |
| Human placental lactogen | Placenta | Stimulates metabolism of glucose and converts it to fat; antagonistic to insulin |
| Human chorionic gonadotropin | Trophoblasts (placenta) | Prevents involution of corpus luteum, thus maintaining production of progesterone until placenta is formed |
| Relaxin | Ovary, placenta | Softens muscles and joints of pelvis |
| Follicle-stimulating hormone | Anterior pituitary | Initiates maturation of ovum, necessary for conception; suppressed during pregnancy |
| Luteinizing hormone | Anterior pituitary | Stimulates ovulation of mature ovum in non-pregnant state |
| Melanocyte-stimulating hormone | Anterior pituitary | Increased during pregnancy; produces hyperpigmentation |
| Oxytocin | Posterior pituitary | Stimulates uterine contractions to initiate labor; stimulates milk-ejection reflex |
| Prolactin | Anterior pituitary | Primary hormone of milk production |
| Aldosterone | Adrenals | Increased during pregnancy to conserve sodium and maintain fluid balance |
| Cortisol | Adrenals | Increased during pregnancy; active in metabolism of glucose and fats; anti-inflammatory effect *may* be helpful in preventing rejection of pregnancy |
| Thyroxine | Thyroid | Increased during pregnancy to stimulate basal metabolic rate |

#### PITUITARY GLAND

Most hormones from the pituitary gland are suppressed during pregnancy. The only hormone from the *anterior* pituitary that increases is prolactin, which prepares the breasts to produce milk. The hormones FSH and LH, normally produced to stimulate ovulation in the non-pregnant woman, are unnecessary during pregnancy, and the growth hormone from the anterior pituitary also appears to decrease during pregnancy.

The *posterior* pituitary secretes oxytocin, a second hormone that is involved in lactation. Oxytocin stimulates the milk-ejection reflex after childbirth. Oxytocin also stimulates contractions of the uterus, but during pregnancy this action is inhibited by progesterone, which relaxes smooth muscle fibers that comprise the uterus. After childbirth, progesterone levels decline, and oxytocin plays an important role in keeping the uterus contracted and thus in preventing excessive bleeding.

#### THYROID GLAND

Early in the first trimester, a rise in total thyroxine ($T_4$) occurs, along with a corresponding gain in thyroxine-binding protein. The increased amounts of $T_4$ bind readily with the thyroxine-binding proteins, and the serum level of unbound $T_4$ remains stable. These changes produce slight enlargement in the size of the thyroid gland and an increase in basal metabolic rate (BMR). The BMR increases by 20 to 25 percent during pregnancy, causing greater cardiac output, pulse rate, and heat intolerance. The BMR returns to normal within a few weeks after childbirth.

#### PARATHYROID GLANDS

Metabolism of calcium and phosphorus depends on the secretion of parathyroid hormone. During pregnancy, fetal demands for calcium and phosphorus increase, and the maternal parathyroid glands respond by producing additional parathyroid hormone. Parathyroid hormone generally acts to improve absorption of calcium from the intestine, to decrease renal losses, and to mobilize bone. During pregnancy, however, no loss of bone density occurs despite the increase in parathyroid activity. The skeleton appears to be protected by increased levels of calcitonin and by estrogen, which interfere with the action of parathyroid hormone on bone.

#### PANCREAS

Significant changes in the pancreas during pregnancy are due to alterations in maternal blood glucose and consequent fluctuations in insulin production. The fetus draws glucose from the maternal supply. In addition, the fetus draws amino acids from maternal circulation and thereby inhibits the mother's ability to synthesize glucose. During the first trimester, the combination of increasing glucose demand by the fetus and a declining supply of glucose results in a fall in maternal blood glucose. Consequently, during this time, the islets of Langerhans produce less insulin.

During the second trimester, maternal tissue sensitivity to insulin begins to decline, mainly because of the effects of hormones, such as human placental lactogen, prolactin, progesterone, and cortisol. By the end of pregnancy, tissue sensitivity to insulin falls by as much as 80 percent (Baker, 1995). As a consequence of the tissue resistance to insulin, postprandial (following a meal) blood glucose levels rise. A higher blood glucose level has two major effects: (1) it makes more glucose available for fetal energy needs and (2) it stimulates the pancreas of a healthy woman to produce additional insulin. Insulin production is closely associated with carbohydrate metabolism. Inadequate insulin production results in gestational diabetes, which is described in Chapter 26.

#### ADRENAL GLANDS

The adrenal glands enlarge only slightly during pregnancy, but they produce a significant increase in two adrenal hormones: cortisol and aldosterone. The unbound level of cortisol is elevated during pregnancy, although the specific plasma protein (transcortin) that binds to cortisol is also elevated. Cortisol regulates carbohydrate and protein metabolism. It stimulates gluconeogenesis (formation of glycogen from noncarbohydrate sources such as amino or fatty acids) whenever the supply of glucose is inadequate to meet the body's needs for energy.

Aldosterone regulates the absorption of sodium from the distal tubules of the kidneys and has been called the "great sodium saver." Aldosterone production is increased during pregnancy to overcome the salt-wasting effects of progesterone, Aldosterone thereby maintains the necessary level of sodium in the greatly expanded blood volume. Aldosterone is closely related to water metabolism (see p. 133).

#### CHANGES CAUSED BY PLACENTAL HORMONES

**Human Chorionic Gonadotropin.** In early pregnancy, human chorionic gonadotropin (hCG) is produced by the trophoblastic cells that surround the developing embryo. The primary function of hCG in early pregnancy is to stimulate the corpus luteum to produce progesterone and estrogen until the placenta is sufficiently developed to assume that function. This hormone is responsible for positive pregnancy tests.

**Estrogen.** Although estrogen is produced by the ovaries during the menstrual cycle and by the corpus luteum for the first few weeks of pregnancy, it is produced primarily by the placenta after the sixth or seventh week of pregnancy. Estrogen has numerous functions during pregnancy: (1) it stimulates uterine growth and increases blood supply to uterine vessels; (2) it aids in developing the ductal system in the breasts in preparation for lactation; and (3) it is associated with hyperpigmentation, vascular changes in the skin, increased activity of the salivary glands, and hyperemia of the gums and nasal mucous membranes.

**Progesterone.** Progesterone is produced first by the corpus luteum and then by the fully developed placenta. Progesterone is the most important hormone of pregnancy. The major functions include the following:

- Maintaining the endometrial layer for implantation of the fertilized ovum
- Preventing spontaneous abortion by relaxing smooth muscles of the uterus
- Stimulating the development of the lobes and lobules in the breast in preparation for lactation
- Facilitating the deposit of maternal fat stores, which provide a reserve of energy for pregnancy and lactation

Progesterone relaxes not only the smooth muscle of the uterus but also all other smooth muscle. As a consequence, progesterone is associated with decreased motility of the bowel, dilation of the ureters, and increased bladder capacity. Progesterone lowers the respiratory sensitivity to carbon dioxide and thus stimulates increased ventilation.

**Human Placental Lactogen.** Also called human chorionic somatomammotropin (hCS), human placental lactogen (hPL) is present in early pregnancy and increases steadily throughout pregnancy. A primary function of hPL is to increase the availability of glucose for the fetus, who needs a constant supply for growth and development. Human placental lactogen does this by decreasing the sensitivity of maternal cells to insulin, which decreases maternal metabolism of glucose, thereby freeing glucose for transport to the fetus. In addition, under the influence of hPL, free fatty acids are quickly metabolized to provide energy for the pregnant woman.

**Relaxin.** Relaxin is produced by the corpus luteum and by the placenta. It is present by the time of the first missed menstrual period. Relaxin inhibits uterine activity, softens connective tissue in the cervix, relaxes pelvic joints, and stimulates growth of the breasts.

#### CHANGES IN METABOLISM

**Weight Gain.** Attitudes about weight gain have changed over the years. At one time, maternal weight gain was restricted as a means of controlling fetal size so that labor would be easier. In recent times, the correlation between infant mortality and low birth weight has been documented. As a result, the number of pounds acceptable for maternal weight gain has increased. (See Table 9–1 for the recommended weight gain for women of normal weight, women who are underweight, and those who are overweight before conception and for women expecting twins.)

The normal composition of weight gain is illustrated in Figure 9–1. The fetus, placenta, and amniotic fluid make up less than half the recommended weight gain. The remainder is found in the increased size of the uterus and breasts, increased blood volume, increased interstitial fluid, and maternal stores of subcutaneous fat.

**Water Metabolism.** Fluid balance depends on adequate concentrations of sodium; therefore, the kidneys must compensate for the many factors that favor excretion of sodium during pregnancy. For example, increased GFR, decreased concentration of plasma proteins, and increased progesterone levels all result in an increase in sodium excretion. On the other hand, increased concentrations of estrogen, cortisol, prolactin, and aldosterone all tend to promote the reabsorption of sodium.

***Dependent Edema.*** The net effect of the combined hormonal action is that sodium balance is maintained. Because of hemodilution, a slight decrease occurs in colloid osmotic pressure, which favors the development of edema during pregnancy. Edema is further increased toward term, when the weight of the uterus compresses the veins of the pelvis. This process delays venous return, causing the veins of the legs to become distended, and increases venous pressure, resulting in additional fluid shifts from the vascular compartment to interstitial spaces.

Edema of the feet and ankles is obvious at the end of the day, particularly if a pregnant woman stands for prolonged periods, and the force of gravity contributes to the pooling of blood in the veins of the legs. Dependent edema is clinically insignificant. If edema of the face or hands is noted, however, further assessment for hypertension or proteinuria is essential to determine whether pregnancy-induced hypertension is developing.

***Carpal Tunnel Syndrome.*** Fluid retention is also associated with carpal tunnel syndrome, believed to result when edema compresses the median nerve at the point where it goes through the carpal tunnel of the wrist. Symptoms include soreness, weakness, and tenderness of the muscles of the thumb. The condition usually resolves when the pregnancy ends.

**Carbohydrate Metabolism.** Carbohydrate metabolism changes markedly during pregnancy because more insulin is required as pregnancy progresses. As hormones such as progesterone and hPL cause maternal tissue to be resistant to insulin, insulinase, an enzyme produced by the placenta, speeds up the breakdown of insulin.

Insulin is essential for the metabolism of glucose and for maintenance of proper blood glucose levels. Decreasing the mother's ability to use insulin is a protective mechanism that allows an ample supply of glucose for transfer to the fetus. The mother's pancreas, however, must produce more insulin so that she can continue to metabolize enough glucose to meet her own energy needs and to prevent hyperglycemia. Hyperglycemia occurs when blood glucose levels exceed available insulin, which is needed to transport glucose into cells.

For most women, hyperglycemia is not a problem, and insulin production is increased, particularly during the second and third trimesters. In some women, however, insulin production cannot be increased, and these women experience periodic hyperglycemia. This condition is called *pregnancy-induced glucose intolerance*, or gestational diabetes (see Chapter 26).

**✓ CHECK YOUR READING**

14. What causes the progressive changes in posture and gait during pregnancy?
15. Why is progesterone called the hormone of pregnancy?
16. Why do maternal needs for insulin change during pregnancy?

## Confirmation of Pregnancy

Confirmation of pregnancy has become much simpler since the development of ultrasonography, which makes it possible to view the fetal outline and to observe the fetal heart beat very early in pregnancy. Traditionally, however, the diagnosis of pregnancy has been based on symptoms experienced by the woman as well as on signs observed by a physician, nurse-midwife, or nurse practitioner. Figure 7–7 summarizes fetal and maternal changes that occur throughout pregnancy. These signs and symptoms are grouped into three classifications: presumptive, probable, and positive indications of pregnancy. A diagnosis of pregnancy cannot be made solely on the presumptive or probable signs. Table 7–2 lists other possible causes for these signs.

### Presumptive Indications of Pregnancy

Presumptive indications can also be termed *subjective* changes because they are what the woman experiences and reports. Presumptive changes are the least reliable indicators of pregnancy because any one of them can be caused by conditions other than pregnancy.

**TABLE 7-2 INDICATIONS OF PREGNANCY AND OTHER POSSIBLE CAUSES**

| Sign | Other Possible Causes |
|---|---|
| PRESUMPTIVE INDICATIONS | |
| Amenorrhea | Emotional stress, strenuous physical exercise, endocrine problems, chronic disease, early menopause |
| Nausea and vomiting | Gastrointestinal virus, food poisoning, emotional stress |
| Fatigue | Illness, stress, sudden changes in lifestyle |
| Urinary frequency | Urinary tract infections |
| Breast and skin changes | Premenstrual changes, use of oral contraceptives |
| Quickening | Abdominal gas, peristalsis, or pseudocyesis (false pregnancy) |
| PROBABLE INDICATIONS | |
| Abdominal enlargement | Abdominal or uterine tumors |
| Cervical changes | Infection or hormonal imbalance |
| Ballottement | Uterine or cervical polyps |
| Braxton Hicks contractions | Soft uterine fibroids (myomas) |
| Palpation of fetal outline | Large myomas may feel like the fetal head; small soft myomas may simulate small parts of the fetus. |
| Pregnancy tests | Certain medications (antianxiety or anticonvulsant drugs), premature menopause, blood in urine, or malignant tumors that produce human chorionic gonadotropin may result in false-positive findings. |
| POSITIVE INDICATIONS | |
| Auscultation of fetal heart sounds | |
| Fetal movements felt by examiner | |
| Visualization of embryo or fetus | |

### AMENORRHEA

Absence of menstruation in a woman who regularly menstruates is one of the first changes noted and strongly suggests that conception has occurred in a sexually active woman. Menses cease after conception because progesterone and estrogen, secreted from the corpus luteum, maintain the endometrial lining in preparation for implantation of the fertilized ovum.

### NAUSEA AND VOMITING

Many women experience nausea and vomiting during early pregnancy, generally beginning about 6 weeks after the last menstrual period. These symptoms generally disappear spontaneously by about 16 weeks (Cunningham et al., 1997). Nausea and vomiting are believed to be caused by the increased levels of hormones (hCG, estrogen), decreased gastric motility (an effect of progesterone), and

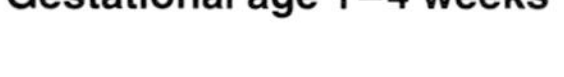
Gestational age 1–4 weeks

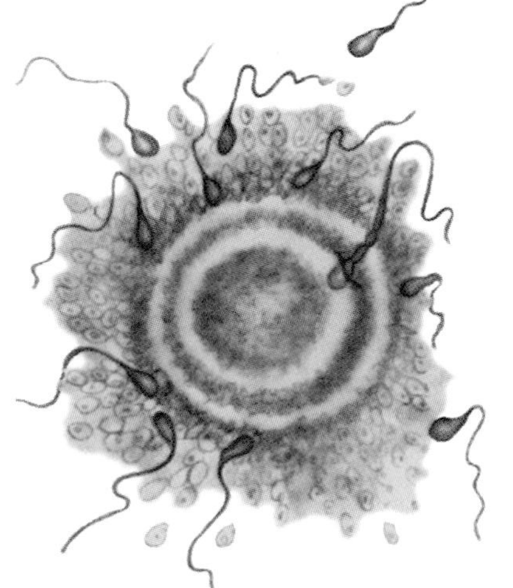

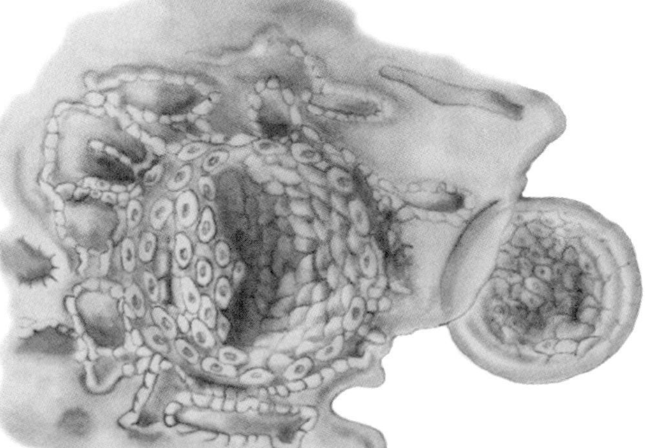

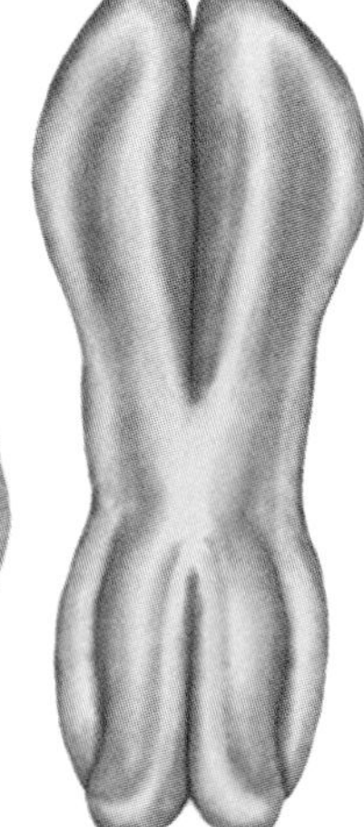

Woman's basal body temperature elevated; hCG elevated; pregnancy tests positive.

Crown-to-rump length 4 mm. Fertilization, implantation. Pre-embryonic stage.

**FIGURE 7-7**

Fetal growth and development and maternal responses based on the date of the last menstrual period.

**Gestational age 5–8 weeks**

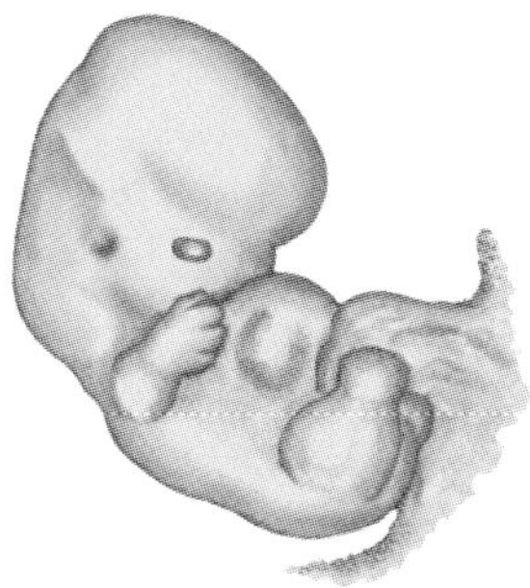

Crown-to-rump length 13 mm. Embryonic stage. Heart developed, beginning to pump. Arm and leg buds present. Head large, with facial features beginning to form.

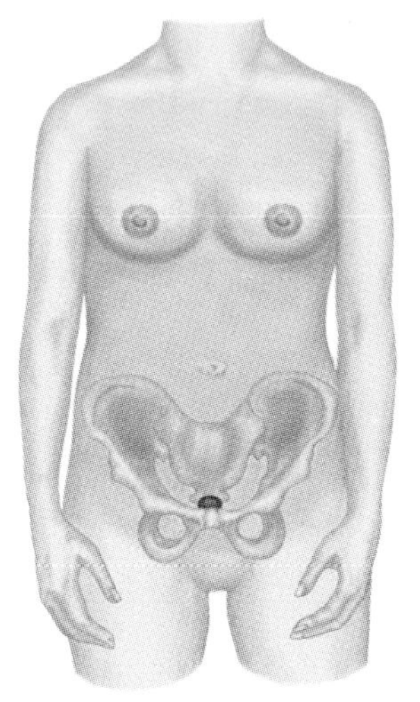

Woman misses menstrual period. Nausea; fatigue. Tingling of breasts. Uterus is size of a lemon; positive Chadwick's, Goodell's and Hegar's sign. Urinary frequency as enlarging uterus presses on the bladder; increased vaginal discharge.

**Gestational age 9–12 weeks**

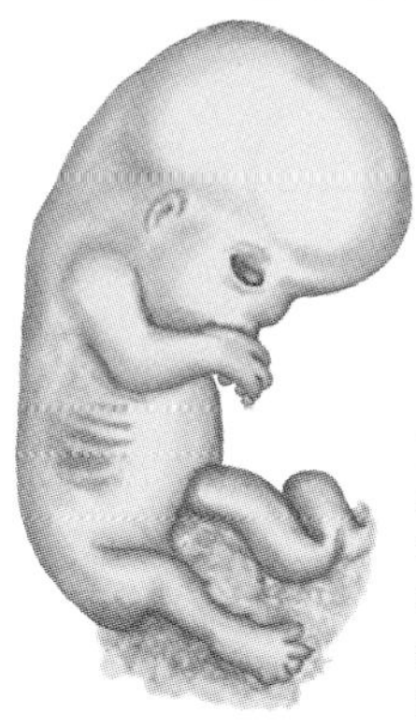

Crown-to-rump length 6–7 cm. Fetal stage begins at 10 weeks after last menstrual period. Extremities developed; fingers and toes differentiated; external genitalia show signs of male or female sex. Weight 14 g (0.5 oz).

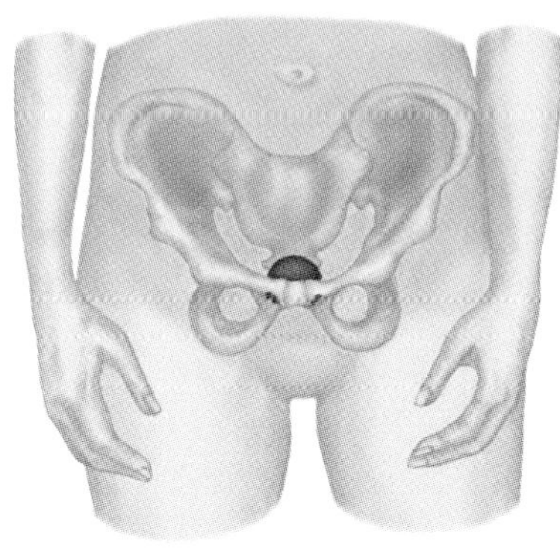

Nausea decreases after 12 weeks. Uterus is size of an orange; palpable above symphysis pubis. Vulvar varicosities may appear.

**Gestational age 13–16 weeks**

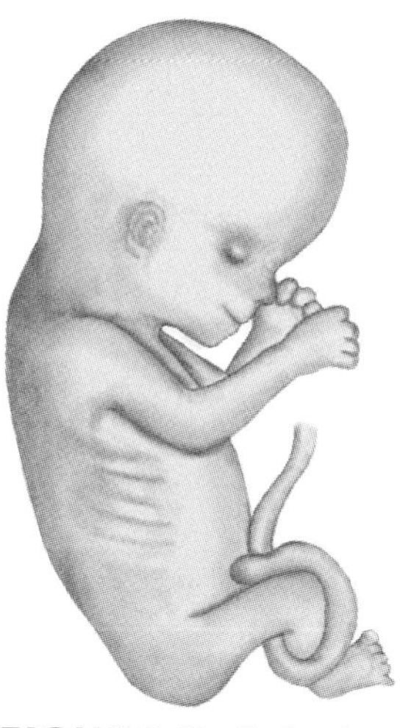

Crown-to-rump length 12 cm. Weight 110 g. Fetus begins to move. Head and thorax can be identified by ultrasound; sexual organs formed. Urine formation begins.

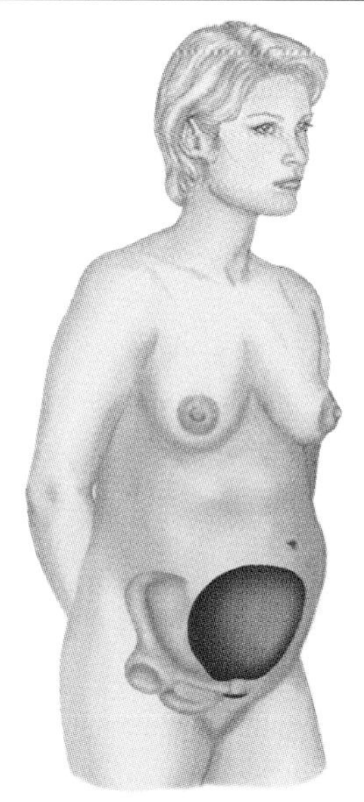

Fetal movements may be felt. Uterus has risen into the abdomen; fundus midway between symphysis pubis and umbilicus. Urinary frequency decreases; blood volume increases; uterine souffle heard.

**FIGURE 7–7** *Continued*

*Illustration continued on following page*

relative hypoglycemia that results from night-long fasting.

### FATIGUE

Many pregnant women experience extraordinary fatigue and drowsiness during the first trimester. The direct cause is unknown. Fatigue may, however, be related to periodic hypoglycemia that occurs because glucose is transferred from the mother to the fetus to provide energy for rapid development.

### URINARY FREQUENCY

Urinary frequency is first noticed by the expectant mother in the first few weeks of pregnancy, when the

**Gestational age 17–20 weeks**

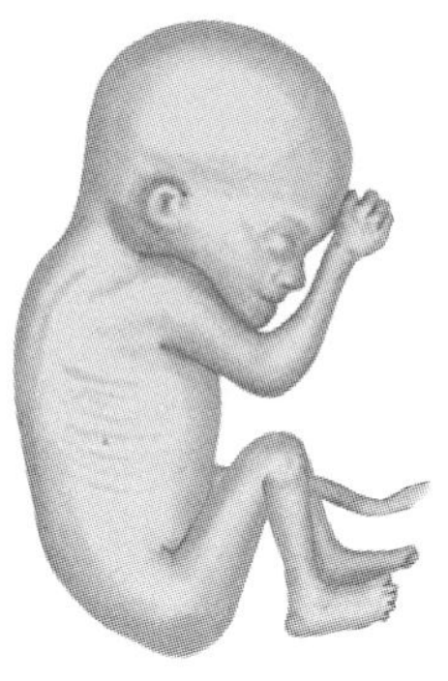

Crown-to-rump length 16 cm. Weight 320 g. Heart beat can be heard with fetoscope or electronic device. Meconium begins collecting in bowel. Period of very rapid growth.

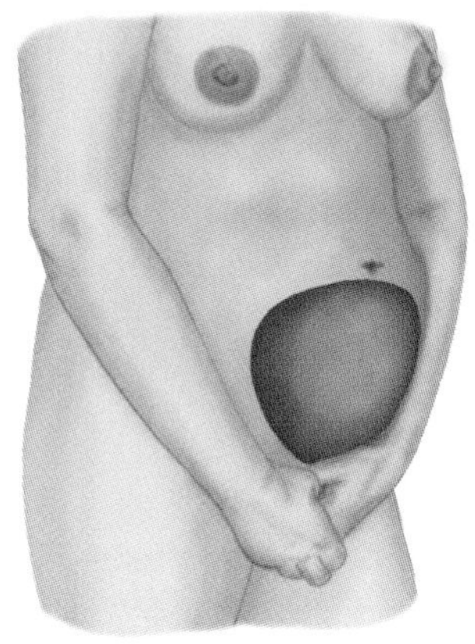

Skin pigmentation increases: areolae darken; chloasma and linea nigra may be obvious. Colostrum may be expressed. Braxton Hicks contractions palpable. Fundus at level of umbilicus.

**Gestational age 21–24 weeks**

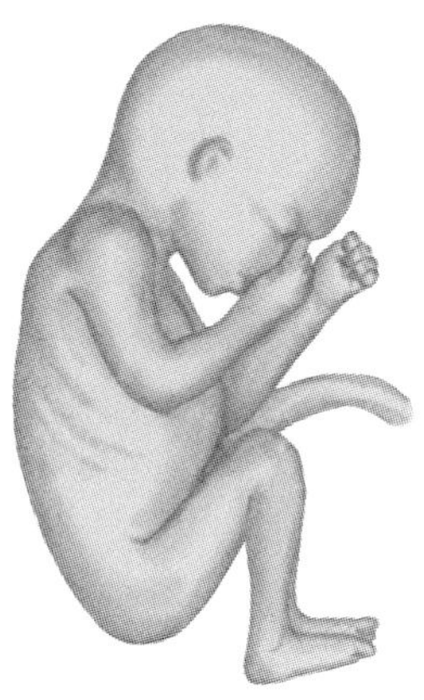

Crown-to-rump length 21 cm. Weight 630 g. Skin wrinkled and red; vernix present; head and body covered with lanugo.

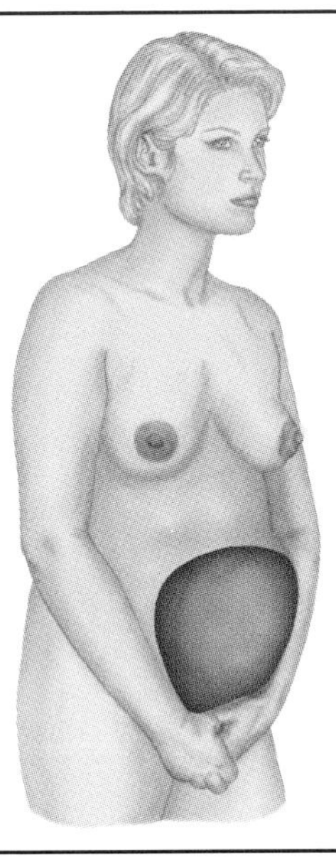

Relaxation of smooth muscles of veins and bladder increases the chance of varicose veins and urinary tract infections. Woman is more aware of fetal movements.

**Gestational age 25–28 weeks**

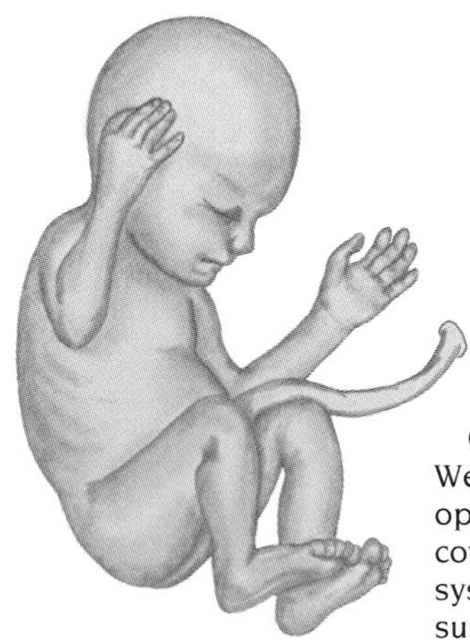

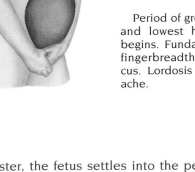

Crown-to-rump length 25 cm. Weight 1000 g. Eyes partially open; eyelashes present. Skin covered with vernix. Respiratory system immature, but fetus may survive if born.

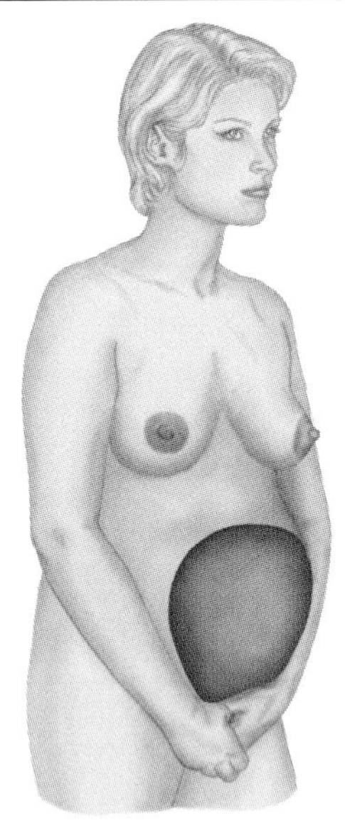

Period of greatest weight gain and lowest hemoglobin level begins. Fundal height is 3 to 4 fingerbreadths above umbilicus. Lordosis may cause backache.

**FIGURE 7–7** *Continued*

urge to void is caused by the pressure exerted on the bladder by the expanding uterus. This symptom abates during the second trimester, when the uterus expands into the abdominal cavity. Late in the third trimester, the fetus settles into the pelvic cavity, and the woman once again experiences frequency and urgency of urination because the uterus presses against the bladder.

**Gestational age 29–32 weeks**

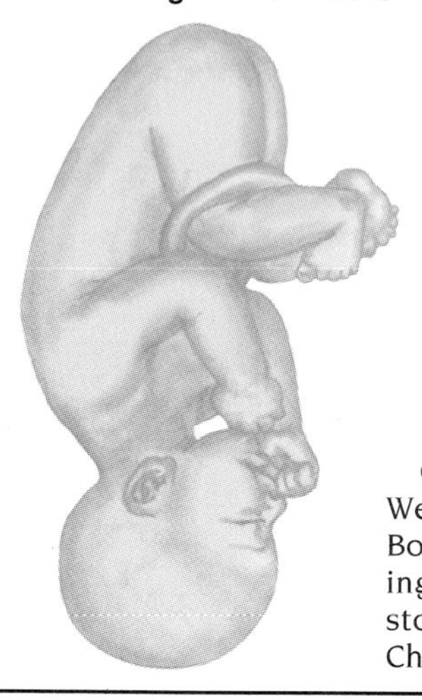

Crown-to-rump length 28 cm. Weight 1700 g. Toenails present. Body filling out, testes descending. Iron, nitrogen, calcium stored. Vernix covers body. Chances of survival improving.

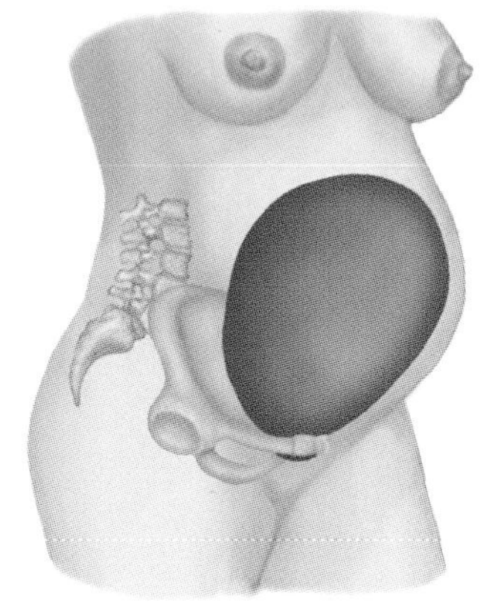

Heartburn common as uterus presses on diaphragm and displaces stomach. Braxton Hicks contractions more noticeable. Lordosis increases; waddling gait develops as relaxin softens pelvic joints.

**Gestational age 33–36 weeks**

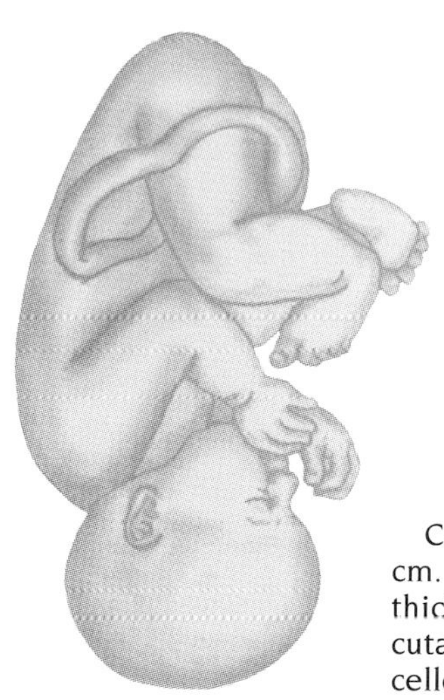

Crown-to-rump length 30–32 cm. Weight 2000–2500 g. Skin thicker, less wrinkled as subcutaneous fat accumulates. Excellent chance for survival.

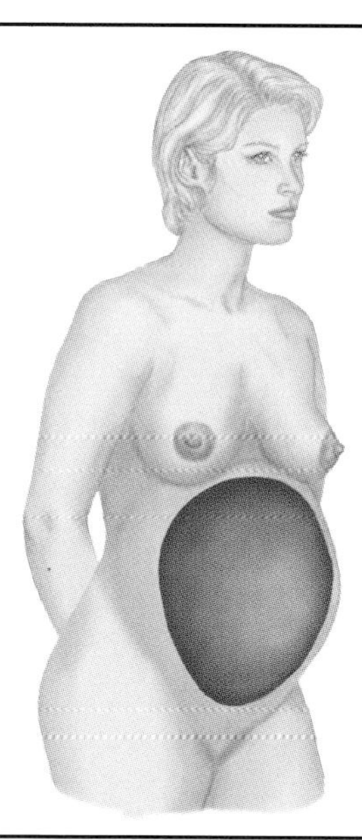

Shortness of breath caused by upward pressure on diaphragm; woman may have difficulty finding a comfortable position for sleep. Umbilicus protrudes. Varicosities more pronounced; pedal or ankle edema may be present. Urinary frequency noted following lightening when presenting part settles into pelvic cavity.

**Gestational age 37–40 weeks**

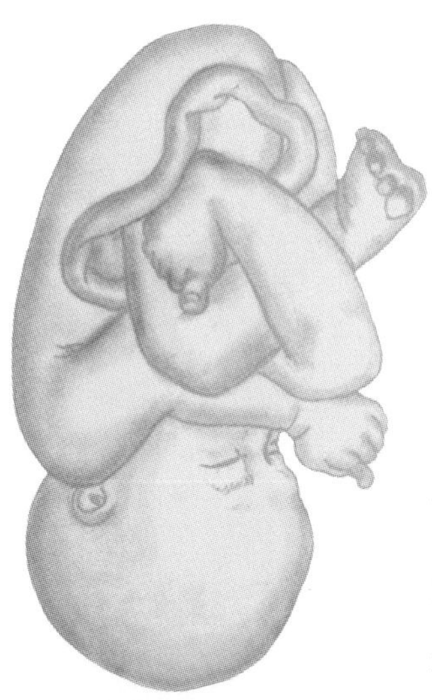

Crown-to-rump length 36 cm. Weight 3400 g. Body plump; lanugo remains only over shoulders; nails extend beyond nail beds; testes within scrotum; female labia well developed; labia majora cover labia minora.

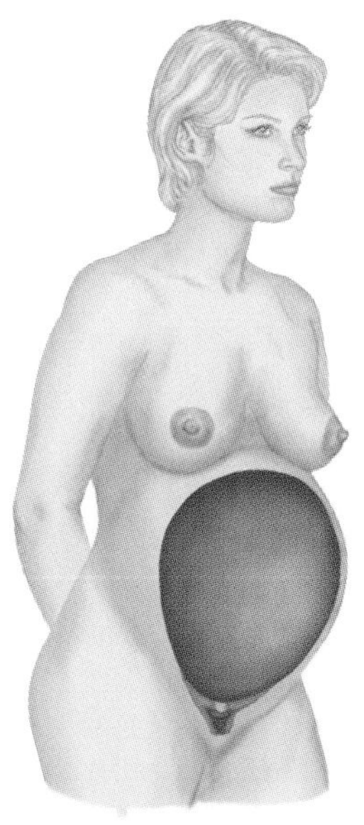

Woman is uncomfortable; looking forward to birth of baby. Cervix softens, begins to efface; mucus plug is often lost.

**FIGURE 7–7** *Continued*

## BREAST AND SKIN CHANGES

Breast changes occur early, at about the sixth week of pregnancy. The expectant mother experiences breast tenderness, feelings of fullness, and increased size and pigmentation of the areolae. Breast changes are due to the influence of estrogen and progesterone, which stimulate the lobes and ducts to prepare for lactation.

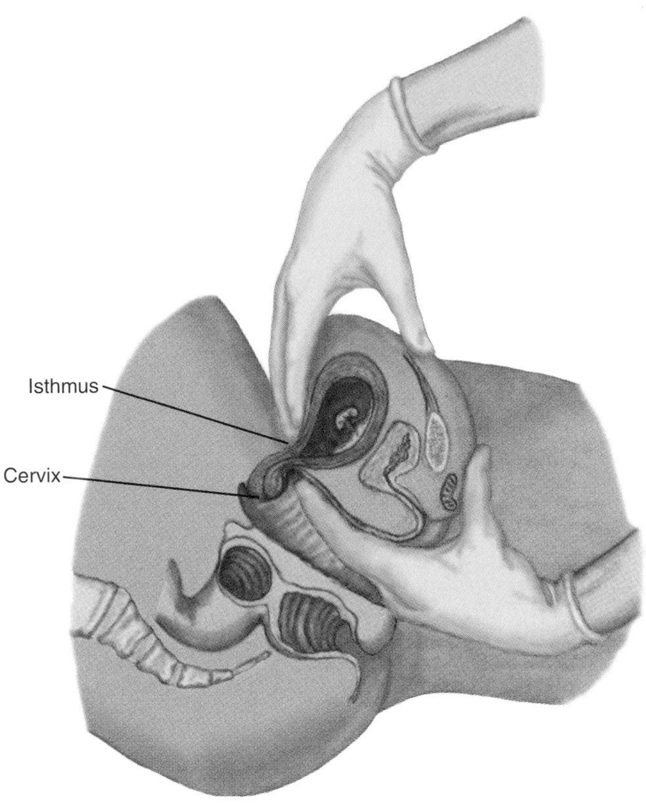


**FIGURE 7–8**

Hegar's sign demonstrates softening of the isthmus of the cervix.

Many women observe increased pigmentation of the skin (chloasma, linea nigra, darkening of the areolae of the breasts) during pregnancy. These skin changes are due to increased levels of melanocyte-stimulating hormone, one of the effects of estrogen.

#### FETAL MOVEMENT

Unlike other presumptive indications of pregnancy, the fetal movement (*quickening*) is not perceived until the second trimester. Between 16 and 20 weeks of gestation, the expectant mother first notices subtle fetal movements, which gradually increase in intensity.

### Probable Indications of Pregnancy

Probable indications of pregnancy are *objective* findings that can be documented by an examiner. They are primarily related to physical changes in the reproductive organs. Although these signs are stronger indicators of pregnancy, a positive diagnosis of pregnancy cannot be made on the basis of objective findings.

#### ABDOMINAL ENLARGEMENT

Enlargement of the abdomen during the childbearing years is a fairly reliable indication of pregnancy, particularly if it corresponds to a slow, gradual increase in uterine growth (see Fig. 7–1). Evidence of pregnancy is even more reliable when uterine growth is accompanied by amenorrhea.

#### CHANGES IN THE CERVIX

**Color.** The cervix changes from pink to a dark bluish violet. The color change, called *Chadwick's sign*, extends to the vagina and labia as well as the cervix. The bluish color is due to increased vascularity of the pelvic organs, and it is one of the earliest signs of pregnancy.

**Consistency.** In the early weeks of pregnancy, the cervix becomes softer as a result of pelvic vasocongestion (which causes Goodell's sign). Cervical softening is noted by the examiner during pelvic examination. At about the sixth week of pregnancy, the lower uterine segment is so soft that it can be compressed to the thinness of paper. This degree of softness is called *Hegar's sign* (Fig. 7–8). Because of the softening, the uterus can be easily flexed against the cervix (leading to *McDonald's sign*).

#### CHANGES IN THE UTERUS

**Ballottement.** Near midpregnancy, a sudden tap on the cervix during vaginal examination may cause the fetus to rise in the amniotic fluid and then rebound to its original position (Fig. 7–9). Ballottement is a strong indication of pregnancy, but it may also be caused by other factors such as uterine or cervical polyps.

**Braxton Hicks Contractions.** Irregular, painless contractions occur throughout pregnancy, although many expectant mothers do not notice them until the third trimester. Braxton Hicks contractions are not positive signs of pregnancy because similar contractions may occur with other conditions, such as soft uterine myomas (fibroids).

**Palpation of the Fetal Outline.** An experienced

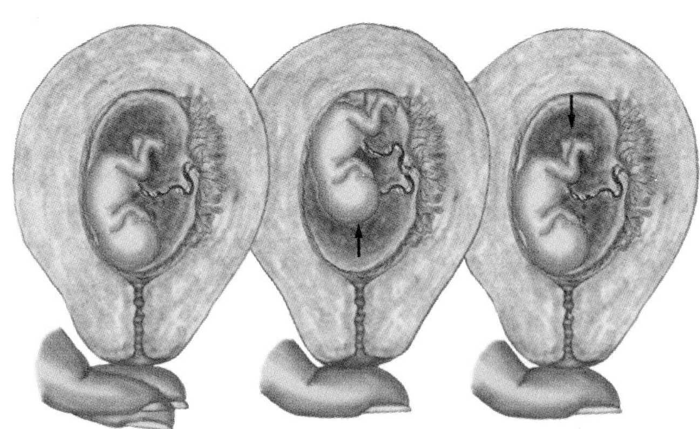


**FIGURE 7–9**

When the cervix is tapped, the fetus floats upward in the amniotic fluid. A rebound is felt by the examiner when the fetus falls back.

practitioner is able to palpate (feel) the outlines of the fetal body by the second half of pregnancy. Outlining the fetus becomes easier as the pregnancy progresses and the uterine walls thin to accommodate the growing fetus. Occasionally, large myomas may feel like the fetal head, or small soft myomas may simulate small parts of the fetus and may result in a false diagnosis of pregnancy.

**Uterine Souffle.** A soft, blowing sound that corresponds to the maternal pulse may be auscultated over the uterus. This sound is due to blood circulating through the placenta, and it corresponds to the maternal pulse. Therefore, to identify uterine souffle, the rate of the maternal pulse must be checked simultaneously. Uterine souffle differs from *funic souffle*, the soft purring sound heard over the umbilical cord and corresponding to the fetal heart rate.

#### PREGNANCY TESTS

**Home Pregnancy Tests.** In recent years, pregnancy tests have been improved greatly. They are based on the presence of hCG in maternal urine, and they may be useful as early as 3 days after a missed menstrual period. Pregnancy tests are available for purchase over the counter, and they are uncomplicated and convenient. Home test kits are capable of greater than 97 percent accuracy, but test kit instructions must be followed precisely to obtain accurate results (Cunningham et al., 1997).

When pregnancy test results are reported as negative and the woman is in fact pregnant, the results are called false negative. Tests with negative results should be repeated in 2 weeks. The primary causes of false-negative results are the following:

- A test performed too soon
- Urine that is too dilute
- Urine that was stored too long at room temperature
- Impending spontaneous abortion
- Ectopic (tubal) pregnancy

When test results are positive and pregnancy has not occurred, the results are called false positive. The major causes of false-positive test results are the following:

- Error in reading
- Test performed at time of ovulation
- Presence of protein or blood in the urine
- Recent pregnancy
- Drug interference (marijuana, methadone, phenothiazine, aspirin in large quantities)

**Radioimmunoassay.** Because radioimmunoassays use radioactively labeled markers to detect antibodies against beta-subunit hCG in blood or urine, they must be performed in a laboratory. They are the most sensitive pregnancy tests available and are accurate as early as 1 week after ovulation.

### Positive Indications of Pregnancy

Only three signs are accepted as positive confirmation of pregnancy: auscultation of fetal heart sounds, fetal movement felt by an examiner, and visualization of the fetus with sonography.

#### AUSCULTATION OF FETAL HEART SOUNDS

Fetal heart sounds can be heard with a fetoscope by 18 to 20 weeks of gestation. The electronic Doppler scan amplifies fetal heart sounds so that they are audible by 10 to 12 weeks. (Both the fetoscope and the Doppler transducer are illustrated in Chapter 14.)

To make a positive diagnosis of pregnancy, it is necessary not only to hear the fetal heart beat but also to distinguish it from the maternal pulse. The fetal heart rate depends on gestational age. The fetal heart rate is in the range of 160 to 170 beats per minute (BPM) in the first trimester (DuBose, 1996). As the fetus grows, the rate becomes slower, and it declines to between 110 and 160 BPM during the third trimester. It should be auscultated while the radial pulse of the expectant mother is being palpated. The fetal heart rate is muffled by amniotic fluid, and the sound has been likened to that of a clock ticking behind a pillow. The location changes because the fetus moves freely in the amniotic fluid.

#### FETAL MOVEMENTS FELT BY EXAMINER

Fetal movements vary from faint flutterings in early pregnancy to the characteristic kick or thrust of later pregnancy. These movements are considered a positive sign of pregnancy when felt by an experienced examiner who is not likely to be deceived by similar sensations produced by peristalsis in the large intestine.

#### VISUALIZATION OF THE FETUS

Transabdominal ultrasound examination is frequently used to confirm pregnancy as early as 5 to 6 weeks of gestation. This procedure involves placing an ultrasound transducer, or "probe," on the lower abdomen to detect the gestational sac, which is readily identifiable in the maternal pelvis; movements of the fetal heart are also discernible. By the 14th week, the fetal head and thorax can be identified. (See Chapter 10 for additional information about sonography.)

Positive confirmation of pregnancy is possible even earlier when transvaginal ultrasonography is used. With an ultrasound probe placed in the vagina, the gestational sac is obvious by 10 days after implantation. This corresponds to 16 days after ovulation (Cunningham et al., 1997).

**CHECK YOUR READING**

17. How do presumptive and probable indications of pregnancy differ?
18. Why is "fetal" movement felt by the pregnant woman not a positive sign of pregnancy?
19. What are the most common causes of false-negative pregnancy tests?

## Antepartum Assessment and Care

The objective of antepartum care is to ensure that every wanted pregnancy culminates in the birth of a healthy infant without impairing the health of the mother. Three basic components of antepartum care are early and continuing risk assessments, health promotion, and medical and psychosocial interventions. Inadequate antepartum care is associated with low birth weight and an increased incidence of prematurity in neonates. A strong correlation has been found between these two complications and increased infant mortality.

Antepartum care is considered adequate when it begins in the first trimester of pregnancy and continues on a regular basis thereafter. In addition to collecting and evaluating laboratory values and physical measurements, prenatal care should also provide health education, counseling, and social support.

Approximately 75 percent of American women begin antepartum care in the first trimester. Six percent do not seek care until the third trimester or obtain no care before childbirth. The United States Public Health Service (1992) goal for the year 2000 is for at least 90 percent of American women to commence antepartum care in the first trimester.

### Terminology Defining Pregnancy

Before beginning antepartum assessment or care, one must be able to define the terms that are unique to maternity nursing.

**abortion** In the United States, abortion refers to spontaneous or elective termination of pregnancy before the 20th week of gestation, based on the date of the last menstrual period. Spontaneous abortion is frequently termed "miscarriage" by the lay public.

**gravida** A woman who is or has been pregnant, regardless of the duration of the pregnancy.

**primigravida** A woman who is pregnant for the first time.

**multigravida** A woman who has been pregnant more than once.

**para** Number of pregnancies that have progressed past 20 weeks. The term does not indicate whether the fetus was born alive or was stillborn. Parity does not reflect the number of fetuses or infants; a multifetal pregnancy (twins, triplets) is considered to be one parous experience.

**nullipara** A woman who has never completed a pregnancy beyond 20 weeks of gestation.

**primipara** A woman who has given birth after a pregnancy of at least 20 weeks of gestation.

**multipara** A woman who has given birth two or more times at more than 20 weeks of gestation.

**preterm** A birth that occurs after the 20th week and before the start of the 38th week of gestation.

**term** A birth that occurs between the 38th and 42nd weeks of gestation.

**postterm** Birth that occurs after 42 weeks of gestation.

**trimester** A division of pregnancy into three equal parts of 13 weeks each.

Knowing how to calculate gravida and para is essential; but incomplete information is obtained when only gravida and para are counted. Use of the TPAL acronym allows description of pregnancy outcomes as term (T), preterm (P), abortions (A), and live (L) births. Table 7–3 lists examples of the TPAL method for obtaining complete information.

**TABLE 7–3 CALCULATION OF GRAVIDA AND PARA**

A useful method for calculating gravida and para is to divide pregnancy outcome into the number of term pregnancies, preterm pregnancies, abortions, and living children. The acronym TPAL is helpful: T = term, P = preterm, A = abortions, L = living children.

The following examples illustrate how to use this method to obtain complete information.

- Sally Elam is pregnant for the fifth time. She had two elective abortions in the first trimester; she has a son who was born at 40 weeks' gestation and a daughter who was born at 36 weeks. She is gravida 5, para 2. T = 1 (the son born at 40 weeks); P = 1 (the daughter born at 36 weeks); A = 2; L = 2. The two abortions are counted in the gravida but are not included in the para because they occurred before 20 weeks.
- Kathleen Eber gave birth to twins at 36 weeks; she gave birth to a stillborn infant at 24 weeks; 2 years later she experienced a spontaneous abortion at 12 weeks. If pregnant now, she is gravida 4, para 2 (the twins count as 1 parous experience, and the stillborn counts as 1). T = 0 (pregnancies did not go to term); P = 2 (the twins, born at 36 weeks, count as 1 preterm birth and the stillborn infant born at 24 weeks also counts as 1); A = 1; L = 2.

**Nurses must exercise caution when discussing gravida and para with the expectant mother in the presence of her family or significant other. Although the antepartum record indicates a previous pregnancy or childbirth, she may not have shared this information with her family, and her right to privacy could be jeopardized by probing questions. The pregnancy may have terminated in elective or spontaneous abortion or in the birth of an infant who was placed for adoption. In either instance, the confidentiality of the pregnant woman must be protected.**

## Initial Visit

A thorough history and physical examination must be completed at the first antepartum visit. Increasing numbers of nurses are prepared to obtain health histories and to perform physical examinations. Nurses who have not fully developed these skills may be responsible for assisting the nurse practitioner, certified nurse-midwife, or physician who is the primary health care provider. Although each agency has its own specific forms, the forms differ only in format because both medical and nursing practices are governed by standards and similar data are obtained by all agencies.

The primary objectives of the first antepartum examination are to do the following:

- Verify or rule out pregnancy
- Evaluate the pregnant woman's physical health relevant to childbearing
- Assess the growth and health of the fetus
- Establish baseline data for comparison with future observations
- Establish trust and rapport with the childbearing family
- Evaluate the psychosocial needs of the woman and her family
- Assess the need for counseling or teaching
- Negotiate a plan of care to ensure a healthy mother and a healthy baby

### HISTORY

**Obstetric History.** The obstetric history provides essential information about prior pregnancies that may alert the physician or nurse-midwife to possible problems in the present pregnancy. The usual components of this history are the following:

- Gravida, para, abortions, living children
- Weight of infants at birth, length of gestation
- Labor experience, type of delivery, location of birth, name of attending physician or midwife
- Type of anesthesia and any difficulties
- Maternal complications, such as hypertension, diabetes, infection, bleeding
- Complications with the infant
- Method of infant feeding planned (breast or formula)
- Special concerns

**Menstrual History.** A complete menstrual history is necessary to establish the EDD. It is common practice to estimate the EDD on the basis of the first day of the last menstrual cycle, although ovulation and conception occur approximately 2 weeks after the beginning of menstruation in a regular 28-day cycle. The average duration of pregnancy from the first day of the last normal menstrual period is 40 weeks, or 280 days. N*agele's rule* is often used to establish EDD. To use this method, one must subtract 3 months, add 7 days to the first day of the last normal menstrual period (LNMP), and correct the year.

For example: LNMP June 30, 1997
Subtract 3 months = March 30, 1997
Add 7 days and change the year = April 6, 1998

Many health care providers also use a gestational calculator, or "wheel," to calculate EDD quickly, although some wheels are prone to error (Cunningham et al., 1997). Newer methods include electronic cal-

### CRITICAL THINKING EXERCISE

Wilma Turner gave birth to twin girls at 38 weeks of gestation 3 years ago. She had a spontaneous abortion last year at 12 weeks of gestation and thinks she may be pregnant now because she has missed a menstrual period and is experiencing morning sickness. Wilma's last normal menstrual period began June 22, 1997.

**Q:**
1. If Wilma is pregnant now, what would be the gravida and para?
2. Explain to Wilma why amenorrhea and morning sickness are not positive indications of pregnancy.
3. Use Nagele's rule to compute the EDD.

**A:**
1. If pregnant now, Wilma is gravida 3, para 1 (the twin birth counts as one parous experience). If the acronym TPAL is used, more complete information can be recorded. T = 1 (twin infants born at term but counted as 1 parous experience); P = 0 (no preterm infants); A = 1 (one pregnancy ended before 20 weeks' gestation); L = 2 (living twins).
2. Amenorrhea and nausea and vomiting are only presumptive (subjective) indications of pregnancy because they can be caused by conditions other than pregnancy.
3. Count back 3 months to March 22, and add 7 days. This brings the date to March 29. Correct the year to 1998. Wilma's EDD is March 29, 1998.

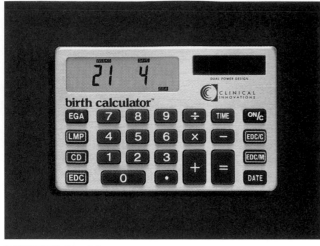


**FIGURE 7–10**

Electronic birth calculator used to compute the estimated due date, appointments, and specific tests. (Used with permission of Clinical Innovations, Murray, Utah.)

culators (Fig. 7–10) that compute the EDD, gestational age, and future dates for procedures, such as ultrasound examinations and Rh immunizations.

**Contraceptive History.** Some forms of contraception may impose a risk on the fetus, the mother, or both; therefore, a detailed history of contraceptive methods is needed. Very recent use of oral contraceptives before pregnancy or continued use during early unrecognized pregnancy remains a source of concern because of the effect of estrogens and some synthetic progestins on the sexual organs of the fetus (Briggs et al., 1994). Some physicians advise women in pre-conception counseling to stop oral contraception and to use alternative methods (condoms, diaphragm) to prevent conception for 3 months before conceiving.

Intrauterine devices, which are not widely used in the United States, can cause complications. If pregnancy occurs with an intrauterine device in place, there are serious risks of abortion, premature delivery, and puncture of the uterus.

**Medical and Surgical History.** Chronic conditions, such as diabetes mellitus, hypertension, and renal disease, can affect the outcome of the pregnancy and must be investigated. Infections, such as hepatitis or pyelonephritis, as well as surgical procedures and trauma that may complicate the pregnancy or childbirth, must be documented. The history includes the following:

- Age, race, ethnic background (relevant for groups at high risk for specific genetic problems, such as sickle cell anemia, thalassemia, and Tay-Sachs disease)
- Childhood diseases and immunizations
- Chronic illnesses, such as asthma and heart disease (onset, treatment)
- Previous illnesses, surgical procedures, injuries (particularly of the pelvis and back)
- Previous infections: hepatitis, sexually transmissible diseases, or tuberculosis
- History of anemia and how it was treated
- Medications: prescription, over the counter; reasons for use
- Bladder, bowel function (problems or changes)
- Amount of caffeine consumed each day (coffee, tea, chocolate, colas)
- Tobacco use (number of years and number of packs per day)
- Use of drugs (name, amount, date and time of last use)
- Overall health and energy
- Appetite, general nutrition, history of eating disorders
- Contact with domestic pets, particularly cats, which increases the risk of infections such as toxoplasmosis
- Allergies and drug sensitivities
- Occupation and related risk factors

**Family History.** A family history provides valuable information about the general health of the family, including chronic diseases, such as diabetes and heart disease, and infections, such as tuberculosis and hepatitis. Moreover, information about patterns of genetic or congenital anomalies may be revealed.

**Partner's Health History.** The partner's history helps determine whether the father of the expected child or his family has a history of significant health problems. These include genetic abnormalities, chronic diseases, and infections. Use of drugs, such as cocaine or alcohol, may affect the ability of the family to cope with pregnancy and childbirth. Tobacco use by the father is important because both the mother and infant are at risk for upper respiratory complications as a result of passive smoking (inhaling smoke that is exhaled by another).

In addition, the blood type and Rh factor of the father are important if the mother is Rh negative and there is the possibility of a blood incompatibility between the mother and the fetus.

**Psychosocial History.** The psychosocial history, which should be completed at the same time, is discussed in Chapter 8.

### PHYSICAL EXAMINATION

Because many women have never had a physical examination until they become pregnant, a thorough evaluation of all body systems is necessary to detect previously undiagnosed physical problems that may affect the pregnancy outcome. A complete examination also allows the examiner to establish baseline levels that will guide the treatment of the expectant mother and fetus throughout pregnancy.

### VITAL SIGNS

**Blood Pressure.** Because position affects blood pressure in the pregnant woman, the method for obtaining blood pressure should be standardized as much as possible. Blood pressure should be obtained in the sitting position with the arm supported in a horizontal position at heart level (Knuppel & Drukker, 1993). Documentation should include the position, the arm used, and the pressures obtained. Ideally, documentation should also indicate whether Korotkoff's fourth phase (muffling) or fifth phase (disappearance of sound) is used because pressures are 5 to 10 mmHg higher if the fourth phase is used.

**Pulse.** The normal pulse rate is 60 to 90 BPM. Tachycardia is associated with anxiety, hyperthyroidism, and infection and should be investigated. Apical pulse should be assessed for at least 1 minute to determine the amplitude and regularity of the heart beat. Pedal pulses are assessed to determine if circulatory problems are present in the legs. Pedal pulses should be strong, equal, and regular.

**Respiratory Effort.** Respiratory rate during pregnancy is in the range of 16 to 24 BPM. Tachypnea may indicate respiratory infection or cardiac disease. Breath sounds should be equal bilaterally; chest expansion should be symmetric, and lung fields should be free of all abnormal breath sounds.

**Temperature.** Normal temperature during pregnancy is 36.2 to 37.6°C (98 to 99.6°F). Increased temperature suggests infection that may require medical management.

### CARDIOVASCULAR SYSTEM

**Venous Congestion.** Additional assessment of the cardiovascular system includes observation for venous congestion, which can develop into varicosities. Venous congestion is most commonly noted in the legs, vulva, or rectum.

**Edema.** Edema of the legs may be a benign condition that reflects pooling of blood in the extremities, which results in a shift of intravascular fluid into interstitial spaces. When pressure, exerted by a finger or thumb, leaves a persistent depression, it is termed *pitting edema* (see Fig. 17–9).

### MUSCULOSKELETAL SYSTEM

**Posture and Gait.** Body mechanics, as well as changes in posture and gait, should be addressed. Body mechanics during pregnancy may produce strain on the muscles of the lower back and legs.

**Height and Weight.** An initial weight is needed to establish a baseline for weight gain throughout pregnancy. Weight should be compared to the ideal-weight-for-height charts to determine whether the expectant mother is underweight or overweight. Preconception weight lower than 45 kg (100 pounds) or height under 150 cm (60 inches) is associated with preterm labor and low-birth-weight infants. Preconception weight higher than 90 kg (200 pounds) is associated with increased incidence of pregnancy-induced glucose intolerance (gestational diabetes) and pregnancy-induced hypertension.

**Pelvic Measurements.** Early in pregnancy, the bony pelvis is evaluated to determine whether the diameters are adequate to permit vaginal delivery. (For pelvic measurements, see Chapter 12.)

**Abdomen.** The contour, size, and muscle tone of the abdomen should be assessed. Fundal height should be measured if the fundus is palpable above the symphysis pubis. For the measurement to be accurate, the bladder must be empty before the measurement is taken. With the MacDonald method of measurement, the woman lies on her back with the knees slightly flexed. The top of the fundus is palpated, and a tape is stretched from the top of the symphysis pubis over the abdominal curve to the top of the fundus (Fig. 7–11).

From 22 weeks until term, the fundal height, measured in centimeters, is roughly equal (±2 cm) to the gestational age of the fetus in weeks (Hobel, 1992). If fundal height exceeds weeks of gestation, additional assessment is necessary to investigate the cause for the unexpected uterine size. It may be that the EDD is incorrect and the pregnancy is further advanced than previously thought; perhaps the EDD is correct, but more than one fetus is present.

If fundal height is less than expected on the basis of gestational age, the EDD must be confirmed. If dates are accurate, further assessment may be nec-

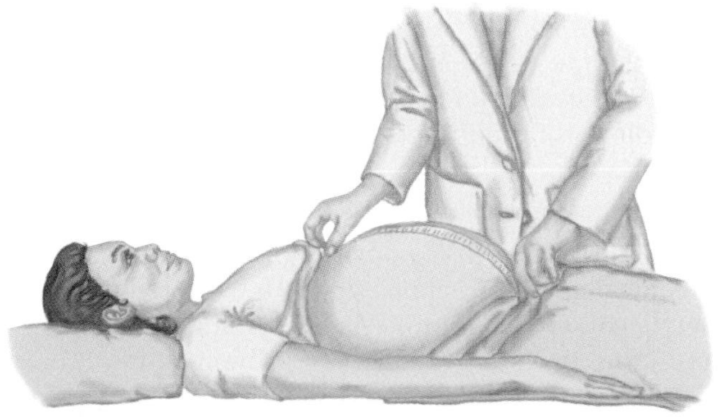

**FIGURE 7–11**

Measuring the uterus includes the distance between the upper border of the symphysis pubis and the top of the fundus.

essary to determine whether the fetus is experiencing inadequate growth.

Fetal heart rate should be counted and documented if the pregnancy is advanced enough to hear fetal heart tones.

#### NEUROLOGIC SYSTEM

A complete neurologic assessment is not necessary for young women who are free of signs or symptoms that indicate a problem. Deep tendon reflexes should be evaluated, however, because hyperreflexia is associated with complications of pregnancy. See Procedure 25–1 for assessment of deep tendon reflexes.

#### INTEGUMENTARY SYSTEM

Skin color should be consistent with racial background. Pallor may indicate anemia. Jaundice may indicate hepatic disease. Lesions, bruising, or areas of hyperpigmentation (chloasma, linea nigra) related to pregnancy, as well as stretch marks (striae), should be noted. Nail beds should be pink, with instant capillary return.

#### ENDOCRINE SYSTEM

The thyroid enlarges slightly during the second trimester. Gross enlargement or tenderness, however, may indicate hyperthyroidism and requires further medical evaluation.

#### GASTROINTESTINAL SYSTEM

**Mouth.** Mucous membranes should be pink, smooth, glistening, and uniform. The lips should be free of ulcerations. The gums may be red, tender, and edematous as a result of the effects of increased estrogen, which produces hyperplasia. The teeth should be in good repair.

**Intestine.** A warm stethoscope for assessing bowel sounds is more comfortable. Bowel sounds may be diminished because of the effects of progesterone on smooth muscle. The examination is an excellent time to ask if there are problems with constipation. Bowel sounds are often increased if a meal is overdue or if diarrhea is present.

#### URINARY SYSTEM

Urine collected for testing should always be a clean-catch midstream sample. Urine is tested to detect signs of urinary tract infection and substances in the urine that may indicate a problem.

**Protein.** Protein should not be present in urine. Its presence may indicate contamination by vaginal secretions. It may also indicate kidney disease or pregnancy-induced hypertension.

**Glucose.** Small amounts of glucose may indicate physiologic "spilling" that occurs during normal pregnancy. Larger amounts require glucose screening of the blood.

**Ketones.** Ketones may be found in the urine after heavy exercise or as a result of inadequate intake of food and fluid.

**Bacteria.** Increased bacteria in the urine is associated with urinary tract infection, which is common during pregnancy.

#### REPRODUCTIVE SYSTEM

**Breasts.** Breast size, symmetry, condition of nipples, and presence of colostrum should be noted. Any lumps, dimpling of the skin, or asymmetry of the nipples requires further evaluation.

**External Reproductive Organs.** The skin and mucous membranes of the perineum, vulva, and anus are inspected for excoriations, growths, ulcerations, lesions, varicosities, warts, chancres, and perineal scars. Enlargement, tenderness, redness, or discharge of Bartholin's glands or Skene's glands may indicate gonorrheal or chlamydial infection. The examiner should obtain a specimen for culture of any discharge from lesions or inflamed glands to determine the causative organisms and to provide effective care.

**Internal Reproductive Organs.** A speculum inserted into the vagina permits the examiner to see the walls of the vagina and the cervix. The cervix should be pink in a non-pregnant woman, but bluish discoloration (Chadwick's sign) may be seen during pregnancy. The external cervical os is closed in primigravidas, but one fingertip may be admitted in multiparas. The cervix feels relatively firm except during pregnancy, when marked softening is noted (Goodell's sign). Routine cervical cultures for gonorrhea and chlamydial infection are standard practice during initial pregnancy examination at most agencies. The examiner also collects a specimen for a Papanicolaou (Pap) smear, a screening test for cervical cancer.

A bimanual examination involves using both hands to palpate the internal genitalia. The examiner palpates the uterus for size, contour, tenderness, and position. The uterus should be movable between the two examining hands and should feel smooth. The ovaries, if palpable, should be about the shape and size of almonds and should not be tender.

#### LABORATORY DATA

Table 7–4 lists laboratory examinations that are commonly performed during pregnancy. The table briefly describes their purpose and the significance of each test.

**TABLE 7–4 COMMON LABORATORY TESTS**

| Test | Purpose | Significance |
|---|---|---|
| Blood grouping | Determine blood type | Should blood replacement be necessary |
| Hemoglobin (Hgb) or hematocrit (Hct) | To detect anemia | Hgb < 11 g/dl or Hct < 32% requires iron supplementation |
| Complete blood count (CBC) | To detect infection or cell abnormalities | 15,000/mm³ or more white blood cells or decreased platelets require follow-up |
| Rh factor and antibody screen | For possible maternal-fetal blood incompatibility | If mother Rh-negative and mate Rh-positive or antibodies present, additional testing and treatment required |
| VDRL or rapid plasma reagin (RPR) | Syphilis screen | Treat if positive<br>Retest at 36 weeks |
| Rubella titer | To determine immunity | If titer is <1:8, mother is not immune; retest during pregnancy, immunize postpartum if not immune |
| Skin test | Screen for tuberculosis | If positive, refer for additional testing or therapy |
| Hemoglobin electrophoresis | To screen for sickle cell trait if client is African-American | If mother is positive, check partner; infant is at risk only if both parents are positive |
| Hepatitis B screen | To detect presence of antigens in maternal blood | If present, infants should be given hepatitis immune globulin and vaccine soon after birth |
| Human immunodeficiency virus (HIV) screen | Offered at first visit to detect HIV antibodies | Positive results require retesting, counseling, and treatment |
| Urinalysis | To detect infection, renal disease, or diabetes | Positive for protein, glucose, ketones, or bacteria |
| Papanicolaou (Pap) test | To screen for cervical neoplasia | Treat and refer if abnormal cells are present |
| Cervical culture | To detect sexually transmissible diseases, such as gonorrhea, group B streptococci | Treat and retest as necessary |
| Maternal serum alpha-fetoprotein | To screen for fetal anomalies | Either low or high levels should be investigated |
| Maternal blood glucose | To screen for gestational diabetes | If elevated, a 3-hour glucose tolerance test is recommended |

**CHECK YOUR READING**

20. Why is a medical-surgical history as well as an obstetric history necessary?
21. How should blood pressure be obtained and documented? Why is documentation of blood pressure important during pregnancy?
22. How does fundal height relate to gestational age?

## RISK ASSESSMENT

Risk assessment begins at the initial visit, when the health care team identifies factors that put the expectant mother or the fetus at risk for complications and thus in need if specialized care. Because not all factors present equal threats, a risk-scoring tool is used by many agencies to determine degree of risk. Although risk scoring is a valuable method for identifying the high-risk pregnancy, it cannot be counted on to predict problems or the absence of complications 100 percent of the time.

Many women identified as high risk give birth to healthy term infants. Furthermore, risk factors change as pregnancy progresses, and risk assessment must be updated throughout pregnancy because gestations that are categorized as low risk at the initial assessment may become high risk later. Table 7–5 lists the major risk factors and identifies maternal and fetal-neonatal implications.

## SUBSEQUENT ASSESSMENTS

Ongoing antepartum care is important to the successful outcome of pregnancy. The recommended schedule for prenatal assessment in an uncomplicated pregnancy is as follows:

Conception to 28 weeks—every 4 weeks
29 to 36 weeks—every 2 to 3 weeks
37 weeks to birth—weekly

**Vital Signs.** To obtain accurate information, blood pressure must be measured in the same arm with the mother in the same position each time. Deviations from the baseline value in blood pressure, pulse, or respiratory rate indicate the need for further assessment. Temperature should remain within normal limits.

**Weight.** Weight should be plotted to document that the expected pattern of weight gain is occurring. Inadequate weight gain may signify that the preg-

**TABLE 7-5 SUMMARY OF HIGH-RISK FACTORS IN PREGNANCY**

| Factors | Implications |
|---|---|
| **DEMOGRAPHIC FACTORS** | |
| <16 years or >35 years | Increased risk for preterm labor, pregnancy-induced hypertension, congenital anomalies |
| Low socioeconomic status or dependent on public assistance | Increased risk for preterm labor, low-birth-weight infants |
| Nonwhite race | Incidence of infant and maternal death twice that of whites |
| Multiparity: >4 pregnancies | Increasing parity increases risk of pregnancy loss, antepartum or postpartum hemorrhage, and cesarean birth |
| **SOCIAL-PERSONAL FACTORS** | |
| Weight <45 kg (100 pounds) | Associated with low-birth-weight infant |
| Weight >90 kg (200 pounds) | Increased risk for pregnancy-induced hypertension, difficult labor, large-for-gestational-age infant, and cesarean birth |
| Height <154 cm (5 feet) | Increased incidence of cesarean birth due to cephalopelvic disproportion |
| Smoking | Associated with low-birth-weight infant, increased risk for preterm birth |
| Use of alcohol or addicting drugs | Increased risk of congenital anomalies, neonatal withdrawal syndrome, and fetal alcohol syndrome |
| **OBSTETRIC FACTORS** | |
| Birth of previous infant >4000 g (8.5 pounds) | Increased need for cesarean birth; increased risk for infant birth injury, neonatal hypoglycemia, and maternal gestational diabetes |
| Previous stillborn infant | Maternal psychological distress |
| Rh sensitization | Fetal anemia, erythroblastosis fetalis, kernicterus |
| **EXISTING MEDICAL CONDITIONS** | |
| Diabetes mellitus | Increased risk of pregnancy-induced hypertension, cesarean birth, infant either small or large for gestational age, neonatal hypoglycemia, fetal or neonatal death; increased incidence of congenital anomalies (see Chapter 26) |
| Thyroid disorder | |
| Hypothyroidism | Increased incidence of spontaneous abortion, congenital anomalies, congenital hypothyroidism |
| Hyperthyroidism | Maternal risk of pregnancy-induced hypertension, thyroid storm, or postpartum hemorrhage; neonatal risk of thyrotoxicosis |
| Cardiac disease | Maternal risk for cardiac decompensation and increased death rate; increased risk for fetal and neonatal death |
| Renal disease | Maternal risk for renal failure and preterm delivery; fetal risk for intrauterine growth retardation |
| **CONCURRENT INFECTIONS** | Severe fetal implications (heart disease, blindness, deafness, bone lesions) if maternal disease occurred in the first trimester<br>Increased incidence of spontaneous abortion or congenital anomalies are associated with some infections (see Chapter 26) |

nancy is not as advanced as first thought or that the fetus is not growing as expected. Sudden, rapid weight gain may indicate fluid retention, and further assessment for pregnancy-induced hypertension is indicated. (See Chapter 9 for a thorough discussion of the desired pattern of weight gain.)

**Urinalysis.** Urine is tested for protein, glucose, and ketones. A screen for bacteria may be repeated at 26 to 30 weeks if the woman has a history of previous urinary tract infections (Aumann & Baird, 1993).

**Glucose Screen.** Blood glucose is screened between 24 and 28 weeks, using a 50-g glucose load followed by a 1-hour plasma glucose determination. Additional testing is indicated if the result is 140 mg/dl or higher (ACOG, 1994a).

**Fundal Height.** Measuring fundal height is an inexpensive and noninvasive method for evaluating fetal growth and confirming gestational age.

**Leopold's Maneuvers.** Leopold's maneuvers provide a systematic method for palpating the fetus through the abdominal wall during the later part of pregnancy. These maneuvers provide valuable information about location and presentation of the fetus (see Chapter 13).

**Fetal Heart Rate.** The fetal heart rate may be

heard in early pregnancy with a Doppler transducer, or, in later pregnancy, with a fetoscope. Figure 14–1 illustrates fetoscopic and Doppler techniques. The site provides information that may help determine in what position the fetus is entering the pelvis. For instance, fetal heart tones heard in an upper quadrant of the abdomen suggest that the fetus is in a breech presentation.

**Fetal Activity.** First noticed by the expectant mother at 16 to 20 weeks of gestation (quickening), fetal movements gradually increase in both frequency and strength. In the last trimester, the woman may be asked to count fetal body movements. These are commonly called "kick counts," and a variety of methods is used. In general, fetal activity indicates that the fetus is physically healthy; fetal activity is therefore a reassuring sign.

Figure 7–12 provides an example of a clinical pathway for prenatal care. This pathway provides guidelines and a time sequence for specific assessments and interventions. A pathway does not detail how to perform assessment or interventions or interpret laboratory or test values, nor the significance of specific data. Instead, a clinical pathway allows a multidisciplinary team—made up of nurses, nurse-midwives, physicians, social workers, nutritionists and counselors—to coordinate care for each woman. Note that the most common family problems and risk factors are listed at the top of the page and alert the team that additional assessments or care may be required.

## Multifetal Pregnancy

A multifetal pregnancy may be defined as any pregnancy in which two or more embryos or fetuses exist simultaneously. (See Chapter 6 for information about conception and prenatal development of twins and other multifetal gestations.)

### DIAGNOSIS

Maternal symptoms of multifetal pregnancy include feeling larger than with previous pregnancies and feeling excessive fetal movements. Excessive weight gain and rapid uterine growth also increase the suspicion that more than one fetus is present. Fundal height is often 4 cm larger than expected on the basis of gestational age computed from the last menstrual period. See Figure 7–11 for fundal height measurement.

Maternal history may be of some help in making the diagnosis. A maternal family history that includes twins slightly increases the chance of twins. Recent administration of fertility drugs such as clomiphene greatly increases the chance of multifetal pregnancy.

When more than one fetus is suspected, diagnosis should be confirmed by sonography. Separate gestational sacs may be seen as early as 6 weeks of gestation. Multiple fetal parts may be visible by the 10th week.

### MATERNAL ADAPTATION TO MULTIFETAL PREGNANCY

The degree of maternal physiologic change is greater with multiple fetuses than with a single fetus. For instance, there is a 500-ml increase in blood volume over that needed for a single fetus. This increase heightens the workload of the heart and may contribute to fatigue and activity intolerance. The additional size of the uterus intensifies the *mechanical* effects of pregnancy. The uterus may achieve a volume of 10 liters or more and weigh more than 20 pounds (Cunningham et al., 1997). The weight increases respiratory difficulty because the overdistended uterus causes greater elevation of the diaphragm.

The uterus may also cause more compression of the large vessels, resulting in more pronounced and earlier supine hypotension. Greater compression of the ureters can occur, and maternal edema and proteinuria are common. Compression of the bowel makes constipation a persistent problem.

### ANTEPARTUM CARE IN MULTIFETAL PREGNANCY

Early diagnosis of multifetal pregnancy allows time for the family to be educated about the many ways in which the pregnancy will differ from those with a single fetus. Special antepartum classes can explain the need for increased nutrition, rest, and fetal monitoring.

Many physicians increase the number of times women with a multifetal pregnancy are seen during the antepartum period. More frequent visits permit extra vigilance in the detection of common complications, such as anemia, hypertension, premature labor, and congenital anomalies.

Diet must also be considered. The need for calories, iron, vitamins, and folate is increased. The Institute of Medicine has recommended that the target (total) weight gain at term for women carrying twins should be 16 to 20.5 kg (35 to 45 pounds).

**✓ CHECK YOUR READING**

23. What are major risk factors during pregnancy?
24. What is the recommended schedule for subsequent antepartum visits?
25. How does maternal adaptation differ in multifetal pregnancies?

*Text continued on page 152*

**YORK HOSPITAL**
YORK, PENNSYLVANIA
**CLINICAL PATHWAY**

**PRENATAL CARE**

| CLINICAL PATH VISITS | | EXPECTED PATIENT/ FAMILY OUTCOMES | MULTIDISCIPLINARY ASSESSMENT (Refer to STD-0011) | TESTS | CONSULTS/PROBLEM MANAGEMENT |
|---|---|---|---|---|---|
| Nurse Interview | Date | ☐ Signed contract for HBP Program–if M.A. [2]<br>☐ Referrals made as indicated following Prenatal Standard of Care [3,4,6]<br>☐ Verbalizes understanding of normal vs. abnormal signs & symptoms of pregnancy [1,3,4,7]<br>☐ Verbalizes agreement to complete labs, obtain prenatal vitamins, and keep scheduled appointments [2]<br>☐ Verbalizes signs & symptoms of preterm labor [7]<br>☐ No risk factors for PTL identified<br>☐ ________ | ☐ Refer to Standard 0011–Nurse Interview<br>☐ Weight, Height<br>☐ Physical, psych/social, behavioral, nutritional risk factors<br>☐ Knowledge of normal vs. abnormal Signs & Symptoms of pregnancy<br>☐ Planned method of infant feeding<br>☐ Premature labor<br>☐ ________ | ☐ **CCMS-UA, for nitr/leuk/glucose C & S if applicable.**<br>☐ Prenatal Group I/II.<br>☐ Sickle cell if applicable<br>☐ Dating Ultrasound scheduled<br>☐ HIV<br>☐ ________ | ☐ Social Service prn<br>☐ Perinatologist for Dating Ultrasound<br>☐ Genetic Counseling prn<br>☐ WIC prn<br>☐ Pastoral Care<br>☐ ________ |
| 1st Doctor | Date | ☐ Prenatal group tests within normal limits. [1]<br>☐ Takes prenatal vitamins. [2,3]<br>☐ Demonstrates measures to relieve normal complaints of pregnancy. [1,5]<br>☐ No change in Preterm Labor risk factors<br>☐ ________ | ☐ Signs & Symptoms of normal physical changes, complications<br>☐ Behavioral Risks<br>☐ BP, Weight<br>☐ Urine dipstick for Sugar, Ketone, Protein<br>☐ Fetal Heart Sounds<br>☐ Fundal Height<br>☐ Pelvimetry<br>☐ ________ | ☐ Pap ☐ GC<br>☐ Chlamydia (if indicated)<br>☐ **Wet smear bacterial/trich./vaginosis**<br>☐ **Vaginal ph & Whiff test**<br>☐ ________ | ☐ Social Service, prn<br>☐ Nutritionist, prn<br>☐ Perinatologist, prn<br>☐ Genetic Counseling, prn<br>☐ Pastoral Care<br>☐ ________ |
| (1-14 Weeks) | Date(s) | ☐☐ Demonstrates measures to relieve the normal complaints of pregnancy during 1st Trimester [1]<br>☐☐ Established exercise routine [5]<br>☐☐ Exhibits minimum weight loss/gain [3]<br>☐☐ 1st Trimester test results within normal limits [7]<br>☐☐ Avoids or demonstrates decrease in risk associated behavior (i.e., smoking) [4]<br>☐☐ No change in Preterm Labor risk factors<br>☐☐ ________ | ☐☐ Signs & Symptoms of normal physical changes, complications<br>☐☐ Behavioral Risks<br>☐☐ BP, Weight<br>☐☐ Urine Dipstick for Sugar, Ketone, Protein<br>☐☐ Fetal Heart Sounds<br>☐☐ Fundal Height<br>☐☐ ________ | ☐☐ Ultrasound for dating or prn<br>☐☐ ________ | ☐☐ Social Service, prn<br>☐☐ Nutritionist, prn<br>☐☐ Perinatologist, prn<br>☐☐ Genetic Counseling, prn<br>☐☐ Pastoral Care<br>☐☐ ________ |

| NAME | INITIALS | NAME | INITIALS |
|---|---|---|---|
| | | | |
| | | | |

MCCL-107 (2/96)

**FIGURE 7–12**

Prenatal clinical pathway that identifies outcomes, assessments, interventions, and consultations performed during pregnancy. (Courtesy of Women and Children Services of the York Health System, York, Pennsylvania. Reprinted with modifications.)

**PRETERM LABOR RISK**
CHECK THOSE THAT APPLY:

| | | |
|---|---|---|
| 1. ☐ Substance abuse | 1. ☐ <90 lb. pre-pregnancy weight | 1. ☐ Multiple gestation |
| 2. ☐ Prior preterm delivery | 2. ☐ Placenatal anomaly | 2. ☐ Persistent bleeding |
| 3. ☐ >2 abortions | 3. ☐ STD current pregnancy | 3. ☐ Incompetent cervix |

**DOCUMENTATION CODES**
Initial= Meets Standard
C = Chronic problems
* = Exception on pathway identified
N = Not applicable
D = Deferred

**PATIENT/FAMILY PROBLEMS**
1. Knowledge deficit r/t normal changes of pregnancy.
2. Noncompliance ________________
3. Alteration in nutritional status.
4. Knowledge deficit r/t risk association behavior on pregnancy. (Dependency)
5. Potential for activity intolerance.
6. Alteration in support system.
7. Knowledge deficit r/t complications of pregnancy.
8. ________________
9. ________________

| TREATMENTS | MEDS | DIET/ NUTRITION | EDUC & DC PLANNING (Refer to STD-0011) |
|---|---|---|---|
| ☐ Prenatal exercise program<br>☐ ________________ | ☐ Prescription for Prenatal Vitamins.<br>☐ ________________ | ☐ Diet to meet needs of pregnancy<br>☐ ________________ | ☐ 24° LOS after delivery concept.<br>☐ Childbirth Ed., Baby Care & Postpartum Classes<br>☐ Exercise during pregnancy.<br>☐ Effects of risk factors on pregnancy.<br>☐ Sexuality during pregnancy.<br>☐ Nutrition education.<br>☐ Normal effects of pregnancy on the body.<br>☐ Fetal Growth/Development.<br>☐ **S & S of complications/pre-term labor.**<br>☐ Pre-admission form.<br>☐ Contraceptives/ STD Prevention/HIV counseling.<br>☐ Schedule Return-to-Clinic Appointment<br>☐ Orient to Clinic hours/physical setup, emergency protocol<br>☐ ________________ |
| ☐ Prenatal exercise program<br>☐ ________________ | ☐ Prenatal Vitamins<br>☐ $FeSO_4$, if needed<br>☐ ________________ | ☐ Diet to meet needs of pregnancy<br>☐ ________________ | ☐ Reinforce STD-0011 (Prenatal Standard of Care)<br>☐ Importance of Compliancy<br>☐ ________________ |
| ☐☐ Activity ad lib<br>☐☐ Prenatal Exercise Program<br>☐☐ ________________ | ☐☐ Prenatal Vitamins<br>☐☐ $FeSO_4$, if needed<br>☐☐ ________________ | ☐☐ Diet to meet needs of pregnancy<br>☐☐ ________________ | ☐ Fetal Growth/Development of 1st Trimester<br>☐ Reinforce STD-0011 (Prenatal Standard of Care)<br>☐ Importance of Compliancy<br>☐ Home Visit Scheduled<br>☐ ________________ |

| NAME | INITIALS | NAME | INITIALS |
|---|---|---|---|
| | | | |
| | | | |

**FIGURE 7–12** *Continued*

*Illustration continued on following page*

| CLINICAL PATH DAY | EXPECTED PATIENT/ FAMILY OUTCOMES | MULTIDISCIPLINARY ASSESSMENT | TESTS | CONSULT |
|---|---|---|---|---|
| (15-28 Weeks) Date(s) | Demonstrates measures to relieve the normal complaints of pregnancy during 2nd Trimester. [1]<br>Exhibits normal weight gain. [3]<br>2nd Trimester test results within normal limits. [7]<br>Continues exercise routine. [5]<br>Avoids risk associated behavior. [4]<br>Responds appropriately to Signs & Symptoms of preterm labor when indicated. [7]<br>**Demonstrates self palpation technique & verbalizes signs & symptoms of preterm labor.**<br>No change in Preterm Labor risk factors. | Signs & Symptoms of normal physical changes, complications.<br>Behavioral Risks.<br>BP, Weight.<br>Urine Dipstick for Sugar, Ketone, Protein<br>Fetal Heart Sounds, Fundal Height.<br>Fetal Movement at 16-20 weeks.<br>Premature Labor. | Triple Screen (16-19 weeks).<br>Ultrasound, as needed.<br>Fibronectin (24-26 weeks).<br>**ORDER at 26 Weeks:**<br>Trutol<br>Antibody Screen (Rh Neg)<br>Repeat WCBC | Social Service, prn<br>Nutritionists, prn<br>Perinatologist, prn<br>Genetic Counseling, prn<br>Pastoral Care |
| (29-41 Weeks) Date(s) | Demonstrates measures to relieve the normal complaints of pregnancy during 3rd Trimester. [1]<br>Exhibits normal weight gain. [3]<br>3rd Trimester test results within normal limits. [7]<br>Continues exercise routine. [5]<br>Normal physical changes of pregnancy w/o complications.<br>Avoids risk associated behavior. [4]<br>Attends Childbirth, Baby Care and Postpartum classes [1,3,7]<br>Responds appropriately to Signs & Symptoms of preterm labor or other complication when indicated. [7]<br>Performing nipple preparation, if needed. [1]<br>No change in Preterm Labor risk factors. | Signs & Symptoms of normal physical changes, complications<br>Behavioral risks.<br>BP, Weight.<br>Urine Dipstick for Sugar, Ketone, Protein.<br>Fetal Heart Sounds, Fundal Height.<br>Fetal Movement.<br>Nipple exam, if planning to breast feed.<br>Premature Labor. | **ORDER at 36 Weeks:**<br>Recto Vaginal Cultures for GBS.<br>**ORDER at 41 Weeks:**<br>NST & AFI Bi-weekly (Amniotic Fluid Index)<br>Ultrasound, as needed. | Social Service, prn<br>Nutritionists, prn<br>Perinatologist, prn<br>Genetic Counseling, prn<br>Lactation Consultant, prn<br>Pastoral Care |

| NAME | INITIALS | NAME | INITIALS |
|---|---|---|---|
| | | | |
| | | | |
| | | | |

NOTE: EACH PATIENT REQUIRES AN INDIVIDUAL ASSESSMENT & TREATMENT PLAN. THIS CLINICAL PATH IS A RECOMMENDATION FOR THE AVERAGE PATIENT WHICH REQUIRES MODIFICATION WHEN NECESSARY BY THE PROFESSIONAL STAFF.

**FIGURE 7–12** *Continued*

| TREATMENTS | MEDS | DIET/NUTR. | EDUC & DC PLANNING |
|---|---|---|---|
| ☐☐☐☐ Activity ad lib.<br>☐☐☐☐ Prenatal Exercise Program.<br>☐☐☐☐<br>__________ | ☐☐☐☐ Prenatal Vitamins<br>☐☐☐☐ $FeSO_4$, if needed<br>☐☐☐☐<br>__________ | ☐☐☐☐ Diet to meet needs of pregnancy.<br>☐☐☐☐<br>__________ | ☐ Fetal Growth/Development for 2nd Tri.<br>☐ Schedule Childbirth, Baby Care, and Postpartum classes.<br>☐ Reinforce STD-0011 (Prenatal Standard of Care).<br>☐☐☐☐ S & S of preterm labor at 24 week appointment.<br>☐☐☐☐ Importance of compliancy.<br>☐ **Home Visit.**<br>☐☐☐<br>__________ |
| ☐☐☐☐☐☐☐ Activity ad lib.<br>☐☐☐☐☐☐☐ Prenatal Exercise Program.<br>☐ Rhogam at 28 weeks, if indicated.<br>☐☐☐☐☐☐☐<br>__________ | ☐☐☐☐☐☐☐ Prenatal Vitamins<br>☐☐☐☐☐☐☐ $FeSO_4$, if needed<br>☐☐☐☐☐☐☐<br>__________ | ☐☐☐☐☐☐☐ Diet to meet needs of pregnancy.<br>☐☐☐☐☐☐☐<br>__________ | ☐ Fetal Growth/Development for 3rd Tri.<br>☐ Review Signs & Symptoms and Admission procedures for normal labor at 36 weeks.<br>☐☐☐☐☐☐☐ Reinforce STD-0011 (Prenatal Standard of Care).<br>☐☐☐☐☐☐☐ S & S of preterm labor.<br>☐☐☐☐☐☐☐ Importance of compliancy.<br>☐ Update Perinatal Risk Assessment.<br>☐ Childbirth Education, Baby Care, and Postpartum classes and 24° LOS concept.<br>☐ Tubal forms, if indicated.<br>☐ Treatment for inverted nipples.<br>☐ **Home Visit.**<br>☐☐☐☐☐☐☐<br>__________ |

| NAME | INITIALS | NAME | INITIALS |
|---|---|---|---|
| | | | |
| | | | |
| | | | |

**FIGURE 7–12** *Continued*

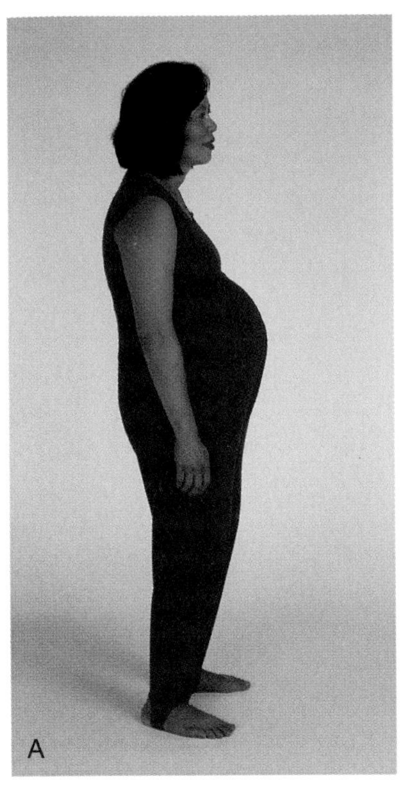


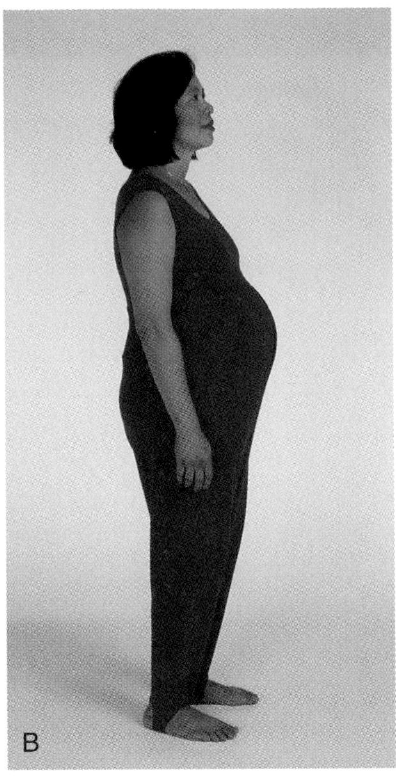


**FIGURE 7–13**

Posture during pregnancy may cause or alleviate backache. A, Incorrect posture. The neck is jutting forward, the shoulders are slumping, and the back is sharply curved, creating back pain and discomfort. B, Correct posture. The neck and shoulders are straight, the back is flattened, and the pelvis is tucked under and slightly upward.

## Common Discomforts of Pregnancy

Many women experience discomforts of pregnancy that are not serious in themselves but detract from the woman's feeling of comfort and well-being.

### NAUSEA AND VOMITING

Nausea and vomiting of pregnancy are frequently called "morning sickness" because these symptoms are more acute on arising. They may, however, occur at any time of the day and may continue throughout the day. Women need reassurance that nausea and vomiting, however distressing, are common and that the condition is temporary. Morning sickness must be distinguished from *hyperemesis gravidarum,* a severe state of vomiting that is accompanied by weight loss, dehydration, electrolyte imbalance, and ketosis (see Chapter 25).

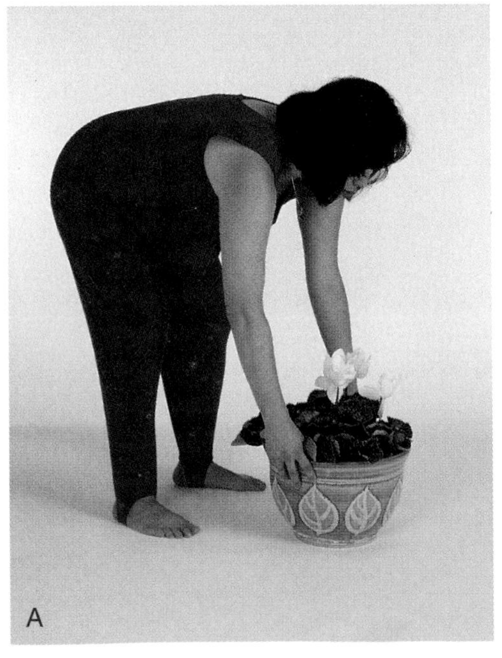


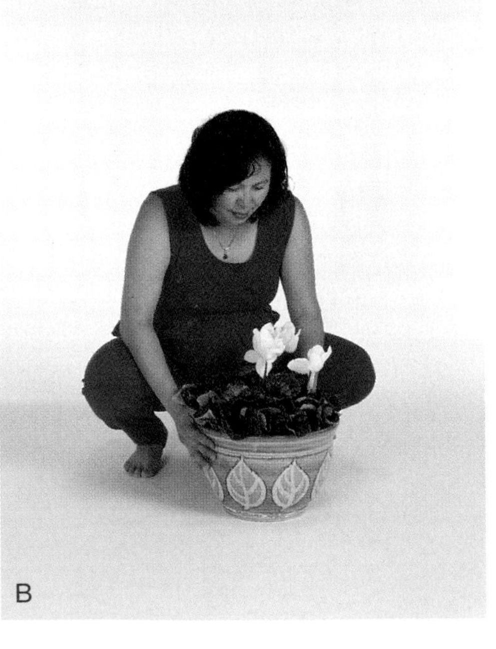


**FIGURE 7–14**

Techniques for lifting. Squatting places less strain on the back. A, Incorrect technique. Stooping or bending places a great deal of strain on muscles of the lower body. B, Correct technique. Squatting and moving the object close permits the stronger muscles of the legs to do the lifting.

Although, the cause of nausea and vomiting is unknown, these symptoms are believed to be related to increased levels of hCG and estrogen, as well as periodic hypoglycemia. Symptoms may be aggravated by cooking odors and fatigue. Emotional factors may also be implicated. Women under emotional stress are more likely to experience nausea.

#### HEARTBURN

Heartburn is described as an acute burning sensation in the epigastric and sternal regions. It may be associated with other gastrointestinal symptoms, such as frequent belching, nausea, and epigastric pressure.

Heartburn occurs when reverse peristaltic waves cause regurgitation of acidic stomach contents into the esophagus. The underlying causes are diminished gastric motility and displacement of the stomach by the enlarging uterus. Improper diet and nervous tension may be precipitating factors. (See Women Want to Know: How to Overcome the Common Discomforts of Pregnancy for measures to relieve heartburn.)

#### BACKACHE

Backache is a common complaint during the third trimester. A primary focus is to prevent backache by teaching correct posture and body mechanics. Figure 7–13 illustrates correct and incorrect posture. Stooping or bending puts a great deal of strain on the muscles of the lower back. Figure 7–14 demonstrates correct and incorrect methods for lifting. In addition, Figure 7–15 suggests exercises that relax the shoulders and thighs and help prevent backache.

#### URINARY FREQUENCY

Although urinary frequency is a common complaint of women during the first trimester and near term, the condition is temporary and is managed by most women without undue distress. Kegel's exercises are sometimes recommended to help maintain bladder control. (See Women Want To Know: How to Overcome the Common Discomforts of Pregnancy.)

#### VARICOSITIES

Varicosities are usually confined to the legs but may involve the veins of the vulva or rectum (hemorrhoids). Varicosities occur most often in women with a family history of varicose veins and are more likely to be a problem in women who are obese or who are multiparas. Symptoms depend on the degree of engorgement—from barely noticeable blemishes with minimal discomfort at the end of the day to large, tortuous veins that produce severe discomfort with any activity.

Varicosities are common in pregnancy because the weight of the uterus partially compresses the veins that return blood from the legs. As blood pools, the vessels dilate and the valves in the veins become stretched and incompetent. This process results in even more pooling, and, in time, the veins may become engorged, inflamed, and painful. Varicose veins are exacerbated by prolonged standing when the force of gravity makes blood return more difficult.

#### HEMORRHOIDS

Hemorrhoids are varicosities of the rectum; they may be external (outside the anal sphincter) or internal (above the sphincter). Some of the most common causes of hemorrhoids are vascular engorgement of the pelvis, constipation, straining at stool, and prolonged sitting or standing. Pushing during the second stage of labor exacerbates the problem, which may continue into the postpartum period.

#### CONSTIPATION

Occasional constipation is not harmful, although it can cause a feeling of abdominal fullness and flatulence and can aggravate painful hemorrhoids. Intestinal motility is reduced during pregnancy as a result of progesterone. This benefits the expectant mother and the fetus by allowing additional time for nutrients to be absorbed. It also adds time for water to be absorbed from the large intestine, which can result in hard, dry stools and decreased frequency of bowel movements. Iron supplementation also causes constipation in some women.

#### LEG CRAMPS

Painful contraction of the muscles of the lower legs occurs most often during sleep, when the muscles are relaxed. Cramps are also likely to occur when the woman stretches and extends her foot. Leg cramps are believed to be caused by an imbalance of serum calcium and phosphorus. A 1-to-1 ratio of calcium to phosphorus is desired, but this ratio is difficult to achieve in pregnancy, when many women consume large amounts of dairy products that are high in calcium. Venous congestion in the legs during the third trimester also contributes to leg cramps.

## Cultural Considerations

Although the physical changes of pregnancy are fairly universal, culture often determines the health beliefs, values, and expectations of the family when a woman becomes pregnant. When a family and the health care professionals are from different cultures, they often hold different health beliefs and rely on health practices that are specific to their culture. Conflict may result from these variations in beliefs about what constitutes appropriate practices. To overcome the conflict and provide effective care,

**Shoulder circling**

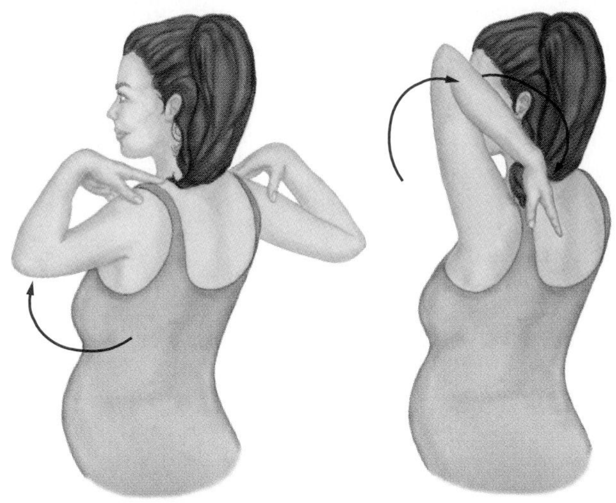

The fingertips are placed on the shoulders, then the elbows are brought forward and up during inhalation, back and down during exhalation. Repeat five times.

**Tailor sitting**

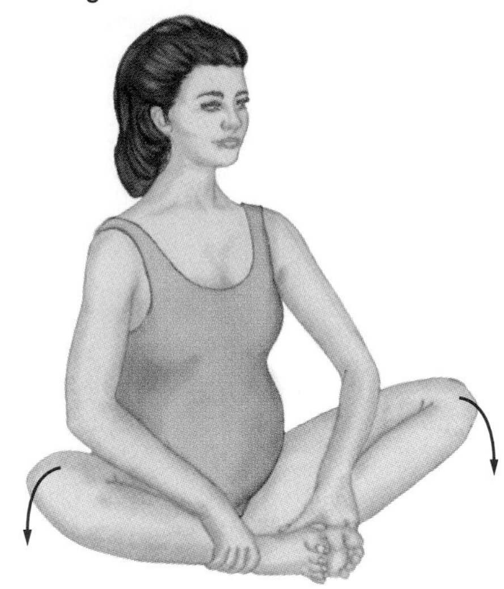

The woman uses her thigh muscles to press her knees to the floor. Keeping her back straight, she should remain in the position for 5 to 15 minutes.

**Pelvic tilt or pelvic rocking**

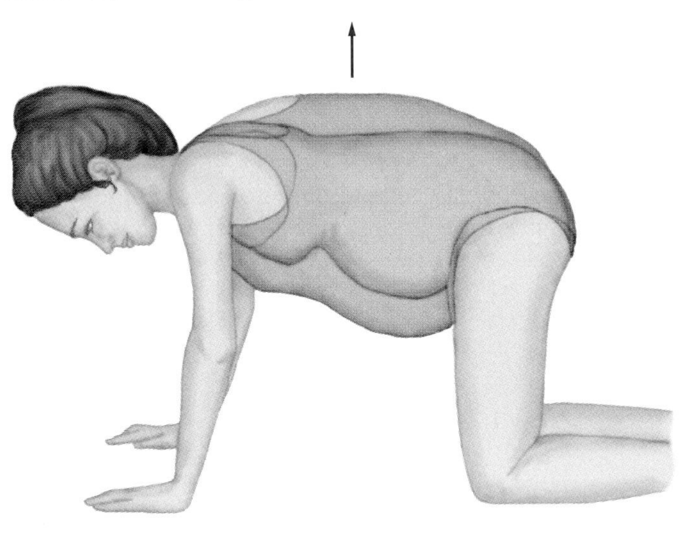

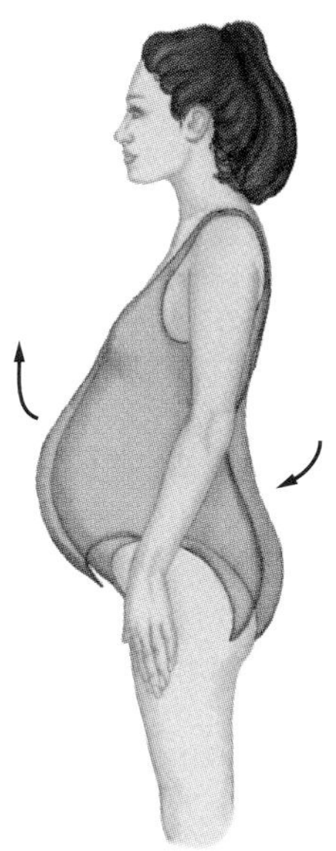

This exercise can be performed on hands and knees, with the hands directly under the shoulders and the knees under the hips. The back should be in a neutral position, not hollowed. The head and neck should be aligned with the straight back. The woman then presses up with the lower back and holds this position for a few seconds, then relaxes to a neutral position. Repeat 5 times. The exercise may also be performed in a standing position when the pelvis is rotated forward to flatten the lower back.

**FIGURE 7–15**

Exercises to prevent backache.

nurses must understand the family's way of thinking, feeling, and acting during pregnancy.

#### CULTURAL ASSESSMENT

Cultures are so diverse that nurses cannot know all the specific aspects of each. Instead, they must be aware of the predominant cultures seen in their practice area and become adept at performing cultural assessment. Some specific questions may elicit information that helps the nurse understand the family's beliefs about appropriate care during pregnancy:

- How will you and your family prepare for the baby?
- What concerns do you have about the pregnancy?
- What would provide the greatest assistance?
- What do you and your family expect from the health care team during pregnancy?

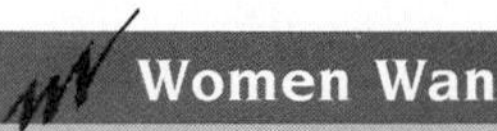

Women Want to Know

## How to Overcome the Common Discomforts of Pregnancy

**Nausea and Vomiting**

Nausea and vomiting are *temporary*. Here are some remedies:

- Eat dry crackers or toast before arising in the morning; then get out of bed slowly.
- Eat dry crackers every 2 hours to prevent an empty stomach, or eat five or six small meals a day rather than three full meals.
- Take fluids separately from meals.
- Avoid fried, greasy, or spicy foods and foods with strong odors, such as onion and cabbage.

**Heartburn**

- Eat several small meals daily, and avoid fatty foods.
- Curtail smoking and coffee drinking, which stimulate acid formation in the stomach.
- Sit upright to reduce reflux and relieve symptoms.
- At night, sleep with an extra pillow under your head and shoulders.
- Try deep breathing and sipping water to help relieve the burning sensation.
- Use antacids, but avoid those that are high in sodium (Alka-Seltzer, baking soda) because excessive sodium may result in fluid retention and electrolyte imbalance. Antacids high in calcium (Tums, Alkamints) provide relief but may cause rebound hyperacidity.

**Backache**

- Maintain correct posture, with head up and shoulders back.
- To pick up objects, squat rather than bend from the waist.
- When sitting, use foot supports, arm rests, and pillows behind your back.
- Exercise. Tailor sitting, shoulder circling, and pelvic rocking strengthen your back and help prepare you for labor.

**Urinary Frequency**

Performing Kegel's exercises helps to maintain bladder control:

- Identify the muscles to be exercised when you stop the flow of urine midstream. Do not, however perform the exercise while urinating because urinary retention increases the risk of urinary tract infection.
- Contract the muscles around the vagina, and hold for 5 seconds. Relax.
- Repeat the contraction-relaxation cycle 10 times, slowly contracting and relaxing the muscles.

**Varicosities**

The key to treatment is to prevent pooling of blood in the large veins of the legs.

- Avoid constricting clothing, and refrain from crossing your legs at the knees because this position impedes blood return from the legs.
- Take frequent rest periods with your legs elevated above the level of your hips.
- Obtain relief by wearing support hose or elastic stockings. Stockings should reach above the varicosities, and they should be applied before you get out of bed each morning. Putting them on later makes them less effective because pooling begins as soon as you arise.
- If you must work in one position for prolonged periods, walk around for a few minutes at least every 2 hours. This stimulates blood flow and relieves discomfort.

**Hemorrhoids**

- To prevent hemorrhoids, try to establish a regular pattern of bowel elimination that does not require straining. Drink plenty of water, eat foods rich in fiber, and exercise regularly.
- To relieve existing hemorrhoids, take frequent, tepid sitz baths or warm soaks; apply cool witch hazel compresses or anesthetic ointments; or lie (on your side) with your hips elevated on a pillow.
- Gently push the hemorrhoids back into the rectum. To do so, put on a latex glove and lubricate your index finger. Maintain pressure for 1 to 2 minutes.
- If you have persistent pain or bleeding, call your physician or midwife.

**Constipation**

Self-care measures generally are as effective as using laxatives, but they are most beneficial because they do not interfere with absorption of nutrients or lead to laxative dependency.

- Drink at least eight glasses of water each day. These should not include coffee, tea, or carbonated drinks because of their diuretic effect. If you do drink one of these beverages, adding a glass of water afterward may counteract its diuretic effect.
- Additional fiber in your diet helps to maintain bowel elimination. Foods high in fiber include unpeeled fresh fruits and vegetables, whole-grain cereals, bran muffins, oatmeal, baked potatoes with skins, and fruit juices. Four pieces of fruit plus a large salad provide enough fiber requirements for 1 day.
- Restrict cheese consumption, which causes constipation.
- Curtail your intake of sweets, which increase bacterial growth in the intestine and can lead to flatulence.
- Do not discontinue taking iron supplements if they have been prescribed. If constipation persists, consult your health care provider for advice about bulk-forming laxatives or fecal wetting agents.
- A brisk walk of at least 1 mile per day is one of the best exercises to stimulate peristalsis and improve muscle tone. Swimming and riding a stationary bicycle are also helpful.
- Establish a regular pattern by allowing a consistent time each day for elimination. One hour after meals is ideal to take advantage of the gastrocolic reflex (the peristaltic wave in the colon that is induced by taking food into the fasting stomach). Using a footrest during elimination provides comfort and decreases straining.

*Women Want to Know continued on following page*

## Women Want to Know *Continued*

## How to Overcome the Common Discomforts of Pregnancy

**Leg Cramps**

Dependent edema increases when the pregnant woman sits or stands for long periods. Periodic elevation of the legs helps to reduce dependent edema.

- To relieve cramps, extend the affected leg, keeping the knee straight; bend your foot toward you, or ask someone to help you flex the foot. If you are alone, stand and apply pressure on the affected leg. Either measure lengthens the affected muscles and relieves cramping.
- To prevent cramps, frequently elevate your legs during the day to improve circulation.
- Restricting milk intake and taking supplemental calcium may provide relief, but these measures should be initiated only with advice of the physician or certified nurse-midwife.
- For frequent leg cramps, your physician or nurse-midwife may suggest aluminum hydroxide gel capsules. These absorb phosphorus and thus raise the level of calcium in the blood.

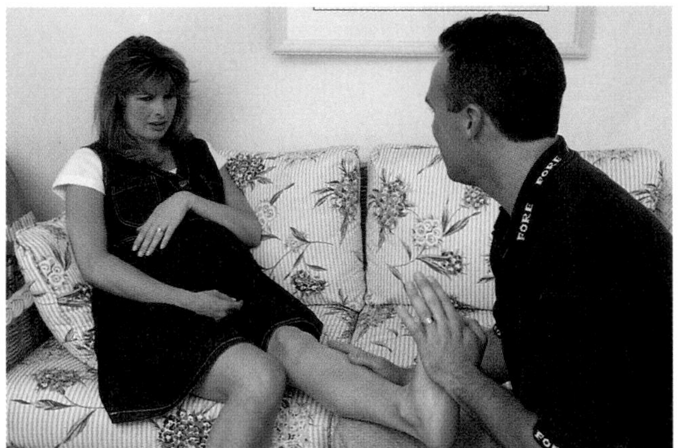

- Where do you obtain most health care information?
- What foods are encouraged? Curtailed?
- Where will the baby be born? Who will assist in the birth of the baby?

### CULTURAL NEGOTIATION

Cultural negotiation involves providing information while acknowledging that the family may hold different views. If the family indicates that the information would be helpful, it can be incorporated into the teaching plan.

**If the family indicates that the information is not helpful or is harmful in their opinion, the conflict must be acknowledged openly and clarified. "I sense that you are unsure of this." "Help me understand your reluctance to try it." The nurse then explains why the recommendation is valid and allows the family to continue to express their beliefs until a compromise is worked out.**

Cultural negotiation also involves being sensitive to specific concerns. For example, nurses must be aware of Islamic laws governing modesty when caring for childbearing Muslim women. Laws of modesty require that a Muslim woman keep her hair, body, arms to the wrist, and legs to the ankles covered at all times when in the presence of a man. Moreover, a Muslim woman is not to be alone in the presence of a man other than her husband or a male relative.

Muslim women prefer a female health care provider and should be informed of the availability of female caregivers. Adequate drapes and covers should be available to allow covering all areas of the body except those that must be exposed for examination. Moreover, the woman's husband, a female friend, or male relative should be allowed to be present during examinations.

### CHECK YOUR READING

26. What is the cause of "morning sickness"?
27. How can backache be alleviated during pregnancy?
28. What is meant by the term *cultural negotiation*?

## Application of Nursing Process: Family Responses to Physical Changes of Pregnancy

Nursing process focuses on identifying each family's unique responses to the physiologic changes of pregnancy, determining factors that might interfere with the ability to adapt to changes that occur, and finding solutions to problems that are identified.

### Assessment

The nurse uses a variety of methods to assess the family's responses to the physiologic processes of pregnancy and to explore the family's preparation for the birth. These methods include structured interviews and planned teaching-learning sessions, as well as more informal discussions that occur spontaneously during the initial or subsequent assessments. Significant information may be obtained by a review of the history and physical examination. Information may come not only from the expectant mother but also from the spouse and other significant family members.

## Analysis

When analyzing data, nurses must use all their critical thinking skills before coming to a conclusion about the most significant nursing diagnoses. One of the most common errors is unexamined *assumptions.* Many nurses assume that all families experience the same concerns and the same discomforts. Such assumptions may lead to diagnoses that are not relevant to the actual problems that a unique family experiences. (See Nursing Care Plans 7–1 through 7–3 for some common, but not universal, nursing diagnoses.) To improve critical thinking skills, questions are posed throughout the nursing care plans.

Nurses must also remember that nursing process must be adapted in maternal-newborn nursing to a generally healthy population experiencing a life event that holds the possibility for growth as well as for problems. Unlike medical-surgical nursing, much maternal-newborn nursing activity is devoted to assessing, diagnosing, and promoting family strengths and healthy functioning.

Many problem-oriented nursing diagnoses provided by the North American Nursing Diagnosis As-

## Nursing Care Plan 7–1
## Discomfort During Early Pregnancy

**ASSESSMENT:** Maria Gomez, a thin, 18-year-old primigravida of 8 weeks' gestation, has dry, cracked lips and a pulse rate of 90 when she arrives at the prenatal clinic. She states that she is experiencing nausea with occasional vomiting throughout the day. She reports that the nausea is intensified by the odor of cooking food and that she has little appetite. Although she is always thirsty, she restricts fluids because "they make me sicker." Her urine sample is concentrated with a specific gravity of 1.030.

**NURSING DIAGNOSIS:** Risk for Altered Nutrition: Less than Body Requirements related to nausea, vomiting, and anorexia

### Critical Thinking

Were all the data considered? Organize the data and develop a second diagnosis. State outcomes for that diagnosis, and identify at least two interventions.

**ANSWER**

No. All data should be grouped and analyzed. For example, nausea throughout the day, occasional vomiting, and anorexia support the stated nursing diagnosis. Dry lips, tachycardia, thirst, and concentrated urine, however, are not analyzed. These data suggest a second nursing diagnosis: Risk for Fluid Volume Deficit related to inadequate intake of fluids and fluid loss through vomiting.

Goals and outcomes include the following:

1. Increase intake of fluids to 2000 ml/day.
2. Maintain urine specific gravity within normal range.
3. Demonstrate no signs or symptoms of dehydration.

Interventions include the following:

1. Suggest alternative fluids, such as jello, popsicles, ice cream, pudding, watermelon.
2. Recommend frequent small amounts of ice chips or clear liquids.
3. Emphasize the importance of taking frequent small amounts of water instead of coffee or tea, which act as diuretics.
4. Ask Maria to return within 2 to 3 days if she is unable to retain recommended amounts of fluid. It would not be prudent to wait until the next scheduled prenatal visit if she is dehydrated.

**GOALS/EXPECTED OUTCOMES**

Maria will do the following:

1. Maintain adequate intake of calories and nutrients to meet her needs, as evidenced by sufficient energy to carry on the activities of daily living, and a continuous pattern of weight gain during pregnancy. (See Chapter 9 for recommended pattern of weight gain.)
2. Report less nausea and a decrease in the episodes of vomiting.

*Nursing Care Plan continued on following page*

## Nursing Care Plan 7–1 *Continued*

# Discomfort During Early Pregnancy

| INTERVENTION | RATIONALE |
|---|---|
| 1. Recommend that she eat two dry crackers half an hour before arising in the morning and that she get out of bed slowly. | 1. Food counteracts hypoglycemia resulting from night-long fasting and prevents an initial episode of nausea that may become difficult to control. |
| 2. Suggest that Maria consume a bedtime snack that is high in protein, such as cottage cheese or half a tuna fish sandwich on whole wheat bread. | 2. Proteins are metabolized at a slower rate, and this helps to prevent morning hypoglycemia. |
| 3. Instruct her to eat small, dry meals five to six times a day rather than three large ones. | 3. Frequent dry meals prevent the stomach from becoming empty, increasing the feeling of nausea. |
| 4. Suggest that fluids be taken separately. | 4. Fluids overstretch the stomach and may precipitate vomiting. |
| 5. Recommend that she eat a dry cracker, unbuttered popcorn, or dry toast every 2 hours. | 5. Nausea is more intense when the stomach is empty. |
| 6. Suggest that she avoid fried or greasy foods, foods that are highly seasoned, and foods that have strong odors. | 6. Odors and greasy textures are associated with nausea and increased episodes of vomiting. |
| 7. Teach Maria to keep a record of daily intake of food and fluids, episodes of vomiting, and measures that reduce nausea. | 7. It is essential to determine whether adequate nutrients and fluids are being retained and to identify the most helpful measures to control nausea. |
| 8. Suggest that she experiment with soups, eggnogs, and vegetable drinks. | 8. These foods are high in nutrients and are often tolerated well when taken separately. |
| 9. Reassure her that nausea and vomiting usually disappear by the second trimester and that they do not indicate a problem with the pregnancy. | 9. It reduces anxiety to know the condition is self-limiting and that it does not threaten the fetus. |
| 10. Assess Maria's weight at each prenatal visit, and compare weight gain with that expected for the weeks of gestation. | 10. If weight gain compares favorably with that expected, the focus remains on relieving the discomfort of nausea and vomiting. If weight gain is less than it should be or if signs of dehydration are present, refer her for medical management. |

### EVALUATION

Periodic nausea and vomiting continued throughout the first trimester but ceased during the second trimester. At 20 weeks, Maria appears well hydrated and has gained 4.5 kg (approximately 10 pounds).

**ASSESSMENT:** Maria also says that she is often very tired during the day even though she is sleeping 8 to 10 hours at night. Fatigue concerns her because she is employed and must keep her mind on her work.

**NURSING DIAGNOSIS:** Fatigue related to inadequate rest periods to accommodate the physiologic demands of pregnancy.

### Critical Thinking

What assumption has the nurse made? What other factors should be considered before this diagnosis is made?

**ANSWER**

Although extraordinary fatigue is common in early pregnancy, nurses must not assume that pregnancy is the only cause. Additional data, such as hemoglobin and hematocrit levels, should be obtained before this diagnosis is made. Information about increasing iron-rich foods or iron supplementation may be necessary.

### GOALS/EXPECTED OUTCOMES

Maria will do the following:

1. Identify methods to cope with fatigue, such as negotiating a flexible work schedule or time for short rest periods while continuing employment during pregnancy.
2. Report increased energy by the end of the first trimester.

## Nursing Care Plan 7–1 *Continued*
## Discomfort During Early Pregnancy

| INTERVENTION | RATIONALE |
|---|---|
| 1. Acknowledge the fatigue and reassure Maria that this is self-limiting and a common experience during the first months because of the change in hormone levels. | 1. Reassurance helps to alleviate the concern that fatigue indicates a problem with her pregnancy. |
| 2. Recommend that she lie down or sit comfortably with feet elevated for a few minutes every 2 hours and consciously relax the muscles of the legs, abdomen, and shoulders. | 2. This position renews energy even though sleep is not possible. |
| 3. Suggest that she try deep breathing, visualizing a favorite location or pastime, whenever possible. Progressive relaxation—conscious tensing and relaxing of groups of muscles beginning with those in the feet and working upward toward the head—may be helpful. | 3. These exercises relieve physical tension that adds to fatigue and also provide mental distraction. |
| 4. Recommend that she get as much sleep as she feels she needs when possible. Adequate rest may involve curtailing social activities and tasks that can be postponed. | 4. Although recreation is important, the need for sleep is overwhelming for some women during the first weeks of pregnancy. |
| 5. Encourage her to explore a flexible schedule or routine with her employer. | 5. Often a very short nap in the morning or afternoon is all that is needed to continue to function effectively. |
| 6. Recommend that she enlist the assistance of family, significant other, and friends with home responsibilities. | 6. Assistance can free her of all but the most essential tasks during this time. |

**Critical Thinking**

What additional interventions are necessary if the hemoglobin and hematocrit are low?

**ANSWER**

If low levels of hemoglobin and hematocrit indicate that the client is anemic, the physician or nurse-midwife should be notified so that iron supplementation can be started.

EVALUATION

Maria was able to negotiate two short rest periods each day and, at 12 weeks' gestation, continues to use learned techniques to renew energy. Maria relates increased energy at the third prenatal visit (16 weeks).

ADDITIONAL NURSING DIAGNOSES TO CONSIDER

Fluid Volume Deficit
Risk for Activity Intolerance
Diversional Activity Deficit
Altered Sexuality Patterns
Altered Family Processes

sociation do not address the healthy family preparing for the birth of a child. Most families express an intense desire to protect the health of the unborn child and the well-being of the mother. Perhaps the most encompassing nursing diagnosis for the prenatal period is Health-Seeking Behaviors: prenatal care and health practices that provide optimum benefit to the fetus and mother.

### Planning

Outcomes for this nursing diagnosis are that the expectant mother (and/or the family) will do the following:

- Demonstrate knowledge of practices that promote the safety and well-being of the mother and fetus throughout pregnancy.

## Nursing Care Plan 7–2

# Self-Care During Pregnancy

**ASSESSMENT:** Paula Orne, a primigravida of 28 weeks' gestation, has numerous questions about self-care. She is a courier and drives many hours each day. She is concerned about safety while driving. She also asks what sexual activity is allowed, and she is concerned because her partner continues to smoke.

**NURSING DIAGNOSIS:** Health-Seeking Behaviors: prenatal care related to travel, sexual activity, and effects of passive smoking.

### Critical Thinking

What are appropriate goals and outcomes for this nursing diagnosis?

**ANSWER**

Goals must be realistic and measurable. For example, Paula will do the following:

1. Describe measures to decrease discomfort and promote safety while traveling by next visit.
2. Continue mutually satisfactory sexual activity during pregnancy.
3. Modify the environment to eliminate exposure to passive smoking by (specific date).

| INTERVENTION | RATIONALE |
|---|---|
| 1. Recommend that she use both the lap and shoulder restraints throughout pregnancy. Suggest that she keep the lap restraint under the abdomen. | 1. Use of restraints prevents ejection from the car in case of an accident. The most serious injuries are sustained when a person is ejected at impact. |
| 2. Suggest that she stop the car at least every 2 hours to walk for a few minutes and perform some gentle shoulder and upper body stretches. She should also empty her bladder at each stop. | 2. Frequent stops improve circulation and relieve the muscles involved in prolonged sitting and driving. Frequent voiding promotes comfort and prevents bladder infection due to stasis of urine. |
| 3. Suggest that she drink a glass of water at each stop but that she avoid sweet drinks and those that contain caffeine. | 3. Sweet drinks increase thirst, and caffeine drinks act as a diuretic and increase thirst. Water refreshes and prevents dehydration. |
| 4. Determine the client's specific concerns about sexuality, and respond to those in particular. | 4. Concerns vary from couple to couple. Some couples worry about harming the fetus or causing discomfort for the mother. |
| 5. Reassure her that sexual activity poses no harm to either the mother or the fetus in a normal pregnancy; explain the anatomy of the vagina, cervix, and uterus; if necessary, use a plastic model; and suggest she bring her partner to the next visit if he has concerns. | 5. Knowledge of the separation between the vagina and the fetus may relieve concern about the safety of vaginal intercourse during pregnancy. |
| 6. Suggest that alternative positions, such as side-lying, woman-superior, or rear-entry, be used during the third trimester. | 6. The male-superior position becomes uncomfortable for the woman when the uterus is large and heavy, and it increases the risk of supine hypotension. |
| 7. Acknowledge the danger of passive smoking, and recommend that the partner curtail smoking in the house, car, and other enclosed areas. This limitation is important during pregnancy and also after the infant is born. | 7. Toxins in cigarette smoke affect those in the vicinity as well as the one who is smoking. |

**EVALUATION**

Paula uses both shoulder and lap restraints and says she feels more comfortable while driving. She relates mutually satisfying sexual experiences. Her partner agrees to curtail smoking in Paula's presence.

**ADDITIONAL NURSING DIAGNOSES TO CONSIDER**

Risk for Injury
Altered Sexuality Patterns
Altered Health Maintenance

## Nursing Care Plan 7–3
# Discomfort During Late Pregnancy

**ASSESSMENT:** Ann Reeves, a multipara of 32 weeks' gestation, states that she has persistent backache and seeks information to alleviate it. She demonstrates marked lordosis and is observed to bend to pick up her toddler. She stands with shoulders slumped and head forward.

**NURSING DIAGNOSIS:** Pain: backache related to muscular strain secondary to change in balance and knowledge deficit of measures to reduce strain.

### GOALS/EXPECTED OUTCOMES

Ann will do the following:

1. Demonstrate body mechanics that prevent muscle strain when lifting.
2. Demonstrate correct posture to relieve muscle strain.
3. Report increased comfort at next clinic visit.

#### Critical Thinking

Interventions should be based on sound principles. Note four interventions listed below and evaluate the rationale for each.

**ANSWER**
See rationales for the listed interventions.

| INTERVENTION | RATIONALE |
|---|---|
| 1. Teach correct posture: Stand erect with shoulders back and neck straight; contract abdominal muscles to flatten the back; tuck pelvis under and slightly forward; and distribute weight through the center of the feet (Fig. 7–14). | 1. Further muscle strain occurs when the shoulders slump forward and the curve in the lower back is exaggerated. |
| 2. Demonstrate proper body mechanics for stooping and lifting: Squat and move the object to be lifted close to the body, and use the thigh muscles to stand and lift (Fig. 7–15). | 2. These motions prevent muscle strain in the lower back by using the stronger muscles of the legs. Squatting lowers the center of gravity and prevents muscle strain that occurs when one bends and lifts. |
| 3. Demonstrate prenatal exercises: pelvic rocking, shoulder circling, and tailor sitting (see Fig. 7–16). | 3. Shoulder circling strengthens muscles of the shoulders and helps to prevent slumping that exacerbates lordosis. Tailor sitting and pelvic rocking strengthen muscles of the thighs and back and help maintain posture as well as relieve discomfort. |
| 4. Recommend that Ann vary activities frequently, avoid prolonged standing, and use a foot rest when sitting. | 4. Prolonged standing or sitting in an unsupported position causes one group of muscles to become fatigued. |

### EVALUATION

Ann demonstrates correct posture and body mechanics to relieve muscle strain, but backache continues. Ann demonstrates pelvic rocking and agrees to practice this prenatal exercise several times a day.

### ADDITIONAL NURSING DIAGNOSES TO CONSIDER

Risk for Activity Intolerance
Risk for Injury
Sleep Pattern Disturbance

- Describe measures that provide relief from the common discomforts of pregnancy.
- Describe a realistic plan during the first trimester to modify behaviors or habits that do not promote the health of the mother and fetus.

## Interventions

Following the initial assessment, the woman is usually not seen by the health care provider for 4 weeks. She and her family must be instructed about

## Critical to Remember

### DANGER SIGNS OF PREGNANCY

- Vaginal bleeding, with or without discomfort
- Rupture of membranes (escape of fluid from the vagina)
- Swelling of the fingers (rings become tight) or puffiness of the face or around the eyes
- Continuous pounding headache
- Visual disturbances (blurred vision, dimness, spots before the eyes)
- Persistent or severe abdominal pain
- Chills or fever
- Painful urination
- Persistent vomiting
- Change in frequency or strength of fetal movements

signs and symptoms that indicate a serious danger; any such signs or symptoms should be reported immediately. (See Critical to Remember: Danger Signs of Pregnancy.)

**Although it is crucial that the expectant mother be made aware of the danger signs of pregnancy, the nurse must take care not to frighten her. Avoid the term "danger signs" when talking to the woman or her family. It is less frightening to say, "The signs I am about to explain to you are rare, but if you see them, notify the physician (or nurse-midwife) at once because they require immediate attention."**

### TEACHING HEALTH BEHAVIORS

**Bathing.** Daily bathing protects pregnant women from potential infection. If bacteria normally present on the skin are allowed to remain and multiply, infection may develop. Bathing also promotes comfort by dissipating heat that is produced by increased metabolism. During the last trimester, when balance is altered by a changing center of gravity, the woman should be cautioned to use nonskid pads in the tub or shower.

**Hot Tubs and Saunas.** Although warm baths and showers help relax tense, tired muscles, saunas and hot tubs should be avoided because they may produce maternal hyperthermia. Maternal hyperthermia, particularly during the first trimester, has been associated with fetal anomalies, such as central nervous system defects (Rogers & Davis, 1995).

**Douching.** Despite increased vaginal discharge, no hygienic need exists for douching before, during, or after pregnancy. The only exception is an order by a physician or nurse-midwife to treat a specific problem. In that case, guidelines must be carefully followed to prevent the possibility of injury (Cunningham et al., 1997).

- Bulb-type syringes have been associated with deaths caused by air embolism and therefore should never be used.
- Douche bags should not be elevated more than 2 feet above the hips to prevent excessive force of the fluid.
- The nozzle should not be inserted more than 3 inches into the vagina.

**Breast Care.** Instruct the expectant mother to wash her breasts and nipples with clear water and to avoid soap, which removes the natural lubricant that forms on the nipples. Advise all clients to wear a well-made bra that supports the breasts and prevents loss of muscle tone that can occur as the breasts become heavier during pregnancy. Wide bra straps distribute the weight evenly across the shoulders and provide greater comfort. Inform the couple that breast stimulation, which increases oxytocin secretion and thus initiates uterine contractions, is unsafe if there has been a history of preterm labor or if signs of preterm labor exist. These signs include uterine contractions that increase in frequency or intensity, rhythmic pelvic pressure, and uterine contractions that assume a regular pattern.

**Clothing.** Recommend practical, comfortable, nonconstricting clothing. Tight jeans or panty hose that may constrict venous circulation should be worn only for short periods. Low heels are preferred because they do not interfere with balance and because high heels increase the curvature of the lower spine (lordosis) that is prevalent during the last trimester.

**Exercise.** Exercise during pregnancy is generally beneficial. The amount and type of exercise recommended, however, depend on the physical condition of the woman and the stage of pregnancy. Walking is perhaps the ideal exercise because it stimulates muscular activity of the entire body, gently increases respiratory and cardiovascular effort, and does not result in fatigue or strain.

A major concern is the possibility that vigorous exercise will divert blood supply from the placenta to maternal muscles and thus deprive the fetus of needed oxygen. Vigorous exercise also increases circulating catecholamines, which cause visceral vasoconstriction and decreased placental circulation.

Women should not *begin* strenuous exercise programs or intensify training during pregnancy. As pregnancy progresses, it may be necessary to reduce the level of exercise to prevent physiologic stress. Teach the client to take her pulse every 10 to 15 minutes and not to exceed a target heart rate that has been determined in consultation with the physician or midwife.

Pregnant women must avoid becoming overheated because heat is transmitted to the fetus. Women should allow a cool-down period of mild activity after exercising. Emphasize the importance of taking liquids before and after exercising to prevent dehydration and the possible need to interrupt the exercise program to replace fluids.

Expectant mothers should curtail any activity that causes undue fatigue or poses the threat of injury. This caution may mean that activity that is safe in the first trimester may not be safe in the third trimester. Suggest that the expectant mother avoid sports that require balance and that she postpone undertaking a totally new sport until after childbirth.

It is also important that pregnant women avoid exercise in the supine position after the first trimester; this position is associated with decreased cardiac output (ACOG, 1994b).

**Sleep and Rest.** Finding a comfortable position for rest becomes a problem in the third trimester. Pillows can be used to support the abdomen and back and to provide the best opportunity for sleep (Fig. 7–16). Emphasize that frequent rest periods are beneficial, even if the woman does not fall asleep.

**Employment.** Most women of childbearing age in the United States are employed outside the home, and most continue to work during pregnancy. Whether the expectant mother can or should work depends on the presence of environmental toxins and industrial hazards and the level of physical activity involved.

***Maternal Safety.*** Work should not lead to undue fatigue. Frequent rest periods, with feet elevated, are essential. Jobs that require constant standing or sitting are very tiring, and it is necessary to plan ways to change positions or to walk briefly to stimulate circulation and reduce fatigue. Tasks that require balance may be hazardous because the uterus enlarges and the center of gravity shifts. Suggest that these jobs be curtailed during the last trimester.

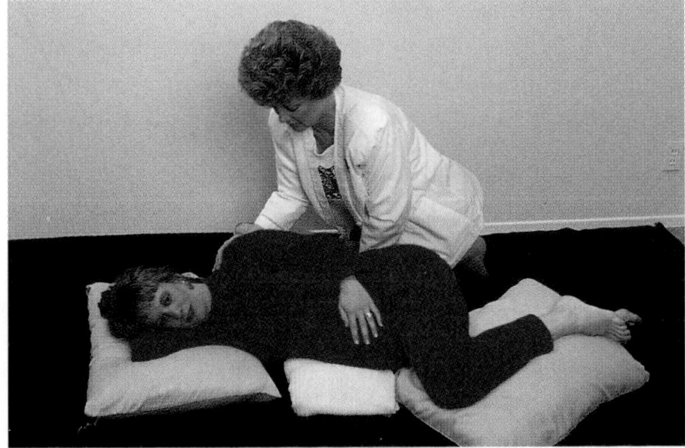

**FIGURE 7–16**

During the third trimester, pillows supporting the abdomen and back provide a comfortable position for rest.

***Exposure to Teratogens.*** The problem of intrauterine exposure to toxic substances is a major concern in many industries. Exposure is a particular concern during the first trimester, which is the period of organogenesis. Advise women to take the initiative to investigate their own occupational hazards. For example, hairdressers are exposed to toxic substances in hair dyes and aerosol sprays; painters and printers may be exposed to benzene, lead, or toluene; nurses and hospital personnel may be exposed to radiation, anesthetic gases, and hexachlorophene; and laundry and dry cleaning workers may be exposed to fetotoxic compounds. In addition, some women are exposed to smoke from other people's cigarettes (called passive smoking) in the workplace. Passive smoking is known to be harmful to both mother and fetus.

**Sexual Activity.** Despite the need for information, most couples are reluctant to initiate a discussion about sexual activity. Furthermore, most health professionals do not introduce the topic for a number of reasons: They may fear offending the client; they may be uncomfortable with their own sexuality and feel embarrassed to begin a discussion; or they may lack time for any but the most pressing assessments. The result may be that an important aspect of care is ignored.

**It may be helpful to use a broad opening statement to initiate a discussion about sexual activity. For example, "Many women tell me that it is difficult to find a comfortable position for intercourse during pregnancy." Or "Sometimes couples are concerned about having sex during pregnancy." Broad opening statements provide a method of introducing the subject in such a way that the woman feels comfortable to pursue it or to let it drop.**

It is generally agreed that sexual intercourse does no harm to the healthy pregnant woman and that maternal comfort is the watchword for couples during pregnancy. Position may need to be altered during the last 4 to 6 weeks, when supine hypotensive syndrome may result from a male-superior position. Alternate positions include side-lying, female-superior, and rear-entry. The side-lying position may be the most comfortable and require the least amount of energy during the third trimester. It is important to view sexuality in its broadest sense because fatigue, ligament pain, urinary frequency, and shortness of breath may also interfere with vaginal intercourse. Hugging, kissing, mutual massage, and cuddling are pleasurable expressions of affection that do not always lead to intercourse.

The nurse should advise the couple to curtail all sexual activity if the client is at risk for preterm labor because uterine contractions may be initiated by orgasm. The nurse also emphasizes that if membranes have ruptured or if bleeding occurs, intercourse should be curtailed.

**Travel.** Although travel by car is generally safe, it may cause discomfort or fatigue. Frequent stops are necessary to allow the expectant mother to empty her bladder and walk around. She must fasten the seat belt snugly, with the lap belt under the abdomen. This position is uncomfortable for some women, and it causes concern about internal injuries should a collision occur. It is much safer to wear the belt, however, than to leave it off and risk being ejected from the car during an accident.

Travel by plane and train is generally safe, although some physicians discourage air travel after 26 weeks. If travel is necessary, women should be advised to walk frequently to maintain adequate peripheral circulation. During travel to remote locations, a major concern is that adequate medical care be available at the destination.

**Immunizations.** In general, immunizations that use live virus vaccines are contraindicated during pregnancy because of teratogenic effects on the fetus. These vaccines include measles, mumps, rubella, and oral polio. The pregnant woman should consult her physician or nurse-midwife about which immunizations are safe during pregnancy. The nurse advises the woman to divulge that she is pregnant before a vaccine is administered.

#### TEACHING ABOUT THE COMMON DISCOMFORTS OF PREGNANCY

Although pregnancy is a state of health, the numerous physiologic changes that occur during pregnancy often cause physical discomfort. No medical care exists for these discomforts. Relief depends on self-help measures that informed nurses are expected to teach. See Figures 7–14, 7–15, and 7–16 for measures that prevent or relieve backache. In addition, measures to prevent or alleviate other discomforts are detailed in Women Want To Know: How to Overcome the Common Discomforts of Pregnancy.

#### TEACHING NECESSARY LIFESTYLE CHANGES

Many expectant parents are willing to make changes in a lifestyle to avoid adversely affecting the fetus. For example, use of tobacco, alcohol, and illegal drugs should be curtailed during pregnancy. Moreover, the use of over-the-counter medications and prescription drugs should be discussed.

**Over-the-Counter Drugs.** The nurse advises the pregnant woman to consult with her health care provider before taking any drugs. This precaution is important for over-the-counter drugs as well as for prescription drugs. Because some common discomforts of pregnancy may require use of medication, the nurse should explain that for some medications on the market inadequate information is available in regard to safe use during pregnancy. In general, the health care provider must weigh the risks against the benefits and decide if a drug can safely be used.

**Tobacco.** The nurse makes every effort to motivate the expectant mother to stop smoking and to avoid contact with others who smoke. It is well documented that pregnant women who smoke have smaller infants and an increased incidence of preterm births. Moreover, developmental problems, such as short attention span and lower cognitive skills, are also more common in children when the mother continues to smoke during pregnancy.

Smoking tobacco affects fetal development for several reasons:

- Nicotine causes vasoconstriction of vessels in the placenta.
- Carbon monoxide, released in tobacco smoke, inactivates maternal and fetal hemoglobin, which is essential to transport oxygen to the fetus.
- Maternal appetite is decreased, causing inadequate intake of calories.
- Plasma volume, needed to transport nutrients and oxygen to the fetus, is decreased.

**Alcohol.** Alcohol is a known teratogen, and maternal alcohol use is one of the leading causes of mental retardation in the United States. Alcohol produces a characteristic cluster of developmental anomalies known as *fetal alcohol syndrome*. Children with fetal alcohol syndrome exhibit a typical pattern of prenatal and postnatal growth retardation with characteristic facial, cardiovascular, and limb defects (see Fig. 24–1). These children also exhibit cognitive and fine-motor dysfunction that is tragic and irreversible.

Some controversy exists about the effects of social or moderate drinking on the fetus, and conclusive data are not available. Therefore, the best advice for women who are pregnant or who plan to become pregnant is to abstain from all alcohol.

**Illegal Drugs.** Use of so-called street drugs, such as cocaine, heroin, and methamphetamines, is harmful to the fetus. Cocaine and crack cocaine use has escalated dramatically in the past decade (Kaye & Chasnoff, 1993). The pregnant woman should be advised to discontinue all illicit drug use. (See Chapter 24 for additional information about substance abuse.)

## Evaluation

Interventions can be judged to be effective in meeting the outcomes established if the mother and her family (1) verbalize or demonstrate knowledge of self-care practices that promote her safety and health and those of the fetus, (2) identify a plan early in pregnancy (first trimester) to modify habits that do not promote health, such as curtailing the use of alcohol or tobacco, and (3) verbalize knowledge of measures that provide relief from the common discomforts of pregnancy. If interventions are ineffective, the nurse collaborates with the family to define new plans and work out additional interventions.

## Antepartum Home Care Nursing

Although guidelines have been developed for antepartum home care nursing for low-risk and at-risk clients (AWHONN, 1994), they define an ideal. Economic constraints in health care often limit or prevent antepartum nursing care for clients in the home setting. Low-risk clients are those who have no obvious complications. At-risk clients are those who have identified risk factors and are being monitored to identify any complications as they develop.

The goal of low-risk antepartum home care nursing is to make certain that no risk factors for pregnancy complications are present and to provide routine maternal and fetal surveillance. Visits ideally begin as soon as the pregnancy is known and include a thorough physical and psychosocial assessment. Nursing interventions emphasize providing information and making appropriate referrals.

## SUMMARY

- Pregnancy causes a predictable pattern of uterine growth that provides information about fetal development and helps to confirm the expected date of birth. In general, the uterus can be palpated at the level of the umbilicus at 20 weeks of gestation and at the xiphoid process by 36 weeks.
- Thick mucus fills the softened connective tissue in the cervical canal and protects the fetus from infection caused by bacteria ascending from the vagina.
- Plasma volume expands faster and to a greater extent than red blood cells, resulting in a dilution of hemoglobin concentration. This condition is referred to as physiologic (pseudo) anemia because the low levels of hemoglobin and hematocrit are due to dilution and do not reflect an inadequate number of red blood cells.
- Blood flow is altered during pregnancy to include the uteroplacental unit. Increased renal plasma flow results in increased glomerular filtration rate, which effectively removes additional metabolic wastes produced by the mother and the fetus but often results in "spilling" of glucose and other nutrients in the urine. Increased blood flow to the skin attempts to reduce the additional heat generated by the fetus and by the increased maternal metabolic rate.
- The gravid uterus partially occludes the vena cava and the descending aorta when the mother rests in a supine position. The occlusion causes supine hypotensive syndrome, which can be prevented or corrected when she assumes a lateral position.
- During the last trimester, the uterus pushes the diaphragm upward, decreasing lung capacity. To compensate, the ribs flare, the substernal angle widens, and the circumference of the chest increases.
- Alterations in hormones during pregnancy may result in discomfort for the mother. Increased hCG and estrogen are associated with nausea in early pregnancy. Increased progesterone is associated with relaxation of all smooth muscles, including those of the ureters, bladder, and bowel. Resulting stasis of urine rich in nutrients increases the risk of urinary tract infections. Decreased bowel motility is a major cause of constipation during pregnancy.
- Alterations in hormones are also responsible for cutaneous changes, such as hyperpigmentation.
- The expanding uterus plus the hormone relaxin result in progressive changes that can lead to muscle strain and backache during the last trimester.
- Progesterone is called the hormone of pregnancy because it maintains the uterine lining for implantation of the blastocyst; prevents uterine contractions during pregnancy, which could result in spontaneous abortion; and helps to prepare the breasts for lactation.
- Presumptive and probable signs of pregnancy may be caused by conditions other than pregnancy and thus cannot be considered positive or diagnostic signs. Positive signs can have no other cause.
- A complete history and physical examination are necessary at the initial antepartum visit to determine the potential risks to the mother and fetus and to obtain baseline data so that a plan of care can be developed.
- Risk assessment begins at the initial visit and continues throughout pregnancy because gestations that are categorized as low risk in early pregnancy may become high risk later.
- Multifetal pregnancies impose greater physiologic changes than a single-fetus pregnancy and require extra vigilance to detect possible complications.
- Families require information related to self-care and health promotion as well as information to deal with the common discomforts of pregnancy, which do not require or respond to medical management.
- Nurses must use nursing-process and critical-thinking skills to assist the parents in making necessary changes in lifestyle.

### References and Readings

American College of Obstetricians and Gynecologists (ACOG) (1994a). *Diabetes and pregnancy*. Washington, D.C.: Technical Bulletin number 200.

American College of Obstetricians and Gynecologists (ACOG) (1994b). *Exercise during pregnancy and the postnatal period*. Washington, D.C.: Technical Bulletin number 189.

American College of Obstetricians and Gynecologists (ACOG) (1996). *Guidelines for women's health care*. Washington, D.C.

Aminoff, M.J. (1994). Neurologic disorders. In R.K. Creasy & R. Resnik, *Maternal-fetal medicine: Principles and practice* (3rd ed., pp. 1071–1100). Philadelphia: W.B. Saunders.

Andres, R.L., & Jones, K.L. (1994). Social and illicit drug use in pregnancy. In R.K. Creasy & R. Resnik, *Maternal-fetal medicine: Principles and practice* (3rd ed., pp. 171–181). Philadelphia: W.B. Saunders.

Association of Women's Health, Obstetric, and Neonatal Nurses (AWHONN) (1994). Didactic content and clinical skills verification for professional nurse providers of perinatal home care. Washington, D.C.

Aumann, G.M-E., & Baird, M.M. (1993). Risk assessment for pregnant women. In R.A. Knuppel & J.E. Drukker, *High-risk pregnancy: A team approach* (2nd ed., pp. 8–35). Philadelphia: W.B. Saunders.

Baker, E.R. (1995). Physiologic adaptations to pregnancy. In P.L. Carr, K.M. Freund, & S. Somani, *The medical care of women* (pp. 294–303). Philadelphia: W.B. Saunders.

Blackburn, S.T., & Loper, D.L. (1992). *Maternal, fetal, and neonatal physiology*. Philadelphia: W.B. Saunders.

Briggs, G.G., Freeman, R.K., & Sumner, J.Y. (1994). *Drugs in pregnancy and lactation*. Baltimore: Williams & Wilkins.

Cunningham, F.G., MacDonald, P.C., Gant, N.F., Leveno, K.J., Gilstrap, L.C., Hankins, G.D.V., & Clark, S.L. (1997). *Williams obstetrics* (20th ed.). Norwalk, Conn.: Appleton & Lange.

DuBose, T.J. (1996). First trimester. In T.J. DuBose, *Fetal sonography* (pp. 389–425). Philadelphia: W.B. Saunders.

Duffy, T.P. (1995). Hematologic aspects of pregnancy. In G.N. Burrow & T.F. Ferris (Eds.), *Medical complications during pregnancy* (4th ed., pp. 62–82). Philadelphia: W.B. Saunders.

Enkin, M.W., Keirse, M.J., Renfrew, M.J., & Neilson, J.P. (1995). Effective care in pregnancy and childbirth: A synopsis. *Birth*, 22(2), 101–111.

Grohar, J. (1994). Nursing protocols for antepartum home care. *Journal of Obstetric, Gynecologic, and Neonatal Nursing*, 23 (8), 687–695.

Hobel, C.J. (1992). Prenatal care. In N.F. Hacker & J.G. Moore, M. *Essentials of obstetrics and gynecology* (pp. 82–92). Philadelphia: W.B. Saunders.

Hutchinson, M.K., & Baqi-Aziz, M. (1994). Nursing care of the childbearing Muslim family. *Journal of Obstetric, Gynecologic, and Neonatal Nursing*, 23(9), 767–771.

Kaye, M.E., & Chasnoff, I.J. (1993). Substance abuse in pregnancy. In R.A. Knuppel & J.E. Drukker, *High-risk pregnancy: A team approach* (2nd ed., pp. 163–179). Philadelphia: W.B. Saunders.

Knuppel, R.A., & Drukker, J.E. (1993). Hypertension in pregnancy. In R.A. Knuppel & J.E. Drukker, *High-risk pregnancy: A team approach* (2nd ed., pp. 468–515). Philadelphia: W.B. Saunders.

MacLennan, A.H. (1994). Multiple gestation: Clinical characteristics and management. In R.K. Creasy & R. Resnik, *Maternal-fetal medicine: Principles and practice* (3rd ed.). Philadelphia: W.B. Saunders.

Matthews, A.K., & Smith, A.C.M. (1993). Genetic counseling. In R.A. Knuppel & J.E. Drukker (Eds.), *High-risk pregnancy: A team approach* (2nd ed., pp. 664–703). Philadelphia: W.B. Saunders.

Mattson, S., & Smith, J.E. (Eds.) (1993). *Core curriculum for maternal-newborn nursing*. The Organization for Obstetric, Gynecologic, and Neonatal Nursing. Philadelphia: W.B. Saunders.

Meikle, S.F., Orleans, M., Leff, M., Shain, R., & Gibbs, R.S. (1995). Women's reasons for not seeking prenatal care: Racial and ethnic factors. *Birth*, 22(2), 81–86.

Mills, J.L. (1993). Moderate caffeine use and the risk of spontaneous abortion and intrauterine growth retardation. *Journal of the American Medical Association* 269(5), 593–597.

Monga, M., & Creasy, R.K. (1994). Cardiovascular and renal adaptation to pregnancy. In R.K. Creasy & R. Resnik, *Maternal-fetal medicine: Principles and practice* (3rd ed., pp. 758–767). Philadelphia: W.B. Saunders.

Newman, R.B., & Ellings, J.M. (1995). Antepartum management of the multiple gestation: The case for specialized care. *Seminars in Perinatology*, 19(5), 387–402.

North American Nursing Diagnosis Association (1995–1996). Nursing diagnoses: Definitions & classification. Philadelphia.

Nurses Association of the American College of Obstetrics and Gynecology (1991). *Standards for the nursing care of women and newborns* (4th ed.). Washington, D.C.

Nuwayhid, B., & Khalife, S. (1992). Medical complications of pregnancy. In N.F. Hacker & J.G. Moore (Eds.), *Essentials of obstetrics and gynecology* (2nd ed., pp. 197–222). Philadelphia: W.B. Saunders.

O'Brien, B., & Zhou, Q. (1995). Variables related to nausea and vomiting during pregnancy. *Birth*, 22(2), 93–100.

Rapini, R.P., & Jordon, R.E. (1994). The skin and pregnancy. In R.K. Creasy & R. Resnik, *Maternal-fetal medicine: Principles and practice* (3rd ed., pp. 1101–1111). Philadelphia: W.B. Saunders.

Resnik, R. (1994). Anatomic alterations in the reproductive tract. In R.K. Creasy & R. Resnik, *Maternal-fetal medicine: Principles and practice* (3rd ed., pp. 128–133). Philadelphia: W.B. Saunders.

Rogers, J., & Davis, B.A. (1995). How risky are hot tubs and saunas for pregnant women? *The American Journal of Maternal/Child Nursing*, 20(3), 137–140.

Simpson, K.R., & Creehan, P.A. (1996). AWHONN *perinatal nursing*. Philadelphia: Lippincott–Raven Publishers.

Spector, R.E. (1991). *Cultural diversity in health and illness* (3rd ed.). Norwalk, Conn.: Appleton & Lange.

Thorpe, K., Greenwood, R., & Goodenough, T. (1995). Does a twin pregnancy have a greater impact on physical and emotional well-being than a singleton pregnancy? *Birth*, 22(3), 148–152.

U.S. Public Health Service (1992). *Healthy people* 2000, *National health promotion and disease preventing objectives*. Washington, D.C.: U.S. Department of Health and Human Services.

Wasserstrum, N. (1992). Maternal physiology. In N.F. Hacker & J.G. Moore (Eds.), *Essentials of obstetrics and gynecology* (2nd ed., pp. 61–81). Philadelphia: W.B. Saunders.

Winn, H.N., Hess, O., Goldstein, I., Wackers, F., & Hobbins, J.C. (1994). Fetal responses to maternal exercise: Effect on fetal breathing and body movement. *American Journal of Perinatology*, 11(4), 263–266.

# 8

# Psychosocial Adaptations to Pregnancy

**OBJECTIVES**

1. Describe the psychological responses of the expectant mother to pregnancy.
2. Identify the process of role transition
3. Explain the maternal tasks of pregnancy.
4. Describe the developmental processes that a man completes to make the transition to the role of father.
5. Describe the responses of prospective grandparents and siblings to pregnancy.
6. Discuss factors that influence psychosocial adaptation to pregnancy such as age, parity, socioeconomic status, and cultural influences.
7. Describe how these factors affect nursing practice.

**DEFINITIONS**

**ambivalence** *Simultaneous conflicting emotions, attitudes, ideas, or wishes.*

**attachment** *Development of strong affectional ties as a result of interaction between an infant and a significant other (mother, father, sibling, caretaker).*

**body image** *Subjective image of one's physical appearance and capabilities; derived from own observations and from the evaluation of significant others.*

**bonding** *Development of a strong emotional tie of a parent to a newborn; also called claiming or binding in.*

**couvade** *Pregnancy-related rituals or a cluster of symptoms experienced by some prospective fathers during pregnancy and childbirth.*

**developmental task** *A necessary step in growth and maturation that one must complete before additional growth and maturation are possible.*

**disturbance in body image** *Negative feelings about characteristics, functions, or limits of one's body.*

**fantasy** *Mental images formed to prepare for the birth of a child.*

**introversion** *Inward concentration on oneself and one's body.*

**mimicry** *Copying the behaviors of other pregnant women or mothers as a method of "trying on" the role of advanced pregnancy or motherhood.*

**narcissism** *Undue preoccupation with oneself.*

**role transition** *Changing from one pattern of behavior and one image of self to another.*

Becoming a parent who is capable of loving and caring for a totally dependent infant is more than a biologic event. It is a process that begins before conception and involves major changes in the expectant mother, her partner, and the entire family. Although each couple adapts to pregnancy in a unique manner, the psychological responses of prospective parents change as the pregnancy progresses. Thus, although the initial reaction may be uncertain, by the time the infant is born, the woman and her partner have completed developmental tasks that make it possible for them to become parents in the true sense of the word. Moreover, both social and cultural factors influence the way the woman adjusts to pregnancy.

# Maternal Psychological Responses

A woman's psychological response to pregnancy changes over time. Initially she may be uncertain or ambivalent about the pregnancy, and her primary focus is on herself. Gradually her focus shifts, and she becomes increasingly concerned about how she can protect and provide for the fetus she is carrying.

## First Trimester

### UNCERTAINTY

During the early weeks, the woman is unsure whether she is pregnant and spends a great deal of time trying to confirm it. She observes her body carefully for changes that indicate she is pregnant. She may confer with family and friends about the probability and may use an over-the-counter pregnancy test kit for validation.

Reaction to the uncertainty of pregnancy depends on the individual. A woman may be eager to find confirming signs, or she may dread the possibility and hope for signs that indicate she is not pregnant at this time. Usually, she seeks confirmation from a physician, certified nurse-midwife, or nurse practitioner within 12 weeks of the first missed menstrual period.

### AMBIVALENCE

Once the pregnancy is confirmed, almost all women have conflicting feelings, or ambivalence, about being pregnant. Many feel that this is not the right time, even if the pregnancy is wanted and planned. Women who had planned to become pregnant often say they thought it would take longer for the pregnancy to become a reality and are unprepared for it. Many pregnancies are desired but unplanned, and these women often say they wish they had not become pregnant until some specific goals were met or plans were completed.

Many women examine what the pregnancy means in terms of changes that must be made in their lives and what they must give up as a result of the pregnancy. If it is a first pregnancy, a woman may worry about the added responsibility and feel unsure of her ability to be a good parent. Some women worry about how this pregnancy will affect their relationship with other children or with the father.

### THE SELF AS PRIMARY FOCUS

Throughout the first trimester, the woman's primary focus is on herself, not the fetus. Early physical responses to pregnancy, such as nausea and fatigue, confirm that something is happening to her, but the fetus remains vague and unreal. Because she has not gained weight that would confirm that a fetus is growing and developing, she probably says, "I am pregnant," rather than, "I am going to have a baby."

Physical changes and increased hormone levels may cause emotional lability (unstable moods). Her mood can change quickly from contentment to irritation or from optimistic planning to an overwhelming need for sleep, when all plans are temporarily abandoned. This may be confusing to her partner, who is accustomed to a more stable relationship. The nurse should tell the couple that mood changes are normal and that they do not necessarily indicate unresolved problems.

## Second Trimester

### PHYSICAL EVIDENCE OF PREGNANCY

During the second trimester, physical changes occur in the expectant mother that make the fetus "real." The uterus grows rapidly and can be palpated in the abdomen; weight increases, and breast changes are obvious. Most importantly, she feels the fetus move ("quickening"). This movement is an important event because the gentle fetal movement confirms that a life is developing within the uterus. As a result, she no longer thinks of the fetus as simply a part of her body but now perceives it as separate, although entirely dependent on her. Now she might say, "I am going to have a baby." (Fig. 8–1).

### THE FETUS AS PRIMARY FOCUS

The woman's major focus during the second trimester becomes the fetus. The pregnant woman usually feels well; the discomforts of the first trimester have usually abated; and her size does not alter her activity. She is now concerned about how she can produce a healthy infant. She generally seeks infor-

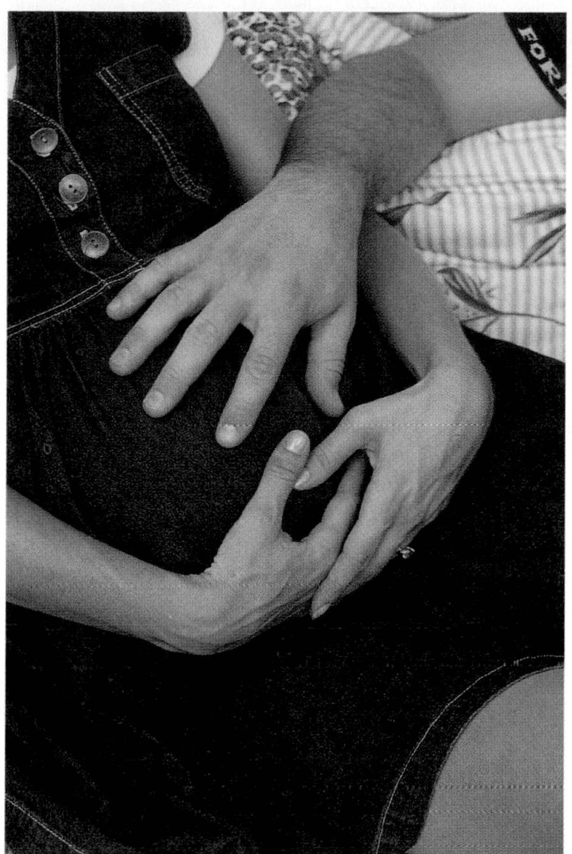

**FIGURE 8–1**

Fetal movement, "quickening," confirms that a separate life is developing.

mation about diet and about how the fetus grows and develops. She experiences a feeling of creative energy and satisfaction.

### NARCISSISM AND INTROVERSION

During this time many women become increasingly concerned about their ability to protect and provide for the fetus. This concern is often manifested as narcissism and introversion. Selecting exactly the right foods to eat, the right clothes to wear, or the most comfortable environment may assume more importance than ever before. Some women may lose interest in their jobs because the work seems alien to the events taking place in their bodies. They may be less interested in current events as they concentrate on their pregnancy, or they may become fearful that world events threaten them and therefore present a danger to the fetus.

If she is a primigravida, the expectant mother wonders what the infant is like. She looks at baby pictures of herself and her mate and wants to hear stories about them as infants. Although multiparas know what infants are like, they are interested in *this* infant and think about how this child will be accepted by siblings and grandparents.

### BODY IMAGE

Rapid and profound changes take place in the body during the second trimester. Changes in body size and contour are noticeable, with obvious bulging of the abdomen, thickening of the waist, and enlargement of the breasts. The changes may be welcomed because they signify growth of the fetus, and this creates pride in the woman and her partner. For some women, however, the change in body size and shape, coupled with hyperpigmentation of the skin and striae gravidarum (stretch marks), may contribute to a negative body image. Moreover, changes in body function, such as altered balance, less physical endurance, and discomfort in the pelvis and lower back areas, may also contribute to a negative body image (Nursing Care Plan 8–1).

### CHANGES IN SEXUALITY

Sexual interest and activity of pregnant women and their partners are unpredictable. They may increase, decline, or remain unchanged. The woman's physical comfort and sense of well-being are closely linked to her interest in sexual activity. During the first trimester physical complaints, such as nausea, fatigue, and breast tenderness, may interfere with erotic feelings. Moreover, fear of miscarriage may cause couples to avoid intercourse, particularly if the woman has previously lost a pregnancy. Guilt and anxiety may develop if sexual activity is curtailed. Nurses can help reassure the couple that there is no evidence that intercourse is related to early pregnancy loss when no other complications are present.

As a result of pelvic vasocongestion, women experience increased sensitivity of the labia and clitoris and increased vaginal lubrication during the second trimester. These changes, coupled with not having to deal with the concern about getting pregnant, may increase the sexual responsiveness of many women.

During the third trimester, the "missionary position" (male on top) may cause discomfort from abdominal pressure. Heartburn and indigestion may also increase in this position. As they become larger, some women feel that their bodies are ugly and may worry about how their partners react to their increased size.

Sexual response varies widely among males. Some report heightened feelings of sexual interest, but some men perceive the woman's body in late pregnancy as unattractive and erotic feelings decrease. Moreover, for some men, fear of harming the fetus or causing discomfort during pregnancy interferes with sexual activity.

The expectant couple should be made aware of the normal changes in sexual desire that occur during pregnancy and the importance of communicating their feelings openly with each other so that solutions to problems can be found. The nurse can sug-

## Nursing Care Plan 8–1

# Body Image During Pregnancy

**ASSESSMENT:** Dolores White is a 34-year-old primigravida in the 26th week of pregnancy. Both she and her husband have been runners for several years. Dolores stopped running 6 months ago and reports that she now walks "like other old ladies." She verbalizes concern about how much bigger she will get and says she feels "awkward and ugly." She states, "I hate the way I look; I can't wait to get back into shape."

**NURSING DIAGNOSIS:** Body Image Disturbance related to changes in body size, contour, and function

### GOALS/EXPECTED OUTCOMES

The client will do the following:

1. Make statements that indicate acceptance of expected body changes during pregnancy.
2. Express her feelings about body changes to her husband as well as to the health care team by (date).
3. Set realistic goals for weight loss and the resumption of a running program following childbirth.

| INTERVENTION | RATIONALE |
|---|---|
| 1. Acknowledge Dolores' feelings. "I can see you are disappointed at not being able to run, and I sense you are concerned about how your body has changed as a result of pregnancy." | 1. Feelings must be acknowledged, reflected, and dealt with before the underlying cause can be addressed. |
| 2. Clarify her concerns. "You have always been an athlete. Are you wondering how much permanent change will result from pregnancy?" | 2. An underlying, unvoiced concern may be that pregnancy and childbirth will change the woman from athlete to mother. This altered perception of herself causes fear and/or grief. |
| 3. Suggest that she share her feelings with her husband and seek his support. It may be necessary to model this interaction. "I am feeling awkward and left out of a big part of our lives. I need some reassurance from you now." | 3. Although one may assume that the partner observes and understands when negative feelings exist, this may not be true. |
| 4. Demonstrate the expected patttern of weight gain from 26 weeks to term gestation, and correlate this with the growth and develoment of the fetus. | 4. Many women achieve satisfaction from the knowledge that weight gain indicates tht the fetus is growing. Moreover, knowledge of how much weight gain is expected may allay unexpressed fears of excessive weight gain. |
| 5. Help Dolores make realistic plans to lose weight and recover her strength and endurance following childbirth.<br>a. Discuss the expected pattern of weight loss following childbirth: an initial weight loss of 4.5 to 5 kg, or 10 to 12 pounds. An additional 2.5 kg, or 5.5 pounds, may be lost in the first few postpartum days. By the end of 8 weeks, many women return to their prepregnancy weight.<br>b. Demonstrate graduated exercises that increase muscle tone and strength.<br>c. Explain the purpose of adipose tissue gained during pregnancy, and discuss a diet that provides sufficient calories to meet the client's needs, taking into account the calories required for breastfeeding. | 5. Adipose tissue provides a needed source of energy after childbirth and during lactation. Many women are relieved to know that there is a purpose and that the added weight will be lost gradually. Breastfeeding requires at least 500 additional calories per day. |

### EVALUATION

Statements by Dolores indicating acceptance of body changes during pregnancy are important signs that the interventions have been successful. Increased communication between the partners about the woman's concerns reduces her frustration. be necessary to monitor her plans for weight loss and for exercise after childbirth so that unrealistic goals are not set.

### ADDITIONAL NURSING DIAGNOSES TO CONSIDER

Risk for Situational Low Self-Esteem
Personal Identity Disturbance
Knowledge Deficit
Altered Family Processes

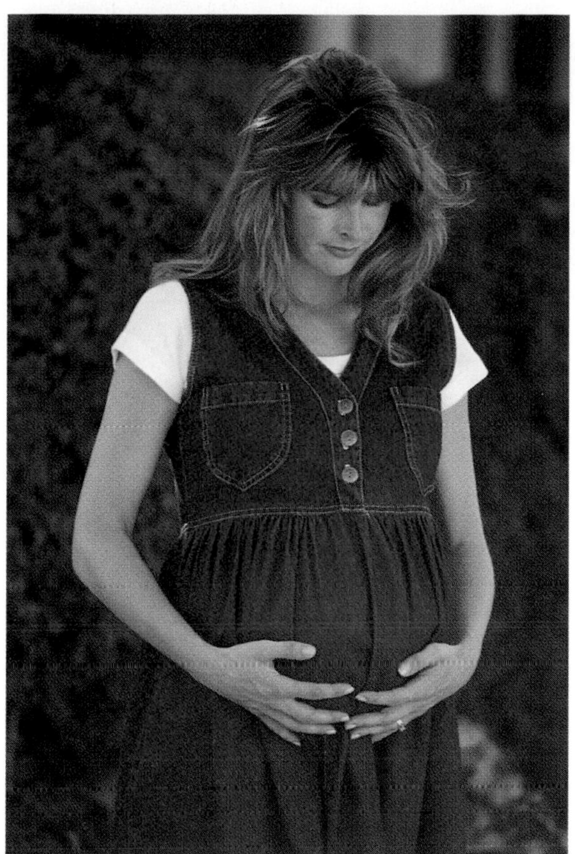

**FIGURE 8–2**

During the third trimester, the mother feels increasingly vulnerable; she cradles her fetus to signify her protectiveness.

gest alternative positions and reassure the couple that their feelings are normal.

## Third Trimester

### VULNERABILITY

The sense of well-being and contentment that dominates the second trimester gives way to increasing feelings of vulnerability during the third trimester, particularly during the seventh month of pregnancy. Pregnant women often feel that the precious baby may be lost or harmed if not protected at all times (Fig. 8–2). Many mothers have fantasies or nightmares about harm coming to the infant and become very cautious as a result. They may avoid crowds because they feel unable to protect the infant from infectious diseases or physical dangers that may be present.

### INCREASING DEPENDENCE

The expectant mother often becomes increasingly dependent on her partner in the last weeks of pregnancy. She may insist that he carry a beeper, or she may call his place of work several times during the day just to be sure that he is available. Her need for love and attention from her partner is even more pronounced in late pregnancy. She needs to be certain of his support and availability. When she is assured of his concern and willingness to provide assistance, she feels more secure and able to cope.

Although the woman may not be able to explain the increasing dependence, she expects her partner to understand the feeling and may become angry if he is not sympathetic. The nurse can encourage couples to discuss their fears and feelings openly so that misunderstandings can be avoided.

### PREPARATION FOR BIRTH

Gradually, the feelings of vulnerability decrease as the woman comes to terms with her situation. The fetus continues to grow, and fetal movements are no longer gentle; pokes, jabs, and kicks are intrusive expressions of the baby's crowded condition and increasing activity. The woman's relationship with the fetus changes as she acknowledges that although she and the fetus are interrelated, the baby is not a part of herself but is a pervasive presence. Although she may not consciously acknowledge the increasing feelings of separateness, she longs to *see* the baby and to become acquainted with her child.

Most pregnant women are concerned with their ability to determine when they are in labor. They review the signs of labor that are taught in childbirth education classes and question friends and family members who have given birth. Many couples worry that they will not get to the hospital or clinic in time for the birth, and they may be concerned about how they will cope with labor.

During the last several weeks, the woman becomes increasingly concerned with her expected date of delivery (EDD) and with the experience of labor and delivery. Some women fear labor and dread the EDD, whereas some are so uncomfortable that they look forward to that day as the *exact* day the birth will occur.

During the third trimester, an expectant mother may say, "I am going to be a mother" as she prepares for the infant. Clothing, a place for the infant to sleep, and negotiating how household tasks will be shared with her partner are among the plans made at this time. In addition, many couples complete childbirth education classes at this time. Table 8–1 summarizes the progressive changes in maternal responses during pregnancy.

**CHECK YOUR READING**

1. Why might an expectant mother say, "I am pregnant" during the first trimester but "I am going to be a mother" late in pregnancy?
2. How might pregnancy affect sexual responses of the mother and the father?

**TABLE 8-1 PROGRESSIVE CHANGES IN MATERNAL RESPONSES TO PREGNANCY**

| First Trimester | Second Trimester | Third Trimester |
|---|---|---|
| **Emotional Response** | | |
| Uncertainty, ambivalence, focus on self | Wonder, increased narcissism, introversion, concern about body and changes in sexuality | Vulnerability<br>Increased dependence<br>Acceptance that fetus is separate but totally dependent |
| **Physical Validation** | | |
| No obvious signs of fetal growth | Quickening<br>Obvious fetal growth | Discomfort<br>Decreased maternal activity |
| **Role** | | |
| May begin to seek safe passage for self and fetus | Seeks acceptance of fetus and her role as mother | Prepares for birth |
| **"Self" Statement** | | |
| "I am pregnant." | "I am going to have a baby." | "I am going to be a mother." |

## Maternal Role Transition

Becoming a mother involves more than giving birth and providing physical care for the newborn. Mothering also involves intense feelings of love, tenderness, and devotion that endure over a lifetime. But how does one learn to be a mother?

The transition into mothering begins during pregnancy and increases with gestational age. An early task of pregnancy is to accept the intrusion of the fetus, then move to developing love for the child as an independent being (Mercer & Ferketich, 1994a). The greatest increase in maternal-fetal attachment seems to occur after quickening, when the mother begins to differentiate herself from the fetus (Bloom, 1995). A pregnant woman prepares for becoming a mother by contemplating her life as a woman with a child. She thinks about what characteristics she wishes to have as a mother and anticipates life changes that will be necessary.

### Steps in Maternal Role Taking

Rubin (1984) observed specific steps that provide a framework for understanding the process of maternal role taking: mimicry, role play, fantasy, looking for a role fit, and grief work.

#### MIMICRY

Mimicry involves observing and copying the behavior of other women who are pregnant or who are already mothers. It is an earnest attempt to discover what it is like to begin the role. Mimicry often begins in the first trimester, when the woman may wear maternity clothes before they are needed to see how women in more advanced pregnancy feel and to see how people react to her. She may also mimic the waddling gait or posture of a woman who is close to delivery long before these changes are necessary for her.

#### ROLE PLAY

Role play consists of acting out some aspect of what mothers actually do. The pregnant woman searches for opportunities to hold infants or to provide care for infants in the presence of another person. She does this to evaluate not only her comfort in the situation but also the response of the observer. Role playing gives her an opportunity to "practice" the expected role and to receive validation from the observer that she has functioned well. She is particularly sensitive to the responses of her partner and her own mother.

#### FANTASY

Fantasy takes place in the mind rather than in behavior. Many fantasies have to do with how the infant will look and what characteristics he or she will have. Fantasies allow the woman to try out a variety of possibilities and to daydream or to "try on" a variety of behaviors. She may daydream about taking her daughter to the park or how she will hold the child and read or play music.

At times, fantasies are fearful. What happens if something is wrong with the infant? What if the baby cries and won't stop? Fearful fantasies often provoke a pregnant woman to respond to the fears by seeking information or reassurance. For instance, she may ask her partner if he will love the baby even if it is not perfect, or she may strive to learn all she can about how to care for a baby that is difficult to console.

#### LOOKING FOR A ROLE FIT

Looking for a role fit is a process that occurs once the woman has built up a set of role expectations for herself and has internalized a view of how a "good" mother behaves. She then observes the behaviors of mothers and compares them with her own expectations of herself. She imagines herself acting in the same way and either rejects or accepts the behaviors, depending on how well they fit her sense of what is right. This process implies that the woman has explored the role of mother long enough to have developed a sense of herself in the role and to be able to select behaviors that reaffirm her sense of how she wants to fulfill the role.

#### GRIEF WORK

At first, grief work seems incongruous with maternal role taking, but women often experience a sense of sadness when they realize that they must give up certain aspects of their previous selves and can never go back. A mother will never again be a carefree girl without a child. She must relinquish some of her old patterns of behavior so that she can move into the new identity as mother of an infant. Even simple things such as going shopping or going to the movies will require planning to include the infant or to find alternative care. Changes may be particularly difficult for the adolescent who is not used to planning and who may have to give up or change school plans as well.

## Maternal Tasks of Pregnancy

To become mothers, pregnant women spend a great deal of time and energy learning new behaviors. Moreover, as a woman works to establish a relationship with the infant, she must also reorder the relationship with her partner and family. This psychological work of pregnancy has been grouped into four maternal tasks of pregnancy (Rubin, 1984): (1) seeking safe passage for self and baby through pregnancy, labor, and childbirth; (2) securing acceptance of the baby and herself by her partner and family; (3) learning to give of herself; and (4) developing attachment and interconnection with the unknown child.

#### SEEKING SAFE PASSAGE

Seeking safe passage for herself and her baby is the woman's priority task. If she cannot be assured of that safety, she cannot move on to the other tasks. Behaviors that ensure safe passage include seeking the care of a physician or certified nurse-midwife and following recommendations about diet, vitamins, rest, and subsequent visits to the office or clinic.

In addition to following advice of health care professionals, the pregnant woman must adhere to cultural practices that ensure the safety of herself and the infant. For instance, some Southeast Asian women avoid contact with scissors and knives because they fear sharp instruments may cause cleft lip or abortion (Mattson & Lew, 1995).

#### SECURING ACCEPTANCE

Securing acceptance is a process that begins in the first trimester and continues throughout pregnancy. The process involves reworking relationships so that the important persons in the family accept the woman in the role of mother and welcome the baby into the family constellation. For example, she and the father of the baby must give up an exclusive relationship and make a place in their lives for a child. When the partner expresses pride and joy in the pregnancy, the woman feels valued and comforted. This feeling is so important that many women retain a memory of the partner's reaction to the announcement of pregnancy for many years.

Women's childhood relationships with their own mothers have been shown to be particularly important to the development of maternal attachment (Mercer & Ferketich, 1994a). The pregnant woman gains energy and contentment when acceptance and support are freely offered by her mother (Fig. 8–3).

Problems may occur if the family strongly desires a child with particular characteristics and the woman feels that the family may reject an infant who does not meet the criteria. For example, if family members wish for a boy, will they accept a girl? Women who gain unconditional acceptance experience the least anxiety (Mercer, 1990).

#### LEARNING TO GIVE OF SELF

Giving is one of the most idealized components of motherhood but one that must be learned. Learning to give begins in pregnancy when the woman allows her body to give space and nurturing to the fetus. She also observes giving in others and then tests her own ability to derive pleasure from giving. This test most often takes the form of providing food or care for her family. Their acceptance and enjoyment of the "gift" enhance her pleasure, so that the role is strengthened. She may explore further by making and giving small gifts to friends, especially those who are pregnant, and she feels pride and delight when the gift is appreciated.

Pregnant women also learn to give by receiving.

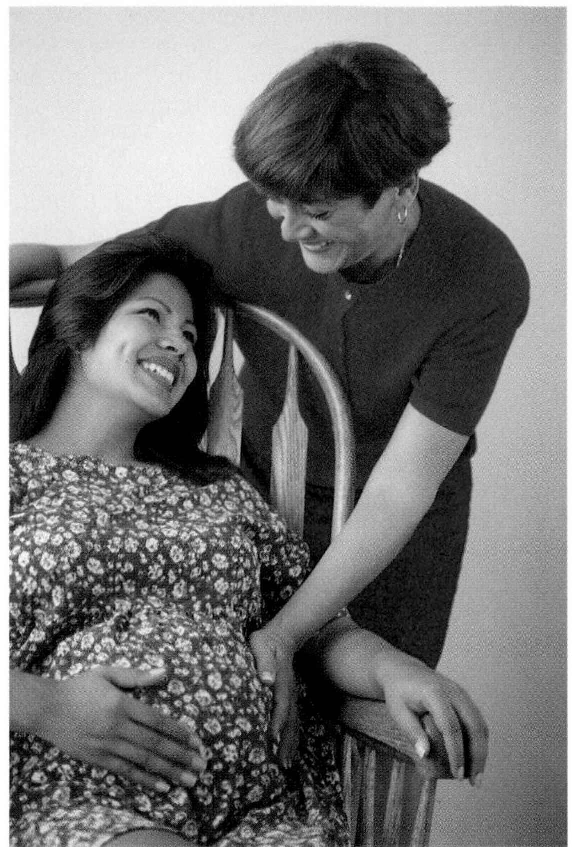

**FIGURE 8–3**

The bond between a pregnant woman and her own mother is particularly important to the young mother.

Gifts received at "baby showers" are more than needed items. They also confirm continued interest and commitment from friends and family and enhance the ability of the woman to give. Intangible gifts from others, such as companionship, attention, and support, help to increase her energy and affirm the importance of giving.

#### COMMITTING HERSELF TO THE UNKNOWN CHILD

Developing attachment to the unborn baby does not end in pregnancy but continues throughout the neonatal period (Mercer & Ferketich, 1994b). The process begins in early pregnancy when the woman accepts or "binds-in" to the idea she is pregnant, although the baby is not yet real to her. During the second trimester, the baby becomes real, and feelings of love and attachment surge. A special, exclusive relationship develops between woman and fetus that simulates a secret, romantic love. Mothers report feedback from their unborn infants during the third trimester and describe unique characteristics of the fetus with regard to sleep-wake cycles, temperament, and communication. Love of the infant becomes possessive and leads to feelings of vulnerability. The woman integrates the role of mother into her image of herself. She becomes comfortable with the idea of herself as mother and finds pleasure in contemplating the new role.

**CHECK YOUR READING**

3. What does "looking for a fit" mean in role transition?
4. Why is grief work part of maternal role transition?
5. How does the pregnant woman seek safe passage for herself and the baby?

## Paternal Adaptation

Although expectant fathers do not experience the biologic processes of pregnancy as women do, they must also make major psychosocial changes to adapt to their new role. Moreover, the changes may be more difficult because the male partner is often neglected by the health care team as well as by his peer group as attention is focused on the woman.

### Variations in Paternal Adaptation

Wide variations exist in how men respond to pregnancy. Some are emotionally invested and comfortable as full partners and wish to explore every aspect of pregnancy, childbirth, and parenting. Others are more task-oriented and see themselves as managers. They may direct the diet and rest periods of the pregnant partner and act as coaches during childbirth but remain detached from the emotional components. Other men are more comfortable as observers and prefer not to participate. Some men are culturally conditioned to see pregnancy and childbirth as "women's work," and they may not be able to express their true feelings about pregnancy and fatherhood.

Research indicates that a stable relationship with their partners, financial security, and a sense of closure to the childless part of the couple's relationship contribute to readiness for fatherhood (Tiller, 1995). Additional factors that influence how a man adapts to pregnancy and childbirth include the relationship with his own father, previous experience with children, and confidence in his ability to care for the infant.

### Developmental Processes

As with the responses of the expectant mother, the responses of the expectant father are not static but progress through phases that are subject to individual variation. Jordan (1990) describes three developmental processes that an expectant father must work through:

- He must grapple with the reality of pregnancy and the new child.
- He must struggle for recognition as a parent from his family and social network.
- He must make an effort to be seen as relevant to childbearing.

#### GRAPPLING WITH THE REALITY OF PREGNANCY AND THE CHILD

The pregnancy and the child must become real before a man can take on the identity of father. The process requires time, and it is often incomplete until the father meets the child face to face at birth. Initially, the pregnancy is a diagnosis only, and changes in the expectant woman's behavior, such as nausea and fatigue, are perceived as symptoms of illness that have little to do with having a baby.

A man's initial reaction to the announcement of pregnancy may be pride and joy, but he often experiences the same ambivalence that his partner experiences, particularly if he is unprepared for the added responsibility or commitment. Various experiences act as catalysts or "reality boosters" that make the child more real (Fig. 8–4). The most frequently mentioned experiences are hearing the baby's heart beat, feeling the infant move, and seeing the fetus on a sonogram. Once they can feel the fetus move, many expectant fathers invent a nickname and talk to the fetus. Almost all describe specific behaviors of their unborn child (Ferketich & Mercer, 1995).

Preparing the nursery or a space in the home and accumulating supplies for the new addition also reinforce the reality of the forthcoming child. These tasks often represent the first time that the expectant father has the opportunity to do something for the child directly. The birth itself is the most powerful "reality booster," and the infant becomes real to the father when he has an opportunity to see and hold the infant.

#### STRUGGLING FOR RECOGNITION AS A PARENT

Men tend not to be perceived as parents in their own right by their mates, co-workers, friends, or family. They are often viewed as helpmates but not as co-parents. As they progress through pregnancy and childbirth, their primary responsibility is to act as a support person for their partner.

Many men find it upsetting that there is often little validation of their feelings or recognition that they want to be considered a parent as well as a helper. Some men accept that the focus should be on the woman, but others find it frustrating that there is so little understanding of what the experience is like for them.

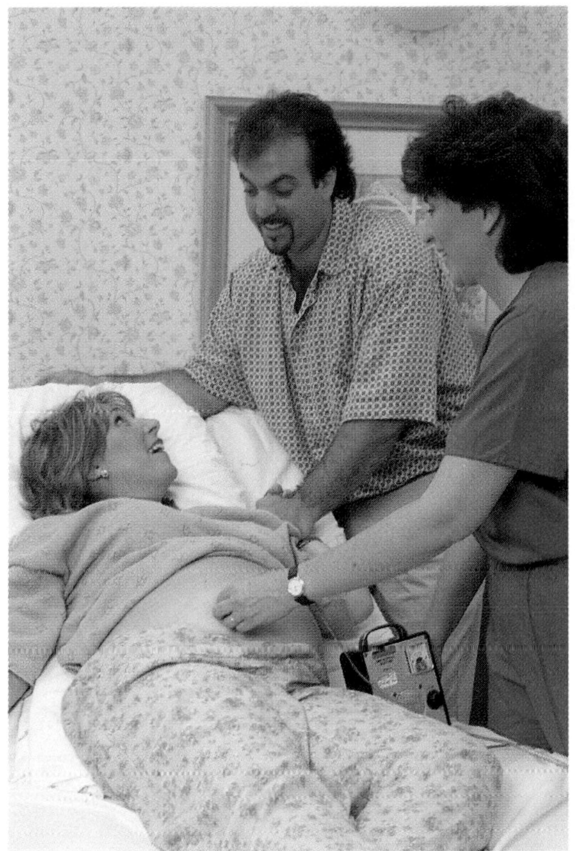

**FIGURE 8–4**

Reality booster: The existence of the fetus becomes real for the father when he hears the fetal heart beat through the transducer.

Expectant mothers play an important role in helping their partners gain recognition as parents. Women who openly share the physical sensations and emotions that they experience help the expectant father to feel that he is part of the process. These women often refer to it as "our" pregnancy and "our" child rather than as "my" pregnancy or "my" child. They also insist that the man be included in all discussions and decisions.

Nurses must learn to view the mother-father-child as the client and not focus exclusively on the mother and fetus. Men are reported to worry more than women about physical symptoms experienced by expectant mothers (Bothamley, 1990). The nurse should encourage the man to ask questions about his partner's pregnancy. These men are entitled to as much advice and reassurance as expectant women (Fig. 8–5).

#### CREATING THE ROLE OF INVOLVED FATHER

Men use various means to create a parenting role that is comfortable for them. They may seek closer ties with their own fathers to reminisce about their own childhood. They also observe men who are al-

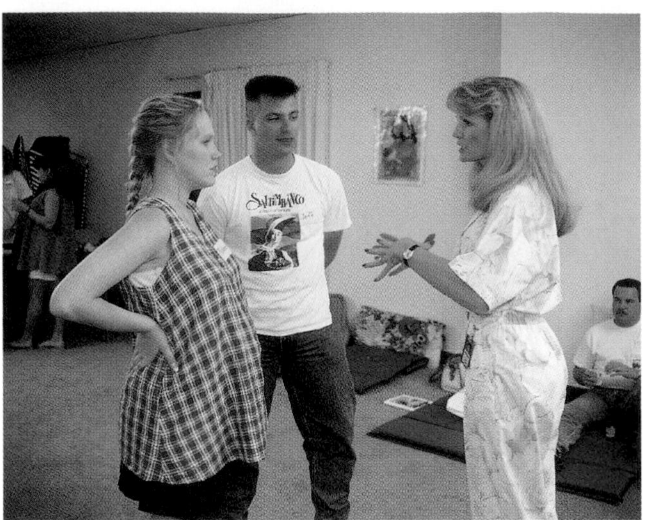

**FIGURE 8-5**

The nurse who views the mother-father-child as a client provides parents with the greatest opportunity to learn infant care and parenting skills.

ready fathers and "try on" fathering behaviors to determine whether they are comfortable and fit their own concept of the father role. Moreover, many men assertively seek information about infant care and growth and development so that they will be prepared when the infant arrives.

#### PARENTING INFORMATION

Studies indicate that fathers believe they receive inadequate parenting information in prenatal classes (Tiller, 1995). Although adequate information is usually presented, fathers may not be ready for the information at the time it is provided. As a result, they may be unprepared to care for their infants and have unrealistic expectations of the newborn. Nurses must review information about infant care and growth and development after the infant is born, when the information is immediately relevant.

#### COUVADE

The term *couvade* refers to pregnancy-related symptoms and behavior in expectant fathers. In primitive cultures, couvade took the form of rituals involving special dress, confinement, limitations of physical work, avoidance of certain foods, sexual restraint, and in some instances performance of "mock labor."

In modern practice, expectant fathers sometimes experience a cluster of physical symptoms similar to those experienced by women during pregnancy: loss of appetite, nausea and vomiting, headache, fatigue, and weight gain (Broude, 1988). Couvade symptoms are more likely to occur in early pregnancy and diminish as the pregnancy progresses. Symptoms may be caused by stress, anxiety, or empathy for the pregnant partner. They are usually harmless but may persist and result in nervousness, insomnia, restlessness, and irritability. Although the symptoms are almost always unobserved by the health care team, anticipatory guidance is believed to be beneficial for both partners.

**CHECK YOUR READING**

6. What are reality boosters? Why are they important for the expectant father's adjustment?
7. How can nurses help men in their struggle for recognition as parents?
8. Why should information relating to newborn care presented in prenatal classes be repeated after the infant is born?

## Adaptation of Grandparents

The initial reaction of grandparents depends on several factors, such as their age, the number and spacing of other grandchildren, and their perceptions of the role of grandparents.

### Age

Age is a major factor in determining the emotional responses of prospective grandparents. By the time they become grandparents, many people have already dealt with their feelings about aging and react with joy when they find that they are to become grandparents. They look forward to being able to love grandchildren, who signify the continuity of life and family.

Grandparents who are in their mid-40s may not be happy with the stereotype of grandparents as old persons. They may experience a great deal of conflict when they must resolve their self-image with the stereotype. Furthermore, people in their 40s and 50s often have career responsibilities and may not be accessible because of the continuing demands of their own lives.

### Number and Spacing of Other Grandchildren

The number and spacing of other grandchildren also determine how grandparents feel. A first grandchild may be an exciting event that creates great joy. If the grandparents already have several young grandchildren, however, the birth of another may be welcomed, but the excitement is often less than that experienced with the birth of the first grandchild. The subdued reaction may be disappointing to the couple, who may desire the same excited reaction as that expressed for the first grandchild.

### Perceptions of the Role of Grandparents

Beliefs about how important grandparents are to grandchildren vary widely. Many grandparents see their relationship with the grandchild as second in importance only to the parent-child relationship. They want to be involved in the pregnancy, and grandmothers often engage in rituals such as shopping and gift-giving showers that confirm their role as important participants. Many grandparents look forward to being intimately involved in child care and offer unconditional love to the child. They offer to care for older children while the mother gives birth, and they assist during the first weeks following childbirth.

In the past, grandparents were often looked to for advice about childbearing and childrearing. Health care workers have now become the "experts," and many grandparents have difficulty adjusting to this change. If the issue is not recognized, distance may develop as the grandparents withdraw, sensing that their participation is no longer valued. Nurses may be able to help defuse a potentially disruptive process by clarifying the situation and assisting the families to verbalize their feelings.

**"It may seem that the grandparents aren't interested in the child; however, that may not be the actual message. Perhaps they are uneasy about being responsible for care of the child. Reassure them that you are responsible but that you want them to share in the joy the child brings."**

On the other hand, some contemporary grandparents hold different beliefs about the role of grandparents and plan much less participation in pregnancy or child care. A comment frequently heard is, "I have raised my children, and I don't plan to do it again." This attitude often results in conflict with the parents, who are hurt and wish that the grandparents were around to help during the third trimester and after the birth.

Parents and grandparents may need to negotiate how the grandparents can be involved without feeling that they must assume care of the child. For instance, the couple may need suggestions that help the grandparents participate in family gatherings that do not involve babysitting or child care. (See Chapter 11 for information about classes for grandparents.)

## Adaptation of Siblings

### Toddlers

How siblings adapt to the birth of an infant depends largely on age and developmental level. Very young children, 2 years or younger, are unaware of the maternal changes that occur during pregnancy and are unable to understand that a new brother or sister is going to be born. Because toddlers have little perception of time, many parents delay telling them that a baby is expected until shortly before the birth.

Although it is difficult to prepare very young children for the birth of a baby, the nurse can make suggestions that may prove helpful. First, any change in sleeping arrangements should be made several weeks before the birth so that the child does not feel displaced by the new baby. Second, parents can prepare family and friends for feelings the toddler may have, such as jealousy and resentment, when the young child must share time and attention with a baby.

Until children feel that their place in the affection of their parents is secure, it is not realistic to expect the 2 year old to welcome the new "stranger." Frequent reassurances of parental love and affection are of primary importance. The parents can be taught to accept strong feelings that the toddler expresses, such as anger, jealousy, or frustration, without judgment and to continue to reinforce the lovability of the child. (See Chapter 18 for additional information.)

### Older Children

The older child, from 3 to 12 years, is more aware of changes in the mother's body and may be aware that a baby is to be born. These children may be interested in observing the mother's abdomen and feeling the fetus move. They enjoy listening to the heart beat and may have questions about how the fetus develops, how it started, and how it will get out of the abdomen. They often understand that the baby will be a brother or sister and look forward to its arrival. They may expect that the infant will be a full-fledged playmate, however, and so are shocked when the infant is small and helpless.

School-aged children benefit from being included in preparations for the new baby. They often enjoy recording the size and development of the fetus on a calendar. They are interested in preparing space for the infant to sleep and accumulating supplies the infant will need. The children should be encouraged to feel the fetus move, and many come close to the mother's abdomen and talk to the fetus. Older children also gain a sense of security and enjoy time alone with parents (Fig. 8–6).

Children as young as 3 years benefit from sibling classes. They are encouraged to bring a doll so that they can simulate care that an infant will need. The classes also provide an opportunity for them to discuss what changes the new baby will mean for the

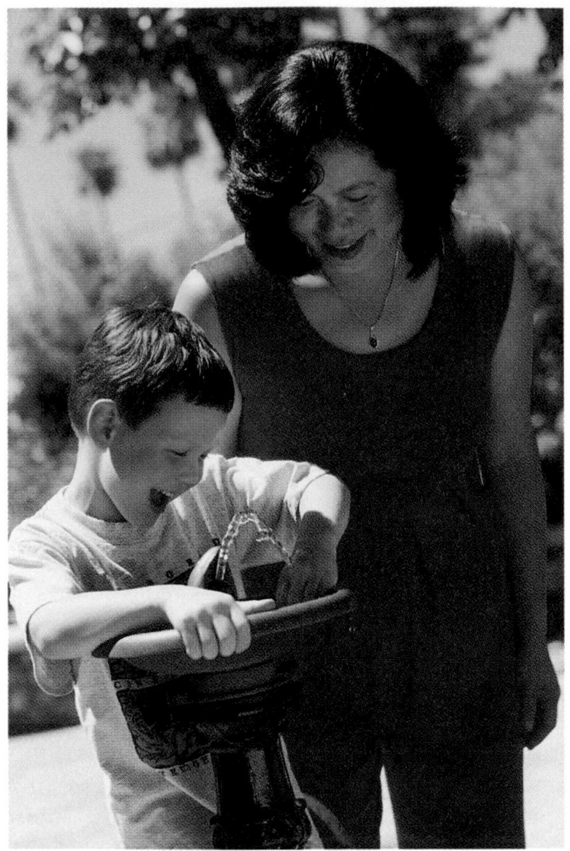

**FIGURE 8-6**

A pregnant woman who spends time with an older child can provide affection and a sense of security.

family. (See Chapter 11 for additional information about sibling classes.)

In some settings, children as young as 3 years are permitted to be with the mother during childbirth. If young children are to be present, they should attend a class that prepares them for the event. A familiar person should be available to explain what is taking place and to comfort them or to remove them if the birth becomes overwhelming.

### Adolescents

The response of adolescents also depends on their developmental level. Some adolescents may be embarrassed because the pregnancy confirms the continued sexuality of their parents. They may be repelled by the obvious physical changes. Many adolescents are immersed in their own developmental tasks that involve loosening ties to their parents and coming to terms with their own sexuality. They may be indifferent to the pregnancy unless it directly affects them or their activities. Some adolescents, on the other hand, become very involved and want to help with preparations for the baby.

**CHECK YOUR READING**

9. What determines the response of grandparents to the pregnancy?
10. How does the effect of pregnancy differ for a toddler, preschool child, and adolescent?
11. How can parents prepare siblings for the addition of a newborn to the family?

## Factors That Influence Psychosocial Adaptations

### Age

Pregnancy presents a challenge for teenagers who, as expectant parents, must cope with the conflicting developmental tasks of pregnancy and adolescence at the same time. The major developmental task of adolescence is to form and become comfortable with a sense of self. On the other hand, one of the major tasks of pregnancy involves learning to "give of self," a process that includes sacrificing personal desires for the benefit of the fetus. Giving is particularly difficult for young adolescents, who may not be able to perceive the fetus as real (Bloom, 1995).

Nurses who work with pregnant teenagers should help the adolescent tune in to her changing body and the increasing presence of the developing fetus. Adolescents also need prompting to follow a lifestyle that promotes the best outcomes for them and for their infants (see also Chapter 24).

### Absence of a Partner

The proportion of single women who become pregnant is increasing. Although some unmarried women have the financial and emotional support of a partner, many do not. These women have unique concerns, especially in the first and second trimesters. For instance, they experience more stress about how to tell their family and friends about the pregnancy. They may have to enlist more social support to substitute for that of a partner. They may have legal concerns such as whom to list as the father on birth records and what arrangements must be made to allow the father contact with the infant.

Single women without partners often live below the poverty level. They are more likely to delay prenatal care until the second or third trimester and are at increased risk for pregnancy complications and delivery of a low-birth-weight infant.

Nurses must recognize the single mother's needs for accessible and affordable prenatal care. Moreover, nurses must be prepared to offer specialized supportive care for single mothers. Needed social services may include Medicaid, food stamps, and transportation to the prenatal clinic.

## Multiparity

One might assume that a multipara needs less help than a first-time mother, but, this is not the case. Pregnancy tasks are actually much more complex for the multipara than they are for the primigravida (Mercer, 1990). When dealing with the task of negotiating safe passage for self and infant, the multipara does not have time to take special care of herself as she did during the first pregnancy. Multiparas report more fatigue, and significantly fewer report feeling very well or excellent. Moreover, more multiparas report having serious worries, such as how the children will accept the infant and how to find time and energy for additional responsibilities. When seeking acceptance of the new baby, the multipara may find the family less excited than they were for the first child. The couple's celebration is also more subdued.

The woman spends a great deal of time working out a new relationship with the first child, who often becomes demanding. This behavior may foster feelings of guilt as she tries to expand her love to include the second child. Developing attachment for the coming baby is hampered by feelings of loss between herself and the first child. She senses that the child is growing up and away from her, and she may grieve for the loss of their special relationship.

Nurses must remember that multiparas may need more help and understanding than primigravidas. The nurse cannot assume that the process is "old hat" and that information about labor, breastfeeding, and infant care is not needed. Special assistance may be necessary to help a multipara integrate an additional infant into the family structure.

## Socioeconomic Status

One of the greatest influences on childbearing practices is the socioeconomic status of the family. Socioeconomic status refers to the resources that the family has to meet the needs for food, shelter, and health care. Socioeconomic status can be divided into the affluent, middle class, working poor, and new poor. Table 8–2 summarizes the impact of socioeconomic status on the family's response to pregnancy.

### THE AFFLUENT

Affluent families have resources to provide for their needs and to purchase health care. They have a good income, secure shelter in a safe neighborhood, and the education and reserves to protect themselves from economic fluctuations. They are

**TABLE 8–2 IMPACT OF SOCIOECONOMIC FACTORS ON FAMILY'S RESPONSE TO PREGNANCY**

| Affluent | Middle Class | Working Poor and Unemployed |
|---|---|---|
| **Resources** | | |
| Confident of ability<br>Financial reserves protect family from economic fluctuations<br>Own or rent home in a safe neighborhood<br>Have health insurance or can pay for health care<br>Able to provide enriched environment | Relative security, but fewer reserves and more debt<br>Own or rent home in relatively safe neighborhood<br>Health insurance depends on employment | Lack skills, bargaining power<br>Most vulnerable to economic fluctuations<br>Struggle for basic needs |
| **Value Placed on Health Care** | | |
| Value preventive care | Value health care but must rely on health insurance related to employment | May value health care but often do not see a way to improve situation |
| **Time Orientation** | | |
| Seek prenatal care early | Future oriented and seek early prenatal care<br>Make plans to provide best possible care and education for children | Priority is to meet needs of present<br>Often seek prenatal care late<br>Uncertain future |

able to provide an enriched environment for children, and they can pay for health care either from private means or through insurance.

The attitudes related to health care reflect the ability of affluent families to pay. They know that they deserve the best in health care and believe that they deserve respect from health care providers. They insist on being active participants in their care and they are future-oriented, so that they value preventive care. In general, they seek early, regular antepartum care and comply with recommendations of the health care providers.

### THE MIDDLE CLASS

The middle class makes up the largest group of families in the United States; indeed, most health care workers fit into this class. Although they do not have the reserves of the affluent, the middle class generally has adequate income to rent or own their homes in relatively safe neighborhoods. They have an adequate supply of good food, and they have either education or skills that assist them in getting and in keeping jobs for long periods. They often share child care with family and neighbors and develop a network of people who can rely on each other for support and assistance.

Middle-class families rely on group insurance, obtained as part of their salaries, to shield themselves from exorbitant costs. A major concern is loss of a job that results in loss of health insurance.

Middle-class families are future-oriented; they seek health care early in pregnancy so that the mother and infant have the best chance for a healthy outcome. They prepare for the birth and make plans to provide as much as possible for their children's security and education.

### THE WORKING POOR AND UNEMPLOYED

The working poor and unemployed are a group composed of unemployed workers or unskilled workers who live with a great deal of uncertainty. They work for low wages and are often the last hired and the first fired. They often live below the poverty level and barely have enough to survive. Many have difficulty meeting the basic needs for food and shelter, and some become homeless families. They have few financial resources, and their limited skills give them little bargaining power.

Attitudes related to health care differ from those of the more affluent (Nursing Care Plan 8–2). Because of economic uncertainty, they place more emphasis on meeting the needs of the present rather than on future goals. As a result, they place less value on preventive care, which requires an orientation toward the future. This attitude is particularly obvious during pregnancy, when prenatal care may be postponed until the second or even the third trimester.

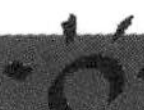

### CRITICAL THINKING EXERCISE

Emma H., a 24-year-old multipara of 32 weeks' gestation, appears apathetic and tired when she arrives at the prenatal clinic. She states that she is concerned about how her 2-year-old son will accept the new baby and sometimes feels guilty that she is having this baby so soon.

**Q:**
1. How does multiparity affect the maternal tasks of pregnancy?
2. How should the nurse respond to her concerns?
3. What measures can the client take to prepare the 2-year-old before the new baby arrives? After the infant is born?

**A:**
1. The tasks of pregnancy are more complex than for a primigravida; there is not enough time; there is more fatigue; there is less excitement; the client must work out a new relationship with the first child, who has had her undivided time.
2. Respond by acknowledging her concerns and reflecting her feelings so that she can fully express how she feels. "You worry that your son will be upset when the new baby is born, and you feel guilty that he will have to share your time and energy with the baby."
3. Suggest that the client make any changes in sleeping arrangements now so that her son will not feel displaced by the infant. Recommend that she plan ways to have time alone with the older child when the baby arrives, and review measures to reduce sibling rivalry. The mother can tell the 2-year-old how much she loves him, hug and cuddle him frequently, and arrange his bedtime to allow time together for favorite activities, such as reading, listening to music, or watching his favorite videos. The mother can remind others to pay attention to him as well as to the baby.

### THE NEW POOR

The new poor comprise an expanding group of individuals and families who were previously self-sufficient but who, because of such circumstances as loss of a job and loss of health care insurance, are now without resources. These people must find their way into a health care system that is unfamiliar and frightening.

The values of the new poor are those of the middle class: self-sufficiency, hard work, and pride in their ability to succeed. It is very difficult for this group to seek public assistance. These families are devastated when they encounter the lack of respect and rudeness that are prevalent among health care workers dealing with families who are unable to pay for health care.

## Barriers to Prenatal Care

The value of prenatal care has been extensively documented. Women who receive inadequate prenatal care are likely to have poor pregnancy outcomes, including higher rates of low-birth-weight babies and increased infant mortality. Women's access to prenatal care, however, is limited by financial, systemic, and attitudinal barriers.

Financial barriers are one of the most important factors that limit prenatal care. Many women either do not have enough insurance or have no insurance to cover maternity care. Although Medicaid finances prenatal care for indigent women, the enrollment process is so burdensome that some women do not register (Maloni et al., 1996).

Systemic barriers include negative institutional practices that interfere with consistent care. For instance, women must often wait 6 to 8 weeks before being seen for their first visit. Prenatal visits are usually scheduled during daytime hours when working women cannot attend. Moreover, child care is rarely available, and women who must find child care are

### *Nursing Care Plan 8–2*
### *Socioeconomic Problems During Pregnancy*

**ASSESSMENT:** Theresa Matheny, a 19-year-old primigravida, is seen for initial prenatal care at 24 weeks of gestation. She took the day off from work in a laundry and rode the bus to the clinic. She is currently living with an unmarried sister who receives Aid to Families with Dependent Children. During the interview, Ms. Matheny states that she will not be able to keep clinic appointments because she cannot afford to take more time off until the baby comes. She is unmarried and states that the father of the baby "Is gone." She says that she is healthy and only needs to find someone to deliver the baby.

**NURSING DIAGNOSIS:** Risk for Altered Health Maintenance related to lack of a plan to obtain regular prenatal care and knowledge deficit of the importance of care

**GOALS/EXPECTED OUTCOMES**

The client will do the following:

1. Verbalize a plan for regular prenatal care at the initial prenatal visit.
2. Describe the benefits of regular prenatal care by the end of the initial prenatal visit.

| INTERVENTION | RATIONALE |
|---|---|
| 1. Emphasize reasons why regular prenatal care is essential to<br>a. Monitor the growth and development of the baby (maternal pattern of weight gain, fundal height, fetal heart tones, fetal activity).<br>b. Evaluate Theresa's health, which directly affects the health of the fetus (blood pressure, urinalysis, weight gain).<br>c. Detect problems, and intervene before they become severe. | 1. Preventive care is often not a priority when the client has conflicting needs for food and shelter. Moreover, many women are unaware that some complications, such as pregnancy-induced hypertension and glucose intolerance (gestational diabetes), which may be detected and treated in early pregnancy, are serious hazards if they remain undetected. |
| 2. Assist Theresa in devising a plan to obtain regular prenatal care.<br>a. Provide her with a list of prenatal clinics near her home or place of work and the hours they are open.<br>b. Provide alternative bus schedules or transportation services.<br>c. Determine whether family members or friends can help her keep prenatal appointments.<br>d. Explore dates, times, and alternatives until she finds a schedule that works for her.<br>e. Obtain a list of phone numbers where she can be reached for follow-up. Include the numbers of friends, family, and the employer. | 2. Some clinics are open weekends and evenings to accommodate working women. Unreliable transportation is a major reason for failure to keep scheduled appointments, and clinic schedules that allow some flexibility are helpful. Moreover, interest in a client's individual situation is highly motivating for her to find a way to continue prenatal care. |

*Nursing Care Plan continued on following page*

## Nursing Care Plan 8–2 *Continued*

## Socioeconomic Problems During Pregnancy

**EVALUATION**

Verbalized knowledge of the benefits of prenatal care, a plan for transportation, and the development of a schedule to attend a prenatal clinic on a regular basis meet the original goals. If a client misses scheduled appointments, follow-up phone calls to arrange alternative appointments may be necessary.

**Critical Thinking**

Although the above diagnosis addresses Theresa's problem with managing prenatal care, what additional assessments should be made to determine how she is managing the psychosocial concerns of pregnancy? What additional nursing diagnosis might be relevant?

**ANSWER**

It is important to determine how she is progressing with the maternal taks of pregnancy. She has made the first step in seeking safe passage, but other tasks need attention, such as securing the acceptance of her family and learning to give of herself. In addition, signs that she is developing attachment for the fetus are particularly important.

An additional nursing diagnosis might be Risk for Altered Parenting related to lack of support from significant others or the presence of financial stress.

**ADDITIONAL NURSING DIAGNOSES TO CONSIDER**

Altered Family Processes
Impaired Home Maintenance Management
Risk for Injury
Altered Role Performance

torn between being a mother and keeping clinic appointments.

An important barrier to health care results from the unsympathetic attitude of some health care workers toward those who are unable to pay for prenatal care. Poor families often experience long delays, hurried examinations, rudeness, and arrogance from members of the health care team who work in public clinics. Many pregnant women report waiting 3 to 4 hours for an examination that lasts only a few minutes. Many never see the same health care provider more than once. Many pregnant women fail to keep clinic appointments because they do not see the importance of the hurried examinations.

In addition to unsympathetic attitudes of health professionals, other attitudinal reasons for not seeking early prenatal include the following:

- Fear of discovering pregnancy
- Advice received from family or friends
- Lack of problems
- Thinking that prenatal care is unimportant
- Consideration of an abortion
- Not wanting anyone to know about the pregnancy (Meikle et al., 1995)

Additional reasons may be that no one is available to watch other children, the woman cannot afford to take time off from work, and no transportation is available. Nurses must understand the importance of treating each family with respect and consideration, and they must insist that poor families who are unable to pay receive the same standard of care as that received by families who can pay.

## Cultural Influences on Childbearing

More different cultural groups live in the United States than anywhere else in the world. Each culture has its own health and healing belief system that offers explanation and provides order during major life events such as pregnancy and childbirth. Belief systems vary from culture to culture, and the success of health care depends on how well it fits in with the beliefs of those being served. Therefore, ignorance of culturally divergent beliefs may lead to failure in health care delivery. Groups with beliefs that differ significantly from those of the dominant culture include Native Americans, Hindus (largely from India), Muslims, and Filipinos.

## Culturally Divergent Groups

The newest large group of immigrants comes from Southeast Asia and includes Cambodians, Vietnamese, Laotians, and Hmong. Latinos—individuals living in the United States and coming directly from or with ancestry from Mexico, Puerto Rico, Cuba, El Salvador, the Dominican Republic, and other Latin American countries—make up another large group. The term *Latino* indicates common background in Spanish language and customs but is not accepted by all groups. Some prefer Hispanic, Mexican-American, Chicano, or La Raza (the race).

The term *African-American* includes those with a common background in African languages and customs. Generalizations about the cultural aspects of pregnancy for African-Americans are particularly difficult. Many have been in the United States for generations, and their health beliefs do not differ significantly from those held by whites. New immigrants from Africa, however, often retain some of the cultural beliefs of their country of origin.

## Differences Within Cultures

Wide variations of beliefs and practices exist within each culture, and nurses must recognize that not everyone who shares a culture has identical beliefs. Those who have lived in Western societies for years or even for generations often do not exhibit behaviors prescribed by their culture. Nurses must be careful not to stereotype families or expect a certain set of behaviors from every family in a particular cultural group. Individual differences are as important as cultural variations.

## Cultural Differences That Can Cause Conflict

Cultural differences that cause conflict between health care workers and families during pregnancy are observed most often in the areas of health care beliefs, communication, and time orientation.

### HEALTH BELIEFS

For many cultures, health is the balance of mind, body, and spirit. Health-promoting behaviors are the actions used in each of these dimensions to maintain health, prevent illness, or restore health (Spector, 1995).

**Health Maintenance.** Practices that maintain health include wearing proper clothing, which is believed by some Latinas to ensure a safe birth. Other examples include eating a specific diet for pregnancy. For instance, women from Southeast Asia may eat rice daily. Many groups also believe that concentration, silence, prayer, and meditation maintain mental and spiritual health.

**Belief in Fate.** Some cultures (Southeast Asian, Middle Eastern) promote a strong belief in fate. Women often believe that the only way in which they can affect the outcome of pregnancy is by eating correctly and observing the taboos of their culture. Because of this belief, it is sometimes difficult to get women to seek early and regular prenatal care.

**Preventing Illness.** Practices that prevent illness include the use of protective religious objects or charms, such as amulets and talismans. Some women also believe that the type of food one eats can prevent illness. For instance, those from many backgrounds eat raw garlic or onion or adhere to numerous food taboos and prescribed combinations of foods. Strict adherence to religious codes, morals, and practices is also believed to prevent illness.

**Modesty.** Fear, modesty, and a desire to avoid examination by men may keep some women from seeking health care during pregnancy. In many cultures (Muslim, Hindu, Latino), exposure of the genitals to men is considered demeaning. Nurses must remember that the reputations of women from these cultures depend on their demonstrated modesty. If necessary, female physicians or female nurse practitioners can perform examinations. If this is not possible, the woman should be carefully draped, with the legs completely covered. A female nurse needs to remain with the woman at all times. It may be necessary to obtain permission from the husband before any examination or treatment can be performed.

**Infibulation.** Female circumcision involves removal of part or all of the clitoris, labia minora, and labia majora and suturing together the lacerations to reduce the size of the introitus. The procedure is widely practiced in parts of northern Africa, Indonesia, Malaysia, and the Mideast (Lightfoot-Klein & Shaw, 1990; Shorten, 1995). The practice has been associated with premarital chastity, and in some African cultures it is a prerequisite for marriage.

Women who have been infibulated and are now living in the United States express hope that physicians and nurses are knowledgeable about the custom and prepared for how the genitals look. Pelvic examination provokes two major concerns: (1) exposure of the genitals and (2) inescapable pain because the introitus is so small and inelastic scar tissue makes the area especially sensitive.

Nurses must make sure that pelvic examinations

## Nursing Care Plan 8–3

# Language Barrier During Pregnancy

**ASSESSMENT:** Ms. Thuy Nguyen, a young Vietnamese primigravida of 26 weeks' gestation, speaks very little English. She listens quietly to the nurse's health care instructions, and although she appears confused, she asks no questions. Her husband has difficulty responding to questions about his wife's health; however, he frequently nods and smiles.

**Critical Thinking**

Why must additional assessments be made before a nursing diagnosis can be formulated?

**ANSWER**

Nodding and smiling do not always mean that persons from Southeast Asia understand health teaching. Instead they may simply indicate the information has been heard or that Mr. Nguyen is polite and does not want the nurse to think she is a poor teacher. Before assuming that Mr. Nguyen can translate health care teaching for his wife, the nurse must validate what he learned by asking him to explain it himself.

**NURSING DIAGNOSIS:** Impaired Verbal Communication related to foreign language barriers

**GOALS/EXPECTED OUTCOMES**

The family will do the following:

1. Keep scheduled appointments, demonstrate ability to follow health care instructions, and verbalize basic needs and concerns.
2. Verbalize feelings of support from the health care team throughout prenatal care and childbirth.

| INTERVENTION | RATIONALE |
|---|---|
| 1. Assess the couple's ability to speak, read, and write in English and determine the languages in which each is fluent. | 1. Although the client may not be fluent in speaking a language, at times she may be more adept at reading. Many Vietnamese also speak Chinese or French; this knowledge is important when you are seeking an interpreter. |
| 2. Obtain the assistance of a fluent interpreter.<br>a. Establish a list of bilingual staff members in all areas of the facility (business office, housekeeping, maintenance) who are willing to interpret and to be educated about the importance of confidentiality and exactness.<br>b. Enlist the aid of family members or friends who can accompany the client and who can interpret for them, if a professional interpreter is not available.<br>c. Engage a translator to develop written material, such as colorful cards that have common questions and answers printed in languages that are most frequently spoken.<br>d. Develop printed instructions in the most commonly spoken languages. | 2. A fluent interpreter is essential because Vietnamese do not always reveal when they do not understand instructions, and it is essential that follow-up questions can be asked. Communication cards convey interest in communicating and provide a means of eliciting basic information. Printed instructions reinforce information that was given verbally and may answer unasked questions. |

are as comfortable as possible, maintaining utmost privacy, draping the woman to provide maximum coverage, and assisting her in locating a health care provider with whom she is comfortable. The infibulated woman may not give any verbal or nonverbal sign of pain, but this lack of response does not indicate an absence of pain.

**Restoring Health.** Traditional ways to restore health include natural folk medicine such as herbs and plants. Charms, holy words, and holy actions as well as traditional healers are often used before other medical advice is sought. Latinas, for instance, often consult with *curanderas* (faith healers), who work with women to keep a balance between hot and cold and to relieve them of their sins, which may be the basis for illness. Some rely on folk medicine that

## Nursing Care Plan 8–3 *Continued*

## Language Barrier During Pregnancy

| | |
|---|---|
| 3. Speak quietly, and use the same interpreter whenever possible. | 3. Soft speech protects the privacy and modesty of the patient. A natural response when people do not understand is to raise the voice; this does not facilitate understanding but may convey impatience or anger. |
| 4. Consider nonverbal factors when communicating.<br>a. Speak slowly and softly; smile.<br>b. Keep an open posture. Avoid crossing the arms over the chest or turning away from the family.<br>c. Determine the client's response to light touch on the arm, and either use or avoid touch, depending on her response.<br>d. Attend carefully to what the family says by nodding, leaning forward, or encouraging continued talk with frequent "uh huhs."<br>e. Avoid foot shuffling or fidgeting.<br>f. Do not expect prolonged eye contact. | 4. Even subtle body language can indicate interest and empathy or impatience, annoyance, or a desire to escape. Touch and eye contact are sensitive cultural variables, and nurses must be aware that they are not always welcomed. |

EVALUATION

Continued regular prenatal care and compliance with recommended health care indicate progress in communication. Continued attempts of the family to share specific concerns indicate a feeling of support from the staff.

ADDITIONAL NURSING DIAGNOSES TO CONSIDER

Knowledge Deficit
Risk for Altered Health Maintenance

includes witchcraft, voodoo, and magic (Africans, Haitians).

**To be certain that all essential information about folk medicine is obtained, nurses should inquire whether the client is taking folk remedies. "What do pregnant women take to protect themselves and the baby?" "How often and how much of this do you take?" "Tell me about special foods and drinks that are important."**

### COMMUNICATION TECHNIQUES

**Language.** Language is a major barrier to health care. Not only are the national languages different, but numerous tribal languages and dialects in most languages can also make it difficult to find competent interpreters. The ideal is to have trained interpreters, preferably a woman. Sometimes others may be used if a well-trained interpreter is not available, but considerations of confidentiality, use of medical jargon, and the possible need to discuss sensitive issues indicate the need for professional interpreters. Adults who came to the United States as children may speak English well and can interpret for their parents and grandparents. Other family members or friends, as well as co-workers in the clinic or hospital, may be helpful, but many are not fluent and can misunderstand instructions, particularly if medical jargon is used (Nursing Care Plan 8–3).

English is spoken by most African-Americans, but variations in pronunciation, grammar, and sentence structure may make communication difficult. The dialect spoken by African-Americans is sometimes labeled "Black English" (Cherry & Giger, 1991). Nurses who work with African-Americans must bear in mind that English as spoken by African-Americans cannot be viewed as an unacceptable form of English, and nurses must avoid labeling and stereotyping those who speak a different dialect. Nurses must also clarify the meaning of slang terms. For example, "tripped out" may be interpreted as related to taking drugs, whereas the term actually means that the woman became excited and energetic.

**Communication Style.** Styles in communication differ among cultures. For example, among Asians, nodding and smiling do not necessarily denote agreement or even understanding but simply, "Yes, I hear you." When presenting information, the nurse should validate how much the person understands by requesting the listener to repeat the information:

"Tell me what you understood, and show me what you learned."

Latinas are traditionally diplomatic and tactful; they frequently engage in "small talk" before bringing up questions they may have about their care. Nurses must remember that small talk is a valuable use of time. It establishes rapport and often helps to accomplish the goals of care.

**Eye Contact.** Southeast Asians believe that eye contact shows disrespect (Mattson & Lew, 1995). Eye avoidance sometimes frustrates health care personnel, who believe that eye contact denotes honesty. Eye behavior is also important when nurses deal with Latino infants and children. *Mal ojo* (evil eye) is a sudden unexplained illness that may occur when an individual with special powers admires a child too openly (Spector, 1991). Eye contact between unmarried men and women is considered taboo by Hindus, who may view prolonged eye contact as seductive.

**Touch.** Touch is also an important component of communication. Some Native Americans avoid shaking hands but lightly touch the hand of the person they are greeting. In some cultures (Hindu and Muslim), touch by a woman other than the wife is offensive. In contrast, women from Haiti find touch supportive and reassuring, and gentle touch is particularly important during labor and birth. Nurses must remain sensitive to the response of the person being touched and should refrain from touching if the person indicates that touch is not welcomed.

#### TIME ORIENTATION

Time orientation can create conflict between health care professionals, who parcel out care in discrete units of time measured in minutes, and groups who keep time by the progress of the sun or even by the seasons. Middle Eastern women, Latinas, and African-American women tend to emphasize the moment rather than the future. This attitude causes conflicts in a health care setting where tests or appointments are scheduled at particular times. If a woman does not place the same importance on keeping appointments, she may encounter anger and frustration in the health care setting that leaves her bewildered and shamed.

**✓ CHECK YOUR READING**

12. Why do many poor women delay seeking health care until the second or third trimester?
13. How do the attitudes of health care workers affect the care of poor families?
14. What are some cultural differences that may cause conflict between health care workers and clients?

## Application of Nursing Process: Psychosocial Concerns

### Assessment

The purpose of a psychosocial assessment is to monitor the adaptation of the family to pregnancy, which has been termed a maturational "crisis" that requires a major transition in role function and relationships. Whether one agrees that pregnancy is a crisis, there is no doubt that it initiates change and stress. How the family copes is a primary concern. For some families, pregnancy offers the potential for growth; for others, an alteration in family processes requires guidance and information. Other women or families have more specific needs that are discovered during a thorough psychosocial assessment.

Some data required for a psychosocial assessment can be obtained from the physical assessment. For example, age, gravida, para, and general health status provide important information in both areas. Table 8–3 identifies areas for assessment, provides sample questions, and indicates nursing implications.

### Analysis

Critical thinking is extremely important when analyzing psychosocial data that may be open to several interpretations. Nurses must be careful to examine their own assumptions and biases about proper responses to pregnancy. They must resist the urge to form an opinion before adequate information is obtained. In addition, they must validate data, particularly when assessing those of different cultural backgrounds.

Nursing diagnoses are based on data obtained during individual assessments and can vary from family to family (see Nursing Care Plans 8–1 through 8–3). Most families strive to maintain the health of the expectant mother and fetus and to complete developmental tasks that allow the couple to become parents of one child or more than one child. The most encompassing nursing diagnosis is probably Family Coping: Potential for Growth related to readiness and desire to meet added family needs and to assume parenting roles.

### Planning

Goals related to family coping as a nursing diagnosis are as follows:

- The family will verbalize emotional responses that are appropriate to each trimester.
- The family will verbalize methods that assist the expectant parents to complete the developmental processes of pregnancy.

**TABLE 8-3 PSYCHOSOCIAL ASSESSMENT**

| Findings (Normal and Unusual)* | Sample Questions | Nursing Implications |
|---|---|---|
| **Psychological Response** | | |
| First trimester: Uncertainty, ambivalence, mood changes, self as primary focus<br>Second trimester: Wonder, joy, focus on fetus<br>Third Trimester: Vulnerability, preparing for birth (fear, anger, apathy, lack of preparation) | "How do you/partner feel about being pregnant?"<br>"How will your lives change as a result of being pregnant?"<br>"How do you feel about the changes in your body?"<br>"What preparations have you made for the baby?" | Use active listening and reflection to establish a sense of trust; re-evaluate negative responses (fear, apathy, anger) in subsequent assessments |
| **Availability of Resources** | | |
| Financial concerns (lack of funds, or insurance) | "What are your plans for prenatal care and birth?" | Determine if there are adequate funds or if family needs help to find a public clinic that will provide care |
| Response and availability of grandparents, friends, family (family geographically or emotionally unavailable) | "How do your parents feel about being grandparents?" "What do they want to be called?" "Who else can you depend on besides the family?" "Who provides strength when there is a conflict?" | It may be necessary to help the couple discover alternative resources if the family is unavailable; early identification of family conflicts allows time for resolution |
| **Changes in Sexual Practices** | | |
| Mutual satisfaction with changes (concern with comfort or safety) | "How have sexual patterns or satisfaction changed?" "How do you cope with the changes?" "What concerns you most?" | Offer reassurance that intercourse is usually safe; suggest alternative positions and open communication |
| **Educational Needs** | | |
| Many questions about pregnancy, childbirth, and infant care (no questions, absence of interest in educational programs) | "How do you feel about caring for an infant?" "What are your major concerns?" "Whom do you count on for information?" "What would be most helpful?" | Respond to priority needs that are expressed; refer couple to appropriate child- and parenting classes |
| **Cultural Influences** | | |
| Either the woman or her family is able to speak English or fluent interpreters are available; cultural influences support a healthy pregnancy and infant (unable to communicate verbally, some cultural beliefs or health practices may prove harmful) | "What foods are recommended during pregnancy?" "What practices are recommended?" "What is forbidden?" "How can we provide the best care?" "What is most important in your care?" "How do your religious beliefs affect pregnancy?" | Locate fluent interpreters if necessary; avoid labeling beliefs as superstitions; reinforce beliefs that promote a good pregnancy outcome; assess accepted source of information; elicit help of this person to overcome practices that may prove harmful |

* Findings that require additional assessment or intervention are shown in parentheses.

- The family will identify cultural factors that may produce conflicts and collaborate to reduce those conflicts.

## Interventions

### PROVIDING INFORMATION

Provide information and anticipatory guidance about the following:

- The emotional changes that occur during pregnancy (ambivalence, introversion, increased feelings of vulnerability)
- The developmental tasks of the mother (seeking safe passage, securing acceptance, forming attachment with the unknown baby)
- Role transition (mimicry, role playing, fantasy, grief work)
- The developmental processes of the prospective

father (grappling with the reality, struggling for recognition as a parent, creating the role of involved father)

Guidance is necessary to prepare prospective parents for the progressive changes that occur during pregnancy and to reassure them that their feelings and behaviors are normal. Guidance also gives them an opportunity to ask questions and explore their feelings.

#### DISCUSSING RESOURCES

Initiate a discussion of the adequacy of the financial situation and support systems. The nurse may have to help couples who have no financial resources or insurance coverage to find the most convenient location to obtain prenatal care and to determine where the client will give birth. This concern is particularly important for the new poor, who have little idea of how to gain access to government-sponsored care. Emotional resources include those that assist the new family to adjust to the demands of pregnancy and parenting.

Discuss the responses and participation of the grandparents. Although emotional responses vary, the family unit is strengthened and the attachment of the grandparents to the child is enhanced when grandparents actively participate in the pregnancy.

If family members who traditionally offer support in times of stress are unavailable, refer the prospective parents to community resources, such as childbirth education classes, support groups, sibling classes, and later to breastfeeding and new parenting classes.

#### HELPING THE FAMILY PREPARE FOR THE BIRTH

During the last trimester, it is helpful to discuss lifestyle changes that will occur when the infant is born. Unanticipated changes that accompany this dramatic life event may add stress and lead to disruption in family processes. Help the prospective parents make practical plans for the infant, such as obtaining clothing, finding a place to sleep, and choosing the method of feeding. Siblings should also be prepared several weeks or even months before the birth. The response of children depends on their ages and developmental levels. Older children (above 3 to 4 years) often benefit from participating in prenatal care and planning for the baby; younger children do not grasp the concept of time and can be prepared for the arrival of a new baby shortly before the birth.

Discuss with expectant parents how they will work out the division of household and parenting tasks. Ask them to consider how they will manage the care of the newborn if the mother must return to work following childbirth. If these issues are not dealt with, the couple can experience frustration and anger as one parent, usually the mother, assumes total care of the infant and attempts to complete all household tasks. Moreover, exhaustion and frustration can overwhelm the joys of parenting when one parent must provide all care.

#### MODELING COMMUNICATION TECHNIQUES

When disagreements are evident, it is often helpful to discuss and model therapeutic communication techniques that include all significant family members as the family prepares for the birth. Techniques that clarify, summarize, and reflect feelings can defuse negative feelings that might result in family disruption (see Chapter 2).

#### IDENTIFYING CULTURAL FACTORS THAT COULD CAUSE CONFLICT

Discuss possible areas of conflict related to cultural beliefs and health practices that affect pregnancy.

**It is reassuring to expectant mothers when nurses support health beliefs that are beneficial before confronting them with health care beliefs that cause concern. For example, "It is so good for you and the baby when you eat so many vegetables, but I am worried because you missed your last appointment."**

If there is conflict as a result of differences in time orientation, acknowledge the problem, convey understanding of the differences, and emphasize the importance of calling when appointments cannot be kept. Many families do not realize that when they miss their appointment, another family misses the opportunity for health care.

### Evaluation

When the family verbalizes concerns and emotions throughout pregnancy, the initial goal is met. Continued interest and involvement of the partner and significant family members are evidence that the family has completed the developmental tasks of pregnancy. Participation of the family with health care workers to find a compromise when differing cultural beliefs cause conflict confirms that the family will identify and initiate measures to reduce conflicts.

## SUMMARY CONCEPTS

- Maternal psychological responses progress during pregnancy from uncertainty and ambivalence to feelings of vulnerability and preparation for the birth of the infant.
- As the fetus becomes real, usually in the second trimester, maternal focus shifts from self to the fetus, and the woman turns inward to concentrate on the processes going on in her body.

- Changes in the maternal body during pregnancy may result in a negative body image that affects sexual responses. This change may be especially troubling if the couple does not discuss emotions and concerns related to the changes in sexuality.
- It takes time for a woman to make the transition to the role of mother, and the process involves mimicking the behavior of other mothers, fantasizing about the baby, grieving for the loss of previous roles, and developing a sense of self as mother.
- To complete the maternal tasks of pregnancy, the woman must take steps to seek safe passage for herself and the infant, gain acceptance of significant persons, and form an interconnection and attachment to the unknown child.
- Paternal responses change throughout pregnancy and depend on the ability to perceive the fetus as real, to gain recognition for the role of parent, and to create a role as involved father.
- The most powerful reality boosters for the expectant father during pregnancy are hearing the fetal heart beat, feeling the fetus move, and viewing the infant on a sonogram.
- In primitive cultures, couvade refers to pregnancy-related rituals performed by the man; in modern society, it often refers to a cluster of pregnancy-related signs and symptoms experienced by the man.
- The response of grandparents to the announcement of pregnancy depends on their age, the number and ages of other grandchildren, and their perception of the role of grandparents.
- The response of siblings to pregnancy depends on their ages and developmental levels. Toddlers may feel displaced in their parents' affection unless measures are taken to reassure them.
- It is more difficult for multiparas to complete the developmental tasks of pregnancy because they have less time, experience more fatigue, and must negotiate a new relationship with the older child or children.
- Socioeconomic status is a major factor in determining health practices during pregnancy. Poor families have competing priorities for food and shelter and seek prenatal care late in pregnancy.
- Cultural differences can create major conflicts between expectant families and health care workers. Language, time orientation, and health beliefs are the areas in which conflicts are most likely to occur.

### References and Readings

Bloom, K.C. (1995). The development of attachment behaviors in pregnant adolescents. *Nursing Research*, 44(5), 284–289.

Bothamley, J. (1990). Are fathers getting a fair deal? *Nursing Times*, 86(36), 68–69.

Broude, G.J. (1988). Rethinking the couvade: Cross-cultural evidence. *American Anthropologist*, 90(6), 902–911.

Callister, L.C. (1995). Cultural meanings of childbirth. *Journal of Obstetric, Gynecologic, and Neonatal Nursing* 24(4), 327–331.

Cherry, B., & Giger, J.N. (1991). Black Americans. In J.N. Giger & R.E. Davidhizar (Eds.), *Transcultural nursing* (pp. 147–182). St. Louis: Mosby–Year Book.

Ferketich, S.L., & Mercer, R.T. (1995). Paternal-infant attachment of experienced and inexperienced fathers during infancy. *Nursing Research*, 44(1), 31–37.

Fortier, J.C., Carson, V.B., Will, S., & Shubkagel, B.L. (1991). Adjustment to a newborn: Sibling preparation makes a difference. *Journal of Obstetric, Gynecologic, and Neonatal Nursing*, 20(1), 73–79.

Fraser, A.M., Brockert, J.E., & Ward, R.H. (1995). Association of young maternal age with adverse reproductive outcomes. *The New England Journal of Medicine*, 332(17), 1113–1117.

Jordan, P.L. (1990). Laboring for relevance: Expectant and new fatherhood. *Nursing Research*, 39(1), 11–16.

Lalonde, A. (1995). Clinical management of female genital mutilation must be handled with understanding, compassion. *Canadian Medical Association Journal*, 152(6), 949–946.

Lightfoot-Klein, H., & Shaw, E. (1990). Special needs of ritually circumcised women patients. *Journal of Obstetric, Gynecologic, and Neonatal Nursing*, 20(2), 102–106.

Maloni, J.A., Cheng, C.Y., Liebl, C.P., & Maier, J.S. (1996). Transforming prenatal care: Reflections on the past and present with implications for the future. *Journal of Obstetric, Gynecologic, and Neonatal Nursing*, 25(1), 17–23.

Mattson, S., & Lew, L. (1995). Culturally sensitive perinatal care for Southeast Asians. *Journal of Obstetric, Gynecologic, and Neonatal Nursing*, 24(4), 335–341.

McClanahan, P. (1992). Improving access to and use of prenatal care. *Journal of Obstetric, Gynecologic, and Neonatal Nursing*, 21(4), 280–284.

Meikle, S.F., Orleans, M., Leff, M., Shain, R., & Gibbs, R.S. (1995). Women's reasons for not seeking prenatal care: Racial and ethnic factors. *Birth*, 22(2), 81–86.

Mercer, R.T. (1990). *Parents at risk*. New York: Springer.

Mercer, R.T., & Ferketich, S.L. (1994a). Maternal-infant attachment of experienced and inexperienced mothers during infancy. *Nursing Research*, 43(6) 344–351.

Mercer, R.T., & Ferketich, S.L. (1994b). Predictors of maternal role competence by risk status. *Nursing Research*, 43(1), 38–43.

Muller, M.E., & Ferketich, S. (1993). Factor analysis of the maternal fetal attachment scale. *Nursing Research*, 42(3), 144–147.

Nance, T.A. (1995). Intercultural communication: Finding common ground. *Journal of Obstetric, Gynecologic, and Neonatal Nursing*, 24(3), 249–255.

Rubin, R. (1975). Maternal tasks in pregnancy. *Maternal Child Nursing Journal*, 4(3), 143–153.

Rubin, R. (1984). *Maternal identity and the maternal experience*. New York: Springer.

Shorten, A. (1995). Female circumcision: Understanding special needs. *Holistic Nurse Practitioner*, 9(2), 66–73.

Spector, R.E. (1991). *Cultural diversity in health and illness* (3rd ed.). Norwalk, Conn.: Appleton & Lange.

Spector, R.E. (1995). Cultural concepts of women's health and health-promoting behaviors. *Journal of Obstetric, Gynecologic, and Neonatal Nursing* 24(3), 241–245.

Thorpe, K., Greenwood, R., & Goodenough, T. (1995). Does a twin pregnancy have a greater impact on physical and emotional well-being than a singleton pregnancy? *Birth*, 22(3), 148–152.

Tiller, C.M. (1995). Father's parenting attitudes during a child's first year. *Journal of Obstetric, Gynecologic, and Neonatal Nursing*, 24(6), 508–514.

Walker, L.O., & Montgomery, E. (1994). Maternal identity and role attainment: Long-term relations to children's development. *Nursing Research*, 43(2), 105–110.

# 9

# Nutrition for Childbearing

## OBJECTIVES

1. Explain the importance of adequate nutrition and weight gain during pregnancy.
2. Compare the nutrient needs of pregnant and non-pregnant women.
3. Describe common factors that influence a woman's nutritional status and choices.
4. Describe how common nutritional risk factors affect nutritional requirements during pregnancy.
5. Compare the nutritional needs of the postpartum woman who is breastfeeding with those of one who is not breastfeeding.
6. Apply the nursing process to nutrition during pregnancy, the postpartum period, and lactation.

## DEFINITIONS

**anorexia nervosa** *Refusal to eat because of a distorted body image and a feeling of obesity.*

**bulimia** *Eating disorder characterized by ingestion of large amounts of food, followed by purging behavior such as induced vomiting or laxative abuse.*

**complete protein food** *Food containing all the essential amino acids.*

**essential amino acids** *Amino acids that cannot be synthesized by the body and must be obtained from foods.*

**gynecologic age** *The number of years since menarche (first menstrual period).*

**heme iron** *Iron obtained from meat, poultry, or fish sources; the form most usable by the body.*

**incomplete protein food** *Food that does not contain all the essential amino acids.*

**kilocalorie** *A unit of heat; used to show the energy value in foods; commonly called calorie.*

**lacto-ovovegetarian** *A vegetarian whose diet includes milk products and eggs.*

**lactose intolerance** *Inability to digest most dairy products because of a lack of the enzyme lactase.*

**lactovegetarian** *A vegetarian whose diet includes milk products.*

**non-heme iron** *Iron obtained from plant sources.*

**nutrient density** *The quality of protein, vitamins, and minerals per 100 calories in foods.*

**ovovegetarian** *A vegetarian whose diet includes eggs.*

**pica** *Ingestion of a nonfood substance, such as laundry starch, dirt, or ice.*

**recommended dietary allowances (RDA)** *Levels of nutrient intake considered to meet the needs of healthy individuals.*

**vegan** *A complete vegetarian who does not eat any animal products.*

**vegetarian** *An individual whose diet consists wholly or mostly of plant foods and who avoids animal food sources.*

At no other point in a woman's life is nutrition as important as it is during pregnancy and lactation. At this time, her food intake must nourish not only her own body but also that of her baby. Nutrition may affect the size of the fetus and whether it has adequate stores of some nutrients after birth. If the woman fails to consume sufficient nutrients, her own stores of some nutrients may be depleted to meet the needs of the fetus, who may be deprived of essential nutrients as well.

The nurse has ongoing contact with women during office or clinic visits throughout the childbearing period and can provide education about nutritional needs on a continuing basis. Nurses are often in a position to offer nutrition counseling even before conception for women who are considering becoming pregnant. This counseling increases the chances that they are nutritionally healthy at the time of conception and continue to practice good nutrition throughout pregnancy. It may also increase the level of nutrition a woman provides her entire family. Therefore, nutritional education is an essential part of nursing care.

Nutritional care is accomplished by a team of health professionals. Although the nurse can do much of the counseling necessary for normal pregnancy, the registered dietitian counsels women who have complex nutritional needs.

## Weight Gain During Pregnancy

Weight gain during pregnancy, especially after the first trimester, is an important determinant of fetal growth. Low birth weight (less than 2500 g), preterm labor, and increased risk of fetal and newborn mortality and morbidity have been associated with insufficient weight gain during pregnancy. Poor maternal weight gain indicates not only lower caloric intake, but low intake of other important nutrients as well.

Excessive weight gain is also a problem. It is associated with higher risk for macrosomia (large babies), labor abnormalities, meconium staining, and cesarean birth (Johnson et al., 1992). The amount of weight gained is important, but the nutrient intake that makes up the gain is even more important. Weight gain from a diet lacking in essential nutrients is not as beneficial as weight gain from a balanced diet.

### Recommendations for Total Weight Gain

Recommendations for weight gain during pregnancy have changed considerably over the years. In the late 19th century, rickets, a disease of the bones from calcium and vitamin D deficiency, caused some women to have small, distorted pelves. Restricted weight gain kept the fetus small so that delivery was easier. Beginning in the 1920s, weight gain was limited because of the belief that large gains caused pregnancy-induced hypertension, a view now known to be inaccurate. Recommendations for weight gain gradually increased from approximately 15 pounds to 20 to 25 pounds during the 1970s.

The recommended weight gain during pregnancy is now 25 to 35 pounds (11.5 to 16 kg) for women who begin pregnancy at normal weight for height. This amount is believed to reduce intrauterine growth restriction caused by inadequate maternal intake. The range allows for individual differences because no precise weight gain is appropriate for every woman. The range provides a target while allowing for variations in individual needs.

Suggested gains vary according to the woman's weight before pregnancy, as shown in Table 9–1. Women who are 10 percent below normal weight for their height should gain more during pregnancy to meet the needs of pregnancy and bring their weight up to normal. Overweight women (20 percent above normal weight for height) can gain somewhat less. In the past, obese women, more than 35 percent over their normal weight, were told to gain little or even to lose weight during pregnancy. The current recommended gain is at least 15 pounds, which is equivalent to the weight of the products of conception

**TABLE 9–1 RECOMMENDED WEIGHT GAIN DURING PREGNANCY**

| Weight Before Pregnancy | Total Gain | Total Gain (First Trimester) | Weekly Gain (Second and Third Trimesters) |
|---|---|---|---|
| Normal weight | 25–35 lb (11.5–16 kg) | 3.5 lb (1.6 kg) | 0.97 lb (0.44 kg) |
| Underweight (10% below normal for height) | 28–40 lb (12.5–18 kg) | 5 lb (2.3 kg) | 1.07 lb (0.49 kg) |
| Overweight (20% over normal for height) | 15–25 lb (7–11.5 kg) | 2 lb (0.9 kg) | 0.67 lb (0.3 kg) |
| Twin pregnancies | 35–45 lb (16–20.5 kg) | 3.5 lb (1.6 kg) | 1.5 lb (0.75 kg) |

Based on data from *Nutrition during pregnancy, Part I: Weight gain.* © 1990 by the National Academy of Sciences. Published by National Academy Press, Washington, D.C.

(e.g., fetus, placenta). This provides sufficient nutrients for the fetus.

Other variations include the woman who is pregnant with more than one fetus. Infants of a multifetal pregnancy are often born before term and tend to weigh less than infants born of single pregnancies. A greater weight gain in the mother may help prevent low birth weight. Women who are shorter than 62 inches (157 cm) may not need to gain as much as taller women and should gain only to the lower limits of the recommended range. Young adolescents need to gain to the upper end of the range to provide for their own growth during pregnancy as well as that of the fetus.

## Pattern of Weight Gain

The pattern of weight gain is as important as the total increase. Inadequate early weight gain may be associated with small-for-gestational age infants, whereas poor gain late in pregnancy is associated with preterm labor. This is true even when total weight gain is within normal range (Scholl & Hediger, 1995). Early and adequate prenatal care allows assessment of weight gain on a week-to-week basis throughout pregnancy. The general recommendation is for an increment of about 3.5 pounds (1.6 kg) during the first trimester, when the mother may be nauseated and the fetus needs fewer nutrients for growth. During the rest of the pregnancy, the expected weight gain is just under 1 pound (0.44 kg) a week.

### CHECK YOUR READING

1. How does weight gain in the mother relate to the birth weight of the infant?
2. How much weight should the average woman gain during pregnancy? What factors might change this?
3. What pattern of weight gain is recommended for the average woman?

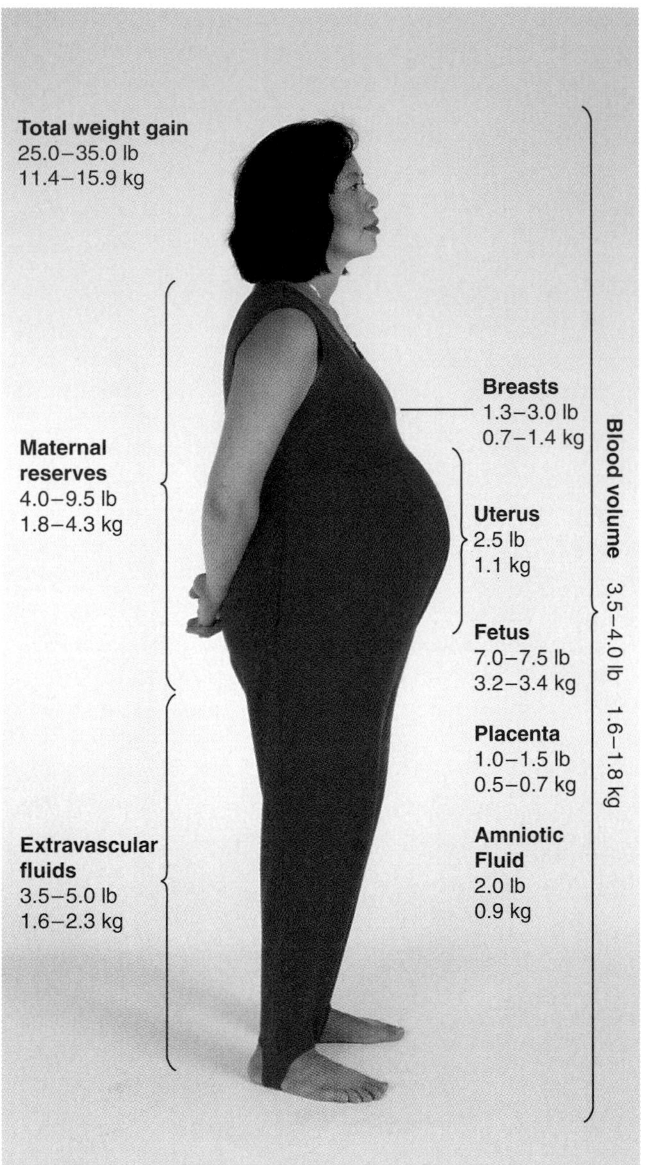


**FIGURE 9–1**

Distribution of weight gain in pregnancy. The numbers represent a general distribution, because there is a great deal of variation among women. The component with the greatest fluctuation is the amount of weight increase attributed to extravascular fluids (edema) and maternal reserves of fat.

## Maternal and Fetal Distribution

Women often wonder why they should gain so much weight when the fetus weighs only 7 to 8 pounds (3 to 3.6 kg). Explaining the distribution of weight helps them understand this (Fig. 9–1). The nurse should also explain the dangers of poor weight gain by the mother.

## Factors That Influence Weight Gain

Factors that may have a positive influence on weight gain include the expectant mother's understanding of the importance of her diet for fetal growth. This is an area in which the nurse may have great influence. Discussing the reasons why maternal intake is important for fetal growth and storage of nutrients often motivates women to improve their nutrition. Knowledge of factors that may have a negative influence on nutrient intake and weight gain helps the nurse devise plans for improving nutrition.

Women at risk for inadequate weight gain include those who are young, unmarried, in a low-income group, poorly educated, of short stature, or in poor general health or who receive insufficient prenatal care. African-American, Southeast Asian, and Latino women are more at risk for low weight gains during pregnancy than are white women. Adequate weight gain is especially important for African-Americans and teenagers, who tend to have smaller infants even when they gain weight in the same amount as whites or older mothers. The reasons for this difference are not fully understood (Institute of Medicine, 1990). Multiparas are at higher risk for low weight gain than women in their first pregnancy. Smoking or substance abuse may interfere with food intake and weight gain.

# Nutritional Requirements During Pregnancy

Nutrient needs during pregnancy increase to meet the demands of the mother and fetus. The amount of increase for each nutrient varies. In most cases, the increases are not large and are relatively easy to obtain through the diet. Table 9–2 gives examples of foods that meet the increases recommended for some of the major nutrients.

## Recommended Dietary Allowances

Studies have determined the amounts of specific nutrients necessary in the diet to meet the needs of people at different ages and during pregnancy and lactation. In the United States, the Food and Nutrition Board of the National Research Council sets these recommended dietary allowances (RDAs). The RDA refers to the intake of major nutrients necessary for healthy individuals to meet daily nutrient needs. Except for calories, the recommendations are about 30 percent higher than amounts essential to maintain health. This provides a safety margin to allow for individual differences and the fact that most people do not meet the need for every nutrient every day.

Tables of recommendations are based on a "reference individual," a hypothetical person of medium size. These tables are used to calculate nutrient needs based on age and size. For example, the reference woman from age 19 to 24 years is 65 inches (164 cm) tall and weighs 128 pounds (58 kg). The reference woman between the ages of 25 and 50 years is slightly shorter at 64 inches (163 cm) and heavier at 138 pounds (63 kg). Actual needs of individuals (particularly for calories and protein) may vary according to body size, previous nutritional status, and usual activity level. Table 9–3 shows the current RDAs.

## Energy

The energy provided by foods for body processes is calculated in kilocalories. Kilocalories (often used interchangeably with the term *calories*) are obtained from carbohydrates and proteins, which provide 4 calories in each gram, and fats, which provide 9 calories in each gram.

### CARBOHYDRATES

Carbohydrates may be simple or complex. The most common simple carbohydrate is sucrose, or table sugar, which is a source of energy but does not provide other nutrients. Fruits and vegetables also contain simple sugars. Complex carbohydrates are present in starches, such as cereals. They supply vitamins, minerals, and fiber. They should be the major source of carbohydrates in the diet because of their value in providing other nutrients.

Another type of carbohydrate is fiber, the nondigestible product of plant foods. It is an important source of bulk in the diet. Fiber absorbs water and stimulates peristalsis, causing food to pass more quickly through the intestines. Fiber helps prevent constipation. It also slows gastric emptying, causing a sensation of fullness.

### FATS

Fats provide energy as well as fat-soluble vitamins. When reduction of calories is necessary, it is important to reduce but not eliminate carbohydrates and fats. If carbohydrate and fat intake provides insufficient calories, the body uses protein to meet energy needs. This use decreases protein available for building and repairing tissue.

### CALORIES

Approximately 85,000 additional calories are needed during pregnancy (Worthington-Roberts, 1997a). These extra calories furnish energy for production and maintenance of the fetus, placenta, added maternal tissues, and increased basal metabolic rate. The RDA for women of childbearing age is approximately 2200 calories per day. Although there is little need for additional calories during the early weeks of pregnancy, another 300 calories are necessary each day after that time. A 300-calorie increase can be achieved relatively easily with a variety of foods. For example, a banana, a carrot, a piece of whole wheat toast, and a glass of low fat milk consumed over one day would provide the extra calories along with other important nutrients.

Nutrient density, the quality of the various nutrients in each 100 calories of food, must be considered when adding calories. Foods of high nutrient density have large amounts of good-quality nutrients per serving. During pregnancy, the increased need for most nutrients may not be met unless calories

**TABLE 9–2 EXAMPLES OF FOOD AMOUNTS NEEDED DAILY TO MEET NUTRIENT NEEDS OF PREGNANCY**

| Adult Female RDA* | Pregnancy RDA | Extra Foods Needed to Meet Pregnancy Needs | Total Food Amounts Needed |
|---|---|---|---|
| **Protein** | | | |
| Age 11–14: 46 g<br>Age 15–18: 44 g<br>Age 19–24: 46 g<br>Age 25–50: 50 g | 60 g | 2 oz meat, fish, poultry or 2 c milk or 2 oz cheddar cheese or ½ c cottage cheese or 1 c rice and 1 c beans or 1 block (4 oz) tofu | 6 oz meat, fish, poultry and 1 oz hard cheese and 1 c noodles and ½ c peas and 1 slice bread |
| **Calcium** | | | |
| Age <25: 1200 mg<br>Age >25: 800 mg | 1200 mg | 1⅓ c milk or 1 c yogurt, or 2 oz hard cheese or 3 oz salmon with bones and 1 c peanuts and 1 c broccoli or 1 oz cheese and 5 corn tortillas | 4 c milk or 1 block tofu (2.5 × 2.75 × 1 inch) and 1 c almonds and 2 T molasses and 1½ c kale and 1½ c broccoli |
| **Iron** | | | |
| 15 mg | 30 mg | 3 oz red meat and 2 eggs and 1 c lima beans and ½ c bran flakes with raisins and ½ c cooked spinach and 2 slices bread | Iron supplements usually needed to meet recommended amounts |
| **Vitamin A** | | | |
| 800 RE (retinol equivalents)<br>1 RE = 3.33 IU | 800 RE | No increase | ⅔ c broccoli or ⅓ raw carrot or ½ c raw spinach or ¼ baked sweet potato or 1⅓ c tomato juice |
| **Thiamine** | | | |
| 1.1 mg | 1.5 mg | 1 c bran flakes or 1 c peanuts or 2 T sunflower seeds or 3 oz pork or 1 c kidney beans and 1 c rice or barley or macaroni | 1 c wheat flakes and 3 oz pork and ¼ c sunflower seeds or 1 c bran flakes and 1 c rice and 1 c blackeye peas and 1 c peanuts |
| **Riboflavin** | | | |
| 1.3 mg | 1.6 mg | ¾ c milk or yogurt or cottage cheese or enriched cereal or 2 eggs or 5 oz poultry or meat or 1 c broccoli or 1 c spinach and ½ c macaroni | 4 c milk and 1 oz cheese or 1 c macaroni and 1 c sunflower seeds and 1 c broccoli and 1 c enriched cereal and 1 c peanuts |
| **Niacin** | | | |
| 15 mg | 17 mg | 1 T peanut butter or 3 slices bread or 1½ oz meat<br>Also made by body from tryptophan | 3 oz meat and 3 oz white poultry or ⅔ c peanuts or 1 c enriched cereal and 1 c noodles and 1 c navy beans and 1 c sunflower seeds. |
| **Vitamin C** | | | |
| 60 mg | 70 mg | ⅓ c cabbage or ⅓ c lima beans or 1 c looseleaf lettuce | ⅔ c orange juice or 1¾ c tomato juice or 1 orange or 1 c strawberries |

* Unless otherwise specified, values are for adult females aged 19–24 years.
Data from Mahan, L.K., & Escott-Stump, S. (1996). *Krause's food, nutrition, and diet therapy* (9th ed.). Philadelphia: W.B. Saunders Co.

are selected carefully. The term *empty calories* refers to foods that are high in calories but low in other nutrients. Many snack foods not only contain excessive calories and low nutrient density but are high in fat and sodium (Table 9–4). Increased calories should be "spent" on foods that provide the nutrients needed in increased amounts during pregnancy.

**TABLE 9–3 RECOMMENDED DIETARY ALLOWANCES**

| | Non-pregnant (15–23 Years) | Non-pregnant (19–24 Years) | Non-pregnant (25–50 Years) | Pregnant | Lactating (1st 6 Months) | Lactating (2nd 6 Months) |
|---|---|---|---|---|---|---|
| Protein (g) | 44 | 46 | 50 | 60 | 65 | 62 |
| Vitamin A (μg RE)* | 800 | 800 | 800 | 800 | 1300 | 1200 |
| Vitamin D (μg)† | 10 | 10 | 5 | 10 | 10 | 10 |
| Vitamin E (mg)‡ | 8 | 8 | 8 | 10 | 12 | 11 |
| Vitamin K (μg) | 55 | 60 | 65 | 65 | 65 | 65 |
| Vitamin $B_6$ (mg) | 1.5 | 1.6 | 1.6 | 2.2 | 2.1 | 2.1 |
| Vitamin $B_{12}$ (μg) | 2.0 | 2.0 | 2.0 | 2.2 | 2.6 | 2.6 |
| Folate (μg) | 180 | 180 | 180 | 400 | 280 | 260 |
| Thiamine (mg) | 1.1 | 1.1 | 1.1 | 1.5 | 1.6 | 1.6 |
| Riboflavin (mg) | 1.3 | 1.3 | 1.3 | 1.6 | 1.8 | 1.7 |
| Niacin (mg NE)§ | 15 | 15 | 15 | 17 | 20 | 20 |
| Vitamin C (mg) | 60 | 60 | 60 | 70 | 95 | 90 |
| Iron (mg) | 15 | 15 | 15 | 30 | 15 | 15 |
| Calcium (mg) | 1200 | 1200 | 800 | 1200 | 1200 | 1200 |
| Phosphorus (mg) | 1200 | 1200 | 800 | 1200 | 1200 | 1200 |
| Zinc (mg) | 12 | 12 | 12 | 15 | 19 | 16 |
| Magnesium (mg) | 300 | 280 | 280 | 300 | 355 | 340 |
| Iodine (μg) | 150 | 150 | 150 | 175 | 200 | 200 |

* Retinol equivalents. 1 retinol equivalent = 1 μg retinol or 6 μg beta-carotene.
† As cholecalciferol. 10 μg cholecalciferol = 400 IU of vitamin D.
‡ Alpha-tocopherol equivalents. 1 mg, *d*-alpha-tocopherol = 1 alpha-TE
§ 1 NE (niacin equivalent) = 1 mg of niacin or 60 mg of dietary tryptophan.
Reprinted with permission from *Recommended Dietary Allowances* (10th ed.). © 1989 by the National Academy of Sciences. Courtesy of the National Academy Press, Washington, D.C.

## Protein

Protein is necessary for metabolism, tissue synthesis, and tissue repair. The RDA for adults is 0.75 g of protein per kg of body weight daily. This requirement averages to a daily need of 44 to 50 g for females, depending on their age and size. During pregnancy, a protein intake of 60 g is recommended each day for expansion of blood volume and growth of maternal and fetal tissues. This increase is 10 to 16 g over non-pregnancy needs.

**TABLE 9–4 HIGH-SODIUM FOODS***

Products that contain the word salt or sodium, such as table salt, onion salt, monosodium glutamate, bicarbonate of soda (baking soda)
Foods that taste salty, including snack foods like popcorn, potato chips, pretzels, crackers
Condiments and relishes, like catsup, horseradish, mustard, soy sauce, bouillon cubes, pickles, green and black olives
Smoked, dried, or processed foods, such as ham, bacon, lunch meats, corned beef
Canned soups, meats, and vegetables unless label states low in sodium
Packaged mixes for sauces, gravies, cakes, and other baked foods

* During pregnancy, foods high in sodium should be consumed in moderation. Expectant mothers should be taught to read labels and to avoid products in which sodium is listed among the first ingredients.

Protein is generally abundant in diets in most industrialized nations, and many women obtain more than the required amount of this nutrient. However, diets low in caloric intake may also be low in protein. If calories are low and protein is used to provide energy, fetal growth may be impaired.

The nurse should counsel women at risk for poor protein diets about how to determine protein intake and ways to increase food sources of protein. When a woman needs to increase her protein intake, she should eat more high-protein foods rather than use high-protein powders or drinks. Protein substitutes increase protein but do not have the other nutrients provided by foods. (See Table 9–2 for examples of protein foods.)

## Vitamins

Although most people do not eat as much of every vitamin each day as they should, true deficiency states are uncommon in North America. During pregnancy, women usually get enough of most vitamins in their diets. However, they may not eat enough foods high in vitamins $B_6$, D, or E and folic acid to obtain the recommended levels.

The fat-soluble vitamins include A, D, E, and K. These vitamins can be stored in the liver, so defi-

**TABLE 9-5 VITAMINS AND MINERALS**

### Fat-Soluble Vitamins

| Sources | Purpose | Importance in Pregnancy |
|---|---|---|
| ***Vitamin A*** | | |
| Green leafy vegetables, dark yellow vegetables, liver, whole or fortified low-fat or skim milk, egg yolk, butter and fortified margarine. | Important for vision and cell reproduction, growth, and functioning in skin and mucous membranes. | Fetal growth and cell differentiation. Stored in liver, so no increase in RDA in pregnancy. Excessive intake causes spontaneous abortions or serious fetal defects. Women taking isotretinoin (Accutane), a vitamin A derivative, for acne should not take it during pregnancy because it causes fetal defects. |
| ***Vitamin D*** | | |
| Fortified milk, margarine, and soy products, butter, egg yolks. Synthesized in skin when exposed to sunlight. Vegans who are not exposed to sun and who do not eat fortified foods need supplements. | Necessary for metabolism of calcium and prevention of rickets. | Inadequate amounts may result in neonatal hypocalcemia, hypoplasia of tooth enamel, and maternal osteomalacia (softening of the bones). Excessive amounts can cause hypercalcemia and possible fetal deformities. Therefore, supplementary vitamin D should be taken cautiously. |
| ***Vitamin E*** | | |
| Vegetable oils, whole grains, nuts, and green leafy vegetables. | Antioxidant, important for tissue growth and integrity of cells, particularly red blood cell membranes. | Deficiency is rare in pregnant women but can cause anemia in mother and fetus. |
| ***Vitamin K*** | | |
| Green leafy vegetables. Also produced by normal bacterial flora in small intestine. | Necessary for clotting. | No increased RDA in pregnancy. Newborns are temporarily deficient in vitamin K and receive one dose by injection at birth to prevent hemorrhage. |

### Water-Soluble Vitamins

| Sources | Purpose | Importance in Pregnancy |
|---|---|---|
| ***Vitamin $B_6$(Pyridoxine)*** | | |
| Chicken, fish, liver, pork, eggs, peanuts, whole grains. Vegans at risk for low intake should take supplements. | Important in amino acid metabolism. Also in blood, hormone, and immune function. | Increased metabolism of amino acids during pregnancy. |
| ***Vitamin $B_{12}$*** | | |
| Meat, fish, eggs, milk, fortified soy and cereal products. | Cell division and protein synthesis. Prevents megaloblastic anemia. | Increased formation of red blood cells and protein synthesis. |
| ***Folic Acid*** | | |
| Raw green leafy vegetables, oranges, whole grains and fortified cereals, liver, dried peas and beans, yeast. May be lost in cooking. | Important for cell replication and metabolism and for prevention of megaloblastic anemia. | Expanded blood volume and tissue growth. Deficiency in first 6 weeks of pregnancy may cause spontaneous abortion and neural tube defects. |
| ***Thiamine*** | | |
| Pork, whole or enriched grain products, milk, legumes, organ meats, corn, seeds, nuts. | Forms coenzymes necessary to release energy. | Increased due to intake of calories. |
| ***Riboflavin*** | | |
| Milk, pork, beef, enriched grain products, and deep green vegetables. | Forms coenzymes necessary to release energy. | Increased due to intake of calories. |

**TABLE 9–5 VITAMINS AND MINERALS** *Continued*

**Water-Soluble Vitamins (continued)**

| Sources | Purpose | Importance in Pregnancy |
|---|---|---|
| *Niacin* | | |
| Meats, legumes, fish, poultry, enriched grains. | Forms coenzymes necessary to release energy. | Increased due to intake of calories. |
| *Vitamin C* | | |
| Citrus fruit, peppers, strawberries, cantaloupe, green leafy vegetables, tomatoes, potatoes. Destroyed by heat and oxidation. | Important in collagen formation, tissue integrity, healing, immune response, and metabolism. Severe deficiency causes scurvy. | Necessary for formation of fetal tissue. Need increased with smoking, drug or alcohol abuse, or aspirin use. |

**Minerals**

| Sources | Purpose | Importance in Pregnancy |
|---|---|---|
| *Iron* | | |
| Meats, green leafy vegetables, eggs, grain products, tofu, legumes, nuts. | Formation of hemoglobin, enzymes for metabolism. | Expanded maternal blood volume, formation of fetal red blood cells, and storage in the fetal liver for use after birth. |
| *Calcium* | | |
| Dairy products, salmon or sardines with bones, legumes, nuts, dried fruits, dark green leafy vegetables, tofu, broccoli. | Needed in bone formation, cell membrane permeability, coagulation, and neuromuscular function. | Mineralization of fetal bones and teeth. |
| *Phosphorus* | | |
| Dairy products, lean meat. High in processed foods, snacks, carbonated drinks. | Needed in 1:1 ratio with calcium for bone formation and cell metabolism. | Mineralization of fetal bones and teeth. Excessive intake causes binding of calcium in intestines and prevents calcium absorption. |
| *Zinc* | | |
| Meat, poultry, seafood, eggs, nuts, seeds, legumes, wheat germ, whole grains, yogurt. | Used in cell differentiation and reproduction, DNA and RNA synthesis, metabolism, acid-base balance. | Fetal and maternal tissue growth. |
| *Magnesium* | | |
| Whole grains, nuts, legumes, dark green vegetables, scallops, oysters, small amounts in many foods. | Important in cell growth and neuromuscular function; activates enzymes for metabolism of protein and energy. | Same as for non-pregnancy state. Excessive intake may interfere with absorption of iron. |
| *Iodine* | | |
| Seafood, iodized salt. | Important in thyroid function. | Deficiency may cause abortion, stillbirth, fetal congenital hypothyroidism, neurologic conditions. |
| *Sodium* | | |
| See Table 9–4. | Important for fluid and electrolyte balance. | Needed for expanded fluid volume of pregnancy. |

ciency states are not as likely to occur as with the water-soluble vitamins ($B_6$, $B_{12}$, and C and folic acid, thiamine, riboflavin, and niacin). However, excessive intakes of fat-soluble vitamins can be toxic. For example, excess vitamin A can cause fetal defects. The nurse should include vitamins when inquiring about medications taken by pregnant women and counsel them about the dangers of taking too much. Further information about the major vitamins is summarized in Table 9–5.

Water-soluble vitamins are easily transferred from food to water in cooking, so foods should be steamed, microwaved, or prepared in only small amounts of water. The remaining water can be used in other dishes, such as soups. Water-soluble vitamins are not stored in the body as well as fat-soluble vitamins. Therefore, they should be included in the daily diet. Excess amounts are excreted in the urine, so there is less chance of toxicity from ingestion of excessive amounts.

Folic acid (also called folate) can decrease the occurrence of neural tube defects in newborns. Adequate intake of folic acid is especially important just before conception and during the first 6 weeks after conception, when the neural tube is closing. Many pregnancies are unplanned, so all women of childbearing age should consume at least 0.4 mg of folic acid each day; this can decrease the incidence of neural tube defects by 50 percent (Rose & Mennuti, 1995). Women who have given birth to an infant with a neural tube defect should take higher doses of folic acid. A national goal is to reduce the incidence of neural tube defects to 3 per 10,000 live births from 6 per 10,000 in 1990 (U.S. Department of Health and Human Services, 1995).

**CHECK YOUR READING**

4. How many more calories should a woman eat each day during pregnancy?
5. How much protein is recommended during pregnancy?
6. Which vitamins are most likely to be low in the diets of pregnant women?
7. Which vitamins are in the fat-soluble and water-soluble groups? What is the difference in the way the body stores them?

## Minerals

Although most minerals (see Table 9–5) are supplied in adequate amounts in normal diets, the intake of iron, calcium, zinc, and magnesium may drop below recommended levels for pregnancy (Institute of Medicine, 1990).

### IRON

Iron is important in the formation of hemoglobin to carry oxygen throughout the body, and it helps form some enzymes necessary for metabolism. During pregnancy, added iron is needed for the 20 to 30 percent increase in maternal red blood cells and for transfer to the fetus for storage and production of red blood cells. Full-term infants are seldom anemic at birth. However, if storage of iron during fetal life is not enough to last 4 to 6 months after birth, the infant may develop anemia later.

Iron is probably the only nutrient that cannot be supplied completely and easily from the diet during pregnancy. Food sources include meats, green leafy vegetables, eggs, whole or enriched grain products, legumes, nuts, blackstrap molasses, tofu (soybean curd), and foods cooked in cast iron pans. Table 9–6 lists the amount of iron that common foods contain.

**TABLE 9–6 FOODS HIGH IN IRON CONTENT**

| Food and Amount | Average Amounts Supplied Iron (mg) |
|---|---|
| **Meats (3 oz)** | |
| Liver | 5.3 |
| Red meats (avg) | 2.5 |
| Poultry | |
| Chicken | 0.9 |
| Turkey | 1.4 |
| **Legumes (1 c)** | |
| Kidney beans | 4.6 |
| Lentils | 4.2 |
| Peanuts | 2.8 |
| Sunflower seeds | 15.2 |
| Chickpeas (garbanzo beans) | 4.9 |
| Blackeyed peas | 3.6 |
| Lima beans, baby | 3.5 |
| Peas | 2.5 |
| **Eggs** | |
| Eggs (each) | 1.0 |
| **Grains (1 c)** | |
| Rice | 1.8 |
| Bran flakes | 6.8 |
| with raisins | 9.0 |
| Oatmeal | 1.6 |
| Bread (slice) | 0.9 |
| **Fruits** | |
| ⅓ c raisins | 1.0 |
| 4 prunes | 1.2 |
| ½ c dried apricots | 3.0 |
| **Vegetables (1 cup)** | |
| Asparagus (frozen) | 1.2 |
| Broccoli | 1.8 |
| Collards | 1.9 |
| Spinach | |
| Raw | 1.5 |
| Cooked (frozen) | 2.9 |
| **Other** | |
| Tofu (2.5 × 2.75 × 1 inch) | 2.3 |

The Recommended Daily Allowance for iron during pregnancy is 30 mg. Although many women do not eat enough iron-containing foods in their daily diet to meet this need and take supplements, iron in foods is often better absorbed. Therefore, the nurse should suggest ways a woman can increase her dietary iron.

Data from Mahan, L.K., & Escott-Stump, S. (1996). *Krause's food, nutrition, and diet therapy* (9th ed.). Philadelphia: W.B. Saunders.

Iron is present in many foods, but it takes large amounts of these foods to provide enough iron for pregnancy needs by diet alone. The average American diet contains only about 6 mg of iron for each 1000 calories of food. The non-pregnant woman would have to eat approximately 2500 calories daily and the pregnant woman would need as much as 5000 calories to meet her iron needs (Worthington-Roberts, 1997b). In addition, some women restrict their intake of meats and grains in an effort to cut down on fat and calories. Thus, many adult women do not meet their daily non-pregnancy requirement for iron and begin pregnancy already anemic or with low iron stores.

Absorption of iron is affected by many other substances. Calcium and phosphorus in milk and tannin in tea decrease iron absorption from plant sources (called non-heme iron) if consumed during the same meal. Coffee binds iron (prevents it from being fully absorbed). Foods cooked in iron pans contain more iron. Foods containing ascorbic acid and meats eaten with other iron-containing foods may increase absorption. Iron from meat (called heme iron) is more readily absorbed than that from plants and is less affected by other foods.

Physicians and nurse practitioners often prescribe iron supplements of 30 mg daily during pregnancy because of the difficulty of obtaining enough iron in the diet. Supplementation should begin during the second trimester, when the need increases. Because morning sickness usually ends by this time, the expectant mother tolerates the iron better. Iron taken on an empty stomach is absorbed more completely, but many women find iron difficult to tolerate without some food. Women should not take iron with milk, but taking it with a vitamin C source such as orange juice may increase absorption. Taking it at bedtime may make it easier to tolerate. Side effects occur more often with higher doses and include nausea, vomiting, heartburn, epigastric pain, constipation, and diarrhea. Women who experience discomfort from side effects when taking iron on an empty stomach may take it 1 to 2 hours after meals more comfortably. (Anemia during pregnancy is discussed on p. 210.)

### CALCIUM

Calcium is necessary for bone formation, maintenance of cell membrane permeability, coagulation, and neuromuscular function. It is transferred to the fetus, especially in the last trimester, and is important for mineralization of fetal bones and teeth. Calcium absorption increases during the second trimester. The pregnant woman's diet must provide enough calcium for her own and the fetus' needs to avoid loss from her bones. Because the total amount of calcium required is only a small part of that stored in the bones, mineralization of her bones is not usually reduced significantly. However, in women with poor diets, more than one fetus, or closely spaced pregnancies, stores may be depleted. A common myth is that calcium is removed from the teeth during pregnancy, leading to excessive decay. Actually, calcium in the teeth is stable and is not affected by pregnancy.

The best source of calcium is dairy products. Whole, low-fat, and skim milk all contain the same amount of calcium and may be used interchangeably to increase or reduce calorie intake. However, women with lactose intolerance (lactase deficiency resulting in gastrointestinal problems when dairy products are consumed) need other sources of calcium.

Calcium is also present in legumes, nuts, dried fruits, dark green leafy vegetables, and broccoli. Although spinach contains calcium, it also contains oxalates that decrease calcium availability; thus, it is not a good source. Canned salmon or sardines with bones also provide calcium. Blackstrap molasses and tofu processed with calcium sulfate are sources for vegans. Caffeine increases the excretion of calcium. Table 9–7 lists foods high in calcium.

The 1200-mg daily calcium requirement for pregnancy is a 50 percent increase over the RDA for the non-pregnant woman older than 25 years but the same as that for the woman younger than 25. Women who do not eat dairy products for cultural reasons, because of lactose intolerance, because they avoid animal products, or for other reasons should receive supplements. Women younger than 25 years with diets low in calcium may need supplements during pregnancy because their bone density is not complete; lack of available calcium may interfere with adequate bone formation in the mother. To ensure absorption of calcium, women should take supplements with meals, separately from when they take iron supplements.

## Pregnant Women Want to Know About Vitamins and Minerals

- Take only vitamin and mineral supplements prescribed by a physician, nurse practitioner, or certified nurse-midwife. Over-the-counter supplements may not be formulated to meet your individual needs and could be harmful to you and your baby.
- Take iron on an empty stomach, if possible. If you have nausea, heartburn, constipation, or diarrhea, try taking your iron at different times of the day, such as at bedtime or 1 to 2 hours after meals. To increase absorption, take it with orange juice or another source of vitamin C. Do not take iron with calcium supplements, milk, tea, or coffee because these substances decrease absorption.

**TABLE 9–7 CALCIUM SOURCES APPROXIMATELY EQUIVALENT TO 1 CUP OF MILK ***

1 c yogurt
1½ oz hard cheese
2 c low-fat cottage cheese
1¾ c ice cream or ice milk
3 c sherbet
11 eggs
2½ c peanuts
1 c almonds
9 oz sunflower seeds
2 c refried beans
3 pieces (2.5 × 2.75 × 1 inch) tofu (soybean curd)
1¾ c broccoli
1½ c cooked kale
1 c cooked collard greens
1⅓ c oysters
4 oz salmon with bones
2½ oz sardines with bones
7 corn tortillas
5 tsp blackstrap molasses

* This list can be used to counsel women who are vegans or lactose-intolerant. Lactose-intolerant women can often tolerate yogurt and cheese without distress. Although the amounts of some foods listed are more than would be likely to be eaten within a day, they serve for comparison.

Data from Mahan, L.K., & Escott-Stump, S. (1996). *Krause's food, nutrition, and diet therapy* (9th ed.). Philadelphia: W.B. Saunders.

## Supplementation

### PURPOSE

Food is the best source for nutrients. The Institute of Medicine Subcommittee on Nutritional Status and Weight Gain During Pregnancy (Institute of Medicine, 1990) states that women do not need routine vitamin and mineral supplements during pregnancy unless there is reason to believe that the diet is inadequate. The exception is iron, which is unlikely to be obtained in adequate amounts through normal food intake. Expectant mothers who are vegetarians or lactose-intolerant or who have special problems in obtaining nutrients through diet alone may need vitamin and mineral supplements. Assessment of each woman's individualized needs determines whether supplementation is appropriate.

### DISADVANTAGES AND DANGERS

Routine supplementation with vitamin-mineral capsules or tablets is very common during pregnancy, but this practice has been questioned because of the problems it may cause. Commonly used supplements provide from 50 percent to 150 percent of the RDA for the vitamins and minerals they contain. In some cases, the interaction between certain nutrients may interfere with their absorption or use. For example, a high calcium intake decreases absorption of iron and zinc. Excessive intake of vitamin C inhibits absorption and metabolism of vitamin $B_{12}$.

Because many people think supplements are a harmless way to improve their diets, some women take them without consulting a physician or take them in addition to those prescribed. Women should be advised that taking extra vitamins and minerals may cause them to be deficient in others. The physician, nurse-midwife, or nurse practitioner can advise them how to increase intake if necessary and still maintain a balance.

The use of supplements, in addition to food, may increase the intake of some nutrients to doses much higher than the recommended amounts. Excessive amounts of some vitamins and minerals may be toxic to the fetus. Vitamin A can cause craniofacial, central nervous system, and cardiac defects in the fetus when taken in large amounts. (Worthington-Roberts, 1997a). High levels of vitamin A are taken by women using the drug isotretinoin (Accutane) for acne. Other nutrients that may cause harm in excessive amounts include vitamins $B_6$, C, and D and the minerals iron and zinc. The consequences of excessive intake of some nutrients on the fetus are not fully understood at this time, and future research may discover other effects.

Another disadvantage of vitamin-mineral supplements is that some women may develop a false sense of security. If they think their nutrient needs can be met in pill form, they may be unconcerned about their food intake. Supplements do not contain protein or calories and may lack many necessary nutrients. Nurses must emphasize that supplements are not food substitutes and do not contain all the nutrients needed during pregnancy. In fact, we may not even know all the nutrients that are important to pregnancy and provided by foods.

## Water

Water is important during pregnancy for the expanded blood volume (see Chapter 7) and as a part of the increased maternal and fetal tissues. Women should drink approximately eight to 10 8-ounce glasses of fluids each day, with water constituting most of the fluid intake. Fluids low in nutrients should be limited because they are filling and replace other more nutritional foods and drinks. These include carbonated beverages, coffee, tea, and "juice" drinks that contain high amounts of sugar and little real juice.

## Food Guide Pyramid

The U.S. Department of Agriculture's (USDA) food pyramid (Fig. 9–2) provides a guide for healthy eating for adults and children. It can be adapted to

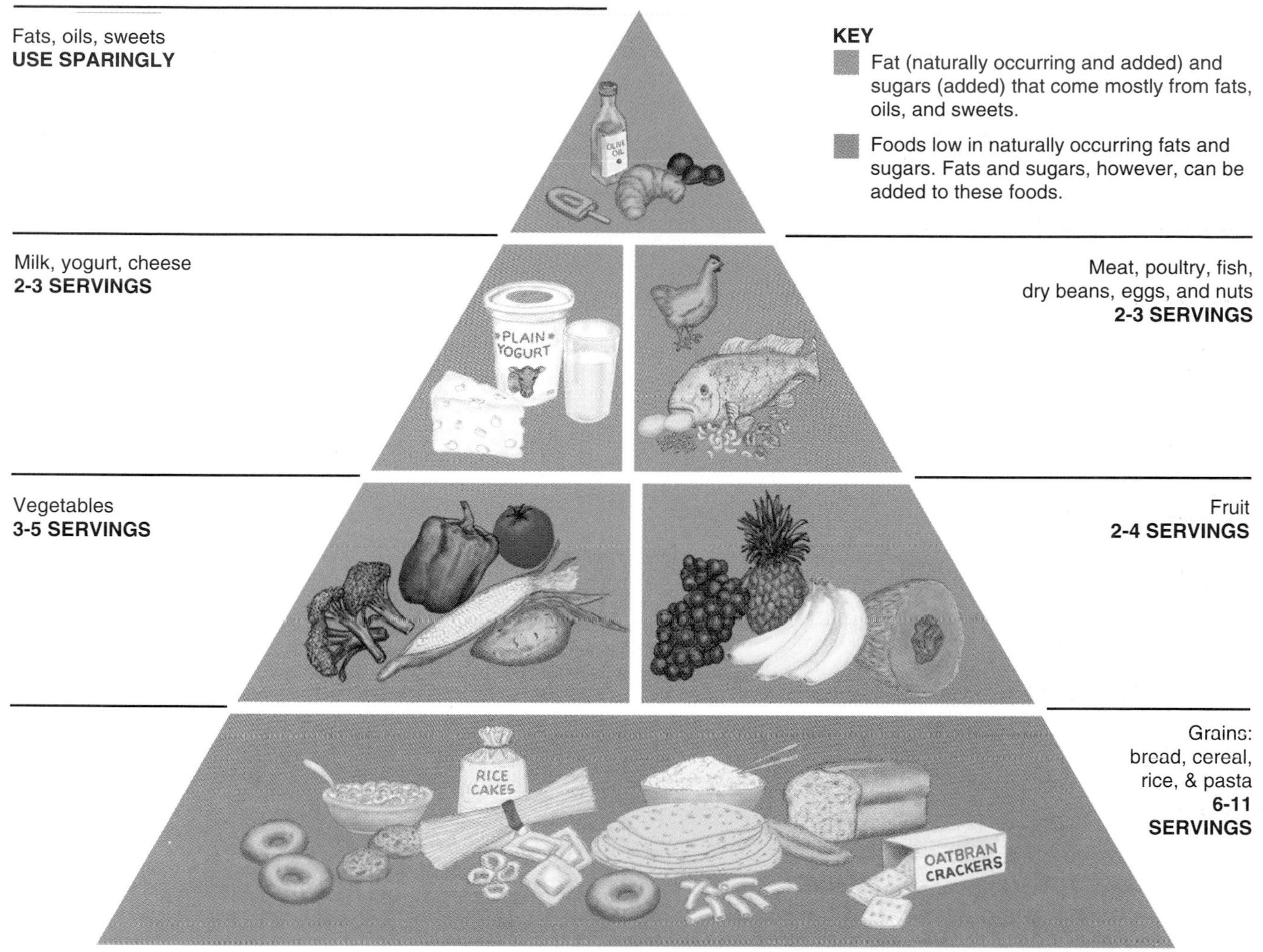


**FIGURE 9–2**

The food guide pyramid. (Adapted from U.S. Department of Agriculture, 1992.)

serve as a guide during pregnancy as well. Table 9–8 lists the servings of each food pyramid group needed during pregnancy.

### WHOLE GRAINS

At the base of the pyramid are breads, cereals, rice, and pastas. They provide complex carbohydrates and fiber as well as vitamins and minerals. Whole grains provide more nutrients than processed grain products. Although foods can be enriched to replace some of the nutrients lost during processing, zinc, vitamin $B_6$, magnesium, and vitamin E may not be replaced by enrichment. The USDA recommends 6 to 11 servings of this group for healthy adults over age 25. Pregnant women should have at least 7 servings.

### VEGETABLES AND FRUITS

Vegetables and fruits form the next two groups of the pyramid and are important sources of vitamins, minerals, and fiber. At least one food that provides vitamin C and one that provides vitamin A are important in selecting from the fruit and vegetable group each day. Healthy adults should have at least five servings of fruits and vegetables with a range of three to five servings of vegetables and two to four of fruits. The pregnant or lactating woman needs the same amount.

### DAIRY FOODS

Dairy foods include foods like milk, yogurt, and cheese. They contain approximately the same nutrient values whether they are whole (4 percent fat), low-fat (2 percent fat), or nonfat (skim), but the calories and fat are lower in the latter two. Dairy products are especially good sources of calcium. Adults older than age 25 need two to three servings from this group. Younger women and those who are pregnant or lactating need at least three servings.

In the past, calcium supplements and decreased milk intake were recommended to prevent leg cramps; this was thought to improve the balance of

**TABLE 9–8 DAILY FOOD PLAN**

| Food Guide Pyramid Group | Typical Food Amounts for One Serving | Number of Servings | |
|---|---|---|---|
| | | Non-pregnant Women | Pregnant and Lactating Women |
| Unsaturated fats | 1 tsp | 3 tsp | 3 tsp |
| Dairy products | 1 c milk or yogurt, 1½ oz or ⅓ c grated hard cheese, 2 c cottage cheese | <Age 25: 3 or more<br>>Age 25: 2 or more | 3 or more |
| Protein sources | 1 oz or ¼ c chopped meat, poultry, fish, ½ c cooked legumes, 1 egg, 3 oz tofu, 2 tbsp peanut butter | 5 ounces | 7 ounces |
| Vegetables and fruits | 1 medium piece or ½ cup cooked or chopped raw, ¾ cup juice, 1 lettuce leaf | | |
| Total servings | | 5 or more | 5 or more |
| Vitamin C source | | 1 | 1 |
| Deep yellow or dark green leafy (vitamin A) | | 1 | 1 |
| Other fruits and vegetables | | 3 | 3 |
| Whole grains | Breads (1 slice), cereals (½–¾ c), rice and pastas (½ c) | 6–11<br><Age 25: 7 or more<br>>Age 25: 6 or more | 7 or more |

Nurses can use this table as a guide to counsel women about nutrient needs during pregnancy and lactation. Eating *at least* the number of servings listed meets the minimum nutrient need for pregnancy. Additional calories may be necessary to meet individual requirements.

Modified from California Department of Health Services, Maternal and Child Health (1990): *Nutrition during pregnancy and the postpartum period: A manual for health care professionals, summary*. Sacramento: Author.

calcium and phosphorus, both occurring in high amounts in milk. However, the effectiveness of this treatment has not been proven. Because milk provides a large number of nutrients, women generally should not limit it during pregnancy (Worthington-Roberts, 1997b; Neuhouser, 1996).

#### PROTEIN

Many adults think of meat, poultry, fish, and eggs as the only sources of protein. However, legumes (dried beans and peas), nuts, and soybean products such as tofu are also good sources. Adults should consume 5 to 6 ounces; pregnant or lactating women need 7 or more ounces of protein foods. A typical serving of meat, fish, or poultry is approximately 3 ounces. Three ounces is about the size of a deck of playing cards.

#### OTHER ELEMENTS

The tip of the pyramid represents fats, oils, and concentrated sugars, which should be used sparingly. They provide calories for energy but few other nutrients. Three teaspoons of unsaturated fats are adequate for this group.

**✓ CHECK YOUR READING**

8. Which minerals are often below the recommended amounts in the diets of pregnant women?
9. Why is routine use of vitamin-mineral supplements unnecessary and possibly dangerous?
10. How much fluid should a woman drink each day during pregnancy?
11. How many servings of each food pyramid group are recommended during pregnancy?

## Factors That Influence Nutrition

Cultural background, age, and knowledge about nutrition influence the food choices women make and their nutritional status. The nurse must consider them when counseling women about their diets.

### Culture

Food is important in all cultures and often has special meaning during pregnancy or childbirth, when certain foods may be favored or discouraged. Nurses need knowledge about the habits of a variety of cultures so that they can provide culturally appropriate nutritional counseling. Before making assumptions about the influence of a woman's culture on her diet, the nurse must assess each woman individually. Not all women follow food practices considered typical for their culture. Variations among members of a culture may be attributable to diverse practices found in different areas of their country of origin.

The nurse should assess the woman's age, her length of time in America, and whether she has adopted prevalent American eating habits. Greater exposure to an American diet may cause younger members of a group to make more dietary changes than older relatives. Some women who follow an American diet may return to some aspects of their culture's traditional diet during pregnancy to "be sure" they do not harm the fetus.

Nurses often use pamphlets as a part of nutritional teaching and may be able to obtain them in various languages.

**The nurse should be certain that the woman can read her own language before giving her written materials. People who cannot read may not readily admit it. In addition, the translation may be too complicated for the woman with little education to understand. Having an interpreter discuss the material with the woman helps to discover whether she can read and aids in other teaching.**

Many cultures believe that certain foods, conditions, and medicines are "hot" or "cold" and that they must maintain a balance to preserve health. In Asian cultures, this is referred to as "yin" (cold) and "yang" (hot) and may influence what the mother eats during pregnancy and the postpartum period. Table 9–9 lists common "hot" and "cold" foods.

Food taboos may influence what some women eat during the childbearing period. For example, Korean women may avoid chicken, pork, and blemished fruits during pregnancy. These foods are thought to have a harmful effect on the infant's physical appearance.

An enormous variety exists in cultural preferences for foods. For instance, some African-Americans may follow a diet that is similar to that of people living in the southeastern United States. This diet includes foods such as okra, collards, mustard greens, ham hocks, black-eyed peas, and hominy or grits. However, the diet of others varies according to the geographic area in which they live. Many African-Americans eat a diet deficient in iron and fresh fruits and vegetables, especially if they have low incomes. Lactose intolerance is common, resulting in lack of calcium if other sources are not present in the diet. Intake of high-sodium and fried foods may present health problems.

Jewish women may follow no dietary restrictions, or they may follow a strictly kosher diet. A kosher diet includes meat processed to remove all blood, meat only from animals with cloven hooves, and avoidance of milk and meat in the same meal. Muslim women do not eat pork and may wish to fast on certain days. However, the religion exempts pregnant and nursing women from obligatory fasting.

The diet of Native American women may contain corn, beans, and squash but lack fresh fruits and vegetables. Lactose intolerance is common, and meat intake is low. Fat, carbohydrate, sodium, and sugar intake are often high. Low-income Native Americans living on reservations may receive foods such as white flour, cornmeal, white rice, and processed meats from federal programs. However some of these families take in less than two thirds the RDA for calories, calcium, iron, iodine, riboflavin, and vitamins A and C (Davis & Sherer, 1994).

Food preferences for two cultures, Southeast Asian and Latino, are discussed in detail as examples of the influence of culture on diet. Immigrants and refugees from Southeast Asia are the newest large group of people to come into the United States. They are likely to continue diets similar to those from their homelands. Latinos are a large minority group in the United States, making up about 11 percent of the population (U.S. Department of Commerce, 1992). Nurses throughout the United States need information about Latino food preferences.

**TABLE 9–9 COMMON "HOT" AND "COLD" FOODS: SOUTHEAST ASIAN AND LATINO DIETS***

**Southeast Asian**

| "Hot" (Yang) Foods | "Cold" (Yin) Foods |
|---|---|
| Peppers, onions | Most fruits and juices |
| Meat and poultry | Flour |
| Fish and fish sauce | Cold fluids |
| Broth | Sour foods |
| Eggs | |
| Spices, sweets | |

**Latino**

| "Hot" Foods | "Cold" Foods |
|---|---|
| Potatoes, peas, onions, chili peppers | Most fruits and vegetables |
| Cheese, evaporated milk | Milk |
| Chicken, lamb | Fish |
| Flour tortillas | Corn tortillas |
| Chickpeas and kidney beans | Green and red beans |

* Although there are variations within cultural groups, foods considered "hot" are used for conditions thought to be "cold" and vice versa. This influences what women are willing to eat during pregnancy or illness, and these customs must be respected as part of nursing care.

### SOUTHEAST ASIAN DIETARY PRACTICES

The term *Southeast Asian* refers to people from Cambodia, Laos, and Vietnam who came to the United States beginning in the mid-1970s. The majority settled in western states, but smaller numbers found homes elsewhere in the country.

Southeast Asian cooking methods include searing fresh vegetables quickly with a small portion of meat, poultry, or fish in a little oil over high heat. Meals cooked in this manner are low in fat and retain vitamins. Most meals are accompanied by rice, which increases the intake of complex carbohydrates. A salty fish sauce called *nuoc mam* and fresh vegetables are part of most meals.

Many Southeast Asians have adapted their dietary habits to more American ways. Increased intake of meats, eggs, fruit, and bread has added nutrients but also fat to the diet. Coffee, soft drinks, and fast foods have been less favorable influences because they are low in nutrients but high in sugar or fat. Southeast Asians have decreased their intake of fish, a low-fat source of protein (Williams, 1993).

#### EFFECT OF CULTURE ON DIET DURING CHILDBEARING

In the Southeast Asian culture, pregnancy, especially the third trimester, is considered "hot," and the woman is encouraged to eat "cold" foods to maintain a balance of hot and cold. During pregnancy she eats more sour foods, fruits, noodles, and sweets and avoids fish, excessively salty or spicy foods, alcohol, and rice. She does not eat unfamiliar foods for fear that they may harm her or her fetus.

The postpartum period is considered "cold," partly because of the loss of blood, which is "hot." Mothers avoid losing more heat, which would have ill effects on their health. They stay warm physically (and may refuse to shower for fear of exposure to cold). They choose "hot" foods to eat, including rice with fish sauce, broth, salty meats, fish, and eggs. They may refuse cold drinks but welcome hot fluids, requesting tea or even plain hot water. Families frequently bring food to the mother while she is in the hospital because hospital food may not meet her preferences.

The diet of Southeast Asians, especially those with low incomes, may be below recommended levels for energy, calcium, iron, zinc, magnesium, and vitamins $B_6$ and D, but high in sodium. These deficiencies may be of special concern during pregnancy. The woman can often increase her intake of needed nutrients without deviating greatly from her usual diet.

#### INCREASING NUTRIENTS WITH TRADITIONAL FOODS

Milk products are not part of the traditional Southeast Asian diet, and lactose intolerance is common. However, increasing intake of commonly used dark green leafy vegetables, such as mustard greens, bok choy, and broccoli, increases levels of calcium, iron, magnesium, and folic acid. Tofu contains good amounts of calcium and iron. A broth made from pork or chicken bones soaked in vinegar (which removes calcium from the bones) is frequently taken. If the mother avoids fortified milk, she may need vitamin D supplementation. Increasing the intake of meats or poultry elevates levels of vitamin $B_6$ and zinc.

### LATINO DIETARY PRACTICES

Spanish-speaking people, such as Mexican-Americans, Puerto Ricans, and Cuban-Americans, are often referred to as Latinos or Hispanics. This major minority group in the United States continues to grow. Mexican-Americans make up the largest share of the group. Although many live in the southwestern United States and Florida, they are located throughout the country. Like Asians, Latinos follow the theories of "hot" and "cold" foods and conditions. They also consider pregnancy to be "hot" and the postpartum period to be "cold" and adjust the diet accordingly.

Dried beans (especially pinto beans) are a staple of the Mexican-American diet and are part of most meals either alone, as refried beans, or mixed with other foods, such as rice. The most common meats are beef, pork, and chicken. The major grain is corn, which is ground and made into a dough called *masa* to make corn tortillas. The corn is treated with lime and is a good source of calcium. Corn or flour tortillas are eaten with most meals. Rice is also an important grain. Although milk is not commonly used except for infants, cheese is part of many dishes.

Chili peppers and tomatoes are the most common vegetables used; others include beets, cabbage, chayotes, bell peppers, and string beans. Green leafy and yellow vegetables are seldom used. Oranges, bananas, canned peaches, pumpkin, and avocado are common fruits.

Foods are often hot and spicy and frequently fried. The diet is high in fiber and complex carbohydrates. However, it tends to be high in calories and fat, leading many Mexican-Americans to become overweight. The diet may be low in iron, calcium, and vitamins A and D, which should be increased through foods or supplements during pregnancy.

Puerto Rican and Cuban diets are similar to that of the Mexican-American, with the addition of tropical fruits and vegetables from the homeland, when available. Viandas (starchy fruits and vegetables like plantain, green bananas, sweet potatoes, yams, and breadfruit) are common. They may be cooked with codfish and onion. Guava, papaya, mango, and eggplant are also used when available.

#### ✓ CHECK YOUR READING

12. When the nurse assesses cultural influences on nutrition during pregnancy, what factors must be considered?
13. Compare the diet of the Southeast Asian woman with that of the Latina woman.

### Age

Extremes of age may have an influence on the nutritional needs of pregnancy. The adolescent who is not fully mature needs nutritional support for her own growth. Older women who are in good health have the same nutritional requirements as younger pregnant women. They may have more knowledge about nutrition through life experiences or may need as much teaching as younger women. They are more likely to be financially secure than very young women.

### Nutritional Knowledge

Information about nutrition is readily available to those who read popular books and magazine articles about the subject. Even women who have not been attentive to their diets before pregnancy often try to learn about the relationship between what they eat and the effect on the fetus, once pregnancy is confirmed. Although women know they should "eat well" during pregnancy, they may have little idea of what that means. Some lack basic understanding about nutrition and have misconceptions based on common food myths that interfere with good nutritional choices. These expectant mothers need help from nurses in learning about nutrition.

## Nutritional Risk Factors

Factors that may interfere with a woman's ability to meet the nutritional needs of pregnancy include poverty, adolescence, vegetarianism, lactose intolerance, nausea and vomiting of pregnancy, anemia, abnormal pre-pregnancy weight, eating disorders, pica, multiparity, and substance abuse.

### Socioeconomic Status

#### POVERTY

Low-income women may have deficient diets because of lack of financial resources and nutritional education. Carbohydrate foods are often less expensive than meats, dairy products, fruits, and vegetables. Therefore, the diet may be high in calories but low in vitamins and minerals. A referral to Aid to Families with Dependent Children or the special supplemental food program for women, infants, and children (WIC) may be helpful if a woman's food intake is inadequate because of lack of money. Vitamin and mineral supplementation may be important for her, especially if her diet is likely to be inconsistent.

#### FOOD SUPPLEMENT PROGRAMS

The WIC program is administered by the USDA to provide nutritional assessment, counseling, and education to low-income women and children up to age 5 years who are at nutritional risk. The program also provides food vouchers or foods such as milk, cheese, eggs, iron-fortified cereal, fruit juice, dried beans, and formula to qualified women and their children. Eligibility is based on an income below 185 per cent of the federal poverty level. Women are eligible throughout pregnancy and for 6 months after birth if formula feeding or 1 year if breastfeeding. However, funding problems may prevent all of those who are entitled to benefits from receiving them. Although the program has been in existence since 1974, changing priorities for government funds often put it at risk.

### Adolescence

Adolescent pregnancies are associated with higher risk for complications for both the expectant mother and the fetus. Adolescents at greatest risk for problem pregnancies are those who are the youngest in terms of gynecologic age (number of years since menarche) and those who are still growing. Girls who become pregnant less than 2 years after menstruation begins are not anatomically and physiologically mature, and they require more nutrients to meet their needs than do older adolescents. Those with a gynecologic age of 4 years are usually physically mature and have nutritional demands similar to those of older women (Worthington-Roberts & Rees, 1997) (see also Chapter 24, p. 645).

However, whether the adolescent is still growing is even more important than her age, because some adolescents may continue to grow as long as 6 years after menarche (Scholl et al., 1994). Growing adolescents continue to add fat to their own bodies in late pregnancy rather than use it for support of the fetus. As a result, they tend to have smaller infants even with good weight gains.

To determine the appropriate gain for an individual teenager, the nurse should consider how much weight the adolescent would gain in the next 9 months if she were not pregnant. (See growth charts for children and adolescents in pediatrics textbooks.) This amount is added to the recommended weight gain for pregnancy. An example of weight gain to meet the girl's growth needs follows.

For a 13-year-old girl:

- *Pre-pregnancy height*: 61.75 inches (157 cm)
- *Pre-pregnancy weight*: 101 pounds (46 kg)
- *Expected weight gain for age over 40 weeks*: 6.5 pounds (3 kg)

- *Weight gain for pregnancy (upper limits suggested for adolescents)*: 35.0 pounds (16 kg)
- *Total during pregnancy*: 41.5 pounds (19 kg)

Just as for the older adult, the underweight teenager should gain more to place her at normal weight for her age and height. The overweight girl must still gain, but 15 to 25 pounds may be adequate for her.

#### NUTRIENT NEEDS

In the past, it was usual to add the RDA for pregnancy to the nutritional requirements for the adolescent. The 1989 RDAs list absolute amounts for each nutrient, based on a woman aged 19 to 24 years. These amounts are adequate for most adolescents, but individualized assessment of gynecologic age, nutritional status, and daily diet may indicate the need for increases in some areas. Energy, protein, iron, and calcium are nutrients that are commonly increased to meet growth needs for the younger teen.

#### COMMON PROBLEMS

The diets of teenagers, both before and during pregnancy, are often low in vitamin A, vitamin D, vitamin $B_6$, folic acid, riboflavin, calcium, iron, and zinc (Mahan & Escott-Stump, 1996). Supplements may be prescribed, but the adolescent may not take them regularly. This combination of poor intake and unreliable supplementation may further deplete nutrient stores and general nutrition.

Peer pressure is an important influence on nutritional status. Adolescents are often concerned about their body image. If weight is a major focus for a teenager and her peers, she is more likely to restrict calories to avoid weight gain during pregnancy. Teenagers tend to skip meals, especially breakfast. The fetus requires a steady supply of nutrients, and the expectant mother's stores may be used if intake is not sufficient to meet energy needs.

Because snacks provide as much as one quarter of the caloric intake of the adolescent girl, they should be rich in nutrients (Worthington-Roberts & Rees, 1997). Fast foods from restaurants or snack machines are a significant part of many teenagers' diets. Although occasional consumption of these foods is not harmful, they are often high in calories, fat, and sodium yet low in vitamins, minerals, and fiber. Choosing fast foods that do not make her appear different to her peers, yet meet her added nutrient needs, is important. The Nursing Care Plan lists strategies for educating and encouraging the pregnant adolescent about nutrition.

#### TEACHING THE ADOLESCENT

Teaching the adolescent about nutrition can be a challenge for nurses. It is essential to establish an accepting, relaxed atmosphere and show willingness to listen to the teenager's concerns. Her lifestyle, pattern of eating, and food likes and dislikes should be explored first. The nurse must consider these factors in determining whether changes are necessary in the diet.

The adolescent's home life may affect her nutritional status. She may live at home with a mother who does the cooking, and the whole family may eat together. Or she may eat with the rest of the family only occasionally because she is often away at mealtimes. Some pregnant adolescents are homeless or in unstable situations. The number of other people in the home and whether enough food is available for all affect the dietary intake.

In making suggestions, the nurse should focus on only those changes that are necessary. If an adolescent believes she must eliminate all her favorite foods, she is likely to rebel. Suggestions should be kept to a minimum, and snacks should be included in the meal plan. Asking for the adolescent's input increases the likelihood that she will follow suggestions. When changes are necessary, the nurse should explain why they are important for the fetus as well

### Pregnant Adolescents Want to Know

### How Can I Eat Fast Foods and Still Maintain a Good Diet?

- Add cheese to hamburgers to increase calcium and protein. Include lettuce and tomato for vitamins A and C.
- Avoid dressings on hamburgers because they tend to be high in calories and fat.
- Choose broiled, roasted, or barbecued foods to reduce fat and calories. Examples are barbecued or broiled chicken breast or roast beef. Cut down on fried foods (French fries, fried zucchini, onion rings) because they are high in fat and the high heat may destroy some of the vitamins. Breaded foods like chicken nuggets or breaded clams are also high in calories and absorb more oil if they are fried.
- Baked potatoes with broccoli, cheese, or meat fillings provide better nutrition than French fries or even baked potatoes with sour cream and butter.
- Pizza is high in calories, but the cheese provides protein and calcium. Ask for vegetable toppings or add a salad to increase vitamins.
- Salad bars are often available at fast food restaurants and provide vitamins and minerals without adding too many calories. Use only a small amount of salad dressing, which is high in fat.
- Milk, milkshakes, and orange juice provide more nutrients than carbonated beverages, which are high in sodium, phosphorus, and calories. Too much sodium may increase swelling of the ankles; too much phosphorus may lead to leg cramps.
- Avoid pickles, olives, and other salty foods. Add only small amounts of salt to foods to prevent or decrease swelling.

## Nursing Care Plan 9–1

# Nutrition for the Pregnant Adolescent

**ASSESSMENT:** Vicki, age 15, is 20 weeks pregnant and has gained 10 pounds. She attends school and lives at home but usually cooks for herself because "I don't like the stuff Mom cooks." She skips breakfast and eats from snack machines during breaks at school. She goes to fast food restaurants for lunch and after school. Vicki says she is disgusted with how heavy she is and wants to go on a diet to lose some weight or "I'm going to look like a blimp!" Her hemoglobin level is 10.4 g/dl. She listens with interest when the nurse discusses nutrition, especially when weight is mentioned. Her statements show concern about her baby's needs. Vicki was at a normal weight before her pregnancy, and a weight gain of approximately 35 pounds is appropriate for her. Her gynecologic age is 2.5 years.

**NURSING DIAGNOSIS:** Altered Nutrition: Less Than Body Requirements related to concern about weight gain and diet choices inadequate to meet nutrient requirements of adolescent pregnancy

### Critical Thinking

What other information does the nurse need to complete the assessment?

**ANSWER**

A 24-hour diet history is necessary for a better understanding of Vicki's diet. The nurse should also ask about her likes and dislikes to make a meaningful diet plan for Vicki.

### GOALS/EXPECTED OUTCOMES

Vicki will do the following:

1. Explain the weight gain pattern and intake from each food group optimal for adolescent pregnancy.
2. List foods she can choose at fast food restaurants that meet her nutrient needs and allow her to feel part of her peer group.
3. Gain approximately 1 to 1 1/4 pounds (0.44 to 0.57 kg) a week for the rest of her pregnancy.
4. Maintain a hemoglobin level above 10 g/dl throughout her pregnancy.

| INTERVENTIONS | RATIONALE |
|---|---|
| 1. Praise Vicki for her interest in nutrition and her concern about gaining too much weight. | 1. Praise helps foster rapport and may focus attention on learning. |
| 2. Discuss the reasons for appropriate weight gain during pregnancy and its effect on the fetus. Explain the needs of the adolescent who is not finished growing and the importance of preventing the problems associated with low birth weight in the infant. | 2. Adolescents may not understand how diet affects the fetus and themselves during pregnancy. Explanation of the potential effects of her actions will increase the expectant mother's interest in nutrition. |
| 3. Assist Vicki in comparing her food intake with the recommended servings from each food group. Point out areas of strength, and praise her for these. | 3. Active involvement of the learner and positive reinforcement help increase motivation. |
| 4. Ask Vicki what problems she sees in her diet. Point out areas she may have missed. Explain the effect that lack of specific nutrients may have on the fetus. | 4. Adolescents learn best when they see how the material applies to them. |
| 5. Discuss the high caloric intake of fast foods in relation to her present diet, and explain the concept of nutrient density in terms of "spending calories" to "buy" nutrients needed during pregnancy. | 5. Relating information to concepts already understood increases understanding. |
| 6. Determine, from Vicki's food likes and dislikes, low-calorie foods she would like that meet her nutrient needs. Point out fruits and vegetables high in vitamins A and C, yet low in calories. | 6. Individualizing the recommended diet to meet the woman's likes and dislikes increases compliance. |
| 7. Suggest nutritional foods that Vicki could choose at fast food restaurants, and ask which ones are acceptable to her. | 7. The adolescent needs to feel that she is part of her peer group. Including her input on what she likes to eat may increase her compliance. |

*Nursing Care Plan continued on following page*

## Nursing Care Plan 9–1 *Continued*

# Nutrition for the Pregnant Adolescent

| | |
|---|---|
| 8. Discuss the importance of breakfast during pregnancy. Explain that the fetus needs a steady supply of nutrients and needs food in the morning after the long fast during the night. | 8. Prolonged periods without maternal food intake can lead to a state of ketosis that is hostile to the fetus. |
| 9. Discuss breakfast foods that Vicki likes. Point out the nutrients found in whole grain breads and cereals (protein, iron, B vitamins) and their importance. | 9. Whole grains are often a part of a well-balanced breakfast. |
| 10. Suggest that Vicki eat foods not usually considered breakfast foods if she prefers. For example, cold pizza provides calcium and protein. | 10. Nontraditional methods of meeting the adolescent's nutritional needs may be very effective. |
| 11. Suggest foods high in nutrient density that are available from snack dispensers. Ask which of these are acceptable to Vicki. | 11. Adolescents are unlikely to give up foods that help them feel part of their peer group. |
| 12. Ask Vicki if she is willing to eat more dairy products after explaining their importance to her and her baby. Ask her to help plan which ones she will eat to meet her needed intake. | 12. Compliance is increased when clients maintain a feeling of control. |
| 13. Ask Vicki if she is taking her vitamin-mineral supplements and how she is tolerating them. Offer suggestions on how to deal with any problems she is having in this area. Reinforce the importance of consistent intake. | 13. Adolescents generally need supplements but may be inconsistent in taking them, especially if they experience side effects. |
| 14. Ask Vicki to bring in another 24-hour diet history on her next visit. | 14. Reassessment of dietary intake identifies new or continuing problems. |
| 15. Ask Vicki to share ways she has found to meet her diet needs that you could tell other teenagers. Ask for feedback on the methods discussed. | 15. It is important for the adolescent to feel that her thoughts and ideas are valued by the nurse. |

### EVALUATION

Vicki gains 4 to 6 pounds a month throughout the rest of her pregnancy, for a total weight gain of 33 pounds. Her reported dietary intake shows that she is meeting the recommendations for each food group. She brings back ideas about how to eat fast foods healthfully and seems to like "educating" the nurse about teenage diet preferences. Her hemoglobin level rises to 11 g/dl. A healthy $7\frac{1}{2}$-pound baby girl is born at term.

### ADDITIONAL NURSING DIAGNOSES TO CONSIDER

Body Image Disturbance
Situational Low Self-Esteem

as for the expectant mother. Teenagers, like other pregnant women, often make changes for the sake of their unborn child that they would not consider for themselves alone.

The need to be like her peers is of major importance to the adolescent, especially when she is going through the changes of pregnancy. With education about what foods to choose, she can eat fast foods with her friends and still maintain a nourishing diet. Giving her plenty of examples of alternatives from which she can choose should be very helpful. Table 9–10 and Pregnant Adolescents Want to Know provide suggestions for foods she can select from snack dispensers or fast food restaurants that are nutritional yet similar to what her peers are eating.

## Vegetarianism

Although the knowledgeable vegetarian may eat a highly nutritional diet, she is at higher risk during pregnancy, when her nutrient intake must nourish the fetus as well as herself. If she is new to vegetarian food practices, uninformed about pregnancy

**TABLE 9–10 NUTRITIOUS CHOICES FROM SNACK MACHINES***

| Food | Nutrients Provided |
|---|---|
| Yogurt, white or chocolate milk | Protein, calcium |
| Fruit juices or fresh fruits (usually apples or oranges) | Vitamins, fiber |
| Popcorn (best without butter or salt) | Fiber |
| Peanuts | Protein |
| Granola or granola bars | Fiber, protein |
| Crackers and cheese | Protein, calcium |
| Crackers and peanut butter | Protein |

* Snack machines generally dispense foods high in calories, fats, and sodium and low in nutrients. The foods listed here, although somewhat high in calories, also provide other worthwhile nutrients.

needs, or careless with her diet, she could fail to meet her nutrient needs.

Vegetarianism occurs in a variety of forms. Vegans avoid all animal products and may have the most difficulty meeting their nutrient needs. Their diet may be lacking in adequate iodine, calcium, iron, zinc, riboflavin, and vitamins D and $B_{12}$ (Peckenpaugh & Poleman, 1995). Vegans must pay particular attention to obtaining these nutrients in food or supplement form. It is easier for lactovegetarians, ovovegetarians, and lacto-ovovegetarians to meet their nutrient needs.

While not true vegetarianism, elimination of red meats from the diet to decrease intake of saturated fats and cholesterol is a growing trend. Women who follow this type of diet usually eat small amounts of chicken, fish, and dairy products. The needs of women who follow any form of vegetarianism are different during pregnancy.

### MEETING THE NUTRITIONAL REQUIREMENTS OF PREGNANCY

**Energy.** Vegetarian diets are low in calories and fat and may not meet energy needs of pregnancy. The diets are high in fiber and may cause a feeling of fullness before enough calories are eaten. A pregnant woman can increase caloric intake by eating between-meal snacks and foods with higher caloric content. If carbohydrate and fat intake are too low, her body may use protein for energy, making it unavailable for other purposes.

**Protein.** Protein intake is a concern in all vegetarian diets. "Complete" proteins, which contain all the essential amino acids the body cannot synthesize from other sources, are an indispensable part of the diet. Animal proteins are complete, but vegetable proteins lack one or more of the essential amino acids. Combining incomplete plant proteins with other plant foods that have complementary amino acids allows intake of all essential amino acids. Knowledge of how to mix foods is required to ensure adequate intake of essential amino acids. Dishes that combine beans or tofu with rice are examples. Table 9–11 lists combinations of foods that provide complete proteins.

Incomplete proteins can also be combined with small amounts of complete protein foods like cheese to provide all amino acids. Therefore, women who include even small amounts of animal products have less difficulty meeting their protein needs.

**Calcium.** Vegetarians who include milk products

**TABLE 9–11 PLANT FOOD COMBINATIONS TO PROVIDE COMPLETE PROTEINS**

| Food | Served with |
|---|---|
| **Grains** | |
| Wheat | Beans |
| | Soybeans and rice |
| | Soybeans and rice and peanuts |
| | Soybeans and sesame |
| Rice | Beans (other types) |
| | Peas |
| | Sesame |
| | Soybeans and rice |
| | Soybeans and peanuts and wheat |
| | Soybeans and wheat |
| Corn | Beans |
| **Legumes** | |
| Soybeans | Peanuts and sesame |
| | Peanuts and wheat and rice |
| | Rice and wheat |
| | Wheat and sesame |
| Beans (other types such as garbanzo, navy, peas) | Rice |
| **Nuts and Seeds** | |
| Peanuts | Soybeans and sesame |
| | Soybeans and wheat and rice |
| | Sunflower seeds |
| Sesame | Beans |
| | Broccoli |
| | Cauliflower |
| | Lima beans |
| | Rice |
| | Soybeans and peanuts |
| | Soybeans and wheat |
| | Sprouts |
| Sunflower | Peanuts |

Based on data from Lappé, F.M. (1991). *Diet for a small planet.* New York: Ballantine.

in their diet may meet their pregnancy needs for calcium. Vegans obtain calcium from vegetables, but their high-fiber diet may interfere with calcium absorption. Calcium-fortified soy products, such as soy milk or tofu, may meet the requirements, or calcium supplements may be necessary. Vitamin D supplementation is especially important if the woman drinks no milk and has little exposure to sunlight. Soy milks may be enriched with vitamin D.

**Iron.** Iron in the vegetarian diet is poorly absorbed because of the lack of heme iron (from meats), which improves absorption. Iron supplementation is particularly important for vegetarian women during pregnancy.

**Zinc.** Because the best sources of zinc are meat and fish, vegans may be deficient in this mineral. They usually need zinc supplements to meet their needs.

**Vitamin $B_{12}$.** Vitamin $B_{12}$ is obtained only from animal products. Because vegetarian diets contain large amounts of folic acid, the development of anemia from inadequate intake of vitamin $B_{12}$ may not be apparent at first. Vegans may eat fortified foods such as soy products or may take supplements.

**Vitamin A.** Vitamin A is generally abundant in vegetarian diets. If a pregnant woman receives a multiple vitamin-mineral supplement, she may take in excessive amounts of vitamin A, causing toxicity with anorexia, irritability, hair loss, and dry skin and damage to the fetus. Supplementation should be individualized for each woman based on her diet and her needs.

Table 9–12 presents guidelines on vegetarian foods during pregnancy. This scheme is similar to the use of food pyramid groups for the non-vegetarian and easy to remember when planning the daily diet.

## Lactose Intolerance

Intolerance to lactose is caused by absence of the small-intestine enzyme lactase, necessary for absorption of the milk sugar lactose. Some degree of lactose intolerance is normal for most of the world's population after early childhood. This includes many African-American, Latina, Asian, Native American, and Middle Eastern women. Although women with lactose intolerance may tolerate cultured or fermented milk products, such as aged cheese, buttermilk, and yogurt, symptoms may occur after drinking as little as a cup of milk. Symptoms include nausea, bloating, flatulence, diarrhea, and intestinal cramping.

Although the ability to tolerate lactose may increase during pregnancy, women who avoid dairy foods are at risk for not meeting the recommended amounts of calcium unless they get enough from other sources. Most women can tolerate small amounts of milk, and they should increase their intake of other foods that provide calcium. Low-lactose milk is available, or the enzyme lactase (LactAid) can be added to milk. Table 9–6 lists additional sources of calcium.

**TABLE 9–12 FOOD PLAN FOR PREGNANT VEGETARIANS**

| Food | No. of Servings |
|---|---|
| Whole and enriched grains | 7 |
| Green and yellow vegetables | 3–5 |
| Fruits, including vitamin C | 3 |
| Dairy products | 3 |
| Legumes, soy products, meat substitutes | 2–3 |

Vitamin and mineral supplements may be necessary according to individual needs. Those who do not use dairy products need to increase sources of calcium and may need supplementation.

## Nausea and Vomiting of Pregnancy

Morning sickness usually occurs during the first trimester and disappears soon afterward, although some women experience nausea at other times of the day and for longer than 12 weeks. However, most women can consume enough food to maintain nutrition sufficiently. They are often able to manage frequent, small meals better than three large meals. Protein and complex carbohydrates are often tolerated best, but fatty foods increase nausea. Drinking liquids between meals instead of with meals often helps. At bedtime, a protein snack, such as cheese, helps to maintain glucose levels through the night. Eating a carbohydrate food like dry toast or crackers before getting out of bed in the morning helps to prevent nausea.

## Anemia

Anemia is a common concern during pregnancy. Although the normal hemoglobin level for non-pregnant women is 13.5 g/dl, hemoglobin values during the second trimester of pregnancy average 11.6 g/dl as a result of the dilution of the blood caused by plasma increases. This is often called *physiologic anemia* because it is normal (see Chapter 7). During the third trimester, hemoglobin levels generally rise to 12.5 g/dl because of increased absorption of iron from the gastrointestinal tract, even though iron is transferred to the fetus primarily during this time.

Fetal iron stores during the third trimester are sufficient to prevent anemia in the newborn for the first 4 to 6 months after birth. However, if the woman's intake of iron is insufficient, her hemoglobin levels may not rise during the third trimester, nutritional anemia may develop, and transfer of iron to the fetus may be decreased. One large nutritional survey among low-income women showed that more than 37 percent of women had hemoglobin levels of less than 11.0 g/dl (Perry et al., 1995).

Iron stores may be measured by determining the serum ferritin level of the blood. A ferritin level less than 12 micrograms per liter ($\mu$g/L) indicates that anemia is caused by iron deficiency. A woman may begin pregnancy with anemia, or it may develop during pregnancy. Pregnant women are considered anemic if the hemoglobin level drops below 10.5 to 11.0 g/dl (Laros, 1994).

Anemic women need help in choosing foods high in iron (see Table 9–5). They should take iron supplements because diet alone is unlikely to provide adequate amounts of iron. Iron supplements are best absorbed if taken between meals with a dietary source of vitamin C to increase absorption. Because high intakes of iron inhibit use of zinc and copper, anemic women may also need to take these minerals.

### Abnormal Pre-pregnancy Weight

The need for adjustments in the caloric intake according to pre-pregnancy weight has been described under weight gain. In addition to teaching about dietary changes, the nurse should be alert for other problems associated with abnormal pre-pregnancy weight. The woman who is below normal weight may not have enough money for food or may have an eating disorder. An obese woman may have other health problems, such as hypertension, that may affect the nurse's nutritional counseling plan.

### Eating Disorders

Eating disorders include anorexia nervosa (refusal to eat because of a distorted body image and feelings of obesity) and bulimia (overeating, sometimes followed by induced vomiting). Some women with these disorders eat normally during pregnancy for the sake of the fetus. In others, old fears about obesity may be reactivated by the normal weight gain of pregnancy. They may return to their previous eating patterns during pregnancy or in the early postpartum period when they do not lose weight immediately. These women need a great deal of individual counseling to be sure that they meet the increased nutrient needs of pregnancy and understand normal postpartum weight loss.

### Pica

The practice of eating substances not normally considered food is called pica. Clay or dirt and solid laundry starch are the most common materials involved, but other items, such as chalk, crushed ice, freezer frost, baking soda, burnt matches, or ashes may be included. Pica is more common in the southeastern United States but is not limited to any one socioeconomic or geographic area.

The cause of pica is unknown, although cultural values may make pica a common practice. Pica may be related to beliefs about the effect of the material eaten on labor or the baby. For example, some women believe that starch gives the skin a lighter tone or helps the baby to be born more easily. Some women may fear that their eating habits are harmful but may be unable to ignore the cravings. They may keep their eating practices secret from caregivers who might disapprove (Cooksey, 1995).

The major concern with pica is that eating nonfood substances decreases the intake of foods and, therefore, essential nutrients. Iron deficiency was once thought to be a cause of pica but is now considered a result. Clay and dirt may decrease absorption of other nutrients, such as iron, and may be contaminated with organisms.

**CRITICAL THINKING EXERCISE**

A woman very hesitantly confides in the nurse that the reason she is not gaining much weight is that she eats large amounts of ice. She buys bags of crushed ice or eats the frost that forms in her freezer. "I know I should be gaining more weight, but I'm just not hungry for anything besides ice," she says.

**Q:** How should the nurse handle this situation?

**A:** It is important to be accepting and nonjudgmental in responding to this woman. It is unlikely that she will end her pica, and she may withdraw and continue to practice it in secret if she feels that the nurse is disapproving. Therapeutic communication techniques are important to explore the woman's feelings about her cravings. A discussion of her feelings can then lead to teaching about nutrition. The nurse should determine how much ice the woman eats each day and whether she has other cravings. A 24-hour diet history assists in identifying deficient areas in the diet. The nurse can work with the woman to find ways to modify the diet to include more of the food groups that are lacking. She should be referred to a dietitian for further counseling, but the nurse should also discuss the diet at each prenatal visit.

### Multiparity

The number and spacing of pregnancies as well as the presence of more than one fetus influence the nutritional requirements. The woman who has had more than five pregnancies may begin a pregnancy with a nutritional deficit. In addition, she may be too busy meeting the needs of her family to be attentive to her own nutritional needs.

Closely spaced pregnancies may not allow a woman to make up any nutritional deficits originating during a previous pregnancy. Thus, she begins a new pregnancy with inadequate nutrient stores to maintain her own needs and fetal requirements. She is not able to draw from those stores, as is usual during pregnancy, and must meet nutritional needs from her daily diet and supplementation alone. The development of morning sickness from a new pregnancy soon after delivery may further interfere with an expectant mother's ability to eat an adequate diet.

The woman with a multifetal pregnancy must provide enough nutrients to meet the needs of each fetus without depleting her own stores. The expectant mother definitely needs more calories to meet her weight gain and energy needs. Suggested weight gain for women pregnant with twins is 10 to 20 pounds more than for women with single pregnancies. Supplementation with calcium, iron, and folic acid may also be necessary.

## Substance Abuse

The damaging effects of smoking, alcohol, and drug use on the fetus are discussed in Chapter 24. Substance abuse often accompanies a lifestyle that is unlikely to promote good eating habits. The expense of supporting a substance abuse habit may decrease money available for the purchase of food. Therefore, nutrition in pregnant women who abuse substances should be explored fully. Usually, more than one substance is involved, and the effects on nutrition of various combinations of substances are not fully understood.

### SMOKING

Cigarette smoking increases maternal metabolic rate and decreases appetite, which may result in a lower weight gain. Infant birth weight decreases in spite of adequate diet as the amount of smoking increases. Smoking causes vasoconstriction that interferes with blood flow through the placenta. The many chemicals found in cigarette smoke may also retard fetal growth. Smokers need more vitamins $B_{12}$ and C, folic acid, iron, zinc, and amino acids because smoking decreases the availability of these nutrients to both the pregnant woman and the fetus. Vitamin-mineral supplements may help meet their needs during pregnancy. Counseling to help the woman stop smoking or at least decrease the number of cigarettes smoked during pregnancy is important.

### CAFFEINE

The effect of caffeine on nutrition during pregnancy is not fully understood, but it may increase the risk of abortion and preterm or small-for-gestational age infants. It also changes calcium, zinc, and iron absorption or excretion. Until more is known about its effects on nutrition and the fetus, caffeine intake should be limited to two drinks a day during pregnancy. Because many women think that caffeine is present only in coffee and tea, the nurse should discuss other sources of caffeine. These include chocolate, some carbonated beverages, and some medications.

### ALCOHOL

Because of the association between drinking and fetal alcohol syndrome (see Chapter 24, p. 650) women should avoid alcohol completely during pregnancy. Alcohol interferes with absorption and use of some nutrients (protein, thiamine, folic acid, and zinc), impairs metabolism, and often takes the place of food in the diet. Vitamin-mineral supplementation may be necessary for women who had large intakes of alcohol before pregnancy, even if they stop drinking after conception, because their nutrient stores may be depleted.

### DRUGS

The use of drugs other than those prescribed during pregnancy increases danger to the fetus and may interfere with nutrition. Abusers often use a combination of various drugs. The interaction of various drugs with nutrients is not fully understood.

Marijuana increases appetite, but women may not satisfy their hunger with foods of good nutrient quality. Heroin interferes with insulin response to glucose and metabolism. Cocaine acts as an appetite suppressant, interfering with nutrient intake. The vasoconstriction that results from cocaine use decreases nutrient flow to the fetus. Cocaine users tend to drink more beverages with alcohol or caffeine. Amphetamines depress appetite. Women who use amphetamines for dieting should be warned that the drugs should be discontinued during pregnancy.

## Other Risk Factors

Women who follow food fads may be at risk for not meeting the requirements for pregnancy. Each diet must be carefully analyzed to determine its nutrient content. Women who have followed a severely restricted diet for a long period of time may have depleted nutrient stores. The nurse can help them understand nutrition during pregnancy and what diet changes they need to make to help ensure a successful pregnancy.

Women with complications of pregnancy, such as diabetes, heart disease, and pregnancy-induced hypertension, may require dietary alterations (see Chapters 25 and 26). Those with other medical conditions, such as extreme obesity, cystic fibrosis, and celiac disease, may need nutritional counseling from a dietitian.

**CHECK YOUR READING**

14. What nutritional problems should the nurse look for and assess when caring for low-income women?
15. What nutritional problems may the adolescent have during pregnancy?
16. What suggestions can the nurse give the vegan about diet during pregnancy?
17. How can lactose-intolerant women increase their intake of calcium?
18. What other conditions present nutritional risk factors during pregnancy?

## Nutrition After Birth

Nutritional requirements after birth depend on whether the mother breastfeeds her infant or gives formula. If she plans to breastfeed, the nurse should teach her how to adapt her diet to meet the needs of lactation. If she plans to use formula, the nurse can review the woman's nutritional knowledge as she returns to her pre-pregnancy diet.

### Nutrition for the Lactating Mother

The lactating mother must nourish both herself and her baby as she did during pregnancy. Therefore, she continues to need a highly nutritious diet. The RDAs for lactating women are significantly increased for calories, protein, magnesium, zinc, and vitamins A and C. They are lower than RDAs for pregnant women for iron and folic acid and remain the same for calcium. They are higher for almost every nutrient compared with the needs of the non-pregnant adult woman (see Table 9–3). These recommendations are based on the assumption that the mother produces approximately 750 to 800 ml of breast milk daily. However, the amount of milk produced varies according to the infant's age and whether the infant is taking formula or solid foods in addition to breast milk.

Lactating women are most likely to consume calcium, zinc, magnesium, vitamin $B_6$, and folic acid in amounts below the RDAs for nursing mothers (Institute of Medicine, 1991). A woman can produce milk that is adequate for her infant for at least the first 4 to 6 months even when her own diet is less than optimal. However, this production depletes her own nutrient stores.

#### ENERGY

During the first 6 months of lactation, a woman needs approximately 640 calories a day more than she required before she became pregnant. The RDA during lactation is 500 calories each day over normal needs for women according to age, weight, and height. The other 140 calories a day needed to produce breast milk are drawn from maternal stores, aiding in weight loss over a period of time. For the average adult woman, this represents a total caloric intake of 2700 calories each day. Women who were underweight before pregnancy and/or had inadequate weight gain during pregnancy need more calories. The recommendation for them is 650 additional calories each day, depending on their overall nutritional status.

#### PROTEIN

The RDA for protein during lactation is 65 g each day during the first 6 months and slightly less during the second 6 months. This is 5 g above that needed during pregnancy and 15 to 21 g above that required by non-pregnant women, depending on age. This small increase is easily met. A small (5-ounce) glass of milk supplies the extra protein needed and provides calcium as well.

#### VITAMINS AND MINERALS

Lactating women who take in at least 1800 calories (which is well below the energy intake recommended) probably consume adequate amounts of other essential nutrients to meet the infant's and their own needs. Although the quality of the milk is not affected by the mother's intake of most minerals, the vitamin content may be decreased if her diet is consistently low in vitamins. Nutrient levels in the milk may remain constant because some nutrients, such as calcium and folic acid, are drawn from the mother's stores if her intake is poor. Routine vitamin-mineral supplements are not necessary unless there is concern that the diet is lacking.

#### SPECIFIC CONCERNS

Some women are unlikely to regularly consume all the nutrients they require, and they need special counseling. This group includes women who are dieting, adolescents, vegans, women who avoid dairy products, and those whose diet is inadequate for other reasons.

##### DIETING

Women who are concerned about losing weight after pregnancy need special consideration. After the initial losses in the first month, the average weight loss for the lactating woman is approximately 1 to 2 pounds each month. This gradual decrease in weight occurs because maternal fat is used to meet a portion of the energy needs of lactation. Gradual weight loss is preferable and should be accomplished by a combination of moderate exercise and a diet high in nutrients with at least 1800 calories per day.

Dieting should be postponed for at least 3 weeks after birth to allow the woman to recover fully from childbirth and establish her milk supply if she is breastfeeding. Weight loss of more than 2 kg (about 4.5 pounds) a month or intakes below 1500 calories per day are likely to interfere with milk production and the mother's nutrient stores (Institute of Medicine, 1991). Although moderate dieting does not affect the quantity of the milk, the mother should evaluate the infant's apparent satisfaction with feedings. She should not use liquid diet drinks or diets that severely restrict any nutrient because she will not meet her needs. Nursing mothers should avoid appetite suppressants, which may pass into the milk and harm the infant.

#### ADOLESCENCE

The problems of the adolescent diet continue to be of concern during lactation. The adolescent may be deficient in the same nutrients listed for other mothers during lactation, and she may also be lacking in iron. If she dislikes or cannot afford fruits and vegetables, she may have an inadequate vitamin A intake.

#### VEGAN DIET

The milk of the vegan mother may contain inadequate vitamin $B_{12}$, and she and her infant need supplementation. Vitamin D and calcium may also be low. Vegans can meet their need for other nutrients during lactation by diet alone with careful planning. Those who are not knowledgeable about nutrition need supplementation.

#### AVOIDANCE OF DAIRY PRODUCTS

The recommendation for calcium remains the same for pregnancy and lactation, and the calcium content of breast milk is not affected by maternal intake. However, prolonged lactation with inadequate calcium intake may cause removal of calcium from the mother's bones. Women who do not eat dairy products should obtain calcium from other sources (see Table 9–6) or take a calcium supplement. Unless they consume foods fortified with vitamin D or have exposure to sunlight, they may also require vitamin D supplementation because it is necessary for calcium absorption.

#### INADEQUATE DIET

Women who have cultural or other food prohibitions may need help choosing a diet adequate for lactation. Those with inadequate income may need referral to agencies such as WIC. If the mother must take medications that interfere with absorption of certain nutrients, her diet should be high in foods containing those nutrients.

#### ALCOHOL

Alcohol intake during lactation is another concern. Although it was once thought that the relaxing effect of alcohol would be helpful to the nursing mother, the deleterious effects of alcohol are too important to consider this suggestion appropriate today. An occasional single glass of an alcoholic beverage may not be harmful, but larger amounts may interfere with the milk-ejection reflex and be harmful to the infant.

#### CAFFEINE

Foods high in caffeine should also be limited. The mother should restrict her caffeine intake to two cups of coffee or the equivalent each day. Caffeine in excessive amounts can make the infant irritable and may decrease the iron content of the milk.

#### FLUIDS

Nursing mothers should drink fluids sufficient to relieve thirst, which often increases in the early breastfeeding period. Eight to ten glasses of fluids, other than those containing caffeine, are adequate. There is no need to drink larger quantities of fluids, as was once recommended.

### FOODS TO AVOID

Lactating mothers are often concerned about whether they should avoid certain foods that might adversely affect the infant. Except for foods to which the mother is allergic, no specific foods must be restricted in every case. Most mothers find that few foods affect the infant and that fussiness is related to other factors.

## Nutrition for the Nonlactating Mother

The postpartum woman who is not breastfeeding can return to her pre-pregnancy diet, provided that it meets the RDA for the adult woman. She should plan her diet so that it contains enough protein and vitamin C foods to promote healing. If the woman was taking prenatal vitamin-mineral supplements, many nurse practitioners and obstetricians suggest that she continue to take them until her supply is finished. This ensures adequate intake during the early weeks, when involution occurs, and helps renew nutrient stores.

The nurse should assess the mother's understanding of the number of servings she needs from each food group. A review of important nutrient sources

## Breastfeeding Mothers Want to Know

### How Can I Tell Which Foods Are Affecting My Baby?

- Keep a list of any new foods you eat (those different from your usual diet).
- Observe for signs that the baby may be reacting to something you ate. Signs are excessive irritability, crying as if in pain, passing gas, diarrhea, or rash. Remember, these signs happen for other reasons besides a reaction to your diet, so consider other causes as well.
- When your baby has a fussy period, note whether you ate anything new during the previous 8 to 12 hours.
- Watch the baby's reaction after you have eaten any of the foods that sometimes cause problems for infants. These include foods in the cabbage family, onions, foods that are highly allergenic (wheat, eggs, cow's milk) or acidic (orange juice), spicy foods, garlic, nuts, chocolate, or large amounts of fresh fruits.
- If you think there may be a connection between something you ate and distress in your baby, avoid that food for several days to a week. Then try a small amount of the food again. If the baby seems to be affected, eliminate that food from your diet.
- Eat all foods in moderation. Babies often tolerate small amounts of any food in the mother's diet but react to large amounts.

for calcium and iron may be relevant. If a woman was anemic during pregnancy, she should continue to take an iron supplement until hemoglobin levels return to normal.

When her baby is born, a woman can expect to lose about 12 pounds immediately. She loses approximately another 8 pounds during the first 6 weeks and probably all but about 2 pounds by the end of the first year if she follows a well-balanced diet. She should take in 300 calories per day less than she did during pregnancy to avoid retaining weight.

Some women are impatient with slow weight loss and disappointed that they do not lose all their pregnancy weight gain soon after the baby is born. New mothers should wait at least 3 weeks to start dieting to lose weight because they need energy to meet the demands of infant care. Suggestions for sensible calorie reduction combined with exercise are appropriate. Women who gain a large amount of weight beyond that recommended during pregnancy may have more difficulty losing it after birth and take a longer time to do so. They may require help from a dietitian in planning a weight loss program.

Mothers are sometimes so involved with the needs of the infant during the early days that they fail to eat properly. They may snack instead of planning meals for themselves, especially if they are home alone with the baby during the day. The nurse should remind them that snacking often involves high caloric intake without meeting nutritional needs. This is a time when a mother needs to ensure her own good health so that she is able to care for her baby. Therefore, meals and snacks should be high in nutrient content.

### CHECK YOUR READING

19. How do the nutritional needs of the lactating mother compare with those of the woman who is not lactating? With those of the woman who is pregnant?
20. What should the breastfeeding woman avoid in her diet?
21. What changes should the woman who is not breastfeeding make after the birth of her baby?

## Application of Nursing Process: Nutrition for Childbearing

The nursing process focuses on determining the factors that might interfere with the woman's ability to meet the nutrient needs of pregnancy, the postpartum period, and lactation and on finding solutions to any problems identified. This process primarily involves education of the woman.

### Assessment

A number of methods are available to assess for nutritional problems. These methods are similar to those used for assessment of other problems.

#### INTERVIEW

The interview provides an opportunity to develop rapport and to determine whether any specific problems are present that affect dietary intake.

**Appetite.** Begin the interview by discussing the woman's appetite. Has it changed during the pregnancy, and how does it compare with her appetite before pregnancy? Morning sickness may decrease food intake during the first trimester. Determine the severity and duration of nausea and vomiting. For some women, the discomfort is mild and occurs only during the morning or when they are fatigued. For others, severe nausea continues throughout the day and beyond the first trimester. Hyperemesis gravidarum is the most serious form of this problem, often requiring intravenous correction of fluid and electrolyte imbalance (see Chapter 25, p. 689).

**Eating Habits.** Assess the usual pattern of meals to discover poor food habits, such as skipping breakfast or eating only snack foods for lunch. Determine who does the cooking for the family. The teenager whose mother cooks for her may have little choice about what she eats when at home. In that case, discuss nutritional needs during pregnancy with her mother. If the woman does the cooking herself, the likes and dislikes of other family members may influence what she serves, especially if she has little understanding of her own needs during pregnancy.

**Food Preferences.** Ask about her food preferences and dislikes. The woman who dislikes all fruits and vegetables needs another source of vitamins. During pregnancy, some women experience an aversion to certain foods, like meats, that they do not have at other times. Careful counseling helps to work around dislikes or aversions to find ways of obtaining the nutrients needed.

Discussing likes and dislikes provides an opening to ask about food cravings and pica. Cravings may be for nutritional foods or for foods low in nutrient density and eaten in amounts that interfere with intake of other foods. Ask about pica in a matter-of-fact way to avoid giving an impression of disapproval. Food items such as ice are sometimes included in pica, so ask about it as well. Also ask if the mother eats large amounts of any one particular food or group of foods.

**In assessing for pica, you might say, "Have you had any cravings for special things to eat during your pregnancy?" This can be followed by, "Women sometimes eat things like clay or starch during pregnancy. Are you fond of those?" Or "Do you have cravings for things that are not usually considered food—like clay or starch?" Some women substitute foods such as nonfat dry milk powder for nonfood items, like laundry starch.**

**Psychosocial Influences.** Ascertain whether cultural or religious considerations affect the diet. Do these apply only during pregnancy, or are they present at all times? Assess whether the woman follows them completely or whether she observes only certain restrictions. Determine the effect on her nutrient intake.

The interview may reveal other factors that interfere with adequate nutrition. Women with low incomes may not know about sources of help. Question the vegetarian to determine how long she has followed the practice and her awareness of changes necessary during pregnancy. A woman's smoking, alcohol intake, and other substance abuse may become obvious during the interview. Ask about prescription drugs, and determine whether she takes medications that interfere with nutrient absorption. Include questions about how much time she has for food preparation and the frequency of eating fast foods.

Ask the woman if she has any special concerns about her diet. This question may bring out fears about weight gain leading to obesity or concerns that specific foods could hurt the fetus. It also allows her to discuss issues that you have not yet addressed.

### DIET HISTORY

Diet histories provide information about a woman's usual intake of nutrients. Twenty-four-hour diet histories, food intake records, and food frequency questionnaires can form a basis for counseling about any changes required to meet pregnancy needs. They also help the woman become more aware of her eating habits.

**Twenty-Four-Hour Diet History.** Ask the woman to recall what she ate at each meal and snack during the previous 24 hours. Use specific questions about the size of portions, ingredients, and how foods were prepared, taking each meal individually. Inquire about beverages, as well as snacks between meals and at bedtime. Determine whether this sample is typical of her usual daily food intake; if not, ask which foods are more representative. Analyze the 24-hour diet history to determine whether the woman has met the recommendations for specific food groups, calories, and protein. Detailed analysis for individual nutrients is unnecessary because it is time-consuming and there may be a daily variation in intake.

The food history may be inaccurate if the woman cannot remember what she ate or is mistaken about the amounts of food. Models of food items and use of measuring utensils may be helpful. The expectant mother may wish to please the nurse and alter her reported intake to make it appear that she is eating better than she is. She may be embarrassed about her inability to follow the diet prescribed because of lack of money or cooking facilities. The atmosphere that you set is important in helping mothers feel free to be honest.

**Food Intake Records.** Food intake records are used to report foods eaten over one or more days. Ask the woman to list everything she eats throughout the day. The list is more accurate if she writes down each food immediately after eating; this avoids the problem of forgetfulness. Some women eat more nutritious foods during the recording period, when they are concentrating on good diet, then go back to a less wholesome diet later.

**Food Frequency Questionnaires.** Food frequency questionnaires may provide information about diet over a longer time. They contain lists of common foods. Review the questionnaire with the woman, and ask her how often she eats each food. Foods consumed daily or weekly are her most common source of nutrients. Analyze the list to determine whether foods from each food group are eaten in adequate amounts to meet pregnancy needs. Determine whether any major groups are omitted.

### PHYSICAL ASSESSMENT

Information about nutritional status can be obtained during the physical assessment that is part of each prenatal checkup. This assessment includes measurement of weight and examination for signs of nutritional deficiency.

**Weight at Initial Visit.** Weigh the woman at the first prenatal visit to get a baseline value for future comparison. Ask if this is her usual weight or if she has gained or lost weight. Measure her height without shoes, rather than asking her how tall she is because she may not have had an accurate recent measurement. Compare her pre-pregnancy weight for height to tables of normal values to help draw conclusions about her nutritional condition. If her weight is low for height, nutritional reserves are marginal. If it is high, she may be overweight or obese.

**Weight at Subsequent Visits.** Assessment of weight gain at each prenatal visit provides an easy method of estimating whether nutrition is adequate and serves as a basis for counseling about nutrition. Weigh the woman at each visit on the same scale with approximately the same amount of clothing. To obtain an accurate measurement, have her remove her shoes and coat.

Record the weight on a weight grid at each visit throughout the pregnancy. This grid allows examination of the pattern as well as the total gain to date. It also helps keep track of the amount of gain between individual visits. Figure 9–3 is an example of a weight gain grid. Measurement of skinfold thickness is often used in research to determine body fat changes, but its use in clinical practice is generally

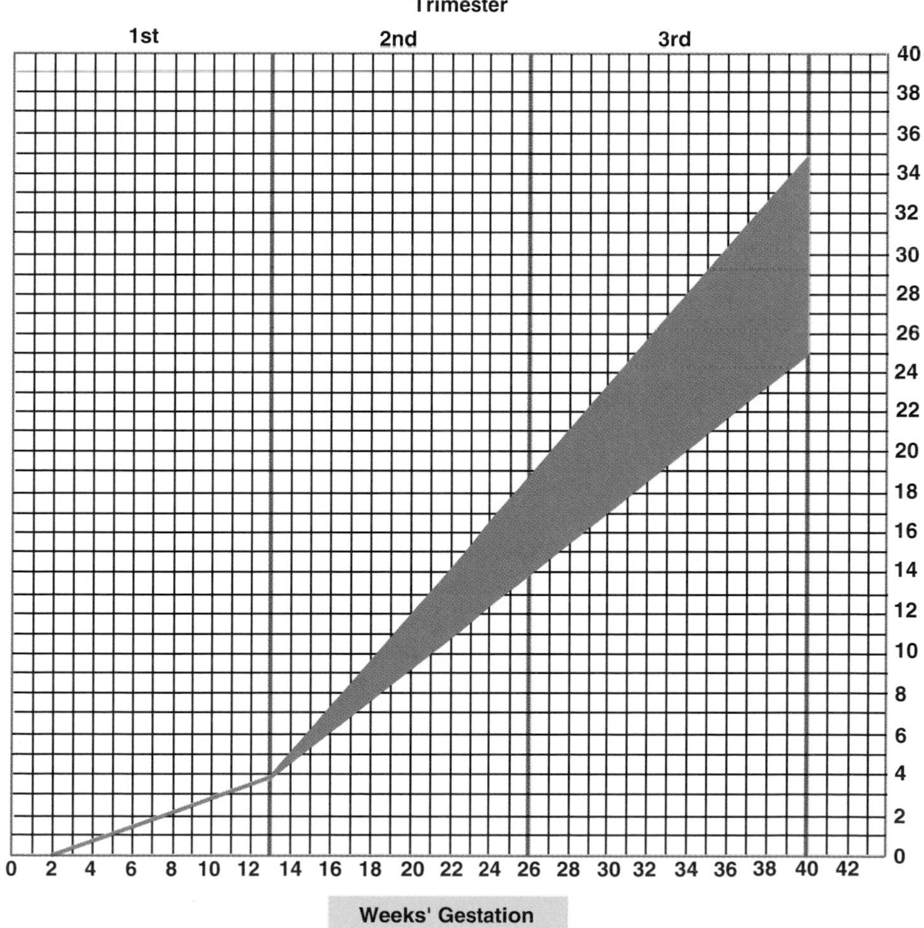


**FIGURE 9–3**

Weight gain grid for pregnancy. The normal range for weight gain is 25 to 35 pounds. Adolescents often need to gain in the higher end of the range. Women who are shorter than 62 inches should gain in the lower portion.

not helpful because there are no standardized recommendations for pregnancy.

**Be careful to avoid overemphasizing weight gain. In some instances, a woman may be afraid that caregivers will be disapproving if she gains weight, and, consequently, she may diet or fast a day or two before her prenatal visit.**

**Signs of Nutrient Deficiency.** Other indications of nutritional status include any signs of deficiency. For example, bleeding gums may indicate inadequate intake of vitamin C. However, actual deficiency states are not likely to occur in women in most industrialized countries. Even though intake may not be enough to allow for optimal health and storage of nutrients, most women obtain enough nutrients to avoid signs of deficiency. The most important exception is iron-deficiency anemia, which is common in a mild form. Signs and symptoms include pallor, low hemoglobin level, fatigue, and increased susceptibility to infection.

#### LABORATORY TESTS

Laboratory tests are generally impractical for in-depth analysis of nutrient intake. Analysis of specific nutrients is expensive and may be inaccurate because physiologic changes of pregnancy, rather than true deficits of nutrients, may be demonstrated. In addition, the normal laboratory values during pregnancy have not been determined for all laboratory tests. Hemoglobin, hematocrit, and in some cases serum ferritin are the tests most often used to determine anemia, particularly iron-deficiency anemia.

### Analysis

Although some women consume more calories than they need during pregnancy and risk obesity as a result, more women are likely to eat fewer nutrients than are recommended. The problem may be related to many factors, but the most common factor is general lack of knowledge. Therefore, the most important nursing diagnosis concerning nutrition is Altered Nutrition: Less Than Body Requirements related to lack of understanding about the nutrient needs of pregnancy.

### Planning

Goals for this nursing diagnosis are the following:

- The woman will consume a diet meeting the RDAs for nutrients throughout her pregnancy.
- The woman (of normal weight for height before pregnancy) will gain approximately 3 to 4 pounds during the first trimester. She will gain a pound a week during the second and third trimesters, for a total gain of 25 to 35 pounds.

### Interventions

#### IDENTIFYING PROBLEMS

After analysis of food likes and dislikes and a 24-hour diet history, identify any obvious areas of potential deficiency. For example, the woman might eat little meat, avoid vegetables, be lactose-intolerant, or follow a vegetarian diet. Determine also the woman's knowledge about the nutrient needs of pregnancy.

#### EXPLAINING NUTRIENT NEEDS

Use the woman's diet history as a basis to introduce information about nutrition during pregnancy. Explain the recommended servings from each food group. Help the woman analyze her own diet so that she understands the process and its importance. Determine whether she meets the number of servings recommended for each food group. Explain which important nutrients are provided in each food group and why they are necessary for her and the fetus.

Make a rough estimate of calories, protein, iron, and calcium in the diet for a general idea of intake of these nutrients. Compare the usual sources of these major nutrients with her diet history and favorite foods to help her determine whether she eats enough of these foods on a regular basis. Suggest ways she can increase nutrients that she is lacking.

#### PROVIDING REINFORCEMENT

Give frequent positive reinforcement when the woman is eating appropriately. Assist her in evaluating where changes in her diet may be necessary, and plan ways to overcome weaknesses in her present diet (Fig. 9–4). Ask her what problems she foresees in obtaining the nutrients she needs. Explore a variety of ideas with her on how she can overcome expected problems. Ask how this change will affect the rest of her family. Perhaps the changes she needs to make for her own needs would be beneficial for the entire family.

If the woman can read, give her written materials on nutrition during pregnancy and review them with her. If she can take the information home, she can review it often to ensure that she is eating what she should. A small pamphlet with pictures might be placed on the refrigerator to help her remember what foods she needs each day.

#### EVALUATING WEIGHT GAIN

Compare the woman's weight to a weight gain grid to ascertain whether she has gained the appropriate

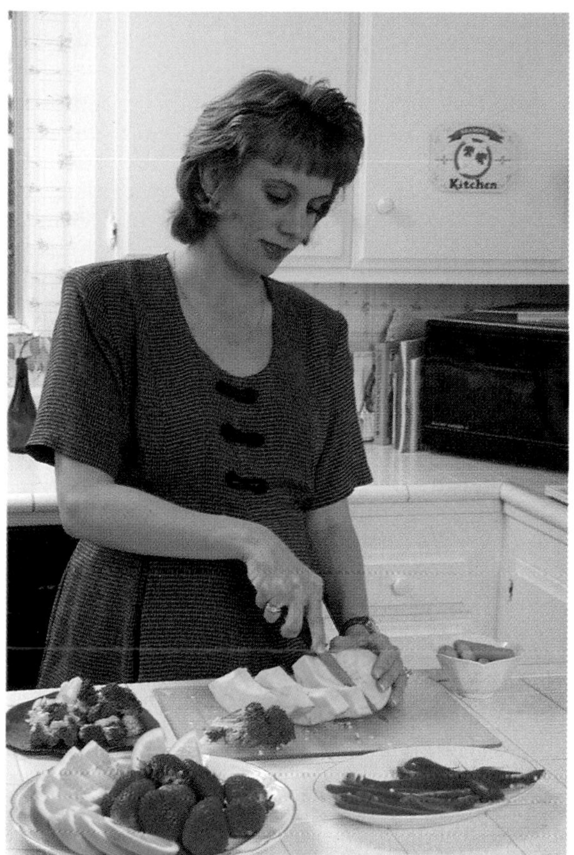

FIGURE 9-4

Women often make changes in their diets for the sake of their unborn child that they would not consider for themselves alone.

amount of weight for this point in her pregnancy. Discuss the importance of weight gain and the expected pattern of weight gain for her. Explain the importance of eating foods high in nutrient density when she is increasing calories. If she is greatly outside of normal ranges, discuss with her primary health care provider what modifications of her diet may be necessary. For example, an obese woman is expected to gain some weight, but the amount must be individualized according to her particular needs.

Although slight variations from the recommended weight gain have little significance, possible reasons for larger differences should be examined carefully. For women of normal weight, a monthly gain of less than 2 pounds (1 kg) should lead to a discussion of diet and possible problems in food intake. A gain of more than 6.5 pounds (3 kg) per month may signify a serious problem such as pregnancy-induced hypertension (see Chapter 25). However, errors in calculation of gestation may also reflect a pattern of weight gain different from that expected.

#### REASSESSING NUTRITIONAL STATUS AT EACH VISIT

At each office or clinic visit for prenatal care, reassess the woman's dietary status. Ask her how she is doing with the diet and if she has had any difficulty. Check her weight gain to see if she is within the expected pattern. Evaluate her hemoglobin and hematocrit levels to detect anemia. Explain what assessments are being made and why.

#### ASSESSING SUPPLEMENT INTAKE

If vitamin-mineral supplements have been prescribed, determine whether she is taking them regularly. If she is not taking the supplements, explore the reasons and possible solutions. Iron supplements often cause constipation, but dietary changes, such as increasing fluids and fiber, can help avoid this problem (Table 9–13). If the problem is forgetfulness, suggest that she take vitamin-mineral supplements with meals or iron supplements with orange juice at bedtime just before she brushes her teeth. If she avoids iron supplements because of side effects such as nausea, suggest that she take them with meals or a snack. Even though taking iron supplements with food decreases the absorption of the iron, it is preferable to not using the supplements at all. Let her know that black stools are a harmless side effect of taking an iron supplement.

#### MAKING REFERRALS

The nurse can provide nutritional counseling that is more than adequate for most women, but some situations may warrant referral to other sources. Women with health problems that affect nutrition may need an initial consultation with a dietitian and follow-up with the nurse. New diabetics, women with celiac disease, and women with extreme weight problems fall within this category. Women with inadequate financial resources to buy food can be referred to public assistance programs such as Aid to Families with Dependent Children or the WIC program. At the next visit, determine if the woman ob-

**TABLE 9–13 COMMON SOURCES OF DIETARY FIBER**

Fruits and vegetables, with skins when possible
- Apples, strawberries, pears, carrots, corn, potato with skin, cabbage, broccoli

Whole grains and whole grain products
- Whole wheat bread, bran muffins, bran cereals, oatmeal, brown rice, whole wheat pasta

Legumes
- Peas, lentils, kidney beans, lima beans, baked beans, peanuts

tained the help needed and whether other assistance is necessary.

### Evaluation

Ongoing evaluation of diet and pattern of weight gain throughout the pregnancy determines whether the goals have been met. The woman should meet the RDA for pregnancy by eating the recommended number of servings of each food group. She should gain 3 to 4 pounds during the first trimester and a pound a week for the second and third trimesters. Total weight gain should fall within 25 to 35 pounds.

## SUMMARY CONCEPTS

- Nutritional education during the childbearing period may have long-term positive effects on the mother, the infant, and the entire family.
- Weight gain during pregnancy is an important determinant of fetal growth. Poor weight gain in pregnant women is associated with low birth weight in infants; however, excessive weight gain may lead to macrosomia and labor complications.
- The recommended weight gain during pregnancy is 25 to 35 pounds. The amount is greater for women who are underweight or who carry more than one fetus, and it is less for obese women.
- The pattern of weight gain is as important as the total increase in weight. The average should be 3 to 4 pounds during the first trimester and a pound a week thereafter.
- The recommended increase in energy intake during pregnancy is 300 calories per day. Calorie increases should be attained by choosing foods high in nutrient density to meet the other needs of pregnancy.
- Protein should be increased to 60 g daily during pregnancy, an increase of 10 to 16 g over nonpregnancy needs. Although most North Americans obtain enough protein, the nurse should teach the woman about high-protein foods if necessary.
- Women may not eat enough foods high in vitamins $B_6$, D, and E and folic acid to meet recommendations. The nurse should encourage clients to eat more foods containing these vitamins.
- Fat-soluble vitamins (A, D, E, and K) are stored in the liver. Excess consumption may result in toxicity.
- Daily intake of water-soluble vitamins (B and C) is necessary because excesses are not stored but excreted.
- Minerals most likely to be consumed below recommended amounts in pregnancy are iron, calcium, zinc, and magnesium. Iron is often added as a supplement, whereas calcium is added for women with low intake. The nurse can suggest foods high in iron and calcium.
- Routine use of vitamin-mineral supplements is unnecessary and may lead to excessive intake and toxicity. Increased intake of some nutrients interferes with use of others and may result in deficiencies.
- Pregnant women should drink eight to ten 8-ounce glasses of fluids each day. They should eat at least seven servings of whole grains, five servings of fruits and vegetables, three servings of dairy products, and the equivalent of seven 1-ounce servings of protein foods.
- Culture can influence diet during pregnancy. The nurse should learn whether a woman follows traditional dietary practices and whether her food practices are consistent with good nutrition.
- Both Southeast Asian and Latino dietary practices include the importance of balancing yin and yang, or cold and hot. The nurse must know which foods are acceptable at what times.
- Low-income women may not have enough money or knowledge to meet the nutrient needs of pregnancy. The nurse should refer them for financial assistance and nutritional counseling.
- Adolescents may skip meals and eat snacks and fast foods of low nutrient density, and they are subject to peer pressure that may decrease their nutritional intake.
- Pregnant vegetarians may need help in choosing an adequate diet that includes non-animal sources of energy, protein, iron, calcium, vitamin $B_{12}$, and other nutrients. Vegetarians may need vitamin-mineral supplements during pregnancy.
- Lactose-intolerant women should increase calcium intake from foods other than milk, like calcium-rich vegetables.
- Abnormal pre-pregnancy weight, anemia, eating disorders, pica, grand multiparity, substance abuse, closely spaced pregnancies, and multifetal pregnancies are all nutritional risk factors that warrant adaptations of diet during pregnancy.
- Lactating women need more of almost every nutrient than women who are not lactating. The increased calories needed for milk production can be met by an added intake of 500 cal, and the rest comes from maternal fat stores.
- During lactation, mothers should avoid alcohol, caffeine, and foods that seem to cause distress in the infant.
- The postpartum woman who does not breastfeed should decrease her calorie intake by 300 calories but should eat a well-balanced diet to enhance recovery from childbirth. Weight loss should be accomplished slowly and sensibly.

#### References and Readings

Abrams, B. (1994). Maternal nutrition. In R.K. Creasy & R. Resnik (Eds.), *Maternal-fetal medicine: Principles and practice* (3rd ed.). Philadelphia: W.B. Saunders.

American Dietetic Association (1994). Position of the American Dietetic Association: Nutrition care for pregnant adolescents. *Journal of the American Dietetic Association, 94*(4), 449–450.

Andrews, M.M., & Boyle, J.S. (1995). *Transcultural concepts in nursing care* (2nd ed.). Philadelphia: J.B. Lippincott.

Brown, H.L., Watkins, K., & Hiett, A.K. (1996). The impact of the Women, Infants and Children Food Supplement Program on birth outcome. *American Journal of Obstetrics and Gynecology*, 174(4), 1279–1283.

California Department of Health Services (1990). *Nutrition during pregnancy and the postpartum period: A manual for health care professionals, summary*. Sacramento: Author.

Cerrato, P.L. (1993). Nutrition support: Suggest diets with a difference. RN, 56(2), 67–72.

Cooksey, N.R., (1995) Pica and olfactory craving of pregnancy: How deep are the secrets? *Birth*, 23(1), 129–137.

Cunningham, F.G., MacDonald, P.C., Gant, N.F., Leveno, K.J., Gilstrap, L.C., Hankins, G.D.V. & Clark, S.L. (1997). *Williams obstetrics* (20th ed.). Norwalk, Conn: Appleton & Lange.

D'Avanzo, C.E. (1992). Bridging the cultural gap with Southeast Asians. MCN: *American Journal of Maternal Child Nursing*, 17(4), 204–208.

Davis, J., & Sherer, K. (1994). *Applied nutrition and diet therapy for nurses* (2nd ed.). Philadelphia: W.B. Saunders.

Dobson, B. (1994). WIC highlights. *Journal of Human Lactation*, 10(3), 199–202.

Herbert, W.N.P., Dodds, J.M., & Cefalo, R.C. (1993). Nutrition in pregnancy. In R.A. Knuppel, & J.E. Drukker (Eds.), *High-risk pregnancy: A team approach* (2nd ed.). Philadelphia: W.B. Saunders.

Hutchinson, M.K., & Bazi-aziz, M. (1994). Nursing care of the childbearing Muslim family. *Journal of Obstetric, Gynecologic, and Neonatal Nursing*, 23(9), 767–771.

Institute of Medicine, National Academy of Sciences, Food and Nutrition Board (1990). *Nutrition during pregnancy*. Part I: *Weight gain*. Part II: *Nutrient supplements*. Washington, D.C.: National Academy Press.

Institute of Medicine, National Academy of Sciences, Food and Nutrition Board (1991). *Nutrition during lactation*. Washington, D.C.: National Academy Press.

Institute of Medicine, National Academy of Sciences, Subcommittee for a Clinical Application Guide (1992). *Nutrition during pregnancy and lactation, an implementation guide*. Washington, D.C.: National Academy Press.

Johnson, J.W.C., Longmate, J.A., & Frentzen, B. (1992). Excessive maternal weight gain and pregnancy outcome. *American Journal of Obstetrics and Gynecology*, 174(4), 1279–1283.

Knuppel, R.A., & Drukker, J.E. (1993). *High-risk pregnancy: A team approach* (2nd ed.). Philadelphia: W.B. Saunders.

Lappé, F.M. (1991). *Diet for a small planet*. New York: Ballantine.

Laros, R.K. (1994). Maternal hematolgic disorders. In R.K. Creasy & R. Resnik (Eds.), *Maternal-fetal medicine: Principles and practice* (3rd ed.). Philadelphia: W.B. Saunders.

Lawrence, R.A. (1994). *Breastfeeding: A guide for the medical profession* (4th ed.). St. Louis: C.V. Mosby.

Lust, K.D., Brown, J.E., & Thomas, W. (1996). Maternal intake of cruciferous vegetables and other foods and colic symptoms in exclusively breastfed infants. *Journal of the American Dietetic Association*, 96(1), 46–48.

Mahan, L.K., & Escott-Stump, S. (1996). *Krause's food, nutrition, and diet therapy* (9th ed.). Philadelphia: W.B. Saunders.

Mattson, S. (1995). Culturally sensitive perinatal care for Southeast Asians. *Journal of Obstetric, Gynecologic, and Neonatal Nursing*, 24(4), 335–341.

Merlin, R. (1992). Understanding bulimia and its implications in pregnancy. *Journal of Obstetric, Gynecologic, and Neonatal Nursing*, 21(3), 199–205.

National Research Council (1989). *Recommended dietary allowances* (10th ed.). Washington, D.C.: National Academy Press.

Neuhouser, M.L.S. (1996). Nutrition during pregnancy and lactation. In L.K. Mahan, & S. Escott-Stump, *Krause's food, nutrition, and diet therapy* (9th ed.). Philadelphia: W.B. Saunders.

Peckenpaugh, N.J., & Poleman, C.M. (1995). *Nutrition essentials and diet therapy* (7th ed.). Philadelphia: W.B. Saunders.

Perry, G.S., Yip, R., & Zyrkowski, C. (1995). Nutritional risk factors among low-income pregnant U.S. women: The Centers for Disease Control and Prevention (CDC) pregnancy nutrition surveillance system 1979 through 1993. *Seminars in Perinatology*, 19(3), 211–221.

Purfield, P., & Morin, K. (1995). Excessive weight gain in primigravidas with low-risk pregnancy: Selected obstetric consequences. *Journal of Obstetric, Gynecologic, and Neonatal Nursing*, 24(5), 434–439.

Romanczuk, A.N., & Brown, J.P. (1994). Folic acid will reduce risk of neural tube defects. MCN: *American Journal of Maternal Child Nursing*, 19(6), 331–334.

Rose, N.C., & Mennuti, M.T. (1995). Periconceptional folic acid supplementation as a social intervention. *Seminars in Perinatology*, 19(4), 243–254.

Scholl, T.O., & Hediger, M.L. (1995). Weight gain, nutrition, and pregnancy outcome. Findings from the Camden study of teenage and minority gravidas. *Seminars in Perinatology*, 19(3), 171–181.

Scholl, T.O., Hediger, M.L., Schall, J.I., Khoo, C., & Fischer, R.L. (1994). Maternal growth during pregnancy and the competition for nutrients. *American Journal of Clinical Nutrition*, 60, 183–188.

Seidman, R.Y., Jacobson, S., Primeaux, M., Burns, P., & Weatherby, F. (1996). Assessing American Indian families. MCN: *American Journal of Maternal/Child Nursing*, 21(6), 274–279.

Springer, N.S., Bischoping, K., Sampselle, C.M., Mayes, F.L., & Petersen, B.A. (1992). Using early weight gain and other nutrition-related risk factors to predict pregnancy outcomes. *Journal of the American Dietetic Association*, 92(2), 217–219.

Stowers, S.L. (1992). Development of a culturally appropriate food guide for pregnant Caribbean immigrants in the United States. *Journal of the American Dietetic Association*, 92(3), 331–336.

U.S. Department of Agriculture (1992, April). USDA's food guide pyramid. *Home and Garden Bulletin*, No. 249.

U.S. Department of Agriculture and U.S. Department of Health and Human Services (1990, November). Nutrition and your health: Dietary guidelines for Americans (3rd ed.). *Home and Garden Bulletin*, No. 232.

U.S. Department of Commerce (1992). *Summary population and housing characteristics—United States*. Washington, D.C.

U.S. Department of Health and Human Services, Public Health Service (1995). *Healthy people 2000: Midcourse review and 1995 revisions*. Washington, D.C.

Werler, M.M., Shapiro, S., & Mitchell, A.A. (1993). Periconceptional folic acid exposure and risk of occurrent neural tube defects. *Journal of the American Medical Association*, 269(10), 1257–1261.

Willett, W.C. (1992). Folic acid and neural tube defect: Can't we come to closure? *American Journal of Public Health*, 82(5), 666–668.

Williams, S.R. (1993). *Nutrition and diet therapy* (7th ed.). St. Louis: Times Mirror/Mosby.

Williams, S.R. (1997). Nutrition assessment and guidance in prenatal care. In B. Worthington-Roberts & S.R. Williams (Eds.), *Nutrition in pregnancy and lactation* (6th ed.). St. Louis: Times Mirror/Mosby.

Worthington-Roberts, B.S. (1997a). Energy and vitamin needs during pregnancy. In B. Worthington-Roberts & S.R. Williams (Eds.), *Nutrition in pregnancy and lactation* (6th ed.). St. Louis: Times Mirror/Mosby.

Worthington-Roberts, B.S. (1997b). Mineral needs during pregnancy. In B. Worthington-Roberts & S.R. Williams (Eds.), *Nutrition in pregnancy and lactation* (6th ed.). St. Louis: Times Mirror/Mosby.

Worthington-Roberts, B.S. (1997c). Nutrition, fertility, and family planning. In B. Worthington-Roberts & S.R. Williams (Eds.), *Nutrition in pregnancy and lactation* (6th ed.). St. Louis: Times Mirror/Mosby.

Worthington-Roberts, B.S., & Rees, J.M. (1997). The pregnant adolescent. Special concerns. In B. Worthington-Roberts & S.R. Williams (Eds.), *Nutrition in pregnancy and lactation* (6th ed.). St. Louis: Times Mirror/Mosby.

# 10

# Fetal Diagnostic Tests

**OBJECTIVES**

1. Identify indications for fetal diagnostic procedures.
2. Discuss the purpose, procedure, advantages, and risks of specific diagnostic procedures:
   Fetal ultrasonography
   Doppler ultrasound blood flow assessment
   Alpha-fetoprotein testing
   Chorionic villus sampling
   Amniocentesis
   Fetal surveillance techniques such as nonstress test, vibroacoustic stimulation test, contraction stress test, and biophysical profile
   Percutaneous umbilical blood sampling
   Maternal assessment of fetal movement
3. Provide information for common questions parents have about procedures.

**DEFINITIONS**

**alpha-fetoprotein** *Plasma protein produced by the fetus.*

**amniocentesis** *Transabdominal puncture of the amniotic sac to obtain a sample of amniotic fluid that contains fetal cells and biochemical substances for laboratory examination.*

**biophysical profile** *Method for evaluating fetal status during the antepartum period based on five variables originating with the fetus: fetal heart rate, breathing movements, gross movements, muscle tone, and amniotic fluid volume.*

**chorionic villus sampling** *Transcervical or transabdominal sampling of chorionic villi (projections of the outer fetal membrane) for analysis of fetal cells.*

**contraction stress test** *Method for evaluating fetal status during the antepartum period by observing response of the fetal heart to the stress of uterine contractions that may induce recurrent episodes of fetal hypoxia.*

**late deceleration** *Slowing of the fetal heart rate after the onset of a uterine contraction and persisting after the contraction ends.*

**lecithin/sphingomyelin ratio (L/S ratio)** *Ratio of two phospholipids in amniotic fluid that is used to determine fetal lung maturity; an L/S ratio greater than 2 : 1 usually indicates fetal lung maturity.*

**neural tube defect** *A congenital defect in closure of the bony encasement of the spinal cord or of the skull. Neural tube defects include anencephaly, spina bifida, meningocele, myelomeningocele, and others.*

**nonstress test** *A method for evaluating fetal status during the antepartum period by observing the response of the fetal heart rate to fetal movement.*

**percutaneous umbilical blood sampling (PUBS or cordocentesis)** *Procedure for obtaining fetal blood through ultrasound-guided puncture of an umbilical cord vessel to detect fetal problems such as inherited blood disorders, acidosis, or infection.*

**phosphatidylglycerol** *A major phospholipid of surfactant; its presence in amniotic fluid indicates fetal lung maturity.*

**phosphatidylinositol** *A phospholipid of surfactant; produced and secreted in increasing amounts as the fetal lungs mature.*

**placenta previa** *Abnormal implantation of the placenta in the lower uterus, at or very near the cervical os.*

**surfactant** *Combination of lipoproteins produced by the lungs of the mature fetus to reduce surface tension in the alveoli, thus promoting lung expansion after birth.*

**triple-marker screening** *Analysis of maternal serum for abnormal levels of alpha-fetoprotein, human chorionic gonadotropin, and estriols that may predict chromosomal abnormalities of the fetus.*

**ultrasonography** *Technique for visualizing deep structures of the body by recording the reflections (echoes) of sound waves directed into the tissue.*

**uteroplacental insufficiency** *Inability of the placenta to exchange oxygen, carbon dioxide, nutrients, and waste products properly between the maternal and fetal circulations.*

**vibroacoustic stimulation test** *Use of sound stimulation to elicit fetal movement and acceleration (speeding up) of the fetal heart rate.*

Until recently, only nonspecific methods were available to assess the condition of the fetus. Fundal height was measured to estimate fetal growth; the fetal heart rate was auscultated; and the mother's perception of fetal movements was noted. In recent years, however, the development of a variety of sophisticated methods has made it possible to detect physical abnormalities in the fetus and to monitor the fetal condition with greater accuracy.

The ability to predict fetal outcome offers reassurance for some parents but not for all. If the fetus is free of anomalies and is determined to be in good condition, the parents experience a feeling of relief and reduced anxiety. If fetal health is uncertain and the tests must be repeated, however, parents may experience anxiety throughout the pregnancy. If fetal anomalies are identified, parents are then faced with the choice of whether to continue or to terminate the pregnancy. This decision can create emotional conflict as well as ethical dilemmas that impose a great deal of stress on the family.

## Indications for Fetal Diagnostic Tests

At this time most fetal diagnostic procedures are reserved for pregnancies in which there is reason to believe the fetus may experience developmental or physical problems. Many physicians, however, believe that certain tests, such as ultrasonography and maternal serum screening, should be offered to all women.

In general, two reasons exist for performing diagnostic procedures: to detect congenital anomalies and to evaluate the condition of the fetus. Some procedures, such as amniocentesis and ultrasonography, are used for both purposes. They are used in early and midpregnancy to detect congenital defects, but they are used in the latter half of pregnancy to determine fetal maturity.

Many factors increase the risk for the fetus during pregnancy. These include maternal medical conditions, such as diabetes and hypertension. Demographic factors such as age and poverty as well as obstetric factors such as prior birth of a stillborn infant or an infant with congenital anomalies increase the risk to the current pregnancy. Table 10–1 provides a more complete list of indications for fetal diagnostic procedures.

## Ultrasonography

When high-frequency sound waves are aimed in a specific direction, they are deflected by objects in their path and return as echoes. The amount of energy returned as an echo depends on the density of the object that deflected the ultrasonic wave. In obstetrics, when ultrasonic waves are directed through the maternal abdomen, they are deflected by tissue and returned as two-dimensional images showing structures of different densities (Fig. 10–1).

Almost all ultrasound procedures in obstetrics now use real-time scanning, so that a rapid sequence of fixed images is displayed on the screen, showing movement as it happens. This technique allows the observer to detect fetal heart beat, fetal breathing activity, and fetal body movement.

### Emotional Responses

As might be expected, the parents' response to ultrasonography varies widely. Some expectant mothers exhibit excitement and pleasure and report feel-

**TABLE 10–1 INDICATIONS FOR FETAL DIAGNOSTIC PROCEDURES**

| |
|---|
| **Medical Conditions** |
| Preexisting diabetes mellitus or gestational diabetes |
| Hypertension (chronic or pregnancy-induced) |
| Chronic infections (such as pyelonephritis) |
| Sexually transmissible diseases |
| Anemia |
| Parents carry or exhibit genetic disorder (such as sickle cell anemia, cystic fibrosis) |
| **Demographic Factors** |
| Maternal age <16 or >35 years |
| Poverty |
| Nonwhite (twice the risk of neonatal or infant death) |
| Inadequate prenatal care (initial visit after 20 weeks' gestation or fewer than five prenatal visits to physician or nurse-midwife) |
| **Obstetric Factors** |
| History of low-birth-weight infant (<2500 g) |
| Multifetal pregnancy |
| Malpresentation (breech, shoulder) |
| Previous fetal loss or birth of infant with congenital anomaly |
| Previous infant >4000 g at birth |
| Hydramnios (>2000 ml at term) |
| Oligohydramnios (<500 ml at term) |
| Decrease or absence in fetal movements |
| Uncertainty about gestational age |
| Suspected intrauterine growth restriction |
| Postmaturity (>42 weeks) |
| Preterm labor (>20 weeks and <38 weeks of gestation) |
| Grand multiparity (>5 pregnancies) |
| **Concurrent Maternal Factors** |
| Less than ideal-weight-for-height at conception |
| More than 20% above ideal-weight-for-height at conception |
| Inadequate weight gain or poor pattern of weight gain |
| Excessive weight gain |
| Use of drugs, alcohol, tobacco |

ings of love and protectiveness when they view the fetus. Others, however, report increased feelings of vulnerability and anxiety about the fetus. Some mothers state that they fear something will be found wrong, and they dread the procedure for this reason.

Expectant fathers are often fascinated by fetal movement and insist that the fetus "waved" at them or that they could see the facial expression as the fetus looked directly at them. Some couples wish to be told if the fetus is male or female and are either disappointed or pleased with the news. Others do not want to know the sex of the child, even if it is obvious, and prefer to wait and "be surprised."

Although ultrasonography is not yet a standard of care for all women, it is widely used because a great deal of information can be obtained with minimum risk to mother or fetus. Ultrasonography may be used during any trimester, but the procedure and the reasons for its use vary.

## First Trimester

During the first trimester, transvaginal ultrasonography is often used because it allows clear visibility of the uterus, gestational sac, embryo, and deep pelvic structures, such as the ovaries and fallopian tubes.

### PROCEDURE

The woman is placed in a lithotomy position for transvaginal ultrasonography. A transvaginal probe, which is encased in a disposable cover and coated with a gel that provides lubrication and promotes conductivity, is inserted into the vagina. The woman may feel more comfortable if she is allowed to insert the probe. The procedure takes about 10 to 15 minutes.

### PURPOSES

During the first trimester, ultrasonography is most frequently used to do the following:

- Confirm pregnancy
- Verify the location of the pregnancy (uterine or ectopic)
- Detect multifetal gestations
- Determine gestational age
- Confirm fetal viability
- Determine the position of the uterus, cervix, and area of placental formation for transcervical chorionic villus sampling
- Guide the needle insertion for transabdominal chorionic villus sampling

During the first trimester, gestational age is based on the appearance of the gestational sac, which can be seen as early as 4 weeks after the last menstrual

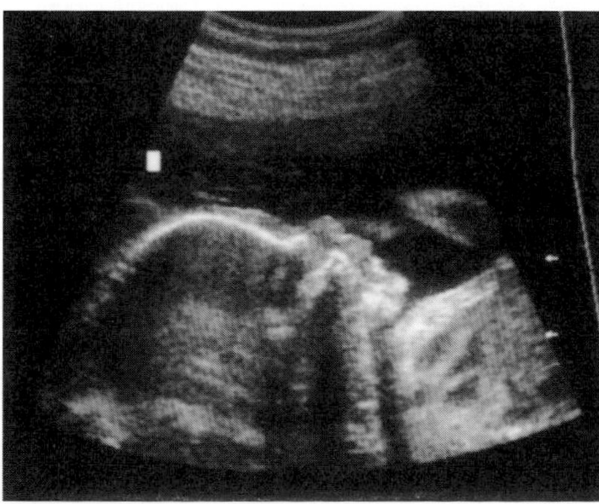

**FIGURE 10–1**

Sonogram showing profile of fetal facial structures. (Courtesy of Karin Buxton.)

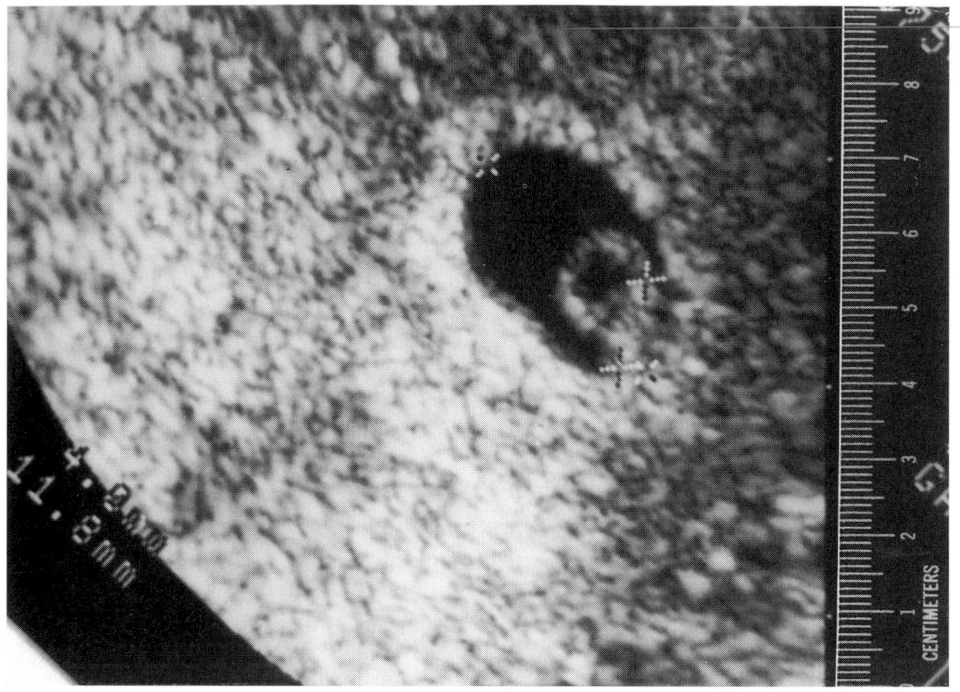


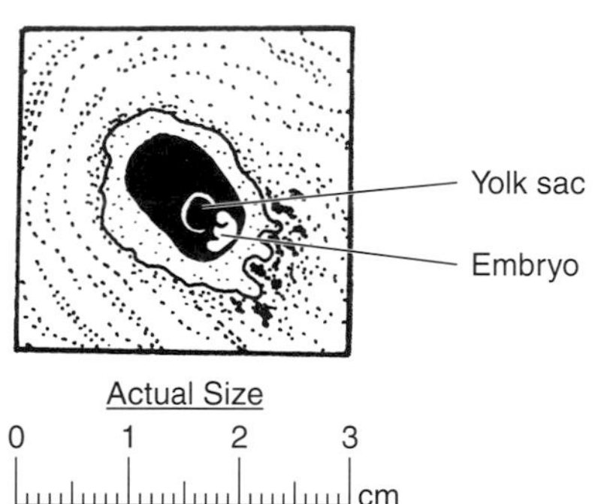


**FIGURE 10–2**

Sonogram showing chorionic cavity, yolk sac, and embryo at 6 weeks' gestation (based on last menstrual period). (From DuBose, T.J. [1996]. *Fetal sonography*. Philadelphia: W.B. Saunders. Sonogram by T.J. DuBose, MS, RDMS.)

period (Berman, 1996). During the sixth week the embryo and adjacent yolk sac are visible. At this time, the crown-to-rump length of the embryo is the most reliable indicator of gestational age (DuBose, 1996) (Fig. 10–2).

Fetal viability is confirmed by observation of fetal heart beat, which is visible by the eighth week following the last menstrual period. The heart beat is rapid, with a normal heart rate of 168 beats per minute (BPM). In addition, embryonic organs can be studied for normal growth and appearance (Berman, 1996). Maternal abnormalities, such as bicornuate uterus, uterine fibroids, and ovarian cysts are also visible.

## Second and Third Trimesters

During the second and third trimesters the uterus extends out of the pelvis, allowing clear views of the fetus and placenta, which are no longer obstructed by pelvic bones. As a result, transabdominal ultrasonography is most often used.

### PROCEDURE

The expectant mother is positioned on her back with the head and knees supported by pillows. If she desires, a display panel can be positioned so that she (and the father) can see the images on the screen. Her head should be elevated, and she should be turned slightly to one side to prevent supine hypotension, which may be caused by compression of the vena cava and aorta by the gravid uterus. A wedge or rolled blanket is placed under one hip to help her maintain this position comfortably. Warm mineral oil or transmission gel is spread over her abdomen, and the sonographer (nurse, physician, or ultrasound technician) slowly moves a transducer over the abdomen to obtain a picture (Fig. 10–3).

The procedure takes 10 to 30 minutes. The sonog-

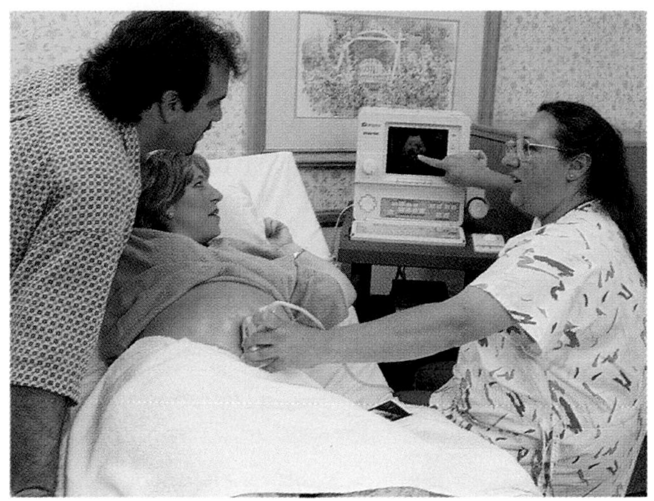

**FIGURE 10-3**

The nurse provides information as she moves an ultrasound transducer over the mother's abdomen to obtain an image.

rapher can "freeze" a picture and copy it for permanent records or for the parents if they wish. Many new ultrasound systems offer video taping of the evaluation, and some facilities provide a small section of video tape for the parents.

During the second trimester a full bladder may make it easier for sound waves to reach the pelvic viscera. A urine-filled bladder displaces the gas-filled intestines and elevates the uterus for better visibility. If a full bladder is necessary, the woman should be instructed to drink 1 to 2 quarts of clear fluid an hour before the time of the examination, and she should be instructed not to void until the examination is completed. Some discomfort may be felt as the transducer is moved over the distended bladder.

#### PURPOSES

Ultrasonography is used throughout the second and third trimesters to do the following:

- Confirm gestational age
- Locate the placenta when there is vaginal bleeding and placenta previa is suspected
- Determine fetal malpresentation (breech, shoulder)
- Evaluate amniotic fluid volume (see biophysical profile, p. 239)
- Monitor and document fetal movements
- Guide needle placement when amniocentesis or percutaneous umbilical blood sampling is necessary

Various measurements are used to determine gestational age during the last half of pregnancy. These include biparietal diameter, femur length, and abdominal circumference. The biparietal diameter is most accurate (±7 days) from 12 to 20 weeks (Manning, 1994). Ultrasonography is usually not used for dating after 30 weeks, but abdominal circumference, biparietal diameter, and femur length provide some data to consider.

Gestational age must be determined accurately when screening for maternal serum alpha-fetoprotein (AFP), which is altered by fetal age. Accurate gestational age is also important if intrauterine growth restriction is suspected or if there is a question about the expected date of delivery.

Assessment of fetal movements is important because coordination of whole-body movement requires complex neurologic control, which indicates that the nervous system is functioning well. On the other hand, a lower-than-expected number of body movements may predict fetal compromise, especially if placental perfusion is suspected to be inadequate, with resulting fetal hypoxia and acidosis.

In the second trimester, ultrasound may be *targeted* toward specific evaluation of fetal anatomy and physiology. Targeted ultrasonography is indicated when an increased risk exists for fetal anomalies. Risk factors include prior birth of an infant with anomalies or abnormal clinical findings, such as *hydramnios* (excessive amniotic fluid), *oligohydramnios* (insufficient amniotic fluid), or abnormal levels of AFP. Fetal anatomy is carefully and systematically examined to identify major system and organ anomalies. Anomalies that can be detected with targeted ultrasonography include neural tube defects, protrusion of intestine through the intestinal wall (gastroschisis), malformed kidneys, hydrocephalus, obstruction in fetal bowel or urinary system, and cleft lip and palate.

Ultrasonography may be also used to evaluate placental maturity on the basis of identification and distribution of calcium deposits within the placenta and the increasing delineations that occur as the placenta matures.

### Advantages

Ultrasonography is one of the most important tools in modern obstetric care. It allows clear visibility of the fetus and surrounding structures, and it is safe. No clinically significant adverse effects have been reported (Veille et al., 1993; Anthony, 1996). Ultrasonography is noninvasive and relatively comfortable; moreover, results are obtained immediately. It is widely available and portable, so that it can be moved to the area of need.

### Disadvantages

The cost of ultrasonography can be a problem for a woman who does not have insurance or who does not have access to prenatal care in the first trimester of pregnancy.

## Doppler Ultrasound Blood Flow Assessment

The ability to study blood flow in the fetus and the placenta is a relatively new advance in perinatal medicine. When an ultrasound wave is directed at an acute angle to a moving target, as with blood flowing through a vessel, the frequency of echoes is changed as the cardiac cycle goes through systole and diastole. This change, referred to as the *Doppler shift*, indicates forward movement of blood within a vessel.

### Purpose

The primary indication for Doppler ultrasonography is to detect or confirm intrauterine growth restriction, which is recognizable because of characteristic blood flow abnormalities (Cartier, 1996). Doppler ultrasonography has been used most extensively to study blood velocity through the umbilical vessels and the placenta. Although a great deal of information may be obtained, Doppler ultrasound investigation is currently not a standard of care. Given the present state of knowledge, Doppler velocity testing should be considered in the context of other abnormal test results in formulating a management plan (ACOG, 1994).

### Color Doppler

The location of any Doppler shift can be imaged as either red or blue, depending on whether the direction of the flow is toward the transducer or away from the transducer, respectively. Figure 10–4 illustrates the use of color Doppler imaging to measure blood flow and velocity in umbilical vessels. Color Doppler imaging is also useful in the study of fetal vessels, such as the aorta, middle cerebral artery, and ductus arteriosus (Farmakides et al., 1994).

**CHECK YOUR READING**

1. What are the major indications for ultrasonography during the first trimester? During the second trimester?
2. How does the procedure for first-trimester ultrasonography differ from that performed during the second trimester?
3. What are the major advantages and disadvantages of ultrasonography?

## Alpha-Fetoprotein Screening

Alpha-fetoprotein is the predominant protein in fetal plasma. It is synthesized by the embryonic yolk sac, the developing fetal liver, and the gastrointestinal tract. Alpha-fetoprotein diffuses from fetal plasma into fetal urine and is excreted into the amniotic fluid. Although a portion of the AFP in amniotic fluid is swallowed and digested by the fetus, the remain-

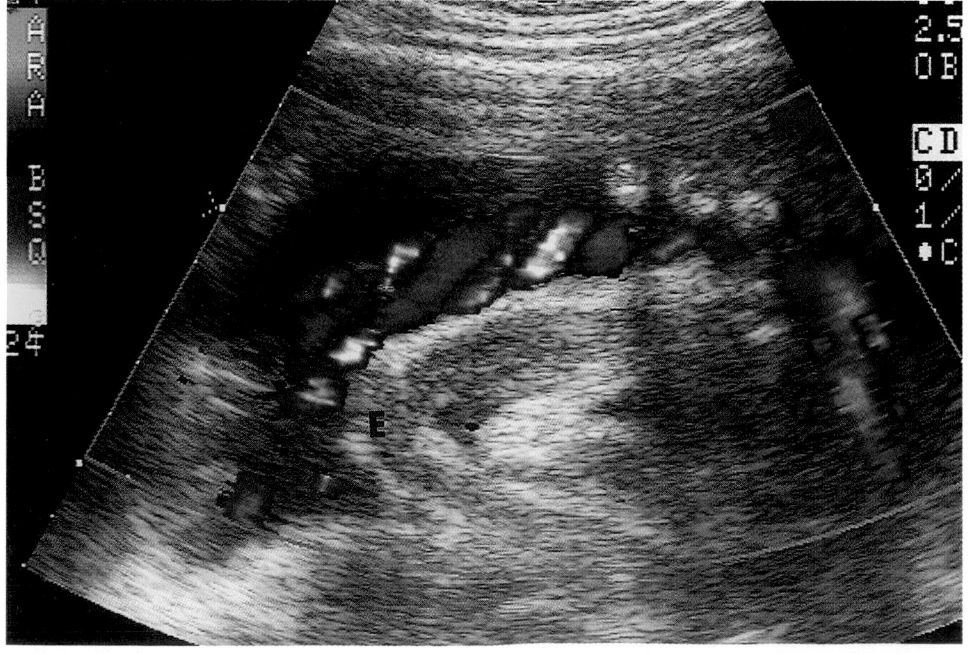


**FIGURE 10–4**

Color Doppler imaging of the umbilical vein and two arteries. Blood flow toward the transducer is shown as blue and the flow away as red. Three fetal fingers can be seen to grasp and press the cord against the other wrist. (From DuBose, T.J. [1996]. *Fetal sonography*. Philadelphia: W.B. Saunders. Sonogram by T.J. DuBose, MS, RDMS.)

der crosses placental membranes into the maternal circulation. Therefore, AFP can be measured in maternal serum (MSAFP) as well as in amniotic fluid (AFAFP). Abnormal concentrations of AFP can be associated with serious fetal anomalies.

## Purpose

Several conditions are associated with abnormal levels of MSAFP. Low levels of MSAFP suggest chromosomal anomalies, such as trisomy 21. The most common cause of elevated MSAFP is failure of the embryonic neural tube to close properly, leaving the neural tube open. In this condition neural tissue is totally exposed or is covered with only a very thin layer of tissue, allowing high levels of AFP to seep into amniotic fluid and enter maternal serum.

The most common open neural tube defects are (1) anencephaly, in which the cranial vault is absent and most of the brain is undeveloped and (2) spina bifida. Spina bifida ranges in severity from spina bifida occulta, which is barely noticeable, to meningocele, in which the meninges protrude from the spinal canal, to myelomeningocele, in which the spinal cord as well as the meninges protrude through the defect and extensive nerve damage may be expected. See Table 10–2 for additional conditions that are associated with abnormal MSAFP.

To avoid inaccurate test results, the clinician must adjust MSAFP values according to multiple factors.

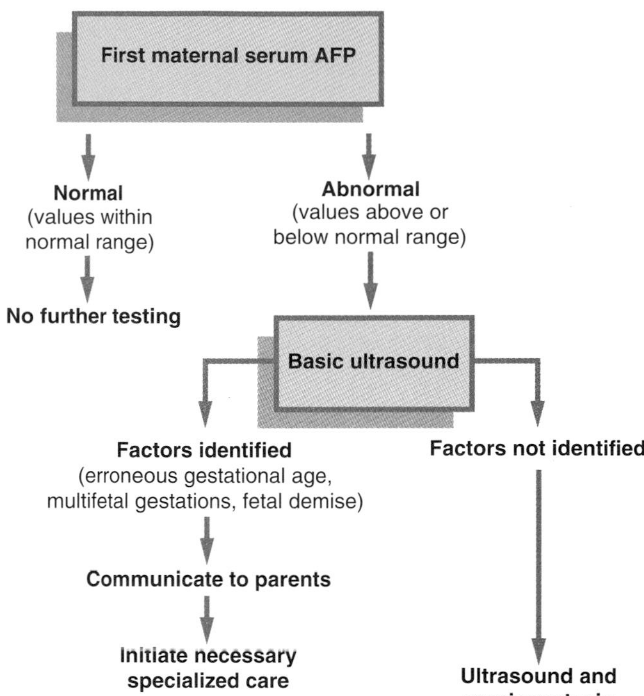


**FIGURE 10–5**

Abnormal levels of maternal serum alpha-fetoprotein (MSAFP) indicate the need for further testing to identify the cause.

For instance, gestational age, maternal weight, multifetal pregnancy, and maternal diabetes can all affect MSAFP. Without appropriate adjustments, such as confirmation of gestational age, the test results are not reliable.

**TABLE 10–2 CONDITIONS ASSOCIATED WITH ABNORMAL MATERNAL SERUM ALPHA-FETOPROTEIN LEVELS**

**Elevated Levels of AFP**

Open neural tube defects
Esophageal obstruction
Abdominal wall defects (omphalocele, gastroschisis)
Increased amount leaked by fetal kidney (hydronephrosis)
Threatened abortion
Undetected fetal demise
Normal fetus in conjunction with one or more of the following:
- Amniotic fluid contaminated with fetal blood
- Underestimation of fetal age
- Multifetal gestation
- Decreased maternal weight
- Maternal insulin-dependent diabetes

**Low Levels of AFP**

Chromosomal trisomies (e.g., Down syndrome)
Gestational trophoblastic disease
Normal fetuses in conjunction with:
- Overestimation of gestational age
- Increased maternal weight

## Procedure

Initial screening is offered between 15 and 20 weeks of gestation, when blood may be drawn to evaluate the concentration of MSAFP. The mother is informed that MSAFP is only a screening test and that further tests will be necessary to investigate abnormal concentrations. Figure 10–5 shows recommended diagnostic procedures associated with abnormal levels of AFP. If MSAFP levels are elevated, basic ultrasonography is recommended to determine whether the abnormal concentration is due to multifetal gestation, inaccurate gestational age, or fetal demise.

If ultrasonography fails to explain the abnormal levels of AFP, amniocentesis is the next step offered. Amniotic fluid is analyzed for elevated levels of AFP and for acetylcholinesterase (AChE). Elevations of AChE have been noted in association with open neural tube defects. Acetylcholinesterase assessment is not a primary diagnostic tool, but it is especially useful for detecting elevated AFAFP levels that result from fetal blood contamination.

### Advantages

Maternal serum AFP evaluation has several advantages:

- It is a simple procedure that requires only a sample of maternal blood.
- It is the least invasive and most economical procedure to screen for an open neural tube defect, a defect that occurs in one in 700 white pregnancies and one in 1000 African-American pregnancies (Evans et al., 1994). Open neural tube defects may produce serious, lifelong neurologic disability.
- Prenatal diagnosis allows parents time to examine their options or to prepare for the birth of an infant who will require special care.

### Limitations

Some major limitations of MSAFP are the following:

- Maternal serum AFP evaluation is a screening test only and must be viewed as the first step in a series of diagnostic procedures that are necessary if abnormal concentrations are found.
- Because many other conditions, such as inaccurate estimation of gestational age, can result in apparently abnormal levels, the parents may experience a great deal of anxiety and expense when follow-up tests are necessary.
- Timing also imposes some limits. Maternal serum AFP evaluation is performed between the 15th and 20th weeks of pregnancy, but many women do not seek prenatal care until after the 18th week and therefore miss the opportunity for MSAFP screening.
- Inaccurate reports of maternal weight can influence the maternal serum value because AFP diffuses into a larger maternal compartment in heavier women. Thus, if a reported weight is 20 pounds lighter than the actual weight, the value reported in the normal range may be high for the actual weight.
- Because closed neural tube defects do not produce elevated levels of AFP, normal levels of AFP do not guarantee a perfect baby.

## Triple-Marker Screening

In recent years two other markers, human chorionic gonadotropin (hCG) and unconjugated estriol, have been added to MSAFP to screen for chromosomal abnormalities. This triple-marker screening has been found to increase detection of trisomy 18 and trisomy 21 (Kellner et al., 1995). Maternal serum samples are taken between 15 and 22 weeks' gestation (based on last menstrual period), and results are considered positive if all three markers are low. In that case, the woman should be offered additional testing, such as amniocentesis for karyotyping.

**CHECK YOUR READING**

4. Why is MSAFP called a screening test?
5. What are the possible causes for an elevation in AFP levels?
6. What are possible causes of low levels of AFP?
7. What is triple-marker screening? Why is it performed?

## Chorionic Villus Sampling

### Purpose

Chorionic villus sampling (CVS) is a first-trimester alternative to amniocentesis for prenatal diagnosis of some conditions. Chorionic villi are microscopic projections from the outer membrane (chorion) that develop and burrow into endometrial tissue as the placenta is formed. The villi are fetal in origin and reflect the chromosomal and genetic makeup of the fetus. Fetal villous tissue can be obtained as early as 10 weeks of gestation and is analyzed directly for chromosomal and genetic abnormalities (ACOG, 1995).

### Indications

Chorionic villus sampling is recommended only for women who are at high risk for giving birth to an infant with diagnosable genetic anomalies. Its use is restricted because of reported complications, such as spotting or bleeding, uterine cramping, and fetal loss. Women past the age of 35 years, those with a history of a previous fetus with anomalies that can be detected with fetal cells, or couples who are carriers or who exhibit genetic defects are at the greatest risk, and CVS is an option to consider.

### Procedure

Chorionic villus sampling can be performed by two techniques. Transcervical aspiration, under direct vision with real-time ultrasonography, is the most widely used technique. The woman is placed in the lithotomy position. Both the vagina and cervix are washed with an antiseptic germicidal agent, and strict aseptic technique is observed to decrease the chance of infection. A flexible catheter is inserted through the cervix, and a sample of chorionic villi is aspirated through the catheter into a syringe (Fig. 10–6).

Transabdominal CVS is performed with the woman in a supine position. Ultrasound examination first

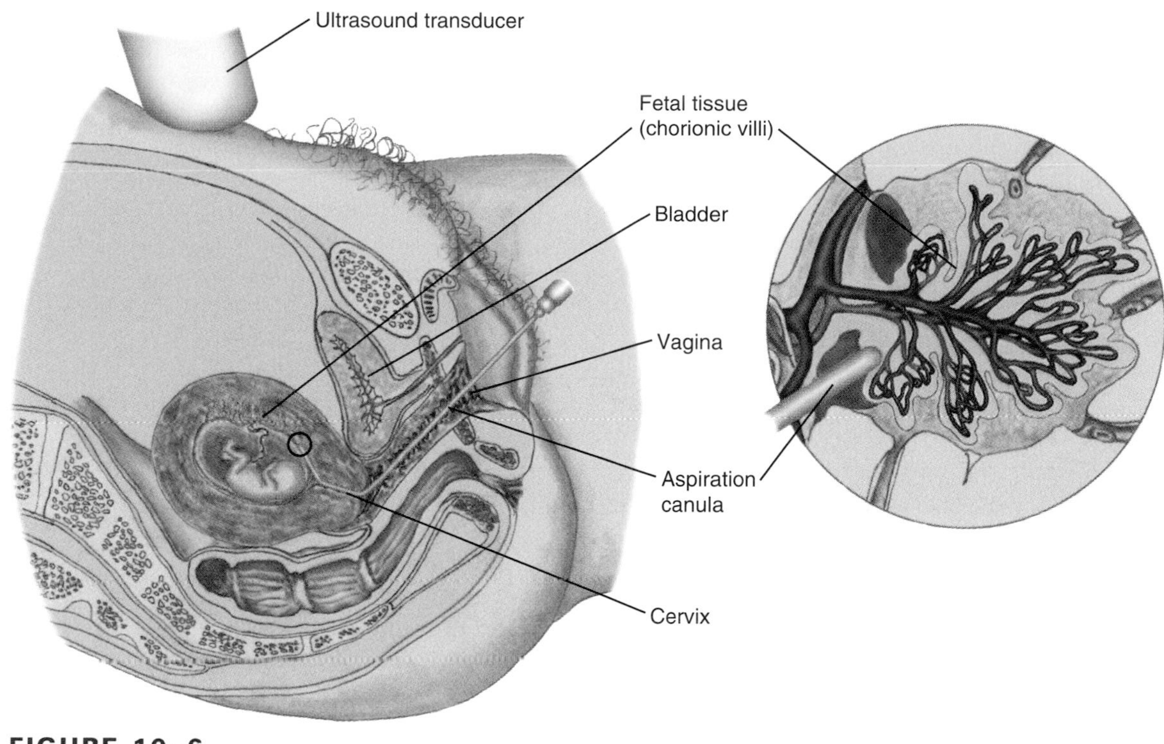


**FIGURE 10-6**

Transvaginal chorionic villus sampling (CVS). Tissue is aspirated to detect the presence of genetic defects in the fetus. Transabdominal aspiration is an alternative method.

determines the entry position and angle of passage of the sampling needle. An area on the abdomen is cleansed with antiseptic solution. With ultrasonography as a guide, the clinician insects a needle through the abdominal wall and myometrium, and the tip is advanced to the longest axis of the placenta. Sufficient tissue is withdrawn for accurate sampling of chorionic villi.

## Advantages

Chorionic villus sampling is most often performed between 10 and 12 weeks of gestation. Because first-trimester cells divide rapidly, results can be known within 24 to 48 hours. Unlike amniocentesis, which is performed during the second trimester and often requires 2 to 3 weeks for culture of fetal cells that have been shed into amniotic fluid, CVS does not impose the burden of a long, anxious wait on the prospective parents before data are available. As a result, CVS offers access to prenatal diagnosis to women who find second-trimester procedures unacceptable. Furthermore, it may save women carrying affected fetuses from the physical and emotional trauma of a second-trimester abortion.

## Risks

Although CVS is now considered a safe and effective technique for first-trimester prenatal diagnosis, prospective parents remain concerned that the risks may outweigh the benefits. The rate of pregnancy loss varies from 0.5 to 1 percent, slightly higher than that of amniocentesis (Pergament, 1994). Factors that decrease the risk of pregnancy loss include an experienced sampling team, an anterior placenta, and ease in obtaining an adequate villus sample. Infection has not proven to be a significant problem. The procedure is contraindicated, however, if endocervicitis, active genital herpes, pelvic inflammatory process, or a positive culture for *Neisseria gonorrhoeae* has been documented.

Reports of limb reduction defects (LRD) at a rate exceeding 1 percent in newborns who underwent CVS at 6 to 8 weeks of gestation have caused concern (Pergament, 1994). Although the cause of LRD is unknown, several mechanisms have been investigated. These include hypoperfusion due to fetomaternal hemorrhage or embolus of chorionic villus material that blocks perfusion of a limb, and limb entrapment during the procedure (Simpson & Elias, 1994). Because of LRD, many medical centers now perform CVS between 10 and 12 weeks' gestation. Families should, however, be informed about reports of LRD before the procedure is performed. Chorionic villus sampling also increases the risk of Rh sensitization, and Rho(D) immune globulin should be administered to all unsensitized Rh-negative women following the procedure.

As with all diagnostic procedures, the family should receive genetic counseling prior to the test. The risks and benefits of the procedure should be carefully explained and a signed consent obtained. The woman should be informed that the actual procedure takes about half an hour, but up to 2 hours should be allotted in case of delays.

After the procedure, maternal vital signs are assessed, and the woman is allowed to void. A small amount of vaginal spotting may appear, but heavy bleeding or the passage of amniotic fluid, clots, or tissue should be reported. The woman needs to rest at home for several hours after the procedure.

**✓ CHECK YOUR READING**

8. What is the major advantage of CVS over amniocentesis?
9. What are the major risks associated with CVS?

## Amniocentesis

Amniocentesis is aspiration of amniotic fluid from the amniotic sac for examination. The procedure is traditionally performed in an ambulatory clinic between 15 and 17 weeks' gestation (Simpson & Elias, 1994).

### Purposes

#### MIDTRIMESTER

The primary purpose for midtrimester amniocentesis is to examine fetal cells present in amniotic fluid to identify any chromosomal abnormalities. Abnormal number and structure of chromosomes are readily identified from the karyotype. (See Chapter 5 for detailed information about karyotyping and specific chromosomal abnormalities.)

In addition to detecting chromosomal abnormalities, amniocentesis is used to evaluate the fetal condition when the woman is sensitized to Rh-positive blood, to diagnose amnionitis, and to investigate AFAFP when MSAFP is elevated. (Indications for midtrimester amniocentesis are listed in Table 10–3.)

#### THIRD TRIMESTER

During the third trimester, amniocentesis is usually performed to determine fetal maturity or to diagnose fetal hemolytic disease, most often caused by Rh incompatibility.

**Tests to Determine Fetal Lung Maturity.** A test for fetal lung maturity is recommended when delivery is contemplated before 38 weeks' gestation. The lecithin/sphingomyelin (L/S) ratio is the best-known test for estimating fetal lung maturity. Lecithin and sphingomyelin are lipoproteins that make up surfactant, which lines the pulmonary alveoli in term infants. Surfactant keeps the alveoli patent by reducing surface tension on their inner walls. The decreased surface tension prevents collapse of the alveoli when the infant exhales and the walls of the alveoli tend to come together. It may be helpful to picture the alveoli as small, inflated balloons and to imagine what happens when the air is let out. Without adequate surfactant, the walls come together and adhere, making it difficult to inflate the alveoli with the next breath.

The proportion of lecithin to sphingomyelin does not differ markedly until about the 30th week of gestation. At this time the level of sphingomyelin plateaus, but lecithin continues to rise. An L/S ratio greater than 2:1 generally indicates that surfactant is adequate and the fetal lungs are mature. These conditions, however, are not always met, particularly if the pregnant woman has diabetes mellitus. Therefore, amniotic fluid is also tested for the presence of phosphatidylglycerol and phosphatidylinositol. These phospholipids boost the properties of lecithin, and their presence confirms fetal lung maturity.

**Test for Fetal Hemolytic Disease.** Amniocentesis is also performed to determine fetal bilirubin concentration if the mother is Rh-negative and is sensitized (that is, has been exposed to the Rh antigen and has developed antibodies); see Chapter 25 for a more complete description of Rh incompatibility. Because spectrophotometers are used to measure the *change* in optical density of bilirubin, the test is referred to as Δ (*delta*) OD (delta means change, and it is shown as a triangle). The level of bilirubin in amniotic fluid reflects the amount of fetal red blood cell destruction that occurs when antibodies destroy Rh-positive fetal red blood cells, leaving the fetus vulnerable to erythroblastosis fetalis and hydrops fetalis.

Erythroblastosis is marked by excessive destruction of *erythrocytes* (mature red blood cells that are capable of carrying oxygen) and the proliferation of

**TABLE 10–3 INDICATIONS FOR SECOND-TRIMESTER AMNIOCENTESIS**

Maternal age 35 years or more
Chromosomal abnormality in close family member
Sex determination for maternal carrier of X-linked disorder (such as hemophilia or Duchenne's muscular dystrophy)
Birth of previous infant with chromosomal abnormalities or neural tube defect
Pregnancy after three or more spontaneous abortions
Elevated levels of maternal serum alpha-fetoprotein
Maternal Rh sensitization

*erythroblasts* (immature red blood cells, incapable of carrying oxygen). Because of the rapid hemolysis of erythrocytes, *bilirubin* (a waste product of red blood cell breakdown) increases markedly. The fetus becomes anemic, jaundiced, and edematous (hydrops fetalis).

## Procedure

Amniocentesis involves aspiration of amniotic fluid from the amniotic sac (Fig. 10–7). Before the examination, the woman is placed in a supine position and is draped with her abdomen exposed. A rolled towel is placed under the right buttock to shift the weight of the uterus slightly to the left and off the vena cava and aorta. Maternal blood pressure and fetal heart tones are assessed for baseline levels.

Ultrasonography is used to locate the fetus and placenta and to identify the largest pockets of amniotic fluid that can safely be sampled. Next, the skin is prepared with antiseptic solution. A small amount of local anesthetic may be injected in the skin. This step causes the only pain the woman experiences, although she may experience the sensation of pressure as the needle is inserted and mild cramping as the needle enters the myometrium.

A 3- to 4-inch, 20- or 21-gauge needle is inserted into the pocket of fluid. Approximately 20 ml of fluid are removed for analysis. An adhesive bandage is applied to the puncture site. The woman rests quietly for 30 to 60 minutes with electronic monitoring of fetal heart rate (FHR). She then may resume normal activities. Strenuous exercise, such as jogging and aerobic exercise, should be deferred for a day or two (Simpson & Elias, 1994). The patient should report to the obstetrician if she experiences persistent uterine contractions, vaginal bleeding, leakage of amniotic fluid, or fever.

As with CVS, Rho(D) immune globulin is administered to nonsensitized Rh-negative women following amniocentesis. The drug is used to prevent sensitization. (See Chapter 25, Drug Guide for Rho(D) immune globulin.)

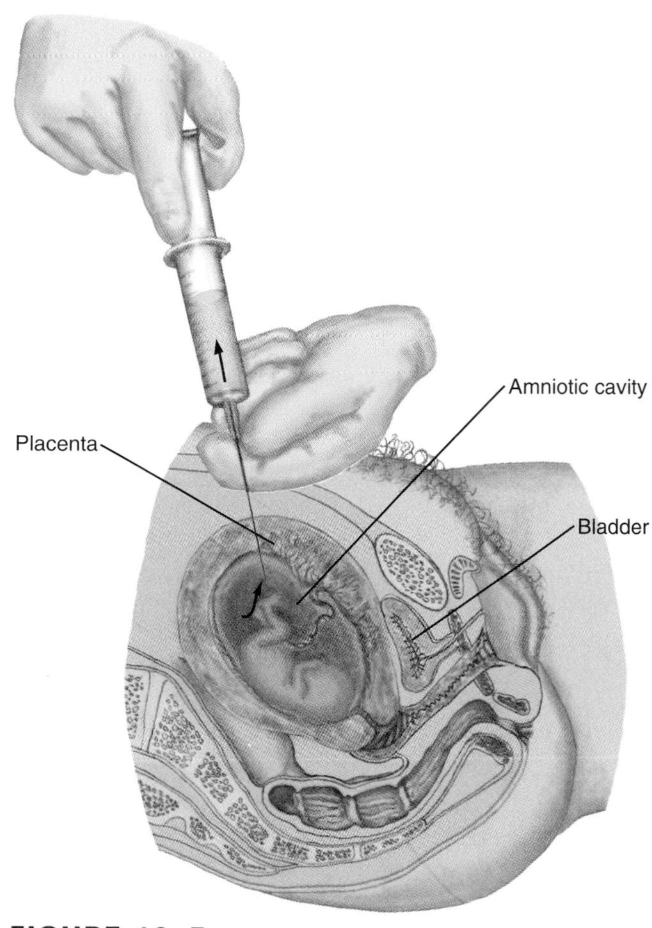


**FIGURE 10–7**

In amniocentesis, a needle is inserted through the expectant mother's abdomen to aspirate fluid from the amniotic sac. The fluid can then be tested to determine fetal maturity, chromosomal abnormalities, or other possible problems.

## Advantages

Amniocentesis has several advantages:

- It is a simple, safe procedure that permits the diagnosis of many fetal anomalies and confirms fetal maturity.
- It is a relatively painless procedure that takes only a short time.
- It has been done for many years with few reported complications.

## Disadvantages

A major disadvantage of amniocentesis has been timing. Until recently, amniocentesis was done between 15 and 17 weeks' gestation, when the uterus is readily accessible and the volume of amniotic fluid permits removal of 20 ml. Cells are allowed to grow in a culture medium for 2 to 3 weeks before they are harvested for karyotyping. New culture techniques, however, may permit faster results. When the cells are grown in an enriched culture, duration is reduced to an average of 9.5 days, and techniques for DNA probing may hasten results even more in the future (Ramsay & Fisk, 1994).

Abnormal results are known in time to allow termination of pregnancy before 20 weeks' gestation. This time frame, however, is unacceptable for many parents. The reluctance of parents to undergo procedures so late in the pregnancy has focused interest on alternatives, such as CVS, early amniocentesis, and improved culture techniques.

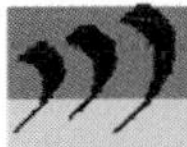

THERAPEUTIC COMMUNICATION

**Responding to Anxiety Related to Fetal Testing**

Margaret Kitchner is a 37-year-old primigravida. She has postponed pregnancy to complete her education and to establish a law practice. The pregnancy is at 16 weeks, and she has been referred for amniocentesis. Counseling has already been provided by a specialist in genetics, and the risks and benefits have been discussed.

**Margaret:** I'm here, but I'm not thrilled to be here.
**Nurse:** You wish you were somewhere else?

*Clarifying without attempting to lead . . .*

**Margaret:** The place isn't the problem really, but what about this test?
**Nurse:** You have some questions you'd like to ask about the amniocentesis?

*Seeking information, staying with the woman's comments by paraphrasing . . .*

**Margaret:** Well, my mother believes that if one thinks bad thoughts, bad things will come to pass.
**Nurse:** Bad thoughts?

*Knowing that the intergenerational belief system is powerful, the nurse focuses and seeks clarification . . .*

**Margaret:** Yes, you know, if we think something could be wrong with the baby, it's more likely to be true.
**Nurse:** I'd like to hear more.

*"I" statement conveys interest and invites more discussion.*

**Margaret:** Well, my mother is not familiar with the tests, and she's just afraid that the test could hurt the baby.
**Nurse:** She must be very anxious about this test. How do you feel?

*Notes that Margaret identifies her mother as the person who is concerned, avoids her own feelings. Acknowledging mother's feeling; focusing on woman's feeling by open-ended question . . .*

**Margaret:** She's anxious, and to tell you the truth, I'm anxious too.
**Nurse:** You would rather not be having the test.

*This makes an assumption; she said only that she was anxious. It might be more therapeutic to say, "Tell me more about that."*

**Margaret:** No, I want the test. I know the reason is my age, but I want this baby so much.
**Nurse:** So the anxiety is really about the test results.

*"Hears" the anxiety that Margaret didn't put into words; summarizes concerns and helps the woman identify and focus on what seems unclear to her . . .*

**Margaret:** That's for sure. It will be so hard to wait for the results, and I don't know what I would do if the news is bad.
**Nurse:** Waiting is difficult, but chances are that the news will be good.

*It is therapeutic to acknowledge the difficulty, but offering reassurance blocks the interaction instead of focusing on the uncertainty expressed. The nurse might have said instead: "And it's very hard to imagine something is wrong with the baby." This response would have kept the interaction going and focused on the patient's feelings. Instead, the blocking comment ended the interaction without allowing a full expression of feelings.*

**Margaret:** You think so? I hope so.

## Early Amniocentesis

Early amniocentesis is generally performed between 11 and 14 weeks' gestation (Cunningham et al., 1997).

### Procedure

The technique is similar to that of traditional amniocentesis except that a smaller volume of fluid (10 to 12 ml) is withdrawn. The safety of early amniocentesis has not yet been established, but when compared with traditional amniocentesis, the pregnancy loss rate was higher (Cunningham et al., 1997).

### Risks

The use of ultrasonography has greatly reduced the risks once associated with amniocentesis. The risk of infection is also minimal, because aseptic technique is used throughout the procedure. The risk of injury to the fetus or umbilical cord is minimal when ultrasound is used to guide needle insertion. A second puncture at a different site, however, may be necessary if enough fluid cannot be obtained for analysis.

The risk of spontaneous abortion associated with amniocentesis is 0.5 percent or less (Simpson & Elias, 1994). Fetal hemorrhage can result from perforation of the placenta or vessels in the umbilical cord, but this is unlikely when ultrasonography is used to guide needle insertion. Accidental transfer of fetal blood to maternal circulation may also occur, resulting in isoimmunization of the Rh-negative mother carrying an Rh-positive fetus.

As with all fetal diagnostic procedures, amniocentesis cannot guarantee the birth of a perfect infant. Parents need to be counseled that not all defects are detectable by amniocentesis.

**CHECK YOUR READING**

10. What factors make a pregnant woman a candidate for amniocentesis?
11. How is fetal lung maturity confirmed?
12. Why is bilirubin in amniotic fluid evaluated?
13. Why is early amniocentesis sometimes preferred?

## Antepartum Fetal Surveillance

Antepartum fetal surveillance has three important goals: (1) to prevent perinatal morbidity and mortality, (2) to determine fetal health or compromise as accurately as possible, and (3) to determine appropriate intervention by the obstetric team. The three most common methods of fetal surveillance are the nonstress test, the contraction stress test, and the biophysical profile.

### Nonstress Test

#### PURPOSE

One way to assess fetal well-being is to evaluate the ability of the fetal heart to accelerate (speed up) in association with fetal movement. An increase in FHR when the fetus moves indicates adequate oxygenation, a healthy neural pathway from the fetal central nervous system to the fetal heart, and the ability of the fetal heart to respond to stimuli. If the fetal heart does not accelerate with movement, however, fetal hypoxemia and acidosis are concerns. In those cases, an additional test, such as the contraction stress test or the biophysical profile, is necessary to determine the metabolic condition of the fetus.

#### PROCEDURE

The nonstress test takes about 30 to 40 minutes. A nurse with special preparation conducts the test in a hospital or in an obstetrician's office. Before the test, the nurse instructs the woman about the test and explains why it is recommended. The test is termed "nonstress" because it consists of monitoring only; the fetus is not challenged or stressed by uterine contractions to obtain the necessary data.

The woman usually sits in a reclining chair in a semi-Fowler's position to prevent supine hypotension. Her blood pressure is checked before the test and every 10 to 15 minutes throughout the test. If hypotension occurs, her position is changed to maintain the baseline pressure.

The nurse applies external electronic monitoring equipment. First, an ultrasound transducer, to record fetal heart activity, is secured over the spot on the woman's abdomen where the fetal heart is heard most clearly. Next, a tocotransducer, which detects uterine activity and fetal movement, is secured to the maternal abdomen (Fig. 10–8). The woman may also be given a remote event marker to press each time she senses movement. Fetal heart activity and fetal movements are recorded on the same moving strip of paper. (See Chapter 14 for more information about fetal monitoring.)

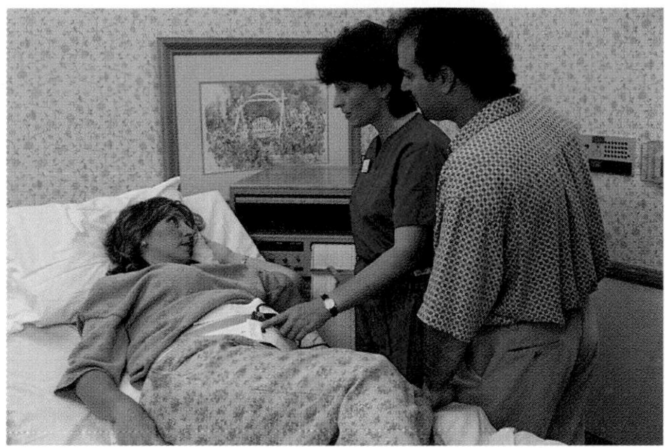

**FIGURE 10–8**

A nonstress test is a noninvasive test that measures the ability of the fetal heart to respond to fetal movements. Here the nurse reassures the parents by pointing to fetal heart rate accelerations detected by the external fetal monitor.

#### INTERPRETATION

Physicians must review and interpret nonstress test results. Results are judged to be reactive (normal), nonreactive (abnormal), or equivocal.

To be considered *reactive*, the baseline rate must be within normal range (110 to 160 BPM with good long-term variability [amplitude of at least 10 BPM]), and there must be two or more FHR accelerations of at least 15 BPM, each with a duration of at least 15 seconds, in a 20-minute interval (Fig. 10–9) (Paul & Miller, 1995). A finding is considered *nonreactive* if it does not meet the criteria in a minimum time of 40 minutes and requires further evaluation.

At times the data are conflicting or difficult to interpret and results are judged to be *equivocal*. For example, a finding is equivocal when fewer than two fetal movements occur in a 20-minute period, accelerations occur with fewer than 15 BPM, and the FHR baseline is abnormal (less than 110 or greater than 160 BPM). In this case, further follow-up is essential. Moreover, if decelerations (slowing down), either late or variable, occur, further testing is necessary (Parer, 1994).

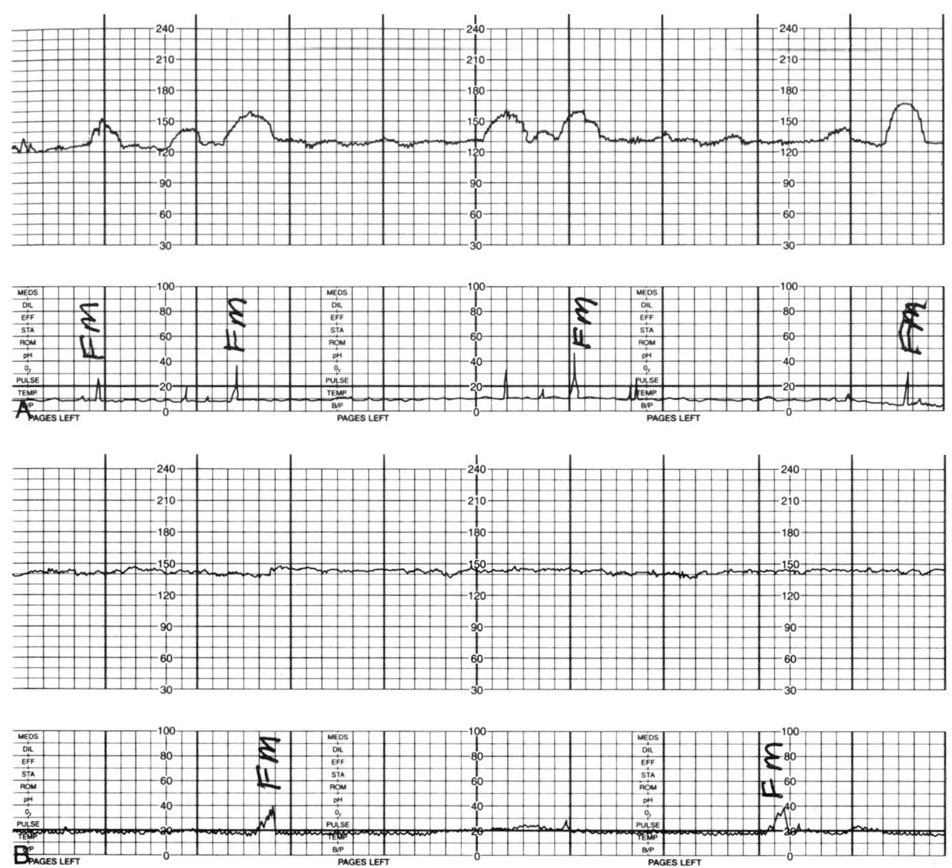


**FIGURE 10–9**

A, In this reactive nonstress test, fetal heart rate accelerates by 25 to 30 beats per minute (BPM) for at least 15 seconds in response to fetal movement. B, In this nonreactive nonstress test, accelerations are absent following fetal movement (FM). (Courtesy of Graphic Controls, Buffalo, New York.)

#### ADVANTAGES

The nonstress test is noninvasive and painless and is believed to be without risk to mother or fetus. As a consequence, it is the primary means of fetal surveillance in pregnancies that are at increased risk for uteroplacental insufficiency and consequent fetal hypoxia. The nonstress test is easy to administer and is often repeated weekly or even daily if necessary. In addition, results are available immediately.

#### DISADVANTAGES

A major disadvantage is the large number (80 percent) of nonreactive findings that are termed false-positive (Parer, 1994). In a false-positive test result, a normal, well-oxygenated fetus may not exhibit movement for more than 20 minutes, primarily because of the sleep-wake cycle. If the test is administered during a sleep cycle, the fetus may not move during the time allotted, and the test result may be interpreted as nonreactive when, in fact, the fetus is healthy but merely asleep. Testing is usually continued for a minimum of 40 minutes before a pattern is called nonreactive (Paul & Miller, 1995).

Waiting for the fetus to awaken prolongs the time required for testing, and efforts may be made to stimulate the fetus to move. No support has been found, however, for the use of juice or glucose to facilitate fetal response in nonstress tests (McCarthy & Narrigan, 1995). Other methods used to stimulate fetal activity, such as transabdominal and transvaginal light, as well as manual manipulation of the maternal abdomen, have also been found to be of little value (Smith, 1994). Only vibroacoustic stimulation has been shown to have a meaningful impact on the outcome of the nonstress test.

## Vibroacoustic Stimulation Test

#### PURPOSE AND PROCEDURE

In recent years, the vibroacoustic stimulation test has been used to confirm nonreactive nonstress test findings or to shorten the time required to obtain nonstress test data of good quality. The procedure for the vibroacoustic stimulation test is similar to that for the nonstress test. Electronic fetal monitoring equipment is used to obtain an FHR baseline. Then an artificial larynx is applied to the maternal abdomen over the area of the fetal head for 1 second. The fetus is stimulated by the sound emitted as well as the vibration created. If no acceleration occurs within 10 seconds, stimulation may be repeated (Smith, 1994). A review of the literature reveals that

FHR accelerations in response to vibroacoustic stimulation indicate fetal health and correlate well with other methods of fetal assessment (Smith, 1994).

#### POTENTIAL RISKS

Although no known risks exist, there is speculation that repeated use of the artificial larynx may cause fetal hearing loss. Preliminary information, however, suggests that the increased intrauterine sound pressure level is unlikely to lead to significant fetal injury (Smith, 1994).

In addition, prolonged fetal tachycardia has been noted in some instances, but the significance is not known. Moreover, if the test is used frequently, the fetus may become habituated to the stimulus and not respond, making the test results unclear.

### ✓ CHECK YOUR READING

14. What is a nonstress test, and why is it so named?
15. How does a vibroacoustic stimulation test differ from a nonstress test?

## Contraction Stress Test

#### PURPOSE

A contraction stress text is indicated if nonstress test findings are nonreactive. The concern is that if fetal oxygenation is only marginally adequate when the uterus is at rest, it may be decreased further during uterine contractions. As the name implies, a contraction stress test involves recording the response of the FHR to stress that is induced by uterine contractions. Uterine contractions compress the arteries supplying the placenta with oxygenated maternal blood. Therefore, uterine contractions routinely cause a recurrent decrease in fetal oxygen levels.

The fetus with adequate oxygen reserves can tolerate the temporary hypoxia induced by uterine contractions, so that the FHR remains unchanged. If the fetus has inadequate reserves, however, and if substantial hypoxia has led to anaerobic metabolism, fetal acidosis may result. This condition leads to myocardial depression and late decelerations in the FHR. Late decelerations are associated with a poor fetal outcome, such as perinatal death, low 5-minute Apgar scores, and late decelerations in labor in about 50 percent of the cases (Parer, 1994). If FHR variability is also decreased in the presence of persistent late decelerations, the correlation with fetal compromise is increased. (Chapter 14 reviews FHR monitoring and abnormal FHR patterns.)

#### PROCEDURE

The nurse is responsible for administering the test and for protecting the safety of the mother and fetus throughout the testing period. In many ways the procedure is similar to that in the nonstress test. The woman is positioned in the same manner, and external electronic fetal monitoring devices are applied to record both uterine activity and FHR. The major difference is that uterine contractions must be initiated. Two methods are used to accomplish this.

The *breast self-stimulation test* is based on the knowledge that stimulation of the breasts and nipples causes the release of oxytocin from the posterior pituitary and that oxytocin causes uterine contractions. To induce contractions, the woman brushes her palm across one nipple through her shirt for 2 to 3 minutes, stopping if a contraction begins. The nipple stimulation continues after a 5-minute rest period, with the same process repeated if no contractions occur. To avoid hyperstimulation (uterine contractions lasting more than 90 seconds or occurring more frequently than every 2 minutes), bilateral stimulation should not be instituted unless unilateral stimulation fails to induce contractions (Halle, 1993).

The *oxytocin challenge test* involves the intravenous infusion of dilute oxytocin to stimulate uterine contractions. This method is used if the breast self-stimulation test is not effective in stimulating contractions. The nurse conducting the test inserts a primary intravenous line plus a "piggyback" line for administration of oxytocin. The objective is to stimulate three recordable uterine contractions, 40 to 60 seconds in duration, in a 10-minute period. Interpretation of data is based on this number of contractions of this duration in this amount of time (Lagrew, 1995).

#### INTERPRETATION

Contraction stress test results may be interpreted as negative (normal), positive (abnormal), or equivocal. (See Figure 10–10 for a summary of contraction stress test interpretations and implications.)

A negative test result indicates that no late decelerations occurred in the FHR, although the fetus was stressed by three contractions of at least 40 seconds duration in a 10-minute period.

Findings are judged to be positive when 50 percent or more of contractions are accompanied by late decelerations (those persisting after the contraction ends).

A result is equivocal when fewer than 50 percent of the contractions have produced late decelerations or when the uterus is hyperstimulated—that is, contractions closer than every 2 minutes or duration longer than 90 seconds (Lagrew, 1995).

| | | |
|---|---|---|
| Negative | No late decelerations | Reassuring that the fetus can tolerate labor |

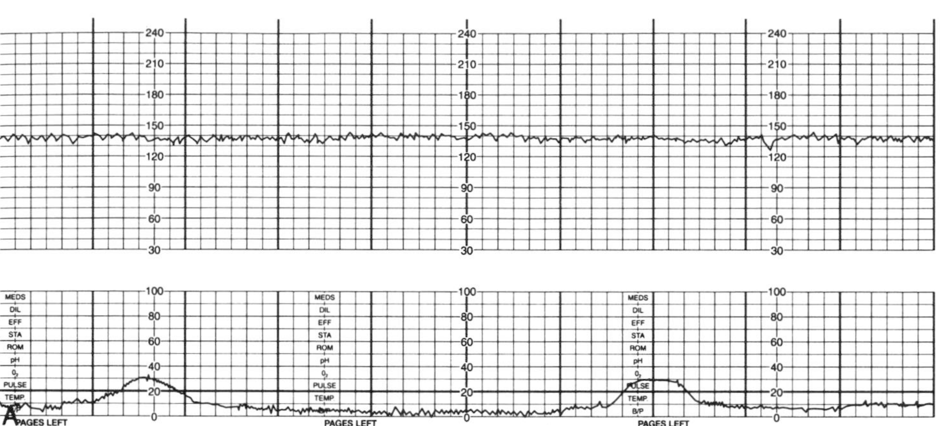

| | | |
|---|---|---|
| Positive | Consistent late decelerations in 50% of the contractions | Indicates UPI and fetal compromise during contractions |

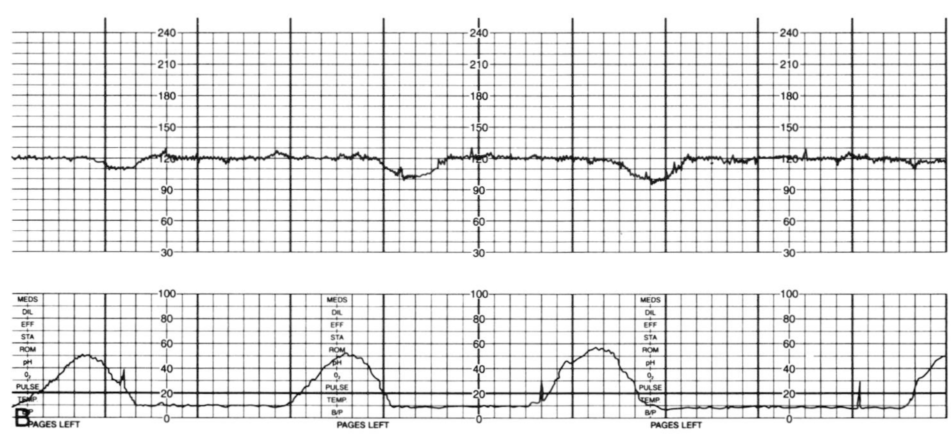

| | | |
|---|---|---|
| Equivocal | Late decelerations with <50% of the contractions | A second CST should be repeated within 24 hours |
| Hyperstimulation | Late decelerations with excessive uterine activity (contractions closer than every 2 minutes or lasting longer than 90 seconds) | Repeat CST within 24 hours with careful monitoring of the situation |
| Unsatisfactory | Test cannot be interpreted; either not enough data or unsatisfactory tracing | Repeat CST with careful attention to maternal position, oxytocin infusion, and placement of tocotransducer |

**FIGURE 10–10**

Interpretation of contraction stress test (CST). UPI, uteroplacental insufficiency. (Courtesy of Graphic Controls, Buffalo, New York.)

#### ADVANTAGES

Contraction stress testing has several advantages:

- The test allows follow-up of a nonreactive nonstress test result.
- If findings are negative, contraction stress test offers reassurance that the uteroplacental unit will continue to support life for at least a week longer (Cunningham et al., 1997).
- A positive contraction stress test result allows the physician to analyze available options and to make plans for the birth of an infant who may be compromised because of decreased placental functioning during labor.

#### DISADVANTAGES

The contraction stress test is associated with four major disadvantages:

- The test is time consuming, usually requiring about 2 hours.
- The contraction stress test is tedious, necessitating either the participation of the woman in breast self-stimulation or careful infusion of oxytocin to obtain an adequate contraction pattern without causing hyperstimulation of the uterus.
- Errors in interpretation are common. These may be due to technical difficulties in obtaining tracings or problems in interpreting the data. For

example, the FHR may accelerate with fetal movement, or late decelerations may occur with contractions (a reactive nonstress test but a positive contraction stress test). Such an interpretation requires further testing, such as a biophysical profile, to confirm the well-being of the fetus.

- The cost is high. A contraction stress test is usually done in a hospital setting, where there is a per-hour charge; equipment and supplies, such as intravenous lines, oxytocin, and infusion pumps, add to the cost. The time spent by a nurse who is educated to administer the test must also be factored into the total cost.

**CHECK YOUR READING**

16. Why is it necessary to initiate contractions in a contraction stress test?
17. In a contraction stress test, what do late decelerations of FHR indicate?

## Biophysical Profile

Predicting the condition of the fetus can be most accurate if several parameters are evaluated. Unlike the nonstress test and contraction stress test, which assess only fetal heart activity, the biophysical profile assesses five parameters of fetal activity: FHR, fetal breathing movements, gross fetal movements, fetal tone, and amniotic fluid volume.

### PURPOSE

The individual components of the examination are a combination of both acute and chronic markers of fetal well-being. The acute markers are the FHR reactivity, fetal breathing movements, gross fetal movements, and fetal tone. The major chronic marker is the amount of amniotic fluid.

The acute markers are controlled by different central nervous system control centers that develop at different stages in gestation. Fetal tone is the earliest to develop, followed by fetal movements, then regular breathing movements. Fetal heart rate reactivity is last to develop, occurring at the end of the second or the beginning of the third trimester.

The fetal central nervous system centers that control each individual parameter of the biophysical profile react differently to hypoxemia. The later-developing control centers require higher oxygen levels than earlier-developing centers. Therefore, FHR reactivity disappears first. Fetal breathing movements are affected next, with fetal movement and finally fetal tone being the last areas affected. Thus, absence of fetal tone indicates advanced asphyxia and acidosis. This progression has been termed the

| HYPOXIA ↓ | | pH ↓ |
|---|---|---|
| | Late decelerations appear (first sign) | |
| | Accelerations disappear (next sign) | |
| | Fetal breathing movement stops | |
| | Fetal movement ceases (late sign) | |
| | Fetal tone absent (fetus already compromised) | |

**FIGURE 10–11**

Cascade effect of gradual hypoxia.

*gradual hypoxia concept.* Figure 10–11 illustrates the cascade effect of gradual hypoxia on the central nervous system of the fetus.

The amount of amniotic fluid provides information about chronic or long-term hypoxia. During periods of hypoxemia, the fetus has a remarkable ability to shunt blood from areas that are not critical to fetal life, such as the kidneys and lungs, toward the vital organs (heart, brain, and placenta). If the hypoxemia is prolonged, blood flow to the fetal kidneys and lungs that help produce amniotic fluid may virtually cease. Therefore, oligohydramnios indicates prolonged fetal hypoxia and is a strong indication of fetal compromise.

### PROCEDURE AND INTERPRETATION

Fetal heart rate reactivity is measured and interpreted from a nonstress test. The other four parameters are measured by real-time ultrasound scanning. The test is administered by nurses who have additional preparation in ultrasonography. A scoring technique is used to interpret the data, with each of the five parameters contributing either 2 or 0 points. A score of 10 is perfect; a score of 0 is the worst possible score. A total score of 8 to 10 is considered normal *unless oligohydramnios is present* (Table 10–4) (Manning, 1995). Oligohydramnios may indicate chronic fetal hypoxia and requires further testing.

## Modified Biophysical Profile

Although biophysical profile is a relatively new procedure, it has already been modified. Some physicians now elect to assess the fetus only by ultrasonography and to omit the nonstress test if all parameters are normal. In other medical centers, the test is modified to include only two parameters: an amniotic fluid index (quantity, in all four quadrants) and a nonstress test. Some physicians, however, now add a sixth parameter, placental grading.

### ADVANTAGES

The modified biophysical profile is noninvasive and is less costly than some tests because it can be done on an outpatient basis. Results are immediately available, and it may decrease the number of

**TABLE 10-4 SCORING THE BIOPHYSICAL PROFILE**

| Criterion | Points: None | Points: Present |
|---|---|---|
| Reactive nonstress test | 0 | 2 |
| Fetal breathing movements (at least one episode of 30 seconds in 30 minutes) | 0 | 2 |
| Gross body movements (at least three body or limb movements in 30 minutes) | 0 | 2 |
| Fetal tone (at least one episode of extension with return to flexion) | 0 | 2 |
| Amniotic fluid volume (at least one pocket of fluid that measures at least 1 cm in two perpendicular planes) | 0 | 2 |

*Key*: Normal = 8 to 10 points (if amniotic fluid volume is adequate); equivocal = 6; abnormal = <4 and delivery may be considered (Manning, 1995).

false-positive nonstress test findings. The biophysical profile allows conservative treatment of high-risk patients because delivery can be delayed if fetal well-being is indicated. The test is often used to monitor for impending signs of fetal infection when membranes rupture prematurely.

#### DISADVANTAGES

Additional research is needed to refine interpretation of the test. For example, each variable is given equal weight, although some variables are more important. At present, not enough research has been done to determine the meaning of low scores to long-term development of the child.

**CHECK YOUR READING**

18. What is the relationship between loss of fetal tone and hypoxia?
19. Why is amniotic fluid volume an important parameter in the biophysical profile?

## Percutaneous Umbilical Blood Sampling

Percutaneous umbilical blood sampling, also called cordocentesis, involves the aspiration of fetal blood from the umbilical cord for prenatal diagnosis or therapy (Fig. 10–12). Major indications for percutaneous umbilical blood sampling include diagnosis and intrauterine management of Rh disease, genetic studies, diagnosis of abnormal blood-clotting factors, and acid-base status of the fetus.

### Procedure

High-resolution ultrasonography is used to locate the fetus, placenta, and umbilical cord. A needle is inserted through the abdomen and into the uterine cavity. The puncture is made into the umbilical cord near the site at which the cord meets the placenta because the cord is almost always stable at this site. The umbilical vein is targeted more commonly than the umbilical arteries because it is larger and is less likely to constrict during the procedure. Although it is not important to know which vessel (vein or artery) was used when simply sampling fetal blood, it is very important to know when testing fetal acid-base parameters. Blood from the umbilical vein contains oxygenated blood and has a lower carbon dioxide content than blood from an umbilical artery that comes directly from the fetus.

### Risks

It is predicted that percutaneous umbilical blood sampling will become a widely used procedure in the future, but it is not risk free. Complications that can occur include cord laceration, cord hematoma,

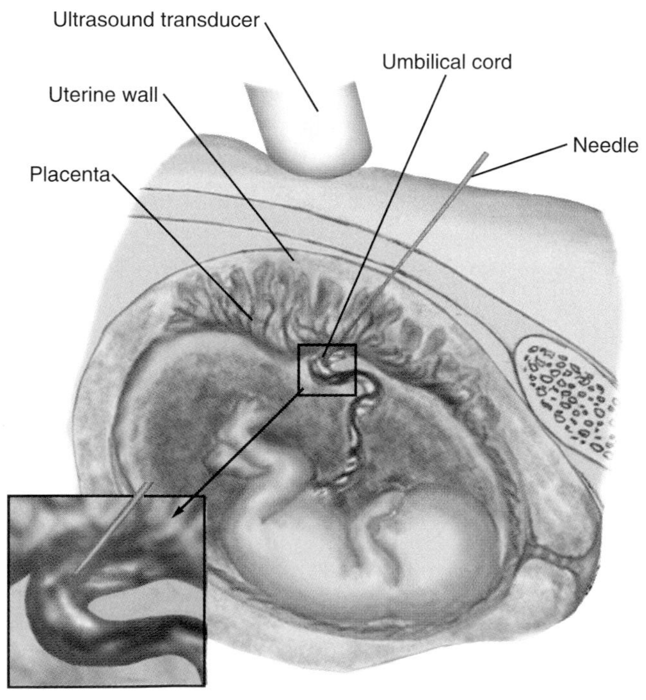


**FIGURE 10–12**

In percutaneous umbilical blood sampling (cordocentesis) a needle is inserted through the expectant mother's abdomen and into an umbilical vessel (vein or artery) to withdraw a sample of fetal blood.

thrombosis, thromboembolism, premature labor, and premature rupture of membranes. After needle withdrawal, the duration of bleeding from the umbilical cord is usually short and can be monitored by ultrasound examination. In addition, the fetal heart can be monitored electronically to confirm that the fetus experienced no ill effects.

## Maternal Assessment of Fetal Movement

Movements by the fetus, as assessed by the mother, are sometimes referred to as "kick counts." Fetal movement is associated with fetal condition, and daily evaluation of these movements provides a way of evaluating the fetus.

### Procedure

Protocols for assessing the mother's perception of fetal movement vary. In general, women are advised to count fetal movements for 30 to 60 minutes three times a day. The woman lies on her side. She places her hands on the largest part of her abdomen and concentrates on fetal movements. She uses a clock or timer and records the number of movements felt during that time (Fig. 10–13).

Women should notify their health care provider if they experience the following:

- They do not feel a movement at least four times in any counting period.
- The number of total movements for the day is fewer than 12.
- She notes any change in the type or character of the movements.

### Advantages

Counting fetal movement is one of the oldest methods for evaluating the condition of the fetus. There are some obvious advantages:

- It is inexpensive.
- It is noninvasive.
- It is convenient for the client.

### Disadvantages

Many variables make interpretation of fetal movement counts difficult:

- Fetal resting state decreases movements.
- Maternal perception of movement may vary.
- Time of day may affect fetal movement (lower in the morning, higher in the evening).
- Drugs (methadone, heroin, cocaine, alcohol, tobacco) may affect fetal activity.

## Application of Nursing Process: Diagnostic Testing

Many perinatal nurses with special education are actively involved in fetal diagnostic procedures. Nurses perform nonstress tests, contraction stress tests, and biophysical profiles. Many nurses who work in ambulatory centers or with physicians in private practice do basic ultrasonographic examinations. Regardless of the level of the nurse's involvement in actual testing, nursing process is the organizing framework for providing care. Nurses are expected to explain both the testing procedures and the information that can be determined from the tests. Nurses also reduce anxiety by providing emotional support when re-

Dates: 11/14/98 to 11/20/98

| Time of day | Sunday | Monday | Tuesday | Wednesday | Thursday | Friday | Saturday |
|---|---|---|---|---|---|---|---|
| Morning 8-9 a.m. | 𝍸 𝍸 | 𝍸 \|\| | 𝍸 \|\|\| | | | | |
| Afternoon 1-2 p.m. | 𝍸 \| | 𝍸 \|\|\| | 𝍸 | | | | |
| Evening 9-10 p.m. | 𝍸 \|\| 𝍸 | 𝍸 \|\|\|\| | | | | | |
| **Total** | 28 | 24 | | | | | |

**FIGURE 10–13**

Daily fetal movement record in use. The mother counts the number of fetal movements, or "kicks," within a specified period several times a day and indicates each movement on a chart. She reports any abnormality to her health care provider.

peated testing or a series of procedures becomes necessary.

## Assessment

Nurses must collect as much information as possible about the woman and her reasons for having the tests. The information may be important to conducting the tests or may be helpful to the physician interpreting the results. Necessary information includes the following:

- Gravida, para, living children, gestation (in weeks)
- Maternal health problems (hypertension, diabetes, heart disease)
- Current obstetric problems (vaginal bleeding, decreased fetal movement, multifetal gestation, intrauterine growth restriction, malpresentation, polyhydramnios, oligohydramnios)
- Prior obstetric problems (birth of stillborn infant or infant with congenital anomalies, birth of low-birth-weight infant or large-for-gestational age infant)
- History of substance abuse, including alcohol and tobacco
- Knowledge of reasons for the test and the procedure to be performed: "Do you have any questions before we start the test?"
- Knowledge of surveillance regimen if additional testing is necessary: "Do you have questions about the need to repeat the test every week?"
- Emotional response to the tests: "What are your major concerns?" "What can we do to make the tests easier for you?"
- Expectations of the diagnostic tests. Many couples think that the tests can guarantee a perfect baby but must be told what the test actually reveals.

## Analysis

Women who are at increased risk for problems during pregnancy require fetal diagnostic procedures. Clients' responses vary, depending on their knowledge and on their usual response to stressful situations. Many women, however, are concerned not only with the tests themselves but also with the condition of the fetus. The nursing diagnosis relevant to this woman is: Anxiety related to lack of knowledge of diagnostic procedures and the uncertain condition of the fetus.

## Planning

Goals for this nursing diagnosis are that the woman (and her family) will do the following:

- Verbalize knowledge of how, when, and why she is to be tested before testing procedures are initiated.
- Verbalize concerns about the condition of the fetus and seek information from health care team at each appointment.

## Interventions

### PROVIDING INFORMATION

Even nurses who do not work in antepartum testing must understand reasons for the tests and should be able to describe in general terms what the procedures entail. Many parents want to know how safe the tests are and how much discomfort they cause. Parents want to know why some of the tests must be repeated. Many parents become very concerned when a screening test result, such as an AFP assessment, is abnormal, and they need to know that the findings may be due to other factors and do not necessarily indicate a problem. Moreover, nurses often need to interpret technical information that may confuse the parents and cause them undue anxiety.

Provide simple, clear explanations of what the tests measure and the purpose and frequency of the tests. Explain how long the test takes, and describe the procedure so that anxiety caused by lack of knowledge can be reduced. Instruct the woman and her family about follow-up care and events that should be reported to the health care team.

### PROVIDING SUPPORT

It is critical that nurses identify and respond to feelings expressed by prospective parents when antepartum testing procedures are recommended or when fetal problems are confirmed. The woman often experiences frustration with the discomfort, limitations, and time-consuming demands of the pregnancy and the regimen of fetal testing. Skill in therapeutic communication is never more important than when counseling about fetal diagnostic tests.

Active listening conveys interest and concern. Paraphrasing allows for interpretation because it expresses in different words what concerns the family. The art of reflecting back to the family what they convey about feelings helps them "hear" what their feelings are. Clarifying helps the woman "see" what the issues are and what options are available. Comforting measures, such as touch, convey empathic concern and are especially important during difficult procedures. Although nurses offer caring concern and careful reflection of feelings, they do not offer advice. The decisions must be made by the family, but nurses frequently help the family contact persons to whom they turn in troubled times, perhaps a member of the clergy or a close relative.

#### HELPING CLIENTS SET REALISTIC GOALS

Women benefit from knowing that compliance with the testing regimen is beneficial for the fetus. Each day in the uterus allows time for growth and development and increases the chance that the infant will be strong and healthy. The fetus has an improved chance of surviving as long as the test results remain reassuring.

#### SUPPORTING THE WOMAN'S DECISION

Nurses must examine their own ethical beliefs before they become involved in fetal diagnostic testing. They must be prepared to support whatever decision a family makes, even if it is not one they would make. For example, whether a woman decides to continue or terminate a pregnancy, she is entitled to compassionate care regardless of the nurse's personal views about the decision.

### Evaluation

Interventions are successful if the woman verbalizes knowledge of why tests are recommended, an idea of how and when they will be performed, and her concerns about the condition of the fetus and whether she actively seeks information to relieve her anxiety.

## SUMMARY CONCEPTS

- Ultrasonography is widely used during pregnancy to determine a variety of fetal and placental conditions and to aid in the performance of other tests, such as amniocentesis.
- Alpha-fetoprotein assessment, a screening test performed on maternal serum or amniotic fluid, is used primarily to detect open neural tube defects and chromosomal abnormalities. Additional tests are required if AFP levels are abnormal. Two other markers, human chorionic gonadotropin and estriol, are assessed along with AFP for chromosomal anomalies.
- Chorionic villus sampling can be performed as early as 10 weeks of gestation. CVS provides parents with information about chromosomal defects in the first trimester of pregnancy. Parents continue to be concerned about risks, such as limb reduction defects, which are associated with chorionic villus sampling.
- Amniocentesis is usually performed in the second or third trimester to identify chromosomal defects and to evaluate fetal maturity or Rh incompatibility problems, but early amniocentesis (12 to 14 weeks) is becoming more common.
- The nonstress test determines whether the FHR accelerates when the fetus moves. Accelerated heart rate is a reassuring sign associated with adequate fetal oxygenation and an intact neural pathway from the fetal brain to the heart.
- Contraction stress tests are used to determine the ability of the fetal heart to respond to uterine contractions that decrease placental blood flow and may result in fetal hypoxemia.
- Percutaneous umbilical blood sampling or cordocentesis involves aspirating blood from umbilical vessels to detect blood disorders, acid-base balance, infection, or fetal disease.
- Maternal assessment of fetal movement ("kick counts") provides an inexpensive and noninvasive method of evaluating the fetus.
- All perinatal nurses must be prepared to offer clear explanations of diagnostic procedures and to provide support for the family requiring fetal diagnostic tests.

#### References and Readings

American College of Obstetricians and Gynecologists (ACOG). (1994). *Antepartum fetal surveillance*, Technical Bulletin No. 188, pp. 1–5. Washington, D.C.

American College of Obstetricians and Gynecologists (ACOG). (1995). *Chorionic villus sampling*, Committee Opinion, No. 160. Washington, D.C.

Anthony, A. (1996). Biological effects and safety. In T.J. Dubose (Ed.), *Fetal sonography* (pp. 27–44). Philadelphia: W.B. Saunders.

Berman, M. (1996). History of fetal sonography. In T.J. DuBose (Ed.), *Fetal sonography* (pp. 11–26). Philadelphia: W.B. Saunders.

Cartier, M.S. (1996). Fetal Doppler. In T.J. DuBose (Ed.), *Fetal sonography* (pp. 275–303). Philadelphia: W.B. Saunders.

Covington, C., Gielghem, P., Board, F., Madison, K., Nedd, D., & Miller, L. (1996). Family care related to alpha-fetoprotein screening. *Journal of Obstetric, Gynecologic, and Neonatal Nursing, 25*(2), 125–130.

Cunningham, F.G., MacDonald, P.C., Gant, N.F., Leveno, K.J., Gilstrap, L.C., Hankins, G.D.V., et al. (1997). *Williams obstetrics* (20th ed.). Norwalk, Conn.: Appleton & Lange.

Devoe, L.D., Youssef, A.E., Croom, C.S., & Watson, J. (1994). Can biophysical profile observations anticipate outcome in preterm labor or preterm rupture of membranes? *Obstetrics and Gynecology, 84*(3), 432–437.

DuBose, T.J. (1996). First trimester. In T.J. DuBose, *Fetal sonography* (pp. 389–425). Philadelphia: W.B. Saunders.

Dubose, T.J. (1996). Second and third trimester. In T.J. DuBose, *Fetal sonography* (pp. 427–471). Philadelphia: W.B. Saunders.

Evans, M.I., Johnson, M.P., & Drugan, A. (1994). Amniocentesis for antenatal diagnosis of genetic disorders. In F.P. Zuspan & E.J. Quilligan, *Current therapy in obstetrics and gynecology* (pp. 199–205). Philadelphia: W.B. Saunders.

Farmakides, G., Weiner, Z., Mammapoulos, M., & Nikolaides, P. (1994). Doppler velocimetry: Where does it belong in evaluation of fetal status? *Clinics in Perinatology, 21*(4), 849–862.

Gebauer, C.L., & Lowe, N.K. (1993). Biophysical profile: Antepartal assessment of fetal wellbeing. *Journal of Obstetrical, Gynecologic, and Neonatal Nursing, 22*(2), 115–127.

Gegor, C.L., Paine, L.L., Costigan, K., & Johnson, T.R. (1994). Interpretation of biophysical profiles by nurses and physicians. *Journal of Obstetric, Gynecologic, and Neonatal Nursing, 23*(5), 405–410.

Halle, J.N. (1993). Diagnostic evaluation of high-risk pregnancies. In S. Mattson & J.E. Smith (Eds.), NAACOG *core curriculum for maternal-newborn nursing* (pp. 157–184). Philadelphia: W.B. Saunders.

Huddleston, J.F., Williams, G.S., & Fabbri, E.L. (1993). Antepartum assessment of the fetus. In R.A. Knuppel & J.E. Drukker (Eds.), *High-risk pregnancy: A team approach* (2nd ed., pp. 62–75). Philadelphia: W.B. Saunders.

Johnson, T.R.B. (1994). Maternal perception and Doppler detection of fetal movement. *Clinics in Perinatology*, 21(4), 765–778.

Kellner, L.H., Weiss, R.R., Weiner, Z., et al. (1995). The advantages of using triple-marker screening for chromosomal abnormalities. *American Journal of Obstetrics and Gynecology*, 172(3), 831–836.

Lagrew, D.C. (1995). The contraction stress test. *Clinical Obstetrics and Gynecology*, 38(1), 11–25.

Manning, F.A. (1994). General principles and applications of ultrasonography. In R.K. Creasy & R. Resnik (Eds.), *Maternal-fetal medicine: Principles and practice* (3rd ed., pp. 201–232). Philadelphia: W.B. Saunders.

Manning, F.A. (1995). Dynamic ultrasound-based fetal assessment: The fetal biophysical profile score. *Clinical Obstetrics and Gynecology*, 38(1), 26–43.

McCarthy, K.E., & Narrigan, D. (1995). Is there scientific support for the use of juice to facilitate the nonstress test? *Journal of Obstetric, Gynecologic, and Neonatal Nursing*, 24(4), 303–306.

Parer, J.T. (1994). Fetal heart rate. In R.K. Creasy & R. Resnik (Eds.), *Maternal-fetal medicine: Principles and practice* (3rd ed., pp. 298–325). Philadelphia: W.B. Saunders.

Paul, R., & Miller, D.A. (1995). Nonstress test. *Clinical Obstetrics and Gynecology*, 38(1), 3–9.

Pergament, E. (1994). Chorionic villus sampling for prenatal diagnosis. In F.P. Zuspan & E.J. Quilligan (Eds.), *Current therapy in obstetrics and gynecology* (pp. 224–226). Philadelphia: W.B. Saunders.

Raines, D.A. (1996). Fetal surveillance: Issues and implications. *Journal of Obstetric, Gynecologic, and Neonatal Nursing*, 25(7), 559–564.

Ramsay, P.A., & Fisk, N.M. (1994). Amniocentesis. In D.K. James, P.J. Steer, C.P. Weiner, & B. Gonik (Eds.), *High-risk pregnancy: Management options* (pp. 735–744). Philadelphia: W.B. Saunders.

Rayburn, W.F. (1995). Fetal movement monitoring. *Clinical Obstetrics and Gynecology*, 38(1), 59–67.

Santalahti, P., Latikka, A.M., Ryynänen, M., & Hemminki, E. (1996). Women's experiences of perinatal serum screening. *Birth*, 23(2), 101–107.

Simpson, J.L., & Elias, S. (1994). Prenatal diagnosis of genetic disorders. In R.K. Creasy & R. Resnik (Eds.), *Maternal-fetal medicine: Principles and practice* (3rd ed., pp. 61–88). Philadelphia: W.B. Saunders.

Smith, C.V. (1994). Vibroacoustic stimulation for risk assessment. *Clinics in Perinatology*, 21(4), 797–809.

Sonek, J., & Nicolaides, K. (1994). The role of cordocentesis in the diagnosis of fetal well-being. *Clinics in Perinatology*, 21(4), 723–742.

Veille, J.C., Deviney, M., & Hanson, R. (1993). Ultrasound in pregnancy. In R.A. Knuppel & J.E. Drukker (Eds.), *High-risk pregnancy: A team approach* (pp. 78–96). Philadelphia: W.B. Saunders.

Vintzileos, A.M., & Knuppel, R.A. (1994). Multiple parameter biophysical testing in the prediction of acid-base status. *Clinics in Perinatology*, 21(4), 823–848.

Ware, D.J., & Devoe, L.D. (1994). The nonstress test: Reassessment of the "gold standard." *Clinics in Perinatology*, 21(4), 779–796.

Wenstrom, K.D., Owen, J., Boots, L., & Ethier, M. (1995). The influence of maternal weight on human chorionic gonadotropin in the multiple-marker screening test for fetal Down syndrome. *American Journal of Obstetrics and Gynecology*, 173(4), 1297–1300.

# 11

# Perinatal Education

**OBJECTIVES**

1. List the goals of perinatal education.
2. Explain choices in childbearing and the effect of education on these choices.
3. Describe the various types of education for childbearing families.
4. Describe techniques for pain relief taught in Lamaze childbirth classes.
5. Describe the support person's role in helping women during labor and birth.
6. Explain the components frequently included in a birth plan.

**DEFINITIONS**

**birth plan** *A plan describing a couple's preferences for their birth experience.*

**cleansing breath** *A deep breath taken at the beginning and end of each labor contraction.*

**effleurage** *Massage of the abdomen or other body part performed during labor contractions.*

**habituation** *Decreased response to a repeated stimulus.*

**paced breathing** *Learned breathing technique used during labor contractions to promote relaxation and increase pain tolerance.*

**psychoprophylaxis** *Method of prepared childbirth that emphasizes mental concentration and relaxation to increase pain tolerance.*

**Valsalva's maneuver** *Increasing pressure within the abdomen and thorax by holding the breath and pushing against a closed glottis.*

Perinatal education has become increasingly important in helping couples learn about pregnancy, birth, and parenting. With shorter birth facility stays, classes that once focused solely on preparing for childbirth are now expanding to include information formerly received during the birth facility stay. Prenatal classes are often included in perinatal clinical pathways (see Figure 1–2).

## Goals of Perinatal Education

The goals of perinatal education are to help parents become knowledgeable consumers, take an active role in maintaining health during pregnancy and birth, and learn coping techniques to deal with pregnancy, childbirth, and parenting. Meeting these goals increases parents' ability to make decisions regarding childbirth and parenting with confidence and satisfaction.

## Providers of Education

Although most perinatal education classes are taught by registered nurses, physical therapists or others who have taken special courses may also become perinatal educators. Many instructors are certified by organizations such as the American Society for Psychoprophylaxis in Obstetrics (ASPO) or the International Childbirth Education Association (ICEA). Certification ensures that the instructors have received special preparation to provide sound education that adheres to the certifying organization's general philosophy. The Association of Women's Health, Obstetric, and Neonatal Nurses has published guidelines for educator competencies and class curricula (AWHONN, 1993). Teachers must be versed in adult education theory and techniques and skillful in handling groups of people from diverse backgrounds.

Classes may be sponsored by community agencies such as schools, health departments, or civic organizations or by health care providers such as medical groups or hospitals. Teachers may be employed by any of these sponsoring agencies or may be self-employed. Classes may also occur in less traditional sites. For example, some companies offer employees free prenatal classes at the work site. Teaching women how to reduce risk factors for complications is a way for employers to reduce costs associated with prematurity and low birth weight.

Education may be presented formally in classrooms. Nurses in offices, clinics, and birth sites also educate women informally. For example, teaching may occur in waiting rooms of clinics before women are called for their appointments or as a part of routine care.

## Class Participants

Participants in classes about childbearing have traditionally been middle-income couples who are older and better educated than those who do not take classes. Low-income women may not have money to pay for classes. Although inexpensive or free classes are available in some areas, women with little or no prenatal care may not know about this form of education. Classes in languages other than English have become more readily available in areas where they are needed.

People take classes for a variety of reasons. Many have a strong desire to participate actively in all aspects of childbearing. For these people, making decisions about what happens to them is important, and they want the education to help them decide wisely. Others are looking for coping strategies to deal with their fear of childbirth or pain. When women feel informed and feel that they have some control over what happens to them, they are more likely to expect birth to be satisfying and fulfilling and to experience it as such. In one large study, women with positive expectations regarding labor and the effectiveness of learned coping strategies like breathing and relaxation were more likely to feel that their experience was positive (Green, 1993).

## Choices for Childbearing

Many of the changes in childbearing practices during the last 40 years have occurred in response to consumer desire for more input and control over the birth experience. The family-centered approach, designed to make birth less institutional and more personal, is one response to this consumer movement. Choices about the setting and interventions used and the inclusion of the father or other support person have resulted from the work of concerned consumers and health care providers.

One purpose of any perinatal education program is to help parents learn what options are available so that they can make appropriate choices. Parents learn that there are many ways of birthing and that no one "right" method exists. Knowledgeable parents can communicate assertively with their health care providers about their needs and desires.

### Health Care Professional

Women contemplating pregnancy and birth may choose a certified nurse-midwife (CNM), nurse practi-

## Parents Want to Know

### What Options Should We Consider for Our Birth Plan?

*Whether or not the following options are available may depend on the policies of the birth facility and the health care provider. Discuss them with your provider to learn more about what is available to you.*

**Monitoring**

Do you have strong feelings about using electronic fetal monitoring? Some women find it reassuring because it provides continuous information about the fetus. Others feel that it interferes with their ability to remain active during labor. Intermittent use of monitoring may be possible if no complications occur.

**Intravenous Fluids**

Some health care professionals consider intravenous fluids necessary to replace fluids lost during labor and for giving pain medications or emergency drugs. Some women find them painful and intrusive, whereas others do not mind them. Alternatives include waiting until active labor to begin intravenous fluids, avoiding them unless complications occur, and using a saline lock so that you can move about more freely.

**Food and Oral Fluids**

Other than ice chips, food and fluids are generally not allowed during active labor because of decreased gastric motility, vomiting, and the possibility of aspiration if general anesthesia is suddenly needed. Clear fluids may be an option.

**Shaving and Enemas**

A very-small-volume enema and shaving just around the episiotomy area may or may not be routine. Enemas may stimulate contractions, but many women dislike them and have loose stools in early labor.

**Position**

Walking, taking a shower, or otherwise remaining active rather than staying in bed throughout labor may or may not be important. Some women prefer a squatting, kneeling, or side-lying position for birth. A birthing bed or chair may allow a comfortable and effective delivery position.

**Episiotomy**

Although an episiotomy is frequently performed, you may wish to avoid it unless absolutely necessary. Discuss the use of massage to stretch the perineal tissue as an alternative to an episiotomy.

**Pain Relief**

You may plan to avoid medication for pain relief completely, use it only if absolutely necessary, or wish to take it as soon as possible to avoid pain. You may expect to use relaxation techniques throughout labor or only until you can receive anesthesia. Specific ideas about kinds of pain relief available should also be considered.

**Support Person**

You may wish only the infant's father, a relative, or a close friend to be with you during labor and birth, or you may prefer a number of people present for some or all of the experience.

**Breastfeeding**

You may wish to begin breastfeeding immediately after birth or within the first hour. You may prefer that no water or formula be given to your baby unless a problem develops. Some mothers ask that the nursery staff feed the baby during the night.

**Siblings**

You may want your other children present at the birth or want them to visit you while you are in the hospital.

**Care of the Newborn**

It may be possible to have your baby stay with you at all times to promote bonding. To get more rest, you may prefer to care for the baby only during the day and evening hours. The infant may spend the night in the nursery or return to you for night feedings.

**Discharge**

Check your insurance coverage, which may influence your discharge time. Expect to go home about 48 hours after a vaginal birth or 96 hours after a cesarean birth. Or you may be discharged earlier with follow-up visits from a home visit nurse, in a clinic, or in your provider's office. Also discuss discharge with your caregiver to learn more about your options. Some women prefer to go home as soon as possible, but others desire a longer stay to rest before assuming full care of the newborn along with their other responsibilities.

---

tioner (NP), obstetrician, or family practice physician to be their health care provider. They need to know what to expect from each of these practitioners.

A CNM cares for women who are at low risk for complications and refers them to a "back-up" physician if problems develop. The CNMs, NPs, and physicians follow women during pregnancy and the postpartum period, but the NPs do not usually perform deliveries. A CNM, NP, or family practice physician may care for the newborn as well. A physician generally arrives for the birth near the end of labor, whereas the CNM is often present through most of labor and birth. Some couples visit several different care providers to discuss their plans for birth before choosing the one they feel is best for them.

## Setting

The woman and her partner must choose a birth setting and select a care provider who practices in that setting. Hospitals are the most frequent setting for birth in North America. They may have birthing suites that provide a home-like atmosphere or traditional labor and delivery rooms. A free-standing birth center provides an atmosphere that is less institutional than that of the hospital. Home birth allows the woman to give birth in her own surroundings with delivery managed by a nurse-midwife. (More information about these birth settings is presented in Chapter 1.)

### Support Person

During labor, the woman needs to have someone with her to help her through the experience. The support person is most often the father of her baby, but a relative or friend may also take this role (Fig. 11–1). Some women wish to share the birth experience with several relatives or close friends. If the birth setting is traditional, only one person is permitted to be present. In less traditional settings, more support people are usually allowed. Some women hire a support person, such as a doula, to provide support during labor. An experienced labor support person (such as a doula) can reduce length of labor and minimize the need for cesarean births and for pain medication (Klaus et al., 1993).

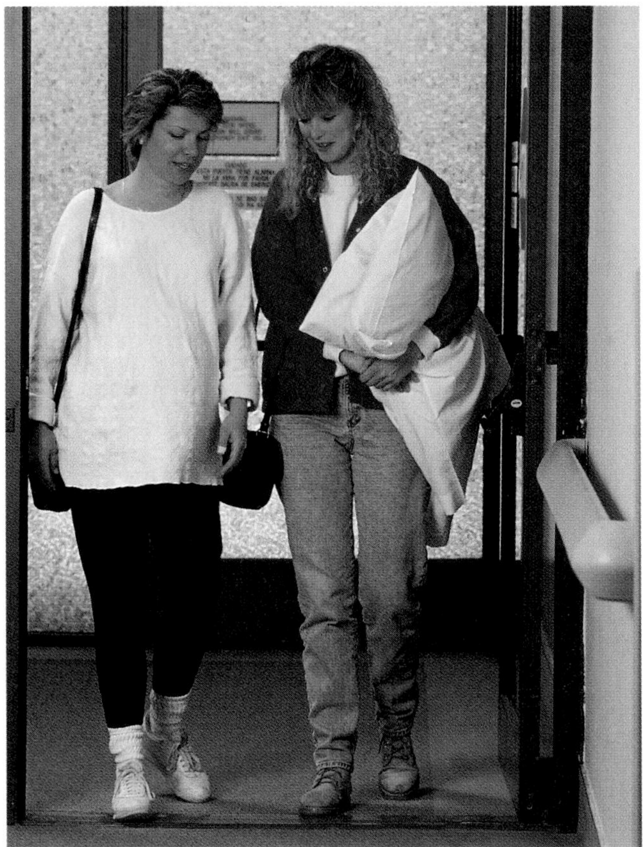

**FIGURE 11–1**

Often an expectant mother will ask a sister or close female friend to be her labor partner and to attend classes with her.

### Siblings

The presence of children at birth is controversial. Some believe that children become closer to their new sibling when they are present at the birth. Others think that seeing the birth process, the blood, and the mother in pain may be too frightening for children. Some of the debate centers on the age of the child attending the birth.

Children who participate in the birth of a sibling may attend all or part of the labor and birth or may join the parents just after the birth to participate in the immediate celebration. An adult support person stays with the child throughout the experience. The support person should have no role other than attending to the child. This role includes gauging the child's response, providing explanations and reassurance, and taking the child out of the room as needed. Because labor generally is lengthy, children often come and go during the labor process but are present when birth is imminent or just after the actual birth.

### Education

Expectant mothers must also decide on prenatal education classes. Their decisions are based on the classes available in the area, the costs, and the kinds of information they need. Some areas have a vast array of classes from which to choose. In others, the selection is limited to childbirth preparation classes only.

Small classes of a few women and their partners are ideal, but they may be too expensive or unavailable. If the class includes more than 10 to 12 couples, the teacher should have an assistant to help with individual instruction. The teacher is usually a registered nurse who has experience in maternity nursing and is often certified by a nationally known organization.

Prepared childbirth classes based in birth facilities include detailed information on what to expect in that particular setting but may not cover options that are unavailable at that agency. Hospital classes have sometimes been criticized for teaching clients to be "good" or compliant patients. A woman may wish to talk to the instructor before taking a class to ask about class size and the teacher's philosophy, background, and teaching methods.

**CHECK YOUR READING**

1. What are the goals of perinatal education?
2. What are some of the major decisions couples must make in preparation for childbirth?

## Types of Classes Available

Although most people think of perinatal education primarily as preparation for the birth experience, classes are available in all areas of pregnancy, childbirth, and parenting.

### Preconception Classes

Classes for couples who are thinking about having a baby are designed to help them have a healthy pregnancy from the beginning. Information about nutrition before conception, signs of pregnancy, healthy lifestyle, and choosing a caregiver are presented. The effect of pregnancy and childbirth on a woman's relationships and career is discussed. Preconception classes emphasize ways to reduce risk factors for poor pregnancy outcome and early and regular prenatal care.

### Early Pregnancy Classes

Early pregnancy classes focus on the first two trimesters (Table 11–1). First-trimester classes are sometimes called "early bird" or "right start" classes. They cover information on adapting to pregnancy, dealing with early discomforts such as morning sickness and fatigue, and understanding what to expect in the months ahead. Emphasis is placed on how to have a healthy pregnancy by obtaining prenatal care and avoiding hazards to the fetus.

Second-trimester classes focus on changes that occur during middle pregnancy and on preparing for birth. Information on body mechanics in relation to an enlarging abdomen, working during pregnancy, and what to expect during the third trimester is included. Teachers discuss childbirth choices and information to help students become more knowledgeable consumers.

Parents may begin to learn about the needs of the mother and infant after birth in these classes or attend other classes to meet this need. This information is especially important because of the short period they stay in the birth facility.

**TABLE 11–1 EARLY PREGNANCY CLASSES**

**Pregnancy**
- Anatomy and physiology
- Physiologic and psychological changes
- Fetal development
- Hazards to the mother or fetus (drugs, alcohol, smoking, environmental)
- Medical care (importance, what to expect at each visit)
- Communicating with the provider
- Prenatal screening tests

**Self-care**
- Hygiene
- Nutrition
- Exercise and body mechanics
- Discomforts of pregnancy
- Danger signs
- Sexuality
- Working and pregnancy

**Infant Care**
- Choosing a pediatrician
- Infant development and care
- Infant feeding
- Preparation for breastfeeding

**Birth**
- Birth options (birth plan, costs)
- Preterm labor

### Exercise Classes

Exercise classes help women keep fit and healthy during pregnancy. Some classes continue into the postpartum period as well. Written consent from the primary caregiver may be required to ensure that the woman can participate safely. The instructor should understand the special needs of pregnancy and teach low-impact exercises preceded by warm-up routines. To prevent diversion of blood away from the uterus, women should avoid excessive heart rate elevation. An added benefit of the classes is the opportunity for women to meet others with similar concerns.

### Childbirth Preparation Classes

Women and their support persons learn self-help measures and what to expect during labor and birth in childbirth preparation classes (Fig. 11–2). Although once referred to as "natural childbirth" classes, they are now called "prepared childbirth" classes to denote that women are prepared for all aspects of childbirth, including complications. Cou-

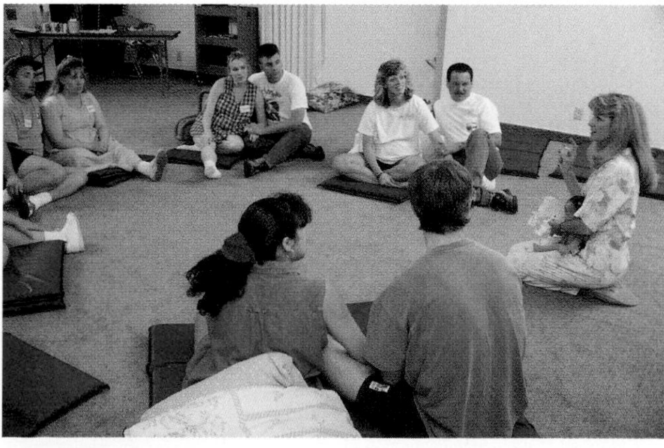

**FIGURE 11–2**

The nurse teaching this class discusses movement of the fetus through the pelvis.

**TABLE 11–2 PREPARED CHILDBIRTH CLASSES**

**Pregnancy**
- Physical and psychological changes of the last trimester
- Common discomforts and concerns
- Nutrition
- Exercise and body mechanics
- Sexuality

**Antepartum Testing**
- Common third-trimester tests

**Labor and Birth**
- Anatomy and physiology of labor
- Planning for the birth (consumerism, options, birth plan)
- Signs of labor and when to go to the hospital
- Hospital admission and procedures
- Physical and emotional aspects of labor
- Labor variations (e.g., back labor, inductions)
- Birthing process
- Recovery
- Tour of maternity unit

**Coping Techniques for Labor**
- Relaxation
- Breathing techniques
- Comfort measures
- Labor rehearsals
- Pain relief: pharmacologic and nonpharmacologic

**Complications**
- Danger signs
- High-risk pregnancy
- Cesarean birth

**Support Person**
- Role of the coach
- Coaching techniques

**Postpartum**
- Physiologic and psychological changes
- Birth agency stay/early discharge
- Role adaptation, postpartum blues
- Family planning

**Normal Newborn**
- Characteristics
- General care and safety
- Feeding (breast and formula)

ples learn coping methods that help them approach childbirth in a positive manner. Teachers do not promise prevention of all pain in labor. The increased confidence gained in prepared childbirth classes is, however, associated with a decreased perception and increased tolerance of pain during labor and lower use of drugs for labor pain (Lowe, 1996).

Classes include information about labor, pharmacologic and nonpharmacologic methods of pain relief, and a tour of the birth setting. Supervised practice of relaxation and coping strategies in "labor rehearsals" is part of every class. Films assist women to develop a realistic picture of the birth process (Table 11–2).

The teacher describes advantages and disadvantages of various options in birthing. For example, couples may learn that epidural anesthesia, which is almost routine in many areas, usually removes most pain but may increase the length of labor, cause less effective pushing, and make catheterization and administration of oxytocin more likely. On the other hand, use of relaxation techniques avoids the disadvantages of analgesic drugs and anesthesia but does not remove all discomfort. When women have a balanced view of their options, they are able to discuss them intelligently with caregivers and make better decisions.

Even women who plan to have epidural anesthesia as soon as possible should learn and practice methods they can use for pain relief. Birth facilities may not admit women into the labor unit until they are in active labor. This timing of admission makes pain relief measures necessary until the woman can receive anesthesia.

Class series range from four to nine meetings, depending on the content included. Because these may be the only classes a woman attends, information about the third trimester of pregnancy is often presented. Some classes also include discussion of the postpartum period, breastfeeding, and infant care.

### Refresher Courses

Women whose last prepared childbirth was more than 2 or 3 years ago often take a refresher class for an update of current practices and review of techniques. Classes consist of one to three sessions in which supervised practice is the major focus. Basic information is omitted or briefly reviewed. Refresher

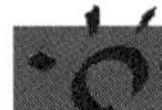

**CRITICAL THINKING EXERCISE**

**Q:** Should women who attended prepared childbirth classes for their first pregnancy go to classes for subsequent pregnancies? Why should women who have had an earlier prepared birth take another course?

**A:** Women and their support people should attend classes before each birth because they may have forgotten some of the information they learned during a previous childbirth class. Birthing care and options may have changed since the last birth. Couples often have concerns and questions about their last experience, and the nurse can discuss these issues and help them feel more positive about the pending birth. The needs of other children can also be addressed, with practical suggestions about easing the transition.

**TABLE 11-3 CESAREAN BIRTH CLASSES**

| |
|---|
| Indications |
| Prenatal tests |
| Preparation (e.g., NPO, shave, Foley catheter) |
| Anesthesia |
| Surgical procedure |
| Role of support person during surgery |
| Options |
| Postsurgical care |
| Postoperative pain relief |
| Relaxation techniques |
| Postpartum course |
| Future birth options |

courses also include discussion of role changes in the family and sibling adjustment.

## Cesarean Birth Preparation Classes

Education about cesarean birth may take place in general childbirth classes or may be conducted separately for those expecting a cesarean birth (Table 11–3).

### GENERAL CESAREAN CLASSES

Approximately one fourth of all births are by cesarean delivery, and women need preparation for this possibility. Cesarean birth is usually discussed during general prepared childbirth classes. Some teachers show films of both vaginal and cesarean births. Topics include indications, options, surgical procedure, and postoperative course.

Reasons for cesarean births should be discussed in detail. A woman might view the terms "failed induction" or "failure to progress" as casting blame on her. She may believe that if she had used relaxation techniques better or been more tolerant of pain, she might have avoided the need for surgery. Teachers often point out that the causes of cesarean births are conditions over which the woman has no control.

**Couples are sometimes inattentive during discussions about cesarean birth because they think that "it can't happen to me." Pointing out the number of couples in the class who may have cesarean births (based on the 1994 rate of 21.2 percent [Guyer et al., 1996]) may catch their attention. Providing written materials may be helpful for later review if the need for surgery develops.**

### PLANNED CESAREAN BIRTH CLASSES

Women who know they will have a cesarean birth may attend planned cesarean birth classes. For those who had a cesarean birth previously, the class offers an opportunity to share experiences and feelings and to clarify misconceptions. Often these women remember little of the preparation for the procedure because they were frightened and exhausted. Couples anticipating their first cesarean birth may appreciate hearing from others who have had the experience.

Class content includes indications for cesarean births, care the woman will receive, and possible options. A woman may want to watch the birth and can ask that a mirror be positioned so that she can see it. A woman who wishes to go into labor to ensure maturity of the fetus or to experience labor should discuss this decision with her caregiver. Class discussion helps couples feel that they have some control over what happens and provides a basis for discussion with caregivers.

## Vaginal Birth After Cesarean Birth

Whenever possible, vaginal birth is encouraged for women who have had a previous cesarean birth. These women may take a vaginal birth after cesarean, or VBAC, class. Content includes explanations of when a VBAC is possible, the extra precautions taken and their reasons, what to expect during labor and birth, and coping techniques. Although the focus is on positive expectations, situations that might make another cesarean birth necessary are also covered. Discussion includes the emotional aspects of a "failed VBAC" as well.

## Breastfeeding Classes

Prenatal breastfeeding education is increasingly important because the time available to help breastfeeding mothers in the birth facility after birth is very short. Classes help increase a woman's confidence in her ability to breastfeed successfully and provide her with sources of help if she encounters difficulties. Women who attend prenatal classes that include breastfeeding information are more likely to breastfeed their infants and to do so for longer than 6 months compared with women who do not attend classes (Piper & Parks, 1996).

Breastfeeding classes include information on physiology of lactation, feeding techniques, establishing a milk supply, and dealing with common problems (Table 11–4). Partners who attend learn methods of providing support during breastfeeding. Some teachers hold additional sessions after the birth to provide ongoing counseling at a time when mothers may experience unexpected problems alone. These sessions allow discussion of problems as they occur. Classes that focus on working mothers may also be available.

## Parenting Classes

Instruction on parenting and newborn care may be included in prepared childbirth classes or provided separately. Content typically includes general care

**TABLE 11-4 BREASTFEEDING CLASSES**

Anatomy and physiology
Preparation for breastfeeding
Positioning
Establishing milk supply
Nutrition
Problems
- Prevention
- Engorgement
- Sore nipples
- Insufficient milk supply
- Mastitis

Use of bottles
- Storing breast milk
- Nipple confusion

Breast pumps
Working and breastfeeding
Weaning

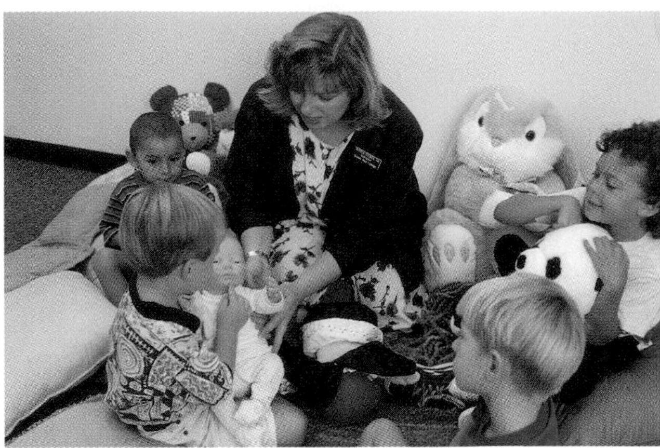

**FIGURE 11-3**
During sibling classes, children learn about the new baby coming into their lives.

and common concerns, such as the crying infant and advantages and disadvantages of circumcision (Table 11–5). Baby equipment, such as various types of infant car seats, is often displayed. Practice with dolls may also be included. Classes may continue after birth of the infant.

## Postpartum Classes

Although the topic of the postpartum period is covered in prepared childbirth classes, the mother can also attend classes after birth. Content includes the physiologic and psychological changes of the postpartum period, role transition, sexuality, and nutrition. Some classes are informal support groups led by a knowledgeable professional. Other classes focus primarily on exercise for the postpartum period. Because so many women return to work soon after childbirth, sessions are often held at night or on weekends and include the concerns of working mothers.

**TABLE 11-5 PARENTING CLASSES**

Normal newborn characteristics: marks, rashes, normal behavior
General care: diapering, cord care, circumcision care, bathing
Feeding methods and problems: schedules, colic
Other concerns: crying, sleeping through the night
Safety: car seats, "baby proofing" the home
Baby equipment: choosing toys appropriate for age
Early growth and development: expectations, infant stimulation, immunization
Illness: signs of common conditions, taking a temperature, calling the physician
Infant cardiopulmonary resuscitation (CPR)

## Classes for Other Family Members

### SIBLINGS

Sibling classes are for children aged 2 to 10 years. The classes help them learn about newborn characteristics and help decrease anxiety about the approaching birth (Fig. 11–3). Parents learn ways of helping children adjust to the birth of a new baby. Such preparation may help improve family interaction and reduce sibling rivalry (see also Chapter 18).

Many young children have never seen a newborn and are expecting an older child to be their playmate. A tour of the nursery or a visit with a newborn infant allows them to see newborns at close range and learn to be safe helpers. Videos or stories promote discussion about normal feelings of jealousy and anger. Emphasis is placed on the important role of big brothers and sisters and the fact that a baby could not take their place.

A separate parent discussion provides suggestions for further preparation and coping with the transition after birth. Concerns about sibling rivalry and meeting the needs of more than one child are common topics. Sibling visitation during hospitalization is another topic. Seeing the mother in the hospital decreases a child's anxiety about why she is not at home.

Special sibling classes may be held for children who will be present at the birth. These help prepare the child for the sights and sounds of birth. The child's support person also attends the class.

### GRANDPARENTS

Classes for grandparents provide an update about recent developments in childbirth and parenting practices. Lack of understanding about new ways of childbearing can cause conflict between young couples and their parents. An explanation of these changes improves communication between the generations. Grandparents compare parenting in the past and present in a supportive environment with others in similar situations.

Topics generally focus on family-centered childbirth and infant care. Infant care discussions review current thinking about care and feeding. Early growth and development and accident prevention are also included. Particularly emphasized are the art of grandparenting and the importance of grandparents.

**✓ CHECK YOUR READING**

3. How are early pregnancy classes different from later pregnancy classes?
4. Why should all women learn about cesarean childbirth?
5. Why are sibling and grandparent classes important?

## Education for Childbirth

Many studies have attempted to determine whether education for childbirth affects the outcome in regard to client satisfaction, pain relief, length of labor, and frequency of complications. The results of these studies vary. Some report shorter labors with fewer complications and less need for pharmacologic pain relief measures, whereas others report no difference between prepared and unprepared women. Most studies agree that couples receiving prenatal preparation for childbirth are more satisfied with their birth experiences and have a greater feeling of control, even when unexpected complications occur.

### Causes of Pain in Labor

The pain of childbirth results from hypoxia of uterine muscle, dilation and stretching of the cervix, pressure and pulling on adjacent organs, and pressure from the presenting part on the vagina and perineum during birth (Blackburn & Loper, 1992). Many other factors can increase pain. Fetal size and position influence length of labor as well as degree of pain. Vaginal examinations and use of oxytocin increase the strength of contractions. A woman's expectations, level of fatigue, anxiety, and the availability and actions of a support person also affect her perception of pain.

### Methods of Pain Management

#### EDUCATION

One of the most important aspects of any childbirth preparation class is education to increase the woman's confidence in her ability to cope with birth. Women who are confident about their coping abilities report less pain during labor than women who lack confidence (Lowe, 1996). Confidence may be increased by attending classes that provide information about what will happen, vicarious experiences such as films or reports of others' births, and techniques to increase coping ability during labor.

By learning what to expect during labor and birth, women and their support persons have a chance to rehearse the experience in their minds to prepare for the actual event. They practice using coping techniques during simulated contractions. It is essential that class information is realistic and valid and that possible variations are discussed so that couples are adequately prepared.

#### RELAXATION

Tension and anxiety during labor cause tightening of abdominal muscles, impeding contractions and increasing pain by stimulation of nerve endings that heighten awareness of pain. Prolonged muscle tension causes fatigue and increased pain perception. When anxiety and tension are high, uterine contractions are less effective and the length of labor increases. A woman who is able to remain relaxed is likely to labor more efficiently and with less pain and to be better able to use other techniques to help herself. A number of different techniques are taught to enhance relaxation during labor.

#### CONDITIONING

Many of the techniques used for prepared childbirth are based partially on theories of conditioned response, in which certain responses to stimuli become automatic through frequent association. Women learn to associate uterine contractions with relaxation by practicing relaxation techniques with a mental image of a contraction. Because conditioning requires a great deal of practice to make it effective, women are encouraged to practice their techniques daily. For some women, the intensity of real uterine contractions is surprisingly different from what they experienced during practice sessions. They may have difficulty with relaxation as a result and need to use other methods along with conditioning.

#### GATE CONTROL THEORY

According to the gate control theory of pain, transmission of nerve impulses is controlled by a neural mechanism in the dorsal horn of the spinal cord. Transmission is affected by stimulation of large- or small-diameter sensory nerve fibers and descending impulses from the brain. This mechanism opens or closes the "gate" to pain sensation by allowing or preventing some impulses from reaching the brain, where they are recognized as pain.

Pain is transmitted through small-diameter sensory nerve fibers. Stimulation of large-diameter fibers in the skin interferes with conduction through small-diameter fibers, thus "closing the gate" and decreasing the amount of pain felt. Massage and pressure on the palms or fingertips stimulate large-diameter nerve fibers. Relief is temporary because stimulation of these fibers results in habituation, or decreased response to stimuli. Periodically changing the type or area of stimulation increases effectiveness (Blackburn & Loper, 1992).

Impulses from the brain have a similar ability to impede transmission through the dorsal horn using visual and auditory stimulation techniques. These include use of a focal point or breathing techniques. Memory and cognitive processes affect the perception of stimuli as painful. Education and support during labor are used to increase the woman's confidence and feeling of control. Although these methods may not completely prevent pain, they may decrease the severity of perceived pain (Creehan, 1996).

## Methods of Childbirth Education

Although all methods of prepared childbirth education use some combination of pain-management techniques, each has some unique aspects. Some differences exist in types of classes and class content, depending on geographic area. Many classes have an eclectic approach, providing a variety of techniques from which couples can choose those that work best for them.

### Dick-Read Childbirth Education

Grantly Dick-Read was an English physician who was one of the first to use education and relaxation techniques to help women through childbirth. His theory was that fear of childbirth results in tension and pain. The method he developed involves slow abdominal breathing in early labor and rapid chest breathing in advanced labor. His methods were the first to be called "natural childbirth."

### Bradley Childbirth Education

The Bradley method was the first to include the father as support person for "husband-coached childbirth." Slow abdominal breathing and relaxation are taught in these classes. They also emphasize avoidance of medication and other interventions.

### LeBoyer Method of Childbirth

LeBoyer childbirth, sometimes called "birth without violence," views birth as a traumatic experience for the neonate. To decrease the trauma at birth, lights are dimmed and noise is decreased to help the newborn adapt to extrauterine life more easily. The infant receives a warm bath immediately after birth to help relaxation.

### Lamaze Childbirth Education

The Lamaze method is often called "psychoprophylaxis" because it uses the mind to prevent pain. It involves the mind in concentration and uses conditioning to help the woman respond to contractions with relaxation and various techniques to decrease pain. The Lamaze method is the most popular method used today.

#### CLASS CONTENT

Content of specific Lamaze classes may differ, but most follow a similar pattern. Although the focus is on the childbirth experience, other topics such as the postpartum period and infant care are often included. Techniques for coping with labor include education to prevent fear of the unknown and activities that promote relaxation during labor.

Lamaze teachers acknowledge that labor is painful and do not promise that techniques will produce a pain-free birth. Instead, the techniques are used to increase the woman's ability to cope with pain by relieving some of the distress that accompanies it.

#### EXERCISES

Women learn toning and conditioning exercises to prepare for childbirth and help prevent discomfort in late pregnancy. Because the classes are taken during the third trimester of pregnancy, selection of exercises must take into consideration the changes in center of gravity and joint stability that occur at that time. (See Chapter 7 for exercises for pregnancy.)

#### RELAXATION TECHNIQUES

The ability to relax during labor is one of the most important components for coping effectively with childbirth. It conserves energy and enhances other pain-relief techniques. Women learn a variety of exercises to help them recognize and release tension. The labor partner or coach assists the woman by providing feedback during exercise sessions as well as during labor. He or she is alert to ways in which the woman shows tension. For example, she may tighten her shoulders, wrinkle her forehead, or jiggle her foot when stressed. The coach helps her focus on areas that she finds difficult to relax.

Relaxation exercises must be practiced frequently to be useful during labor. Couples begin practice sessions in a quiet, comfortable setting. Later they practice in other places that simulate the noise and unfamiliar setting of the hospital. Relaxation exercises may also be combined with other techniques such as imagery or massage (Fig. 11–4).

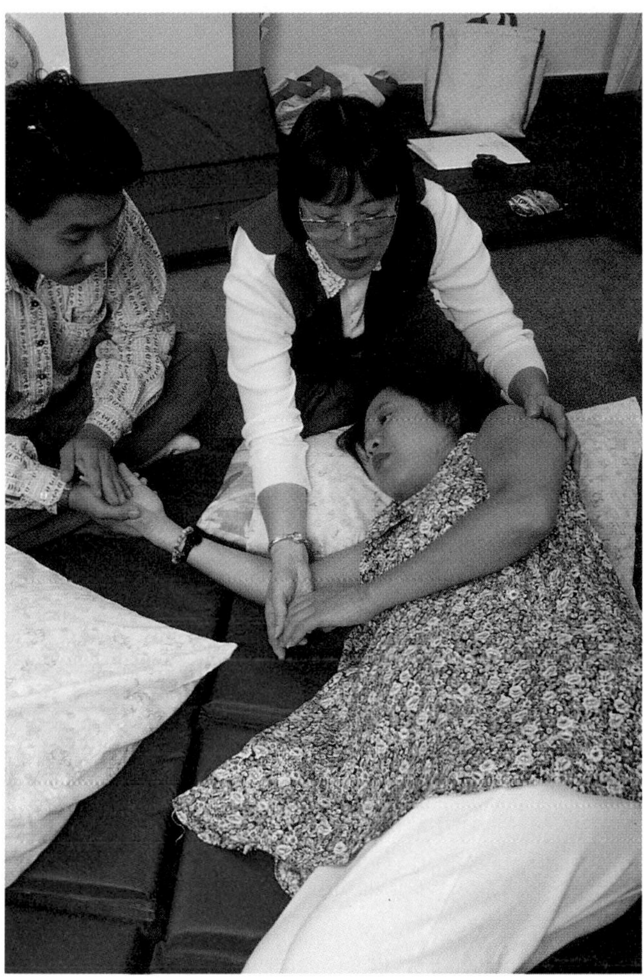

**FIGURE 11–4**

As the woman practices relaxation techniques for labor, the coach massages her hand, and the nurse checks for muscle tension.

**Progressive Relaxation.** Progressive relaxation involves contracting and then consciously releasing different muscle groups. The exercise is repeated throughout the body until all voluntary muscles are relaxed. By doing this, the woman learns to differentiate the feeling of tense muscles from that of relaxation. With this knowledge, she can systematically assess and then free muscle tension throughout her body.

**Neuromuscular Dissociation.** Neuromuscular dissociation (also called differential relaxation) helps the woman learn to relax her body even when one group of muscles is strongly contracted. This process helps prepare her to relax during the powerful uterine contractions of labor. The woman contracts an area such as an arm or leg, then concentrates on letting tension go from the rest of her body. After a short time of contracting one area, she relaxes it and moves on to another. Her coach checks for unrecognized tension by gently moving areas to see that they are limp.

**Touch Relaxation.** The purpose of touch relaxation is to help the woman learn to loosen taut muscles when they are touched by her partner. The woman tenses an area and then relaxes it as her partner strokes or massages it. By frequent practice of this exercise, the woman becomes conditioned to respond to touch with relaxation. During labor, her partner's touch is a signal for release of tension.

**Relaxation Against Pain.** Because it is difficult for the first-time mother to imagine the pain and strength of labor contractions, women may occasionally practice use of relaxation against pain. The pain is caused by her partner, who exerts pressure against a tendon or large muscle of the arm or leg. The pressure is applied gradually to simulate the gradual increase, peak, and decrease of a uterine contraction.

### OTHER TECHNIQUES

Other techniques to aid the woman in relaxation include cutaneous or mental stimulation. Touch stimulates large-diameter sensory nerve fibers and interferes with transmission of pain impulses to the brain through small-diameter sensory nerve fibers. Mental focusing or distraction also interferes with pain messages reaching the brain.

#### CUTANEOUS STIMULATION TECHNIQUES

**Effleurage.** Effleurage is massage of the abdomen during contractions (Fig. 11–5). Women learn to do effleurage using both hands in a circular motion. If fetal monitor belts cover the abdomen during labor, the woman can massage between the belts. When she lies on her side, she uses only one hand to massage her abdomen. In the side-lying position, she may find it more comfortable to make smaller movements on her abdomen or to massage her thigh so that her arm and shoulder can remain relaxed.

Because habituation results in loss of effectiveness, effleurage should be varied periodically. The woman and her coach may alternate effleurage to provide more variety in sensory input and decrease habituation. The woman can massage her thigh instead of her abdomen or use her fingertips to trace circles or a figure-8 on the bed. When a specific pattern of effleurage is used, it provides a source of concentration and increased input to the brain. This exercise may also interfere with transmission of pain impulses.

**Other Massage.** Massage of the temples or shoulders by the labor partner may help relax these areas. The palms and soles of the feet are particularly sensitive to touch, and firm massage of these areas may be helpful. Types of stimuli should be changed whenever they no longer seem effective, generally every 15 to 30 minutes.

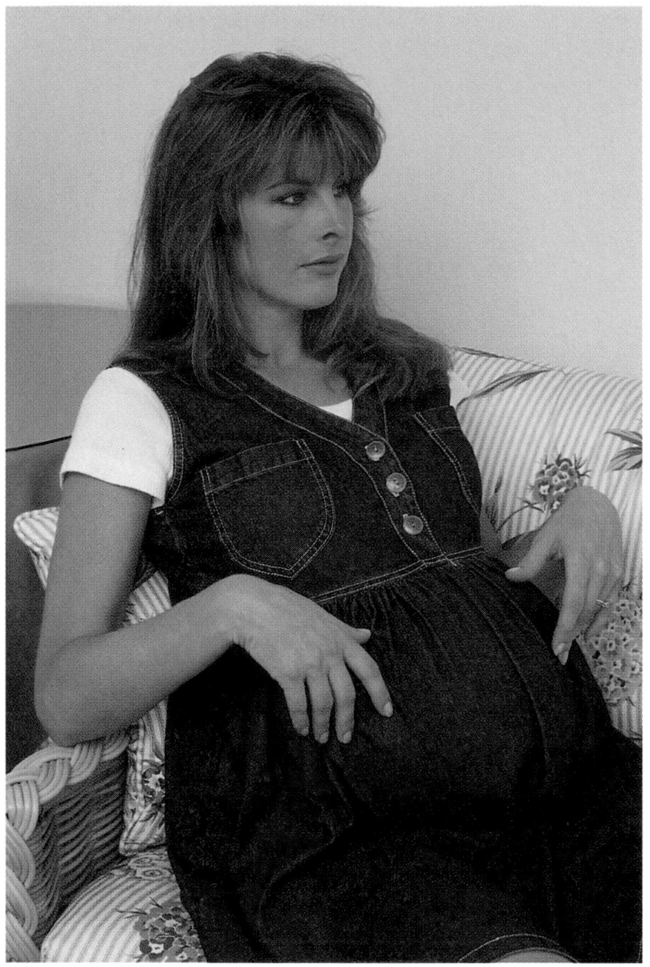

**FIGURE 11–5**

The woman begins effleurage with the hands at the symphysis and then slowly moves around the sides and down the center to the symphysis again. As an alternative, she can go up the center of the abdomen and around the sides.

**Sacral Pressure.** Firm pressure against the sacral area may help relieve strain on the sacroiliac joint from a fetal occiput posterior position (Simpkin, 1995). During contractions, the coach begins to increase pressure on the sacrum as soon as the contraction begins. If a fetal monitor is in place, the coach can watch the line depicting the contraction to determine when to begin and end the pressure. The hand may be moved slowly over the area or remain positioned directly over the sacrum, but pressure should be continuous and firm throughout the contraction.

The coach should place the other hand over the woman's hip and hold her steady during sacral pressure. Care should be taken not to jiggle the woman, as this may be irritating. Between contractions, the woman gives her coach feedback about hand placement. Often moving the hands a fraction of an inch increases effectiveness. This technique can be combined with thermal stimulation to increase effectiveness. Tennis balls may also be used to apply pressure to the back.

**Thermal Stimulation.** Application of heat or cold stimulates thermoreceptors and may decrease pain sensation. Cool cloths used to wipe the woman's face, ice in a glove covered with a washcloth applied to the woman's lower back, or even ice chips offered to the woman for eating may be effective. Alternating cold with heat prevents habituation. In early labor, a whirlpool bath or shower with warm water directed against the back may be soothing. A warm bath blanket or a glove filled with warm water can be held against the sacrum for pressure and warmth. Heat and cold should never be applied to any area that is anesthetized, as injury could result.

**Positioning.** Position changes during labor also provide cutaneous stimulation. Women are taught to practice their techniques using a variety of positions and to change position frequently during labor. Ambulation and upright position make contractions more efficient yet less painful. Position changes approximately every 30 to 60 minutes increase comfort and decrease muscle fatigue.

MENTAL STIMULATION TECHNIQUES

A variety of methods decrease pain by increasing mental concentration. These may modify pain perception as a result of interference with pain impulses in the spinal cord or in the brain itself.

**Focal Point.** A focal point is an object on which the woman centers her attention during contractions (Fig. 11–6). It helps her direct her thoughts away from the contractions. During the contraction, she looks at the focal point and thinks about its shape, size, and gradations of colors. Women often use pictures of infants or a restful scenic landscape for a

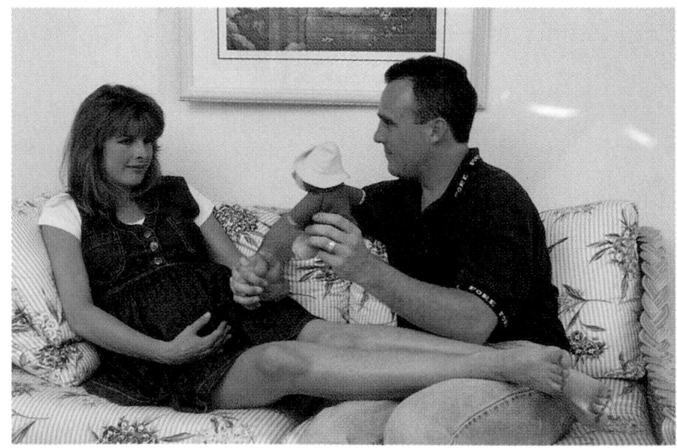

**FIGURE 11–6**

A stuffed toy or any other object can serve as a focal point on which the expectant mother can fix her attention during labor.

focal point. If a video player is available during labor, a video tape of scenery, perhaps combined with music, may increase interest in the focal point.

Women who do not bring a focal point to the birth setting may use anything in their line of vision, such as a pattern on the wallpaper or the support person's face. Because the fetal monitor is directly next to the bed, many women focus on it. Watching the contraction pattern on the monitor is usually not soothing and tends to increase attention to the strength of the contraction. Focusing on a button or knob may be more helpful.

Some women prefer closing their eyes and using an internal focal point during contractions. Closing their eyes allows them to shut out light and movement around them and to focus on a mental picture. Women who are familiar with meditation techniques may be more comfortable with this method of focusing.

**Imagery.** Another technique to enhance relaxation is imagery. During imagery exercises, childbirth educators often talk about a pleasant scene or experience while the woman imagines herself in that setting. A walk through a meadow is portrayed by describing the flowers, the warmth of the sun, the sound of birds, and a feeling of peacefulness. Couples are encouraged to practice imagery with scenes of their own choosing. While practicing breathing techniques, the woman can picture oxygen entering her body to nourish her baby every time she inhales and tension leaving each time she exhales.

Other imagery suggestions are given for use during labor. The woman might picture a flower opening from a bud into full bloom to simulate opening of the cervix. She can imagine the cervix pulling over the infant's head or the infant moving lower in the pelvis with each contraction. Teachers usually advise women to save images of cervical dilation and childbirth until labor actually begins.

**Music.** Some women find that music or other sounds, like rainfall or waves at the seashore, help them relax. They may use tapes during practice and bring them, with headphones, when they come to the birth setting in labor. Headphones have the added benefit of obscuring surrounding noise. The rhythm of the music may assist the woman in pacing her breathing.

#### SPECIAL TECHNIQUES

Special techniques may be discussed briefly in classes. Some techniques require further preparation elsewhere. Acupressure is pressure over acupuncture points, which may raise endorphin levels in the area to reduce pain. Biofeedback may lower pain by reducing tension of abdominal muscles. Some women find transcutaneous electrical nerve stimulation helpful. This process provides pain relief through the use of electrodes on the lower back to deliver low-intensity, high-frequency electrical stimulation of the nerves.

In hydrotherapy the woman is immersed in a tub of water, with or without whirlpool jets. The water helps the woman relax, decreases muscle tension and pressure on the abdomen, and helps labor progress more quickly. A tub bath after rupture of membranes does not seem to increase infection (Waldenstrom & Nilsson, 1992; Simpkin, 1995). Apgar scores for infants of women who use tub baths in labor, however, may be lower if more than 24 hours passes after rupture of membranes.

### BREATHING TECHNIQUES

As with other coping strategies, the primary purpose of breathing techniques is to enhance relaxation and decrease the number of pain impulses recognized by the brain. Although no research proves that breathing techniques decrease pain perception, many women feel that learning the techniques is important and helpful during labor (Hodnett, 1996). As with other techniques, the woman should use breathing as one of many tools to help her cope with labor.

The woman and her partner must practice the techniques frequently to gain comfort with them. If they become too complicated or if the woman has not practiced, they may not be helpful during labor. In labor, breathing techniques should not be used until they are actually needed, usually when the woman can no longer walk or talk during a contraction. If breathing techniques are used too early, the woman tends to move through the different techniques too quickly, and she may stop using them.

#### FIRST-STAGE BREATHING

Breathing in the first stage of labor consists of a cleansing breath and various breathing techniques known as paced breathing. The method begins with a very simple technique used as long as possible. When it is no longer effective, breathing that requires more concentration is added.

**Cleansing Breath.** Each contraction begins and ends with a deep inspiration and expiration known as the cleansing breath. Like a sigh, a cleansing breath helps the woman release tension. It provides oxygen to help prevent myometrial hypoxia, one cause of pain in labor. The cleansing breath also helps the woman clear her mind to focus on relaxing and signals her labor partner that the contraction is beginning or ending. The woman may inhale through the nose and exhale through the mouth or take her cleansing breath in any way comfortable for her.

**Slow-Paced Breathing.** The first breathing is slow-paced breathing—a slow, deep breathing that increases relaxation (Fig. 11–7). The woman should

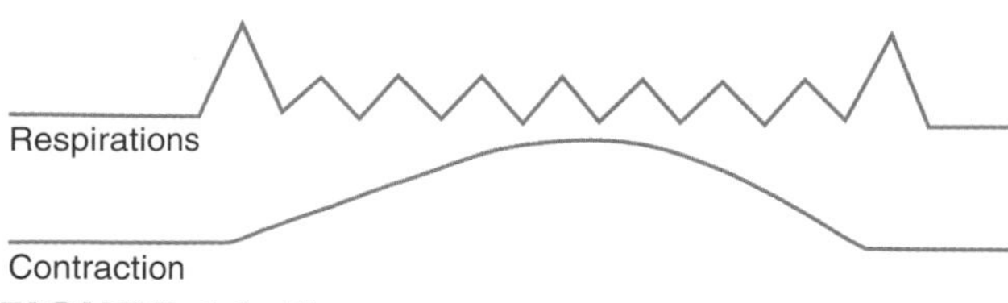


**FIGURE 11–7**

Slow-paced breathing. Although a specific rate may or may not be taught, slow-paced breathing should be *no slower than half* the woman's usual respiratory rate to ensure adequate oxygenation. This pace is generally about six to nine breaths per minute.

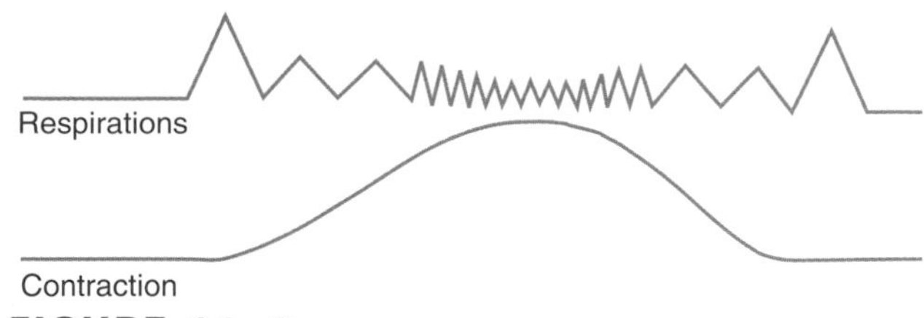


**FIGURE 11–9**

Combining techniques. Slow- and modified-paced breathing can be combined by using the slower breathing at the beginning and end of the contraction and the more rapid breathing over the peak of the contraction.

concentrate on relaxing her body rather than on regulating the rate of her breathing. Relaxation naturally brings about slower breathing, similar to that which occurs during sleep. She can use nose, mouth, or combination breathing, depending on which is most comfortable.

The woman uses slow-paced breathing as long as possible during labor because it promotes relaxation and sufficient oxygenation. Labor nurses often teach the technique to women who enter labor unprepared. It is easy to learn between contractions and, with the support of the nurse, helps even a frightened woman become calm and able to work with her contractions.

As with all techniques, introducing variety prevents habituation. Adding other pain-relief approaches such as effleurage may help prolong the effectiveness of slow-paced breathing. Using another type of breathing for a short time may allow the woman to return to slower breathing again later.

**Modified-Paced Breathing.** When slow-paced breathing is no longer effective, the woman begins modified-paced breathing (Fig. 11–8). This chest breathing at a faster rate matches the natural tendency to use more rapid breathing during stress or physical work, such as labor. Although modified-paced breathing is more shallow than slow-paced breathing, the faster rate allows oxygen intake to remain about the same. As with slow-paced breathing, the focus is on release of tension rather than on the actual number of breaths taken.

Women sometimes learn to combine slow- and modified-paced breathing during the course of a contraction (Fig. 11–9). They begin slowly and use shallow, faster breathing over the peak of the contraction. During labor, women often do this naturally. The most important concern is that the breathing not interfere with relaxation but enhance it.

**Patterned-Paced Breathing.** Patterned-paced breathing (sometimes called pant blow, "hee hoo," or "hee blow" breathing) involves focusing on the pattern of breathing (Fig. 11–10). It is similar to modified-paced breathing. After a certain number of breaths, however, the woman exhales with a slight emphasis or blow and then begins the modified-paced breathing again. This addition causes her to focus more on her breathing and reduces habituation. Some educators teach women to make a sound such as "hee" during this breathing and to blow through pursed lips with a "hoo" sound. Others avoid special sounds, which tighten the vocal cords and may decrease relaxation.

The number of breaths before the blow may remain constant (usually between two and six) or may change in a pattern. Variations include a set pattern such as "3-1, 5-1, 3-1" or a decreasing pattern such as "6-1, 5-1, 4-1, 3-1." Some couples use a random pattern determined by the coach, who uses hand signals to show the number of breaths the woman should take before each blow. The coach holds up fingers to show the total breaths to be taken or a

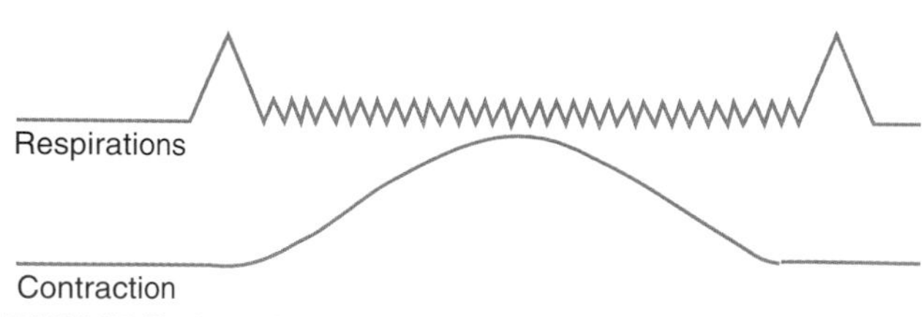


**FIGURE 11–8**

Modified-paced breathing. The pattern for modified-paced breathing should be comfortable to the woman and *no faster than twice* her normal respiratory rate to prevent hyperventilation or interference with relaxation.

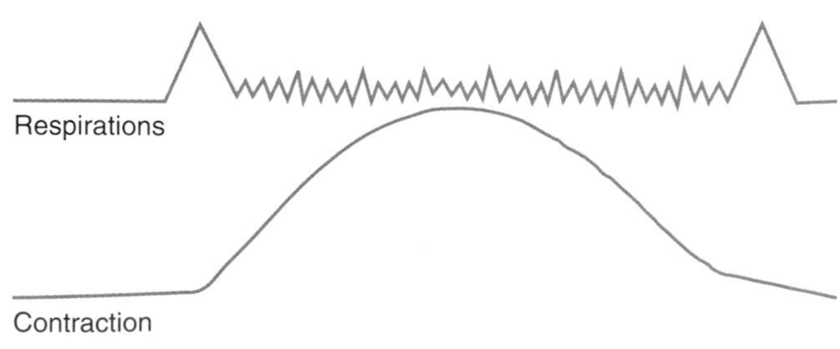


**FIGURE 11–10**

Patterned-paced breathing. Patterned-paced breathing adds a slight emphasis or "blow" on the exhalation in a pattern. The diagram shows the emphasis after every third inhalation.

single finger for each breath. Use of the random pattern, however, may be ineffective without sufficient practice to enable the couple to work together well.

**Breathing to Prevent Pushing.** If a woman pushes strenuously before the cervix is completely dilated, she risks injury to the cervix and the fetal head. Instructors teach women to blow when they have a premature urge to push. Blowing prevents closure of the glottis and breath holding, which are a part of strenuous pushing. The woman blows repeatedly using short puffs when the urge to push is strong. The support person may learn to blow along with her to help the woman concentrate. Some women vary the blowing by using one short breath and one blow.

**Common Problems.** Hyperventilation and mouth dryness may occur during breathing techniques. Hyperventilation shows that breathing is being performed incorrectly. It is due to rapid deep breathing that causes excessive loss of carbon dioxide, eventually resulting in respiratory alkalosis. The woman may feel dizzy or lightheaded and have impaired thinking. Vasoconstriction leads to tingling and numbness in fingers and lips. If hyperventilation continues, tetany due to decreased calcium in tissues and blood may result in stiffness of the face and lips and carpopedal spasm.

Women are taught to blow into a paper bag or their own cupped hands if they begin to feel dizzy. This kind of blowing increases carbon dioxide levels. Coaches learn that hyperventilation is a sign of incorrect breathing and help the woman make changes in her breathing as necessary.

Dryness of the mouth occurs when the woman uses prolonged mouth breathing. To avoid dryness, she can place her tongue gently against the roof of her mouth to moisturize entering air. The support person can offer ice, mouthwash, sour suckers, or liquids if they are allowed.

### SECOND-STAGE BREATHING

Breathing in the second stage of labor includes the traditional method of pushing, as well as methods that involve less breath holding. The childbirth educator should be knowledgeable about the methods practiced in the surrounding communities so that the mother and her support person can learn those that they will actually use during labor (Fig. 11–11). The couple is encouraged to discuss second-stage breathing techniques with the physician or nurse-midwife.

**Traditional Pushing.** In traditional pushing, the woman takes one or more cleansing breaths at the beginning of the contraction and then holds her breath, pushing as hard as she can for as long as possible. Generally, the coach counts slowly to 10 while the woman holds her breath. She then quickly exhales, takes another breath, and pushes again, repeating the process until the contraction is over. The concern of those who oppose this method is that pushing against a closed glottis, Valsalva's maneuver, results in an increase in intrathoracic pressure and a decrease in blood pressure and blood return to the heart. The final result may be impaired blood flow to the uterus. Proponents believe that breath holding is important to complete the second stage as quickly as possible, because this may be a time of danger for the fetus.

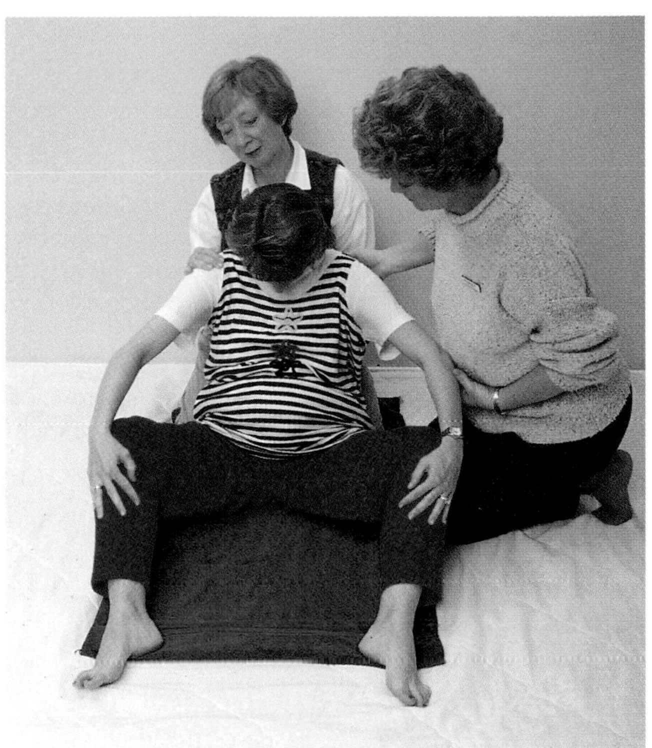

**FIGURE 11–11**
The teacher helps each couple, individually and together, with pushing.

**Other Pushing Methods.** Other methods of pushing involve exhalation of small amounts of air through an open glottis during pushing. The woman may push in short bursts only when the urge is very strong instead of using prolonged expulsive efforts. If she holds her breath at all, it is for very short intervals (5 to 6 seconds) only. Proponents believe that this method allows better oxygenation of both expectant mother and fetus.

**CHECK YOUR READING**

6. How can education, relaxation, and conditioning decrease pain?
7. How do cutaneous stimulation and imagery help reduce pain?
8. What is the purpose of breathing methods in labor?

## The Support Person

Almost all methods of childbirth preparation encourage participation of someone who remains with the woman throughout labor. This person may be called a support person, coach, labor partner, or labor companion. The terms are often used interchangeably. Having someone with the woman during labor has been shown to help her cope more effectively and to decrease distress, duration of labor, and need for medication. The overall result is greater satisfaction with the childbirth experience. Emotional support has also been shown to reduce hospital stay and need for cesarean birth (Kennell et al., 1991).

The person who takes on this role may be the father of the baby, a friend or relative, or even a hired professional labor coach. The support person generally attends classes with the mother to learn about labor and birth as well as techniques of coaching. By practicing together, the woman and her support person learn to work smoothly as a team during labor. Classes may increase confidence for support persons, who learn specific techniques to use during labor. When the support person is the father, practice sessions and working together may enhance communication and a sense of closeness between the expectant parents.

### Role of the Support Person

Not all support persons play identical roles during labor. Some take a major part in assisting the mother with relaxation and breathing techniques, but others provide support in less active ways. They may con-

## Nursing Care Plan 11–1
## Planning for Childbirth

ASSESSMENT: Carmen Sanchez, age 19, is 4 months pregnant with her first baby and in good health. She and her husband, Ramon, "want to be the best parents possible." Carmen works as a bilingual teacher's aide in a primary school. Ramon, age 26, manages a small restaurant. Both Carmen and Ramon are the youngest in their families and have little actual experience with infants. Carmen plans to have her baby at the local hospital in a labor, delivery, recovery room.

Carmen tells the nurse that Ramon tends to favor the "old ways" and is unsure whether or not he should be involved during childbirth. She is most anxious for him to participate during her labor. Ramon seems embarrassed and says, "Having a baby is for women." He seems very loving toward Carmen and later says, "I want to help Carmen, but I don't know anything about these things. I'd just be in the way."

NURSING DIAGNOSIS: Decisional Conflict related to father's ambivalence toward his anticipated role in childbirth

**Critical Thinking**

Is this an appropriate use of a nursing diagnosis? If Carmen is the client, should the nurse make a nursing diagnosis that focuses on her husband?

**ANSWER**

Although Carmen is the primary client, family-centered nursing involves care of all family members, especially when their needs affect the needs of the primary client. If the nurse can help Carmen and Ramon resolve this problem, Carmen will be able to focus more positively on preparing for the birth of their baby.

GOALS/EXPECTED OUTCOMES

Ramon will do the following:

1. Explore various options regarding his role during Carmen's labor and the birth of his baby.
2. Make a decision about his role during childbirth by 1 month before the baby is expected.

| INTERVENTION | RATIONALE |
|---|---|
| 1. Explore Ramon's concerns before beginning discussion of educational opportunities with Carmen. | 1. In some cultures, the man is the head of the family and makes many of the decisions. It is important to show respect for his authority if health teaching is to be accepted. |
| 2. Use therapeutic communication techniques (such as reflection or paraphrasing) to help Ramon discuss his feelings about participating in childbirth. | 2. Use of therapeutic communication shows that the nurse is willing to listen and thinks that the client's feelings are important. |

fine their coaching to verbal encouragement or to giving physical care such as back rubs only when asked. Still others feel most comfortable with passive support—"being there" but not participating actively. Even with education, the support person may feel somewhat helpless and look to others to provide help to the laboring woman.

Some men believe that active involvement in labor is not an acceptable role for them, perhaps because of cultural values. For example, Latino couples often expect the partner to offer support more by being present and encouraging during labor than by taking a more active role (Khazoyan & Anderson, 1994). Nurses should encourage whatever role support persons choose. Nursing Care Plan 11–1 is an example of helping couples decide on the role of the support person.

It is important that labor partners do not feel responsible for more than is included in the role. Teachers should discuss the duties of the labor nurse and encourage coaches to seek assistance when they are uncertain. The labor nurse may have suggestions or adaptations of techniques that are very helpful. Class discussion of complications should include the role of the support person. For example, coaches should understand circumstances that would allow or preclude their presence during a cesarean birth.

### Support Techniques

Support persons need practical methods to help the woman in labor. They learn how to time contractions at home and how to work with the fetal monitor, if used, in the hospital. Telling the woman when the monitor shows that the peak of the contraction is

## Nursing Care Plan 11–1 *Continued*
## Planning for Childbirth

| | |
|---|---|
| 3. Ask Ramon how he pictures childbirth and the role of the support person during labor and birth. | 3. Teaching should begin at the client's level of knowledge. |
| 4. Explain various labor support roles. Include the options of acting as "coach" or merely being present for the labor, the birth, both, or neither. | 4. The nurse must encourage and accept whatever role the support person chooses. |
| 5. Ask Ramon what the advantages and disadvantages of each role might be. Clarify misinformation and discuss additional advantages and disadvantages if necessary. | 5. Participation increases learning. |
| 6. Present all information in a nonjudgmental atmosphere. | 6. If the nurse remains nonjudgmental, the client does not feel pressured to make a particular decision. |
| 7. Encourage Ramon to discuss this new information with his friends and family. If possible, refer him to other men who have played various roles during labor and birth. | 7. Discussion with family and friends is important when making decisions and provides a source for other viewpoints. |
| 8. Suggest that Ramon think about his options and make a decision at a later date. Provide written information for Ramon and Carmen to review at home. | 8. It takes time to process new information and make decisions. Written information provides a readily available source for review. |
| 9. Include Carmen throughout the discussion. | 9. A couple may be unaware of each other's concerns and feelings. Hearing the partner talk about them helps each understand the other's point of view. |

#### EVALUATION

Ramon reports 2 months later that he had decided to go with Carmen to classes to learn more about childbirth. He is unsure about how much he will participate during labor and birth and says that he will decide when the time arrives. Carmen says that she feels comfortable with Ramon's decision and is glad he will go to prepared childbirth classes with her.

#### ADDITIONAL NURSING DIAGNOSES TO CONSIDER

Health-Seeking Behavior related to desire for information about pregnancy and birth
Anxiety related to lack of knowledge about childbirth
Ineffective Individual Coping related to extreme worry about childbirth

over can be particularly helpful. In advanced labor, the monitor may show a contraction beginning before the woman feels it. The coach can alert her to begin her breathing techniques before the contraction becomes strong. The coach suggests ways to make the environment less stressful, such as listening to tapes with headphones to obscure surrounding noise and turning down the lights to promote rest between contractions.

Coaches often learn a "panic technique" to use when the woman is finding coping with labor particularly difficult. This includes making eye contact and breathing along with her to help pace the breathing, helping her move to a more advanced level of breathing, and remaining calm. Having some direction for what to do if the woman loses control may make the support person feel more secure.

Providing comfort measures is an important role of the support person. These measures include offering ice chips, wiping the woman's face with a cold cloth, and helping her change positions. The coach applies sacral pressure or gives back rubs or other types of massage. During classes, couples learn breathing and relaxation techniques together. Coaches learn how to provide feedback and make suggestions during practice sessions as well as in labor. They discover the importance of encouragement and giving directions in a positive manner.

The woman and her support person may pack a "goodie bag" of things that may help to comfort the expectant mother during labor (Table 11–6). As labor progresses, the couples use each article as it seems appropriate.

**TABLE 11–6 ITEMS TO BE INCLUDED IN THE "GOODIE BAG"**

Focal point
Lotion or powder to make massage more comfortable
Warm socks for cold feet
Several washcloths for washing face (colored, not white, because white ones might get lost)
Hand-held fan
Rubber bands or clips for hair
Tennis balls in a sock for sacral pressure
Sugarless sour lollipop for a dry mouth
Mouthwash
Lip balm, unflavored
Instruction sheets or reminder checklists
Paper and pencil
Playing cards or simple games for early labor
Camera
Snack for coach
Tape player with headphones and tapes
Change and telephone numbers for calls after birth
Pillows

**CHECK YOUR READING**

9. How does having someone with her help the woman in labor?
10. What are the various roles that the support person might take?
11. What specific techniques do coaches learn to help the woman in labor?

## Application of Nursing Process: Education for Childbirth

The nursing process focuses on assisting the woman and her partner to obtain the knowledge necessary to plan for a birth experience that is realistic and meets their individual needs. Preparation ensures that each family progresses through the childbearing experience as knowledgeable consumers and full participants in their own health care.

### Assessment

Assess the educational needs of the woman and her partner. The nurse may find that the couple is quite knowledgeable about available prenatal classes and childbirth options or that they need direction. They may need help in choosing classes that are right for them. The couple may come to the nurse with a birth plan already made or may need help in thinking through their expectations and desires.

Determine whether special factors require adaptation of the usual educational approaches. Examples are the pregnant adolescent and the woman with a high-risk pregnancy. Cultural factors may be very influential in determining individual educational needs.

Assess the needs of support persons as well as the degree of participation they wish to have in the birth. They may have concerns about their role, especially during labor and birth. These must be addressed to decrease their anxiety and to help them to be more effective in supporting their partner.

### Analysis

The nursing diagnosis that pertains to the couple that is not unusually anxious about childbirth but desires more information is Health-Seeking Behaviors related to desire for education about pregnancy, childbirth, and/or parenting.

## Planning

The goals for this nursing diagnosis are that the woman and her partner will do the following:

- Write a birth plan that is realistically based on available options and meets their needs.
- Verbalize a plan for obtaining education for pregnancy, childbirth, and parenting.
- Report a feeling of increased confidence in their ability to cope with pregnancy, childbirth, and parenting after educational preparation is completed.

## Interventions

### MAKING A BIRTH PLAN

Help couples write out a plan for their birth experience if they wish. The birth plan, sometimes called a family preference plan, helps women and their partners look at the options they have and take an active part in planning their birth experience. The plan is a tool for expanding communication with health professionals. It ensures that the couple's wishes are known before labor begins. The plan may help the couple choose a provider, a setting, and classes that are most conducive to meeting specific needs.

Help the couple learn about what choices are actually available in the locale. A plan to have a midwife assist at the birth in a free-standing birth center is unrealistic if this facility is unavailable near the couple's home. Explain any other restrictions that may be placed on choices. For example, insurance coverage may dictate which facility a woman must use. Those without insurance are concerned about the cost of various options. In addition, the health care provider or birth agency may have set policies on certain issues. Complications during labor or birth may necessitate changes in the plan.

Some couples interview several physicians or nurse-midwives to learn about the provider's usual practices and whether exceptions are possible. With discussion, the couple and the provider can work out a plan that all find satisfactory.

### CHOOSING CLASSES

Help the woman and her partner find classes suited to their educational needs. Give them a list of classes in the community and a description of each. Suggest that they talk with others who have taken various classes to learn how well their needs were satisfied. They may wish to interview teachers to learn about their preparation and philosophy. Some couples may want classes that make avoidance of medication a primary goal of childbirth. Many prefer those that consider a variety of tools, including medication, for coping with pain.

### SUGGESTING CLASSES FOR SPECIAL NEEDS

Women with special needs may need referral to courses specifically for them. If none is available, make suggestions about how they can adapt what they learn in regular classes to their own situation.

**Adolescents.** Although adolescents may attend regular prenatal classes, those designed especially to meet their needs are most effective. High schools with programs for school-aged mothers, hospitals, clinics, or community agencies may offer courses. Separating teenagers from adults results in a more comfortable environment in which teenagers can learn with peers who have similar problems and concerns. Fathers or other support persons may also attend.

Education for pregnant adolescents is similar to that for adults, but it focuses on the teenager's perceptions of childbearing. Clarification of misconceptions in a nonjudgmental manner makes classes more meaningful. The young women need information about the importance of prenatal care, nutrition, weight gain, body image, and contraception as well as labor and birth. The effects of substance abuse and sexually transmissible diseases on pregnancy and the fetus are important topics for discussion.

Although the decision about whether to keep or relinquish the infant is often made before classes begin, options may be discussed. Because of their lack of experience and unrealistic expectations of infants, adolescents have a greater need for information about infant care than do older mothers. Classes provide an opportunity for discussion of how an infant will affect their lives, future goals, and schooling.

Teenagers with academic problems may have difficulty with reading material or understanding abstract concepts. The effective teacher uses concrete terms and simple language to ensure understanding. Models, videos, and hearing from those who have previously taken classes make the course more relevant.

**Mature Women.** Although women older than age 35 may have special needs, classes specifically for them are seldom available. They generally take regular prenatal classes, but they may feel "different" from the younger women in their class as well as isolated from their friends who have completed childbearing. Yet because delaying parenthood is quite common today, classes may provide an opportunity to make friends with others with similar backgrounds. Older couples may want more sophisticated information than is usually included in regular prenatal classes, and they have many questions about the chances of complications related to age. Offer realistic reassurance, and direct them to books and articles that meet their need for in-depth information.

**Women with High-Risk Pregnancies.** The woman with a high-risk pregnancy has needs in addition to those of other women. Those in jeopardy of preterm labor or with gestational diabetes may attend special classes that emphasize their needs.

A woman on restricted activity may not be able to attend regular perinatal classes. If possible, help her arrange for individual instruction. Audio and video tapes, written materials, or phone contact with an instructor are ways for her to learn and practice techniques without attending classes. In addition to helping her to prepare for childbirth, these measures may decrease the boredom of bedrest and reduce her anxiety about what lies ahead.

**Women Who Must Make Cultural Adaptations.** Women from other cultures, especially those who do not speak English, are at a disadvantage when they enter birth settings in the United States. Classes in other languages are often available in communities in which there are large groups with this need. They contain the same basic information as the English versions, with the content and process adapted to meet the cultural needs of the students. The teacher usually has the same cultural background as the students. This cultural match ensures fluency in their language and understanding of their needs and increases the likelihood that the instructor will be accepted.

The instructor discusses childbirth in the United States and compares it with that in the couples' country of origin. Students learn the importance of prenatal care, which may not have been emphasized in their own culture. They discuss what to expect of health care providers and what is expected of them during the birthing experience. Misconceptions about needs and care throughout the childbearing period are clarified. It is important that the instructor not disparage customs that may seem very different from those practiced in the United States.

**Women with Other Needs.** Refer the woman and her support person to classes that address other specific needs if necessary. Classes for adoptive couples or for women with multifetal pregnancies or handicaps may be available. Women who have concerns about continuing their careers after birth may enroll in courses for working mothers to help them choose child care and learn to balance the needs of family and work. Classes for fathers only may provide a comfortable environment for discussion of fathering, sexuality, and role during labor and birth, breastfeeding, and the postpartum period in the company of other men with similar concerns.

### Evaluation

If goals have been achieved, the woman and her partner will do the following:

- Write a realistic birth plan and attend classes that are appropriate for their needs.
- Verbalize satisfaction with the education they have received.
- Verbalize increased confidence in coping with pregnancy, childbirth, and parenting.

## SUMMARY CONCEPTS

- Education for childbearing helps couples become knowledgeable consumers and active participants in pregnancy and childbirth.
- Women must make many decisions about childbirth. Some of the most important include choosing a birth attendant, a birth setting, a support person for labor, and the type of educational classes to attend.
- Many classes are available for pregnant women and their support persons. Early pregnancy classes emphasize having a healthy pregnancy. Those conducted in later pregnancy focus on preparing for childbirth, breastfeeding, and early parenting.
- Because more than 20 percent of all births are cesarean, women in all prepared childbirth classes should be made aware of this possibility and learn about the procedure.
- Classes for siblings and grandparents help all family members prepare for the birth. Classes are designed to improve communication by discussing feelings and role change.
- Education, relaxation, and conditioning are used to increase coping ability for childbirth. Other techniques act to decrease transmission of pain impulses from the spinal cord to the brain; these are based on the gate control theory.
- Exercises in relaxation help women recognize and learn to reduce tension during labor.
- Cutaneous and mental stimulation techniques act to reduce pain perception. Techniques need to be varied to prevent habituation.
- Women learn a variety of breathing techniques for labor. Their purpose is to increase relaxation. Lamaze breathing should be no slower than half a woman's normal respiratory rate and no faster than twice her normal rate.
- Having a support person increases a woman's satisfaction with childbirth. The educated support person may find labor less stressful and feel increased confidence.
- The support person may participate in labor actively, minimally, or only by being present. All roles taken by the support person should be accepted by the nurse.
- Specific support techniques include assisting with relaxation and breathing, encouragement, sacral pressure, massage, and comfort measures.

### References and Readings


Association of Women's Health, Obstetric, & Neonatal Nurses (AWHONN) (1993). *Competencies and program guidelines for nurse providers of perinatal education.* Washington, D.C.: Author.

Bernat, S.H., Powhatan, J.W., Marecki, M., & Snell, L. (1992). Biofeedback-assisted relaxation to reduce stress in labor. *Journal of Obstetric, Gynecologic, and Neonatal Nursing,* 21(4), 295–303.

Biasella, S. (1993). A comprehensive perinatal education program. AWHONN's *Clinical Issues in Perinatal and Women's Health Nursing,* 4(1), 5–19.

Blackburn, S.T., & Loper, D.L. (1992). *Maternal, fetal, and neonatal physiology: A clinical perspective.* Philadelphia: W.B. Saunders.

Chapman, L.L. (1992). Expectant fathers' roles during labor and birth. *Journal of Obstetric, Gynecologic, and Neonatal Nursing,* 21(2), 114–119.

Cook, A., & Wilcox, G. (1997). Pressuring pain. AWHONN *Lifelines,* 1(2), 36–41.

Creehan, P.A. (1996). Pain relief and comfort measures during labor. In K.R. Simpson & P.A. Creehan (Eds.), AWHONN's *perinatal nursing.* Philadelphia: J.B. Lippincott.

Creehan, P.A. (1996). Ask the experts. AWHONN *Voice,* 4(7), 4.

Dick-Read, G. (1959). *Childbirth without fear.* New York: Harper & Row.

Green, J.M. (1993). Expectations and experiences of pain in labor: Findings from a large prospective study. *Birth,* 20(2), 65–72.

Guyer, B., Strobino, D.M., Ventura, S.J., MacDorman, M., & Martin, J.A. (1996). Annual summary of vital statistics—1995. *Pediatrics,* 98(6), 1007–1019.

Hodnett, E. (1996). Nursing support of the laboring woman. *Journal of Obstetric, Gynecologic, and Neonatal Nursing,* 25(3), 257–264.

Humenick, S.S. (1996). Commentary: Childbirth education groups should collaborate more to inform parents about birth alternatives. *Birth,* 23(4), 204–205.

Jeffers, D.F. (1993). Outreach childbirth education classes for low-income families: A strategy for program development. AWHONN's *Clinical Issues in Perinatal and Women's Health Nursing,* 4(1), 95–101.

Kennell, J., Klaus, M., McGrath, S., Robertson, S., & Hinkley, C. (1991). Continuous emotional support during labor in a U.S. Hospital: A randomized controlled trial. *Journal of the American Medical Association,* 265(17), 2197–2202.

Khazoyan, C.M., & Anderson, N.L.R. (1994). Latinas' expectations for their partners during childbirth. *American Journal of Maternal-Child Nursing,* 19(4), 226–229.

Klaus, M.H., Kennell, J.H., & Klaus, P.H. (1993). *Mothering the mother.* New York: Addison-Wesley.

Koehn, M.L. (1993). The psychoeducational model of prepared childbirth education. AWHONN's *Clinical Issues in Perinatal and Women's Health Nursing,* 4(1), 66–71.

Lothian, J.A. (1993). Critical dimensions in perinatal education. AWHONN's *Clinical Issues in Perinatal and Women's Health Nursing,* 4(1), 20–27.

Lowe, M., Millea, D., & Simpson, K.R. (1996). Discharge planning. In K.R. Simpson & P.A. Creehan (Eds.), AWHONN's *perinatal nursing.* Philadelphia: J.B. Lippincott.

Lowe, N.K. (1996). The pain and discomfort of labor and birth. *Journal of Obstetric, Gynecologic, and Neonatal Nursing,* 25(1), 82–92.

Monto, M.A. (1996). Lamaze and Bradley childbirth classes: Contrasting perspectives toward the medical model of birth. *Birth,* 23(4), 193–201.

Moore, M., & Hopper, U. (1995). Do birth plans empower women? Evaluation of a hospital birth plan. *Birth,* 22(1), 29–36.

Mullaly, L.M. (1993). Preparation for childbirth. In S. Mattson & J.E. Smith (Eds.), NAACOG *core curriculum for maternal-newborn nursing.* Philadelphia: W.B. Saunders.

Nichols, F. (1993). Issues in perinatal education. AWHONN's *Clinical Issues in Perinatal and Women's Health Nursing,* 4(1), 55–59.

Nichols, F.H., & Humenick, S.S. (Eds.) (1988). *Childbirth education: Practice, research, and theory.* Philadelphia: W.B. Saunders.

Nichols, M.R. (1995). Adjustment to new parenthood: Attenders versus nonattenders at prenatal education classes. *Birth,* 22(1), 21–26.

Peterson, K.J., & Peterson, F.L. (1993). Family-centered perinatal education. AWHONN's *Clinical Issues in Perinatal and Women's Health Nursing,* 4(1), 1–4.

Piper, S., & Parks, P. (1996). Predicting the duration of lactation: Evidence from a national survey. *Birth,* 23(1), 7–12.

Shapiro, H.R. (1993). Prenatal education in the work place. AWHONN's *Clinical Issues in Perinatal and Women's Health Nursing,* 4(1), 113–121.

Shearer, E.L. (1995). Commentary: Many factors affect the outcome of prenatal classes. *Birth,* 22(1), 27–28.

Simpkin, P. (1995). Reducing pain and enhancing progress in labor: A guide to nonpharmacologic methods for maternity caregivers. *Birth,* 22(3), 161–171.

Simpkin, P. (1996). The experience of maternity in a woman's life. *Journal of Obstetric, Gynecologic, and Neonatal Nursing,* 25(3), 247–252.

Waldenstrom, U., & Nilsson, C. (1992). Warm tub bath after spontaneous rupture of the membranes. *Birth,* 19(2), 57–63.

Zwelling, E. (1996). Childbirth education in the 1990's and beyond. *Journal of Obstetric, Gynecologic, and Neonatal Nursing,* 25(5), 425–432.

# Part III

# The Family During Birth

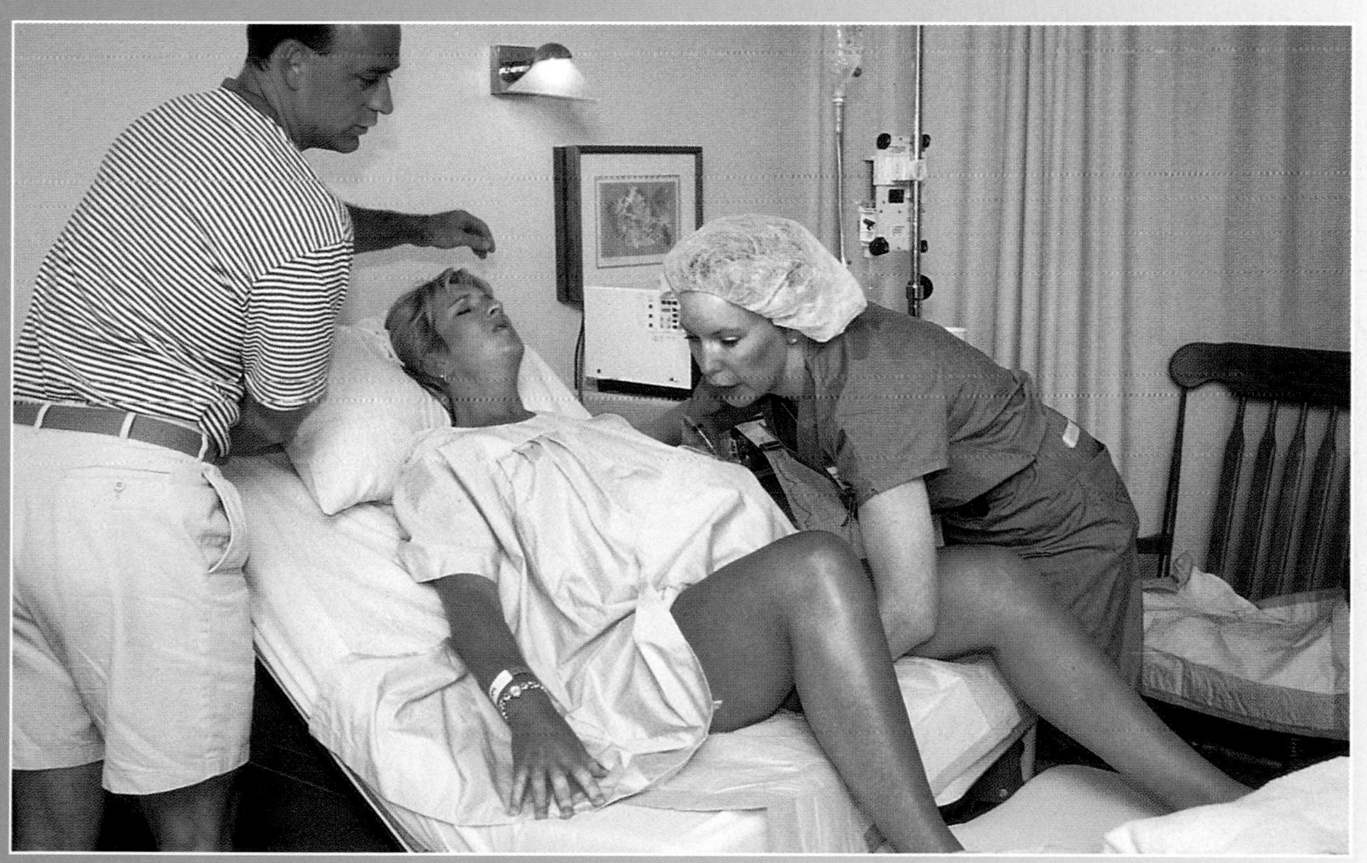

# 12

# The Processes of Birth

**OBJECTIVES**

1. Describe the woman's physiologic and psychological responses to labor.
2. Describe fetal responses to labor.
3. Explain how each component of the birth process affects the course of labor and birth and how the components are interrelated.
4. Relate each mechanism of labor to the process of vaginal birth.
5. Explain premonitory signs of labor.
6. Compare true labor with false labor.
7. Describe common differences in the labors of nulliparous and parous women.
8. Compare each stage of labor and the phases within the first stage.

**DEFINITIONS**

**acme** *Peak, or period of greatest strength, of a uterine contraction.*

**attitude** *Relationship of fetal body parts to one another.*

**bloody show** *Mixture of cervical mucus and blood from ruptured capillaries in the cervix; often precedes labor and increases with cervical dilation.*

**Braxton Hicks contractions** *Irregular, mild uterine contractions that occur throughout pregnancy; they become stronger in the last trimester.*

**decrement** *Period of decreasing strength of a uterine contraction.*

**duration** *Period from the beginning of a uterine contraction to the end of the same contraction.*

**engagement** *Descent of the widest diameter of the fetal presenting part to at least a zero station (the level of the ischial spines in the maternal pelvis).*

**fontanelle** *Space at the intersection of sutures connecting fetal or infant skull bones.*

**frequency** *Period from the beginning of one uterine contraction to the beginning of the next.*

**increment** *Period of increasing strength of a uterine contraction.*

**intensity** *Strength of a uterine contraction.*

**interval** *Period between the end of one uterine contraction and the beginning of the next.*

**lie** *Relationship of the long axis of the fetus to the long axis of the mother.*

**lightening** *Descent of the fetus toward the pelvic inlet before labor.*

**lochia** *Vaginal drainage after birth.*

**molding** *Shaping of the fetal head during movement through the birth canal.*

**nullipara** *A woman who has not completed a pregnancy to at least 20 weeks' gestation.*

**para** *A woman who has given birth after a pregnancy of at least 20 weeks' gestation. Also designates the number of pregnancies that end after at least 20 weeks of gestation. (A multifetal gestation, such as twins, is considered one birth when calculating parity.)*

**position** *Relation of a fixed reference point on the fetus to the quadrants of the maternal pelvis.*

**presentation** *Fetal part that enters the pelvic inlet. Also, the presenting part.*

**station** *Measurement of fetal descent in relation to the ischial spines of the maternal pelvis. See also* ***Engagement.***

**sutures** *Narrow areas of flexible tissue that connect fetal skull bones, permitting slight movement during labor.*

**VBAC** *Acronym for vaginal birth after cesarean.*

An understanding of the physiologic and psychological components of the birth process helps the nurse to better care for the childbearing family during the intrapartum period. Awareness of expected changes allows the nurse to reassure the laboring woman and provides a basis for identifying abnormal occurrences. This chapter focuses on the changes that occur during birth. Nursing care of the normal childbearing family is discussed in Chapter 13.

# Physiologic Effects of the Birth Process

The process of birth affects the physiologic systems of both the pregnant woman and her fetus. These effects occur in several body systems but are striking in the maternal reproductive system and those related to fetal and neonatal oxygenation.

## Maternal Response

The most obvious changes of pregnancy and birth occur in the woman's reproductive system, but her other systems respond in various ways as well. Significant changes during labor also occur in her cardiovascular, respiratory, gastrointestinal, urinary, and hematopoietic systems.

### REPRODUCTIVE SYSTEM

#### CHARACTERISTICS OF CONTRACTIONS

Normal labor contractions are coordinated, involuntary, and intermittent.

**Coordinated.** The uterus can contract and relax in a coordinated way, as can other smooth muscles such as the heart. Contractions during pregnancy are of low intensity and uncoordinated. As the woman approaches full term, contractions become organized and gradually assume a regular pattern of increasing frequency, duration, and intensity during labor. Coordinated labor contractions begin in the uterine fundus and spread downward toward the cervix to propel the fetus through the pelvis.

**Involuntary.** Uterine contractions are involuntary, in that they are not under conscious control as are skeletal muscles. The mother cannot cause labor to start or stop by conscious effort. However, walking or other activity may stimulate existing labor contractions. Anxiety and excessive stress can diminish them.

**Intermittent.** Labor contractions are intermittent rather than sustained, allowing relaxation of the uterine muscle and resumption of blood flow to and from the placenta to permit gas, nutrient, and waste exchange for the fetus.

#### CONTRACTION CYCLE

Each contraction consists of three phases (Fig. 12–1). The *increment* occurs as the contraction begins in the fundus and spreads throughout the uterus. The *peak* or *acme* is the period during which the contraction is most intense. The *decrement* is the period of decreasing intensity as the uterus relaxes.

The contraction cycle and the overall pattern of contractions are also described in terms of frequency, duration, and intensity. *Frequency* is the period from the beginning of one uterine contraction to the beginning of the next; it is usually expressed in minutes and fractions of minutes. For example, "Contractions are 3½ to 4 minutes apart."

*Duration* is the length of each contraction from beginning to end; it is usually expressed in seconds. For example, the nurse might say, "Her contractions last 55 to 65 seconds."

*Intensity* is the strength of the contractions. The terms "mild," "moderate," and "strong" describe contraction intensity as palpated by the nurse. Different descriptions of intensity may apply when the electronic fetal monitor is used to record contractions (see Chapter 14).

The *interval* is the period between the end of one contraction and the beginning of the next. The interval is the time when most fetal exchange of oxygen, nutrients, and waste products occurs.

#### UTERINE BODY

Uterine activity during labor is characterized by opposing features. The upper two thirds of the

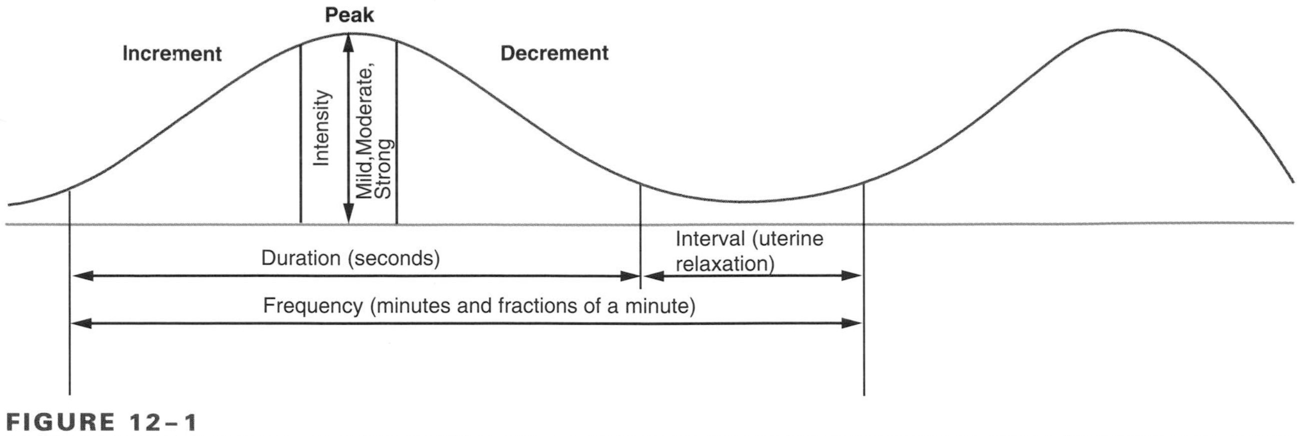


**FIGURE 12–1**

Contraction cycle.

uterus contracts actively to push the fetus down. The lower one third of the uterus remains less active, promoting downward passage of the fetus. The cervix is similar to the lower uterine segment in that it is also passive. The net effect of labor contractions is enhanced because the downward push from the upper uterus is accompanied by reduced resistance to fetal descent in the lower uterus.

Myometrial (uterine muscle) cells in the upper uterus remain shorter at the end of each contraction rather than returning to their original length. In contrast, myometrial cells in the lower uterus become longer with each contraction. These two characteristics enable the upper uterus to maintain tension between contractions to preserve the cervical changes and downward fetal progress made with each contraction.

The opposing characteristics of myometrial contraction in the upper and lower uterine segments cause changes in the thickness of the uterine wall during labor. The upper uterus becomes thicker while the lower uterus becomes thinner and pulled upward during labor. The physiologic retraction ring marks the division between the upper and lower segments of the uterus (Fig. 12–2).

The opposing characteristics of contractions in the upper and lower uterine segments change the shape of the uterine cavity to become more elongated and narrower as labor progresses. This change in uterine shape straightens the fetal body and efficiently directs it downward in the pelvis.

### CERVICAL CHANGES

*Effacement* (thinning and shortening) and *dilation* (opening) are the major cervical changes during labor. Effacement and dilation occur concurrently during labor but at different rates. The nullipara completes most cervical effacement early in the process of cervical dilation. In contrast, the parous woman's cervix is usually thicker than a nullipara's cervix at any point during labor.

**Effacement.** Before labor, the cervix is a cylindric structure, about 2 cm long, at the lower end of the uterus. Labor contractions push the fetus downward against the cervix as they pull the cervix upward. If the membranes are intact, hydrostatic (fluid) pressure of the amniotic sac adds to the force of the presenting part on the cervix. The cervix becomes shorter and thinner as it is drawn over the fetus and amniotic sac (Fig. 12–3). The cervix merges with the thinning lower uterus rather than remaining a distinct cylindric structure. Effacement is estimated as a percentage of the original cervical length, with a fully thinned cervix being 100 percent effaced. Effacement also may be documented as cervical length estimated during vaginal examination.

**Dilation.** As the cervix is pulled upward and the fetus is pushed downward, the cervix dilates. Dilation is expressed in centimeters, with approximately 10 cm being full dilation, large enough to allow passage of the average-sized term fetus. The action during effacement and dilation can be likened to pushing a ball out the cuff of a sock.

### CARDIOVASCULAR SYSTEM

During each uterine contraction, blood flow to the placenta gradually decreases, causing a relative increase in the woman's blood volume. This temporary change increases her blood pressure slightly and slows her pulse. Therefore, *the mother's vital signs are best assessed during the interval between contractions because of slight alterations in her blood pressure and pulse that may occur during a contraction.* Although it is more likely to occur during the antepartum period, supine hypotension (see p. 126) also may occur during labor if the mother lies on her back. *The mother should be encouraged to rest in positions other than the supine to promote blood return to her heart and therefore enhance blood flow to the placenta and promote fetal oxygenation.*

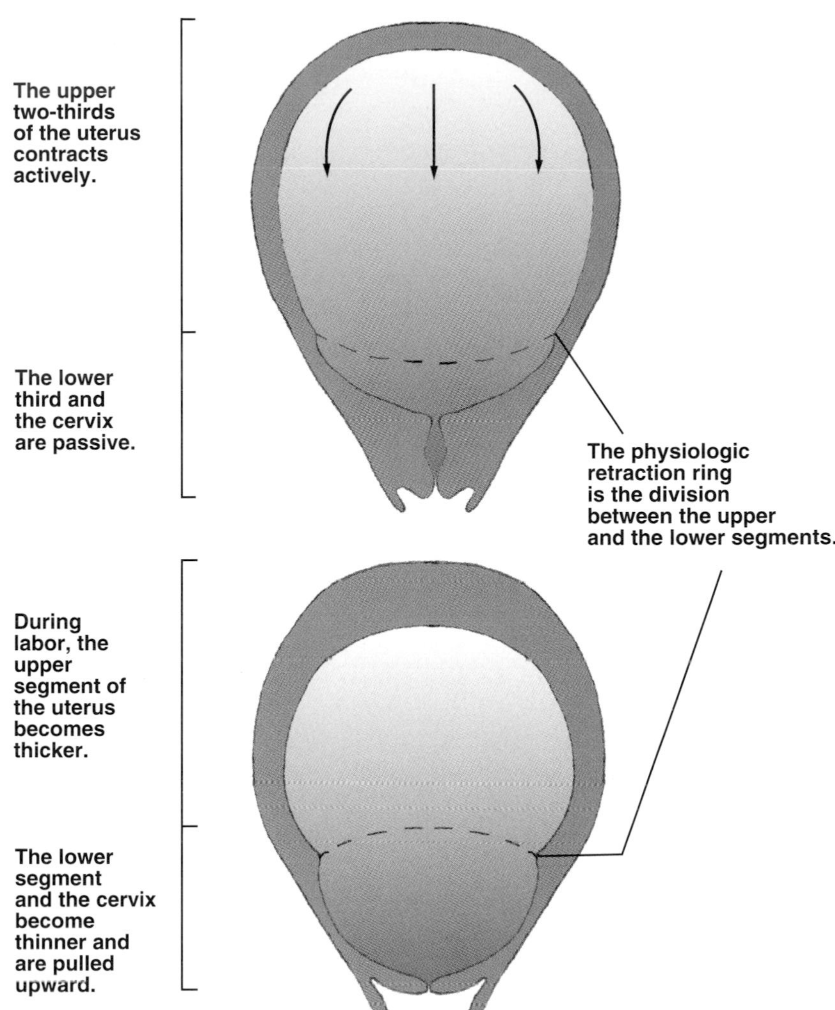
The upper two-thirds of the uterus contracts actively.
The lower third and the cervix are passive.
The physiologic retraction ring is the division between the upper and the lower segments.
During labor, the upper segment of the uterus becomes thicker.
The lower segment and the cervix become thinner and are pulled upward.

**FIGURE 12-2**

Opposing characteristics of uterine contraction in the upper and lower segments of the uterus.

#### RESPIRATORY SYSTEM

The depth and rate of respirations increase, especially if the woman is anxious or in pain. A woman who breathes rapidly and deeply may experience symptoms of hyperventilation if respiratory alkalosis occurs as she exhales too much carbon dioxide. She may feel tingling of her hands and feet, numbness, and dizziness. Helping her to slow her breathing and to breathe into a paper bag or her cupped hands can restore normal blood levels of carbon dioxide and relieve these symptoms.

#### GASTROINTESTINAL SYSTEM

Gastric motility is reduced during labor to varying degrees. Most women are not actually hungry but are often thirsty and have a dry mouth. General anesthesia is rarely needed for birth, but it is occasionally required. Food and large volumes of liquids are therefore withheld to reduce the risk of vomiting and aspiration. Ice chips are commonly provided, and small amounts of other clear liquids or juices, popsicles, or hard candy on a stick also may be permitted.

#### URINARY SYSTEM

The most common change in the urinary system during labor is reduced sensation of a full bladder. Because of intense contractions or effects of regional anesthesia, the woman may be unaware that her bladder is full. Yet it may contribute to discomfort, especially that which persists after regional anesthesia. A full bladder can inhibit fetal descent because it occupies space in the pelvis.

After birth, fluid retention that is normal during pregnancy is quickly reversed, and large quantities of urine are excreted. The bladder may fill rapidly during the first few days after birth.

#### HEMATOPOIETIC SYSTEM

Most authorities recognize 500 ml as the maximum normal blood loss during vaginal birth. Women usually tolerate this loss well because the blood volume

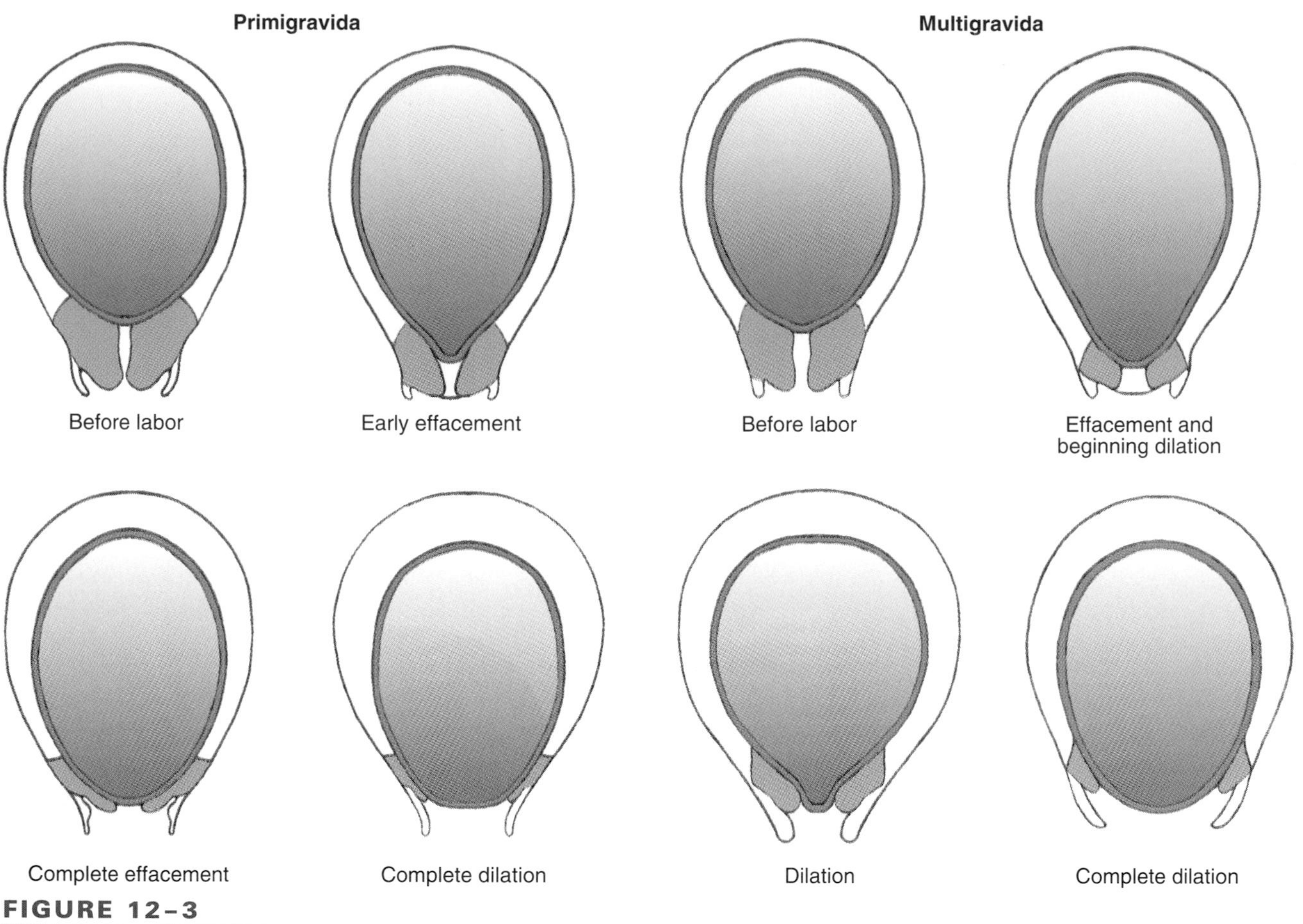


**FIGURE 12-3**

Cervical dilation and effacement. During labor, the multigravida's cervix remains thicker than the nullipara's.

increases during pregnancy by 1 to 2 liters (Guyton & Hall, 1996). A woman who is anemic at the beginning of labor has less reserve for normal blood loss and a poor tolerance for excess bleeding. A hemoglobin of 11 g/dl and a hematocrit of 33 percent or higher give most women an adequate margin of safety for blood loss associated with normal birth. The leukocyte count averages 14,000 to 16,000 per cubic millimeter but may be as high as 25,000 to 30,000 per cubic millimeter during active labor, a level that might otherwise suggest infection (Blackburn & Loper, 1992; Cunningham et al., 1997).

Levels of several clotting factors, especially fibrinogen, are elevated during pregnancy and continue to be higher during labor and after delivery. Although the increase of clotting factors provides protection from hemorrhage, it also increases the mother's risk for a venous thrombosis during pregnancy and after birth.

## Fetal Response

Fetal systems are also affected by labor. Responses are most notable in the placental circulation, the cardiovascular system, and the pulmonary system.

### PLACENTAL CIRCULATION

Chapter 6 explains the functions of the placenta during prenatal life. Exchange of oxygen, nutrients, and waste products between mother and fetus occurs in the intervillous spaces without mixing of maternal and fetal blood. During strong labor contractions, the maternal blood supply to the placenta decreases and eventually stops temporarily as the spiral arteries supplying the intervillous spaces are compressed by the uterine muscle. Therefore, most placental exchange occurs during the interval between contractions.

The placental circulation usually has enough reserve over fetal basal needs to tolerate the intermittent interruption of blood flow. The fetus has protective mechanisms, such as fetal hemoglobin, which more readily takes on oxygen and releases carbon dioxide, a high hematocrit, and a high cardiac output. The fetus may not tolerate labor contractions well in conditions associated with reduced placental function, such as maternal diabetes or hypertension, or in conditions associated with reduced fetal oxygen-carrying capacity, such as fetal anemia.

#### CARDIOVASCULAR SYSTEM

The fetal cardiovascular system reacts quickly to events during labor. Alterations in the rate and rhythm of the fetal heart may result from normal labor effects, or they may suggest that the fetus is not tolerating the stress of labor. The fetal heart rate is rapid, ranging from 110 to 160 beats per minute (BPM) at term (Menihan, 1996; NAACOG [now AWHONN], 1990). In general, the preterm fetus has a higher heart rate than the term fetus.

#### PULMONARY SYSTEM

Before birth, the fetal lungs are filled with fluid to allow normal development of the airways. This fluid must be cleared to allow normal air breathing. As term approaches, production of fetal lung fluid decreases and its absorption into the interstitium of the lungs increases. Labor intensifies the absorption of lung fluid. Some fluid is expelled from the upper airways as the fetal head and thorax are compressed during passage through the birth canal. The remaining fluid is absorbed into the newborn's pulmonary and lymphatic circulations after birth.

Catecholamines, primarily epinephrine and norepinephrine, produced by the fetal adrenal glands in response to the stress of labor, appear to contribute to the infant's adaptation to extrauterine life. They stimulate cardiac contraction and breathing, speed clearance of remaining lung fluid, and aid in temperature regulation. Infants born by cesarean birth not preceded by labor are more likely to have transient breathing difficulty (see p. 848).

### ✓ CHECK YOUR READING

1. How do labor contractions cause the cervix to efface and dilate? How do they cause fetal descent?
2. What differences in effacement are expected between the parous woman and the woman who has not previously given birth?
3. What changes occur in the maternal cardiovascular, respiratory, gastrointestinal, renal, and hematopoietic systems during labor?
4. Why is it important that uterine contractions be intermittent rather than sustained?
5. How does the normal process of vaginal birth benefit the newborn after birth?

## Components of the Birth Process

Four major factors interact during normal childbirth. These factors are often called the "four P's." They are the powers, the passage, the passenger, and the psyche.

### Powers

The two powers of labor are uterine contractions and maternal pushing efforts.

**Uterine Contractions.** During the first stage of labor (onset through full cervical dilation), uterine contractions are the primary force that moves the fetus through the maternal pelvis.

**Maternal Pushing Efforts.** During the second stage of labor (full cervical dilation through birth of the baby), uterine contractions continue to propel the fetus through the pelvis. In addition, the woman feels an urge to push or bear down as the fetus distends her vagina and puts pressure on her rectum. She adds her voluntary pushing efforts to the force of uterine contractions in second-stage labor.

### Passage

The passage for birth of the fetus consists of the maternal pelvis and the soft tissues. The bony pelvis is usually more important to the outcome of labor than the soft tissue because the bones and joints do not readily yield to the forces of labor. However, softening of the cartilage linking the pelvic bones occurs at term owing to an increase in the hormone relaxin.

The bony pelvis is divided by the linea terminalis (or pelvic brim) into the false pelvis above and the true pelvis below (see Chapter 4). The true pelvis is most important in childbirth. The true pelvis has three subdivisions: (1) the *inlet*, or upper pelvic opening; (2) the *midpelvis*, or pelvic cavity; and (3) the *outlet*, or lower pelvic opening. During birth, the true pelvis functions like a curved cylinder with different dimensions at different levels. Figure 12–4 illustrates important pelvic measurements.

### Passenger

The passenger is the fetus plus the membranes and placenta. Several fetal anatomic and positional variables influence the course of labor.

#### FETAL HEAD

The fetus enters the birth canal in the cephalic presentation 96 percent of the time. The fetal shoulders are also important because of their width, but they are usually movable to adapt to the pelvis.

**Bones, Sutures, and Fontanelles.** The bones of the fetal head involved in the birth process are the two frontal bones on the forehead, the two parietal bones at the crown of the head, and the occipital bone at the back of the head (Fig. 12–5). The five major bones are not fused but are connected by sutures, composed of strong but flexible fibrous tissue. The fontanelles are wider spaces at the intersections of the sutures.

## INLET

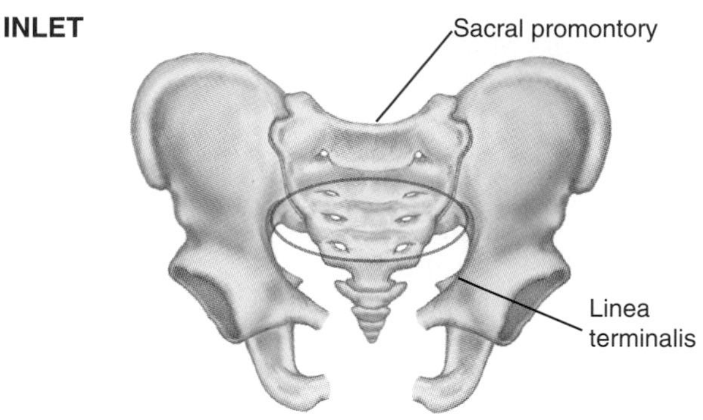


Frontal view, cutaway

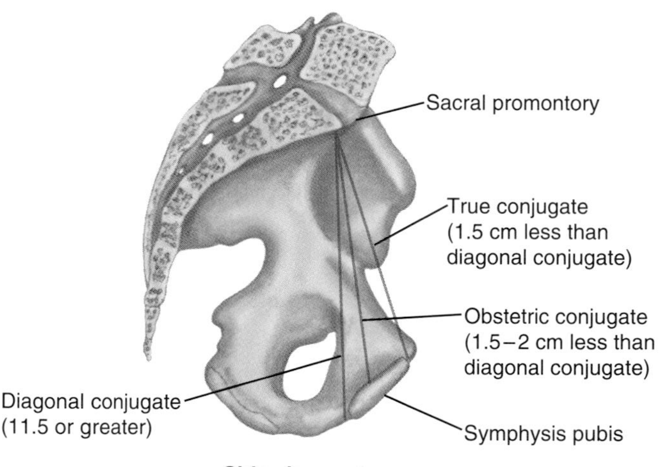


View from above



Side view, cutaway

The boundaries of the inlet are the symphysis pubis anteriorly, the sacral promontory posteriorly, and the linea terminalis on the sides. The inlet is slightly wider in its transverse diameter (13.5 cm) than in its anteroposterior (diagonal conjugate) diameter (11.5 cm or greater).

The diagonal conjugate is slightly larger than both the obstetric and true conjugates. The obstetric conjugate is the narrowest of the three conjugate diameters but cannot be measured directly. The obstetric conjugate is estimated by first measuring the diagonal conjugate and then subtracting 1.5 to 2 cm.

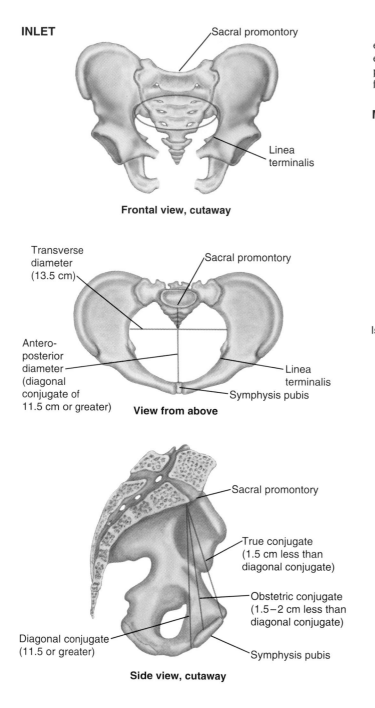

If the inlet is small, the fetal head may not be able to enter it. Because it is almost entirely surrounded by bone, except for cartilage at the sacroiliac joint and symphysis pubis, the inlet cannot enlarge much to accommodate the fetus. The bony measurements are essentially fixed.

## MIDPELVIS

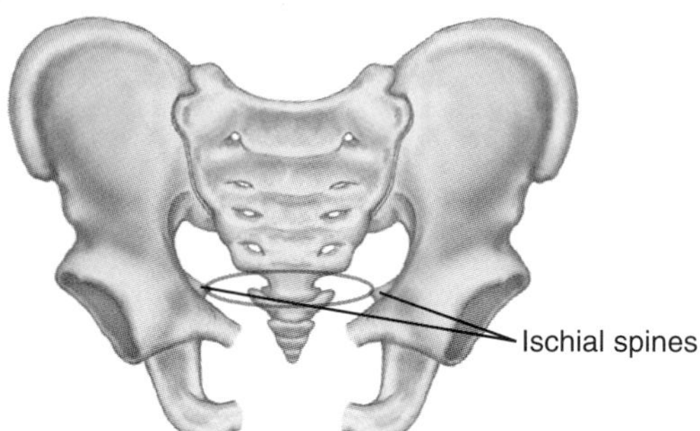


Frontal view, cutaway

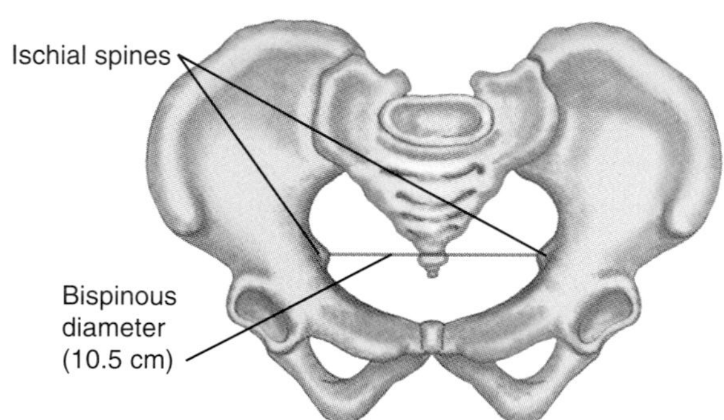


View from above, with pelvis tilted anteriorly

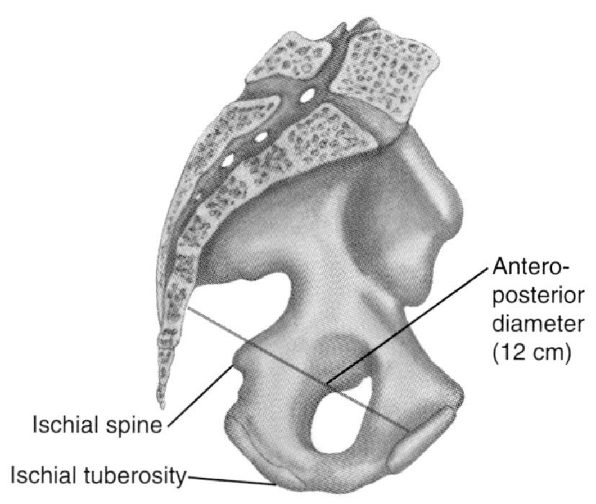


Side view, cutaway

The midpelvis, or pelvic cavity, is the narrowest part of the pelvis through which the fetus must pass during birth. Midpelvic diameters are measured at the level of the ischial spines. The anteroposterior diameter averages 12 cm.

The transverse diameter (bispinous or interspinous) averages 10.5 cm. Prominent ischial spines that project into the midpelvis can reduce the bispinous diameter.

**FIGURE 12–4**

Pelvic divisions and measurements.

**OUTLET**

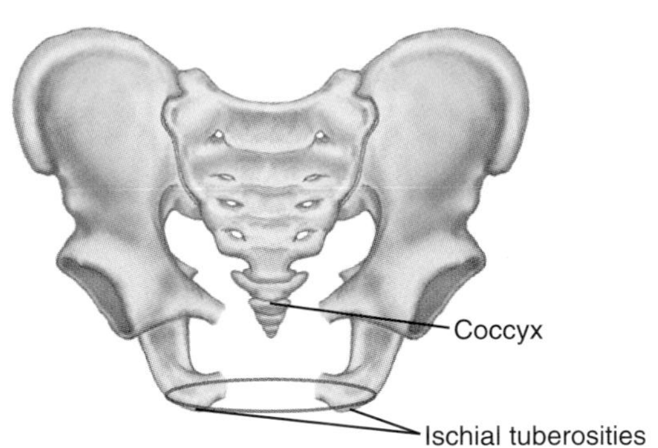


**Frontal view, cutaway**

Three important diameters of the pelvic outlet are (1) the anteroposterior, (2) the transverse (bi-ischial or intertuberous), and (3) the posterior sagittal. The angle of the pubic arch is also an important pelvic outlet measure.

The anteroposterior diameter ranges from 9.5 to 11.5 cm, varying with the curve between the sacrococcygeal joint and the tip of the coccyx. The anteroposterior diameter can increase if the coccyx is easily movable.

The transverse diameter is the bi-ischial, or intertuberous, diameter. This is the distance between the ischial tuberosities ("sit bones"). It averages 11 cm.

The posterior sagittal diameter is normally at least 7.5 cm. It is a measure of the posterior pelvis. The posterior sagittal diameter measures the distance from the sacrococcygeal joint to the middle of the transverse (bi-ischial) diameter.

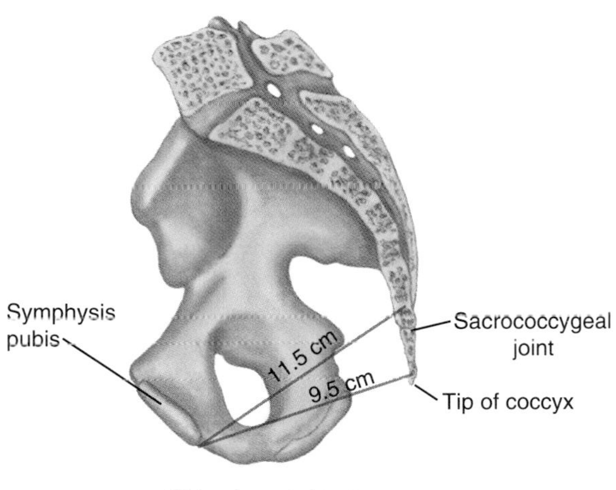


**Side view, cutaway**

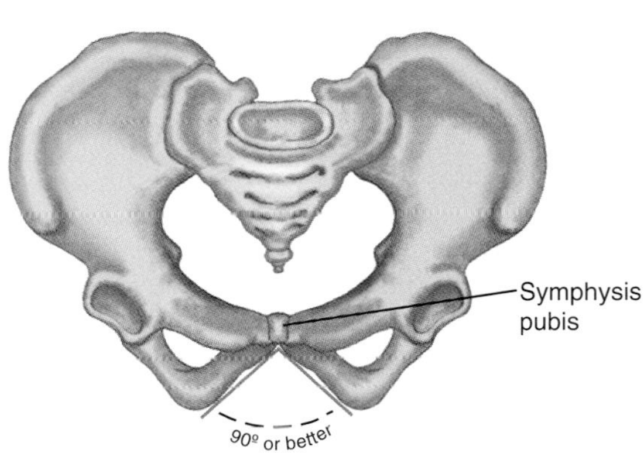


**Frontal view, with pelvis tilted anteriorly**

The angle of the pubic arch is important because it must be wide enough for the fetus to pass under it. The angle of the pubic arch should be at least 90 degrees. A narrow pubic arch displaces the fetus posteriorly toward the coccyx as it tries to pass under the arch.

Ischial tuberosity
Symphysis pubis
Posterior sagittal diameter (7.5 cm or greater)
Bi-ischial or intertuberous diameter (11 cm)
Tip of coccyx

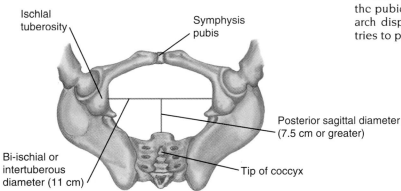

**View from below (woman is in lithotomy position)**

**FIGURE 12–4** *Continued*

The *anterior fontanelle* is diamond shaped and formed by the intersection of four sutures: the two coronal, the frontal, and the sagittal, which connect the two frontal and the two parietal bones. The *posterior fontanelle* has a triangular shape formed by the intersection of three sutures: one sagittal and two lambdoid, which connect the two parietal bones and the occipital bone. The posterior fontanelle is very small, often more like a slight indentation in the skull. The sutures and fontanelles allow the bones to move slightly, changing the shape of the fetal head so that it can adapt to the size and shape of the pelvis by molding. *The sutures and the different shapes of the fontanelles provide important landmarks to determine fetal position and head flexion during vaginal examination.*

**Fetal Head Diameters.** Most fetuses enter the

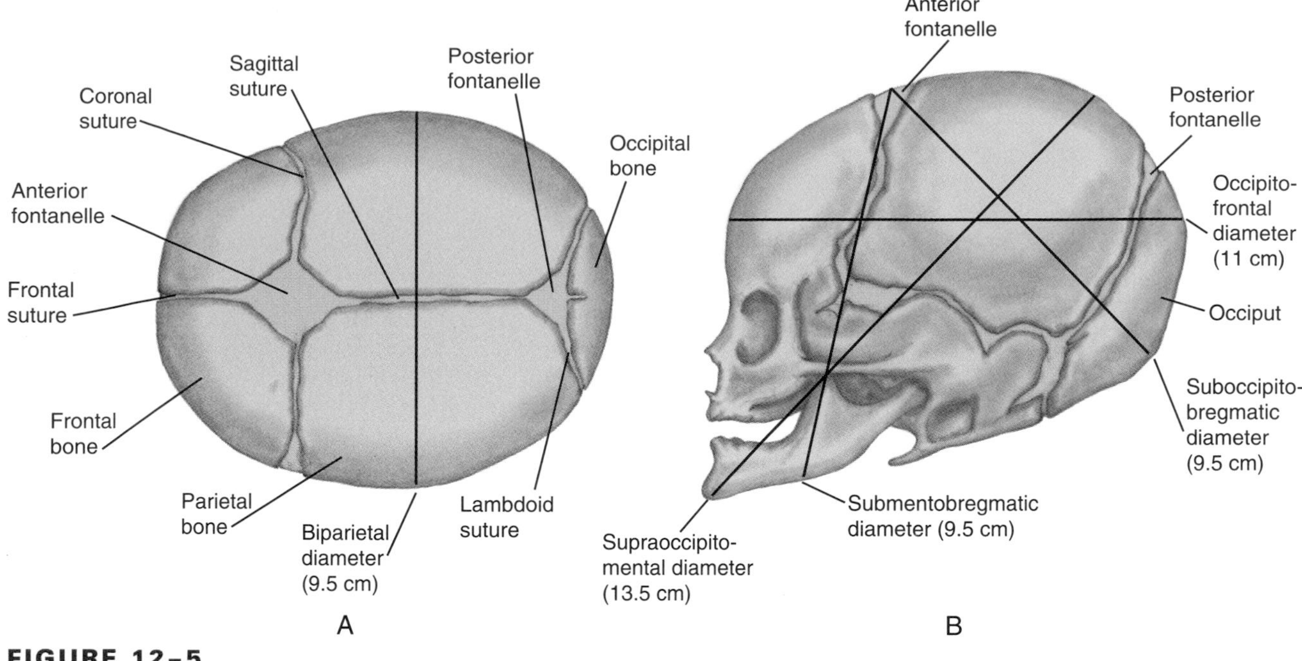


**FIGURE 12–5**

A, Bones, sutures, and fontanelles of the fetal head. Note that the anterior fontanelle has a diamond shape, whereas the posterior fontanelle is triangular. B, Lateral view of the fetal head demonstrating how anteroposterior diameters vary with the amount of flexion or extension.

pelvis in the cephalic presentation, but several variations are possible. The major transverse diameter of the fetal head is the biparietal, measured between the two parietal bones. The biparietal diameter averages 9.5 cm in a term fetus.

The anteroposterior diameter of the head varies with the degree of flexion. In the most favorable situation, the head becomes fully flexed during labor and the anteroposterior diameter is the suboccipitobregmatic, averaging 9.5 cm. See Figure 12–5*B* for anteroposterior head diameters in different degrees of head flexion and extension.

### VARIATIONS IN THE PASSENGER

#### FETAL LIE

The orientation of the long axis of the fetus to the long axis of the woman is the fetal lie (Fig. 12–6). In more than 99 percent of pregnancies, the lie is longitudinal, or parallel to the long axis of the woman. In the *longitudinal lie*, either the head or buttocks of the fetus enters the pelvis first. A *transverse lie* exists when the long axis of the fetus is at right angles to the woman's long axis; it occurs in fewer than 1 percent of pregnancies. An *oblique lie* is one that is at some angle between the longitudinal and the transverse lie.

#### ATTITUDE

The relation of fetal body parts to each other is the attitude of the fetus (Fig. 12–7). The normal fetal attitude is one of flexion, with the head flexed toward the chest and the arms and legs flexed over the thorax. The back is curved in a convex C shape. Flexion remains a characteristic feature of the term newborn.

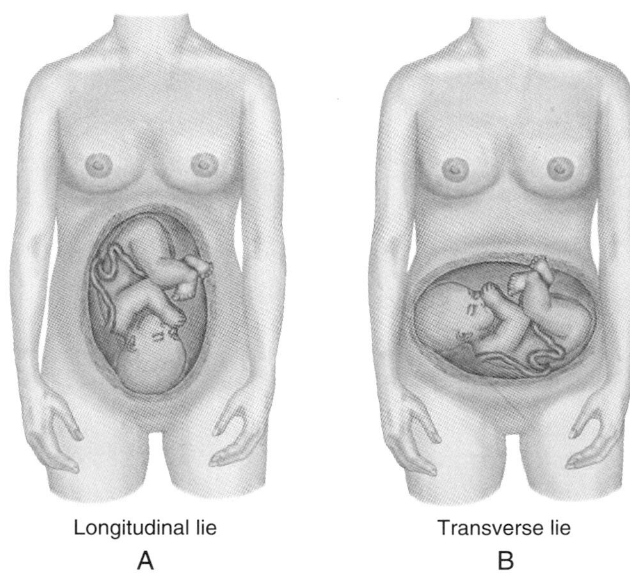


**FIGURE 12–6**

A, Lie. In a longitudinal lie, the long axis of the fetus is parallel to the long axis of the woman. B, In a transverse lie, the long axis of the fetus is at right angles to the long axis of the mother. The woman's abdomen has a wide, short appearance.

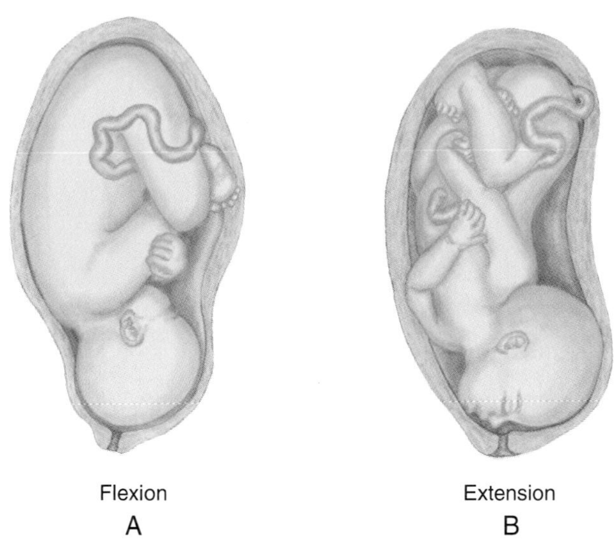


**FIGURE 12-7**

A, Attitude. The fetus is in the normal attitude of flexion, with the head, arms, and legs flexed tightly against the trunk. B, The fetus is in an abnormal attitude of extension. The head is extended, and the right arm is extended. A face presentation is illustrated.

### PRESENTATION

The fetal part that enters the pelvis first is the presenting part. Presentation falls into three categories (1) cephalic, (2) breech, and (3) shoulder. The cephalic presentation with the fetal head flexed is the most common (Fig. 12–8). Other presentations are associated with prolonged labor or other problems and are more likely to require cesarean birth.

**Cephalic Presentation.** The cephalic presentation is more favorable than others for several reasons:

- The fetal head is the largest single fetal part, although the breech (buttocks), with the legs and feet flexed on the abdomen, is collectively larger than the head. After the head is born, the smaller parts follow easily as the extremities unfold.
- During labor, the fetal head can gradually change shape, molding to adapt to the size and shape of the maternal pelvis.
- The fetal head is smooth, round, and hard, making it a more effective part to dilate the cervix, which is also round.

Cephalic presentation has four variations (Fig. 12–8).

***Vertex.*** This is the most common type of cephalic presentation, with the fetal head fully flexed. It is simply called a "vertex (or occiput) presentation" in everyday usage. This presentation is the most favorable for normal progress of labor because the smallest suboccipitobregmatic diameter is presenting.

***Military.*** The head is in a neutral position, neither flexed nor extended. The occipitofrontal diameter is presenting.

***Brow.*** The fetal head is partly extended. The brow presentation is unstable, converting to a vertex presentation if the head flexes or to a face presenta-

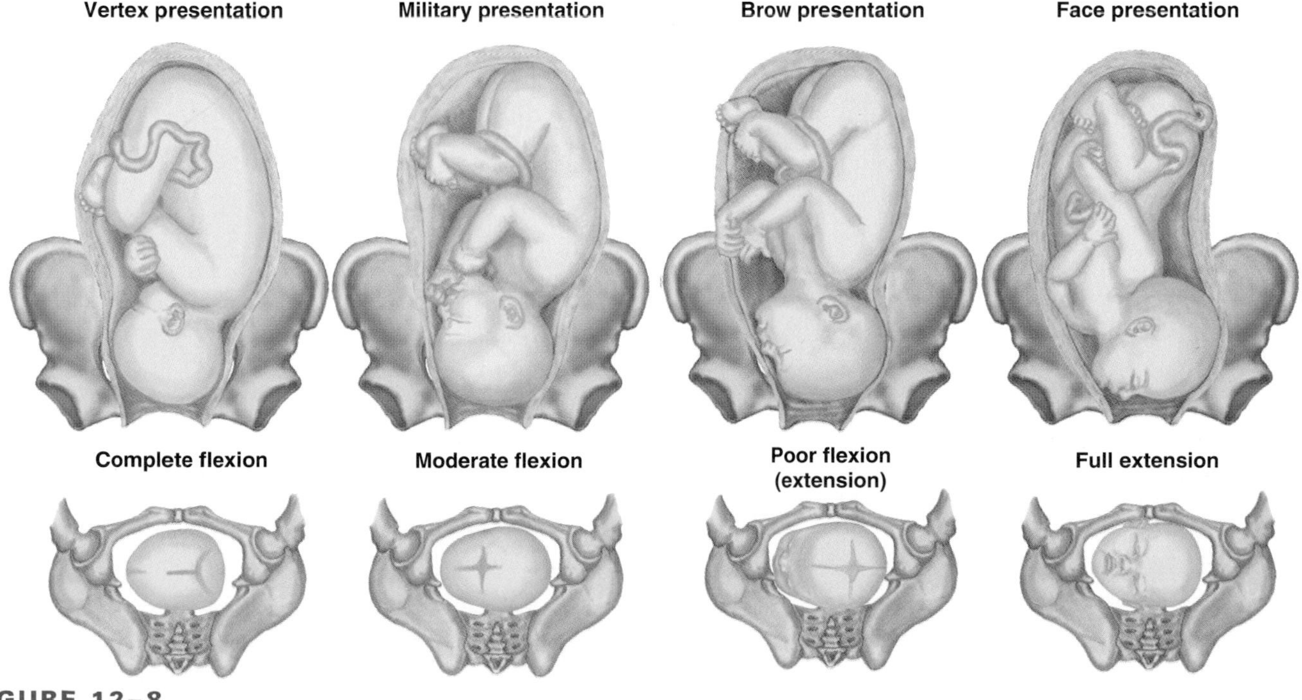


**FIGURE 12-8**

Four types of cephalic presentation. The vertex presentation is normal. Note positional changes of the anterior and posterior fontanelles in relation to the maternal pelvis.

tion if it extends. The longest supraoccipitomental diameter is presenting.

***Face.*** The head is fully extended, and the fetal occiput is near the fetal spine. The submentobregmatic diameter is presenting.

**Breech Presentation.** A breech presentation occurs when the fetal buttocks enter the pelvis first. Breech presentation is more common in preterm births or when a fetal abnormality such as hydrocephalus (enlargement of the head with fluid) prevents the head from entering the pelvis. Breech presentation is also more likely to occur with abnormalities of the maternal uterus or pelvis.

Breech presentations are associated with several disadvantages:

- The buttocks are not smooth and firm like the head and are less effective at dilating the cervix.
- The fetal head is the last part to be born. By the time the fetal head is deep in the pelvis, the umbilical cord is outside the mother's body and is subject to compression between the head and maternal pelvis.
- Because the umbilical cord can be compressed after the fetal chest is born, the head must be delivered quickly to allow the infant to breathe. This does not permit gradual molding of the fetal head as it passes through the pelvis.

The breech presentation has three variations, depending on the relationship of the legs to the body (Fig. 12–9):

***Frank Breech.*** This is the most common variation, occurring when the fetal legs are extended across the abdomen toward the shoulders.

***Full (or Complete) Breech.*** This is a reversal of the usual cephalic presentation. The head is flexed, and the knees and hips are flexed but the buttocks are presenting.

***Footling Breech.*** This occurs when one or both feet are presenting.

**Shoulder Presentation.** The shoulder presentation is a transverse lie and accounts for only 0.2 percent of births (Cunningham et al., 1997). It is more likely with preterm birth, high parity, prematurely ruptured membranes, hydramnios, and placenta previa (placenta low in the uterus). A cesarean birth is almost always necessary.

**CHECK YOUR READING**

6. What are the two powers of labor?
7. What are the three divisions of the true pelvis?
8. Why is the vertex presentation best during birth?

POSITION

Fetal position describes the location of a fixed reference point on the presenting part in relation to the four quadrants of the maternal pelvis (Fig. 12–10). The four quadrants are the right and left anterior and the right and left posterior. The fetal

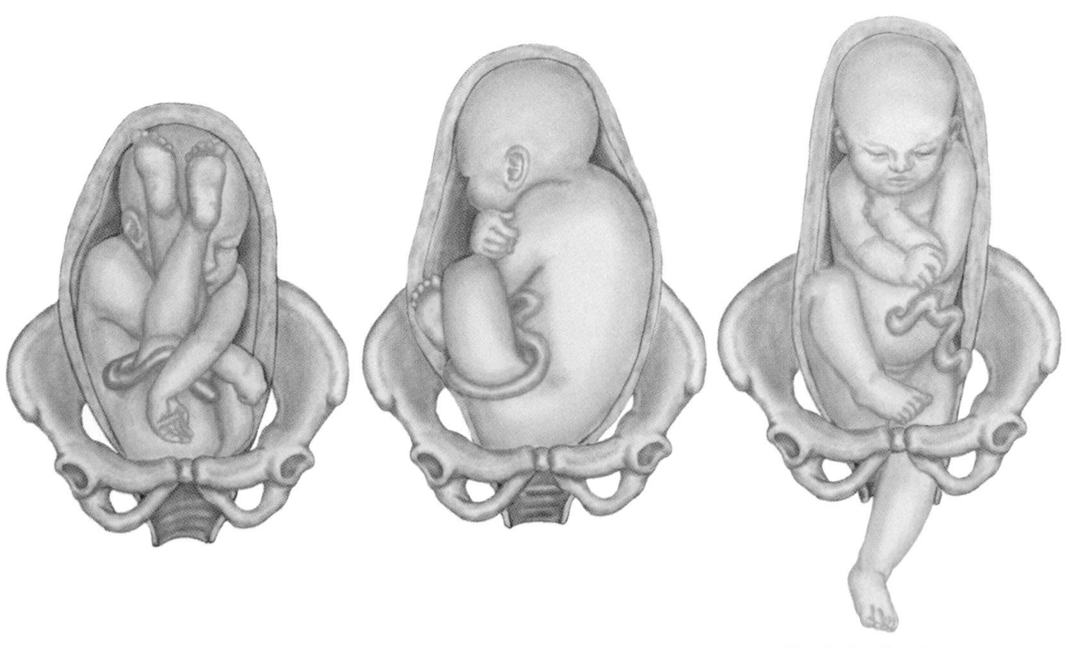


**FIGURE 12–9**

Three variations of a breech presentation. Frank breech is the most common variation. Footling breeches may be single or double.

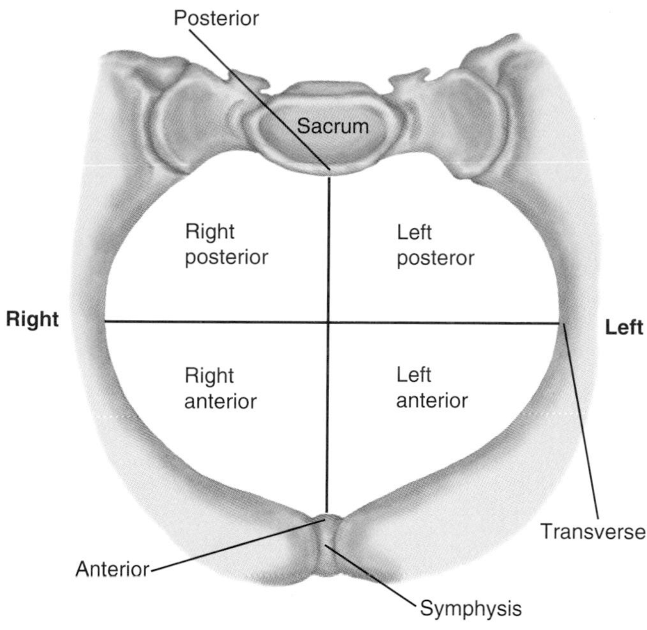


**FIGURE 12-10**

Four quadrants of the maternal pelvis, used to describe fetal position.

position is not fixed but rather changes during labor as the fetus moves downward and adapts to the pelvic contours. Abbreviations indicate the relationship between the fetal presenting part and the maternal pelvis.

**Right (R) or Left (L).** The first letter of the abbreviation describes whether the fetal reference point is in the right or left of the mother's pelvis. If the fetal point is neither to the right nor to the left of the pelvis, this letter is omitted.

**Occiput (O), Mentum (M), or Sacrum (S).** The second letter of the abbreviation refers to the fixed fetal reference point, which varies with the presentation. The occiput is used in a vertex presentation. The chin, or mentum, is the reference point in a face presentation. The sacrum is used for breech presentations. Letters may also designate the less common brow (F for fronto-) and shoulder (Sc for scapula) presentations.

**Anterior (A), Posterior (P), or Transverse (T).** These letters describe whether the fetal reference point is in the anterior or posterior quadrant of the mother's pelvis. If the fetal reference point is in neither the anterior nor the posterior quadrant, it is described as transverse.

If the fetal occiput is located in the left anterior quadrant of the mother's pelvis, the position is described as left occiput anterior (LOA). If the occiput is in the mother's anterior pelvis, neither to the right nor to the left, it is described as occiput anterior (OA). If the fetal sacrum is located in the mother's right posterior pelvis, the abbreviation is R (right) S (sacrum) P (posterior). See Figure 12–11 for different fetal presentations and positions.

**CHECK YOUR READING**

9. For each fetal position listed, describe the fetal landmark. Where is this landmark located in relation to the mother's pelvis: ROP? OA? RSA? LMA?
10. If the fetus is in a face presentation, why is it not possible to use the occiput to determine position within the pelvis?

## Psyche

The psyche is a crucial part of childbirth. Marked anxiety or fear decreases a woman's ability to cope with pain in labor. Maternal catecholamines secreted in response to anxiety or fear can inhibit uterine contractility and placental blood flow. Relaxation, however, augments the natural process of labor. Preparation for childbirth can enhance a woman's ability to work with her body's efforts rather than resisting the natural forces. Much of the nurse's care during labor involves promoting relaxation and reducing anxiety and fear.

### INDIVIDUAL AND CULTURAL VALUES

A woman in childbirth is more than a physical being. She is a blend of her experiences, her present state, and her future expectations. She is an individual, a member of a family and cultural group, and part of her larger society.

A family's culture affects its members' views of birth and the practices that surround it. Culture shapes the values that people hold, their expectations of the birth experience, and their responses to birth. A woman's culture gives her cues about how she should behave and react to labor and how she should interact with her newborn. If the woman, her family, and caregivers have similar viewpoints, little conflict in their values and expectations is likely. However, if these individuals hold markedly different viewpoints, they may be confused because each expects something different of the other. Cultural differences are most obvious when newly immigrant women give birth. After time and exposure to other cultural groups, the distinctive cultural practices and values often become blurred.

Within a culture, people are individuals. Knowledge of the values and practices of cultural groups that the nurse encounters provides a framework to assess and care for the woman and her family. The nurse must assess the personal expectations and values of each woman and her family related to birth within this general framework. Cultural assessment

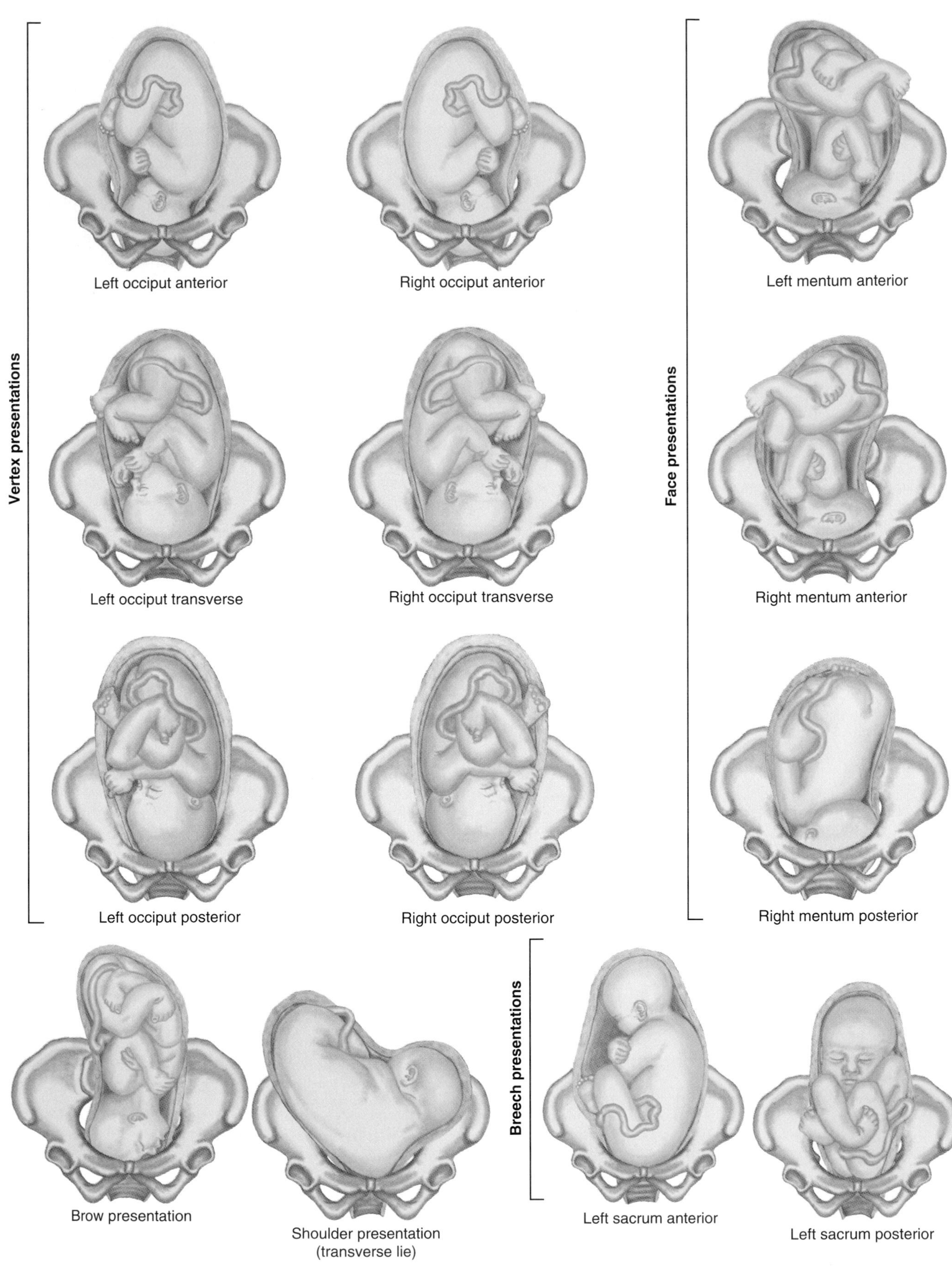


**FIGURE 12–11**

Fetal presentations and positions.

questions for the intrapartum period might include the following:

- How long has the family been in the area? Are they recent immigrants, or have their relatives and friends lived in the area for generations?
- What is the family's primary language? Are they comfortable communicating in the nurse's language if the two are different? If an interpreter is needed, are there people the family considers unacceptable?
- Who is the woman's primary support person for labor? What is that person's role? How extensively will that support person interact with the laboring woman?
- If the woman's primary support is to be her husband, how does the couple view his role? Will he actively support the woman (e.g., coaching her breathing) or will he take a less active role?
- Is a caregiver of the same gender and cultural group essential?
- What are the woman's feelings about touch? Is she comfortable telling the nurse when she does or does not welcome touch?
- Are specific symbols, practices, or ceremonies used during the birth period? Who will conduct any ceremonies?

Other cultural assessments are needed as labor progresses and birth occurs. The impact of culture on pain expression and pain relief and on food choices after birth are covered in the relevant chapters (see Chapters 15 and 17).

#### BIRTH AS AN EXPERIENCE

Childbirth is both a physical and an emotional experience. It is an irrevocable event that changes a woman forever. Families describe the births of their children as they describe other pivotal events in life: marriages, anniversaries, religious events, and even deaths. They do not talk about childbirth in the factual way they might discuss an illness or surgery. With the prevalence of smaller families, parents have greater expectations about the *experience* of childbirth than in the past. The more realistic a woman's expectations about the birth are, the more likely she is to have a positive experience.

Nurses should promote a positive childbirth experience for the woman and her family. Nursing measures that increase their sense of control and mastery during birth help them perceive the birth as a positive event. Nursing measures to empower families include teaching them about their choices in childbirth in an unbiased way and supporting the choices they make.

#### IMPACT OF TECHNOLOGY

The goal of maternity care is to protect the health of the mother, the fetus, and the newborn and to support and enrich family ties. Technology helps caregivers identify problems and intervene quickly to protect the health of mother and fetus. However, use of sophisticated technology can make maternity care less personal. Women may feel that they are less important than the monitors and infusion pumps attached to them.

Childbirth is a natural process that does not warrant routine use of complex technology. Indeed, interventions during birth often lead to other interventions that can inhibit the natural process. For example, epidural analgesia requires that the woman receive large amounts of intravenous fluids and confines her to bed. Her bladder fills quickly, but she may not feel the urge to void, leading to urinary catheterization. Confining her to bed removes the gravitational advantage of walking, squatting, and other upright positions for much of her labor.

Although normal labor and birth do not warrant sophisticated technology, many women subordinate their desire for a peak emotional experience to their desire for what they believe offers maximum safety for their baby. They may accept and even seek interventions that they believe best assure them of having a healthy child. The intrapartum nurse can be the bridge between the technology and the humanness of the birth experience.

The opposite situation may occur. Some women and their partners choose a low-intervention birth rather than a high-tech version. They may find themselves at odds with caregivers if they decline use of available technology and interventions. The nurse must respect their choices and remember that these families are doing what they believe offers them and their baby the best possible outcome.

### Interrelationships of Components

The four "P's" have been described separately, but they are actually an interrelated whole. For instance, a woman with a small pelvis (passage) and a large fetus (passenger) can have a normal labor and birth if the fetus is ideally positioned and the uterine contractions and maternal bearing down efforts (powers) are vigorous. The nurse's supportive attitude strengthens positive psychological elements (psyche) and enhances the processes of birth. The nurse can act as an advocate for the laboring woman and her family to increase their sense of control and mastery of labor, often reducing anxiety and fear.

## Normal Labor

### Theories of Onset

The factors that initiate labor remain unknown despite much research on the subject. Labor normally starts when the fetus is mature enough to adjust easily to extrauterine life but before it grows so large that vaginal birth is impossible. This stage (term gestation) occurs between 38 and 42 weeks after the first day of the woman's last menstrual period.

Labor begins when forces favoring continuation of pregnancy are offset by forces favoring its end. Factors that have a role in starting labor are the following:

- Increased fetal adrenal gland production of glucocorticoids and androgens, which reduces placental progesterone secretion and increases prostaglandin production. When progesterone levels decline, the uterus becomes more easily stimulated to contract.
- A change in the ratio of maternal estrogen to progesterone so that estrogen levels are higher than progesterone levels. Progesterone promotes uterine muscle relaxation during most of pregnancy. Relatively higher estrogen levels enhance uterine sensitivity to substances that stimulate uterine contractions: prostaglandins from the fetal membranes and oxytocin from the maternal posterior pituitary gland.
- Stretching, pressure, or irritation of the uterus and cervix.

## Premonitory Signs

Before labor begins, women usually notice one or more premonitory, or warning, signs that labor is about to begin.

### BRAXTON HICKS CONTRACTIONS

The contractions are irregular and mild, occurring throughout pregnancy. As term approaches, contractions become more noticeable and even painful. Parous women often describe more uterine activity preceding labor than do nulliparous women.

Increased perception of Braxton Hicks contractions often makes sleep difficult at the end of pregnancy. The contractions may become regular at times, only to decrease spontaneously. Because contractions are often uncomfortable and at times regular, the woman may be confused about whether labor has really begun.

### LIGHTENING

As the fetus descends toward the pelvic inlet ("dropping"), the woman notices that she breathes more easily because upward pressure on her diaphragm is reduced. However, increased pressure on her bladder causes her to urinate more frequently. Pressure of the fetal head in the pelvis also may cause leg cramps and edema. Lightening is most noticeable in nulliparas, occurring about 2 to 3 weeks before the onset of labor.

### INCREASED VAGINAL MUCOUS SECRETIONS

An increase in clear and nonirritating vaginal secretions occurs as fetal pressure causes congestion of the vaginal mucosa. The woman may need to wear a perineal pad because of the quantity of mucus.

### BLOODY SHOW

As full term approaches, the cervix begins to soften, dilate, and efface slightly ("ripening") so that it yields more easily to labor contractions. These cervical changes cause expulsion of the mucus plug that sealed the cervix during pregnancy, rupturing small

### CRITICAL THINKING EXERCISE

Alan Lindsey phones you as you are working in the birth unit of your hospital one night. He says, "My wife's baby is due. She's been having some contractions off and on all day, and they are keeping her awake now." Should we come to the hospital?

**Q:** 1. Do you need any other information? If so, what information do you need?

You next speak to Heather Lindsey about her symptoms. You find out that her first baby is due the following week and that she has had no leaking of fluid from her vagina. She says, "My contractions are coming every 2 to 10 minutes, and most of them last about 30 seconds. They didn't bother me much till I tried to go to sleep, but now they are keeping me awake. I'm so tired of all this!"

**Q:** 2. What should you tell Heather about her symptoms? What advice should you give her?

**A:**

1. First, you need to speak directly to the woman who is having the contractions. You need some additional information as well: which baby this is for her, what her due date is, whether her membranes have ruptured, and the characteristics of her contractions (frequency, duration, intensity, effect of activity).
2. Heather's symptoms sound like those typical of false labor: irregular contractions, mild, fairly short, and more annoying than truly painful. Although not harmful, these frequent contractions in late pregnancy interrupt the woman's rest. You should tell Heather that these contractions do not sound like true labor, then review with her the typical signs and symptoms of true labor. Advise her to come to the hospital if her contractions intensify and become more consistent, if her "water breaks," if the baby seems to move much less, or if she has bleeding. And, because it is impossible to diagnose labor over the phone, tell her to come to the hospital for evaluation if she has any continuing concern.

cervical capillaries in the process. Bloody show is a mixture of thick mucus and pink or dark brown blood. It may begin several days to a few weeks before labor's onset, especially in the nulliparous woman.

A recent vaginal examination or sexual intercourse also may result in small amounts of bloody show because it disrupts these small vessels. Bloody show increases during labor as the cervix completes dilation and effacement. Women who have previously had a vaginal birth often have less bloody show than do nulliparas.

#### ENERGY SPURT

Some women have a sudden increase in energy ("nesting"). They should be cautioned to conserve their energy so that they are not exhausted when labor actually begins.

#### WEIGHT LOSS

A small weight loss of about 1 to 3 pounds may occur because of changing levels of estrogen and progesterone. These hormone changes cause excretion of some of the extra fluid that accumulates during pregnancy.

## True Labor and False Labor

False labor, also called prodromal labor, is common because the exact time of labor's onset is rarely known and is usually a gradual process. False labor often causes women to go to the birth center, thinking that labor has started, only to be disappointed when it has not. The term *false labor* is discouraging to women, because they do not realize that these "false" contractions are preparation for the main event of true labor.

Several characteristics distinguish true labor from false labor: contractions, discomfort, and cervical change. The best distinction between the two is that contractions of true labor cause *progressive change in the cervix*. Effacement and dilation occur with true labor contractions.

Some women experience membrane rupture as their first sign of labor's onset. If this occurs, the woman should go to the birth center for evaluation. Infection and compression of the fetal umbilical cord are possible complications.

### Women Want to Know

### How to Know Whether Labor Is "Real"

True labor differs from false labor in three categories.

| FALSE LABOR | TRUE LABOR |
|---|---|
| **Contractions** | |
| Inconsistent in frequency, duration, and intensity. | A consistent pattern of increasing frequency, duration, and intensity usually develops. |
| A change in activity, such as walking, does not alter contractions, or activity may decrease them. | Walking tends to increase contractions. |
| **Discomfort** | |
| Felt in the abdomen and groin | Begins in lower back and gradually sweeps around to lower abdomen like a girdle. |
| May be more annoying than truly painful. | Back pain may persist in some women.<br>Early labor often feels like menstrual cramps. |
| **Cervix** | |
| No significant change in effacement or dilation of the cervix. | Effacement and/or dilation of cervix occurs.<br>Progressive effacement and dilation of cervix are most important characteristics. |

## Mechanisms of Labor

The mechanisms (cardinal movements) of labor occur as the fetus is moved through the pelvis during birth. The fetus undergoes several positional changes to adapt to the size and shape of the mother's pelvis at different levels (Fig. 12–12). Although the mechanisms of labor are described separately in this figure, some occur concurrently. In a vertex presentation, the mechanisms are the following:

- *Descent* of the fetal presenting part through the true pelvis.
- *Engagement* of the fetal presenting part as its widest diameter reaches the level of the ischial spines of the mother's pelvis.
- *Flexion* of the fetal head so that the smallest head diameters pass through the pelvis.
- *Internal rotation* to allow the largest fetal head diameters to match with the largest maternal pelvic diameters.
- *Extension* of the fetal head as the head passes beneath the mother's symphysis pubis.
- *External rotation* of the fetal head to allow the shoulders to rotate internally to best fit the mother's pelvis.
- *Expulsion* of the fetal shoulders and fetal body.

The mechanisms of labor are different in presentations other than the vertex, but the reason is the same: effective use of available space in the maternal pelvis.

**CHECK YOUR READING**

11. What are some of the signs and symptoms that a woman might experience before labor begins?
12. What are the differences between true and false labor? Which difference is the most significant?
13. Why does the fetus enter the pelvis with the sagittal suture aligned with the transverse diameter of the woman's pelvic inlet?
14. Why does the fetal head turn during labor until the sagittal suture aligns with the anteroposterior diameter of the mother's pelvic outlet?

### Descent, Engagement, and Flexion

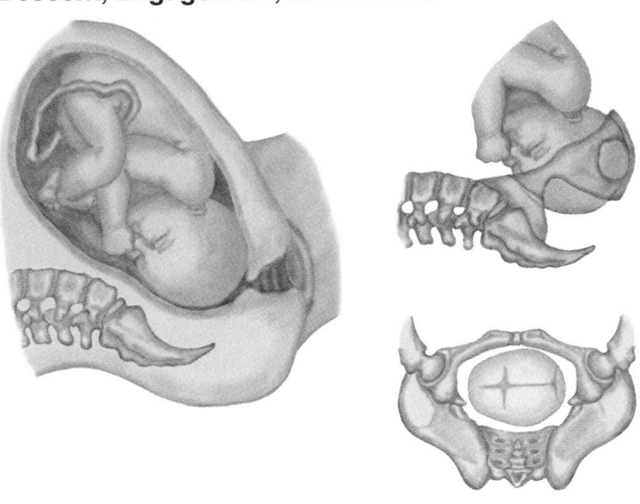

Descent of the fetus is a mechanism of labor that accompanies all the others. Without descent, none of the mechanisms will occur.

### Station

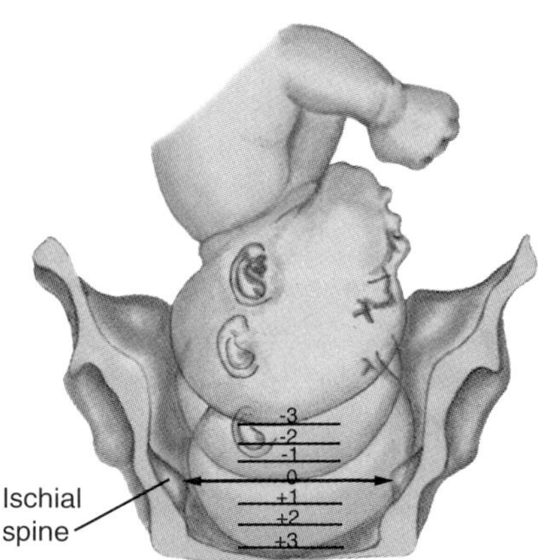


Station describes the descent of the fetal presenting part in relation to the level of the ischial spines. The level of the ischial spines is a zero station. Other stations are described with numbers representing the approximate number of centimeters above (negative numbers) or below (positive numbers) the ischial spines. As the fetus descends through the pelvis, the station changes from higher negative numbers(−3, −2, −1) to zero to higher positive numbers (+1, +2, +3, etc.) Sometimes the terms *floating* or *ballottable* may describe a fetal presenting part that is so high that it is easily displaced upward during abdominal or vaginal examination, similar to tossing a ball upward.

### Engagement

Engagement occurs when the largest diameter of the fetal presenting part (normally the head) has passed the pelvic inlet and entered the pelvic cavity. Engagement is presumed to have occurred when the station of the presenting part is zero or lower. Engagement often takes place before onset of labor in nulliparous women. In many parous women and in some nulliparas, it does not occur until after labor begins.

### Flexion

As the fetus descends, the fetal head is flexed further as it meets resistance from the soft tissues of the pelvis. Head flexion presents the smallest anteroposterior diameter (suboccipitobregmatic) to the pelvis.

### Internal Rotation

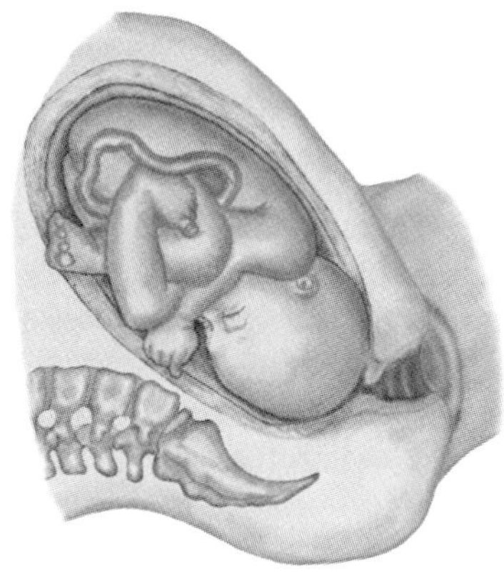

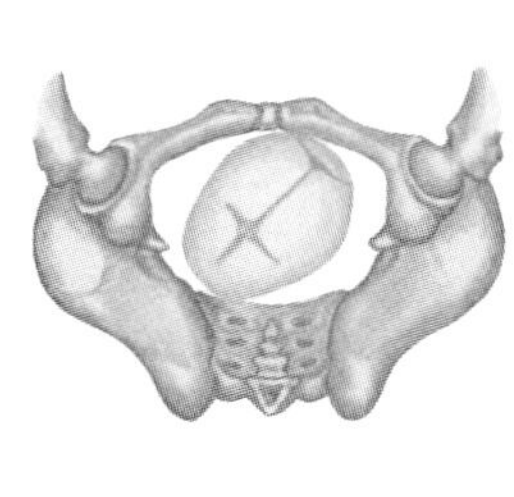

The fetus enters the pelvic inlet with the sagittal suture in a transverse or oblique orientation to the maternal pelvis because that is the widest inlet diameter. Internal rotation allows the longest fetal head diameter (the anteroposterior) to conform to the longest diameter of the maternal pelvis.

The longest pelvic outlet diameter is the anteroposterior. As the head descends to the level of the ischial spines, it gradually turns so that the fetal occiput is in the anterior of the pelvis (OA position, directly under the maternal symphysis pubis). When internal rotation is complete, the sagittal suture is oriented in the anteroposterior pelvic diameter (OA). Less commonly, the head may turn posteriorly so that the occiput is directed toward the mother's sacrum (OP).

**FIGURE 12–12**

Mechanisms (cardinal movements) of labor.

## Extension

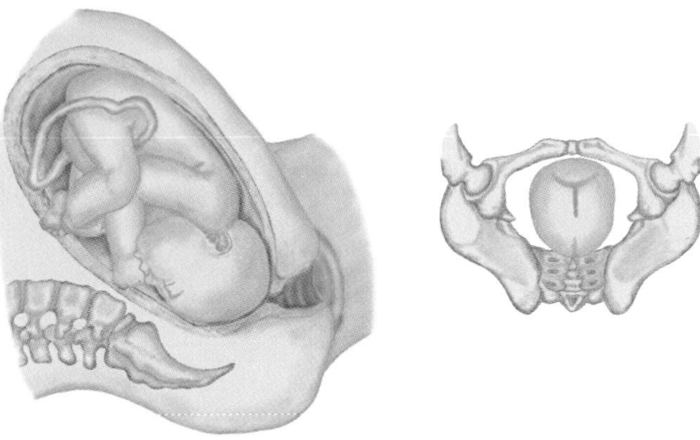

Extension beginning (internal rotation complete)

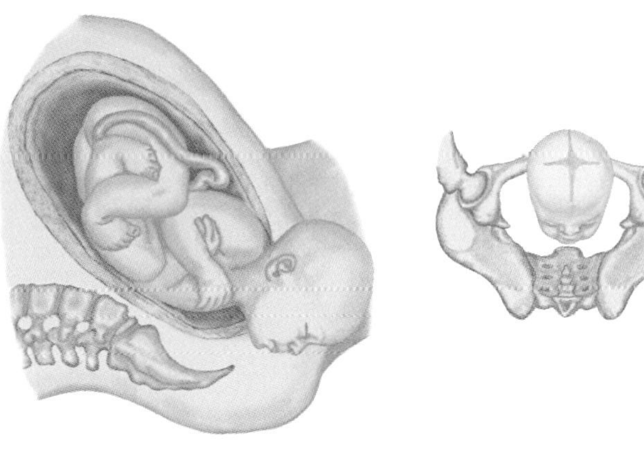

Extension complete

Because the true pelvis is shaped like a curved cylinder, the fetal head is directed posteriorly toward the rectum as it begins its descent. To negotiate the curve of the pelvis, the fetal head must change from an attitude of flexion to one of extension.

While still in flexion, the fetal head meets resistance from the tissues of the pelvic floor. At the same time, the fetal neck stops under the symphysis, which acts as a pivot. The combination of resistance from the pelvic floor and the pivoting action of the symphysis causes the fetal head to swing anteriorly, or extend, with each maternal pushing effort. The head is born in extension, with the occiput sliding under the symphysis and the face directed toward the rectum. The fetal brow, nose, and chin slide over the perineum as the head is born.

## External Rotation

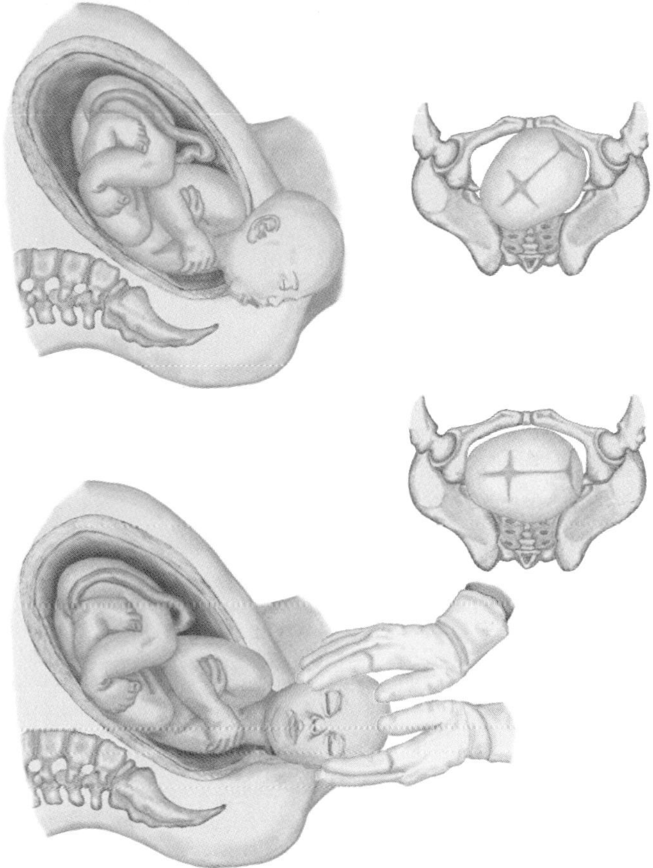

When the head is born with the occiput directed anteriorly, the shoulders must rotate internally so that they align with the anteroposterior diameter of the pelvis.

After the head is born, it spontaneously turns to the same side as it was in utero as it realigns with the shoulders and back (through a process called restitution). The head then turns further to that side in external rotation as the shoulders internally rotate and are positioned with their transverse diameter in the anteroposterior diameter of the pelvic outlet. External rotation of the head accompanies internal rotation of the shoulders.

## Expulsion

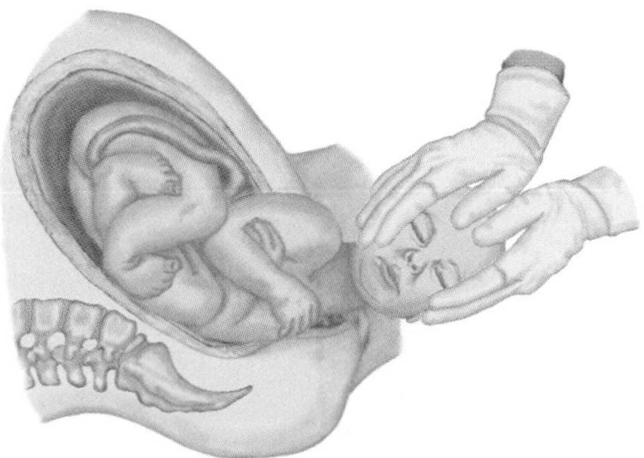

Expulsion occurs first as the anterior, then the posterior, shoulder passes under the symphysis. After the shoulders are born, the rest of the body follows.

## TABLE 12-1 CHARACTERISTICS OF NORMAL LABOR

| | First Stage | Second Stage | Third Stage | Fourth Stage |
|---|---|---|---|---|
| Work accomplished | Effacement and dilation of cervix | Expulsion of fetus | Separation of placenta | Physical recovery and bonding with newborn |
| Forces | Uterine contractions | Uterine contractions and voluntary bearing-down efforts | Uterine contractions | Uterine contraction to control bleeding from placenta site |
| Average duration | | | | |
| Nullipara | 8–10 hr after reaching active phase; dilation averages 1 cm/hr | Average 50 min (range 30 min–3 hr) | 5–10 minutes; up to 30 minutes is normal for unassisted placental separation | 1–4 hr after birth |
| Multipara | 6–7 hr (range 2–10 hr) after reaching active phase; dilation averages 1.2 cm/hr | Average 20 min (range 5–30 min) | Same as for nullipara | Same as for nullipara |
| Cervical dilation | Latent phase: 0–3 cm<br>Active phase: 4–7 cm<br>Transition phase: 8–10 cm | 10 cm (complete dilation) | Not applicable | Not applicable |
| Uterine contractions | *Latent phase*<br>Initially mild and infrequent; progress to moderate strength, every 5 min with a regular pattern; duration increases to 30–40 sec by end of latent phase<br>*Active phase*<br>Increase in frequency, duration, and intensity until every 2–5 min, 40–60 sec, and moderate to strong intensity<br>*Transition phase*<br>Strong, every 1½ to 2 min, 60 sec | Strong, every 2–3 min, lasting 40–60 sec; may be slightly less intense than during transition phase of first stage; may pause briefly as second stage begins | Firmly contracted | Firmly contracted |
| Discomfort | Often begins with a low backache and sensations similar to those of menstrual cramps; back discomfort gradually sweeps to the lower abdomen in a girdle-like fashion, discomfort intensifies as labor progresses | Urge to push or bear down with contractions, which becomes stronger as fetus descends; distention of vagina and vulva may cause a stretching or splitting sensation | Little discomfort; sometimes slight cramp is felt as placenta is passed | Discomfort varies; some women have afterpains, more common in multigravidas or those who have had a large baby; as anesthesia wears off, perineal discomfort may become noticeable |
| Maternal behaviors | Sociable, excited, and somewhat anxious during early labor; becomes more inwardly focused as labor intensifies; may lose control during transition | Intense concentration on pushing with contractions; often oblivious to surroundings and appears to doze between contractions | Excited and relieved after baby's birth; usually very tired; often cries | Tired, but may find it difficult to rest because of excitement; eager to become acquainted with her newborn |

## Stages and Phases of Labor

Labor is divided into four stages. Each stage has qualities that set it apart from the others. These descriptions of the typical physiologic characteristics and maternal behaviors are approximate. Individual women vary in their labor patterns and responses to labor. Use of regional anesthetics, such as the epidural block, is likely to modify the typical maternal behaviors. Table 12–1 summarizes characteristics of each stage of labor.

### FIRST STAGE

Cervical effacement and dilation occur in the first stage, or *stage of dilation*. It begins with the onset of true labor contractions and ends with complete dilation (10 cm) and effacement (100 percent) of the cervix.

The first stage of labor is the longest for both nulliparous and parous women. Average duration of first stage labor is 8 to 10 hours (range 6 to 18 hours) for the nullipara and 6 to 7 hours (range 2 to 10 hours) for the parous woman. The rate of labor progress is also important. Once the active phase begins, the cervix of the nullipara usually dilates about 1 cm per hour and that of the multipara about 1.2 cm per hour. Labor progress is often plotted on a graph, often called a Friedman curve (Fig. 12–13).

First-stage labor differs from the other stages because it has three phases within it: latent (early), active, and transition. Each phase is characterized by changing maternal behaviors. These behaviors vary with the woman's preparation, use of coping skills, and use of medication.

**Latent Phase.** The latent, or early, phase lasts from the beginning of labor until about 3 cm of cervical dilation. Its length is quite variable among women. Despite being called "latent," much cervical effacement and fetal positional change occur during this phase, preparing for more rapid changes during active labor.

Contractions gradually increase in frequency, duration, and intensity. The interval between contractions shortens until contractions are about 5 minutes apart as the woman progresses to the active phase. Duration increases to about 30 to 40 seconds by the end of the latent phase. Intensity begins with mild contractions, when the contracting uterus can be easily indented with the fingertips, progressing to moderate contractions, in which the uterine muscle is indented with more difficulty. The contractions gradually build to their peak intensity and remain at the peak briefly before they diminish.

During early labor, the woman may notice discomfort in her back with each contraction. As labor progresses, back discomfort encircles the lower abdo-

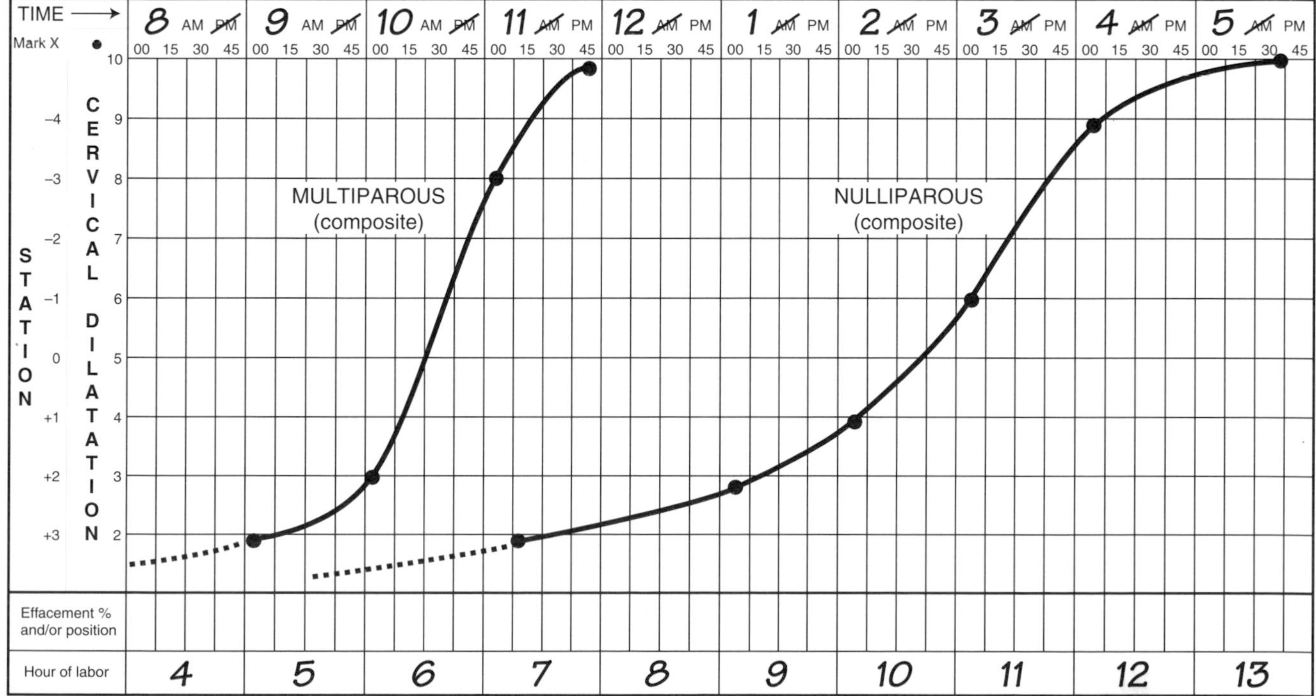


**FIGURE 12–13**

A labor curve, often called a Friedman curve, may be used to identify whether a woman's cervical dilation is progressing at the expected rate.

## CRITICAL THINKING EXERCISE

After examining a woman in labor with her first baby, the nurse-midwife gives you the following information:

"Carmelita Saenz is about 2 to 3 cm, 75 percent, and 0. The baby is vertex and ROP."

**Q:** What is the correct interpretation of this information? What behaviors would be expected for Mrs. Saenz at this time? What behaviors should suggest to you that she has begun making very rapid labor progress?

**A:** Mrs. Saenz's cervix is about 2 to 3 cm dilated and has effaced to about one fourth of its original length (now about 0.5 cm long, or 75% effaced). The widest part of the fetal head (the biparietal diameter) is at the level of the ischial spines (0 station) and has passed the pelvic inlet.

The vertex presentation means that the fetal head is well flexed, which is most favorable because it presents the smallest anterior-posterior diameter to the maternal pelvis. ROP means that the fetal occiput is in Mrs. Saenz's right posterior pelvic quadrant.

During the early part of first-stage labor (latent phase), you would expect Mrs. Saenz to be relatively comfortable. She may be visiting with her husband and other family or friends. Although rapid progress is unlikely with the first baby, be alert to behaviors such as sudden grunting or bearing down (usually accompanied by a marked increase in bloody show); crying out that "The baby's coming" or "I've got to push"; or inability to maintain control with techniques that have previously been helpful. Summon an experienced nurse or her nurse-midwife by using the call signal at once if any of these behaviors occur. Do not leave her unattended in case the baby arrives unexpectedly.

men with each contraction. Many women describe the discomfort as similar to menstrual cramps, especially during early labor.

The woman is usually sociable and excited but cooperative. She is anxious as she realizes that this is the "real thing" and there is no turning back. Yet she is usually relieved that pregnancy is about to end and she can hold her baby.

**Active Phase.** The active phase of labor is aptly named because the pace of labor increases. The cervix dilates from 4 to 7 cm and at a more rapid rate than in the latent phase. Effacement of the cervix is completed. The fetus descends in the pelvis, and internal rotation begins.

Contractions average 2 to 5 minutes apart, with a duration of about 40 to 60 seconds, and range from moderate to strong intensity. Active labor contractions reach their peak intensity more quickly and stay at the peak longer than during the latent phase.

As contractions intensify, discomfort also increases. The site of discomfort during the active phase is similar to the location during the latent phase.

The woman's behavior changes. She becomes more anxious and may feel helpless as the contractions intensify. The sociability that characterized early labor is gone, replaced with a serious, inward focus. She is less likely to initiate interactions with others unless she has specific requests. Her behaviors are typical of one concentrating intently on a demanding task, which birth certainly is. The nurse helps her maintain her concentration, supports her coping techniques, and helps her find alternatives for methods that do not work for her.

**Transition Phase.** The cervix dilates from 8 to 10 cm, and the fetus descends further into the pelvis. Bloody show often increases with completion of cervical dilation. Transition is a short but intense phase.

Contractions are very strong. They may be as frequent as 1½ to 2 minutes apart, and their duration is 60 to 90 seconds. Strong contractions combined with fetal descent may cause the woman to have an urge to push or bear down during contractions. If she pushes before cervical dilation is complete, the cervix may swell and labor may be prolonged. Leg tremors, nausea, and vomiting are common.

The woman often finds the transition phase to be the most difficult. She may be irritable and lose control. Her partner may be confused because actions that were helpful just a short time ago now bother her. The nurse can encourage the partners that the end of labor is near and support the coping techniques they are using. If premature bearing down is a problem, the nurse can help her blow outward with each breath until the urge passes.

### SECOND STAGE

The second stage (*expulsion*) begins with complete (10 cm) dilation and full (100 percent) effacement of the cervix and ends with the birth of the baby. The duration is about 50 minutes (range 30 minutes to 3 hours) in nulliparas and about 20 minutes (range 5 to 30 minutes) in parous women.

Contractions may diminish slightly, or even pause briefly, as the second stage begins. They are still strong, about 2 to 3 minutes apart, with a duration of 40 to 60 seconds.

As the fetus descends, pressure of the presenting part on the rectum and the pelvic floor causes the mother to have an involuntary pushing response. She may say that she needs to have a bowel movement or "the baby's coming" or "I have to push." Her voluntary pushing efforts augment involuntary uterine contractions. As the fetus descends low in the pelvis and the vulva distends with crowning of the fetal head, she may feel a sensation of stretching or splitting even if no trauma occurs.

The woman often regains a feeling of control during the second stage of labor. Contractions are strong, but she may feel more in control, knowing that she is doing something to complete the process by pushing with them. "Labor" is a fitting word to describe the second stage. The woman exerts intense physical effort to push her baby out. Between contractions, she may be oblivious to her surroundings and may appear asleep. She feels tremendous relief and excitement as the second stage ends with the birth of the baby.

### THIRD STAGE

The third (*placental*) stage begins with the birth of the baby and ends with the expulsion of the placenta (Fig. 12–14). This stage is the shortest, lasting up to 30 minutes, with an average length of 5 to 10 minutes. There is no difference in duration for nulliparas and parous women.

When the infant is born, the uterine cavity becomes much smaller. The reduced size decreases the size of the placenta site, causing it to separate from the uterine wall. Four signs suggest placenta separation:

- The uterus has a spheric shape.
- The uterus rises upward in the abdomen as the placenta descends into the vagina and pushes the fundus upward.
- The cord descends further from the vagina.
- A gush of blood appears as blood trapped behind the placenta is released.

The placenta may be expelled in one of two ways. In the more common *Schultze* mechanism, the placenta is expelled with the shiny fetal side first (see Fig. 12–14*B*). The *Duncan* mechanism is less common, with the rough maternal side presenting (see Fig. 12–14*A*).

The uterus must contract firmly and remain contracted after the placenta is expelled to compress open vessels at the implantation site. Inadequate uterine contraction after birth may result in hemorrhage.

Pain during the third stage of labor results from uterine contractions and brief stretching of the cervix as the placenta passes through it.

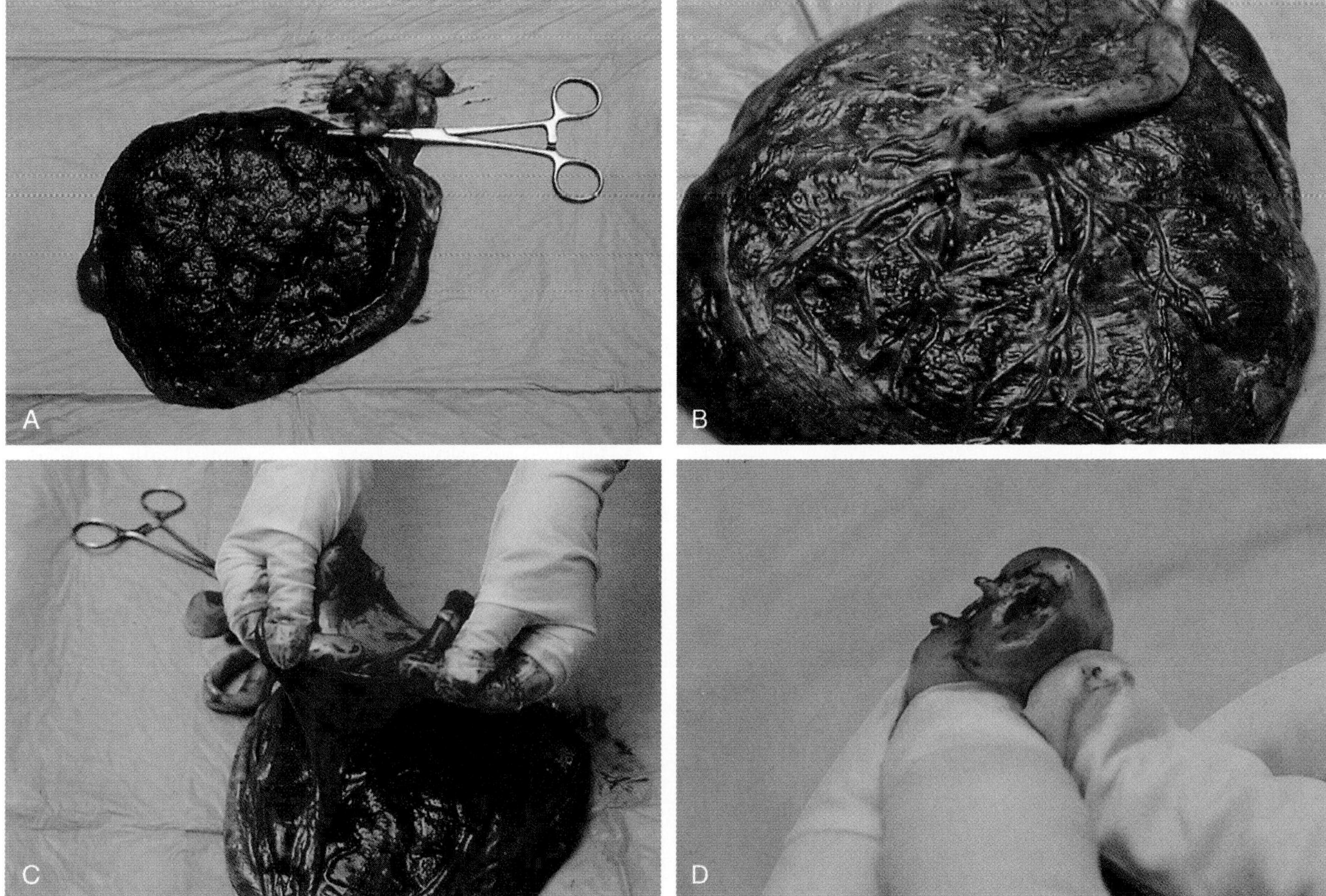

**FIGURE 12–14**

A, Maternal side of the placenta. B, Fetal side of the placenta. C, Separating membranes. D, Umbilical cord vessels, two arteries, and one vein.

#### FOURTH STAGE

The fourth stage of labor is the *stage of physical recovery* for the mother and infant. It lasts from the delivery of the placenta through the first 1 to 4 hours after birth.

Immediately after birth, the firmly contracted uterus can be palpated through the abdominal wall as a firm, rounded mass about 10 to 15 cm (4 to 6 inches) in diameter at or below the level of the umbilicus. Uterine size varies with the size of the infant and parity of the mother, being larger when the infant is large or the mother is a multipara. A full bladder or a blood clot in the uterus interferes with uterine contraction, increasing blood loss. A soft (boggy) uterus and increasing uterine size are associated with postpartum hemorrhage because large blood vessels at the placenta site are not compressed (see Chapter 28).

The vaginal drainage after childbirth is called *lochia*. There are three stages: lochia rubra, lochia serosa, and lochia alba (see p. 428). Lochia rubra, consisting mostly of blood, is present in the fourth stage of labor.

Many women have a chill after birth. The cause of this reaction is unknown but probably relates to the sudden decrease in effort, loss of the heat produced by the fetus, a decrease in intra-abdominal pressure, and fetal blood cells that enter the maternal circulation. The chill lasts for about 20 minutes and subsides spontaneously. A warm blanket, hot drink, or soup may help shorten the chill and make the woman more comfortable.

Discomfort during the fourth stage usually results from birth trauma or afterpains. Localized discomfort from birth trauma such as lacerations, an episiotomy, edema, or a hematoma is evident as the effects of local or regional anesthetics diminish. Ice packs on the perineum limit this edema and hematoma formation.

Afterpains are intermittent uterine contractions that occur after birth as the uterus begins its return to the pre-pregnancy state. The discomfort is similar to that of menstrual cramps. Afterpains are more common in multiparas, in women who breastfeed, in women who have large babies or other uterine overdistention during pregnancy, or in cases when something interferes with uterine contraction such as a full bladder or a blood clot that remains in the uterus.

The mother is simultaneously excited and tired after birth. She may be exhausted but too excited to rest. The fourth stage of labor is an ideal time for bonding of the new family because the interest of both parents and newborn is high. It is the best time to initiate breastfeeding if no maternal or infant problems are present. The baby is alert and seeks to make eye contact with the new parents, giving powerful reinforcement for the parents' attachment to their newborn.

#### ✓ CHECK YOUR READING

15. How do maternal behaviors change during each phase of first-stage labor and during the second stage?
16. What are the typical characteristics of contractions during each phase of first-stage labor and second-stage labor?
17. What four signs may indicate that the placenta has separated?
18. What complications may occur if the uterus does not contract firmly and remain contracted after the placenta is expelled?

## Duration of Labor

Total duration of labor is significantly different for women who have never given birth and for those who have previously given birth vaginally. The parous woman usually delivers more quickly than does the nulliparous woman. However, women are individuals. Some nulliparas progress through labor quickly, whereas labor for some parous women resembles that of women who have never given birth. A woman who experienced a long labor with her first child may not have a long labor with every baby. If she has a history of rapid labor, however, later births are often rapid as well.

Because vaginal birth after cesarean (VBAC) is common, a parous woman may have had no vaginal births. In this situation, the woman is likely to have a labor more like that of the nullipara, particularly if she did not labor before her previous cesarean birth.

## SUMMARY CONCEPTS

- Labor contractions are intermittent, allowing placental blood flow and exchange of oxygen, nutrients, and waste products between maternal and fetal circulations during the interval.
- The upper uterus contracts actively during labor, maintaining tension to pull the more passive lower uterus and cervix over the fetal presenting part. These actions bring about cervical effacement and dilation.
- Maternal vital signs are best assessed between contractions because slight alterations in the woman's blood pressure and pulse may occur during a contraction.
- Hyperventilation may occur if the woman breathes deeply and rapidly. Its manifestations include tingling of the hands and feet, numbness, and dizziness.
- The fetal heart rate and rhythm respond rapidly to events that occur during labor.

- Several occurrences during late pregnancy and labor aid the newborn in making adaptations to extrauterine life: reduced production of fetal lung fluid and increased absorption of lung fluid into the interstitium of the fetal lungs; expulsion of fluid from upper airways during the compression forces of labor; and increased catecholamine secretion by the fetal adrenals to stimulate cardiac contraction and breathing, speed clearance of remaining lung fluid, and aid in temperature regulation.
- Four interrelated components affecting the process of birth are the powers, the passage, the passenger, and the psyche. Presentation and position further describe the relation of the fetus (passenger) to the maternal pelvis.
- The mechanisms of labor favor the most efficient passage of the fetus through the mother's pelvis.
- The exact reasons labor begins are unknown, but several maternal and fetal factors seem to have a role. These include fetal adrenal gland production of glucocorticoids and androgens, changes in ratios of estrogen and progesterone production so that estrogen is higher than progesterone, increased uterine sensitivity to prostaglandins and oxytocin, and stretching of the uterus and cervix.
- As labor approaches, the woman may notice one or more premonitory signs that precede its onset: increase in frequency and intensity of Braxton Hicks contractions, lightening, increased vaginal secretions, bloody show, a spurt of energy, and weight loss.
- The conclusive difference between true labor and false labor is progressive effacement and dilation of the cervix.
- The four stages and phases of labor are characterized by different physiologic events and maternal behaviors: first stage, cervical dilation and effacement; second stage, expulsion of the fetus; third stage, expulsion of the placenta; fourth stage, maternal physiologic stabilization and parent-infant bonding.
- Normal labor is characterized by consistent progression of uterine contractions, cervical dilation and effacement, and fetal descent.

### References and Readings


Albers, L.L., Schiff, M., & Gorwoda, J.G. (1996). The length of active labor in normal pregnancies. *Obstetrics and Gynecology*, 87(3), 355–359.

Bachman, J., & Kendrick, J.M. (1996). Childbirth. In K.R. Simpson & P.A. Creehan, AWHONN'S *perinatal nursing* (pp. 151–186). Philadelphia: J.B. Lippincott.

Blackburn, S.T., & Loper, D.L. (1992). *Maternal, fetal, and neonatal physiology: A clinical perspective*. Philadelphia: W.B. Saunders.

Bowes, W.A. (1994). Clinical aspects of normal and abnormal labor. In R.K. Creasy & R. Resnik (Eds.), *Maternal-fetal medicine: Principles and practice* (3rd ed., pp. 527–557). Philadelphia: W.B. Saunders.

Challis, J.R.G. (1994). Characteristics of parturition. In R.K. Creasy & R. Resnik (Eds.), *Maternal-fetal medicine: Principles and practice* (3rd ed., pp. 482–493). Philadelphia: W.B. Saunders.

Creehan, P.A. (1996). Pain relief and comfort measures during labor. In K.R. Simpson & P.A. Creehan, AWHONN'S *perinatal nursing* (pp. 227–245). Philadelphia: J.B. Lippincott.

Cunningham, F.G., MacDonald, P.C., Gant, N.F., Leveno, K.J., Gilstrap, L.C., Hankins, G.D.V., & Clark, S.L. (1997). *Williams obstetrics* (20th ed.). Norwalk, Conn.: Appleton & Lange.

Gennaro, S. (1988). The childbirth experience. In F.H. Nichols & S.S. Humenick (Eds.), *Childbirth education: Practice, research and theory* (pp. 52–68). Philadelphia: W.B. Saunders.

Guyton, A.C., & Hall, J.C. (1996). *Textbook of medical physiology* (9th ed.). Philadelphia: W.B. Saunders.

Haddad, G.G., & Pérez Fontán, J.J. (1996). Development of the respiratory system. In W.E. Nelson, R.E. Behrman, R.M. Kliegman, & A.M. Arvin (Eds.), *Nelson textbook of pediatrics* (15th ed., pp. 1165–1167). Philadelphia: W.B. Saunders.

Kilpatrick, S.J., & Laros, R.K. (1989). Characteristics of normal labor. *Obstetrics and Gynecology*, 74(1), 85–87.

Lowe, N.K., & Reiss, R. (1996). Parturition and fetal adaptation. *Journal of Obstetric, Gynecologic, & Neonatal Nursing*, 25(4), 339–349.

Menihan, C.A. (1996). Intrapartum fetal monitoring. In K.R. Simpson & P.A. Creehan, AWHONN'S *perinatal nursing* (pp. 187–225). Philadelphia: J.B. Lippincott.

NAACOG (now AWHONN) (1990). *Fetal heart rate auscultation*. Washington, D.C.: Author.

Parer, J.T. (1994). Fetal heart rate. In R.K. Creasy & R. Resnik (Eds.), *Maternal-fetal medicine: Principles and practice* (3rd ed., pp. 298–325). Philadelphia: W.B. Saunders.

Petrie, R.H., & Williams, A.M. (1993). Labor. In R.A. Knuppel & J.E. Drukker (Eds.), *High-risk pregnancy: A team approach* (2nd ed., pp. 281–302). Philadelphia: W.B. Saunders.

Resnik, R. (1994). Anatomic alterations in the reproductive tract. In R.K. Creasy & R. Resnik (Eds.), *Maternal-fetal medicine: Principles and practice* (3rd ed., pp. 128–132). Philadelphia: W.B. Saunders.

Ross, M.G., & Hobel, C.J. (1992). Normal labor, delivery, and the puerperium. In N.F. Hacker & J.G. Moore (Eds.), *Essentials of obstetrics and gynecology* (2nd ed., pp. 119–133). Philadelphia: W.B. Saunders.

Steer, P.J., & Danielian, P.J. (1994). Fetal distress in labor. In D.K. James, P.J. Steer, C.P. Weiner, & B. Gonik (Eds.), *High risk pregnancy: Management options* (pp. 1077–1100). London: W.B. Saunders Ltd.

# The Childbirth Story

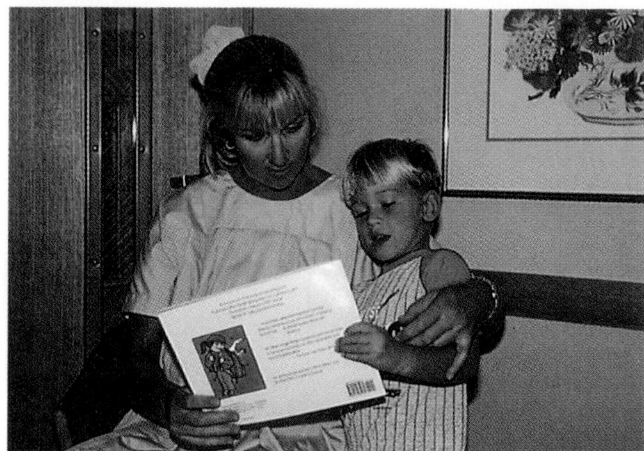

1. Shari, in early labor with her second child, spends time with her 5-year-old son in the labor-delivery-recovery room.

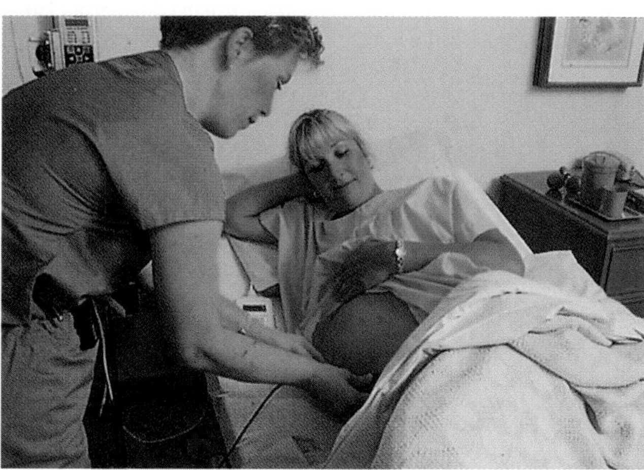

2. The nurse frequently assesses the condition of both the mother and the fetus. Here she listens to fetal heart tones.

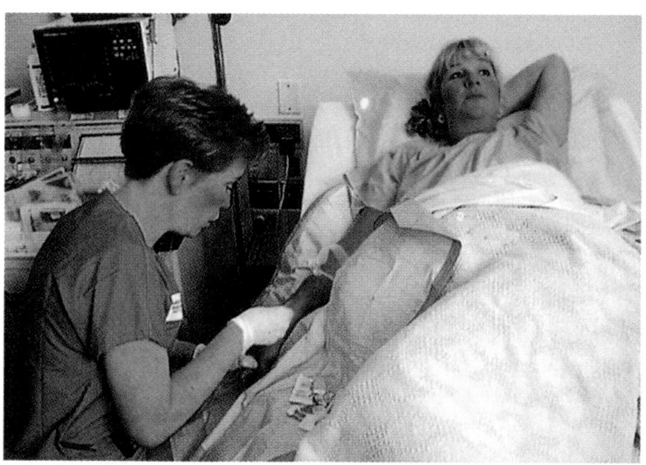

3. Although intravenous fluids are not always necessary, most physicians order them to prevent dehydration and for access to a vein in case an emergency develops.

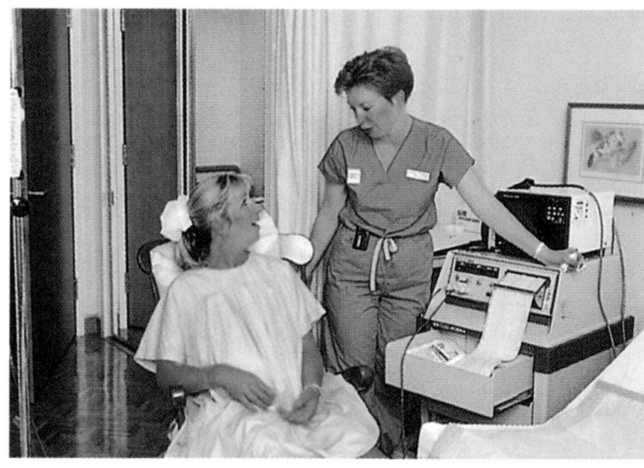

4. The nurse establishes a relationship of trust by assisting Shari into a position of comfort and explaining information obtained by electronic monitoring.

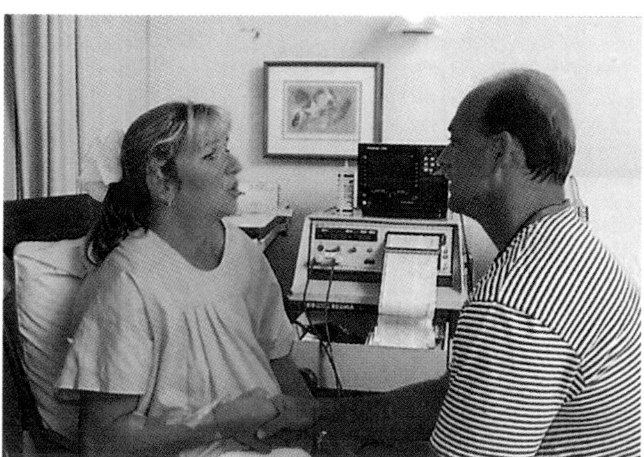

5. Shari plans a childbirth without anesthesia, and the father, Darren, uses skills learned in childbirth education classes to help her cope with discomfort.

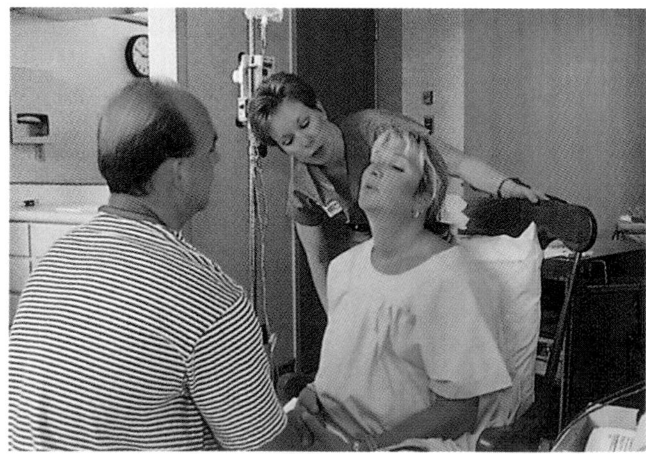

6. It is more difficult for the couple to maintain control as the contractions become stronger. The nurse praises their efforts and reviews measures to reduce discomfort.

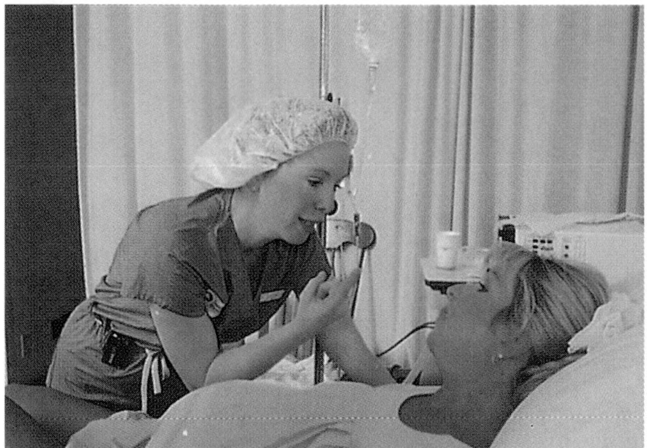
7. During transition, often the most painful phase of labor, the nurse remains in close contact with Shari and assists her through each contraction.

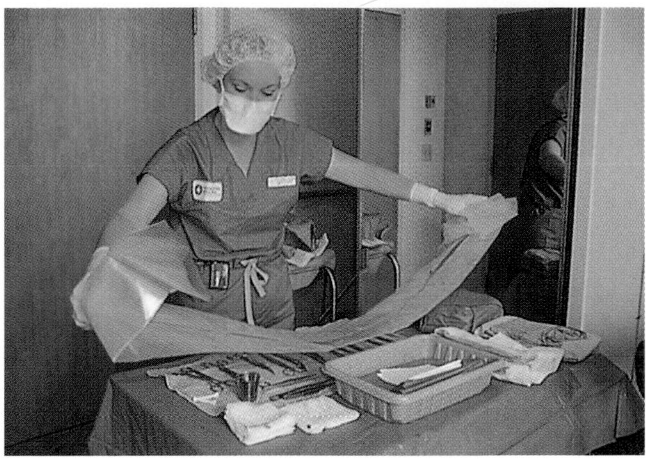
8. The nurse prepares the sterile instruments that will be used during the birth.

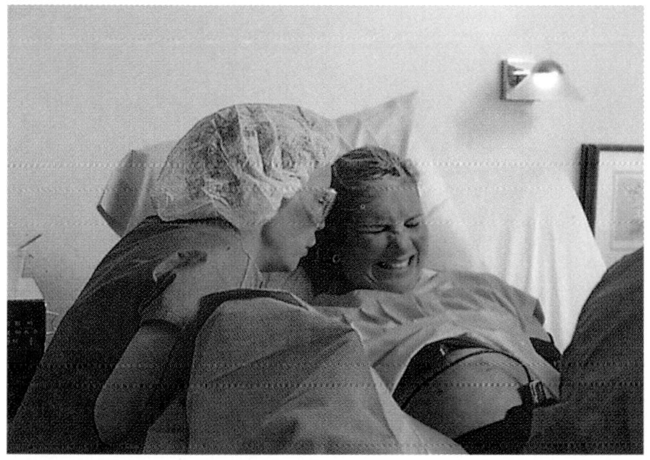
9. As birth approaches, the nurse positions Shari and assists her to push with each contraction. Note the nurse now wears protective glasses.

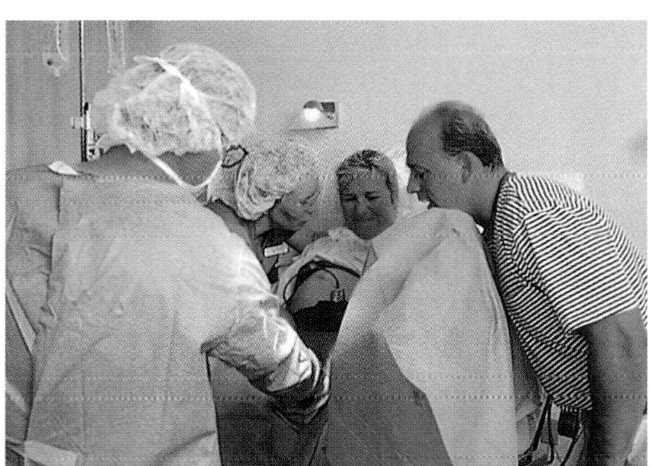
10. The nurse also encourages Darren to remain in close contact with the mother and continue to participate in the birth.

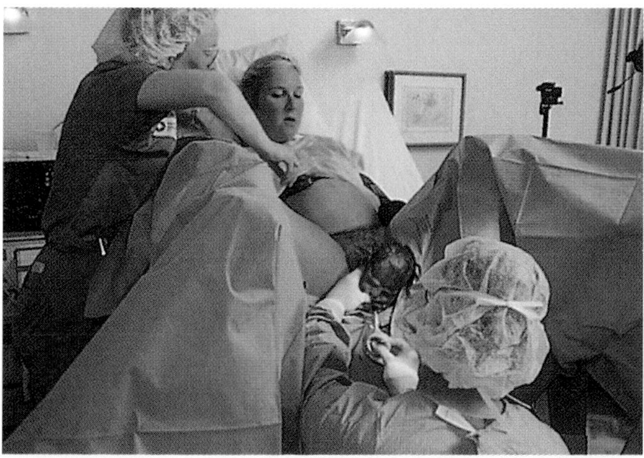
11. The physician suctions secretions from the nose and mouth of the infant when the head is delivered.

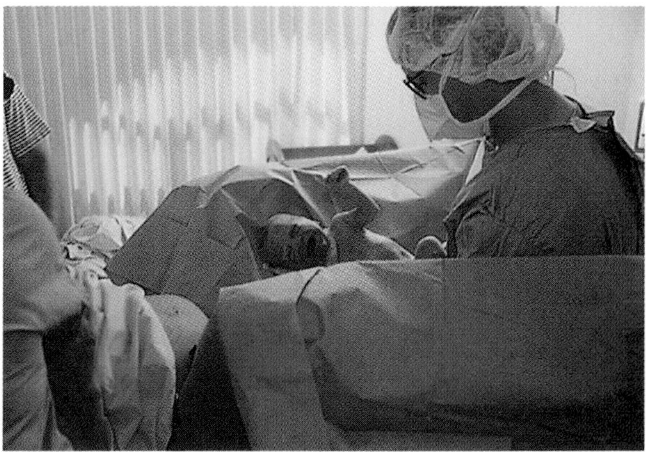
12. The physician holds the infant so the parents can get their first look at their newborn son.

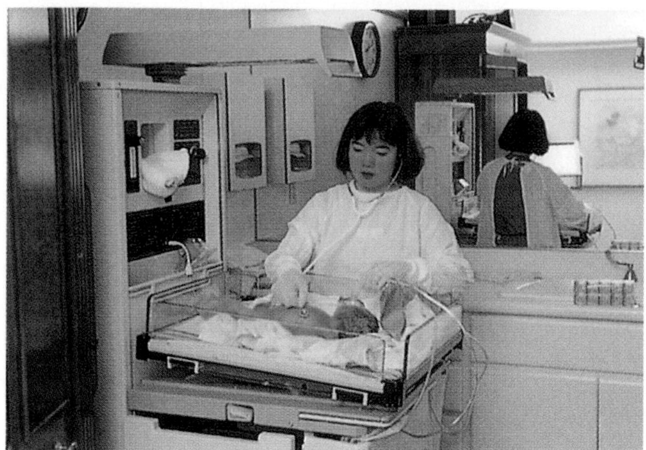

13. A nurse counts the apical pulse and observes the newborn's pink color, which makes the administration of oxygen unnecessary.

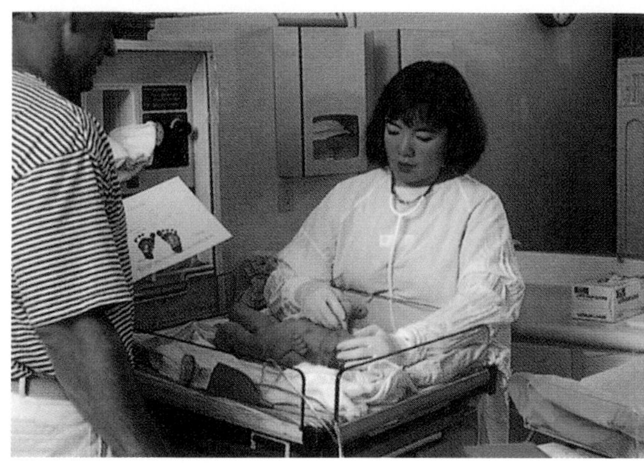

14. The father observes as the nurse suctions secretions from the newborn's nose and mouth and completes identification procedures, such as footprinting.

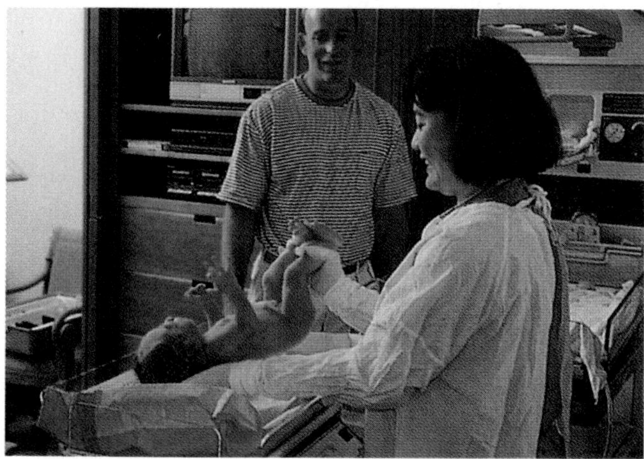

15. The father is an interested observer as the nurse weighs and measures the newborn.

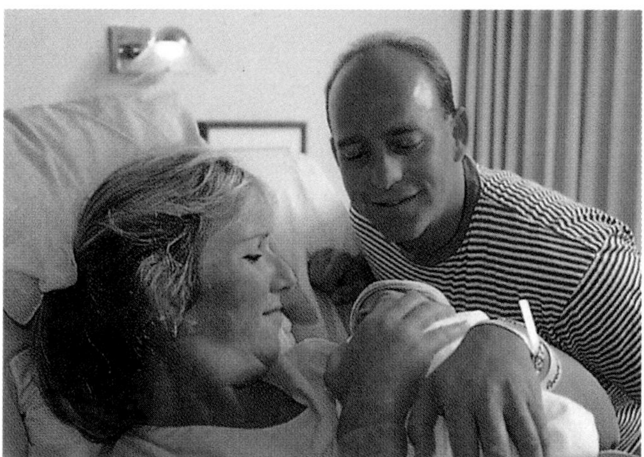

16. Nurses are aware of the importance of early contact, and as soon as possible after birth, the mother, father, and newborn are brought together.

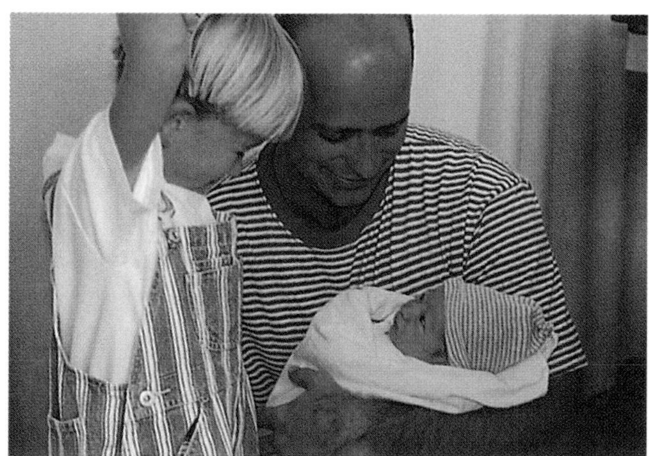

17. Although Adam was not present at the birth, within a short time he meets the wide-eyed baby who gazes intently at his older brother.

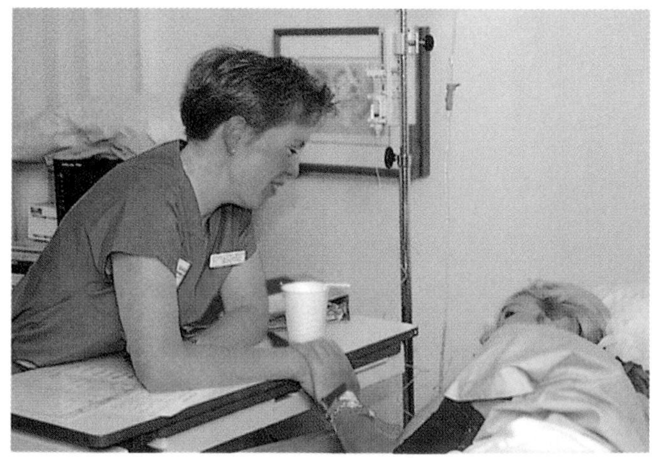

18. Shari and the nurse demonstrate the mutual regard that developed as they shared the intense experience of labor and birth.

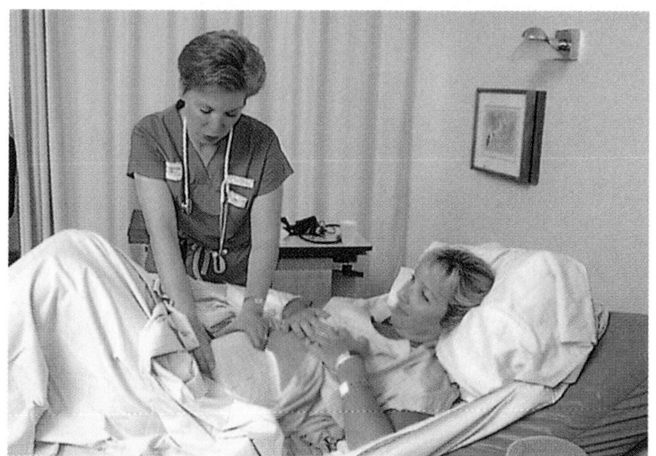

19. The nurse palpates the fundus frequently the first hour following childbirth to confirm that the uterus is firmly contracted and thus to prevent excessive bleeding.

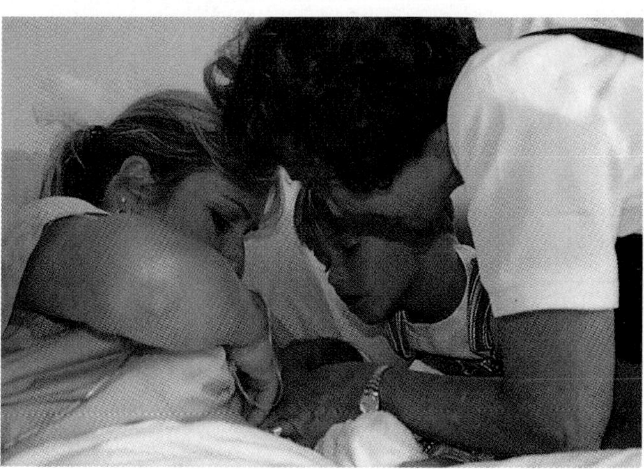

20. Adam watches intently as his mother and grandmother put the baby to breast for the first time.

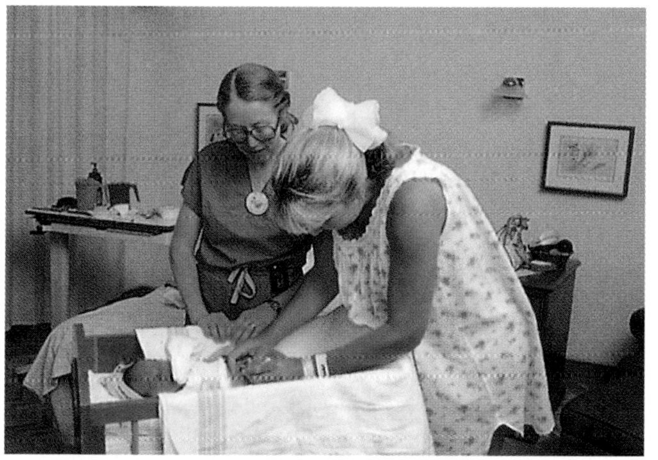

21. Nurses must teach mothers how to care for themselves and the infant within a very short time. Here the nurse instructs Shari in cord care.

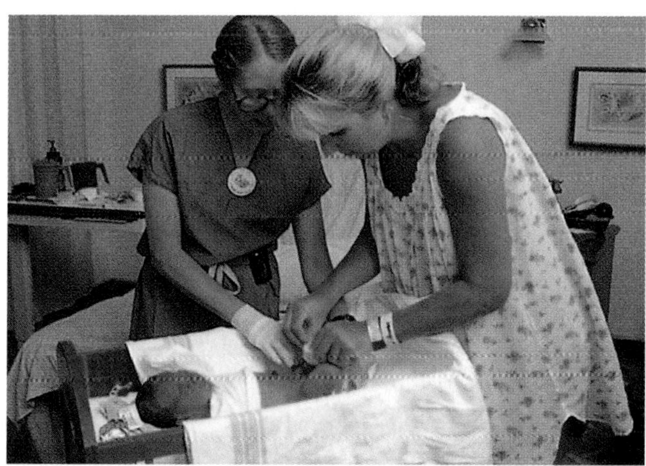

22. Shari gains confidence in circumcision care when the nurse allows for a return demonstration.

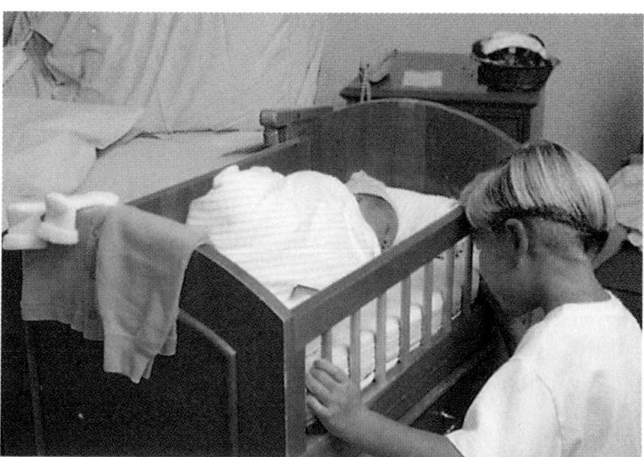

23. Adam peeks at his baby brother while the family receives additional instructions.

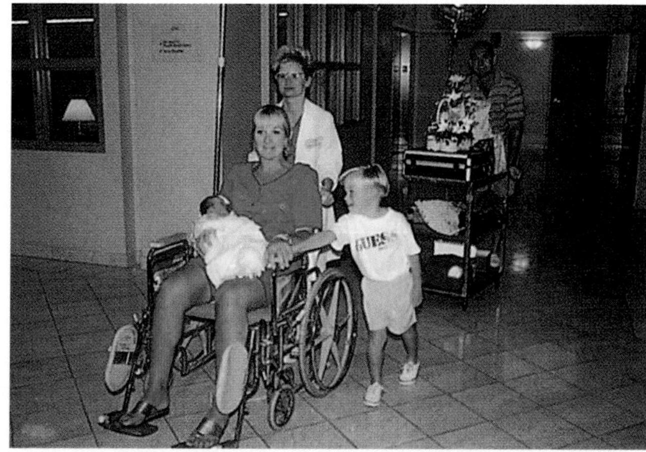

24. Twenty-four hours after her admission, Shari and the infant are discharged from the postpartum unit.

# 13

# Nursing Care During Labor and Birth

## OBJECTIVES

1. Analyze issues that may face the new nurse who cares for women during the intrapartum period.
2. Explain guidelines for going to the hospital or birth center.
3. Describe admission and continuing intrapartum nursing assessments.
4. Describe common nursing procedures used when caring for women during the intrapartum period.
5. Identify nursing priorities when assisting the woman to give birth under emergency circumstances.
6. Relate therapeutic communication skills to care of the intrapartum family.
7. Apply the nursing process to care of the woman experiencing false labor.
8. Apply the nursing process to care of the woman and her family during the intrapartum period.

## DEFINITIONS

**abortion** *A pregnancy that ends before 20 weeks' gestation, either spontaneously or electively. Miscarriage is a lay term for a spontaneous abortion.*

**amniotomy** *Artificial rupture of the amniotic sac (fetal membranes).*

**caput succedaneum** *Area of edema over the presenting part of the fetus or newborn resulting from pressure against the cervix. Usually called simply caput.*

**crowning** *Appearance of the fetal scalp or presenting part at the vaginal opening.*

**EDD** *Abbreviation for estimated date of delivery; this date may also be abbreviated EDB (estimated date of birth).*

**episiotomy** *Surgical incision of the perineum to enlarge the vaginal opening.*

**ferning (or fern test)** *Microscopic appearance of amniotic fluid that resembles fern leaves when the fluid is allowed to dry on a microscope slide.*

**gravida** *A pregnant woman. Also refers to a woman's total number of pregnancies, including the one in progress, if applicable.*

**multipara** *A woman who has given birth after two or more pregnancies of at least 20 weeks' gestation. Also informally used to describe a pregnant woman before the birth of her second child.*

**Nitrazine paper** *Paper to determine pH; helps to determine whether the amniotic sac has ruptured.*

**nuchal cord** *Umbilical cord around the fetal neck.*

**nullipara** *A woman who has not completed a pregnancy to at least 20 weeks' gestation.*

**para** *A woman who has given birth after a pregnancy of at least 20 weeks' gestation. Also designates the number of a woman's pregnancies that have ended after at least 20 weeks of gestation.*

**primipara** *A woman who has given birth after a pregnancy of at least 20 weeks of gestation. Also used informally to describe a pregnant woman before the birth of her first child.*

Care of the woman and her family during labor and birth is a rewarding field of nursing. The birth of a baby is more than a physical event; it has deep personal and social significance for the family. Their roles and relationships are forever altered by this event.

Caring for women who are giving birth is also demanding. The nurse must support natural physical processes, promote a meaningful experience for the family, and be alert for complications. Additionally, the nurse cares for two clients—and the fetus cannot be directly observed.

The intrapartum area is typically a happy place, and good outcomes for mothers and infants are usual. Most women have accepted their pregnancy and look forward to meeting their infant. Yet some women have had stressful pregnancies because of physical or substance abuse, economic hardship, nonsupportive personal relationships, or other problems. Added nursing care for women with special needs is described in Chapter 24.

## Issues for New Nurses

New nurses and nursing students often approach care of laboring women with apprehension. Several common issues may face them when caring for families during birth.

### Pain Associated with Birth

Working with people in pain is difficult; most nurses feel compelled to relieve pain promptly. Yet pain is an expected part of labor and cannot be eliminated. Helping the woman to manage the pain of birth is a crucial part of nursing care.

### Inexperience or Negative Experiences

The nurse who has never given birth may feel inadequate to care for laboring women, although he or she rarely feels it necessary to experience a fracture to care for someone with that problem. Nursing skills needed by the intrapartum nurse are basic: observation, critical thinking, problem solving, therapeutic communication, comfort promotion, empathy, and common sense.

Nurses may be anxious because of their own difficult experiences during birth. They must be careful not to convey negative attitudes to the laboring woman and her partner.

### Unpredictability

Some nurses find the uncertain nature of an intrapartum area troubling, whereas others find it exciting. Labor is a natural process that follows its own timetable. Some occurrences simply are not easily predicted or explained. In addition, the number of women needing care and the level of care they need can change quickly.

### Intimacy

The intimate nature of intrapartum care and its sexual overtones make some nurses uncomfortable. They may feel that they are intruding on a private time.

The male nurse often finds this aspect of intrapartum care most anxiety provoking. Although he may have cared for other female clients, his care has not been this focused on the reproductive system. He often wonders how a woman's male partner will accept him as a care provider.

The best approach for both male and female nurses is to maintain professional conduct and take cues from the couple. If they want privacy, the nurse should intervene only as needed to assess the woman and fetus. In more advanced labor, both partners often welcome the presence of a competent, caring nurse of either sex.

## Admission to the Birth Center

### The Decision to Go to the Hospital or Birth Center

During the last trimester, the woman needs to know when she should go to the hospital or birth center. Many factors are considered:

- Number and duration of any previous labors
- Distance from the hospital
- Available transportation
- Child care needs

Nurses teach women differences between false labor and true labor and offer guidelines for going to the birth center (see Women Want to Know: When to

Go to the Hospital or Birth Center). Not everyone has a typical labor, so a woman should be encouraged to go to the birth center if she is uncertain or has other concerns.

### Nursing Responsibilities During Admission

The nurse has two priorities when the woman arrives at the birth center: (1) establishing a therapeutic relationship and (2) assessing the condition of the mother and fetus.

#### ESTABLISHING A THERAPEUTIC RELATIONSHIP

The nurse must quickly establish a therapeutic relationship with the woman and her partner or family. A family's first impression influences how they feel about the quality of their birth experience.

##### MAKING THE FAMILY FEEL WELCOME

A warm greeting conveys to the woman and her family that they are valued. Even if the unit is busy, the nurse should communicate interest, friendliness, caring, and competence. Families understand if the nurse is busy; they do not understand rudeness or insensitivity to their needs.

**Women Want to Know**

**When to Go to the Hospital or Birth Center**

*These are guidelines for providing individualized instruction to women about when to enter the hospital or birth center.*

**Contractions**

A pattern of increasing regularity, frequency, duration, and intensity.

- *Nullipara*: Regular contractions, 5 minutes apart, for 1 hour
- *Multipara*: Regular contractions, 10 minutes apart, for 1 hour

***Ruptured Membranes*:** A gush or trickle of fluid from the vagina should be evaluated, whether or not you have contractions.

***Bleeding*:** Bright-red bleeding that is not mixed with mucus should be evaluated promptly. Normal bloody show is thicker, pink or dark red, and mixed with mucus.

***Decreased Fetal Movement*:** If you notice a substantial decrease in the baby's movement, notify your physician or nurse-midwife or come to the labor unit.

***Other Concerns*:** These guidelines cannot cover all situations. Therefore, please go to the hospital for evaluation of any concerns or feelings that something may be wrong.

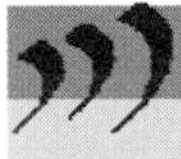

**THERAPEUTIC COMMUNICATION**

**Establishing a Therapeutic Relationship**

Sandra Hall is a nursing student assigned to the intrapartum unit. A woman walks to where Sandra is standing. The woman is leaning on her partner and breathing rapidly. She says to Sandra, "I think I'm in labor, and my water broke on the way to the hospital."

**Sandra:** It sounds like today's the day! Let's find you a room.

Sandra asks the woman's name (Amy James) and that of her birth attendant (Donna Moore, CNM, a nurse-midwife) as they walk to a room.

**Sandra:** I'm Sandra Hall, a nursing student. What names do you want us to call each of you?

*Questioning for information. Shows respect by not assuming how the couple wants to be addressed or that they are married.*

**Amy:** Amy, and my husband is Jeff.

**Sandra:** Is this your first baby, Amy, or have you had others?

*Questioning in a way that avoids yes or no answers.*

**Amy:** It's my second, but the first took forever! I've been having contractions since midnight, but they didn't get regular till about 6:00 this morning. They are coming every 3 minutes now and starting to hurt a lot.

Sandra prepares to check the FHR with the external fetal monitor, but she does not follow up on Amy's implied concern about having a long labor.

**Amy:** Oh no . . . the monitor . . .

**Sandra:** You have a problem about the monitor?

*Clarifying the nonspecific remark that Amy made about the monitor.*

**Amy:** I hated having that thing on with my last baby. I had to lay the same way all the time or they couldn't hear the baby. I know it's best for the baby, though.

**Sandra:** You seem to have mixed feelings about the monitor.

*Reflecting what Amy seems to be feeling.*

**Amy:** Yes, I didn't like it, but I do feel better knowing the baby's OK.

**Sandra:** We can usually find ways so it doesn't bother you so much. We don't want you to feel tied down because that will make you more uncomfortable.

*Giving information without promising that Amy will be totally comfortable with the external fetal monitor.*

Sandra observes that Amy's contractions are every 3 minutes and strong. She finds an experienced nurse to help evaluate Amy. Sandra used critical thinking and wisely sought help from an experienced nurse because Amy seems to be in active labor and this is her second baby. The fact that Amy's first labor "took forever" does not necessarily mean that this labor will be long.

**When caring for the woman who has not had prenatal care or childbirth classes—behaviors most nurses value—one must not be judgmental in either words or actions. The woman's priorities and values may not be the same as those of the nurse, but she deserves the same respect, support, and care as the woman who made every preparation for her baby's birth.**

Nurses often encounter women who speak a language other than English. Arranging for a culturally acceptable interpreter who is fluent in the woman's language makes the woman and family feel more welcome and promotes safety because it enhances understanding among the woman, her family, and the nurse.

DETERMINING FAMILY EXPECTATIONS ABOUT BIRTH

Regardless of how many children they have, women and their partners have expectations about the birth experience. The partners have often studied their options extensively and planned a birth that best fits their ideals. Those who have not made specific plans also have expectations, shaped by contact with relatives and friends or by previous birth experiences. A couple may want to repeat a previous satisfying experience, or they may want to avoid repeating a poor experience. Sometimes only one part of a past birth has negatively colored their impression of the entire process.

CONVEYING CONFIDENCE

From the first encounter, the nurse should convey confidence in the woman's ability to give birth and her partner's ability to support her. Contractions and discomfort intensify as labor progresses. Women having their first baby may find the power of normal labor contractions overwhelming. The nurse can reassure a woman that intense contractions are normal in active labor while helping her deal with them and watching for problems.

**Consider the different perspective implied by the phrases "give birth" and "be delivered." The woman who *gives birth* is an active and able participant; she is the principal action figure. However, when her baby *is delivered*, the language implies that she is passive. The nurse might ask, "Who will attend you as you give birth?" rather than, "Who will deliver your baby?"**

ASSIGNING A PRIMARY NURSE

Having one nurse give care during all of labor is ideal but often unrealistic. However, the number of different caregivers should be limited as much as possible. The woman should know who each caregiver is and what to expect from each. For example, the primary nurse might explain the role of a nursing student in her care. Common roles of nursing students in the intrapartum area include promoting comfort, giving emotional support, and helping the primary nurse observe for maternal or fetal problems.

USING TOUCH FOR COMFORT

Touch can communicate acceptance and reassurance and can provide physical and emotional comfort to many laboring women. Women who do not usually welcome touch may appreciate it during labor. Cultural norms and personal history influence whether a woman is comfortable with touch from a stranger such as a nurse. One should not assume that the woman desires touch but should ask her if she welcomes or benefits from touch. As labor progresses, her desire for touch may change; during late labor, it may become an irritant rather than a comfort measure.

RESPECTING CULTURAL VALUES

Cultural beliefs and practices give structure and meaning to the birth experience. They influence behavior of both the childbearing family and the professional staff. Most cultural groups have specific practices related to childbearing. The nurse should incorporate a family's cultural practices into care as much as possible if they are beneficial or neutral.

**People naturally believe that their own cultural values are best. The nurse should avoid using a superior attitude or one that diminishes the validity of another's cultural beliefs. Trust in technology is a common value of many caregivers in the United States, but this high-tech focus is considered unnecessary, or even harmful, by many people.**

**CHECK YOUR READING**

1. What communication skills can the nurse use to establish a therapeutic relationship when the woman and her family enter the hospital or birth center?
2. How can the nurse incorporate a couple's cultural practices into intrapartum care?

## ASSESSMENTS AT THE TIME OF ADMISSION

A record of prenatal care is sent to the center where the woman plans to give birth and is added to her chart when she is admitted. Information can be obtained from the prenatal record and verified or updated as needed. Women who have not had prenatal care need a more extensive assessment by the nurse and physician. See Table 13–1 for common intrapartum assessments, usual findings, significant

*Text continued on page 306*

## TABLE 13–1 INTRAPARTUM ASSESSMENT GUIDE

Women who have had prenatal care have much of this information available on their prenatal record. The nurse need only verify it or update it as needed.

| Assessment, Method (Selected Rationales) | Common Findings | Significant Findings, Nursing Action |
|---|---|---|
| **Interview** | | |
| *Purpose*: To obtain information about the woman's pregnancy, labor, and conditions that may affect her care. The interview is curtailed if she seems to be in late labor. | | |
| *Introduction*: Introduce yourself and ask the woman how she wants to be addressed. Ask her if she wants her partner and/or family to remain during the interview and assessment. (Shows respect for the woman and gives her control over those she wants to remain with her.) | Many women prefer to be addressed by their first names during labor. | The surname (family name) precedes the given name in some cultures. Clarify which name is used to properly address the woman and to properly identify both mother and newborn. |
| *Culture/language*: If she is from another culture, ask what her preferred language is and what language(s) she speaks, reads, or verbally understands. (Enables the most accurate data collection.) | Common non-English languages of women in the United States are Spanish or one of the Asian dialects. The most common non-English language varies with location. | Try to secure an interpreter fluent in the woman's primary language. Ask her if there are people who are not acceptable to her as interpreters (e.g., males or one from a group in conflict with her culture). Family members may not be the best interpreters because they may interpret selectively, adding or subtracting information as they see fit. |
| *Communication*: Ask the woman to tell you when she has a contraction, and pause during the interview and physical assessment. (Shows that the nurse is sensitive to her comfort and allows her to concentrate more fully on the information the nurse requests.) | Women in active labor have difficulty answering questions or cooperating with a physical examination while they are having a contraction. | If contractions are very frequent, assess the woman's labor status promptly rather than continuing the interview. Ask only the most critical questions. |
| *Nonverbal cues*: Observe the woman's behaviors and interactions with her family and the nurse. (Permits estimation of her level of anxiety. Identifies behaviors indicating that she should have a vaginal examination to determine whether birth is imminent.) | *Latent phase*: Sociable and mildly anxious.<br>*Active phase*: Concentrating intently with contractions; often uses prepared childbirth techniques. | The unprepared or extremely anxious woman may breathe deeply and rapidly, displaying a tense facial and body posture during and between contractions.<br>These behaviors suggest that birth is imminent:<br>1. Her statement that the baby is coming.<br>2. Grunting sounds (low-pitched, guttural sounds).<br>3. Bearing down with abdominal muscles.<br>4. Sitting on one buttock.<br>Euphoria, combativeness, or sedation suggest recent illicit drug ingestion. |
| *Reason for admission*: "What brings you to the hospital/birth center today?" (Open-ended question promotes more complete answer.) | Labor contractions at term are the usual reason. Observation for false labor is another common reason for admission. | Bleeding, preterm labor, pain other than labor contractions. Report these findings to the physician or nurse-midwife promptly. |

## TABLE 13–1 INTRAPARTUM ASSESSMENT GUIDE *Continued*

Women who have had prenatal care have much of this information available on their prenatal record. The nurse need only verify it or update it as needed.

| Assessment, Method (Selected Rationales) | Common Findings | Significant Findings, Nursing Action |
|---|---|---|
| **Interview** | | |
| *Prenatal care*: "Did you see a doctor or nurse-midwife during your pregnancy?" "Who is your doctor or nurse-midwife?" "How far along were you in your pregnancy when you saw the physician or nurse-midwife?" (Enables location of prenatal record.) | Early and regular prenatal care promotes maternal and fetal health. | No prenatal care or care that was irregular or begun in late pregnancy means that complications may not have been identified. |
| *Estimated date of delivery* (EDD): "When is your baby due?" (Determines if gestation is term.) "When did your last menstrual period begin?" (For estimation of EDD if woman did not have prenatal care.) | *Term gestation*: 38–42 weeks. The woman's gestation may have been confirmed or adjusted during pregnancy with an ultrasound or other clinical examination. | Gestations earlier than 38 weeks (preterm) or later than the end of the 42nd week (postterm) are associated with more fetal or neonatal problems. |
| *Gravidity, parity, abortions*: "How many times have you been pregnant?" "How many babies have you had? Were they full-term or premature?" "How many children are now living?" "Have you had any miscarriages or abortions?" "Were there any problems with your babies after they were born?" (Helps estimate probable speed of labor and anticipate neonatal problems.) | Labor may be faster for the woman who has given birth before than for the nullipara. Miscarriage is used to describe a spontaneous abortion because many lay people associate the term "abortion" with only induced abortions. | Parity of 5 or more (grand multiparity) may be associated with placenta previa (see p. 682) or postpartum hemorrhage (see p. 783). Women who have had several spontaneous abortions or who have given birth to infants with abnormalities may face a higher risk for an infant with a birth defect. |
| *Pregnancy history* (identifies problems that may affect this birth) | | |
| Present pregnancy: "Have you had any problems during this pregnancy, such as high blood pressure, diabetes, or bleeding?" | Complications are not expected. | Women having diabetes or hypertension may have poor placental blood flow, possibly resulting in fetal compromise. Some complications of past pregnancies, such as diabetes, may recur in another pregnancy. The woman who plans a VBAC may need more support and reassurance to give birth vaginally. |
| Past pregnancies: "Were there any problems with your other pregnancy(ies)?" "Were your other babies born vaginally or by cesarean birth?" | Women who had previous cesarean birth(s) often have a trial of labor and vaginal birth (VBAC). A woman who previously had a difficult labor may be more anxious than one who had an uncomplicated labor and birth. | |
| Other: "Is there anything else you think we should know so that we can better care for you?" | This open-ended question gives the woman a chance to share information that may not be elicited by other questions. | |
| *Labor status*: "When did your contractions become regular?" "What time did you begin to think you might really be in labor?" (Facilitates a more accurate estimation of the time labor began.) | Varies among women. Many women go to the birth facility when contractions first begin. Others wait until they are reasonably sure that they are really in labor. | Women who say they have been "in labor" for an unusual length of time (for example, "for two days") have probably had false labor. These women may be very tired from the annoying, nonproductive contractions. |

*Table continued on following page*

**TABLE 13–1 INTRAPARTUM ASSESSMENT GUIDE** *Continued*

Women who have had prenatal care have much of this information available on their prenatal record. The nurse need only verify it or update it as needed.

| Assessment, Method (Selected Rationales) | Common Findings | Significant Findings, Nursing Action |
|---|---|---|
| **Interview** | | |
| *Contractions*: "How often are your contractions coming?" "How long do they last?" "Are they getting stronger?" "Tell me if you have a contraction while we are talking." (Obtains the woman's subjective evaluation of her contractions. Alerts the nurse to palpate contractions that occur during the interview.) | Varies according to her stage and phase of labor. Labor contractions are usually regular and show a pattern of increasing frequency, duration, and intensity. | Irregular contractions or those that do not increase in frequency, duration, or intensity are more likely to represent false labor. Contractions with a duration of longer than 90 seconds or intervals of full uterine relaxation shorter than 60 sec can reduce placental blood flow. |
| *Membrane status*: "Has your water broken?" "What time did it break?" "What did the fluid look like?" "About how much fluid did you lose—was it a big gush or a trickle?" (Alerts the nurse of the need to verify whether the membranes have ruptured if it is not obvious. Identifies possible prolonged rupture of membranes.) | Most women go to the birth facility for evaluation soon after their membranes rupture. If a woman is not already in labor, contractions usually begin within a few hours after the membranes rupture at term. | If the woman's membranes have ruptured and she is not in labor or if she is not at term, a vaginal examination is often deferred. Labor may be induced if she is at term with ruptured membranes. |
| *Allergies*: "Are you allergic to any foods or medicines?" "What kind of reaction do you have?" "Have you ever had a problem with anesthesia when you had dental work?" (Determines possible sensitivity to drugs that may be used.) | Record any known allergies to food and medication. As needed, describe how they affected the woman. | Allergy to seafood, iodized salt, or x-ray contrast media may indicate iodine allergy. Because iodine is used in many "prep" solutions, alternative ones should be used. Allergy to dental anesthetics may indicate possible allergy to the drugs used for local or regional anesthetics. These drugs usually end in the suffix *-caine*. |
| *Food intake*: "When was the last time you had something to eat or drink?" "What did you have?" (Helps evaluate risk for regurgitation and aspiration of stomach contents during general anesthesia.) | Record the time of the woman's last food intake and what she ate. Include both liquids and solids. | If the woman says she has not had any intake for an unusual length of time, question her more closely: "Is there any food you may have forgotten, such as a snack or a drink of water?" |
| *Recent illness*: "Have you been ill recently?" "What was the problem?" "What did you do for it?" "Have you been around anyone with a contagious illness recently?" | Most pregnant women are healthy. An occasional woman may have had a minor illness such as an upper respiratory infection. | Untreated urinary tract infections are associated with preterm labor. The woman who has had contact with someone having a communicable disease may become ill and possibly infect others in the facility. |
| *Medications*: "What drugs do you take that your doctor or nurse-midwife has prescribed?" "Are there any over-the-counter drugs that you use?" "I know this may be uncomfortable to discuss, but we need to know about any illegal substances that you use to more safely care for you and your baby." (Permits evaluation of the woman's drug intake and encourages her to disclose nonprescribed use.) | Prenatal vitamins and iron are commonly prescribed. Record all drugs the woman takes, including time and amount of last ingestion. Women who use illegal substances often conceal or diminish the extent of their use because they fear reprisals. | Drugs may interact with other medications given during labor, especially analgesics and anesthetics. Substance abuse is associated with complications for the mother and infant (see Chapter 24). If the woman discloses that she uses illegal drugs, ask her what kind and the last time she ingested them (often referred to as a "hit"). A nonjudgmental approach is more likely to result in honest information. |

**TABLE 13-1 INTRAPARTUM ASSESSMENT GUIDE** *Continued*

Women who have had prenatal care have much of this information available on their prenatal record. The nurse need only verify it or update it as needed.

| Assessment, Method (Selected Rationales) | Common Findings | Significant Findings, Nursing Action |
|---|---|---|
| **Interview** | | |
| *Tobacco or alcohol*: "Do you smoke or use tobacco in any other form? About how many cigarettes a day?" "Do you use alcohol? About how many drinks do you have each day (or week)?" (Evaluates use of these legal substances.) | As in substance abuse, women may underreport the extent of their use of tobacco or alcohol. | Infants of heavy smokers are often smaller and may have reduced placental blood flow during labor. Infants of women who use alcohol may show fetal alcohol effects (see Chapter 24). |
| *Birth plans* (shows respect for the woman and her family as individuals and promotes achievement of their expectations. Enables more culturally appropriate care): | | |
| Coach or primary support person: "Who is the main person you want to be with you during labor?" Ask that person how he or she wants to be addressed, such as "Mr. Smith" or "Bob." | This is usually the woman's husband or the baby's father, but it may be her mother, sister, or a friend, especially if she is single. | The woman who has little or no support from significant others probably needs more intense nursing support during labor and after the birth. These clients are more likely to have problems with parent-infant attachment. |
| Other support: "Is there anyone else you would like to be present during labor?" | Women often want another support person present. | |
| Preparation for childbirth: "Did you attend prepared childbirth classes?" "Did someone go with you?" | Ideally, the woman and a partner have had some preparation in classes or self-study. Women who attended classes during previous pregnancies do not always repeat the classes during subsequent pregnancies. | The unprepared woman may need more support with simple relaxation and breathing techniques during labor. Her partner may need to learn techniques to assist her. |
| *Preferences*: "Are there any special plans you have for this birth?" "Is there anything you want to avoid?" "Did you plan to record the birth with pictures or video?" | Some women or couples have strong feelings regarding certain interventions. Common ones are: (1) analgesia or anesthesia; (2) intravenous lines; (3) fetal monitoring; (4) shave prep or enema; or (5) use of episiotomy or forceps. | Conflict may arise if the woman has not previously discussed her preferences with her physician or nurse-midwife or if she is unaware of what services are available where she gives birth. |
| *Cultural needs*: "Are there any special cultural practices that you plan when you have your baby?" "How can we best help you to fulfill these practices?" | Women from Asian and Hispanic cultures often subscribe to the "hot/cold" theory of illness and want specific foods after birth, such as soft-boiled eggs. They may not want their water iced. | Try to incorporate all positive or neutral cultural practices. If a practice is harmful, explain why and try to find a way to work around it if the family does not want to give it up. |
| **Fetal Evaluation** | | |
| *Purpose*: To determine if the fetus seems to be healthy and tolerating labor well. | | |
| *Fetal heart rate* (FHR): Assess by intermittent auscultation, or apply an external fetal monitor if that is the facility's policy (most common in the United States). Document FHR at least this often for the fetus at low risk for complications:<br>1. Every hour during the latent phase<br>2. Every 30 min during active and transition phases<br>3. Every 15 min during second stage | Average at term is a lower limit of 110–120 BPM and an upper limit of 150–160 BPM. Rate should increase when the fetus moves. | These signs may indicate fetal stress and should be reported to the physician or nurse-midwife:<br>1. Rate outside the normal limits<br>2. Slowing of the rate that persists after the contraction ends<br>3. No increase in rate when the fetus moves<br>More frequent assessments should be made of the FHR. |

*Table continued on following page*

**TABLE 13–1 INTRAPARTUM ASSESSMENT GUIDE** *Continued*

Women who have had prenatal care have much of this information available on their prenatal record. The nurse need only verify it or update it as needed.

| Assessment, Method (Selected Rationales) | Common Findings | Significant Findings, Nursing Action |
|---|---|---|
| **Labor Status** | | |
| *Purpose*: To identify whether the woman is in labor and if birth is imminent. If she displays signs of imminent birth, this assessment is done as soon as she is admitted. | | |
| *Contractions* (Yields objective information about labor status): In addition to asking the woman about her contraction pattern, assess the contractions by palpation with the fingertips of one hand. A guideline is to assess:<br>1. Hourly during the latent phase<br>2. Every 30 min during the active phase<br>3. Every 15 min during transition and second stage | See interview section earlier in table | See interview section earlier in table. Women who have intense contractions or who are making rapid progress need to be assessed more frequently. |
| *Vaginal examination* (Determines cervical dilation and effacement; fetal presentation, position, and station; bloody show; and status of the membranes) | Varies according to the stage and phase of labor. It may not be possible to determine fetal position by vaginal examination when membranes are intact and bulging over the presenting part. | A vaginal examination is not performed if the woman reports or has evidence of active bleeding (not bloody show). Report reasons for omitting a vaginal examination to the physician or nurse-midwife. |
| *Status of membranes*: During a vaginal examination a flow of fluid suggests ruptured membranes. A Nitrazine test and/or fern test may be done. (Test needed only if it is not obvious that the membranes have ruptured.) | Amniotic fluid should be clear, possibly containing flecks of white vernix. Its odor is distinctive but not offensive. Nitrazine test with a color change to blue-green to dark blue (pH $> 6.5$) suggests true rupture of the membranes but is not conclusive.<br>Fern test is more diagnostic of true rupture of membranes. | A greenish color indicates meconium staining, which may be associated with fetal compromise or postterm gestation. Thick meconium with much particulate matter ("pea soup") is most significant (see p. 850). Thick green-black meconium may be passed by the fetus in a breech presentation and is not necessarily associated with fetal compromise.<br>Cloudy, yellowish, strong- or foul-smelling fluid suggests infection.<br>Bloody fluid may indicate partial placental separation (p. 684). |
| *Leopold's maneuvers*: Often done before assessing the FHR because they help locate the best place to assess the FHR. (Identifies fetal presentation and position. Most accurate when combined with information from vaginal examination.) | A cephalic presentation with the head well flexed (vertex) is normal.<br>The fetal head is often easily displaced upward ("floating") if the woman is not in labor. When the head is engaged, it cannot be displaced upward with Leopold's maneuvers. | A hard, round, freely movable object in the fundus suggests a fetal head, meaning the fetus is in a breech presentation. Less commonly, the fetus may be cross-wise in the uterus: a transverse lie. |
| *Pain*: Note discomfort during and between contractions. Note tenderness when palpating contractions. (Distinguishes between normal labor pain and abnormal pain that may be associated with a complication.) | There may be verbal or nonverbal evidence of pain with contractions, but the woman should be relatively comfortable between contractions. The skin around the umbilicus is often sensitive. | Constant pain or a tender, rigid uterus suggests a complication, such as abruptio placentae (separated placenta) (see p. 684) or, less commonly, uterine rupture (see p. 775). |

**TABLE 13–1 INTRAPARTUM ASSESSMENT GUIDE** *Continued*

Women who have had prenatal care have much of this information available on their prenatal record. The nurse need only verify it or update it as needed.

| Assessment, Method (Selected Rationales) | Common Findings | Significant Findings, Nursing Action |
|---|---|---|
| **Physical Examination** | | |
| *Purpose*: To evaluate the woman's general health and identify conditions that may affect her intrapartum and postpartum care. | | |
| *General appearance*: Observe skin color and texture, nutritional state, and appearance of rest or fatigue. Examine the woman's face, fingers, and lower extremities for edema. Ask her if she can take her rings off and on. | Women are often fatigued if their sleep has been interrupted by Braxton Hicks contractions, fetal activity, or frequent urination.<br>Mild edema of the lower extremities is common in late pregnancy. | Pallor suggests anemia.<br>Edema of the face and fingers or extreme (pitting) edema of the lower extremities is associated with pregnancy-induced hypertension (see p. 690). |
| *Vital signs*: Take the woman's temperature, pulse, respirations, and blood pressure. Reassess the temperature every 4 hr (every 2 hr after membranes rupture or if elevated); repeat blood pressure, pulse, and respirations every hour. | *Temperature*: 35.8°–37.3°C (96.4°–99.1°F).<br>*Pulse*: 60–100/min<br>*Respirations*: 12–20/min, even and unlabored.<br>Blood pressure near baseline levels established during pregnancy. Transient elevations of blood pressure are common when the woman is first admitted, but they return to baseline levels within about ½ hour. | Report abnormalities to physician or nurse-midwife. Temperature of 38°C (100.4°F) or higher suggests infection. Pulse and respirations may also be elevated. Pulse and blood pressure may be elevated if the woman is extremely anxious or in pain. A blood pressure of 140/90 or higher is considered hypertensive. For women who did not have prenatal care, there is no baseline to compare. |
| *Heart and lung sounds*: Auscultate all areas with a stethoscope. | Heart sounds should be clear with a distinct $S_1$ and $S_2$. A physiologic murmur is common because of the increased blood volume and cardiac output. Breath sounds should be clear, with respirations even and unlabored. | The woman who is breathing rapidly and deeply may have symptoms of hyperventilation: tingling and spasm of the fingers, numbness around the lips. |
| *Breasts*: Palpate for a dominant mass. | Breasts are full and nodular. Areola is darker, especially in dark-skinned women. Breasts may leak colostrum (clear, sticky, straw-colored fluid) during labor. | Report a dominant mass to the physician or nurse-midwife. |
| *Abdomen*: Observe for scars at the same time Leopold's maneuvers and the FHR are assessed. It is usually sufficient to assess the fundal height by observing its relation to the xiphoid process. | Striae (stretch marks) are common. If scars are noted, ask the woman what surgery she had. The fundus at term is usually slightly below the xiphoid process. | Report a previous cesarean birth to the physician or nurse-midwife. Transverse uterine scars are least likely to rupture if the woman is in labor (see p. 412). Measure the fundal height (see p. 143) if the fetus seems small or if the gestation is questionable. |
| *Deep tendon reflexes*: Assess patellar reflex (see p. 698). Upper extremity deep tendon reflexes should be used after epidural block analgesia. | Brisk knee jerk without spasm or sustained muscle contraction is normal. Some women normally have hypoactive reflexes. | Report absent (uncommon unless the woman is receiving magnesium sulfate) or hyperactive reflexes. Hyperactive reflexes and clonus (repeated tapping when the foot is dorsiflexed) are associated with pregnancy-induced hypertension and often precede a seizure (see p. 699). |
| *Midstream urine specimen*: Assess protein and glucose levels with a dipstick. Follow instructions on the package for waiting times. Send for urinalysis if ordered. | Negative or trace of protein; negative glucose. | Proteinuria is associated with pregnancy-induced hypertension but may also be associated with urinary tract infections or a specimen that is contaminated with vaginal secretions. Glucosuria is associated with diabetes. |

*Table continued on following page*

**TABLE 13–1 INTRAPARTUM ASSESSMENT GUIDE** *Continued*

Women who have had prenatal care have much of this information available on their prenatal record. The nurse need only verify it or update it as needed.

| Assessment, Method (Selected Rationales) | Common Findings | Significant Findings, Nursing Action |
|---|---|---|
| **Physical Examination** | | |
| *Laboratory tests*: Women who have had prenatal care may not need additional tests. Common tests include: | | |
| 1. Complete blood count (or hematocrit done on unit) | 1. Hemoglobin at least 11 g/dl; hematocrit at least 33% | 1. Values lower than these reduce maternal reserve for normal blood loss at birth. |
| 2. Blood type and Rh factor | 2. The woman who is Rh-negative usually has received Rh immune globulin at about 28 weeks' gestation to prevent formation of anti-Rh antibodies | 2. Rh-negative mothers need Rh immune globulin if their infant is Rh-positive. |
| 3. Serologic tests for syphilis | 3. Negative | 3. A positive test may indicate that the baby is infected and needs treatment after birth. The mother should be treated if she has not been treated already. |

findings, and appropriate nursing actions.

FOCUS ASSESSMENT

In the intrapartum unit, a focus assessment is done before the broader data base assessment, opposite of the usual order. Assessment priorities are to determine the condition of the mother and fetus and to determine whether birth is imminent.

**Fetal Heart Rate.** Use Leopold's maneuvers (Procedure 13–1) to locate the best place to assess the fetal heart rate (FHR). Procedure 13–2 explains assessment of the FHR with the fetoscope or Doppler transducer. In Chapter 14, the procedure for application of the electronic fetal monitor is explained. For a term fetus, these guidelines are considered reassuring (ACOG, 1995b; Menihan, 1996; Murray, 1997):

- A lower limit of 110 to 120 beats per minute (BPM) and an upper limit of 150 to 160 BPM. (Some sources state that 120 BPM is the lower limit of normal.)
- Presence of variability in the electronically monitored fetal heart rate.
- Presence of accelerations, usually associated with fetal movement, in the fetal heart rate of 15 BPM above the baseline rate.
- Absence of decelerations following contractions.

See Chapter 14 for added information about the fetal heart's response to labor and electronic fetal monitor patterns.

**Maternal Vital Signs.** Assess maternal vital signs primarily for signs of hypertension or infection. Hypertension during pregnancy is defined as a sustained blood pressure increase to 140 mmHg systolic or 90 mmHg diastolic. An elevation of 30 mmHg systolic or 15 mmHg diastolic from second-trimester levels is no longer considered diagnostic of hypertension (ACOG, 1996). A temperature of 38°C (100.4°F) or higher suggests infection.

**Impending Birth.** Occasionally a woman enters the intrapartum unit almost ready to give birth. Grunting sounds, bearing down, sitting on one buttock, or saying urgently, "The baby's coming," suggests imminent birth. The nurse abbreviates the initial assessment and collects other information after birth.

Vital information to obtain if birth is imminent includes the following:

- Mother's name
- Support person's name
- Whether the woman had prenatal care
- Physician's or nurse-midwife's name
- Number of pregnancies and prior births, including whether vaginal or cesarean birth
- Status of membranes
- Estimated date of delivery
- Any problems during this pregnancy
- Allergies to medications
- Time and type of last oral intake
- Maternal vital signs and FHR

## Procedure 13–1
# Leopold's Maneuvers

**PURPOSE:** To determine presentation and position of the fetus. To aid in location of the fetal heart sounds.

**1. Explain procedure to woman and the rationale for each step as it is done. Tell her what is found at each step.** *Gives information, teaches woman, and reassures her when the assessment findings are normal.*

**2. Ask the woman to empty her bladder if she has not done so recently. Have her lie on her back with her knees flexed slightly. Place a small pillow or folded towel under one hip.** *Decreases discomfort of a full bladder during palpation and improves ability to feel fetal parts in the suprapubic area. Knee flexion helps the woman relax her abdominal muscles to enhance palpation. Uterine displacement prevents aortocaval compression, which could reduce blood flow to the placenta.*

**3. Wash your hands with warm water. Wear gloves if contact with secretions is likely.** *Prevents transmission of microorganisms. Warm hands are more comfortable during palpation and prevent tensing of abdominal muscles.*

**4. Stand beside woman, facing her head, with your dominant hand nearest her.** *First three maneuvers are most easily performed in this position.*

### FIRST MANEUVER

**5. Palpate the uterine fundus. The breech (buttocks) is softer and more irregular in shape than the head. Moving the breech also moves the fetal trunk. The head is harder, with a round, uniform shape. The head can move without moving the entire fetal trunk.** *Distinguishes between a cephalic and a breech presentation. If the fetus is in a cephalic presentation, the breech is felt in the fundus. If the presentation is breech, the head is felt in the fundus.*

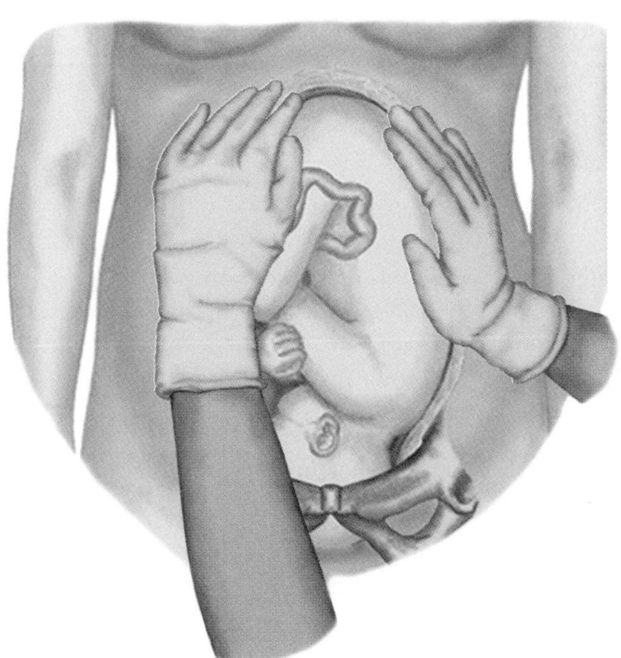

### SECOND MANEUVER

**6. Hold the left hand steady on one side of the uterus while palpating the opposite side of the uterus with the right hand. Then hold the right hand steady while palpating the opposite side of the uterus with the left hand. The fetal back is a smooth convex surface. The fetal arms and legs feel nodular, and the fetus often moves them during palpation.** *Determines which side of the uterus the back is on and which side the fetal arms and legs ("small parts") are on.*

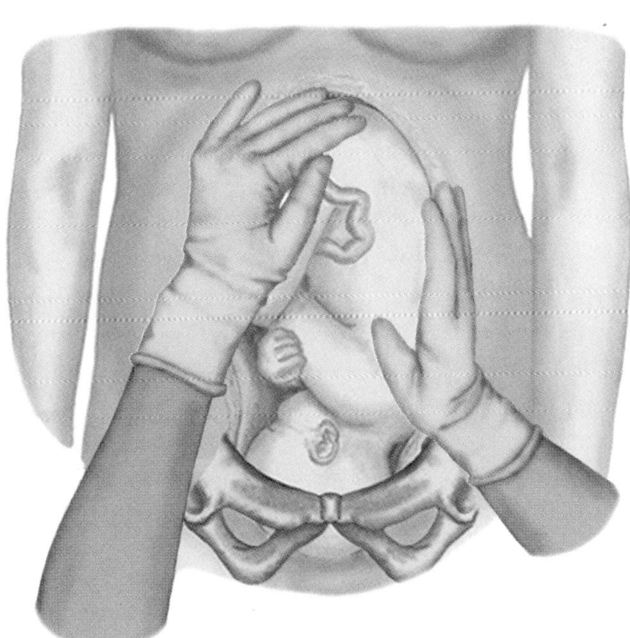

### THIRD MANEUVER

**7. Palpate the suprapubic area. If a breech was palpated in the fundus, expect a hard, rounded head in this area. Attempt to grasp the presenting part gently between the thumb and fingers. If the presenting part is not engaged, the grasping movement of the fingers moves it upward in the uterus.** *Confirms the presentation determined in the first maneuver. Determines whether the presenting part is engaged (widest diameter at or below a zero station) in the maternal pelvis.*

*Procedure continued on following page*

## Procedure 13–1 *Continued*

# Leopold's Maneuvers

**PURPOSE:** To determine presentation and position of the fetus. To aid in location of the fetal heart sounds.

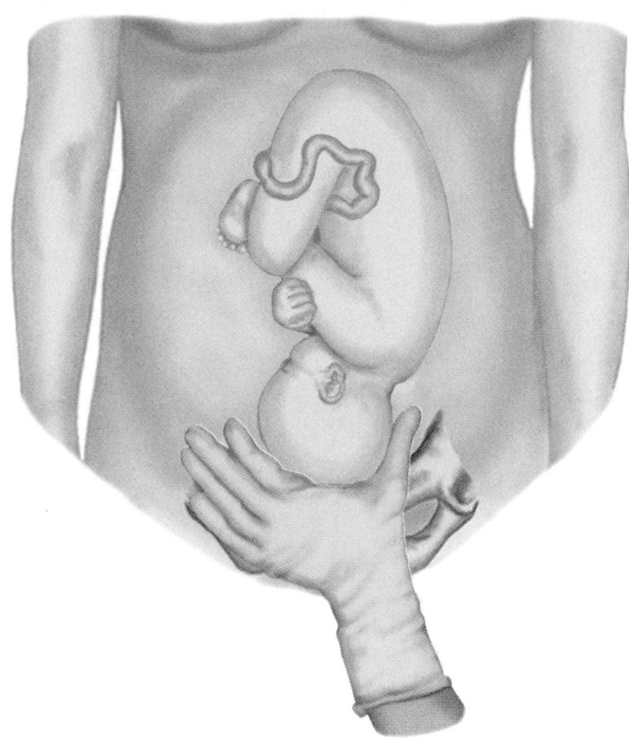

**8. Omit the fourth maneuver if the fetus is in a breech presentation.** *Is done only in cephalic presentations to determine if the fetal head is flexed.*

FOURTH MANEUVER

**9. Turn so that you face the woman's feet.** *Is most easily performed in this position.*

**10. Place your hands on each side of the uterus with fingers pointed toward the pelvic inlet. Slide hands downward on each side of the uterus. On one side, your fingers easily slide to the upper edge of the symphysis. On the other side, your fingers meet an obstruction, the cephalic prominence.** *Determines whether the head is flexed (vertex) or extended (face). The vertex presentation is normal. If the head is flexed, the cephalic prominence (the forehead in this case) is felt on the opposite side from the fetal back. If the head is extended, the cephalic prominence (the occiput in this case) is felt on the same side as the fetal back.*

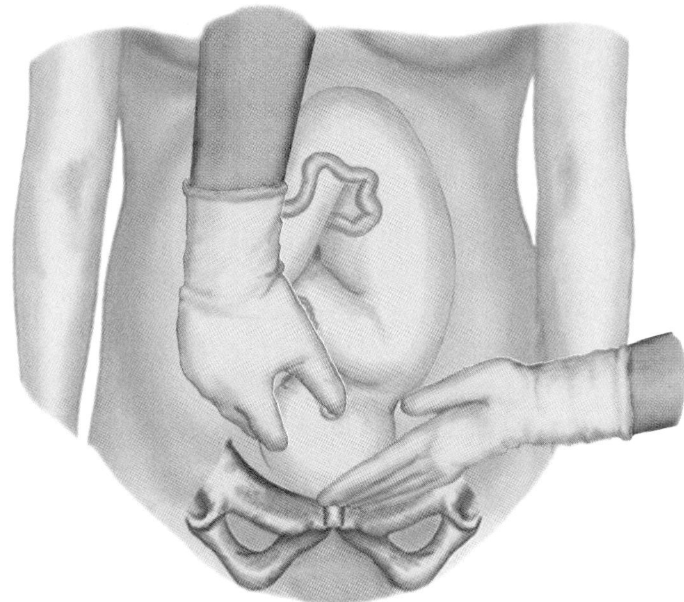

If focus assessments of mother and fetus are normal and birth is not imminent, the admission assessment is completed. If the initial assessments are not normal or birth is near, the physician or nurse-midwife is notified promptly.

### CHECK YOUR READING

3. What are the major assessment priorities when a woman comes to the intrapartum unit?
4. What is the average FHR at term? What other FHR characteristics are reassuring of fetal well-being?
5. What observations suggest that a woman is about to give birth very soon? What should the nurse do in that case?

#### DATA BASE ASSESSMENT

In addition to the focus assessment, assess the mother and fetus and available maternal support.

**Basic Information.** Most intrapartum admission forms guide the nurse to ask for essential information. Typical information includes the following:

- Her reason for coming to the hospital or birth center (e.g., contractions or rupture of membranes)
- Whether she has had prenatal care
- Her estimated date of delivery
- Number of pregnancies, births, and abortions
- Medical, surgical, and pregnancy history
- Allergies
- Food intake: what food and when it was eaten

## Procedure 13–2

# Auscultating Fetal Heart Rate

**PURPOSE:** To evaluate the fetal condition and tolerance of labor.

**1. Explain the procedure, and wash hands with warm water.** *Gives information to the woman and partner. Reduces transfer of microorganisms. Warm hands are more comfortable.*

**2. Use Leopold's maneuvers to identify the fetal back (Procedure 13–1). Illustrations show approximate locations of the FHR in different presentations and positions.** *The FHR is most easily heard through the fetal back because it usually lies closest to the surface of the maternal abdomen.*

**3. Assess the FHR with a fetoscope, Doppler transducer, or external fetal heart monitor. (Application of the external fetal monitor is discussed in Chapter 14.)** *The FHR can be assessed using any of these instruments.*

**4.** ***Fetoscope*** **(see Fig. 14–1): Place the bell of the fetoscope over the fetal back with the head plate pressed against your forehead. Move the fetoscope until you locate where the sound is loudest. Use your forehead to maintain pressure during auscultation.** *The head plate adds bone conduction to the sound coming through the earpieces. The FHR is faint with the fetoscope because sounds pass through several layers of maternal and fetal tissue.*

**5.** ***Doppler transducer*** **(see Fig. 14–1): Review manufacturer's instructions for operating the Doppler device. Place water-soluble conducting gel over the transducer, and turn it on. Place the transducer over the fetal back, and move it until you clearly hear the double sounds of the fetal heart.** *The Doppler transducer uses sound waves reflected off the moving fetal heart to create an audible signal. Gel makes a liquid interface for clear signal transmission.*

**6. With one hand, palpate the mother's radial pulse. If her pulse is synchronized with the sounds from the fetoscope or Doppler transducer, try another location for the fetal heart.** *The nurse must be sure that the FHR is what is actually heard. Other sounds that may be heard are the funic souffle (blood flowing through the umbilical cord) or uterine souffle (blood flowing through the uterine vessels). The funic souffle is synchronized with the fetal heart; the uterine souffle is synchronized with the mother's pulse.*

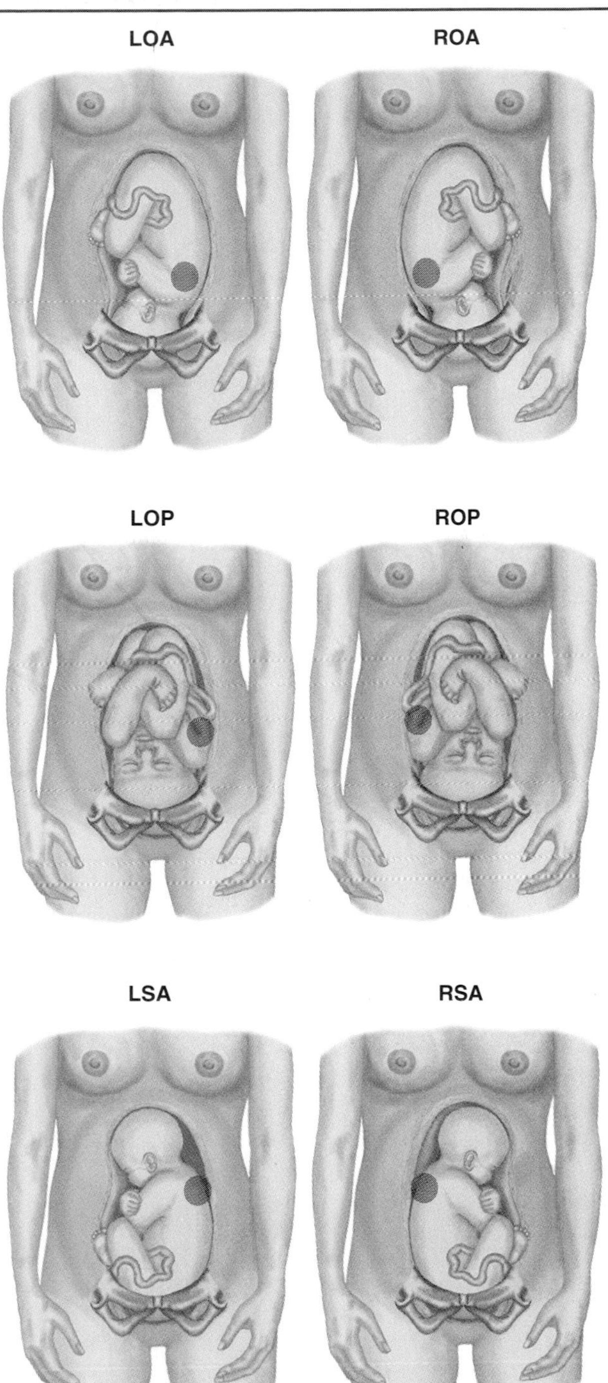


AUSCULTATING FETAL HEART RATE

**7. Assess the FHR before, during, and after a contraction. Count the baseline FHR for 30 to 60 seconds between contractions. Note accelerations and slowing of the rate.** *Allows fetal assessment through a contraction cycle: increment, peak, decrement, and interval. It is more difficult to hear the FHR with a fetoscope during contractions, especially if the mother is moving.*

**8. Note reassuring signs:**

**a. Average rate of 110 to 120 BPM at the lower limit and 150 to 160 BPM at the upper limit for a term fetus.**

**b. Accelerations of at least 15 BPM, usually with fetal movement.**

**c. Presence of variability (electronic monitoring).** *These signs indicate that the fetus seems to be tolerating labor well.*

**9. Note non-reassuring signs, and make more frequent assessments. Notify the physician or nurse-midwife.**

**a. FHR outside normal limits.**

**b. Slowing of the FHR after the contraction ends.** *These signs do not necessarily indicate fetal compromise but should be further evaluated by the nurse and physician or nurse-midwife. (See Chapter 14 for discussion of fetal response and appropriate nursing actions.)*

- Recent illness, including treatment
- Medications, including prescription and over-the-counter drugs, tobacco, alcohol, and abused substances
- Her subjective evaluation of her labor
- Birth plans, including expected pain management methods
- Support persons: who they are and the role of each

**Be careful when asking about prior pregnancies and births when a woman's family is present. She may have had an abortion or relinquished a baby for adoption, and her family may not know about it. Even if her partner knows about previous pregnancies, her family and friends may not.**

**Fetal Assessments.** The fetal presentation and position and the FHR (see Procedures 13–1 and 13–2) are assessed. The nurse documents the color of the amniotic fluid and the time of rupture if the membranes have ruptured.

**Labor Status.** The woman's labor status is determined by assessing her contraction pattern, performing vaginal examination, and determining whether her membranes have ruptured. Contractions are assessed by palpation (Procedure 13–3) or the fetal monitor or both. Cervical dilation and effacement and the fetal station, presentation, and position are

### CRITICAL THINKING EXERCISE

During a labor admission assessment, a woman quickly denies her use of drugs other than her prescribed prenatal vitamins. She becomes quiet, answering each of the nurse's questions in a terse manner.

**Q:** What might explain the woman's change in behavior? Should the nurse alter the assessment interview?

**A:** The woman's behavior may have changed for any of several reasons, so the nurse must not make assumptions. For example, she may have felt insulted that the nurse found it necessary to ask her questions about illicit drug use. Or she may use other drugs (licit or illicit) but prefer not to admit it. However, she may simply have been surprised at the question about drug use. Women often want their family to remain during the admission assessment but may not admit substance or physical abuse in their presence. Nonverbal cues, such as a too-quick denial, avoidance of eye contact, or vague responses, are clues that the woman may not be answering these questions truthfully. The nurse should follow up on maternal behaviors privately to clarify the facts that underlie them.

## Procedure 13–3
# Palpating Contractions

**PURPOSE:** To determine whether a contraction pattern is typical of true labor. To identify abnormal contractions that may jeopardize the health of the mother or fetus.

**1. Assess at least three contractions in a row. Guidelines for minimum frequency of assessments are:**

**a. Hourly during latent phase.**

**b. Every 30 minutes during active phase and transition.**

**c. Every 15 minutes during second stage.**

**Assess more frequently if abnormalities are identified.** *Assessment of at least three sequential contractions permits better evaluation of the pattern. Palpate contractions periodically when an external fetal monitor is used because it is less accurate for intensity as a result of thickness of the abdominal fat pad, maternal position, and fetal position.*

**2. Place fingertips of one hand on uterine fundus, using light pressure. Keep fingertips relatively still rather than moving them over uterus. The fingertips are more sensitive to the first tightening of the uterus.** *Contractions usually begin in the fundus, although the mother usually feels them in her lower abdomen and back. Moving the hand over the uterus may stimulate contractions and give an inaccurate assessment of their true pattern.*

**3. Note the time when each contraction begins and ends.**

**a. Determine frequency by noting average time that elapses from beginning of one contraction to beginning of the next one.**

**b. Determine duration by noting average time in seconds from beginning to end of each contraction.**

**c. Determine interval by noting average time between end of one contraction and beginning of the next one.** *Contractions are expected to increase in frequency, duration, and intensity as labor progresses. False labor is usually characterized by contractions that are irregular and do not increase in frequency, duration, and intensity.*

**4. Estimate the average intensity of contractions by noting how easily the uterus can be indented during the peak of the contraction:**

**a. Mild contractions are easily indented with the fingertips. They feel similar to the tip of the nose.**

**b. Moderate contractions can be indented with more difficulty. They feel similar to the chin.**

**c. Firm contractions feel "woody" and cannot be readily indented. They feel similar to the forehead.** *Contractions during labor are expected to intensify progressively. If they do not, the woman may not be in true labor, or she may be experiencing dysfunctional labor (see Chapter 27).*

**5. Report hypertonic contractions:**

**a. Durations longer than 90 seconds**

**b. Intervals shorter than 60 seconds**

**c. Incomplete relaxation of the uterus between contractions.** *Hypertonic contractions reduce placental blood flow by prolonged compression of the vessels that supply the intervillous space.*

evaluated by vaginal examination. The vaginal examination may also reveal whether the membranes have ruptured or are still intact. *Vaginal examination is not performed if the woman has active bleeding (other than bloody show) because the procedure may increase bleeding.*

**Physical Examination.** If birth is not imminent, a brief physical examination evaluates the woman's overall health. Important general observations that relate to birth include presence and location of edema, abdominal scars, and height of the fundus.

## CHECK YOUR READING

6. Which tests may be done if the nurse is not certain whether the woman's membranes have ruptured? (See Table 13–1.)
7. Which characteristics of contractions may reduce blood flow to the placenta? (See Procedure 13–3.)

### ADMISSION PROCEDURES

#### NOTIFYING THE BIRTH ATTENDANT

After assessment, the nurse notifies the woman's birth attendant to report on her status and obtain orders. The nurse includes the following data in the report:

- Gravidity, parity, and abortions
- Estimated date of delivery
- Contraction pattern
- Fetal presentation and position
- Cervical dilation and effacement; station of the presenting part
- FHR
- Maternal vital signs
- Any identified abnormalities or concerns about the maternal or fetal condition
- Pain, anxiety, or other reactions to labor

If the birth attendant admits the woman, any of several procedures may be done.

#### CONSENT FORMS

The woman signs consent for care during labor, anesthesia, vaginal birth, and possible cesarean birth. Consent for newborn care is often completed as well.

#### LABORATORY TESTS

Women who had regular prenatal care may need laboratory tests only for specific indications. Simple tests are often done on the unit, such as the following:

- Hematocrit obtained by finger stick
- Midstream urine specimen for measurement of protein and glucose levels, usually obtained before notifying the birth attendant

#### INTRAVENOUS ACCESS

If used, intravenous access is started with at least an 18-gauge catheter. A saline or heparin lock may be used, or the woman may receive continuous infusion of fluids. The lock eases walking during early labor and is less associated with illness but still provides quick access if fluids or drugs are needed. Continuous fluid infusion helps prevent or relieve dehydration and is needed if epidural block analgesia is used. Intravenous solutions containing electrolytes, such as lactated Ringer's solution, are often used.

#### PERINEAL PREPARATION

If necessary, hair in the immediate area of an episiotomy is removed by shaving or by clipping the hair near the skin with a shaver or disposable scissors.

#### ENEMA

The woman may need an enema if stool in her rectum causes discomfort or interferes with fetal descent. Small-volume enemas (such as Fleet enemas) are most common. Extra lubricant on the enema tip reduces discomfort from hemorrhoids.

### ASSESSMENTS AFTER ADMISSION

The woman is usually observed if it is unclear after the initial assessment whether she is in true labor. After 1 or 2 hours, progressive cervical change (effacement, dilation, or both) strongly suggests true labor. The woman and fetus are assessed during the observation period as if she were in early labor.

After the admission assessment, laboring women and their fetuses need regular assessments based on their risk status and whether they have interventions such as epidural analgesia. General guidelines for continuing assessments are listed here.

#### FETAL ASSESSMENTS

Fetal assessments are done to identify signs of well-being and signs that suggest compromise. The principal fetal assessments include the FHR and patterns and the character of the amniotic fluid. Abnormalities revealed in these assessments may be associated with impaired fetal gas exchange or infection.

**Fetal Heart Rate.** The FHR is assessed using either intermittent auscultation or electronic fetal monitoring. Intermittent auscultation is done with a Doppler transducer or a fetoscope. Electronic fetal monitoring may be continuous or intermittent. (See Chapter 14 for discussion of fetal monitoring.)

For the fetus at low risk for complications, guidelines for assessment (by either intermittent auscultation or continuous monitoring) and documentation are presented in Table 13–2.

**Amniotic Fluid.** The membranes may rupture spontaneously (SROM, or spontaneous rupture of membranes), or the birth attendant may perform an amniotomy (AROM, or artificial rupture of membranes). The FHR is assessed for at least 1 minute when the membranes rupture. The umbilical cord could be displaced in a large fluid gush, resulting in compression and interruption of blood flow through it (prolapsed cord; see p. 773). Charting related to membrane rupture includes the time, FHR, and character of the fluid.

Amniotic fluid should be clear and may include bits of vernix, the creamy fetal skin lubricant. Cloudy, yellow, or foul-smelling amniotic fluid suggests infection. Green fluid indicates that the fetus passed meconium before birth. Meconium passage may have been in response to transient hypoxia, although the cause may remain unknown. The newborn may need extra respiratory suctioning at birth if the fluid is heavily stained with meconium.

Describe quantity in approximate terms; for example, at term, a "large" amount is more than 1000 ml; a "moderate" amount is about 500 to 1000 ml; and "scant" amniotic fluid is only a trickle, barely enough to detect. If the fetus is well down into the pelvis when the membranes rupture, a small amount of fluid in front of the fetal head may be discharged (forewaters), with the rest lost at birth.

#### MATERNAL ASSESSMENTS

Several maternal assessments also relate to the health of the fetus, such as vital signs and contractions.

**Vital Signs.** Guidelines for maternal vital signs assessment are listed in Table 13–1. Hypotension, hypertension, elevated pulse and respiratory rates, and elevated temperature should be reported.

**Contractions.** Contractions can be assessed by palpitation or with the electronic fetal monitor. Guidelines appear in Table 13–1.

**Progress of Labor.** A vaginal examination is done periodically to determine cervical dilation and effacement and fetal descent (Fig. 13–1). The frequency of vaginal examinations depends on the woman's parity, the status of her membranes, and the overall speed of her labor. Vaginal examinations are limited to avoid introducing microorganisms from the perineal area into the uterus.

**Intake and Output.** Oral and intravenous intake is recorded. Each voiding is recorded. Labor may reduce a woman's urge to void, so her suprapubic area should be checked every 2 hours to identify bladder distention.

Pressure of the fetal head on the rectum in late labor makes many women feel the need to defecate. Look at the woman's perineum for crowning of the

### TABLE 13–2 ASSESSMENT AND DOCUMENTATION OF FETAL HEART RATE

| Low-Risk Patients | High-Risk Patients |
|---|---|
| First stage of labor | First stage of labor |
| Every 1 hr in latent phase | Every 30 min in latent phase |
| Every 30 min in active phase | Every 15 min in active phase |
| Second stage of labor | Second stage of labor |
| Every 15 min | Every 5 min |

**Labor Events**

**Assess fetal heart rate before:**
- Initiation of labor-enhancing procedures (such as artificial rupture of membranes)
- Periods of ambulation
- Administration of medications
- Administration or initiation of analgesia or anesthesia

**Assess fetal heart rate following:**
- Rupture of membranes
- Recognition of abnormal uterine activity patterns, such as increased basal tone or tachysystole (excessive frequency)
- Evaluation of oxytocin (maintenance, increase, or decrease of dosage)
- Administration of medications (at time of peak action)
- Expulsion of enema
- Urinary catheterization
- Vaginal examination
- Periods of ambulation
- Evaluation of analgesia and/or anesthesia (maintenance, increase, or decrease in dosage)

From NAACOG. (1990). *Fetal heart rate auscultation*. Washington, D.C.: Author.

### CRITICAL THINKING EXERCISE

Chloe Green is in labor with her second baby. The baby is in a left occiput anterior (LOA) position, and Chloe's cervix is 5 cm dilated and completely effaced. Her membranes rupture at the end of a strong contraction. You note that the fluid is green and watery.

**Q:** What are the most important nursing actions at this time? Why?

**A:** Assess the fetal heart rate for at least 1 minute to identify any abnormal rate or pattern. Note the time of rupture, odor, and approximate amount of amniotic fluid. Report the findings to the physician or nurse-midwife because green, meconium-stained amniotic fluid may be associated with fetal compromise. A foul or strong odor is associated with infection. The FHR should be assessed more often, and an electronic fetal monitor is usually applied if it is not already in place.

**Purposes**

To determine whether membranes have ruptured.
To determine cervical effacement and dilation.
To determine fetal presentation, position, and station.

**Method**

Vaginal examination is not performed by the inexperienced nurse except when training for graduate nursing practice in the intrapartum area.

***Equipment***

Sterile gloves, sterile lubricant. If Nitrazine paper is being used to test for ruptured membranes, lubricant is not used to avoid altering the test paper.

***Hand Position***

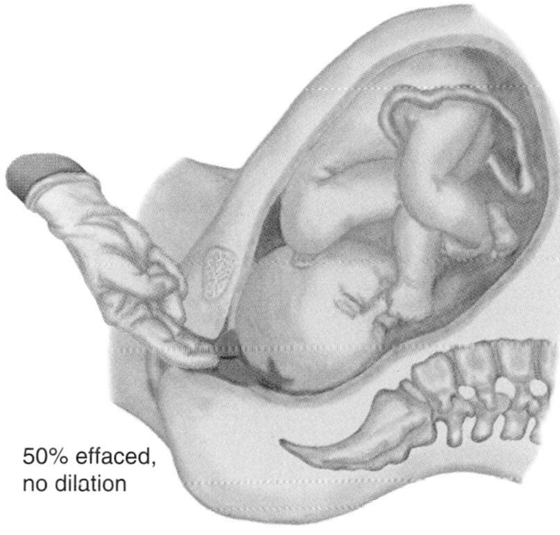


The nurse usually uses the index and middle fingers of the dominant hand for vaginal examination. The thumb and other fingers are kept out of the way to avoid carrying microorganisms into the vagina.

***Determining Whether Membranes Have Ruptured***

*Intact* membranes feel like a slippery membrane over the fetal presenting part.

If the membranes are *bulging*, they feel like a slippery, fluid-filled balloon over the presenting part. It may be difficult to feel the fetal presentation clearly if the membranes are bulging tensely.

If the membranes have ruptured, fluid will often drain from the vagina as the nurse manipulates the cervix and presenting part.

***Determining Cervical Effacement and Dilation***

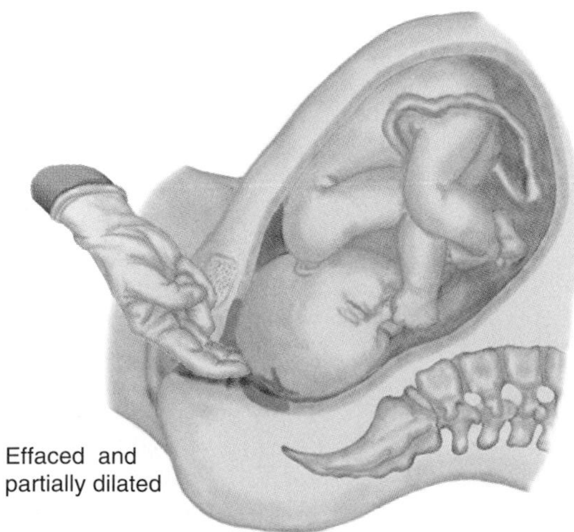


The nurse determines *effacement* by estimating the thickness of the cervix. The uneffaced cervix is about 2 cm long. If it is 50% effaced, it is about 1 cm long. Effacement is expressed as a percentage of 0% to 100%, or it may be described as the length in centimeters.

*Dilation* is determined by sweeping the fingertips across the cervical opening. The average woman's index finger is about 1.5 cm in diameter.

***Determining the Presenting Part***

The fetal skull feels smooth, hard, and rounded in a cephalic presentation. The fetal buttocks are softer and more irregular in a breech presentation. If the membranes are ruptured, the fetus in a breech presentation may expel thick, green-black meconium. (Presence of meconium in a breech presentation is *not* necessarily a sign of fetal compromise. The nurse must evaluate other signs of fetal condition.)

***Determining the Fetal Position***

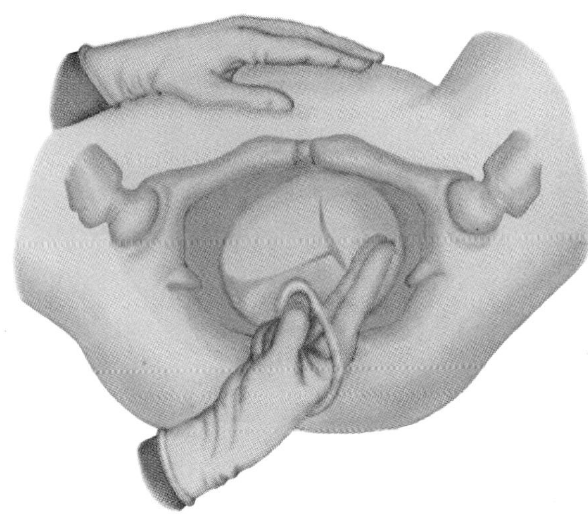

In a cephalic presentation, the nurse feels for the distinctive features of the fetal skull. The posterior fontanelle is usually felt in a vertex presentation and is triangular with three suture lines (two lambdoid and one sagittal) leading into it. The anterior fontanelle is not felt unless the head is poorly flexed or is in the mechanism of extension in late labor. It feels like a diamond-shaped depression with four suture lines (one frontal, two coronal, and one sagittal) leading into it.

***Determining the Station***

The nurse locates the the ischial spines on either side of the pelvis and estimates how far the leading edge of the fetal presenting part is above or below them. If the leading edge is at the same level as the ischial spines, the station is zero (0).

***Documenting the Examination***

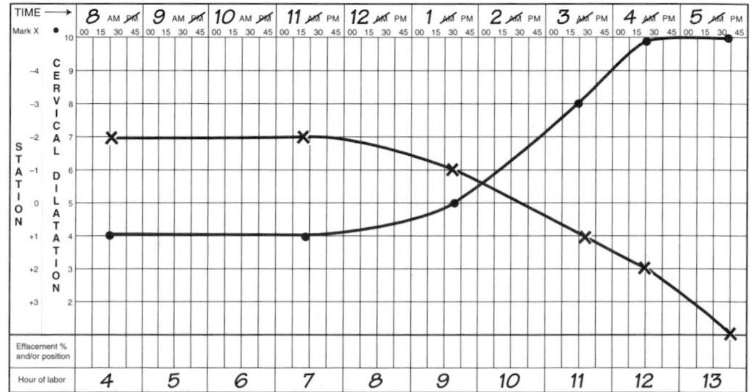


Findings of the vaginal examination may be recorded on a labor flow sheet, narrative, or on a graph. The graph may be termed a Friedman curve, a partogram, or a labor curve.

**FIGURE 13–1**

Vaginal examination during labor.

fetal head if she abruptly expresses a need to defecate.

**Response to Labor.** The woman's behavioral responses change as labor intensifies. She withdraws from interactions but needs more nursing presence and reassurance. She may become more anxious because of pain and fear of bodily injury, unknown outcome, loss of control, unresolved psychological issues that influence her readiness to give birth (such as sexual abuse or previous birth experiences), or unexpected occurrences during labor.

Women vary in how they handle the pain of labor. The nurse must constantly assess whether added pain control measures are needed. Behaviors that suggest the woman needs help with pain management include the following:

- Expressing that nonpharmacologic measures are ineffective.
- Tensing her muscles or arching her back during contractions.
- Persistence of muscle tension between contractions.
- A tense facial expression.
- Expressions such as "I can't take it anymore."
- Specific requests for medication or other pain control.

THE SUPPORT PERSON'S RESPONSE

Labor is stressful for the woman's support person, often the baby's father. He may become anxious, fearful, or tired. He feels a responsibility to protect and support the woman but may have limited resources for doing so. It is difficult for him to watch the woman he loves in pain, even if the pain is normal. He may respond to stress in many ways: quiet, suffering silently, or reacting with pacing or anger. Some fathers respond by leaving the room frequently or for long periods of time, whereas others resist taking even short breaks.

Nurses encourage and value the father's presence during labor and birth. However, this may conflict with a couple's cultural norms, which dictate that birth is a strictly female activity. The father may be pulled in two directions, wanting to be included but hesitant because it is not customary to be part of birth in his culture. The nurse should respect the values of each couple and their wishes about father involvement.

The support person also may be a parent or other relative, a friend of either gender, or a homosexual partner. The nurse must remember that anyone who assists the woman during labor may have feelings of anxiety and helplessness at times. Reassurance and care for the labor partner strengthen that person's ability to support the woman and enhance the likelihood that both will view the birth experience as positive.

**CHECK YOUR READING**

8. What is the routine frequency for FHR assessment in uncomplicated labor? Why should the FHR be assessed after the membranes rupture?
9. What is the significance of greenish amniotic fluid? Of cloudy, yellowish, or foul-smelling amniotic fluid?
10. Why are frequent vaginal examinations undesirable during labor?
11. What observations suggest that the woman may need added help with pain management during labor?

## Application of Nursing Process: False or Early Labor

### Assessment

After assessment, it may be apparent that the woman is not in true labor. If findings are normal and her membranes are intact, she is usually discharged home. The woman who is in very early labor may be discharged to await active labor, especially if she is a nullipara and does not live far away.

### Analysis

A woman may be frustrated because she cannot tell whether labor is real. She may resist returning to the birth center, possibly causing needless delay of care. A nursing diagnosis that applies to many women with false labor contractions is Knowledge Deficit: Characteristics of True Labor.

### Planning

A goal or expected outcome for this nursing diagnosis is that before discharge home, the woman and her support person will describe reasons for returning to the birth center for evaluation.

### Interventions

#### PROVIDING REASSURANCE

A woman sent home after observation often feels foolish and frustrated. Reassure her that even professionals cannot always identify true labor and that false labor and early true labor have similar characteristics. Tell her that important preparation occurs during late pregnancy, such as softening of her cervix, even if obvious progress like cervical dilation has not yet occurred.

#### TEACHING

Review with her guidelines for returning to the birth center. Explain that these are only guidelines and that she should call or return if she has any concerns. It is better for her to return with another false alarm than to arrive at the birth center in advanced labor or to develop complications at home.

### Evaluation

The woman and her support person should be able to describe guidelines for returning to the birth center. These include regular contractions, leaking of amniotic fluid, bleeding other than bloody show, and decreased fetal movement.

# Application of Nursing Process: True Labor

The admission assessment may confirm that the woman is in true labor, or true labor may be evident after observation. Nursing diagnoses and collaborative problems change during labor because the intrapartum period is an evolving process. Those covered in this chapter relate to fetal oxygenation, maternal discomfort, and maternal injury.

Nursing diagnoses are often interrelated during labor. For example, anxiety or fear can impact pain-relief measures. A fluid volume deficit can alter fetal oxygenation because less blood is available to circulate to the placenta.

## Fetal Oxygenation

### Assessment

Refer to assessments listed in Tables 13–1 and 13–2 for intrapartum assessments. The main assessments related to fetal well-being are the following:

- FHR
- Character of amniotic fluid and time of rupture
- Maternal vital signs
- Contractions: frequency, duration, intensity, resting interval

### Analysis

Several factors can reduce fetal oxygen, nutrient, and waste exchange, such as maternal hypotension or hypertension, maternal fever, excessively strong or long contractions (*tetanic*), and compression of the umbilical cord. The healthy fetus usually tolerates labor well, and the nurse simply needs to be alert for problems. Therefore, a valid collaborative problem is Potential complication: fetal compromise. The focus of this chapter is normal labor. For further discussion of this collaborative problem, see Chapter 14.

### Planning

Client-centered goals are not made for collaborative problems as they are for nursing diagnoses. Planning includes nursing responsibilities to (1) promote normal placental function and (2) observe for and report problems to the physician or nurse-midwife.

### Interventions

#### PROMOTING PLACENTAL FUNCTION

Maternal positioning is the primary measure to promote placental function during normal labor. The woman can choose any position other than the supine. The supine position may cause her heavy uterus to compress her aorta and inferior vena cava (aortocaval compression), reducing blood flow to the placenta. If she must be in the supine position for a procedure such as catheterization, a small pillow under one hip shifts her uterus to maintain good placental blood flow.

#### OBSERVING FOR CONDITIONS ASSOCIATED WITH FETAL COMPROMISE

Determine whether any conditions associated with fetal compromise exist (see Critical to Remember). If any are identified, assess the fetus more frequently and notify the birth attendant.

**Critical to Remember**

**CONDITIONS ASSOCIATED WITH FETAL COMPROMISE**

- FHR outside the normal range for a term fetus: lower limit of 110 to 120 BPM and upper limit of 150 to 160 BPM
- Little or no variability in the electronically monitored FHR
- Slowing of the FHR persisting after contraction ends
- Meconium-stained (greenish) amniotic fluid
- Cloudy, yellowish, or foul odor to amniotic fluid (suggests infection)
- Contractions lasting longer than 90 seconds
- Incomplete uterine relaxation or intervals shorter than 60 seconds between contractions
- Maternal hypotension (may divert blood flow away from the placenta to ensure adequate perfusion of the maternal brain and heart)
- Maternal hypertension (may be associated with vasospasm in spiral arteries, which supply the intervillous spaces of the placenta)
- Maternal fever (38°C [100.4°F] or higher)

### Evaluation

Evaluation of client goals or expected outcomes does not apply to a collaborative problem. Throughout labor, the nurse compares actual data with the norms for the mother and fetus.

## Discomfort

### Assessment

See Table 13–1 for continuing assessments of the laboring woman.

### Analysis

Labor is painful. Women vary in how they respond to pain and in the pain management methods they choose. Providing choices for pain management and supporting the woman's choices increase her sense of control over her birth experience. The woman who successfully masters the pain and other physical demands of labor is more likely to view her experience as positive. Her support person is likely to feel more satisfaction with the experience as well.

Nursing diagnoses that are often related are pain and anxiety. Excess anxiety intensifies pain perception, and pain worsens anxiety. The nurse clusters assessment data to determine which of the two is the primary client problem. For example, several cues suggest that anxiety is the primary problem: a previous poor experience during birth or expressions of worry and concern. However, if contractions are intense and labor is progressing quickly, pain would be the primary nursing diagnosis. Of these two, the nursing diagnosis selected for this discussion is Pain related to effects of uterine contractions.

### Planning

Elimination of the laboring woman's pain is not realistic. Appropriate goals or expected outcomes that address the needs of the woman and her partner are as follows:

1. During labor, the woman will state that she is able to tolerate the pain satisfactorily.
2. The woman will use breathing and relaxation techniques during labor.
3. By the end of labor, the woman's partner will express satisfaction with his ability to support her.

### Interventions

Labor pain management includes measures to promote comfort as well as specific methods, such as breathing techniques or medication. (See Chapters 11 and 15 for other pain management techniques.)

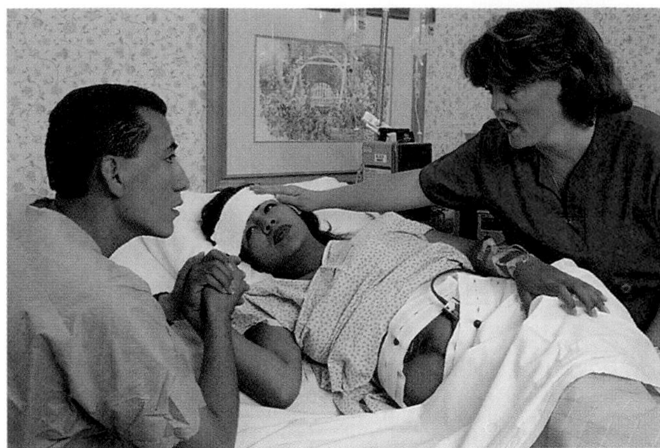

**FIGURE 13–2**

Cool, damp washcloths placed where the woman finds them most comforting helps her to relax during each contraction. Several washcloths should be kept near to maintain their cool dampness.

#### PROVIDING COMFORT MEASURES

Ordinary measures reduce irritating surroundings that impair a woman's ability to relax and use coping skills.

**Lighting.** Soft, indirect lighting is soothing, whereas a bright overhead light is an irritant. Bright lights imply a hospital ("sick") atmosphere rather than the normal life event that birth is. Use the overhead light only when needed. A small flashlight is handy if the woman wants her room dark.

**Temperature.** Labor is work. Women in labor are often hot and perspiring. Cool, damp washcloths on the woman's face and neck promote comfort (Fig. 13–2). Keep an ample supply of damp washcloths available, and change them often to keep them cool. An electric fan circulates air in the labor room and directs a breeze on the woman. Be sure that the fan does not blow on the infant after birth, which might lead to hypothermia.

Have the woman wear socks if her feet are cold.

**Cleanliness.** Bloody show and amniotic fluid leak from the woman's vagina during labor. Change the sheets and gown as needed to keep her dry and comfortable. Let her preferences be the guide because she may not want to be disturbed during late labor. Change the disposable underpad regularly to reduce microorganisms that may ascend into the vagina. A folded towel absorbs larger quantities of amniotic fluid than the pad alone.

**Mouth Care.** Ice chips (Fig. 13–3), popsicles, or hard candy on a stick reduces the discomfort of a

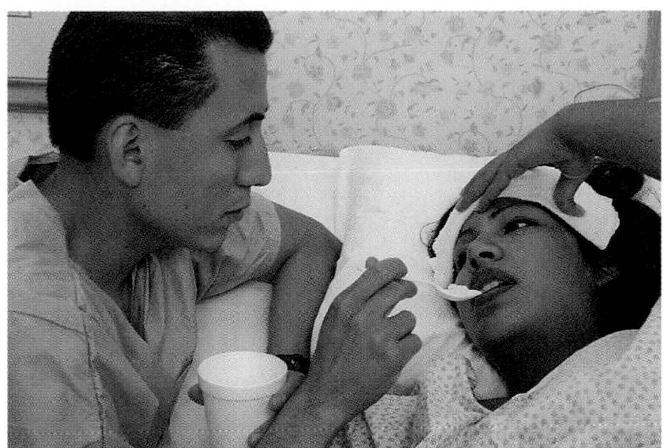

**FIGURE 13–3**

Most laboring women welcome ice chips to ease their dry mouth.

dry mouth. If oral intake is contraindicated, brushing the teeth (without swallowing water) or simply rinsing the mouth helps. Many women appreciate a moist washcloth to their lips.

**Bladder.** A full bladder intensifies pain during labor and can delay fetal descent. Remind the woman to empty her bladder at least every 2 hours.

**Positioning.** Occasionally, a specific maternal position is recommended to reduce discomfort or to assist the labor process. Otherwise, encourage the woman to assume any position she finds comfortable (other than the supine). Frequent changes reduce discomfort from constant pressure, help the fetus adapt to the pelvic contours, and promote fetal descent. Figure 13–4 illustrates various maternal positions for labor.

The woman may have "back labor" if the back of the fetal head puts pressure on her sacral promontory (occiput posterior position). The discomfort of back labor is difficult to relieve with medication. Positions that encourage the fetus to fall away from the sacral promontory, such as those in which the mother leans forward or uses the hands-and-knees position, promote her comfort and enhance the internal rotation mechanism of labor.

**Water.** Water in the form of a shower, tub, or whirlpool is relaxing and helps many women tolerate contractions. Nipple stimulation by water currents causes release of oxytocin by the posterior pituitary gland, which increases contractions and promotes labor progress. If contractions become too strong, she simply moves her breasts from the water steam.

#### TEACHING

Teaching the woman in labor is a constant and changing task.

##### FIRST STAGE

Many women become discouraged because several hours are needed to reach 4 or 5 cm cervical dilation. They believe that the last 5 cm will take as long as the first 5 cm. From a time standpoint, 5 cm is more like two thirds of the way to full dilation rather than half of the way because the rate of dilation increases during the active phase.

A woman's urge to push usually occurs when her cervix is fully dilated and effaced and when the fetus descends deep into the pelvis and internally rotates. However, as she nears the second stage, her baby may descend enough to give her an urge to push before full cervical dilation. If her cervix, which is usually 8 or 9 cm dilated at this time, yields easily to downward pressure, pushing in response to her spontaneous urge rarely causes problems.

Either of two problems may occur if she pushes against a cervix that does not easily yield to pressure from the fetal presenting part:

- The cervix may become edematous, which can block progress.
- The cervix may be lacerated.

Teach the woman to blow out in short breaths if she should not push.

##### SECOND STAGE

The woman may need help to trust the sensations from her body and to push most effectively during second-stage labor.

**Time Limit.** Two hours was once considered the upper limit for the duration of the second stage. It is now recognized that a second stage longer than 2 hours is safe as long as the mother and fetus show no signs of compromise.

Women push most effectively when they feel the reflex urge to do so. Many women do not immediately feel the urge to push when their cervix is fully dilated. If maternal and fetal assessments are reassuring, the woman does not need to push before she feels the urge. Pushing vigorously sooner than this time may contribute to birth canal injury because her vaginal tissues are stretched more forcefully and rapidly than they would be if she pushed spontaneously and in response to her body's signals.

**Positions.** The mother can push in any position she prefers. Position changes promote her natural pushing efforts. Many women prefer semi-sitting and side-lying positions. Squatting enlarges the pelvic outlet slightly and adds the force of gravity to the mother's efforts; this is an advantage if she has a small pelvis or the fetus is large. Some women push most effectively while sitting on the toilet because that is where they are accustomed to giving in to that sensation.

STANDING

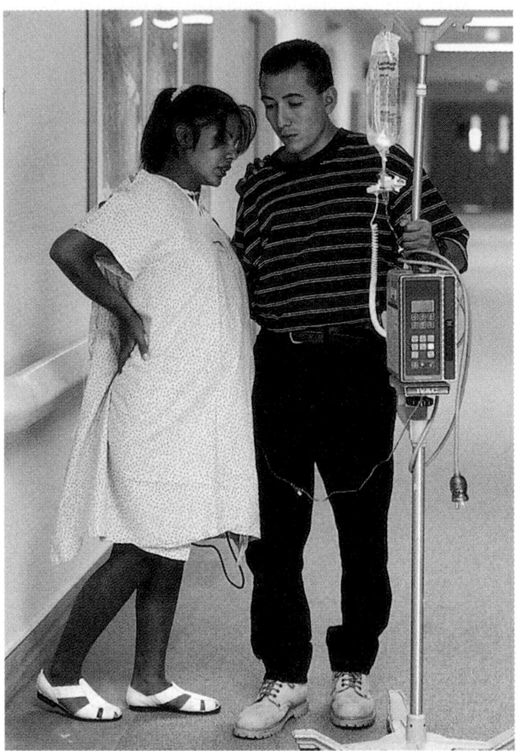

*Advantages*

Adds gravity to force of contractions to promote fetal descent.
Contractions are less uncomfortable and more efficient.
Variation: Standing, leaning forward with support reduces back pain because fetus falls forward, away from the sacral promontory.

*Disadvantages*

Tiring over long periods.
Continuous electronic fetal monitoring is not possible without telemetry.

*Nursing Implications*

If the woman has intravenous fluid running, give her a rolling pole. Encourage her to alternate walking with other positions whenever she tires or desires to do so.
Remind the woman and her partner when she should return to the labor area for evaluation of the fetal heart rate and her labor status.

SITTING UPRIGHT

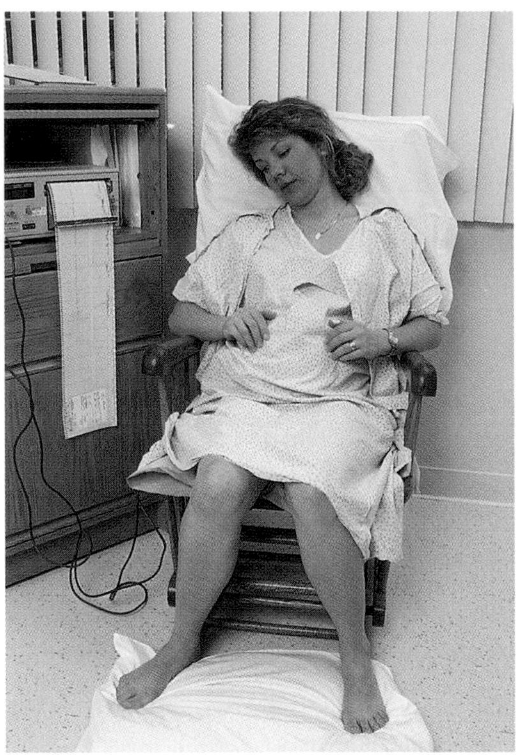

*Advantages*

Uses gravity to aid fetal descent.
Can be done when sitting on side of bed, in a chair, or on the toilet.
Can be used with continuous fetal monitoring.
Avoids supine hypotension.

*Disadvantages*

May increase suprapubic discomfort.
Contractions are the most efficient when the woman alternates sitting with other positions.

*Nursing Implications*

A rocking chair is soothing.
Place a pillow on a chair with a disposable underpad over the pillow to absorb secretions.
Use pillows or a foot stool to keep the short woman's legs from dangling.
Encourage the woman to alternate positions periodically; for example, she can alternate walking with sitting or sitting with side lying.

**FIGURE 13-4**

Maternal positions for labor.

When the mother pushes, teach her to curve her body around her uterus in a C shape rather than arching her back. For most effectiveness, teach her to pull on her knees, hand-holds, or a squatting bar while pushing. Women often find that pulling on something from above is efficient.

**Method and Breathing Pattern.** If she is pushing effectively and safely, do not interfere, but support the woman's spontaneous techniques. She should push with her abdominal muscles while relaxing her perineum. Teach her to take a breath and exhale to begin. Have her take another breath and exhale

SITTING, LEANING FORWARD WITH SUPPORT

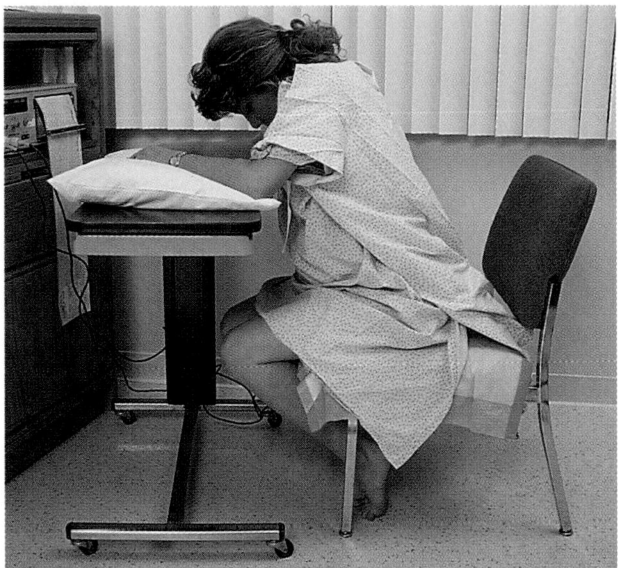

*Advantages*

Same as for sitting.
Reduces back pain because fetus falls forward, away from sacral promontory.
Partner or nurse can rub back or give sacral pressure to relieve back pain.

*Disadvantages*

Same as for sitting.

*Nursing Implications*

Same as for sitting.

SEMI-SITTING

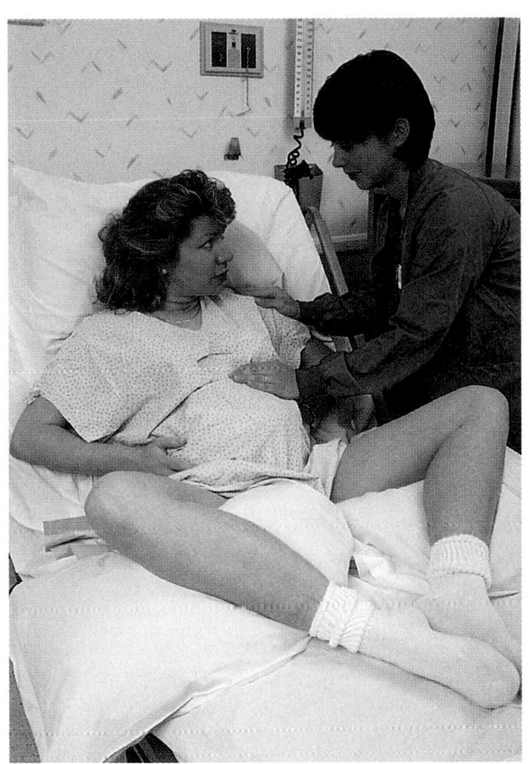

*Advantages*

Same as for sitting.
Aligns long axis of uterus with pelvic inlet, which applies contraction force in the most efficient direction through pelvis.

*Disadvantages*

Same as for sitting.
Does not reduce pain as well as the forward-leaning positions.

*Nursing Implications*

Same as for sitting.
Raise bed to about a 30- to 45-degree angle.
Encourage the woman to use sitting (leaning forward) or side lying if she has back pain so that the caregiver can rub her back or apply sacral pressure.

**FIGURE 13–4** *Continued*

*Illustration continued on following page*

while pushing strongly for about 4 to 6 seconds at a time. Sustained pushing while breathholding (the Valsalva maneuver) reduces blood flow to the placenta and is fatiguing. Another deep breath helps her relax at the end of the contraction.

**A woman who is modest or fears losing control may inhibit her best pushing efforts if she is instructed to push as if she were having a bowel movement, particularly if she is in a bed or chair. An anatomically correct image is to teach the woman to push down and out under her symphysis ("pubic bone"), following the pelvic curve. Seeing a diagram of the pelvis helps her to visualize the curve.**

**PROVIDING ENCOURAGEMENT**

Success breeds success. Tell the woman when her labor is progressing. If she can see that her efforts

SIDE-LYING

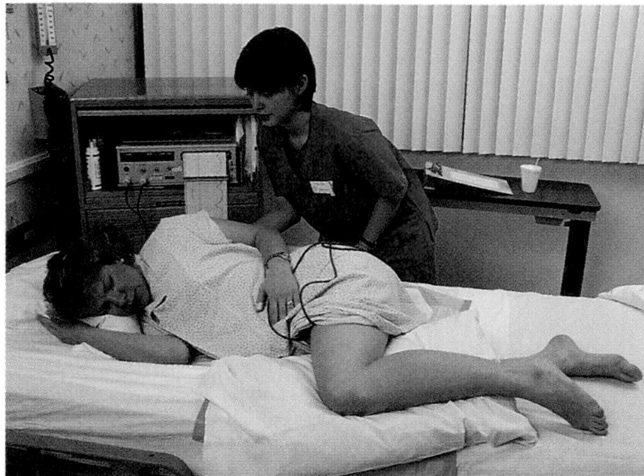

*Advantages*

Is a restful position.
Prevents supine hypotension and promotes placental blood flow.
Promotes efficient contractions, although they may be less frequent than with other positions.
Can be used with continuous fetal monitoring.

*Disadvantages*

Does not use gravity to aid fetal descent.

*Nursing Implications*

Teach the woman and her partner that although the contractions are less frequent, they are more effective.
This position offers a break from more tiring positions.
Use pillows for support and to prevent pressure: at her back, under her superior arm, and between her knees.
Use disposable underpads to protect the pillow between the woman's knees from secretions.
Some women like to put their superior leg on the bed rail. If the woman wants this variation, pad the bed rail with a blanket to prevent pressure.
If she wants to remain recumbent, she should use this position to promote placental blood flow.

KNEELING, LEANING FORWARD WITH SUPPORT

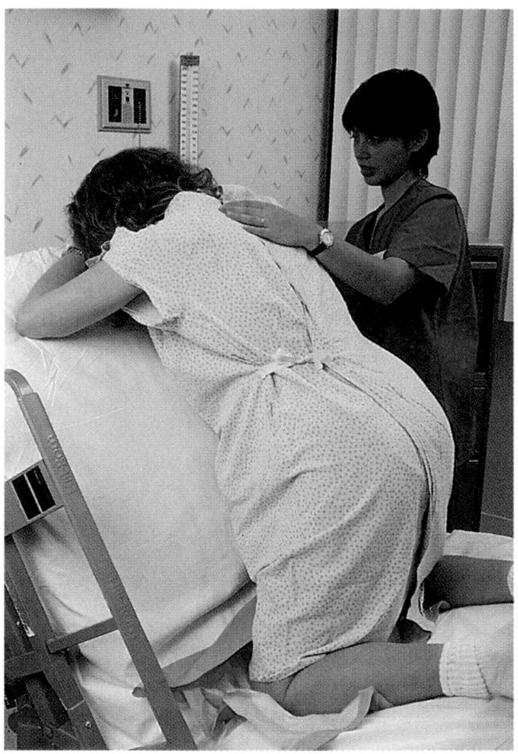

*Advantages*

Reduces back pain because fetus falls forward, away from sacral promontory.
Adds gravity to force of contractions to promote fetal descent.
Can be used with continuous fetal monitoring.
Caregivers can rub her back or apply sacral pressure.
Promotes normal mechanisms of birth.

*Disadvantages*

Knees may become tired or uncomfortable.
Tiring if used for long periods.

*Nursing Implications*

Raise the head of the bed, and have the woman face the head of the bed while she is on her knees.
Another method is for the partner to sit in a chair, with the woman kneeling in front, facing her partner, and leaning forward on him or her for support.
Use pillow under the knees and in front of the woman's chest, as needed, for comfort.
Encourage her to change positions if she becomes tired.

**FIGURE 13–4** *Continued*

are effective, she has more courage to continue. Help her touch or see the baby's head with a mirror as crowning occurs.

Praise the woman and her labor partner when they use breathing or other coping techniques effectively. This reinforces their actions, gives them a sense of control, and conveys the respect and support of the nurse. If one technique is not helpful after a reasonable trial (at least three to five contractions), encourage them to try other techniques.

### GIVING OF SELF

The nurse's caring presence is a crucial element in labor support. Even women who are very indepen-

HANDS AND KNEES

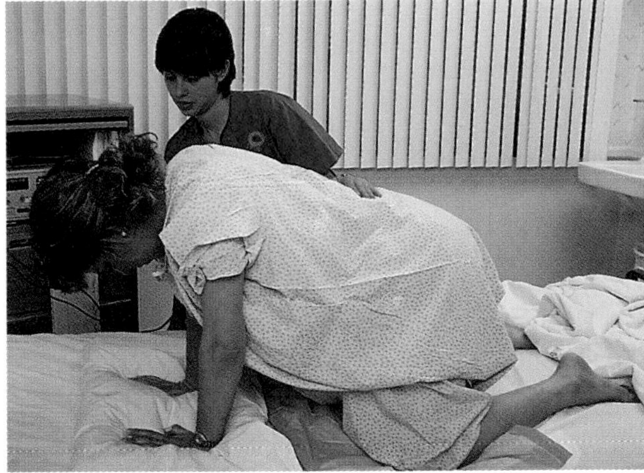

*Advantages*

Reduces back pain because the fetus falls forward, away from the sacral promontory.
Promotes normal mechanisms of birth.
The woman can use pelvic rocking to decrease back pain.
Caregivers can rub the woman's back or apply sacral pressure easily.

*Disadvantages*

The woman's hands (especially wrists) and knees can become uncomfortable.
Tiring when used for a long time.
Some women are embarrassed to use this position.

*Nursing Implications*

Encourage the woman to change to less tiring positions occasionally
Ensure privacy when encouraging the reluctant woman to try this position if she has back pain.
A second hospital gown with the opening in front covers her back and hips but may be too warm.

POSITIONS FOR PUSHING IN SECOND STAGE

ADAPTATIONS OF POSITIONS FOR PUSHING

*Standing*

This position may be tiring, and access to the woman's perineum is difficult. Because the infant could fall to the ground if birth occurs rapidly, provide padding under the mother's feet. Gravity aids fetal descent.

*Hands and Knees*

Advantages and disadvantages are similar to those during first-stage labor. In addition, caregivers must reorient themselves because the landmarks are upside down from their usual perspective.

A variation is for the mother to kneel and lean forward against a beanbag or the side of the bed. This variation reduces some of the strain on her wrists and hands.

SQUATTING

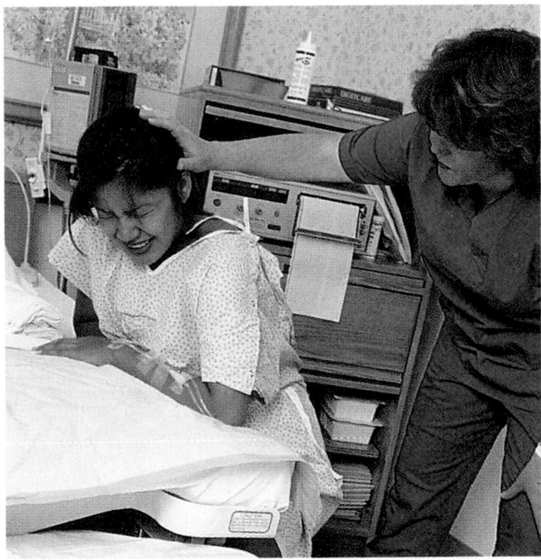

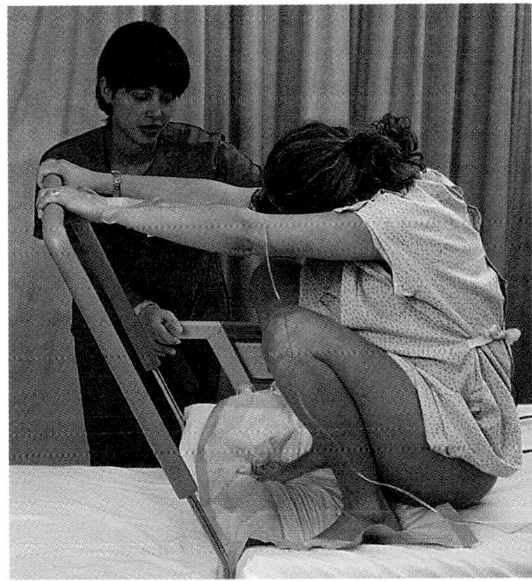

*Advantages*

Adds gravity to force of contractions to promote fetal descent.
Straightens the pelvic curve slightly for more direct fetal descent.
Increases dimensions of pelvis slightly.
Promotes effective pushing efforts in the second stage.
Caregivers can rub back or provide sacral pressure.

*Disadvantages*

Knees and hips may become uncomfortable because of prolonged flexion.
Tiring over a long time.

*Nursing Implications*

Provide support with a squat bar attached to the bed or by two people standing on each side of the woman.
If she becomes tired, or between contractions, she can lean back into the sitting position.
Variation: Have the woman squat beside the bed as she pushes.

**FIGURE 13–4** *Continued*

*Illustration continued on following page*

SEMI-SITTING

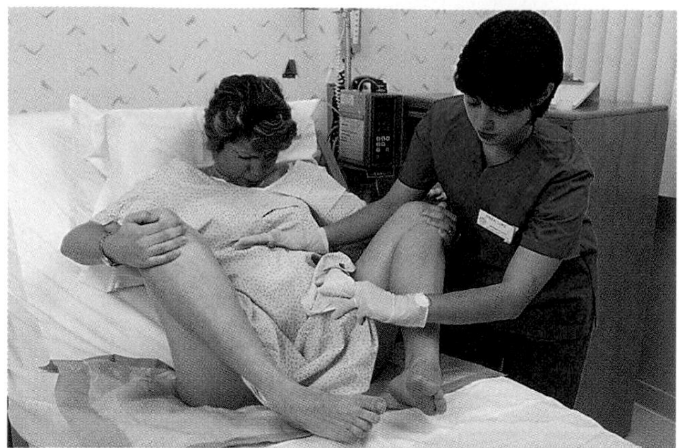

Many woman prefer this because they have the security of a back rest; it is also familiar to caregivers and allows easy observation of the perineum. Elevate the woman's back at least 30 to 45 degrees so that gravity aids fetal descent. The woman pulls on her flexed knees (behind or in front of them) as she pushes. She should keep her head flexed and her sacrum flat on the bed to straighten the pelvic curve.

SIDE-LYING

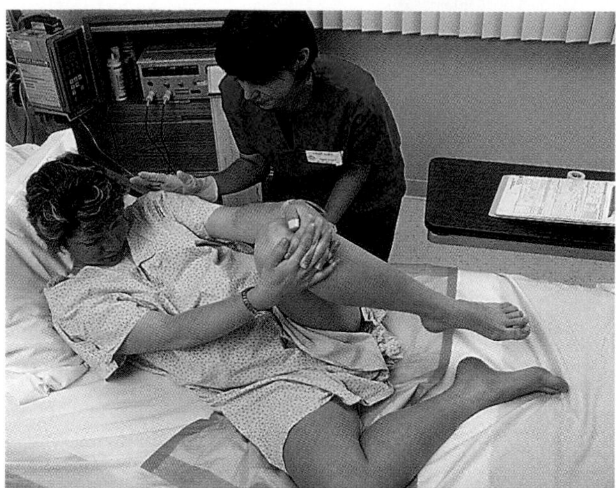

The woman flexes her chin on her chest and curls around her uterus as she pushes. She pulls on her flexed knees or the knee of the superior leg as she pushes.

**FIGURE 13–4** *Continued*

dent may become dependent during labor and need human contact. Many times the woman simply needs reassurance that all is going well and that the nurse is there for her. The nurse's presence helps to allay her fears of abandonment and conveys safety, acceptance, support, and comfort.

Although the woman and her support person may have prepared for childbirth, they often welcome suggestions and affirmation from the nurse. The nurse who is familiar with the techniques they are using can better support them and avoid contradicting what they have learned and practiced. The nurse's presence, gentle coaching, and encouragement help her to have confidence in her own body and her fitness to give birth.

#### OFFERING PHARMACOLOGIC MEASURES

Some women do not need pharmacologic pain relief during labor. Birth is usually a normal process, and the prepared woman and labor partner can deliver their infant without medication. However, many do choose to have pharmacologic pain management. Inform the woman about medications available to her without pressuring her to take them.

Most women have an open mind about using analgesia or anesthesia, but some may have a firm goal of avoiding all pain medication during labor. They may then feel let down or guilty if they need medication. Other women may plan to use a specific pain-relief method, such as epidural analgesia. If something prevents use of their chosen method, they may be upset about this unexpected development in their birth experience. In either case, allow the woman to ventilate her feelings about her experience. Although the event may not be what she wanted, expressing her feelings helps her put it into perspective.

#### CARING FOR THE BIRTH PARTNER

The woman's support person is an integral part of her labor care. Her labor partner can provide care and comfort, which support the woman's ability to give birth. However, do not expect too much of the partner or make assumptions about the type and amount of involvement desired.

Some partners are coaches in the true sense of the word, actively assisting the woman through labor. Others want the woman and nurse to lead them and tell them how to help. They are eager to do what they can but expect instructions about how and when to do it. Many couples see the partner's role as one of encouragement, moral support, and just being there for the woman. Moreover, not every woman wants her partner to take an active role; she may expect only nearness and concern (Chapman, 1992).

To impose unrealistic expectations of leadership, care, and comfort on the partner makes the birth experience unnecessarily stressful. To ensure a positive experience for both, accept whatever pattern of support the partner is able and willing to provide and whatever the couple finds comfortable. Without taking over or diminishing this role, provide support that the partner cannot.

Encourage the partner to conserve physical strength. The partner may have missed sleep during the hours of early labor or may need a break. The nurse may need to encourage the partner to eat or bring a snack. Remind the partner that he can be a more effective support if his own needs are met. Support persons who do not eat for a long time are more likely to faint during the birth.

### Evaluation

Achievement of the three goals or expected outcomes occurs if the following conditions are met:

1. The woman indicates that she is able to tolerate the pain of labor satisfactorily.
2. The woman uses the breathing and relaxation techniques that she was taught.
3. Her partner expresses satisfaction with his support during labor.

This nursing diagnosis and its goals are constantly reevaluated during labor.

## Preventing Injury

### Assessment

Nursing assessments of the mother and fetus continue as the woman nears birth. During the second stage, observe the woman's perineum to determine when to make final birth preparations.

The exact time for final birth preparations varies according to the woman's parity, the overall speed of labor, and the fetal station. Preparations are usually completed when crowning in the nullipara reaches a diameter of about 3 to 4 cm. The multipara is prepared sooner, usually when her cervix is fully dilated and the fetal head is well down in the pelvis but before much crowning has occurred.

### Analysis

The woman is vulnerable to injury immediately before and after birth for several reasons: (1) altered physical sensations, such as intense pressure or effects of medication, (2) positional changes for birth, and (3) unexpectedly rapid progress. The nursing diagnosis selected for the laboring woman near the time of birth is Risk for Injury (maternal) related to altered sensations and positional or physical changes.

### Planning

The nurse's primary objective is to avoid or minimize injuries that can occur during final birth preparations or because of a sudden birth. The goal or expected outcome for this nursing diagnosis is that the woman does not have an avoidable injury, such as muscle strains, thrombosis, or lacerations, during birth.

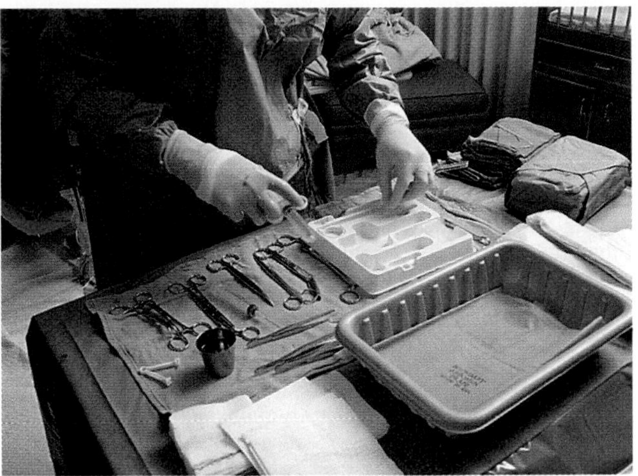

**FIGURE 13-5**

The nurse makes final preparations for birth. Included on the sterile table are anesthesia trays (if needed), instruments for birth and repair of maternal injury or episiotomy, and infant care materials.

### Interventions

Transfer of the woman to the delivery site or positioning her in the birthing bed is the first step in the sequence of events that culminates in birth of the baby (Figs. 13-5 through 13-7).

During the period surrounding birth, the nurse reduces factors that contribute to maternal injuries.

#### TRANSFER TO A DELIVERY ROOM

Most births occur in a combination labor, delivery, and recovery room. In some facilities, or with some client conditions, the woman must be transferred to a separate room for birth. Transfer her early enough to avoid rushed, last-minute preparations that cause anxiety for everyone.

#### POSITIONING FOR BIRTH

Raise the woman's back, shoulders, and head to promote effective pushing and take advantage of gravity.

Stirrups or foot rests support the woman's legs and feet and make her perineum more accessible. To reduce strain on muscles and ligaments, raise and lower her legs together (if anesthesia limits her movement) and do not separate them too widely. Pad surfaces that contact the popliteal space behind the knee because veins are near the surface there, and pressure on them could lead to thrombus formation.

**Transfer and Positioning for Birth**
*Action*: When the woman is almost ready to give birth, transfer her to the delivery room or position the birthing bed. The exact time varies with several factors (such as overall speed of labor and rate of fetal descent). *Rationale*: Rushed, last-moment preparations are anxiety-producing for the woman, her partner, and the nurse. Remaining in the birth position for a long time can be tiring.

*Action*: Continue observing her perineum while making final preparations for birth. *Rationale*: Birth may occur unexpectedly, and the nurse should be prepared to "catch" the infant if the attendant (physician or nurse-midwife) is not in the room.

*Action*: Continue observing the fetal heart rate (FHR) with continuous monitoring or intermittent auscultation. *Rationale*: Detects changes in fetal condition that may require interventions by the attendant to speed birth.

*Action*: Elevate the woman's back, shoulders, and head with a wedge (on a delivery table) or by raising the head of the birthing bed. *Rationale*: Allows more effective maternal pushing and uses gravity to aid fetal descent.

*Action*: Stirrups or foot rests to support the woman's legs and feet may be used on a birthing bed. Pad the surface. *Rationale*: Padding reduces pressure, preventing venous stasis and possible thrombus formation.

*Action*: When placing the woman's legs in stirrups, elevate them and remove them simultaneously. Do not separate her legs widely. *Rationale*: Reduces strain on muscles and ligaments.

**Prepping and Draping**
*Action*: After the woman is in position, cleanse the perineal area with a sterile iodophor and water preparation unless she is allergic. Use warm water to dilute the iodophor scrub. *Rationale*: Removes secretions and feces from perineal area.

*Action*: After handwashing, apply sterile gloves for the prep procedure. Take a fresh sponge to begin each new area, and do not return to a clean area with a used sponge. Six sponges are needed. The proper order and motions are as follows:

1. Use a zig-zag motion from clitoris to lower abdomen just above the pubic hairline.

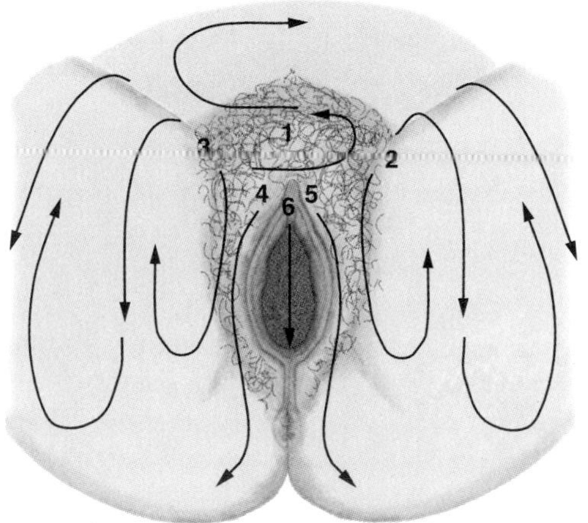


2., 3. Use a zig-zag motion on the inner thigh from the labia majora to about halfway between the hip and knee. Repeat for the other inner thigh.

4., 5. Apply a single stroke on one side from clitoris over labia, perineum, and anus. Repeat for the other side.

6. Use a single stroke in the middle from the clitoris over the vulva and perineum.

*Rationale*: Prevents cross-contamination or recontamination of an area that is already clean.

*Action*: The attendant may apply sterile drapes if desired. *Rationale*: A vaginal birth is a clean procedure rather than a sterile one because the vagina is not sterile. Sterile drapes are unnecessary, but some attendants may prefer to use them.

**Birth of the Head**
*Action*: If an episiotomy is needed, the attendant will perform it when the head is well crowned (see Chapter 16). *Rationale*: Minimizes blood loss from the episiotomy.

*Action*: As the vaginal orifice encircles the fetal head, the attendant applies gentle pressure to the woman's perineum with one hand while applying counterpressure to the fetal head with the other hand (Ritgen's maneuver). The attendant may ask the mother to blow so that she avoids pushing, or to push gently. *Rationale*: Controls the exit of the fetal head so that it is born gradually rather than popping out; this minimizes trauma to the maternal tissues.

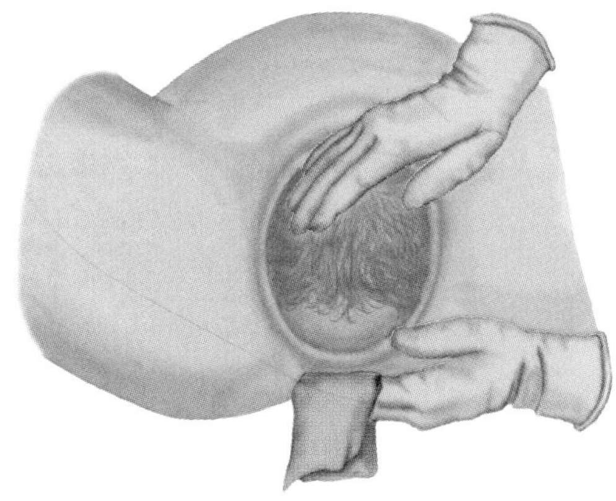

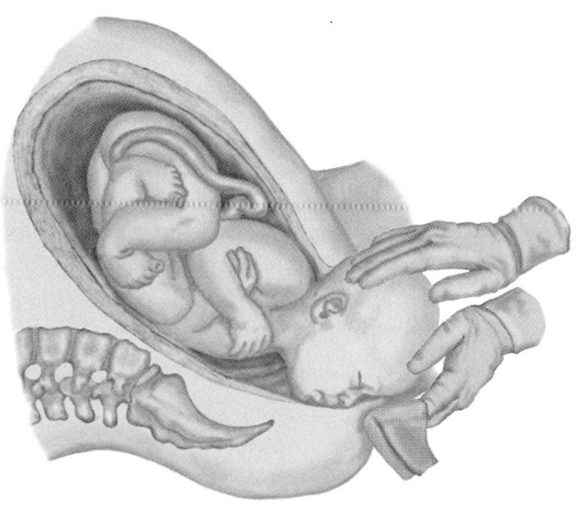

**FIGURE 13–6**
Sequence for delivery.

*Action*: The attendant wipes secretions from the infant's face and suctions the nose and mouth with a bulb syringe. *Rationale*: Removes blood and secretions, preventing the infant from aspirating them with the first breaths.

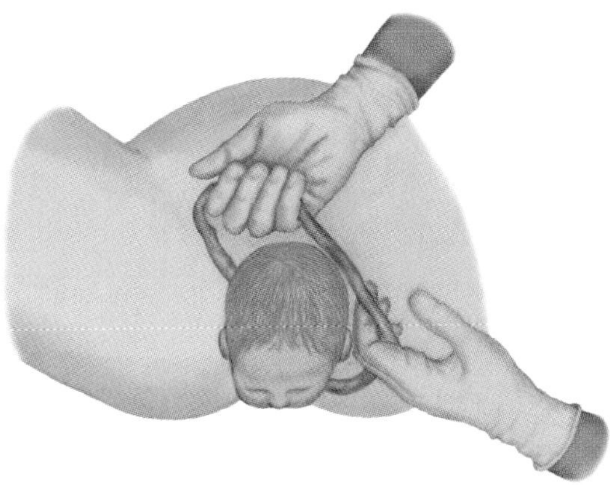

*Action*: The attendant feels for a cord around the fetal neck (nuchal cord). If it is loose, it is slipped over the head. If tight, it is clamped and cut between two clamps before the rest of the baby is born. *Rationale*: Allows the rest of the birth to occur and prevents stretching or tearing the cord.

**Birth of the Shoulders**

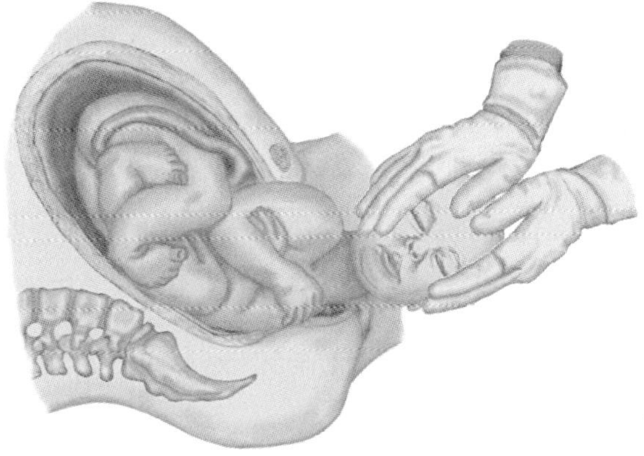

*Action*: After external rotation, the attendant applies gentle traction on the fetal head in the direction of the mother's perineum. *Rationale*: External rotation allows the shoulders to rotate internally and aligns their transverse diameter with the anteroposterior diameter of the mother's pelvic outlet. Traction on the head in the direction of her perineum allows the anterior fetal shoulder to slip under the symphysis pubis.

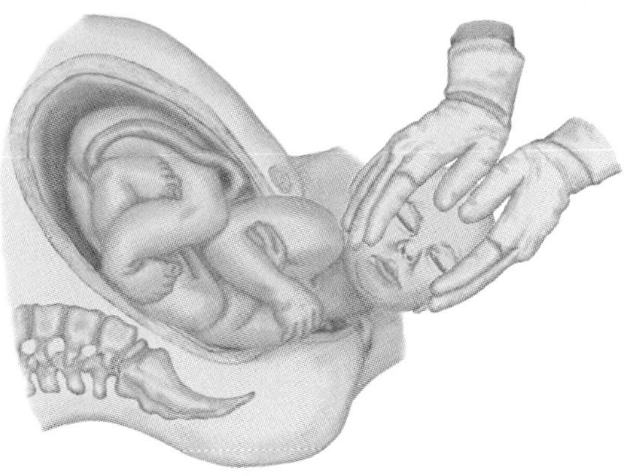

*Action*: The attendant then lifts the head toward the mother's symphysis pubis. *Rationale*: Permits the posterior fetal shoulder to be eased over the perineum, minimizing trauma to the maternal tissues.

**Clearing the Infant's Airway and Cutting the Cord**

*Action*: The rest of the infant's body is born quickly after the shoulders are born. The attendant maintains the infant in a slightly head-dependent position while suctioning excess secretions with a bulb syringe. The infant is often placed on the mother's abdomen. *Rationale*: Gravity aids spontaneous drainage of secretions and prevents aspiration of oral mucus and secretions.

*Action*: The attendant clamps the cord. Either the father or the attendant cuts the cord above the clamp. *Rationale*: Allows parents to interact more freely with their infant. Prevents flow of blood between placenta and infant, which might result in anemia (if infant is higher than placenta) or polycythemia (if infant is below the placenta).

**Delivery of the Placenta**

*Action*: After the placenta separates, it can be usually delivered if the mother bears down. The attendant may pull gently on the cord. *Rationale*: Excess traction on the cord may cause it to break, making the placenta harder to deliver.

*Action*: The attendant inspects both sides of the placenta. *Rationale*: Ensures that no fragments remain inside the uterus that might cause hemorrhage and infection.

After the infant and placenta are born, the attendant inspects the birth canal for injuries. If needed, any injuries and the episiotomy (if one was done) are repaired.

**FIGURE 13-6** *Continued*

## OBSERVING THE PERINEUM

The exact time at which a woman is ready to give birth is an educated guess. A woman who has been having a slow labor may suddenly make rapid progress. Birth is near when the fetal head swings anteriorly in the mechanism of extension as the occiput slips under the symphysis pubis. Observe the woman's perineum, especially during late second-stage labor.

As birth nears, perineal massage or warm applications to the perineum may be used. These techniques relax the perineum, allowing it to stretch and better accommodate the baby's head during expulsion, minimizing the need for an episiotomy and reducing the risk of a large laceration.

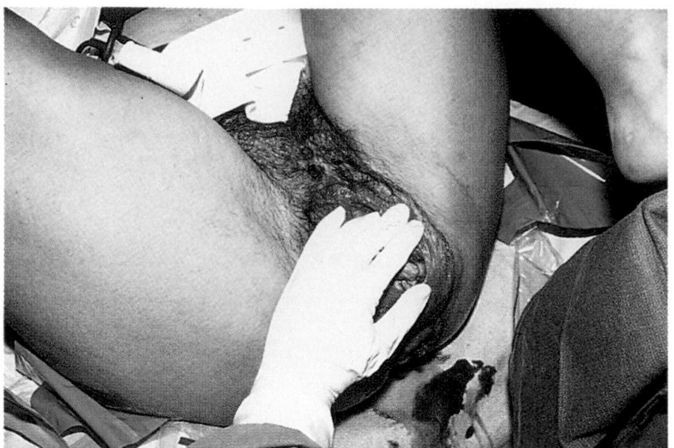

A. **Crowning.** The fetal head distends the labial and perineal tissues. The anus is stretched wide, and it is not unusual to see the woman's anterior rectal wall at this time. Any feces expelled are wiped posteriorly to avoid contaminating the vulva. The attendant (physician or nurse-midwife) is not holding the fetal head back but rather controlling its exit by using gentle pressure on the fetal occiput.

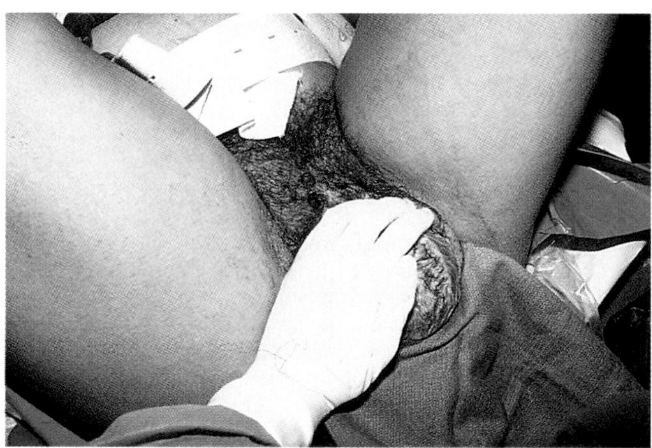

B. **Ritgen maneuver.** Pressure is applied to the fetal chin through the perineum at the same time pressure is applied to the occiput of the fetal head. This action aids the mechanism of extension as the fetal head comes under the symphysis.

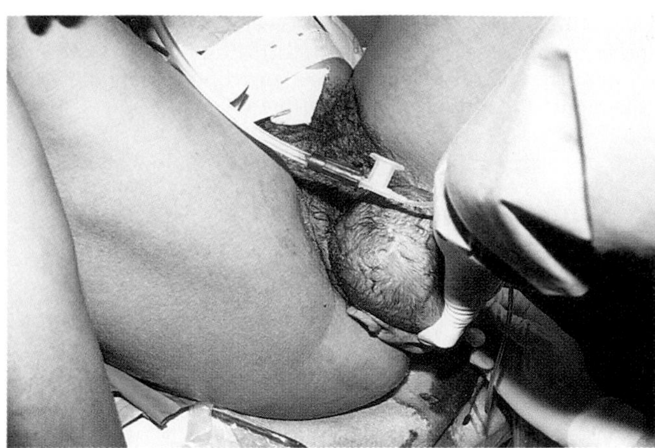

C. **Birth of the head.** As the head emerges, the attendant prepares to suction the nose and mouth to avoid aspiration of secretions when the infant takes the first breath.

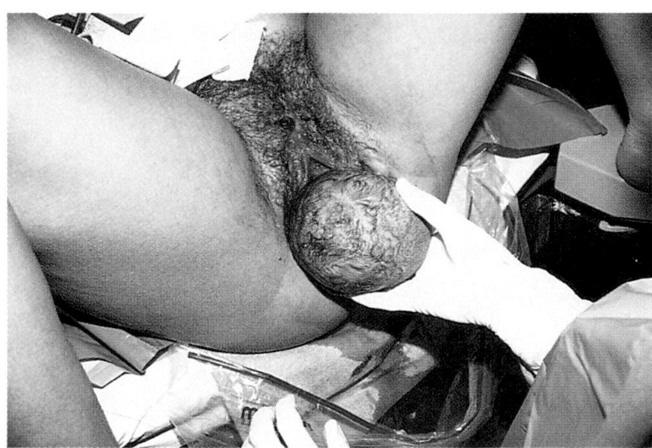

D. **Restitution and external rotation.** After the head emerges, it realigns with the shoulders (restitution). External rotation occurs as the fetal shoulders internally rotate, aligning their transverse diameter wirh the anteroposterior diameter of the pelvic outlet.

**FIGURE 13–7**

Vaginal birth.

A *classic sign of imminent birth is the mother's urgent cry, "The baby's coming!"* Look at her perineum, and if the baby will be born before the physician or nurse-midwife arrives, remain calm and support the infant's head and body with gloved hands as it emerges (Table 13–3).

## Evaluation

The goal or expected outcome for this nursing diagnosis is evaluated throughout the postpartum period because muscle strains or thrombus formation is not evident until later. The birth attendant notes lacerations after the baby's birth. See Chapter 17 for postpartum assessments to evaluate this goal.

### ✓ CHECK YOUR READING

12. How may maternal hypotension or hypertension affect the fetus?
13. What position should the woman avoid during labor? Why? What if the woman must be in this position temporarily?
14. What are some general measures that can make the woman more comfortable during labor? How can the nurse support the woman's labor partner?

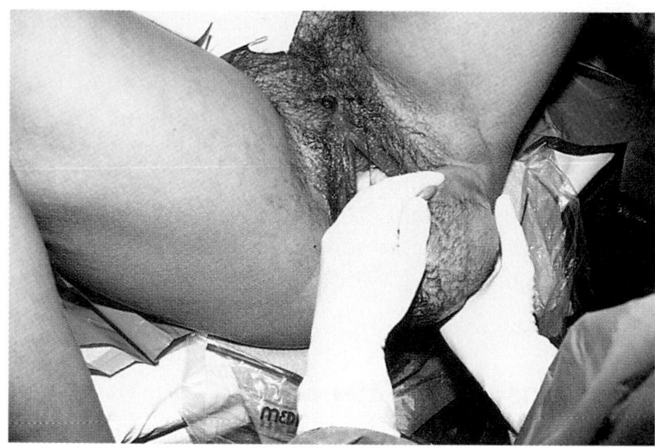

E. **Birth of the anterior shoulder.** The attendant gently pushes the fetal head toward the woman's perineum to allow the anterior shoulder to slip under her symphysis. The bluish skin color of the fetus is normal at this point; it becomes pink as the infant begins air breathing.

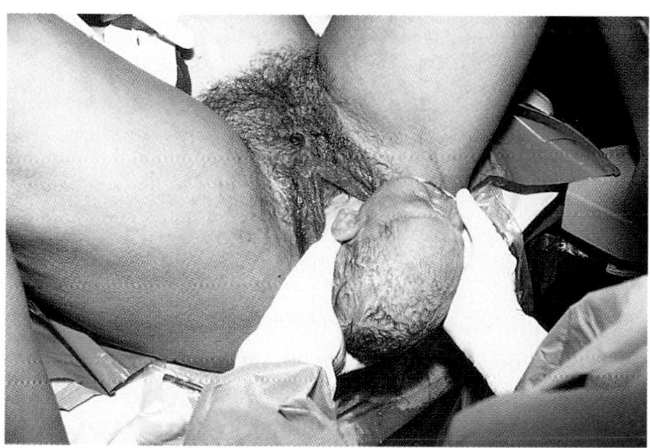

F. **Birth of the posterior shoulder.** The attendant now pushes the fetal head upward toward the woman's symphysis to allow the posterior shoulder to slip over her perineum.

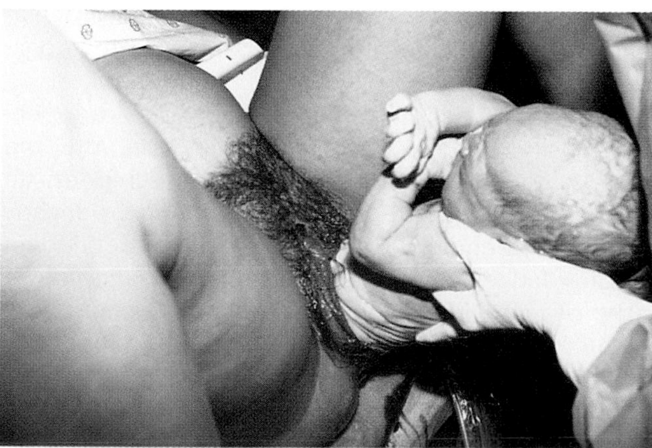

G. **Completion of the birth.** The attendant supports the fetus during expulsion. Note that the fetus has excellent muscle tone, as evidenced by facial grimacing and flexion of the arms and hands.

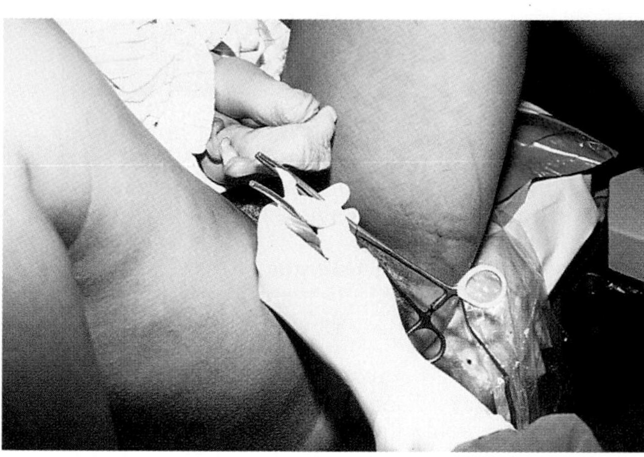

H. **Cord clamping.** While the infant is in skin-to-skin contact on the mother's abdomen, the attendant doubly clamps the umbilical cord. The cord is then cut between the two clamps. Samples of cord blood are collected after it is cut.

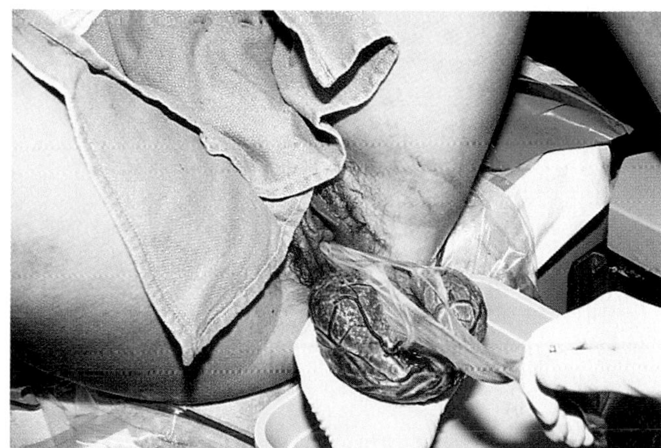

I. **Birth of the placenta.** The attendant applies gentle traction on the cord to aid expulsion of the placenta. This placenta is expelled in the more common Schultze mechanism, with the shiny fetal surface and membranes emerging. Note the fetal membranes that surrounded the fetus and amniotic fluid during pregnancy. The chorionic vessels that branch from the umbilical cord are readily visible on the fetal surface of the placenta.

**FIGURE 13–7** *Continued*

**TABLE 13–3 ASSISTING WITH AN EMERGENCY BIRTH**

The inexperienced nurse rarely must deliver a baby in the hospital or birth center but occasionally helps the more experienced nurse do so. Unplanned out-of-hospital births are not common, but they do occasionally occur.

**Nursing Priorities for an Emergency Birth in Any Setting**
Prevent or reduce injury to the mother and infant.
Maintain the infant's airway and temperature after birth.

**Preparing for an Emergency Birth**
Study the delivery sequence in Figures 13–6 and 13–7.
Locate the emergency delivery tray ("precip" tray) on the unit.

**During the Birth**
Remain with the woman to assist her in giving birth. Use the call bell, or ask her partner to call for help. Stay calm to reduce the couple's anxiety.
Put on gloves, preferably sterile, to prevent contamination with blood and other secretions. Sterile gloves reduce transmission of environmental organisms to the mother and infant. The nurse will be "catching" the infant in this situation. No invasive procedure is done.

**After the Birth**
Observe the infant's color and respirations for distress. Suction excess secretions with a bulb syringe.
Dry the infant, and place skin-to-skin with the mother or cover with warmed blankets to maintain warmth.
Put the infant to the mother's breast, and encourage suckling to promote uterine contraction, facilitating expulsion of the placenta and controlling bleeding.

15. Why is it important to watch the perineum as a woman pushes?
16. How can perineal massage and heat applications reduce the risk for maternal birth injury?

# Nursing Care During the Late Intrapartum Period

## Responsibilities During Birth

The nurse has added responsibilities during the birth. These may include the following:

- Preparation of a sterile delivery table with gowns, gloves, drapes, solutions, and instruments (see Fig. 13–5)
- Perineal cleansing preparation
- Initial care and assessment of the newborn
- Administration of medications, usually oxytocin, to contract the uterus and control blood loss (see Drug Guide 16–1)

An anesthesiologist or nurse-anesthetist may give maternal medications. A nurse from the nursery is often present if the newborn is at risk for problems such as respiratory depression.

Eye shields should be worn to protect from fluid splashing or blood spurting as the cord is cut. At birth, the newborn is covered with blood, amniotic fluid, vernix, and other body substances. All personnel involved in infant care should wear gloves and other protective equipment until after the first bath to avoid contact with potentially infectious secretions.

## Responsibilities After Birth

Intrapartum nursing care extends through the fourth stage of labor and includes care of the infant, the mother, and the family unit. Nursing care during the immediate recovery period is presented in this chapter. The discussion of later postpartum care of the mother and infant is found in Chapters 17 through 23.

### CARE OF THE INFANT

Nursing care of the newborn includes supporting cardiopulmonary and thermoregulatory function and placing an identifying band on the infant. In addition, the nurse assesses the infant for approximate gestational age (see p. 538) and examines for obvious anomalies or birth injuries.

#### MAINTAINING CARDIOPULMONARY FUNCTION

Assess the infant's Apgar score (Table 13–4) at 1 and 5 minutes after birth for rapid evaluation of early cardiopulmonary adaptation. If the Apgar score is 8 or higher, usually no intervention other than promoting normal respiratory efforts is needed. If the infant is obviously in distress (i.e., no or low heart rate and/or respirations, limp muscle tone, lack of response to stimulation, blue or pale color), interventions to correct the problem are instituted immediately rather than awaiting the 1-minute Apgar score.

Keep the infant in a flat or slightly head-dependent position briefly while secretions drain. After the infant has a vigorous cry and minimal secretions, tilt the baby to one side with the head flat or slightly elevated. Keeping the infant in a head-dependent position longer than needed limits diaphragm movement because of pressure from the intestines. Suction secretions from the infant's mouth and nose with a bulb syringe as needed, and teach parents how to use the bulb syringe (see p. 560).

#### SUPPORTING THERMOREGULATION

Dry the infant to reduce evaporative heat loss. Dry the head well because substantial heat loss can occur from the head, which is about one fourth of the neonate's body surface area.

## TABLE 13–4 APGAR SCORE*

| Assessment | Points 0 | 1 | 2 |
|---|---|---|---|
| Heart rate | Absent | Below 100/min | 100/min or higher |
| Respiratory effort | No spontaneous respirations | Slow respirations or weak cry | Spontaneous respirations with a strong, lusty cry |
| Muscle tone | Limp | Minimal flexion of extremities; sluggish movement | Flexed body posture; spontaneous and vigorous movement |
| Reflex response | No response to suction or gentle slap on soles | Minimal response (grimace) to suction or gentle slap on soles | Responds promptly to suction or a gentle slap to the sole with cry or active movement |
| Color | Pallor or cyanosis | Bluish hands and feet | Pink (light-skinned) or absence of cyanosis (dark-skinned) |

* The Apgar score is a method of rapid evaluation of the infant's cardiorespiratory adaptation after birth. The nurse scores the infant at 1 minute and 5 minutes in each of five areas. The assessments are arranged from most important (heart rate) to least important (color). The infant is assigned a score of 0 to 2 in each of the five areas and the scores are totaled. General guidelines for the infant's care are based on three ranges of 1 minute scores:

| 0 1 2 3 | 4 5 6 7 | 8 9 10 |
|---|---|---|
| Infant needs resuscitation. | Gently stimulate by rubbing the infant's back while administering oxygen. Determine whether mother received narcotics, which may have depressed infant's respirations. Have naloxone (Narcan) available for administration. | Provide no action other than support of the infant's spontaneous efforts and continued observation. |

Place the infant in a prewarmed radiant warmer to limit heat loss while giving initial care (see p. 561). Skin-to-skin contact with a parent has the same effect and also promotes bonding. Avoid coming between the infant and the heat source. Wrap the infant in warm blankets when he or she is not in the warmer or making skin-to-skin contact. A stockinette cap further reduces heat loss if placed on the baby's *dry* head. A cap is not worn in the radiant warmer because the cap slows transfer of heat to the baby.

#### IDENTIFYING THE INFANT

Bands having matching imprinted numbers and identifying information are the primary means to ensure that the right baby goes to the right mother after any separation (Fig. 13–8). Apply two bands on the infant, one on an arm and another on an ankle, or one on each ankle to prevent facial scratching. Infant bands are applied more snugly than they would be if worn by an adult: about one adult fingerwidth of slack in the bands. Apply the longer band to the mother's wrist. A fourth band is usually worn by the father or other primary support person. Check that imprinted numbers and names are identical on each set of bands. A set is needed for each baby in a multiple birth.

### CARE OF THE MOTHER

Nursing care of the mother during the fourth stage of labor focuses on observing for hemorrhage and relieving discomfort. Table 13–5 summarizes problems during the fourth stage of labor.

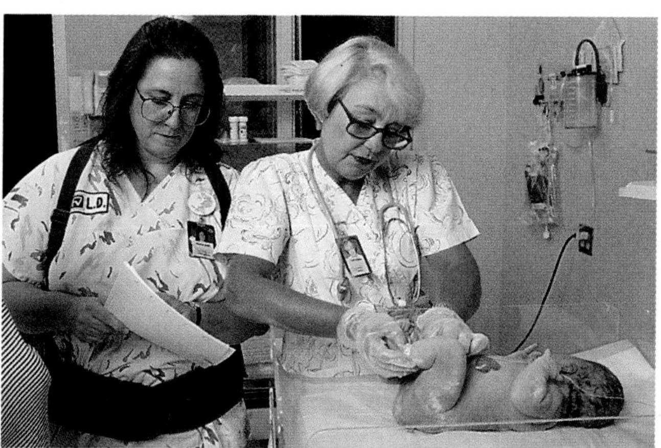

**FIGURE 13–8**

When the birthing room nurse turns care of the newborn over to the nursery nurse, both check the identification bands and record for the same information.

**TABLE 13–5 PROBLEMS DURING THE FOURTH STAGE OF LABOR**

| Sign | Potential Problem | Immediate Nursing Action |
|---|---|---|
| Rising pulse rate and/or falling blood pressure | An early sign of hypovolemia due to excessive blood loss (visible or concealed) | Identify the probable cause of the blood loss, usually a poorly contracted uterus. Take steps to correct it (see below). |
| Soft (boggy) uterus | A poorly contracted uterus does not adequately compress large open vessels at the placental site, resulting in hemorrhage. | With one hand securing the uterus just above the symphysis, and the other on the fundus, massage the uterus until firm. Push downward on the *firm* uterus to expel any clots. Empty the woman's bladder (by voiding or catheterization) if that is contributing to the uterine atony. |
| High uterine fundus, often displaced to one side | Suggests a full bladder that can interfere with uterine contraction and result in hemorrhage | Massage the uterus if it is not firm. Help the woman urinate in the bathroom or on the bedpan. If she cannot void, catheterize her. |
| Lochia exceeding one *saturated* perineal pad per hour during the fourth stage | Suggests hemorrhage; however, perineal pads vary in their absorbency, and this must be considered. | Identify cause of hemorrhage, usually uterine atony, which is manifested by a soft uterus. Correct the cause. If lacerations are the suspected cause (excess bleeding with a firm fundus), notify the birth attendant. Keep the woman NPO until the birth attendant evaluates her. |
| Intense perineal or vaginal pain, poorly relieved with analgesics | Hematoma, usually of vaginal wall or perineum; signs of hypovolemia may occur with substantial blood loss into tissues. | If the hematoma is visible, apply cold packs to the area to slow bleeding into tissues. Notify the birth attendant, and anticipate possible surgical drainage. Keep the woman NPO. |

OBSERVING FOR HEMORRHAGE

Important assessments related to hemorrhage are the woman's vital signs, uterine fundus, bladder, and lochia. For detailed information about these assessments, see Chapter 17.

**Vital Signs.** Assess the woman's temperature when fourth-stage care begins. Assess her blood pressure, pulse, and respirations every 15 minutes during the first hour. A rising pulse is an early sign of excessive blood loss because the heart pumps faster to compensate for reduced blood volume. The blood pressure may fall as the blood volume diminishes.

**Fundus.** The most common reason for excessive postpartum bleeding is that the uterus does not firmly contract and compress open vessels at the placental site. Assess the firmness, height, and positioning of the uterine fundus with each vital sign assessment. The fundus should be firm, in the midline, and below the umbilicus (about the size of a large grapefruit). If the fundus is firm, no massage is needed; if it is soft (boggy), massage it until it is firm. Nipple stimulation from the infant's sucking releases natural oxytocin from the mother's posterior pituitary gland to maintain firm uterine contraction. Oxytocin in the intravenous solution or intramuscularly has the same effect.

**Bladder.** A full bladder interferes with contraction of the uterus and may lead to hemorrhage. Suspect a full bladder if the fundus is above the umbilicus or is displaced to one side, usually the right. If there is no contraindication, such as altered sensation, the mother can walk to the bathroom (with assistance the first few times). The first two voidings are often measured until it is evident that she voids without difficulty and empties her bladder completely. Each voiding is usually at least 300 to 400 ml if she is emptying her bladder.

**Lochia.** Assess lochia with each vital sign and fundal assessment. The amount of lochia seems large to the inexperienced nurse and the new mother. Perineal pads vary in their absorbency, but *saturation* of one pad within the first hour is a guideline for the maximum normal lochia flow. Observe for lochia that pools under the mother's buttocks and back. Small clots may be present, but the presence of large clots is not normal and the physician or nurse-midwife should be notified. A continuous trickle of bright red blood when the fundus is firm suggests a laceration in the birth canal. A hematoma causes bleeding into the tissues, but the visible bleeding is unusual.

#### RELIEVING DISCOMFORT

Uterine contractions (afterpains) and perineal trauma are common causes of pain after birth. A postpartum chill often adds to discomfort. Pain is usually mild and readily relieved by simple measures. Notify the birth attendant if pain is intense or does not respond to common relief measures.

**Ice Packs.** Apply an ice pack to the perineum promptly after birth to reduce edema and limit hematoma formation. Small hematomas are common, but a rapidly enlarging hematoma causes significant concealed blood loss and pain. Some perineal pads have chemical cold packs incorporated in them. These pads absorb less lochia than ordinary pads, so this should be considered when estimating pad saturation.

**Analgesics.** Afterpains and perineal pain respond well to mild oral analgesics. Regular urination reduces the severity of afterpains because the uterus contracts more effectively.

**Warmth.** A warm blanket is soothing and can shorten the chill that is common after birth. A portable radiant warmer provides warmth to both the mother and infant. The mother may enjoy warm drinks.

### PROMOTING EARLY FAMILY ATTACHMENT

The first hour after birth is an ideal time for parent-infant attachment because the healthy neonate is alert and responsive. Provide privacy while unobtrusively observing the parents and infant. The infant can remain in the parent's arms to take vital signs or suction small amounts of secretions.

Assist the mother to breastfeed during the recovery period if she desires. The infant is usually attentive and nurses briefly. Early nipple stimulation helps initiate milk production.

When the parents are ready, allow siblings, other family members, and friends to visit. Help siblings to see and touch their new brother or sister by putting a stool at the bedside or letting them sit on the bed.

Toddlers are often upset by separation from their mother and may not be interested in the new baby. With supervision, children of preschool age or older may sit in a chair and hold the baby. School-aged children are often fascinated by the new baby and surroundings and ask many questions. Adolescents react in various ways. They may be excited and eager to be a substitute parent, or they may be embarrassed about their parents having a new baby "at their age."

Observe for signs of early parent-infant attachment. Parent behaviors are tentative at first, progressing from fingertip touch to palm touch to enfolding of the infant. Expect parents to make eye contact with the infant and talk to a baby in higher-pitched, affectionate tones.

Cultural variations should be considered when assessing early attachment. The nurse should be knowledgeable about the typical practices of the populations commonly served. In some cultures, great attention to the newborn is considered unlucky ("evil eye"). See Chapter 18 for further discussion of parent-infant attachment and the variations a nurse might encounter.

## Nursing Care Plan 13–1

## Normal Labor and Birth

**ASSESSMENT:** Cathy Taggart, 17 years old, is a gravida I, para 0, who has just been admitted in early labor. Her cervix is 3 cm dilated and completely effaced, and the fetus is at a 0 station. Her membranes are intact. Cathy's husband Tim is with her. They did not attend childbirth classes. Cathy is holding Tim's hand tightly and breathing rapidly with each contraction. She says in a shaky voice, "I'm so scared. I've never been in a hospital before. I just don't know if I can do this."

**Critical Thinking**

Are there any assumptions or biases that the nurse must avoid in this situation?

**ANSWER**

The nurse should not assume that a 17-year-old girl is not married to the baby's father. He or she should not assume that because the parents are young and did not attend childbirth classes they are not interested in the baby or Cathy will tolerate labor's demands poorly. The nurse should consider Cathy's age and non-attendance in childbirth classes when supporting her during birth but should assess her needs individually, as with all clients.

**NURSING DIAGNOSIS:** Anxiety related to unfamiliar environment and lack of birth preparation

*Nursing Care Plan continued on following page*

## Nursing Care Plan 13–1 *Continued*
# Normal Labor and Birth

### Critical Thinking

What cues led the nurse to choose this nursing diagnosis?

**ANSWER**

Several objective facts relate to the nursing diagnosis: (1) Cathy is having her first baby; (2) she has never been in the hospital; (3) she and Tim did not attend childbirth classes; (4) she is in early labor; (5) she has physical signs of anxiety—holding tightly to Tim, breathing rapidly, and talking shakily; (6) she says she is "scared"; (7) she expresses doubt about her ability to tolerate labor. Although Cathy is probably having pain with contractions, anxiety is her dominant problem at this time.

**GOALS/EXPECTED OUTCOMES**

Cathy will do the following:

1. Express a reduction in her anxiety after admission procedures are completed.
2. Have a relaxed facial and body posture between contractions.

| INTERVENTION | RATIONALE |
|---|---|
| 1. Maintain a calm and confident manner when caring for Cathy. Express confidence in her ability to give birth. | 1. Provides nonverbal and verbal reassurance that labor is normal and that she has the resources within her to manage it. |
| 2. Use therapeutic communication when talking with Cathy. Adapt communication to the changing situation, simplifying explanations and directions as labor intensifies. | 2. Identifies dominant concerns so that they can be properly addressed. Intense physical sensations reduce the ability to comprehend complex information. |
| 3. Determine the couple's plans for birth and work within them as much as possible. | 3. Enhances their sense of control and helps them to have a satisfying birth experience. |
| 4. Stay with Cathy as much as possible during labor. | 4. Provides reassurance of human contact and reduces fears of abandonment. |
| 5. Orient Cathy to the labor room and explain procedures and equipment she will encounter. | 5. Reduces fear of the unknown. |

**EVALUATION**

Cathy relaxes a bit after talking with the nurse and slows her breathing. She still holds Tim's hand, but not as tightly. Cathy says, "I feel a little better now. I hope I can have my baby before you go home."

**ASSESSMENT:** Cathy's admission vital signs are all normal: Temperature 98.8°F, pulse 88, respirations 20, and blood pressure 112/70. The FHR averages 140 to 150. Her contractions are every 4 minutes, duration of 50 seconds, and of moderate intensity.

**POTENTIAL COMPLICATION:** Fetal compromise.

**GOALS/EXPECTED OUTCOMES**

Goals are not formulated for a potential complication because the nurse cannot independently manage fetal compromise. The nurse will do the following:

1. Take actions to promote normal placental function.
2. Observe for and report signs associated with fetal compromise.

| INTERVENTION | RATIONALE |
|---|---|
| 1. Encourage Cathy to use any position she desires except the supine. | 1. The supine position can cause aortocaval compression, reducing blood flow to the placenta. |

## *Nursing Care Plan 13–1 Continued*
# *Normal Labor and Birth*

| INTERVENTION | RATIONALE |
|---|---|
| 2. Assess and document the FHR using the guidelines in Table 13–2. Report rates outside the normal 110 to 160 BPM or slowing that persists after contractions. Assess the FHR more frequently if deviations from normal are identified. | 2. Allows prompt identification of changes in the rate or of abnormal rates. FHR assessments that are outside expected limits should be reported for possible medical intervention. |
| 3. When the membranes rupture, observe the color, odor, and approximate amount of fluid; note the time of rupture. | 3. Normal amniotic fluid is clear and does not have a strong or foul odor. Meconium-stained fluid may be associated with fetal compromise and should be reported. Cloudy, yellow, or foul-smelling fluid suggests infection. Prolonged rupture of membranes increases the risk of infection. |
| 4. Assess contractions using guidelines in Table 13–1. Report contraction durations longer than 90 seconds, intervals shorter than 60 seconds, or incomplete uterine relaxation between contractions. | 4. Most placental exchange occurs during the interval between contractions. Contractions that are too long or an inadequate interval between them decreases the time available for the intervillous spaces of the placenta to eliminate wastes and refill with oxygenated blood and nutrients. |
| 5. Assess Cathy's blood pressure, pulse, and respirations every hour. Assess her temperature every 4 hours until her membranes rupture, then every 2 hours. | 5. Maternal hypotension or hypertension can decrease blood flow to the placenta. Maternal fever can increase the fetus' demand for oxygen beyond the mother's ability to supply it. A rising maternal pulse or FHR may precede the temperature elevation. |
| 6. See Nursing Care Plan 14–1 for additional interventions if signs of fetal compromise occur. | 6. This nursing care plan addresses only basic actions to promote fetal oxygenation and identify possible problems. |

**EVALUATION**

Because no client goal is established for a potential complication, evaluation is not done. The FHR remains at approximately the same rate, and no signs of fetal compromise occur. Cathy finds that sitting in a rocking chair is most comfortable.

**ASSESSMENT:** In 1½ hours, Cathy's cervical dilation progresses to 5 cm, and the fetus descends to a +1 station. Her contractions are every 3 minutes, 60 seconds long, and of strong intensity. The FHR remains near its admission level. Cathy is having difficulty relaxing between contractions and is complaining of back pain. She is relieved that her labor is progressing normally.

**NURSING DIAGNOSIS:** Pain related to effects of uterine contractions

**GOAL/EXPECTED OUTCOME**

Cathy will express that she can manage labor pain satisfactorily.

| INTERVENTION | RATIONALE |
|---|---|
| 1. Encourage Cathy to try positions such as standing/sitting and leaning forward, side-lying, leaning over the back of the bed, or hands and knees. Remind her to change positions about every half hour or when she feels the need for a change. | 1. These positions shift the weight of the fetus away from the sacral promontory, reducing back pain. Alternating positions relieves strain and constant pressure and also helps the fetus to adapt to the pelvis. |
| 2. Teach Tim to rub or to apply firm pressure to Cathy's back. Ask her where the best place is and how hard to press. Apply powder to the area rubbed. | 2. Back rubs or firm pressure counteracts some of the back pain. Powder decreases friction and promotes skin comfort. |

*Nursing Care Plan continued on following page*

## Nursing Care Plan 13–1 *Continued*
# Normal Labor and Birth

| INTERVENTION | RATIONALE |
| --- | --- |
| 3. Offer thermal pain management options:<br>a. Warm blanket or hot pack to her back<br>b. Cold packs to her back<br>c. Alternate warm and cold packs, or use them for 20 minutes on and 20 minutes off<br>d. Warm water in a shower or whirlpool | 3. Thermal stimulation interferes with transmission of pain impulses. Changing the thermal stimulation prevents habituation. Nipple stimulation in a shower or whirlpool causes release of oxytocin from the posterior pituitary and enhances contractions. |
| 4. Teach Cathy simple breathing and relaxation techniques (see Chapters 11 and 15). | 4. Provides distraction from pain and gives her a sense of control. Relaxation enhances a woman's ability to manage pain and enhances normal labor processes. |
| 5. Observe Cathy's suprapubic area and palpate for a full bladder every 2 hours. Remind her to void if she has not done so recently. | 5. A full bladder contributes to discomfort and can prolong labor by obstructing fetal descent. |
| 6. Tell Cathy about her progress in labor. Explain that she will probably begin to dilate faster now that she has entered active labor. | 6. Encouragement and the knowledge that her efforts are having the desired results increases a woman's willingness to continue. |
| 7. Tell Cathy what pharmacologic pain relief measures are available to her. | 7. Knowing available options gives the woman a sense of control because she can choose whether she wants these measures. (This action may be done during early labor to give a woman more time to consider her options.) |
| 8. See Nursing Care Plan 15–1 for additional interventions. | 8. Provides guidance about several non-pharmacologic and pharmacologic pain management measures. |

EVALUATION

Cathy continues to have back pain but says that she is more comfortable sitting on the side of the bed with her head on a pillow on the overbed table. Tim rubs her back during contractions. She says she is able to manage the pain and does not want medication yet.

ASSESSMENT: After another 2 hours, Cathy is quite uncomfortable and requests pain medication. She is occasionally feeling an urge to push. Cathy cries and says she is "losing it" and "can't take it anymore." Tim asks anxiously, "What's wrong? Is Cathy OK? Why is she acting this way?" The FHR remains near the admission range and shows no signs suggesting fetal compromise. Contractions are every 2 minutes, 70 seconds, and strong.

**Critical Thinking**

What do these observations suggest? Does the nurse need more data?

**ANSWER**

Cathy's behaviors and the characteristics of her contractions suggest that she has entered the transition phase of first-stage labor, but her urge to push could indicate that she is in second-stage labor. The nurse usually does a vaginal examination at this point to determine whether to discourage or encourage Cathy's pushing and to identify the most appropriate pain-relief methods.

ASSESSMENT: A vaginal examination reveals that Cathy's cervix is 8 cm dilated and the station is +1. Butorphanol (Stadol), 0.5 mg IV, gives her enough analgesia to regain control and work with her contractions. She avoids pushing by blowing out at the peak of each contraction.

Cathy is fully dilated in 45 minutes, and the fetal station is +2. She pushes spontaneously several times with each contraction, but tends to stiffen her back and push on the bed with her arms with each push. She pushes for about 10 to 15 seconds at a time, holding her breath each time. She prefers a semi-sitting position.

NURSING DIAGNOSIS: Knowledge Deficit: Effective pushing techniques

GOAL/EXPECTED OUTCOME

After instruction in more effective pushing techniques, Cathy will use the techniques until the birth occurs.

## Nursing Care Plan 13–1 *Continued*
## Normal Labor and Birth

| INTERVENTION | RATIONALE |
|---|---|
| 1. Observe Cathy's perineum for fetal crowning with each push. | 1. A woman having her first baby can still give birth rapidly. Observation permits the nurse to maintain her safety and that of the baby should rapid birth occur. |
| 2. Encourage Cathy to exhale as she pushes strongly for about 4 to 6 seconds at a time. | 2. Prolonged pushing against a closed glottis reduces blood return to the heart and maternal oxygen saturation and decreases placental blood flow, especially if it is done with every contraction. |
| 3. Teach Cathy techniques to make each push more effective:<br>a. Flex head slightly with each push.<br>b. Pull against her flexed knees (or hand holds on the bed) as she pushes, curving her body around her uterus. Encourage upright positions, including squatting.<br>c. Push toward the vaginal outlet.<br>d. Relax her perineum as she pushes down.<br>e. Keep her sacrum flattened against the bed when she pushes. | 3. a. Directs each push downward into the pelvic cavity.<br>b. Provides leverage to gain more effective push from abdominal muscles. Upright positions take advantage of gravity, and squatting enlarges the pelvic outlet slightly.<br>c. Anatomically correct direction.<br>d. Reduces soft tissue resistance to fetal descent.<br>e. Straightens pelvic curve somewhat (similar to squatting). |
| 4. Do not talk to Cathy unnecessarily between contractions. | 4. Allows her to conserve her energy for pushing efforts. |

**EVALUATION**

Cathy pushes more effectively with the nurse coaching her during each contraction. In another hour, she gives birth to a 7-pound, 6-ounce (3346-g) boy. The baby's Apgar scores are 9 at both 1 and 5 minutes. Cathy has a small first-degree laceration that is sutured with a local anesthetic. The new family gets acquainted during the recovery period.

**ADDITIONAL NURSING DIAGNOSES TO CONSIDER**

Impaired Verbal Communication
Ineffective Family or Individual Coping
Fluid Volume Deficit
Risk for Injury
Powerlessness
Sensory/Perceptual Alterations

## SUMMARY CONCEPTS

- Some women do not have symptoms typical of true labor. They should enter the birth center for evaluation if they are uncertain or have concerns other than those listed in the guidelines.
- The childbearing family's first impression on admission to the intrapartum unit is important to promote a therapeutic relationship with caregivers and a positive birth experience.
- The initial intrapartum assessments are to quickly evaluate maternal and fetal health and labor status.
- The fetus is the more vulnerable of the maternal-fetal pair because of complete dependence on the mother's physiologic systems.
- The normal FHR at term averages 110 to 120 BPM at the lower limit and 150 to 160 BPM at the upper limit. Other reassuring findings include the presence of variability in the electronically monitored fetus, accelerations of at least 15 BPM, and absence of decelerations following contractions.
- Persistent contraction durations of longer than 90 seconds or intervals shorter than 60 seconds may reduce placental blood flow and fetal oxygen, nutrient, and waste product exchange.
- A maternal supine position can reduce placental blood flow because the uterus compresses the aorta and inferior vena cava.
- General comfort measures promote the woman's ability to relax and cope with labor.
- Regular changes in position during labor promote maternal comfort and help the fetus adapt to the pelvis.
- The nurse must be alert for signs of impending

birth: The woman may state, "The baby's coming"; she may make grunting sounds; or she may be bearing down.
- The priority nursing care of the newborn immediately after birth is to promote normal respirations, maintain normal body temperature, and promote attachment.
- The priority nursing care of the mother after birth is to assess for hemorrhage, promote firm uterine contraction, and promote parent-infant attachment.

### *References and Readings*

American Academy of Pediatrics and American College of Obstetricians and Gynecologists. (1992). *Guidelines for perinatal care* (3rd ed.). Elk Grove Village, Ill. & Washington, D.C.: Author.

American College of Obstetricians and Gynecologists (ACOG). (1995a). ACOG *practice patterns: Vaginal delivery after previous cesarean birth.* Washington, D.C.: Author.

American College of Obstetricians and Gynecologists (ACOG). (1995b). ACOG *technical bulletin number* 207: *Fetal heart rate patterns: Monitoring, interpretation, and management.* Washington, D.C.: Author.

American College of Obstetricians and Gynecologists (ACOG). (1996). ACOG *technical bulletin number* 219: *Hypertension in pregnancy.* Washington, D.C.: Author.

Arrabal, P.P., & Nagey, D.A. (1996). Is manual palpation of uterine contractions accurate? *American Journal of Obstetrics and Gynecology,* 174(1, part 1), 217–219.

Bachman, J., & Kendrick, J.M. (1996). Childbirth. In K.R. Rice & P.A. Creehan (Eds.), *Perinatal nursing* (pp. 151–186). Philadelphia: J.B. Lippincott.

Biancuzzo, M. (1993). Six myths of maternal posture during labor. MCN: *American Journal of Maternal-Child Nursing,* 18(5): 264–269.

Bowes, W.A. (1994). Clinical aspects of normal and abnormal labor. In R. Creasy & R. Resnik (Eds.), *Maternal-fetal medicine: Principles and practice* (3rd ed., pp. 527–557). Philadelphia: W.B. Saunders.

Bryanton, J., Fraser-Davey, H., & Sullivan, P. (1994). Women's perceptions of nursing support during labor. *Journal of Obstetric, Gynecologic, and Neonatal Nursing,* 23(3), 638–644.

Burian, J. (1995). Helping survivors of sexual abuse through labor. MCN: *American Journal of Maternal/Child Nursing,* 20(5), 252–256.

Callister, L.C. (1995). Cultural meanings of childbirth. *Journal of Obstetric, Gynecologic, and Neonatal Nursing,* 24(4), 327–331.

Chapman, L.L. (1992). Expectant fathers' roles during labor and birth. *Journal of Obstetric, Gynecologic, and Neonatal Nursing,* 21(2), 114–120.

Creehan, P.A. (1996). Pain relief and comfort measures during labor. In K.R. Rice & P.A. Creehan (Eds.), *Perinatal nursing* (pp. 227–245). Philadelphia: J.B. Lippincott.

Cunningham, F.G., MacDonald, P.C., Gant, N.F., Leveno, K.J., Gilstrap, L.C., Hankins, G.D.V., et al. (1997). *Williams obstetrics* (20th ed.). Norwalk, Conn.: Appleton & Lange.

Enkin, M.W., Keirse, M.J., Renfrew, M.J., & Neilson, J.P. (1995). Effective care in pregnancy and childbirth: A synopsis. *Birth,* 22(2), 101–110.

Evans, S., & Jeffrey, J. (1995). Maternal learning needs during labor and delivery. *Journal of Obstetric, Gynecologic, and Neonatal Nursing,* 24(3), 235–240.

Gagnon, A.J., & Waghorn, K. (1996). Supportive care by maternity nurses: A work sampling study in an intrapartum unit. *Birth* 23(1):1–6.

Hodnett, E. (1996). Nursing support of the laboring woman. *Journal of Obstetric, Gynecologic, and Neonatal Nursing,* 25(3), 257–264.

Hutchinson, M.K., & Baqi-Aziz, M. (1994). Nursing care of the childbearing Muslim family. *Journal of Obstetric, Gynecologic, and Neonatal Nursing,* 23(9), 767–771.

Jackson, M.M., & Rymer, T.E. (1995). Nurses: At special risk. *Journal of Obstetric, Gynecologic, and Neonatal Nursing,* 24(6), 533–540.

Khazoyan, C.M., & Anderson, N.L.R. (1994). Latinas' expectations for their partners during childbirth. MCN: *American Journal of Maternal-Child Nursing,* 19(4), 226–229.

Kliegman, R.M. (1994). Fetal and neonatal medicine. In R.E. Behrman & R.M. Kliegman (Eds.), *Nelson essentials of pediatrics* (2nd ed., pp. 157–213). Philadelphia: W.B. Saunders.

Letko, M.D. (1996). Understanding the Apgar score. *Journal of Obstetric, Gynecologic, and Neonatal Nursing,* 25(4), 299–303.

Mackey, M.C., & Flanders-Stephans, M.E. (1994). Women's evaluations of their labor and delivery nurses. *Journal of Obstetric, Gynecologic, and Neonatal Nursing,* 23(5), 413–420.

Mattson, S. (1995). Culturally sensitive perinatal care for Southeast Asians. *Journal of Obstetric, Gynecologic, and Neonatal Nursing,* 24(4), 335–341.

Menihan, C.A. (1996). Intrapartum fetal monitoring. In K.R. Rice & P.A. Creehan (Eds.), *Perinatal nursing* (pp. 187–225). Philadelphia: J.B. Lippincott.

Murray, M. (1997). *Antepartal and intrapartal fetal monitoring* (2nd ed.). Albuquerque, N.Mex.: Learning Resources International.

NAACOG (now AWHONN). (1990). *Fetal heart rate auscultation.* Washington, D.C.: Author.

Nelsson-Ryan, S. (1988). Positioning: Second stage labor. In F.H. Nichols & S.S. Humenick (Eds.), *Childbirth education: Practice, research, & theory* (pp. 256–274). Philadelphia: W.B. Saunders.

Pavlik, M. (1988). Positioning: First stage labor. In F.H. Nichols & S.S. Humenick (Eds.), *Childbirth education: Practice, research, & theory* (pp. 234–254). Philadelphia: W.B. Saunders.

Roberts, J., & Woolley, D. (1996). A second look at the second stage of labor. *Journal of Obstetric, Gynecologic, and Neonatal Nursing,* 25(5), 415–423.

Rothman, B.K. (1996). Women, providers, & control. *Journal of Obstetric, Gynecologic, and Neonatal Nursing,* 25(3), 253–256.

Rush, J., Burlock, S., Lambert, K., Loosley-Millman, M., Hutchison, B., & Enkin, M. (1996). The effects of whirlpool baths in labor: A randomized controlled trial. *Birth,* 23(3), 136–143.

Simkin, P. (1996). The experience of maternity in a woman's life. *Journal of Obstetric, Gynecologic, and Neonatal Nursing,* 25(3), 247–252.

Supplee, R.B., & Vezeau, T.M. (1996). Continuous electronic fetal monitoring: Does it belong in low-risk births? MCN: *American Journal of Maternal and Child Nursing,* 21(6), 301–306.

Tomlinson, P.S., & Mattson Bryan, A.A. (1996). Family centered intrapartum care: Revisiting an old concept. *Journal of Obstetric, Gynecologic, and Neonatal Nursing,* 25(4), 331–337.

Waymire, V. (1997). A triggering time: Childbirth may recall sexual abuse memories. *Lifelines,* 1(2), 47–50.

# 14

# Intrapartum Fetal Monitoring

**OBJECTIVES**

1. Identify the purposes of fetal surveillance during labor.
2. Explain the normal and pathologic mechanisms that influence fetal heart rate.
3. Identify the advantages and limitations of each method of intrapartum fetal surveillance: auscultation and electronic monitoring.
4. Explain the types of equipment used for electronic fetal monitoring during labor, including the advantages and limitations of each.
5. Describe the interpretation of electronic fetal monitoring data.
6. Explain the methods that may be used in addition to electronic fetal monitoring to judge fetal well-being.
7. Describe appropriate responses to nonreassuring fetal heart rate patterns.
8. Use the nursing process to plan care for a woman having intrapartum electronic fetal monitoring.

**DEFINITIONS**

**acidosis** *A condition resulting from accumulation of acid (hydrogen ions) or depletion of base (bicarbonate). The pH measures acid-base balance.*

**amnioinfusion** *Infusion of lactated Ringer's solution or isotonic saline into the uterine cavity during labor to reduce umbilical cord compression; also done to dilute meconium in amniotic fluid, reducing the risk that the infant will aspirate thick meconium at birth.*

**asphyxia** *Insufficient oxygen and excess carbon dioxide in the blood and tissues.*

**baroreceptors** *Cells that are sensitive to blood pressure changes.*

**chemoreceptors** *Cells that are sensitive to chemical changes in the blood, specifically changes in oxygen and carbon dioxide levels, and in acid-base balance.*

**hypercapnia** *Excess carbon dioxide in the blood, evidenced by an elevated* $Pco_2$.

**hypertonic contractions** *Uterine contractions that are too long or too frequent, have too short a resting interval, or have an inadequate relaxation period to allow optimal uteroplacental exchange.*

**hypoxemia** *Reduced oxygenation of the blood, evidenced by a low* $Po_2$.

**hypoxia** *Reduced availability of oxygen to the body tissues.*

**intermittent monitoring** *A variation of electronic fetal monitoring in which an initial strip is obtained on admission. If patterns are reassuring, the woman is remonitored for 15 minutes at regular intervals (about every 30 to 60 minutes).*

**nuchal cord** *Umbilical cord around the fetal neck.*

**telemetry** *Transmission of electronic fetal monitoring data to the bedside monitor unit with radio signals.*

**tocolytic** *A drug that inhibits uterine contractions.*

**transducer** *A device that translates one physical quantity to another, such as fetal heart motion to an electrical signal for rate calculation or generation of sound or of a written record.*

**uterine resting tone** *Degree of uterine muscle tension when the woman is not in labor or during the interval between labor contractions.*

Intrapartum fetal monitoring is the process of fetal surveillance to identify signs associated with well-being and with compromise. Accurate assessment of these signs permits appropriate and timely care to reduce hazards to the fetus. At a minimum, intrapartum fetal monitoring includes assessment of the fetal heart rate (FHR) and the mother's uterine activity. More comprehensive monitoring may add assessment of fetal activity, fetal response to stimulation, and evaluation of fetal blood gases and pH.

During labor there are two clients: the expectant mother and her fetus. The purposes of intrapartum fetal monitoring are to evaluate how the fetus tolerates labor and to identify hypoxic insult to the fetus during labor. Fetal monitoring cannot identify every compromised fetus.

Two basic approaches are taken to intrapartum fetal monitoring: a low-technology approach and electronic fetal monitoring. Each has advantages and limitations. The nurse may use either or both of these approaches to assess a fetus during labor, depending on the woman's wishes, risk status, and facility policy.

The low-technology approach uses auscultation of the FHR and palpation of uterine activity. In the United States, this type of fetal observation is more often used in home births and birth centers. It may be used during hospital births as well.

Electronic fetal monitoring is the second approach to intrapartum fetal surveillance. Although it is the more commonly used method in U.S. hospital births, its routine use remains controversial because its benefits to the fetus are not always clear.

# Fetal Oxygenation

Adequate fetal oxygenation requires five related factors:

1. Normal maternal blood flow and volume to the placenta
2. Normal oxygen saturation in maternal blood
3. Adequate exchange of oxygen and carbon dioxide in the placenta
4. An open circulatory path between the placenta and the fetus through vessels in the umbilical cord
5. Normal fetal circulatory and oxygen-carrying functions

Labor is stressful on a fetus, but several mechanisms exist to compensate for these stresses. One must understand the dynamics of uteroplacental exchange and fetal circulation to understand fetal responses to labor. (Also see Chapter 6 for discussion of fetal circulation and placental functions.)

## Uteroplacental Exchange

Oxygen-rich and nutrient-rich blood from the mother enters the intervillous spaces of the placenta via the spiral arteries (see Fig. 6–7). Oxygen and nutrients in the maternal blood pass into the fetal blood that circulates within capillaries in the intervillous spaces. Carbon dioxide and other waste products pass from the fetal blood into the maternal blood at the same time. Maternal blood carrying fetal waste products drains from the intervillous spaces through endometrial veins and returns to the mother's circulation for elimination by her body. Substances pass back and forth between mother and fetus without mixing of maternal and fetal blood.

During labor, contractions gradually compress the spiral arteries, temporarily stopping maternal blood flow into the intervillous spaces. The fetus depends on the oxygen supply already present in body cells, fetal erythrocytes, and the intervillous spaces during contractions. The oxygen supply in these areas is enough for about 1 to 2 minutes. As each contraction relaxes, fresh oxygenated maternal blood reenters the intervillous spaces and carbon dioxide–laden blood drains out.

## Fetal Circulation

The fetal heart circulates oxygenated blood from the placenta throughout the body and returns deoxygenated blood to the placenta. The umbilical vein carries oxygenated blood to the fetus, and the two umbilical arteries carry deoxygenated blood from the fetus to the placenta (see Fig. 6–7).

## Regulation of Fetal Heart Rate

Mechanisms that regulate the heart rate are balanced to maintain cardiac output at a level that keeps the fetal heart and brain oxygenated. Fetal cardiac output increase is primarily accomplished by an increase in the heart rate. Conversely, a marked decrease in FHR decreases the cardiac output.

Five fetal factors interact to regulate the FHR: (1) autonomic nervous system, (2) baroreceptors, (3) chemoreceptors, (4) central nervous system, and (5) adrenal glands. The balance among forces that increase and those that slow the heart rate result in the characteristic fluctuations in FHR during the latter one third of pregnancy.

#### AUTONOMIC NERVOUS SYSTEM

The sympathetic and parasympathetic branches of the autonomic nervous system are balanced forces that regulate the FHR. Sympathetic stimulation increases the heart rate and strengthens myocardial contractions through release of epinephrine and norepinephrine. The net result of sympathetic stimulation is an increase in cardiac output.

The parasympathetic nervous system, through stimulation of the vagus nerve, reduces the FHR and maintains short-term variability (see p. 361). The parasympathetic branch gradually exerts greater influence as the fetus matures, beginning between 28 and 32 weeks of gestation. Therefore, the average FHR in the term fetus is lower than in the preterm fetus.

#### BARORECEPTORS

Cells in the carotid arch and major arteries respond to stretching when the fetal blood pressure increases. The baroreceptors stimulate the vagus nerve to slow the FHR and decrease the blood pressure, thus lowering cardiac output.

#### CHEMORECEPTORS

Cells that respond to changes in oxygen, carbon dioxide, and pH are found in the medulla oblongata and in the aortic and carotid bodies. Decreased oxygen, increased carbon dioxide content, or a lower pH in the blood or cerebrospinal fluid triggers an increase in the heart rate. However, prolonged hypoxia, hypercapnia, and acidosis depress the FHR.

#### ADRENAL GLANDS

The adrenal medulla secretes epinephrine and norepinephrine in response to stress, causing a sympathetic response that accelerates the FHR. The adrenal cortex responds to a fall in the fetal blood pressure with release of aldosterone and retention of sodium and water, resulting in an increase in the circulating fetal blood volume.

#### CENTRAL NERVOUS SYSTEM

The fetal cerebral cortex causes the heart rate to increase during fetal movement and decrease when the fetus sleeps. The hypothalamus coordinates the two branches of the autonomic nervous system. The medulla oblongata maintains the balance between stimuli that speed and stimuli that slow the heart rate.

### Pathologic Influences on Fetal Oxygenation

Compromise of fetal oxygenation may occur because of alterations in any of the placental or fetal factors or those of the pregnant woman.

#### MATERNAL CARDIOPULMONARY ALTERATIONS

Actual or relative reductions in the mother's circulating blood volume impair perfusion of the intervillous spaces with oxygenated maternal blood. Hemorrhage causes an actual decrease in her blood volume. Relative reductions in maternal circulating volume involve altered distribution of the blood volume without blood loss. For example, epidural block analgesia may result in vasodilation, which increases the capacity of the maternal vascular bed. However, the amount of blood available to fill the vessels is unchanged. Hypotension then results, with reduction of placental blood flow.

Aortocaval compression can occur when a pregnant woman lies in the supine position and the weight of the uterus compresses the aorta and inferior vena cava. Aortocaval compression reduces blood return to her heart, lowers her cardiac output (supine hypotension), and can reduce placental perfusion.

Maternal hypertension may reduce blood flow to the placenta because of vasospasm and narrowing of the spiral arteries. Hypertension may be pregnancy-induced or chronic or may result from ingestion of drugs such as cocaine.

A lowered oxygen level in the mother's blood reduces the amount available to the fetus. Maternal acid-base alterations that often accompany respiratory abnormalities also can compromise exchange in the placenta. A lower maternal oxygen tension may result from respiratory disorders, such as asthma, or from smoking.

#### UTERINE ACTIVITY

Hypertonic uterine activity can reduce the time available for exchange of oxygen and waste products in the placenta. Contractions may be too long (over 90 seconds) or too frequent (closer than every 2 minutes) or have too short an interval (less than 60 seconds). The uterus may not fully relax between contractions, applying continuous compression to the spiral arteries and reducing maternal-fetal exchange in the intervillous spaces. Hypertonic uterine activity may occur spontaneously or with oxytocin administration.

#### PLACENTAL DISRUPTIONS

Conditions such as abruptio placentae (partial separation before birth) and infarcts reduce the placental surface area available for exchange. The amount and location of placental disruption relate to the degree of impairment in uteroplacental exchange.

#### INTERRUPTIONS IN UMBILICAL FLOW

The usual cause of interrupted blood flow through the umbilical cord is compression. Blood flow through the umbilical cord may be reduced by compression between the fetal presenting part and the pelvis, a nuchal cord or one that is wrapped around the fetal body, or a knot in the cord. It may occur with oligohydramnios because the amount of amniotic fluid is inadequate to cushion the cord. The umbilical cord also may become entangled between fetal body parts.

The thin-walled umbilical vein is compressed initially, resulting in a reduced inflow of more highly oxygenated blood to the fetus. This results in initial hypoxia with hypotension. Baroreceptors and chemoreceptors respond by accelerating the FHR. Flow through the firmer-walled umbilical arteries is reduced as cord compression continues, resulting in hypertension. Baroreceptors respond to hypertension by stimulating the vagus nerve, thus reducing blood pressure and slowing the fetal heart. The FHR again accelerates as pressure is relieved on the arteries and then on the vein.

#### FETAL ALTERATIONS

Fetal cells may be hypoxic despite adequate oxygen supply from the woman and adequate exchange within the placenta. A low circulating fetal blood volume, fetal hypotension, or fetal anemia may result in cellular hypoxia. Central nervous system or cardiac abnormalities may cause an abnormal rate or rhythm. For example, a fetus with complete heart block may not respond to stimuli that would normally cause a rate increase.

A prolonged rate lower than 50 beats per minute (BPM) may reduce fetal cardiac output enough to impair brain and heart perfusion. However, a persistent heart rate faster than 200 BPM also decreases cardiac output because the ventricles do not have time to fill with oxygenated blood during diastole.

### Risk Factors

When conditions associated with reduced fetal oxygenation exist (Table 14–1), assessments by either intermittent auscultation and palpation or electronic fetal monitoring are done more often. *No absolute indications, including the presence of risk factors, demand the use of electronic fetal monitoring during labor.* Properly performed intermittent auscultation is equivalent to continuous electronic monitoring in assessing fetal condition (ACOG, 1995a).

**TABLE 14–1 CONDITIONS ASSOCIATED WITH DECREASED FETAL OXYGENATION**

**Antepartum Period**

*Maternal history*
- Prior stillbirth
- Prior cesarean birth
- Chronic diseases, such as cardiac disease, hpertension, and diabetes
- Drug abuse

*Problems identified during pregnancy*
- Fetal growth restriction
- Gestation >42 weeks
- Marked decrease in fetal movement
- Multifetal gestation
- Pregnancy-induced hypertension
- Gestational diabetes
- Placenta previa
- Maternal severe anemia
- Maternal infection

**Intrapartum Period**

*Maternal problems*
- Hypotension
- Hypertonic uterine contractions
- Abnormal labor: preterm or dysfunctional
- Prolonged ruptured membranes
- Chorioamnionitis
- Fever

*Fetal or placental problems*
- Abnormal fetal heart rate
- Meconium-stained amniotic fluid
- Abnormal presentation or position
- Prolapsed cord
- Abruptio placentae

**✓ CHECK YOUR READING**

1. What five factors influence fetal oxygenation?
2. What changes in the FHR occur when the umbilical cord is compressed?
3. How is the FHR related to fetal cardiac output?
4. What risk factors indicate that fetal monitoring should be done more frequently (see Table 14–1)?

## Auscultation and Palpation

The nurse may use intermittent auscultation of the FHR and palpation of uterine activity for intrapartum fetal surveillance. This approach allows the woman greater freedom to move around during labor. Intermittent auscultation of the FHR can be done using either the fetoscope or Doppler ultrasound trans-

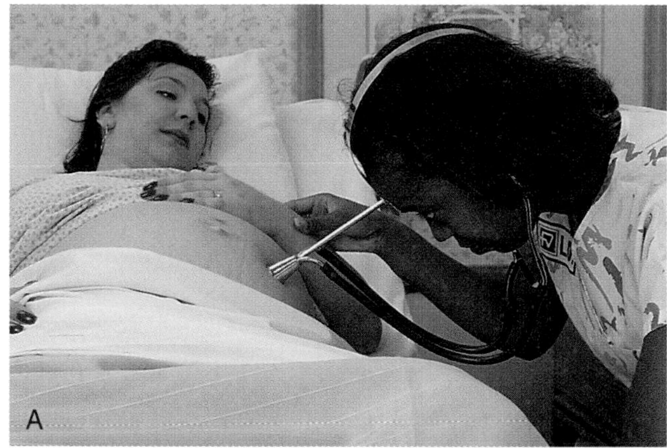

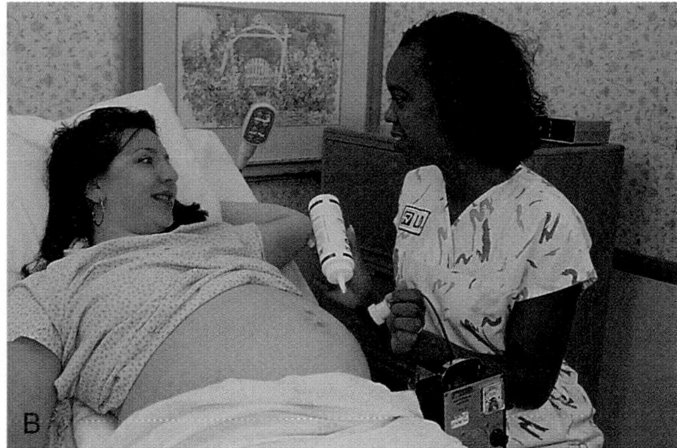

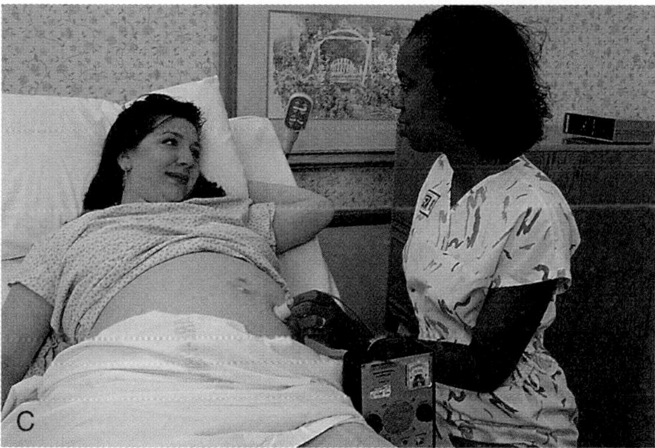

**FIGURE 14–1**

Low-intervention methods for evaluating the fetal heart rate during labor. A, Fetoscope, showing the head attachment to enhance conduction of faint fetal heart sounds. B, Transmission gel improves the clarity of the fetal heart movement sensed by the Doppler ultrasound transducer. C, The nurse moves the transducer until the fetal heart sounds are heard clearly. This location is usually over the fetal back, which is most likely to be located in the woman's right or left lower abdomen.

ducer (Fig. 14–1). Because fetal assessment is an important part of nursing care during labor, several aspects are addressed in Chapter 13.

### Advantages

Mobility is the primary advantage of auscultation and palpation for intrapartum fetal monitoring. The woman is free to change position and walk around, which is especially helpful during early labor. She can use water-based methods of pain management, such as whirlpool baths or showers. The atmosphere is more natural than technologic, which is important to some families during their birth experience.

### Limitations

One disadvantage of auscultation and palpation as the primary method of fetal assessment is that FHR and uterine activity are assessed for a small percentage of the total labor. The fetus is most stressed during contractions because of normal reduction of blood flow to the placenta at that time. Although the FHR is assessed during some contractions, it is not recorded during every contraction. Moreover, no continuous printed record is available to show the fetal response throughout labor or to identify subtle trends in the response.

Some women find that interruptions for auscultation are distracting. The pressure of the instrument on the abdomen is uncomfortable for some, and it may require several moves to locate the best place for auscultation.

Intermittent auscultation is more staff-intensive than electronic monitoring. For example, the nurse must check the FHR before, during, and after a contraction. When many clients are present for the number of nurses, auscultation may not be a realistic option as the primary method of intrapartum fetal surveillance.

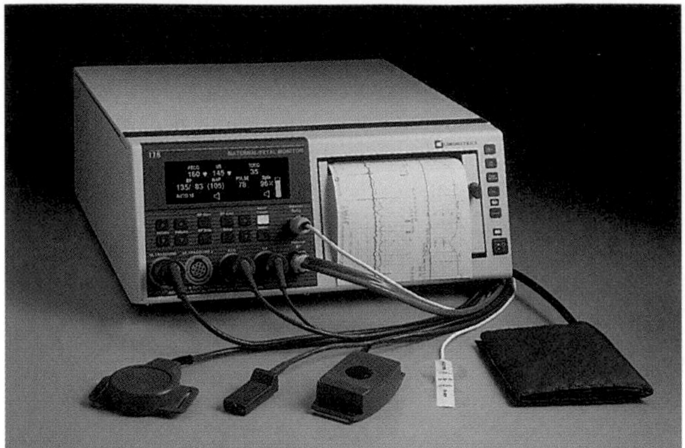

**FIGURE 14–2**

Bedside unit for electronic fetal monitoring. This unit can measure and record several maternal and fetal signs. In addition to fetal heart rate and uterine activity, the unit can help the nurse evaluate the woman's pulse, blood pressure, and saturation of oxygen in her blood. Both fetuses in a twin gestation can be assessed. (Courtesy of Corometrics Medical Systems, Inc., Wallingford, Conn.).

## Electronic Fetal Monitoring

Electronic fetal monitoring may be continuous, starting shortly after the woman is admitted, or intermittent, with a strip taken at regular intervals during labor.

### Advantages

The electronic monitor supplies more data about the fetus than auscultation and prints a permanent record (Fig. 14–2). Gradual trends that suggest problems may be identified because the strip provides a graphic record for review. Continuous electronic fetal monitoring shows how the fetus responds before, during, and after each contraction rather than only occasional contractions.

Many women in the United States expect electronic monitoring and find the constant sound of the fetal heart beat comforting. The coach can use the tracing of contractions on the monitor strip to help the woman anticipate the beginning and end of each contraction.

Electronic monitoring allows one nurse to observe two laboring women, primarily during uncomplicated early labor. A 1-to-1 nurse-client ratio is needed during the second stage, regardless of the monitoring method used. Electronic monitoring can give the nurse more time for teaching and supporting the laboring woman with breathing and relaxation techniques if the nurse maintains the primary focus on the woman, not on the monitor.

### Limitations

Reduced mobility is a limitation of electronic fetal monitoring. Telemetry or intermittent monitoring gives the woman more freedom of movement than continuous electronic monitoring without telemetry.

Frequent maternal position changes or an active fetus sometimes requires constant adjustment of equipment. The belts or stockinette used to keep sensors positioned properly for external monitoring are uncomfortable for some women.

The electronic fetal monitor imparts a more technical air to the surroundings and may be objectionable to a woman and her partner.

## Electronic Fetal Monitoring Equipment

Electronic fetal monitoring equipment consists of the bedside monitor unit and sensors for FHR and uterine activity. Sensors for each function may be either internal or external. Additional equipment may include data entry devices, remote units, and computer interfaces.

### Bedside Monitor Unit

The bedside monitor unit receives information about the FHR and uterine activity from the sensors. It processes the information and provides output in the form of a numerical display and a printed strip

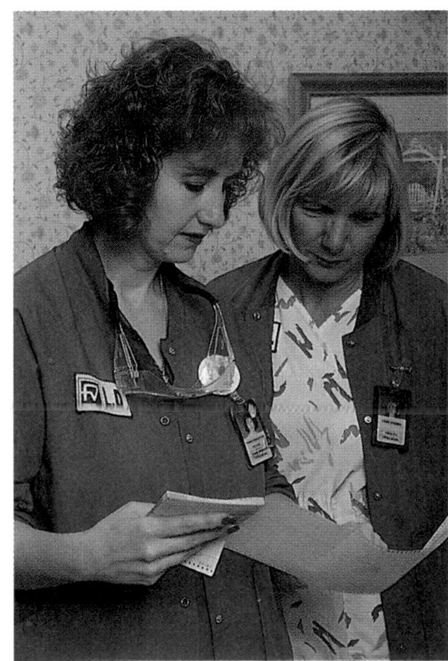

**FIGURE 14–3**

Electronic fetal monitoring can be continuous and provides nurses with monitor strips on which uterine activity and fetal heart rate are permanently recorded.

(Fig. 14–3). Most units can record rates for both fetuses in a twin pregnancy.

## Paper Strip

Data about the FHR and uterine activity are printed on a paper strip having a horizontal grid for the FHR and another for the uterine activity (Fig. 14–4). Each segment of paper between perforations is numbered for identification and reassembly of a multipart strip. The FHR is recorded on the upper strip. The range of rates is from 30 to 240 BPM.

Uterine activity is recorded on the lower grid as bell-shaped curves. Contraction intensity and uterine resting tone from 0 to 100 mmHg are recorded on the lower grid.

Vertical lines on both upper and lower grids are time divisions. At a paper speed of 3 cm/minute, dark vertical lines are 1 minute apart. Lighter lines subdivide the 1-minute divisions into six 10-second segments. The vertical lines are used to time contraction frequency and duration and to identify the fetal response in relation to the contractions.

## Data Entry Devices

Most monitors print some notations automatically, such as the date, time, paper speed, and devices being used to detect the FHR and uterine activity. Some also have data entry devices to enter data and print it on the strip. Small keypads or full keyboards allow information such as vital signs, labor data, or procedures such as vaginal examinations to be printed rather than handwritten on the strip.

## Remote Surveillance

Many facilities have display units at the nursing station or other locations to allow surveillance when the nurse is not at the bedside. These units display the tracing on a screen and have settings for alerts, such as range of the heart rate, decelerations, and end of the paper.

## Computer Interface

Computers are used increasingly with electronic fetal monitoring to help nurses manage the large amount of data generated during birth. Computer systems can help alert the nurse to suspicious patterns and can store recordings.

## Devices for External Fetal Monitoring

Both the FHR and uterine activity can be monitored by external sensors, or transducers. External devices

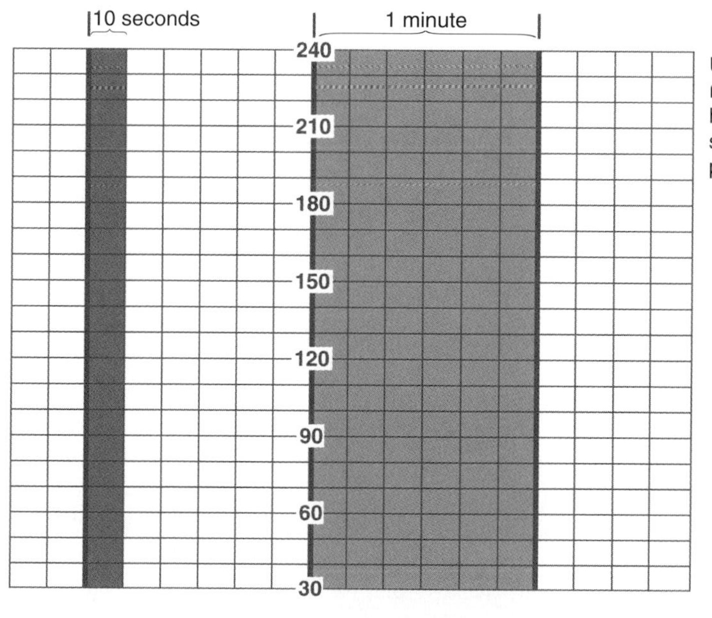


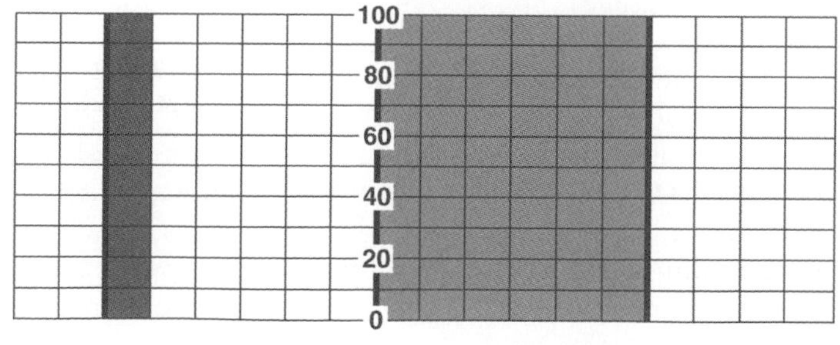


**FIGURE 14–4**

Paper strip for recording electronic fetal monitoring data. Each dark vertical line represents 1 minute, and each lighter vertical line represents 10 seconds.

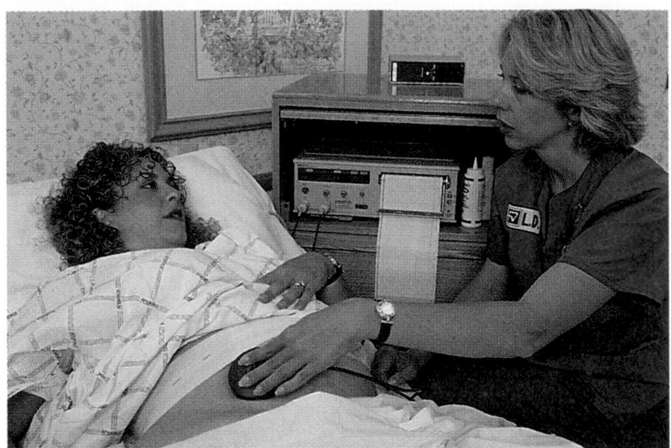

**FIGURE 14–5**

The nurse applies the uterine activity transducer on the woman's upper abdomen, in the fundal area. The Doppler transducer for sensing the fetal heart rate is usually placed on her lower abdomen when the fetus is in the cephalic presentation.

are secured on the mother's abdomen by elastic straps, a tube of wide stockinette, or an adhesive ring (Fig. 14–5). External devices are somewhat less accurate than internal ones but are noninvasive; they do not require ruptured membranes or cervical dilation. Procedure 14–1 contains instructions for using the external electronic fetal monitor.

#### FETAL HEART RATE MONITORING WITH AN ULTRASOUND TRANSDUCER

A Doppler ultrasound transducer detects fetal heart movement for rate calculation. The transducer sends high-frequency sound waves into the uterus. The sound waves are reflected, and the monitor's computer calculates the FHR based on the movement sensed.

Fetal heart motion does not always correlate with electrical heart activity. Other movements such as fetal or maternal activity or blood flow through the umbilical cord and the woman's aorta also can be detected. Most monitors today ignore these extraneous sounds to provide a clean tracing.

The Doppler transducer produces a two-part muffled sound resembling galloping horses. The two closely linked sounds represent closure of the heart valves during systole (mitral and tricuspid valves) and diastole (aortic and pulmonic valves). Fetal or maternal activity produces a rough, erratic sound rather than the crisp, rhythmic sound characteristic of the fetal heart.

#### UTERINE ACTIVITY MONITORING WITH A TOCOTRANSDUCER

A tocotransducer (also called a tocodynamometer or simply a "toco") with a pressure-sensitive area detects changes in abdominal contour to measure uterine activity. The uterus pushes outward against the mother's anterior abdominal wall with each contraction. The monitor calculates changes in this signal and prints them as bell shapes on the lower grid of the strip.

Movement other than uterine activity also registers on the monitor. For example, maternal respirations cause the uterine activity line to have a zigzag appearance. Other fetal or maternal movements appear as spikes on the uterine activity tracing.

Because uterine activity is sensed through the woman's abdomen, it is useful for observing the frequency and duration of contractions. It does not reliably measure actual contraction intensity and uterine resting tone. Several factors affect apparent intensity as printed on the strip.

- *Fetal size.* A small fetus prevents the uterus from pushing firmly against the abdominal wall with each contraction, making contractions appear less intense.
- *Abdominal fat thickness.* A thick layer of abdominal fat absorbs energy from uterine contractions, reducing the apparent intensity on the printed strip. The uterine activity recording of a thin woman whose uterus rotates sharply forward with each contraction may appear to be more intense than it actually is.
- *Maternal position.* Different maternal positions may increase or decrease the pressure against the transducer.
- *Location of the transducer.* Uterine activity is best detected where it is strongest and where the fetus lies close to the uterine wall. This is usually over the fundus. Changes during contractions may not be detectable if the transducer is located elsewhere.

### Devices for Internal Fetal Monitoring

Accuracy is the main advantage of using internal devices for electronic fetal monitoring. However, their use requires ruptured membranes and about 2 cm of cervical dilation. The devices are invasive, and the risk of infection is slightly increased. As with external devices, the FHR is printed in the upper grid and the uterine activity is printed in the lower grid of the monitor paper.

#### FETAL HEART RATE MONITORING WITH A SCALP ELECTRODE

The fetal scalp electrode (or spiral electrode) detects electrical signals from the fetal heart (Fig. 14–6). Fetal or maternal movement does not interfere with accuracy because the rate is calculated from electrical events in the fetal heart. The monitor

## Procedure 14-1

# External Fetal Monitor

**PURPOSE:** To properly apply the electronic fetal monitor. To perform a basic evaluation of the fetal heart rate (FHR) and uterine activity patterns to identify data needing further assessment by the experienced nurse, physician, or nurse-midwife.

1. **Read instruction manual for equipment.** *To become familiar with proper operation of the equipment and identify equipment.*

2. **Perform a function test following manufacturer's instructions. Press TEST button and observe for result. Common correct test results are:**
   a. **Fetal heart rate: The monitor prints a line at 120, 150, or 200 BPM, depending on the model.**
   b. **Uterine activity: The monitor adds 50 to uterine activity display.** *A correct function test ensures that the bedside monitor unit is calibrated properly so that caregivers are assured of accurate data to interpret. Each manufacturer sets standards for indicators of proper function.*

3. **Explain the basic procedure of electronic fetal monitoring to the woman and her partner or family. Vary instructions according to equipment being used and hospital protocols. A sample is:**
   a. **Using the electronic fetal monitor does not mean that you or the baby has a problem. It is the way we normally assess the baby's response to labor contractions.**
   b. **Two belts go around your abdomen, one for the fetal heart rate sensor and one for contractions.**
   c. **Feel free to move with the monitor on. If the tracing is poor, we can adjust the sensors.** *Knowledge decreases the woman's fear of the unknown. Teaching her that she can move with the monitor in place enhances her comfort and promotes normal labor.*

4. **Apply belts or stockinette if an adhesive ring is not used:**
   a. **Slide both belts under the woman's back without the sensors attached. Be sure to keep the belts smooth under her back.**
   b. **Cut a length of stockinette tubing about 15 to 18 inches long for the average-sized woman. Cut a longer length of wide stockinette for a heavier woman. Slide the stockinette up from her feet to her abdomen.** *Smooth application of straps or stockinette enhances a woman's comfort and improves contact of external sensors with her abdomen. Good contact improves the quality of the tracing and may reduce the number of adjustments needed.*

5. **Use Leopold's maneuvers (see Procedure 13-1) to locate the fetus' back. During early labor, this is usually in the left or right lower quadrant of the woman's abdomen. During later labor, the fetal back is usually nearer the woman's abdominal midline.** *The FHR is best detected through the back of the fetus. If the fetus is not engaged or is in a breech presentation, the FHR is probably found higher on the woman's abdomen.*

6. **Apply ultrasound gel to the Doppler ultrasound transducer and place it on the woman's abdomen at the approximate location of the fetus' back. Move the transducer until a clear signal is heard. Most bedside units have a green light or flashing heart shape to indicate a good signal.** *Gel improves transmission and reception of the ultrasound waves to provide more accurate data.*

7. **Place the uterine activity sensor in the fundal area or the area where contractions feel the strongest when palpated. This is often slightly above the umbilicus. When the woman has a contraction, observe the tracing for the bell shape. The line for uterine activity is jagged because it also senses the rise and fall of the abdomen with breathing. Fetal or maternal movement causes a spike in the line. Observe through several contractions.** *The external uterine activity monitor senses the change in the abdominal contour as the uterus rotates forward with each contraction. Contractions are usually strongest in the fundus of the uterus. Observation of the uterine activity line (on the lower paper grid) through several contractions verifies correct placement and identifies needed position changes.*

8. **Observe the strip for baseline FHR, presence of long-term variability, periodic changes, and uterine activity (contraction duration and frequency). Palpate contractions for intensity and relaxation between contractions. Notify the physician or nurse-midwife of nonreassuring patterns.** *Identifies reassuring and nonreassuring FHR patterns (see Table 14-2). Contractions having a frequency greater than every 2 minutes, duration longer than 90 seconds, or incomplete uterine relaxation between contractions may reduce maternal blood flow into the intervillous spaces and impair exchange of oxygen and waste products. The external uterine activity sensor is useful only for contraction frequency and duration. It is not accurate for actual intensity or uterine resting tone.*

unit generates a beeping sound with each fetal heart beat, but this sound can be silenced.

Although called a fetal scalp electrode, the device may be applied to the buttocks in a breech presentation. Areas to avoid for electrode application are the fetal face, fontanelles, and genitals. Two wires from the electrode protrude from the mother's vagina and are attached to a leg plate to secure them.

Because it barely penetrates the fetal skin (about 1 mm), the electrode is easily displaced. The tracing then becomes erratic or stops if the electrode is fully detached. Secure attachment of the electrode is often difficult if the fetus has thick hair. The electrode

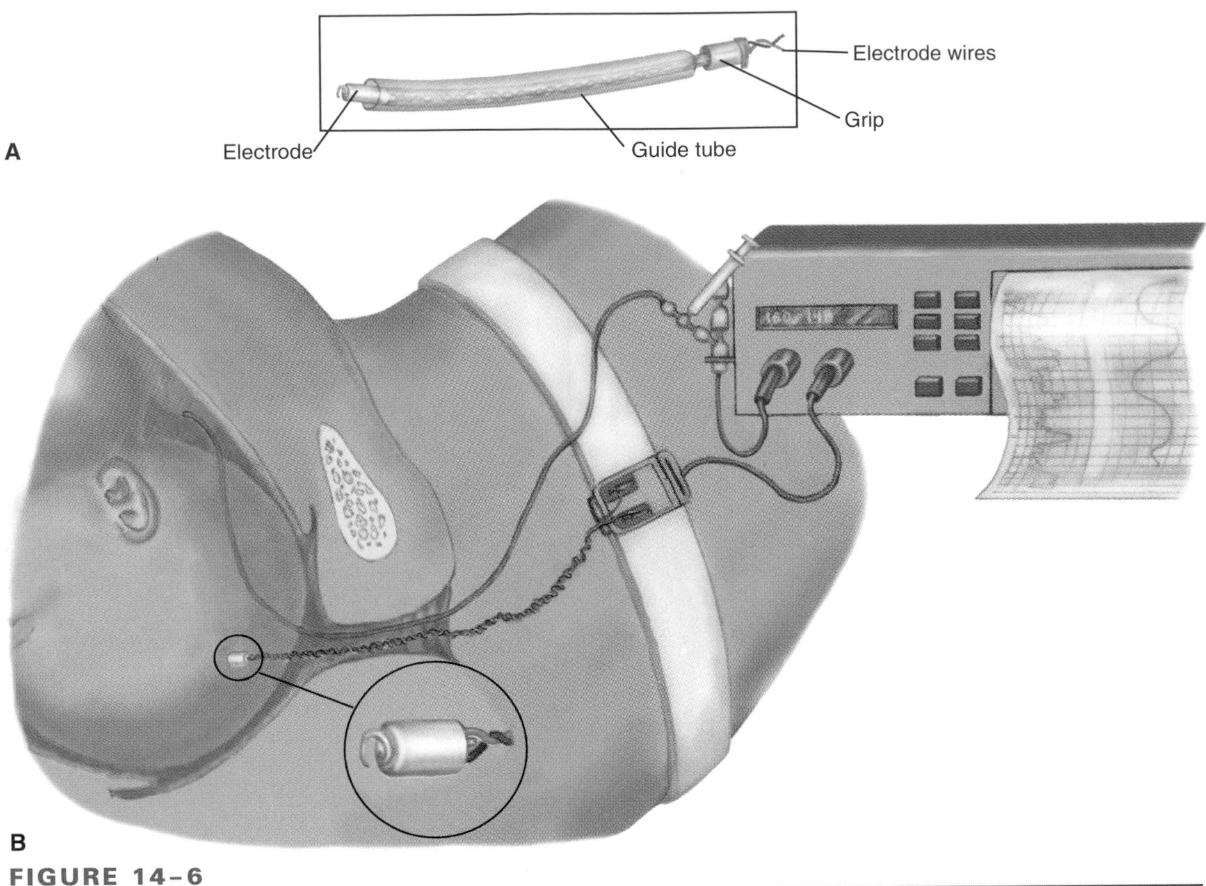


FIGURE 14-6

Internal spiral electrode and intrauterine pressure catheter. A, parts of the fetal scalp electrode before it is applied. B, Fetal scalp electrode and intrauterine pressure catheter in place and connected to the bedside monitor unit.

is removed by turning it counterclockwise about one and one-half turns until it detaches.

### UTERINE ACTIVITY MONITORING WITH AN INTRAUTERINE PRESSURE CATHETER

Two kinds of intrauterine pressure catheters can be used to measure uterine activity, including contraction intensity and resting tone:

- A solid catheter with a pressure transducer in its tip (Fig. 14–7); this catheter may have an additional lumen for amnioinfusion.
- A hollow, fluid-filled catheter that connects to a pressure transducer on the bedside monitor unit.

Both types sense intrauterine pressure and increases in intra-abdominal pressure, such as with coughing or vomiting.

The solid catheter is not affected by height because its transducer is in the catheter. However, the sensor in its tip measures hydrostatic pressure from the amniotic fluid above the fetal presenting part as well as the pressure from uterine activity. Therefore, recorded intrauterine pressures from the solid catheter are higher than those from the fluid-filled catheter, and the nurse must consider this fact when assessing whether uterine activity is normal or hypertonic.

The tip of the fluid-filled catheter in the uterus should be at the level of the transducer on the outside for best accuracy. If the tip is lower than the transducer, the recorded pressure is lower than the actual intrauterine pressure. If the tip is higher, the recorded pressure may be artificially high. Changes in the mother's position may alter the height of the catheter tip, requiring adjustment of the transducer's height.

#### CHECK YOUR READING

5. What are the advantages and limitations of each fetal monitoring method?
6. Which grid on the paper strip of the electronic fetal monitor is used to record the FHR? Uterine activity?
7. Which electronic fetal monitoring sensor uses heart motion to measure FHR?

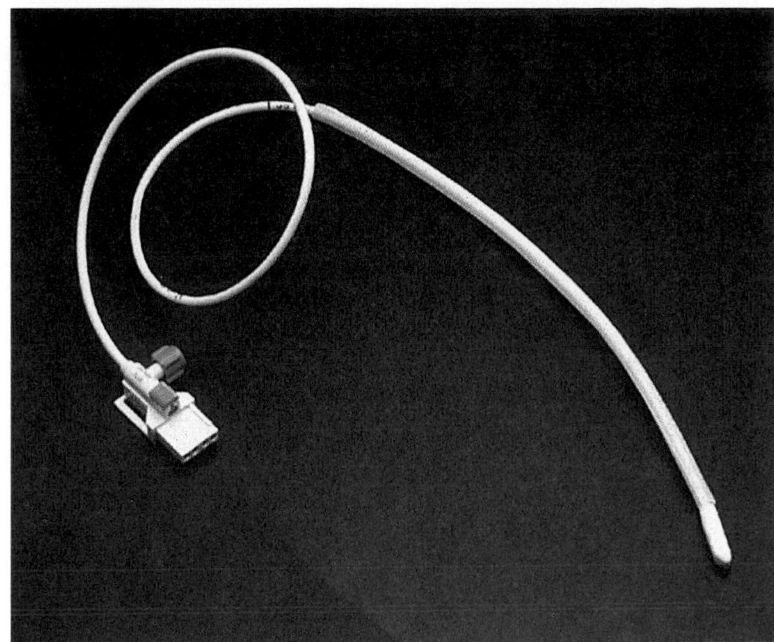

**FIGURE 14-7**

Solid intrauterine pressure catheter with transducer in its tip. This model also has a lumen for amnioinfusion and is shown with its introducer over the catheter. (Courtesy of Utah Medical Products, Midvale, Utah.)

8. What are some variables that can affect the accuracy of the external uterine activity sensor?
9. What are the two types of internal uterine activity catheters? Which one tends to record higher intrauterine pressures? Which one is affected by its height in relation to the mother's position?

## Evaluating Electronic Fetal Monitoring Strips

A consistent, organized approach to analyzing fetal monitor patterns ensures completeness. The nurse evaluates the FHR tracing for baseline rate, variability, and presence of periodic changes. Uterine activity is evaluated by determining the frequency, duration, and intensity of contractions and by assessing uterine resting tone. Fetal heart rate and uterine activity patterns must be evaluated together.

Other data are relevant to strip interpretation, such as maternal vital signs, maternal position, drug or oxygen administration, character of the amniotic fluid, labor status, and procedures performed. These are customarily recorded on the strip as well as in the labor record.

### Fetal Heart Rate Baseline

The FHR baseline is the most consistent heart rate when the uterus is at rest (Fig. 14–8). The baseline excludes periodic (temporary and recurrent) changes. It is composed of rate and variability. The baseline rate is classified as follows (Murray, 1997; Menihan, 1996; West et al., 1993; NAACOG, 1990):

- *Normal*: for the term fetus, a lower limit of 110 to 120 BPM, and an upper limit of 150 to 160 BPM (some sources say that 120 BPM is the lower limit of normal)
- *Bradycardia*: less than 110 to 120 BPM, persisting at least 10 minutes
- *Tachycardia*: greater than 150 to 160 BPM, persisting at least 10 minutes

Some healthy term fetuses have bradycardia between 100 and 110 BPM with no other signs of compromise. A normal preterm fetus may have a baseline rate slightly higher than that of a term fetus (about 130 to 170 BPM) because the parasympathetic nervous system is immature.

### Baseline Fetal Heart Rate Variability

*Variability* denotes the fluctuations in the baseline FHR that cause the printed line to have an irregular rather than a smooth appearance (Fig. 14–9). Two types of variability are evaluated together:

- Short-term variability—changes in the FHR from one beat to the next (beat-to-beat). It is most accurately assessed with an internal spiral electrode.
- Long-term variability—broader fluctuations that are apparent over 1-minute intervals. About three to six of these cycles occur each minute.

Short-term variability may be decreased by several non-pathologic and pathologic factors, such as the following:

- Narcotics or other sedative drugs given to the woman, including those given with epidural analgesia

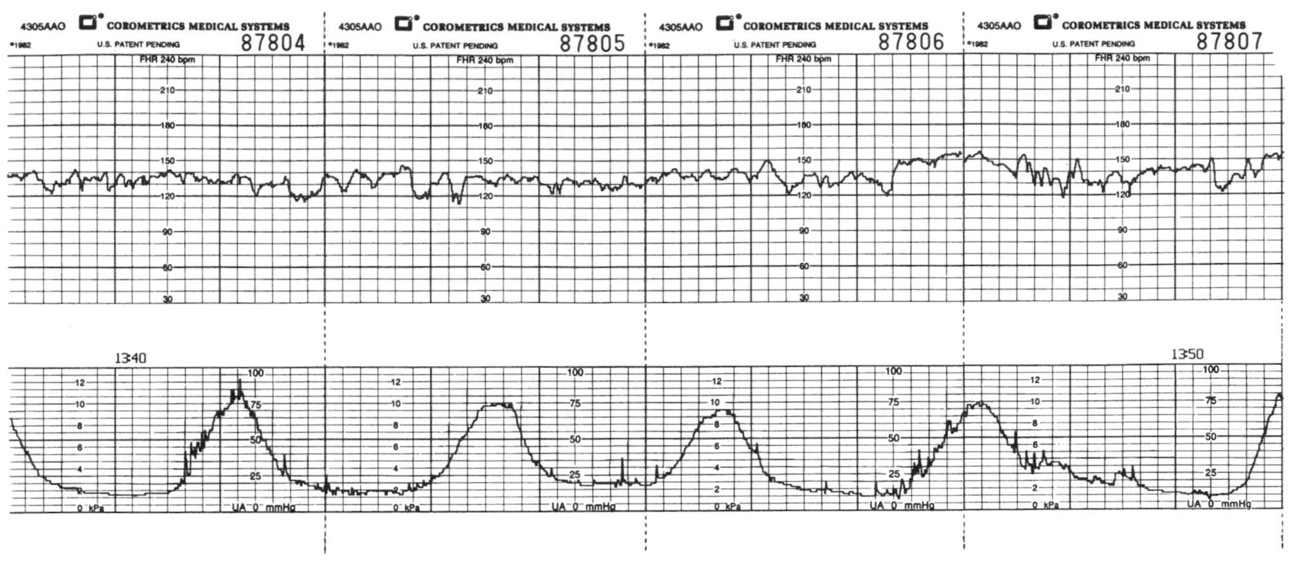


**FIGURE 14–8**

Electronic fetal monitor strip showing a reassuring pattern of fetal heart rate (FHR) and uterine activity. The FHR baseline is 130 to 140 beats per minute (BPM), variability is about 10 BPM. There are no periodic changes in this strip. Contraction frequency is approximately every 2 to 3 minutes, duration is about 50 to 60 seconds, intensity is 75 to 90 mmHg with the internal spiral electrode, and uterine resting tone is approximately 10 mmHg. (Courtesy of Corometrics Medical Systems, Inc., Wallingford, Conn. Redrawn with permission.)

- Fetal sleep
- Tachycardia
- Prematurity
- Decreased oxygenation of the central nervous system
- Abnormalities of the central nervous system, heart, or both

Long-term variability varies with fetal sleep. It is often reduced as the fetus sleeps (about 20 to 30 minutes at a time) and increases when the fetus awakens.

Both kinds of variability occur because multiple factors constantly speed and slow the fetal heart in a push-and-pull manner. Evaluation of variability helps to clarify how a fetus is tolerating the stress of labor, including factors that cause hypoxia. Variability is a significant component of the FHR tracing on the electronic monitor for two reasons:

- Adequate oxygenation promotes normal function of the autonomic nervous system and helps the fetus adapt to the stress of labor
- Variability evaluates the function of the fetal autonomic nervous system, especially the parasympathetic branch

No consensus exists on terms to describe variability. Some sources describe short-term and long-term variability separately, whereas others describe the two as a unit. Some use two levels (absent or present), whereas others use as many as five.

Variability of 6 to 25 BPM is considered reassuring by most authorities. For short-term variability, this means that the beat-to-beat rate changes that occur over 1 minute of *baseline* FHR are at least 6 BPM but lower than 25 BPM. For long-term variability, it means that there are three to six broad cycles of rate changes within the 6 to 25 BPM range.

## Periodic Patterns in the Fetal Heart Rate

Periodic patterns are transient and recurrent changes from the baseline rate associated with uterine contractions. They include accelerations and decelerations. Periodic patterns are evaluated with baseline characteristics (rate and variability).

### ACCELERATIONS

An acceleration is a brief, temporary increase in the FHR of at least 15 beats above the baseline, lasting at least 15 seconds (Fig. 14–10). Accelerations usually occur with fetal movement. They may be nonperiodic (having no relation to contractions) as well as periodic. They may occur with vaginal examinations, uterine contractions, and mild cord compression and when the fetus is in a breech presentation. Accelerations are usually a reassuring sign, reflecting a responsive, non-acidotic fetus.

### DECELERATIONS

Periodic decelerations are classified into three types based on their shape and relationship to uterine contractions.

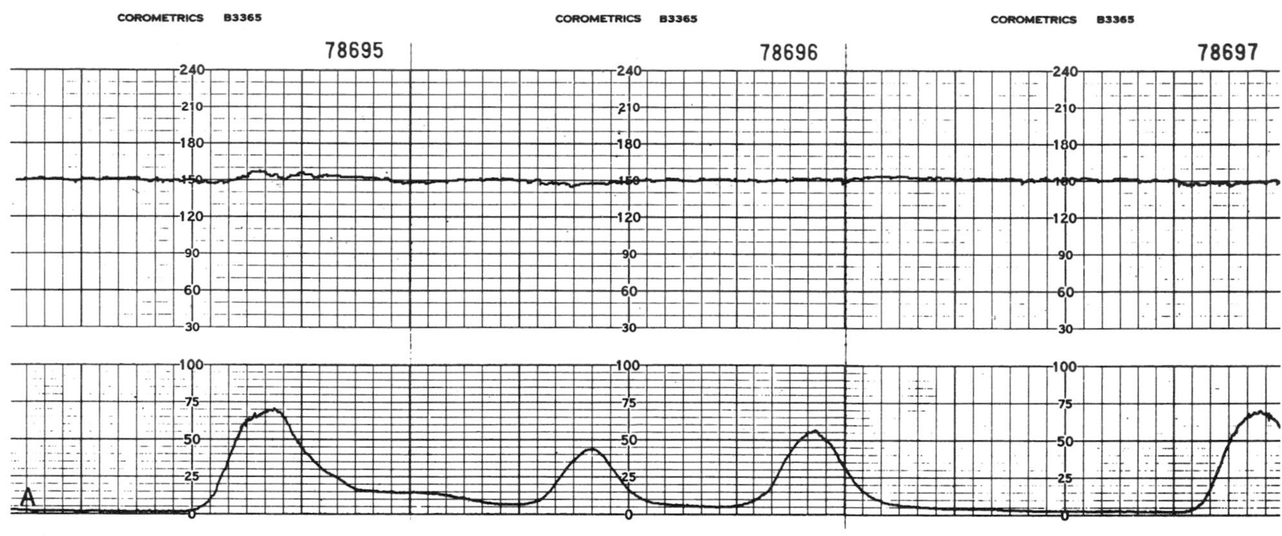


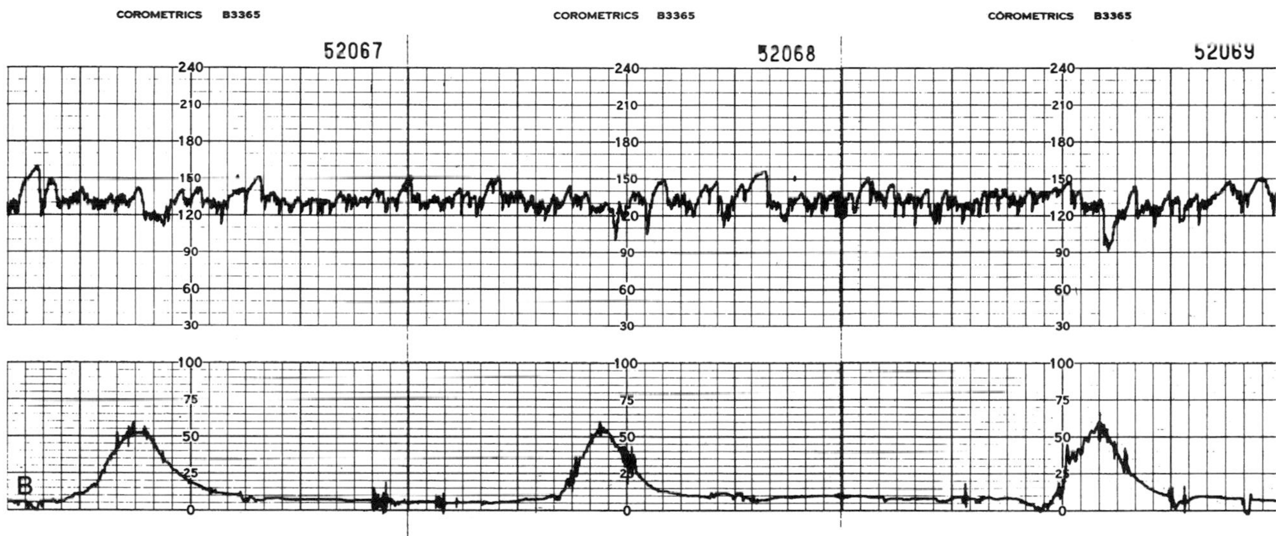


**FIGURE 14–9**

Contrasts in fetal heart rate variability. A fetal scalp electrode is being used. A, Minimal to absent variability (less than 3 BPM). Note the smooth, flat line in the FHR channel. B, Increased variability (about 20 BPM). Note the marked zigzag appearance of the fetal heart rate line. (Courtesy of Corometrics Medical Systems, Inc., Wallingford, Conn. Redrawn with permission.)

**Early Decelerations.** Fetal head compression briefly increases intracranial pressure, causing the vagus nerve to slow the heart rate. Early decelerations are not associated with fetal compromise and require no intervention. They occur *during* contractions as the fetal head is pressed against the woman's pelvis or soft tissues, such as the cervix.

Early decelerations are consistent in appearance; they are uniform in that one early deceleration looks similar to others. They mirror the contraction, beginning near its onset and returning to the baseline by the end of the contraction (Fig. 14–11). The rate at the lowest point of the deceleration usually remains above 100 BPM.

**Late Decelerations.** Deficient exchange of oxygen and waste products in the placenta (uteroplacental insufficiency) may result in a pattern of late (delayed) decelerations. This nonreassuring pattern suggests that the fetus has reduced reserve to tolerate the recurrent reductions in oxygen supply that normally occur with contractions. The cause of uteroplacental insufficiency may be acute, such as maternal hypotension. It may also occur with chronic conditions that impair placental

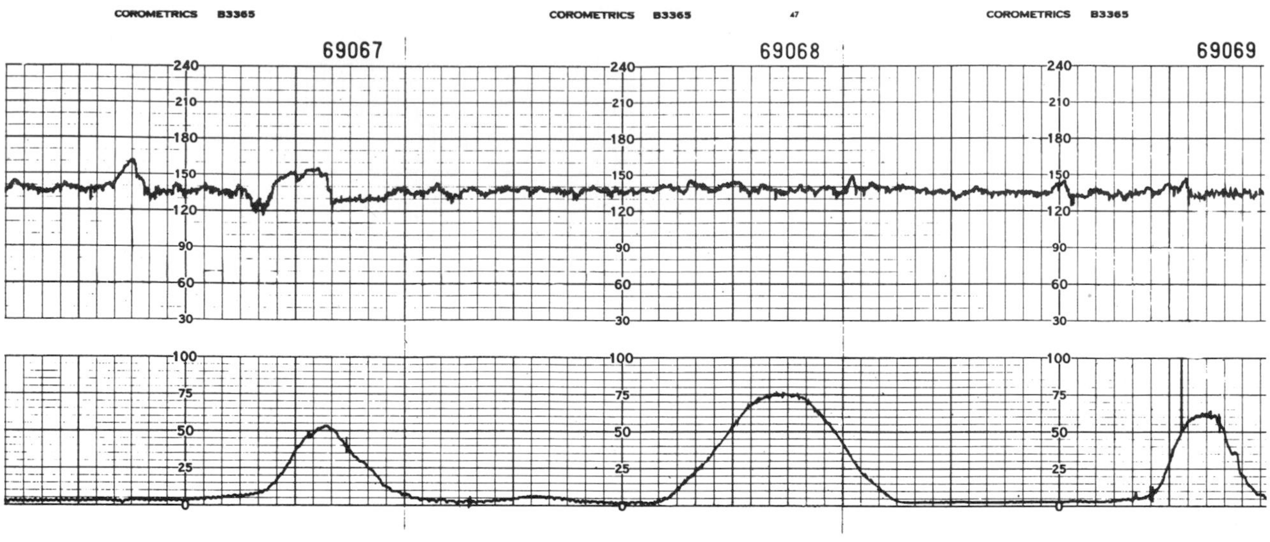


**FIGURE 14–10**

Accelerations of the fetal heart rate. (Courtesy of Corometrics Medical Systems, Inc., Wallingford, Conn. Redrawn with permission.)

exchange, such as maternal hypertension or diabetes.

Late decelerations look similar to early decelerations but are shifted to the right in relation to the contraction. They often begin after the peak of the contraction. The rate returns to the baseline *after* the contraction ends (Fig. 14–12). They have a consistent appearance. The FHR may remain in the normal range and may not fall much below its baseline level. The amount of rate decrease from the baseline does not indicate how much uteroplacental insufficiency exists.

Late decelerations are evaluated with baseline characteristics. For example, late decelerations that occur with a normal rate and variability are of less concern than late decelerations that occur with an abnormal rate or in conjunction with absent variability. However, prompt action to correct the uteroplacental insufficiency is taken for any nonreassuring pattern, whether it occurs alone or is combined with others.

**Variable Decelerations.** Conditions that restrict flow through the umbilical cord may result in variable decelerations. These decelerations do not have the uniform appearance of early and late decelerations. Their shape, duration, and degree of fall below baseline rate are variable. They fall and rise abruptly with the onset and relief of cord compression, unlike the gradual fall and rise of early and late decelerations (Fig. 14–13). Variable decelerations also may be nonperiodic, occurring at times unrelated to contractions.

Several methods are used to classify variable decelerations according to depth and duration, but no uniform agreement exists. One guideline suggests that variable decelerations are significant when the FHR repeatedly decreases to less than 70 BPM and persists at that level for at least 60 seconds before

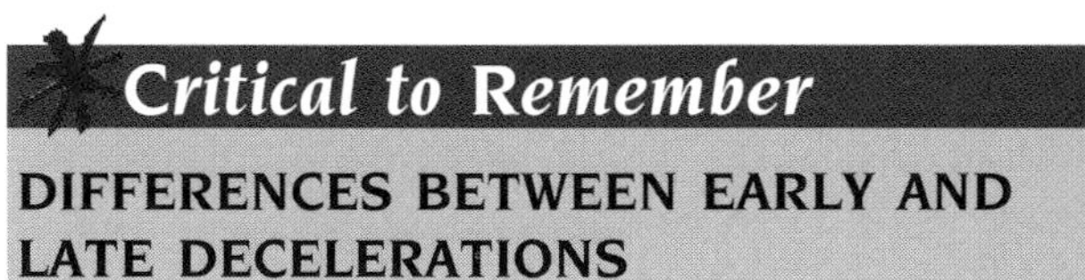

## Critical to Remember

### DIFFERENCES BETWEEN EARLY AND LATE DECELERATIONS

**Early Decelerations**

- Occur only during contractions as the fetal head is compressed
- Return to the baseline fetal heart rate by the end of the contraction
- Are mirror images of the contraction (fetal heart rate line goes down as contraction line goes up)
- Are not associated with fetal compromise and require no added interventions

**Late Decelerations**

- Look similar to early decelerations but begin well after the contraction begins (often near the peak)
- Return to baseline after the contraction ends
- Reflect impaired placental exchange or uteroplacental insufficiency
- The degree of fall in rate from baseline is not related to the amount of uteroplacental insufficiency
- Should be addressed by nursing interventions to improve placental blood flow and fetal oxygen supply

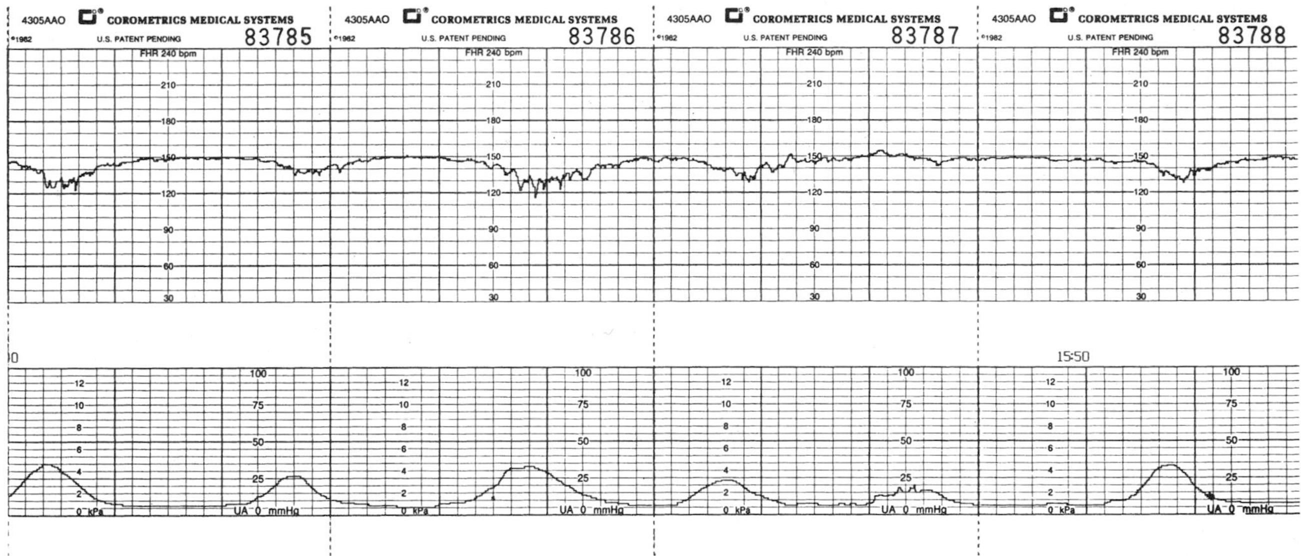

FIGURE 14–11

Early decelerations. Note that the slowing of the fetal heart rate mirrors the contraction. It begins near the beginning of the contraction and returns to the baseline by the end of the contraction. Cause: fetal head compression. (Courtesy of Corometrics Medical Systems, Inc., Wallingford, Conn.)

returning to the baseline (ACOG, 1995a). Baseline rate and variability are also considered when evaluating variable decelerations.

## Uterine Activity

Assessment of uterine activity has four components: frequency, duration, and intensity of the contractions, and uterine resting tone. Contraction frequency may be measured with the electronic monitor the same way as with palpation (beginning of one contraction to beginning of the next) or from peak to peak. Duration is calculated from the beginning to end of each contraction.

Palpation is used to estimate contraction intensity and uterine resting tone when an external uterine activity monitor is used (see Procedure 13–3). Contraction intensity is described as mild, moderate, or strong. The uterus should relax between contractions for 60 seconds or longer.

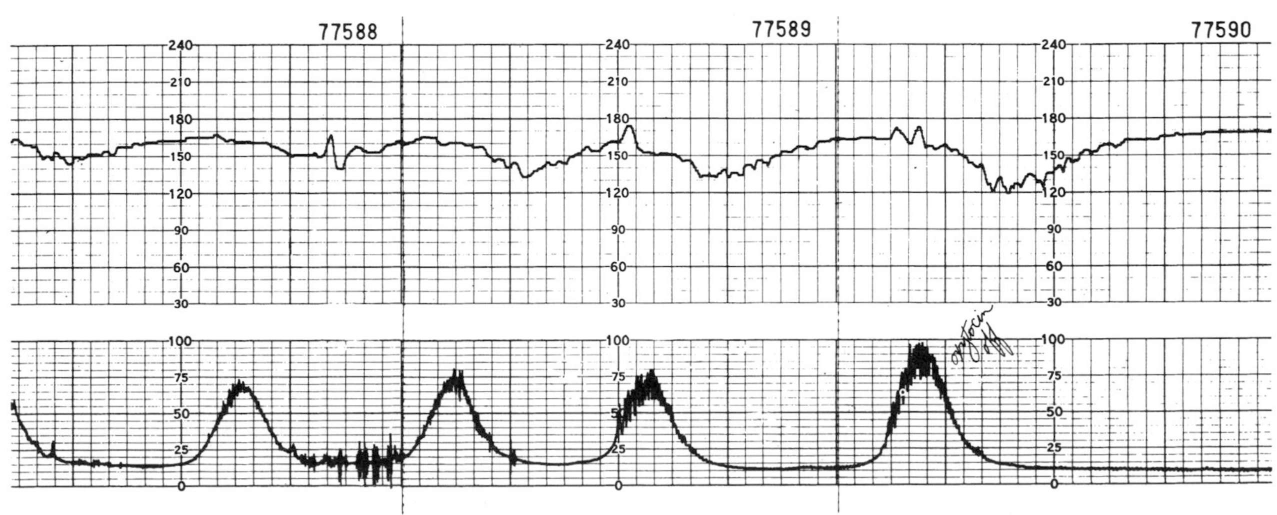

FIGURE 14–12

Late decelerations. Note that the decelerations look similar to early decelerations but are offset to the right. They begin at about the peak of the contraction and do not return to the baseline until after the contraction ends. Cause: uteroplacental insufficiency. (Courtesy of Corometrics Medical Systems, Inc., Wallingford, Conn. Redrawn with permission.)

## CRITICAL THINKING EXERCISE

Nancy Joe is having her labor induced with oxytocin and is having internal electronic fetal monitoring. Her contractions occur every 2.5 minutes, are 90 seconds in duration, and reach 75 mmHg on the scale for the intrauterine pressure catheter. Uterine resting tone between contractions is 20 mmHg. The baseline fetal heart rate is 135 to 145 BPM with about 7 BPM variability.

Her nurse, Jackie Brown, notes a pattern of uniform decelerations that begin at the peak of each contraction. The rate falls to 125 BPM before returning to the previous baseline about 30 seconds after the contraction ends.

**Q:** 1. What pattern does this describe?
2. What is the most appropriate nursing response?

**A:** The pattern described is one of late decelerations, probably caused by excess uterine activity secondary to the use of oxytocin. Jackie's initial action should be to stop the oxytocin infusion and increase the rate of Nancy's nonadditive intravenous fluid. Oxygen should be given through a snug face mask at about 8 to 10 liters per minute. Nancy should be placed on her side, if she is not already in this position, to increase placental blood flow. After the immediate corrective actions are completed, Jackie should contact Nancy's physician or nurse-midwife, documenting her interventions and the content of the call.

With the intrauterine pressure catheter, the scale on the paper is used to describe intensity and resting tone. Intensity increases as labor progresses. Uterine contraction intensity with the intrauterine pressure catheter is about 50 to 75 mmHg during labor, although it may reach 110 mmHg with pushing during the second stage. Average resting tone is 5 to 15 mmHg.

## CHECK YOUR READING

10. What is the significance of FHR accelerations?
11. What are the differences between early and late decelerations? Which pattern is nonreassuring?
12. What do variable decelerations look like? What is their cause?

# Significance of Fetal Heart Rate Patterns

Fetal heart rate patterns on the electronic monitor are classified as either "reassuring" or "nonreassuring." Between these two classifications are patterns that are "equivocal"—neither clearly reassuring nor clearly nonreassuring. For equivocal (ambiguous) patterns, several methods may be used to further evaluate the fetal condition. Table 14–2 summarizes reassuring and nonreassuring patterns.

## Reassuring Patterns

Reassuring patterns, such as accelerations with fetal movement, are associated with fetal well-being. No intervention is required because the pattern suggests that the fetus is tolerating intrapartum stressors.

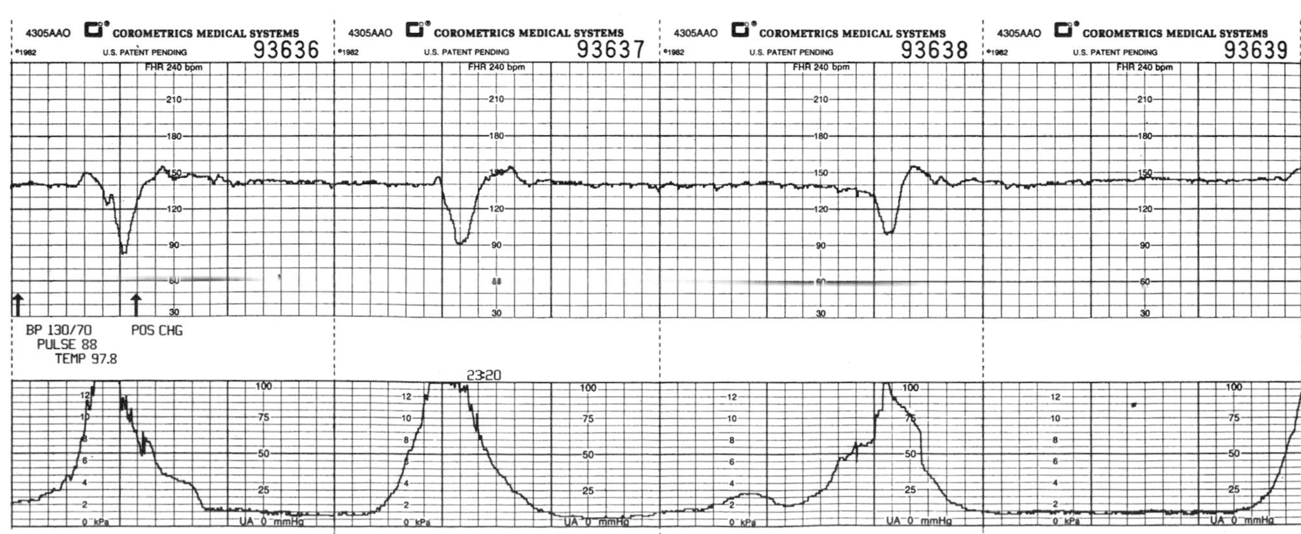


**FIGURE 14–13**

Variable decelerations. The decelerations are sharp in onset and offset. Note slight rate accelerations (shoulders) after each variable deceleration. Cause: umbilical cord compression. (Courtesy of Corometrics Medical Systems, Inc., Wallingford, Conn. Redrawn with permission.)

### CRITICAL THINKING EXERCISE

LaShonda Blair is in active labor and is having external electronic fetal monitoring for fetal assessment. LaShonda has not had medication, and her labor has been normal so far. Her membranes ruptured about 1 hour ago, and the amniotic fluid was clear. Contractions are every 3 minutes, 60 seconds in duration, and of moderate intensity. Her uterus fully relaxes between each contraction.

The new graduate nurse who is supporting LaShonda notes abrupt slowing of the fetal heart rate to 90 BPM during the next two contractions, each time lasting about 30 seconds.

**Q:**
1. Are any nursing actions needed?
2. If nursing actions are needed, what are they and in what order should they be done?

**A:**

The pattern described is one of variable decelerations, usually associated with cord compression. The novice nurse should use the call bell to summon a more experienced nurse. At the same time, LaShonda should be asked to change her position; if she is on her left side, she should turn to the right. Changing position may relieve pressure on the cord. The experienced nurse will further evaluate LaShonda and her baby and may perform other interventions.

The physician or nurse-midwife should be contacted if the variable decelerations persist or worsen. However, attempting to correct the cause of the variable decelerations is the first priority.

## Nonreassuring Patterns

Nonreassuring patterns occur if favorable signs are absent or if signs that are associated with fetal hypoxia or acidosis are present. Nonreassuring patterns do not necessarily indicate that fetal hypoxia or acidosis has occurred. Electronic fetal monitoring best identifies the well-oxygenated fetus; it less reliably identifies the compromised fetus. Thus, electronic fetal monitoring is a screening rather than a diagnostic tool.

Nonreassuring patterns are more significant if they occur together and are persistent. For example, bradycardia with short-term variability of less than 3 BPM and late decelerations suggests greater fetal stress than bradycardia alone. The healthy fetus may demonstrate an occasional late deceleration, but a persistent pattern of late decelerations is more likely to represent compromise in a fetus. Nonreassuring patterns include but are not limited to the following:

- Tachycardia
- Bradycardia
- Decreased or absent variability
- Late decelerations
- Variable decelerations falling to less than 70 BPM for longer than 60 seconds
- Prolonged decelerations
- Hypertonic uterine activity

Nonreassuring patterns do not always indicate that labor should end immediately. Several interventions may be used to clarify the fetal condition and to determine the best course of action. Other interventions can increase fetal oxygenation.

#### CLARIFICATION OF DATA

Any of four methods may clarify data to better understand the fetal condition. Three methods are used during the intrapartum period: (1) fetal scalp stimulation, (2) vibroacoustic stimulation, and (3) fetal scalp blood sampling. A fourth method, analysis of umbilical cord blood gases and pH, is used immediately after birth.

**Fetal Scalp Stimulation.** Scalp stimulation evaluates the fetus' response to tactile stimulation (Fig. 14–14). It may be done by the nurse, physician, or nurse-midwife. The examiner applies pressure to the scalp (or other presenting part) with a gloved finger or fingers and sweeps the fingers in a circular motion. An FHR acceleration of 15 BPM for at least 15 seconds is a reassuring response, suggesting a fetus in normal oxygen and acid-base balance. The

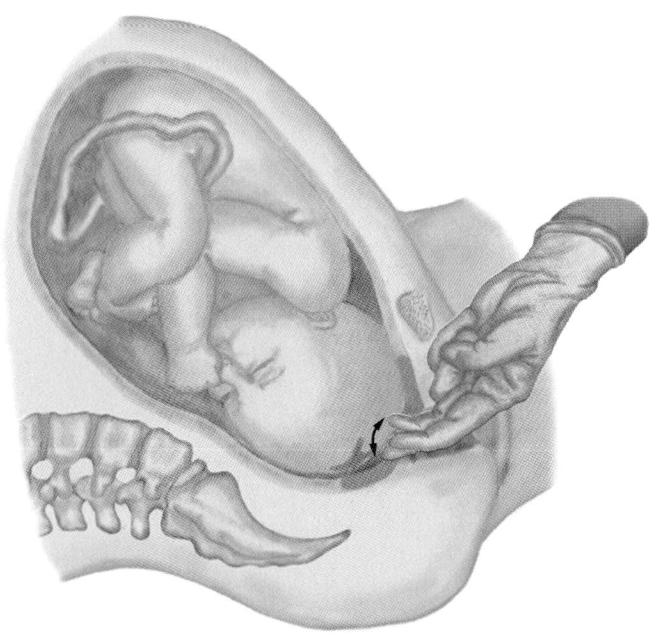

**FIGURE 14–14**

Fetal scalp stimulation helps identify whether the fetus responds to gentle massage. An acceleration in the FHR of 15 BPM for 15 seconds suggests that the fetus is in normal oxygen and acid-base balance.

## TABLE 14–2 REASSURING AND NONREASSURING FETAL HEART RATE PATTERNS

### Reassuring Patterns

Baseline rate: Stable, with a lower limit of 110–120 BPM and an upper limit of 150–160 BPM at term
Variability of 6–25 BPM
Accelerations with fetal movement: At least 15 BPM above the baseline for at least 15 sec
Uterine activity:
- Contraction frequency: no more frequent than every 2 min
- Contraction duration: no longer than 90 sec
- Interval between contractions: at least 60 sec
- Uterine resting tone: uterus relaxed between contractions (with external monitor); uterine resting tone <20 mmHg (with intrauterine pressure catheter)

### Nonreassuring Patterns

| Pattern and Description | Possible Cause |
|---|---|
| **TACHYCARDIA** | |
| Baseline FHR >160 BPM for at least 10 min<br>Mild: 161–180 BPM<br>Severe: >181 BPM | Maternal fever (fetal tachycardia may be the first sign of an intrauterine infection)<br>Maternal dehydration<br>Maternal or fetal hypoxia<br>Fetal acidosis<br>Maternal or fetal hypovolemia<br>Fetal cardiac arrhythmias<br>Maternal severe anemia<br>Maternal hyperthyroidism<br>Drugs administered to mother (such as terbutaline) |
| **BRADYCARDIA** | |
| Baseline FHR <110 BPM for at least 10 min<br>Baseline rates between 100 and 110 BPM are usually not associated with fetal compromise if there are no nonreassuring patterns | Fetal head compression<br>Fetal hypoxia<br>Fetal acidosis<br>Fetal heart block<br>Umbilical cord compression<br>Second-stage labor with maternal pushing |
| **DECREASED OR ABSENT VARIABILITY** | |
| FHR baseline has a smooth, flat appearance | Fetal sleep (usually lasts no longer than 30 min at a time)<br>Fetal hypoxia with acidosis<br>Drug effects:<br>CNS depressants<br>Local anesthetic agents |
| **LATE DECELERATIONS** | |
| Recurrent decelerations with a uniform appearance and a consistent relation to the contraction; begin after the contraction starts (usually at the peak) and do not return to baseline until after the contraction ends | Uteroplacental insufficiency, which may be secondary to:<br>Maternal hypotension<br>Excess uterine activity<br>Placental interruption, such as abruptio placentae or placenta previa<br>Pregnancy-induced or chronic hypertension<br>Maternal diabetes<br>Maternal severe anemia<br>Maternal cardiac disease |
| **VARIABLE DECELERATIONS** | |
| Sharp in onset and offset<br>Appearance and relationship to contractions is not consistent, may occur as a non-periodic pattern (randomly) | Umbilical cord compression, which may be secondary to:<br>Prolapsed cord<br>Nuchal cord (around fetal neck)<br>Oligohydramnios (abnormally small amount of amniotic fluid)<br>Cord between fetus and mother's uterus or pelvis, without obvious prolapse<br>Cord between fetal body parts<br>Knot in cord |

*Abbreviations*: BPM, beats per minute; FHR, fetal heart rate.

acceleration may be delayed rather than immediate.

Fetal scalp stimulation is not done in some cases. These situations are essentially those in which vaginal examination would be restricted:

- Preterm fetus (may cause contractions)
- Prolonged rupture of membranes (higher risk of infection)
- Chorioamnionitis (intrauterine infection)
- Placenta previa
- Maternal fever of unknown origin (with the possibility of introducing microorganisms into the uterus)

**Vibroacoustic Stimulation.** Acoustic, or vibroacoustic, stimulation may be used by the nurse, physician, or nurse-midwife to supplement fetal scalp stimulation or if scalp stimulation is contraindicated.

An artificial larynx is applied to the mother's lower abdomen, and it is turned on for up to 3 seconds. The reassuring response is the same as with fetal scalp stimulation: acceleration of 15 BPM for 15 seconds or more. An absent response, however, does not necessarily mean that the fetus is hypoxic or acidotic.

Concerns about the loudness of the electronic larynx have led to the use of other methods to induce FHR accelerations. Methods that have been used include vibration with an electric toothbrush and playing music through radio speakers placed on the woman's abdomen.

**Fetal Scalp Blood Sampling.** Occasionally, the physician may obtain a sample of fetal scalp blood to evaluate the pH. This procedure is more complex than scalp stimulation or vibroacoustic stimulation. It requires rupture of membranes, which is not always desirable. Normal scalp pH is 7.25 to 7.35. Acidosis is present if the pH is less than 7.20, and the clinician may hasten the birth by using forceps or cesarean delivery. The scalp sample may be repeated for a borderline pH of 7.20 to 7.24.

**Cord Blood Gases and pH.** Umbilical cord blood analysis is used to assess the infant's status immediately after birth for oxygenation and acid-base balance. The samples are analyzed for pH, $Pco_2$, $Po_2$, and bicarbonate and for base deficit. This information helps identify whether acidosis exists and whether it is respiratory (short-term), metabolic (prolonged), or mixed. Normal cord blood gases and pH can confirm that the fetus was adjusting normally to the stresses of labor, although the fetal monitoring pattern may have been nonreassuring.

The cord is promptly double clamped (within 20 to 30 seconds of birth) and cut to isolate a 10- to 20-cm (4 to 8 inches) segment. Blood samples from an umbilical artery provide the most accurate information about the newborn's acid-base status. The sample can also be obtained from a fetal artery on the surface of the placenta. Blood is drawn into heparinized syringes to prevent coagulation, and the syringes are capped to avoid altering values by exposure to room air (Fig. 14–15). Samples kept at room temperature are reliable for 30 to 60 minutes (ACOG, 1995b). Samples should be kept in ice if there is a delay beyond this time.

### INTERVENTIONS FOR NONREASSURING PATTERNS

Any of several nursing or medical interventions, or both, may be indicated if a nonreassuring FHR pattern is present. All are directed toward identifying the cause of the nonreassuring pattern and improving fetal oxygenation.

**Identifying the Cause of a Nonreassuring Pattern.** Careful examination of the strip may suggest a cause for the nonreassuring FHR pattern and direct the most appropriate interventions. For example, a pattern of late decelerations suggests uteroplacental insufficiency. However, uteroplacental insufficiency may be secondary to a variety of causes, such as maternal hypotension and excessive uterine activity. Different causes require different corrective interventions. Checking the mother's vital signs identifies hypotension, hypertension, and fever. Maternal medications such as narcotics may alter variability.

A vaginal examination may identify a prolapsed cord, which may cause variable decelerations, bradycardia, or both, as it is compressed. A vaginal examination also evaluates the woman's labor status, which helps the birth attendant decide if labor should continue. For example, labor may be allowed to continue, or it may be ended with forceps or a vacuum extractor if a nonreassuring pattern occurs during late labor. If the same nonreassuring pattern

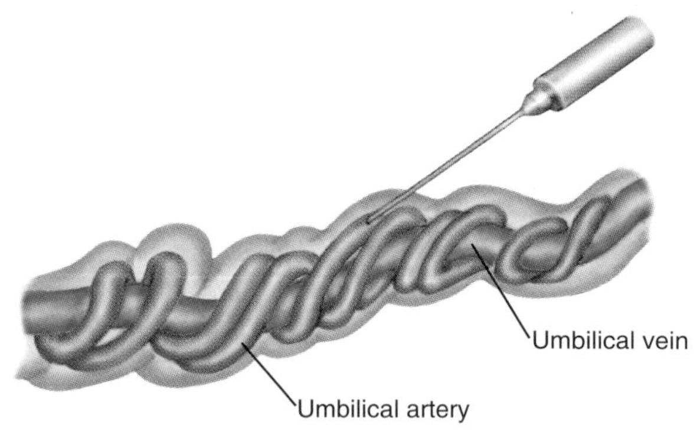


**FIGURE 14–15**

Obtaining a blood sample for umbilical cord blood gases and pH. Samples are drawn from the umbilical cord blood gases and pH. Samples are drawn from the umbilical artery, vein, or both. The samples in capped syringes may be kept for up to 60 minutes at room temperature and 3 hours on ice.

## Critical to Remember

### NURSING RESPONSES TO NONREASSURING FETAL HEART RATE PATTERNS

1. Identify the cause of the nonreassuring pattern to plan the best interventions:
   - Evaluate the pattern for probable cause (late or variable decelerations, bradycardia or tachycardia, absent variability).
   - Evaluate maternal vital signs to identify hypotension, hypertension, or fever.
   - Perform vaginal examination to identify a prolapsed umbilical cord.
2. Stop oxytocin infusion if the drug is being administered.
3. Reposition the woman, avoiding the supine position, for patterns associated with cord compression; repositioning may improve other nonreassuring patterns as well.
4. Increase the rate of a nonadditive intravenous fluid to expand the mother's blood volume and improve placental perfusion.
5. Administer oxygen by face mask at 8 to 10 liters per minute to increase her blood oxygen saturation, making more oxygen available to the fetus.
6. Initiate continuous electronic fetal monitoring with internal devices if no contraindication exists.
7. Notify physician or nurse-midwife as soon as possible. Report and document the following:
   - The pattern that was identified
   - Nursing interventions taken in response to the pattern
   - The fetal response after nursing interventions
   - The response of the physician or nurse-midwife (orders, other response)
8. If the nonreassuring pattern is severe, other staff members should begin preparing for immediate delivery (usually cesarean birth unless vaginal birth is imminent).

prevailed during early labor, a cesarean birth would be more likely.

Internal monitoring is needed for greater accuracy if a nonreassuring pattern develops when external devices are used. The fetal scalp electrode gives a true picture of variability, which is a strong indicator of fetal condition.

**Increasing Placental Perfusion.** The woman is positioned on her side to eliminate aortocaval compression, which can reduce placental blood flow. Increasing nonadditive intravenous fluids such as lactated Ringer's solution increases the maternal blood volume to better perfuse the placenta.

Uterine activity reduces blood flow into the intervillous spaces, and a fetus with little reserve for stress may be unable to tolerate even normal contractions. Persistent hypertonic uterine activity may compromise a fetus with normal reserves. If a woman is receiving oxytocin, it is discontinued so that uterine activity is not stimulated. A tocolytic drug, such as terbutaline (0.125 to 0.25 mg intravenously or 0.25 mg subcutaneously), may be given to reduce uterine activity.

**Increasing Maternal Blood Oxygen Saturation.** Administration of 100 percent oxygen through a snug face mask makes more oxygen available for transfer to the fetus. A commonly suggested rate is 8 to 10 liters per minute.

**Reducing Cord Compression.** If cord compression is suspected, the woman is repositioned. She may be turned from side to side, or her hips may be elevated to shift the fetal presenting part toward her diaphragm. Several position changes may be required before the pattern improves or resolves.

Amnioinfusion increases the fluid around the fetus and cushions the cord. Lactated Ringer's solution or normal saline is infused into the uterus through an intrauterine pressure catheter. The underpads must be changed regularly because fluid leaks out constantly. Possible complications include overdistention of the uterus and increased uterine resting tone. These complications are relieved by releasing some of the fluid. Amnioinfusion also may be used to wash out and dilute fluid that is stained heavily with meconium so that the infant does not aspirate it at birth.

### CHECK YOUR READING

13. What is the rationale for performing fetal scalp stimulation or vibroacoustic stimulation? What is the expected fetal response to these actions?
14. What is the purpose of blood gas and pH determinations on cord blood samples?
15. What nursing actions are appropriate for a nonreassuring FHR pattern? Why are they done?
16. Why might a tocolytic drug increase oxygen supply to the fetus?
17. What are the two purposes of amnioinfusion?

## Application of Nursing Process: Electronic Fetal Monitoring

Interpretation of electronic fetal monitoring patterns requires additional education after entering the intrapartum nursing specialty. The novice nurse or student usually provides care in the form of applying the external monitor, recording maternal vital signs, and assisting in position changes and ambulation. The experienced nurse should be notified promptly if questionable or basic nonreassuring patterns, such as bradycardia, occur.

The nurse may identify any of several problems if a woman has electronic fetal monitoring. The woman or couple who prefer a nontechnical environment for birth may encounter a decisional conflict if electronic fetal monitoring is recommended. Anxiety is likely if the woman does not understand the electronic monitor or if complications develop. Pain may be increased if mobility is restricted during labor.

Two nursing care needs related to intrapartum fetal monitoring are the woman's (or couple's) learning needs and an expansion of nursing care related to fetal oxygenation. Care related to fetal monitoring by either electronic means or auscultation should be combined with that for normal or complicated intrapartum nursing as needed.

## Learning Needs

### Assessment

Determine what the woman and her partner already know about the electronic fetal monitor (Fig. 14–16). Women who have attended prepared childbirth classes or have given birth before may have a basic understanding of the purpose and limitations of the fetal monitor. Identifying what they already know allows the nurse to build on their knowledge appropriately and allows correction of inaccurate information.

If the woman is not familiar with electronic fetal monitoring, assess her perception of it. For example, does she believe that use of the monitor indicates the development of a complication, or does she expect its use? Is the woman comfortable with intermittent auscultation for fetal assessment?

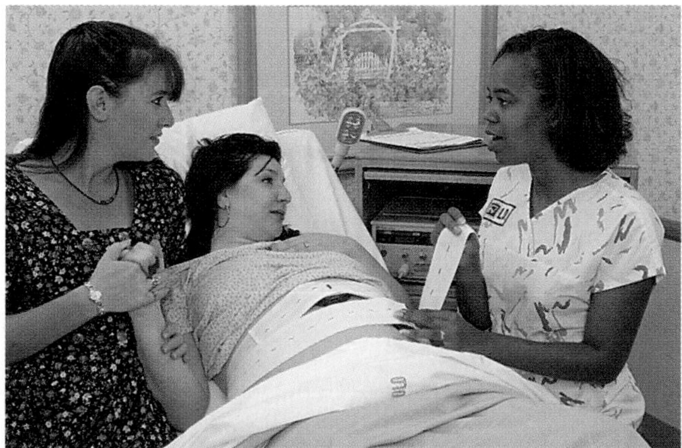

**FIGURE 14–16**

The nurse teaches the woman and her partner about electronic fetal monitoring to limit her anxiety and promote her comfort during labor. The nurse should help the woman understand that the electronic fetal monitor is only one method used to evaluate the fetal well-being during labor.

Lack of knowledge contributes to anxiety. Note the anxiety level of the woman and her partner when the monitor is used. For example, is the woman afraid to move because the fetal heart sounds and tracing skip at that time? Does she place the monitor's data above her own comfort? Note questions about the monitor and its data. Reassess after teaching to identify information that is still unclear or causing anxiety.

### Analysis

Many women expect to have continuous electronic fetal monitoring during labor, and they have often been introduced to it during prepared childbirth classes. Most women have additional questions, however, and some women know little about this mode of fetal surveillance.

The nursing diagnosis is Knowledge Deficit: Fetal Monitoring.

### Planning

A goal for this nursing diagnosis is that, after being taught about the fetal monitor, the woman and her partner express understanding of the following:

- The equipment
- The procedures
- The expected data

### Interventions

#### EXPLAINING THE ELECTRONIC FETAL MONITOR

Teaching is continuous as circumstances change. Explain the purposes of the monitor and the equipment to be used. A simple explanation is to tell the parents that the monitor is a tool to assess how the fetus reacts to labor, especially during contractions. If true, assure the woman that its use does not mean something is wrong with her baby. Explain why changes in the monitoring mode (external to internal) are done. It may be helpful to explain that her physician or nurse-midwife evaluates many factors during labor and that the monitor strip is only one of those factors.

#### ADDRESSING PARENTS' SAFETY CONCERNS

Explain how the equipment functions. Some women are afraid of being attached to an electrical device, especially because cords and electrodes are wet with amniotic fluid and vaginal secretions. Reassure the woman that the connections to her and those to the wall current are isolated from each other.

## Parents Want to Know
## About Electronic Fetal Monitoring

When women have electronic fetal monitoring during labor, they often have questions that the nurse may answer. Here are some commonly asked questions and answers the nurse might use.

*Can I move around with the monitor?*

You can move freely with the monitor. If you notice that the machine isn't picking up the fetal heart sounds or contractions as well, call me and I'll readjust it. Make yourself comfortable; then we'll adjust the machine if necessary.

*What if I need to go to the bathroom?*

If you need to go to the bathroom, we'll unplug the cords from the machine and you can walk in there, or we can roll the monitor to the door of the bathroom.

*Will the monitor shock me? I don't know if I want to be hooked to an electrical outlet, especially since my water has broken.*

The part of the monitor that is attached to you and your baby only transmits information into the machine for processing. The sensors on your body are isolated from electrical parts in the monitor.

*Why is the baby's heart beating so fast?*

A baby's heart normally beats faster than an adult's, both before and after birth. The normal rate is about 110 to 160 beats per minute. A rate outside these boundaries does not necessarily mean that the baby has a problem, but we do look at the monitor strip closely to see how he or she is doing.

*Why do those numbers for the baby's heart rate change so much?*

The heart rate of a healthy baby who is awake changes constantly. When the baby moves, the heart speeds up, just as yours does.

*What do those numbers for contractions (external monitor) mean? They change all the time.*

The numbers reflect a change in the pressure that the monitor senses. The monitor senses many changes in pressure other than those from contractions, such as changes from breathing, coughing, or movement of you or the baby.

*My contractions don't look very strong, but they sure seem strong to me!* (External uterine activity monitor is being used.)

The external monitor senses contractions indirectly, rather than sensing the actual pressure within the uterus. Their appearance on the tracing varies because of many factors, such as your position, the position of the sensor on your abdomen, and the thickness of your abdominal wall.

*Will the internal monitor hurt my baby?*

The spiral electrode attaches only to the outer layer of skin on the baby's head. We are careful to avoid sensitive areas on the head, such as the fontanelles (soft spots), or the face. The uterine catheter slides up beside the baby.

---

Parents may be concerned about attachment of the scalp electrode to the fetal presenting part. Show them that the electrode is a very fine wire that penetrates the outer layer of skin only (about 1 mm, or the thickness of a dime). If she is concerned about the intrauterine pressure catheter, tell her that it lies beside the fetus, next to the inner wall of the uterus.

### COPING WITH MISLEADING DATA

Teach the woman that the monitor sometimes gives data that suggest a problem when no problem exists. For example, the FHR may suddenly fall to zero and the audible tone stop if the sensor (external or scalp electrode) is displaced. Tell her to call the nurse for adjustment or replacement of the sensor.

The woman may be discouraged because the curves representing contractions do not look as strong on the strip as they feel to her. This situation is more likely if an external transducer is used. Explain the many factors that may cause the contraction curves to appear stronger or weaker than they really are. Tell her that the strip is used mainly to assess the timing of contractions and the fetus' reaction when an external tocotransducer is used. Explain that an intrauterine pressure catheter may be recommended if knowledge of intrauterine pressure is crucial.

Reassure the woman that her perception of her contractions and discomfort is important. Value the woman-generated data as well as the machine-generated data. Palpate contractions at intervals as well as evaluating their appearance on the monitor strip.

It is natural for the nurse's attention to be drawn to the electronic fetal monitor when he or she enters a woman's room. Stay focused on the woman and her family rather than devoting excessive attention to the monitoring equipment.

### INCLUDING THE LABOR PARTNER

Tell the partner how to identify the onset and peak of contractions. During active labor, some women discover that contractions become intense before they can prepare for them. If this is the case, have the coach tell the woman when each contraction begins. The coach also can tell her when the peak has passed to encourage her.

**ENHANCING COMFORT**

Some women feel tied to the electronic fetal monitor and are reluctant to make themselves more comfortable. Nursing care involves finding ways to make the mother comfortable and the monitor as nonintrusive as possible. Teach her ways to improve comfort while still obtaining an adequate tracing.

Explain that staying in one position is uncomfortable and does not promote normal labor. The woman may assume any other position than supine unless a specific position is needed. Encourage her to find the position in which she is most comfortable; then adjust the external devices to best detect contractions and the fetal heart beat. Internal devices may be an option if external devices cannot be adjusted to provide useful data.

If the woman finds the sound produced by the electronic fetal monitor distracting or inconsistent with the atmosphere she desires, turn the sound off. Remember that the auditory cues for rate accelerations and decelerations are absent.

If no other contraindications to walking exist, the woman may go to the bathroom to urinate or defecate. Unplug the sensors at the machine and let her walk to the bathroom. Reconnect and adjust them when she returns. Alternatively, you may roll the machine to the door of the bathroom; the cords are usually long enough to remain connected. Document ambulation and any interruption in monitoring on the strip. If the fetus has a nonreassuring pattern, it is preferable not to interrupt the recording.

### Evaluation

The evaluation of parental knowledge is continuous because most parents think of questions after initial explanations and as conditions change. Achievement of the goal is evident if the partners indicate their understanding after each explanation. Their understanding may be accompanied by a decrease in anxiety as well.

## Fetal Oxygenation

### Assessment

Use a systematic approach when evaluating a fetal monitoring strip. Assess the FHR for baseline, variability, and periodic changes. Assess uterine activity for frequency, duration, and intensity of contractions and for uterine resting tone. Assessment and documentation intervals are the same as those recommended for intermittent auscultation:

- *Low-risk women*: every 30 minutes during the active phase and every 15 minutes during the second stage
- *High-risk women*: every 15 minutes during the active phase and every 5 minutes during the second stage

See Table 13–2 for other times when the FHR should be evaluated and documented.

Take the woman's temperature every 4 hours (every 2 hours after membranes rupture). Maternal fever increases the fetal temperature and fetal oxygen requirements. Assess the woman's pulse, respirations, and blood pressure hourly. Hypotension or hypertension may reduce maternal blood flow to the intervillous spaces.

Assessment of mother and fetus is continuous during the dynamic process of labor. Compare data about FHR patterns, uterine activity, and maternal vital signs with baseline data and normal ranges. Observe for subtle trends in the data. Distinguish between patterns having similar appearances, such as early and late decelerations.

Vaginal examination may be performed to evaluate specific FHR patterns—for example, to check for a prolapsed cord if a pattern of variable decelerations occurs (see p. 773).

### Analysis

The collaborative problem Potential Complication: Fetal distress is selected for nursing care related to fetal oxygenation when electronic fetal monitoring is used.

### Planning

Because the nurse cannot manage fetal distress independently, client (fetal) goals are not made. The nurse's responsibility includes planning to do the following:

- Promote adequate fetal oxygenation.
- Take corrective actions to increase fetal oxygenation if nonreassuring patterns are identified.
- Report nonreassuring patterns to the physician or nurse-midwife.
- Support the woman and her partner if a complication develops.
- Document assessments and care.

### Interventions

Measures to promote fetal oxygenation are discussed with the care of the woman in normal labor (see Chapter 13) and of the woman having an epidural or subarachnoid block (see Chapter 15).

#### TAKING CORRECTIVE ACTIONS

If a nonreassuring pattern is noted, take actions to identify its cause and improve fetal oxygenation (see p. 356). Birth facilities should have protocols to give nurses a framework for interventions if nonreassuring patterns develop. Nursing interventions may include both independent and delegated actions.

#### REASSURING PARENTS

Parents understandably become anxious when a nonreassuring pattern occurs. Remain at the bedside, and use a calm manner to avoid increasing their anxiety. Use the call bell to summon other nurses to help with corrective actions and to notify the physician or nurse-midwife.

Explain the problem that was identified and the reason for corrective actions in simple, concise language. Severe anxiety reduces the parents' ability to understand information. Inform them if the FHR returns to a reassuring pattern. Some corrective actions, such as oxygen administration and positioning, may continue after a reassuring pattern returns. Tell the woman that she may talk with the oxygen mask on.

#### REPORTING NONREASSURING PATTERNS

Notify the birth attendant of nonreassuring patterns as soon as possible after taking corrective actions. The priority of nursing care is to improve fetal oxygenation. Document the time and content of all consultations with the physician or nurse-midwife about the mother or fetus and the birth attendant's response.

#### DOCUMENTING ASSESSMENTS AND CARE

Record data related to fetal well-being in the labor record and on the monitor strip. Both are permanent records and should be complete and able to document care independently of the other. Table 14–3 shows guidelines for documentation on the monitor strip and labor record. Documentation can demonstrate good nursing care and show that the standard of care has been met.

Write the woman's name, the date, and the time on the strip when electronic fetal monitoring begins. If a break in the strip occurs, such as to change paper, label the new strip with the woman's name, the date, and the time. Record the last panel number of the previous strip on the new strip so that the entire record can be reassembled sequentially.

Continue documenting the heart rate and maternal observations until vaginal birth occurs. If a cesarean birth is needed, continue monitoring by auscultation or electronic means as long as practical while preparing the woman for surgery. Remove internal devices before securing her legs to the operating table with a strap. Document the time at which monitoring is stopped and the time of abdominal incision.

**TABLE 14–3 DOCUMENTING ELECTRONIC FETAL MONITORING**

**Documentation When Monitoring Initiated**

*Monitor Strip*

Woman's name
Physician's or nurse-midwife's name
Date and time of admission
Date and time electronic monitoring is begun (verify date and time if this information is automatically printed by monitor)
Gravidity, parity, abortions, living children
Gestation in weeks
Presence of identified risk factors
Character of amniotic fluid (if membranes are ruptured)
Function test of monitor accuracy
Initial mode of monitoring (external or internal devices)

*Labor Record*

Same information as on monitor strip
First panel number when strip is begun

**Continuing Documentation**

*Monitor Strip*

Maternal vital signs
Vaginal examinations, including cervical dilation and effacement and fetal station
Rupture of membranes (spontaneously or artificially)
Color, quantity, and character (such as foul odor or cloudiness) of amniotic fluid
Maternal position changes
Maternal or fetal movement
Maternal vomiting, coughing, or other movement that affects tracing
Adjustment of equipment
Medication and anesthesia, including related interventions
Changes of equipment mode (such as external to internal device)
Interventions for nonreassuring patterns
Temporary interruptions in strip, such as woman walking

*Labor Record*

Same information as on monitor strip
Periodic summary of the baseline rate, variability, periodic changes, and uterine activity (frequency, duration, and intensity of contractions and uterine resting tone)

## Evaluation

Client-centered goals are not formulated for a collaborative problem. The nurse compares data with established standards to determine whether they are within normal limits. If nonreassuring patterns are identified, the nurse does the following:

- Takes measures to increase fetal oxygenation
- Notifies the physician or nurse-midwife
- Documents all relevant data

## Nursing Care Plan 14–1
# Intrapartum Fetal Compromise

**ASSESSMENT:** Glenda Brown is a 30-year-old African-American woman. She is a gravida IV, para I who has had two spontaneous abortions. Glenda has been an insulin-dependent diabetic since the age of 15 years. Glenda began seeing Dr. Terry Bloomquist before she became pregnant and has had regular, frequent prenatal care. She had several fetal diagnostic tests during her pregnancy, including two normal biophysical profiles. Glenda's labor is being induced with oxytocin (Pitocin) today at 39 weeks' gestation because she had a blood pressure elevation at today's antepartum care appointment. Baseline pregnancy blood pressure averaged 110 to 120 mmHg systolic and 70 to 75 mmHg diastolic. Today's blood pressure was 146/94, and repeat assessments have been about the same level. Glenda's fetus is to be monitored with electronic fetal monitoring. Glenda is accompanied by her husband, Paul. Glenda said they did not take classes because she was afraid this pregnancy would be "another disappointment." Chris Lowe is Glenda's intrapartum nurse.

### Critical Thinking

What nursing diagnosis is appropriate at this time? Does the nursing diagnosis apply only to Glenda, or should the nurse include Paul when considering the appropriate nursing diagnosis?

**ANSWER**

Although the Browns have had one successful pregnancy, the nurse should not assume that they know about fetal monitoring. The fact that they did not attend classes also increases the likelihood that they need teaching about the electronic fetal monitor and its advantages and limitations.

**NURSING DIAGNOSIS:** Knowledge deficit: Electronic fetal monitoring

**GOALS/EXPECTED OUTCOMES**

Glenda and Paul will state that they understand the reason for electronic monitoring, related equipment and procedures, and the data that are expected.

| INTERVENTION | RATIONALE |
|---|---|
| 1. Assess the parents' present knowledge about electronic fetal monitoring. | 1. Allows the nurse to build on existing accurate knowledge and to correct misunderstandings. |
| 2. Explain information about the monitor to Glenda and Paul:<br>a. Purposes: To provide an audible and written record of the fetal response to labor and to guide caregivers in appropriate interventions if nonreassuring patterns are identified.<br>b. Safety: The monitoring sensors are electrically isolated from the wall current. The fetal scalp electrode (if used) penetrates the outer layer of skin, about a dime's thickness. The intrauterine pressure catheter lies between the baby and the wall of the uterus.<br>c. Misleading data: Encourage Glenda to call for assistance if she cannot hear the fetal heart beat or if she notices that her contractions do not seem to be evident on the strip.<br>d. Encourage Glenda to move about freely. Tell her that a nurse will readjust her monitor if it stops recording properly. Explain that she should urinate about every 2 hours and that the nurse can help her roll the monitor to the bathroom door or temporarily disconnect the sensors. | 2. Reassure Glenda and Paul that the use of the electronic fetal monitor does not mean something is wrong with Glenda or the baby.<br>a. Provides a realistic explanation of how the monitor is used.<br>b. Answers safety concerns that parents often express.<br>c. Sensors, especially external devices, can easily be displaced and stop picking up data. Preparing Glenda and Paul for this possibility reduces their fears if they should stop hearing the fetal heart beat.<br>d. Maternal movement and regular urination enhance normal labor processes. A woman is likely to become anxious and uncomfortable if she concentrates more on maintaining data from the monitor than on coping with labor. |

**EVALUATION**

Glenda and Paul say that they did not go to classes but expected electronic fetal monitoring during labor. Glenda is familiar with the external monitor because it was used for the biophysical profile. She agrees to have internal monitoring if needed, saying that she understands that greater accuracy is important because of her higher risk status.

*Nursing Care Plan continued on following page*

## Nursing Care Plan 14–1 *Continued*

# Intrapartum Fetal Compromise

**ASSESSMENT:** Chris applies the external fetal monitor because Glenda's membranes are intact. She is having irregular spontaneous contractions. The fetal heart rate (FHR) baseline averages 125 to 135 BPM and accelerates when the fetus moves. The nurse begins an oxytocin infusion to induce labor. Glenda's blood pressure is 154/94.

### Critical Thinking

Does the nurse need other data at this point?

**ANSWER**

Added information would help clarify whether the elevation in Glenda's blood pressure is in response to anxiety or pain or reflects a complication such as pregnancy-induced hypertension. The nurse should assess Glenda for hyperactive reflexes and edema, particularly of her face and fingers. See Chapters 13 and 26 for further discussion of these assessments.

**POTENTIAL COMPLICATION:** Fetal compromise

**GOALS/EXPECTED OUTCOMES**

Client goals for the fetus are inappropriate because nurses cannot independently manage fetal distress. Chris' planning for Glenda should reflect the need to do the following:

1. Compare FHR and uterine activity data with baseline levels before oxytocin induction.
2. Promote normal fetal oxygenation.
3. Take corrective actions for nonreassuring patterns.
4. Notify Glenda's physician if nonreassuring patterns develop.

| INTERVENTION | RATIONALE |
|---|---|
| 1. Identify relevant risk factors for fetal compromise. | 1. Women who have risk factors that could reduce fetal oxygenation should have fetal assessments more frequently. In this case, Glenda has three identified risk factors: diabetes mellitus, pregnancy-induced hypertension, and labor induced with oxytocin. |
| 2. Encourage Glenda to assume any comfortable position other than the supine position. | 2. The supine position can reduce blood return to the heart by compressing the inferior vena cava. Compression of the aorta and reduced cardiac output reduce placental perfusion. |
| 3. Evaluate the tracing at the following times, signing or initialing the strip each time. Document a summary of the evaluation on the labor record.<br>a. Every 15 minutes during the first stage and every 5 minutes during the second stage.<br>b. Before and after procedures such as amniotomy, medications, epidural anesthesia.<br>c. With changes of activity, such as urination and repositioning. | 3. Documents that assessment was done. Documenting on both strip and labor record allows each to stand alone.<br>a. Provides a framework for regular assessment of the fetal response to labor. This situation describes a high-risk pregnancy, and the fetus should be evaluated by those guidelines.<br>b. Rupture of membranes (spontaneously or by amniotomy) may result in cord compression. Medications may alter the rate or variability of the fetal heart beat. Epidural anesthesia may cause hypotension, which can decrease uteroplacental perfusion.<br>c. Changes in activity or position could alter the uterine or umbilical cord blood flow. Also, external sensors may slip and need adjustment. |
| 4. Use a four-step approach to evaluate the strip:<br>a. Baseline FHR<br>b. Variability (primarily if fetal scalp electrode is used)<br>c. Periodic changes: Accelerations, decelerations. Note relationship of periodic changes to fetal movement, contractions, and the woman's status and activity. Note nonperiodic (random) accelerations or variable decelerations. | 4. Provides a systematic framework to evaluate the fetal response to labor.<br>a. Tachycardia may be an early response to hypoxia. Bradycardia may occur in response to vagal stimulation or prolonged hypoxia.<br>b. Normal variability (6 to 25 BPM) suggests that the fetus is well oxygenated and not in acidosis. Variability is most accurate with a fetal scalp electrode. |

## Nursing Care Plan 14–1 *Continued*

# Intrapartum Fetal Compromise

**INTERVENTION**

d. Uterine activity: Evaluate frequency and duration using either external or internal devices. Estimate intensity with an external device by palpating three or more contractions. Note whether the uterus relaxes between contractions for at least 60 seconds. If an intrauterine pressure catheter is used, reach contraction intensity and uterine resting tone from scale on strip.

5. If nonreassuring patterns develop, take appropriate corrective actions such as discontinuing the oxytocin, increasing the rate of the nonadditive intravenous solution, positioning Glenda on her side, and administering oxygen. Notify Dr. Bloomquist of nonreassuring patterns, corrective actions taken, and the fetal response. Document Dr. Bloomquist's response and any orders.

**RATIONALE**

c. Accelerations are a reassuring sign of fetal well-being and are accompanied by fetal movement. Early decelerations are a normal response to head compression. Late (uteroplacental insufficiency) and variable (umbilical cord compression) decelerations are nonreassuring. The nurse should attempt to identify their cause, correct it if possible, and take steps to improve fetal oxygenation.

d. Contractions that are too long (more than 90 seconds duration) or too frequent (closer than every 2 minutes), a resting interval of less than 60 seconds, or intrauterine pressure of more than 20 mmHg can reduce the time available for normal uteroplacental exchange. Because of high-risk problems (specifically diabetes and pregnancy-induced hypertension), uteroplacental exchange may be reduced before labor begins. Oxytocin stimulates uterine activity.

5. The first priority is to identify the cause of the nonreassuring pattern and increase fetal oxygenation. The physician should be notified to keep abreast of the maternal-fetal status for needed medical orders or interventions.

**EVALUATION**

Goals are not established for collaborative problems. Chris compared data from the fetal monitor and other nursing evaluations with the baseline data before Glenda started having oxytocin or contractions. For the first 4 hours of the oxytocin induction, the FHR continued near its baseline of 125 to 135 RPM, with long-term variability averaging 10 BPM. Fetal heart rate accelerations with fetal movement continue. No nonreassuring patterns were noted.

**ASSESSMENT:** Dr. Bloomquist ruptures Glenda's membranes and inserts internal devices for the FHR and uterine activity. Glenda's blood pressure remains near 145/90, and her oxytocin infusion continues. She is having contractions every 4 minutes; they are of 50 seconds' duration and 50 mmHg intensity, and she has a uterine resting tone of 10 mmHg. One hour after Glenda's membranes are ruptured, Chris notes that the baseline FHR has risen to approximately 145 to 150 BPM with variability averaging 3 BPM. A pattern of repeated late decelerations develops. Chris stops the oxytocin infusion and increases the rate of nonadditive intravenous fluid, positions Glenda on her left side, and administers oxygen at 10 liters per minute with a snug face mask. Dr. Bloomquist is notified. Baseline variability improves to 5 BPM, but repeated late decelerations continue. Glenda is holding Paul's hand tightly and breathing rapidly. Her vital signs are blood pressure, 145/90; pulse, 90; respirations, 32. Uterine activity is unchanged.

**Critical Thinking**

What new nursing diagnosis or collaborative problem seems apparent based on the latest assessment data? Why?

**ANSWER**

Glenda displays several behaviors typical of anxiety: rapid pulse and respiratory rates and holding her husband's hand. Also, because of the development of complications and the minimal improvement in the fetal status superimposed on her higher-risk status, anxiety seems appropriate. Helping her control her anxiety can promote a more normal labor as well as make her more comfortable.

**NURSING DIAGNOSIS:** Anxiety related to unexpected development of complications

**GOALS/EXPECTED OUTCOMES**

1. Glenda will have a reduced respiratory rate (14 to 22/minute) after interventions.
2. Glenda will have a more relaxed face and body posture after interventions.

*Nursing Care Plan continued on following page*

## Nursing Care Plan 14–1 *Continued*
# Intrapartum Fetal Compromise

| INTERVENTION | RATIONALE |
|---|---|
| 1. Maintain calm behavior while performing corrective actions and notifying Dr. Bloomquist. | 1. Nonverbally communicates to Glenda and Paul that mother and fetus are receiving competent care. Anxious behavior on the part of caregivers tends to increase the parents' anxiety. |
| 2. Use simple, concise language for all explanations. | 2. High anxiety or intense physical sensations impair one's ability to comprehend explanations. |
| 3. Explain the following to Glenda and Paul:<br>a. The problem that was identified<br>b. The usual cause of the problem<br>c. Reasons for corrective actions<br>d. Expected results<br>e. That Glenda can talk with oxygen mask on | 3. If Glenda and Paul understand what is happening and why the corrective actions are taken, they are more likely to comply with the care. Knowledge decreases fear of the unknown. Assuring Glenda that she can talk with the oxygen mask on allows her to ask questions and ventilate feelings to reduce anxiety and fear. |
| 4. Inform Glenda and Paul if the pattern improves or is resolved. For example, tell them when baseline variability improves. | 4. Decreases anxiety about the fetus' condition. |
| 5. Allow Glenda and Paul to ventilate their feelings about the labor and birth during the postpartum period. Explain any gaps in their understanding about what happened. | 5. Helps the couple accept and put unexpected occurrences in perspective. Decreases the possibility that one or both parents feel like "a failure" if emergency intervention (cesarean birth) becomes necessary. |

**EVALUATION**

Over the next hour, the FHR pattern gradually improves. The baseline rate becomes lower (130 to 140 BPM), and late decelerations are sporadic. Baseline short-term variability improves to about 8 BPM. Glenda gradually relaxes her grip on Paul's hand and her body relaxes. Her respiratory rate slows to 22 breaths per minute. Glenda requires a cesarean birth, however, because her cervix does not dilate to greater than 7 cm, despite adequate contractions for 2 hours.

## SUMMARY CONCEPTS

- The purpose of intrapartum fetal surveillance is to identify fetal well-being and to identify the fetus who may be having hypoxic stress beyond the ability to compensate for it.
- The two approaches to intrapartum fetal monitoring are intermittent auscultation with palpation of uterine activity and electronic fetal monitoring. Because each type has distinct advantages and limitations, neither approach is superior to the other.
- Fetal oxygenation depends on a normal flow of oxygenated maternal blood into the placenta, normal exchange within the placenta, patent umbilical cord vessels, and normal fetal circulatory and oxygen-carrying function.
- Stimulation of the sympathetic nervous system increases the FHR and strengthens the heart contraction. Stimulation of the parasympathetic nervous system slows the heart rate and maintains short-term variability.
- External electronic fetal monitoring is less accurate for FHR and uterine activity patterns than internal monitoring, but it is noninvasive.
- Greater accuracy is the main advantage of internal electronic fetal monitoring devices.
- Nursing responsibilities related to intrapartum fetal monitoring include promoting fetal oxygenation, identifying and reporting nonreassuring findings, supporting parents, communicating with the physician or nurse-midwife, and documenting all care.

### *References and Readings*

Albers, L.L. (1994). Clinical issues in electronic fetal monitoring. *Birth* 21(2):108–110.

American Academy of Pediatrics and American College of Obstetricians and Gynecologists. (1992). *Guidelines for perinatal care* (3rd ed.). Elk Grove Village, Ill.: Author.

American College of Obstetricians and Gynecologists (ACOG). (1995a). *ACOG technical bulletin*, No. 207. Fetal heart rate patterns: Monitoring, interpretation, & management. Washington, D.C.: Author.

American College of Obstetricians and Gynecologists (ACOG). (1995b). *ACOG technical bulletin*, No. 216. Umbilical artery blood acid-base analysis. Washington, D.C.: Author.

Barnes, J. (1996). Fetal communication: Calling the placenta (Cassette Recording No. OGN-619). Anaheim, Calif. AWHONN.

Blackburn, S.T., & Loper, D.L. (1992). *Maternal, fetal, & neonatal physiology: A clinical perspective*. Philadelphia: W.B. Saunders.

Boylan, P., & Parisi, V. (1994). Fetal acid-base balance. In R. Creasy & R. Resnik (Eds.), *Maternal-fetal medicine: Princi-*

*ples and practice* (pp. 349–358). Philadelphia: W.B. Saunders.

Committee on Obstetric Practice and AAP Committee on Fetus and Newborn. (1996). ACOG Committee opinion number 174: Use and Abuse of the Apgar score. *International Journal of Gynecology and Obstetrics*, 54, 303–305.

Cunningham, F.G., MacDonald, P.C., Gant, N.F., Leveno, K.J., Gilstrap, L.C., Hankins, G.D.V., et al. (1997). *Williams obstetrics* (20th ed.). Norwalk, Conn.: Appleton & Lange.

Cusick, W., Smulian, J.C., & Ventzileos, A.M. (1995). Intrapartum use of fetal heart rate monitoring, contraction monitoring, and amnioinfusion. *Clinics in Perinatology*, 22(4), 875–906.

Davis, L.K. (1992). Protocol for fetal heart rate monitoring. In L.K. Mandeville & N.H. Troiano (Eds.), *High-risk intrapartum nursing* (pp. 305–308). Philadelphia: J.B. Lippincott.

Flamm, B.L. (1994). Electronic fetal monitoring in the United States. *Birth*, 21(2), 105–106.

Folsom, M.S. (1997). Amnioinfusion for meconium: Does it help? MCN: *American Journal of Maternal-Child Nursing*, 22(2), 74–79.

Grossman, S.Z. (1993). The nature of lawsuits related to obstetric care. In R.A. Knuppel & J.E. Drukker (Eds.), *High-risk pregnancy: A team approach* (2nd ed., pp. 733–742). Philadelphia: W.B.Saunders.

Guyton, A.C., & Hall, J.E. (1996). *Textbook of medical physiology*. Philadelphia: W.B. Saunders.

Helwig, J.T., Parer, J.T., Kilpatrick, S.J., & Laros, R.K. (1996). Umbilical cord blood acid-base state: What is normal? *American Journal of Obstetrics and Gynecology*, 174(6), 1807–1814.

Inturrisi, M. (1996). Amnioinfusion (Cassette Recording No. OGN-631). Anaheim, Calif.: AWHONN.

Ladebauche, P. (1994). Limiting liability to avoid malpractice litigation. MCN: *American Journal of Maternal-Child Nursing*, 20(5), 243–248.

Low, J.A., Simpson, L.L., Tonni, G., & Chamberlain, S. (1995). Limitations in the clinical prediction of intrapartum fetal asphyxia. *American Journal of Obstetrics and Gynecology*, 172(3), 801–804.

Menihan, C.A. (1996). Intrapartum fetal monitoring. In K.R. Simpson & P.A. Creehan (Eds.), AWHONN *perinatal nursing* (pp. 187–225). Philadelphia: J.B. Lippincott.

Miller, D.A. (1994). Fetal distress in the intrapartum period. In F. Zuspan & E. Quilligan (Eds.), *Current therapy in obstetrics and gynecology*, 4 (pp. 349–353). Philadelphia: W.B. Saunders.

Miller, F. (1994). Fetal scalp stimulation. In F. Zuspan & E. Quilligan (Eds.), *Current therapy in obstetrics and gynecology*, 4 (pp. 355–356). Philadelphia: W.B. Saunders.

Murray, M. (1997). *Antepartal and intrapartal fetal monitoring* (2nd ed.) Albuquerque, N.Mex.: Learning Resources International.

NAACOG (1990). *Fetal heart rate auscultation*. Washington, D.C.: Author.

Neilson, J.P. (1994). Electronic fetal heart rate monitoring during labor: Information from randomized trials. *Birth*, 21(2), 101–104.

Parer, J. (1994). Fetal heart rate. In R. Creasy & R. Resnik (Eds.), *Maternal-fetal medicine: Principles and practice* (pp. 298–325). Philadelphia: W.B. Saunders.

Rosen, M.G., & Dickinson, J.C. (1993). The paradox of electronic fetal monitoring: More data may not enable us to predict or prevent infant neurologic morbidity. *American Journal of Obstetrics and Gynecology*, 162(3), 745–751.

Schifrin, B.S. (1995). Medicolegal ramifications of electronic fetal monitoring during labor. *Clinics in Perinatology*, 22(4), 837–854.

Supplee, R.B., & Vezeau, T.M. (1996). Continuous electronic fetal monitoring: Does it belong in low-risk births? MCN: *American Journal of Maternal-Child Nursing*, 21(6), 301–306.

Wallerstedt, C., Higgins, P., Kasnic, T., & Curet, L.B. (1994). Amnioinfusion: An update. *Journal of Obstetric Gynecologic, and Neonatal Nursing*, 23(7), 573–578.

West, J., Chez, B.F., & Miller, F.C. (1993). Fetal heart rate. In R.A. Knuppel & J.E. Drukker (Eds.), *High-risk pregnancy: A team approach* (2nd ed., pp. 317–336). Philadelphia: W.B. Saunders.

Woods, J.R., & Glantz, J.C. (1994). Significance of amniotic fluid meconium. In R. Creasy & R. Resnik (Eds.), *Maternal-fetal medicine: Principles and practice* (pp. 413–422). Philadelphia: W.B. Saunders.

# 15

# Pain Management During Childbirth

**OBJECTIVES**

1. Compare childbirth pain with other types of pain.
2. Describe how excessive pain can affect the laboring woman and her fetus.
3. Examine how physical and psychological forces interact in the laboring woman's pain experience.
4. Describe use of nonpharmacologic pain management techniques in labor.
5. Describe how medications may affect a pregnant woman and the fetus or neonate.
6. Identify benefits and risks of specific pharmacologic pain control methods.
7. Explain nursing care related to different types of intrapartum pain management.

**DEFINITIONS**

**agonist** *A substance that causes a physiologic effect.*

**analgesic** *A systemic agent that relieves pain without loss of consciousness.*

**anesthesia** *Loss of sensation, especially to pain, with or without loss of consciousness.*

**anesthesiologist** *A physician who specializes in administration of anesthesia.*

**antagonist** *A drug that blocks the action of another drug or of body secretions.*

**aspiration pneumonitis** *A chemical injury to the lungs that may occur with regurgitation and aspiration of acidic gastric secretions.*

**endorphins** *Morphine-like substances that occur naturally in the central nervous system and modify pain sensations.*

**epidural space** *The area outside the dura, between the dura mater and the vertebral canal.*

**general anesthesia** *Systemic loss of sensation with loss of consciousness.*

**motor block** *Loss of voluntary movement caused by regional anesthesia.*

**nurse anesthetist** *A registered nurse who has advanced education and certification in administration of anesthetics. Also certified registered nurse anesthetist (CRNA).*

**pain threshold (or pain perception)** *The lowest level of stimulus one perceives as painful. Pain threshold is relatively constant under different conditions.*

**pain tolerance** *Maximum pain one is willing to endure. Pain tolerance may increase or decrease under different conditions.*

**regional anesthesia** *Anesthesia that blocks pain impulses in a localized area without loss of consciousness.*

**sensory block** *Loss of sensation caused by regional anesthesia.*

**subarachnoid space** *Space between the arachnoid mater and the pia mater containing cerebrospinal fluid.*

Each woman has unique expectations about birth, including expectations about pain and her ability to manage it. The woman who successfully handles the pain of labor is more likely to view her experience as a positive life event. A woman's experience with labor pain varies with several physical and psychological elements, and each woman responds differently.

Management of labor pain motivates many pregnant women and their partners to attend childbirth classes. This chapter provides an overview of techniques to help laboring women manage pain successfully. Nonpharmacologic and pharmacologic methods give the nurse and laboring woman a selection of pain management techniques to choose from.

## Unique Nature of Pain During Birth

Pain is a universal experience but is difficult to define. It is an unpleasant sensation of distress resulting from stimulation of sensory nerves. Pain involves two components:

- A physiologic component that includes reception by sensory nerves and transmission to the central nervous system
- A psychological component, which involves recognizing the sensation, interpreting it as painful, and reacting to the interpretation

Pain is subjective and personal; no one can feel another's pain. One must simply believe what another person says about his or her pain experience.

Childbirth pain, however, differs from other pain in several important respects:

- *It is part of a normal process.* Childbirth pain is part of a normal process, whereas other types of pain usually indicate an injury or illness. Pain may cause a woman to assume different positions in labor, favoring descent of the fetus through her pelvis.
- *There is time for preparation.* The pregnant woman has several months to prepare for labor, including acquiring skills to help manage pain. Realistic preparation and knowledge about the birth process help her develop skills to cope with labor pain.
- *It is self-limiting.* Labor pain has a foreseeable end. A woman can expect her labor to end in hours, rather than days, weeks, or months. Other kinds of pain may also be brief, but the baby's birth brings a rapid decrease in pain.

  Labor pain is not constant but intermittent. A woman may describe little discomfort with contractions during early labor. Even during late labor, a woman may be relatively comfortable during the short rest periods between contractions.
- *Labor ends with the birth of a baby.* The emotional significance of her child's birth cannot be ignored when trying to understand a woman's response to pain. Concern about her fetus often motivates a woman to tolerate more pain during labor than she otherwise might be willing to endure.

## Adverse Effects of Excessive Pain

Although expected during labor, pain that exceeds a woman's tolerance can have harmful effects on her and the fetus.

### Physiologic Effects

A woman may react to pain with fear and anxiety, which increase sympathetic nervous system activity and result in increased secretion of catecholamines (epinephrine and norepinephrine). Catecholamines stimulate $\alpha$ and $\beta$ receptors. Epinephrine stimulates both $\alpha$ and $\beta$ receptors, whereas norepinephrine stimulates primarily $\alpha$ receptors.

Stimulation of the $\alpha$ receptors causes uterine and generalized vasoconstriction and an increase in the uterine muscle tone. These effects reduce uterine blood flow as they increase the maternal blood flow and maternal blood pressure.

Stimulation of the $\beta$ receptors relaxes the uterine muscle and causes vasodilation. However, uterine vessels are already dilated, so dilation of other maternal vessels allows her blood to pool in them. The pooling of blood reduces the amount of blood available to perfuse the placenta.

The combined effects of excessive catecholamine secretion are therefore the following:

- Reduced blood flow to and from the placenta, restricting fetal oxygen supply and waste removal
- Reduced effectiveness of uterine contractions, slowing labor progress

The work of labor increases a woman's metabolic rate and her demand for oxygen. Pain and anxiety escalate her already high metabolic rate. She breathes fast to obtain more oxygen, exhaling too much carbon dioxide in the process. Significant changes, more than those expected during labor, can occur in the woman's $PaO_2$ and $PaCO_2$ and in her arterial pH. These maternal respiratory and metabolic changes alter placental exchange. The fetus may have less oxygen available for uptake and be less able to unload carbon dioxide to the mother. The net result is that the fetus shifts to anaerobic metabolism, with buildup of hydrogen ions (acidosis). This type of acidosis is metabolic and does not resolve as quickly after birth as respiratory acidosis.

### Psychological Effects

Poorly relieved pain lessens the pleasure of this extraordinary life event for both partners. The mother may find it difficult to interact with her infant because she is depleted from a painful labor. Unpleasant memories of the birth may affect her response to sexual activity or another labor. Her partner may feel inadequate as a support person during birth.

**CHECK YOUR READING**

1. How does the pain of childbirth differ from other kinds of pain?
2. How can excessive pain adversely affect a laboring woman and her fetus?

## Variables in Childbirth Pain

To intervene effectively, the nurse must identify factors that modify childbirth pain and influence a woman's response. Physical and psychosocial factors contribute to her response.

### Physical Factors

Childbirth pain is of two types—visceral and somatic. Visceral pain is a slow, deep pain that is poorly localized. It is often described as dull or aching. Visceral pain dominates during first-stage labor as the uterus contracts and the cervix dilates.

Somatic pain is a faster, sharp pain. It can be precisely localized. Somatic pain is most prominent during late first-stage labor and during second-stage labor as the descending fetus puts direct pressure on maternal tissues.

#### SOURCES OF PAIN

Four potential sources of labor pain exist in most labors. Other physical factors may modify labor pain, increasing or decreasing it.

**Tissue Ischemia.** The blood supply to the uterus decreases during contractions, leading to tissue hypoxia and anaerobic metabolism. Ischemic uterine pain has been likened to ischemic heart pain.

**Cervical Dilation.** Dilation and stretching of the cervix and lower uterus are a major source of pain. Pain stimuli from cervical dilation travel through the hypogastric plexus, entering the spinal cord at the T10, T11, T12, and L1 levels (Fig. 15–1).

**Pressure and Pulling on Pelvic Structures.** Some pain results from pressure and pulling on pelvic structures, such as ligaments, fallopian tubes, ovaries, bladder, and peritoneum. The pain is a visceral pain; a woman may feel it as referred pain in her back and legs.

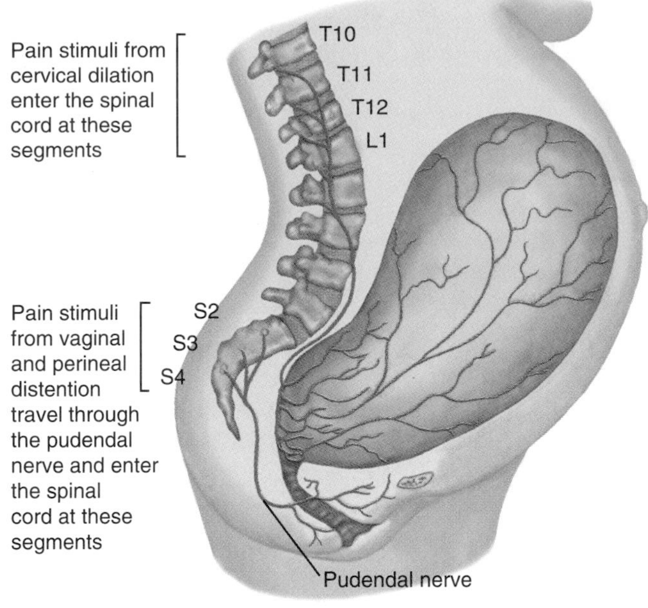
Pain stimuli from cervical dilation enter the spinal cord at these segments
T10
T11
T12
L1
Pain stimuli from vaginal and perineal distention travel through the pudendal nerve and enter the spinal cord at these segments
S2
S3
S4
Pudendal nerve

**FIGURE 15–1**

Pathways of pain transmission during labor.

**Distention of the Vagina and Perineum.** Marked distention of the vagina and perineum occurs with fetal descent, especially during the second stage. The woman may describe a sensation of burning, tearing, or splitting (somatic pain). Pain from vaginal and perineal distention and pressure and pulling on adjacent structures enters the spinal cord at the S2, S3, and S4 levels (see Fig. 15–1).

#### FACTORS INFLUENCING PERCEPTION OR TOLERANCE OF PAIN

Although physiologic processes cause labor pain, a woman's tolerance of pain may be affected by other physical influences.

**Intensity of Labor.** The woman who has a short, intense labor often complains of severe pain because each contraction does so much work (effacement, dilation, and fetal descent). A rapid labor may limit her options for pharmacologic pain relief as well.

**Cervical Readiness.** If pre-labor cervical changes (softening, with some dilation and effacement) are incomplete, the cervix does not open as easily. More contractions are needed to achieve dilation and effacement, resulting in a longer labor and greater fatigue in the laboring woman.

**Fetal Position.** Labor is likely to be longer and more uncomfortable when the fetus is in an unfavorable position. An occiput posterior position is a common variant seen in otherwise normal labors. In this position, each contraction pushes the fetal occiput against the woman's sacrum. She experiences intense back discomfort (*back labor*) that persists between contractions. Often a woman cannot deliver her infant in the occiput posterior position. The fetal head must therefore rotate a wider arc before the mechanisms of extension and expulsion occur, so labor is often longer (see p. 749). Back pain may decrease dramatically when a fetus rotates into the more favorable occiput anterior position. The rate of labor progress usually increases as well.

**Characteristics of the Pelvis.** The size and shape of a woman's pelvis influence the course and length of her labor. Abnormalities may cause a difficult and longer labor and may contribute to fetal malpresentation or malposition.

**Fatigue.** Fatigue reduces a woman's ability to tolerate pain and to use coping skills she has learned. She may be unable to focus on relaxation and breathing techniques that would otherwise help her tolerate labor. An extremely fatigued woman may have an exaggerated response to contractions, or she may be unable to respond to sensations of labor such as the urge to push.

Many women find that sleep is difficult during the last weeks of pregnancy. A woman's shortness of breath when lying down, frequent urination, and fetal activity interrupt sleep so that she often begins labor with a sleep deficit. If labor begins late in the evening, she may have been awake well over 24 hours by the time she gives birth. Even if a woman begins labor well rested, slow progress may exhaust her.

**Intervention of Caregivers.** Although they may be appropriate for the well-being of a woman and fetus, some interventions add discomfort to the natural pain of labor.

Intravenous lines cause pain when they are inserted and remain noticeable to many women during labor. Fetal monitoring equipment is uncomfortable to some women. Both may hamper a woman's mobility, which she might use to assume a more comfortable position.

A woman whose labor is induced or augmented often reports more pain and increased difficulty coping with it because contractions reach peak intensity quickly. Vaginal examinations and amniotomy also increase a woman's discomfort briefly because of vaginal and cervical stretching.

## Psychosocial Factors

Several psychosocial variables influence a woman's experience of pain.

### CULTURE

A woman's sociocultural roots influence how she perceives, interprets, and responds to pain during childbirth. Some cultures encourage loud and vigorous expression of pain, whereas others value self-control. However, women are individuals within their cultural groups. The experience of pain is personal, and one should not make assumptions about how a woman from a specific cultural or ethnic group will behave during labor.

Women should be encouraged to express themselves in any way they find comforting, and the diversity of their expressions must be respected. *Accepting a woman's individual response to labor and pain promotes a therapeutic relationship.*

The nurse should avoid praising some behaviors (such as stoicism) while belittling others (such as noisy expression). This restraint is difficult because noisy women are challenging to work with and may disturb others.

The unique nature of childbirth pain and women's diverse responses to it make nursing management complex. The nurse can miss important cues if the woman is either stoic, having little outward expression of pain, or expresses herself loudly and con-

### CRITICAL THINKING EXERCISE

Truc Pham is a Vietnamese-American in labor with her first baby. Her cervix is dilated 6 cm, effacement is 100 percent, and the fetus is at a +1 station. Truc's contractions are every 3 minutes, 50 to 60 seconds, and of strong intensity. She smiles at the nurse each time the nurse talks to her but does not talk much herself. Truc stiffens her body during contractions and interacts little with her husband or the nurse at those times.

**Q:**
1. How should the nurse interpret Truc's assessment and behavior?
2. Does the nurse need additional data?
3. What nursing actions are appropriate?

**A:**
1. Truc's labor progress and pattern of contractions plus her tension suggest that she may need medication. However, the nurse should not assume that she needs or wants medication either. Breathing techniques or other non-pharmacologic measures may be adequate for Truc.

   The nurse must not assume that Truc does not need pain relief because she smiles and has not requested pain medication. Asian women often value stoicism and are concerned with harmonious relationships. Truc may be smiling to please the nurse rather than because she is comfortable.
2. The nurse needs additional data about Truc's needs and plans for pain relief.
3. The nurse can share observations about Truc's body posture during contractions. If Truc does not speak English well, an interpreter may improve assessment of her need for pain relief. The nurse can demonstrate non-pharmacologic actions, such as breathing techniques, for Truc to use with or without medication.

stantly. With either extreme, the nurse may not readily identify critical information such as impending birth or symptoms of a complication.

### ANXIETY AND FEAR

Mild or moderate anxiety can have a positive effect on birth by heightening attention and enhancing learning. However, extreme anxiety and fear magnify sensitivity to pain and impair a woman's ability to tolerate it. They consume energy she needs to cope with the birth process, including its painful aspects.

Anxiety and fear increase muscle tension, diverting oxygenated blood to the brain and skeletal muscles. Tension in pelvic muscles counters the expulsive forces of uterine contractions and the laboring woman's pushing efforts during the second stage. Prolonged tension results in general fatigue, increased pain perception, and reduced ability to use skills to cope with pain.

If a previous pregnancy had a poor outcome, such as a stillborn infant or one with abnormalities, a woman is probably more anxious during labor and for a time after birth. She is likely to examine and reexamine her infant to assure herself that this baby is normal.

### PREVIOUS EXPERIENCES WITH PAIN

Early in life a child learns that pain is a symptom of bodily injury. Consequently, fear and withdrawal are a woman's natural reactions to pain during labor. Learning about the normal sensations of labor, including pain, helps a woman suppress her natural reactions of fear and withdrawal, allowing her body to do the work of birth.

A woman who has given birth previously has a different perspective. If she has had a vaginal delivery, she is probably aware of normal labor sensations and is less likely to associate them with injury or abnormality. Also, time has a way of blunting the memory of painful experiences.

A woman who had a child by caesarean birth and has never experienced labor may be particularly anxious. The experience of cesarean birth is known to her, whereas labor is unknown. A repeat cesarean birth may seem like the quicker and less painful option. She may have difficulty yielding to the normal forces of birth.

A woman who has had a previous long and difficult labor is more likely to be anxious about the outcome of the present one. If she had a cesarean birth following the difficult labor, she may doubt her ability to give birth vaginally. Her anxiety often intensifies when she reaches the point at which her prior labor ended with the cesarean birth.

Previous experiences do not always adversely affect a woman's ability to deal with pain. She may have learned ways to cope with pain during other episodes of pain or during other births and use these skills adaptively during labor.

### PREPARATION FOR CHILDBIRTH

Preparation for childbirth does not ensure a pain-free labor. A woman should be prepared for pain realistically, including reasonable expectations about analgesia and anesthesia. She may feel that her entire preparation is invalid if what she expects does not happen when she is in labor.

Preparation reduces anxiety and fear of the unknown. It allows a woman to rehearse for labor and learn a variety of skills to master pain as labor progresses. She and her partner learn about expected behavioral changes during labor, and their knowledge decreases their anxiety when those changes occur.

### SUPPORT SYSTEM

An anxious partner is less able to provide the support and reassurance that the woman needs during labor. In addition, anxiety in others can be contagious, increasing her anxiety. She may assume that if others are worried, something is probably wrong.

The birth experiences of a woman's family and friends cannot be ignored. Those individuals can be an important source of support if they convey realistic information about labor pain and its control. If they describe labor as intolerable, however, she may have needless distress. It is equally detrimental for a woman to hear that labor is painless. No two labors are alike, even in the same woman.

**CHECK YOUR READING**

3. How may physical and psychological factors interact in a woman's labor pain experience?
4. What four sources of pain are present in most labors?
5. How can each of these physical factors influence the pain a woman experiences during childbirth? (a) Labor intensity? (b) Cervical readiness? (c) Fetal position? (d) Maternal pelvis? (e) Fatigue?
6. How do psychosocial factors influence a woman's experience with labor pain?

## Nonpharmacologic Pain Management

The nurse who cares for women in labor and birth can offer nonpharmacologic and pharmacologic pain management methods. Nonpharmacologic methods require no medical order. Education about nonpharmacologic pain management is the foundation of prepared childbirth classes.

The intrapartum nurse should know methods that are taught in local childbirth classes to be most helpful to women and their labor partners. Teaching techniques that conflict with what a woman learned and practiced may confuse her. Other techniques can be reserved for use if a woman finds learned techniques ineffective.

## Advantages

Nonpharmacologic methods have several advantages over pharmacologic methods *if* pain control is adequate. They do not slow labor and have no side effects or risk of allergy.

Nonpharmacologic techniques are both an alternative and an adjunct to drugs. Many women use a combination of the two. The woman who chooses analgesia needs alternate pain management until it is given, usually after labor is established. Also, pharmacologic methods may not eliminate labor pain, and a woman needs nonpharmacologic methods to control the pain that remains.

Nonpharmacologic methods may be the only realistic option for a woman who enters the hospital in advanced, rapid labor. In this case, drugs might not have enough time to take effect. Also, the newborn might have respiratory depression if a systemic opioid narcotic reaches its peak action about the time of birth.

## Limitations

Nonpharmacologic methods also have limitations, especially as the sole method of pain control. Women do not always achieve their desired level of pain control using these methods alone. Because of the many variables in labor, even a well-prepared and highly motivated woman may have a difficult labor and need analgesia or anesthesia.

## Preparation for Pain Management

The ideal time to learn nonpharmacologic pain control is before labor. During the last few weeks of pregnancy, the woman learns about labor, including its painful aspects, in childbirth classes. She can prepare to confront the pain, learning a variety of skills to use during labor. Her support person learns specific methods to encourage and support her. After admission, the nurse can review and reinforce what the partners learned in class.

The nurse can teach the unprepared woman and her support person nonpharmacologic techniques. The latent phase of labor is the best time for intrapartum teaching because the woman is usually anxious enough to be attentive and interested, yet comfortable enough to understand. Late labor is a difficult time to teach because the woman cannot focus well on learning.

No one method or combination of methods helps every woman. Many methods may become less effective (habituation) after prolonged use. Changing techniques counters habituation. The nurse who knows a variety of methods can select those that are most helpful to an individual woman.

## Application of Nonpharmacologic Techniques

Four kinds of techniques discussed in Chapter 11 that can be applied to intrapartum care are addressed in this chapter: relaxation, cutaneous stimulation, mental stimulation, and breathing.

### RELAXATION

Promoting relaxation provides a base for all other methods, both nonpharmacologic and pharmacologic, because it does the following:

- Promotes uterine blood flow, improving fetal oxygenation.
- Promotes efficient uterine contractions.
- Reduces tension that increases pain perception and decreases pain tolerance.
- Reduces tension that can inhibit fetal descent.

**Environmental Comfort.** Comfortable surroundings support relaxation. The nurse can reduce irritants such as bright lights and can adjust the room temperature.

Music masks outside noise and provides a background for use of imagery and breathing techniques. It is a distraction that shifts the woman's attention from bodily sensations. Television may have the same effect for some women.

**General Comfort.** Promoting the woman's personal comfort helps her focus on pain management techniques during labor (Fig. 15–2). This includes actions to increase comfort and reduce the effect of irritants.

**Reducing Anxiety and Fear.** The nurse may reduce a woman's anxiety and increase her self-control by providing accurate information and focusing on the normality of birth. Hospitals are typically associated with illness or injury, situations that are anxiety provoking. Yet hospitals are the most common site for the physiologically and emotionally unique event of birth.

Simple nursing actions keep the focus on the normality of childbirth, regardless of the setting. For example, referring to a woman as a patient reinforces the atmosphere of illness associated with being in a hospital, whereas calling her by name helps her to see birth as a normal process. Empowerment of the woman and her partner by giving them choices

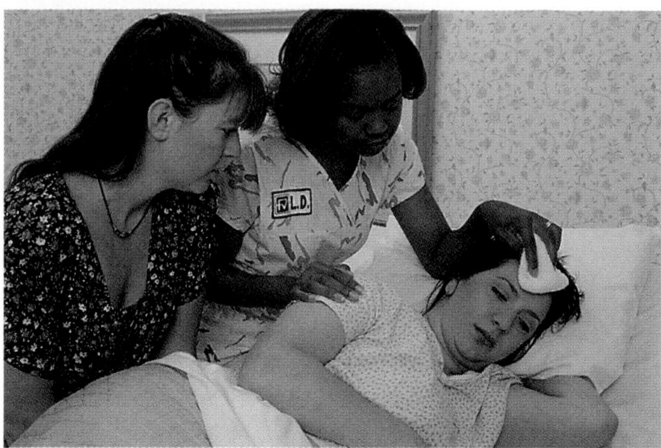


**FIGURE 15–2**

General comfort measures such as the nurse's reassuring presence or a cool cloth to the face supplement other methods of nonpharmacologic and pharmacologic pain control.

whenever possible helps them to see themselves as competent people who can accomplish the task of giving birth.

**Implementing Specific Relaxation Techniques.** The techniques discussed in Chapter 11 are most successful if practiced before labor. However, during labor, caregivers can watch a woman for signs of tension and help her focus on relaxing tense muscles. Her partner often recognizes subtle signs of tension and can be taught to massage the area or call attention to the tension and guide the laboring woman to release it.

### CUTANEOUS STIMULATION

Cutaneous stimulation has several variations that are often combined with each other or with other techniques.

**Self-massage.** The woman may rub her abdomen, legs, or back during labor (effleurage) to counteract discomfort. Some women find abdominal touch irritating, especially near the umbilicus. Women in labor may find firm stroking more helpful than very light stroking (see Fig. 11–5).

Some women benefit from firm palm or sole stimulation during labor. They may like to have their palms rubbed vigorously by another, rub their hands or feet together, or bang their palms on, or grip, a cool surface. They may hold another's hand tightly during a contraction. The nurse should determine if these actions indicate excess pain or if they are a woman's way of countering pain and therefore useful.

**Massage by Others.** The partner or the nurse can rub the woman's back, shoulders, legs, or any area where she finds massage helpful. Sacral pressure is a variation that may help when the woman has back pain, which is usually most intense when the fetus is in an occiput posterior position. Sacral pressure may be applied, using the palm of the hand, the fist or fists, or a firm object such as two tennis balls in a sock (Fig. 15–3).

Nonclinical touch by the nurse is a powerful tool if the woman does not object to it. Holding her hand, stroking her hair, or similar actions convey caring, comfort, affirmation, and reassurance at this vulnerable time.

**Thermal Stimulation.** Many women appreciate warmth to their back, abdomen, or perineum during labor. A warm shower, tub bath, or whirlpool bath is relaxing and provides thermal stimulation.

Cool, damp washcloths may be comforting, especially if a woman is hot. She may put them on her head, throat, abdomen, or any place she wants. She also may want to put them in her mouth to relieve dryness.

### MENTAL STIMULATION

Mental techniques occupy the woman's mind and compete with pain stimuli. They also aid relaxation by providing a tranquil imaginary atmosphere.

**Imagery.** If the woman has not practiced a specific imagery technique, the nurse can help her create a relaxing mental scene. Most women find images of warmth, softness, security, and total relaxation most comforting.

Imagery can help the woman dissociate herself from the painful aspects of labor. For example, the nurse can help her visualize the work of labor: the cervix opening with each contraction or the fetus

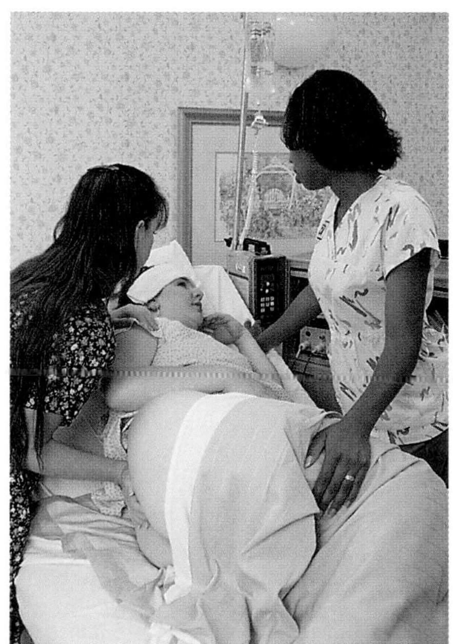

**FIGURE 15–3**

The coach applies sacral pressure to counter back pain that is common in many women's labors.

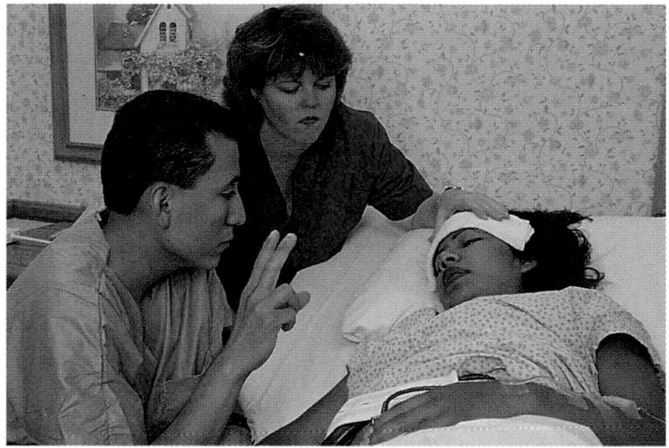

**FIGURE 15–4**

A woman and her partner who are prepared for labor have learned a variety of skills to master pain as labor progresses. The coach uses hand signals to tell the woman how to change her pattern of paced breathing.

moving down toward the outlet each time she pushes. This technique is like visualizing success or movement toward a goal with each contraction.

**Focal Point.** When using nonpharmacologic techniques, a woman may prefer to close her eyes or may want to concentrate on an external focal point. She may bring a picture of a relaxing scene or an object to use as a focal point and to aid in the use of imagery. She can use any point in the room as a focal point.

#### BREATHING

Breathing techniques give a woman a different focus during contractions, interfering with pain sensory transmission (Fig. 15–4). They begin with simple patterns and progress to more complex ones as needed. There is no single right time to change patterns during labor. However, complex patterns are fatiguing to use for a prolonged time.

### CHECK YOUR READING

7. Why should the nurse promote relaxation during labor?
8. What are some nursing actions to encourage relaxation during labor?
9. How can the nurse reduce a laboring woman's anxiety or fear?
10. What touch techniques may help the woman during labor? What action may reduce back pain during labor?

## Pharmacologic Pain Management

Pharmacologic methods for pain management include systemic drugs, regional pain management techniques, and general anesthesia.

### Special Considerations When Medicating a Pregnant Woman

Medicating a woman when she is pregnant is not as straightforward as when she is not pregnant:

- Any drug taken by the woman may affect her fetus.
- Drugs may have unusual effects in pregnancy.
- Drugs can affect the course and length of labor.
- Complications may limit the choice of pharmacologic pain management methods.
- Women who require other therapeutic drugs or who practice substance abuse may have fewer safe choices for pain relief.

#### EFFECTS ON THE FETUS

Effects on the fetus of drugs given to the mother may be direct, resulting from passage of the drug or its metabolites across the placenta to the fetus. An example of a direct effect on the fetus is decreased fetal heart rate (FHR) variability following administration of an analgesic to the woman.

Effects on the fetus may be indirect, or secondary to drug effects in the mother. For example, if a drug causes maternal hypotension, blood flow to the placenta is reduced. Fetal hypoxia and acidosis may result.

#### MATERNAL PHYSIOLOGIC ALTERATIONS

Normal pregnancy changes in four body systems have the greatest implications for pharmacologic pain management methods.

**Cardiovascular Changes.** Compression of the aorta and inferior vena cava (aortocaval compression) by the uterus can occur when a woman lies in the supine position. However, some anesthetics require that she assume the supine position temporarily. In such a case, the uterus is displaced to one side with the hands or with a small wedge under one hip.

**Respiratory Changes.** A pregnant woman's full uterus reduces her respiratory capacity. To compensate, she breathes more rapidly and deeply. As a result, she is more vulnerable to reduced arterial oxygenation during induction of general anesthesia and is more sensitive to inhalational anesthetic agents.

**Gastrointestinal Changes.** A pregnant woman's stomach is displaced upward by her large uterus; the stomach's interior also has a higher pressure. Progesterone slows peristalsis and reduces the tone of the sphincter at the junction of the stomach and esophagus. These changes make a pregnant woman more vulnerable to regurgitation and aspiration of acidic gastric contents during general anesthesia.

**Nervous System Changes.** During pregnancy and labor, circulating levels of endorphins are high. Endorphins modify pain perception and reduce requirements for analgesia and anesthesia.

The epidural and subarachnoid spaces are smaller during pregnancy, enhancing the spread of anesthetic agents used for epidural or subarachnoid blocks. Cerebrospinal fluid (CSF) pressure is higher, reaching a peak during the second stage of labor. Nerve fibers are more sensitive to local anesthetic agents, probably because of acid-base or hormonal alterations. High intra-abdominal pressure causes engorgement of the epidural veins, increasing the risk for intravascular injection of anesthetic agents. The net result of these changes is that a reduced volume of local anesthetic is needed to achieve satisfactory epidural or subarachnoid block.

#### EFFECTS ON THE COURSE OF LABOR

Most analgesics are not given until labor is well established because they may slow progress if given too early. However, caregivers must consider the adverse effects of excessive pain on labor's progress when helping a woman choose methods of pain relief. Regional anesthetics, primarily the epidural block, can slow progress during the second stage if they impair the laboring woman's natural urge to push.

#### EFFECTS OF COMPLICATIONS

Complications during pregnancy may limit the choices of analgesia or anesthesia. For example, infusion of large volumes of intravenous fluids is done to prevent hypotension with regional anesthesia. If a pregnant woman has heart disease, this fluid load could be detrimental. Yet without it, she is vulnerable to hypotension.

#### INTERACTIONS WITH OTHER SUBSTANCES

A woman who ingests drugs (therapeutic, over-the-counter, or illicit) or other substances may have fewer options because of interactions between these substances and analgesics or anesthetics. For example, alcohol increases the depressant effects of opioid analgesics, making both the mother and newborn susceptible to respiratory depression.

#### CHECK YOUR READING

11. How can drugs taken by the expectant mother affect the fetus?
12. How do changes in these maternal body systems affect pharmocologic pain management? (a) Cardiovascular? (b) Respiratory? (c) Gastrointestinal? (d) Nervous system?
13. How do endorphins influence the mother's need for pharmacologic pain relief during labor?
14. Why is it important to know all drugs or abused substances that a laboring woman has ingested?

## Systemic Drugs for Labor

Systemic drugs are those that have effects on multiple systems because they are distributed throughout the body. These intrapartum drugs include opioid analgesics and adjunctive drugs. Although general anesthesia is also systemic, it is discussed separately because it is used only at birth.

#### OPIOID ANALGESICS

Opioid analgesics reduce perception of pain without loss of consciousness. Injectable opioid analgesics are the systemic drugs of choice in labor. Common analgesics for intrapartum use are meperidine (Demerol), butorphanol (Stadol) (Drug Guide 15–1), and nalbuphine (Nubain). Table 15–1 summarizes common drugs used for intrapartum pain relief.

#### DRUG GUIDE

### BUTORPHANOL (Stadol)

***Classification:*** Opioid analgesic.

***Action:*** Opioid analgesic with some agonist-antagonist effects. Exact mechanism of action is unknown. Produces respiratory depression that does not increase markedly with larger doses.

***Indications:*** Systemic pain relief during labor.

***Dosage and Route:*** Intravenous: 1 mg every 3 to 4 hours; range 0.5 to 2 mg. May be given undiluted.

***Absorption:*** Onset of analgesia almost immediate with intravenous administration, peaks about 30 minutes, and lasts about 3 hours. Faster onset and shorter duration of action than meperidine or morphine.

***Excretion:*** Excreted in urine. Crosses placental barrier. Secreted in breast milk.

***Contraindications and Precautions:*** Contraindicated in persons who are hypersensitive. Do not use in opiate-dependent persons because antagonist activity of the drug may cause withdrawal symptoms in the woman or newborn. Use cautiously during birth of preterm infant. Drug actions are potentiated (enhanced) by barbiturates, phenothiazines, cimetidine, and other tranquilizers.

***Adverse Reactions:*** Respiratory depression or apnea (woman or newborn), anaphylaxis. Dizziness, lightheadedness, sedation, lethargy, headache, euphoria, mental clouding, fainting, restlessness, excitement, tremors, delirium, insomnia. Nausea, vomiting, constipation, increased biliary pressure, dry mouth, anorexia. Flushing, altered heart rate and blood pressure, circulatory collapse. Urinary retention. Sensitivity to cold.

***Nursing Considerations:*** Assess for allergies and opiate dependence. Observe vital signs and respiratory function in woman (12 per minute or more) and newborn (30 per minute or more). Have naloxone and resuscitation equipment available for respiratory depression in woman and neonate. Report nausea or vomiting to the birth attendant for a possible order for an antiemetic. Antiemetics or other central nervous system depressants may enhance the respiratory depressant effects of butorphanol.

**TABLE 15-1 DRUGS COMMONLY USED FOR INTRAPARTUM PAIN MANAGEMENT**

| Drug/Dose | Comments |
|---|---|
| **Opioid Analgesics** | |
| Meperidine (Demerol) 12.5–50 mg every 2–4 hr IV | Respiratory depression (primarily in the neonate) is the main side effect |
| Butorphanol (Stadol) 1 mg every 3–4 hr; range 0.5–2 mg IV | Has some narcotic antagonist effects; should not be given to the opiate-dependent woman (may precipitate withdrawal) or after other narcotics such as meperidine (may reverse their analgesic effects); also a respiratory depressant |
| Nalbuphine (Nubain) 10 mg every 3–6 hours IV | Same as butorphanol |
| **Adjunctive Drugs** | |
| Promethazine (Phenergan) 12.5–25 mg every 4–6 hr IV | Duration of action is longer than most narcotics; enhances respiratory depressant effects of narcotics |
| Diphenhydramine (Benadryl) 10–50 mg every 4–6 hr IV | Given to relieve pruritus from epidural narcotics |
| Hydroxyzine (Atarax, Vistaril) 25–100 mg IM Z-track only | See promethazine. |
| **Narcotic Antagonists** | |
| Naloxone (Narcan) Adult: 0.4–2 mg IV To reverse pruritus from epidural opioids: 0.04–0.2 mg IV or IV infusion 5–10 μg/kg/hr | Action shorter than most narcotics it reverses; must observe for recurrent respiratory depression and be prepared to give additional doses |
| Neonate: 0.1 mg/kg IV (umbilical vein) or intratracheal | For neonatal resuscitation |
| Naltrexone (Trexan): 3–6 mg p.o. × 1 dose | Long-acting drug to relieve pruritus from epidural narcotics (investigational when used for this purpose) |

IV = intravenously; p.o. = orally; IM = intramuscularly.

Meperidine is a pure opioid agonist, but butorphanol and nalbuphine have mixed opioid agonist and antagonist effects. These agonist-antagonist drugs should not be given to a woman who is opiate-dependent (such as heroin) to avoid withdrawal effects. They should not be given if she has already received a pure opioid such as meperidine because some analgesic effect of the first drug will be reversed.

The primary side effect of opioid analgesics is respiratory depression, which is more likely to occur in the newborn. Timing of administration is important to reduce neonatal respiratory depression. An infant who is born at the peak of the drug's action is more likely to have respiratory depression than if born earlier or later. Drugs such as meperidine have metabolites that are active for a long time in the newborn and can cause delayed respiratory depression.

Opioid analgesics are usually given in small, frequent doses by the intravenous route during labor to provide a rapid onset of analgesia and a predictable duration of action. A woman benefits from rapid pain control, with less likelihood of neonatal respiratory depression. Starting the injection at the beginning of the contraction, when blood flow to the placenta is normally reduced, limits transfer to the fetus. When placental blood flow resumes, much of the drug is in maternal tissues.

### OPIOID ANTAGONISTS

Naloxone (Narcan) reverses opioid-induced respiratory depression. Naloxone does not reverse respiratory depression from other causes, such as barbiturates, anesthetics, non-opioid drugs, or pathologic conditions. Naloxone has a shorter duration of action than most of the opioids it reverses. In an opiate-dependent woman or newborn, naloxone may induce withdrawal symptoms. Naloxone is used with other measures as needed to support cardiopulmonary function. (See Chapter 30 for discussion of neonatal resuscitation.)

Naloxone is most often given to the neonate. The recommended neonatal route for administration is intravenous or intratracheal for the most reliable absorption. The neonatal and pediatric resuscitation dose is 0.1 mg/kg by the intravenous or intratracheal route (American Academy of Pediatrics, 1992). Intravenous naloxone is given to the neonate through the umbilical vein. The adult dose is 0.4 to 2 mg.

Naltrexone (Trexan) is an opioid antagonist that is usually prescribed for opioid dependence. In the intrapartum setting, naltrexone may be given orally to relieve pruritus that often occurs when intrathecal or epidural opioid analgesics are used.

### ADJUNCTIVE DRUGS

Adjunctive drugs during the intrapartum period include those with antiemetic and tranquilizing effects and sedatives. These drugs are given to reduce nausea and anxiety and to promote rest (see Table 15–1).

Promethazine (Phenergan) relieves nausea and vomiting, which may occur when opioid drugs are given. Promethazine may be given by either the intramuscular or intravenous route. Use of promethazine allows a lower total opioid dose, but it does not potentiate the opioid's effects.

Hydroxyzine (Atarax, Vistaril) is an antihistamine with antiemetic effects. Parenteral hydroxyzine can be given only into a large muscle with a deep Z-track technique. *Hydroxyzine is not given by the intravenous route.*

### SEDATIVES

Sedatives such as barbiturates are not routinely given because they have prolonged depressant effects on the neonate. However, a small dose of a short-acting barbiturate may be given to promote rest if a woman is fatigued from false labor or a prolonged latent phase.

### ✓ CHECK YOUR READING

15. What is the primary adverse effect of opioid administration? How can this effect be reduced?
16. What should the nurse watch for after birth in the infant who received naloxone?
17. What is the correct dose of naloxone for an infant weighing 7 pounds (3178 g)?

## Regional Pain Management Techniques

Regional pain control methods may be used for intrapartum analgesia, anesthesia, or both. These methods provide pain relief without loss of consciousness. Depending on the specific technique, it may be used only for labor, only for the birth, or for both labor and birth.

Epidural block analgesia or anesthesia provides pain control during much of labor and for the birth itself. Intrathecal opioids are used for pain control during labor; additional measures are needed during late labor and for the birth. Regional anesthetics that are used only during the birth include the local, pudendal, and subarachnoid blocks.

The major advantage of regional pain management methods is that the woman can participate in birth yet still have good pain control. The woman usually feels some pressure and discomfort, although these sensations are greatly reduced. She can interact with her infant and partner and does not lose her protective airway reflexes, as can happen with general anesthesia. Disadvantages depend on the specific technique. The effects on the fetus depend on how the woman responds rather than on direct drug effects.

### EPIDURAL BLOCK

The lumbar epidural block is a popular regional block that provides pain relief for labor and birth without sedation of the woman and fetus. It is used for both vaginal and cesarean births.

The epidural space is outside the dura mater, between the dura and the spinal canal. It is loosely filled with fat, connective tissue, and epidural veins that are dilated during pregnancy (Fig. 15–5).

The epidural block is done by injecting local anesthetic into the tiny epidural space. It provides substantial relief of pain from contractions and birth canal distention. The level of the epidural block can be extended upward to provide anesthesia for a cesarean birth or tubal ligation after birth. The woman usually retains motor function and some sensation when lower concentrations of anesthetic are used. Higher concentrations of the anesthetic agent that are used for abdominal surgery result in loss of both motor and sensory functions.

**Technique.** The epidural block is started after labor is established or just before a scheduled cesarean birth. The epidural space is entered at about the L3–L4 interspace (below the end of the spinal cord), and a catheter is passed through the needle into the epidural space (Fig. 15–6). The catheter allows continuous infusion or intermittent injection of medication to maintain pain relief during labor and vaginal or cesarean birth.

Epidural anesthesia requires a larger amount of anesthetic agent than the subarachnoid block because it is outside the meninges. A small (3 ml) test dose of local anesthetic is injected before giving the full dose and before subsequent intermittent doses. If the catheter is in the subarachnoid space instead of the epidural space, the woman experiences rapid, intense motor and sensory block. The test dose also can detect accidental intravascular injection. The woman has numbness of the tongue and lips, lightheadedness, dizziness, and tinnitus with intravascular injection. Epinephrine in the test dose produces tachycardia if injected intravascularly.

Local anesthetic drugs are usually combined with a very small dose of an opioid analgesic such as fentanyl (Sublimaze), sufentanyl (Sufenta), or morphine (Duramorph). *All drugs injected into the epidural or subarachnoid spaces are preservative-free.* The drug combination provides quicker and longer-lasting pain relief for labor with a lower total dose of local anesthetic

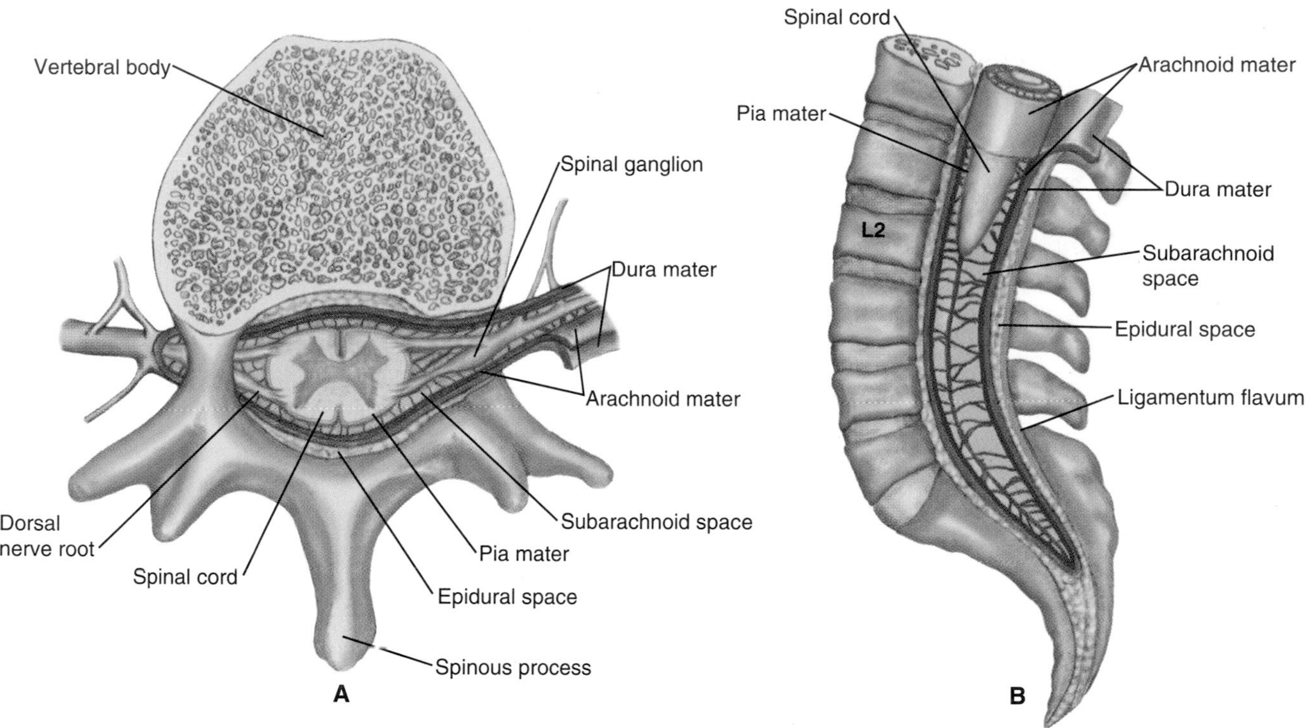


**FIGURE 15-5**

A, Cross section of spinal cord, meninges, and protective vertebra. The dura and arachnoid lie close together. The pia mater is the innermost of the meninges and covers the brain and spinal cord. The subarachnoid space is between the arachnoid and pia mater. B, Sagittal section of spinal cord, meninges, and vertebrae. The epidural and subarachnoid spaces are illustrated. Note that the spinal cord ends at the L2 vertebra.

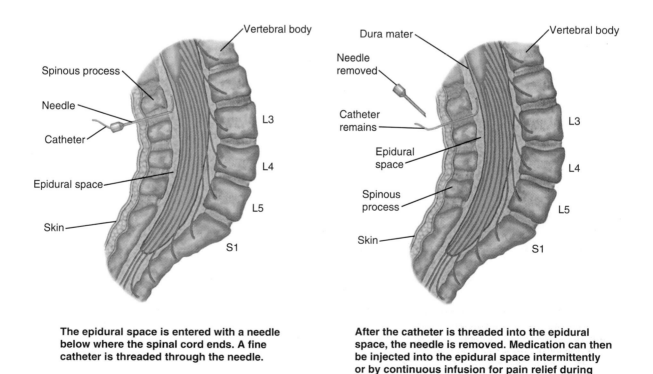

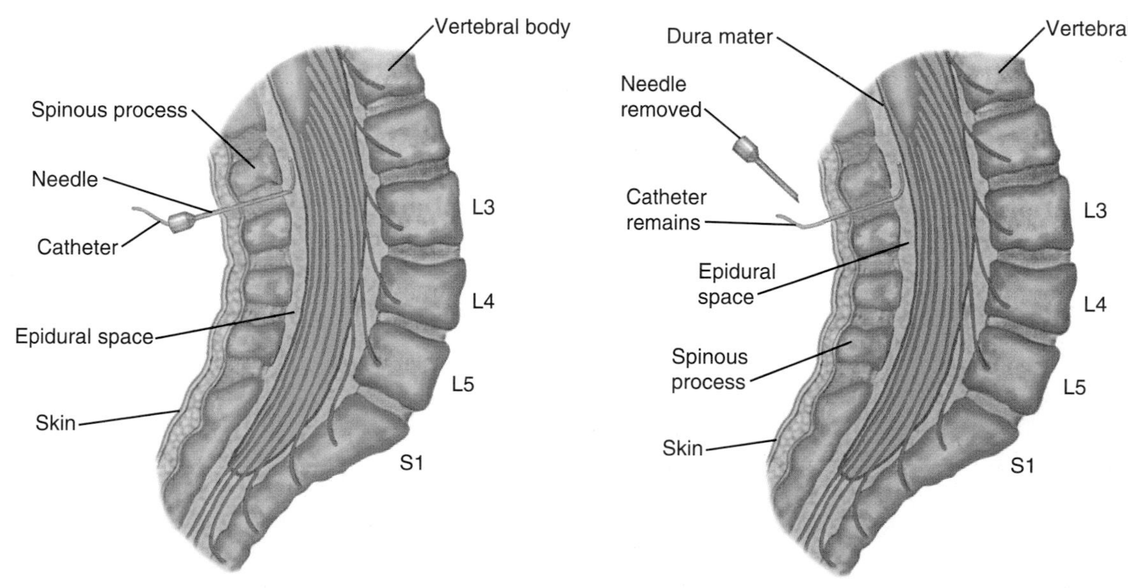


**The epidural space is entered with a needle below where the spinal cord ends. A fine catheter is threaded through the needle.**

**After the catheter is threaded into the epidural space, the needle is removed. Medication can then be injected into the epidural space intermittently or by continuous infusion for pain relief during labor and birth.**

**FIGURE 15-6**

Technique for epidural block.

and less motor block. Epidural analgesics also are given after cesarean birth to provide long-acting pain relief with a low dose. The mother is comfortable enough to have good interaction with her infant and family. She may require no added analgesics, or oral ones may be sufficient.

For vaginal birth, the anesthetized area is usually from the T10 to the S5 level (Cunningham et al., 1997). For cesarean birth, a higher block is needed, up to T4 to T6 (Zuspan, 1994a).

**Dural Puncture.** Because the tough dura and the fragile web-like arachnoid membranes lie close together, dural puncture also punctures the arachnoid. If the dura is unintentionally punctured with the large-gauge needle used to introduce the catheter, substantial leakage of CSF can occur, which may result in a spinal headache (see p. 381). Dural puncture and spinal headache also can occur without obvious CSF leakage.

**Contraindications and Precautions.** Epidural block is not suitable for all laboring women. Contraindications include the woman's refusal, coagulation defects, uncorrected hypovolemia, an infection in the area of insertion or a severe systemic infection, allergy, or a fetal condition that demands immediate birth.

**Adverse Effects of Epidural Block.** Epidural block can have adverse effects.

***Maternal Hypotension.*** Sympathetic nerves are blocked along with pain nerves, which may result in vasodilation and hypotension. Rapid infusion of warmed intravenous solution such as lactated Ringer's solution offsets vasodilation by filling the vascular system. The amounts infused are large compared with those given in other settings: often 500 to 1000 ml or more are rapidly infused (Creehan, 1996). If hypotension occurs, intravenous ephedrine in 5- to 10-mg increments promotes vasoconstriction to raise the blood pressure.

***Bladder Distention.*** A woman's bladder may fill quickly because of the large quantity of intravenous solution, yet her sensation to void is often reduced. Bladder distention may cause pain that remains after initiation of the block.

***Prolonged Second Stage.*** The urge to push is often less intense than if a woman does not have an epidural block. Forceps- or vacuum extractor–assisted births are more likely because of the reduced urge to push.

***Catheter Migration.*** After accurate placement, the catheter may move. A woman may then have symptoms of intravascular injection, an intense block or one that is too high, absence of anesthesia, or a unilateral block.

**Adverse Effects of Epidural Opioids.** Adverse effects associated with epidural opioids may include nausea and vomiting, pruritus, and delayed respiratory depression.

***Nausea and Vomiting.*** As when opioids are given by other routes, nausea and vomiting may occur. Adjunctive drugs such as promethazine (Phenergan) reduce nausea and vomiting.

***Pruritus.*** Itching of the face and neck is an annoying side effect of many epidural opioids. Although she may not specifically complain of itching, a woman may rub or scratch her face and neck frequently. Diphenhydramine (Benadryl), naloxone (Narcan), or naltrexone (Trexan) may relieve pruritus (see Table 15–1).

***Delayed Respiratory Depression.*** The possibility of late respiratory depression exists for up to 24 hours after the administration of an epidural opioid, depending on the drug used.

**Nursing Care.** The nurse should record baseline vital signs for comparison after the block is begun. Intravenous access is ensured, and the prescribed preload of fluid is given. The nurse supports the woman in the correct position for instituting the block and tells the anesthesia clinician when the woman is having a contraction. The woman may feel a brief "electric shock" sensation as the catheter is passed. The nurse should assist her in remaining still while the block is completed. After the test dose, the nurse observes for signs of subarachnoid puncture or intravascular injection.

There are currently no national standards for frequency of monitoring of maternal vital signs after epidural block is begun, and standards for fetal assessment are based on risk status (see Chapters 13 and 14). Facility protocols and the maternal-fetal status should guide the frequency of vital signs and fetal assessments. Pulse oximetry is often used to observe blood oxygenation. Maternal respiratory monitoring may continue for up to 24 hours after birth, depending on the drugs given.

The woman's bladder must be assessed frequently because of the large intravenous fluid load and her reduced sensation to void. The nurse should observe for signs associated with catheter migration from the epidural space and for adverse effects, such as nausea and vomiting and pruritus.

### INTRATHECAL OPIOID ANALGESICS

Intrathecal injection of an opioid analgesic is an option for labor pain management that is gaining acceptance. The drug is injected into the subarachnoid space, where it binds to opiate receptors, allowing much smaller doses than would be adequate if given systemically. The woman can feel her contractions but not the pain they would otherwise bring.

Advantages of intrathecal analgesics include the following:

- Rapid onset of pain relief without sedation
- No motor block, enabling the woman to ambulate during labor
- No sympathetic block, with its hypotensive effects

Disadvantages may include the following:

- Limited duration of action, possibly requiring another procedure for continued pain relief
- Inadequate pain relief for late labor and the birth itself, requiring added measures to manage pain at that time

**Technique.** The subarachnoid space is entered with a spinal needle, as in the subarachnoid block. A preservative-free opioid analgesic is then injected.

The drug chosen depends on the expected duration of labor at the time it is given. Drugs that may be used by this route include fentanyl, sufentanyl, and morphine. Fentanyl and sufentanyl have a rapid onset of action and last up to 3 hours. Morphine has a slightly longer onset but lasts longer.

**Adverse Effects of Intrathecal Opioids.** As with epidural opioids, nausea, vomiting, and pruritus may occur. Delayed respiratory depression may occur, depending on the drug used.

**Nursing Care.** Vital signs and fetal heart rate are taken at the usual intervals for the woman's stage of labor. Side effects, such as nausea and vomiting or pruritus, are reported and managed similarly to those occurring with the epidural block. Reduced effectiveness suggests that the drug's duration of action is ending or that the woman is in late labor. Other pain management methods may be needed for the remainder of labor and for birth.

#### LOCAL INFILTRATION ANESTHESIA

Infiltration of the perineum with a local anesthetic is done by the physician or nurse-midwife just before performing an episiotomy or suturing a laceration (Fig. 15–7). Local infiltration does not alter pain from uterine contractions or distention of the vagina. The local agent provides anesthesia in the immediate area of the episiotomy or laceration. There is a short delay between anesthetic injection and onset of numbness, and the drug burns before its anesthetic action begins. Local infiltration rarely has adverse effects on either mother or infant.

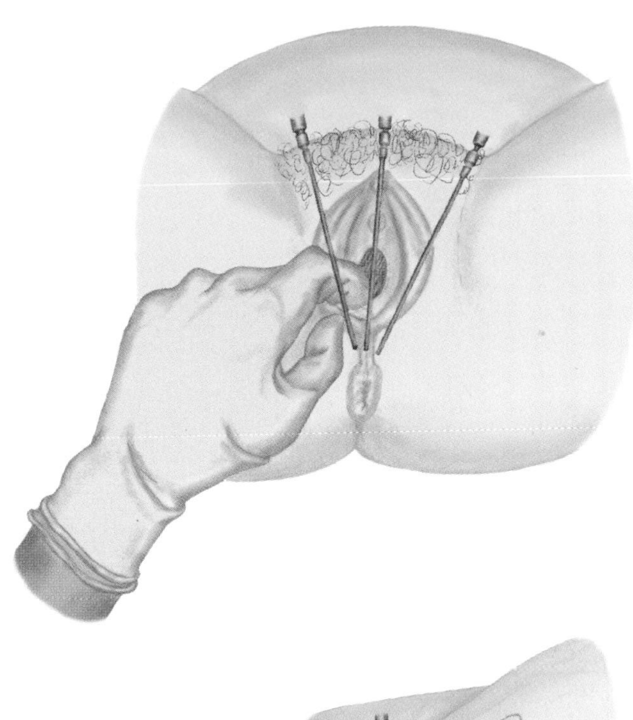

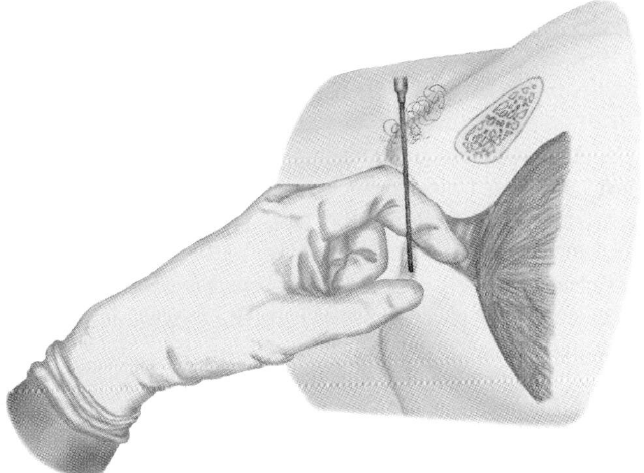

**FIGURE 15–7**

Local infiltration anesthesia numbs the perineum just before birth for an episiotomy or after birth for suturing of a laceration. The birth attendant protects the fetal head by placing a finger inside the vagina while injecting the perineum in a fan-like pattern.

#### PUDENDAL BLOCK

A pudendal block anesthetizes the lower vagina and part of the perineum to provide anesthesia for an episiotomy and vaginal birth, using low forceps if needed. A pudendal block does not block pain from uterine contractions, and the mother feels pressure.

The physician or nurse-midwife injects the pudendal nerves near each ischial spine with about 10 ml of local anesthetic (Fig. 15–8). The perineum is infiltrated with local anesthetic because the pudendal block does not fully anesthetize this area. As in local infiltration, a delay occurs between injection and onset of numbness. Possible maternal complications include a toxic reaction to the anesthetic, rectal puncture, hematoma, and sciatic nerve block. If maternal toxicity is avoided, the fetus is usually not affected.

#### SUBARACHNOID (SPINAL) BLOCK

A subarachnoid block is a simpler procedure than the epidural block and may be done when a quick cesarean birth is necessary and an epidural catheter is not in place. It is similar to local infiltration and

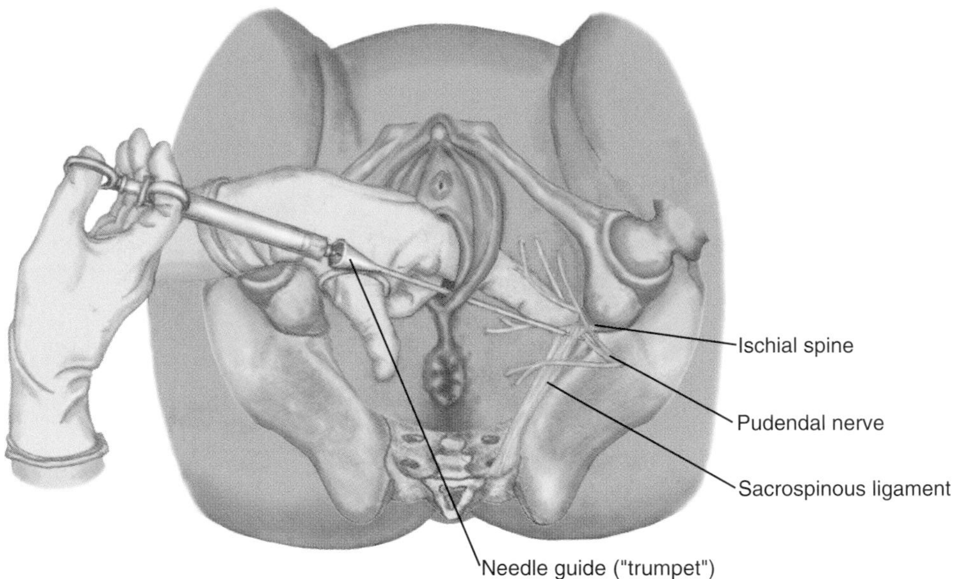


**FIGURE 15–8**

Pudendal block provides anesthesia for an episiotomy and use of low forceps. A needle guide ("trumpet") protects the maternal and fetal tissues from the long needle needed to reach the pudendal nerve.

pudendal block in that it is done just before birth and so provides no pain relief during most of labor.

The physician or nurse-anesthetist injects local anesthetic into the subarachnoid space in a single dose. The woman loses both sensory and motor function below the level of the subarachnoid block, with complete relief of pain from contractions.

**Technique.** A 25- to 27-gauge spinal needle is placed in the subarachnoid space. Appearance of CSF at the needle hub assures correct placement, and the local anesthetic is injected (Fig. 15–9).

The level of anesthesia for both epidural and subarachnoid blocks is determined by the volume, concentration, and density of the drug (Fig. 15–10).

**Contraindications and Precautions.** Contraindications and precautions are similar to those for epidural block: the woman's refusal, coagulation defects, uncorrected hypovolemia, infection in the area of in-

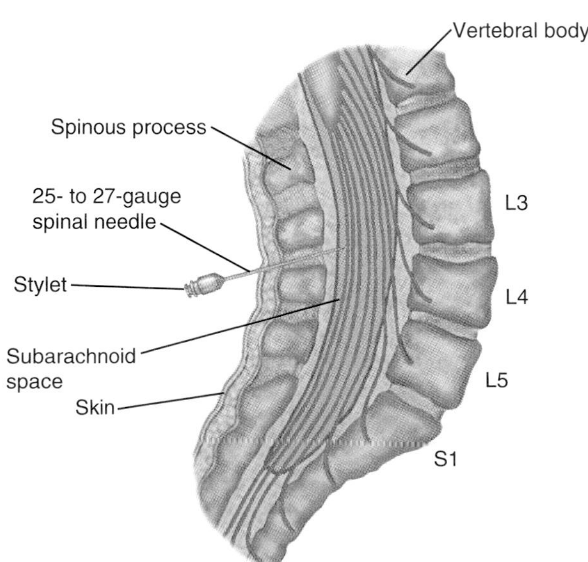


**A 25- to 27-gauge spinal needle with a stylet occluding its lumen is passed into the subarachnoid space below where the spinal cord ends.**

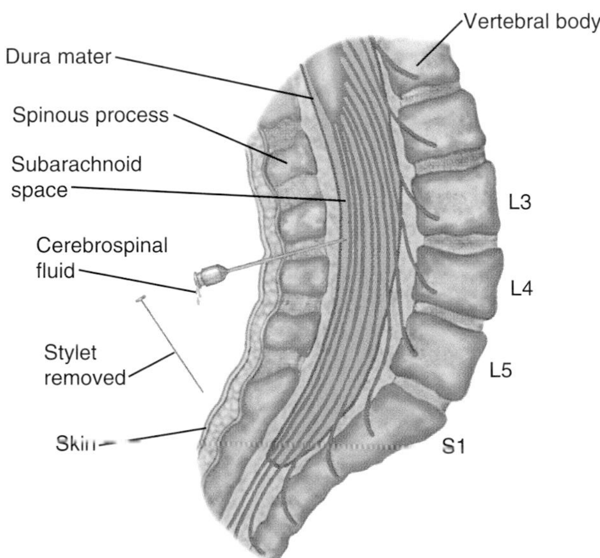


**The stylet is removed, and one or more drops of clear cerebrospinal fluid at needle hub confirm correct needle placement. Medication is then injected, and the needle is removed.**

**FIGURE 15–9**

Technique for subarachnoid block.

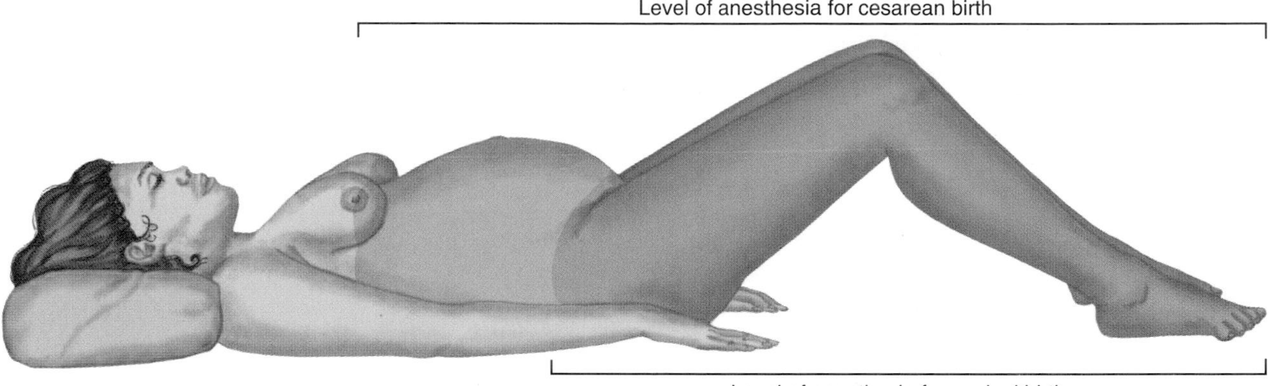


**FIGURE 15-10**

Levels of anesthesia for epidural and subarachnoid blocks. A level of T10 through S5 is adequate for vaginal birth. A higher level to T4–6 is needed for cesarean birth.

sertion, systemic infection, and allergy. Subarachnoid block can be done more quickly than an epidural block if prompt birth is necessary.

**Adverse Effects.** Three adverse effects of a subarachnoid block are maternal hypotension, bladder distention, and spinal headache. Hypotension is more likely with the subarachnoid block than with the epidural block.

Post-spinal headache may occur after subarachnoid block in some women because of CSF leakage at the site of dural puncture. A spinal headache is postural; it is worse when a woman is upright and may disappear when she is lying flat. The incidence of spinal headache is lower if a small-gauge needle is used.

Bedrest with oral or intravenous hydration helps relieve the postspinal headache. A blood patch often gives dramatic, definitive relief. The blood patch is done by injecting 10 to 15 ml of the woman's blood (obtained with sterile technique) into the epidural space. The blood forms a gelatinous seal over the hole in the dura, stopping spinal fluid leakage (Fig. 15–11). The blood patch can be repeated if needed. Epidural injection of sterile saline also has had some success.

### GENERAL ANESTHESIA

General anesthesia is systemic pain control that involves loss of consciousness. It is rarely used for vaginal births, but it still has a place in cesarean birth. Some women either refuse or are not good candidates for epidural or subarachnoid block. In other cases, it may be necessary to perform a cesarean birth so quickly that no time is available to establish either type of regional block.

**Technique.** Before induction of anesthesia, a woman breathes oxygen for 3 to 5 minutes, or at least four deep breaths, to increase her oxygen stores and those of her fetus for the short period of apnea during anesthesia induction. The woman has a wedge under her right side (or the operating table is tilted toward her left side) to reduce aortocaval compression and increase placental blood flow.

**Adverse Effects.** Major adverse effects are possible with the use of general anesthesia.

***Maternal Aspiration of Gastric Contents.*** Regurgitation with aspiration of acidic gastric contents is a potentially fatal complication of general anesthesia. Aspiration of food particles may result in airway obstruction. Aspiration of acidic secretions results in a

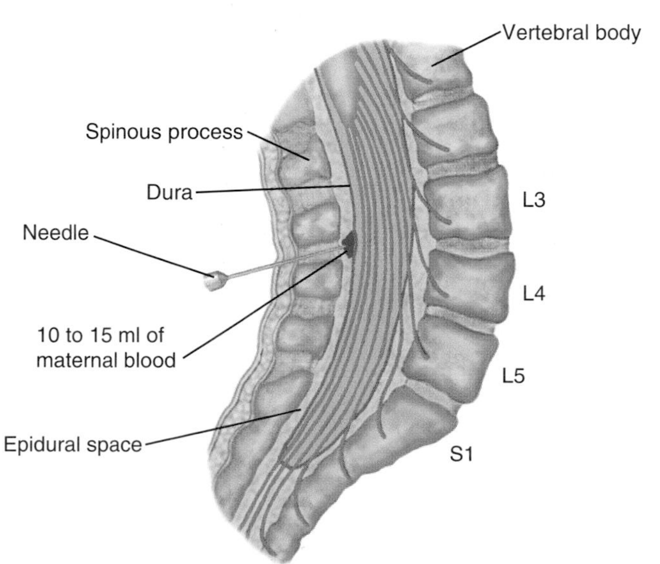


**FIGURE 15-11**

Blood patch for relief of spinal headache. Ten to 15 ml of the woman's blood is injected into the epidural space to seal a dural puncture.

chemical injury to the airways—aspiration pneumonitis. Infection often occurs after the initial lung injury.

***Respiratory Depression.*** Respiratory depression may occur in either the mother or the infant but is more likely in the baby.

***Uterine Relaxation.*** Some inhalational anesthetics may cause uterine relaxation. This characteristic is desirable for some complications, such as replacing an inverted uterus (see p. 777). However, postpartum hemorrhage may occur if the uterus relaxes after birth.

**Methods to Minimize Adverse Effects.** Measures to reduce the risk of maternal aspiration or of lung injury if aspiration occurs include the following:

- Restricting intake to clear fluids or nothing by mouth if surgery is anticipated.
- Administering drugs to raise the gastric pH and make secretions less acidic, such as sodium citrate and citric acid (Bicitra), ranitidine (Zantac), cimetidine (Tagamet), or famotidine (Pepcid).
- Administering drugs to reduce secretions, such as glycopyrrolate (Robinul).
- Administering drugs to speed gastric emptying, such as metoclopramide (Reglan).
- Use of cricoid pressure (Sellick's maneuver) to block the esophagus by pressing the rigid trachea against it (Fig. 15–12).

Neonatal respiratory depression may be averted by doing the following:

- Reducing the time from induction of anesthesia until the umbilical cord is clamped.
- Keeping the anesthesia level as light as possible until the cord is clamped.

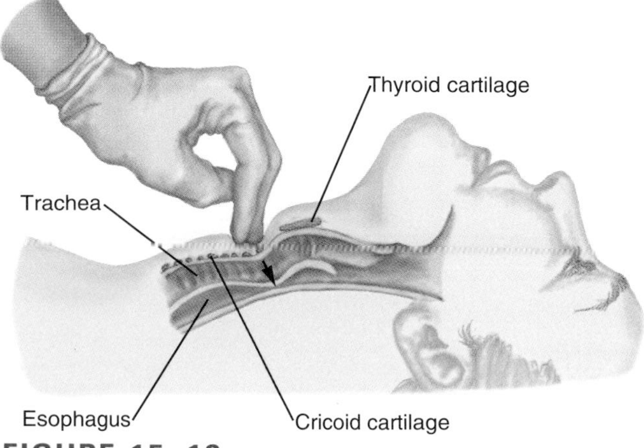


**FIGURE 15–12**

Sellick's maneuver to prevent vomitus from entering the woman's trachea while she is being intubated for general anesthesia. An assistant applies pressure to the cricoid cartilage to obstruct the esophagus. Once the woman is successfully intubated with a cuffed endotracheal tube, gastric secretions cannot enter the trachea.

To reduce the time from induction of anesthesia to cord clamping, the woman is prepared and draped and the physicians are ready before anesthesia is begun. Before cord clamping, the anesthesia is so light that it is more accurately described as amnesia with profound analgesia. The woman may move on the operating table as the incision is made, but she rarely remembers the experience. If a hazy memory remains, she does not usually remember the experience as painful. The anesthesia level is deepened after the cord is clamped.

**CHECK YOUR READING**

18. What are two major advantages of using regional pain management techniques during childbirth?
19. What is the major adverse effect of the epidural or subarachnoid block? How can the fetus be affected? How may this effect be reduced?
20. What are common side effects of epidural or intrathecal opioid analgesics, and how are these managed?
21. What are the major adverse effects of general anesthesia? What measures reduce the risks?

## Application of Nursing Process: Pain Management

The nurse assists laboring women with both nonpharmacologic and pharmacologic methods of pain control as needed (Nursing Care Plan 15–1). Nursing care related to pain management should be combined with that for normal labor and any complications that arise. Care of the fetus remains a priority and is discussed in Chapters 13 and 14. Two problems that commonly affect the woman are pain and her potential for respiratory compromise if she needs general anesthesia.

## Pain

### Assessment

Pain assessment begins at admission and continues throughout labor. The assessments discussed in Table 13–1 guide the nurse in obtaining data related to pain management. Pain-related assessments include the following:

- Preferences for pain management
- Maternal vital signs
- Fetal heart rate and monitor patterns
- Allergies, focusing especially on allergy to opioid analgesics, dental anesthetics, and iodine (used in most prep solutions)

## Nursing Care Plan 15–1

# Intrapartum Pain Management

**ASSESSMENT:** Beth Anderson is a 28-year-old gravida I, para 0 who was admitted 1 hour ago in early labor. Vaginal examination reveals that Beth is 3 cm dilated and 100 percent effaced, and the station is −2. Her membranes are intact. Contractions are every 3 minutes, last 40 to 50 seconds, and are of moderate intensity. The fetal heart rate averages 135 to 145 beats per minute and has no abnormal patterns on the monitor. Although relatively comfortable when admitted. Beth is becoming more uncomfortable. She says that back pain is most troubling. Beth and her husband, Sam, attended prepared childbirth classes and are using breathing techniques they learned.

**NURSING DIAGNOSIS:** Pain related to effects of uterine contractions and pressure on pelvic structures

### GOALS/EXPECTED OUTCOMES

During labor, Beth will do the following:

1. Continue to use techniques she learned in prepared childbirth classes.
2. Have a relaxed facial and body posture between contractions.

### Critical Thinking

At this time, what methods for pain management are most appropriate to suggest, nonpharmacologic or pharmacologic?

**ANSWER**

If not already done, the nurse should explore Beth's preferences for pain relief with her before labor becomes more intense. At this time, nonpharmacologic methods are most appropriately suggested because she is in early labor and has not specifically requested medication. Walking or other upright positions often ease back discomfort and aid fetal descent, but Beth's ability to use these would be less if she receives some pharmacologic methods of pain control, such as systemic analgesics. Her labor pattern is normal, membranes are intact, and the fetal heart rate is stable and within normal limits, so there is no apparent contraindication to walking.

| INTERVENTION | RATIONALE |
|---|---|
| 1. Adjust the environment for comfort:<br>a. Adjust room thermostat.<br>b. Add warm blankets and socks for warmth.<br>c. Offer small electric fan or hand fan if Beth is hot. | 1. A comfortable environment is conducive to relaxation. Relaxation underlies all other interventions because it increases a woman's ability to use her coping skills to tolerate discomfort. |
| 2. Reduce distractions:<br>a. Close door to reduce outside noise.<br>b. Play music of Beth's choice to mask external noise.<br>c. Do not stand in front of her focal point.<br>d. Try to delay assessments or questions until after a contraction is over. | 2. Distractions interfere with use of the skills for pain management that are taught in prepared childbirth classes. |
| 3. Reduce irritating stimulants.<br>a. Keep sheets and underpads dry.<br>b. Lower lights as Beth desires. Use bright lights only when necessary.<br>c. Do all procedures and nursing interventions as gently as possible.<br>d. Avoid bumping the bed. | 3. Irritating stimulants are distractions that decrease the woman's ability to use learned childbirth skills and add to her discomfort. |
| 4. Encourage Beth to assume positions she finds most comfortable and to change positions regularly (about every 30 to 60 minutes). If there is no contraindication, she may walk around or sit in a chair at the bedside. She should avoid the supine position. | 4. Frequent position changes favor fetal descent by encouraging the fetal head to adapt to the pelvic diameters most efficiently. Position changes also reduce muscle tension and unrelieved pressure.<br>• Upright positions enhance descent with gravity.<br>• The supine position is uncomfortable to most women and may cause aortocaval compression with decreased placental perfusion. |

*Nursing Care Plan continued on following page*

## Nursing Care Plan 15–1 *Continued*

# Intrapartum Pain Management

| INTERVENTION | RATIONALE |
|---|---|
| 5. Check for bladder distention hourly, and encourage Beth to void at least every 2 hours. With an order, catheterize her if her bladder is full and she cannot void. | 5. The sensation to void may be decreased during labor. A full bladder contributes to overall discomfort and may impede fetal descent and prolong labor. |
| 6. If permitted, give Beth small amounts of clear fluids such as ice chips. If oral intake is prohibited, moisten her mouth with a damp washcloth or have her rinse her mouth with water. | 6. Women often use rapid mouth breathing during labor, resulting in a dry mouth. These methods may relieve some of the discomfort associated with a dry mouth. Clear liquids limit the risk of aspiration if general anesthesia is needed. |
| 7. Offer a back rub or firm, constant sacral pressure. Ask Beth where and how firm pressure should be. Use baby powder when rubbing back. Have her tell caregivers if this technique becomes uncomfortable or if the location on her back needs to be changed. If Sam is rubbing her back, offer to relieve him occasionally and encourage him to take a break. | 7. Back rubs may reduce discomfort associated with back labor somewhat by stimulating large-diameter fibers and interfering with transmission of the pain impulse to the brain. As labor continues, back rubs may become less effective or even uncomfortable. Powder reduces friction, which could be another source of discomfort. The partner needs a break to conserve energy and better help the woman in later labor. |
| 8. Keep Beth and Sam informed about the progress of labor and their baby's condition. | 8. Reduces anxiety and fear of the unknown. Anxiety and fear increase pain perception and reduce pain tolerance. |

### EVALUATION

Beth concentrates on her breathing techniques with each contraction but has a relaxed body posture between them. She continues to use learned skills effectively for about 2 hours, when she begins to have more difficulty coping with her contractions. Interventions for pain continue but are revised to include those for pharmacologic pain management.

**ASSESSMENT:** Three hours after admission, Beth's cervix is 4 cm dilated and 100 percent effaced, and the fetal station is −1. Membranes have ruptured and the amniotic fluid is clear. Contractions are every 2 to 3 minutes, last 50 seconds, and are firm. Fetal heart rate and monitor patterns are essentially unchanged. Back discomfort persists, and she is having difficulty relaxing between contractions and is discouraged that labor is not progressing as quickly as she expected. She is no longer able to use prepared childbirth techniques effectively. Beth reluctantly requests an epidural block, which will be given by continuous infusion.

### Critical Thinking

Should the nurse discourage Beth from having an epidural block? At this point, what are some advantages and disadvantages related to having an epidural? Are added measures needed to safeguard the fetus because of an epidural block?

**ANSWER**

The nurse should not discourage Beth's request for an epidural block, although she has reluctantly requested it. An epidural may slow labor if done earlier than this, but labor progress may benefit from the relief of pain and tension. One disadvantage of the epidural block is that she is more likely to be restricted to bed; upright positions, including ambulation, promote labor progress.

To safeguard the fetus, the nurse gives Beth 500 ml or more of ordered intravenous solution before the block begins, which offsets its hypotensive effects. Fetal monitoring, usually by continuous electronic means, helps identify nonreassuring patterns that may occur. If Beth must remain on her back for any reason, a small pillow or wedge is placed beneath one hip to tilt her uterus and prevent aortocaval compression.

**NURSING DIAGNOSIS:** Risk for injury related to altered sensation in her lower extremities

### GOALS/EXPECTED OUTCOMES

1. Beth will not fall or suffer other injury while experiencing the effects of epidural block.
2. The fetus will not be born in an uncontrolled manner.

## Nursing Care Plan 15–1 *Continued*

# Intrapartum Pain Management

| INTERVENTION | RATIONALE |
|---|---|
| 1. Assist Beth to change positions regularly. Keep Beth in bed as long as she has any motor block. | 1. Changing positions reduces constant pressure on one area and helps prevent muscle strain. The epidural block causes a varying degree of motor block, so ambulation is generally contraindicated. |
| 2. Observe for signs of labor progress:<br>a. Contractions increase in frequency, duration, and intensity<br>b. Increase in bloody show<br>c. Statement reflecting urge to push (may *not* be present) | 2. Sensation is altered, and rectal pressure associated with fetal descent may not be felt. The fetus could be born unattended because of reduced sensation. |
| 3. If Beth cannot feel a strong urge to push during the second stage, tell her when to push during each contraction. | 3. Epidural block may alter the reflex urge to push. Coaching about when to push aids fetal descent. |
| 4. After birth, do not allow Beth to ambulate until sensation and movement have returned to her lower extremities. Ask another nurse to assist when she first ambulates. | 4. Prevents falls due to weakness and inability to sense where her feet are. Having assistance prevents injury if a woman is unexpectedly weak when she ambulates. |

### EVALUATION

Beth is satisfied with her pain relief after the epidural block. She has little motor block. Her blood pressure and the fetal heart rate remain within expected limits. Vaginal dilation progresses to 10 cm (complete) without injury to Beth or her fetus. However, despite her vigorous pushing efforts, the fetal station remains at 0. Beth has a cesarean birth, delivering an 8-pound, 10-ounce girl.

### ADDITIONAL NURSING DIAGNOSES* AND COLLABORATIVE PROBLEM TO CONSIDER

Anxiety
Risk for Aspiration
Powerlessness
Situational Low Self-esteem
Urinary Retention
Potential Complication: Fetal compromise

* Only nursing diagnoses related to pain relief during and immediately after surgery are discussed here. For related care plans, see Nursing Care Plans 13–1, 14–1, and 16–1. See Chapter 17 for related postpartum nursing care.

- Oral intake—time and type of intake
- Evidence of pain: verbal—statement, requests for pain relief measures, crying, moaning; and nonverbal—tense, guarded posture or facial expression
- Labor status

In addition to these routine assessments, ask the woman if she needs help with pain management. A stoic woman may give little outward evidence of pain yet may say she wants medication or other pain control if asked.

When assessing pain, clarify the words a woman uses. When asked if she has "pain," the woman may deny it. Yet changing the word used to "discomfort," "aching," "pulling," "pressure," or other words that may describe labor pain may bring a different response. Do not assume that everyone uses the same words to describe their pain. Just as pain is an individual experience, so also is the expression of pain, including verbal expression.

Asking a woman to rate her pain on a scale of 0 to 10 or a similar scale helps clarify her pain's intensity. Zero represents no pain, whereas 10 is the worst possible pain. Ask the woman to rate her pain on this scale before and after pain relief measures to evaluate their effectiveness.

The woman who remains tense between contractions may be having difficulty coping with pain. Moaning, crying, thrashing, and an inability to use nonpharmacologic techniques suggest that she needs pharmacologic pain relief.

Evaluate the woman's labor status to help her

choose the most appropriate method of pain control. If she has reached a point in labor at which she needs to decide for or against a specific pharmacologic method, inform her. This is not an exact time or an exact amount of cervical dilation but is estimated according to when she is likely to give birth, the time needed to establish a specific method, and the pharmacology of the drug or drugs.

Avoid making assumptions about the amount of pain a woman is having on the basis of her rate of labor progress, cervical dilation, or apparent intensity of contractions. It is tempting to assume that a woman whose cervix is 2 cm dilated has little pain and that a woman whose cervix is dilated 8 cm has intense pain. An obese woman's contractions may be strong, but they may seem mild if they are assessed by palpation or an external monitor because of her thick abdominal fat pad. *Labor progress or contraction intensity cannot be equated with a woman's pain perception or tolerance.*

Neither should a woman's need for pain relief be based on her outward expression only. A quiet woman may need medication but may be reluctant to ask, whereas the expressive woman may be quite satisfied with only nonpharmacologic measures. Because women who do not speak the prevailing language may not know what is available, seek an interpreter to communicate accurately.

Observe for pain that is not typical of labor. Although labor pain is often intense, it should not be constant but should come and go with each contraction. The uterus should not be tender or board-like between contractions. Report atypical pain to the physician or nurse-midwife.

## Analysis

Because pain is an expected part of normal childbirth, most laboring women have nursing needs that relate to its management. The nursing diagnosis is: Pain related to effects of uterine contractions and fetal descent.

## Planning

Because pain is a subjective experience and labor is not expected to be painless, two goals are realistic. The woman will do the following:

1. Describe pain relief measures as satisfactory during labor.
2. Use learned breathing and relaxation techniques during labor.

## Interventions

The main points of nursing care related to intrapartum pain management are to reduce factors that hinder the woman's pain control and to enhance those that benefit it. Refer to Chapter 13 for nursing measures that should be included in the care of all laboring women, such as positioning, teaching, encouragement, and care of the partner.

### PROMOTING RELAXATION

Simple attention to details can help the woman relax. Adjust her environment so that it is more comfortable. If noise is a problem, suggest music or television to mask it.

A warm blanket or a cool cloth provides tangible comfort and conveys the nurse's caring attitude. Change the linens or underpads as needed to keep the woman reasonably clean and dry.

Offer the woman a warm shower or bath, especially if she is tense and if no contraindications exist (Table 15–2). In general, walking is good during early labor, and water therapy is better during active labor. The mild nipple stimulation that occurs in a whirlpool or shower may intensify contractions in a

**TABLE 15–2 USE OF WATER THERAPY DURING LABOR**

Use of water therapy has accompanied trends toward a low-intervention approach to intrapartum care. Water therapy can be delivered in several ways:
Shower
Standard tub
Whirlpool

**Benefits**

Associated with a more natural, home-like atmosphere
Gives a woman greater control over her labor
Upright position facilitates progress of labor
Faster labor progress if contractions are frequent when entering the tub
Buoyancy relieves tired muscles
Facilitates fetal rotation from occiput posterior or transverse positions to the occiput anterior; the woman can also assume different positions to aid rotation
Many women report a perception of less pain
Reduction in the mean arterial pressure, edema, and increased diuresis; this is especially helpful if the woman has pregnancy-induced hypertension

**Disadvantages**

May reduce frequency of contractions and dilation during the latent phase of labor
Fetus must be assessed with intermittent auscultation rather than electronic fetal monitoring

**Contraindications-Precautions**

No specific contraindications if the woman can safely be out of bed
Thick meconium in the amniotic fluid is an indication for continuous electronic fetal monitoring in most birth facilities and would preclude use of water therapy
Bleeding
Oxytocin induction or augmentation; use of both oxytocin and water therapy could cause excess uterine activity

woman whose labor has slowed because it causes her posterior pituitary gland to secrete oxytocin.

Reduce intrusions as much as possible. For example, wait until a contraction is over before asking questions or doing a procedure. Longer assessments and procedures may span several contractions, but try to stop during each contraction.

#### REDUCING OUTSIDE SOURCES OF DISCOMFORT

Anesthetize the intravenous site with lidocaine (Xylocaine) before inserting the line if the woman is not allergic and if facility policy permits. Normal saline infiltration of the site has a similar effect. Remind her to change position regularly to reduce tension and discomfort from constant pressure. Support her with pillows.

Observe the woman's bladder for distention hourly, and encourage her to void every 2 hours or more often if she has received a large quantity of intravenous fluids. Obtain an order to catheterize her if she cannot void and her bladder is full.

#### REDUCING ANXIETY AND FEAR

Accurate information reduces the negative psychological impact of the unknown. Tell the woman about her labor and its progress. It is impossible to predict when she will give birth, but tell her if labor progress is or is not on course. Sometimes she needs only the reassurance from an experienced nurse that her intense contractions are indeed normal. The woman may be willing to endure more discomfort than she otherwise would if she is making progress.

Be honest if problems do occur. A woman usually knows if there is a problem and is more anxious if she does not know what it is. Explain all measures taken to correct the problem, and keep her informed about the results.

#### HELPING THE WOMAN USE NONPHARMACOLOGIC TECHNIQUES

*If the nonpharmacologic method is safe for the woman and fetus and if it is effective, do not interfere with its use.* Try not to distract the woman from whatever technique she is using.

**Massage.** Fetal monitor belts hinder abdominal effleurage. Encourage the woman to do effleurage on uncovered areas of her abdomen or to stroke her thighs. Consider using intermittent fetal monitoring if this method is appropriate.

During massage, baby powder reduces friction and skin irritation. The woman needs to tell the person who is providing sacral pressure or other massage how much pressure helps and the best location for it. Because this information may change during labor or massage may become uncomfortable rather than helpful, seek the woman's feedback regularly.

**Mental Stimulation.** Use a low, soothing voice when helping a woman use imagery. It is often helpful to speak close to her ear when trying to create a tranquil imaginary scene or to calm her. Music can enhance mental stimulation techniques.

**Breathing.** Women learn a variety of breathing techniques in prepared childbirth classes and often modify them or invent some of their own during labor. Encourage the woman to change techniques when she needs to, avoiding the complex ones during early labor. If she has trouble maintaining her concentration, the nurse or her partner can make eye contact (if culturally appropriate) and breathe the pattern with her.

Symptoms of hyperventilation (dizziness, tingling and numbness of the fingers and lips, carpopedal spasm) are likely if a woman breathes fast and deep, whether or not she is using patterned breathing techniques. If she hyperventilates, have her breathe into her cupped hands, a paper bag, or a washcloth placed over her nose and mouth.

Teach breathing techniques to the unprepared woman when she is admitted. Review them when she seems to need a different method. Many women make up their own breathing techniques.

When teaching the woman who is in advanced labor non-pharmacologic pain management techniques, follow these guidelines:

- Teach one method at a time.
- Demonstrate the method between contractions.
- Use breathing techniques with the woman while maintaining eye contact.
- Allow her control over her labor: who is present, what technique she will use, and the like.

#### INCORPORATING PHARMACOLOGIC METHODS

All pharmacologic methods require collaboration with medical personnel for orders. Tell the woman soon after admission what medication is available if she needs it. This is done not to undermine her self-confidence but so that she can better understand when she needs to make a choice about medication. Also, analgesia is most effective if it is given before pain is severe.

Tell her that her preferences about pain relief methods will be honored if possible, but it is impossible to predict the course of her labor. Her preferred method of pain management may be inappropriate if labor has unexpected developments. Assure her that no pharmacologic method will be given without her understanding and consent (see Parents Want to Know: How Will This Medicine Affect Our Baby?).

If a woman finds nonpharmacologic methods inadequate, try other ones or offer her available medication. When contacting the birth attendant for medication orders, report the fetal and maternal status and vital signs, labor status, and her request for medication. If she has a continuous epidural block, contact the person who inserted it if problems occur. Observe special nursing considerations associated with the method used (Table 15–3).

### Evaluation

Labor is not expected to be painless, even with the most effective pharmacologic methods. The first goal is achieved if the woman is satisfied with her ability to manage her pain. Many women have occasional difficulty using breathing or other techniques, even if they have practiced faithfully. They achieve the second goal if they use coping skills somewhat consistently during labor.

## Respiratory Compromise

### Assessment

General anesthesia may be needed any time during birth, most often for cesarean birth. Document the type (solids or liquids) and time of the woman's last food intake. Question her closely if she reports an unusually long interval since her last oral intake. Anesthesia clinicians can anticipate and prevent problems better if they know the actual oral intake.

**Parents Want to Know**

**How Will This Medicine Affect Our Baby?**

*Women and their partners often ask whether pain medication or anesthesia will harm their baby. The nurse can help parents to choose wisely from available options by providing honest information.*

- Pain that is beyond your ability to tolerate is not good for you or your baby, and it reduces the pleasure of this special event.
- Some risk is associated with every type of pain medication or anesthesia, but careful selection and use of preventive measures minimize this risk. If complications occur, corrective measures can reduce the risk to you and your baby.
- Pain relievers can cause your baby to be slow to breathe at birth, but carefully controlling the timing and dose of the medication reduces the likelihood that this will occur. We can use another medication to reverse this effect if needed.
- Epidural or spinal anesthesia can cause your blood pressure to fall, which can reduce the blood flow to your baby. However, we give you lots of intravenous fluids to reduce this effect. We have other medications to increase your blood pressure if the fluids are not enough.
- General anesthesia can cause your baby to be slow to breathe at birth. To reduce this risk, the anesthesia will not be started until everything is ready for the surgery, and the doctors will clamp the baby's umbilical cord as quickly as possible.

**TABLE 15–3 PHARMACOLOGIC METHODS OF INTRAPARTUM PAIN MANAGEMENT**

| Method and Uses | Nursing Considerations |
|---|---|
| **Opioid Analgesics** | |
| Systemic analgesia during labor and for postoperative pain after cesarean birth. May be combined with adjunctive drug such as promethazine to reduce nausea and vomiting that sometimes occur with narcotic use. | 1. Assess the woman for drug use at admission. Women who are opiate-dependent should not receive analgesics having mixed agonist and antagonist actions (butorphanol and nalbuphine).<br>2. Observe neonate for respiratory depression, especially if the mother had narcotics within 4 hours of birth:<br>Delay in initiating or sustaining respirations<br>Rate <30/min<br>Poor muscle tone: limp, floppy<br>3. Use of adjunctive drugs, such as promethazine, enhances respiratory depressant effects.<br>4. Have naloxone available. Observe for recurrent respiratory depression after administration of naloxone. Repeat at 20- to 60-minute intervals as needed. |
| **Epidural Opioids** | |
| *Labor*: Mixed with a local anesthetic agent to give better pain relief with less motor block.<br>*Postoperatively*: Gives long-acting analgesia without sedation, allowing the mother and infant to interact more easily. | 1. Observe same nursing implications as with epidural block.<br>2. Do not give additional opioids or other CNS depressants except as ordered by the anesthesia clinician.<br>3. Respiratory depression may be delayed up to 24 hr. Observe respiratory rate, depth, and arousability hourly for 24 hr. Notify anesthesia clinician for rate <12/min, oxygen saturation <95% on pulse oximeter, reduced respiratory effort, or difficulty arousing. Cyanosis is a late sign.<br>4. Have naloxone, 0.4 mg, readily available.<br>5. Observe for pruritus or rubbing of the face and neck. Notify anesthesia clinician for relief measures. |

| TABLE 15–3 PHARMACOLOGIC METHODS OF INTRAPARTUM PAIN MANAGEMENT *Continued* | |
|---|---|
| **Method and Uses** | **Nursing Considerations** |
| **Epidural Opioids** | |
| | 6. Urinary retention may occur. Observe for adequate voiding if the woman does not have a catheter<br>7. Notify anesthesia clinician for relief of nausea or vomiting.<br>8. Assess sensation and mobility before allowing ambulation. |
| **Intrathecal Opioid Analgesics** | |
| Provides analgesia for most of first-stage labor without maternal sedation. A very small dose of the drug is needed because it is injected very near the spinal cord where sensory fibers enter. Usually not adequate for late labor or the birth itself. | 1. Observe for the common side effects of nausea, vomiting, and pruritus. Notify the anesthesia clinician if these occur, and have an antagonist such as naloxone or naltrexone available.<br>2. Observe for delayed respiratory depression, depending on the drug given. Use a pulse oximeter as indicated. |
| **Local Infiltration Anesthesia** | |
| Numbs perineum for episiotomy or repair of laceration at vaginal birth. No relief of labor pain. Not adequate for forceps-assisted birth. | 1. Assess for drug allergies, especially to dental anesthetics because they are related to those used in maternity care.<br>2. Apply ice to perineum to reduce edema and hematoma formation and to increase comfort. |
| **Pudendal Block** | |
| Numbs the lower vagina and perineum for vaginal birth. No relief of labor pain because it is done just before birth. Provides adequate anesthesia for many forceps-assisted births. | 1. Same as local infiltration. A woman may be alarmed by the long needle (about 6 inches). Teach her that it must be long to reach the pudendal nerve and that it will be inserted only about 0.5 inch into her tissue. Tell her that a guide ("trumpet") will be used to avoid damaging her or her fetus' tissue. |
| **Epidural Block** | |
| *Labor*: Insertion of catheter provides pain relief for labor and vaginal birth (T10–S5 levels).<br>*Cesarean birth*: If epidural was used during labor, level of block can be extended upward (T4–T6 level). Also used for planned cesarean birth and post-birth tubal ligation. | 1. Prehydrate the woman with warmed non-glucose crystalloid solution such as Ringer's lactate. Common amounts: 500–1000 ml for labor and vaginal birth; 1500–2000 ml for cesarean birth.<br>2. Displace uterus to left manually or with a wedge under woman's right side to enhance placental perfusion.<br>3. Assess for hypotension at least every 5 min after block is begun and with each new dose until vital signs are stable. Report to anesthesia clinician: systolic BP $<110$ mmHg or a fall of 20% or more from baseline levels, pallor, or diaphoresis.<br>4. Assess FHR for signs of of impaired placental perfusion and report to anesthesia clinician and nurse-midwife: Tachycardia ($>150$–160/min) bradycardia $<110$–120/min) late decelerations (see Table 14–2).<br>5. If hypotension or signs of impaired placental perfusion occur: increase rate of nonadditive IV fluid; turn woman to her left side, administer oxygen by face mask 8–10 L/minute. Have ephedrine available (usually included in epidural tray).<br>6. Observe for bladder distention. Get an order to catheterize woman if she cannot void.<br>7. Turn woman from side to side hourly when a continuous infusion is used to avoid unilateral block.<br>8. If block is being given by intermittent injection, notify anesthesia clinician for reinjection when pain recurs.<br>9. Observe progress of labor. Coach woman to push if she cannot feel the urge during second stage.<br>10. Observe for signs of catheter migration: unilateral or absent pain relief, too intense motor and sensory block, signs of intravascular injection (numbness of tongue and lips, lightheadedness, dizziness, and tinnitus).<br>11. Transfer carefully because the woman may not have full use of her legs. Assess for return of sensation and movement before ambulation. |

*Table 15–3 continued on following page*

**TABLE 15-3 PHARMACOLOGIC METHODS OF INTRAPARTUM PAIN MANAGEMENT** *Continued*

| Method and Uses | Nursing Considerations |
|---|---|
| **Subarachnoid Block** | |
| *Cesarean birth.* Is simpler and can be established more quickly than epidural block.<br>May rarely be used for complicated vaginal birth.<br>Does not provide pain relief for labor because it is done just before birth. | 1. See Epidural Block for these interventions:<br>a. IV prehydration<br>b. Uterine displacement<br>c. Observation of blood pressure and FHR<br>d. Care for hypotension or signs of impaired placental perfusion<br>e. Bladder distention<br>f. Transfer and ambulation precautions<br>2. Observe for post-spinal headache: a headache that is worse when woman is upright and that may disappear when she is lying flat. Notify anesthesia clinician if it occurs (a blood patch may be done).<br>3. Nursing interventions for post-spinal headache: bedrest, increase oral fluids if not contraindicated, oral caffeine, and give analgesics as ordered. |
| **General Anesthesia** | |
| Cesarean birth if epidural or spinal block is not possible or if the woman refuses regional anesthesia. May be required for emergency procedures such as replacement of inverted uterus. | 1. Determine type and time of last food intake on admission.<br>2. Restrict oral intake to clear liquids or as ordered. Consult with physician or nurse-midwife if surgical intervention is likely.<br>3. Report to anesthesia clinician: oral intake before and during labor, vomiting.<br>4. Displace uterus (see Epidural Block).<br>5. Give ordered drugs such as sodium citrate and citric acid (Bicitra).<br>6. Maintain cricoid pressure (Sellick's maneuver) during intubation.<br>7. Maintain in a side-lying position (after surgery) until protective (gag) reflexes have returned.<br>8. Interventions for postoperative respiratory depression: give oxygen by face mask; observe oxygen saturation with pulse oximeter until woman is awake and alert; have woman take several deep breaths if oxygen saturation falls below 95%. |

*Abbreviations:* CNS, central nervous system; BP, blood pressure; FHR, fetal heart rate; IV, intravenous.

## Analysis

Aspiration is a short-term risk if the woman has general anesthesia. Nursing care of laboring women includes this risk because it is impossible to predict every woman who will require general anesthesia. The nursing diagnosis is: Risk for Aspiration related to impaired protective laryngeal reflexes.

## Planning

The goal for this nursing diagnosis is that the woman will not aspirate gastric contents into her trachea during the perioperative period.

## Interventions

Aspiration of gastric contents may occur despite careful medical and nursing interventions to prevent it. Nursing interventions relate to identifying factors that increase a woman's risk for aspiration, and collaborative and nursing measures to reduce the risk of aspiration or lung injury.

### IDENTIFYING RISK FACTORS

Report oral intake both before and after admission to the anesthesia clinician. In general, oral intake during labor is restricted to medications, clear liquids (usually ice chips), Popsicles, or hard candies. Chart all oral intake during labor.

Vomiting is a common discomfort during normal labor, regardless of the mother's oral intake. If vomiting occurs, chart the time, quantity, and character (amount, color, presence of undigested food).

### REDUCING RISK OF ASPIRATION OR LUNG INJURY

Nursing and medical personnel collaborate to reduce a woman's risk for pulmonary complications.

**Perioperative Care.** Discontinue the woman's oral intake until consulting the physician or nurse-midwife if surgical intervention seems likely because the woman may need general anesthesia. Give ordered medications such as sodium citrate and citric acid (Bicitra). Either the nurse or anesthesia clinician may give parenteral drugs, such as glycopyrrolate (Robinul), depending on when they are administered.

An experienced nurse or a trained anesthesia assistant provides cricoid pressure (Sellick's maneuver) to block the esophagus until the woman is intubated and the cuff of the endotracheal tube is inflated. Successful intubation with the cuffed endotracheal tube blocks passage of any gastric contents into the trachea.

**Postoperative Care.** Following general anesthesia, the woman is extubated after her protective laryngeal reflexes have returned. Position her on her side until she is awake to allow gravity to drain her secretions or emesis.

Birth facility protocols guide postoperative care. Administer oxygen by mask or face tent until the woman is awake and alert because general anesthesia is a respiratory depressant. Monitor oxygen saturation with a pulse oximeter. If her oxygen saturation falls below 95 percent, have her take several deep breaths. Deep breathing also helps her eliminate inhalational anesthetics and reduces stasis of pulmonary secretions.

Assess the woman's pulse, respiration, and blood pressure every 15 minutes for 1 hour or until stable, then according to policy. Observe her color for pallor or cyanosis, which suggests shock or hypoventilation.

## Evaluation

Interventions for this nursing diagnosis are preventive and short-term because it is a temporary high-risk situation. The goal is met if the woman does not aspirate gastric contents during the perioperative period.

## SUMMARY CONCEPTS

- Childbirth pain is unique because it is normal and self-limiting, can be prepared for, and ends with a baby's birth.
- Excess or poorly relieved pain may be harmful to the mother and fetus.
- Pain is a complex physical and psychological experience. It is subjective and personal.
- Four sources of pain are present in most labors, but other physical and psychological factors may increase or decrease the pain felt from these sources. These sources are cervical dilation, uterine ischemia, pressure and pulling on pelvic structures, and distention of the vagina and perineum.
- Relaxation enhances other pain management techniques.
- Physiologic alterations of pregnancy may affect a woman's response to medications.
- Any drug that the expectant mother takes, whether therapeutic or abused, also may affect the fetus. Fetal effects may be direct or indirect.
- The nurse should observe for respiratory depression, primarily in the newborn, when the mother has received opioid analgesics during labor.
- The major advantages of regional pain management methods are that the woman can participate in the birth and that she retains her protective airway reflexes.
- The nurse should observe for and take actions to prevent maternal hypotension with the epidural or subarachnoid block.
- The nurse should observe for fetal heart rate changes associated with impaired placental perfusion if the woman is at risk for hypotension, such as with epidural or subarachnoid blocks.
- The main nursing observations for the woman who receives epidural or intrathecal opioids are for nausea and vomiting, pruritus, and delayed respiratory depression.
- Regurgitation with aspiration of acidic gastric contents is the greatest risk for a woman who receives general anesthesia.

### References and Readings

American Academy of Pediatrics and American College of Obstetricians and Gynecologists. (1992). *Guidelines for perinatal care* (3rd ed.) Washington, D.C.: Author.

American College of Obstetricians and Gynecologists. (1996). ACOG technical bulletin no. 225: Obstetric analgesia and anesthesia. *International Journal of Gynecology and Obstetrics*, 54, 281–292.

Association of Women's Health, Obstetric, and Neonatal Nurses (AWHONN). (1996a). Clinical commentary: Obstetric epidural analgesia and the role of the professional registered nurse. AWHONN *Voice*, 4(8).

Association of Women's Health, Obstetric, and Neonatal Nurses (AWHONN). (1996b). *Position statement: Role of the registered nurse (RN) in the management of the patient receiving analgesia by catheter techniques (epidural, intrathecal, intrapleural, or peripheral nerve catheters)*. Washington, D.C.: Author.

Baram, D.A. (1995). Hypnosis in reproductive health care: A review and case reports. *Birth*, 22(1), 37–42.

Blackburn, S.T., & Loper, D.L. (1992). *Maternal, fetal, and neonatal physiology: A clinical perspective*. Philadelphia: W.B. Saunders.

Creehan, P.A. (1996). Pain relief and comfort measures during labor. In K.R. Simpson & P.A. Creehan (Eds.), AWHONN'S *perinatal nursing* (pp. 227–245). Philadelphia: J.B. Lippincott.

Cunningham, F.G., MacDonald, P.C., Gant, N.F., Leveno, K.J., Gilstrap, L.C., Hankins, G.D.V., et al. (1997). *Williams obstetrics* (20th ed.). Norwalk, Conn.: Appleton & Lange.

Dewan, D.M., & Hood, D.D. (1997). *Practical obstetric anesthesia*. Philadelphia: W.B. Saunders.

Dick, M.J. (1995). Assessment and measurement of acute pain. *Journal of Obstetric, Gynecologic, and Neonatal Nursing*, 24(9), 843–848.

Goer, H. (1995). *Obstetric myths versus research realities: A guide to the medical literature*. Westport, Conn.: Bergin & Garvey.

Hueston, W.J., McClaflin, R.R., Mansfield, C.J., & Rudy, M. (1994). Factors associated with the use of intrapartum epidural analgesia. *Obstetrics and Gynecology*, 84(4), 579–582.

Kendrick, J. (1996). *Controversies in decision-making for pain control in* L & D (Cassette recording M1). Anaheim, Calif.: MCN Convention.

Lowe, N.K. (1996). The pain and discomfort of labor and birth. *Journal of Obstetric, Gynecologic, and Neonatal Nursing*, 25(1), 82–92.

MacArthur, C. (1994). Commentary: More evidence against the routine use of epidurals. *Birth*, 21(3), 172–174.

Manning, J. (1996). Intrathecal narcotics: New approach for labor analgesia. *Journal of Obstetric, Gynecologic, and Neonatal Nursing*, 25(3), 221–224.

Newton, E.R., Schroeder, B.C., Knape, K.G., & Bennett, B.L. (1995). Epidural analgesia and uterine function. *Obstetrics and Gynecology*, 85(5), 749–755.

Simkin, P. (1995). Reducing pain and enhancing progress in labor: A guide to nonpharmacologic methods for maternity caregivers. *Birth*, 22(3), 161–171.

Thorp, J., & Breedlove, G. (1996). Epidural analgesia in labor: An evaluation of risks and benefits. *Birth*, 23(2), 63–83.

Weber, S.E. (1996). Cultural aspects of pain in childbearing women. *Journal of Obstetric, Gynecologic, and Neonatal Nursing*, 25(1), 67–72.

Youngstrom, P.C., Baker, S.W., & Miller, J.L. (1996). Epidurals redefined in analgesia and anesthesia: A distinction with a difference. *Journal of Obstetric, Gynecologic, and Neonatal Nursing*, 25(4), 350–354.

Zuspan, K. (1994a). Anesthesia for obstetrics. In F.P. Zuspan & E.J. Quilligan (Eds.), *Current therapy in obstetrics and gynecology* (pp. 211–217). Philadelphia: W.B. Saunders.

Zuspan, K. (1994b). Control of postpartum pain. In F.P. Zuspan & E.J. Quilligan (Eds.), *Current therapy in obstetrics and gynecology* (pp. 233–235). Philadelphia: W.B. Saunders.

# 16

# Nursing Care During Obstetric Procedures

**OBJECTIVES**

1. Identify clinical situations in which specific obstetric procedures are appropriate.
2. Explain risks, precautions, and contraindications for each procedure.
3. Identify nursing considerations for each procedure.
4. Identify methods to provide effective emotional support to the woman having an obstetric procedure.
5. Apply the nursing process to plan care for the woman having a cesarean birth.

**DEFINITIONS**

**abruptio placentae** *Premature separation of a normally implanted placenta.*

**amniotomy** *Artificial rupture of the amniotic sac (fetal membranes).*

**augmentation of labor** *Artificial stimulation of uterine contractions that have become ineffective.*

**cephalopelvic disproportion** *Fetal head size that is too large to fit through the maternal pelvis at birth. Also called fetopelvic disproportion.*

**cesarean birth** *Surgical birth of the fetus through an incision in the abdominal wall and uterus.*

**chignon** *Newborn scalp edema created by a vacuum extractor.*

**chorioamnionitis** *Inflammation of the amniotic sac (fetal membranes); usually caused by bacterial or viral infections. Also called amnionitis.*

**dystocia** *Difficult or prolonged labor; often associated with abnormal uterine activity and cephalopelvic disproportion.*

**episiotomy** *Surgical incision of the perineum to enlarge the vaginal opening.*

**hydramnios** *Excessive volume of amniotic fluid (more than 2000 ml at term). Also called polyhydramnios.*

**iatrogenic** *An adverse condition resulting from treatment.*

**induction of labor** *Artificial initiation of labor.*

**nuchal cord** *Umbilical cord around the fetal neck.*

**oligohydramnios** *Abnormally small quantity of amniotic fluid (less than 500 ml at term).*

**placenta previa** *Abnormal implantation of the placenta in the lower uterus.*

**premature rupture of the membranes** *Spontaneous rupture of the membranes before the onset of labor. The gestation may be term, preterm, or postterm.*

**version** *Turning the fetus from one presentation to another before birth, usually from breech to cephalic.*

Although labor is a normal process, some women require special procedures to help them or their fetus. A physician or nurse-midwife performs these procedures; nursing considerations for each are addressed.

## Amniotomy

### Indications

Amniotomy may be performed to induce labor, augment labor, or allow internal electronic fetal monitoring and fetal scalp blood sampling (see Chapter 14). Although amniotomy is often used for induction or stimulation of labor, its actual effectiveness for these purposes is not always supported by research (Busowski & Parsons, 1995).

### Risks

Amniotomy is performed by the physician or nurse-midwife. The nurse must observe for three risks associated with amniotomy and assist in emergency procedures.

**Prolapse of the Umbilical Cord.** The primary risk is that the umbilical cord will slip down in the gush of fluid. The cord can be compressed between the fetal presenting part and the woman's pelvis, obstructing blood flow to and from the placenta and reducing fetal gas exchange.

**Infection.** With interruption of the membrane barrier, vaginal organisms have free access to the uterine cavity and may cause chorioamnionitis. The risk is low at first but increases as the interval between membrane rupture and birth increases. Birth within 24 hours of amniotomy is desirable, although there is no absolute time when infection occurs.

**Abruptio Placentae.** Abruptio placentae may occur if the uterus is distended with excessive amniotic fluid when the membranes rupture. As the uterus collapses with discharge of the amniotic fluid, the area of placental attachment shrinks. The placenta then no longer fits its implantation site and partially separates. A large area of placental disruption re-

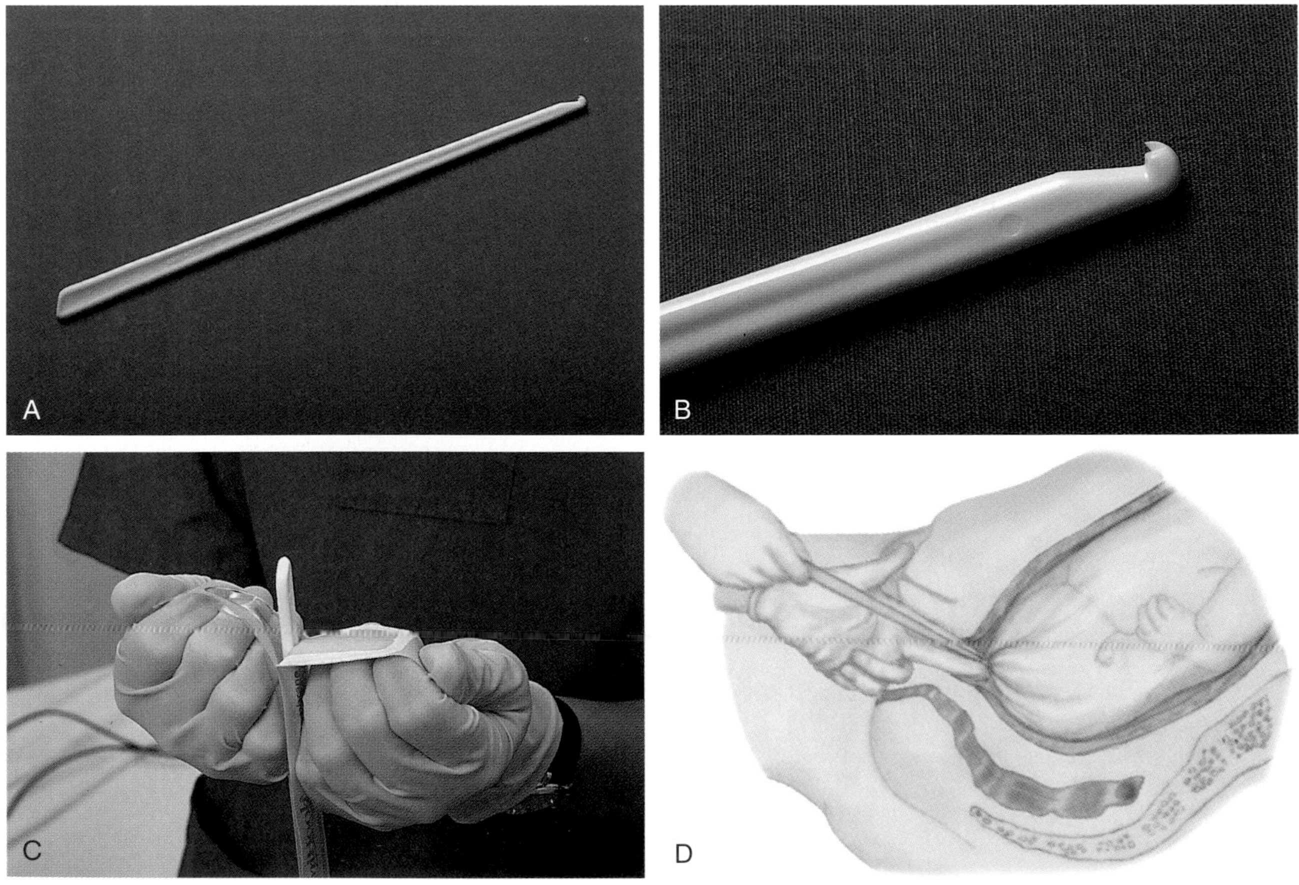


**FIGURE 16–1**

A, Disposable plastic membrane perforator. B, Close-up of hook end of plastic membrane perforator. C, Correct method to open the package. D, Technique for artificial rupture of membranes.

duces fetal oxygenation, nutrition, and waste disposal.

## Technique

A disposable plastic hook (Amnihook) is commonly used to perforate the amniotic sac (Fig. 16–1). The birth attendant does a vaginal examination to determine cervical dilation and effacement, fetal station, and fetal presenting part. Amniotomy is deferred if the fetal presenting part is high or if the presentation is not cephalic. The risk of a prolapsed cord is higher in these situations because more room is available for the cord to slip down.

The hook is passed through the cervix, and the membranes are snagged. The hole is enlarged with the finger, allowing fluid to drain.

## Nursing Considerations

### OBTAINING BASELINE INFORMATION

The fetal heart rate is assessed with auscultation or electronic monitoring to identify a reassuring rate and pattern before amniotomy is done. The initial fetal assessment provides a baseline to compare later assessments. A minimum of 20 to 30 minutes is needed for adequate baseline fetal evaluation.

### ASSISTING WITH AMNIOTOMY

Before amniotomy, two or three underpads should be placed under the woman's buttocks to absorb the fluid, overlapping them to extend from her waist to her knees. A folded bath towel under the buttocks absorbs a large quantity of amniotic fluid.

Other supplies needed are a disposable plastic hook, a sterile glove, and a packet of sterile lubricant. Peel the package containing the plastic hook partly open at the handle end, holding the package ends back until the birth attendant takes the hook.

### PROVIDING CARE AFTER AMNIOTOMY

Nursing care after amniotomy is the same as that following spontaneous membrane rupture.

**Identifying Complications.** The fetal heart rate is assessed for at least 1 full minute following amniotomy. Nonreassuring monitor patterns or significant changes from previous assessments are reported promptly to the birth attendant. Cord compression is usually accompanied by a rate less than 100 beats per minute (BPM), which worsens during contractions.

The quantity, color, and odor of the amniotic fluid are charted. The fluid should be clear (sometimes with bits of vernix) and have a mild odor. A large amount of vernix in the fluid suggests that the fetus may be preterm. Greenish meconium-stained fluid may be seen in postterm gestation or placental insufficiency. Fluid having a foul or strong odor, cloudy appearance, or a yellow color suggests chorioamnionitis. Hydramnios is associated with some fetal abnormalities. Oligohydramnios may be associated with placental insufficiency or fetal urinary tract abnormalities.

The woman's temperature should be assessed every 2 to 4 hours after the membranes rupture. Report elevations above 38°C (100.4°F). Fetal tachycardia (above 160 BPM) may precede maternal fever.

**Promoting Comfort.** Amniotic fluid continues to leak from the woman's vagina. Regularly changing the underpads keeps her drier and reduces the moist environment that favors bacterial growth.

### CRITICAL THINKING EXERCISE

A physician performs an amniotomy on a laboring woman whose cervix is dilated to 5 cm. The amniotic fluid is pale yellow and moderate in amount and has a strong odor. The fetal heart rate is 164 and accelerates when the fetus moves. Maternal vital signs are temperature 37.6°C (99.7°F), pulse 92, respirations 22, blood pressure 116/80. Contractions are moderate to firm intensity, every 3 to 4 minutes, with a duration of 50 to 60 seconds and complete uterine relaxation between contractions.

**Q:**

1. Which of these observations should the nurse regard as normal? Which factors are abnormal?
2. Should the nurse modify routine labor care based on the postamniotomy assessments?

**A:**

1. a. The amount of amniotic fluid is normal, but the pale yellow color and strong odor suggest chorioamnionitis, or infection of the amniotic sac. The risk for chorioamnionitis increases as the duration of ruptured membranes increases, but it can be apparent at any time, including at initial rupture.
   b. The fetal heart rate is slightly elevated from the normal maximum rate at term of 160 BPM. Accelerations with fetal movement are a reassuring sign. The maternal temperature, pulse, and respirations are slightly elevated. It is difficult to accurately interpret these values because the baseline values are not stated.
   c. These contractions are typical for a woman entering the active phase of first-stage labor.
2. The nurse should continue to assess the fetus for tachycardia, which often precedes maternal fever. Assess the woman's temperature at least every 2 hours for temperature of 38°C (100.4°F) or higher. Report abnormalities to the physician. Observe also for fetal tachycardia and signs of fetal compromise that may occur with maternal infection.

**CHECK YOUR READING**

1. What are three risks associated with amniotomy?
2. Why is the fetal heart rate assessed before and after the membranes rupture?
3. What is the significance of green amniotic fluid?
4. What maternal and fetal signs are associated with chorioamnionitis?

# Induction and Augmentation of Labor

Induction and augmentation of labor use artificial methods to stimulate uterine contractions. Techniques and nursing care are similar for both induction and augmentation.

## Indications

Induction of labor is considered when continuing the pregnancy may jeopardize the health of the woman or fetus and when labor and vaginal birth are considered safe. Labor induction is not done if the fetus must be delivered more quickly than the process permits; a cesarean birth would be performed instead. Induction may be done for these specific conditions:

- Pregnancy-induced hypertension, which is associated with reduced placental blood flow
- Spontaneous rupture of the membranes at or near term without onset of labor
- Chorioamnionitis (inflammation of the amniotic sac)
- Maternal medical conditions that are worsening with continuation of the pregnancy (e.g., diabetes, renal disease, pulmonary disease)
- Conditions in which the intrauterine environment is hostile to fetal well-being (such as intrauterine fetal growth restriction, postterm gestation, maternal-fetal blood incompatibility)
- Fetal death

Induction solely for convenience is not recommended. However, factors such as a history of rapid labors or living a long distance from the hospital are valid reasons to induce labor because of the real possibility that the baby would be born in uncontrolled circumstances.

Prenatal diagnosis sometimes identifies a fetal anomaly that will need specialized neonatal care at a distant facility. The mother may be transported to that facility for labor induction with needed equipment and specialists assembled there to care for the newborn.

Augmentation of labor with oxytocin is considered when labor has begun spontaneously, but progress has slowed or stopped because of poor contractions.

## Contraindications

Any contraindication to labor and vaginal birth is a contraindication to induction or augmentation of labor. These conditions may include the following:

- Placenta previa, which may result in hemorrhage during labor
- Umbilical cord prolapse
- Abnormal fetal presentation (vaginal birth is often more hazardous; also, the fetus may turn to a normal position by the time spontaneous labor occurs)
- Fetal presenting part above the pelvic inlet, which may be associated with cephalopelvic disproportion or a preterm fetus
- Active genital herpes infection, which can cause serious consequences if the fetus acquires it during birth
- Maternal pelvic structural abnormalities that contribute to cephalopelvic disproportion
- Previous classic (vertical) cesarean incision, which is more likely to rupture during labor than the more common low transverse incision

## Risks

Induction and augmentation of labor are associated with risks, as is spontaneous labor. These risks include the following:

- Hypertonic (excessive) uterine activity that can reduce placental perfusion and fetal oxygenation
- Uterine rupture
- Maternal water intoxication, which is more likely if a dextrose and water intravenous solution is used to dilute the oxytocin and with rates greater than 20 mU per minute (Cunningham et al., 1997).

## Technique

Surgical and medical methods may be used for labor induction or augmentation. Amniotomy is the method of surgical induction and augmentation because rupturing membranes stimulates uterine contractions if the cervix is favorable. Medical methods for induction or augmentation use drugs such as prostaglandin or intravenous oxytocin (Pitocin), or both, to stimulate contractions.

### DETERMINING WHETHER INDUCTION IS INDICATED

The birth attendant evaluates whether labor and birth are safer for the woman or fetus than continuing the pregnancy. Labor is not induced if the fetus is younger than 39 weeks' gestational age unless there is a compelling reason. Also, induction is more likely to be successful at term because pre-labor cervical changes favor dilation.

Cervical assessment estimates how favorable the cervix is for induction. The Bishop scoring system (Table 16–1) is used to estimate cervical readiness for labor with five factors: cervical dilation, effacement, consistency, position, and fetal station. Induction is likely to be successful with a Bishop score higher than six.

Because accuracy of the Bishop score is subjective and depends on the experience of the examiner, more objective methods to evaluate a woman's readiness for induction of labor are being explored. One method being studied is assessment of fetal fibronectin in the cervical and vaginal secretions. Studies have noted that this fetal protein is rarely present in the cervical and vaginal secretions from 21 weeks until 37 weeks but that it is present and increases as labor nears. Fetal fibronectin appears to be a marker for the pre-labor changes in the cervix and amniotic membranes at any gestation and thus may be valuable for predicting women who are at risk for preterm labor (Blanch et al., 1996).

**TABLE 16–1 BISHOP SCORING SYSTEM* TO EVALUATE THE CERVIX**

| Factor | Score | | | |
|---|---|---|---|---|
| | 0 | 1 | 2 | 3 |
| Dilation | 0 cm | 1–2 cm | 3–4 cm | 5–6 cm |
| Effacement | 0–30% | 40–50% | 60–70% | 80% or more |
| Station | −3 | −2 | −1 or 0 | +1 or +2 |
| Cervical consistency | Firm | Medium | Soft | |
| Cervical position | Posterior | Middle | Anterior | |

*This system is used to estimate how easily a woman's labor can be induced. Higher scores are associated with a greater likelihood of successful induction because her cervix has undergone prelabor changes, often called ripening. A woman who has given birth before usually has a successful induction when her Bishop score is 5 or higher. A woman who is having her first baby is most successfully induced if her score is 7 or higher.
Adapted from Bishop, E.H. (1964). Pelvic scoring for elective induction. *Obstetrics and Gynecology*, 24(2), 266–268.

### CERVICAL RIPENING

Procedures to ripen (soften) the cervix and make it more likely to dilate with the forces of labor are a common adjunct to induction. Most are done the day before the scheduled induction. If there are no complications, the woman may go home afterward and return for induction the following morning.

**Chemical Methods.** Preparations containing prostaglandin $E_2$ ($PGE_2$) may be used to facilitate cervical ripening. $PGE_2$ may be given as an intravaginal gel, an intracervical gel, or a timed-release vaginal insert (Table 16–2). It is administered in a setting in which fetal monitoring and emergency care are immediately available.

The major adverse reaction to $PGE_2$ is hypertonic uterine contractions. Prostaglandin should be given cautiously to women who have asthma, glaucoma, or pulmonary, hepatic, or renal disease. The woman should lie flat for 15 to 20 minutes after the gel is inserted to reduce leakage. The fetal heart rate should be monitored for at least 30 minutes for changes, and the uterus should be assessed for excessive contractions.

**TABLE 16–2 PROSTAGLANDIN $E_2$ PREPARATIONS FOR CERVICAL RIPENING**

| Hospital-Prepared Gel | Commercially Prepared Gel | Commercially Prepared Vaginal Insert |
|---|---|---|
| **Dosage** | | |
| For vaginal application: up to 5 mg<br>For intracervical application: 0.5 mg. Repeat up to three times in 24 hr at 4- to 6-hr intervals. | For intracervical application: 0.5 mg. Repeat up to three times in 24 hr at 6-hr intervals. | 10 mg in a time-released vaginal insert. Rate of release is 0.3 mg/hr. Remove at onset of active labor or 12 hr after insertion. |
| **Actions for Uterine Hyperstimulation** | | |
| Side-lying position<br>Oxygen by face mask at 8–10 L/min<br>Tocolytic drug such as terbutaline or magnesium sulfate | Same as for hospital-prepared gel | Remove insert. Implement actions as for hospital-prepared gel if necessary. |
| **When Oxytocin for Induction May Begin** | | |
| 4 hr after last dose | 6–12 hr after last dose | 30 min after removal of insert |

**Mechanical Methods.** The most common mechanical method for cervical ripening involves placement of hydrophilic (moisture-attracting) inserts into the cervical canal, where they absorb water and swell, gradually dilating the cervix. Examples of these dilators are the following:

- Dilapan, a synthetic material
- Lamicel, a synthetic sponge containing 450 mg of magnesium sulfate
- Laminaria tents, sterile cone-shaped preparations of dried seaweed

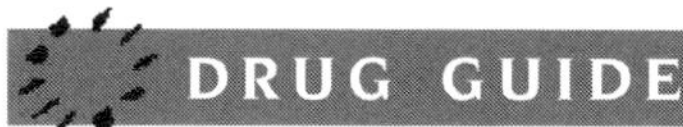


## OXYTOCIN (Pitocin)

***Classification:*** Oxytocic.

***Action:*** Synthetic compound identical to the natural hormone from the posterior pituitary. Stimulates uterine smooth muscle, resulting in increased strength, duration, and frequency of uterine contractions. Uterine sensitivity to oxytocin increases gradually during gestation. Has vasoactive and antidiuretic properties.

***Indications:*** Induction or augmentation of labor at or near term. Maintenance of firm uterine contraction after birth to control postpartum bleeding. Management of inevitable or incomplete abortion.

**Dosage and Route:**

*Induction or Augmentation of Labor*

1. *Intravenous infusion* via a secondary (piggyback) line. Dilute 10 units (1 ml) of oxytocin in 1000 ml of a balanced electrolyte solution such as lactated Ringer's solution, resulting in a concentration of 10 milliunits (mU) of oxytocin per milliliter. Other mixtures of oxytocin and solution may be used, such as 15 units of oxytocin (1.5 ml) plus 250 ml intravenous solution, resulting in a concentration of 60 mU/ml. Oxytocin infusion is controlled with a pump. The drug may also be given in 10-minute pulsed infusions rather than continuously.
2. Administration protocols vary, but guidelines from the American College of Obstetricians and Gynecologists (1995) suggest (a) starting dosages of 0.5 to 2 mU/minute, and (b) increasing dosage by 1 to 2 mU/minute increments every 30 to 60 minutes. The actual oxytocin dose is based on uterine response and absence of adverse effects. Shorter intervals between dose increases may result in uterine hyperstimulation. A lower starting dose is usually required to augment labor.
3. After an adequate contraction pattern is established and the cervix is dilated 5 to 6 cm, the oxytocin may be reduced by similar increments.

*Control of Postpartum Bleeding*

*Intravenous infusion*—Dilute 10 to 40 units in 1000 ml of intravenous solution. Rate of infusion must control uterine atony. Begin at a rate of 20 to 40 mU/minute, increasing or decreasing rate according to uterine response and rate of postpartum bleeding.

*Intramuscular injection*—10 units after delivery of placenta.

*Inevitable or Incomplete Abortion*

Dilute 10 units in 500 ml of intravenous solution, and infuse at 10 to 20 mU/minute.

***Absorption:*** Intravenous, immediate; intramuscular, 3 to 5 minutes.

***Excretion:*** Liver and urine.

***Contraindications and Precautions:*** Include, but are not limited to, placenta previa, vasa previa, nonreassuring fetal heart rate patterns, abnormal fetal presentation, prolapsed umbilical cord, presenting part above the pelvic inlet, previous classic uterine incision, active genital herpes infection, pelvic structural deformities, invasive cervical carcinoma.

***Adverse Reactions:*** Most result from hypersensitivity to drug or excessive dosage. Adverse reactions include hypertonic uterine activity, impaired uterine blood flow, uterine rupture, and abruptio placentae. Uterine hypertonicity may result in fetal bradycardia, tachycardia, reduced fetal heart rate variability, and late decelerations. Fetal asphyxia may occur with diminished uterine blood flow. Fetal or maternal trauma, or both, may occur from rapid birth. Prolonged administration may cause maternal fluid retention, leading to water intoxication. Hypotension (seen with rapid intravenous injection), tachycardia, cardiac dysrhythmias, and subarachnoid hemorrhage are rare adverse reactions.

**Nursing Considerations**

*Intrapartum*

Assess fetal heart rate for at least 20 minutes before induction to identify reassuring or nonreassuring patterns. Perform Leopold's maneuvers, a vaginal examination, or both to identify fetal presentation. Do not begin induction and, notify physician if nonreassuring fetal heart rate patterns are identified or if fetal presentation is other than cephalic.

Observe uterine activity for establishment of effective labor pattern: contraction frequency every 2 to 3 minutes, duration 40 to 90 seconds, intensity 50 to 80 mmHg (using intrauterine pressure catheter). Observe for hypertonic uterine activity: contractions less than 2 minutes apart, rest interval shorter than 60 seconds, duration longer than 90 seconds, or an elevated resting tone greater than 20 mmHg with an intrauterine pressure catheter. Observe fetal heart rate for nonreassuring patterns such as tachycardia, bradycardia, decreased variability, and late decelerations.

If uterine hypertonicity or a nonreassuring fetal heart rate pattern occurs, intervene to reduce uterine activity and increase fetal oxygenation: stop oxytocin infusion; increase rate of nonadditive solution; position woman in side-lying position; administer oxygen by snug face mask at 8 to 10 L/minute. Notify physician of adverse reactions, nursing interventions, and response to interventions. Record maternal blood pressure every 30 to 60 minutes or with each dosage increase. Record intake and output.

*Postpartum*

Observe uterus for firmness, height, and deviation. Massage until firm if uterus is soft ("boggy"). Observe lochia for color, quantity, and presence of clots. Notify birth attendant if uterus fails to remain contracted or if lochia is bright red or contains large clots. Assess for cramping. Assess vital signs every 15 minutes or according to protocol. Monitor intake and output to identify fluid retention or bladder distention.

*Inevitable or Incomplete Abortion*

Observe for cramping, vaginal bleeding, clots, and passage of products of conception. Observe maternal vital signs, intake, and output as noted under postpartum nursing implications.

The woman usually goes home overnight, and oxytocin induction of labor begins the following morning.

### OXYTOCIN ADMINISTRATION

Oxytocin is a powerful drug (see Drug Guide, p. 398), and it is impossible to predict a woman's response to it. Several precautions reduce the chance of adverse reactions in the mother and fetus.

- Oxytocin is diluted in a physiologic electrolyte-containing fluid and given as a secondary (piggyback) infusion so it can be stopped quickly if complications develop (Fig. 16–2).
- The oxytocin line is inserted into the primary (nonadditive, or maintenance) intravenous line as close as possible to the venipuncture site (the proximal port) to limit the amount of drug infused after changing to the nonadditive fluid.
- Oxytocin is started slowly, increased gradually, and regulated with an infusion pump.
- Uterine activity and fetal heart rate and patterns are monitored when oxytocin is given.

The woman's uterus becomes more sensitive to oxytocin as labor progresses. Therefore, the rate of oxytocin infusion may be gradually reduced when she is in the active phase of labor, about 5 to 6 cm cervical dilation. It may be stopped or reduced after her membranes rupture. When labor is augmented with oxytocin, a lower total dose is usually needed to achieve adequate contractions.

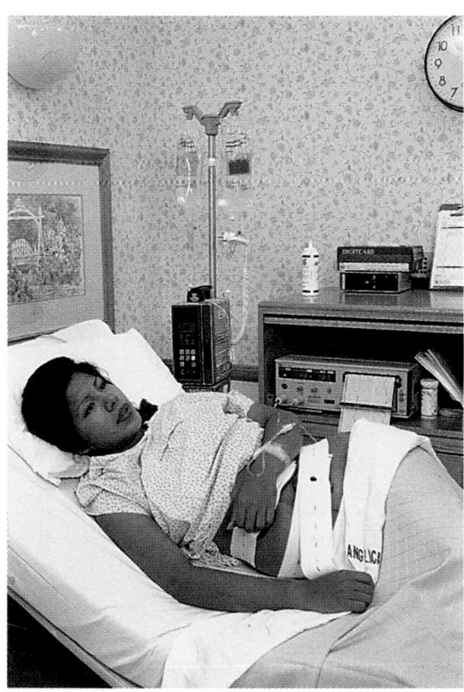

**FIGURE 16–2**

Intravenous oxytocin setup for induction or augmentation of labor. The primary line (nonadditive, or maintenance line) on the left side of the pole contains no medication. The secondary line with the orange "medication added" label contains oxytocin. The secondary oxytocin line is regulated by the infusion pump and is inserted into the lowest port in the primary fluid line. An external fetal monitor is used to assess the fetal response to oxytocin-stimulated contractions. The woman lies on her side to promote uterine blood flow.

### SERIAL INDUCTION OF LABOR

Serial induction of labor is a variation of oxytocin initiation of labor. Serial induction may be done when the woman's cervix is not favorable but same-day birth is not essential. Postdate pregnancy (gestation past the expected delivery date) is a common situation in which serial induction may be done.

Oxytocin solution is given over a 2- to 3-day period for about 8 to 10 hours each day. If the woman has not made progress in her labor during the day, the oxytocin is stopped, she is given a light meal, and the infusion is resumed the next morning. At the end of the third day, the woman is reevaluated if she is not yet in labor.

### ACTIVE MANAGEMENT OF LABOR

Active management of labor is a protocol for labor augmentation first used in Ireland. It applies only to nulliparous women in spontaneous labor at term and is aimed at reducing the cesarean birth rate in this group. The goal of active labor management is to achieve birth within 12 hours of admission. Criteria for diagnosing labor and defining abnormal labor progress are strict.

If the membranes remain intact, amniotomy is performed within 1 hour of admission. Oxytocin augmentation is begun if the rate of progress is less than 1 cm per hour after amniotomy. Oxytocin dosages given by the Irish protocol are higher than those typical in the United States. Cesarean delivery may be performed 12 hours after admission if birth is not imminent.

Variations of the Irish protocol may be used in U.S. hospitals. An example of a care map for active management of labor is presented in Figure 16–3.

## Nursing Considerations

In addition to basic intrapartum care, the nurse observes the woman and fetus for complications and takes corrective actions if abnormalities are noted. The same nursing care applies if a woman has a cervical ripening procedure until she is discharged home.

The nurse has a great responsibility when administering oxytocin to a pregnant woman. The nurse must decide, within the facility's protocols and medical orders, when to start, change, or stop the oxytocin infusion. This responsibility requires additional education and refinement of the nurse's critical thinking skills.

**LONG BEACH MEMORIAL MEDICAL CENTER**
**MULTIDISCIPLINARY ACTION PLAN**
**Active Management of Labor**

| | 1ST STAGE | 2ND STAGE | IMMEDIATE RECOVERY | POSTPARTUM |
|---|---|---|---|---|
| **DATE** | | | | |
| **PATIENT LOCATION** | ☐ LDR | ☐ LDR | ☐ LDR | ☐ Postpartum |
| **PATIENT OUTCOMES** | ☐ Meets criteria for inclusion<br>☐ VS WNL<br>☐ Reassuring FHR<br>☐ H + H, platelets WNL<br>☐ Cervical change of 1 cm/hr<br>☐ Adequate pain control | ☐ VS WNL<br>☐ Reassuring FHR<br>☐ Progressive descent/delivery<br>☐ Adequate pain control | ☐ Fundus firm midline, < u + 2<br>☐ VS WNL<br>☐ Lochia WNL<br>☐ Bladder not full<br>☐ Moving legs<br>☐ Minimal discomfort<br>☐ Breastfeeding initiated | ☐ OB checks WNL<br>☐ VS WNL<br>☐ Voids without difficulty, bladder empty after void<br>☐ Able to walk w/out weakness/fainting<br>☐ H + H WNL<br>☐ Minimal discomfort<br>☐ Breastfeeding progressing<br>☐ Able to care for self and infant |
| **VS/CRITICAL ASSESSMENTS** | ☐ VS Q 1 hr or Q 30 min if epidural<br>☐ FHR Q 30 min or continuous monitoring<br>☐ Vaginal exam Q 1 hr x first 3 hours, or up to initiation of oxytocin protocol<br>☐ Vaginal exam within 1 hour following epidural placement<br>☐ I + O | ☐ VS Q 1 hr or Q 30 min if epidural<br>☐ FHR Q 5 min or continuous monitoring<br>☐ Vaginal exam Q 30 min<br>☐ I + O | ☐ VS Q 15 min x 1 hr, then Q 30 min x 1 hr<br>☐ OB check Q 15 min x 1 hr, then Q 30 min x 1 hr<br>☐ NB VS at birth and Q 1 hr<br>☐ Motor function if epidural<br>☐ I + O | ☐ VS Q 1 hr x 3, then Q shift<br>☐ OB check Q 1 hr x 3 then Q shift<br>☐ Bladder empty post void |
| **CONSULTS** | ☐ Anesthesiologist prn<br>☐ Notify anesthesiologist of platelets <100,000 | ☐ Anesthesiologist prn | | ☐ Lactation specialist prn<br>☐ Social worker, prn |
| **DIAGNOSTIC TESTS** | ☐ Antenate<br>☐ VDRL, HBSAG, Rubella results on prenatal record or drawn | | | ☐ H + H first AM after delivery |
| **TREATMENT/ INTERVENTION** | ☐ AROM within 1–2 hrs of admission to protocol<br>☐ Epidural protocol, prn<br>☐ $O_2$ prn<br>☐ Cath prn | ☐ Delivery<br>☐ Epidural protocol, prn<br>☐ $O_2$ prn<br>☐ Cath prn | ☐ Perineal ice pack<br>☐ Pericare<br>☐ Remove epidural catheter<br>☐ Cath prn | ☐ Perineal ice pack<br>☐ Pericare<br>☐ DC IV<br>☐ Sitz bath<br>☐ Cath prn |

10/95 ©LBMMC

✓ Indicates achievement of outcome/performance or intervention. • Indicates an unachieved outcome or intervention not performed. ☐ Indicates an intervention that was not applicable.

**FIGURE 16–3**

Care map for management of labor.

**LONG BEACH MEMORIAL MEDICAL CENTER**
**MULTIDISCIPLINARY ACTION PLAN**

**Active Management of Labor**

| | 1ST STAGE | 2ND STAGE | IMMEDIATE RECOVERY | POSTPARTUM |
|---|---|---|---|---|
| **MEDICATIONS** | ☐ Stadol 1–2 mg IVP Q 1–2 hr prn<br>☐ Terbutaline 0.25 mg S Q prn<br>☐ Oxytocin per protocol if progress < 1 cm/hr | ☐ Oxytocin per protocol if progress < 1 cm/hr | ☐ Oxytocin added to IV, 20 units/liter<br>☐ Analgesic prn | ☐ Rubella vaccine prn<br>☐ RhoGAM prn<br>☐ Analgesic prn<br>☐ PNV<br>☐ Perineal meds prn |
| **ACTIVITY** | ☐ Ambulate/standing<br>☐ Rocking chair<br>☐ Shower<br>☐ BRP<br>☐ Bedrest, if epidural | ☐ Bedrest<br>☐ Lateral positioning<br>☐ Squatting/kneeling | ☐ Bedrest > 1 hr<br>☐ To postpartum via wheelchair or gurney | ☐ Ambulate<br>☐ Shower |
| **NUTRITION** | ☐ Ice chips<br>☐ IV RL @ 125 cc/hr<br>☐ Clear liquids | ☐ Ice chips<br>☐ IV RL @ 125 cc/hr | ☐ Regular diet<br>☐ IV RL @ 125 cc/hr | ☐ Regular diet |
| **ELIMINATION** | ☐ Empty bladder at least Q 4 hr | ☐ Empty bladder at least Q 4 hr | ☐ Empty bladder at least Q 4 hr | |
| **PATIENT/FAMILY EDUCATION** | ☐ Breathing/relaxation techniques<br>☐ Review analgesic/anesthesia options<br>☐ Progress of normal labor | ☐ Pushing technique and positioning | ☐ Breastfeeding instruction | ☐ Breastfeeding instruction<br>☐ Educational assessment per teaching sheet<br>☐ Self care<br>☐ Infant care<br>☐ Sibling interaction |
| **DISCHARGE PLANNING** | | | ☐ Transfer to postpartum | ☐ 6 week OB appointment<br>☐ Parent to parent support group referral |
| **BEHAVIORAL** | | | ☐ Initial bonding | ☐ Bonding<br>☐ Involved in care of infant |
| **DATE** | | | | |
| **RN SIGNATURES** | ______<br>______<br>______ | ______<br>______<br>______ | ______<br>______<br>______ | ______<br>______<br>______ |



✓ Indicates achievement of outcome/performance or intervention. • Indicates an unachieved outcome or intervention not performed. ☐ Indicates an intervention that was not applicable.

**FIGURE 16–3**

### OBSERVING THE FETAL RESPONSE

Oxytocin stimulates uterine contractions, and they may become too strong (hypertonic). Hypertonic contractions can reduce placental blood flow (uteroplacental insufficiency) and therefore reduce exchange of fetal oxygen and waste products. Before induction or augmentation of labor, the nurse determines whether the fetal heart rate and patterns are reassuring. The fetal heart rate is charted in the labor record every 15 minutes during first-stage labor and every 5 minutes during the second stage (Menihan, 1996).

The nurse remains alert for fetal heart patterns that suggest reduced placental exchange secondary to hypertonic contractions. Examples of these patterns are fetal bradycardia (rate less than 110 to 120 BPM at term), tachycardia (rate more than 150 to 160 BPM at term), late decelerations (slowing after the peak of the contraction), and decreased fetal heart rate variability (reduced rate fluctuations). Reduced placental exchange also may have causes other than excess uterine activity, such as maternal hypotension. The nurse must assess the woman and fetus carefully to identify the most likely cause of the problem and the indicated corrective actions.

If nonreassuring patterns occur or if contractions are hypertonic, the nurse takes steps to reduce uterine activity and increase fetal oxygenation:

1. Reduce or stop the oxytocin infusion and increase the rate of the primary nonadditive infusion.
2. Keep the woman on her side to prevent aortocaval compression and increase placental blood flow.
3. Give 100 percent oxygen by snug face mask at 8 to 10 liters per minute to increase the woman's oxygen saturation, making more available for the fetus.

The physician may order a drug to reduce uterine activity such as terbutaline (Brethine) or magnesium sulfate.

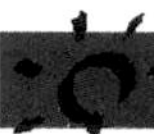

## CRITICAL THINKING EXERCISE

A woman is having labor induced with oxytocin. Her cervix is 4 cm dilated and fully effaced, and the fetal head is at station 0. The nurse notes that the fetal heart rate (internal monitor) is near its baseline of 120 to 130 BPM, with variability of 10 BPM. Contractions are firm (100 mmHg with intrauterine pressure catheter), occur every 2 to 2.5 minutes, and typically last 95 to 100 seconds.

**Q:**
1. What is the correct interpretation of these assessments?
2. What are appropriate nursing actions in this situation, and why are they done?

**A:**
1. The woman is having hypertonic uterine activity because the duration of contractions is longer than 90 seconds and the rest interval is no longer than 55 seconds. Her peak intrauterine pressure during contractions is 10 mmHg higher than expected for first-stage labor. Oxytocin stimulation is the probable cause of the excessive contractions. The normal fetal heart rate suggests that the fetus is now tolerating the excessive contractions.
2. Fetal oxygenation may be compromised if the excessive contractions continue. Reduce or stop the oxytocin infusion to decrease uterine stimulation. Increase the primary (nonadditive) intravenous infusion as needed to maintain adequate circulating volume and ensure maximum uterine blood flow. Keep the woman in a lateral position to reduce aortocaval compression and increase placental blood flow. Oxygen at 8 to 10 L/minute with a snug face mask increases her blood oxygen saturation, making more available to the fetus. (See Chapter 14 for further information about fetal responses to reduced placental perfusion.)

### OBSERVING THE MOTHER'S RESPONSE

The woman who has a laminaria or prostaglandin for cervical ripening may begin labor before her scheduled induction. The signs of labor's onset should be reviewed (see p. 283), and she should be instructed to return to the birth facility if these signs occur.

## Critical to Remember

### SIGNS OF HYPERTONIC UTERINE ACTIVITY

- Contraction duration longer than 90 seconds
- Contractions occurring less than 2 minutes apart or relaxation of less than 60 seconds between contractions
- Uterine resting tone above 20 mmHg (with intrauterine pressure catheter)
- Peak pressure higher than 90 mmHg during first stage labor (with intrauterine pressure catheter)
- A fetal heart rate pattern of late decelerations may accompany hypertonic uterine activity

**Nursing Actions for Hypertonic Uterine Activity**

- Reduce or stop the oxytocin infusion.
- Increase the rate of the primary non-additive infusion.
- Keep the laboring woman in a lateral position.
- Give oxygen by face mask, 8 to 10 mL/minute.
- Notify the physician or nurse-midwife.

Uterine activity must be assessed for hypertonus that may reduce fetal oxygenation and contribute to uterine rupture. Contractions are assessed for frequency, duration, and intensity, and uterine resting tone is assessed for relaxation of at least 60 seconds between contractions. Uterine activity observations are charted at the same intervals as the fetal heart rate. Corrective actions for hypertonic uterine activity are the same as those listed in the discussion of the fetal response. Additionally, a tocolytic drug such as terbutaline may be given.

The woman's blood pressure and pulse are taken every 30 to 60 minutes or with each oxytocin dose increase to identify changes from her baseline. Her temperature is checked every 2 to 4 hours to identify infection that can occur with ruptured membranes.

Recording intake and output identifies fluid retention, which may precede water intoxication. Signs and symptoms of water intoxication include headache, blurred vision, behavioral changes, increased blood pressure and respirations, decreased pulse, rales, wheezing, and coughing. Water intoxication is more likely when larger doses of oxytocin are given, such as a multiday serial induction or higher infusion rates.

After birth, the mother is observed for postpartum hemorrhage caused by uterine relaxation, as is the mother who had spontaneous labor. Postpartum uterine atony is more likely if she has received oxytocin for a long time because the uterine muscle becomes fatigued and does not contract effectively to compress vessels at the placental site. It is manifested by a soft uterine fundus and excess amounts of lochia, usually with large clots. Hypovolemic shock may occur with hemorrhage.

**CHECK YOUR READING**

5. What precautions are taken to enhance the safety of oxytocin administration for the woman and fetus?
6. How may oxytocin administration differ if labor is being augmented rather than induced?
7. What signs may indicate an abnormal fetal response to oxytocin?
8. What are the signs of hypertonic uterine activity?
9. How can induction of labor with oxytocin contribute to postpartum hemorrhage?

# Version

Either of two methods may be used to change fetal presentation: external or internal version. Each has different indications and technique. External version is much more common.

## Indications

**External Version.** The fetus may be changed from a breech, shoulder (transverse lie), or oblique presentation to a cephalic presentation using external version. Successful version may allow the woman to avoid a cesarean birth. One study found that version was successful in 51 percent of the women in whom it was attempted but that more of these women than expected (31 percent) eventually had a cesarean birth (Laros et al., 1995). The reasons for cesarean birth in the version group were primarily induction failure and abnormal labor progress.

**Internal Version.** Malpresentation in twin gestations is usually managed by cesarean birth, but internal version is sometimes used for the vaginal birth of the second twin.

## Contraindications

Version is not done if a woman is unlikely to have vaginal birth because that is the goal of the procedure. Contraindications are similar for both internal and external version. Maternal conditions that may contraindicate external version or reduce its success include the following:

- Uterine malformations that limit the room available to perform the version and may be the reason for the abnormal fetal presentation.
- Previous cesarean birth with a vertical uterine incision. Manipulation of the fetus within the uterus may strain and rupture the old incision.
- Disproportion between fetal size and maternal pelvic size.

Fetal conditions also may contraindicate the use of version:

- Placenta previa. Manipulation of the fetus within the uterus may cause hemorrhage, endangering both mother and fetus. Placenta previa other than marginal is an indication itself for cesarean birth.
- Multifetal gestation, which reduces available room to turn the fetus or fetuses. External version may be done after the first twin is born.
- Oligohydramnios, ruptured membranes, or a cord around the fetal body or neck (nuchal cord). These conditions limit the room to turn the fetus and may lead to cord compression and fetal hypoxia.
- Uteroplacental insufficiency. Uterine contractions occurring during the version or during labor may worsen the insufficiency and cause fetal compromise.
- Engagement of the fetal head into the pelvis.

## Risks

There are few risks to the woman. The principal risk is that the fetus may become entangled in the umbilical cord, compressing its vessels and resulting in hypoxia. Abruptio placentae also may occur if fetal manipulation disrupts the placental site. Fetal and maternal blood could become mixed because of small breaks in placental vessels, possibly resulting in maternal sensitization to the fetal blood type. Cesarean birth may be needed for fetal compromise at the time of version or later if the fetus returns to an abnormal presentation.

## Technique

**External Version.** A nonstress test (see p. 235) is done before external version to evaluate fetal health and placental function. If the test is nonreactive or other nonreassuring signs are present, the version is not done. Version would add stress to the fetus already functioning with reduced physiologic reserve. An ultrasound examination confirms fetal gestational age and fetal presentation and identifies adequacy of amniotic fluid.

External version is usually attempted after 37 weeks of gestation but before the woman is in labor for the following reasons:

- As term nears, the fetus may spontaneously turn to a cephalic presentation.
- The fetus is more likely to return to an abnormal presentation if version is attempted before 37 weeks.
- If fetal compromise or onset of labor occurs, a fetus born after 37 weeks is unlikely to have major problems associated with preterm birth, such as respiratory distress syndrome.

The woman is usually given a tocolytic drug such as terbutaline to relax the uterus while the version is performed.

Ultrasonography guides fetal manipulations during external version and helps monitor the fetal heart rate. The physician gently pushes the breech out of the pelvis in a forward or backward roll (Fig. 16–4).

If indicated, Rh immune globulin is given to the Rh-negative woman after external version to prevent Rh sensitization.

**Internal Version.** Internal version is an unexpected and urgent procedure. The physician reaches into the uterus with one hand and, with the other hand on the maternal abdomen, maneuvers the fetus into a longitudinal lie (cephalic or breech) (Fig. 16–5) to allow delivery.

## Nursing Considerations

When caring for the woman having external version, the nurse provides information, assesses the woman and fetus, and helps to reduce her anxiety.

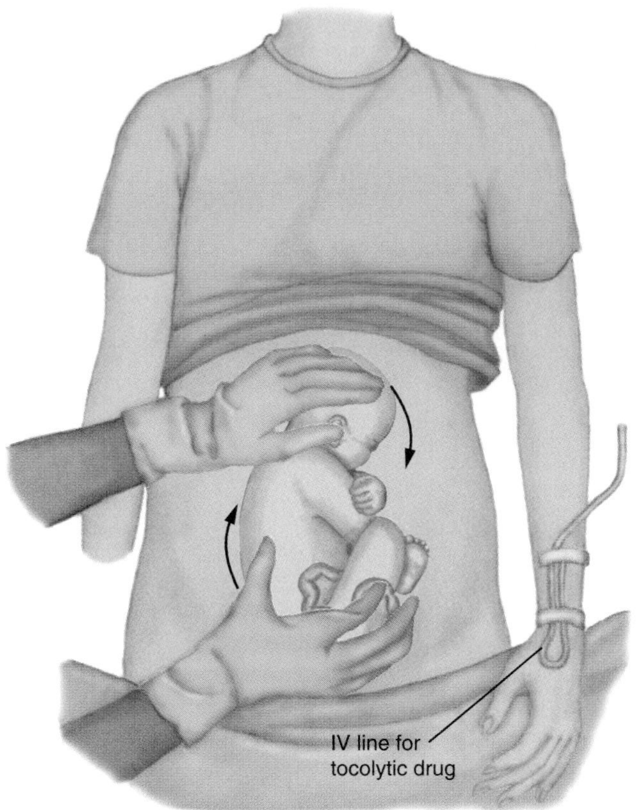


**FIGURE 16–4**

External version.

#### PROVIDING INFORMATION

The birth attendant explains the indications and risks for external version to the woman before she signs an informed consent. The nurse verifies the woman's understanding of the purposes, risks, and limitations of version.

The purposes and side effects of any planned tocolytic drug are reviewed. Tachycardia and tremors are common side effects of tocolytics such as terbutaline and stop shortly after the medication is discontinued at the end of the procedure.

#### PROMOTING MATERNAL AND FETAL HEALTH

Admission information is collected as if the woman were in labor or having a cesarean birth because the need for operative intervention may arise suddenly. The woman should have nothing by mouth during this short procedure.

Maternal vital signs are assessed, and fetal monitoring is begun to obtain baseline values and to evaluate the initial nonstress test. Abnormalities and nonreassuring fetal heart rate patterns should be reported promptly.

The nurse administers the tocolytic drug. The blood pressure and pulse are checked every 5 minutes with Doppler or real-time ultrasonography used to guide the version. Fetal bradycardia may occur

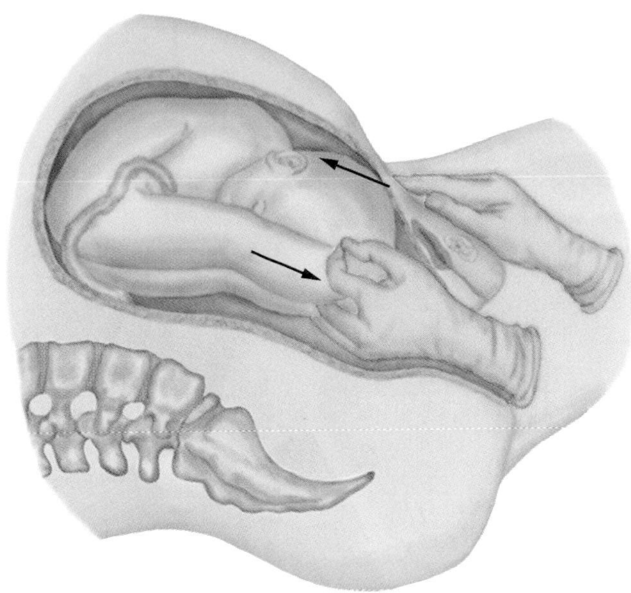

**FIGURE 16–5**

Internal version for vaginal birth of a second twin.

during the procedure, but the fetal heart rate usually returns to normal when manipulation ends.

After the version, the tocolytic drug is discontinued. The mother and fetus are observed for at least 1 hour after the version for a return of their vital signs to baseline values. Reassuring fetal signs are a heart rate about the same range as on admission, resolution of bradycardia, and the presence of rate accelerations with fetal movement.

Maternal vital signs are taken every 15 minutes until they return to their baseline level. The presence of regular contractions suggests onset of labor. Spontaneous rupture of membranes sometimes occurs, with leakage of fluid from the mother's vagina. Rh immune globulin is given if indicated.

The woman usually has some discomfort during the version, but it should diminish quickly afterward. Persistent or continuous pain suggests a complication such as abruptio placentae.

Because the woman having external version is near term, the nurse should review the signs of true labor with her and explain guidelines for returning to the hospital (see Chapter 13).

#### REDUCING ANXIETY

The woman may be anxious before version because its success is not certain, and complications may require rapid cesarean delivery. After version, she may still be anxious because the fetus can return to its previous position. The nurse should keep her informed about what is occurring during the version to reduce her fear of the unknown.

The expectant mother is probably concerned about the fetal condition. Pointing out reassuring fetal monitor patterns, such as a normal rate and rate accelerations, can help reduce her anxiety about her baby. If problems develop, such as bradycardia, the nurse should explain what has happened, what steps are being done to relieve it, and the result of these interventions.

**✓ CHECK YOUR READING**

10. Why is it important to observe the fetal heart rate during and after external version?
11. Why should the uterine activity be monitored after external version?

## Forceps and Vacuum Extraction

The physician may use forceps or vacuum extraction to apply traction to the fetal head during birth, aiding the woman's expulsive efforts. Both techniques assist descent only or descent and rotation of the fetal head from an occiput posterior or occiput transverse position to the occiput anterior position.

Forceps are curved metal instruments having two curved blades that can be locked in the center. Many styles are available for different needs. The blades may be closed or open and are shaped to grasp the fetal head (Fig. 16–6). Disposable foam pads are available to cushion the fetal head from the blades. Piper forceps are a special type used to assist birth of the head as it is born last in a vaginal breech birth. Forceps or a vacuum extractor also may be used during cesarean birth.

A vacuum extractor uses suction to grasp the fetal head while traction is applied (Fig. 16–7). It is not used to deliver the fetus in a nonvertex presentation, such as breech or face; otherwise, its use is similar to that of forceps.

### Indications

Forceps or vacuum extraction is considered if the second stage should be shortened for the well-being of the woman, fetus, or both and if vaginal birth can be accomplished quickly without undue trauma. Maternal indications may include exhaustion, inability to push effectively, cardiac or pulmonary disease, and intrapartum infection. Fetal indications may include a prolapsed cord, premature separation of the placenta, and nonreassuring fetal heart rate patterns.

### Contraindications

Cesarean birth is preferable if the maternal or fetal condition mandates a more rapid birth than can be accomplished with forceps or vacuum extractor or if the procedure would be too traumatic. Examples of

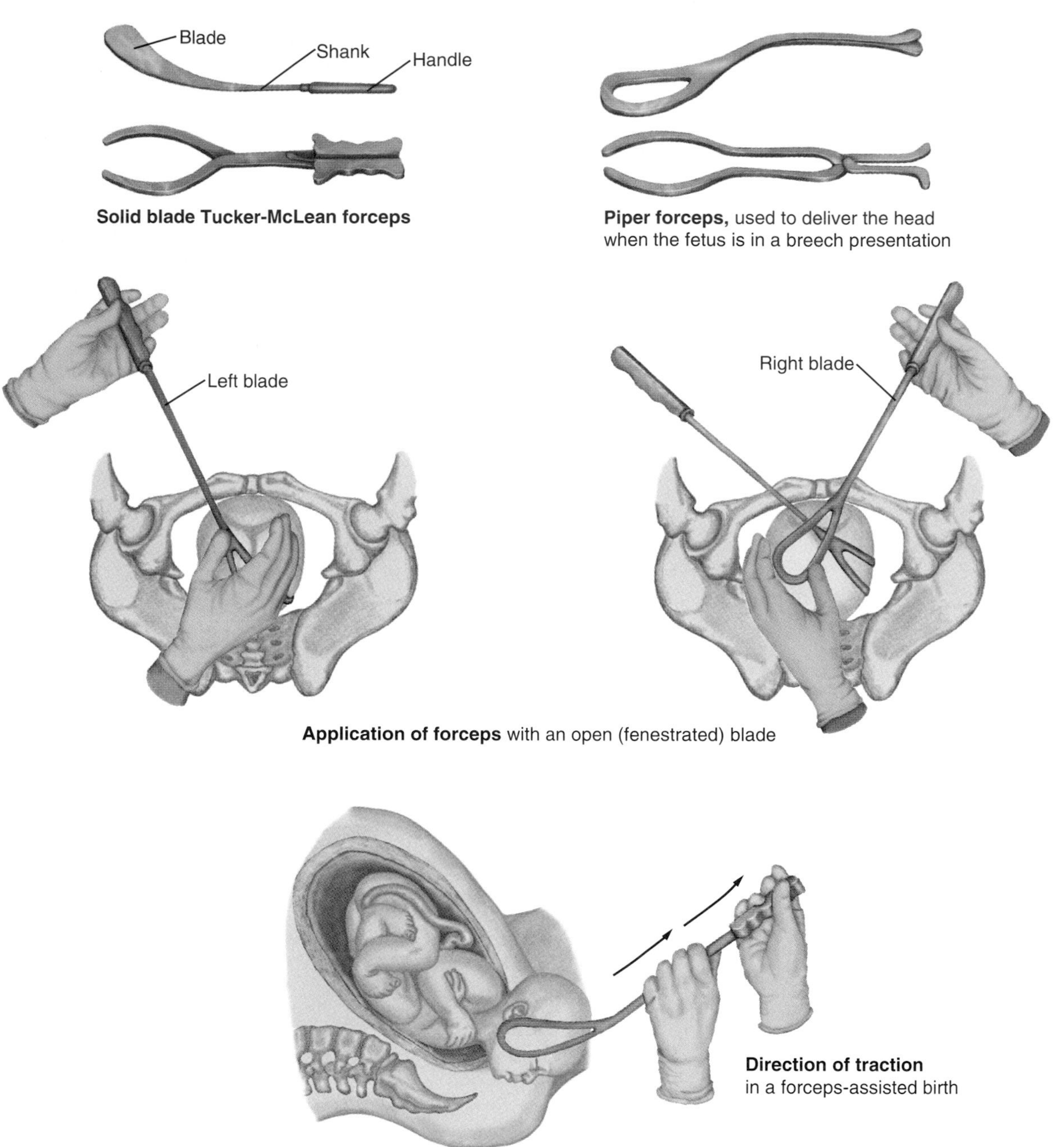


**FIGURE 16–6**

Obstetric forceps and their application.

these conditions are severe fetal compromise, acute maternal conditions such as congestive heart failure and pulmonary edema, a high fetal station, and disproportion between the size of the fetus and the maternal pelvis.

## Risks

The main risk of forceps or vacuum extraction is trauma to maternal or fetal tissues. Because of the relative safety of cesarean birth, the attempt at an instrumental birth is usually abandoned if the fetal head does not descend easily.

Maternal risks include laceration or hematoma of the vagina. The infant may have ecchymoses, facial and scalp lacerations or abrasions, facial nerve injury, cephalhematoma, subgaleal hemorrhage, and intracranial hemorrhage. A vacuum extractor may create scalp edema called a *chignon* at the application area (see Fig. 16–7).

## Technique

Preparation for forceps or vacuum extraction is the same as for any vaginal birth. In addition, the woman is often catheterized to provide more room in the

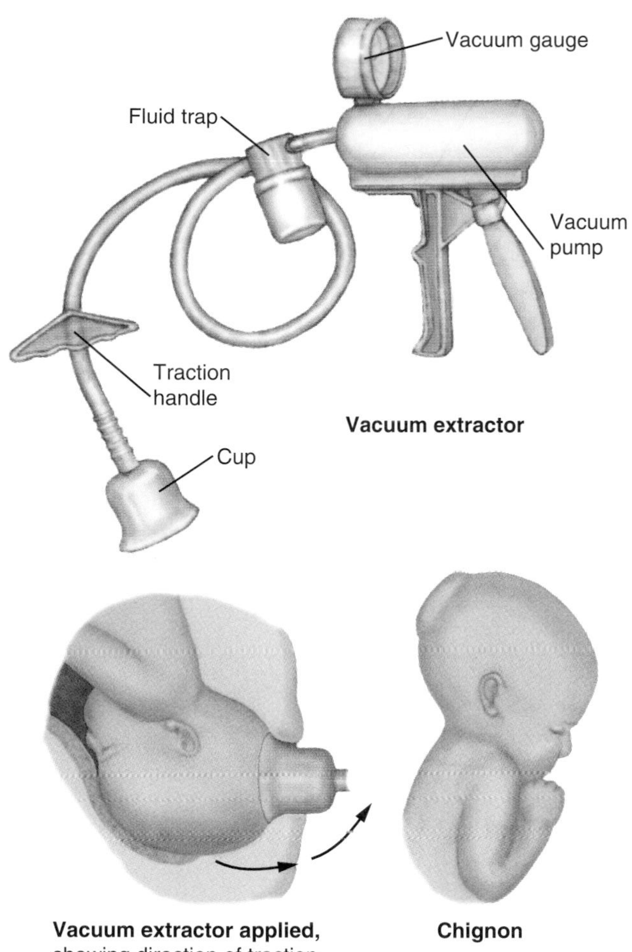


**FIGURE 16-7**

Birth assisted with a vacuum extractor. The chignon is scalp edema that often forms under the suction cup when the vacuum extractor is used.

pelvis and limit bladder trauma. Membranes must be ruptured and the cervix completely dilated for forceps or vacuum extraction birth. The woman needs adequate anesthesia, usually a regional block such as pudendal or epidural. An episiotomy is often done.

Forceps- and vacuum extractor–assisted births are classified according to how far the fetal head has descended into the pelvis when they are applied (American College of Obstetricians and Gynecologists, 1994).

**Outlet** The fetal head is on the perineum, with the scalp visible at the vaginal opening without separating the labia. The position is OA, ROA, LOA, or OP.

**Low** The leading edge of the fetal skull is at station +2 (about 2 cm below the level of the mother's ischial spines) or lower.

**Midforceps** The leading edge of the fetal skull is between a 0 (at the level of the ischial spines) and a +2 station.

The physician determines the presentation, position, and station of the fetal head and the amount of cervical dilation. When correctly applied, the long axis of the blades lies over the fetal cheeks and parietal bones. After checking for proper application, the physician locks the two blades in the center and pulls gently, following the curve of the pelvis. An episiotomy is often done as the fetal head distends the perineum. The physician may keep the forceps on until the head is born or may remove the blades just before expulsion. The rest of the fetus is born in the usual way.

For vacuum extraction, the cup is connected to a machine that creates a vacuum to hold the cup on the fetal head in the midline of the occiput. The physician applies traction intermittently, as in forceps birth.

## Nursing Considerations

When a forceps or vacuum extraction birth is anticipated, a catheter is added to the instrument table for the birth. The physician specifies the type of forceps or vacuum cup. The fetal heart rate should be assessed, and any rate lower than 100 BPM should be reported.

After birth, the mother and infant are observed for trauma. The mother may have vaginal wall lacerations or hematoma. Vaginal wall lacerations bleed brighter red than normal lochia and more or less continuously. The fundus is usually firm unless uterine atony is also present. Women with vaginal wall hematomas complain of severe and unrelenting pain and may have edema and discoloration of the labia and perineum. Cold applications for the first 12 hours reduce pain by numbing the area and limit bruising and edema of the tissues. Heat applications after 12 hours aid resolution of the edema and bruising.

The infant often has reddening and mild bruising of the skin where the forceps were applied. These areas do not need treatment. Cold treatment is not done for an infant because of possible hypothermia. Observe for skin breaks that allow entry of microorganisms; keep skin breaks clean. Facial asymmetry, most obvious when the infant cries, suggests facial nerve injury.

**After a forceps birth, a parent may ask why the baby's cheeks are reddened or bruised. A good response is to explain that the pressure of the forceps on the baby's delicate skin may cause minor bruising that usually resolves without treatment. Point out improvement in the area during the postpartum stay.**

## Episiotomy

Ideally, the physician or nurse-midwife has discussed the possibility of episiotomy with the woman during her antepartum care. Routine performance of an episiotomy remains controversial, despite several research studies. The decision about whether an episiotomy is needed must be made just before birth, however, and indications are not always clear.

### Indications

Fetal indications for episiotomy are similar to those for forceps or vacuum extraction. Episiotomy may be done to reduce pressure on the head when a small preterm infant is born.

Maternal indications are also similar to those for forceps or vacuum extraction. Other maternal indications may include the following:

- Control of the direction and extent that the vaginal opening is enlarged. This is an advantage if a laceration is likely to disrupt the anal sphincter.
- A straight, clean-edged incision that can be simpler to repair than a large perineal laceration. However, a small perineal laceration would be easier to repair and would heal better.

### Risks

Infection is the primary risk of episiotomy. Perineal pain occurs with both episiotomy and spontaneous tears. However, perineal pain may last longer with episiotomy, mainly because of its tendency to extend into deeper lacerations. Prolonged perineal pain impairs resumption of sexual intercourse.

### Technique

An episiotomy is done when the fetal presenting part has crowned to a diameter of about 3 to 4 cm. The two types of episiotomies have different advantages and disadvantages: *median* or midline and *mediolateral* (Fig. 16–8).

### Nursing Considerations

An episiotomy can sometimes be avoided (or its length limited) with nursing measures. Assuming an

**Median or Midline**

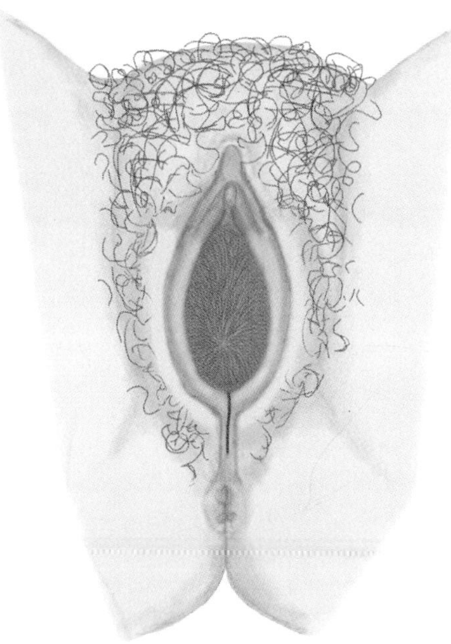

***Advantages***
Minimal blood loss
Neat healing with little scarring
Less postpartum pain than the mediolateral episiotomy

***Disadvantages***
An added laceration may extend the median episiotomy into the anal sphincter
Limited enlargement of the vaginal opening because perineal length is limited by the anal sphincter

**Mediolateral**

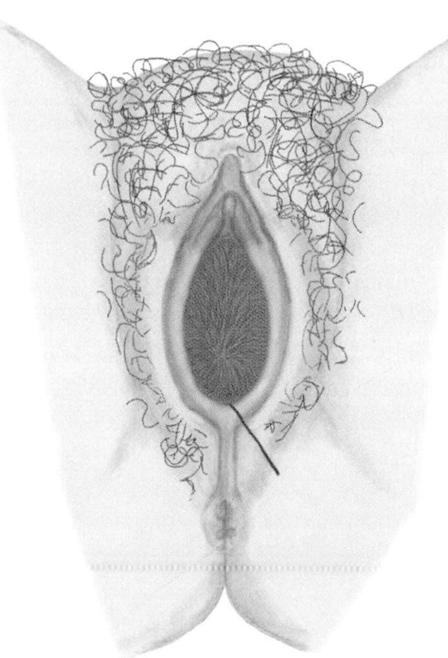

***Advantages***
More enlargement of the vaginal opening
Little risk that the episiotomy will extend into the anus

***Disadvantages***
More blood loss
Increased postpartum pain
More scarring and irregularity in the healed scar
Prolonged dyspareunia (painful intercourse)

**FIGURE 16–8**

Types of episiotomies.

upright position while pushing gently promotes gradual stretching of the woman's perineum. Warm perineal compresses and perineal massage may relax perineal muscles so that the birth canal more readily accommodates the fetal head as it emerges. Further research needs to be done to clarify whether warm compresses, perineal massage, or other techniques are truly effective in reducing the need for episiotomy.

Nursing interventions during the recovery and postpartum periods are similar for episiotomy and perineal laceration. Observe the perineum for hematoma and edema. As with forceps use, perineal cold applications are done for the first 12 hours, followed by perineal heat after 12 hours.

**CHECK YOUR READING**

12. What are the similarities in the uses of forceps and vacuum extractors? What are the differences?
13. Why should the nurse add a urinary catheter to the instrument table if a forceps-assisted birth is expected?
14. A woman has a forceps birth with a median episiotomy. What nursing interventions can make her more comfortable?
15. What injury is suggested by an asymmetric facial appearance when the infant cries?

## Cesarean Birth

In 1965, the cesarean birth rate in the United States was 4.5 percent of all births, rising to 24 percent in the late 1980s. The 1994 rate was 22 percent of all births. Of 1994 births, 15.8 percent were primary (first) cesareans and 6.2 percent were repeat cesareans (Clark & Miller, 1996).

Several factors led to the high U.S. cesarean birth rate. Paul and Miller (1995) describe several:

- Greater safety of the surgery for the woman makes the surgery a reasonable option in more circumstances.
- Improved survival of very small preterm infants makes use of cesarean birth reasonable.
- High consumer expectations of a good fetal outcome cause physicians to intervene with a surgical birth quickly.
- Greater threat of litigation if outcomes are not good causes physicians to opt for surgery quickly if the maternal or fetal condition, or both, seems to be at risk.

A national goal for the Healthy People 2000 initiative is to reduce the rate of cesarean births to no more than 15 percent, with the rate of primary cesarean births being no more than 12 percent of total births. Efforts to accomplish the goal include (1) promoting vaginal birth after cesarean (VBAC) (Table 16–3), (2) careful evaluation of dystocia, and (3) selection of some women to deliver their infants in the breech presentation. Because previous cesarean birth and dystocia contribute substantially to the current rate, promotion of VBAC and critical evaluation of dystocia can reduce the total rate.

Experience with electronic fetal monitoring has improved knowledge of normal fetal responses to labor, promoting interventions for fetal benefit that may avoid cesarean delivery. Nurses and birth attendants increasingly recognize that simple interventions, such as walking or squatting during the second stage, may promote normal labor progress.

### Indications

Cesarean birth is performed when awaiting vaginal birth would compromise the mother, fetus, or both. Possible indications for cesarean birth include, but are not limited to, the following:

- Dystocia
- Cephalopelvic (fetopelvic) disproportion

**TABLE 16–3 VAGINAL BIRTH AFTER CESAREAN BIRTH (VBAC)**

- Sixty to 80 percent of women with one low transverse uterine incision from a previous cesarean birth have successful vaginal births.
- Women whose previous cesarean birth was done for breech presentation or a nonreassuring FHR appear to have more success with VBAC than if the primary cesarean birth was for cephalopelvic disproportion or failure to progress in labor.
- The benefits of a trial of labor outweigh its risks.
- About 40 to 50 percent of women who are candidates for a trial of labor refuse it and undergo a repeat cesarean birth.
- Candidates for VBAC include the following:
  - A woman who has one previous low transverse uterine incision should be encouraged to attempt labor in her current pregnancy.
  - A woman who has two or more low transverse uterine incisions should not be discouraged from laboring in her current pregnancy.
- Estimated fetal weight greater than 4000 g by itself is not a contraindication if the woman is not diabetic.
- VBAC is contraindicated if a woman has a previous classic uterine incision.
- Insufficient data are available about risks and benefits of a trial of labor in a (1) multifetal gestation, and (2) breech presentation.
- Normal activity should be encouraged during latent labor.
- Epidural analgesia and anesthesia may be used.
- Oxytocin induction and augmentation of labor may be done. Risks and benefits of prostaglandin gel have not been thoroughly researched, although there are reports of success using this drug.

Data from American College of Obstetricians and Gynecologists & American Academy of Pediatrics. (1995). ACOG *practice patterns: Vaginal delivery after previous cesarean birth, number* 1. Washington, D.C.: Author.

- Pregnancy-induced hypertension, if prompt delivery is necessary
- Maternal diseases such as diabetes, heart disease, or cervical cancer, if labor is not advisable
- Active genital herpes
- Some previous uterine surgical procedures, such as a classic cesarean incision
- Persistent nonreassuring fetal heart rate patterns
- Prolapsed umbilical cord
- Fetal malpresentations, such as breech or transverse lie
- Hemorrhagic conditions, such as abruptio placentae or placenta previa

A prior cesarean birth is not by itself an indication for another cesarean birth. Repeating the cesarean birth should be based on specific indications, as was the primary surgery (American Academy of Pediatrics & American College of Obstetricians and Gynecologists, 1992).

## Contraindications

There are few absolute contraindications to cesarean birth, but there are conditions in which it is not desirable because the risks to the woman are too great compared with the potential benefit to mother or fetus. These conditions include fetal death, a fetus that is too immature to survive, and maternal coagulation defects.

## Risks

Cesarean birth is one of the safest major surgical procedures; however, it poses greater risk for the mother than does vaginal birth. Maternal risks include the following:

- Infection
- Hemorrhage
- Urinary tract trauma
- Thrombophlebitis
- Paralytic ileus
- Atelectasis
- Anesthesia complications, such as aspiration of gastric contents

Cesarean delivery poses added risks to the infant, which may include the following:

- Inadvertent preterm birth
- Transient tachypnea of the newborn caused by delayed absorption of lung fluid (see p. 848)
- Persistent pulmonary hypertension of the newborn (see p. 852)
- Injury, such as laceration, bruising, or other trauma

Diagnostic studies are often done to ensure that the fetal lungs are mature when a cesarean birth is planned (see Chapter 10). These include the amniotic fluid lecithin/sphingomyelin (L/S) ratio, and assessment for presence of phosphatidylglycerol (PG) and phosphatidylinositol (PI).

## Technique

### PREPARATION

Regional anesthesia, such as epidural block, is commonly used for cesarean birth. However, general anesthesia, with its risk for vomiting and aspiration of gastric contents, may be needed unexpectedly. Placement of the regional block may not be possible, or an inadequate block may require supplemental general anesthesia. Therefore, the woman receives nothing by mouth. A drug such as famotidine (Pepcid) or sodium citrate with citric acid (Bicitra) is given to reduce gastric acidity before surgery. The woman does not have routine premedication other than drugs to control gastric and respiratory secretions.

The fetus is monitored for 20 to 30 minutes after admission if the woman is having a scheduled cesarean birth. Monitoring may be discontinued if the initial monitor strip shows reassuring patterns. If she is in labor when a cesarean birth becomes necessary, fetal monitoring continues as long as possible before the surgery. It is important to remove a fetal scalp electrode so that it is not pulled from the vagina through the uterus as the infant is delivered. A wedge under one hip prevents aortocaval compression and promotes placental blood flow.

Routine laboratory studies vary with the mother's condition and type of anesthesia but often include complete blood count, clotting studies such as prothrombin and partial thromboplastin times, and blood typing and screening. The physician may order 1 or more units of blood typed and crossmatched to have available for transfusion if the woman's hemoglobin and hematocrit values are low or if she is at greater risk for hemorrhage, such as grand multiparity (five or more births).

A single intravenous dose of a prophylactic antibiotic such as ampicillin or a cephalosporin is often ordered. Additional antibiotic doses are given to a woman who has an increased risk for infection, such as one who has had prolonged rupture of membranes.

If a Pfannenstiel (transverse, or "bikini") skin incision is planned, the woman's abdomen is shaved from about 3 inches above the pubic hairline to the mons pubis, about where her legs come together. For a vertical skin incision, the upper border of the shave is just above the umbilicus.

An indwelling catheter inserted before the surgery keeps the bladder away from the operative area, reducing the risk for injury. The catheter allows accurate observation of urine output during and after surgery, which helps evaluate circulatory status. Insertion may be delayed until an epidural block has taken effect.

Preoperative preparations are completed before a general anesthetic is begun to reduce neonatal exposure to anesthesia. The team scrubs, dons gowns and gloves, and drapes the woman before general anesthesia is induced.

An abdominal scrub is done just before sterile draping. As in other surgical skin preparations, the direction is circular, from the center of the operative area outward.

### INCISIONS

Two incisions are made: one in the abdominal wall (skin incision) and the other in the uterine wall. Either of two skin incisions is used: a midline vertical incision between the umbilicus and the symphysis or a Pfannenstiel incision just above the symphysis. Figure 16–9 presents advantages and disadvantages of each type.

Three types of uterine incisions are possible (Fig. 16–10), each with different indications and limitations: (1) low transverse, (2) low vertical, and (3) classic, a vertical incision into the upper uterus. The low transverse uterine incision is preferred. The uterine incision does not always match the skin incision. For example, a woman may have a vertical skin incision and a low transverse uterine incision.

The low transverse uterine incision may not be suitable if the fetus is very large. The length of this incision is limited because the uterine artery and vein enter the uterus at its lower right and left sides. The low transverse incision may not be large enough to deliver a large fetus through without tearing these large vessels. Sometimes a vertical uterine incision must be added to a transverse one (making an inverted T) to deliver a very large baby.

A classic uterine incision must occasionally be used when the other two incisions are not possible, such as a placenta previa located in the lower anterior uterus. The vertical uterine incision, especially the classic one, is more likely to rupture during later pregnancies.

### SEQUENCE OF EVENTS IN CESAREAN BIRTH

The sequence of events in cesarean birth is similar to that in a vaginal birth. When the woman is anesthetized and draped, the physician makes the skin incision. If the woman has general anesthesia, she may move on the operating table during the early part of surgery because the anesthesia level is kept very light to limit transfer of anesthetic to the fetus. The anesthesia level is deepened after the umbilical cord is clamped.

After the bladder is separated from the uterine wall, it is held downward with a wide bladder retractor. The uterus is incised, usually in a low transverse incision. If the membranes are intact, they are ruptured with a sharp instrument, and amniotic fluid is suctioned from the operative field. As in vaginal

Vertical

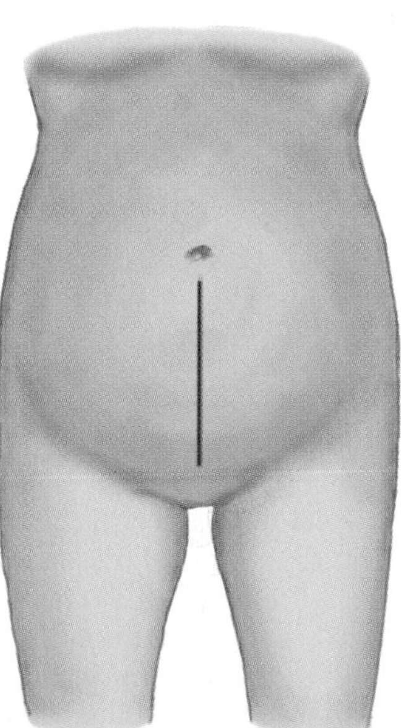

*Advantages*
Quicker to perform
Better visualization of the uterus
Can quickly extend upward for greater visualization if needed
Often more appropriate for obese women

*Disadvantages*
Easily visible when healed
Greater chance of dehiscence and hernia formation

Pfannenstiel

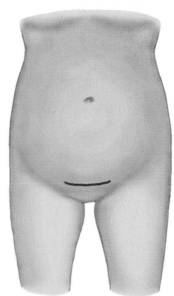

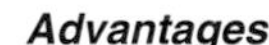

*Advantages*
Less visibility when healed and the pubic hair grows back
Less chance of dehiscence or formation of a hernia

*Disadvantages*
Less visualization of the uterus
Cannot be done as quickly, which may be important in an emergency cesarean birth
Cannot easily be extended to give greater operative exposure
Re-entry at a subsequent cesarean birth may require more time

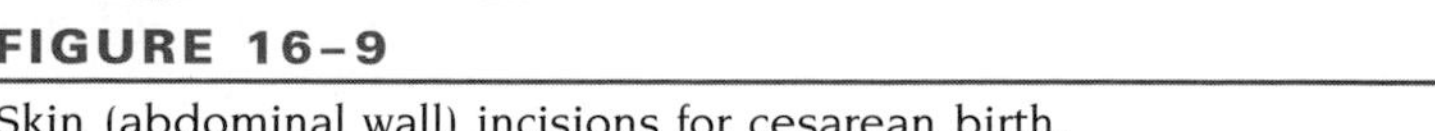

**FIGURE 16–9**

Skin (abdominal wall) incisions for cesarean birth.

| Low Transverse | Low Vertical | Classic |
|---|---|---|
| 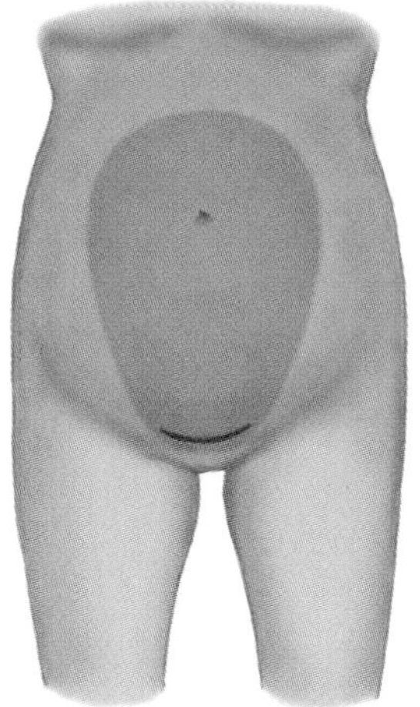 | 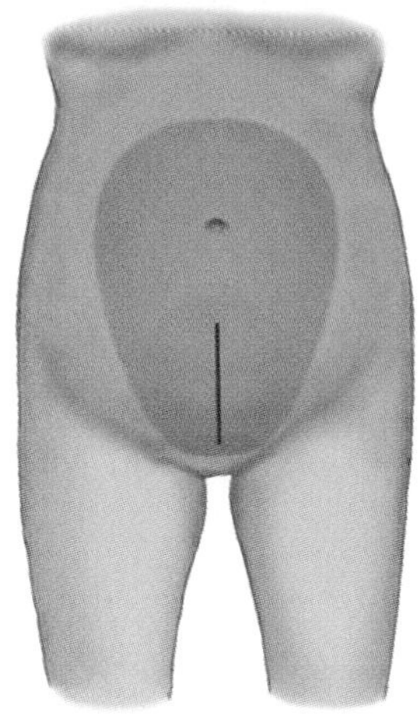 | 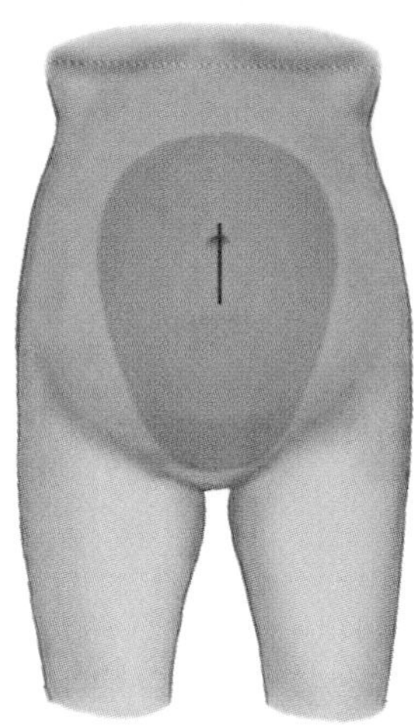 |
| ***Advantages***<br>Unlikely to rupture during a subsequent birth<br>Makes VBAC possible for subsequent pregnancy<br>Less blood loss<br>Easier to repair<br>Less adhesion formation | ***Advantage***<br>Can be extended upward to make a larger incision if needed | ***Advantage***<br>May be the only choice in these situations:<br>Implantation of a placenta previa on the lower anterior uterine wall<br>Presence of dense adhesions from previous surgery<br>Transverse lie of a large fetus with the shoulder impacted in the mother's pelvis |
| ***Disadvantage***<br>Limited ability to extend laterally to enlarge the incision | ***Disadvantages***<br>Slightly more likely to rupture during a subsequent birth<br>A tear may extend the incision downward into the cervix | ***Disadvantages***<br>Most likely of the uterine incisions to rupture during a subsequent birth<br>Eliminates VBAC as an option for birth of a subsequent infant |

**FIGURE 16–10**

Uterine incisions for cesarean birth. The abdominal and uterine incisions do not always match. VBAC, vaginal birth after cesarean.

births, the color, odor, and quantity of the amniotic fluid are noted and the time of rupture is recorded.

The physician lifts the fetal presenting part through the uterine incision. An assistant may push on the uterine fundus to help deliver the fetus through the abdominal incision. Forceps or a vacuum extractor may be needed to facilitate birth of the fetal head.

The infant's face is wiped, and the mouth and nose are suctioned to remove secretions that would impair breathing. The cord is quickly clamped and cut. The physician collects cord blood for analysis.

Following the infant's birth, the physician removes the placenta. Oxytocin is given intravenously to contract the uterus firmly. The physician then closes the uterine and abdominal incisions, approximating each layer separately. Some physicians flush the operative area with saline or an antibiotic solution before abdominal closure.

Nursing care for the infant is similar to that following vaginal birth. Resuscitation equipment should be readied for use. Professional personnel who care for the infant born by cesarean vary with the baby's anticipated condition and facility policy. A pediatrician, neonatal nurse-practitioner, or neonatal nurse usually attends the infant at the time of cesarean birth.

## Nursing Considerations

Nursing care for a woman who has a cesarean birth varies according to the situation. She may be planning a cesarean birth, or a surgical birth may be unexpected. Even within these two situations, women differ. For example, is the planned cesarean her first, or has she had a cesarean birth before? Was her previous cesarean planned? An unplanned cesarean birth may occur after hours of unsuccessful labor or may be needed quickly in an emergency.

**TABLE 16–4 SUMMARY OF NURSING CARE FOR A WOMAN HAVING CESAREAN BIRTH**

**Before the Cesarean Birth**

1. Assess time of last oral intake and what was eaten.
2. Assess for allergies.
3. Have woman sign an informed consent form.
4. Obtain ordered laboratory work.
5. Do preoperative teaching: what to expect in the operating and recovery rooms.
6. Start ordered intravenous infusion.
7. Do abdominal shave.
8. Insert an indwelling catheter.
9. Administer ordered medication to control gastric secretions.
10. Assist woman to operating table, positioning her with a wedge under her hip (or tilt table).
11. Apply grounding pad for electrocautery.
12. Do cleansing prep of abdomen.

**During the Recovery Period**

1. Begin anesthesia-related interventions: pulse oximeter, oxygen administration, cardiac monitor.
   a. Assess for return of sensation and movement if regional anesthesia was used.
   b. Assess level of consciousness if general anesthesia was used.
2. Do routine assessments every 15 min the first hour, every 30 min the second hour, and hourly until she is transferred to the postpartum unit.
   a. Vital signs
   b. Uterine fundus for firmness, height, and deviation. Massage if poorly contracted.
   c. Lochia for color, quantity, and presence of large clots
   d. Urine output for color, quantity, and patency of the catheter and tubing
   e. Abdominal dressing for drainage
3. Assess need for analgesia and administer as ordered.
4. Change position hourly if no contraindication exists. Have her breathe deeply and cough at each routine assessment time. Provide a small pillow to support her incision when coughing or turning.

Nursing care for women having cesarean childbirth is similar, but the approach in each situation is different. For example, although preoperative teaching is important, it must be abbreviated or even omitted in a true emergency. Table 16–4 presents a summary of nursing care for a woman having cesarean birth.

### PROVIDING EMOTIONAL SUPPORT

Emotional support may begin well before the birth and extend well after it. A mother who has had a previous cesarean birth may harbor unresolved feelings of grief, guilt, or inadequacy because she perceives that she somehow failed in her expected birth experience. Therapeutic communication techniques help identify stressors and misunderstandings to promote a positive childbirth experience.

**The nurse in the prenatal setting can open the subject of a woman's previous cesarean birth with a broad lead such as, "Tell me about when you had your other baby."**

Anxiety is an expected and normal reaction to surgery and, within limits, is useful. For example, mild to moderate anxiety may prompt the woman who expects a cesarean birth to learn more about her upcoming experience. If anxiety is high, however, she has difficulty concentrating. The woman who has an unplanned cesarean birth is more likely to have high levels of anxiety, but the woman who expects the surgery is also vulnerable.

The staff's behavior can either reduce or increase the woman's anxiety. A calm and confident manner helps her feel that she is being cared for by competent professionals. A quiet, low voice is calming. There is little reason to shout, even in an emergency.

The nurse and the woman's significant others are important sources of emotional support. The nurse should remain with her and let her express her fears. Therapeutic communication helps clarify her concerns, so explanations to reduce her fear of the unknown can be most effective.

The father or other support person should be encouraged to remain with her during surgery if she has regional anesthesia. In some hospitals, the support person may come into the operating room after the woman is intubated for general anesthesia to foster attachment with the infant and help the mother integrate her birth experience.

Nurses also support a woman's partner and significant others during the cesarean birth. The partner may be as anxious as the woman but may be afraid to express it because she needs so much support. The partner may be physically exhausted after hours of labor coaching. The staff should not expect more support from the partner than he or she can provide.

**Although cesarean births are routine in the intrapartum unit, they are not routine to women who undergo them or to their families. Avoid belittling their fears by telling women and their families not to worry or that everything will be all right.**

After birth, visiting the mother and her family allows the nurse to answer questions about the surgery and fill in any gaps in their understanding. This helps them understand the experience and promotes a positive perception of the birth.

## Nursing Care Plan 16–1
# Cesarean Birth

**ASSESSMENT:** Christina Cole is 22 years old and is expecting her first baby. Her due date is 1 week from today. The baby is in a complete (full) breech presentation. A previous attempt at version was unsuccessful, and the fetus did not turn spontaneously. She is in early labor and expecting a cesarean birth. Although her physician discussed cesarean birth with her, Christina is anxious and has many questions about what will happen to her and her baby. She says she is very nervous about the upcoming surgery. She has never been a patient in a hospital before. Christina's mother and husband Bruce are with her.

**NURSING DIAGNOSIS:** Anxiety related to unfamiliarity with the setting and procedures for cesarean birth

### GOALS/EXPECTED OUTCOMES

After interventions, Christina will do the following:

1. State that she feels less apprehensive.
2. Verbalize understanding of preoperative and postoperative care.
3. Demonstrate postoperative techniques for coughing and deep breathing.

| INTERVENTION | RATIONALE |
|---|---|
| 1. Assess Christina's level of anxiety. Mild to moderate levels of anxiety are expected. | 1. Assessment enables the nurse to approach preoperative care of the woman in the most appropriate manner. Mild to moderate anxiety may facilitate learning, but higher levels impair learning. |
| 2. Remain with Christina as much as possible. Allow her to express her fears. Encourage her mother and Bruce to remain with her. | 2. Provides support from significant others and a caring nurse. Enables the nurse to answer the woman's concerns specifically. |
| 3. Elicit Christina's feelings about surgery by using broad leads, such as: "What were your thoughts when you found out you might have your baby by cesarean?" | 3. Identifies expectations of the birth experience so that actions can be taken to make it a positive one. If a woman's expected and actual experience closely match, she is likely to be more satisfied with it. Identifies misunderstandings and possible feelings of inadequacy or anger. |
| 4. Explain the following preoperative preparations using simple language, verifying Christina's understanding and giving her the opportunity to ask questions.<br>a. Visit by anesthesiologist or nurse anesthetist to explain anesthesia. The epidural anesthetic will be given in the operating room.<br>b. Shave prep (a Pfannenstiel incision is planned): from about 3 inches above the pubic hair to the level where the thighs meet. Other preparation if ordered, such as cleansing enema.<br>c. Indwelling urinary catheter, which is usually inserted after shave prep and epidural anesthesia is begun.<br>d. Operating room: appearance, narrow table, wedge under one hip (or tilted table), cool temperature, equipment.<br>e. People who will be in the operating room: circulating nurse, scrub nurse, surgeon's assistant, neonatal nurse, pediatrician. | 4. Knowledge decreases anxiety and fear of the unknown. Simple language facilitates understanding when a woman's attention is narrowed from anxiety. Shows respect and gives the woman a greater sense of control. |
| 5. Explain what to expect postoperatively, demonstrating as needed.<br>a. Oxygen mask may be used.<br>b. Pulse oximeter on finger. Automatic blood pressure cuff. | 5. Reduces anxiety and fear of the unknown. Promotes understanding and acceptance of care that will be painful while providing reassurance of pain control. Return demonstration verifies learning and identifies the need for additional teaching. |

## Nursing Care Plan 16–1 *Continued*
# Cesarean Birth

| INTERVENTION | RATIONALE |
|---|---|
| c. Frequent checks of her vital signs, fundus, lochia; anesthesia-related assessments. Emphasize that nurses will be as gentle as possible when palpating her fundus.<br>d. Catheter usually remains in place up to 24 hours.<br>e. She will be kept as comfortable as possible with analgesics.<br>f. She will be asked to move and change position several times.<br>g. Demonstrate effective coughing (splinting the abdomen with a pillow) and deep breathing techniques; have Christina demonstrate each. | |
| 6. Reduce unnecessary stimulation:<br>a. Keep lights low and noise to a minimum.<br>b. Limit unnecessary visitors and staff.<br>c. Plan operative preparations so that they are done efficiently.<br>d. Maintain calm and friendly behavior. | 6. Avoids adding to her anxiety. Emphasizes that a cesarean delivery is a birth, not just a surgical procedure. |

**EVALUATION**

Christina discusses her disappointment that the baby did not turn before she went into labor. However, she believes that a cesarean birth is best for her baby. Christina asks a few other questions, then states that she understands preoperative and postoperative care. She demonstrates effective coughing and deep breathing techniques.

**ASSESSMENT:** Christina had soup and a sandwich about 2 hours before admission. She will have epidural anesthesia for her birth. Her vital signs are temperature 37.2°C (99°F), pulse 90 BPM, respirations 22 breaths per minute, blood pressure 122/70. The fetal heart rate is 130 to 140 BPM and accelerates with fetal movement.

**Critical Thinking**

Does this assessment suggest another nursing diagnosis? What interventions should the nurse institute for the nursing diagnosis?

**ANSWER**

Risk for Aspiration would apply during the intraoperative period because general anesthesia might be needed unexpectedly and Christina has food in her stomach that might be vomited and aspirated. The woman is given nothing by mouth if general anesthesia is a possibility. The nurse should expect orders for a drug to reduce gastric acidity.

**EVALUATION**

Christina does not need general anesthesia and does not aspirate.

**ASSESSMENT:** Christina is transferred to the operating room, and epidural anesthesia is begun. She gives birth to an 8-pound, 8-ounce (3856 g) baby. Christina is transferred to the recovery room for postoperative care.

**NURSING DIAGNOSIS:** Risk for injury related to altered sensation from epidural anesthesia and use of electrical equipment during surgery

**GOALS/EXPECTED OUTCOMES**

Christina will not have injury, such as pressure areas, muscle strains, and electrical injury, during the perioperative period.

| INTERVENTION | RATIONALE |
|---|---|
| 1. Pad the operating table carefully, particularly under Christina's bony prominences. Avoid obstructing her popliteal area. | 1. Reduces potential for tissue damage caused by pressure. Reduces venous stasis with possible thrombus formation. |
| 2. Transfer Christina to and from the operating table carefully, using enough staff members to keep her body in alignment. Brace the bed and operating table to keep them from separating. | 2. Reduces risk of fall or muscle strains in both Christina and the staff. |

*Nursing Care Plan continued on following page*

## Nursing Care Plan 16–1 *Continued*
# Cesarean Birth

| | |
|---|---|
| 3. After anesthesia is begun, position Christina on the operating table and secure her legs with a safety strap. She should have a wedge under one hip, or the table should be tilted. | 3. Prevents falls or displacement of legs, which have lost sensation. A hip wedge or tilting the table reduces aortocaval compression, which might reduce placental blood flow. |
| 4. Apply grounding pad if electrocautery is to be used. | 4. Prevents electrical shock or burn. |

**EVALUATION**

During surgery, Christina's body was secured in proper alignment, with proper padding of all her bony prominences. The grounding pad ensured electrical safety when the electrocautery was used. Christina was transferred to the recovery room without incident. During the recovery period, she showed no signs of pressure, electrical, or musculoskeletal injury.

**ADDITIONAL NURSING DIAGNOSES TO CONSIDER**

Pain
Risk for Altered Respiratory Function
Hypothermia
Family Coping: Potential for Growth

*Note:* Only nursing diagnoses related to the preoperative and intraoperative care of the woman are discussed here. See Chapter 14 for nursing care related to fetal oxygenation. See Chapter 15 for care related to anesthesia. See Chapters 13 and 17 for nursing care of the mother during recovery and postpartum period.

### TEACHING

Knowledge helps to reduce fear of the unknown and increases a woman's sense of control over her infant's birth. The nurse cannot assume that a woman who had a previous cesarean birth already knows what will happen and why. If her previous surgery was done after a long labor or in an emergency, she may recall only bits and pieces and may not understand what she does remember. Teaching should be given in simple language and should include her partner.

The nurse explains preoperative procedures and their purposes, such as the abdominal shave, indwelling catheter, intravenous lines, and dressings. The catheter and intravenous lines usually remain in place no longer than 24 hours after birth. The nurse may need to reinforce anesthetic information provided by the anesthesia clinician.

Women who have regional anesthesia, such as epidural or subarachnoid block, often fear that they will feel pain during surgery. They do feel pressure and pulling, but these sensations do not mean that the anesthesia is wearing off. The nurse reassures her that her pain management is regularly assessed by the anesthesia clinician.

If a woman is having general anesthesia, the nurse explains why operative preparations are completed before she is anesthetized. She should be reassured that her surgery will not begin until she is asleep and that she will not wake up during the procedure.

The nurse describes the operating room and everyone who will be present to make it less intimidating to her. The operating room is very cool, and the surgery table is narrow. Her labor nurse is often the circulating nurse during surgery, reassuring her with a familiar face and voice.

The support person should be told when he or she can expect to come into the operating room. If it is not already in place, an epidural block is often established after the woman goes to the operating room. Bringing the partner in may be delayed until the regional block and other preparations, such as the indwelling catheter, are complete. These preparations may take 30 to 45 minutes if there is no rush. The support person should be told that he or she will not be forgotten and that the apparent delay does not indicate a problem.

The recovery room and any equipment that will be used, such as a pulse oximeter and automatic blood pressure cuff, are explained to the couple. The nurse reviews routine assessments and interventions such as fundus and lochia checks, coughing, and deep breathing. Simple exercises to promote normal circulation in her legs are taught. The nurse reassures her that every effort will be made to promote her comfort with medication, positioning, and other interventions.

### PROMOTING SAFETY

Although the need for general anesthesia occurs infrequently, the nurse must assume that it will be needed. The woman's food intake is assessed for type and time on admission. Oral intake and emesis during labor are recorded and reported to the anesthesia clinician. Oral intake other than ordered medications should be discontinued if a cesarean birth becomes very likely. Anesthesia-related drugs to control gastric and respiratory secretions are administered as ordered.

The woman is transferred and positioned carefully to prevent injury, especially if she has received regional anesthesia that reduces motor control and sensation. Her bony prominences are well padded. A safety strap placed across her thighs secures her on the narrow operating table. A wedge under one hip or tilting the operating table avoids aortocaval compression and reduced placental blood flow. During positioning, the drain tube of the indwelling catheter should be routed under her leg to promote drainage and keep the tube away from the operative area. The catheter bag is placed near the head of the table so that the anesthesia clinician can monitor urine output.

The nurse verifies proper function of machines such as suction devices, monitors, and electrocautery. Leads for the cardiac monitor and pulse oximeter are placed to observe heart and respiratory functions. A grounding pad permits safe use of the electrocautery.

After the surgery, the incision area is cleansed with sterile water and a sterile dressing is applied. Blood and amniotic fluid are cleaned from the woman's abdomen, buttocks, and back before transferring her to a bed. Smooth transfers reduce pain and hypotension.

#### PROVIDING POSTOPERATIVE CARE

Postoperative care for the mother who has had a cesarean birth is similar to that for one who has had a vaginal birth, with added interventions. Her temperature is assessed on admission and according to protocol thereafter. If her condition is stable, other assessments are done every 15 minutes during the first 1 to 2 hours, progressing to every 30 minutes to 1 hour until transfer to her postpartum room. In addition to temperature, routine postoperative assessments include the following:

- Return of motion and sensation (if a regional block was given)
- Level of consciousness (particularly if general anesthesia or sedating drugs were given)
- Vital signs and respiratory character
- Abdominal dressing
- Uterine firmness and position (midline or deviated)
- Lochia
- Urine output (quantity, color, other characteristics)
- Intravenous infusion
- Pain relief needs

The nurse observes for return of motion and sensation if she had epidural or subarachnoid block anesthesia. The level of consciousness and respiratory status (skin or mucous membrane color; rate and quality of respirations) are important observations if she had general anesthesia. Respiratory observations are also important if the woman received epidural opioid narcotics, which can cause delayed respiratory depression. Have naloxone (Narcan) available to reverse opioid-induced respiratory depression. (See Chapter 15 for more information about anesthesia and analgesia for cesarean birth.)

The pulse, respirations, and blood pressure provide important clues to the woman's circulatory and respiratory status. If oxygen saturation falls below 95 percent, having her take several deep breaths usually raises it. A respiratory rate of less than 12 breaths per minute suggests respiratory depression. Deep breathing and coughing move secretions out of the lungs. A small pillow to support her incision reduces pain when she coughs. Position changes every 2 hours improve ventilation and decrease discomfort from constant pressure.

As with vaginal birth, the fundus is assessed for height, firmness, and position. This examination is painful after regional anesthesia wears off, but the postcesarean mother can also have uterine atony. To relax her abdominal muscles, thus reducing pain from fundus checks, the nurse has her flex her knees and take slow deep breaths. The fingers are gently "walked" toward her fundus to determine uterine firmness. The woman who has a Pfannenstiel skin incision usually has less pain with fundus checks than the woman with a vertical skin incision. A firm fundus does not need massage. The dressing is checked for drainage with each fundus check.

The nurse assesses the lochia and urine output with other assessments. Lochia may pool under the mother's buttocks and lower back. Urine may be bloody temporarily if the cesarean delivery was done after a long labor or an attempted forceps delivery. The urine drain tubing should be observed for gradual clearing of the blood. Urine should drain freely to prevent bladder distention, which worsens pain and increases the risk for postpartum hemorrhage. The nurse must remember that falling urine output is an early sign of hypovolemia.

The woman's needs for pain relief should be regularly assessed. The woman who received an epidural analgesic may not need other analgesia during the early postpartum period. If she needs added pain relief while the epidural analgesic is still in effect, the dose ordered is often lower than if she had not had that form of analgesia. Early analgesia is usually given by a patient-controlled analgesia pump or intermittent injections. Oral analgesics usually replace parenteral ones the day after surgery.

### PRESENTING VAGINAL BIRTH AFTER CESAREAN

Teaching the woman about VBAC presents a challenge to nurses. Women have often heard the outdated saying, "once a cesarean, always a cesarean," and are anxious about attempting vaginal birth in a later pregnancy. They may know the facts about VBAC but find it impossible to disregard what they have heard for years. Scheduling a repeat cesarean often seems simpler and something the woman can count on. The prospect of laboring and perhaps still needing a cesarean birth is unattractive as well. Also, the nurse cannot promise the woman that she will not ultimately need a cesarean birth after hours of labor.

The physician discusses VBAC during prenatal care, and the nurse reinforces these explanations and identifies misunderstandings. The nurse should reinforce the appropriateness of attempting VBAC and the advantages of a vaginal birth, such as fewer overall complications. Vaginal birth after cesarean should be presented in a positive way, at the same time acknowledging that a cesarean delivery may be needed.

### ✓ CHECK YOUR READING

16. Why is the low transverse uterine incision preferred for cesarean birth?
17. What should a woman who expects a cesarean birth be taught about the operating room? The recovery room?
18. How should the nurse modify recovery room care of the mother who had a cesarean birth from that of the mother who had a vaginal delivery?

## SUMMARY CONCEPTS

- Prolapse and compression of the umbilical cord are the primary risks of amniotomy. As the fluid gushes out, the cord can become compressed between the fetal presenting part and the expectant woman's pelvis.
- Infection is more likely to occur when membranes have been ruptured for a long time, usually thought to be about 24 hours.
- Induction of labor may be done if continuing the pregnancy is more hazardous to the maternal or fetal health than is the induction. It is not done if a maternal or fetal contraindication exists to labor or vaginal birth.
- Oxytocin-stimulated uterine contractions may be hypertonic, decreasing placental perfusion.
- External version is done to promote vaginal birth by changing the fetal presentation from a breech or transverse lie to cephalic. Internal version is sometimes used to change presentation of a second twin following the birth of the first twin.
- The median episiotomy is less painful but more likely to extend into the rectum. The mediolateral episiotomy is more painful but is not likely to extend into the rectum.
- Trauma to maternal and fetal tissue is the primary risk associated with use of forceps or vacuum extractor. Possible trauma to the mother includes vaginal wall laceration and hematoma. Trauma to the infant may include ecchymoses, lacerations, abrasions, facial nerve injury, and intracranial hemorrhage.
- The preferred uterine incision for cesarean birth is the low transverse incision because it is least likely to rupture in a subsequent pregnancy. The skin incision does not always match the uterine incision and is unrelated to the risk of later uterine rupture.
- Some women have feelings of guilt or inadequacy if they have a cesarean birth. Therapeutic communication and sensitive, family-centered care are essential to help them achieve a positive perception of their birth experience.

### References and Readings

Ahner, R., Egarter, C., Kiss, H. et al. (1995). Fetal fibronectin as a selection criterion for induction of term labor. *American Journal of Obstetrics and Gynecology* 170(2), 1513–1517.

American Academy of Pediatrics & American College of Obstetricians and Gynecologists (1992). *Guidelines for perinatal care* (3rd ed.). Elk Grove Village, Ill.: Author.

American College of Obstetricians and Gynecologists (1994). Operative vaginal delivery. ACOG *technical bulletin no.* 196. Washington, D.C.: Author.

American College of Obstetricians and Gynecologists (1995a). ACOG practice patterns: Vaginal delivery after previous cesarean birth. ACOG *technical bulletin no.* 217. Washington, D.C.: Author.

American College of Obstetricians and Gynecologists (1995b). Dystocia and the augmentation of labor. ACOG *technical bulletin no.* 217. Washington, D.C.: Author.

American College of Obstetricians and Gynecologists (1995c). Induction of labor. ACOG *technical bulletin no.* 218. Washington, D.C.: Author.

Annibale, D.J., Hulsey, T.C., Wagner, C.L., & Southgate, W.M. (1995). Comparative neonatal morbidity of abdominal and vaginal deliveries after uncomplicated pregnancies. *Archives of Pediatric and Adolescent Medicine*, 149(8), 862–867.

Association of Women's Health, Obstetric, & Neonatal Nurses (AWHONN). (1993). *Practice resource: Cervical ripening and induction and augmentation of labor.* Washington, D.C.: Author.

Bachman, J., & Kendrick, J.M. (1996). Childbirth. In K.R. Simpson & P.A. Creehan (Eds.), AWHONN's *perinatal nursing* (pp. 151–245). Philadelphia: J. B. Lippincott.

Bishop, E.H. (1964). Pelvic scoring. *Obstetrics and Gynecology*, 24(2), 266–268.

Blackburn, S.T., & Loper, D.L. (1992). *Maternal, fetal, and neonatal physiology: A clinical perspective.* Philadelphia: W.B. Saunders.

Blanch, G., Oláh, K.S.J., & Walkinshaw, S. (1996). The presence of fetal fibronectin in the cervicovaginal secretions of women at term: Its role in the assessment of women before labor induction and in the investigation of the physiologic mechanisms of labor. *American Journal of Obstetrics & Gynecology*, 174(1), Part 1: 262–266.

Bowes, W.A. (1994). Clinical aspects of normal and abnormal labor. In R. Creasy & R. Resnik (Eds.), *Maternal-fetal medicine: Principles and practice* (3rd ed., pp. 527–537). Philadelphia: W.B. Saunders.

Boyle, J.G., & Gabbe, S.G. (1996). T and J vertical extensions in low transverse cesarean births. *Obstetrics and Gynecology*, 87(2), 238–243.

Brisson-Carroll, G., Fraser, W., Bréart, G., Krauss, I., & Thornton, J. (1996). The effect of routine early amniotomy on spontaneous labor: A meta-analysis. *Obstetrics and Gynecology*, 87(5): Part 2, 891–896.

Busowski, J.D., & Parsons, M.T. (1995). Amniotomy to induce labor. *Clinical Obstetrics and Gynecology*, 38(2), 246–258.

Centers for Disease Control and Prevention. (1995). Rates of cesarean delivery—United States, 1993. *Morbidity and Mortality Weekly Report*, 44(15), 303–307.

Clarke, S.C., & Taffel, S.M. (1996). Rates of cesarean and VBAC delivery, United States, 1994. *Birth*, 22(3), 166–168.

Cunningham, F.G., MacDonald, P.C., Gant, N.F., Leveno, K.J., Gilstrap, L.C., Hankins, G.D.V., et al. (1997). *Williams obstetrics* (20th ed.). Norwalk, Conn.: Appleton & Lange.

Friesen, C.D., Miller, A.M., & Rayburn, W.F. (1995). Influence of spontaneous or induced labor on delivering the macrosomic fetus. *American Journal of Perinatology*, 12(1), 63–66.

Fuentes, A., & Williams, M. (1995). Cervical assessment. *Clinical Obstetrics and Gynecology*, 38(2), 224–231.

Goer, H. (1995). *Obstetric myths versus research realities: A guide to the medical literature*. Westport, Conn.: Bergin & Garvey.

Hannah, M.E., Huh, C., Hewson, S.A., & Hannah, W.J. (1996). Postterm pregnancy: Putting the merits of a policy of induction of labor into perspective. *Birth*, 23(1), 13–19.

Krammer, J., Williams, M.C., Sawai, S.K., & O'Brien, W.F. (1995). Pre-induction cervical ripening: A randomized comparison of two methods. *Obstetrics and Gynecology*, 85(4), 614–618.

Laros, R.K., Flanagan, T.A., & Kilpatrick, S.J. (1995). Management of term breech presentation: A protocol of external cephalic version and selective trial of labor. *American Journal of Obstetrics and Gynecology*, 172(6), 1916–1925.

Lucas, M.J. (1994). The role of vacuum extraction in modern obstetrics. *Clinical Obstetrics and Gynecology*, 37(4), 794–805.

Lydon-Rochelle, M. (1995a). Cesarean delivery rates in women cared for by certified nurse-midwives in the United States: A review. *Birth*, 22(4), 211–219.

Lydon-Rochelle, M.T., Albers, L., & Teaf, D. (1995b). Perineal outcomes and nurse-midwifery management. *Journal of Nurse-Midwifery*, 40(1), 13–18.

Maier, J.S., & Maloni, J.A. (1997). Nurse advocacy for selective versus routine episiotomy. *Journal of Obstetric, Gynecologic, and Neonatal Nursing*, 26(2), 155–161.

Menihan, C.A. (1996). Intrapartum fetal monitoring. In K.R. Simpson & P.A. Creehan (Eds.), *AWHONN's perinatal nursing* (pp. 187–225). Philadelphia: J.B. Lippincott.

Naef, R.W., Ray, M.A., Chauhan, S.P., Roach, H., Blake, P.G., & Martin, J.N. (1995). Trial of labor after cesarean delivery with a lower-segment, vertical uterine incision: Is it safe? *American Journal of Obstetrics and Gynecology*, 172(6), 1666–1675.

O'Brien, W.F. (1995). The role of prostaglandins in labor and delivery. *Clinics in Perinatology*, 22(4), 973–984.

Paul, R.H., & Miller, D.A. (1995). Cesarean birth: How to reduce the rate. *American Journal of Obstetrics and Gynecology*, 172(6), 1903–1911.

Porreco, R.P., & Thorp, J.A. (1996). The cesarean birth epidemic: Trends, causes, and solutions. *American Journal of Obstetrics and Gynecology*, 175(2), 369–374.

Reichert, J.A., Baron, M., & Fawcett, J. (1993). Changes in attitudes toward cesarean birth. *Journal of Obstetric, Gynecologic, and Neonatal Nursing*, 22(2), 159–167.

Shyken, J.M., & Petrie, R.H. (1995). Oxytocin to induce labor. *Clinical Obstetrics and Gynecology*, 38(2), 232–245.

Thompson, J.P. Forcep deliveries. (1995). *Clinics in Perinatology*, 22(4), 953–972.

Torgersen, K. (1996). Ask the experts: Please compare prostaglandin $E_2$ preparations used to ripen the cervix in preparation for induction. AWHONN *Voice*, 4(3), 4.

U.S. Department of Health and Human Services, Public Health Service (1995). *Healthy people 2000: Midcourse review and 1995 revisions*. Washington, D.C.: Author.

Willcourt, R.J., Pager, D., Wendel, J., & Hale, R.W. (1994). Induction of labor with pulsatile oxytocin by a computer-controlled pump. *American Journal of Obstetrics and Gynecology*, 170(2):603–608.

Williams, M.C. (1995). Vacuum-assisted delivery. *Clinics in Perinatology*, 22(4), 907–931.

Xenakis, E.M.-J., Langer, O., Piper, J.M., Conway, D., & Berkus, M.D. (1995). Low-dose versus high-dose oxytocin augmentation of labor: A randomized trial. *American Journal of Obstetrics and Gynecology* 173(6):1874–1878.

Yeomans, E.R., & Gilstrap, L.C. (1994). The role of forceps in modern obstetrics. *Clinical Obstetrics and Gynecology*, 37(4), 785–793.

# The Cesarean Birth Story

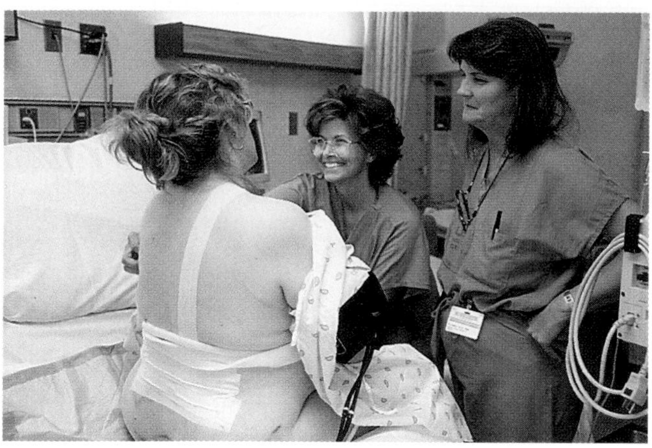

1. Vicky is in active labor. An epidural catheter allows injection of medications to provide analgesia during labor. Additional epidural medications can be used to provide anesthesia if surgery becomes necessary. An intravenous infusion precedes placement of the epidural block to offset the tendency of the block to cause hypotension.

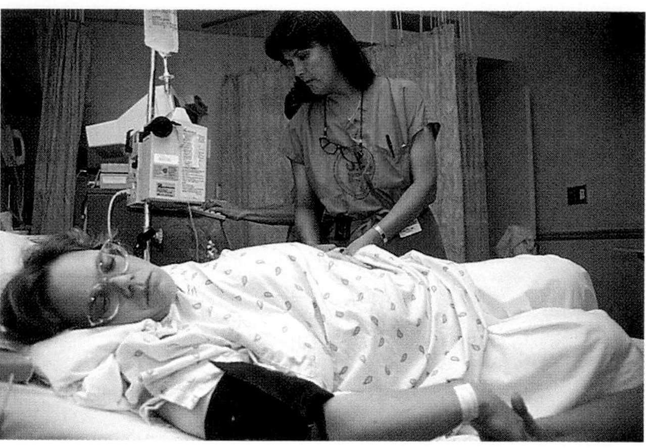

2. Support under her left hip displaces Vicky's uterus, thus avoiding pressure on her inferior vena cava and aorta and enhancing placental circulation. An automatic blood pressure cuff helps keep up with the frequent blood pressure assessments that are necessary when an epidural block is first begun.

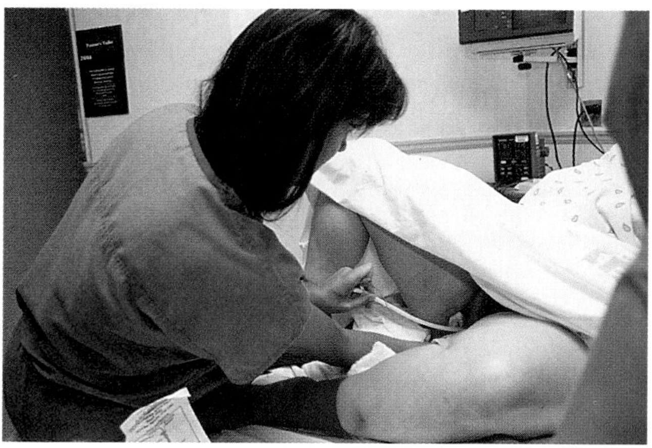

3. After rupturing the membranes, the nurse-midwife applies a spiral electrode to the fetal scalp to improve the accuracy of the fetal heart tracing on the monitor.

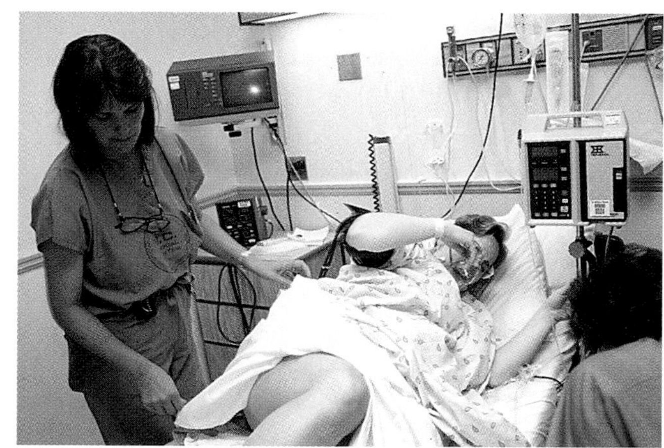

4. Because the fetal monitor shows patterns that suggest fetal compromise, Vicky will need a cesarean birth. Monitors for her blood pressure, pulse, and cardiac rhythm help to identify if there are maternal factors contributing to the fetal heart rate patterns. She receives oxygen by face mask to provide the maximum amount to her fetus.

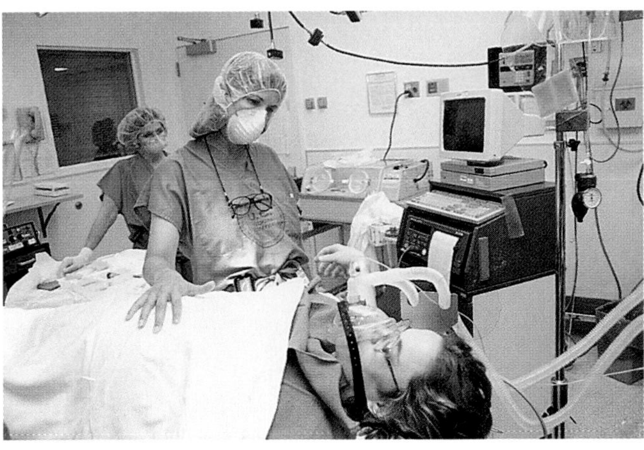

5. While Vicky is prepared for surgery, fetal monitoring and maternal oxygen administration continue. If possible, the same nurses accompany a woman to the operating room so that she has a continuing relationship during the cesarean birth as she would have for most vaginal births.

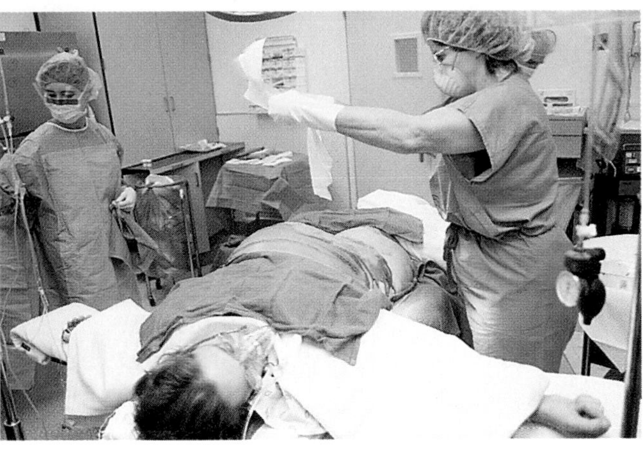

6. Vicky's abdomen is shaved to prepare for the surgery and is then cleansed with an antimicrobial prep solution. Shaving extends from just above the umbilicus to the point where the legs come together if a vertical incision is expected. If a Pfannenstiel (transverse) incision is expected, the top border can be about 3 inches above the upper pubic hairline.

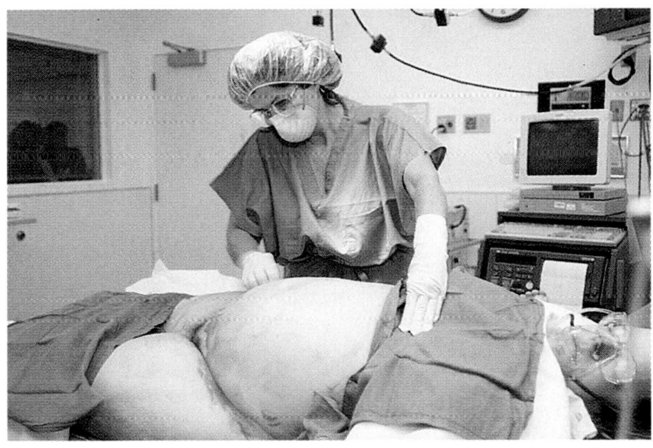

7. An iodine-based prep solution is used to cleanse the abdomen using a circular motion beginning at the incisional area and extending outward. The cleansing sponge should not be returned toward the center. During preparations for surgery, Vicky's trunk is tilted slightly toward her left side by a wedge under her right hip to promote circulation to the placenta. The internal fetal scalp electrode is removed before the incision is made so it is not brought from the unsterile vagina through the incision as the baby is born.

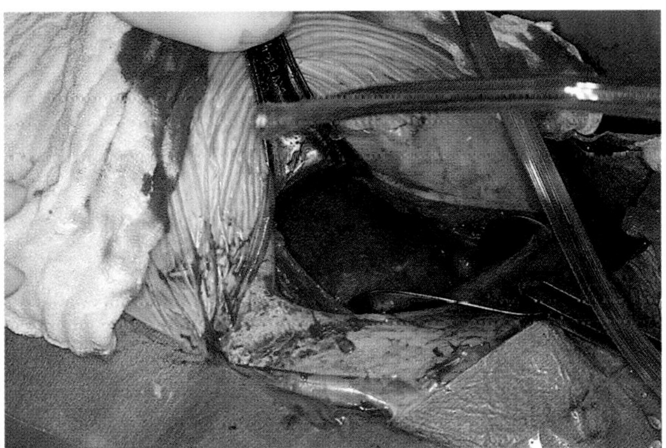

8. After making a Pfannenstiel skin incision, the physician separates the layers until the uterus is reached. The uterus is then opened in a low transverse incision. Wide retractors hold the mother's tissues back to expose an area large enough to allow the fetus to emerge. A suction device is available to suction blood and amniotic fluid from the uterus when it is incised.

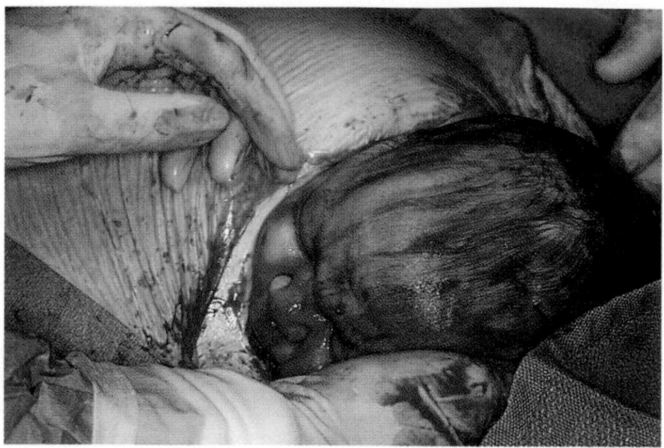

9. The fetal head is first brought through the incision. The bluish skin color is normal at this point.

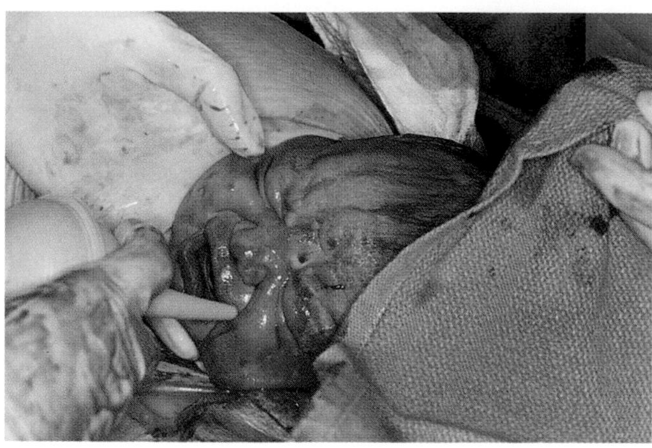

10. After birth of the head, the mouth and nose are suctioned to remove blood and other secretions before the infant takes his first breath. This baby is grimacing with the suction, which is usually associated with adequate oxygenation.

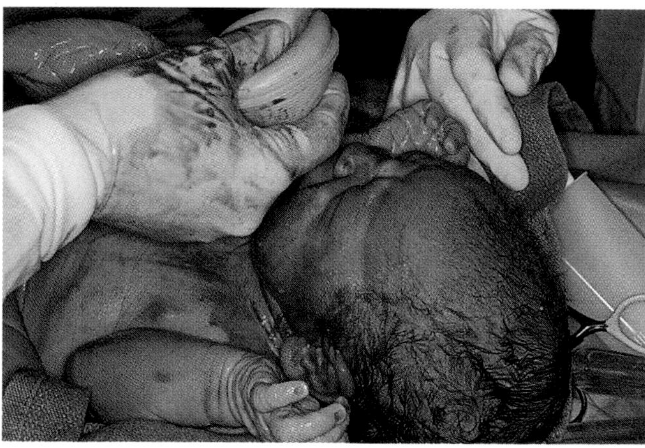

11. Further infant suctioning is done after the baby emerges.

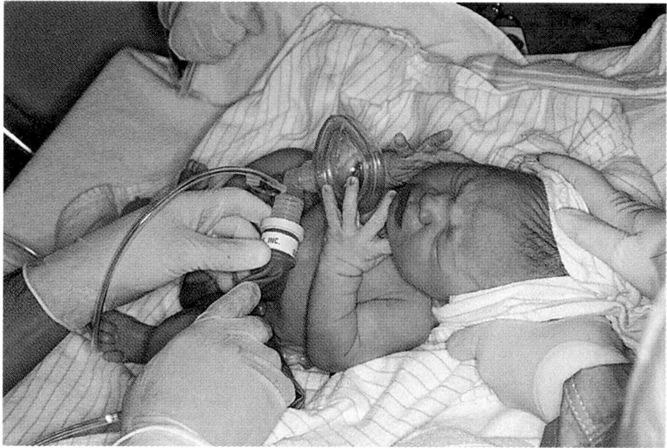

12. The infant is briefly given supplemental oxygen by face mask. His color is becoming pinker than it was immediately after birth because he has a larger proportion of oxygenated hemoglobin. At the same time, another nurse dries the baby to prevent cold stress, which could increase his oxygen needs. Note that nurses handling the baby wear gloves to protect them from blood and other secretions.

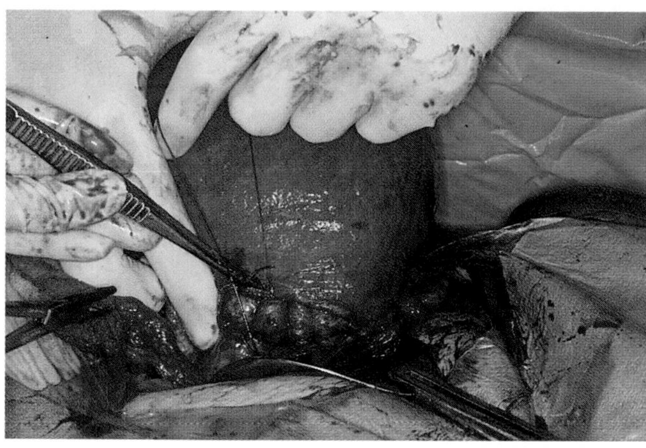

13. Heavy sutures are used to close the muscular layers of the transverse uterine incision.

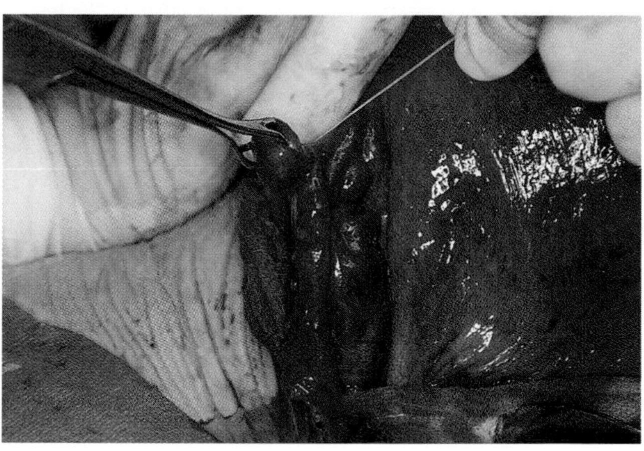

14. Vicky is having a bilateral tubal ligation for sterilization. One fallopian tube is identified by its connection to the uterus to distinguish it from her ureter. It is then doubly tied, and a segment of the tube is cut away and sent to the pathology laboratory for analysis.

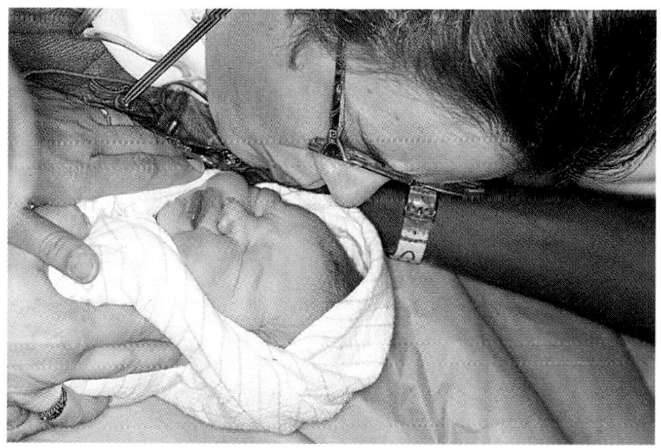

15. As her surgery continues and the infant's condition is stable, Vicky sees her baby up close for the first time.

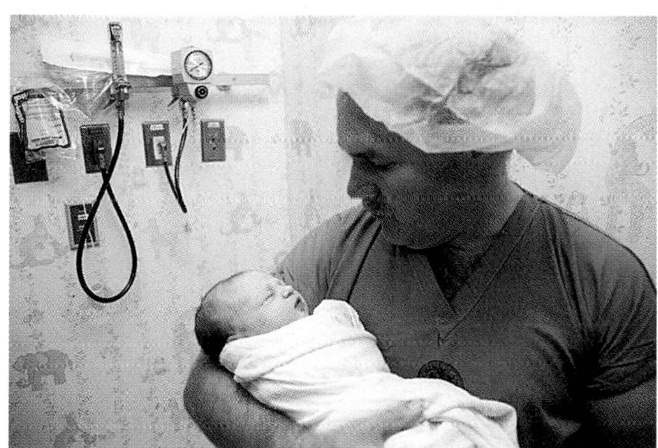

16. Vicky's husband, Greg, holds his newborn son shortly after birth.

# Part IV

# The Family Following Birth

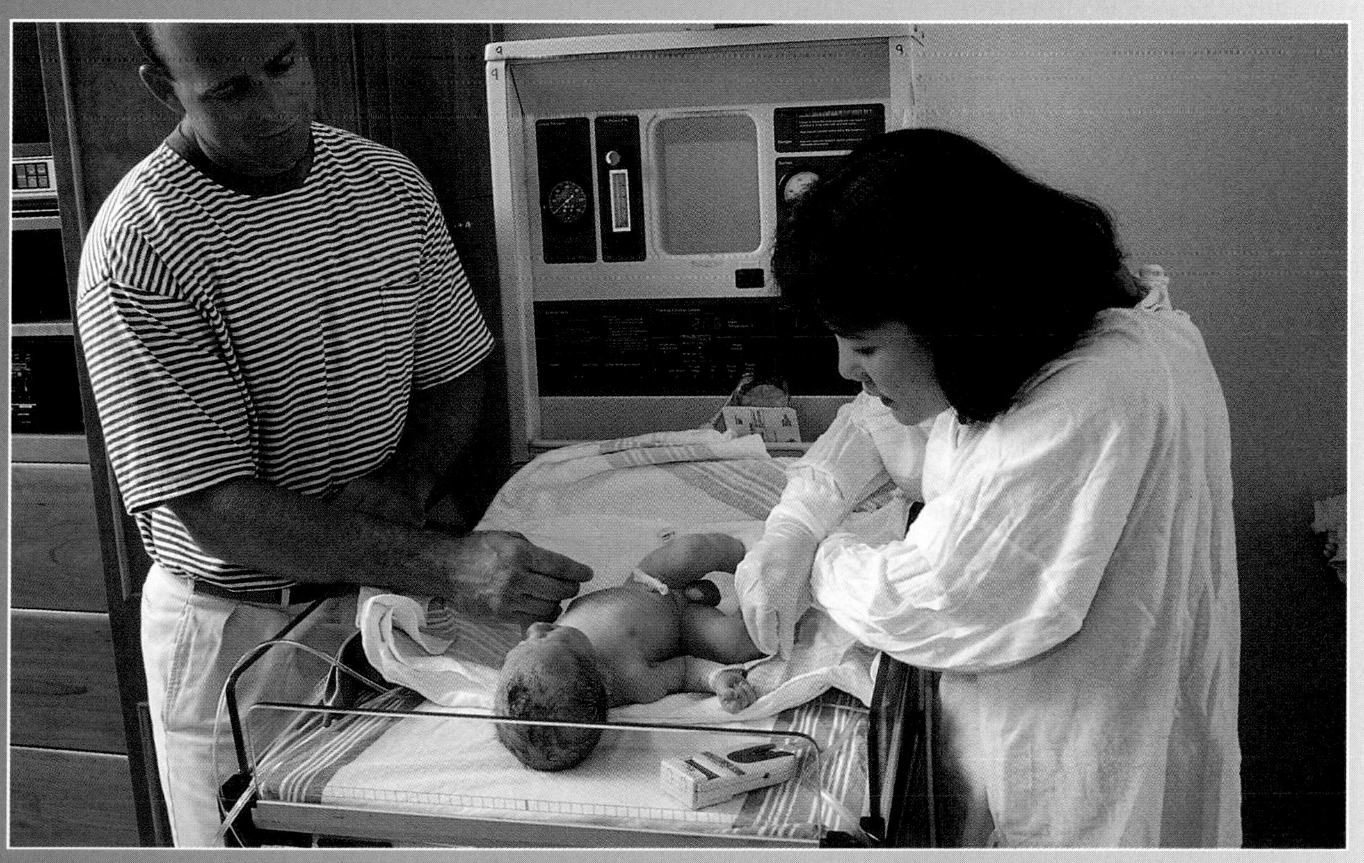

# 17

# Postpartum Physiologic Adaptations

**OBJECTIVES**

1. Explain the physiologic changes that occur during the postpartum period.
2. Identify the purpose of clinical pathways in postpartum care.
3. Describe nursing assessments and nursing care during the postpartum period.
4. Recount goals (outcomes) and interventions for the most common nursing diagnoses.
5. Discuss the role of the nurse in health education, and identify important areas of teaching.
6. Describe postpartum home care in terms of criteria for discharge, common problems, and available health care services.
7. Compare cesarean birth and vaginal birth in terms of nursing assessments and care.
8. Use critical thinking exercises to improve selected nursing care plans.

**DEFINITIONS**

**afterpain** *Cramping pain following childbirth caused by alternate relaxation and contraction of uterine muscles.*

**atony** *Absence or lack of usual muscle tone.*

**catabolism** *A destructive process that converts living cells into simpler compounds; process involved in involution (changes) of the uterus after childbirth.*

**decidua** *Name applied to the endometrium during pregnancy; all except the deepest layer is shed after childbirth.*

**diastasis recti** *Separation of the longitudinal muscles of the abdomen (rectus abdominis) during pregnancy.*

**dyspareunia** *Difficult or painful coitus in women.*

**engorgement** *Swelling of the breasts resulting from increased blood flow and presence of milk.*

**episiotomy** *Surgical incision of the perineum to enlarge the vaginal opening.*

**fundus** *Part of the uterus that is farthest from the cervix, above the openings of the fallopian tubes.*

**involution** *Retrogressive changes that return the reproductive organs, particularly the uterus, to their pre-pregnancy size and condition.*

**Kegel exercises** *Alternate contracting and relaxing of the pelvic muscles; these movements strengthen the pubococcygeal muscle, which surrounds the urinary meatus and vagina.*

**lactation** *Secretion of milk from the breasts; also describes the time when a child is breastfed.*

**lochia alba** *Whitish or clear vaginal discharge that follows lochia serosa; occurs when the amount of blood is decreased and the number of leukocytes is increased.*

**lochia rubra** *Reddish vaginal discharge that occurs immediately after childbirth; composed mostly of blood.*

**lochia serosa** *Pinkish or brown-tinged vaginal discharge that follows lochia rubra and precedes lochia alba; composed largely of serous exudate, blood, and leukocytes.*

**milk-ejection reflex** *Release of milk from the alveoli into the ducts; also known as the let-down reflex.*

**oxytocin** *Posterior pituitary gland hormone that stimulates uterine contractions and the milk-ejection reflex; also prepared synthetically.*

**prolactin** *Anterior pituitary hormone that promotes growth of breast tissue and stimulates production of milk.*

**puerperium** *Period from the end of childbirth until involution of the uterus is complete; approximately 6 weeks.*

**REEDA** *Acronym for redness, ecchymosis, edema, discharge, and approximation; useful for assessing wound healing or the presence of inflammation or infection.*

The first 6 weeks following the birth of an infant are known as the postpartum period, or puerperium. During this time, mothers experience numerous physiologic and psychosocial changes. To clarify the presentation, psychosocial changes and their implications are presented separately in Chapter 18, although in actual practice physiologic and psychosocial care occur at the same time.

Many of the physiologic changes are retrogressive in nature; that is, changes that occurred in body systems during pregnancy are reversed as the body returns to the pre-pregnancy state. Progressive changes also occur, most obviously in the initiation of lactation and the restoration of normal menstrual cycles.

## Reproductive System

### Involution of the Uterus

Involution refers to the changes that the reproductive organs, particularly the uterus, undergo after childbirth to return to their pre-pregnancy size and condition. Involution depends on three processes: (1) contraction of muscle fibers, (2) catabolism, and (3) regeneration of uterine epithelium. Involution begins immediately following delivery of the placenta, when uterine muscle fibers contract firmly around maternal blood vessels at the area where the placenta was attached. This contraction controls bleeding from the area left denuded when the placenta separated. Moreover, the uterus decreases in size when muscle fibers, which have been stretched for many months, contract and gradually regain their former contour and size.

Although the total number of cells remains unchanged, the enlarged muscle cells of the uterus undergo catabolic changes in protein cytoplasm that cause a reduction in individual cell size. The products of the catabolic process are absorbed by the blood stream and are excreted in urine as nitrogenous waste.

Regeneration of the uterine epithelial lining begins soon after childbirth. The outer portion of the endometrial layer is expelled with the placenta. Within 2 to 3 days, the remaining decidua separates into two layers. The first layer is superficial and is shed in lochia. The basal layer remains intact and is the source of new endometrium. Regeneration of the endometrium, except at the site of placental attachment, occurs by 2 to 3 weeks.

The placental site, which is about 7 cm (2.7 inches) in diameter, heals by a process of *exfoliation* (scaling off of dead tissue). New endometrium is generated at the site from glands and tissue that remain in the lower layer of the decidua after separation of the placenta (Cunningham et al., 1997). This process leaves the endometrial layer smooth and spongy, as it was before pregnancy, and leaves the uterine lining free of scar tissue, which would interfere with implantation of future pregnancies. Healing at the placental site occurs more slowly and requires approximately 6 to 7 weeks.

#### DESCENT OF THE UTERINE FUNDUS

The location of the uterine fundus helps to determine if involution is progressing normally. Immediately following delivery, the uterus is about the size of a large grapefruit and the fundus can be palpated midway between the symphysis pubis and umbilicus. Within a few hours, the fundus rises to the level of the umbilicus and should remain at this level for about 24 hours. Although individual differences occur related to body size and type, the uterus now weighs approximately 1000 g (2.2 pounds).

After 24 hours, the fundus begins to descend by approximately 1 cm, or one fingerbreadth, per day, so that by the 10th day it is in the pelvic cavity and cannot be palpated abdominally. Descent is documented in relation to the umbilicus. For instance, U − 1 indicates that the fundus is palpable one fingerbreadth below the umbilicus. Within a week, the weight of the uterus decreases to about 500 g (1 pound); at 6 weeks, the uterus weighs 60 g (2 ounces), which is roughly the pre-pregnancy weight. Figure 17–1 illustrates normal descent of the uterine fundus as involution occurs.

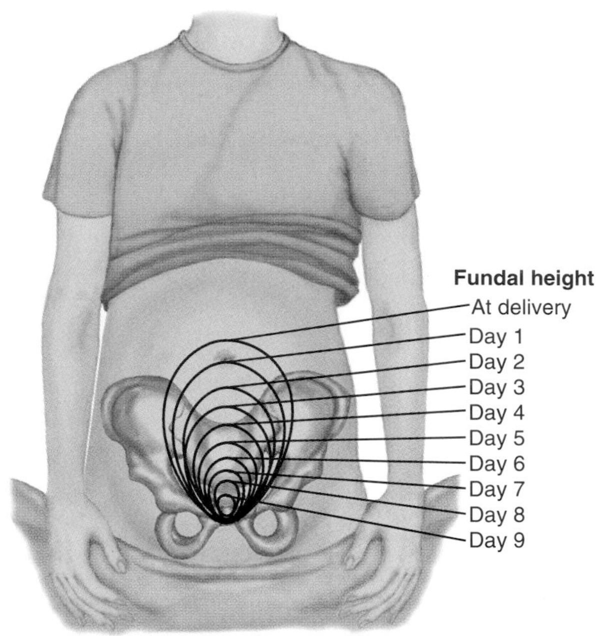


**FIGURE 17–1**

Involution of the uterus. Height of the uterine fundus decreases by approximately 1 cm per day.

#### AFTERPAINS

Intermittent contractions, known as afterpains, are a source of discomfort for many women. The discomfort is more acute for multiparas because repeated stretching of muscle fibers leads to loss of muscle tone that results in alternate contraction and relaxation of the uterus. The uterus of a primipara tends to remain contracted; however, a primipara may also experience severe afterpains if the uterus has been overdistended by twins, a large infant, hydramnios (excess of amniotic fluid), or retained blood clots.

**Severity.** Afterpains are particularly severe during breastfeeding, when oxytocin, released from the posterior pituitary to stimulate the milk-ejection reflex, also stimulates strong contractions of uterine muscles.

**Nursing Considerations.** Analgesics are frequently used to lessen the discomfort of afterpains. If the mother is breastfeeding, she achieves maximum relief by taking the medication at least 30 minutes before nursing the infant. Many breastfeeding mothers are reluctant to take medication for fear that the infant will get the medication in breast milk. There is general agreement, however, that analgesics may be used for short-term pain relief without harm to the infant. The benefits of pain relief, such as comfort and relaxation that facilitate the milk-ejection reflex, usually outweigh the negligible effects of the medication on the infant. Some mothers also find that lying in a prone position, with a small pillow or folded blanket under the abdomen, helps keep the uterus contracted and provides relief. It is also beneficial to reassure the mother that afterpains are self-limiting and that they decrease rapidly after 48 hours.

#### LOCHIA

Changes in the color and amount of lochia also provide information about whether involution is progressing normally.

**Changes in Color.** For the first 3 days following childbirth, lochia consists almost entirely of blood, with small particles of decidua and mucus. Because of its red color it is termed *lochia rubra*. The amount of blood decreases by about the fourth day, when leukocytes begin to invade the area, as they do any healing surface. The color of lochia then changes from red to pinkish (*lochia serosa*). Lochia serosa is composed of serous exudate, erythrocytes, leukocytes, and cervical mucus. By about the 11th day, the erythrocyte component decreases. The discharge becomes clear and colorless or white (*lochia alba*). Lochia alba contains leukocytes, decidual cells, epithelial cells, fat, cervical mucus, and bacteria. It is present in most women until the third week following childbirth but may persist for 6 weeks.

**Amount.** Because it is difficult to estimate the amount of lochia, nurses frequently document lochia in terms that are difficult to quantify, such as "scant," "moderate," and "heavy." Luegenbiehl and colleagues (1990) proposed the following terms, which include a description as well as an estimation in milliliters for the amount of lochia in 1 hour:

**Scant** Less than a 2-inch (5-cm) stain on the peripad (~ 10 ml).
**Small** Less than a 4-inch (10-cm) stain (~ 10 to 25 ml).
**Moderate** Smaller than a 6-inch (15-cm) stain (25 to 50 ml).
**Large** Larger than a 6-inch stain (50 to 80 ml).

Figure 17–2 illustrates lochial discharge for 1 hour and quantifies the amount in milliliters.

Lochia is often heavier when the new mother first gets out of bed because gravity allows blood that pooled in the vagina during the hours of rest to flow freely when she stands. Table 17–1 summarizes the characteristics of normal and abnormal lochial discharge.

### Cervix

Immediately after childbirth, the cervix is formless, flabby, and open wide enough to admit the entire hand. This allows manual extraction of the placenta, if necessary, and manual examination of the uterus. Small tears or lacerations may be present, and the cervix is often edematous. Rapid healing takes place, and by the end of the first week the cervix feels firm

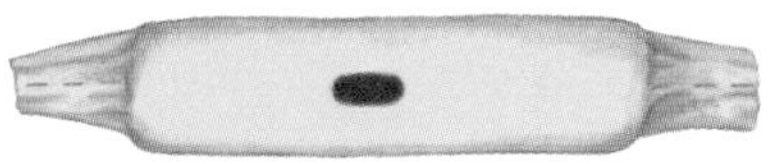

**Scant:** 2-inch stain (10 ml)

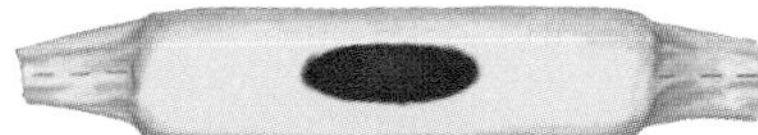

**Small:** 4-inch stain (10 to 25 ml)

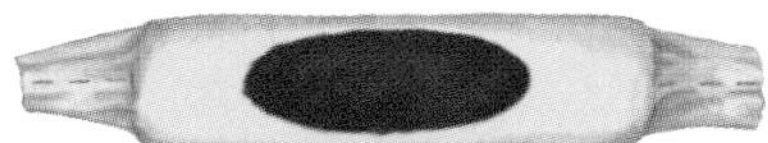

**Moderate:** 6-inch stain (25 to 50 ml)

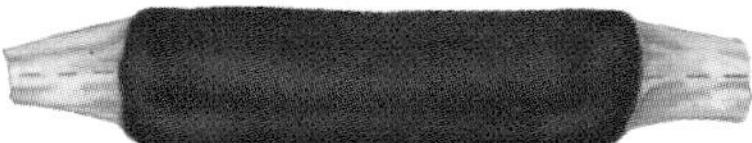

**Large:** >6-inch stain (50 to 80 ml)

**FIGURE 17–2**

Guidelines for assessing the volume of lochia based on amount of stain on the perineal pad.

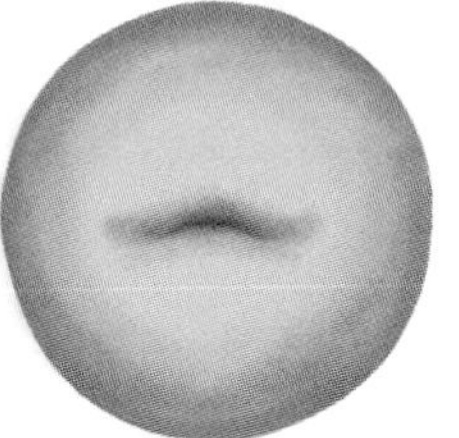

**Nulliparous cervix with round os**

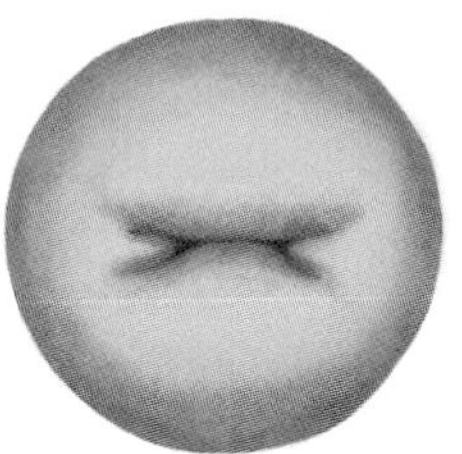

**Parous cervix with slit os**

**FIGURE 17–3**

A permanent change occurs in the cervical os following childbirth.

and the external os is the width of a pencil. The internal os closes as before pregnancy, but the shape of the external os is permanently changed. It remains slightly open and appears slit-like rather than round, as in the nulliparous woman (Fig. 17–3).

## Vagina

The vagina and vaginal introitus are greatly stretched during birth to allow passage of the fetus. Soon after childbirth, the vaginal walls appear edematous, and multiple small lacerations may be present. Very few vaginal rugae (folds) are present. The hymen is permanently torn and heals with small, irregular tags of tissue visible at the vaginal introitus.

Although the vaginal mucosa heals and rugae are regained by 3 weeks, it takes the entire postpartum period (6 weeks) for the vagina to complete involution and to gain approximately the same size and contour it had before pregnancy; however, the vagina does not entirely regain the nulliparous size.

During the postpartum period, vaginal mucosa becomes atrophic and vaginal walls do not regain their thickness until estrogen production by the ovaries is reestablished. Because ovarian function, and therefore estrogen production, is not well established during lactation, breastfeeding mothers are likely to experience vaginal dryness and may experience discomfort during intercourse (dyspareunia) for 4 to 6 months (Blackburn & Loper, 1992). Although many of the concerns about changes in the vagina are unexpressed, a woman and her sexual partner may have numerous questions. Nurses must be sensitive to unasked questions and should try to provide anticipatory guidance. Nursing Care Plan 17–1 presents interventions for the nursing diagnosis Altered Sexuality Patterns.

## Perineum

The muscles of the pelvic floor stretch and thin greatly during the second stage of labor, when the fetal head applies pressure as it descends, rotates, and then extends to be delivered. After childbirth, the perineum may be edematous and bruised. In the United States, many women who give birth also have a surgical incision (episiotomy) of the perineal area.

Generally, the episiotomy is median or midline; that is, it extends straight back from the lower edge of the introitus toward the anus. Occasionally, mediolateral incisions, begun at the introitus and directed laterally and downward away from the rectum to either the right or left side, are made to provide additional room for birth of the infant.

Lacerations of the perineum may also occur during delivery. Lacerations and episiotomies are classified

**TABLE 17–1 CHARACTERISTICS OF LOCHIA**

| Time and Type | Normal Discharge | Abnormal Discharge |
|---|---|---|
| Days 1–3: lochia rubra | Bloody; small clots; fleshy, earthy odor | Large clots; saturated perineal pads; foul odor |
| Days 4–10: lochia serosa | Decreased amount; serosanguineous; pink or brown | Excessive amount; foul smell; continued or recurrent reddish color |
| Days 11–21: lochia alba | Creamy, yellowish color; decreasing amounts | Persistent lochia serosa; return to lochia rubra, foul odor; discharge continuing |

## Nursing Care Plan 17–1

# Postpartum Hypotension, Fatigue, and Pain

**ASSESSMENT:** Jacqueline Tilden, gravida II, para II, gave birth to a baby girl weighing 3400 g (7.5 pounds) 4 hours ago. She became weak and dizzy and mentioned that "everything was going black" when she attempted to ambulate the first time. Her gait was unsteady, and the nurse had to lower her back to bed to prevent her from fainting. Her color was pale, and her pulse was rapid.

**NURSING DIAGNOSIS:** Risk for Injury related to physiologic effects of orthostatic hypotension

### Critical Thinking

Does the nurse have enough data to make this diagnosis? If not, what other data are necessary? Why?

**ANSWER**

Although dizziness and feeling faint may indicate orthostatic hypotension, they may also indicate hypovolemia. The nurse must also assess Jacqueline for signs of excessive blood loss, such as the location and firmness of the uterine fundus, the amount of lochia, the pulse rate at rest, and hemoglobin and hematocrit levels. If these data are within expected levels, a diagnosis of Risk for Injury related to the effects of orthostatic hypotension is appropriate.

### GOAL/EXPECTED OUTCOME

Jacqueline will remain free of injury caused by fainting and falling during the postpartum period.

| INTERVENTION | RATIONALE |
|---|---|
| 1. Check the mother's blood pressure while she is in a supine position and in a sitting position; check her blood pressure in the same arm. | 1. A decrease of 20 mmHg in systolic pressure in the upright position indicates orthostatic hypotension (a sudden decrease in blood pressure when one moves from a supine to a standing position). Measuring from the same arm provides more accurate information because the reading may differ slightly in each arm. |
| 2. Instruct the mother in measures to overcome the sudden drop in blood pressure:<br>a. Elevate the head of the bed for a few minutes before she attempts to stand.<br>b. Help her sit on the side of the bed for several minutes before standing, and help her to stand slowly. | 2. Allows time for blood pressure to stabilize before she is fully upright, thus maintaining circulation to the brain. |
| 3. Instruct the mother to move her feet constantly when she first stands. | 3. Increases venous return from the lower extremities; this maintains cardiac output and increases cerebral circulation. |
| 4. Suggest that she take brief, tepid (not hot) showers and that she bend her knees and "march" during the shower. | 4. Hot water dilates peripheral blood vessels, allowing additional blood to remain in the vessels of the legs. Moving the feet and legs increases blood return from the legs and increases blood to the brain. |
| 5. Initiate measures to prevent injuries that could be sustained if she fainted:<br>a. Stay with the mother when she ambulates, and be prepared to assist her in sitting down or in lowering her gently to the floor if she becomes faint.<br>b. Call for assistance before attempting to return her to bed.<br>c. Remind her to call for assistance before trying to ambulate. Check to see that the call light is conveniently located. | 5. Gravity increases blood flow to the brain when the head is lowered and thus prevents fainting. Adequate assistance prevents falling and possible injury during a fainting episode. |

### EVALUATION

Jacqueline has participated in self-care and has sustained no injury during her hospital stay.

**ASSESSMENT:** Jacqueline demonstrates skill in breastfeeding but wonders how she will be able to care for the baby and her 18-month-old boy when she gets home. She states he "is busy every minute." She has a third-degree episiotomy and asks what can be done to prevent the pain she experienced during intercourse for several months after the last child was born.

**NURSING DIAGNOSIS:** Anxiety related to anticipated fatigue and discomfort

## Nursing Care Plan 17–1 *Continued*

# Postpartum Hypotension, Fatigue, and Pain

**Critical Thinking**

What assumption is the nurse making? How might the nurse validate the assumption? Can you identify another diagnosis that is more specific?

**ANSWER**

The nurse makes an assumption that the client is anxious. Neither signs nor symptoms of anxiety are part of the assessment data. The nurse can validate the assumption by asking Jacqueline if she is anxious. Anxiety is a very broad diagnostic category. Based on the data available, a more specific and therefore more helpful nursing diagnosis might be Risk for Altered Sexuality Patterns related to fatigue and pain.

### GOALS/EXPECTED OUTCOMES

The couple will do the following:

1. Verbalize measures to promote comfort during sexual activity by (date).
2. Verbalize a plan to reduce fatigue, which interferes with interest in and energy for sexual activity by (date).

| INTERVENTION | RATIONALE |
|---|---|
| 1. Recommend that the parents postpone vaginal intercourse until the perineum is well healed, usually about 3 weeks. Suggest that the mother continue perineal care, sitz baths, and the use of topical agents until the perineum is healed. | 1. These measures promote rapid healing and reduce pain or fear of pain when sexual activity is resumed. |
| 2. Suggest the use of a water-soluble vaginal lubricant (KY Jelly, Lubrin, Replens) if the mother is planning to breastfeed for longer than 6 weeks. | 2. Breastfeeding delays the resumption of ovarian hormones, including estrogen, which may result in vaginal dryness that is most noticeable after 6 weeks of breastfeeding. |
| 3. Prior to vaginal intercourse, as part of foreplay, suggest that one finger be inserted into the vaginal introitus to determine areas of tenderness or pain. | 3. Locates areas of discomfort and stretches the perineal scar gently. |
| 4. Suggest that the woman assume the superior position during intercourse. | 4. The woman controls the depth and location of penetration; thus, she can reduce her discomfort. |
| 5. Remind parents that sexual arousal may be slower because of decreased hormones and fatigue; more stimulation may be required before the mother is sexually aroused. | 5. Knowledge of the physiologic changes reduces the anxiety and tension that occur if the parents are unprepared for them. |
| 6. Remind the mother to perform Kegel exercises until she can comfortably do 50 each day. She may gradually work up to performing 100 repetitions twice each day. | 6. Strengthens the muscles around the vagina and promotes increased sexual satisfaction. |
| 7. Suggest that the infant be breastfed just before initiating sexual activity. | 7. Reduces the chance of leaking milk, which interferes with sexual pleasure for some couples; may also allow uninterrupted time while the infant sleeps. |
| 8. Suggest measures that may lessen fatigue:<br>a. Recommend that each partner nap for 30 minutes sometime during the day or evening.<br>b. Suggest that sexual activity be resumed in the morning or afternoon rather than at the end of a tiring day.<br>c. Suggest that parents rest when the infant has long periods of sleep and that they postpone additional home projects that will increase fatigue until the infant is older and is sleeping through the night. | 8. Lessens fatigue, which is cited by both mothers and fathers as one of the major causes of decreased interest in sexual activity following childbirth. |

*Nursing Care Plan continued on following page*

## Nursing Care Plan 17–1 *Continued*

## Postpartum Hypotension, Fatigue, and Pain

| INTERVENTION | RATIONALE |
|---|---|
| 9. Encourage frank communication between partners about measures that reduce discomfort as well as specific concerns and needs. | 9. Facilitates understanding and fosters a feeling of closeness that can enhance sexual interest. |

**EVALUATION**

The couple expresses interest in learning measures that reduce fatigue and discomfort; they verbalize a plan to use the instructions provided.

**ADDITIONAL NURSING DIAGNOSES TO CONSIDER**

Altered Family Processes
Risk for Altered Health Maintenance
Risk for Altered Parenting
Health Seeking Behaviors
Sleep Pattern Disturbance

according to tissue involved (Table 17–2). (See further discussions of episiotomy and lacerations in Chapters 13 and 16.)

**Discomfort.** Although the episiotomy is relatively small, the muscles of the perineum are involved in many activities (walking, sitting, stooping, squatting, bending, defecating). An incision in this area can cause a great deal of discomfort. In addition, many pregnant women are affected by hemorrhoids (distended rectal veins), which are pushed out of the rectum during the second stage of labor.

**Nursing Considerations.** Hemorrhoids, as well as perineal trauma, episiotomy, or lacerations, can make physical activity or bowel elimination difficult during the postpartum period. Relief of perineal discomfort is a nursing priority that includes teaching self-care measures, such as sitz baths, perineal care, and topical anesthesia.

**TABLE 17–2 LACERATIONS OF THE BIRTH CANAL**

**Perineum**

Perineal lacerations are classified in degrees to describe the amount of tissue involved. Some physicians or nurse-midwives also use degrees to describe the extent of median episiotomies.

*First-degree*: Involves the superficial vaginal mucosa or perineal skin.

*Second-degree*: Involves the vaginal mucosa, perineal skin, and deeper tissues, which may include muscles of the perineum.

*Third-degree*: Same as second-degree lacerations but involves the anal sphincter.

*Fourth-degree*: Extends through the anal sphincter into the rectal mucosa.

**Periurethral Area**

A laceration in the area of the urethra. Women with periurethral lacerations may have difficulty urinating after birth. They may require an indwelling catheter for a day or two.

**Vaginal Wall**

A laceration involving the mucosa of the vaginal wall.

**Cervix**

Tears in the cervix may be a source of significant bleeding after birth.

**CHECK YOUR READING**

1. Which three processes are involved in involution?
2. How is the fundus expected to descend following childbirth?
3. Which mothers are most likely to experience afterpains? How are they treated?
4. What are the differences between lochia rubra, lochia serosa, and lochia alba in terms of appearance and expected duration?

## Cardiovascular System

Hypervolemia, which produces a 50 percent increase in blood volume at term, allows the woman to tolerate a substantial blood loss during childbirth without ill effect. On the average, 500 ml of blood is lost in vaginal deliveries and 1000 ml is lost in cesarean births (Cunningham et al., 1997).

### Cardiac Output

Despite the blood loss, a transient increase in maternal cardiac output occurs following childbirth. This increase is caused by (1) increased flow of blood back to the heart when blood from the uteroplacental unit returns to central circulation, and (2) mobilization of excess extracellular fluid into the vascular compartment.

The rise in cardiac output, which persists for about 48 hours after childbirth, is probably caused by an increase in stroke volume because bradycardia is often noted during the postpartum period. Bradycardia is defined as a pulse rate of 50 to 60 beats per minute. Gradually cardiac output decreases and returns to normal levels by 12 weeks after childbirth (Resnik, 1994).

### Plasma Volume

The body rids itself of excess plasma volume, which was necessary during pregnancy, by two methods: diuresis and diaphoresis.

- *Diuresis* (increased excretion of urine) is facilitated by a decline in the adrenal hormone aldosterone, which is increased during pregnancy to counteract the salt-wasting effect of progesterone. As aldosterone production decreases, sodium retention declines and fluid excretion accelerates. A decrease in oxytocin, which promotes reabsorption of fluid, also contributes to diuresis. A urinary output of 3000 ml per day is not uncommon for the first few days of the postpartum period.
- *Diaphoresis* (profuse perspiration) also rids the body of excess fluid. Although it is not clinically significant, diaphoresis can be uncomfortable and unsettling for the mother who is not prepared for it. Explanations of the cause and comfort measures, such as showers and dry clothing, are generally sufficient.

### Coagulation

Significant changes that occur during pregnancy also affect the body's ability to coagulate blood and form clots. During pregnancy, plasma fibrinogen (necessary for coagulation) increased as a protection against postpartum hemorrhage. As a result, the mother's body has a greater ability to form clots and thus prevent excessive bleeding. She does not, however, have an increased ability to eliminate clots because a corresponding increase in plasminogen (necessary for lysis of clots) has not occurred during pregnancy. The net result is that during pregnancy and the postpartum period she is at risk for thrombus (clot) formation.

Although the incidence of thrombophlebitis has declined greatly in recent years, probably as a result of early postpartum ambulation, new mothers are still at increased risk for thrombus formation. Women who have varicose veins, who have a history of thrombophlebitis, or who have experienced a cesarean birth are at further risk, and the lower extremities should be monitored closely. Antiembolism hosiery is often applied before a cesarean birth or if the mother is at particular risk because of a history of previous phlebitis or the presence of varicosities. (See Chapter 28 for further discussion of thromboembolic disorders.)

### Blood Values

Besides clotting factors, other components of the blood change during the postpartum period. Marked leukocytosis occurs, with the white blood cell count increasing from the non-pregnancy normal range of 5000 to 10,000/mm$^3$ up to 20,000 or even 30,000/mm$^3$ (Cunningham et al., 1997). Neutrophils, which increase in response to inflammation, pain, and stress to protect against invading organisms, account for the major increase in white blood cells.

Maternal hemoglobin and hematocrit values are difficult to interpret during the first few days after birth because of the remobilization and rapid excretion of excess body fluid. The hematocrit is low when plasma (the liquid part of blood) increases and dilutes the concentration of blood cells and other substances carried by the plasma. As excess fluid is excreted, the dilution is gradually reduced. Hematocrit should return to normal limits within 3 to 7 days unless excessive blood loss has occurred.

## Gastrointestinal System

Soon after childbirth, digestion begins to be active and the new mother is usually hungry because of the energy expended in labor. Moreover, she is usually thirsty because of the long period of fluid restriction during labor, the fluid loss from exertion, and early diaphoresis. Nurses anticipate the mother's needs and provide a refreshing drink and a nourishing meal soon after childbirth.

Constipation is a common problem during the postpartum period for a variety of reasons. First, bowel tone, which was diminished during pregnancy as a result of progesterone, remains sluggish for several days. Second, restricted food and fluid intake during labor often results in small, hard stools. Third, perineal trauma, episiotomy, and hemorrhoids cause discomfort and interfere with effective bowel elimination. In addition, many women anticipate pain when they attempt to defecate and are unwilling to exert pressure on the perineum.

Temporary constipation is not harmful, although it can cause a feeling of abdominal fullness and flatulence. Many women become extremely concerned about constipation, and stool softeners and laxatives are frequently prescribed to prevent or treat consti-

**TABLE 17-3 COMMONLY RECOMMENDED LAXATIVES FOR THE POSTPARTUM PERIOD**

| Types | Examples | Comments |
|---|---|---|
| Fecal wetting agents | Docusate calcium (Surfak)<br>Docusate sodium (Colace) | Detergent-like action, permit easier mixing of fats and fluids with fecal mass; produce softer, more easily passed stools |
| Saline laxatives | Milk of magnesia | Work by osmotic action, drawing water through the intestinal wall to soften stool |
| Stimulant laxatives | Bisacodyl (Dulcolax) | Should not be taken within 1 hour of taking antacid or milk products |
| Suppositories | Glycerine, bisacodyl | Chill and moisten with cold water prior to insertion. |

Data from Hodgson, B.B., Kizior, R.J., & Kingdon, R.T. (1995). *Nurse's drug handbook* 1995. Philadelphia: W.B. Saunders.

pation. Table 17–3 summarizes the most commonly recommended laxatives.

## Urinary System

### Physical Changes

As a result of many changes that occur during pregnancy, the bladder of the postpartum woman has an increased capacity and has lost some of its muscle tone. Moreover, during childbirth the urethra, bladder, and tissue around the urinary meatus may become edematous and traumatized as the fetal head passes beneath the bladder. This often results in diminished sensitivity to fluid pressure, and many mothers have no sensation of needing to void even when the bladder is distended.

The bladder fills rapidly because of the diuresis that follows childbirth. As a consequence, the mother is at risk for overdistention of the bladder, incomplete emptying of the bladder, and retention of residual urine. Women who have received regional anesthesia are at particular risk for bladder distention and for difficulty voiding until feeling returns.

Urinary retention and overdistention of the bladder may cause two complications: urinary tract infection and postpartum hemorrhage. Urinary tract infection occurs when urinary stasis allows time for bacteria to multiply. Risk of postpartum hemorrhage increases because uterine ligaments, which were stretched during pregnancy, allow the uterus to be displaced upward and laterally by the full bladder. The displacement results in an inability of the uterine muscles to contract (uterine atony); this is a primary cause of excessive bleeding (Fig. 17–4).

### Chemical Changes

Both protein and acetone may be present in the urine in the first few postpartum days. Acetone suggests dehydration that often occurs during the exertion of labor. Mild proteinuria is usually the result of the catabolic processes involved in uterine involution.

## Musculoskeletal System

### Muscles and Joints

In the first 1 to 2 days following childbirth, many women experience muscle fatigue and aches, particularly of the shoulders, neck, and arms, because of exertion during labor. Warmth and gentle massage increase circulation to the area and provide comfort and relaxation.

During the first few days, levels of the hormone relaxin gradually subside, and ligaments and cartilage of the pelvis begin to return to their pre-preg-

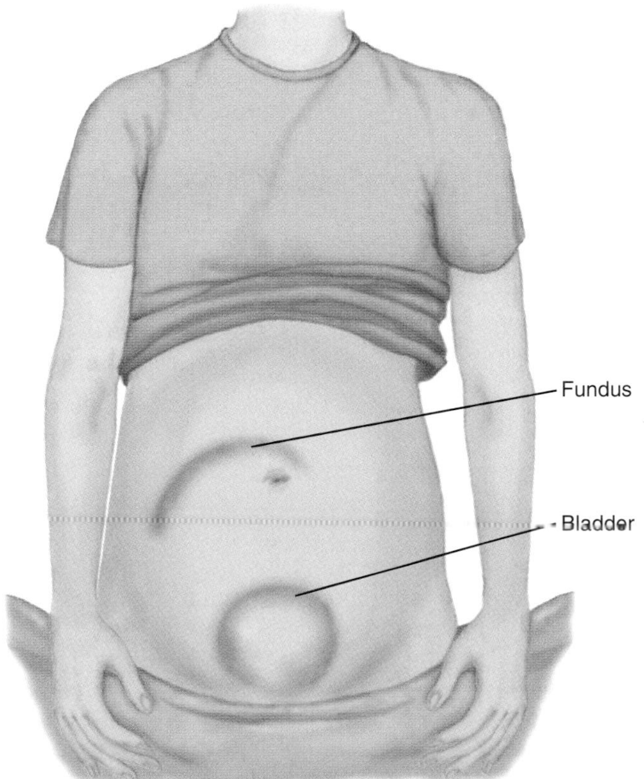


**FIGURE 17–4**

A full bladder displaces and prevents contraction of the uterus.

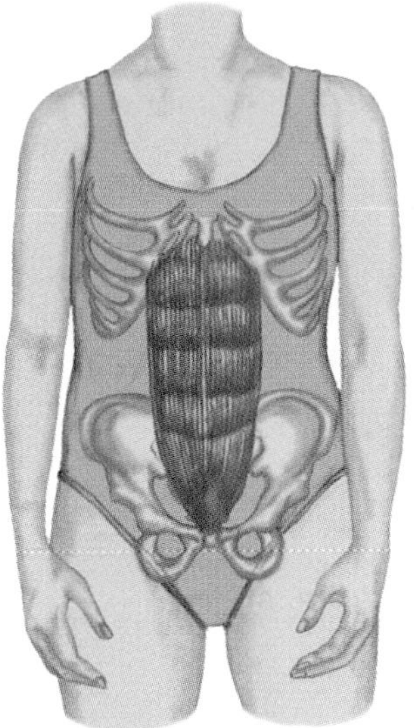
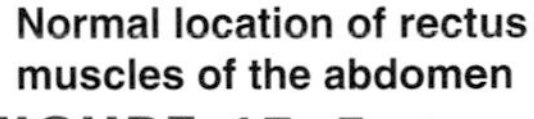
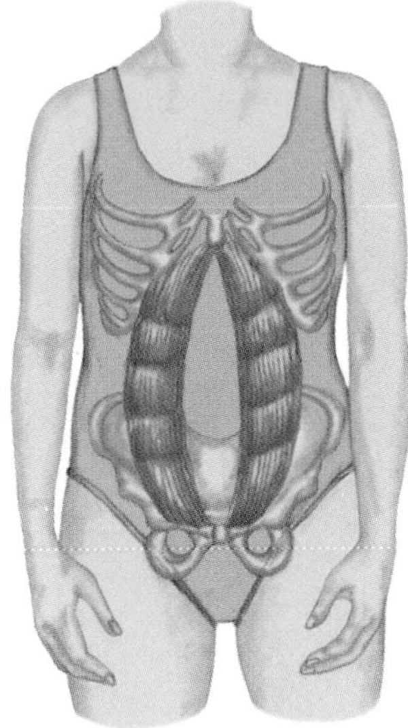


**FIGURE 17–5**

Diastasis recti occurs when the longitudinal muscles of the abdomen separate during pregnancy.

nancy position. These changes can cause hip or joint pain that interferes with ambulation and exercise. It is helpful if the mother understands that the discomfort is temporary and does not indicate a medical problem. Good body mechanics and correct posture are extremely important during this time to prevent low back pain and injury to the joints. (See Figs. 7–13 and 7–14 for correct and incorrect posture and body mechanics.)

### Abdominal Wall

During pregnancy, the abdominal walls stretch to accommodate the growing fetus, and muscle tone is diminished. Many women, expecting that the abdominal muscles will return to the pre-pregnancy condition immediately after childbirth, are dismayed to find the abdominal muscles weak, soft, and flabby.

The longitudinal muscles of the abdomen may also separate (diastasis recti) during pregnancy (Fig. 17–5). The separation may be minimal or severe. The mother may benefit from special exercises to strengthen the abdominal wall. Figure 17–6 illustrates exercises that help to correct diastasis recti.

## Integumentary System

Many skin changes that occur during pregnancy are caused by an increase in hormones; when the hormone levels decline following childbirth, the skin gradually reverts to the pre-pregnancy state. For example, levels of melanocyte-stimulating hormone, which caused hyperpigmentation during pregnancy, decrease rapidly after childbirth, and pigmentation begins to recede. This change is particularly noticeable when the "mask of pregnancy" (*chloasma*) and linea nigra disappear. In addition, spider nevi and palmar erythema, which may develop during pregnancy as a result of increased estrogen levels, gradually disappear.

Striae gravidarum (stretch marks), which develop during pregnancy when connective tissue in the abdomen and breasts is stretched, gradually fade to silvery lines but do not disappear.

## Neurologic System

Many women experience discomfort and fatigue following childbirth. Afterpains, discomfort from episiotomy or incisions, muscle aches, and breast engorgement may contribute to a woman's discomfort and inability to sleep. Anesthesia or analgesia may produce temporary neurologic changes such as lack of feeling in the legs and dizziness. During this time, prevention of injury that could occur as a result of falling is the priority.

Complaints of headache require careful assessment. Although they are uncommon, postpuncture

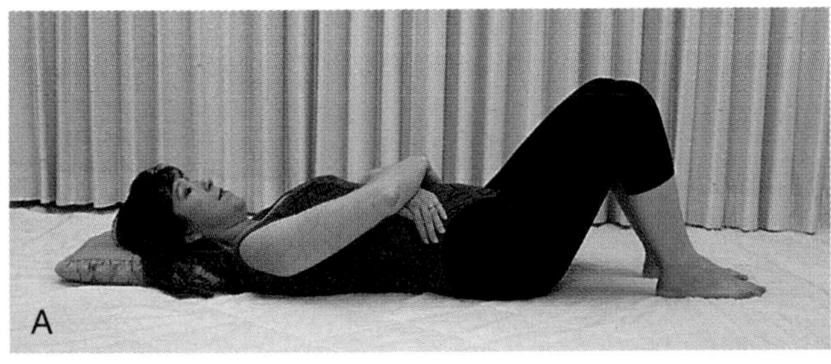

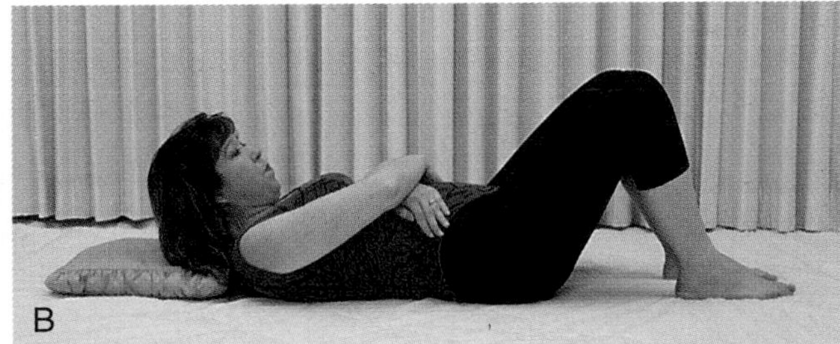


**FIGURE 17–6**

Abdominal exercises for diastasis recti. A, The woman inhales and supports the abdominal wall firmly with her hands. B, Exhaling, the woman raises her head as she pulls the abdominal muscles together.

headaches following regional anesthesia may occur. They may be most severe when the woman is in an upright position and are relieved by a supine position. They should be reported to the appropriate health care provider, usually an anesthesiologist. Headache, along with blurred vision, photophobia, and abdominal pain, may also indicate development or worsening of pregnancy-induced hypertension. See Chapter 25 for a more complete description of the assessments and care for pregnancy-induced hypertension.

## Endocrine System

Following expulsion of the placenta, a fairly rapid decline occurs in placental hormones such as estrogen, progesterone, human placental lactogen, and human chorionic gonadotropin. Adrenal hormones, such as aldosterone, return to pre-pregnancy levels. If the mother is not breastfeeding, the pituitary hormone prolactin, which stimulates milk secretion, disappears in about 2 weeks.

### Resumption of Ovulation and Menstruation

Most nonnursing mothers resume menstruation within 7 to 9 weeks after childbirth, although times vary widely. Of these women, approximately one half ovulate during the first cycle (Resnik, 1994).

Breastfeeding delays return of both ovulation and menstruation. The length of the delay depends on the duration of lactation and the frequency of breastfeeding. Women who breastfeed for less than 28 days ovulate at approximately the same time as nonnursing mothers. The longer the period of lactation, the longer the average time to the first menstrual period. Women who breastfeed six or more times daily are also likely to ovulate and menstruate later than women who breastfeed less often.

Most lactating women resume menstruation within 12 weeks, although a few do not menstruate for the entire lactation period. Breastfeeding is not an effective form of contraception because ovulation may occur before menstrual cycles are established.

### Lactation

During pregnancy, estrogen and progesterone prepare the breasts for lactation. Although prolactin levels also rise during pregnancy, lactation is inhibited at this time by the high levels of estrogen and progesterone. Following expulsion of the placenta, levels of estrogen and progesterone decline rapidly, and prolactin initiates milk production within 2 to 3 days following childbirth. Once milk production is established, it continues because of frequent removal of milk from the breast. That is, the more the infant nurses, the more milk the mother produces.

Whereas prolactin is essential for initiating milk production, oxytocin is necessary for milk ejection or "let down." Oxytocin is a hormone from the posterior pituitary gland that causes milk to be expressed from the alveoli into the lactiferous ducts during suckling. The process of lactation and measures to aid in breastfeeding are described in detail in Chapter 22.

### Weight Loss

Approximately 5.5 kg (12 pounds) are lost during childbirth. This includes the weight of the fetus, placenta, and amniotic fluid and blood lost during the birth. An additional 4 kg (8.8 pounds) is lost during the first 2 weeks following childbirth. This includes the weight lost by diuresis and diaphoresis during the first few postpartum days as well as weight lost as the reproductive organs undergo the process of involution (Cunningham et al., 1997).

Adipose (fatty) tissue that was gained during pregnancy to meet the energy requirements of breastfeeding is not lost initially, and the usual rate of loss is quite slow. Most women approach their pre-pregnancy weight about 6 months after childbirth; however, it may be a year before all weight is lost. This may be frustrating for many mothers, who desire an immediate return to pre-pregnancy weight. Nurses must be prepared to provide information about diet and exercise that will produce an acceptable weight loss but does not deplete the energy or impair the health of the mother. See Chapter 9 for additional information about weight loss and dietary recommendations.

**✓ CHECK YOUR READING**

5. Why is the mother at risk for urinary retention? Which two complications may result?
6. Why does hyperpigmentation decrease following childbirth?
7. How does breastfeeding affect the resumption of ovulation and menstruation?
8. How is lactation suppressed when the mother elects not to breastfeed (see p. 453)?

## Postpartum Assessments

Providing essential, cost-effective postpartum care to new families is a challenge for maternity nurses. Legislation now mandates that a longer length of stay (LOS) be allowed than the 24-hour stay that was previously allowed by many insurance companies. However, the trend for early discharge continues. Women with an uncomplicated vaginal birth generally leave the birth facility within 48 hours. Those who gave birth by cesarean remain in the facility for 96 hours.

Although the LOS is short, the family's need for care and information remains the same. This causes nurses a great deal of concern for families who are discharged without adequate preparation or support. Nurses are actively involved in developing ways to provide continuing care in the home. Moreover, they use innovative measures, such as clinical pathways, to structure assessments and care during the hours following childbirth.

## Clinical Pathways

Many institutions use clinical pathways (also called critical pathways, care maps, or multidisciplinary action plans) to provide necessary care while reducing the LOS. Clinical pathways identify expected outcomes and establish time frames for specific assessments and interventions that prepare the mother and infant for discharge. The clinical pathway is a guideline and documentation tool. It does not teach students how to perform assessments or care. Nor does it identify normal values or exact teaching that must be done. Therefore, students and nurses who are new to perinatal nursing must accumulate a fund of information about the postpartum period before they can use clinical pathways independently. Moreover, they must also be prepared to identify nursing diagnoses and to plan nursing interventions when mothers and infants do not move along the pathway at the expected rate. See Figure 17–7 for an example of a clinical pathway for normal spontaneous vaginal birth.

## Initial Assessments

*Because of the high risk for coming into contact with body fluids (colostrum, breast milk, amniotic fluid, and lochia from the mother as well as urine, stool, and blood from the infant), when caring for postpartum patients, the recommendations of the Centers for Disease Control and Prevention for standard blood and body fluid precautions must be maintained diligently (see Appendix A).*

Postpartum assessments begin during the fourth stage of labor (1 to 2 hours following childbirth). During this time the mother is examined to determine whether she is physically stable. Initial assessments include the following:

- Vital signs
- Skin color
- Location and firmness of the fundus
- Amount and color of lochia
- Presence and location of pain
- Intravenous infusions (type of fluid and rate)
- Added medications (type and amount)
- Patency of intravenous line
- Intravenous site for redness, pain, or edema
- Time and amount of last voiding
- Presence of urinary catheter
- Level of feeling and ability to move if regional anesthesia was administered

## Chart Review

When the initial assessments confirm that the mother's physical condition is stable, nurses should review the chart to obtain pertinent information and to determine if factors are present that increase the risk of complications during the postpartum period. Relevant information includes the following:

- Gravida, parity
- Time and type of delivery (use of forceps, vacuum extractor)
- Anesthesia or medications administered during labor
- Significant medical and surgical history, such as diabetes, heart disease, or hypertension
- Medications routinely taken and reasons why they are needed
- Food and drug allergies
- Chosen method of infant feeding
- Condition of the baby
- Perineum for episiotomy or lacerations

Laboratory data are also examined. Of particular interest are the prenatal hemoglobin and hematocrit values, the blood type and Rh factor, hepatitis B surface antigen, and a syphilis screen.

**Need for $Rh_0$(D) Immune Globulin.** Prenatal and neonatal records are checked to determine whether $Rh_0$(D) immune globulin should be administered. $Rh_0$(D) immune globulin may be necessary if the mother is Rh-negative and the newborn is Rh-positive. *$Rh_0$(D) immune globulin should be administered within 72 hours after childbirth to prevent the development of maternal antibodies that would affect subsequent pregnancies.* (See also Chapter 25 for a discussion of maternal-fetal Rh incompatibility.)

**Need for Rubella Vaccine.** A prenatal rubella antibody screen is done on each pregnant woman to determine if she is immune to rubella. If she is not immune, rubella vaccine is offered following childbirth to prevent her from acquiring rubella during subsequent pregnancies, when it can cause serious fetal anomalies. Rubella vaccine is a live virus that can produce serious consequences for the fetus if the mother becomes pregnant soon after it is administered. Before administration, some agencies require that she sign a statement indicating that she under-

CARELINE:

**LONG BEACH MEMORIAL MEDICAL CENTER**
**MULTIDISCIPLINARY ACTION PLAN**

MAP Coordinator: ____________
DRG: 373 DIAGNOSIS: Vaginal Birth Without Complications
EST. LOS: ____ M.D. ____________

| RECOVERY PERIOD (Birthcare Center) | | BY END OF 3rd HR PP & END OF 1st BABY VISIT | BY END OF 2nd SHIFT AFTER ADMISSION | BY END OF 3rd SHIFT | DISCHARGE SHIFT |
|---|---|---|---|---|---|
| ☐ VS WNL<br>Post del: ☐ bladder not full,<br>☐ fundus midline at correct level, ☐ lochia WNL,<br>☐ moving legs, ☐ minimal discomfort, ☐ breast feeds if desired | **PATIENT OUTCOMES** | ☐ VS WNL<br>☐ OB checks WNL<br>☐ Adequate pain relief<br>☐ Able to stand/walk w/out leg weakness/ fainting<br>☐ Bladder empty after void<br>Demo: ☐ pericare, ☐ infant positioning<br>☐ Verbalize involution | ☐ VS WNL<br>☐ OB checks WNL<br>☐ Adequate pain relief<br>☐ Ambulates w/out assist<br>☐ Bladder empty with each void<br>☐ H&H WNL | ☐ Return demo: newborn char., diaper change, feeding, circ. care, sitz bath | ☐ Able to care for self & baby with minimal assist |
| Post del: ☐ OB check Q 15 min. (incl VS)<br>☐ Assessment of motor/ sensory function post epidural | **VS/CRITICAL ASSESSMENTS** | ☐ VS Q 1° x 3<br>☐ OB check Q 1° x 3<br>☐ Educational needs assessment | ☐ VS Q shift<br>☐ OB checks Q shift | ☐ VS Q shift<br>☐ OB checks Q shift | ☐ VS Q shift |
| | **CONSULTS** | | ☐ MSW as needed<br>☐ Lactation Specialist as needed | ☐ MSW as needed<br>☐ Lactation Specialist as needed | |
| ☐ H&H, ☐ T&S before del.,<br>☐ VDRL, $HBSA_g$, Rubella on prenatal record or drawn | **DIAGNOSTIC TESTS** | ☐ H&H, T&S results in chart | ☐ PP H&H done if AM | | |
| ☐ Pericare<br>☐ Ice pack to perineum | **TREATMENT/ INTERVENTION** | ☐ Apply bra | | ☐ Sitz bath (if ordered) | ☐ Sitz bath (if ordered) |

✓ Indicates achievement of outcome/performace or intervention.
• Indicates an unachieved outcome or intervention not performed.
▫ Indicates an intervention that was not applicable.

This document is not a permanent part of the record.
When MAP is complete/patient discharged, remove from record and send to MAP Coordinator.

**FIGURE 17–7**

Clinical pathway for uncomplicated vaginal birth. Note outcomes and the recommended time frame for assessments and interventions. (Courtesy of Long Beach Memorial Medical Center, Long Beach, California.)

CARELINE:

**LONG BEACH MEMORIAL MEDICAL CENTER**
**MULTIDISCIPLINARY ACTION PLAN**

**Vaginal Birth Without Complications**

| RECOVERY PERIOD (Birthcare Center) | | BY END OF 3rd HR PP & END OF 1st BABY VISIT | BY END OF 2nd SHIFT AFTER ADMISSION | BY END OF 3rd SHIFT | DISCHARGE SHIFT |
|---|---|---|---|---|---|
| ☐ Pitocin added to IV<br>☐ Analgesic prn | **MEDICATIONS** | ☐ Pitocin may be D/C'd<br>☐ Analgesic prn<br>☐ Stool softener/laxative<br>☐ PNV<br>☐ Perineal meds | ☐ Analgesic prn<br>☐ Stool softener/laxative<br>☐ PNV<br>☐ Perineal meds | ☐ RhoGAM/rubella prn<br>☐ Stool softener/laxative<br>☐ PNV<br>☐ Perineal meds | ☐ RhoGAM/rubella prn<br>☐ Rx given to take home or filled in OP Pharm |
| ☐ Transfer to PP via gurney or w/c | **ACTIVITY** | ☐ Assit amb x 1 (☐ x 2 if post-epidural)<br>☐ Positioned for holding baby | | | |
| ☐ IV | **NUTRITION** | ☐ IV may be D/C'd<br>☐ Reg. diet | ☐ Reg. diet | ☐ IV may be D/C'd<br>☐ Reg. diet | |
| ☐ Urinates at least Q 4°<br>☐ I&O | **ELIMINATION** | ☐ Urinates at least once<br>☐ Cath prn | ☐ PP H&H done if AM | | |
| ☐ Positioning for breast-feeding (if baby to breast in BCC) | **PATIENT/FAMILY EDUCATION** | ☐ Teach peri-care<br>☐ Assist with infant feeding, burping<br>☐ Support parent/infant bonding | ☐ Initiate maternal/newborn education<br>☐ Record/teach infant care (cord, bath, diaper) | ☐ Completion of maternal-newborn education<br>☐ Record physician's discharge instructions | |
| ☐ Transfer to PP unit | **DISCHARGE PLANNING** | | | | ☐ Provide follow-up instructions<br>☐ Schedule home visit plan |
| | **BEHAVIORAL** | ☐ Bonding behaviors observed | ☐ Bonding behaviors observed | ☐ Bonding behaviors observed | ☐ Bonding behaviors observed |

✓ Indicates achievement of outcome/performace or intervention.
• Indicates an unachieved outcome or intervention not performed.
▫ Indicates an intervention that was not applicable.

This document is not a permanent part of the record.
When MAP is complete/patient discharged, remove from record and send to MAP Coordinator.

**FIGURE 17–7** *Continued*

## Critical to Remember
### POSTPARTUM HIGH-RISK FACTORS

**Hemorrhage**

- Multiparity (greater than 3)
- Overdistention of the uterus (large baby, twins, hydramnios)
- Precipitous labor (less than 3 hours)
- Retained placenta
- Placenta previa or abruptio placentae
- Induction or augmentation of labor
- Administration of tocolytics to stop uterine contractions
- Operative procedures (vacuum extraction, forceps, cesarean birth)

**Infection**

- Operative procedures (cesarean birth, forceps, vacuum extraction)
- Multiple cervical examinations
- Prolonged labor (>24 hours)
- Manual extraction of placenta
- Diabetes
- Indwelling catheter
- Anemia (hemoglobin <10 mg/dl)

stands the risks of becoming pregnant again within 3 months following the injection.

**Risk Factors for Hemorrhage and Infection.** Nurses must be aware of conditions that increase the risk of *hemorrhage* and *infection*, the two most common complications of the puerperium. See Critical to Remember: Postpartum High-Risk Factors.

## Focus Assessments Following Vaginal Birth

Nurses perform postpartum assessments according to facility protocol or as follows:

- First hour: every 15 minutes
- Second hour: every 30 minutes
- First 24 hours: every 4 hours
- After 24 hours: every 8 hours (Bond, 1993).

Although assessments vary, depending on the particular problems experienced by the mother, in general a focus assessment for a vaginal delivery includes the fundus, lochia, bladder elimination, perineum, vital signs, breasts, and lower extremities. The assessment for women whose infants were born vaginally differs from that performed for postcesarean mothers. (See p. 447 for the more complete assessment required for cesarean birth.)

### FUNDUS

The fundus should be assessed for consistency and location. It should be firmly contracted and at or near the level of the umbilicus. If the uterus is above the expected level or is shifted from the midline position (usually to the right), the bladder may be distended. The location of the fundus should be rechecked after the woman has emptied her bladder. Procedure 17–1 illustrates how to locate and palpate the fundus. If the fundus is difficult to locate or is soft or "boggy," the nurse stimulates the uterine muscle to contract by gently massaging the uterus. *The nondominant hand must support and anchor the lower uterine segment if it is necessary to massage an uncontracted uterus. Uterine massage is not necessary if the uterus is firmly contracted.*

The uterus can contract only if it is free of intrauterine clots. To expel clots, the nurse must support the lower uterine segment as described earlier and as illustrated in Procedure 17–1. This support prevents inversion of the uterus (turning inside out) when the nurse applies firm pressure downward toward the vagina to express clots that have collected in the uterus. Nurses should observe the perineum for the number and size of clots expelled. Table 17–4 describes normal and abnormal findings of the uterine fundus and includes follow-up nursing actions for abnormal findings. The Critical Thinking

**TABLE 17–4 OBSERVATIONS OF THE UTERINE FUNDUS REQUIRING NURSING ACTIONS**

| Normal Findings | Abnormal Findings | Nursing Actions |
|---|---|---|
| Fundus firmly contracted | Fundus soft, "boggy," uncontracted, or difficult to locate | Support lower uterine segment; massage until firm |
| Fundus remains contracted when massage is discontinued | Fundus becomes soft and uncontracted when massage is stopped | Continue to support lower uterine segment; massage until firm and apply pressure to fundus to express clots that may be accumulating in uterus; notify health care provider and begin oxytocin administration, as prescribed, to maintain a firm fundus |
| Fundus located at level of umbilicus and midline | Fundus above umbilicus and/or displaced from midline | Assess bladder elimination; assist mother in urinating or catheterize, if necessary, to empty bladder |

Procedure 17–1

## Assessing the Uterine Fundus

**PURPOSE:** To determine the location and firmness of the uterus.

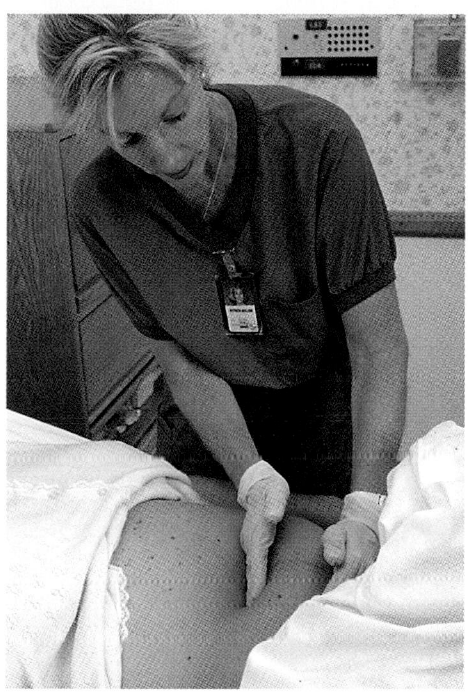

1. **Explain the procedure and rationale for each step before beginning the procedure.** *Reduces anxiety and elicits cooperation.*

2. **Have the mother empty her bladder if she has not voided recently.** *A distended bladder lifts and displaces the uterus.*

3. **Place the mother in a supine position with her knees slightly flexed.** *Relaxes the abdominal muscles and permits accurate location of the fundus.*

4. **Put on clean gloves, and lower the perineal pads to observe lochia as the fundus is palpated.** *Gloves are recommended whenever the possibility exists of coming into contact with body fluids.*

5. **Place your nondominant hand above the woman's symphysis pubis.** *Supports and anchors the lower uterine segment during palpation or massage of the fundus.*

6. **Use the flat part of your fingers (not the fingertips) for palpation** (see illustration). *The larger surface provides more comfort; palpation is essential, but it may be painful, particularly for the mother who had a cesarean birth; locating the fundus is more difficult if the woman is obese or if the abdomen is distended.*

7. **Begin palpation at the umbilicus, and palpate gently until the fundus is located. Notice how the hand "cups" the uterus to determine firmness and location of the fundus. The fundus should be firm, in midline, and approximately at the level of the umbilicus.** *The most common cause of uterine displacement is a distended bladder, which lifts the uterus and promotes uterine atony (loss of muscle tone) that could result in excessive bleeding.*

8. **If the fundus is difficult to locate or is soft or "boggy," keep your nondominant hand above the woman's symphysis pubis and massage the fundus with your dominant hand until the fundus is firm.** *The nondominant hand anchors the lower segment of the uterus and prevents trauma while the uterus is massaged. The uterus contracts in response to tactile stimulation; contraction is essential to control excessive bleeding.*

9. **Document the consistency and location of the fundus. Consistency is recorded as "fundus firm," "firm with massage," or "boggy." Fundal height is recorded in fingerbreadths above or below the umbilicus. For example, "fundus firm, midline, U−2" (two fingerbreadths below umbilicus). As another example, "fundus firm with light massage, U+2" (two fingerbreadths above umbilicus), displaced to right.** *Promotes accurate communication and identifies deviations from expected so that potential problems can be identified early.*

Exercise describes a woman at risk for excessive bleeding (p. 443).

Drugs are sometimes needed to maintain contraction of the uterus and thus to prevent postpartum hemorrhage. The most commonly used drugs are methylergonovine (Methergine) and oxytocin (Pitocin) (see Table 17–5). In addition, a drug guide for methylergonovine is presented on page 785 and for oxytocin on page 398.

### LOCHIA

Important assessments include the amount, color, and odor of lochia. Nurses observe the amount and color of lochia on peripads and while checking the perineum. They also watch vaginal discharge while palpating or massaging the fundus so that the amount of lochia as well as the number and size of any clots expressed during these procedures can be observed. Refer to Figure 17–2 for criteria to determine the amount of lochia and to Table 17–1 for the normal characteristics of lochia as well as abnormal observations that must be reported. Note these important guidelines:

- A constant trickle of lochia indicates excessive bleeding and requires immediate attention.

**TABLE 17–5 COMMONLY USED DRUGS DURING THE POSTPARTUM PERIOD**

| Indications | Usual Dosage | Nursing Considerations |
|---|---|---|
| **Methylergonovine Maleate (Methergine)** | | |
| Prevention and treatment of hemorrhage due to uterine atony | 0.2 mg IM or p.o. q 6–12 hr | Monitor and record blood pressure, pulse rate, and uterine response; report any sudden change in vital signs, continued uterine relaxation, or excessive lochia. |
| **Oxytocin (Pitocin, Syntocinon)** | | |
| Reduction of bleeding after expulsion of the placenta | 10–40 units in 1000 ml of 5% dextrose in normal saline solution IV at a rate to control bleeding (usually 20 to 40 mU/minute, or 10 units IM) | Administer by infusion, not by bolus (a concentrated mass); monitor and record uterine contraction, heart rate, and blood pressure every 15 minutes; assess and record amount of lochia. |
| **Simethecone (Mylicon)** | | |
| Flatulence, abdominal distention | Chewable tablets 40–80 mg after each meal and at bedtime | Assess for bowel activity, relief of distention. |
| **Ibuprofen (Motrin, Advil)** | | |
| Mild to moderate pain | 400 mg p.o. q 4–6 hr | Assess for nausea, vomiting, diarrhea. |
| **Acetaminophen (Tylenol, Panadol)** | | |
| Mild to moderate pain | 325–650 mg p.o. q 4–6 hr | Side effects rare; assess for allergic reaction, such as skin rash. |
| **Percocet (325 mg Acetaminophen and 5 mg Oxycodone)** | | |
| Moderate pain | 1–2 tablets p.o. q 4 hr | Determine sensitivity to acetaminophen or oxycodone; observe for signs of respiratory depression; do not administer with sedatives. |
| **Empirin No. 3 (325 mg of Aspirin with 30 mg Codeine)** | | |
| Moderate pain | 1–2 tablets q 4 hr | Assess for sensitivity to aspirin or codeine; administer with food to prevent gastric upset. |
| **$Rh_0$(D) Immune Globulin (RhoGAM, Gamulin Rh, HypRho-D)** | | |
| Prevention of sensitization to Rh factor in Rh-negative mothers who gave birth to Rh-positive infants | One vial IM within 72 hr following childbirth | Confirm that administration is necessary; check with second licensed personnel that medication is cross-matched for the specific woman. |
| **Rubella Virus Vaccine, Live (Meruvax II)** | | |
| To stimulate active immunity against rubella virus | Single-dose vial; administer SC in outer aspect of upper arm | Advise the mother to avoid pregnancy for 3 months; signed informed consent usually required; do not administer if mother is sensitive to neomycin or if she has had a transfusion within the last 3 months. |

*Abbreviations:* q, every; p.o., orally (per os); IM, intramuscularly; IV, intravenously; mU, milliunit; SC, subcutaneously.

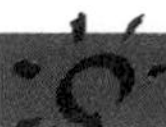

### CRITICAL THINKING EXERCISE

Linda Welker, a 22-year-old multipara, was admitted from the labor, delivery, and recovery unit 2 hours following the birth of an 8-pound (3600 g) baby boy. Her fundus is firm, located three fingerbreadths above the umbilicus, and displaced to the right; her perineal pads, which were changed just before transfer, are saturated.

**Q:**

1. What do these data suggest? Why?
2. What nursing action should be taken first? What follow-up assessments are necessary?
3. Why is it necessary to remind and assist Linda to void?

**A:**

1. The birth of a large infant increases the risk of postpartum hemorrhage. Saturation of pads in a short time suggests excessive bleeding. Location of the fundus above the umbilicus and displaced to the side indicates that the cause of excessive bleeding might be a distended bladder.
2. Assisting the mother to void is the most appropriate nursing action. If, after voiding, the fundus is located at the level of the umbilicus and firmly contracted, the nurse can be relatively certain that the cause of the bleeding was a distended bladder, which made it difficult for the uterus to contract firmly.

   The location and consistency of the uterus, amount of lochia, blood pressure, and pulse should be assessed frequently so that further excessive bleeding can be controlled.
3. Linda does not experience the urge to void because the bladder has not regained the muscle tone lost during pregnancy and the sensitivity to pressure is decreased.

- Excessive lochia in the presence of a contracted uterus suggests lacerations of the birth canal, and the health care provider must be notified so that the laceration can be located and repaired.

The odor of lochia is usually described as "fleshy," "earthy," or "musty." A foul odor suggests endometrial infection, and assessments should be made for additional signs of infection. These signs include maternal fever, tachycardia, and uterine tenderness and pain.

Absence of lochia, like the presence of a foul odor, may also indicate infection. Lochia may be scant, particularly if the birth was cesarean when the cavity of the uterus was wiped by sponges, removing some of the endometrial lining; however, lochia should not be entirely absent.

#### BLADDER ELIMINATION

Because the mother may not experience the urge to void even if the bladder is full, nurses must rely on physical assessment to determine whether the bladder is distended. Bladder distention often produces an obvious or palpable bulge that feels like a soft, movable mass above the symphysis pubis. Other signs include an upward and lateral displacement of the uterine fundus and increased lochia. Frequent voidings of less than 150 ml suggest urinary retention with overflow. Signs of an empty bladder include a firm fundus in the midline and a nonpalpable bladder. Critical to Remember: Signs of a Distended Bladder lists other signs.

Some facilities measure the first two voidings to determine whether normal bladder function has returned. When the mother can void at least 300 to 400 ml, the bladder is usually empty. Regardless of the amount voided, however, the fundus must be assessed to confirm that the bladder is empty. Subjective symptoms of urgency, frequency, or dysuria suggest urinary tract infection and should be reported to the health care provider.

#### PERINEUM

The acronym REEDA is used as a reminder that the site of an episiotomy or a perineal laceration should be assessed for five signs: redness (R), edema (E), ecchymosis (bruising) (E), discharge (D), and approximation (A) (the edges of the wound should be close, as though stuck or glued together).

Redness of the wound may indicate the usual inflammatory response to injury. If accompanied by pain or tenderness, however, it may indicate the beginning of localized infection. Ecchymosis or edema indicates soft tissue damage that can delay healing. There should be no discharge from the wound. Rapid healing necessitates that the edges of the wound be closely approximated. Procedure 17–2 describes the perineal examination.

#### VITAL SIGNS

**Blood Pressure.** Blood pressure varies with position, and to obtain accurate results it should be measured with the mother in the same position each

### *Critical to Remember*

#### SIGNS OF A DISTENDED BLADDER

- Location of fundus above *baseline* level, which is obtained when the bladder is empty
- Fundus displaced from midline
- Excessive lochia
- Bladder discomfort
- Bulge of bladder above symphysis
- Frequent voidings of less than 150 ml of urine, which indicates urinary retention with overflow

Procedure 17-2

## Assessing the Perineum

**PURPOSE:** To observe perineal trauma and the state of healing.

1. **Provide privacy, and explain the purpose of the procedure.** *Elicits cooperation and reduces anxiety about the procedure.*
2. **Put on clean gloves.** *Implement standard precautions to provide protection from possible contact with body fluids.*
3. **Ask the mother to assume a Sims position and flex her upper leg. Lower the perineal pads and lift her superior buttocks. If necessary, use a flashlight to inspect the perineal area.** *Position provides an unobstructed view of the perineum; light allows better visualization.*
4. **Note the extent and location of edema or bruising.** *Extensive bruising or asymmetric edema may indicate formation of a hematoma. (See also Chapter 28.)*
5. **Examine the episiotomy or laceration for redness, ecchymosis, edema, discharge, and approximation (REEDA).** *Redness, edema, or discharge may indicate infection of the wound; extensive bruising may delay healing; wound edges must be in direct contact for uncomplicated healing to occur.*
6. **Note the number and size of hemorrhoids.** *Swollen, painful hemorrhoids interfere with activity and bowel elimination.*

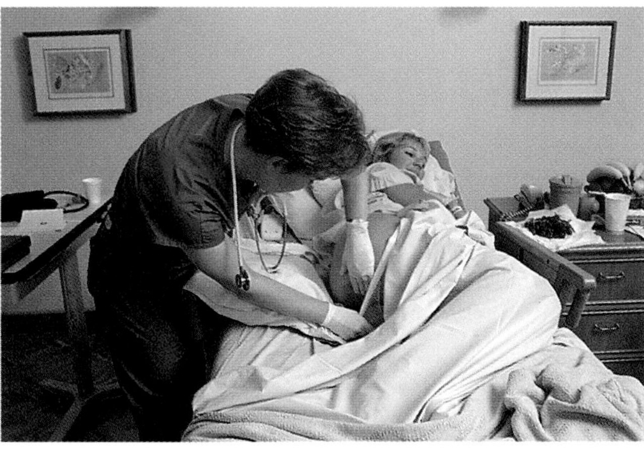

time. Therefore, nurses must document both the mother's position when taking blood pressure and the pressure obtained. Postpartum blood pressure should be compared with that of the predelivery period so that deviations from the parameters that are normal for the mother can be quickly identified. An increase from the baseline suggests pregnancy-induced hypertension; a decrease may indicate dehydration or hypovolemia resulting from excessive bleeding.

**Orthostatic Hypotension.** After birth, a rapid decrease in intra-abdominal pressure results in dilation of blood vessels supplying the viscera. The resulting engorgement of abdominal blood vessels contributes to a rapid fall in blood pressure of 15 to 20 mmHg when the woman moves from a recumbent to a sitting position. As a result of the sudden drop in blood pressure, mothers often say that they feel dizzy or lightheaded, or they faint when they stand. The nursing diagnosis Risk for Injury applies to women with orthostatic hypotension. (See Nursing Care Plan 17–1 for application of this nursing diagnosis.)

Hypotension may also indicate hypovolemia. Careful assessments for hemorrhage (location and firmness of the fundus, amount of lochia, pulse rate for tachycardia) should be made if the postpartum blood pressure is significantly less than the prenatal baseline blood pressure.

**Pulse.** Bradycardia, defined as a pulse rate of 50 to 60 per minute, is expected and reflects the large amount of blood that returns to the central circulation following delivery of the placenta. The increase in central circulation results in increased stroke volume and allows a slower heart rate to provide adequate maternal circulation.

Tachycardia may indicate excitement, fatigue, dehydration, hypovolemia, or infection. If tachycardia is noted, additional assessments should include blood pressure, location and firmness of the uterus, amount of lochia, estimated blood loss at delivery, hemoglobin, and hematocrit values. The objective of the additional assessments is to rule out excessive bleeding and to intervene at once if hemorrhage is suspected.

**Respirations.** A normal respiratory rate of 16 to 20 per minute should be maintained. It is not necessary to assess breath sounds if the mother has had a normal vaginal delivery, is ambulatory, and is without signs of respiratory distress. Breath sounds should always be auscultated if the birth has been cesarean, if the mother is a smoker, if she has a history of frequent or recent upper respiratory infections, or if she has a history of asthma.

**Temperature.** A temperature of 38°C (100.4°F) is common during the first 24 hours following childbirth and may be caused by dehydration or normal postpartum leukocytosis. If the elevated temperature persists for longer than 24 hours or if it exceeds 38°C, infection should be suspected and the fever reported to the physician or nurse-midwife.

### BREASTS

For the first day or two after delivery, the breasts should be soft and nontender. After that, breast changes depend largely on whether the mother is breastfeeding or is taking measures to prevent lactation. The breasts should be examined even if she chooses formula feeding because the breasts may become engorged despite preventive measures. The size, symmetry, and shape of the breasts should be observed. Some mothers need reassurance that breast size has no relationship to successful breastfeeding. The skin should be inspected for dimpling or thickening, which, although rare, can indicate breast tumor.

The areola and nipple should be carefully examined for potential problems such as flat or retracted nipples; these problems sometimes make breastfeeding more difficult. Signs of nipple trauma (redness, blisters, or fissures) are often noted during the first days of breastfeeding, especially if the mother needs assistance in positioning the infant correctly. (For full details, see Chapter 22.)

The breasts should be palpated for firmness and tenderness, which indicate increased vascular and lymphatic circulation that may precede milk production. The breasts may feel "lumpy" as various lobes begin to produce milk.

The breast assessment is an excellent opportunity to provide information or reassurance about breast care and breastfeeding techniques.

#### LOWER EXTREMITIES

The legs are examined for signs or symptoms of thrombophlebitis. These indications include localized areas of redness, heat, edema, and tenderness. Pedal pulses may be obstructed by thrombophlebitis and should be palpated with each assessment.

#### HOMANS' SIGN

Discomfort in the calf with sharp dorsiflexion of the foot (Fig. 17–8) may indicate deep vein thrombosis. Although the sign is of limited value (Cunningham et al., 1997), it continues to be part of the assessment of the lower extremities in the postpartum period. A negative Homans' sign indicates the absence of discomfort. A positive Homans' sign indicates the presence of discomfort and should be reported to the physician or nurse-midwife.

#### EDEMA AND DEEP TENDON REFLEXES

Pedal or pretibial edema may be present for the first day or two, until excess interstitial fluid is remobilized and excreted. Figure 17–9 shows how to assess for pitting edema.

Deep tendon reflexes should be 1+ to 2+. Report brisker-than-average and hyperactive reflexes (3+ to 4+), which suggest pregnancy-induced hypertension. The reflexes are defined as follows (Petree & Mattson, 1993):

0 = no response
1+ = low normal; somewhat diminished
2+ = average, normal
3+ = brisker than average; possible indication of disease
4+ = very brisk, hyperactive; often associated with clonus (sustained muscle contraction)

(See p. 698 for a description of how to assess deep tendon reflexes.)

#### COMFORT LEVEL

Comfort is essential to postpartum recovery; however, some new mothers are too excited by the birth of their child to complain of discomfort. Nurses must remain alert to covert signs of afterpains, perineal discomfort, and breast tenderness. Signs of discomfort include an inability to relax or sleep, a change in

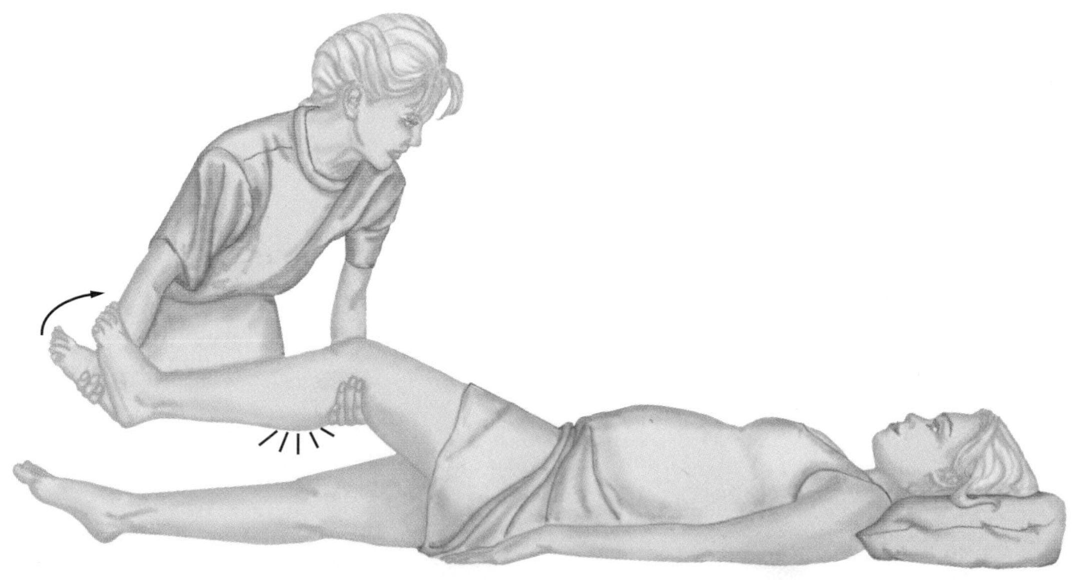

**FIGURE 17–8**

Homans' sign is positive when the mother experiences discomfort in the calf on sharp dorsiflexion of the foot.

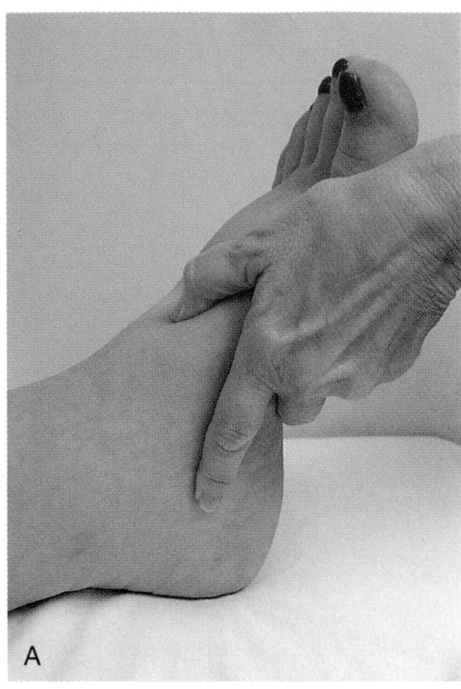


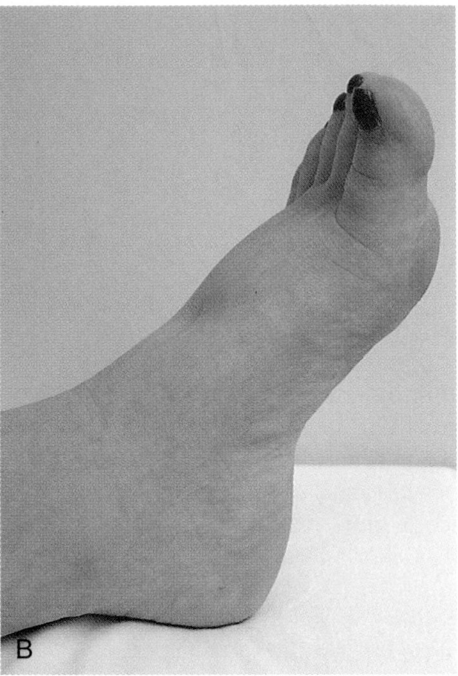


**FIGURE 17–9**

Pedal edema. A, Apply pressure to foot. B, "Pit" appears when fluid moves into adjacent tissue and away from point of pressure.

vital signs, restlessness, irritability, and facial grimaces.

Analgesics, such as acetaminophen (Tylenol, Panadol), and nonsteroidal anti-inflammatory drugs, such as ibuprofen (Motrin, Advil) are frequently prescribed to provide relief for mild to moderate discomfort. Tylenol No. 3, Empirin No. 3, and Percocet are often prescribed for more severe discomfort. Table 17–5 lists usual dosages and nursing considerations for drugs commonly used in the postpartum period.

Adequate fluids help restore the balance altered by fluid loss during labor and the birth process. Women should be encouraged to drink approximately 3000 ml of fluids each day. If a woman is unable to tolerate oral fluids, intravenous administration may be necessary. Women are usually able to have ice chips soon after cesarean birth, and, although protocols vary, most are able to progress to a regular diet after passing flatus.

Women generally have a hearty appetite after normal childbirth, and nurses should encourage healthy food choices with respect for ethnic background. Meals and snacks should be available at all times, not only at regular mealtimes.

**CHECK YOUR READING**

9. When is uterine massage necessary? How is the uterus supported during massage?
10. What does excessive bleeding suggest when the uterus is firmly contracted?
11. What additional assessments are necessary when tachycardia is noted? Why?
12. What are the typical cause, onset, and symptoms experienced by the mother with orthostatic hypotension?

## Care in the Immediate Postpartum Period

The postpartum period is often divided into three periods. The first 24 hours is called the immediate postpartum period, the first week is referred to as the early postpartum period, and the second to the sixth week is the late period. Most mothers remain in the birth facility only during the immediate postpartum period. Care of the mother during this time focuses on the following:

- Maintaining the physiologic safety of the mother through frequent assessments described above
- Providing comfort measures
- Establishing bladder elimination
- Providing health education

### Providing Comfort Measures

**Ice Packs.** Both cold and warmth are used to alleviate perineal pain following childbirth. Ice causes vasoconstriction and is most effective if applied soon after the birth to prevent edema and to numb the area. Chemical ice packs or a glove filled with ice and tied at the cuff is often used during the first 12 hours following a vaginal birth. The ice pack is wrapped in a disposable paper before applying it to the perineum. It should be left in place until the ice melts. It is then removed for 10 minutes before a fresh pack is applied. Some peripads have cold packs incorporated in them, but they do not absorb as much lochia as other peripads.

**Perineal Care.** Perineal care consists of squirting warm water over the perineum after each voiding or bowel movement. Perineal care cleanses, provides comfort, and prevents infection of an area that often has an episiotomy or lacerations. The perineum is gently patted rather than wiped to dry.

**Topical Medications.** Anesthetic sprays decrease surface discomfort and allow more comfortable ambulation. The mother is instructed to hold the nozzle of a benzocaine spray, such as Americaine or Dermoplast, 6 to 12 inches from her body and to direct it toward the perineum. The spray should be used following perineal care and before clean pads are applied.

**Sitting.** The mother should be advised to squeeze her buttocks together before sitting and to lower her weight slowly onto her buttocks. This measure prevents stretching of the perineal tissue and avoids sharp impact on the traumatized area. Many mothers also benefit from an air cushion or "doughnut," which relieves pressure on the perineum when sitting.

**Sitz Baths.** Sitz baths, which provide continuous circulation of water, cleanse and comfort the traumatized perineum. Cool water reduces pain caused by edema and may be most effective within the first 24 hours. Warm water increases circulation and promotes healing and may be most effective after 24 hours. *Nurses must be sure that the emergency bell is within easy reach in case the mother feels faint during the sitz bath.*

**Oral and Parenteral Medications.** As described previously, mothers should be encouraged to take prescribed medications for afterpains and perineal discomfort.

### Promoting Bladder Elimination

Many new mothers have difficulty voiding because of edema and trauma of the perineum as well as diminished sensitivity to fluid pressure in the bladder. As soon as they are able to ambulate safely, mothers should be assisted to the bathroom. It is important to provide privacy and to allow adequate time for the first voiding. Moreover, nurses can use a variety of measures to promote relaxation of the perineal muscles and to stimulate the sensation of needing to void. Some of the most common measures include the following:

- Running water, placing the mother's hands in water, and pouring water over the vulva
- Asking the mother to blow bubbles through a straw
- Encouraging urination in the shower or sitz bath
- Providing hot tea or fluids of choice. The recommended fluid intake is at least 2500 ml per day.

*A nonpalpable bladder and a firm fundus at or below the level of the umbilicus and in the midline confirm that the bladder is empty and rule out urinary retention with overflow.*

A distended bladder lifts and displaces the uterus, making it difficult for the uterus to remain contracted. Thus, urinary retention is a major cause of uterine atony (loss of tone), which permits excessive bleeding. Moreover, stasis of urine in the bladder predisposes the woman to urinary tract infection. Therefore, the mother must be catheterized if:

- She is unable to void
- The amount voided is less than 150 ml
- The fundus is elevated or displaced from the midline

Repeated catheterizations increase the chance of urinary tract infection because bacteria may be pushed into the bladder despite scrupulous aseptic technique. To decrease the risk of infection, an indwelling catheter is usually inserted for 24 hours if catheterization is necessary for the third time.

## Nursing Care Following Cesarean Birth

The length of stay for mothers after a cesarean birth has decreased. Most now leave the hospital within 72 to 96 hours following surgery. Many facilities have developed clinical pathways or care maps that are similar to those used for uncomplicated vaginal births. The clinical pathway identifies outcomes and establishes a time frame for assessments and interventions for postcesarean mothers and their infants. Figure 17–10 shows a clinical pathway for cesarean birth. It is important to remember that pathways or care maps are guidelines only. If a problem arises, sometimes called a variance, additional assessments and interventions are necessary.

### Assessment

In addition to the usual postpartum assessments, the postcesarean mother also must be assessed as any other postoperative patient.

#### RESPIRATIONS

Many mothers receive epidural narcotics for postoperative pain relief. The analgesic effect lasts for approximately 24 hours. During this time respirations must be assessed frequently because narcotics depress the respiratory center. In some facilities an apnea monitor is used for 24 hours to detect a decreased respiratory rate. If an apnea monitor is not used, the respiratory rate and depth should be checked every 15 minutes for the first hour, every 30 minutes for 3 to 6 hours, and every 30 minutes to 1 hour for the remainder of the first 24 hours.

If the respiratory rate begins to decline or if the respiratory rate is less than 12 per minute, the nurse should do the following:

- Notify the anesthesiologist immediately.
- Elevate the head of the bed to facilitate lung expansion.
- Administer oxygen and apply a pulse oximeter to measure oxygen saturation.
- Follow facility protocol to administer narcotic antagonists, such as naloxone hydrochloride (Narcan).
- Be aware that the duration of naloxone is approximately 30 minutes and that respiratory depression may recur.
- Recognize that naloxone reduces the level of pain relief.

In addition to observing respiratory rate and depth, the mother's breath sounds should be auscultated because depressed respirations as well as a longer period of immobility allow secretions to pool in the bronchioles. To counteract this risk, the mother must be assisted to turn, cough, and expand the lungs by breathing deeply. Incentive spirometers are also used to expand the lungs and thus to prevent hypostatic pneumonia that can result from immobility and shallow, slow respirations.

#### ABDOMEN

Nurses assess gastrointestinal function by auscultating for bowel sounds until normal peristalsis is noted in all abdominal quadrants. Although paralytic ileus (lack of movement in the bowel) is rare following cesarean birth, nurses must be aware of the signs, which include abdominal distention, absent or decreased bowel sounds, and no excretion of flatus or stool.

The surgical dressing should be observed for intactness and discharge. When the dressing is removed, nurses observe the incision, which should be approximated, and use the acronym REEDA to assess for signs of infection, such as redness and edema (Fig. 17–11).

The fundus must be palpated gently because of increased discomfort caused by the uterine incision.

#### INTAKE AND OUTPUT

The intravenous infusion should be monitored for the rate of flow and the condition of the intravenous site. Any signs of infiltration, such as edema or coolness at the site, as well as signs of infection, such as edema, redness, and pain, should be reported. The amount as well as the color and clarity of urine should be monitored.

### Interventions

#### THE FIRST 24 HOURS

The mother who gave birth by cesarean is cared for as one would care for other postoperative clients.

**Overcoming Effects of Immobility.** The new mother is on bedrest for the first 8 to 12 hours. To prevent pooling of secretions in the airway, she must be helped every 2 hours to turn, cough, and breathe deeply. Splinting the abdomen with a small pillow reduces incisional discomfort when she coughs. She should be encouraged to flex her legs and to move her feet and legs frequently to improve peripheral circulation. She needs assistance to sit and to dangle her feet for the first few times.

**Providing Comfort.** Placing a pillow behind her back and one between her knees when the mother is in a side-lying position prevents strain and discomfort. Excellent physical care (oral hygiene, perineal care, a sponge bath, and clean linen) comforts and refreshes her.

Postcesarean clients differ from typical postoperative clients in three important ways. First, they are typically anxious to be alert in order to interact with their newborn infants. Second, they are concerned about the type and quantity of analgesics they receive and that they could potentially pass them on in their breast milk. Third, compared with other postoperative patients, postcesarean clients tend to desire more input and control of their care.

At one time, intramuscular injection of narcotics for postcesarean pain was common. This regimen has some limitations, such as discomfort caused by intramuscular injections, drowsiness that interferes with the mother's ability to care for the infant, and side effects such as nausea and vomiting. Periodic injections to control pain thus have been replaced in many institutions by patient-controlled analgesia, administered by continuous intravenous infusion of a low-concentration narcotic solution using a pump specifically designed for that purpose. If analgesia is insufficient, the woman can self-administer intermittent small doses of narcotic from the infusion pump.

A single dose of narcotic (usually morphine) injected into the epidural or subarachnoid space also provides 18 to 24 hours of postcesarean analgesia. Side effects of both patient-controlled analgesia and epidural narcotics include respiratory depression, itching (pruritus), nausea and vomiting, and urinary retention.

#### AFTER 24 HOURS

**Reinstating Normal Activities.** After 24 hours, several normal functions return as postcesarean women are able to participate more actively in their own care:

**Long Beach Memorial Medical Center**
**Multidisciplinary Action Plan**
**Cesarean Birth**

**Patient Problems/Nursing Diagnoses**

**Patient/Diagnosis incorporated into MAP:**

**#1 Pain R/T Childbirth**

**Potential Problems/Diagnoses (Initiate actual problems only)**

# ____ **Urinary Retention R/T** ____
**Expected Outcomes:** The patient shall regain/maintain pattern of urinary elimination as evidenced by:
____ fundus midline, <FU+2 ____ ability to void without difficulty

# ____ **Hyperthermia R/T** ____
**Expected Outcomes:** The patient shall regain/maintain near normal body temperature as evidenced by:
____ oral temperature <100°F ____ vital signs WNL

# ____ **Anxiety R/T** ____
**Expected Outcomes:** The patient/family shall relate decreased level of anxiety as evidenced by:
____ verbal communication ____ non-verbal communication

# ____ ____
Expected outcomes: ____

# ____ ____
Expected outcomes: ____

**Education Assessment**

Interpreter utilized: ☐ Yes ☐ No ☐ Interpreter Service ☐ Family ☐ Other: ____

Desire/Motivation to learn: ☐ High ☐ Medium ☐ Low

Learning method preference: ☐ Visual ☐ Explanation ☐ Demonstration ☐ Handout

**Learning needs assessment key: S–Satisfactory, N–needs education, NA–not applicable**

| **Postpartum Care** | | **Infant Care** | | **Teaching Aids** (written material, videos to be used, initial when provided) | |
|---|---|---|---|---|---|
| TCDB/splinting | ____ | Newborn characteristics | ____ | Newborn Channel | ____ |
| Pain management | ____ | Feeding TB/NTB | ____ | Infant Security | ____ |
| Pericare/Involution | ____ | Diaper changing | ____ | Newborn Screening | ____ |
| Handwashing | ____ | Bathing | ____ | Caring for Yourself & Your Baby | ____ |
| Diet | ____ | Cord care | ____ | The Art of Breastfeeding | ____ |
| Elimination | ____ | Circumcision care | ____ | California Car Seat Law | ____ |
| Activity/rest | ____ | Safety | ____ | ____ | ____ |
| Emotional concerns | ____ | ____ | ____ | ____ | ____ |
| Complications | ____ | ____ | ____ | | |
| ____ | ____ | | | | |
| ____ | ____ | | | | |

ADDRESSOGRAPH AREA

**Multidisciplinary Action Plan–Cesarean Birth**

(05/96)

**FIGURE 17–10**

Clinical pathway (care map) for cesarean birth. Note expected outcomes and time frame for length of stay (LOS) of 72 hours. (Courtesy of Memorial Women's Hospital, Long Beach Memorial Medical Center, Long Beach, California.)

*Illustration continued on following page*

**MAP: Cesarean Birth**
**Care Line: OB/GYN/Newborn**
**MAP Coordinator:** Bev Vander Wal, MN, RN
**DRG:** 371 **Estimated LOS:** 2–3 days

☐ **MAP assigned in TDS**
✔ Indicates achievement of outcome/performance of intervention
* Indicates outcome not achieved/intervention not performed
N/A Indicates intervention not applicable

| Pre-Op | | PP First 12 HRS |
|---|---|---|
| | **Date** | |
| ☐ AMU ☐ LDR ☐ 2E ☐ Pre-op ☐ 2S | **Patient Location** | ☐ LDR ☐ 2S ☐ 2E |
| ☐ Verbalizes indication for C/S<br>☐ Verbalizes understanding of procedure and anesthesia<br>☐ Consent signed<br>☐ Verbalizes plan of care | **Patient Outcomes** | ☐☐ VS WNL (temp <100) ☐☐ Dressing D/I<br>☐☐ OB checks WNL ☐☐ Alert/easily aroused<br>☐☐ UO adequate ☐☐ Moves extremities<br>☐☐ Pain controlled ☐☐ Hypoactive BS<br>☐☐ Nausea controlled ☐☐ Bonding begins |
| ☐☐ Review prenatal record<br>☐☐ Review Admission H&P | **VS/Critical Assessments** | ☐☐ VS/OB check Q 1° x 3, per protocol<br>☐☐ Bowel sounds<br>☐☐ Educational Assessment<br>☐ Postpartum care ☐ Infant care<br>☐☐ Pain Assessment |
| ☐ Social worker ☐ CNS ☐ CM<br>☐ Anesthesia ☐ NICU<br>☐ ________ | **Consults (PRN)** | ☐ Social worker ☐ CNS ☐ CM<br>☐ Lactation Specialist<br>☐ ________ |
| ☐ Antenate ☐ ________ | **Diagnostic Tests** | |
| ☐ Insert Foley catheter<br>☐ Abdominal prep/shave | **Treatment/ Intervention** | ☐☐ Turn/cough/deep breathe Q 2° ☐☐ I & O<br>☐☐ Pericare by caregiver<br>☐☐ Order breastpump, prn |
| ☐ NaCitrate 30 min before surgery<br>☐ ________ | **Medications** | ☐☐ MS epidural<br>☐☐ Demerol 50-100 IM Q 3–4°<br>☐☐ Vistaril 50 mg IM Q 4°<br>☐☐ ________<br>☐☐ Compazine 10 mg IV Q 4–6° |
| | **Functional Level** | ☐☐ Bed rest x 8° ☐☐ Turn Q 1–2°<br>☐☐ Out of bed with assist by 12 hrs<br>☐☐ Initiate breastfeeding |
| ☐☐ NPO x 8° before surgery<br>☐☐ IV RL/D5RL © 125 cc/hr<br>☐☐ 1000 cc RL pre-epidural | **Fluids/Nutrition** | ☐☐ D5RL 125 cc/hr ☐☐ Sips of water/ice, if no N&V<br>☐☐ ________ ☐☐ Clear liquids |
| | **Eliminations** | ☐☐ Foley to gravity drainage |
| P F Method M R Initial<br>Indication for C/S ☐☐ ___ ☐☐ ___<br>C/S procedure ☐☐ ___ ☐☐ ___<br>Anesthesia ☐☐ ___ ☐☐ ___<br>Post-op care ☐☐ ___ ☐☐ ___<br>Postpartum routine ☐☐ ___ ☐☐ ___<br>LOS ☐☐ ___ ☐☐ ___<br>Pain control ☐☐ ___ ☐☐ ___<br>Future VBAC ☐☐ ___ ☐☐ ___ | **Patient/Family Education**<br>**LEARNER:**<br>P=patient<br>F=family<br>**METHOD:**<br>V=video/film<br>E=explanation<br>D=demonstration<br>H=handout/booklet<br>**EVALUATION:**<br>M=mastered<br>R=requires additional instruction | P F Method M R Initial<br>TCDB/splinting ☐☐ ___ ☐☐ ___<br>Pain control ☐☐ ___ ☐☐ ___<br>Self care ☐☐ ___ ☐☐ ___<br>pericare ___ ☐☐ ___<br>involution/lochia ___ ☐☐ ___<br>hand washing ___ ☐☐ ___<br>breast care ___ ☐☐ ___<br>Feeding ☐☐ ___ ☐☐ ___<br>frequency/timing ___ ☐☐ ___<br>positioning ___ ☐☐ ___<br>latch-on/removal ___ ☐☐ ___<br>burping ___ ☐☐ ___ |
| | **Discharge Planning** | ☐☐ ID home maintenance problems<br>☐☐ Identify support system |
| | **Behavioral** | ☐☐ Touches/explores infant |
| ☐ ________<br>☐ ________<br>☐ ________ | **Additional Interventions** | ☐☐ ________<br>☐☐ ________<br>☐☐ ________ |
| ________<br>________<br>________ | **Signatures** | ________<br>________<br>________ |

**FIGURE 17–10** *Continued*

Date of Admission: ____________________

Date of Surgery: ______________ Time: ______ Anticipated DC Date: __________

Infant: ☐ Normal Newborn ☐ NICU ☐ IUFD Anticipated Newborn DC to: ☐ Home ☐ Foster Home

Functional Ability Anticipated at Discharge: ____ Independent/Normal Newborn ____ Dependent/Special Needs

Describe: ________________________________

| Day 2/POD 1 | Day 3/POD 2 | Discharge (POD 2 or 3) |
|---|---|---|
| | | |
| ☐ LDR ☐ 2S ☐ 2E | ☐ LDR ☐ 2S ☐ 2E | ☐ 2S ☐ 2E |
| ☐☐☐ VS WNL (temp <100)<br>☐☐☐ OB checks WNL<br>☐☐☐ Emptying bladder<br>☐☐☐ Pain controlled<br>☐☐☐ BS present<br>☐☐☐ Bonding progressing | ☐☐☐ VS WNL (temp <100)<br>☐☐☐ OB checks WNL<br>☐☐☐ Pain controlled<br>☐☐☐ BS normal<br>☐☐☐ Tol regular diet<br>☐☐☐ Incision site w/o signs of infection | ☐ Satisfactory wound healing<br>☐ Verbalizes & demonstrates ability to care for self & baby with minimal assist<br>☐ Verbalizes & understands discharge instructions |
| ☐☐☐ VS Q 4°<br>☐☐☐ OB check Q shift<br>☐☐☐ Bowel sounds<br>☐☐☐ Flatus<br>☐☐☐ Bladder empty after first 2 voids (normal fundal exam)<br>☐☐☐ Pain Assessment | ☐☐☐ VS Q shift<br>☐☐☐ OB check Q shift<br>☐☐☐ Bowel sounds<br>☐☐☐ Flatus<br>☐☐☐ Pain assessment | ☐☐ VS Q shift<br>☐☐ OB check Q shift<br>☐☐ Bowel sounds<br>☐☐ Flatus |
| ☐ Social worker ☐ CNS ☐ CM<br>☐ Lactation Specialist<br>☐ __________ | ☐ Social worker ☐ CNS ☐ CM<br>☐ Lactation Specialist<br>☐ __________ | ☐ Lactation Specialist ☐ CM<br>☐ __________ |
| | | |
| ☐☐☐ TCDB Q 2°, min. assist<br>☐☐☐ Pericare by Pt<br>☐☐☐ DC Foley<br>☐☐☐ Remove Dsg<br>☐☐☐ Breast pump | ☐☐☐ Staples removed<br>☐☐☐ Breast pump, prn | |
| ☐☐☐ RhoGAM as indicated<br>☐☐☐ Rubella vaccine if indicated<br>☐☐☐ Tylenol #3, 1-2 PO Q 3-4°<br>☐☐☐ Vicodin, 1-2 PO Q3°<br>☐☐☐ __________<br>☐☐☐ Compazine 10 mg IM Q4-6°<br>☐☐☐ Simethicone 80 mg PO TID<br>☐☐☐ Dulcolax Supp prn<br>☐ Benadryl 50 mg PO HS | ☐☐☐ Tylenol #3, 1-2 PO Q 3 4°<br>☐☐☐ Vicodin 1-2 PO Q 3°<br>☐☐☐ __________<br>☐☐☐ Compazine 10 mg IM Q4-6°<br>☐☐☐ Simethicone 80mg PO TID<br>☐☐☐ Dulcolax Supp prn<br>☐ Benadryl 50 mg PO HS | ☐☐ Tylenol #3, 1-2 PO Q 3-4°<br>☐☐ Vicodin 1-2 PO Q 3°<br>☐☐ __________<br>☐☐ Simethicone 80 mg TID<br>☐☐ Prescription for discharge meds |
| ☐☐☐ Chair<br>☐☐☐ Amb with assist<br>☐☐☐ Shower/shampoo | ☐☐☐ Amb w/o assist<br>☐☐☐ Shower/shampoo | ☐☐☐ Amb w/o assist<br>☐☐☐ Shower/shampoo |
| ☐☐☐ Heg diet, if + bowel sounds<br>☐☐☐ Clear liquids<br>☐☐☐ DC IV if adequate PO fluids | ☐☐☐ Reg diet | ☐☐☐ Reg diet |
| | | |
| P F Method M R Initial<br>CDB reinforced ☐☐ ___ ☐☐ ___<br>Self care reinforced ☐☐ ___ ☐☐ ___<br>Diet ☐☐ ___ ☐☐ ___<br>Elimination ☐☐ ___ ☐☐ ___<br>Newborn characteristics ☐☐ ___ ☐☐ ___<br>Feeding reinforced ☐☐ ___ ☐☐ ___<br>Diaper changing ☐☐ ___ ☐☐ ___<br>Cord care ☐☐ ___ ☐☐ ___<br>Circ care ☐☐ ___ ☐☐ ___<br>Bathing ☐☐ ___ ☐☐ ___ | P F Method M R Initial<br>Activity/Rest ☐☐ ___ ☐☐ ___<br>Emotional concerns ☐☐ ___ ☐☐ ___<br>Calif law regarding car seats ☐☐ ___ ☐☐ ___<br>Infant safety ☐☐ ___ ☐☐ ___<br>Feeding reinforced ☐☐ ___ ☐☐ ___<br>Infant care reinforced ☐☐ ___ ☐☐ ___ | P F Method M R Initial<br>Self care reviewed ☐☐ ___ ☐☐ ___<br>Infant care reviewed ☐☐ ___ ☐☐ ___<br>Review discharge instruction & meds ☐☐ ___ ☐☐ ___<br>Complications requiring follow-up ☐☐ ___ ☐☐ ___ |
| ☐☐☐ Home Health referral<br>Home equipment/supplies<br>__________ | ☐☐☐ Home Health referral/follow-up<br>☐☐☐ Has car seat<br>☐☐☐ Community resources | ☐☐☐ Postpartum appointment<br>☐☐☐ Infant appointment<br>☐☐☐ Postpartum support group |
| ☐☐☐ Involve in infant care | ☐☐☐ Caring for infant with minimal assist | |
| ☐☐☐ __________<br>☐☐☐ __________<br>☐☐☐ __________ | ☐☐☐ __________<br>☐☐☐ __________<br>☐☐☐ __________ | ☐☐ __________<br>☐☐ __________<br>☐☐ __________ |
| __________<br>__________<br>__________ | __________<br>__________<br>__________ | __________<br>__________<br>__________ |

**FIGURE 17–10** *Continued*

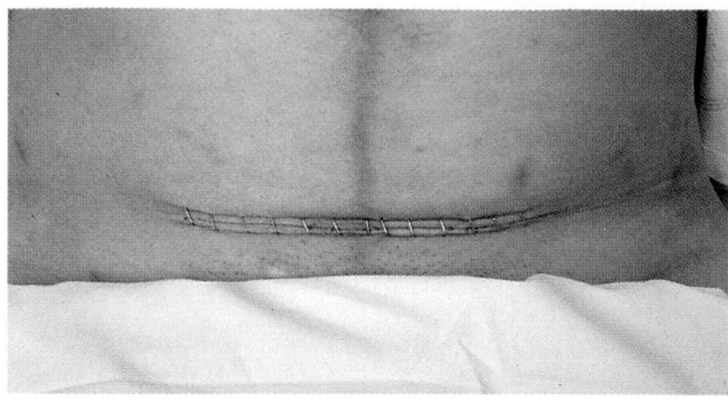

**FIGURE 17–11**

The incision after cesarean birth is closed with staples. Note the absence of all signs of infection, such as redness, edema, bruising (ecchymosis), or discharge.

- Both the indwelling catheter and intravenous infusion are usually discontinued.
- The dressing is usually removed, and often staples or clamps are removed also. Steri-Strips or a small nonstick dressing may be used to cover the incision.
- Mothers are usually helped to ambulate on the first postpartum day and are comfortable sitting in a chair for brief periods of time.
- Clear liquids are allowed once bowel sounds are audible. If abdominal distention is minimal, the diet progresses to soft foods and then to a regular regimen.

Nurses must encourage the mother to increase her activity and ambulation each postpartum day. By the second day, she is usually allowed to shower. Some health care providers request that the incision be covered with plastic; others permit showering without covering the incision.

**Assisting the Mother with Infant Feeding.** It is important to help the mother find a comfortable position for holding and feeding her infant. A side-lying position may be most comfortable; however, some mothers prefer sitting with a pillow on the lap to protect the incisional area. The football hold is often the most comfortable position for breastfeeding because the infant is not on the lap and thus does not cause incisional discomfort. (Chapter 22 discusses breastfeeding in detail.)

**Preventing Abdominal Distention.** Abdominal distention is a major source of discomfort, and measures should be taken to prevent or minimize it. Early, frequent ambulation is perhaps the best method; however, there are some additional measures:

- Pelvic lifts (a flat, supine position with knees bent, lifting the pelvis from the bed) may be repeated up to 10 times several times each day.
- Tightening and relaxing the abdominal muscles may also be helpful.
- Carbonated beverages as well as the use of straws, which increase the accumulation of intestinal gas, should be restricted.
- Simethecone may disperse upper gastrointestinal flatulence.
- Rectal suppositories stimulate peristalsis and passage of flatus.

**CHECK YOUR READING**

13. What additional assessments are necessary for the postcesarean mother?
14. How can hypostatic pneumonia be prevented?
15. Which measures are used to prevent or minimize abdominal distention?

## Application of Nursing Process: Knowledge of Self-Care

### Assessment

Nurses are responsible for providing health education about a long list of subjects before the family is discharged from the birth facility. This task causes a great deal of concern because so much must be taught during a short time and because this is not the best time to teach mothers who are not fully recovered from the birth process.

Before beginning teaching, determine the learning needs and the major concerns of each family. For example, multiparas may remember some aspects of self-care but would benefit from a review. On the other hand, primiparas may be anxious about self-care measures and all aspects of infant care. They may require more thorough teaching and more practice. Be aware of the most common barriers to learning: age and developmental level, cultural factors, and difficulty understanding the language.

### Analysis

In general, mothers adapt to the physiologic changes following childbirth, and most nursing care is wellness oriented. Some new mothers, however, lack knowledge of self-care and thus are at risk for a disruption in health. For example, mothers are expected to know how to assess the fundus and lochia so that they can recognize signs of excessive bleeding or infection. They must know how to promote healing and comfort of the perineum and how to establish normal patterns of elimination. Perhaps the greatest challenge for nurses is to help the mother achieve competence and confidence in her ability to breastfeed. This task often requires more than 24 hours and requires consistent follow-up care.

Because of the need for health education, a nursing diagnosis that applies to many women and forms the basis for nursing interventions is Risk for Altered Health Maintenance related to insufficient knowledge of self-care, signs of complications, and preventive measures. Additional diagnoses include Risk for Injury and Altered Sexuality Patterns. They appear in Nursing Care Plan 17–1.

## Planning

Goals for the nursing diagnosis Risk for Altered Health Maintenance related to insufficient knowledge of self-care, signs of complications, and preventive measures are that the mother will do the following:

- Verbalize or demonstrate understanding of self-care instructions by hour of discharge.
- Verbalize understanding of practices that promote maternal health by (date).
- Describe plans for follow-up care and signs and symptoms that should be reported to the physician, nurse-midwife, or nurse practitioner by day of discharge.

## Interventions

### TEACHING THE PROCESS OF INVOLUTION

Provide the mother with basic information about involution, including how to assess lochia and how to locate and palpate the fundus. This information allows her to recognize abnormal signs, such as prolonged lochia or uterine tenderness, which should be reported to the health care provider. If the mother is a very young adolescent, another family member may also need the information.

### TEACHING SELF-CARE

**Hand Washing.** Emphasize the importance of thorough hand washing before touching the breasts, after diaper changes, after bladder and bowel elimination, and always before handling the infant.

**Breast Care for Lactating Mothers.** Instruct the breastfeeding mother to wash her nipples with clear water and to avoid soaps that remove the natural lubrication secreted by Montgomery's glands. Advise her to feed the infant when the breasts feel full or when the infant indicates hunger rather than to follow a schedule. Explain that she should not restrict the duration of breastfeeding but should allow adequate time for both breasts to be emptied at each feeding. Keeping the nipples dry between feedings helps to prevent tissue damage, and wearing a good bra provides necessary support as breast size increases. (For additional information about breastfeeding, see Chapter 22.)

**Measures to Suppress Lactation.** If the mother chooses not to breastfeed, measures should be initiated to suppress lactation. The safest method is to prevent breast distention by either binding the breasts or having the mother wear a tight-fitting bra 24 hours per day until the breasts become soft. Discomfort can usually be managed by application of ice, which reduces vasocongestion, and by administration of analgesics. The woman should be advised to refrain from doing anything to stimulate milk production, such as allowing warm water to fall on the breasts during showers and pumping or massaging the breasts.

**Perineal Care.** Nurses are responsible for teaching some form of perineal cleansing as soon as possible after childbirth. The most common method is to fill a squeeze bottle with warm water and spray the perineal area from the front toward the back. In some facilities, a small amount of cleansing solution is added; in others, only clear warm water is used. Remind the new mother not to separate the labia during this procedure so that water does not enter the vagina. If a commercial product that includes a nozzle attached to the faucet is used, teach the

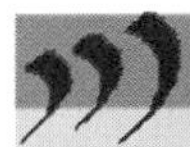

**THERAPEUTIC COMMUNICATION**

**Teaching Self-Care Measures**

Clare Beauchamp gave birth to a baby boy 48 hours ago. Terry Meyer is a nurse preparing to teach Clare self-care measures before discharge from the birth facility.

**Clare:** Look at me; I still look pregnant, and my husband calls me Tubby.

**Terry:** You were looking forward to your abdomen being flat after the baby was born?

*Clarifying the woman's concern by reflecting content.*

**Clare:** Well, I was always so flat; I am really disappointed.

**Terry:** Remember it took 9 months for those muscles to stretch. You can't expect them to snap back in a few days.

*Blocking communication by ignoring the feeling expressed. A more helpful response would be to acknowledge the disappointment and to delay giving information until feelings have been expressed. For example: "It is upsetting, and when you are ready, we can discuss some exercises that will help."*

mother that the nozzle should not touch the perineum during use.

Moist antiseptic towelettes or toilet paper is used in a patting motion to dry the perineum. Teach the mother to dry from front to back to prevent fecal contamination of the vaginal introitus from the anal area. She should perform perineal cleansing after each voiding or defecation, and she should change perineal pads (peripads) at the same time.

Many women do not use peripads for menstrual protection and must be taught how to use them correctly. Careful handling of the pads is important to prevent localized perineal infection:

- Thorough hand washing is a must before and after changing the pads.
- Unused pads should be stored inside their package.
- Pads should be applied without touching the side that comes into contact with the perineum.
- Mesh panties and adhering pads are used in most facilities.
- The pads should be applied and removed in a front-to-back direction to prevent contamination of the vagina and perineum.
- Used pads must be disposed of properly.

**Kegel Exercises.** All mothers should become familiar with Kegel exercises. These movements strengthen the pubococcygeal muscle, which surrounds the vagina and urinary meatus. This exercise helps to prevent the loss of muscle tone that can occur following childbirth.

The exercise, which may be started in the postpartum period, involves contracting muscles around the vagina (as though stopping the flow of urine), holding tightly for a few seconds, and then relaxing. The contraction-relaxation cycle is repeated 10 times, and the series is repeated five times a day during the postpartum period.

### PROMOTING REST AND SLEEP

The mother who is fatigued appears worn out and lethargic, with slumping posture, and often verbalizes a generalized decrease in energy and strength. The extreme fatigue that mothers experience in the puerperium has several reasons. For one thing, they are tired when they begin the postpartum period; women often do not sleep well during the third trimester, and many are further exhausted by the exertion of labor. Women commonly experience feelings of excitement and euphoria for some time following childbirth and are unable to rest. Numerous visitors during the first few days interfere with long periods of rest. Hospital routines, an unfamiliar environment, and physical discomfort also make it difficult for the new mother to rest.

Most mothers are discharged from the facility within 24 to 48 hours after childbirth, and most go home with a tremendous deficit in sleep and energy. Yet new parents may be unprepared for the conflict between their need for sleep and the infant's need for care and attention. The joys of parenting can easily be overshadowed by the exhaustion and frustration that result.

**Rest at the Birth Facility.** Hospital routines continue around the clock, making uninterrupted rest difficult and increasing the probability that the mother is fatigued when she is discharged. Make every attempt to allow the mother adequate time for uninterrupted rest periods. Group assessments and care, and try to correlate them with times when the mother would be awake, such as just before or after meals, feeding times, or visiting hours. If the room is shared, providing care for both women at the same time also reduces activities that interrupt sleep.

Try to persuade the mother to select a time when phone calls and visitors are restricted so that she can use this time for napping. A quiet, softly lit environment also promotes sleep.

**Rest at Home.** Help the mother to understand the impact that her physical discomfort and the demands of the newborn will have on her energy during the first few weeks. Many nurses emphasize measures that conserve energy, such as the following:

- A relaxed, flexible routine that focuses on care of the mother and infant
- Simple meals and flexible meal times
- Accepting assistance with food shopping and meal preparation
- Postponing major household projects
- Involving friends and family to provide care for other children

Explain to the mother that she should delay her return to employment, if possible, until the infant sleeps through the night (usually by 4 months). Advise all mothers to restrict coffee, tea, colas, and chocolate (which all contain the stimulant caffeine) for the first few weeks and to rest whenever the infant sleeps rather than to use that time to catch up on housecleaning tasks.

**Infant Sleep and Feeding Schedules.** Many families require information about infant sleep cycles, frequency of feeding, and probable crying episodes during the first weeks. Although newborns sleep 16 to 20 hours per day, they may awaken every 2 to 3 hours for feeding. Some infants (particularly those who are small or who have colic) may need to be fed more often, and they are often fussier than other infants. (See Chapter 23 for a discussion of parenting during the first weeks.)

**Relaxation Exercises.** Total relaxation exercises (lying quietly, alternately tightening and relaxing the muscles of the neck, shoulders, arms, legs, and feet) are helpful when a nap is not possible. Emphasize to the mother the importance of asking for help when she begins to feel exhausted or overwhelmed. Encourage her to share these feelings with family, friends, and other new mothers.

### PROVIDING NOURISHMENT AND NUTRITION COUNSELING

**Food Supply.** It is sometimes appropriate to determine the amount and type of food that is available to the mother and her family. This is particularly true for families of low socioeconomic status, who might benefit from referral to government-sponsored programs, such as food stamps or Women, Infant, and Children (WIC). It may also be necessary to determine the facilities that are available for cooking and storing food. Sometimes the new family must be referred to a social worker so that the best solutions for their unique problems can be found.

**Lactating Mothers.** Although many women are not satisfied with the slow rate of weight loss, emphasize that moderate to severe restriction of caloric intake during lactation interferes with the ability to synthesize milk (Lawrence, 1994). About 85 calories are required to produce 100 ml of milk. See Chapter 9 for additional information about nutrition required for breastfeeding.

**Nonlactating Mothers.** A mother who has chosen formula feeding should not restrict calories severely. Advise her to select foods that provide adequate calories to meet her energy needs, taking into account the time and energy required to care for a newborn. Strict dieting can leave the mother feeling tired and can lower her immunity. A balanced, low-fat diet with adequate protein, complex carbohydrates, fruits, and vegetables provides the energy needed.

### PROMOTING REGULAR BOWEL ELIMINATION

Progressive exercise, adequate fluid, and dietary fiber are effective means of preventing constipation. Walking is perhaps the best exercise, and the distance can be increased as strength and endurance increase. At least eight glasses of water daily help to maintain normal bowel elimination. Dietary fiber is present in fruits and vegetables, particularly when they are unpeeled. Prunes act as a natural laxative. Additional fiber is found in whole grain cereals, bread, and pasta.

A regular schedule of bowel elimination is also important in overcoming constipation. For instance, bowel elimination following breakfast allows the mother to take advantage of the gastrocolic reflex (stimulation of peristalsis induced in the colon when food is consumed on an empty stomach). Moreover, measures that reduce perineal and hemorrhoidal pain, such as sitz baths, prepackaged witch hazel astringent compresses, and ointments facilitate bowel elimination.

### PROMOTING GOOD BODY MECHANICS

**Exercise.** Teach exercises in the early postpartum period to strengthen the abdominal muscles and to firm the waist. The exercises can be started soon after childbirth; to begin, each can be repeated five times twice each day. Gradually, the number of exercises is increased as the mother gains strength. Figure 17–12 illustrates recommended postpartum exercises that may begin with approval of the physician, nurse-widwife, or nurse practitioner.

Postcesarean mothers should follow the instructions of their health care provider. Generally they should not begin an exercise program for at least 4 to 6 weeks.

**Preventing Back Strain.** Back strain often can be prevented if the mother and father find a location for infant care, such as a kitchen table or bathroom counter, that does not require bending or leaning forward. For lifting objects, teach parents to hold the back straight as they squat and use the legs rather than bending at the waist (see Fig. 7–14).

### COUNSELING ABOUT SEXUAL ACTIVITY

The couple may have concerns about the resumption of sexual intercourse and contraceptive choices. Cultural or religious convictions may restrict the choice of method for some couples, whereas availability of health care or inadequate finances may dictate the choice for others. Discuss previous experience with contraceptives and the satisfaction with that method.

**Many new parents are reluctant to ask about when to resume sexual activity and about potential alterations in sexuality resulting from pregnancy and childbirth. If couples do not indicate such concerns, introduce the topic in a general, nonspecific manner, such as "You have an episiotomy that may cause some discomfort with intercourse until it is completely healed" or "Sometimes couples are not aware that some vaginal dryness occurs as a result of breastfeeding." Such broad opening statements permit the family to pursue the topic as they desire.**

Nursing Care Plan 17–1 describes interventions for the nursing diagnosis Risk for Altered Sexuality Patterns related to perineal discomfort, dryness of vaginal mucosa, or fatigue.

### INSTRUCTING ABOUT FOLLOW-UP APPOINTMENTS

Remind the new mother to make an appointment with her physician or nurse-midwife for postpartum examination at 2 weeks and 6 weeks following childbirth. Emphasize that examination at those times al-

**ABDOMINAL BREATHING**

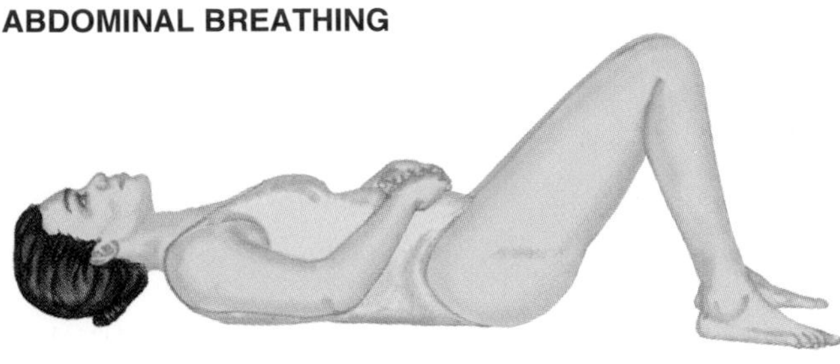

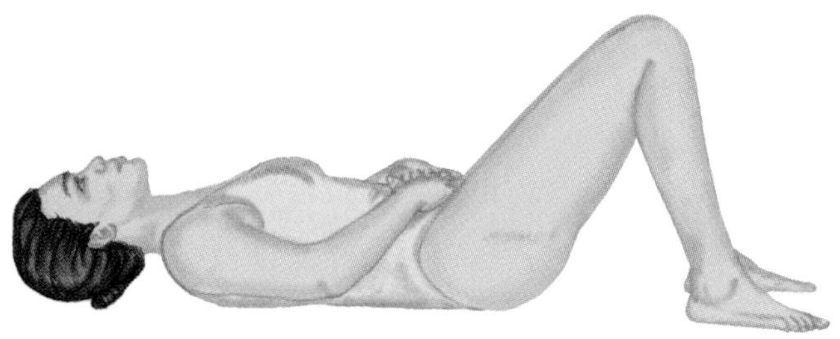

This is one of the simplest exercises and can be started on the first postpartum day. The woman assumes a supine position with knees bent. She inhales through the nose, keeps the rib cage as stationary as possible, and allows the abdomen to expand. She then contracts the abdominal muscles as she exhales slowly through the mouth.

**HEAD LIFT**

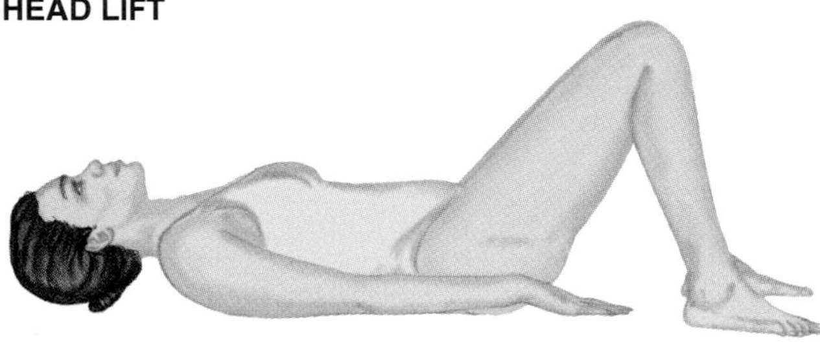

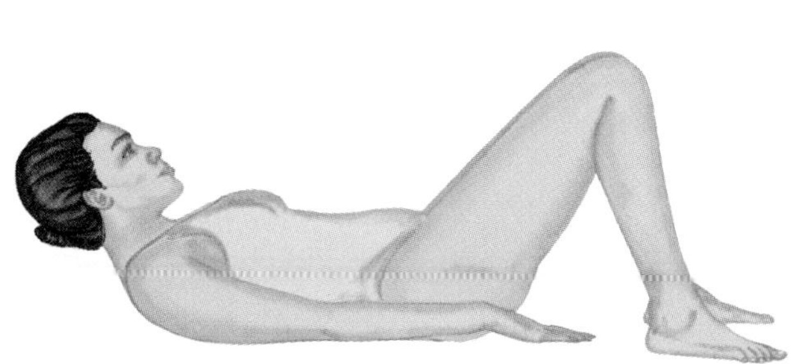

This exercise can be started within a few days after childbirth. The mother is supine with knees bent and arms outstretched at her side. She inhales deeply to begin, then exhales while lifting the head slowly; she holds the position for a few seconds and relaxes.

**MODIFIED SIT-UPS**

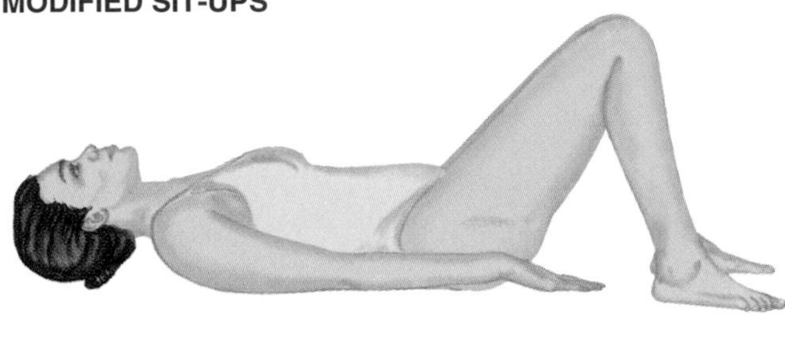

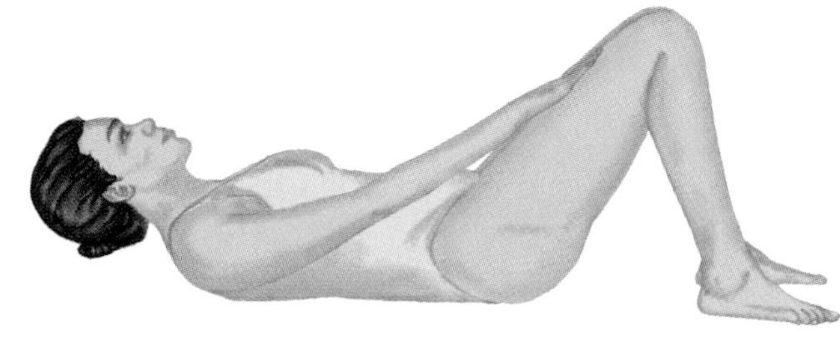

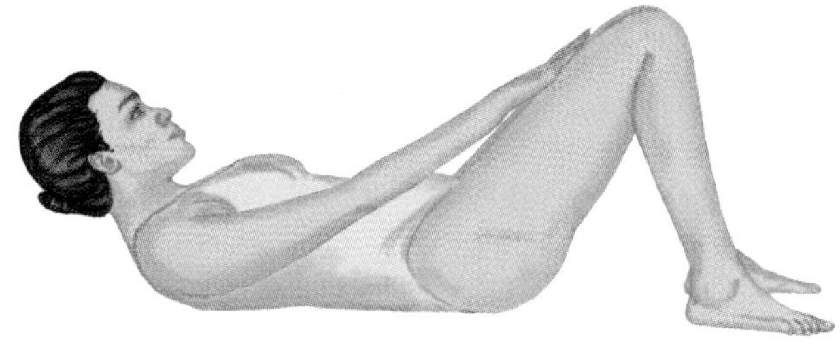

Head lifts may progress to modified sit-ups with the approval of the health care provider; the mother should follow the advice of the health care provider about the number of repetitions.

The exercise begins with the mother supine with arms outstretched and the knees bent. She raises her head and shoulders as her hands reach for her knees. She raises the shoulders only as far as the back will bend; her waist remains on the floor.

**FIGURE 17–12**

Postpartum exercises.

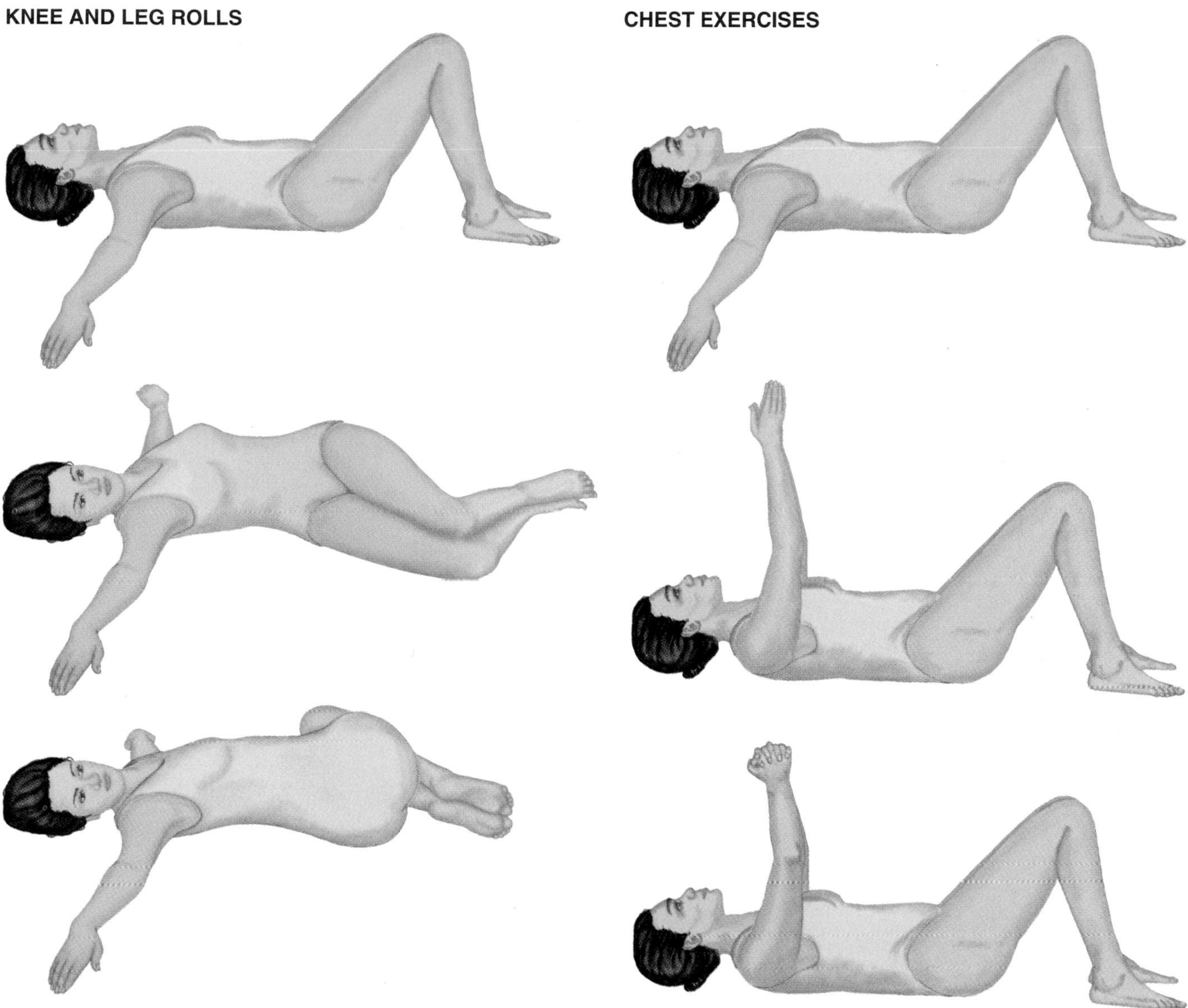


This is an excellent exercise to begin firming the waist. The mother lies flat on her back with knees bent and feet flat on the floor or bed; she keeps the shoulders and feet stationary and rolls the knees to touch first one side of the bed, then the other. She maintains a smooth motion as the exercise is repeated five times. Later, as flexibility increases, the exercise can be varied by the rolling of one knee only. The mother rolls her left knee to touch the right side of the bed, returns to center, and rolls the right knee to touch the left side of the bed.

This is an excellent exercise to strengthen the chest muscles. The mother lies flat with arms extended straight out to the side; she brings the hands together above the chest while keeping the arms straight; she holds for a few seconds and returns to the starting position. She repeats the exercise five times initially and follows the advice of the health care provider for increasing the number of repetitions.

Isometric exercises also increase strength and tone; the mother bends her elbows, clasps her hands together above her chest, and presses her hands together for a few seconds. This is repeated at least five times.

**FIGURE 17–12** *Continued*

lows early identification and treatment of problems that may be developing.

#### TEACHING ABOUT SIGNS AND SYMPTOMS THAT SHOULD BE REPORTED

Teach new mothers and at least one member of the family which physical signs and symptoms should be reported to the health care provider right away. These signs and symptoms include the following:

- Fever
- Localized area of redness, swelling, or pain in either breast that is not relieved by support or analgesics
- Persistent abdominal tenderness or feelings of pelvic fullness or pelvic pressure
- Persistent perineal pain
- Frequency, urgency, or burning on urination
- Change in character of lochia (increased amount,

resumption of bright red color, passage of clots, foul odor)
- Localized tenderness, redness, or warmth of the legs

#### ENSURING THAT ALL ELEMENTS HAVE BEEN TAUGHT

Group instruction and hospital classes, such as those that demonstrate infant care and provide breastfeeding instructions, are returning to the postpartum environment. Nurses streamline and organize information so that it can be presented in the time available.

To prevent omissions, many hospitals use teaching "check-off" sheets listing the areas that must be covered. For example, care of the umbilical cord and circumcision site, using a bulb syringe, and taking a temperature are part of the infant care teaching that must take place before the mother leaves the hospital.

### Evaluation

- The mother's demonstration of correct breast and perineal hygiene provides evidence of her ability to perform self-care measures.
- The mother's ability to verbalize practices that promote health in the areas of diet, exercise, rest, and sleep confirm understanding of these measures.
- Her ability to describe a plan for future appointments for examination with the health care provider increases the likelihood that she will experience an uncomplicated recovery.

## Postpartum Home Care

#### CRITERIA FOR DISCHARGE

Most women must leave the hospital when they are just beginning to recover from giving birth and to learn how to care for themselves and their infants. Both mothers and infants should meet specific criteria before discharge:

- The mother had an uncomplicated vaginal birth following a normal term antepartum course and a normal immediate postpartum course. For instance, she must be able to empty her bladder; lochia and the location and consistency of the fundus must be within normal limits; and she must be free of signs of infection.
- Pertinent laboratory data, as selected by the practitioner, are within normal limits for both mother and newborn.
- The newborn is stable and able to eat and maintain thermal homeostasis.
- The infant must have a lusty, robust cry and normal reflexes.
- The infant must have voided before discharge.
- The infant's vital signs must be within normal limits.
- Family members or other support persons are available to the mother for the first few days following discharge.
- The mother is aware of possible complications and has been instructed to notify the appropriate practitioner, as necessary.
- The institution has in place mechanisms to address client questions that arise after discharge.

These criteria were developed by the American Academy of Pediatrics and the American College of Obstetricians and Gynecologists (1992).

#### COMMON PROBLEMS OF THE POSTPARTUM PERIOD

The most common problems encountered by new mothers are discomfort, such as perineal, incisional, and nipple pain and uterine cramping. Additional problems include fatigue, constipation, and breastfeeding difficulties (Williams & Cooper, 1993). Infants who leave the birth facility within the first 24 hours are at risk for a variety of problems that include feeding difficulties, jaundice, significant weight loss or inadequate weight gain, rashes, and conjunctivitis (Keppler, 1995).

#### HOME CARE SERVICES

New parents must be made aware of the services offered for home care. These services include information lines, follow-up telephone calls, home visits, and nurse-managed postpartum outpatient clinics. In addition, some facilities offer breastfeeding and parenting classes as well as "baby and me" walks or exercise sessions.

**Information Lines.** Ideally, information lines should be open 24 hours a day, 7 days a week. They should be staffed by qualified nurses who use agency protocols to respond to the family's questions. Moreover, these nurses must be prepared to "triage." That is, they must be skilled at soliciting information to identify problems and to determine the priority of the problems identified. For instance, does the information obtained indicate that the family should come to the office or clinic for a more thorough assessment by their health care provider? Should they come now or can they wait? Can their problem be solved by information or advice?

Legal liability is a concern for all agencies and personnel who identify problems, set priorities, and provide information by telephone. Not only must the staff be educated and evaluated for the task, but protocols must be devised, a documentation system must be developed, and adequate consultation or "back-up" support must be available.

A major disadvantage of information lines is that

they rely on families to initiate a request for assistance. Not all families recognize when a problem begins to develop and, as a result, may delay in seeking information.

**Telephone Calls.** Some facilities initiate telephone interviews to assess new families and to provide information to families at home. The calls are usually made 1 to 3 days following discharge. As with information lines, a qualified nurse, following the facility protocol, conducts a systematic assessment of the mother and infant. The nurse solicits questions and reinforces important information. Telephone calls are relatively inexpensive; however, they have the major disadvantage that the nurse cannot confirm the data but must rely on observations made by the family.

**Home Visits.** Home visits allow physical examination of the mother and infant as well as the home environment. Maternal assessment should include the breasts, fundus, and lochia (Fig. 17–13). If possible, nurses should allow time to observe breastfeeding and to provide encouragement and reassurance that is badly needed during the first days before lactation is well established. The newborn's weight, color, and elimination pattern are important parts of the home visit. Ample time should be allowed to reinforce previous learning, to answer questions, and to introduce new topics. Although home visits are expensive, some agencies believe that they are less expensive than readmissions of the mother or infant to the hospital for problems that could be prevented by follow-up care.

**Outpatient Clinics.** Nurse-managed outpatient clinics offer another option for postpartum care. Although transportation is a problem for some families, clinic visits are less costly for the agency than home visits. Clinic visits may be used either to replace or to supplement home visits. Like home care, clinic visits include an examination of the mother and infant. There should be time to answer questions about maternal self-care, to provide assistance with infant feeding, and to deal with special concerns, such as care of the umbilical cord or circumcision (Keppler, 1995).

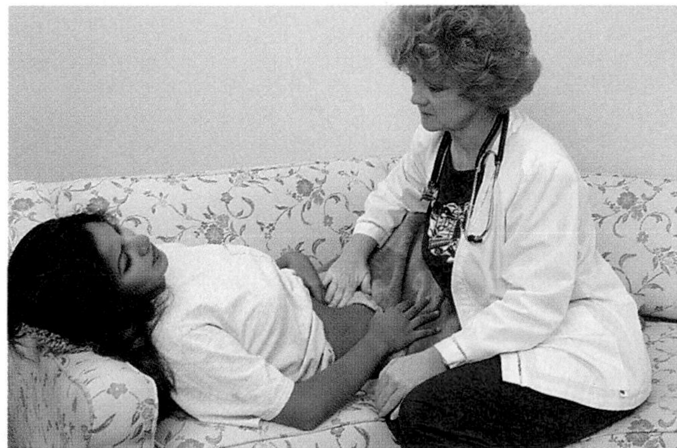

**FIGURE 17–13**

Postpartum home visits include assessments and health education. Here the nurse evaluates involution while teaching the mother how to palpate her fundus.

### ✓ CHECK YOUR READING

16. What is the major challenge that early discharge presents for the nurse? How do clinical pathways affect nursing care?
17. What are the criteria for early discharge from the standpoint of the mother? Of the baby?
18. What are the advantages and disadvantages of information lines, telephone calls, home visits, and nurse-managed outpatient clinics?

## SUMMARY CONCEPTS

- Following childbirth, the uterus returns to its prepregnancy size and condition by involution, which involves contraction of stretched muscle fibers, catabolic processes that reduce enlarged muscle cells, and regeneration of uterine epithelium.
- The site of placental attachment heals by a process of exfoliation, which leaves the endometrium smooth and without scars.
- Involution can be evaluated by measuring the descent of the fundus (about 1 cm/day): by the 10th day after childbirth, the fundus should be located in the pelvic cavity and should no longer be palpable abdominally.
- Afterpains, or intermittent uterine contractions, cause discomfort for many women, particularly multiparas who breastfeed.
- Vaginal discharge (lochia) progresses from lochia rubra (containing mostly blood), to lochia serosa (containing serous exudate, blood, and leukocytes), to lochia alba (containing increased amounts of leukocytes and decidual cells) in a predictable time frame. Lochia should be assessed for volume, type, and odor; foul odor suggests endometrial infection.
- Although vaginal mucosa heals within 3 weeks, it takes 6 weeks for the vagina to regain the same size and contour.
- Perineal trauma, including edema, bruising, episiotomy, and lacerations, as well as hemorrhoids can cause a great deal of discomfort and interfere with bladder and bowel elimination.
- As blood from the uteroplacental unit returns to central circulation and extracellular fluid is mobilized into the vascular compartment, the cardiac output increases and excess fluid is excreted by diuresis and diaphoresis.
- Increased clotting factors predispose the postpar-

tum woman to thrombus formation. Early, frequent ambulation is the best method for preventing thrombophlebitis.

- Constipation may occur as a result of inadequate fluid intake during labor, reduced activity, decreased muscle tone, or fear of pain during defecation.
- Increased bladder capacity and decreased sensitivity to fluid pressure may result in urinary retention. Stasis of urine allows time for bacteria to grow and can lead to urinary tract infection.
- A distended bladder lifts and displaces the uterus; this can interfere with uterine contraction and result in excessive bleeding.
- Exercises to strengthen the abdominal muscles as well as good posture and body mechanics may reduce musculoskeletal discomfort.
- As hormone levels decline, the skin gradually reverts to its pre-pregnancy state.
- Breastfeeding may delay the return of ovulation and menstruation; however, it is not a reliable method of family planning. Both lactating and nonlactating mothers need information about family planning.
- Breastfeeding mothers are more likely to experience dyspareunia as a result of vaginal dryness that results from inadequate estrogen.
- Lactation may be suppressed by wearing a snug bra, by binding the breasts, and by avoiding stimulation of the breasts.
- The postpartum woman should be afebrile; however, her temperature may be higher during the first 24 hours after delivery because of exertion, dehydration, and leukocytosis.
- Bradycardia is expected; tachycardia may be caused by excitement, dehydration, or hypovolemia. Additional assessments (of lochia, fundus) are required to determine whether excessive bleeding is the cause.
- Orthostatic hypotension occurs when the mother goes from a supine to a standing position quickly. It may result in injury if precautions to protect her are not initiated.
- The common practice of early discharge challenges nurses to streamline information and to develop a plan for teaching self-care and infant care in a short amount of time.
- The postcesarean woman requires postoperative as well as postpartum assessments and care. She is at increased risk for problems associated with immobility and discomfort.

### References and Readings

American Academy of Pediatrics & American College of Obstetricians and Gynecologists. (1992). *Guidelines for perinatal care.* Elk Grove Village, Ill.: Author.

Blackburn, S.T., & Loper, D.L. (1992). *Maternal, fetal, and neonatal physiology: A clinical perspective.* Philadelphia: W.B. Saunders.

Bond, L. (1993). Physiological changes. In S. Mattson & J.E. Smith (Eds.), NAACOG *core curriculum for maternal-newborn nursing* (pp. 315–324). Philadelphia: W.B. Saunders.

Brooten, B., Knapp, H., Jacobsen, B., & Arnold, L. (1996). Early discharge after unplanned cesarean birth: Nursing care time. *Journal of Obstetric, Gynecologic, and Neonatal Nursing*, 25(7), 595–600.

Callister, L.C. (1995). Cultural meanings of childbirth. *Journal of Obstetric, Gynecologic, and Neonatal Nursing*, 24(4), 327–334.

Clark, R.A. (1995). Infections during the postpartum period. *Journal of Obstetric, Gynecologic, and Neonatal Nursing*, 24(6), 542–549.

Cunningham, F.G., MacDonald, P.C., Gant, N.F., Leveno, K.J., Gilstrap, L.C., Hankins, G.D.V., et al. (1997). *Williams obstetrics* (20th ed.). Norwalk, Conn.: Appleton & Lange.

Dahlberg, N.L., & Koloroutis, M. (1994). Hospital-based perinatal home-care. *Journal of Obstetric, Gynecologic, and Neonatal Nursing*, 23(8), 682–686.

Evans, C.J. (1995). Postpartum home care in the United States. *Journal of Obstetric, Gynecologic, and Neonatal Nursing*, 24(2), 180–186.

Fawcett, J., Pollio, N., Tully, A., Baron, M., Henklein, J.C., & Jones, R.C. (1993). Effects of information on adaptation to cesarean birth. *Nursing Research*, 42(1), 49–53.

Gupton, A., & McKay, M. (1995). The Canadian perspective on postpartum home care. *Journal of Obstetric, Gynecologic, and Neonatal Nursing*, 24(2), 173–179.

Hodgson, B.B., Kizior, R.J., & Kingdon, R.T. (1995). *Nurse's drug handbook* 1995. Philadelphia: W.B. Saunders.

Keppler, A.B. (1995). Postpartum care center: Follow-up care in a hospital-based clinic. *Journal of Obstetric, Gynecologic, and Neonatal Nursing*, 24(1), 17–21.

Kramer, R.L., Van Someren, J.K., Qualls, C.R., & Curet, L.B. (1996). Postoperative management of cesarean patients: The effect of immediate feeding on the incidence of ileus. *Obstetrics and Gynecology*, 88(1), 29–32.

Lawrence, R. (1994). *Breastfeeding: A guide for the medical profession* (4th ed.). St. Louis: C.V. Mosby.

Luegenbiehl, D., Brophy, G., Artigue, G., Phillips, K., & Flack, R. (1990). Standardized assessment of blood loss. *MCN: American Journal of Maternal Child Nursing*, 15(4), 241–244.

Lukacs, A. (1991). Issues surrounding early postpartum discharge: Effects on the caregiver. *Journal of Perinatal Neonatal Nursing*, 5(1), 33–42.

Martel, L.K. (1995). Response to change: Maternity nursing after World War II. *The American Journal of Maternal/Child Nursing*, 20(3), 131–134.

McGregor, L.A. (1994). Short, shorter, shortest: Improving the hospital stay for mothers and newborns. *The American Journal of Maternal/Child Nursing*, 19(3), 91–96.

Miovech, S.M., Knapp, H., Pugh, L.C., et al. (1994). Major concerns after cesarean delivery. *Journal of Obstetric, Gynecologic, and Neonatal Nursing*, 23(1), 46–52.

Petree, B., & Mattson, S. (1993). Hypertensive states in pregnancy. In S. Mattson & J.E. Smith (Eds.), NAACOG *core curriculum for maternal-newborn nursing* (pp. 412–433). Philadelphia: W.B. Saunders.

Reichert, J.A., Baron, M., & Fawcett, J. (1993). Changes in attitudes toward cesarean birth. *Journal of Obstetric, Gynecologic, and Neonatal Nursing*, 22(2), 159–167.

Resnik, R. (1994). The puerperium. In R.K. Creasy & R. Resnik (Eds.), *Maternal-Fetal medicine: Principles and practice* (pp. 140–144). Philadelphia: W.B. Saunders.

Sheil, E.P., Bull, M.J., Moxon, B.E., et al. (1995). Concerns of childbearing women: A maternal concerns questionnaire as an assessment tool. *Journal of Obstetric, Gynecologic, and Neonatal Nursing*, 24(2), 149–155.

Simpson, K.R., & Creehan, P.A. (Eds.) (1996). AWHONN *perinatal nursing.* Philadelphia: Lippincott-Raven Publishers.

Stolte, K., Myers, S.T., & Owen, W.L. (1994). Changes in

maternity care and the impact on nurses and nursing practice. *Journal of Obstetric, Gynecologic, and Neonatal Nursing*, 23(7), 603–608.

Stover, A.M., & Marnejon, J.G. (1995). Postpartum care. *American Family Physician*, 52(5), 1465–1472.

Stringer, M., Spatz, D., & Donahue, D. (1994). Maternal-fetal physical assessment in the home setting: Role of the advanced practice nurse. *Journal of Obstetric, Gynecologic, and Neonatal Nursing*, 23(8), 720–725.

Valaitis, R., Tuff, K., & Swanson, L. (1996). Meeting parents postpartal needs with a telephone information line. *American Journal of Maternal Child Nursing*, 21(2), 90–95.

Weber, S.E. (1996). Cultural aspects of pain in childbearing women. *Journal of Obstetric, Gynecologic, and Neonatal Nursing*, 25(1), 67–72.

Weinberg, S.H. (1994). An alternative to meet the needs of early discharge: The tender beginnings postpartum visit. *American Journal of Maternal/Child Nursing*, 19(6), 339–342.

Wild, L., & Coyne, C. (1992). Epidural anesthesia: The basics and beyond. *American Journal of Nursing*, 92(4), 26–37.

Williams, L.R., & Cooper, M.K. (1993). Nurse-managed postpartum home care. *Journal of Obstetric, Gynecologic, and Neonatal Nursing*, 22(1), 25–32.

Williams, L.R., & Cooper, M.K. (1996). A new paradigm for postpartum care. *Journal of Obstetric, Gynecologic, and Neonatal Nursing*, 25(9), 745–749.

Zuspan, K. (1994). Control of postpartum pain. In F.P. Zuspan & E.J. Quilligan, *Current therapy in obstetrics and gynecology* (pp. 333–335). Philadelphia: W.B. Saunders.

# 18

# Postpartum Psychosocial Adaptations

## OBJECTIVES

1. Explain the process of bonding and attachment, including maternal touch and verbal interactions.
2. Describe the progressive phases of maternal adaptation to childbirth and the stages of maternal role attainment.
3. Identify maternal concerns and how they change over time.
4. Discuss postpartum blues in terms of cause, manifestations, and interventions.
5. Describe the processes of family adaptation (father, siblings, grandparents) to the birth of a baby.
6. Discuss factors that affect family adaptation.
7. Discuss cultural influences on family adaptation.
8. Describe assessments and interventions for specific nursing diagnoses related to postpartum psychosocial adaptations.
9. Discuss the need for additional care following discharge of the mother and infant from the birth facility.

## DEFINITIONS

**attachment** *Development of strong affectional ties as a result of interaction between an infant and a significant other (mother, father, sibling, caretaker).*

**bonding** *Development of a strong emotional tie of a parent to a newborn; also called claiming or binding in.*

**en face** *Position that allows eye-to-eye contact between the newborn and a parent; optimal distance is 20 to 22 cm (8 to 9 inches).*

**engrossment** *Intense fascination and close face-to-face observation between father and newborn.*

**entrainment** *Newborn movement in rhythm to adult speech, particularly high-pitched tones, which are more easily heard.*

**finger-tipping** *First tactile (touch) experience between mother and newborn; the mother explores the infant's body with her fingertips only.*

**fourth trimester** *First 12 weeks following birth; a time of transition for parents and siblings.*

**letting-go** *A phase of maternal adaptation that involves relinquishment of previous roles and assumption of a new role as a parent.*

**postpartum blues** *Temporary, self-limiting period of weepiness experienced by many new mothers within the first few days following childbirth.*

**reciprocal bonding behaviors** *Repertoire of infant behaviors that promote attachment between parent and newborn.*

**sibling rivalry** *Feelings of jealousy and fear of replacement when a young child must share the attention of the parents with a newborn infant.*

**taking-hold** *Second phase of maternal adaptation during which the mother assumes control of her own care and initiates care of the infant.*

**taking-in** *First phase of maternal adaptation during which the mother passively accepts care, comfort, and details of the newborn.*

Perhaps no other event requires such rapid change in family structure and function as the birth of a baby. The mother progresses through restorative phases to replenish the energy lost during labor and childbirth and to gain confidence in her role as mother. Both mother and father begin the process of attachment with the newborn. Siblings must adapt to a new standing in the family structure and deal with feelings of jealousy and rivalry that may result from the birth of an infant. Numerous factors, such as previous experience and the availability of a strong support system, influence family adaptation. Moreover, culture is among the most significant variables that influence a family's perception of childbearing.

The role of maternity nurses has gradually expanded from the care of the mother-infant dyad to include the well-being of the entire family. Nurses are concerned about the family's adjustment to childbearing, not only during the hospital stay but also during the early weeks at home as they make the transition to parenthood.

## The Process of Becoming Acquainted

A great deal of information has appeared in nursing literature in recent years that describes how parents and newborns become acquainted and progress to develop feelings of love, concern, and deep devotion that last throughout life. The terms *bonding* and *attachment* are commonly used to describe the initial steps. Although the terms are sometimes used interchangeably, their meanings do differ.

### Bonding

Researchers in the 1970s and 1980s coined the term *bonding* to describe the rapid process of attachment that they observed soon after childbirth. Bonding describes the initial attraction felt by parents. It is unidirectional, from parent to child, and is enhanced when parent and infant are permitted to touch and interact during a so-called *sensitive period* that extends through the first 30 to 60 minutes following birth. During this time the infant is in a quiet, alert stage. The eyes are open, and he or she seems to gaze directly at the parents (Fig. 18–1).

Nurses frequently delay procedures that can interfere with this time between parents and newborns. Instillation of prophylactic eye medication, administration of vitamin K injections, and measurements of the head, chest, and length are often postponed so that the parents can have this time with their newborn baby.

Unfortunately, information about a sensitive period was misinterpreted by many parents and health care workers, who believed it to be the critical time for the process of attachment to begin. This misunderstanding resulted in unfounded fears that bonding would not occur if contact between parent and infant was limited at this time because of an obstetric emergency or illness in a neonate. There are many routes to attachment, however, and no period of time is critical for beginning the attachment process (Mercer & Ferketich, 1994a).

### Attachment

*Attachment* is the process by which an enduring bond to a child is developed through pleasurable, satisfying parent-child interaction. The process begins in pregnancy and extends for many months following childbirth. The infant receives warmth, food, and security from the parent. The parent (usually the mother) accepts responsibility for the infant's care and places the child's needs above her own for years to come. In return, she receives enjoyment and

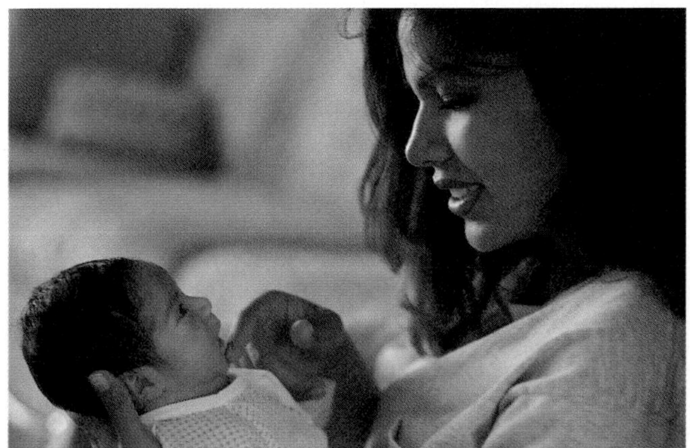

**FIGURE 18–1**

The infant is quiet and alert during the initial sensitive period. The newborn gazes at the mother and responds to her voice and touch.

## Critical to Remember

### RECIPROCAL ATTACHMENT BEHAVIORS

Newborn infants have the ability to do the following:

- Make eye contact and engage in prolonged, intense, mutual gazing
- Move their eyes and attempt to "track" the parent's face
- Grasp the parent's finger and hold on
- Move synchronously in response to rhythms and patterns of the parent's voice; synchronized movement is called *entrainment*
- Root, suckle, and finally latch on to the breast
- Be comforted by the parent's voice or touch

establishes her identity as a mother. Both benefit from the formation of irreplaceable links that continue long after the child ceases to be dependent.

Three important concepts regarding attachment are the following:

- Attachment is a process that follows a progressive or developmental course that changes over time. It is rarely instantaneous. Attachment behaviors of inexperienced or first-time mothers do not differ significantly from those of experienced mothers (Mercer & Ferketich, 1994b).
- Attachment is facilitated by positive feedback, either real or perceived; thus, an infant's grasp reflex around a parent's finger means "I love you" to the parent.
- Attachment occurs through mutually satisfying experiences; therefore, if the newly delivered mother is in severe pain or is physically exhausted, she needs pain relief, assistance, or both, for her to enjoy the early experiences with the baby (Mercer & Ferketich, 1990b).

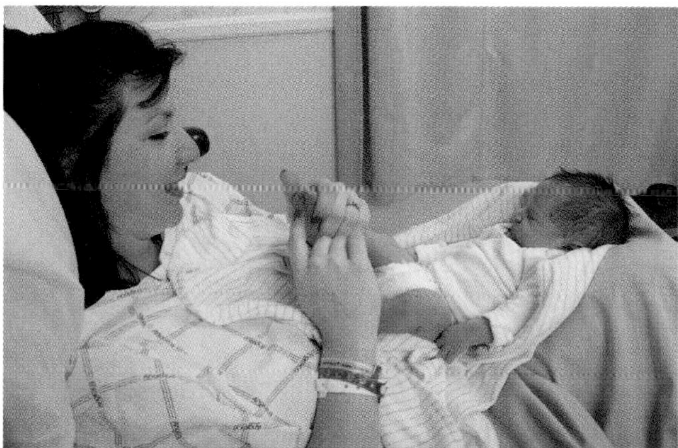

**FIGURE 18–2**

The mother's initial touch includes *finger-tipping*, whereby she becomes acquainted with her infant by touching only with her fingertips.

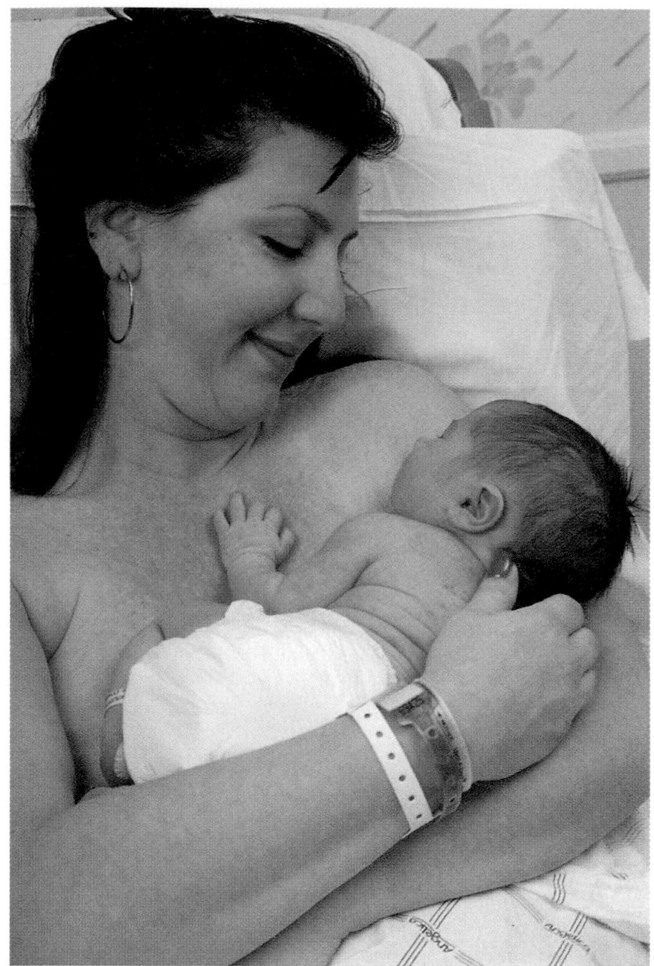

**FIGURE 18–3**

Mothers progress from exploratory touching to enfolding the infant. Their pleasure is enhanced by skin-to-skin contact.

Unlike bonding, attachment is reciprocal; that is, it goes in both directions between parent and infant. For attachment to occur, there must be some response from the infant to parental signals. Alert infants have a whole repertoire of responses called *reciprocal attachment behaviors*. They are the infant's part in the process of early attachment that progresses to lifelong mutual devotion.

### Maternal Touch

Maternal behavior, particularly maternal touch, changes rapidly as the mother progresses through a discovery phase with her infant. Initially, the mother may not reach for the infant, but if the infant is placed in her arms, she holds the baby in an *en face* position, with the infant's face in the same vertical plane as her own. When the infant is awake, the two engage in prolonged mutual gazing, as illustrated in Figure 18–1.

The mother needs time to get acquainted with the tiny stranger. She may gently explore the infant's face, fingers, and toes with her fingertips only. Figure 18–2 illustrates finger-tipping, which is common during the early minutes.

Although some mothers "finger-tip" the infant for a few minutes, others begin to stroke the baby's chest and legs with the palm. Next, the mother uses her entire hand to enfold the infant and to bring him or her close to her body. She holds the newborn closer, strokes the baby's hair, presses her cheek against the infant's cheek, and finally feels comfortable enough to engage in a full range of consoling behaviors (Fig. 18–3).

The mother next begins to identify specific features of the newborn. "Look at his little pink mouth." Then she begins to relate features to family members. "He has his father's chin and nose (Fig. 18–4)."

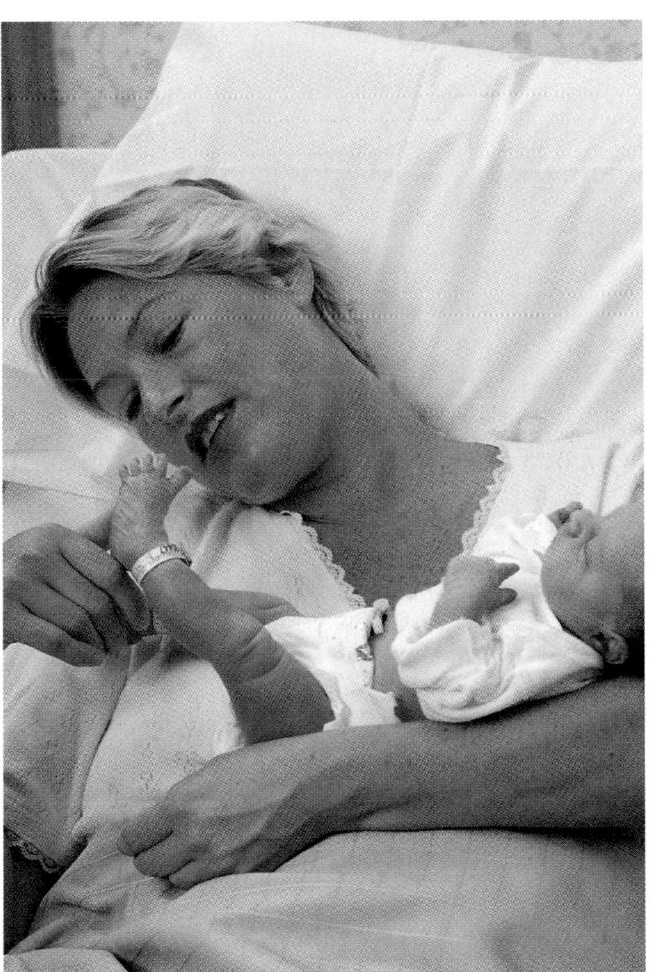

**FIGURE 18–4**

The *binding-in* or *claiming* process includes the mother's identification of her baby's specific features, relating them to other family members. This mother states, "his long toes are exactly like mine."

This identification process has been termed *claiming* or *binding-in* (Rubin, 1977).

### Verbal Behaviors

Verbal behaviors are also important indicators of maternal attachment. Most mothers speak to the infant in a high-pitched voice and progress from calling the baby "it" to "he or she" and then to using the given name. "I cannot believe it is here" rapidly becomes "Michele is such a good girl." Verbal behaviors may provide clues to a mother's early psychological relationship to her infant. Mothers who show the most nonverbal attachment behaviors have been found also to be considerably more active in verbal behaviors (Tomlinson, 1990). Nurses are in a position to observe interactions of mothers and their infants and, if necessary, to teach and model interactions that foster early attachment between them.

**CHECK YOUR READING**

1. How do bonding and attachment differ?
2. How does maternal touch change over time?
3. How does verbal interaction change over time?

## The Process of Maternal Adaptation

### Puerperal Phases

In the early 1960s, Rubin identified restorative phases that the mother must go through to replenish the energy lost during labor and to attain comfort in the role of mother. The puerperal phases are called *taking-in, taking-hold, and letting-go,* and for 35 years they have been used to plan and implement nursing care during the postpartum period.

Although many aspects of maternity care have changed and Rubin's original study has been questioned, contemporary investigators tend to support the concept that mothers do progress through fairly discrete phases of recovery, although at a more rapid rate than was first thought (Martell & Mitchell, 1984; Ament, 1990). The three phases may provide a useful method to observe progressive change in maternal behavior but should not be used as strict guidelines for maternal assessment; rather, they can be used to anticipate maternal needs and to intervene to meet those needs.

#### TAKING-IN PHASE

During the taking-in phase, the mother is focused primarily on her own need for fluid, food, and deep restorative sleep. Inexperienced nurses may be puzzled by the mother's passive behavior as she takes in or receives attention and physical care. She also takes in or absorbs every detail of the neonate, but she seems content to allow others to make decisions.

A major task for the mother during this time is to integrate her birth experience into reality. To do this she recounts the details of her labor and delivery over and over. She may spend a great deal of time on the telephone describing her labor and the birth of this child. She repeats her experiences for visitors and attempts to piece together all the details from those who were involved. This process helps the mother realize that the pregnancy is over; the infant is born, and he or she is now an individual separate from her. Although Rubin believed that the taking-in phase lasted for approximately 2 days, later investigators observed the behaviors for 24 hours or less (Ament, 1990).

The taking-in phase may be prolonged when a cesarean birth—especially an emergency cesarean delivery—has been necessary. Many women have difficulty assimilating the unfamiliar and intrusive procedures that occurred in rapid succession, and they express negative perceptions of the birth experience (Miovech et al., 1994). Studies suggest that women who have had a cesarean birth require continued attention and sensitive care that takes into account their special needs for pain relief and sustained contact with their newborn (Reichert et al., 1993).

#### TAKING-HOLD PHASE

The mother becomes more independent in the taking-hold phase. She exhibits concern about managing her own body functions and assumes responsibility for her own self-care. When she feels more comfortable and in control of her body, she shifts her attention from her own needs to the performance of the infant. She compares her infant with other infants to validate wellness and wholeness. She welcomes information about the wide variety of behaviors exhibited by newborns.

During the taking-hold phase, the mother may verbalize a great deal of anxiety about her competence as a mother. She may compare her caretaking skills unfavorably with those of the nurse. *Nurses must be careful not to assume the mothering role but instead to allow the mother to perform as much of the caretaking as possible and to praise each attempt, even if the mother's early care is awkwardly performed.*

The taking-hold phase, which extends over several days, has been called the "teachable, reachable, referrable moment." Nurses who provide home care can take advantage of this ideal time to review previously taught material and to provide additional instructions and demonstrations.

#### LETTING-GO PHASE

The letting-go phase is a time of relinquishment for the mother and often for the father. If this is a first child, the couple must give up their previous role as a childless couple and acknowledge the loss of a carefree lifestyle. Many mothers must also give up idealized expectations of the birth experience. For example, they may have planned to have a vaginal birth with minimal or no anesthesia, but instead they required a cesarean birth or regional anesthesia. In addition, some mothers (and fathers) are disappointed in the size, sex, or characteristics of the infant who does not "match up" with the fantasy baby of pregnancy. They must relinquish the infant

### THERAPEUTIC COMMUNICATION

## Anxiety About Caretaking Skills

Fawn Jackson is a nurse in the postpartum unit. When she enters the room of Tamara Bradley, a new mother, she finds the woman crying.

**Tamara** (crying): I can't do anything right. The pediatrician just asked me a bunch of questions, and I couldn't answer any of them.

**Fawn:** In fact, you are doing a lot right, but it is distressing when you feel you don't have all the answers.

*Offering reassurance and acknowledging feelings*

**Tamara:** Well, he just fired the questions at me and I couldn't think so fast.

**Fawn:** You feel that you're not measuring up because you couldn't answer the questions?

*Paraphrasing and focusing on Tamara's feelings*

**Tamara:** Well, I want to be a good mother, but I'm so worried that I won't know what to do.

**Fawn:** You're concerned that you don't have all the answers.

*Reflecting feelings without leading*

**Tamara:** There is just so much to caring for a baby. I don't know where to start.

**Fawn:** You don't feel confident about how to take care of the baby. What concerns you most?

*Reflecting feelings and inviting the mother to describe specific concerns*

*By allowing Tamara to express her feelings, Fawn has helped dissipate the feelings and set the stage for effective teaching.*

of their fantasies and accept the real infant. These losses often provoke feelings of grief that may be so subtle that they are unexamined or unacknowledged. Both parents may benefit, however, if given the opportunity to verbalize unexpected feelings and to realize that these feelings are common. If the mother is very young or the pregnancy was unplanned, the feelings of loss and grief may be acute.

## Maternal Role Attainment

Role attainment is a process in which the mother achieves confidence in her ability to care for her infant and becomes comfortable with her identity as a mother. The process begins during pregnancy and continues for several months following childbirth.

The transition to the maternal or paternal role follows four stages (Mercer, 1985):

1. *The anticipatory stage* begins during the pregnancy when pregnant women choose a physician or nurse-midwife and the location for the infant's birth. Many attend childbirth classes in order to be prepared and to have some control over the birth experience. Expectant mothers seek out role models for learning how to assume the role of mother.
2. *The formal stage* begins with the birth of the infant and continues for approximately 6 to 8 weeks (Mercer, 1990). During this stage, behaviors are largely guided by others: health professionals, close friends, or parents. A major task during this stage is for mothers (and fathers) to become acquainted with their infant so that they can mesh their parenting activities with cues from the infant.
3. *The informal stage* begins once the parents have learned appropriate responses to their infant's cues or signals. They begin to respond according to the unique needs of the infant rather than following textbook or health professionals' directives.
4. *The personal stage* is attained when the parent feels a sense of harmony in the role, enjoys the infant, sees the infant as a central person in his or her life, and has internalized the parental role. The mother or father accepts the role of parent and feels comfortable in this role. The range of time for achieving the parental role is highly variable, but most parents feel that they have achieved it by 4 months (Mercer, 1986).

## Redefining Roles

The mother is particularly concerned about redefining roles and focuses on maintaining a strong, adaptive relationship with her partner. She observes him carefully for any change in behavior and is acutely sensitive to his interaction with the infant. From the father's perspective, anxieties about succeeding in his new role put added pressure on the family. Conflicting demands between work and home, feelings of exclusion, and concerns about his relationship with his partner present additional challenges.

It may be essential for the new parents to agree on a division of tasks and responsibilities that was not necessary before the birth of the infant. This process is accomplished quickly and with very little discord in some families. Role assignment in other families is much less flexible, and any change can be a source of tension and frustration.

Although nurses are not actively involved in redefining family roles, they can use their skills in communication to assist the family in expressing their feelings and concerns so that the changes can be accomplished with minimum stress.

## Role Conflict

Role conflict occurs when one's perception of role responsibilities differs significantly from reality. For example, if the mother perceives that her responsibility is to provide the most care and comfort for the infant, but reality dictates that she must place the infant with another caregiver and return to full-time employment, role conflict may occur. Nearly 2 million women in the United States face this conflict each year, and many report feelings of guilt for leaving the infant and experience intense "separation grief" when they first leave the infant with a caregiver. Some report feeling jealous of the caregiver and fear that they will be supplanted by him or her in the infant's affection.

Acknowledging these feelings and reassuring the mother that her emotions are normal may be helpful. The mother also needs time to reestablish feelings of closeness when she comes home from work, and she needs to develop a schedule that allows maximum time with the infant when she is at home. She may have to negotiate with another family member to take over some of the household tasks until she feels more comfortable with the situation. Nursing Care Plan 18–1 describes additional interventions.

## Major Maternal Concerns

Nurses must plan follow-up care based on the knowledge that after childbirth mothers have major concerns that change over time. For instance, during the first month concerns about feeding, infant behavior, and physical care of the infant predominate. Maternal concerns related to the self include discomfort and fatigue. Concerns about family relationships include having less time with older children and not being interested in sex (Sheil et al., 1995). Mothers

## Nursing Care Plan 18–1

# Adaptation of the Working Mother

**ASSESSMENT:** Rebecca Sanders, a 30-year-old single mother, gave birth to a baby boy by cesarean delivery 4 days ago. She cares for herself with minimal assistance and demonstrates confidence in breastfeeding. Rebecca must return to work as a sales executive in 6 weeks. She states that she does not want to leave the baby with someone else while she works. "My mother was always there for me and I want to be with Derrek, but it is just impossible. How can I be a mother and work full time?"

**NURSING DIAGNOSIS:** Anticipatory Grieving related to inability to perform role of mother as she wishes because of the need to place the infant with another care provider and return to full-time employment

**Critical Thinking**

Grieving is related to loss. What has Rebecca lost or what must she give up?

**ANSWER**

Rebecca must give up her idealized picture of motherhood. She must also give up mothering tasks and time with the infant to another caregiver. She will have to modify her self-concept based on the perception of these losses.

### GOALS/EXPECTED OUTCOMES

Rebecca will do the following:

1. Describe the concerns and feelings that result from her need to leave her infant with a secondary caregiver by (specific date).
2. Verbalize plans to achieve maximum satisfaction in her role as mother by the time she returns to work.

| INTERVENTION | RATIONALE |
|---|---|
| 1. Allow Rebecca to describe her perception of her role as mother and to express concerns about how employment will interfere with her ability to fulfill this role. | 1. Role conflict, stress, and grief can result when a mother, who envisions her role as the primary caregiver and always available, must leave the infant with another caregiver and return to her job. |
| 2. Recommend free expression of feelings to significant others and to the care provider who is selected. Many mothers experience intense "separation grief" as well as anxiety, guilt, and jealousy when they leave the infant with a care provider. | 2. Candid expression of feelings helps to resolve them and opens the way for a discussion of measures that will help to overcome the intense feelings that cause so much mental conflict. |
| 3. Acknowledge the feelings Rebecca expresses, and reassure her that the feelings are common. | 3. Knowledge that the feelings are not trivial and that they are common reinforces their validity and importance. |
| 4. Help Rebecca develop a schedule that allows her maximum time with the infant:<br>a. Make a list of errands and supplies needed to avoid frequent stops that delay getting home from work.<br>b. Double the recipe when cooking, and freeze half for future use.<br>c. Pick up nutritious take-out meals to avoid cooking each evening.<br>d. Schedule appointments on the same day when possible.<br>e. Work out plans that include the baby in daily walks, exercise, or social visits. | 4. Feelings of frustration and stress can be alleviated if the mother has a plan that allows her long periods of uninterrupted time with the infant. |
| 5. Recommend that Rebecca allow 30 to 45 minutes when she first gets home to hold the infant. Delay all other activities until this need is satisfied for both mother and infant. | 5. Time is needed to re-establish feelings of closeness, comfort, and attachment. |

## Nursing Care Plan 18–1 *Continued*
## Adaptation of the Working Mother

| INTERVENTION | RATIONALE |
|---|---|
| 6. Suggest that Rebecca delay her return to employment, if possible, until the infant is at least 16 weeks old. | 6. By 16 weeks most infants are able to sleep through the night; this reduces the chance that sleep deprivation will add to the stress of working, caring for the infant, and leaving the infant with a secondary care provider. |
| 7. Recommend that Rebecca investigate several daycare providers before choosing and that she check references, make unannounced visits, insist on seeing required licenses and certification, discuss the number and ages of children cared for, request a schedule of planned care, determine the provider's philosophy of infant care (rigid schedule, predictable environment, or no planned schedule), determine whether the care provider is trained in cardiopulmonary resuscitation (CPR), and know what plans are in place if a fire or disaster occurs. | 7. A great deal of stress is eliminated if parents feel confident that a competent and nurturing daycare provider has been found. |
| 8. Suggest that Rebecca leave the infant with the chosen daycare provider for 2 to 3 days before resuming full-time employment. | 8. Allowing both mother and infant to "practice separating" while there is still some flexibility in their schedules makes the first day back at work less traumatic. |
| 9. Recommend that Rebecca pump her breasts and feed the infant by bottle at least once a day before returning to work. | 9. Becoming proficient at pumping the breasts and introducing the infant to bottle feeding prepares both the mother and infant for all-day separation. |

**EVALUATION**

Rebecca freely expressed her feelings of guilt, anxiety, and concern about leaving her infant. She has organized a plan to investigate daycare in her area and verbalized plans to reorganize her work and social schedule so that she can spend as much time as possible with her son.

**ADDITIONAL NURSING DIAGNOSES TO CONSIDER**

Diversional Activity Deficit
Parental Role Conflict
Altered Role Performance

who had a cesarean birth also express concerns about limited activity and incisional healing (Miovech et al., 1994).

### BODY IMAGE

As women gain confidence in their ability to care for the infant and as their physical discomfort decreases, emotional concerns related to the self become more intense. In particular, women express concern about regaining their normal figure. Some mothers have unrealistic expectations about weight loss and the time it takes for the body to regain its pre-pregnancy shape.

Nurses must emphasize that weight loss should be gradual and that about 6 months is usually required to lose the weight gained during pregnancy. Rigid restriction of calories can lead to depleted energy, decreased immunity, and decreased production of milk.

Moreover, nurses should teach the importance of safe activities such as walking and the importance of graduated exercises to regain muscle tone. Mothers should seek the advice of a health care professional before initiating a rigorous exercise program. See Chapter 17 for additional information about postpartum exercises.

### POSTPARTUM BLUES

Mild depression, also known as postpartum blues or maternity blues, is a frequently expressed concern. This mild, transient condition affects 75 to 80 percent of American women who have just given birth. The condition has an early onset (1 to 10 days after a woman has given birth) and usually lasts no longer than 2 weeks (Ugarriza, 1992). It is characterized by fatigue, weeping, mood instability, and anxiety. The symptoms are usually unrelated to events, and the condition does not seriously affect the ability of the mother to care for the infant. Typically, the mother says, "I do not know why I am crying; I do not feel sad." Although the direct cause is unknown, it is generally accepted that postpartum blues is related to the wide hormonal fluctuations that occur during labor, delivery, and the immediate postpartum period. Although postpartum blues is self-limiting, mothers benefit greatly when unsolicited empathy and support are freely given by the family and the health care team.

Postpartum blues must be distinguished from *postpartum depression* and *postpartum psychosis*. These separate entities are disabling and require therapeutic management for full recovery. (Chapter 28 provides a more detailed discussion of postpartum depression and postpartum psychosis.)

**CHECK YOUR READING**

4. How do maternal behaviors in the taking-in phase differ from those in the taking-hold phase?
5. What does the mother (and the father) relinquish in the letting-go phase?
6. How do the parents progress through the stages of role attainment?
7. What causes postpartum blues? How can nurses intervene for this common emotional response?

## The Process of Family Adaptation

The birth of an infant requires that roles and relationships within the family be reorganized. The previously childless couple now must integrate a new member into the family unit. Fathers learn new skills and often adjust to new roles as they share responsibilities with their partners. Siblings must adapt to a new standing in the family structure. Expectations and involvement of grandparents vary widely and may be a source of support or of increased stress for the family.

### Fathers

The father's developing bond to his newborn has been called *engrossment*. It is characterized by intense interest in how the infant looks and responds, along with a desire to touch and hold the baby. Many fathers comment on the baby's distinctive features and view the baby as perfect. They experience strong attraction to the infant and express elation described as a "high" following the baby's birth. Attachment behaviors of the father parallel behaviors of the mother; they increase when the infant is awake, makes eye contact, and responds to the father's voice (Fig. 18–5).

It has been thought that fathers who were active participants in the birth experienced early bonding and developed stronger ties to the newborn. Research indicates, however, that other factors such as relationship with his own parents, previous experience with children, and relationship with the mother are more important variables (Ferketich & Mercer, 1995b).

Many fathers eagerly look forward to co-parenting with their mate; however, they may lack confidence in providing infant care and are sensitive to being left out of instructions and demonstrations of infant care. Many report that they receive the pervasive message that their major role is to support the

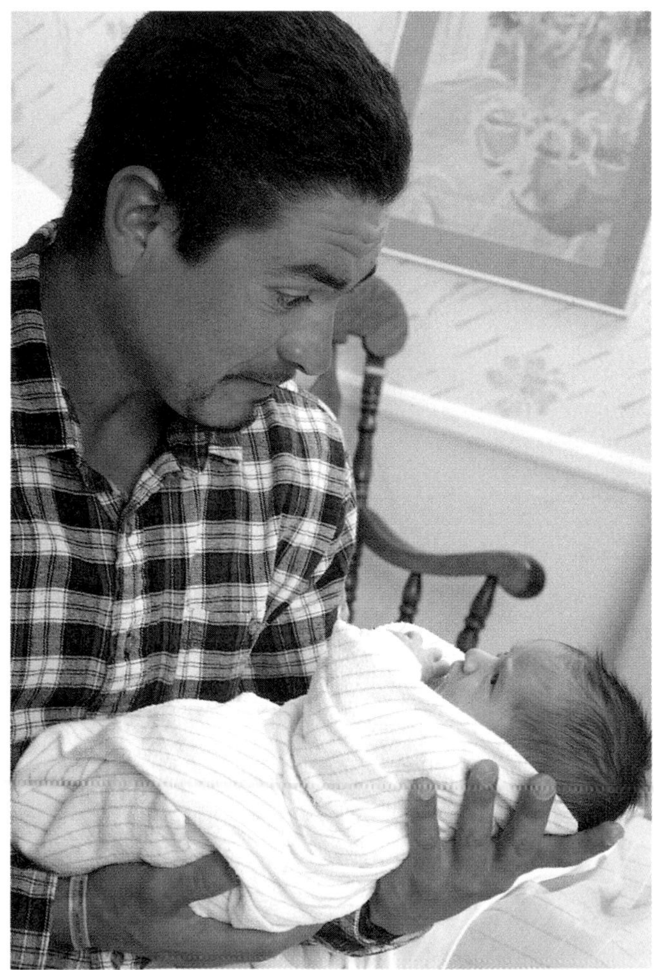

**FIGURE 18–5**

Fathers' behaviors at initial contact with their infants often correspond to maternal behaviors. The intense fascination that fathers exhibit is called *engrossment*. Note eye-to-eye contact between father and infant.

mother (Jordan, 1990). One father said he had been treated as a "fifth wheel" and resented patronizing remarks about his awkwardness when he handled the infant.

Research indicates that fathers need more parenting information than that provided in prenatal classes. In particular, fathers often do not know what to expect from infants during the first 3 months of life. Fathers would benefit from additional information about normal growth and development during infancy. Moreover, information about child care, presented in the prenatal period, should be reviewed after the child is born—when the information is relevant and the father is ready to learn (Tiller, 1995).

## Siblings

Sibling response to the birth of a new brother or sister depends on age and developmental level. Toddlers are usually not completely aware of the impending birth. They may view the infant as competition or fear that they will be replaced in the parents' affection. Negative behaviors may surface and indicate the degree of stress the youngster feels. These behaviors include sleep problems, an increase in attention-seeking efforts, and regression to more infantile behaviors, such as renewed bed-wetting or thumb-sucking. Some may exhibit hostile behaviors toward the mother, particularly when she holds or feeds the newborn. These behaviors are manifestations of the jealousy and frustration that young children feel as they observe the mother's attention being given to another. Parents must find opportunities to affirm their continued love and affection for the very vulnerable sibling.

Preschool siblings engage in more looking than touching. The majority spend at least some time in proximity to the infant and talk to the mother about the infant (Fig. 18–6).

A relaxed, natural setting, without time constraints,

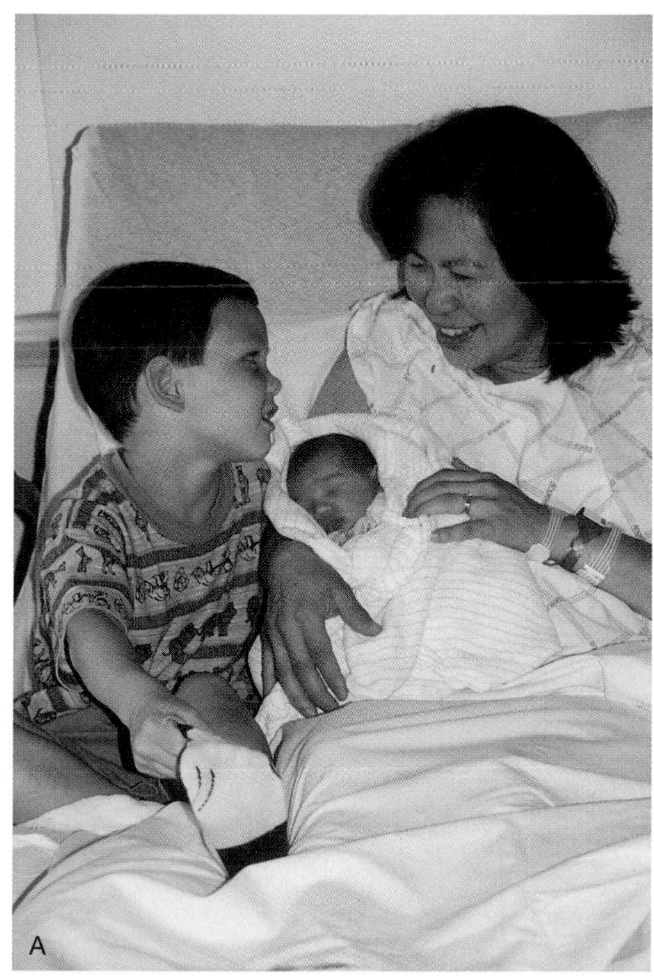


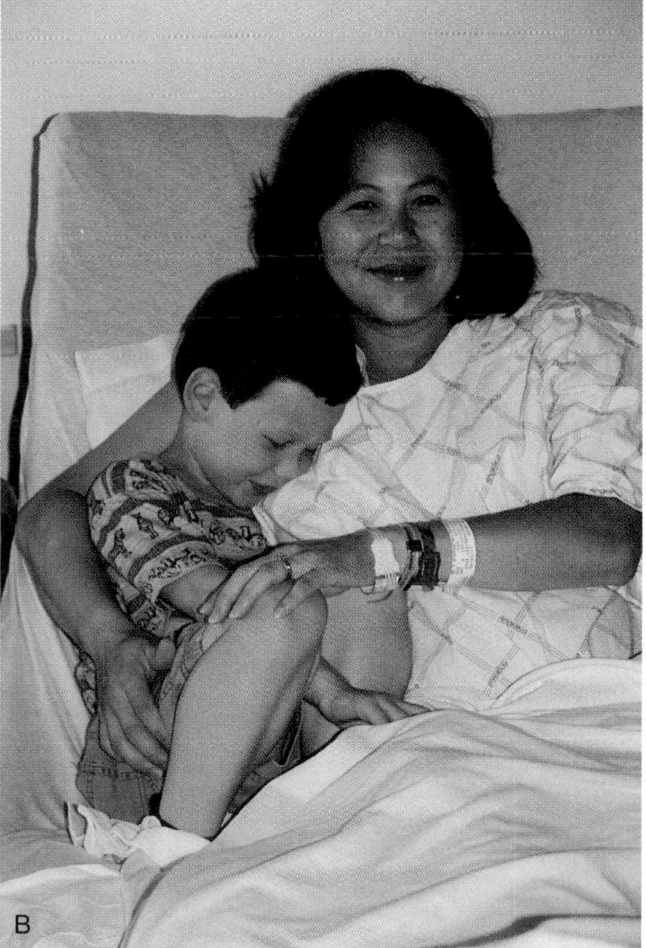


**FIGURE 18–6**

A, Although they may hesitate to touch the infant, children often want to be close. B, This boy's relief and joy are obvious as he reclaims a favorite spot.

may make it easier for young children to interact with the infant. Special care must be taken by the parents, visitors, and nurses to pay as much attention to the sibling as to the new baby.

### Grandparents

The involvement of grandparents with grandchildren depends on many factors. One of the most important factors is proximity. Grandparents who live near enough to see the child frequently develop strong attachment that evolves into unconditional love and a special relationship that brings joy to the grandparents and an added sense of security to the grandchildren.

Often grandparents live many miles from grandchildren, and their contact is, of necessity, sporadic. It is more difficult to form a close attachment when contact is infrequent, and many grandparents spend time trying to devise ways to foster a relationship with grandchildren they seldom see.

Expectations of the role of grandparents are also a factor in how the grandparents adapt to the birth of a grandchild. Many grandparents feel that their role is second in importance to the role of parents, and they strive to be fully involved in the care and upbringing of the child. Others desire less involvement; this may cause some conflict with parents, or it may be a comfortable arrangement with both families.

Grandparents are often a major part of the support system that new parents need. Grandmothers, in particular, provide assistance with household tasks and infant care, which allows the mother to recover from childbirth and make the transition to parenthood. The birth of a grandchild allows grandfathers the opportunity to nurture (Fig. 18–7). They may have been too busy providing for their own children to fully enjoy this aspect of parenting and may want to participate more fully with grandchildren.

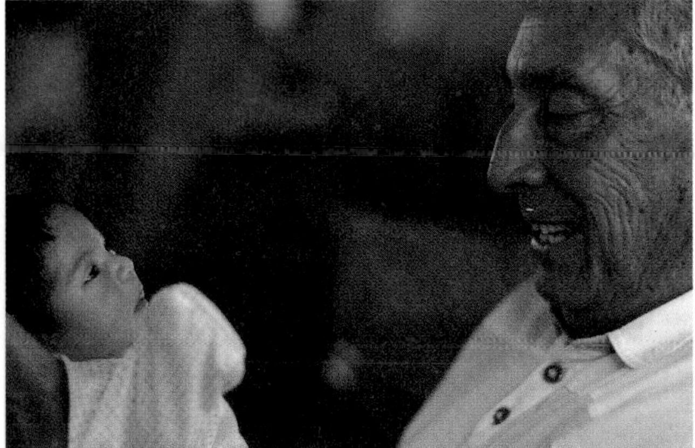

**FIGURE 18–7**

Grandfathers may develop strong bonds with grandchildren.

## Factors Affecting Family Adaptation

Numerous factors influence the family's adjustment. Some can be anticipated because they are so common; lingering discomfort and chronic fatigue in the mother are almost universal. Additional factors include knowledge of infant needs, expectations of the infant, previous experience, age of the parents, and the temperaments of the mother and the infant. Unanticipated events, such as cesarean birth, birth of a preterm or ill infant, or birth of twins also affect the ease and speed with which the family adjusts.

### Lingering Discomfort and Fatigue

Normally, discomfort associated with childbirth, such as perineal pain or afterpains, resolve within the first days following the birth. Discomfort may make it difficult, however, to focus on the needs of the newborn. Fatigue often remains a problem during the first few weeks, when the infant's schedule is erratic and the chance for uninterrupted sleep is minimal. When the infant begins to sleep through the night (at about 16 weeks), the parents can once again establish familiar patterns, and fatigue becomes less of a factor.

### Knowledge of Infant Needs

Parents experience powerful feelings of protectiveness when they discover that they can console their infants and that the infants respond to their care. First-time parents, however, are often unsure of how to care for the newborn and become very anxious if they are unable to console a crying infant. Moreover, many are concerned about specific procedures, such as care of the umbilical cord or the circumcision. They want to know if the infant is receiving adequate nutrition. Breastfeeding benefits both mother and infant; however, initially it adds to the stress that par-

**Critical to Remember**

**FACTORS THAT AFFECT ADAPTATION**

- Lingering discomfort or pain
- Chronic fatigue
- Knowledge of infant needs
- Available support system
- Expectations of the newborn
- Previous experience with infants
- Maternal temperament
- Infant characteristics
- Unanticipated events: cesarean birth, preterm or ill infant, or birth of more than one infant (twins)

ents experience. Is the infant getting enough milk? What happens until the milk comes in? How often should one nurse? (Chapter 22 provides detailed information about breastfeeding, and Chapter 23 discusses early parenting.)

Some parents have concerns about spoiling the infant. They are particularly concerned about responding each time the infant cries and believe that this causes the child to cry to get his or her way. It may be necessary to remind parents that infants cry to indicate a need: they are hungry, cold, or wet or they need to be cuddled or gently stimulated. It is important to reassure the parents that responding to infant crying does not spoil the child. Prompt, gentle response when the infant cries helps him or her to develop trust that the world is a safe, secure place. Trust is a basic developmental task of infancy that depends on the child's learning that caregivers respond consistently and gently.

### Previous Experience

Previous experience with newborns may also affect family adjustment. As expected, multiparas are more comfortable with infants and exhibit attachment behaviors earlier than do primiparas, who may spend many more hours in the early discovery phase of attachment. Mothers who have previously given birth to infants with anomalies or to infants who did not survive may need more time to feel comfortable with this infant.

### Expectations for the Newborn

Unrealistic expectations of the infant may also influence adjustment. Many parents have very little experience with newborns and are disappointed at the way a newborn looks. They are unprepared for the normal characteristics of newborns, such as cranial molding, blotchy skin, and blue hands and feet. They may have anticipated that the infant would be able to smile and would sleep through the night.

Nurses must be prepared to teach normal growth and development and to assist the parents in working through their misconceptions. For instance, the capacity of an infant's stomach is small, and the infant must be fed frequently. Also, infants are neurologically unable to sleep through the night for several weeks. They begin to smile in about 5 to 6 weeks, but they are able to see and hear from the time of birth.

Some mothers may be very disappointed in the sex of the child, or they may sense that their partners are disappointed. These feelings must be acknowledged and dealt with before attachment can take place. One mother, who already had four sons, was so disappointed when the fifth child turned out to be a boy that she cried for several hours and refused to see the infant. Her grief continued until she held the baby and began to observe differences and make comparisons with her other sons. This interaction began her discovery period with this unique child.

### Maternal Age

Adjustment to parenthood is a challenge for teenagers who have not achieved a strong sense of their own identity. In general, teenagers tend to talk less, respond less, appear more passive, and sometimes appear less affectionate with their children than do adult parents. Clearly, teenaged mothers and fathers need special assistance to develop necessary parenting skills that promote optimal development of the infant. (Additional information regarding teenaged parenting is presented in Chapter 24.)

### Maternal Temperament

Maternal personality traits are a major influence on attachment. Mothers who are calm, secure in their ability to learn, and free from unnecessary anxiety adjust more easily to the demands of motherhood. Conversely, mothers who are excitable, insecure, and anxious have more difficulty. Mothers who are aware that it takes time for the body to return to its prepregnancy weight and who do not insist on rigorous dieting or an unrealistic exercise regimen adjust more easily.

### Temperament of the Infant

The infant also affects maternal adjustment. Infants who are calm, easily consoled, and enjoy cuddling increase parental confidence and feelings of competence. Conversely, irritable infants who are difficult to console and who do not need or respond to cuddling increase parental frustration and interfere with attachment.

### Availability of a Strong Support System

A strong, consistent support system is a major factor in the adjustment of the new mother. She needs assistance with household tasks such as meal preparation, laundry, and shopping. In addition, she needs encouragement, praise, and reassurance that she is a good mother. It is very important to her that others see that the baby is special and that they demonstrate love and affection.

### Unanticipated Events

#### CESAREAN BIRTH

Unanticipated events can make parental adjustment more difficult. For example, an unplanned cesarean birth may result in financial strain, a longer recovery time for the mother, additional discomfort, and increased stress for the family. Birth of a preterm or ill infant results in additional concern about the condition of the infant and may necessitate prolonged separation of parents and child. This separation may delay the process of attachment and create stress on the normally functioning family.

### BIRTH OF TWINS

Even if expected, the birth of more than one infant may present problems of attachment. It is believed the process of attachment is structured so that the parents become attached to only one infant at a time. Therefore, parents should be encouraged to interact with each child individually, especially in the early getting-acquainted period. Nurses must help the parents to relate to each infant as an individual rather than as part of a unit by pointing out the individual responses and uniqueness of each infant. Early, frequent contacts or rooming-in helps the parents gain confidence in caretaking and facilitates the attachment process. Mothers are sometimes overwhelmed at the prospect of breastfeeding twins. They need reassurance that they will produce an ample supply of milk for each infant because supply increases with demand. Additional information is provided in Nursing Care Plan 18–2 (Adaptation to the Birth of Twins) and in Chapter 22.

## Nursing Care Plan 18–2
## Adaptation to the Birth of Twins

**ASSESSMENT:** Maureen Parry, a 32-year-old primipara, gave birth to twin girls 22 hours ago. Her labor was induced at term, and she was able to deliver vaginally. She and her husband knew for several months that they were expecting twins; however, neither has experience with infants. Maureen took breastfeeding classes, and both she and her husband attended parenting classes during her pregnancy. Both infants are in the room, and she moves anxiously from one to the other. She has examined both infants; however, she has not had individual time with each infant. She touches the infants cautiously and asks, "How in the world will I be able to care for two babies?"

**NURSING DIAGNOSIS:** Risk for Altered Parenting related to inadequate time with individual infants and lack of confidence in ability to provide care for two infants

**Critical Thinking**

What data (behaviors) led to this diagnosis?

What other data would confirm the diagnosis?

**ANSWER**

It is believed that parents can become attached to only one child at a time, and Maureen has not had time with each child individually. Observing how she touches and interacts verbally with each child and noting that names have not been selected might confirm the diagnosis.

**GOALS/EXPECTED OUTCOMES**

Maureen will do the following:

1. Demonstrate progressive bonding behaviors with each infant before discharge.
2. Collaborate with nursing staff and with her husband to devise a plan for caring for the infants during the early weeks at home.
3. Verbalize increased confidence in her ability to care for the infants before discharge.

| INTERVENTION | RATIONALE |
|---|---|
| 1. Promote bonding and attachment with individual infants by allowing separate time with each infant and pointing out the unique characteristics of each child. For instance, Baby Girl A is larger, she has less hair, and she looks directly at her mother. Baby Girl B is small but alert, and she enjoys cuddling. | 1. It is believed that parents can become attached to only one infant at a time. They must go through the getting-acquainted phases separately and progress with individual infants rather than with both twins at the same time. |

## *Nursing Care Plan 18–2 Continued*
# *Adaptation to the Birth of Twins*

| INTERVENTION | RATIONALE |
|---|---|
| 2. Make sure that the parents have contact with the infant who is awake and responsive. | 2. The infant must respond to the parent by some signal, such as eye contact, gazing, or responding to the parent's voice (entrainment) for attachment to occur. |
| 3. Foster a relaxed atmosphere that permits unlimited contact between the parents and the twins; use some of the time to model behaviors such as holding, consoling, and talking to the infants. | 3. A relaxed atmosphere and prolonged contact with the twins provide the best opportunity for interaction that promotes bonding. Modeling is one of the most effective teaching strategies for demonstrating appropriate interactions. |
| 4. Encourage participation in infant care. Model infant care, and praise all maternal efforts to provide care. | 4. Caring for the infant or successfully consoling a crying infant elicits powerful feelings of nurturing and responsibility and greatly increases feelings of confidence and competence. |
| 5. Assist Maureen in making a plan for caring for the twins.<br>a. Provide instruction and encouragement with breastfeeding; if necessary, refer parents to a lactation educator for continuing support. (See Chapter 22 for detailed information about breastfeeding twins.)<br>b. Suggest that the parents keep a record of care for each baby for the first few days at home so that they do not become confused; include feeding times, elimination, and baths.<br>c. Reassure parents that it is not necessary to bathe and shampoo the infants each day; bathing every other day is adequate because the face, neck, and buttocks are bathed as necessary. | 5. Breastfeeding is usually established within 2 weeks, and during this time the mother needs information and encouragement. Collaborating on a plan for providing and recording care increases the parents' confidence in their ability to care for the infants. This is particularly true when the parents receive reassurance that care does not have to be on a strict schedule. |
| 6. Emphasize the importance of obtaining adequate rest. Suggest that the mother sleep when the infants sleep, and suggest that the parents take turns caring for the infants. Recommend that they accept assistance with all household tasks from family and friends so that they can concentrate on care of the twins. | 6. Sleep deprivation and chronic fatigue can interfere with the joys of parenting unless the parents anticipate the problem and make plans to deal with it. |

### EVALUATION

Maureen progressed from finger-tipping to a full range of consoling behaviors with the twins and selected names for the baby girls. By discharge on the second postpartum day, she was breastfeeding with some confidence but continued to need encouragement. Both parents participated in infant care and collaborated to identify family members they could count on for support and assistance during the early weeks at home. Maureen verbalized increased confidence in their ability to provide care.

**ASSESSMENT:** During discharge teaching, Maureen states that she does not work outside the home and has always assumed total responsibility for household tasks. She reveals that a perfectly maintained home is important to her and especially to her husband. She wonders how he will react to the disruption that the twins will create.

**NURSING DIAGNOSIS:** Risk for Altered Family Processes related to the impact of the twins on family functioning

### GOALS/EXPECTED OUTCOMES

The couple will do the following:

1. Share concerns with each other and identify family strengths by (specific date).
2. Identify measures that reduce stress and promote family adjustment to the birth of twins by discharge.
3. Renegotiate responsibilities for the first few weeks at home by (specific date).

*Nursing Care Plan continued on following page*

## Nursing Care Plan 18–2 *Continued*

# Adaptation to the Birth of Twins

| INTERVENTION | RATIONALE |
|---|---|
| 1. Determine whether Maureen has shared her concerns with her husband; if she has not, advise her to tell him that she is worried that he does not understand how much the twins will disrupt the routine and make meticulous housekeeping impossible during the first weeks at home. | 1. Open communication is the first step in identifying stressors and clarifying feelings. |
| 2. Attempt to determine overlooked family strengths, such as the availability of funds to hire help with the housework for a few weeks. Family members are often willing to shop, do laundry, and help with other household tasks. | 2. Many families develop a higher level of functioning during times of stress, and individual members participate actively for as long as they are needed. Many families also overlook community resources, such as neighbors and friends. |
| 3. Assist the family in identifying measures to reduce stress that may occur when family patterns are disrupted:<br>a. Recommend simple meals that are easy to prepare, and suggest using disposable dishes for a few weeks.<br>b. Emphasize the importance of good nutrition; a supply of fruits, vegetables, whole grain breads, and cereals is particularly important. Also emphasize the need for daily exercise and recreation.<br>c. Review measures to obtain rest; however, fatigue is likely to persist until the twins sleep through the night.<br>d. Recommend that both parents continue to participate in activities that provide recreation and relaxation; Maureen enjoys walking and listening to music, and her husband plays tennis. | 3. During times of stress, many parents overlook the benefits of good nutrition, exercise, and recreation; even a few moments of listening to music or indulging in a favorite pasttime can refresh the spirits and replenish energy. |
| 4. Suggest that the couple negotiate sharing household tasks for the first few weeks, although this is not part of their usual responsibilities. This is particularly important for tasks that must be done daily, like meal preparation and some housecleaning. | 4. It will take both partners to maintain the home and to care for the twins without undue stress on either. Sharing tasks reduces fatigue and helps to prevent frustration and arguments during this time of stress. |

### EVALUATION

Maureen shared her concerns about the effect of the twins on the usual pattern of family life and was surprised to learn that her husband had made plans to assume many of the household tasks while the infants require so much care. Maureen's mother is available to babysit, so the couple can have some time for exercise and recreation.

### ADDITIONAL NURSING DIAGNOSES TO CONSIDER

Ineffective Breastfeeding
Risk for Parental Role Conflict
Diversional Activity Deficit

### ✓ CHECK YOUR READING

8. What does a father mean when he says he feels like a "fifth wheel"?
9. What feelings may siblings experience when a new baby is born into the family?
10. How does the birth of twins affect parental attachment?

## Cultural Influences on Adaptation

A major goal of nursing practice in the postpartum period is to provide nursing care that is culture-specific; that is, it fits the health beliefs, values, and practices of a particular culture. This is difficult because of the increasing ethnic diversity in countries such as the United States and Canada. A major challenge for nurses is to be aware of cultural beliefs and to acknowledge their importance in family adaptation. Many cultural factors that are relevant to the postpartum period can be grouped into communication, dietary practices, and health beliefs.

### Communication

Verbal communication may be difficult because of the numerous dialects and languages spoken. An interpreter should be fluent in the language, of the same religion, and of the same country of origin if possible. This compatibility is particularly important for Middle Eastern families, whose religious orientation may vary widely and who have long-standing social and religious conflicts.

Respecting the privacy and modesty of all families is important, but modesty is especially important to Latinas (ancestry from Mexico, Central America, and South America) and to Middle Eastern and Asian women. If a private room is not possible, privacy screens or curtains should be used. Laws of modesty require that Muslim women keep their hair, body, arms to the wrist, and legs to the ankles covered.

Health care workers who place a premium on efficiency and feel that they must come directly to the point must remember that tactfulness and warmth are important. Direct communication can be distressing, particularly for Latinas and Native Americans, who approach a subject only after polite and gracious comments have been exchanged.

**When the nurse and the family speak different primary languages, it is important to verify that the family has understood what is being said. An affirmative nod may be a sign of courtesy rather than of understanding or agreement. To be certain the message has been received, the nurse should ask the family to repeat in their own words what they have been told.**

### Dietary Practices

Some dietary practices that must be considered center on the hot-cold theory of health and diet. Hot-cold has nothing to do with temperature but with intrinsic properties of certain foods. For example, Southeast Asians (Cambodians, Vietnamese, Hmong, and Laotians) believe that after childbirth the woman should eat only "hot" foods such as eggs, chicken, and rice. They believe "hot" foods help to replace blood that was lost during childbirth (Mattson, 1995).

Some Chinese believe that a combination of yin and yang maintains balance. Yin foods include bean sprouts, broccoli, carrots, and cauliflower. Yang foods include broiled meat, chicken, soup, and eggs.

### Health Beliefs

Cultural beliefs and practices provide a sense of security for new mothers. For example, Muslims believe that the first sounds a child hears should be from the Koran in praise and supplication to God (Allah), and parents want to say a prayer in the newly born child's ears at the time of birth. Facilitating this practice goes a long way toward building trust in the relationship with the family.

Many Middle Eastern families believe that compliments should be directed to Allah rather than to the newborn. The compliment thus is converted into a blessing so that mistrust or jealousy does not occur. Some Southeast Asians believe the spirit resides in the head and are troubled if someone pats or rubs the head of the newborn.

Health beliefs having to do with breastfeeding and hygiene cause the most conflict in the postpartum period. Southeast Asians and Latinas believe that the mother should be kept warm to avoid upsetting the balance of hot and cold. Some women do not wish to take baths or wash their hair during the postpartum period. This practice is upsetting for nurses who are concerned about hygiene. A great deal of tact and sensitivity is required to find a compromise. Many Southeast Asian women believe that colostrum is "unclean" and that they should not breastfeed until the milk comes in. This belief conflicts with the theory that breastfeeding should start as soon after birth as possible. It may be helpful to determine when the woman believes the milk comes in and how the infant is fed until the supply of breast milk is adequate.

Specific religious practices should be accepted and supported. For instance, Muslim mothers are exempted from their obligation to pray while they are bleeding. However, the father and other family members kneel, place their heads on the floor, and pray five times a day. If possible, a clean, quiet room where this obligation can be fulfilled without having to leave the birthing center should be provided.

## Home Care

Because many mothers and infants are discharged from the birth facility a few hours after childbirth, most of the assessments and interventions described in this chapter occur in the home. Many mothers leave the birth facility while still in the taking-in phase. Many still have discomfort and are not fully recovered from the childbirth experience. Consequently, most psychosocial concerns, such as family adaptation and postpartum blues, surface later when support from health care professionals is inadequate.

A variety of methods are currently being tried to

provide care for mothers and infants who leave the birth facility within hours after childbirth. These methods include telephone calls, nurse-managed postpartum clinics, home visits, and "baby" lines staffed by nurses who provide information and guidance for families who call. All methods have advantages and disadvantages. See Chapters 1 and 17.

The overlap between nursing care in the birth facility and that needed in the home makes communication among nurses extremely important. Nurses in the birth facility, who perform the initial assessments, should make information such as nursing care plans or nursing diagnoses available to nurses who give follow-up care. This communication is particularly important when there has not been time to evaluate the nursing care plan and when possible problems have been identified.

## Application of Nursing Process: Maternal Adaptation

### Assessment

Several factors, such as how the mother progresses through the puerperal phases, her mood, interaction with the infant, and unanticipated events, affect maternal adaptation to the birth. Table 18–1 summarizes the psychosocial assessment of the mother and nursing considerations related to each assessment.

### Analysis

Parenting involves the ability of the parents to create an environment that nurtures the growth and development of the infant. Parenting may be altered when one or more caregivers experience difficulty creating or continuing a nurturing environment. This difficulty occurs most often when factors such as maternal discomfort, fatigue, and lack of knowledge or confidence in infant care come into play. Therefore, a common nursing diagnosis is Risk for Altered Parenting related to multiple factors, such as fatigue, discomfort, and lack of knowledge of infant care.

### Planning

Goals or outcomes for this nursing diagnosis are that the mother will do the following:

- Verbalize feelings of comfort and support as she progresses through the phases of recovery.
- Demonstrate progressive attachment behaviors by (specific date).
- Participate in care of the newborn by (date) or by the first home visit.

### Interventions

#### ASSISTING THE MOTHER THROUGH RECOVERY PHASES

**"Mother" the Mother.** The early taking-in phase is a time to mother the mother so that she can move on to more complex tasks of maternal adjustment. During the first few hours following childbirth, she has a great need for physical care and comfort. Provide ample fluids and favorite foods. Keep linens dry, tuck warm blankets around her until chilling has stopped, and use warm water for perineal care. A warm bath not only cleanses the skin following labor but also induces a feeling of being cared for and comforted.

**Monitor and Protect.** The new mother is dependent on nurses to monitor and protect her. She must be reminded of the need to void and should be assisted to ambulate. At the first signs of fatigue, she should be positioned for sleep and reassured that this is necessary for her body to recover from the exertion of labor. Nurses must also assess her level of comfort and offer analgesia before discomfort is severe and analgesia is less effective.

**Listen to the Birth Experience.** Be prepared to listen to details of the birth experience and to offer sincere praise for her efforts during labor.

**Many mothers spend so much time on the telephone that it is difficult to complete assessments and care. Students are reluctant to interrupt; however, the mother's physical safety is a priority, and a request to make an assessment is seldom refused. It is often helpful to offer a choice. "Excuse me for a moment. You do not have to hang up, I just need to check you soon. I can do it now or come back in 5 minutes."**

#### FOSTERING INDEPENDENCE

As the mother becomes more independent, allow her to schedule her care as much as possible. Collaborate with her to plan when procedures, such as sitz baths, will be done. Encourage her to assume responsibility for self-care, and emphasize that the nurse's role at this point is to assist and to teach.

#### PROMOTING BONDING AND ATTACHMENT

Early, unlimited contact between parents and infants is of primary importance to facilitate the attachment process (Fig. 18–8). Many hospitals and almost all birth centers provide for rooming-in, which means that the infant remains in the room with the parents at all times. Research emphasizes the value of rooming-in. Prolonged contact between mothers and infants leads to more touching as well as touching in more intimate places (face and head). Moreover, rooming-in mothers use less arousing stimulation (less moving of limbs, less tickling) (Prodromidis et

**TABLE 18–1 ASSESSING MATERNAL ADAPTATION**

| Assessments | Nursing Considerations |
|---|---|
| **Progression Through Puerperal Phases** | |
| Taking-in (passive, dependent)<br>Taking-hold (autonomous, seeks information)<br>Letting-go (relinquishes fantasy baby, begins to see self as mother) | Behaviors that should be noted include the mother's need to rest, her need to recount the details of her labor and childbirth, and her readiness to learn infant care and assume control of her own care. |
| **Maternal Mood** | |
| Mood and energy level, eye contact, posture, and comfort | Tense body posture, crying, or anxiety may indicate the beginning of postpartum blues, fatigue, or discomfort. |
| **Factors That Affect Maternal Adaptation** | |
| Age of mother | May need additional support if under 18 years of age |
| Previous experience | Primiparas often progress through puerperal phases at a slower pace and may require additional assistance.<br>Multiparas often have more experience and knowledge of infant care.<br>Previous birth of a child with anomalies or death of an infant may delay adaptation. |
| Maternal/infant temperament | Mothers who are calm, secure in their ability to learn, and free from anxiety adjust more easily to the demands of motherhood.<br>Infants who are easily consoled and enjoy cuddling increase parental confidence.<br>Infants who are difficult to console increase parental frustration. |
| Unanticipated events | Cesarean birth may result in increased discomfort and longer recovery.<br>Birth of more than one infant can create problems of attachment. |
| **Interaction with Infant** | |
| Maternal touch | Mother progresses from "finger-tipping" to enfolding and a full range of comforting behaviors. |
| Verbal interaction | Mother may call infant "it" initially but progresses quickly to using given name and identifying specific characteristics. |
| Response to infant cues or signals | Prompt, gentle, consistent response indicates progressive adaptation to parenting role. |
| **Preparation for Parenting** | |
| Classes in breastfeeding, parenting, or infant care | Many mothers feel more prepared after completing classes and participate in care sooner. |

al., 1995), perhaps because they have more time to learn their newborns' needs. Some hospitals have a modified rooming-in plan in which infants are with the mothers for long periods but may be returned to a central nursery at night or when the mother wishes to rest. Specific nursing measures to promote bonding and attachment are the following:

- Assist the parents in taking the baby out of the blanket and inspecting the toes, fingers, and body. Inspection fosters identification and allows the parents to become acquainted with the "real" baby that must replace the fantasy baby that many parents imagined during the pregnancy.
- Position the infant in an *en face* position; point out that the eyes are open and the infant can see the parent's face; face-to-face and eye-to-eye contact is a first step in establishing mutual interaction between the infant and the parent.
- Point out the reciprocal bonding activities of the infant. "Look how she holds your finger." "He has not taken his eyes off you." "See how the baby moves when you speak in a high-pitched voice."
- Allow the infant to remain with the parents as long

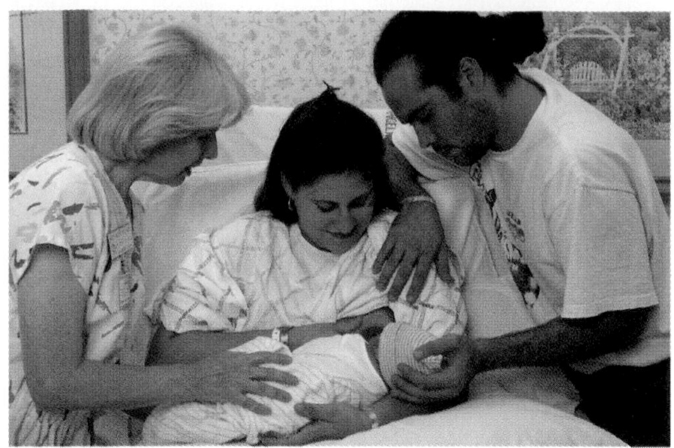

**FIGURE 18–8**

By teaching about the newborn and family, the nurse helps parents develop confidence in their ability to provide care for the infant.

as they wish so that they can progress at their own speed through the discovery or getting-acquainted phase.

- Teach parents that infants exhibit a variety of signals that indicate distress. These include changes in heart rate, respiratory rate, or color. Regurgitation, hiccoughs, tremors, splaying of fingers, sneezing, yawning, and gaze aversion are also cues that the infant needs support, such as a decrease in lights and noise and swaddling.
- Assist the mother in putting the infant to the breast if she plans to breastfeed. If necessary, reassure her that many infants do not latch on to the breast right away. If she is formula feeding, assist her in positioning the infant securely and reassure her that holding and cuddling the infant provides comfort and security.
- Model behaviors by holding the infant close and speaking in high-pitched, soothing tones.
- Point out the positive characteristics of the infant: "She has the tiniest pink ears and such a lot of dark hair."
- Provide comfort and ample time for rest because the mother must replenish her energy and be relatively free of discomfort before she can progress to initiating care of the infant.

#### INVOLVING PARENTS IN INFANT CARE

Providing care for the infant fosters feelings of responsibility and nurturing and is an important component of attachment. Moreover, it allows parents to develop confidence in their ability to care for an infant before they go home.

Although teaching begins during pregnancy, information should be reviewed and demonstrations should be repeated if time allows. Demonstrations should begin with the simpler tasks such as care of the cord and progress to more complicated procedures such as bathing. When the parents receive positive reinforcement for the simple tasks, they are more willing to try the more complicated ones. (See Chapters 21 and 23 for detailed information about the infant care that should be taught before the mother is discharged.)

It is important for the entire staff to agree on how basic care is to be taught. Mothers seek confirmation of information, and they become confused and lose faith in the credibility of the staff if information varies.

- Allow time for practice; mothers become easily discouraged if they think they have failed at some attempt to care for their infants.
- Offer repeated praise and encouragement. Remember, parents are especially vulnerable to criticism.

**Suggestions for care must be tactfully phrased to avoid the implication that the parents are inept. "You burped that baby like a professional. There are a couple of little hints I can share about diapering."**

### Evaluation

- Independent self-care confirms the mother's progression through the phases of recovery.
- Progressive attachment behaviors include enfolding the infant, calling the infant by name, and responding gently when the infant cries.
- Participation in infant care includes diapering, feeding, and care of the umbilical cord and circumcision.

## Application of Nursing Process: Family Adaptation

### Assessment

#### FATHERS

The father's emotional status and interaction with the infant are particularly important because he usually serves as the mother's primary support person. Is the father available? Is he involved with mother and infant? How does he interact with the infant? Does he respond to infant cues? How much information does he have about infant characteristics and care? What are his expectations about his partner's recovery? Unrealistic expectations of the infant (will sleep through the night, smile, be easily consoled) may lead to problems. Moreover, if he expects the mother to recover her energy and libido rapidly, he may become resentful if her recovery takes longer than anticipated.

### SIBLINGS

It is important to note the ages of siblings and how they react to the newborn. Are they interested and helpful? Are they hostile and aggressive? How do the parents react to sibling behaviors?

### SUPPORT SYSTEM

Family members often provide a powerful support system, and their involvement is important to the adaptation of the family. Are grandparents available and involved? Are there sisters or brothers who live nearby? Are they available to help the new parents? If the family is unavailable, who provides support? What arrangements have been made for assistance?

### NONVERBAL BEHAVIOR

Nonverbal behavior is equally important. Are the parents' words congruent with what they do? For example, does the mother verbalize satisfaction with her infant's characteristics but respond slowly to infant signals?

Table 18–2 summarizes the family assessment and briefly indicates nursing considerations.

**Validate impressions and conclusions that are arrived at during a psychosocial assessment. One of the best ways to do this is to ask, for example, "How much experience have you had with newborns?" "You really**

**TABLE 18–2 ASSESSING FAMILY ADAPTATION**

| Assessment | Nursing Considerations |
|---|---|
| **Characteristics of Infant That May Affect Family Adaptation** | |
| Sex and size of infant | The sex of an infant is a factor for some families; disappointment in the sex or concern about the small size may interfere with bonding. |
| Unusual characteristics (cephalhematoma, jaundice, cranial molding, newborn rash) | Be prepared to explain unexpected appearance or behavior in words parents can comprehend. |
| Infant behavior (irritable, easily consoled, cuddles) | Easily consoled, cuddly infant increases bonding and attachment. |
| **Paternal Adaptation** | |
| Response to mother and to infant | Mate often provides the most important support for the mother, and his involvement with the infant indicates acceptance of parenting role. |
| Knowledge of infant care | Useful in planning teaching that includes the father |
| Response to infant cues or signals (crying, fussing) | Many fathers feel awkward handling the infant but want to become proficient in infant care so that they can co-parent. |
| **Ages and Developmental Levels of Siblings** | |
| Reaction of siblings | Young children often fear that the newborn will replace them in the affection of parents; anticipatory guidance about sibling rivalry may be needed. |
| **Support System** | |
| Interest and availability of family or friends to assist during early weeks | Families benefit from active, nurturing support during the weeks following childbirth; families sometimes need assistance in identifying available support. |
| Plans for first few days at home | How much support will parents have? Plans for obtaining adequate rest? Many hospitals have telephone service to answer questions and give reassurance. |
| Follow-up plans | Appointments should be scheduled at 2 weeks and 6 weeks with clinic or health care provider. |
| **Cultural Factors** | |
| Ask family to describe practices that are part of their cultural heritage and beliefs that may affect nursing care; determine expectations of health care team | To determine hygienic practices, dietary preferences, usual care and feeding of infants, and role of mate and family in child care so that culture-specific care can be planned |

**thought you were having a girl and a boy is a big surprise?" "How are newborns fed in Vietnam until the mother's milk comes in?" "What are your plans when you go home? How long can your mother stay?"**

## Analysis

The purpose of the family assessment is to identify family strengths as well as areas in which nursing interventions could promote family adaptation or prevent disruptions in family functioning. Sometimes a family that usually functions effectively is unable to cope because of a specific event. In this case, the event is the birth of a baby and the necessity of the family to integrate a newborn into the existing family structure. Therefore, this common nursing diagnosis is Altered Family Processes related to lack of knowledge of infant needs and behaviors, stress during the early weeks at home, and sibling rivalry.

## Planning

Goals or outcomes for this nursing diagnosis often cannot be evaluated before discharge from the birth facility and overlap with home care.

By (specific date) the family will do the following:

- Verbalize understanding of infant needs and behaviors.
- Identify methods for reducing stress during the early weeks at home.
- Describe measures to reduce sibling rivalry.
- Identify external resources and support system.

## Interventions

### TEACHING THE FAMILY ABOUT THE NEWBORN

**Infant Needs.** Some new parents have unrealistic expectations of the newborn, and nurses are in the best position to provide information about what the infant is capable of doing and what the infant needs to thrive. Parents are often thrilled to learn that the infant can see and hear them. They are sometimes surprised to hear that infants sleep 16 to 20 hours a day but must be fed every 2 to 4 hours and that they will not sleep through the night for 12 to 16 weeks. Besides physical care, infants also need cuddling and gentle stimulation. They enjoy looking at mobiles or being with the family. Some infants respond to soothing music or a rocking motion.

**Infant Signals.** Discuss the importance of responding promptly and gently to cues such as crying or fussing that indicate the infant needs attention. Reassure parents that responding to cues does not "spoil" their child but helps her or him learn to trust that the world is a safe, secure place.

Parents also need to recognize signals that indicate when their infant has had enough and wants to avoid further stimulation. The so-called avoidance cues, such as looking away, splaying the fingers, arching the back, and fussiness, indicate that the infant is ready for quiet time.

### HELPING THE FAMILY ADAPT

**Providing Anticipatory Guidance About Stress Reduction.** Nurses can do a great deal by providing anticipatory guidance about the first weeks at home, when the family must adjust to the demands of a newborn. This is a time when the need for rest is great but when the opportunity for uninterrupted sleep is minimal. As a result, fatigue is a common problem.

- Recommend that mothers establish a relaxed home atmosphere and a flexible meal schedule because attempts to maintain a rigid schedule or meticulous environment increase tension within the family.
- Emphasize that the priority during the first 4 to 6 weeks should be caring for mother and baby; encourage the family to accept assistance with shopping and meal preparation.
- Recommend that the mother sleep when the infant sleeps and that she conserve her energy for care of the baby.
- Encourage family members to let friends and relatives know sleep and nap times and request that they telephone or visit at other times. Adequate rest is necessary for mental restoration, release of tension, and integration of new information into the memory.
- Advise parents to place a "Do Not Disturb" sign on the door and an answering machine on the telephone.
- Instruct the family about the need to restrict coffee, tea, colas, and chocolate because they contain the stimulant caffeine.
- Teach breathing exercises and progressive relaxation to reduce stress and to energize and refresh, especially when a nap is not possible.
- Encourage both parents to delay tiring projects until the infant is older. Remind them that although schedules are chaotic for a while, the infant's behavior is generally more predictable by 12 to 16 weeks.
- Encourage open expression of feelings between parents as a first step in coping with stress.
- Remind parents of the need for healthy nutrition and for favorite recreation. It is easy for fatigue and tension to overwhelm the anticipated joys of parenting if no respite is available from constant care.
- Suggest that new parents enlist grandparents, other relatives, and friends to help with meal preparation and shopping.

**Providing Ways to Reduce Sibling Rivalry.** Suggest that parents plan time alone with the older child and that they praise and reassure the child frequently of his or her place in the family. The parents should try to offer frequent expression of love and affection. It is also helpful if visitors and family do not focus exclusively on the infant but also include the older child in their gift giving and exclamations about the newborn.

Emphasize the importance of responding calmly and with understanding when the child regresses to more infantile behaviors or expresses hostility toward the infant. Acknowledging the child's feelings and offering prompt reassurance of continued love are most valuable.

Some children, particularly those older than 3 years of age, enjoy being a big brother or big sister and respond well when they are included in infant care. This participation may not be possible with younger children, and it may be more worthwhile for the parents to set aside separate time to participate in a favorite activity with them.

**Identifying Resources.** In many homes, women assume the major responsibilities of day-to-day homemaking. With the birth of an infant, this task becomes more difficult. A division of labor must be negotiated to prevent undue stress and fatigue. This division of labor is particularly important if there are other children whose needs for time, attention, and comfort must also be met.

The mother's primary support is often the father of the baby; however, extended family members, particularly grandmothers and sisters, also provide valuable support. Community resources, such as daycare

## CRITICAL THINKING EXERCISE

Carol, a 35-year-old primipara, had an infant daughter by cesarean birth after failure to progress in labor. Carol is very tired, although she is relatively comfortable. Her husband was present during the labor and birth and is excited about being a father. He has no experience with children, and his job requires almost constant travel. Although Carol has two nephews, she has never taken care of a newborn.

The day of delivery, Carol readily accepts attention and assistance with hygiene. She passively follows the nurse's suggestions to turn, cough, and breathe deeply. She recounts the details of her labor and wonders why the physician did not proceed with a cesarean birth earlier. She examines her baby girl closely and touches the face and hands gently with her fingertips. She remarks that she plans to breastfeed and is surprised that the infant sleeps so much.

**Q:**
1. What are Carol's priority needs at this time?
2. What phase of recovery is she manifesting? Why does she "finger-tip" the infant?

The first postoperative day, Carol's indwelling catheter is removed and intravenous fluids are discontinued. Carol ambulates with minimal assistance and announces proudly that she is able to urinate without difficulty. She asks about bowel function and requests the prescribed stool softener. She asks that the infant be left with her and spends a great deal of time getting the baby to breastfeed. She is very frustrated that the infant does not breastfeed well and asks for assistance from the lactation educator.

**Q:**
3. What are Carol's priority needs now?
4. How have her behaviors changed?

Before discharge, Carol is breastfeeding well. The infant latches on and nurses for 10 to 15 minutes, and Carol's nipples are free of tenderness or signs of trauma. Carol has no relatives in the area, and her husband is home for the weekend only. She states that she will just have to get along by herself after that.

**Q:**
5. What anticipatory guidance should Carol receive about her own care? About the infant's care?
6. What further nursing interventions would be most helpful to her and the baby?

---

**A:**

1. Carol's priority needs are for physical care and comfort. She also needs to make the experience of childbirth part of her reality; she does this by recounting the details of her birth experience to anyone who will listen and by trying to fill in the missing pieces about the cesarean birth.
2. Carol is in the taking-in phase. She is getting acquainted with her "real" baby by exploring with her fingertips. This is usually the first maternal touch observed.
3. Carol's priorities are to assume control of her own body functions and to manage her care so that she can "take hold" and assume care of the baby.
4. Carol has become more independent and now initiates breastfeeding. She demonstrates readiness to learn by requesting the assistance of the lactation educator.
5. Anticipatory guidance should focus on how she can manage the care of the infant while still getting adequate rest and nutrition. A flexible schedule, resting while the infant rests, and preparing simple meals are some of the most important items to emphasize.
6. It would be most helpful to assist her in identifying other individuals who could provide some support while her husband is away, perhaps a friend or neighbor. If this is not possible, she should have telephone numbers for community resources, such as the hospital "baby line."

   A follow-up telephone call initiated by the nurse or, if possible, a home visit by an experienced perinatal nurse would be most helpful. The nurse could assess both the mother and the infant and reinforce teaching and provide encouragement.

centers, parenting classes, and breastfeeding support, are available in many areas. In addition, close friends and neighbors often share solutions they have found for specific problems. Remind the mother that resources are available when she begins to feel isolated and exhausted.

### Evaluation

A prompt, gentle response to infant crying or fussing indicates a parent's understanding of the infant's need. Devising a plan for obtaining rest and for reducing anxiety in siblings is a first step in reducing stress. Identifying external resources in the family, neighborhood, and community may help the family function to meet its needs during the early weeks at home.

## SUMMARY CONCEPTS

- Bonding and attachment are gradual processes that begin before childbirth and progress to feelings of love and deep devotion that last all through life. Nurses foster bonding and attachment by providing early, unlimited contact between the parents and infant and by modeling attachment behaviors.
- For bonding and attachment to occur, interaction between parents and the infant is required. Contact is particularly important when the infant is awake and alert and able to interact with the parents. Nurses often delay care that can be postponed so that the parents and infant can have this time together.
- Maternal touch changes over time as many mothers progress from exploratory "finger-tipping" to enfolding and finally demonstrating a full range of comforting behaviors.
- Verbal behaviors are important indicators of maternal attachment as mothers progress from referring to the infant as "it" to calling the infant by name and finally to identifying his or her unique characteristics. Nurses often model how to speak to the infant and point out the infant's response to the verbal stimulation.
- Maternal adjustment to parenthood is a gradual process that involves restorative phases that allow the mother to replenish her energy, relinquish her role as a woman without a child, and develop attachment to the infant. Nurses play a valuable role in the process by first "mothering the mother" and fostering independence as the mother becomes ready.
- Postpartum blues, a temporary, self-limiting period of weepiness, is often ignored by the health care team. Explanations and support are generally all that are required to assist the mother through this distressing episode.
- Mothers (and fathers) usually progress through four stages of role attainment (anticipatory, formal, informal, and personal) before they attain a sense of harmony and structure their parenting behaviors to mesh with the unique needs of their child.
- Many women experience role conflict when they must leave the infant with a caregiver and return to work. Nurses can offer anticipatory guidance that makes the conflict less difficult.
- The birth of a baby necessitates reorganization of family structure and renegotiation of family responsibilities; nurses can make the process easier by assisting the father in co-parenting the infant and helping the new parents identify family resources.
- Siblings feel jealousy and fear that they will be replaced by the newborn in the affection of the parents. Nurses can reduce the negative feelings by providing information about how to reduce sibling rivalry.
- Nurses recognize that families leave the birth facility with unmet needs and that nursing care in the facility overlaps with follow-up care that is provided in the home.

#### References and Readings


Affonso, D.D., Mayberry, L., Inaba, A., Matsuno, R., & Robinson, E. (1996). Hawaiian-style "talkstory": Psychosocial assessment and intervention during and after pregnancy. *Journal of Obstetric, Gynecologic, and Neonatal Nursing, 25*(9), 737–742.

Affonso, D.D., Mayberry, L.J., Lovett, S.M., & Paul, S. (1994). Cognitive adaptation to stressful events during pregnancy and postpartum: Development and testing of CASE instrument. *Nursing Research, 43*(6), 338–343.

Ament, L.A. (1990). Maternal tasks of the puerperium reidentified. *Journal of Obstetric, Gynecologic, and Neonatal Nursing, 19*(4), 330–335.

Anderson, J.M. (1990). Health care across cultures. *Nursing Outlook, 36*(3), 136–139.

Atkinson, L.S., & Baxley, E.G. (1994). Postpartum fatigue. *American Family Physician, 50*(1), 113–118.

Beck, C.T., Reynolds, M.A., & Rutowski, P. (1992). Maternity blues and postpartum depression. *Journal of Obstetric, Gynecologic, and Neonatal Nursing, 21*(4), 287–293.

Callister, L.C. (1995). Cultural meanings of childbirth. *Journal of Obstetric, Gynecologic, and Neonatal Nursing, 44*(4), 327–331.

Comfort, M., Wulff, L.M., & Smeriglio, V.L. (1987). Adolescent parenthood: Implications for care of the mother and child. *Maryland Medical Journal, 36*(11), 955–959.

Cusson, R.M. (1993). Instruments in neonatal research: Measuring attachment behavior. *Neonatal Network, 12*(4), 69–71.

Fawcett, J., Pollio, N., Tully, A., Baron, M., Henklein, J.C., & Jones, R.C. (1993). Effects of information on adaptation to cesarean birth. *Nursing Research, 42*(1), 49–53.

Ferketich, S.L., & Mercer, R.T. (1995a). Predictors of role competence for experienced and inexperienced fathers. *Nursing Research, 44*(2), 89–95.

Ferketich, S.L., & Mercer, R.T. (1995b). Paternal-infant attachment of experienced and inexperienced fathers during infancy. *Nursing Research, 44*(1), 31–37.

Fortier, J.C., Carson, V.B., Will, S., et al. (1991). Adjustment to a newborn: Sibling preparation makes a difference. *Journal of Obstetric, Gynecologic, and Neonatal Nursing, 20*(1), 73–79.

Gullicks, J.N., & Crase, S.J. (1993). Sibling behavior with a newborn: Parents expectations and observations. *Journal of Obstetric, Gynecologic, and Neonatal Nursing*, 22(5), 438–444.

Higley, A.M., & Miller, M.A. (1996). The development of parenting: Nursing resources. *Journal of Obstetric, Gynecologic, and Neonatal Nursing*, 25(9), 707–713.

Hutchinson, M.K., & Baqi-Aziz, M. (1994). Nursing care of the childbearing Muslim family. *Journal of Obstetric, Gynecologic, and Neonatal Nursing*, 23(9), 767–771.

Jordan, P.L. (1990). Laboring for relevance: Expectant and new fatherhood. *Nursing Research*, 39(1), 11–16.

Klaus, M., & Kennell, J. (1982). *Maternal-infant bonding*. St. Louis: C. V. Mosby.

Martell, L.K. (1990). Postpartum depression as a family problem. *Maternal-Child Nursing Journal*, 15(2), 90–93.

Martell, L.K., & Mitchell, S.K. (1984). Rubin's puerperal change reconsidered. *Journal of Obstetric, Gynecologic, and Neonatal Nursing*, 13(3), 145–148.

Mattson, S. (1995). Culturally sensitive perinatal care for Southeast Asians. *Journal of Obstetric, Gynecologic, and Neonatal Nursing*, 24(4), 335–341.

May, K., & Perrin, S. (1985). The father in pregnancy and birth. In S. Hanson & F. Bozett (Eds.), *Dimensions of fatherhood*. Beverly Hills, Calif.: Sage Publishing.

Mercer, R.T. (1985). The process of maternal role attainment. *Nursing Research*, 34(4), 198–204.

Mercer, R.T. (1986). Predictors of maternal role attainment at one year postbirth. *Western Journal of Nursing Research*, 8(1), 932.

Mercer, R.T. (1990). *Parents at risk*. New York: Springer Publishing.

Mercer, R.T., & Ferketich, S.L. (1990a). Predictors of family functioning eight months following birth. *Nursing Research*, 39(2), 76–82.

Mercer, R.T., & Ferketich, S.L. (1990b). Predictors of parental attachment during early parenthood. *Journal of Advanced Nursing*, 15, 268–280.

Mercer, R.T., & Ferketich, S.L. (1994a). Predictors of maternal role competence by risk status. *Nursing Research*, 43(1), 38–43.

Mercer, R.T., & Ferketich, S.L. (1994b). Maternal-infant attachment of experienced and inexperienced mothers during infancy. *Nursing Research*, 43(6), 344–351.

Miovech, S.M., Knapp, H., Borucki, L., Roncoli, M., Arnold, L., & Brooten, D. (1994). Major concerns of women after cesarean delivery. *Journal of Obstetric, Gynecologic, and Neonatal Nursing*, 23(1), 53–59.

Nance, T.A. (1995). Intercultural communication: Finding common ground. *Journal of Obstetric, Gynecologic, and Neonatal Nursing*, 24(3), 249–255.

Prodromidis, M., Field, T., Arendt, R., Singer, L., Yando, R., & Bendell, D. (1995). Mothers touching newborns: A comparison of rooming-in versus minimal contact. *Birth*, 22(4), 196–200.

Reichert, J.A., Baron, M., & Fawcett, J. (1993). Changes in attitude toward cesarean birth. *Journal of Obstetric, Gynecologic, and Neonatal Nursing*, 22(2), 159–167.

Rubin, R. (1961). Puerperal change. *Nursing Outlook*, 9(12), 743–755.

Rubin, R. (1977). Binding-in in the postpartum period. *Maternal-Child Nursing Journal*, 6(1), 65–75.

Rubin, R. (1984). *Maternal identity and the maternal experience*. New York: Springer Publishing.

Schneiderman, J.U. (1996). Postpartum nursing for Korean mothers. *American Journal of Maternal-Child Nursing*, 21(3), 155–158.

Sheil, E.P., Bull, M.J., Moxon, B.E., et al. (1995). Concerns of childbearing women: A maternal concerns questionnaire as an assessment tool. *Journal of Obstetric, Gynecologic, and Neonatal Nursing*, 24(2), 149–155.

Thorpe, K., Greenwood, R., & Goodenough, T. (1995). Does a twin pregnancy have greater impact on physical and emotional well-being than a singleton pregnancy? *Birth*, 22(3), 148–152.

Tiller, C.M. (1995). Fathers' parenting attitudes during a child's first year. *Journal of Obstetric, Gynecologic, and Neonatal Nursing*, 24(6), 508–514.

Tomlinson, P.S. (1990). Verbal behavior associated with indicators of maternal attachment with the neonate. *Journal of Obstetric, Gynecologic, and Neonatal Nursing*, 19(1), 76–81.

Ugarriza, D.N. (1992). Postpartum affective disorders: Incidence and treatment. *Journal of Psychosocial Nursing*, 30(5), 29–32.

Waldenström, U., Borg, I.M., Olsson, B., Sköld, M., & Wall, S. (1996). The childbirth experience: A study of 295 new mothers. *Birth*, 23(3), 144–153.

Walker, L.O., & Montgomery, E. (1994). Maternal identity and role attainment: Long-term relations to children's development. *Nursing Research*, 43(2), 105–110.

Weinberg, S.H. (1994). An alternative to meet the needs of early discharge: The tender beginnings postpartum visit. *American Journal of Maternal Child Nursing*, 19(6), 339–342.

Williams, L.R., & Cooper, M.K. (1993). Nurse-managed home care. *Journal of Obstetric, Gynecologic, and Neonatal Nursing*, 22(1), 25–31.

# 19

# Normal Newborn: The Processes of Adaptation

## OBJECTIVES

1. Explain the physiologic changes that occur in the respiratory and cardiovascular systems during the transition from fetal to neonatal life.
2. Describe thermoregulation in the newborn.
3. Compare gastrointestinal functioning in the newborn and adult.
4. Explain the causes and effects of hypoglycemia.
5. Describe the steps in normal bilirubin excretion and the development of physiologic, pathologic, and breast milk jaundice.
6. Describe kidney functioning in the newborn.
7. Explain the functioning of the newborn's immune system.
8. Describe the periods of reactivity and the six behavioral states of the newborn.

## DEFINITIONS

**acrocyanosis** *Bluish discoloration of the hands and feet due to reduced peripheral circulation.*

**asphyxia** *Insufficient oxygen and excess carbon dioxide in the blood and tissues.*

**bilirubin** *Unusable component of hemolyzed erythrocytes.*

**brown fat (or brown adipose tissue)** *Highly vascular specialized fat found in the newborn that provides more heat than other fat when metabolized.*

**choanal atresia** *Abnormality of the nasal septum that obstructs one or both nasal passages.*

**fetal lung fluid** *Fluid that fills the fetal lungs, expanding the alveoli and promoting lung development.*

**first period of reactivity** *Period beginning at birth in which newborns are active and alert. It ends when the infant first falls asleep.*

**hyperbilirubinemia** *Excessive amount of bilirubin in the blood.*

**jaundice** *Yellow discoloration of the skin and sclera caused by excessive bilirubin in the blood.*

**neutral thermal environment** *Environment in which body temperature is maintained without an increase in metabolic rate or oxygen use.*

**nonshivering thermogenesis** *Process of heat production, without shivering, by oxidation of brown fat.*

**polycythemia** *Abnormally high number of erythrocytes.*

**second period of reactivity** *Period of 4 to 6 hours after the first sleep following birth when the newborn may have an elevated pulse and respiratory rate and excessive mucus.*

**surfactant** *Combination of lipoproteins produced by the lungs of the mature fetus to reduce surface tension in the alveoli, thus promoting lung expansion after birth.*

**tachypnea** *Respiratory rate above 60 breaths per minute in the newborn after the first hour of life.*

**thermogenesis** *Heat production.*

**thermoregulation** *Maintenance of body temperature.*

At birth, neonates must make profound physiologic changes to adapt to extrauterine life to meet their own respiratory, digestive, and regulatory needs. Nurses must be aware of the normal physiologic changes occurring during the early hours and days after birth so that they can identify behaviors signifying problems or abnormalities.

The focus of this chapter is the physiologic changes for adaptation that occur at birth. This provides a basis for discussion of nursing assessment and care related to those changes in Chapters 20 and 21.

## Initiation of Respirations

The first vital task the newborn must accomplish is the initiation of respirations. Forces occurring throughout pregnancy and during birth bring about this change.

### Development of the Lungs

During fetal life, the respiratory tract produces a fluid within the lungs. Fetal lung fluid expands the alveoli and is essential for normal development of the lungs. Some of the fluid empties from the lungs into the amniotic fluid. As the fetus nears term, an increase in sodium in the lung epithelium causes the lung fluid to begin to move into the interstitial spaces. The fluid shift continues during normal labor and after birth. This helps reduce the pulmonary resistance to blood flow that was present before birth and enhances the advent of air breathing (Lowe & Reiss, 1996).

As the lungs mature, they begin to produce surfactant, a slippery, detergent-like lipoprotein. Surfactant reduces surface tension within the alveoli. This allows them to remain partially open when the infant begins to breathe at birth. Without surfactant, the alveoli collapse as the infant exhales and must be reopened with each breath. This greatly increases the work of breathing. Sufficient surfactant is usually produced between 34 and 36 weeks of gestation for most infants born at that time to breathe without difficulty.

### Causes of Respirations

At birth, the infant's first breath must force fetal lung fluid into the interstitial spaces around the alveoli so that air can enter the respiratory tract. This requires a much larger negative pressure (suction) for the first breath than for subsequent breathing. Breathing is initiated by chemical, thermal, and mechanical factors that stimulate the respiratory center in the medulla of the brain and trigger respirations (Fig. 19–1).

#### CHEMICAL FACTORS

Chemoreceptors in the carotid arteries and the aorta respond to changes in blood chemistry brought about by the hypoxia that occurs with normal birth. A decrease in the blood oxygen level ($Po_2$) and the pH of the blood and an increased blood carbon dioxide level ($Pco_2$) cause impulses from these receptors to stimulate the respiratory center in the medulla. In addition, occlusion of the vessels in the cord may end flow of a chemical from the placenta that inhibits respirations (Lowe & Reiss, 1996). A forceful contraction of the diaphragm results, causing air to enter the lungs. However, stimulation of the respiratory center and breathing do not occur if prolonged hypoxia causes central nervous system depression.

#### THERMAL FACTORS

The temperature change that occurs with birth is an important stimulus to the initiation of respirations. At birth, the infant moves from the warm, fluid-filled uterus into an environment where the temperature is more than 20°F cooler. Sensors in the skin respond to this sudden change in temperature by sending impulses to the brain that stimulate the respiratory center and breathing.

#### MECHANICAL FACTORS

During a vaginal birth, the fetal chest is compressed by the narrow birth canal. A small amount of the fetal lung fluid is forced out of the lungs into the upper air passages during birth. The fluid passes out of the mouth or nose or is suctioned as the head emerges from the vagina. When the pressure against the chest is released, it recoils, drawing a small amount of air into the lungs.

Tactile stimuli that occur during birth stimulate skin sensors. Nurses hold, dry, and wrap infants in blankets, providing further stimulation to skin sensors. The stimulation of the sounds and lights at delivery may also aid in initiating respirations.

### Continuation of Respirations

Once the alveoli expand, surfactant acts to keep them partially open between respirations. About half of the air from the first breath remains in the lungs to become the functional residual capacity. Because the alveoli remain partially expanded with this residual air, subsequent breaths require much less effort than the first one. With each of the first few respirations, more alveoli are opened.

The remaining fetal lung fluid moves into the interstitial spaces, where it is absorbed by the circulatory and lymphatic systems. Absorption is accelerated by the process of labor and may be delayed after cesarean birth. Although most fluid is absorbed within a few hours, complete absorption may take as

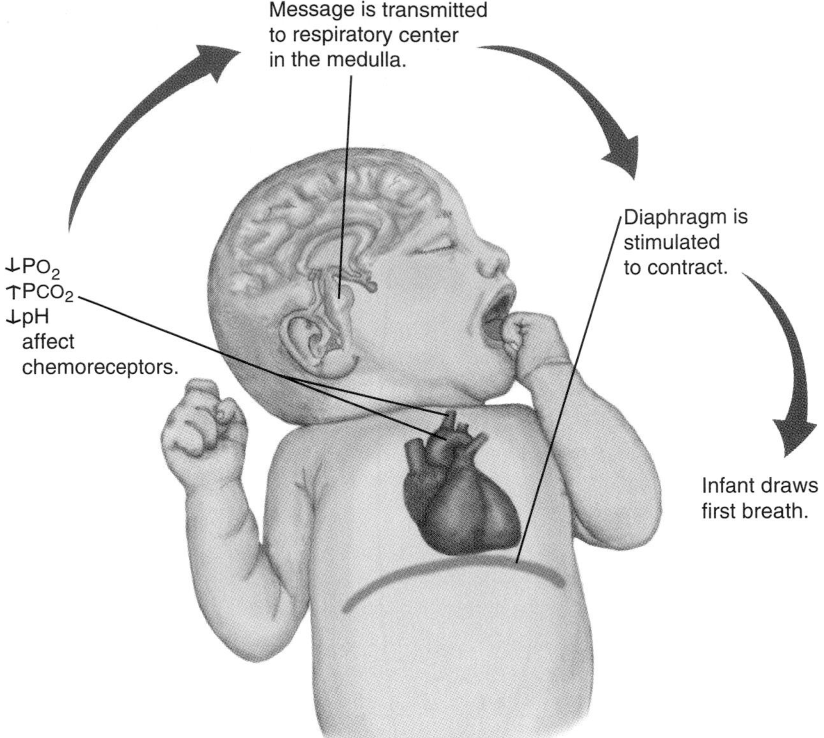
Message is transmitted
to respiratory center
in the medulla.
Diaphragm is
stimulated
to contract.
↓$PO_2$
↑$PCO_2$
↓pH
affect
chemoreceptors.
Infant draws
first breath.
Internal stimuli

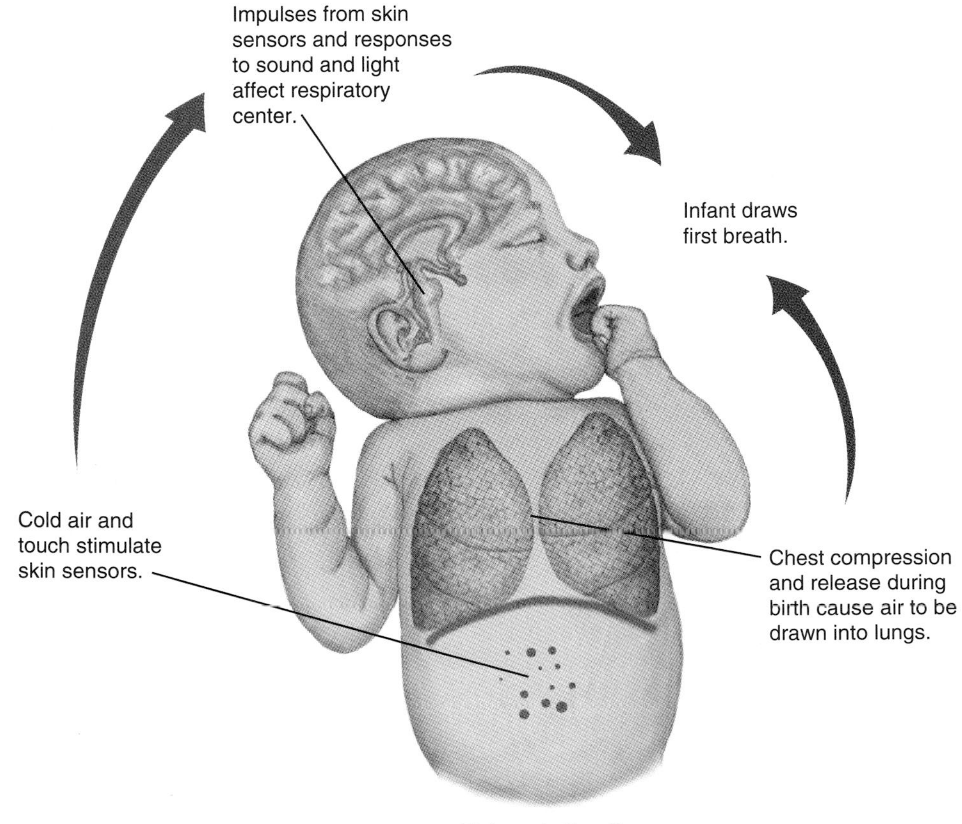
Impulses from skin
sensors and responses
to sound and light
affect respiratory
center.
Infant draws
first breath.
Cold air and
touch stimulate
skin sensors.
Chest compression
and release during
birth cause air to be
drawn into lungs.
External stimuli

**FIGURE 19–1**

Internal causes of the initiation of respirations are the chemical changes that take place at birth. External causes of respirations include thermal and mechanical factors.

long as 24 hours. This explains why the lungs may sound moist when first auscultated but become clear a short time later.

**CHECK YOUR READING**

1. How do hypoxia during birth, a cool delivery room, and handling at birth stimulate the newborn to breathe?
2. Why is surfactant important to the newborn's ability to breathe easily?
3. How is fetal lung fluid removed before and after birth?

## Cardiovascular Adaptation: Transition from Fetal to Neonatal Circulation

During fetal life, most of the fetal blood flow bypasses the nonfunctional lungs and liver. This is due to three structures: the *ductus arteriosus, foramen ovale,* and *ductus venosus,* that shunt blood away from the lungs and liver. It is also due to high pressures within the lungs that permit only a small amount of blood flow into the pulmonary vessels. At birth, the infant's blood must begin to circulate to the lungs for oxygenation and to the liver for filtration (see Chapter 6, pp. 115–117).

For these changes to occur after birth, the shunts must close and the pulmonary vessels must dilate. This occurs in response to increases in the blood oxygen level, shifts in pressure within the heart and pulmonary and systemic circulations, and the end of blood flow through the umbilical vessels. The changes necessary for transition from fetal to neonatal circulation occur simultaneously within the first few minutes after birth. They are discussed separately below. Table 19–1 summarizes these changes.

### Ductus Arteriosus

In the fetus, the ductus arteriosus connects the pulmonary artery and the aorta. Prostaglandin $E_2$ from the placenta and low blood oxygen levels keep the ductus arteriosus widely dilated during fetal life. The vessel directs most of the blood that enters the pulmonary artery into the aorta. This causes the majority of blood flow to bypass the nonfunctioning lungs.

As the newborn takes the first breaths of air at birth, the ductus arteriosus, which responds to a rise in oxygen by constricting, begins to close. At the same time, resistance within the pulmonary circulation decreases and resistance throughout the systemic circulation increases. This change in resistance, along with the constriction of the ductus arteriosus, causes blood to flow from the pulmonary artery into the lungs for oxygenation.

The ductus arteriosus closes gradually as the flow of prostaglandin $E_2$ from the placenta ends and oxygenation improves. Functional closure occurs within 15 to 24 hours. Until closure is complete, the blood that does flow through the vessel reverses, moving from the aorta to the pulmonary artery and increasing blood flow to the lungs. This is because pressure in the aorta is now higher than that in the pulmonary artery. A murmur may be heard as a result of blood flow through the partially open vessel.

The ductus arteriosus closes permanently by 3 to 4 weeks (Lott, 1993). Once closed, it is called the ligamentum arteriosum. Until permanent closure occurs, low levels of oxygen in the blood may cause the ductus arteriosus to dilate and the pulmonary vessels to constrict. This may cause a return to fetal blood flow patterns and is a serious complication. A patent ductus arteriosus may occur in the infant who experiences asphyxia at birth, becomes hypoxic, or is preterm (see Chapter 30, p. 847).

### Pulmonary Blood Vessels

The blood vessels in the lungs must be able to accommodate the large increase in blood flow they receive once the ductus arteriosus closes. They can do this because the vessels dilate in response to the increased oxygenation that occurs when the neonate takes the first breaths. At the same time, fetal lung fluid is shifting into the interstitial spaces and is removed by the blood and lymph system, allowing more room for dilation of the pulmonary blood vessels. This decreases pulmonary vascular resistance and allows the vessels within the lungs to expand to hold the suddenly increased blood flow from the pulmonary artery.

### Foramen Ovale

The foramen ovale is a flap in the septum between the right and the left atria of the fetal heart. As blood returns to the heart, most of the oxygenated blood from the inferior vena cava enters the right atrium and crosses the foramen ovale to the left side of the heart. There is little mixing with the less oxygenated blood that enters from the superior vena cava and continues to the right ventricle. Thus, most of the better-oxygenated blood travels away from the nonfunctioning lungs before birth.

The foramen ovale opens only from right to left. The right-to-left shunting of blood through the foramen ovale operates because the pressure in the right atrium is higher than that in the left atrium. Resistance to blood flow through the constricted pulmonary artery and pulmonary blood vessels causes the elevated pressure in the right side of the heart. Pressure is low on the left side of the heart because there is little resistance to blood leaving the left

## TABLE 19-1 CIRCULATORY CHANGES AT BIRTH

| Structure | Purpose in Fetal Life | Change at Birth | Cause of Change at Birth | Results of Change at Birth | Time of Functional and Permanent Change |
|---|---|---|---|---|---|
| Ductus arteriosus | Widely dilated; carries blood from PA to aorta and avoids nonfunctioning lungs | Reversal of blood flow and constriction | Increased pressure in aorta and increased oxygen level in blood | Blood in PA directed to lungs for oxygenation | Functional: begins within minutes after birth. Complete closure in 15–24 hr.<br>Permanent: 3–4 weeks. Becomes ligamentum arteriosum. |
| Pulmonary blood vessels | Narrowed vessels increase resistance in lungs to blood flow. | Dilation of all vessels in lungs | Elevated blood oxygen level and removal of fetal lung fluid | Decreased pulmonary resistance allows blood to enter freely to be oxygenated. | Begins with first breath |
| Foramen ovale | Provides opening between RA and LA so blood can avoid nonfunctioning lungs and go directly to LV and aorta.<br>Opens only in R to L direction because of high RA pressure and low LA pressure. | Closes when pressure in LA becomes higher than pressure in RA. | Cord occlusion elevates systemic resistance. Blood returns from PV to LA. Both increase L heart pressure. Decreased pulmonary resistance allows free flow of blood into lungs and decreased pressure in RA. | Blood entering RA can no longer pass through to LA. Instead, it goes to RV and through PA to the lungs. | Functional: within minutes<br>Permanent: 3 months. Becomes fossa ovale. |
| Ductus venosus | Shunts 50% of blood from umbilical vein to inferior vena cava and away from immature liver. | Blood flow occluded with end of umbilical circulation. | Occlusion of cord stops flow of blood from placenta through umbilical vein to ductus venosus. | Blood travels through liver to be filtered as in adult circulation. | Functional: when cord is occluded.<br>Permanent: 1 week. Becomes ligamentum venosum. |

*Abbreviations*: R, right; L, left; PA, pulmonary artery; PV, pulmonary veins; RV, right ventricle; LV, left ventricle; RA, right atrium; LA, left atrium.

ventricle. Blood from the left ventricle travels to the rest of the body and into the placental vessels, which are widely dilated. This ensures adequate blood flow into the intervillous spaces during fetal life.

At birth, pressures are reversed between the right and the left atria. Blood flows freely from the right ventricle to the dilated vessels of the lungs. Blood return to the right atrium decreases after occlusion of the umbilical vessels. These two events combine to decrease pressure in the right side of the heart.

Pressure in the left side of the heart builds as blood enters the left atrium from the pulmonary veins. When blood flow to the placenta ceases, the resistance to blood leaving the left ventricle increases, further elevating the pressure in the left side of the heart. In addition, cooling of the skin causes vasoconstriction of the peripheral vessels, further increasing the systemic vascular resistance. Because the foramen ovale opens only from right to left, it closes when the pressure in the left heart is higher than that in the right heart.

Closure of the foramen ovale prevents blood flow from the right to the left atrium and forces the blood into the right ventricle and pulmonary artery. Be-

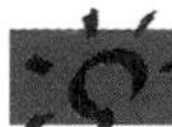

### CRITICAL THINKING EXERCISE

Understanding the changes that occur during the transition from fetal to neonatal circulation helps in predicting the effect on blood flow of various defects in the heart.

**Q:** What would be the effect on blood flow of an opening in the septum of the atria of the heart?

**A:** If there were an opening between the right and left atria after birth, blood would flow from the left atrium, where pressures are high, into the right atrium, where pressures are low. This is the reverse of the blood flow through the foramen ovale during fetal life. The blood would then flow to the right ventricle, the pulmonary artery, and to the lungs. This would cause an increased workload on the lungs and could lead to serious complications.

cause the ductus arteriosus is also closing, the blood continues on into the lungs for oxygenation and returns to the left atrium through the pulmonary veins. It enters the left ventricle and leaves through the aorta to circulate to the rest of the body. Thus, blood flow through the heart and lungs changes from fetal to neonatal circulation and is similar to that in the normal adult (see Fig. 6–9, p. 116, and Table 19–1).

The foramen ovale is functionally closed soon after birth because the pressure changes within the heart prevent it from opening. However, conditions such as asphyxia may reverse the pressures in the heart and cause the foramen ovale to reopen. The foramen ovale becomes permanently closed several months after birth. It is then called the fossa ovale.

### Ductus Venosus

During fetal life, it is not necessary for the liver to filter the blood as it does after the infant is born. The ductus venosus directs about half of the blood flow from the umbilical vein away from the liver and directly to the inferior vena cava. Once the vessels in the umbilical cord are occluded, very little blood enters the ductus venosus. Fibrosis of the ductus venosus occurs by the end of the first week of life, and it is then called the ligamentum venosum.

### CHECK YOUR READING

4. What brings about the closure of the ductus arteriosus, foramen ovale, and ductus venosus at birth?
5. What causes the pulmonary blood vessels to dilate?

## Neurologic Adaptation: Thermoregulation

An important task that the infant must take on at birth is thermoregulation, the maintenance of body temperature. Although the fetus produces heat in utero, the consistently warm temperature of the amniotic fluid makes thermoregulation unnecessary. However, the temperature of the delivery room may be more than 20°F lower than that of the uterus. Neonates must produce and maintain enough heat to prevent cold stress, which can have serious and even fatal effects.

### Newborn Characteristics Leading to Heat Loss

Some characteristics of newborns predispose them to lose heat. The skin is thin, and blood vessels are close to the surface. There is little subcutaneous fat to serve as a barrier to heat loss. Heat is readily transferred from the warmer internal areas of the body to the cooler skin surfaces and then to the surrounding air. Newborns have three times more surface area to body mass than the adult, which provides more area for heat loss. They lose heat at a rate four times greater than adults do (Behrman et al., 1996).

To conserve heat, the healthy full-term infant remains in a position of flexion. This reduces the amount of skin surface exposed to the surrounding temperatures and decreases heat loss. This is not the case for the sick or preterm infant, who has decreased muscle tone and does not maintain a flexed position. Preterm infants also have thinner skin and less subcutaneous fat than the full-term infant. Thus, they are at increased risk for cold stress (see Chapter 29).

### Methods of Heat Loss

There are four methods of heat loss in the neonate: evaporation, conduction, convection, and radiation (Fig. 19–2). The nurse can prevent heat loss by each method and must be watchful for situations in which intervention is needed.

**Evaporation.** Evaporation occurs when wet surfaces are exposed to air. As the surfaces dry, heat is lost. At birth, the infant loses heat when amniotic fluid on the skin evaporates. Evaporation also occurs during bathing. Drying the infant as quickly as possible at birth and after bathing helps prevent excessive heat loss. Insensible water loss from the skin and respiratory tract increases heat loss by evaporation.

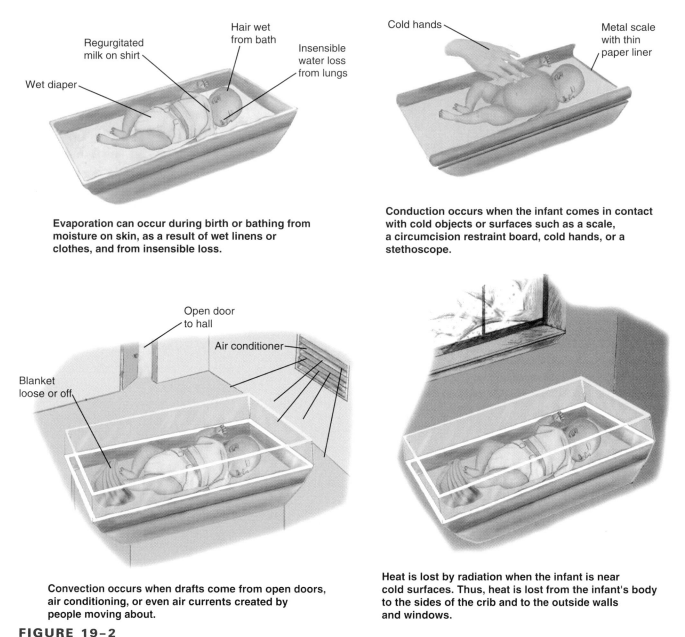

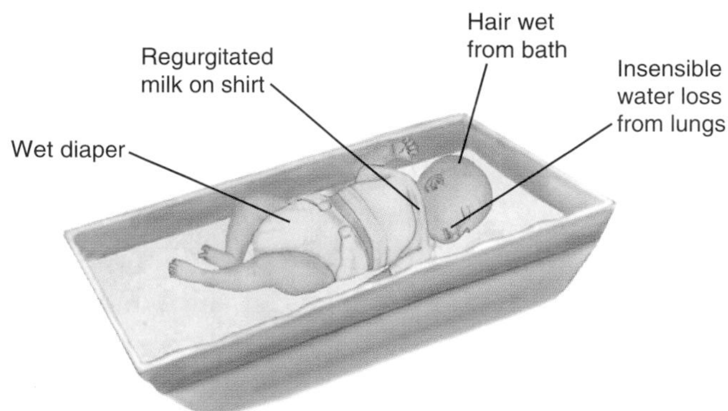


Evaporation can occur during birth or bathing from moisture on skin, as a result of wet linens or clothes, and from insensible loss.

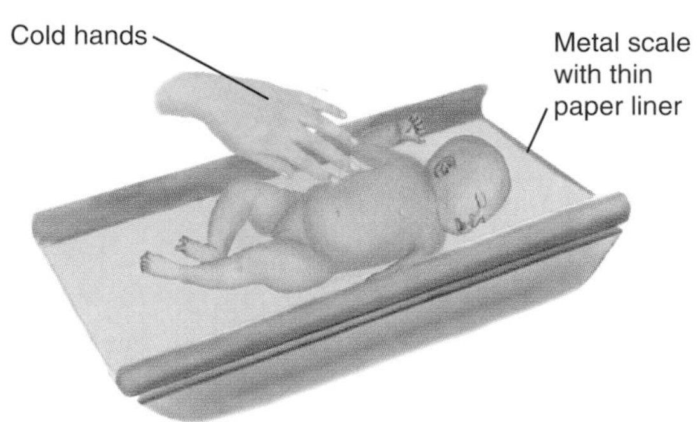


Conduction occurs when the infant comes in contact with cold objects or surfaces such as a scale, a circumcision restraint board, cold hands, or a stethoscope.

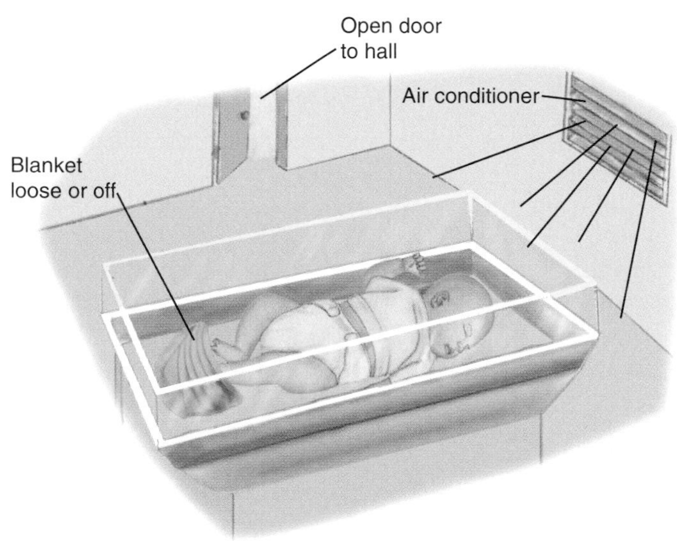


Convection occurs when drafts come from open doors, air conditioning, or even air currents created by people moving about.

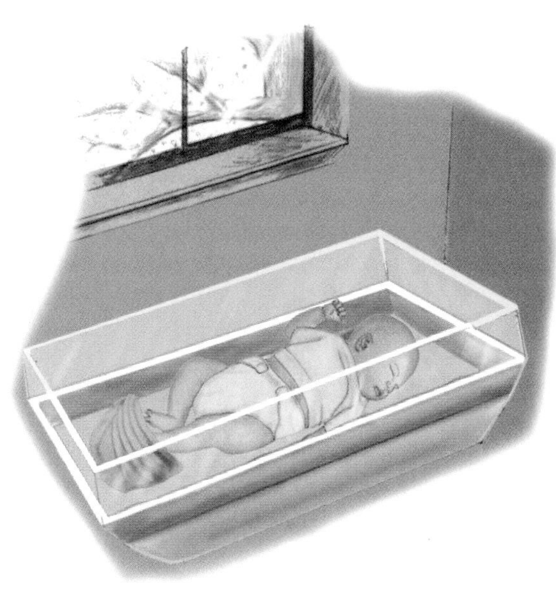

Heat is lost by radiation when the infant is near cold surfaces. Thus, heat is lost from the infant's body to the sides of the crib and to the outside walls and windows.

**FIGURE 19–2**

Methods of heat loss.

**Conduction.** Conduction of heat away from the body occurs when newborns come in direct contact with objects that are cooler than their skin. Placing infants on cold surfaces, such as scales or circumcision restraint boards, or touching them with cold hands or a cold stethoscope causes this type of heat loss. The reverse is also true. That is, wrapping newborns in warm blankets or placing them against the mother's skin can warm them.

**Convection.** Convection occurs when heat is transferred to air surrounding the infant. Air currents from air conditioning or people moving around increase the loss of heat. Keeping the newborn out of drafts and maintaining warm environmental temperatures help prevent this type of heat loss. Oxygen should be warmed before administration. Newborns are often placed in radiant warmers or incubators for a short time after birth so that the surrounding temperature can be controlled to prevent convective heat loss (Fig. 19–3). Once the temperature is stable, infants can be dressed and moved to open cribs.

**Radiation.** Radiation is the transfer of heat to cooler objects that are not in direct contact with the infant. For example, infants placed near cold windows lose heat by radiation. Infants in incubators transfer heat to the walls of the incubator. If the walls of the incubator are cold, the infant is cooled, even when the temperature of the air inside the incubator is warm. Therefore, cribs and incubators

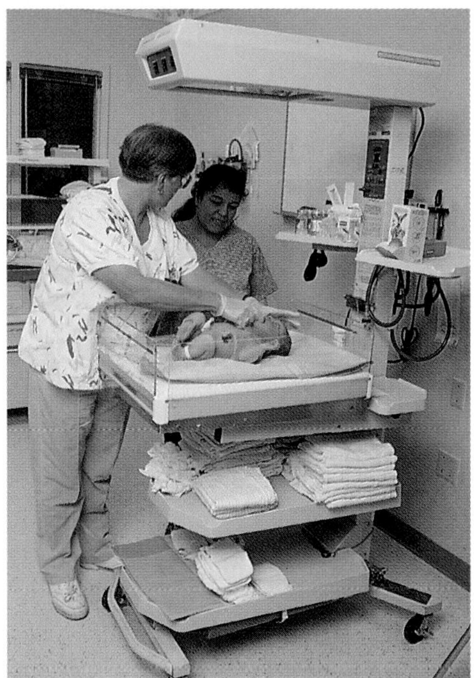

**FIGURE 19–3**

Radiant warmers allow easy access to the infant without increasing heat loss due to exposure. The nurse should be careful not to come between the infant and the overhead source of heat when caring for the infant.

should be kept away from windows and outside walls to minimize radiant heat loss.

## Nonshivering Thermogenesis

When adults are cold, they shiver, increasing muscle activity to produce heat. Newborns rarely shiver except at very low temperatures (Bruck, 1992), and shivering is not an effective method of heat production for them. Although they may become restless or cry when they are cold, newborns have no voluntary control of their muscles. Instead, a neonate's metabolic rate increases in response to falling skin temperature. Heat is a by-product of metabolic activity. Thus, increased metabolism leads to greater production of heat.

If a higher metabolic rate does not provide enough heat to raise the infant's temperature adequately, nonshivering thermogenesis begins. Nonshivering thermogenesis is the oxidation of brown fat to produce heat. Brown fat (also called brown adipose tissue) is a special kind of highly vascular fat found only in newborns. It contains an abundant supply of blood vessels, which cause the brown color. Brown fat is located primarily around the back of the neck; in the axillae; around the kidneys, adrenals, and sternum; between the scapula; and along the abdominal aorta (Fig. 19–4). As brown fat is me-

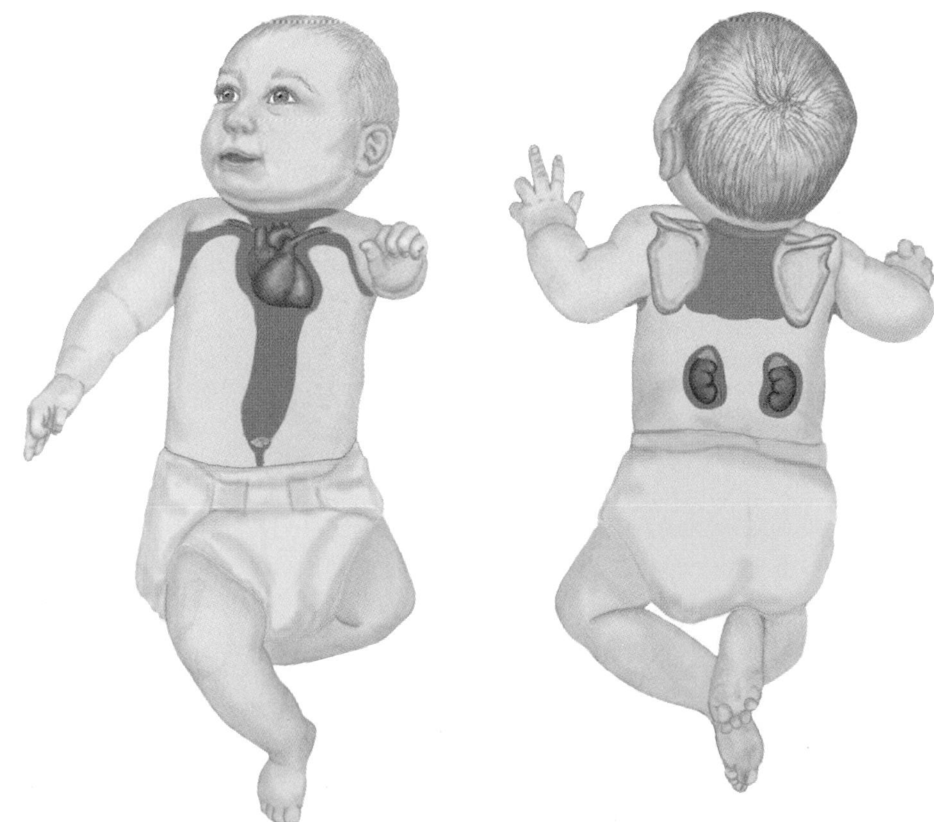

**FIGURE 19–4**

Sites of brown fat in the neonate.

tabolized, it generates more heat than other fats. Blood passing through brown fat is warmed and carries heat to the rest of the body.

Some infants have inadequate brown fat stores. The preterm infant may have been born before stores of brown fat could accumulate. Newborns with intrauterine growth restriction may have depleted brown fat stores before birth. The fat may be consumed in newborns exposed to prolonged cold stress. These infants are not able to raise their body temperature if they are subjected to further episodes of cold stress and may have serious complications. Brown fat is used up during the early weeks after birth and is not present in the older infant.

Nonshivering thermogenesis begins when thermal receptors in the skin detect a drop in skin temperature. It goes into effect even before a change occurs in core or interior body temperature, as measured with a rectal thermometer. Activating thermogenesis before core temperature decreases allows the body to maintain internal heat at an even level. Therefore, nonshivering thermogenesis may begin in an infant when skin temperature is cool, even though a temperature taken rectally shows a normal reading.

### Effects of Cold Stress

When newborns experience a drop in body temperature, their metabolism increases to produce heat (Fig. 19–5). This results in the need for more oxygen and glucose. A small increase in metabolic rate can lead to a significant rise in the need for oxygen. Even during mild respiratory distress, the infant may experience severe hypoxia as oxygen is used for heat production. The infant may not have sufficient oxygen for the metabolic rate to increase. Prolonged cold stress can cause respiratory difficulty even in a healthy full-term infant. Another result of cold stress is decreased production of surfactant, which impedes the expansion of the lungs and leads to more respiratory distress.

Glucose is necessary in larger amounts when the metabolic rate rises to produce heat. When the infant's temperature drops, glycogen stores are converted to glucose. The stores may be quickly depleted, causing hypoglycemia. Metabolism of glucose in the presence of insufficient oxygen causes increased production of acids.

Metabolism of brown fat also releases fatty acids. This can cause metabolic acidosis, which can be a life-threatening condition. Elevated fatty acids in the blood stream can also interfere with transport of bilirubin to the liver, increasing the risk of jaundice.

As the infant's body attempts to conserve heat, vasoconstriction of the peripheral blood vessels occurs. This helps reduce heat loss from the skin's surface. However, decreased oxygen levels in the blood may also cause vasoconstriction of the pulmonary vessels and a return to fetal circulation patterns, further increasing respiratory distress.

**Critical to Remember**

**HAZARDS OF COLD STRESS**

- Increased oxygen need
- Respiratory distress
- Decreased surfactant production
- Hypoglycemia
- Metabolic acidosis
- Jaundice

### Neutral Thermal Environment

A neutral thermal environment helps prevent heat loss in newborns. This is an environment in which the infant can maintain a stable body temperature without an increase in oxygen or metabolic rate. The range of environmental temperature that allows this is called the thermoneutral zone. In healthy, unclothed, full-term newborns, an environmental temperature of 32 to 34°C (89.6 to 93.2°F) provides a thermoneutral zone (Bruck, 1992).

### Hyperthermia

Infants also respond poorly to hyperthermia. With an elevated temperature, the metabolic rate rises, causing an increased need for oxygen and glucose. In addition, vasodilation leads to increased insensible fluid losses. Sweating may occur but is often delayed because sweat glands are immature.

The most frequent cause of hyperthermia in newborns is overheating by poorly regulated equipment designed to keep them warm. When infants are under radiant warmers, warming lights, or in warmed incubators, the temperature mechanism must be set to vary the heat according to the infant's skin temperature and thus prevent heat that is too high or too low. Alarms to signify that the infant's temperature is too high or too low should be functioning properly.

**CHECK YOUR READING**

6. Why are neonates more prone to heat loss than older children or adults?
7. What are the effects of low temperature in newborns?

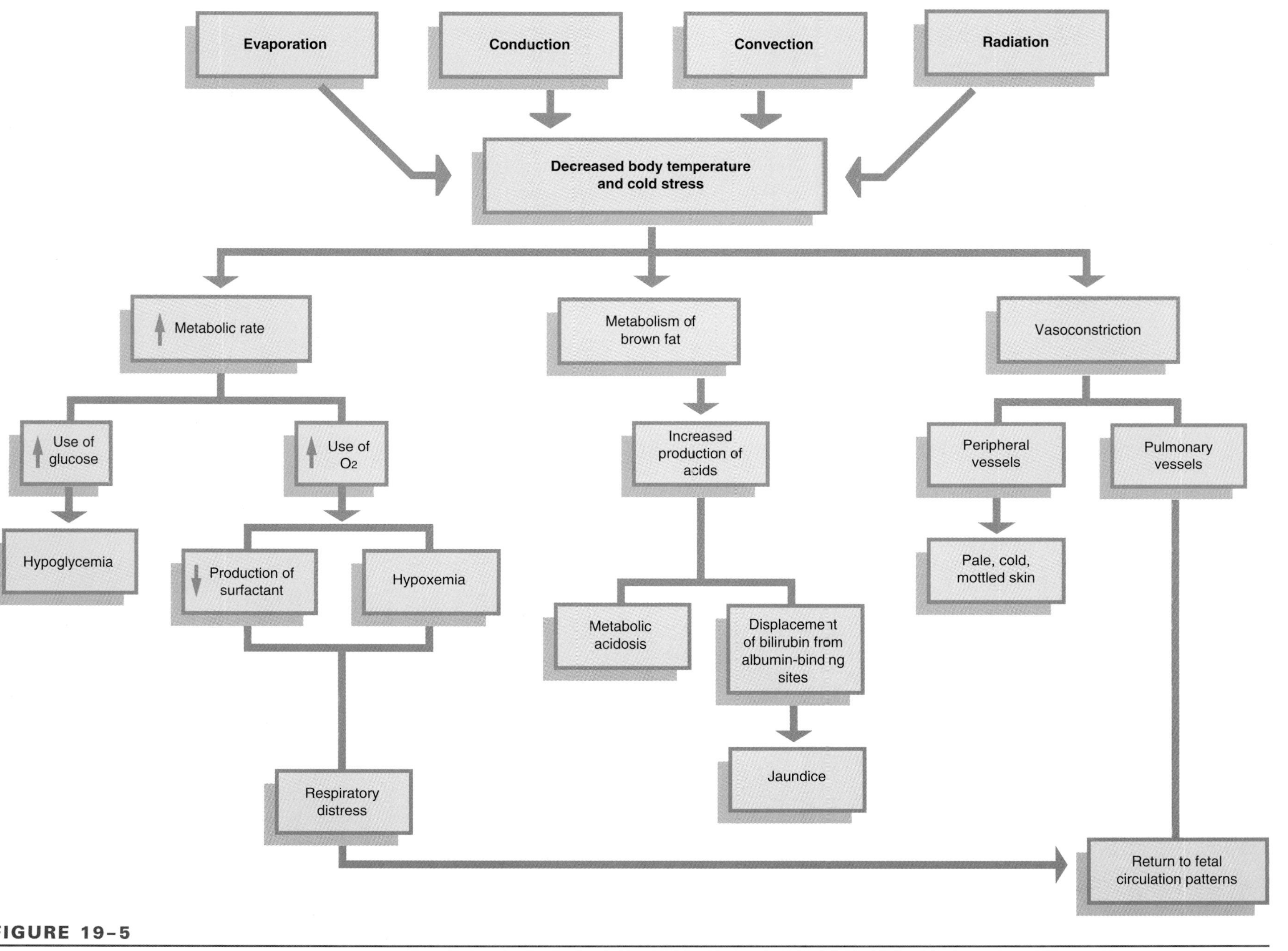


**FIGURE 19–5**
Effects of cold stress.

# Hematologic Adaptation

## Factors Affecting the Blood

In the newborn, the volume of the blood depends on whether clamping of the cord occurs immediately after birth or is delayed. It also depends on the position of the infant just before the cord is clamped. The average blood volume of the newborn is 80 to 85 ml/kg. The placenta contains approximately 100 ml of fetal blood, which can enter the infant's circulation at birth before the cord is clamped. If the cord is not clamped for a few minutes, the infant may have a 75-ml increase in blood volume (Guyton & Hall, 1996). The extra blood volume increases the workload of the heart excessively. In addition, as the added red blood cells break down, bilirubin is released, increasing the risk of jaundice.

The various components found in the blood also depend on the time of cord clamping as well as the site from which the blood is drawn. The erythrocyte count and the hemoglobin level are higher after a delay in cord clamping. Blood samples drawn from the heel, where the circulation is sluggish, indicate higher levels of hemoglobin and hematocrit than samples taken from central areas. Venous blood samples are more accurate and are taken when precise measurement is essential. (Newborn laboratory values are listed in Appendix B, p. 974.)

## Blood Values

### ERYTHROCYTES AND HEMOGLOBIN

At birth, the infant has comparatively more erythrocytes (red blood cells) and higher hemoglobin and hematocrit levels than the adult. This is necessary because the partial pressure of oxygen of fetal blood in the umbilical vein is only about 30 mmHg, much lower than the normal adult level (Guyton & Hall, 1996). The large number of erythrocytes (4 to 6.6 million/mm$^3$) and higher hemoglobin level (14.5 to 22.5 g/dl) enable the fetal cells to receive enough oxygen. Adequate oxygenation to the cells is also possible because fetal hemoglobin (hemoglobin F) carries 20 to 50 percent more oxygen than adult hemoglobin (Guyton & Hall, 1996).

Erythrocytes in the newborn have a shorter life span than those of the adult and break down soon after birth. When this happens, hemoglobin is broken down, releasing bilirubin. Excess bilirubin due to the hemolysis of large numbers of red blood cells may lead to jaundice.

### HEMATOCRIT

The hematocrit level in the normal infant is 48 to 69 percent from peripheral sites (Nicholson & Pesce, 1996). A level above 65 percent from a central site indicates polycythemia, an abnormally high erythrocyte count. Polycythemia increases the risk of jaundice and damage to the brain and other organs as a result of blood stasis. Respiratory distress and hypoglycemia are more common in these infants.

### LEUKOCYTES

The leukocyte count in the newborn is 9000 to 30,000/mm$^3$. In newborns, an elevated white blood cell count does not necessarily indicate infection. In fact, the white blood cell count may decrease in infections. Increased numbers of immature leukocytes are a sign of infection or sepsis in the neonate. Platelets may also decrease as a result of infections.

## Risk of Clotting Deficiency

Newborns are at risk for clotting deficiency during the first few days of life because they lack vitamin K, which is necessary to activate several of the clotting factors (Factors II, VII, IX, and X.) Vitamin K is synthesized in the intestines, but food and normal intestinal flora are necessary for this process. At birth, the intestines are sterile and therefore unable to produce vitamin K. To decrease the risk of hemorrhagic disease of the newborn, vitamin K is administered intramuscularly to most infants during the initial assessment and care. Drugs such as phenytoin (Dilantin), phenobarbital, and aspirin taken by the mother during pregnancy interfere with clotting ability in the infant after birth.

# Gastrointestinal System

Newborns must begin to take in, digest, and absorb food after birth, as the placenta no longer performs these functions for them.

## Stomach

The newborn's stomach capacity is about 6 ml/kg at birth (Blackburn & Loper, 1992) but expands to about 90 ml within the first few days of life. The stomach begins to empty during feeding and is completely empty within 2 to 4 hours. Peristalsis is rapid and is increased by feeding. The gastrocolic reflex is stimulated when the stomach fills, causing increased intestinal peristalsis. Infants frequently pass a stool during or following a feeding. The cardiac sphincter between the esophagus and the stomach is relaxed in the newborn, which explains the tendency to regurgitate feedings easily.

### Intestines

The intestines of the newborn are long in proportion to the infant's size and compared with those of the adult. The added length allows more surface area for absorption. However, it makes infants more prone to water loss should diarrhea develop. Air enters the gastrointestinal tract soon after birth, and bowel sounds are present within the first hour.

The digestive tract is sterile at birth. Once the infant is exposed to the external environment and begins to take in fluids, bacteria enter the gastrointestinal tract. Normal intestinal flora is established within the first few days of life.

### Digestive Enzymes

The enzymes necessary to digest simple carbohydrates, proteins, and fats are present by 36 to 38 weeks of gestation. Pancreatic amylase is deficient for the first 3 to 6 months after birth. As a result, the newborn cannot digest complex carbohydrates such as those in cereals. Amylase is also produced by the salivary glands. However, saliva is not secreted in adequate amounts until about the third month of life.

The newborn is also deficient in pancreatic lipase. Lipase in breast milk may make it more digestible for the newborn than formula. Protein and lactose, the major carbohydrate in the infant's milk diet, are both well digested.

### Stools

Meconium is the first stool excreted by the newborn. It consists of particles from amniotic fluid such as skin cells and hair, along with cells shed from the intestinal tract, bile, and other intestinal secretions. Meconium, which is greenish black in color with a thick, sticky, tar-like consistency, accumulates in the fetus's intestines throughout gestation. The first meconium stool is usually passed within the first 24 hours of life. If meconium is not passed within 36 to 48 hours, obstruction is suspected.

The second type of stool excreted by the newborn is called transitional stool. It is greenish brown and of a looser consistency than meconium. These stools are a combination of meconium and milk stools. They are followed by the stool that is characteristic of the type of feeding that the infant receives.

The stools of infants fed with breast milk are seedy, the color and consistency of mustard with a sweet-sour smell. The breastfed infant generally has more frequent stools than the infant who is formula-fed. Breastfed newborns excrete as many as 10 small stools each day, although some older infants pass only one stool every 2 to 3 days. The normal breastfed newborn should have at least three stools daily.

The formula-fed infant excretes pale yellow to light brown stools. They are firmer in consistency than those of the breastfed infant. The infant may excrete several stools daily, or only one or two. The stools have the characteristic odor of feces.

**✓ CHECK YOUR READING**

8. Why do newborns have higher levels of erythrocytes, hemoglobin, and hematocrit than adults?
9. How do the stools change over the first few days after birth?

## Hepatic System

The liver assumes many different functions after birth. Some of the most important include maintenance of blood glucose levels, conjugation of bilirubin, production of factors necessary for blood coagulation, storage of iron, and metabolism of drugs.

### Blood Glucose Maintenance

Throughout gestation, glucose is supplied to the fetus by the placenta. During the last 4 to 8 weeks of pregnancy, glucose is stored in the fetal liver as glycogen for use after birth. Glucose is used more rapidly in the newborn than in the fetus because energy is needed during the stresses of delivery and for breathing, heat production, movement against gravity, and activation of all the functions that the neonate must take on at birth. In addition, glucose must be readily available for use by the brain, which needs a constant supply. Without adequate glucose, the brain may be damaged. Therefore, the liver's ability to convert glycogen to glucose is essential.

Until newborns begin regular feedings and their intake is adequate to meet energy requirements, the glucose that is present in the body is used. As the blood glucose level falls, the liver begins to convert glycogen to glucose, which is made available for the rest of the body. In the term infant, glucose levels should stabilize at 50 to 60 mg/dl during the early hours after birth (Blackburn & Loper, 1992). A blood glucose level below 40 mg/dl in the term infant indicates hypoglycemia (Behrman et al., 1996). For screening tests on capillary blood, a glucose level below 45 mg/dl is often used as an indicator for hypoglycemia because these tests are less accurate.

Many newborns are at increased risk for hypoglycemia. The newborn may have inadequate glycogen stores, and early needs cannot be met. In the preterm and small-for-gestational age infant, adequate stores of glycogen or even fat for metabolism may not have accumulated. Stores of glycogen may be used up before birth in the postterm infant because of poor intrauterine nourishment from a deteriorating placenta.

Large-for-gestational age newborns may produce excessive insulin that consumes available glucose quickly. This is particularly true if the mother is diabetic. Infants of diabetic mothers receive large amounts of glucose from the mother throughout pregnancy and must produce enough insulin to use the glucose. Although the supply of glucose is cut off at birth, the infants may continue to produce more insulin than needed, which results in hypoglycemia soon after birth (see p. 861 for discussion of the infant of a diabetic mother).

Almost any stress can predispose a newborn to hypoglycemia. When infants are exposed to such stressors as asphyxia or infection, the glycogen in the liver may quickly be exhausted, and signs of hypoglycemia appear. In newborns who are not kept warm, all available glucose may be depleted to increase metabolism and raise body temperature. (See Chapter 20, Critical to Remember: Signs of Hypoglycemia, p. 525.)

## Conjugation of Bilirubin

A major function of the liver is the conjugation of bilirubin (Fig. 19–6). Although the newborn's liver is able to perform this function, it may not be mature enough to prevent the development of jaundice during the first week of life. Jaundice occurs in 60 percent of term newborns and 80 percent of preterm infants (Behrman et al., 1996).

### SOURCE AND EFFECT OF BILIRUBIN

The principal source of bilirubin is the hemolysis of erythrocytes. This is a normal occurrence after birth, when fewer erythrocytes are needed than during fetal life. The breakdown of red blood cells releases their components into the blood stream to be reused by the body. Only bilirubin remains as an unusable residue in the blood. This substance is toxic to the body and must be excreted.

Bilirubin is released in an unconjugated form. Unconjugated bilirubin, also called indirect bilirubin, is not soluble in water. The liver must change it to a water-soluble form by a process called conjugation before excretion can occur. The bilirubin is then known as conjugated or direct bilirubin.

Because unconjugated bilirubin is fat-soluble, it may be absorbed by the subcutaneous fat, causing the yellowish discoloration of the skin called jaundice. If enough unconjugated bilirubin accumulates in the blood, staining of the tissues in the brain may occur. This is known as kernicterus and may result in bilirubin encephalopathy, which may cause severe brain damage.

### NORMAL CONJUGATION

When unconjugated bilirubin is released into the blood stream, it attaches to binding sites on albumin in the plasma and is carried to the liver. There, the enzyme glucuronyl transferase changes the bilirubin to the conjugated form. Conjugated bilirubin is excreted into the bile and then into the duodenum. In the intestines, the normal flora acts on bilirubin to reduce it to urobilinogen, which is excreted in the stool.

A small percentage of conjugated bilirubin may be converted back to the unconjugated state by the intestinal enzyme $\beta$-glucuronidase. This enzyme is important in fetal life because bilirubin is transported to the placenta for conjugation by the mother's liver. The placenta can clear only unconjugated bilirubin. In the newborn, deconjugated bilirubin in the intestines is reabsorbed into the blood stream and carried back to the liver, where it once again undergoes the conjugation process. This recirculation of bilirubin is called the enterohepatic circuit, and it is added work for the liver.

### FACTORS IN INCREASED BILIRUBIN

A number of factors lead to the production of excessive amounts of bilirubin or interfere with the normal process of conjugation, resulting in an increased incidence of jaundice in the first week of life.

**Excess Production.** Bilirubin is produced in infants during the first 2 weeks of life at a rate twice that in adults (Maisels, 1994). Newborns have more red blood cells per kilogram of weight than do adults. This is because oxygen levels are low during fetal life and more erythrocytes are needed to carry enough oxygen to the cells.

**Red Blood Cell Life.** Fetal red blood cells break down more quickly than do adult erythrocytes. They last only two thirds as long as adult erythrocytes before hemolysis occurs. For their size, neonates have more red blood cells breaking down faster and producing greater amounts of bilirubin to excrete than adults.

**Critical to Remember**

**FACTORS THAT INCREASE HYPERBILIRUBINEMIA**

- Hemolysis of excessive erythrocytes
- Short red blood cell life
- Liver immaturity
- Lack of intestinal flora
- Delayed feeding
- Trauma resulting in bruising or cephalhematoma
- Fatty acids from cold stress or asphyxia

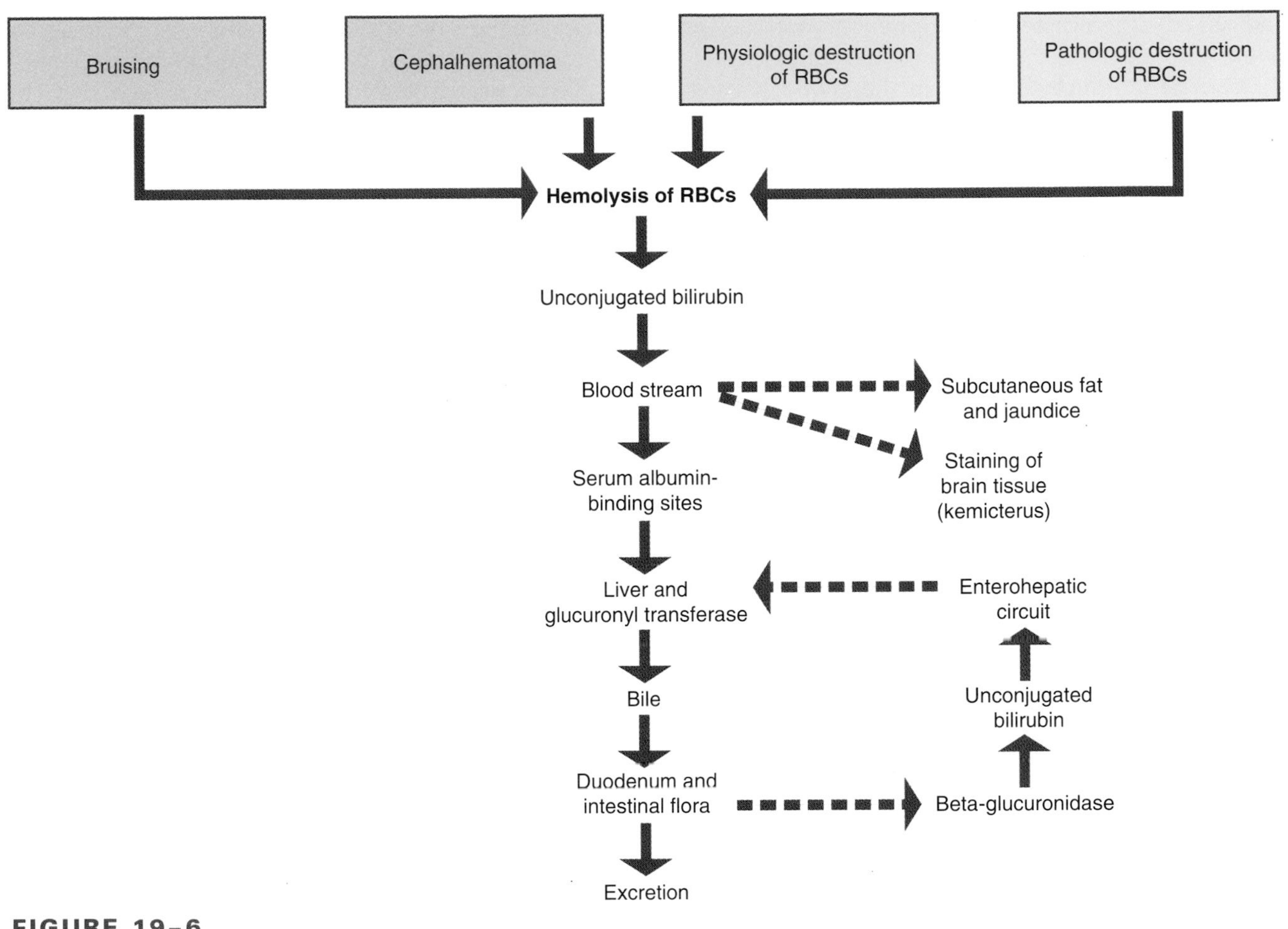


**FIGURE 19–6**

Sources of bilirubin and how it is removed from the body.

**Liver Immaturity.** The newborn's immature liver may not produce adequate amounts of glucuronyl transferase. Insufficient availability of this enzyme limits the amount of bilirubin that can be conjugated. The liver usually matures after the first few days of life and is then able to perform this function adequately for normal needs.

**Intestinal Factors.** At birth, the intestines of the newborn are sterile. Conjugated bilirubin cannot be reduced to urobilinogen for excretion without the action of intestinal flora. In addition, the newborn intestines have a large amount of the enzyme $\beta$-glucuronidase, which changes bilirubin back to the unconjugated state. These two factors may result in high levels of unconjugated bilirubin, which is reabsorbed into the blood circulation.

**Delayed Feeding.** Feeding the newborn helps establish the normal intestinal flora and promotes passage of meconium, which is high in bilirubin. When feeding is delayed or stools are not passed, the chance of conversion of conjugated bilirubin to the unconjugated state and absorption into the blood increases.

**Trauma.** Trauma during birth may result in increased hemolysis of red blood cells. This is particularly true when there is bruising, which may be caused by use of forceps or the vacuum extractor. The infant born in a breech position may also have bruising. A cephalhematoma contains a large number of erythrocytes. As the red blood cells in the bruised areas break down, they add to the bilirubin load.

**Fatty Acids.** Fatty acids have a greater affinity than bilirubin for the binding sites on albumin and bind to albumin in place of bilirubin. Fatty acids are released when brown fat is used to increase heat during cold stress. During asphyxia, anaerobic metabolism also produces fatty acids. Thus, in infants who suffer cold stress or asphyxia, unbound unconjugated bilirubin is in the circulation and jaundice may develop.

## Hyperbilirubinemia

### PHYSIOLOGIC JAUNDICE

Physiologic jaundice is due to the transient hyperbilirubinemia that occurs for any of the reasons already discussed. It is never present during the first 24 hours of life but appears on the second or third day after birth. Physiologic jaundice becomes visible when the bilirubin in the serum reaches 5 to 7 mg/dl and is considered a normal phenomenon in newborns.

The rate at which bilirubin in the blood rises and falls is important because it helps determine whether the rate for a particular infant is following the expected curve for age and birth weight. Cord blood has an average bilirubin level of less than 2 mg/dl. In physiologic jaundice, the serum bilirubin rises rapidly, peaking at 5 to 6 mg/dl between the second and fourth day of life. The bilirubin then begins to fall, declining below 2 mg/dl by the end of the first week (Behrman et al., 1996).

Physiologic jaundice may be treated with phototherapy when the bilirubin levels rise faster or to higher levels than expected. Because preterm and low-birth-weight infants are more susceptible to kernicterus at lower bilirubin levels, phototherapy may be used earlier than in the full-term infant (see p. 853).

#### PATHOLOGIC JAUNDICE

Physiologic jaundice must be differentiated from pathologic jaundice, which is abnormal and requires further investigation. One of the most important differences is the time at which the jaundice appears. Pathologic jaundice occurs during the first 24 hours after birth, whereas physiologic jaundice never occurs that early. A direct bilirubin level above 1 mg/dl or a total bilirubin concentration that increases by more than 5 mg/dl per day, is higher than 12 mg/dl in a full-term infant or 10 to 14 mg/dl in a preterm infant, or persists after the second week of life is considered pathologic (Behrman et al., 1996).

Pathologic jaundice is due to abnormalities causing excessive destruction of erythrocytes. These include incompatibilities between the mother's and infant's blood types (see p. 703), infection, and metabolic disorders (see discussion of pathologic jaundice, p. 852).

#### BREAST MILK JAUNDICE

**Inadequate Intake.** Approximately one of every three normal breastfed infants has jaundice at 2 weeks of age (Maisels, 1995). The most common cause of jaundice in breastfed infants is insufficient intake. A sleepy infant, one who has a poor suck, or one who nurses on an infrequent schedule may not receive enough colostrum, the substance that precedes true breast milk, to take advantage of its normal laxative effect. This delays the elimination of meconium, which is high in bilirubin. When meconium is not eliminated, the bilirubin may be deconjugated by $\beta$-glucuronidase in the intestine, absorbed, and recirculated to the liver.

Lack of adequate suckling also depresses production of breast milk and increases the problem further. Helping the mother with breastfeeding to increase the infant's intake and to stimulate milk production may be the most important treatment.

**True Breast Milk Jaundice.** Jaundice due to inadequate intake is different from true breast milk jaundice. In true breast milk jaundice, bilirubin levels begin to rise between the fourth and seventh day of life, after the time of onset of physiologic jaundice. Bilirubin levels peak at 15 to 20 mg/dl 2 weeks after birth and take as long as 16 weeks to fall to normal levels (de Steuben, 1992).

The exact cause of breast milk jaundice is unknown. Substances such as pregnanediol, free fatty acids, and $\beta$-glucuronidase in the breast milk have been suspected to interfere with conjugation or to increase absorption of bilirubin from the intestine, but none is a proven cause. The most likely cause is a combination of several factors that act together to cause jaundice in some infants (Ince et al., 1995).

Treatment of breast milk jaundice includes close monitoring of bilirubin levels in the blood and at least 8 to 10 feedings each 24 hours. Although the levels are higher and last longer than in physiologic jaundice, reported cases of bilirubin encephalopathy from this type of jaundice are very rare (Maisels & Newman, 1995). If bilirubin levels become too high, treatment includes phototherapy, discontinuation of breastfeeding for 24 to 48 hours, or both. This causes a rapid drop in bilirubin. The level may rise again when breastfeeding is resumed but generally not high enough to interfere with further breastfeeding.

## Blood Coagulation

Prothrombin and coagulation factors II, VII, IX, and X are produced by the liver and activated by vitamin K, which is deficient in the newborn. This is discussed under hematologic adaptation (p. 496).

## Iron Storage

Iron is stored in the liver during the last weeks of pregnancy. If the infant is born at full term and the mother's diet was adequate in iron, enough stored iron is available to prevent anemia during the infant's early months, when the diet is poor in iron. By 4 to 6 months, the iron supply may be depleted and the infant needs to begin iron-containing foods or an iron supplement. The infant whose prenatal stores are inadequate needs iron-fortified formula.

## Metabolism of Drugs

The liver metabolizes drugs inefficiently in the newborn. This must be taken into consideration when drugs are given to the neonate. In addition, a breastfeeding mother should alert her primary caregiver before taking medications, as harmful amounts may be transferred to the infant via the breast milk.

CHECK YOUR READING

10. Why is hypoglycemia a problem for the newborn?
11. What are the differences among physiologic, pathologic, and breast milk jaundice?

## Urinary System

### Kidney Development

The kidneys begin to produce urine at about the 12th week of gestation. Fetal urine is not actually a waste product because the placenta eliminates wastes for the fetus. The kidneys become the major source of amniotic fluid by the second half of pregnancy. Failure to produce urine causes oligohydramnios, or lack of sufficient amniotic fluid.

The kidneys are completely developed at 35 weeks of gestation. However, full kidney function does not occur until after birth, when the kidneys take over the elimination of wastes from the blood. Blood flow to the kidneys increases after birth because of decreased resistance in the renal vessels. The improved perfusion results in a steady improvement in kidney function during the first few days of life.

### Kidney Function

Although the formation of nephrons is complete by birth, kidney function is immature compared with that of the adult. The ability of the glomeruli to filter and the renal tubules to reabsorb is considerably less than in adults. The glomerular filtration rate doubles during the first weeks of life but does not reach adult levels until 1 to 2 years of age (Ferris et al., 1993). Therefore, infants have a decreased ability to filter waste products from the blood.

Substances such as glucose and protein may escape into the urine of the neonate. They disappear within the first 3 days of life as kidney function improves. Urate crystals may give a pink color to the urine that is sometimes mistaken for blood.

The first voiding occurs within 24 hours of birth in most newborns. The newborn who does not void within 48 hours may have hypovolemia due to inadequate intake of fluids. Absence of kidneys or anomalies that interfere with excretion of urine are usually discovered before birth. In these situations, lack of urine excretion causes oligohydramnios, a deficiency of amniotic fluid. This generally prompts investigation into the cause during pregnancy. Only two to six voidings may occur during the first 2 days of life. However, urine output then increases to five to 25 voidings daily (Anand, 1991).

***Critical to Remember***

**INTAKE AND OUTPUT IN THE NEWBORN**

First 2 days of life
  Intake: 65 ml/kg (30 ml/pound) a day
  Output: 2 to 6 voids
After the first 2 days
  Intake: 100 to 150 ml/kg (45 to 68 ml/pound) a day
  Output: 5 to 25 voids

### Fluid Balance

Newborns have a lower tolerance for changes in total volume of body fluid than do older infants. This is because of the location of water within the newborn's body and the inability of the kidneys to adapt to large changes in body fluids. In addition, the fluid turnover rate is greater than that in adults. To maintain fluid balance, newborns need 65 ml/kg (30 ml/pound) daily during the first 2 days of life and then 100 to 150 ml/kg (45 to 68 ml/pound) a day (DeMarini et al., 1993). For example, an infant who weighs 3.4 kg (7.5 pounds) on the third day of life needs 340 to 510 ml of fluid each day.

#### WATER DISTRIBUTION

A large percentage of the infant's body is composed of water, which is distributed differently than it is in the adult (Table 19–2). Water constitutes 78 percent of the infant's body weight. It takes approximately 1 year for body fluid to decrease to the adult level of 55 to 60 percent of body weight (Behrman et al., 1996).

In the adult, 20 percent of body weight is composed of extracellular water located in the interstitial or intravascular spaces. The percentage of extracellular water in newborns is more than twice as high as in adults. Although fluid within the cells is relatively stable, extracellular water is easily lost from the body. Because infants have more fluid for their size than adults, and because a larger proportion of it is located outside the cells, total body water is easily depleted. Conditions such as vomiting and diarrhea can quickly result in life-threatening dehydration.

**TABLE 19–2 DISTRIBUTION OF WATER IN NEWBORNS AND ADULTS**

| | Newborn | Adult |
|---|---|---|
| Total body water | 78% | 55–60% |
| Extracellular water | 45% | 20% |
| Intracellular water | 33% | 40% |

Comparison of distribution of body water in newborns and adults as a percent of body weight.

#### INSENSIBLE WATER LOSS

Water lost from the skin and respiratory tract contributes to insensible water loss. Insensible water losses are increased in the newborn because of the large surface area of the body and the rapid respiratory rate. Fluid losses increase greatly when infants are placed under radiant heaters, which accelerate evaporation from the skin. An elevated respiratory rate or low humidity in the air surrounding the infant raises insensible water losses even further.

#### URINE DILUTION AND CONCENTRATION

The ability of a newborn's kidneys to dilute urine is relatively good, to a specific gravity of 1.001 to 1.005 (Ferris et al., 1993). However, a newborn's kidneys cannot handle large increases in fluids, which result in fluid overload. This is most likely to happen when infants receive too much intravenous fluid. Normal urine output is 1 to 3 ml/kg per hour.

Newborns have more difficulty preventing loss of fluid in the urine than do adults because they have only half the adult's ability to excrete concentrated urine (Guyton & Hall, 1996). Neonates can concentrate urine only to a specific gravity of 1.015 to 1.020 (Ferris et al., 1993), compared with the adult level of 1.040. It takes 3 to 6 months for urine concentrations to reach adult levels. When abnormal conditions such as diarrhea cause excessive loss of fluid, the newborn's limited ability to conserve water may result in dehydration more quickly than in the older infant or child.

### Acid-Base and Electrolyte Balance

The maintenance of acid-base and electrolyte balance is a primary function of the kidneys and may be precarious in neonates. Newborns tend to lose bicarbonate at lower levels than adults, increasing their risk for acidosis. The excretion of solutes is less efficient in newborns as well. Although newborns conserve needed sodium well, they are less able to excrete sodium efficiently if they receive excessive amounts (Brion et al., 1994).

**✓ CHECK YOUR READING**

12. How does the distribution of fluid in the newborn compare with that in the adult?

## Immune System

The neonate is less effective in fighting off infection than the older infant or child. The various white blood cells respond slowly and inefficiently when the body is invaded by organisms. Leukocytes are delayed in moving to the site of invasion and are not efficient in destroying the invader. Fever and leukocytosis, which normally occur during infection of the older child, are often not present in the newborn with infection. This is because the hypothalamus and inflammatory response are immature.

Full-term newborns received antibodies from the mother during the last trimester of pregnancy. The mother continues to give the infant antibodies in breast milk, if she chooses that method of feeding. This transfers passive immunity to the infant. Immunoglobulins (serum globulins with antibody activity) help protect the newborn from infection. The major immunoglobulins are IgG, IgM, and IgA. Each immunoglobulin performs a different function.

### IgG

IgG crosses the placenta readily and provides the fetus with passive temporary immunity to bacteria and viruses to which the mother has developed immunity. IgG also protects the fetus from bacterial toxins. It begins to cross the placenta during the first trimester, but most of the transfer occurs in the third trimester. A preterm infant born before 32 weeks of gestation has received less than half the IgG of an infant born at full term.

Although the fetus begins to make its own IgG at 20 weeks of gestation, very little is produced until 3 to 4 weeks after birth. The infant gradually produces larger quantities of the immunoglobulin to replace IgG from the mother, which is being catabolized. The passive immunity lasts for varying amounts of time. Although much of the passive immunity is gone by about 3 months of age, the antibodies to measles may last much longer. Administration of measles vaccine is delayed until about 12 to 15 months so that the passive immunity does not interfere with the infant's ability to form active immunity to measles.

### IgM

IgM is the first immunoglobulin produced by the body when the newborn is challenged. This immunoglobulin helps protect against gram-negative bacteria. Small amounts of IgM are produced beginning at 20 weeks of gestation, and it is rapidly produced beginning a few days after birth. IgM cannot cross the placenta because the molecules are too large. If IgM is found in larger than normal amounts, exposure to infection in utero is probable.

### IgA

IgA does not cross the placenta and must be produced by the infant. It is not produced in adequate amounts until 6 to 12 weeks after birth, and production gradually increases throughout childhood. Because IgA is important in protection of the gastrointestinal and respiratory systems, newborns are particularly susceptible to infections of those systems. A form of IgA is included in colostrum and breast milk. Therefore, breastfed infants receive protection that formula-fed infants do not.

# Psychosocial Adaptation

## Periods of Reactivity

In the early hours after birth, the infant goes through changes called the periods of reactivity. There are two periods of reactivity separated by a period of sleep.

### FIRST PERIOD OF REACTIVITY

The first period of reactivity begins at birth. Infants are very active at this time and appear wide awake, alert, and interested in their surroundings. Parents enjoy this phase, as the infant gazes directly at them when held in the *en face* (face-to-face) position. Infants move their arms and legs energetically, root, and appear hungry. If allowed to nurse, many infants latch on to the nipple and suck well.

Respirations during the first period of reactivity may be as high as 80 breaths per minute. The heart rate may be elevated to 180 beats per minute. There may be crackles, retractions, nasal flaring, and increased mucous secretions. The pulse and respirations gradually slow, and the infant becomes sleepy after about 30 minutes.

### PERIOD OF SLEEP

After the first period of reactivity, infants become quiet and eventually fall into a deep sleep, which lasts 2 to 4 hours. During this time, the pulse and respirations drop to the normal range but the temperature may be low.

### SECOND PERIOD OF REACTIVITY

When infants waken from the period of sleep, they enter the second period of reactivity. Infants are alert, and parents may enjoy the opportunity to get to know them at this time. Infants become interested in feeding and may pass meconium. The pulse and respiratory rates may increase, and some infants become cyanotic or have periods of apnea. Mucous secretions increase, and infants may gag or regurgitate.

The second period of reactivity may last 4 to 6 hours, although individual variation is great. Many infants pass through all stages within 8 hours. Once the second period of reactivity is over, the infant is usually stable.

## Behavioral States

Six gradations in the behavioral state of the infant have been identified, ranging from deep sleep to crying. The amount of time infants spend in the different sleep-wake states varies and is a key to their individuality. Infants tend to move from one state to the next in the following sequence.

### QUIET SLEEP STATE

In the quiet sleep state, the infant is in a deep sleep with closed eyes and no eye movements. Respirations are quiet, regular, and slower than in the other states. Although startles occur at intervals, the infant's body is quiet. Little or no response to noise or stimuli occurs, and the infant returns to deep sleep quickly if not disturbed.

### ACTIVE SLEEP STATE

In the active sleep state, infants move their extremities, stretch, change facial expressions, and may fuss briefly. During this period, respirations tend to be more rapid and irregular and rapid eye movements (REM) occur. Infants are more likely to startle from noise or disturbances and may return to sleep or move to an awake state.

### DROWSY STATE

The drowsy state is a transitional period between sleep and waking similar to that experienced by adults as they awake. The eyes may remain closed or, if open, appear glazed and unfocused. Infants startle and move their extremities slowly. They may go back to sleep or, with gentle stimulation, gradually awaken.

### QUIET ALERT STATE

The quiet alert state should be pointed out to parents because it is an excellent time to increase bonding. Infants focus on objects or people, respond to the parents with intense gazing, and seem bright and interested in their surroundings. Body movements are minimal, as infants seem to concentrate on the environment.

### ACTIVE ALERT STATE

In the active alert state infants are often fussy. They seem restless, have faster and more irregular respirations, and seem more aware of feelings of discomfort from hunger or cold. Although their eyes are open, infants seem less focused on visual stimuli than during the quiet alert state.

### CRYING STATE

The crying state may quickly follow the active alert state if no intervention occurs to comfort the infant. The cries are continuous and lusty, and the infant does not respond positively to stimulation. It may take a period of comforting to move the infant to a state in which feeding or other activities can be accomplished.

## ✓ CHECK YOUR READING

13. Why are IgG, IgM, and IgA important to the newborn?
14. What are newborns like during the first and second periods of reactivity?
15. How do infant behavioral states vary?

## SUMMARY CONCEPTS

- Chemical, thermal, and mechanical factors combine to stimulate the respiratory center in the brain and initiate respirations at birth.
- Surfactant lines the alveoli and reduces surface tension to keep the alveoli open. Fetal lung fluid moves into the interstitial spaces before, during, and after birth and is absorbed by the lymphatic and vascular systems.
- Increases in blood oxygen levels, shifts in pressure in the heart and lungs, and closing of the umbilical vessels cause closure of the ductus arteriosus, foramen ovale, and ductus venosus at birth.
- Infants are predisposed to heat loss because they have thin skin with little subcutaneous fat, blood vessels close to the surface, and a large skin surface area. They lose heat by evaporation, conduction, convection, and radiation.
- Heat is produced in newborns by an increase in metabolism, vasoconstriction, and nonshivering thermogenesis. These factors increase oxygen and glucose consumption and may cause respiratory distress, hypoglycemia, acidosis, and jaundice.
- Laboratory values for erythrocytes, hemoglobin, and hematocrit are higher for newborns than for adults because oxygen available to them in fetal life was less than after birth.
- After birth, the stools progress from thick, greenish black meconium to loose greenish brown transitional stools to milk stools. Stools of breastfed infants are frequent, soft, seedy, and mustard-colored, whereas those of formula-fed infants are pale yellow to light brown, firmer, and less frequent.
- The brain needs a constant supply of glucose and may be damaged without it.
- Physiologic jaundice occurs in normal newborns after the first 24 hours of life as a result of hemolysis of red blood cells and immaturity of the liver. Pathologic jaundice is abnormal, begins within the first 24 hours, and often requires treatment with phototherapy. Breast milk jaundice begins later than physiologic jaundice and may be due to substances in the milk.
- The ability of the newborn's kidneys to filter, reabsorb, and monitor fluid and electrolyte balance is less than that of the adult's kidneys. The newborn's body is composed of a greater percentage of water, with more located in the extracellular compartment, than the adult's.
- Newborns receive passive immunity when IgG crosses the placenta in utero. After birth, IgM and IgA are produced to protect against infection.
- During the first and second periods of reactivity, newborns are active and alert and may be interested in feeding. Their pulse and respiratory rates may be elevated, and they may show some transient signs of respiratory distress.
- Newborns progress through six behavioral states: quiet sleep, active sleep, drowsy, quiet alert, active alert, and crying.

### References and Readings


American Academy of Pediatrics and American College of Obstetricians and Gynecologists (1992). *Guidelines for perinatal care* (3rd ed.). Elk Grove, Ill.: American Academy of Pediatrics.

Anand, S.K. (1991). Clinical evaluation of renal disease. In H.W. Taeusch, R.A. Ballard, & M.E. Avery (Eds.), *Schaffer's diseases of the newborn* (6th ed.). Philadelphia: W.B. Saunders.

Avery, G.B., Fletcher, M.A., & MacDonald, M.G. (Eds.). (1994). *Neonatology: Pathophysiology and management of the newborn* (4th ed.). Philadelphia: J.B. Lippincott.

Behrman, R.E., Kliegman, R.M., & Arvin, A.M. (Eds.). (1996). *Nelson textbook of pediatrics* (15th ed.). Philadelphia: W.B. Saunders.

Blackburn, S. (1995). Hyperbilirubinemia and neonatal jaundice. *Neonatal Network*, 14(7), 15–25.

Blackburn, S.T., & Loper, D.L. (1992). *Maternal, fetal, and neonatal physiology: A clinical perspective*. Philadelphia: W.B. Saunders.

Brion, L.P., Satlin, L.M., & Edelmann, C.M. (1994). Renal disease. In G.B. Avery, M.A. Fletcher, & M.G. Macdonald (Eds.), *Neonatology: Pathophysiology and management of the newborn* (4th ed.). Philadelphia: J.B. Lippincott.

Brooks, C. (1997). Neonatal hypoglycemia. *Neonatal Network*, 16(2), 15–21.

Brown, L.P., Arnold, L., Allison, D., Klein, M.E., & Jocobsen, B. (1993). Incidence and pattern of jaundice in healthy breastfed infants during the first month of life. *Nursing Research*. 42(2), 106–110.

Bruck, K. (1992). Neonatal thermal regulation. In R.A. Polin & W.W. Fox (Eds.), *Fetal and neonatal physiology* (Vol. 1). Philadelphia: W.B. Saunders.

Crockett, M. (1995). Physiology of the neonatal immune system. *Journal of Obstetric, Gynecologic, and Neonatal Nursing*, 24(7), 627–634.

DeMarini, S., Tsang, R.C., Rath, L.L. (1993). Fluids, electrolytes, vitamins, and trace minerals: Basis of ingestion, digestion, elimination, and metabolism. In C. Kenner, A. Brueggemeyer, & L.P. Gunderson (Eds.), *Comprehensive neonatal nursing: A physiologic perspective*. Philadelphia: W.B. Saunders.

de Steuben, C. (1992). Breast-feeding and jaundice: A review. *Journal of Nurse-Midwifery*, 37(Suppl. 2), 59S–66S.

Fanaroff, A.A., & Martin, R.J. (1997). *Neonatal-perinatal medicine* (Vols. 1 and 2, 6th ed.). St. Louis: Mosby–Year Book.

Ferris, M.E., Brannan, P., & Portman, R. (1993). Neonatal nephrology. In G.B. Merenstein & S.L. Gardner (Eds.), *Handbook of neonatal intensive care* (3rd ed.). St. Louis: C.V. Mosby.

Guyton, A.C., & Hall, J.E. (1996). *Textbook of medical physiology* (9th ed.). Philadelphia: W.B. Saunders.

Ince, Z., Coban, A., Peker, I., & Can, G. (1995). Breast milk β-glucuronidase and prolonged jaundice in the neonate. *Acta Paediatrics, 84*, 3237–3239.

Klaus, M.H., & Fanaroff, A.A. (1993). *Care of the high-risk neonate* (4th ed.). Philadelphia: W.B. Saunders.

Lott, J.W. (1993). Assessment and management of cardiovascular dysfunction. In C. Kenner, A. Brueggemeyer, & L.P. Gunderson (Eds.), *Comprehensive neonatal nursing: A physiologic perspective*. Philadelphia: W.B. Saunders.

Lowe, N.K., & Reiss, R. (1996). Parturition and fetal adaptation. *Journal of Obstetric, Gynecologic, and Neonatal Nursing, 25*(4), 339–349.

Maisels, M.J. (1994). Jaundice. In G.B. Avery, M.A. Fletcher, & M.G. Macdonald (Eds.), *Neonatology: Pathophysiology and management of the newborn* (4th ed.). Philadelphia: J.B. Lippincott.

Maisels, M.J. (1995). Clinical rounds in the well-baby nursery: Treating jaundiced newborns. *Pediatric Annals, 25*(10), 548–552.

Maisels, M.J., & Newman, T.B. (1995). Kernicterus in otherwise healthy, breast-fed term newborns. *Pediatrics, 96*(4), 730–733.

Martinez, J.C., Maisels, M.J., Otheguy, L., et al. (1993). Hyperbilirubinemia in the breast-fed newborn: A controlled trial of four interventions. *Pediatrics, 91*(2), 470–473.

Nelson, N. (1994). Physiology of transition. In G.B. Avery, M.A. Fletcher, & M.G. Macdonald (Eds.), *Neonatology, Pathophysiology and management of the newborn* (4th ed.). Philadelphia: J.B. Lippincott.

Nicholson, J.F., & Pesce, M.A. (1996). Laboratory medicine and reference tables. In R.E. Behrman, R.M. Kliegman, & A.M. Arvin (Eds.), *Nelson textbook of pediatrics* (15th ed.). Philadelphia: W.B. Saunders.

Philip, A. (1996). *Neonatology, a practical guide* (4th ed.) Philadelphia: W.B. Saunders.

Reimann, D., & Coughlin, M. (1996). Newborn physical assessment. In K.R. Simpson & P.A. Creehan (Eds.), *AWHONN's perinatal nursing*. Philadelphia: Lippincott-Raven.

Sansoucie, D.A., & Cavaliere, T.A. (1997). Transition from fetal to extrauterine circulation. *Neonatal Network, 16*(2), 5–12.

# 20

# Assessment of the Normal Newborn

**OBJECTIVES**

1. Describe initial assessments of the newborn.
2. Explain the nurse's responsibility in cardiorespiratory and thermoregulatory assessments.
3. Describe nursing assessments of body systems.
4. Explain the importance and the components of gestational age assessment.
5. Describe newborn behavior, including periods of reactivity and behavior states.

**DEFINITIONS**

**café-au-lait-spots** *Light brown birthmarks.*

**caput succedaneum** *Area of edema over the presenting part of the fetus or newborn resulting from pressure against the cervix. Often called simply "caput."*

**cephalhematoma** *Bleeding between the periosteum and skull from pressure during birth. It does not cross suture lines.*

**craniosynostosis** *Premature closure of the sutures of the infant's head.*

**cryptorchidism** *Failure of one or both testes to descend into the scrotum.*

**epispadias** *Abnormal placement of the urinary meatus on the dorsal side of the penis.*

**erythema toxicum** *Benign rash of unknown cause in newborns, with blotchy red areas that may have white or yellow papules in the center.*

**hypospadias** *Abnormal placement of the urinary meatus on the ventral side of the penis.*

**lanugo** *Fine, soft hair covering the fetus.*

**milia** *White cysts, 1 to 2 mm in size, from distended sebaceous glands.*

**molding** *Shaping of the fetal head during movement through the birth canal.*

**mongolian spots** *Bruise-like marks that occur mostly in newborns with dark skin tones.*

**nevus flammeus** *Permanent purple birthmark. Also called port wine stain.*

**nevus vasculosus** *Rough red collection of capillaries with a raised surface that disappears with time.*

**periodic breathing** *Cessation of breathing lasting no more than 10 seconds without changes in color or heart rate.*

**point of maximum impulse** *Area of the chest in which the heart sounds are loudest when auscultated.*

**polydactyly** *More than 10 digits on the hands or feet.*

**pseudomenstruation** *Vaginal bleeding in the newborn, resulting from withdrawal of placental hormones.*

**strabismus** *A turning inward ("crossing") or outward of the eyes due to poor muscle tone.*

**syndactyly** *Webbing between fingers or toes.*

**telangiectatic nevi (stork bites, nevus simplex)** *Flat pink areas on the nape of the neck and over the eyelids resulting from dilation of the capillaries.*

**vernix caseosa** *Thick white substance that protects the skin of the fetus.*

This chapter focuses on the very important role of the nurse in assessing the newborn to identify abnormalities or problems in adapting to life outside the uterus. The first complete assessment of the newborn is often called an "admission assessment." Subsequent assessments are not as comprehensive. Table 20–1 summarizes newborn assessments. Keys to Clinical Practice (Appendix D) describes the order of initial assessments and care.

Text continued on page 513

**TABLE 20–1 SUMMARY OF NEWBORN ASSESSMENT**

| Normal | Abnormal (Possible Causes) | Nursing Considerations |
|---|---|---|
| **Initial Assessment** | | |
| Assess for obvious problems first. If infant is stable and has no problems that require immediate attention, continue with complete assessment. | | |
| **Vital Signs** | | |
| *Temperature* | | |
| 36.5–37.5°C (97.7–99.5°F) axillary, 36.5–37.6°C (97.7–99.7°F) rectal. Axilla is preferred site. | Decreased (hypoglycemia, CNS problem, infection, cold environment). Increased (infection, environment too warm). | Decreased: Institute warming measures and check in 30 min. Check blood glucose. Increased: Remove excessive clothing. Check warmer temperature setting. Check for dehydration. Decreased or increased: Look for signs of infection. Check radiant warmer temperature setting. Check thermometer for accuracy if skin is warm or cool to touch. Report abnormals to physician. |
| *Pulses* | | |
| Heart rate at 120–160 BPM (100 sleeping, 180 crying). Rhythm regular. Point of maximum impulse (PMI) at third to fourth intercostal space, slightly to left of midclavicular line, may be visible. Brachial, femoral, and pedal pulses present and equal bilaterally. | Tachycardia (respiratory problems, anemia, infection, cardiac conditions). Bradycardia (asphyxia, increased intracranial pressure). PMI to right (dextrocardia, pneumothorax). Murmurs (functional or congenital heart defects) and arrhythmias should be assessed by skilled practitioners. Absent or unequal pulses (coarctation of the aorta). | Note location of murmurs. Refer abnormal rates, rhythms and sounds, pulses. |
| *Respirations* | | |
| Rate 30–60 (average 30–40) per min. Respirations irregular, shallow, unlabored. Chest movements symmetric. Breath sounds present and clear bilaterally. | Tachypnea especially after the first hour. Slow respirations (maternal medications). Nasal flaring. Grunting (respiratory distress syndrome). Gasping (respiratory depression). Periods of apnea more than 20 sec or with change in heart rate or color (respiratory depression, sepsis, cold stress). Asymmetry or decreased chest expansion (pneumothorax). Intercostal, xyphoid, subcostal, or supraclavicular retractions or seesaw respirations (respiratory distress). Moist, coarse breath sounds (rales, crackles, rhonchi), fluid in lungs. Bowel sounds in chest (diaphragmatic hernia). | Mild variations require continued monitoring and usually clear in early hours after birth. If persistent or more than mild, suction, give oxygen, call physician, and initiate more intensive care. |

Table 20–1 continued on following page

**TABLE 20–1 SUMMARY OF NEWBORN ASSESSMENT** *Continued*

| Normal | Abnormal (Possible Causes) | Nursing Considerations |
|---|---|---|
| **Vital Signs** *(continued)* | | |
| ***Blood Pressure*** | | |
| Average 70 mmHg systolic and 45 mmHg diastolic. Varies with activity and gestational age. | Hypotension (hypovolemia, shock, sepsis). Difference of 20 mmHg between arms and legs (coarctation of the aorta). | Refer abnormal blood pressures. Prepare for intensive care if very low. |
| **Measurements** | | |
| ***Weight*** | | |
| Weight 2500–4000 g (5 pounds, 8 ounces to 8 pounds, 13 ounces). Weight loss up to 10% in early days. | Above normal range (LGA, maternal diabetes). Below normal range (SGA, preterm, multifetal pregnancy, medical conditions in mother that affect intrauterine growth). Weight loss above 10% (dehydration, feeding problems). | Determine cause. Monitor for complications common to cause. |
| ***Length*** | | |
| 48–53 cm (19–21 inches). | Below normal range (SGA, congenital dwarf). Above normal range (LGA, maternal diabetes). | Determine cause. Monitor for complications common to cause. |
| ***Head Circumference*** | | |
| 33–35.5 cm (13–14 inches). Head approximately one fourth of infant's length. | Small (SGA, microcephaly, anencephaly). Large (LGA, hydrocephalus, increased intracranial pressure). | Determine cause. Monitor for complications common to cause. |
| ***Chest Circumference*** | | |
| 30.5–33 cm (12–13 inches). Generally 2–3 cm less than head circumference. | Large (LGA). Small (SGA). | Determine cause. Monitor for complications common to cause. |
| **Posture** | | |
| Flexed extremities resist extension, return quickly to flexed state. Hands usually clenched. Movements symmetric. Slight tremors on crying. Breech—extended, stiff legs. "Molds" body to caretaker's when held, responds by quieting when needs met. | Limp, flaccid, "floppy," or rigid extremities (preterm, hypoxia, medications, CNS trauma). Hypertonic (fetal abstinence syndrome, CNS damage). Jitteriness or tremors (low glucose or calcium level). Opisthotonus, seizures, stiff when held (CNS damage). | Seek cause, refer abnormalities. |
| **Cry** | | |
| Lusty, strong. | High-pitched (increased intracranial pressure). Weak, absent, irritable, cat-like "mewing" (neurologic problems). Hoarse or crowing (laryngeal irritation). | Observe for changes, report abnormalities. |

**TABLE 20–1 SUMMARY OF NEWBORN ASSESSMENT** *Continued*

| Normal | Abnormal (Possible Causes) | Nursing Considerations |
|---|---|---|
| **Skin** | | |
| Color pink or tan (according to race) with acrocyanosis. Vernix caseosa in creases. Small amounts of lanugo over shoulders, sides of face or forehead, upper back. Skin turgor good with quick recoil. Some cracking and peeling of skin. **Normal variations:** Milia. Erythema toxicum (flea bite rash). Puncture on scalp (from electrode). Mongolian spots. Telangiectatic nevi (nevus simplex or "stork bites"). | **Color:** Cyanosis of mouth and central areas (hypoxia). Pallor (anemia, hypoxia). Gray (hypoxia, hypotension). Red, sticky, transparent skin (very preterm). Ruddy (polycythemia). Greenish brown discoloration of skin, nails, cord (possible fetal compromise, postterm). Yellow vernix (blood incompatibilities). Jaundice (pathologic if first 24 hours). Thick vernix (preterm). **Delivery marks:** Bruises on body (pressure), scalp (vacuum extractor), or face (cord around neck). Petechiae (pressure, low platelets, infection). Forceps marks. **Birthmarks:** Nevus flammeus (port wine stain). Nevus vasculosus (strawberry hemangioma). Café-au-lait spots (>6 or >1.5 cm, neurofibromatosis). **Other:** Excessive lanugo (preterm). Excessive peeling, cracking (postterm). Skin tags. Pustules or other rashes (infection). "Tenting" of skin (dehydration). | Differentiate facial bruising from cyanosis. Central cyanosis requires suction, oxygen, and further treatment. Refer jaundice in first 24 hr. Watch for respiratory problems in infants with meconium staining. Look for other signs and complications of preterm or postterm birth. Record location, size, shape, color, type of rashes and marks. Check for facial movement with forceps marks. Watch for jaundice with bruising. Point out and explain normal skin variations to parents. |
| **Head** | | |
| Sutures palpable with small separation between each. Anterior fontanelle diamond shaped, 4 to 5 cm across, soft and flat. May bulge slightly with crying. Posterior fontanelle triangular, 0.5–1 cm in size. Hair silky and soft with individual hair strands. **Normal variations:** Overriding sutures (molding). Caput succedaneum or cephalhematoma (pressure during birth). | Head large (hydrocephalus, increased intracranial pressure) or small (microcephaly). Widely separated sutures (hydrocephalus) or sutures not palpable (craniosynostosis). Anterior fontanelle depressed (dehydration, molding), full or bulging at rest (increased intracranial pressure). Woolly, bunchy hair (preterm). Unusual hair growth (chromosomal abnormalities). | Seek cause of variations. Observe for signs of dehydration with depressed fontanelle, increased intracranial pressure with bulging of fontanelle and wide separation of sutures. Refer for treatment. Differentiate caput succedaneum from cephalhematoma and reassure parents of normal outcome. Observe for jaundice with cephalhematoma. |
| **Ears** | | |
| Ears well formed and complete. Area where upper ear meets head even with imaginary line drawn from inner to outer canthus of eye. Startle response to loud noises. Alert to high-pitched voices. | Low-set ears (chromosomal disorders). Skin tags, preauricular sinuses, dimples (kidney anomalies). No response to sound (deafness). | Check voiding if ears abnormal. Look for signs of chromosomal abnormality if position abnormal. Refer for evaluation if no response to sound. |

*Table 20–1 continued on following page*

**TABLE 20–1 SUMMARY OF NEWBORN ASSESSMENT** *Continued*

| Normal | Abnormal (Possible Causes) | Nursing Considerations |
|---|---|---|
| **Face** | | |
| Symmetric in appearance and movement. Parts proportional and appropriately placed. | Asymmetry of jaw (pressure and position in utero). Drooping of mouth or one side of face, "one-sided cry" (facial nerve damage). Abnormal appearance (chromosomal abnormalities). | Seek cause of variations. Check delivery history for possible cause of damage to facial nerve. |
| **Eyes** | | |
| Symmetric. Eyes clear. Transient strabismus. Scant or absent tears. Pupils equal, react to light. Alerts to interesting sights. Follows objects 180 degrees. Doll's-eye sign present. Red reflex present. May have subconjunctival hemorrhage or edema of eyelids from pressure during delivery. | Inflammation or drainage (chemical or infectious conjunctivitis). Constant tearing (plugged lacrimal duct). Unequal pupils. Failure to follow objects (blindness). White areas over pupils (cataracts). Setting-sun sign (hydrocephalus). | Clean and monitor any drainage; seek cause. Reassure parents that subconjunctival hemorrhage and edema will clear. Refer other abnormalities. |
| **Nose** | | |
| Both nostrils open to air flow. May have slight flattening from pressure during birth. | Blockage of one or both nostrils (choanal atresia). Malformations (congenital conditions). Flaring, mucus (respiratory distress). | Observe for respiratory distress; report malformations. |
| **Mouth** | | |
| Mouth, gums, tongue pink. Tongue normal in size and movement. Lips and palate intact. Sucking pads. Sucking, rooting, swallowing, gag reflexes present.<br>**Normal variations:** Precocious teeth, Epstein's pearls. | Cyanosis (hypoxia). White patches on cheeks or tongue (candidiasis). Protruding tongue (Down syndrome). Diminished movement of tongue, drooping mouth (facial nerve paralysis). Unilateral or bilateral cleft lip or palate, or both. Absent or weak reflexes (preterm, neurologic problem). Excessive drooling (tracheoesophageal fistula, esophageal atresia). | Oxygen for cyanosis. Expect loose teeth to be removed. Obtain order for nystatin medication for candidiasis. Check mother for vaginal or breast infection. Refer anomalies. |
| ***Feeding*** | | |
| Good suck/swallow coordination. Retains feedings. | Poorly coordinated suck and swallow. Duskiness or cyanosis during feeding (cardiac defects). Choking, gagging, excessive drooling (tracheoesophageal fistula, esophageal atresia). | Feed slowly. Stop frequently if difficulty occurs. Suction and stimulate if necessary. Remove stomach contents if infant has distended upper abdomen and may have swallowed blood, amniotic fluid, or meconium. Refer infants with continued difficulty for further investigation. |

**TABLE 20–1 SUMMARY OF NEWBORN ASSESSMENT** *Continued*

| Normal | Abnormal (Possible Causes) | Nursing Considerations |
|---|---|---|
| **Neck/Clavicles** | | |
| Short neck turns head easily side to side. Infant raises head when prone. Clavicles intact. | Weakness, contractures, or rigidity (muscle abnormalities). Webbing of neck or large fat pad at back of neck (chromosomal disorders). Crepitus, lump, or crying when clavicle palpated, with diminished or absent movement of arm on that side (fractured clavicle). | Fracture of clavicle occurs especially in large infants with shoulder dystocia at birth. Immobilize arm. Look for other injuries. Refer abnormalities. |
| **Chest** | | |
| Cylinder shape. Xyphoid process may be prominent. Symmetric. Nipples present and located properly. May have engorgement, white nipple discharge (maternal hormone withdrawal). | Asymmetry (diaphragmatic hernia, pneumothorax). Supernumerary nipples. Redness (infection). | Report abnormalities. |
| **Abdomen** | | |
| Rounded, soft. Bowel sounds present soon after birth. Liver palpable 1–3 cm below costal margin. Skin intact. Three vessels in cord. Clamp tight and cord drying. Meconium passed within 24–48 hr. Urine passed within 24 hr. Normal variation: Brick dust staining of diaper (urate crystals). | Sunken abdomen (diaphragmatic hernia). Distended abdomen or loops of bowel visible (obstruction, infection, enlarged organs). Absent bowel sounds after first hr (paralytic ileus). Masses palpated (kidney tumors, distended bladder). Enlarged liver (infection, heart failure, hemolytic disease). Abdominal wall defects (umbilical or inguinal hernia, omphalocele, gastroschisis, extrophy of bladder). Two vessels in cord (other anomalies). Bleeding (loose clamp). Redness, drainage from cord (infection). No passage of meconium (imperforate anus, obstruction). Lack of urinary output (kidney problems) or inadequate amounts (dehydration). | Refer abnormalities. Look for other anomalies if only two vessels in cord. Tighten or replace loose cord clamp. If stool and urine output abnormal, check to see none was unrecorded, increase feedings, report. |
| **Genitals** | | |
| ***Female*** | | |
| Labia majora dark, cover clitoris and labia minora. Small amount of white mucous vaginal discharge. Urinary meatus and vagina present. **Normal variations:** Vaginal bleeding (pseudomenstruation). Hymenal tags. | Clitoris and labia minora larger than labia majora (preterm). Large clitoris (ambiguous genitalia). Edematous labia (breech birth). | Check gestational age for immature genitalia. Refer anomalies. |

*Table 20–1 continued on following page*

**TABLE 20–1 SUMMARY OF NEWBORN ASSESSMENT** *Continued*

| Normal | Abnormal (Possible Causes) | Nursing Considerations |
|---|---|---|
| **Genitals** *(continued)* | | |
| ***Male*** | | |
| Testes within scrotal sac, rugae on scrotum, prepuce nonretractable. Meatus at tip of penis. | Testes in inguinal canal or abdomen (preterm, cryptorchidism). Lack of rugae on scrotum (preterm). Edema of scrotum (pressure in breech birth). Enlarged scrotal sac (hydrocele). Small penis, scrotum (preterm, ambiguous genitalia). Urinary meatus located on upper side of penis (epispadias), underside of penis (hypospadias), or perineum. | Check gestational age for immature genitalia. Refer anomalies. Explain to parents why no circumcision can be performed with abnormal placement of meatus. |
| **Extremities** | | |
| ***Upper and Lower Extremities*** | | |
| Equal and bilateral movement of extremities. Correct number and formation of fingers and toes. Nails to ends of digits or slightly beyond. Flexion, good muscle tone. | Crepitus, redness, lumps, swelling (fracture). Diminished or lack of movement, especially during Moro reflex (fracture, nerve damage, paralysis). Polydactyly (note presence or absence of bone in extra digits). Syndactyly (webbing) or fused or absent digits. Poor muscle tone (preterm, neurologic damage, hypoglycemia, hypoxia). | Refer all anomalies, look for others. |
| ***Upper Extremities*** | | |
| Two transverse palm creases. | Simian crease (single transverse palm crease) (Down syndrome). Diminished movement of arm with extension and forearm prone (Erb-Duchenne paralysis). | Refer all anomalies, look for others. |
| ***Lower Extremities*** | | |
| Legs equal in length, abduct equally, gluteal and thigh creases and knee height equal, no hip click. Normal position of feet. | Resistance when one leg is abducted, unequal thigh or gluteal creases, hip click, movement of head of femur (Ortolani and Barlow tests), unequal leg length (developmental dysplasia of the hip). Malposition of feet, which may or may not be manually manipulated into normal position (position in utero, talipes equinovarus). | Refer all anomalies, look for others. |
| **Back: Vertebral Column** | | |
| No openings observed or felt. Anus patent. | Failure of vertebra to close (spina bifida), with or without sac with spinal fluid and meninges (meningocele) and/or cord (myelomeningocele) enclosed. Tuft of hair over spina bifida occulta. Pilonidal dimple or sinus. Imperforate anus. | Refer abnormalities. Observe for movement below level of defect. If sac, cover with sterile dressings wet with sterile saline. Protect from injury. |

**TABLE 20–1 SUMMARY OF NEWBORN ASSESSMENT** *Continued*

| Normal | Abnormal (Possible Causes) | Nursing Considerations |
|---|---|---|
| **Reflexes** | | |
| Moro, palmar and plantar grasp, rooting, sucking, swallowing, tonic neck, Babinski, Galant, and stepping reflexes present (see Table 20–2). | Absent, asymmetric, or weak reflexes | Observe for signs of fractures, nerve damage, or injury to CNS. |

CNS, central nervous system; BPM, beats per minute; LGA, large for gestational age; SGA, small for gestational age.

# Early Assessments

## Assessing for Anomalies

Immediately after birth, the infant is examined quickly for respiratory problems and obvious anomalies. The nurse determines whether resuscitation (p. 849) or other immediate intervention is necessary. When the infant is stable and oxygenating well, a more thorough assessment can be performed.

**It is important for the nurse to wear gloves when handling newborns until they are bathed and all blood is removed from their skin and hair. This helps protect the nurse from blood-borne infections.**

If major abnormalities are present at birth, it is important for the nurse to maintain a calm, quiet demeanor to avoid frightening the parents. The physician should be quietly alerted and will explain the condition and possible plan of treatment to the parents.

### HEAD

The newborn's head constitutes one fourth of the body size (Lepley et al., 1993). It is much larger in proportion to the rest of the body than in the adult. The head is palpated to assess the shape and to identify abnormalities. The newborn who was in a breech position or was delivered by cesarean has a round head, whereas the infant born vaginally usually has some molding. The degree of molding, size of the fontanelles, and presence of caput succedaneum or later development of a cephalhematoma are noted.

The hair should be fine with a consistent hair pattern. Abnormal hair growth patterns may indicate genetic abnormalities. The nurse separates the hair, if necessary, to display bruises, rashes, or other marks on the scalp. A small red mark is apparent if a fetal monitor electrode was inserted into the skin of the scalp. Later a small scab forms. Occasionally, this area becomes infected.

**Molding.** Molding refers to changes in the shape of the head that allow it to pass through the birth canal. It is caused by overriding of the cranial bones at the sutures and is common, especially following a long second stage of labor. The condition generally resolves within a few days to a week after birth. Often dramatic improvement is seen by the end of the first day of life. Parents may need reassurance that the infant's head is normal.

All suture lines should be palpated. Widening of the sutures may indicate increased intracranial pressure. If no space is found between suture lines, it may be due to molding and overriding of the bones. However, lack of space between suture lines may indicate premature closure. This condition, called craniosynostosis, may impair brain growth and the shape of the head and requires surgery.

**Fontanelles.** The fontanelles are the areas of the head where sutures between the bones meet. In the newborn, the areas are not calcified but are covered by membrane. This allows space for the brain to grow.

The nurse palpates the fontanelles and notes the position in relation to the other bones of the skull (Fig. 20–1). Each fontanelle should be flat or level with the surrounding bones and should feel soft. Although the anterior fontanelle may bulge slightly when the infant cries, bulging at rest may indicate increased intracranial pressure. A fontanelle that is between flat and bulging is termed "full." A larger-than-normal fontanelle may be a sign of increased pressure within the skull. A depressed fontanelle is unusual in a newborn unless it is due to molding. After molding resolves, a depressed fontanelle is a sign of dehydration. Abnormal signs are reported to the primary care provider.

The anterior fontanelle is a diamond-shaped area where the frontal and parietal bones meet (see Fig. 12–5, p. 276). It measures 4 to 5 cm across and should be measured across the sides instead of be-

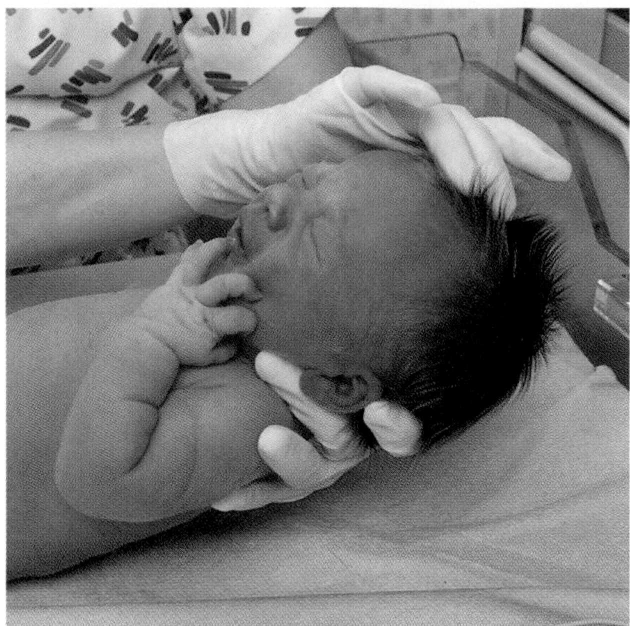

**FIGURE 20–1**

Palpation of the anterior fontanelle. Note elevation of the head.

tween the points. Molding may alter the size and shape of the anterior fontanelle for the first few days. The fontanelle closes between 12 and 18 months of age. When the anterior fontanelle is palpated, the infant's head is elevated for accurate assessment. The infant can be placed in a semisitting position or held in an upright position. The fontanelle should be palpated when the infant is quiet, as vigorous crying may cause it to protrude.

The posterior fontanelle is a triangular area where the occipital and parietal bones meet. It is much smaller than the anterior fontanelle, measuring 0.5 to 1 cm. This fontanelle closes by the time the infant is 2 to 3 months of age.

Molding may make it difficult to identify the fontanelle because the overlapping bones impinge on that space. The posterior fontanelle feels like a dimple at the juncture of the occipital and parietal bones. Careful palpation is necessary.

**Caput Succedaneum.** A caput succedaneum often appears over the vertex of the newborn's head as a result of pressure against the mother's cervix during labor (Fig. 20–2). The pressure interferes with blood flow from the area, causing localized edema at birth. The edematous area crosses suture lines, is soft, and varies in size. It resolves quickly and disappears within 12 hours to several days after birth. Caput may also occur when a vacuum extractor is used to hasten second-stage labor. When a vacuum is used, the caput corresponds to the area where the extractor was placed on the skull. The amount of edema and presence of bruising are assessed.

**Cephalhematoma.** A cephalhematoma occurs when bleeding occurs between the periosteum and the skull as a result of pressure during birth (Fig. 20–3). It occurs on one or both sides of the head over the parietal bones, although occasionally it forms over the occipital bone. The firm swelling is not present at birth but develops within the first 24 to 48 hours.

The area is carefully palpated to determine whether the swelling crosses suture lines. A cephalhematoma has clear edges that end at the suture lines. It does not cross the suture lines like a caput succedaneum because the bleeding is held between the bone and its covering, the periosteum. A cephalhematoma reabsorbs slowly and is generally gone within a few weeks after birth. Because of the breakdown of the red blood cells within the hematoma, affected infants are at greater risk for jaundice.

Both caput succedaneum and cephalhematoma may be frightening to parents. During the assessment the nurse can reassure parents that the conditions are not harmful to the infant. Parents need information, even if they do not ask, about the causes and how long it takes for the areas to resolve.

#### NECK AND CLAVICLES

The nurse assesses the infant's neck visually and by noting the infant's ability to turn the head easily from side to side. The neck is very short. Webbing and an unusually large fat pad between the occiput and the shoulders may indicate a chromosomal anomaly. When lying in a prone position, the newborn should be able to raise and turn the head.

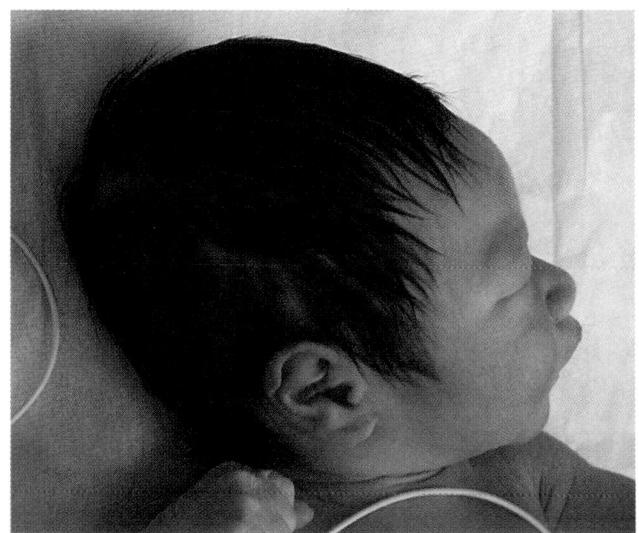

**FIGURE 20–2**

Caput succedaneum is an edematous area on the head from pressure against the cervix. It may cross suture lines.

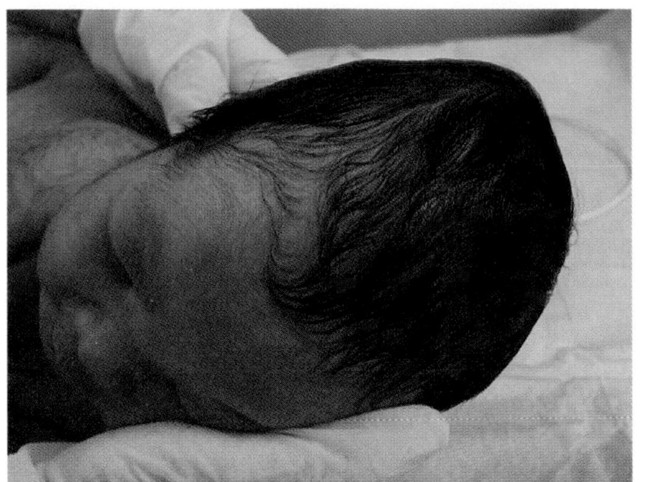

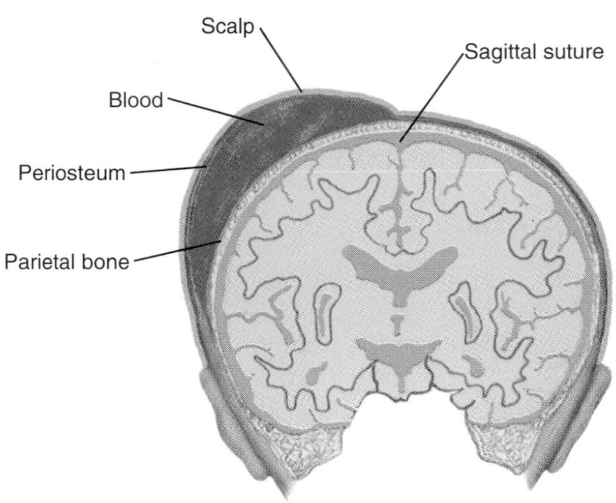


**FIGURE 20-3**

A cephalhematoma is characterized by bleeding between the bone and its covering, the periosteum. It may occur on one or both sides and does not cross suture lines.

Fractures of the clavicle are more likely to occur in large infants, especially when shoulder dystocia occurred. If a fracture is present, a lump or tenderness over the area of the fracture may be observed. Crepitus (grating of the bone) may be felt during palpation. There may also be swelling of the area and decreased movement of the arm on the affected side. A difference in the movement of the arms is especially noticeable when the Moro reflex is elicited. Damage to the brachial plexus may cause paralysis of the arm on the side of the fracture. Treatment of a fractured clavicle includes immobilization of the affected arm (Fig. 20–4).

### CORD

The umbilical cord should contain three vessels. The two arteries are small and may stand up at the cut end. The single vein is larger than the arteries and resembles a slit because its walls are more easily compressed. If only one artery is present, the infant is carefully assessed for other anomalies. A two-vessel cord is associated with chromosomal and

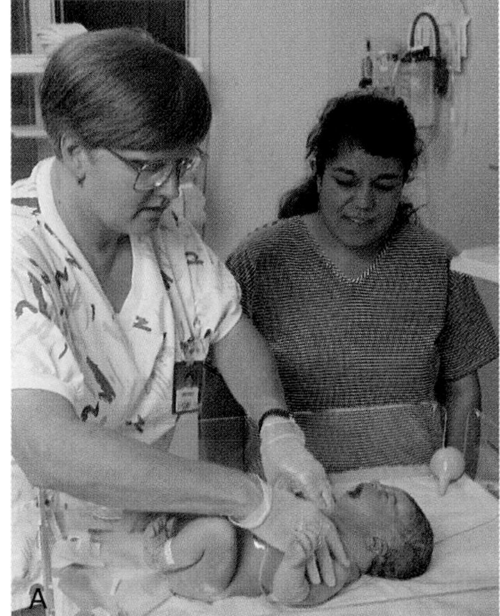


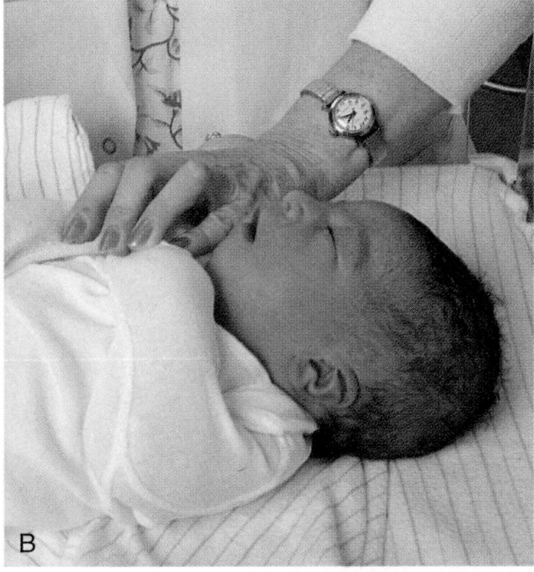


**FIGURE 20-4**

A, The nurse palpates the clavicles to identify fracture. A fracture of the left clavicle is present. B, The arm on the side of the fractured clavicle is immobilized by pinning the sleeve to the shirt.

renal defects. The amount of Wharton's jelly in the cord is noted. If the cord appears thin, the infant may have been poorly nourished in utero. A yellow-brown or green tinge to the cord indicates that meconium was released at some time before birth, perhaps as a result of fetal compromise.

### EXTREMITIES

The normal infant should actively move the extremities equally in a random manner. The extremities of a term infant should remain sharply flexed and resist extension during examination. Poor muscle tone results in a limp or "floppy" infant. This may be due to inadequate oxygen during birth but should resolve within a few minutes as oxygen intake increases. Continued poor muscle tone may be due to prematurity or neurologic damage. Infants with previously good muscle tone may show decreased flexion if they become hypoglycemic or experience respiratory difficulty.

All extremities are examined for signs of fractures such as crepitus, redness, lumps or swelling, and lack of use. It should be determined that each extremity moves independently to identify possible damage to nerves that may occur with or without fractures.

Injury to the brachial nerve plexus may result in Erb's palsy (Erb-Duchenne paralysis), paralysis of the shoulder and arm muscles. Instead of the usual flexed position, the affected arm is extended at the infant's side with the forearm prone. Movement of this arm is diminished during the Moro reflex. The condition is treated by exercise, splinting, or both.

**Hands and Feet.** The fingers and toes are examined for extra digits (polydactyly) or webbing between digits (syndactyly). Extra digits are often small and may not have a bone. Tying the extra digits with sutures causes them to atrophy. Presence of a bone in the extra digit requires surgical removal. Webbed fingers or toes may be corrected by surgery. Nails in a term infant should extend to the end of the fingers or slightly beyond.

Normally, there are two long transverse creases that extend most of the way across the palm. The hands are examined for a simian crease or line. This is a single crease that crosses the palm without a break parallel with the base of the fingers. It may be seen with an incurving of the little finger in Down syndrome. The simian line alone is not diagnostic of Down syndrome, however, and may occur in normal infants.

The feet are assessed for talipes equinovarus, or clubfoot, a common malformation of the feet. If a foot looks abnormal, it should be gently manipulated. If it moves to a normal position, the abnormality is probably temporary, resulting from the position of the infant in the uterus. In true clubfoot, the foot turns inward and cannot be moved to a midline position. Casting is the usual treatment, but sometimes surgery is necessary.

**Hips.** The hips are examined for developmental dysplasia of the hip. This is an incomplete development of the acetabulum, which may allow the head of the femur to slip out of the acetabulum and become dislocated.

Ortolani and Barlow tests are methods of assessing for hip instability in the newborn period. They are described in Figure 20–5. Both legs should abduct equally when the test is performed. It may be more difficult to abduct the affected hip. A hip click may

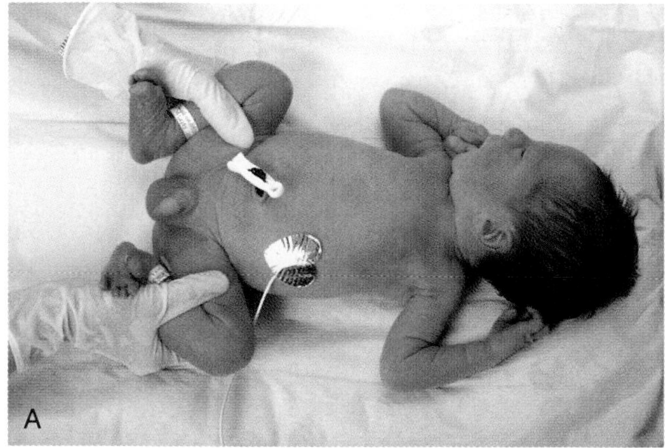


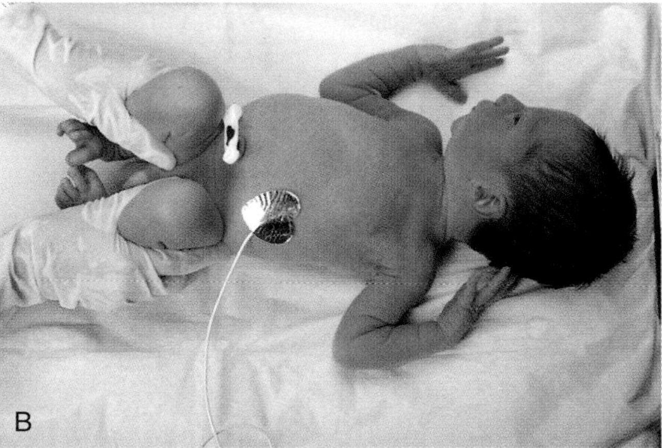


**FIGURE 20–5**

Assessment of the hips. Place the fingers over the infant's greater trochanter and thumbs over the femur. Bend the knees and hips at a 90-degree angle. A, Ortolani test: Abduct the thighs, and apply gentle pressure forward over the greater trochanter. A "clunking" sensation indicates a dislocated femoral head moving into the acetabulum. A hip click may be felt or heard but is usually normal. B, Barlow test: Adduct the hips and apply gentle pressure down and back with the thumbs. In hip dysplasia, the examiner can feel the femoral head move out of the acetabulum.

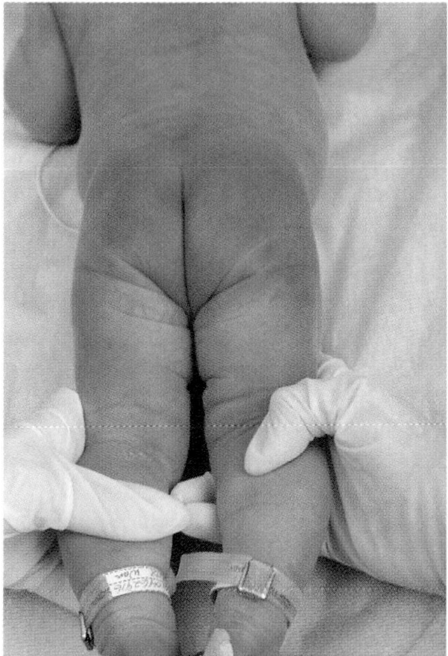

**FIGURE 20-6**

Note the symmetry of gluteal and thigh creases.

be felt or heard but is usually normal and is different from the "clunk" of hip dysplasia (Behrman et al., 1996).

The legs are extended to determine if they are equal in length and if thigh and gluteal creases are symmetric (Fig. 20–6). If the hip is dislocated, the leg on the affected side is shorter and the creases are asymmetric. The infant's knees should be bent with the feet flat on the bed to compare their height. If the hip is dislocated, the knee on the affected side is lower. Because the hip may be unstable but not yet dislocated, these signs are not always present at birth.

Treatment of developmental dysplasia of the hip involves immobilizing the leg in a flexed, abducted position, usually with a harness. Sometimes the use of double or triple diapers is sufficient. Early identification and treatment provide the best results in correcting the problem.

#### VERTEBRAL COLUMN

The nurse palpates the entire length of the newborn's vertebral column to discover any defects in the vertebrae. An indentation is a sign of spina bifida occulta, failure of a vertebra to close. The defect is not obvious on visual inspection because it is covered with skin, but sometimes a tuft of hair grows over the area. Other, more obvious neural tube defects include a meningocele or myelomeningocele. These are protrusions of nerves or the spinal cord, or both, through the defect in the vertebrae. They appear as a sac on the back and may be covered by skin or only the meninges. The tissue should be covered with moist, sterile saline dressings immediately after birth (p. 872).

A pilonidal dimple may be present at the base of the spine. It should be examined for a sinus and the depth noted.

## Measurements

Measurements provide information about the infant's growth in utero. The weight, length, and head and chest circumference are part of the initial assessment (Procedure 20–1). The measurements are compared with the norms for the infant's gestational age. When a difference is noted between what is expected and what is found, expanded assessments are necessary. For example, a newborn may be larger or smaller than expected because there was an error in calculating the length of the pregnancy.

#### WEIGHT

The newborn's weight ranges between 2500 and 4000 g (5 pounds, 8 ounces and 8 pounds, 13 ounces) (Glenn, 1993). The average weight of a full-term newborn is 3400 g (7.5 pounds). If the infant's weight is outside the average range, possible causes are assessed. Factors affecting weight include gestational age, placental functioning, maternal diabetes, and genetic factors such as race and parental size.

Infants are weighed each day they are in the birth facility and at follow-up visits. They can be expected to lose 5 to 10 percent of their birth weight during the first few days of life (Bell & Oh, 1994). This weight loss is due to excretion of meconium from the bowel and normal loss of extracellular fluid. Newborns generally do not take in enough calories to maintain their weight during this period, and this also contributes to early weight loss. Infants normally regain birth weight by the 10th day of life. Thereafter, they gain about 680 g (1.5 pounds) a month for the first 5 months (Wong, 1995).

#### LENGTH

The infant's length is measured from the top of the head to the end of the outstretched leg. The average length of a full-term newborn is 48 to 53 cm (19 to 21 inches) (Glenn, 1993). Some agencies record the crown-to-rump measurement as well, which is approximately equal to the head circumference.

#### HEAD AND CHEST CIRCUMFERENCE

The diameter of the head is measured around the occiput and just above the eyebrows. The average

Procedure 20–1

# Weighing and Measuring the Newborn

**PURPOSE:** To obtain accurate measurements of the newborn.

## WEIGHT

1. **Cover the scale with a blanket. Place a paper cover over the blanket if desired.** *Prevents conductive heat loss from contact between the infant and a cold surface, helps prevent cross-contamination, and makes cleaning easier.*

2. **Balance or adjust the scale to zero after the covering is placed. Electronic scale: push the "on" button and check to see that the digital readout is at zero. The electronic scale is usually self-adjusting. Balance scale: Adjust until the balance arm is horizontal.** *Results in accurate weighing of the infant without including weight of the scale covering.*

3. **Place the infant in supine position on the scale. Keep one hand just above the infant and watch the infant carefully throughout the procedure.** *Infants often are upset when first placed on the scale, and the startle or Moro reflex may occur. There is a danger that they might slide off the scale.*

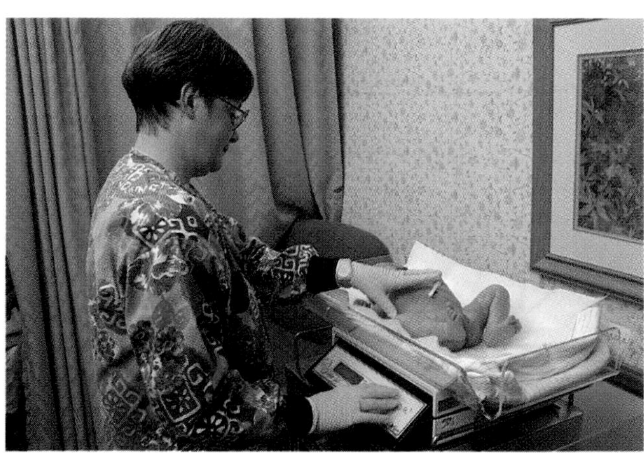

4. **Wait until the infant is somewhat quiet. The electronic scale displays weight in pounds and ounces or in grams. Some electronic scales display "stable" when an accurate weight has been obtained. For a balance scale, move weights slowly until the arm is level.** *Waiting until the infant is quiet increases accuracy.*

5. **Write the numbers down immediately. If the scale is covered with paper, the weight can be written on the paper and taken with the infant to the warmer. Write it on the nurses' notes when the infant is safely settled.** *Prevents forgetting the weight.*

6. **Compare weight with the normal range for term infants: 2500 to 4000 g (5 pounds, 8 ounces to 8 pounds, 13 ounces).** *Shows whether or not the infant is within expected range.*

## LENGTH

*Ruler Printed on Scale or Crib*

1. **Place the infant in supine position with his or her head at the upper edge of the ruler on the scale.** *Places the infant in the proper position.*

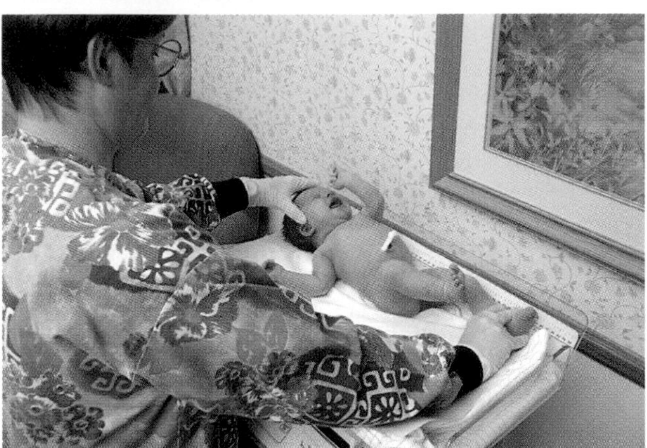

2. **While holding the infant with one hand so that the head does not move, use the other hand to extend the infant's leg along the ruler. Note the length at the bottom of the heel.** *Holding the infant firmly ensures safety and allows an accurate measurement.*

*Tape Measure*

1. **When using a paper tape, be sure that it has no partial tears in it.** *A torn measuring tape would give an inaccurate measurement.*

2. **Place tape beside the infant, with the upper end at the top of the head. Tuck it beneath the shoulder, and extend it down to the feet.** *Prevents movement of the tape and helps ensure accurate measurements.*

3. **Hold the tape straight alongside the infant's body while extending one leg full length. Be sure tape has not moved from the top of the head.** *Careful attention to tape placement ensures accurate measurement.*

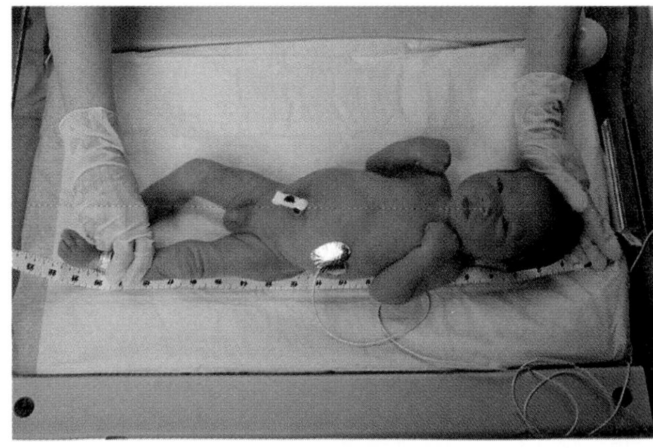

4. **Another method is to mark the paper on which the infant is lying at the top of the head and the end of the extended leg. Then measure the distance between the two marks.** *Makes it easier to measure accurately when the infant is very active.*

## Procedure 20–1 *Continued*

# Weighing and Measuring the Newborn

**PURPOSE:** To obtain accurate measurements of the newborn.

5. **Compare with normal range of 48 to 53 cm (19 to 21 inches).** *Helps determine abnormalities.*

**HEAD AND CHEST CIRCUMFERENCE**

1. **Measure around the fullest part of the head with the tape placed around the occiput and just over the eyebrows.** *Allows measurement of the largest diameter of the head.*

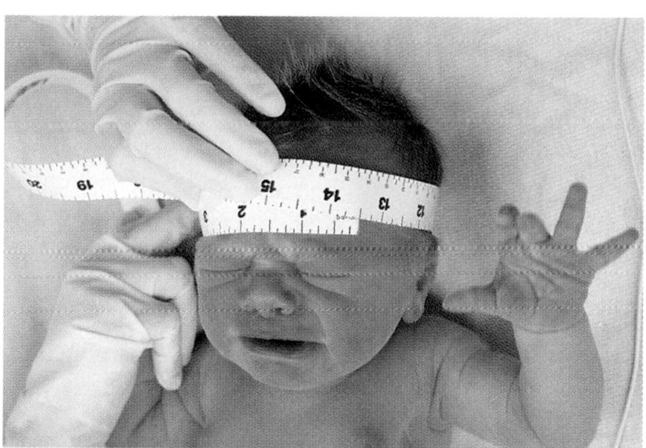

2. **Move tape down to measure the chest at the level of the nipples. Be sure that tape is even and taut.** *Ensures accurate measurement.*

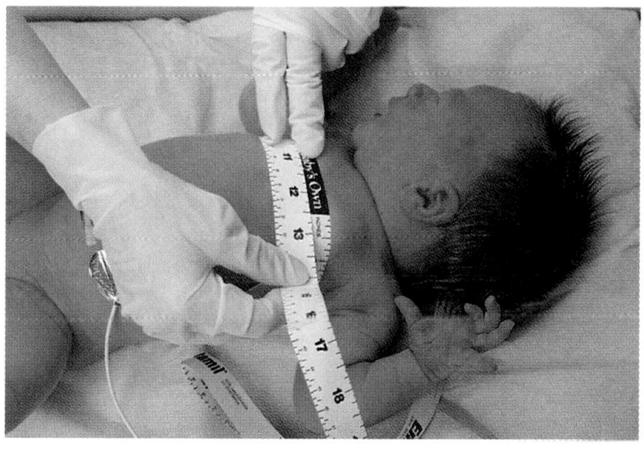

3. **Remove tape by lifting or rolling the infant instead of pulling the tape.** *Pulling tape can cut the infant's skin.*
4. **Compare measurements with normal range. Head: 33 to 35.5 cm (13 to 14 inches). Chest: 30.5 to 33 cm (12 to 13 inches).** *Determines whether the infant's measurements are normal.*

head circumference of the term newborn is 33 to 35.5 cm (13 to 14 inches) (Glenn, 1993). The measurement may be affected by molding of the skull during the birth process. If a large amount of molding occurred, the head is remeasured when it regains its normal shape. An abnormally small head may indicate poor brain growth and microcephaly. A very large head may be a sign of hydrocephalus.

The chest is measured at the level of the nipples. It is usually 2 to 3 cm smaller than the head. The average circumference of the chest is 30.5 to 33 cm (12 to 13 inches) (Glenn, 1993). If molding of the head is present, the head and chest measurement may be equal at birth.

**CHECK YOUR READING**

1. What is the difference between molding, caput succedaneum, and cephalhematoma?
2. What is the purpose of the quick initial assessment of the infant after birth?
3. Why are measurements of the neonate important?

## Assessment of Cardiorespiratory Status

Assessments of respiratory and cardiovascular status are performed together because transitional changes take place in both systems at birth. Problems of adaptation in one system most likely result in problems in the other system as well.

### History

Information about the pregnancy, labor, and delivery is important in assessing the infant's cardiovascular and respiratory status and the likelihood of problems at birth. For example, if the mother received narcotic analgesics late in labor, depression of the fetal central nervous system may interfere with initiation of respirations in the neonate. Although a certain amount of hypoxia enhances the stimulation of respirations, severe asphyxia throughout labor or delivery results in respiratory depression at birth. Infants who are preterm may not produce adequate

## Critical to Remember

### NORMAL VITAL SIGNS IN THE NEWBORN

- Temperature: 36.5–37.5°C (97.7–99.5°F) axillary, 36.5–37.6°C (97.7–99.7°F) rectal
- Apical pulse: 120–160/BPM (100 sleeping, 180 crying)
- Respirations: 30–60 breaths/minute (average 30–40/minute)

amounts of surfactant, and atelectasis occurs because the alveoli do not remain open.

## Airway

During birth, some fetal lung fluid is forced into the upper airway. Excessive fluid or mucus in the infant's respiratory passages may cause respiratory difficulty for several hours after birth.

### RESPIRATORY RATE

The nurse assesses respirations at least once every 30 minutes until the infant has been stable for 2 hours after birth (AAP, 1992). If abnormalities are noted, respirations are assessed more often. The normal respiratory rate is 30 to 60 breaths per minute, with an average rate of 30 to 40. The infant may breathe faster immediately after birth, during crying, and during the first and second periods of reactivity. Respirations should not be labored, and the chest movements should be symmetric. Because the pattern and depth of respirations are irregular, they must be counted for a full minute for accuracy.

Counting the rapid, shallow, irregular respirations of a newborn can be difficult at first. Some nurses count while observing the infant's chest. It may be hard to differentiate the respirations from other movement if the newborn is very active. Observation, palpation, or auscultation, alone or in combination, may be used to obtain an accurate respiratory rate (Procedure 20–2).

Observe for periodic breathing, pauses in breathing lasting up to 10 seconds without other changes. This occurs is some full-term infants during the first few days but most often in preterm infants. Apnea lasting longer than 20 seconds, or accompanied by cyanosis, heart rate changes, or other signs of difficult breathing, is abnormal (Hagedorn et al., 1993).

### BREATH SOUNDS

The entire anterior and posterior lung fields are auscultated for breath sounds, which should be present equally throughout. Breath sounds should be clear over most areas. However, it is not unusual to hear sounds of moisture in the lungs during the first hour or two after birth because fetal lung fluid has not been completely absorbed. Infants born by cesarean birth do not receive pressure on the chest that removes a small amount of lung fluid. Therefore, coarse breath sounds are more likely to occur in infants after cesarean birth.

When the listener is not experienced in assessing the lungs of a newborn, distinguishing between clear breath sounds and coarse or moist sounds is less difficult than trying to describe crackles or wheezes. Abnormal or diminished sounds should always be reported to the primary care provider if they continue. They may indicate a pneumothorax. Bowel sounds in the chest may indicate a diaphragmatic hernia.

### CHOANAL ATRESIA

Assessment for choanal atresia is important because newborns are obligate nose breathers for approximately the first 3 weeks of life. This means that they breathe mostly through the nose, except when crying. If the nose becomes obstructed, the infant has difficulty getting enough oxygen. In choanal atresia, one or both nasal passages are blocked by an abnormality of the septum.

The nurse can assess for choanal atresia by closing the infant's mouth and occluding one nostril at a time. The infant is observed for breathing, and breath sounds are auscultated while each nostril is occluded. Another method of assessment for choanal atresia is to pass a catheter (No. 5 to 8 French in size) through each nostril to check for patency. Infants with choanal atresia may become cyanotic when quiet but pink when crying, as air is then drawn in through the mouth.

Bilateral choanal atresia causes severe respiratory distress and requires surgery. Blockage of one side puts the infant at risk for respiratory distress if the other side becomes occluded by mucus or edema.

### SIGNS OF RESPIRATORY DISTRESS

Throughout the assessment, the nurse must be alert for signs of respiratory distress, which may be present at birth or develop later. They include tachypnea, retractions, flaring nares, central cyanosis, grunting, moaning, and seesaw respirations. Whenever one sign of labored breathing is present, the assessment must be carefully expanded to identify others.

**Tachypnea.** Tachypnea is the most common sign of respiratory distress. Tachypnea, a respiratory rate above 60 breaths per minute, is not unusual during the first hour after birth and during the second period of reactivity. However, continued tachypnea is abnormal.

Procedure 20–2

# Assessing Vital Signs in the Newborn

**PURPOSE:** To obtain an accurate measurement of newborn vital signs.

## RESPIRATIONS

1. **Assess respirations when the infant is quiet or sleeping if possible. Count the respirations (and apical pulse) before disturbing the infant for other assessments.** *Allows the lung sounds to be heard more clearly.*

2. **Assess respirations by observing, palpating, and/or auscultating the chest and abdomen.** *Counting the rapid, shallow, irregular respirations of a newborn can be difficult at first. It is sometimes difficult to differentiate rapid, shallow, irregular respirations from other movements in an active newborn. A combination of methods increases accuracy of the assessment.*

3. **To observe respirations, lift the infant's blanket and shirt to visualize the chest and abdomen. Observe the pattern of respirations before beginning to count.** *Respirations are often irregular, but there is a basic pattern. Observation of the pattern makes it easier to count the rate.*

4. **If desired, place a hand lightly over the infant's chest or abdomen to feel the movement.** *Palpation helps keep track of the rate.*

5. **To auscultate respirations, place a stethoscope on the right side of the infant's chest.** *Allows the sounds of the lungs to be heard with less interference from heart sounds. The assessment of breath sounds on both sides of the chest can be performed as soon as respirations are counted.*

6. **Count for a full minute.** *Respirations are normally irregular in the newborn. Counting for a full minute increases accuracy.*

7. **If the infant is crying, continue to count. Allow the infant to suck on a pacifier or gloved finger.** *Sucking may quiet the infant. Although it is easiest to assess respirations on a quiet infant, they can be counted when the infant is crying. (Remember, the infant breathes while crying!) The rate may be faster than when the infant is quiet and should be charted as crying.*

8. **Observe the infant for signs of respiratory distress, including tachypnea, retractions, flaring, cyanosis, grunting, seesawing, apneic periods, and asymmetry of chest movements. Expect the respiratory rate to be 30 to 60 breaths/minute when the infant is at rest.** *Allows identification and follow-up of abnormalities.*

## PULSE

1. **Listen to the apical pulse on a quiet or sleeping infant if possible. Begin with this assessment before disturbing the infant for other assessments and care.** *Allows the nurse to hear heart sounds more clearly.*

2. **Use a pediatric head on the stethoscope to listen to apical pulse.** *Although the larger head may be used if necessary, the small head allows better contact between the stethoscope and the chest wall and eliminates some of the sounds from the lungs and intestines.*

3. **If the infant is crying, insert a pacifier or a gloved finger into his or her mouth.** *Sucking often quiets infants.*

4. **If the infant cannot be quieted, increase concentration and time spent listening.** *Helps to separate the sounds heard and to focus in on the heart beat.*

5. **Listen briefly before beginning to count. Tapping a finger in rhythm with the beat may be helpful. Expect the heart rate to be 120 to 160 BPM at rest.** *Listening to the pattern of the rapid heart beat allows time to get used to it before counting.*

6. **Move stethoscope over the entire heart area to listen to all sounds. Assess for arrhythmias, murmurs, or other abnormal sounds. Refer any abnormal sounds for follow-up.** *Listening over the entire area increases chances of hearing abnormal sounds. Reporting abnormalities to the pediatrician allows further investigation.*

## TEMPERATURE

*Axillary*

1. **Place the thermometer vertically along the chest wall in the center of the axillary space with the infant's arm firmly over it.** *If the thermometer is held horizontally, it may protrude behind the axilla and give an inaccurate reading. Holding the arm keeps the thermometer positioned correctly and prevents accidental injury if the infant moves unexpectedly.*

2. **Read thermometer at the proper time: glass, 5 minutes; plastic strip, 1 to 1.5 minutes (with a 10-second wait before reading); electronic, when indicator sounds. Normal range: 36.5 to 37.5°C (97.7 to 99.5°F).** *Ensures an accurate reading.*

*Rectal*

1. **Take a rectal temperature when birth facility policy states that this method is to be used for the first temperature or to confirm abnormal axillary measurements. Use the axillary method whenever possible.** *Rectal and axillary readings are very similar. Rectal temperature involves the potential risk of perforation of the rectum, which can be life-threatening.*

2. **Lubricate the tip of the thermometer with water-soluble lubricant.** *Allows the thermometer to be inserted without irritation to sphincter. Water-soluble lubricant dissolves and washes away.*

3. **Place the infant in a supine position and hold the ankles firmly in one hand. Bend the infant's knees against the abdomen and raise the legs to expose the anus. Or place the infant prone or on the side and separate the buttocks.** *Provides visualization and prevents excessive movement that might dislodge the thermometer or cause it to break (if glass), resulting in injury to delicate tissues.*

4. **Insert the thermometer carefully and gently no more than 0.5 inch into the rectum.** *The rectum turns to the right 1 inch from the sphincter. Inserting the thermometer farther may cause perforation.*

*Procedure continued on following page*

Procedure 20–2 *Continued*

## Assessing Vital Signs in the Newborn

**PURPOSE:** To obtain an accurate measurement of newborn vital signs.

5. **Do *not* force the thermometer if it does not insert easily.** *An obstruction may be preventing insertion of the thermometer.*

6. **Hold the thermometer securely throughout the time it remains in the rectum.** *Maintains control over the thermometer to avoid inserting it too far and prevents injury if the infant moves.*

7. **Read thermometer at the proper time: glass, 5 minutes; electronic, when indicator sounds. Normal range: 36.5 to 37.6°C (97.7 to 99.7°F).** *Ensures accurate reading.*

**Retractions.** When the infant's weak chest wall muscles are used to help draw air into the lungs, retractions result. The soft tissue around the bones of the chest is drawn in with the effort of pulling air into the lungs. Substernal or xyphoid retractions occur when the area under the sternum retracts each time the infant inhales. When the muscles between the ribs are pulled in so that each rib is outlined, intercostal retractions are present. The muscles above the sternum and around the clavicles may also be used to aid in respirations (supraclavicular retractions). Retractions may be mild or severe, depending on the degree of respiratory difficulty. Occasional mild retractions are common immediately after birth but should not continue after the first hour.

**Flaring of the Nares.** A reflex widening of the nostrils occurs when the infant is receiving insufficient oxygen. This helps to decrease airway resistance and increase the amount of air entering the lungs. Intermittent flaring may occur in the first hour after birth. Continued flaring indicates a more serious respiratory problem.

**Cyanosis.** Cyanosis is a purplish blue discoloration that indicates that the infant is not getting enough oxygen. It may be preceded by a dusky or gray hue to the skin. Central cyanosis involves the lips, tongue, and trunk and indicates true hypoxia. It indicates that not enough oxygen is reaching the vital organs and requires immediate attention. Central cyanosis must be differentiated from peripheral cyanosis, or acrocyanosis, which involves just the extremities. Acrocyanosis is normal in the first few hours after birth or if the infant becomes cold. It is due to poor perfusion of blood to the periphery of the body (Fig. 20–7).

Cyanosis may be present at birth or may become apparent later. It is not unusual to see a purplish blue discoloration at birth that quickly turns pink as the infant begins to breathe. Cyanosis occurs whenever the infant's breathing is impaired. It may occur during feedings because of difficulty in coordinating sucking and swallowing with breathing. Infants who become cyanotic on exertion or crying may have a congenital heart defect.

**Grunting.** Grunting describes a noise made on expiration when pressure is increased within the alveoli to help keep them open. Grunting may be very mild and heard only with a stethoscope, or it may be loud enough to hear unaided in an infant having severe respiratory difficulty. Grunting is a common sign of respiratory distress syndrome and necessitates expanded assessment and referral for treatment.

**Seesaw Respirations.** Normally, the chest and abdomen rise and fall together during respiration. When the infant is having severe respiratory difficulty, the chest falls when the abdomen rises and the chest rises when the abdomen falls, causing a seesaw effect. This is a sign of severe respiratory difficulty.

**Asymmetry.** Chest expansion should be equal on both sides. Asymmetry or decreased movement on one side may indicate the collapse of a lung (pneumothorax).

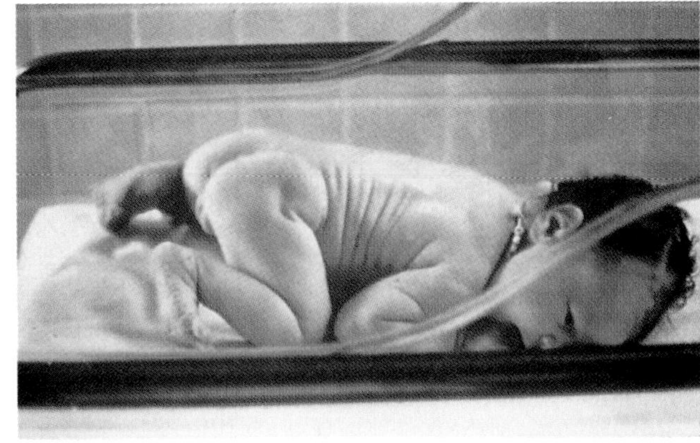

**FIGURE 20–7**

Acrocyanosis. (Courtesy of Jane Deacon, M.S., R.N., N.N.P., The Children's Hospital, Denver, Colorado.)

### Color

In addition to cyanosis, assess for pallor and ruddiness.

**Pallor.** Some infants have a pale skin color. Pallor can indicate that the infant is slightly hypoxic or anemic. A laboratory examination of hemoglobin and hematocrit or a complete blood count may be ordered by the physician.

**Ruddy Color.** In contrast to pallor, a ruddy color occurs in some infants. This reddish color of the skin may indicate polycythemia, an excessive number of red blood cells. A hematocrit determination confirms polycythemia. Infants with elevated hematocrits are at increased risk for jaundice from the normal destruction of excessive red blood cells that occurs after birth. Jaundice may occur in infants with hematocrits above 65 percent.

### Heart Sounds

The heart is auscultated for rate, rhythm, and the presence of murmurs or abnormal sounds. The nurse should count the apical pulse for a full minute for accuracy and listen for abnormalities. The rate should range between 120 and 160 beats per minute (BPM) with normal activity. It may elevate to 180 BPM when infants are crying or drop as low as 100 BPM when they are in a deep sleep.

If there are no problems at birth, the heart rate should be recorded at least once every 30 minutes until the infant has been stable for 2 hours after birth (AAP, 1992). Monitoring is more frequent if there are abnormalities. Once stable, the heart rate is checked once every 8 hours unless a reason exists to assess it more frequently.

**Position.** An experienced examiner can determine the position of the heart in the chest by the location of the heart sounds and the point of maximum impulse. The apex of the heart is located at the point of maximum impulse, where the pulse is most easily felt and the sound is loudest. This is at the third or fourth intercostal space, slightly left of the midclavicular line (a line drawn from the middle of the left clavicle). It may be slightly lower in some newborns and at the fifth intercostal space (Vargo, 1993). Conditions that affect the position of the heart include pneumothorax and dextrocardia (in which the heart position is reversed from normal).

**Rhythm and Murmurs.** The rhythm of the heart should be regular, and the first and second sounds (the lub and dub) should be heard clearly. Abnormalities in rhythm or sounds such as murmurs should be noted. Murmurs are sounds of abnormal blood flow through the heart and may indicate openings in the septum of the heart or problems with blood flow through the valves. Most murmurs in the newborn are temporary and are due to incomplete transition from fetal to neonatal circulation. A murmur is not uncommon until the ductus arteriosus is functionally closed. Although it may be a "normal" or functional murmur, any abnormal sounds of the heart are investigated further because they may be signs of cardiac defects.

### Brachial and Femoral Pulses

The brachial and femoral pulses should be present and equal bilaterally. The brachial pulse is located over the antecubital space, and the femoral pulse is located at the groin. Differences between the brachial and femoral pulses may be due to impaired blood flow in coarctation of the aorta, a congenital heart defect. In this condition, a narrowed area of the aorta impedes blood flow to the lower part of the body and causes pulses in the lower extremities to be weaker.

### Blood Pressure

Measurement of blood pressure is not a necessary part of a routine assessment of the newborn according to the American Academy of Pediatrics (1993). However, the blood pressure is taken on all extremities if the infant shows signs such as unequal pulses or murmurs. Doppler ultrasonography or other electronic measurement (such as Dynamap) makes it easier to obtain an accurate blood pressure. To ensure accurate measurement, the infant should be quiet when the blood pressure is taken, as crying elevates the blood pressure. The width of the blood pressure cuff should be 20 percent greater than the diameter of the extremity and the bladder of the cuff should cover two thirds of the upper arm or thigh (Smith et al., 1996).

The average blood pressure for full-term newborns is 70 mmHg systolic and 45 mmHg diastolic, although there is some variation according to the infant's weight (Anand, 1991). Hypotension may occur in the sick infant. The blood pressure of the lower extremities should be the same as or slightly higher than that of the upper extremities. If there is a difference of as much as 20 mmHg, coarctation of the aorta may be present.

## Assessment of Thermoregulation

Early identification of problems of thermoregulation is an essential nursing role in care of the newborn.

The neonate's temperature is taken soon after birth while the infant is being held by the mother or

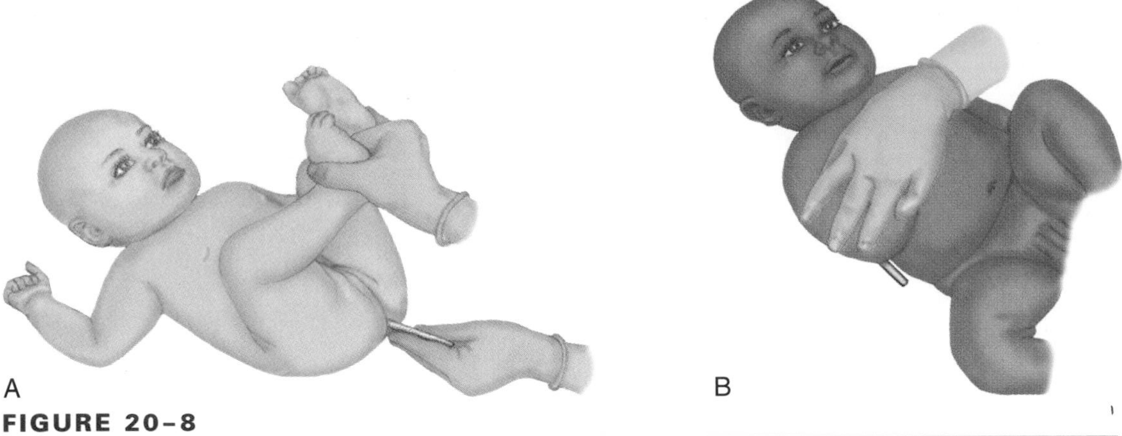


**FIGURE 20–8**

A rectal (A) or axillary (B) temperature may be taken. The infant is held securely to prevent injury and obtain an accurate reading.

is in a radiant warmer with a skin probe attached to the abdomen. The probe allows the warmer to measure and display the infant's temperature continuously. The temperature control is set to regulate the amount of heat produced according to the infant's skin temperature. The temperature should be assessed at least once every 30 minutes until the infant has been stable for 2 hours after birth (AAP, 1992). It is often checked again at 4 hours and then once every 8 hours as long as it remains stable.

In some agencies, the first temperature is taken rectally (Fig. 20–8 and Procedure 20–2). This provides information about the neonate's core temperature as well as patency of the anus. The nurse should insert the thermometer no more than 0.5 inch into the anus when taking a rectal temperature. The colon turns at a sharp right angle approximately 1 inch from the anal sphincter. Inserting the thermometer farther might result in potentially fatal perforation of the intestinal wall. A thermometer should never be forced into the rectum because there could be an imperforate (closed) anus. The normal range of rectal temperature is 36.5 to 37.6°C (97.7 to 99.7°F) (Wong, 1995).

Taking axillary temperatures is safer than taking rectal temperatures because it avoids the possibility of damaging the rectum. Axillary temperatures provide a reading very close to rectal measurements. The normal range for axillary temperature is 36.5 to 37.5°C (97.7 to 99.5°F) (Blake & Murray, 1993).

Temperatures can be measured with an electronic or glass thermometer or a disposable plastic strip. Disposable plastic strips change color to indicate temperature change. Tympanic thermometers are generally not used because they are less accurate in newborns.

## Assessment of Hepatic Function

The major early assessments of the hepatic system are related to blood glucose and bilirubin conjugation.

### Blood Glucose

The nurse must be alert for newborns at increased risk for hypoglycemia, which can cause brain damage. Factors that might have caused the infant to deplete available glucose are noted. A quick estimate to determine whether the newborn appears to be near term and of appropriate size for gestational age is performed at birth.

Observing for signs of hypoglycemia is necessary throughout routine assessment and care. Early signs include jitteriness, poor muscle tone, and sweating. Other signs include respiratory difficulty, such as tachypnea, dyspnea, apnea, and cyanosis. A de-

**Critical to Remember**

**RISK FACTORS FOR HYPOGLYCEMIA**

- Prematurity
- Postmaturity
- Intrauterine growth restriction
- Asphyxia
- Cold stress
- Large for gestational age
- Small for gestational age
- Maternal diabetes
- Maternal intake of ritodrine or terbutaline

## Critical to Remember

### SIGNS OF HYPOGLYCEMIA

- Jitteriness
- Poor muscle tone
- Sweating
- Tachypnea
- Dyspnea
- Apnea
- Cyanosis
- Low temperature
- Poor suck
- High-pitched cry
- Lethargy
- Seizures, coma
- Some infants may be asymptomatic.

crease in temperature may result when not enough glucose is available to maintain a metabolic rate sufficient to maintain body temperature. The infant may suck poorly. Central nervous system signs of lack of glucose include high-pitched cry, lethargy, seizures, and eventually coma. Some infants with hypoglycemia show no signs at all.

In some facilities, all infants are screened for hypoglycemia shortly after birth. However, the American Academy of Pediatrics states that screening for the blood glucose level is necessary only for infants in risk categories or those showing early signs of hypoglycemia (AAP, 1993). Normal blood glucose during the first day of life is 40 to 60 mg/dl (Nicholson & Pesce, 1996). Because capillary blood is used in screening tests, these tests are less accurate than laboratory tests using venous blood. Therefore, a laboratory analysis (per agency policy) should be used to verify readings below 45 mg/dl on glucometers or glucose strips.

It is important to avoid injuring the infant's foot when taking blood from the heel. If the lancet goes into the calcaneus bone, osteomyelitis may result. The site chosen must avoid the major nerves and arteries in the area (Procedure 20–3).

### Bilirubin

The nurse assesses for jaundice and watches for its development, particularly in infants at risk. Pressing the infant's skin over a firm surface, such as the end of the nose or the sternum, helps identify jaundice. The skin blanches as the blood is pressed out of the tissues, making it easier to see the yellow color that remains. Because jaundice begins at the head and moves down the body, one can make a rough estimate of the severity of the problem. Jaundice of the face and neck occurs at levels up to 8 mg/dl and of the upper trunk up to 12 mg/dl (Philip, 1996).

In physiologic jaundice, the bilirubin level peaks at 5 to 6 mg/dl between the second and fourth days of life and then begins to drop. Jaundice becomes visible when the bilirubin level reaches 5 to 7 mg/dl. Therefore, jaundice that appears before the second day of life may indicate that the bilirubin is rising more quickly and to higher levels than normal and may not be physiologic. The physician or nurse practitioner may order laboratory determinations of the bilirubin level based on the nurse's assessment. If serial bilirubin assays are ordered, the nurse notes changes from one reading to the next and correlates the results with the infant's age.

## Procedure 20–3

## Assessing Blood Glucose in the Newborn

**PURPOSE:** To accurately measure the infant's blood glucose by heel puncture using the Accu-Chek or One Touch glucometer or Dextrostix or Chemstrip reagent strips.

1. **Wash hands.** *Helps prevent spread of infection.*
2. **Gather supplies needed: gloves, alcohol wipe, 2 × 2 inch gauze, lancet, adhesive bandage, diaper or commercial warming pack to warm heel, glucometer and/or glucose screening reagent strips. Chemstrip and Accu-Chek: add cotton ball. One Touch: add pipette.** *Having all supplies ready allows efficient performance of procedure.*
3. **Calibrate or program glucometer according to manufacturer's guidelines.** *Ensures proper functioning of machine.*
4. **If the infant's mother has a blood-borne disease such as hepatitis B or human immunodeficiency virus, bathe the infant before puncturing the skin.** *Avoids contamination of the puncture site with maternal blood on the infant's skin.*
5. **Warm the infant's foot for a few minutes if it is cold or if blood is needed for several tests. Dampen a disposable diaper with warm water and fasten it over the heel, or use a heel warming pack according to directions.** *Warming causes vasodilation and allows blood to flow more easily. This avoids having to make more than one puncture because of insufficient blood flow.*
6. **Apply gloves.** *Prevents contamination of hands with blood and is part of standard precautions.*
7. **Hold heel in one hand and locate site. Feel the**

*Procedure continued on following page*

Procedure 20–3 *Continued*

## Assessing Blood Glucose in the Newborn

**PURPOSE:** To accurately measure the infant's blood glucose by heel puncture using the Accu-Chek or One Touch glucometer or Dextrostix or Chemstrip reagent strips.

**bone of the heel. Place the thumb or finger over the walking surface to shield this area. Choose site for puncture.** *Stabilizes heel to prevent movement and inadvertent injury from lancet. Locating the bone helps avoid puncturing the calcaneus bone, which could result in infection. Covering the walking surface avoids damage to nerves and arteries of this area.*

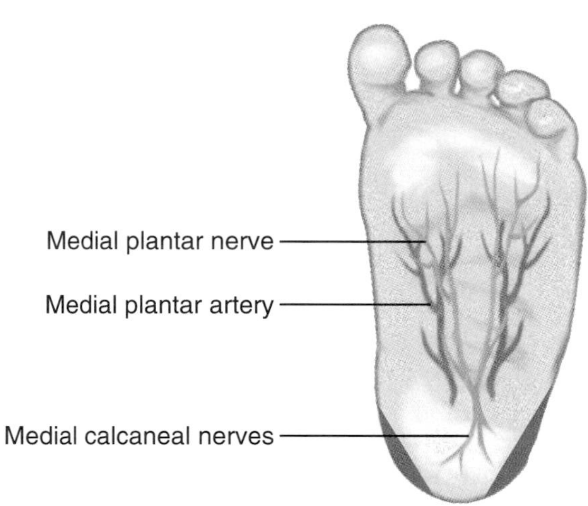


8. **Clean lateral heel with alcohol. Wipe dry with sterile gauze.** *Alcohol removes contaminants. Drying prevents diluting specimen with alcohol and increases accuracy of results.*

9. **Puncture side of heel with lancet. Place lancet in sharps container immediately. If container cannot be placed at bedside, place lancet in a safe place until the test is completed; then dispose of it in sharps container.** *Prevents injury to infant and injury or unnecessary exposure of nurse and others to infant's blood.*

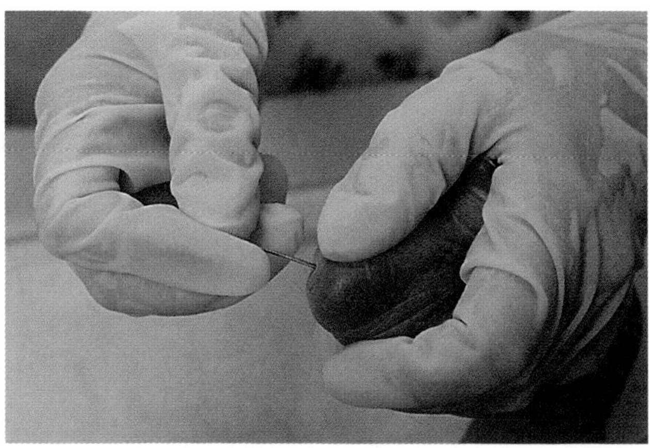

10. **If automatic puncture device is used, place over appropriate site and activate according to manufacturer's directions.** *Ensures proper use of device.*

11. **Dextrostix and Chemstrip: Wipe away first drop of blood with gauze.** *First drop may be diluted with fluid from the area of the puncture.*

12. **Collect a large "stand-up" drop of blood at the puncture site. Avoid excessive squeezing of the foot. Accu-Chek, Dextrostix, and Chemstrip: Place the drop of blood on the treated area of the reagent strip. Cover the entire treated area of the strip and do not smear it. One Touch: Draw blood into pipette and place on reagent strip that has been placed in glucometer.** *An adequate sample size ensures that the blood does not dry during the waiting time and increases accuracy. Excessive squeezing causes dilution of the sample with fluid from the tissues.*

13. **Accu-Chek, Dextrostix, and Chemstrip: Remove blood from the strip at the exact time recommended by manufacturer.** *More or less time affects accuracy of reading.*

14. **Remove blood by the method appropriate for the type of reagent strip used. Dextrostix: Run cold water slowly over the end of the strip to wash away the blood. Accu-Chek and Chemstrip: Wipe blood completely away with cotton ball.** *Correct procedure promotes accuracy. Water flowing with too much force can wash away color change. Warm water may affect color.*

15. **Obtain results. Glucometers: Read the glucometer when sound indicates results ready. Dextrostix and Chemstrip: Compare reagent strips with color chart on bottle. Dextrostix: Read immediately. Chemstrip: Read after 60 seconds.** *Gives accurate results.*

16. **Apply adhesive bandage.** *Prevents bleeding and infection of site.*

17. **Record results. Report readings below 45 mg/dl. Have laboratory draw blood for verification of abnormal results according to agency policy. Feed infant if screening shows a reading below 45 mg/dl. More intensive treatment may be necessary for more abnormal results.** *Feeding is often given at a higher glucose level when screening tests are used because they are less accurate than laboratory analysis. Feeding infants with low glucose level provides calories needed for metabolism and prevents further decrease in glucose levels.*

## Critical to Remember

### COMMON RISK FACTORS FOR HYPERBILIRUBINEMIA

- Prematurity
- Cephalhematoma
- Bruising
- Delayed or poor intake
- Cold stress
- Asphyxia
- Rh incompatibility
- ABO incompatibility
- Sepsis
- Sibling with jaundice
- Breastfeeding

## CHECK YOUR READING

4. What is included in assessment of the newborn's cardiovascular status?
5. Why is it dangerous to take a rectal temperature in an infant?
6. What are some signs of hypoglycemia?
7. Why is it important for the nurse to use the correct site for heel punctures to obtain blood samples?

# Assessment of Body Systems

## Neurologic System

### REFLEXES

Assessment of the presence and strength of the reflexes is important to determine the health of the newborn's central nervous system. The nurse notes the strength of the reflexes and whether both sides of the body respond symmetrically (Fig. 20–9). A diminished overall response occurs in preterm or ill infants. Absence of reflexes may indicate a serious neurologic problem. Asymmetric responses may indicate that trauma during birth caused nerve damage, paralysis, or fracture. For example, trauma to the facial nerve from forceps or pressure during birth may cause drooping of the mouth. The infant may appear to have a one-sided cry and may have no rooting reflex on the affected side. Some of the newborn reflexes gradually weaken and disappear during the early months (Table 20–2).

### SENSORY ASSESSMENT

**Ears.** The ears are assessed for placement, overall appearance, and maturity. An imaginary line drawn from the inner to the outer canthus of the eye should be even with the area where the upper ear joins the head (Fig. 20–10). Ears that are low set may indicate chromosomal abnormalities.

The nurse examines the ears for skin tags and preauricular sinuses or dimples. If abnormalities of the ear are present, the newborn may have chromosomal abnormalities, mental retardation, or kidney defects. The stiffness of the cartilage and the degree of incurving of the pinna are checked as part of the gestational age assessment.

Infants can hear by the last trimester of pregnancy, and their hearing is very good after birth. Hearing is assessed by noting the infant's reaction to sudden loud noises, which should cause a startle response. The infant should respond to the sound of voices, particularly if it is a high-pitched tone of voice or the sound of the mother's voice.

**Eyes.** The eyes should be symmetric and the same size. The usual slate gray-blue color gradually changes to the true color by 3 to 12 months of age. Infants with dark skin may have brown eyes. The eyes are examined for abnormalities and signs of inflammation. Edema of the eyelids or subconjunctival hemorrhages (reddened areas of the sclera) result from pressure on the head during birth, which causes capillary rupture in the sclera. The edema diminishes in a few days, and the hemorrhages take a week or two to resolve.

Conjunctivitis may result from infection or a chemical reaction to medications. *Staphylococcus*, *Chlamydia*, and *Neisseria gonorrhoeae* are common organisms that cause infection. Gonorrhea in the mother can cause infection of the infant during birth. The resulting ophthalmia neonatorum may cause blindness. To prevent this condition, all infants are treated prophylactically with antibiotics to the eyes. Any discharge from the eyes is reported for possible culture and treatment.

## CRITICAL THINKING EXERCISE

**Q:** What might be the effect on normal development if reflexes are retained beyond the age when they should disappear?

**A:** Failure of the reflexes to fade on schedule may interfere with normal development. For example, the palmar grasp reflex must disappear so that the infant can learn to grasp voluntarily and later to release objects at will. Persistence of the plantar reflex would interfere with walking. Retention of reflexes beyond the age when they should disappear indicates pathology and should prompt further investigation.

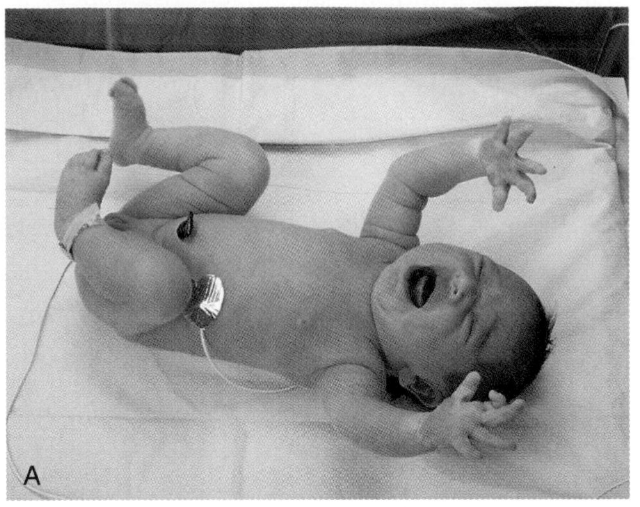


A. **Moro Reflex.**
The Moro reflex is the most dramatic reflex. It occurs when the infant's head and trunk are allowed to drop back 30 degrees when the infant is in a slightly raised position. The infant's arms and legs extend and abduct, with the fingers fanning open and thumbs and forefingers forming a C position. The arms then return to their normally flexed state with an embracing motion. The legs may also extend and then flex.

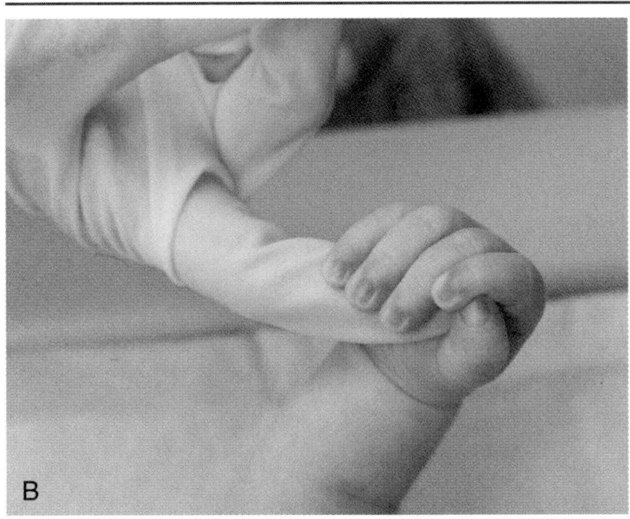


B. **Palmar grasp reflex.**
The palmar grasp reflex occurs when the infant's palm is touched near the base of the fingers. The hand closes into a tight fist. The grasp reflex may be weak or absent if the infant has damage to the nerves of the arms.

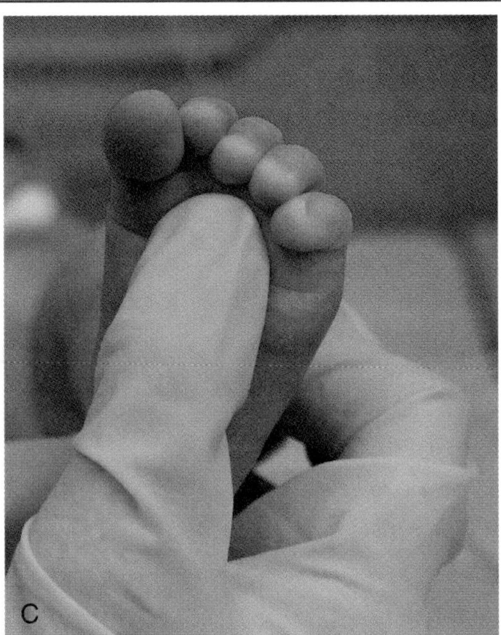


C. **Plantar grasp reflex.**
The plantar grasp reflex is similar to the palmar grasp reflex. When the area below the toes is touched, the infant's toes curl over the nurse's finger.

**FIGURE 20–9**

Reflexes.

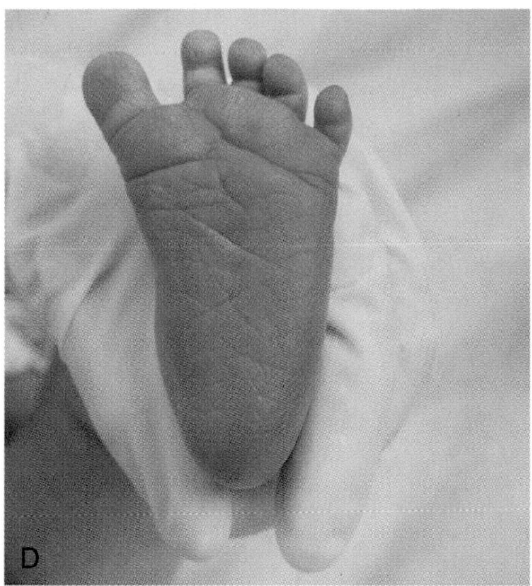


D. **Babinski reflex.**
The Babinski reflex is elicited by stroking the lateral sole of the infant's foot from the heel forward and across the ball of the foot. This causes the toes to flare outward and the big toe to dorsiflex.

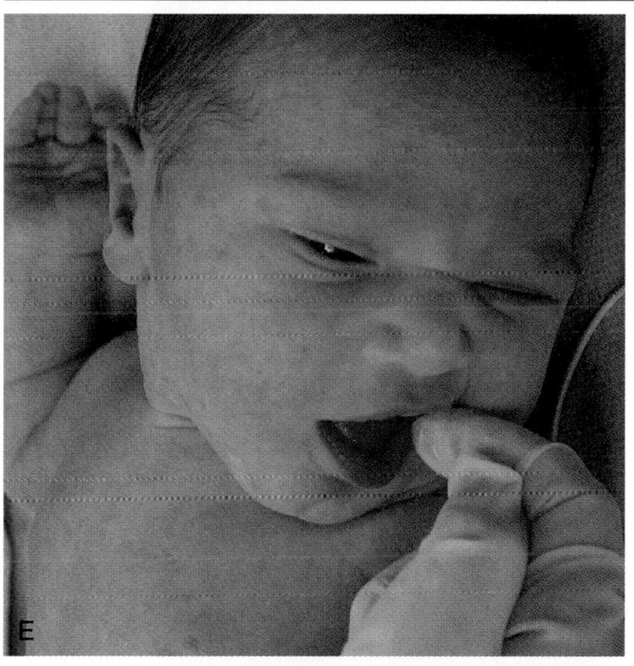


E. **Rooting reflex.**
The rooting reflex is important in feeding and is most often demonstrated when the infant is hungry. When the infant's cheek is touched near the mouth, the head turns toward the side that has been stroked. This helps the infant find the nipple for feeding. The reflex occurs when either side of the mouth is touched. Touching the cheeks on both sides at the same time confuses the infant.

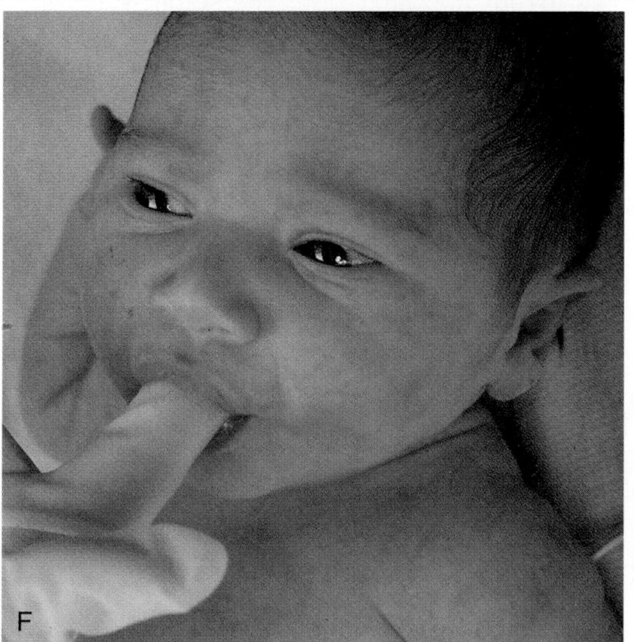


F. **Sucking reflex.**
The sucking reflex is essential to normal life. When the mouth or palate is touched by the nipple or a finger, the infant begins to suck. The sucking reflex is assessed for its presence and strength. Feeding difficulties may be related to problems in the infant's ability to suck and to coordinate sucking with swallowing.

**FIGURE 20–9** *Continued*

*Illustration continued on following page*

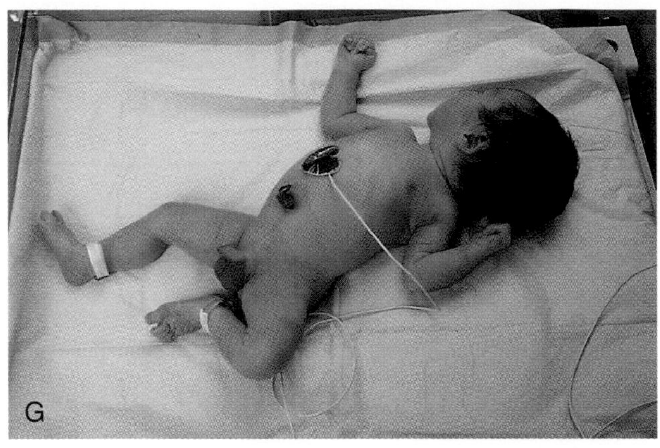


G. **Tonic neck reflex.**
The tonic neck reflex refers to the posture assumed by newborns when in a supine position. The infant extends the arm and leg on the side to which the head is turned and flexes the extremities on the other side. This is sometimes referred to as the "fencing reflex" because the infant's position is similar to that of a person engaged in a fencing match.

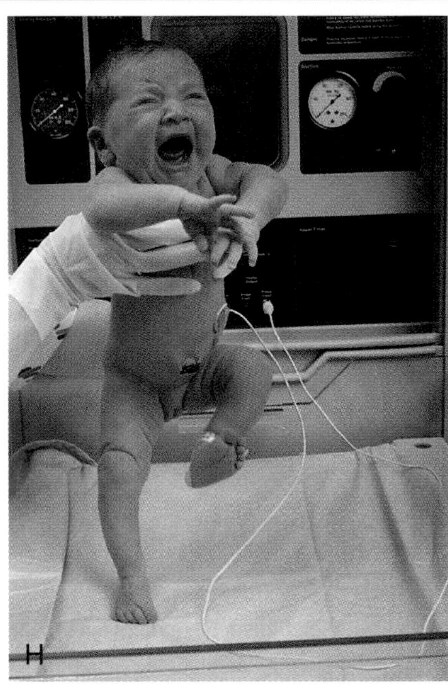


H. **Stepping reflex.**
The stepping reflex occurs when infants are held upright with their feet touching a solid surface. They lift one foot and then the other, giving the appearance that they are trying to walk.

**FIGURE 20–9** *Continued*

Transient strabismus ("crossed eyes") is common for the first 3 to 4 months after birth because infants have poor control of their eye muscles. The doll's-eye sign is a normal finding in the newborn: When the head is turned quickly to one side, the eyes move toward the other side. The setting-sun sign—the iris appears low in the eye and part of the sclera can be seen above the iris—may be an indication of hydrocephalus.

The pupils should be equal in size and react to

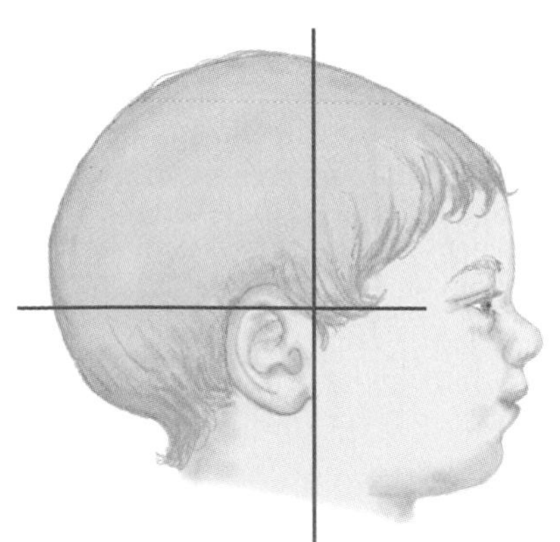


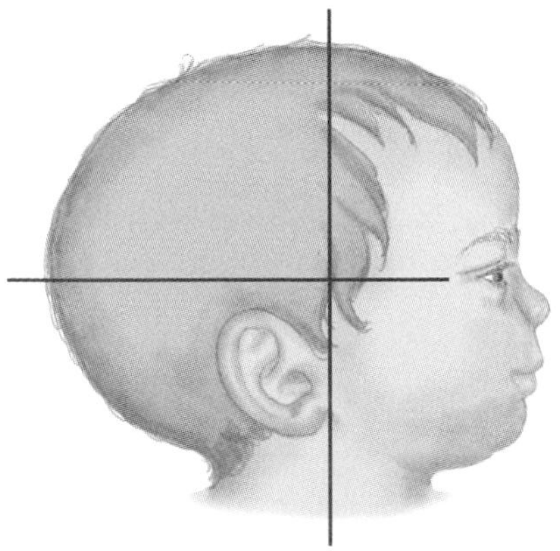


**FIGURE 20–10**
An imaginary line is drawn from the inner to the outer canthus of the eye and then to the ear. The line should intersect with the area where the upper ear joins the head.

**TABLE 20–2 SUMMARY OF NEONATAL REFLEXES**

| Reflex | Method of Testing | Expected Response | Abnormal Response/ Possible Cause | Time Reflex Disappears |
|---|---|---|---|---|
| Babinski | Stroke lateral sole of foot from heel to across base of toes. | Toes flare with dorsiflexion of the big toe. | No response<br>Bilateral: CNS deficit<br>Unilateral: Local nerve damage. | 12 months |
| Galant (trunk incurvation) | Lightly stroke the back lateral to the vertebral column. | Entire trunk flexes toward side stimulated. | No response: CNS deficit | 1 month |
| Grasp reflex (palmar and plantar) | Press finger against base of fingers or toes. | Fingers curl tightly; toes curl forward. | Weak or absent: Neurologic deficit or muscle damage | Palmar grasp lessens 3–4 months, disappears by 5–6 months. Plantar grasp disappears by 8–9 months. |
| Moro | Let infant's head drop back approximately 30 degrees. | Sharp extension and abduction of arms with thumbs and forefingers in "C" position. Followed by flexion and adduction to "embrace" position. Legs follow similar pattern. | Absent: CNS dysfunction. Asymmetry: Brachial plexus injury, paralysis, or fractured clavicle or bone of extremity.<br>Exaggerated: Maternal drug use. | 6 months |
| Rooting | Touch or stroke side of cheek near mouth. | Infant turns to side touched. Difficult to elicit if infant sleeping or just fed. | Weak or absent: Prematurity, neurologic deficit, depression from maternal drug use | 3–4 months |
| Startle | Make a loud noise. | Similar to Moro but hands remain clenched. | Weak or absent: Neurologic damage, deafness | 4 months |
| Stepping | Hold infant so feet touch solid surface. | Infant lifts alternate feet as if walking. | Asymmetry: Fracture of extremity, neurologic deficit | 4–7 months |
| Sucking | Place nipple or finger in mouth, rub against palate. | Infant begins to suck. Weak if recently fed. | Weak or absent: Prematurity, neurologic deficit, maternal drug use | Well coordinated with swallow by 34–36 weeks' gestation. Disappears by 1 yr. |
| Swallowing | Place fluid on the back of the tongue. | Infant swallows fluid. Should be coordinated with sucking. | Coughing, gagging, choking, cyanosis. Tracheoesophageal fistula, esophageal atresia, neurologic deficit | Present throughout life |
| Tonic neck reflex | Gently turn head to one side while infant is supine. | Extension of extremities on side to which head turned, with flexion on opposite side. | Prolonged period of time in position: Neurologic deficit | May be weak at birth and increase to 1 month, then disappears by 4 months. |

CNS, central nervous system.

light. Cataracts (opacities of the lens) appear as white areas over the pupils. They may develop in infants of mothers who had rubella or other infections during the pregnancy. When a light is directed into the eyes, the normal red reflex may not be seen if large cataracts are present. Tears are scant or absent for the first 2 to 4 weeks of life. Excessive tearing may indicate a plugged lacrimal duct, which is treated with massage or surgery.

Although visual acuity is not well developed and the eyes cannot accommodate for distance, newborns should show a visual response to the environment. They should make eye contact when held in a cradle position during a period of alertness and focus on objects that are 8 to 9 inches away. Newborns can follow interesting objects horizontally 180 degrees and vertically 30 degrees. They should respond well to human faces and geometric patterns of black and white or medium-bright colors but show little interest in pastel colors.

Newborns should blink or close their eyes in response to bright lights. Any infant who does not respond to visual stimuli should be reported to the physician or nurse practitioner for further investigation.

**Sense of Smell.** Newborns have a good sense of smell, and discrimination develops quickly. They can identify the odor of the mother's breast milk within 5 days after birth (Brazelton, 1994). The ability of infants to distinguish taste is shown by their increased suck when given sweet liquids and rejection of those that are sour, salty, or bitter.

#### OTHER NEUROLOGIC SIGNS

The newborn is assessed for jitteriness or tremors. If jitteriness is present, the blood glucose level should be checked because hypoglycemia is the most common cause. If blood glucose is within normal range, the cause may be low calcium levels or prenatal exposure to drugs. Tremors increase each time the infant is touched or moved but stop briefly if the extremity is flexed and held firmly.

Seizures indicate central nervous system abnormality. To differentiate jitteriness from seizures, the infant's extremities are held in a flexed position. This causes tremors to stop, but a seizure continues. Seizure activity may also include abnormal movements of the eyes or mouth and other subtle signs. Any infant thought to be having seizures is referred for further assessment and treatment.

The pitch of the cry is important. A shrill or high-pitched cry, a cat-like "mewing," or a hoarse cry is abnormal. These cries may indicate a neurologic disorder or other problem.

Normal infants are quiet and appear content when their needs are met. Infants should respond to soothing, gentle touch and holding. Rocking motions are often effective in quieting an irritable infant. Most infants "mold" their body to that of the person holding them, making them easy to hold and cuddle. The neonate who stiffens the body, seems to pull away from contact, or arches the back when held is showing signs of central nervous system damage. Infants should react to painful stimuli with crying and an increase in vital signs. Excessive irritability or a high-pitched cry may also be a sign of damage to the nervous system. All such abnormal signs are reported for further neurologic assessment.

### Critical to Remember

**DIFFERENTIATING JITTERINESS AND SEIZURES**

**Jitteriness or Tremors**

- Stop when the extremities are held firmly in a flexed position
- Low glucose or calcium levels common cause

**Seizures**

- Continue even if extremities are held
- May have abnormal mouth or eye movements
- Indicate central nervous system abnormality

## Gastrointestinal System

The initial assessment of the gastrointestinal tract occurs during the first hours after birth, as the nurse visualizes the parts that can be seen and the infant takes the initial feeding. Abnormalities and normal variations in structure and function are identified.

#### MOUTH

The mouth is inspected visually and by palpation. Some infants are born with precocious teeth, usually incisors (Fig. 20–11). If the teeth are loose, the physician usually removes them to prevent aspiration. Epstein's pearls may be present on the hard palate. These small, white, hard cysts disappear without treatment.

The nurse examines the tongue for size and movement. A large protruding tongue is present in some chromosomal disorders such as Down syndrome. Paralysis of the facial nerve causes drooping of the mouth and affects the movement of the tongue. The tongue may appear to be tongue-tied because of the short frenulum, but this is normal and usually has no effect on the infant's ability to feed. Clipping of the frenulum is seldom practiced because of the potential for infection.

Although candidiasis (thrush) is not apparent in the mouth immediately after birth, it may appear a

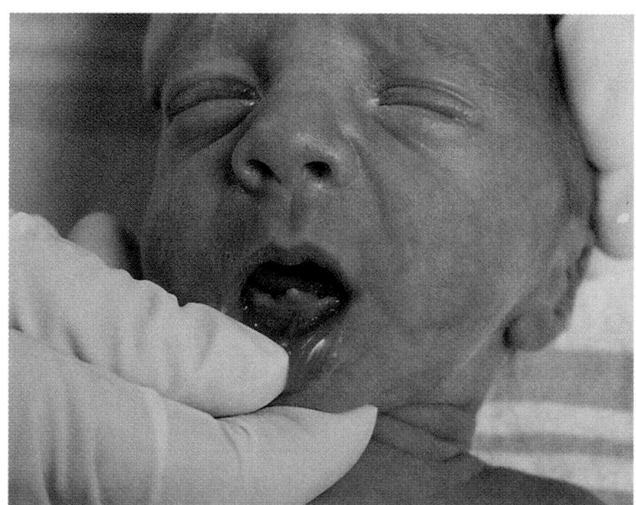

**FIGURE 20–11**

A precocious tooth.

day or two later. The lesions resemble milk curds on the tongue and cheeks that bleed if attempts are made to wipe them away. Newborns may become infected with *Candida albicans* during passage through the birth canal if the mother has a candidal vaginal infection. The infant is treated with nystatin suspension.

A cleft lip or palate results if the lip or palate fails to close. Cleft palate may involve the hard or the soft palate, or both, and may appear alone or with a cleft lip. The palate is inspected when the infant cries. A gloved finger is inserted into the mouth to palpate both the hard and the soft palate. A very small cleft of the soft palate may be missed if only a visual examination is done (see cleft lip and palate, p. 869).

### SUCK

The normal full-term infant should have a strong suck reflex, which is elicited when the lips or palate is stimulated. The reflex is weaker in the neonate who is preterm, ill, or has just been fed. The newborn's cheeks have well-developed muscles and sucking pads that enhance the ability to suck. These fatty sucking pads last until late in infancy, when sucking is no longer essential. There may be blisters on the newborn's hands or arms due to strong sucking before birth.

### ABDOMEN

The abdomen should be rounded and protrude slightly but should not be distended. A distended abdomen with stretched, shiny skin may indicate obstruction. Loops of bowel should not be visible through the abdominal wall. Visible bowel could indicate that air or meconium, or both, is not passing through the intestines normally.

A sunken or scaphoid appearance of the abdomen occurs in diaphragmatic hernia, in which the intestines are located in the chest cavity instead of the abdomen. This condition interferes with development of the lungs, resulting in respiratory difficulty at birth. The nurse listens over the abdomen for bowel sounds, which usually appear within the first hour after birth. Bowel sounds heard in the chest may indicate diaphragmatic hernia.

The stomach may be distended by mucus, blood, or amniotic fluid swallowed during birth, especially after a cesarean birth. If meconium is swallowed in the amniotic fluid, it may be regurgitated and aspirated, causing lung inflammation. In some agencies, it is routine to empty the stomach soon after birth by feeding tube to prevent aspiration. In other facilities, the procedure is performed only if necessary.

An umbilical hernia occurs when the intestinal muscles fail to close around the umbilicus, allowing the intestines to protrude through the weak area. The condition is more common in African-American infants. By the time the infant is walking well, the muscles are usually strong enough that the hernia is no longer present. Some umbilical hernias require surgical repair.

Palpating the abdomen is easiest when the infant is relaxed and quiet. The abdomen should feel soft because the muscles are not yet well developed. Masses may indicate tumors of the kidneys. Palpation of the liver and kidneys usually is not part of the usual nursing assessment of the abdomen. When palpated, the liver is normally felt no more than 1 to 3 cm below the right costal margin. If the organ seems large, it should be reported to the physician or nurse practitioner because it may be a sign of congestive heart failure or congenital infection.

### INITIAL FEEDING

The initial feeding is an opportunity to further assess the newborn. The nurse observes for choking, coughing, and cyanosis, indicating a connection between the trachea and the esophagus, such as tracheoesophageal fistula. The infant's ability to suck, swallow, and breathe in a coordinated manner is evaluated. Although the fetus sucks and swallows in utero, these acts may not have been performed together. The addition of breathing to sucking and swallowing is a new experience.

If the mother is breastfeeding, the nurse can observe the infant's response unobtrusively while assisting the mother to position the infant. A LATCH score should be given to all breastfeeding infants to identify problems with feeding (see Chapter 22, p. 589).

In some facilities the newborn may be given a small amount of sterile water before the first formula feeding. Plain water is less irritating to the lungs than dextrose water or formula, should aspiration occur. Formula is given if the infant tolerates a few sips of water without difficulty. Other facilities give breast milk or formula for all feedings. The initial feeding should be no more than 1 ounce to decrease regurgitation from overdistention of the stomach.

Some newborns choke or gag during the first feeding. Others may become dusky or cyanotic because they become apneic while they are feeding. In either case, the nurse should stop the feeding immediately, suction if necessary, and stimulate the infant to cry by rubbing the back.

Most infants learn to coordinate sucking, swallowing, and breathing by the time the first feeding is finished. Neonates who continue to have difficulty may have a cardiac anomaly, tracheoesophageal fistula, or esophageal atresia (see p. 870). Infants with tracheoesophageal fistula or esophageal atresia may also drool excessively. Further assessment and referral are necessary.

#### STOOLS

Observe the stools for normal color and consistency. Meconium stools are dark greenish black. They are soft but thick and tend to adhere to the skin. The infant may pass meconium at delivery, when a rectal temperature is taken, or after the initial feeding. Meconium stools are followed by transitional loose greenish brown stools.

Breastfed infants pass very soft, seedy, mustard-yellow stools after transitional stools. Formula-fed infants excrete stools that are more solid and pale yellow to light brown. There should never be a "water ring" around the solid part of any stool. This indicates diarrhea, with the watery part absorbed into the diaper.

The nurse should be aware of when the infant's last stool occurred and whether any stools have been passed since birth. Most newborns pass the first meconium stool within 24 hours of birth. If there is a question about whether the infant has excreted a stool, the nurse must investigate further. Feeding may cause the infant to have a stool. Although rectal temperatures are not recommended, a thermometer may be inserted into the rectum gently to determine patency and stimulate stool passage.

### CRITICAL THINKING EXERCISE

You are caring for an infant who was born 20 hours ago and you hear on report that the infant has not passed meconium yet.

**Q:** What should you do?

**A:**

Begin by expanding your assessment of the facts. First, check through the chart to be sure that no stool is recorded. Did the infant pass meconium at delivery? Check the delivery notes. Ask the mother if she has changed a diaper with stool in it. Instruct her to inform the nurse if she does. If the first temperature performed on the infant was rectal, the anus is patent. If it is not clear whether a rectal temperature was done, take one to check patency. Taking a rectal temperature may stimulate peristalsis and passage of meconium. However, even with a patent anus, obstruction of the intestine above the anus is possible.

Consider the infant's intake. How much is the infant feeding and how well are feedings being taken? If the infant has been sleepy and has fed poorly, increase the feedings. Asking a nursing mother to feed more often or offering the neonate extra formula may make the difference.

Keep in mind that most infants pass a stool by 24 hours and that 4 hours remain. If the infant has not had a stool within 24 hours, in spite of extra feedings and normal assessments, alert the pediatrician. Some infants do not have a stool for 48 hours. Be sure other caregivers are alerted. Let the mother know that the infant is being watched for stools without alarming her.

### CHECK YOUR READING

8. Why is assessment of newborn reflexes important?
9. Why is it important for the nurse to observe the first feeding carefully?
10. When do newborns pass the first stool? What can be done to stimulate stool passage?

## Genitourinary System

Assess the genitourinary system for kidney function and anomalies of the genitalia.

#### KIDNEY PALPATION

Palpation of the kidneys is not usually part of the routine nursing assessment of the newborn. However, the kidneys may be felt just above the level of the umbilicus on each side of the abdomen during the first hours after birth. Abdominal masses may indicate enlargement or tumors of the kidneys. Anomalies of the kidney may accompany other defects because an insult early in fetal development often affects all organs being formed at that time. For example, an infant with only one umbilical artery or defects involving the ears may have renal anomalies. The nurse should observe carefully for urinary output in these infants to determine if the kidneys are functioning.

#### URINE

Most newborns void within 24 hours of birth, and almost all void by 48 hours. Because absence of urine output during this time may indicate anomalies, the time of the first void is recorded on the chart. The newborn's bladder empties as little as two to six times during the first 2 days, and the first void may be missed. Sometimes it occurs in the delivery room but goes unnoticed because attention is focused on the infant's overall condition.

If there is concern over whether the newborn has urinated, the delivery notes should be carefully read to see if the infant voided at birth. The nurse should ask the mother if she has changed a wet diaper. Increasing the infant's fluid intake can often initiate urination. If there is no void in the expected time, the physician or nurse practitioner is alerted.

After the first 2 days of life, the newborn's bladder empties 5 to 25 times each day. Each void is recorded in the infant's chart, including diapers the mother changes. The total number is correlated with what is appropriate for the age of the infant. Mothers should be taught that approximately six to 10 wet diapers, after the first 2 days, indicate the infant is taking adequate fluid.

If an infant is having feeding difficulties, it is especially important to note the number of wet diapers. Disposable diapers are very absorbent, and it is sometimes difficult to tell whether the diaper is wet. The pale color of the newborn's urine may cause very little color change on the diaper. Wet diapers generally feel heavier than dry ones. If necessary, the nurse can put on gloves and take the diaper apart to examine it. The absorbent inner lining is damp if urine is present. Cotton balls or tissue placed in the diaper may be used also to make small amounts of urine more visible.

The newborn's urine may contain urate crystals that cause a reddish or pink stain on the diaper. This is known as "brick dust staining" and may be frightening to parents, who may think the infant is bleeding. It does not continue beyond the first few days as the kidneys mature.

#### GENITALIA

The nurse examines the newborn's genitalia for size, maturation, and presence of any abnormalities.

**Female.** In the full-term female infant, the labia majora should be large and completely cover the clitoris and labia minora. The labia may be darker than the surrounding skin, especially in infants with dark skin tones. This pigmentation is a normal response to exposure to the mother's hormones before birth. Edema of the labia and white mucous vaginal discharge are normal. A small amount of vaginal bleeding, known as pseudomenstruation, may occur from the sudden withdrawal of the mother's hormones at birth. Hymenal or vaginal tags are small pieces of tissue at the vaginal orifice. These are normal and disappear in a few weeks. The urinary meatus and vagina should be present.

**Male.** The scrotum should be pendulous at term and may be dark brown from maternal hormones. Pressure during a breech delivery may cause it to be edematous. Rugae (creases in the scrotum) are deep and cover the entire scrotum in the full-term infant.

Enlargement of one or both sides of the scrotum may be due to a hydrocele. This collection of fluid around the testes may make palpating the testes difficult. Placing a flashlight against the sac may outline the testes. Parents should be told that hydroceles are not painful and often reabsorb within a year. Some require later surgery.

The testes begin to descend through the inguinal canal at about 30 weeks of gestation and should be within the scrotal sac at 36 weeks. Palpation of the scrotum determines if the testes have descended. (Fig. 20–12). Testes feel like small, round, movable objects that "slip" between the fingers. If the testes are not present in the scrotal sac, they may be felt in the inguinal canal. Undescended testis (cryptorchidism) occurs on one or both sides in approximately 3.4 percent of full-term newborns (Behrman et al., 1996). An empty scrotal sac appears smaller than one with testes. If the testes do not descend within the first year, the condition must be treated surgically to preserve fertility.

The meatus should be at the tip of the glans penis. It may be abnormally located on the underside of the penis (hypospadias), on the upper side (epispadias), or on the perineum. The prepuce, or foreskin, of the penis covers the glans and is adherent to it. Attempts to retract it in the newborn are unnecessary and can cause damage. Abnormal placement of the meatus may not be visible because it is covered by the prepuce, but often the prepuce in these infants is incompletely formed. Hypospadias may be accompanied by chordee, a condition in which fibrotic tissue causes the penis to curve downward. These abnormalities are later corrected by surgery.

Parents are very concerned about any abnormalities of the genitalia. If the meatus is abnormally positioned, they need an explanation of the condition and why the infant may not be circumcised. The foreskin may be needed for later plastic surgery to repair the defect.

### Integumentary System

#### SKIN

The skin of the newborn is fragile and easily shows marks, especially in infants with fair coloring. Because the skin is so sensitive, reddened areas or rashes may develop during the early days of life.

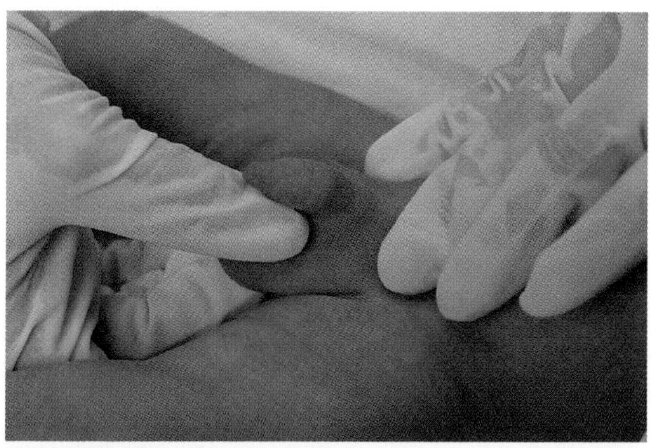

**FIGURE 20–12**

The testes are palpated from front to back with the thumb and forefinger. Placing a finger over the inguinal canal holds the testes in place for palpation.

The nurse must examine every inch of skin surface carefully during the initial assessment and at the beginning of each shift.

**Color.** The color of the newborn's skin should be pink or tan. Red thin skin occurs in preterm infants. Redness (ruddy color) in the full-term infant may indicate polycythemia. Acrocyanosis is common during the first day or two as a result of poor peripheral circulation. The infant's mouth and central body areas should not be cyanotic at any time. Blanching the skin over the nose or chest shows the presence of jaundice. Jaundice is abnormal during the first day of life but common during the first week.

A greenish brown discoloration of the skin, nails, and cord results if meconium was passed before birth. This may indicate that the infant was compromised at some time before birth, and it is more common in the postterm infant. These infants must be watched for other complications, such as respiratory difficulty.

**Vernix Caseosa.** Vernix, a thick white substance, resembles cream cheese and provides a protective covering for the fetal skin in utero. The full-term infant has little vernix left on the body except small amounts in the creases. A thick covering of vernix may indicate a preterm infant, but a postterm infant may have none at all. Most of the vernix is removed when the infant is dried at birth or during the first bath. The rest is absorbed by the skin. Yellow-tinged vernix may indicate elevated bilirubin levels in utero, and green-tinged vernix is due to meconium staining.

**Lanugo.** Lanugo is fine hair that covers the fetus during intrauterine life (Fig. 20–13). As the fetus nears term, the lanugo becomes thinner. Observe the amount of lanugo on the newborn's body. The term infant may have a small amount of lanugo on the shoulders, forehead, sides of the face, and upper back. Dark-skinned infants have more lanugo than infants with lighter coloring, and their darker hair is more visible.

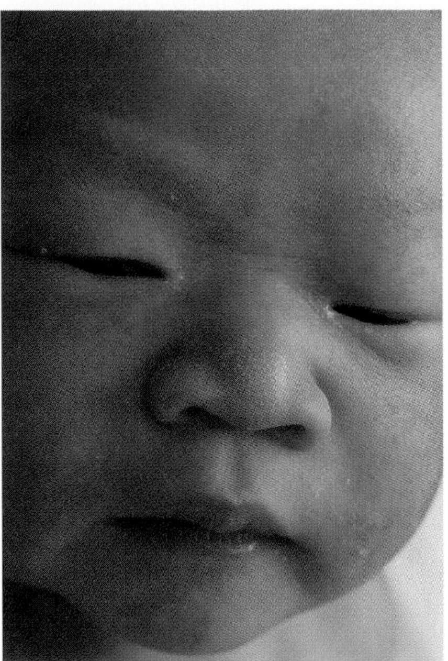

**FIGURE 20–14**

Milia.

**Milia.** Milia are white cysts, 1 to 2 mm in size, due to distention of sebaceous glands (oil glands) that are not yet functioning properly. They occur on the face over the forehead, nose, and chin and disappear within 2 months without treatment (Fig. 20–14).

**Erythema Toxicum.** The nurse notes the presence of erythema toxicum, red blotchy areas that may have white or yellow papules in the center (Fig. 20–15). It is commonly called "flea bite" rash or newborn rash and resembles small bites or acne. The

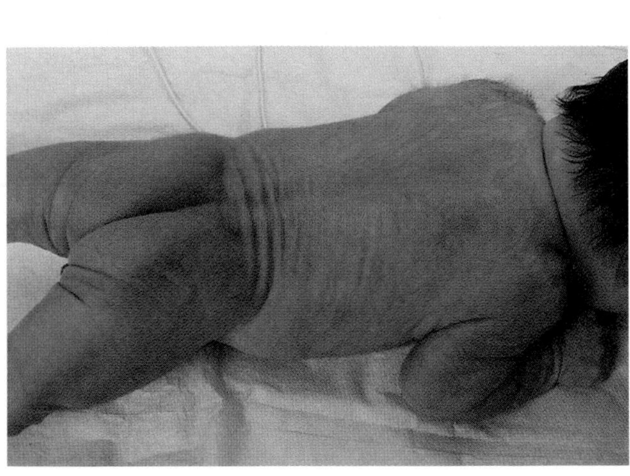

**FIGURE 20–13**

Lanugo is abundant on this slightly preterm infant.

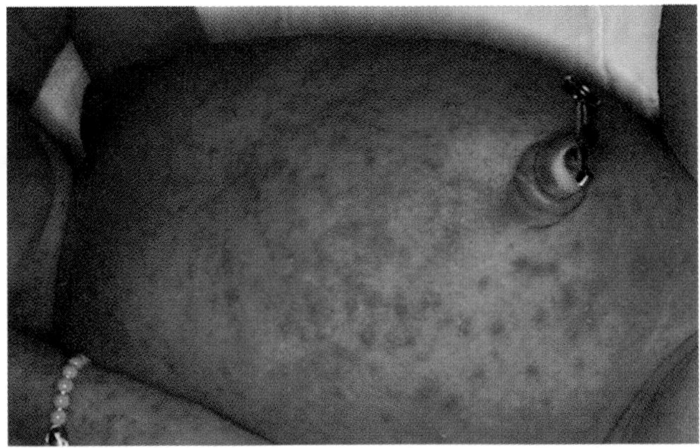

**FIGURE 20–15**

Erythema toxicum. (From Hurwitz, S. [1993]. *Clinical pediatric dermatology* (2nd ed., p. 13). Philadelphia: W.B. Saunders.)

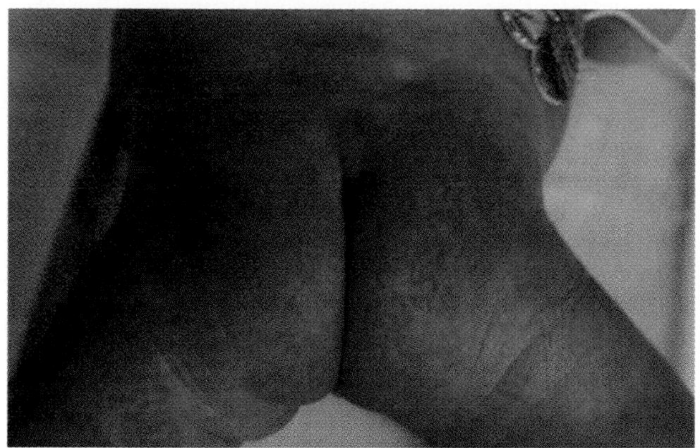

**FIGURE 20–16**

Mongolian spots. (Courtesy of Jane Deacon, M.S., R.N., N.N.P., The Children's Hospital, Denver, Colorado.)

rash appears during the first 24 to 48 hours after birth, although occasionally not until 1 to 2 weeks. It is most common over the back, shoulders, and chest. The condition is not due to infection but should be differentiated from a pustular rash caused by staphylococcal infection. The cause of erythema toxicum is unknown, and it disappears within hours or up to 10 days.

**Birthmarks.** The size and location of all birthmarks should be carefully documented. Some of the more common birthmarks are listed here.

- Mongolian spots are bluish black marks that resemble bruises (Fig. 20–16). They usually occur in the sacral area but may appear on the buttocks, arms, shoulders, or other areas. Mongolian spots occur most frequently in newborns with dark skin and usually disappear after the first few years of life. Some continue into adulthood.
- A telangiectatic nevus is sometimes called nevus simplex or a "stork bite" (Fig. 20–17). It is a flat pink or reddish discoloration from dilated capillaries that occur over the eyelids, above the bridge of the nose, or at the nape of the neck. The color blanches when pressed and is more prominent during crying. Stork bites disappear by age 2 years, although those at the nape of the neck may persist.
- Nevus flammeus (port wine stain) is a permanent, flat, dark reddish purple mark (Fig. 20–18). It varies in size and location and does not blanch with pressure. If it is large and in a visible area, it can be removed by laser surgery.
- Nevus vasculosus (strawberry hemangioma) consists of enlarged capillaries in the outer layers of skin. It is dark red and raised with a rough surface, giving a strawberry-like appearance. The hemangioma is usually located on the head. It may grow larger for 5 to 6 months but usually disappears by the early school years. No treatment is necessary.
- Café-au-lait spots are permanent, light brown areas that may occur anywhere on the body. Although they are harmless, the number and size are important. More than six spots or spots larger than 1.5 cm are associated with neurofibromatosis, a genetic condition of neural tissue.

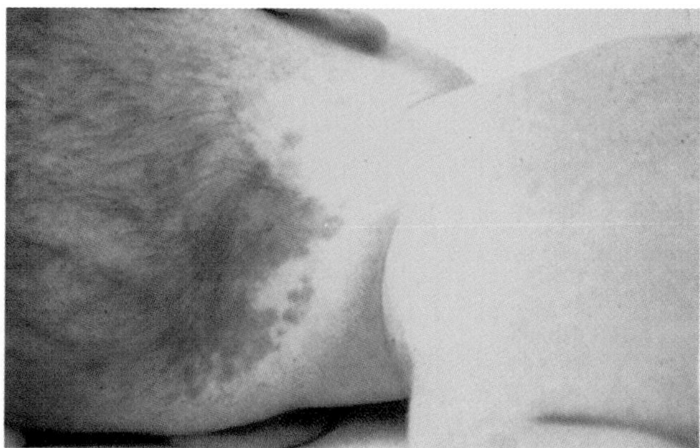

**FIGURE 20–17**

Stork bite. (Courtesy of Jane Deacon, M.S., R.N., N.N.P., The Children's Hospital, Denver, Colorado.)

**Marks from Delivery.** Inspect the infant for marks that may have occurred from injury or pressure during labor or delivery.

- Bruises may occur on any part of the body where there was pressure during delivery. This is especially true when second-stage labor was difficult. Bruising of the face may be present if the cord was wrapped around the neck during birth. Bruising on

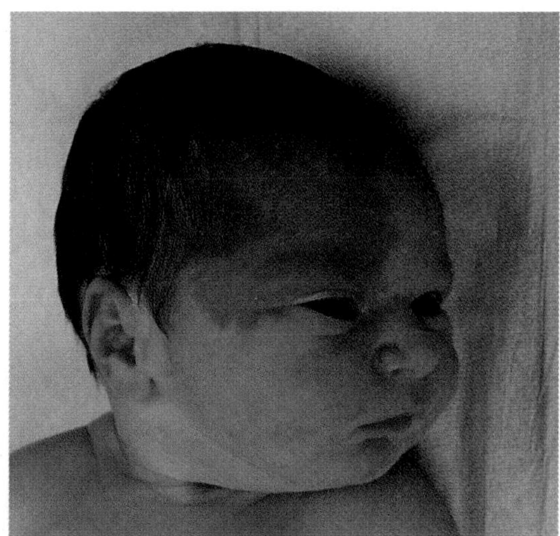

**FIGURE 20–18**

Port wine stain.

the head may occur from use of a vacuum extractor.

- Petechiae, pinpoint bruises that resemble a rash, may appear over areas such as the back or face. They are due to increased intravascular pressure during the birth process, such as occurs when there is a nuchal cord during delivery. Widespread petechiae or continued formation of petechiae may indicate infection or a low platelet count.
- A small puncture mark is present on the newborn's head if a fetal monitor scalp electrode was attached. The area should scab and heal normally but should be observed for signs of infection.
- Forceps marks occur over the cheeks and ears where the instruments were applied. They are carefully documented as to size, color, and location. Lack of movement or symmetry of the face may indicate damage to the facial nerve.

**Other Aspects.** The nurse notes other aspects of the skin that may indicate abnormalities. Localized edema may be due to trauma of delivery. Generalized edema indicates more serious conditions, such as heart failure. Peeling of the skin is normal in full-term newborns. Excessive amounts of peeling may indicate a postterm infant.

#### BREASTS

The nurse notes the placement of the nipples and looks for extra (or supernumerary) nipples, which may appear on the chest or in the axilla. Occasionally, the breasts become engorged 2 or 3 days after birth and secrete a small amount of white fluid (sometimes called "witch's milk") a few days later. This condition is due to hormones from the mother. The condition resolves within a few weeks without treatment. The breasts should not be expressed or manipulated, as this could cause infection.

#### HAIR AND NAILS

The hair on the full-term infant should be silky and soft, whereas that on the preterm infant is woolly or fuzzy. The nails come to the end of the fingers or beyond. Very long nails may indicate a postterm infant.

#### DOCUMENTATION

All marks, bruises, rashes, or other abnormalities of the skin must be recorded in the nurses' notes. A description of the location, size, color, elevation, and texture of each mark is included. Subsequent changes in appearance from previous descriptions are also noted on the chart.

One may not always know the proper name for each of the different types of marks. Most agencies have books with pictures of the common skin variations.

**When in doubt about the name of a mark, a description is sufficient. For example, a stork bite (telangiectatic nevus) might be described as a "flat, reddened area 1 × 2 cm in size over right eyelid that blanches with pressure."**

## Assessment of Gestational Age

The gestational age assessment is an examination of the newborn to determine the number of weeks from conception to birth. The determination is based on physical and neurologic characteristics. It is important because neonates born before or after term and those whose size is not appropriate for gestational age are at increased risk for complications. Both medical care and nursing care are affected by the gestational age of the infant. The gestational age may also be calculated from the mother's last menstrual period and by ultrasonography during the pregnancy. However, the date of the last menstrual period is not always accurate, and ultrasonography is not always performed.

Because it is known when various characteristics develop in the fetus, their presence or absence can help to estimate gestational age. The estimated age can then be compared with the newborn's weight, length, and head circumference to determine whether the neonate is large, appropriate (or average), or small in size for gestational age. It is important to understand that it is the total score of all assessed characteristics that determines the gestational age. One or two characteristics alone cannot be used to assign a gestational age.

### Assessment Tools

Several different tools are used to assess gestational age. The Dubowitz scoring system is an in-depth, detailed assessment tool that includes examination of physical, neurologic, and behavioral characteristics. The New Ballard Score (Fig. 20–19) is a simplified adaptation of the Dubowitz tool that has been revised to include characteristics of very preterm infants. It can be performed quickly yet provides a fairly accurate estimate of the gestational age. The Ballard tool focuses on physical and neuromuscular characteristics, eliminating the behavioral characteristics. With each tool, a score is given to each assessment, and the total score is used to determine the gestational age of the infant. The New Ballard Score is described below.

# NEWBORN MATURITY RATING & CLASSIFICATION

ESTIMATION OF GESTATIONAL AGE BY MATURITY RATING
Symbols: X - 1st Exam O - 2nd Exam

Gestation by Dates__________wks

Birth Date________ Hour________ am pm

APGAR________ 1 min________ 5 min

## NEUROMUSCULAR MATURITY

| | -1 | 0 | 1 | 2 | 3 | 4 | 5 |
|---|---|---|---|---|---|---|---|
| Posture | | | | | | | |
| Square Window (wrist) | >90° | 90° | 60° | 45° | 30° | 0° | |
| Arm Recoil | | 180° | 140°-180° | 110°-140° | 90-110° | <90° | |
| Popliteal Angle | 180° | 160° | 140° | 120° | 100° | 90° | <90° |
| Scarf Sign | | | | | | | |
| Heel to Ear | | | | | | | |

## PHYSICAL MATURITY

| | -1 | 0 | 1 | 2 | 3 | 4 | 5 |
|---|---|---|---|---|---|---|---|
| Skin | sticky friable transparent | gelatinous red, translucent | smooth pink, visible veins | superficial peeling &/or rash, few veins | cracking pale areas rare veins | parchment deep cracking no vessels | leathery cracked wrinkled |
| Lanugo | none | sparse | abundant | thinning | bald areas | mostly bald | |
| Plantar Surface | heel-toe 40-50 mm: -1 <40 mm: -2 | >50mm no crease | faint red marks | anterior transverse crease only | creases ant. 2/3 | creases over entire sole | |
| Breast | imperceptible | barely perceptible | flat areola no bud | stippled areola 1-2mm bud | raised areola 3-4mm bud | full areola 5-10mm bud | |
| Eye/Ear | lids fused loosely: -1 tightly: -2 | lids open pinna flat stays folded | sl. curved pinna; soft; slow recoil | well-curved pinna; soft but ready recoil | formed &firm instant recoil | thick cartilage ear stiff | |
| Genitals male | scrotum flat, smooth | scrotum empty faint rugae | testes in upper canal rare rugae | testes descending few rugae | testes down good rugae | testes pendulous deep rugae | |
| Genitals female | clitoris prominent labia flat | prominent clitoris small labia minora | prominent clitoris enlarging minora | majora & minora equally prominent | majora large minora small | majora cover clitoris & minora | |

## MATURITY RATING

| score | weeks |
|---|---|
| -10 | 20 |
| -5 | 22 |
| 0 | 24 |
| 5 | 26 |
| 10 | 28 |
| 15 | 30 |
| 20 | 32 |
| 25 | 34 |
| 30 | 36 |
| 35 | 38 |
| 40 | 40 |
| 45 | 42 |
| 50 | 44 |

## SCORING SECTION

| | 1st Exam=X | 2nd Exam=O |
|---|---|---|
| Estimating Gest Age by Maturity Rating | ______ Weeks | ______ Weeks |
| Time of Exam | Date______ Hour______ am pm | Date______ Hour______ am pm |
| Age at Exam | ______ Hours | ______ Hours |
| Signature of Examiner | ______ M.D. | ______ M.D. |

**FIGURE 20–19**

New Ballard score. (Courtesy of Bristol-Myers Company, Evansville, Indiana. From Ballard, J.L., Khoury, J.C., Wedig, K., Wang, L., Eilers-Walsman, B.L., & Lipp, R. [1991]. New Ballard score, expanded to include extremely premature infants. *Journal of Pediatrics*, 19(3), 417–423.)

## Neuromuscular Characteristics

### POSTURE

The posture and degree of flexion of the extremities are scored before disturbing the quiet infant to perform the remainder of the examination (Fig. 20–20). Preterm neonates have little energy or muscle tone and immature flexor muscles. Therefore, they have extended, limp arms and legs that offer little resistance to movement by the examiner. Full-term infants hold their arms close to the body with the elbows sharply flexed. The legs should be flexed

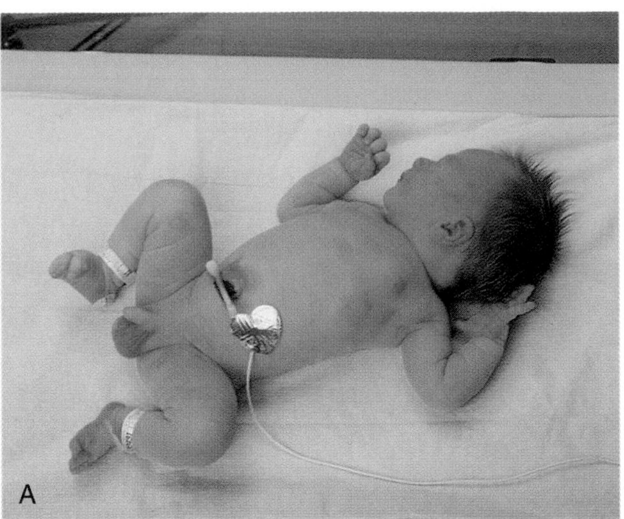

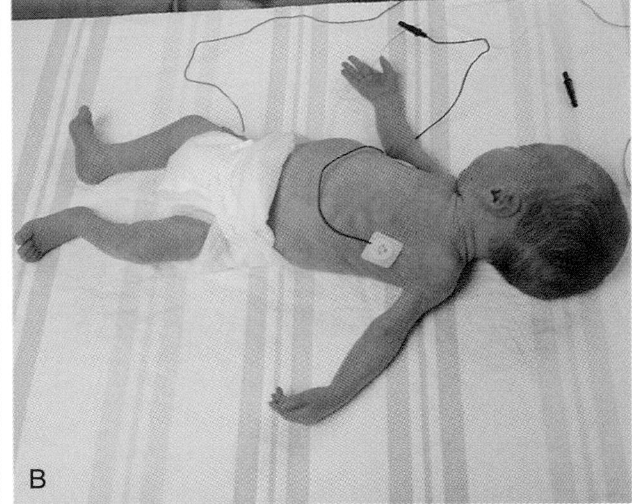

**FIGURE 20–20**

Posture in newborns. A, The healthy full-term infant remains in a strongly flexed position. B, The preterm infant's extremities are extended.

at the hips, knees, and ankles. Posture is scored from zero (0) for a limp, flaccid posture to 4 if the newborn demonstrates good flexion of all extremities.

### SQUARE WINDOW

The square window sign is elicited by bending the hand at the wrist until the palm is as flat against the forearm as possible with gentle pressure (Fig. 20–21). The angle between the palm and the forearm is measured. If the palm bends only 90 degrees (which is the extent of flexion of the adult wrist and looks like a square window), the score is 0. The gestational age of the infant is probably 32 weeks or less. If the infant's wrist does not flex to 90 degrees, the score is −1. The more mature the neonate, the smaller the angle, until the palm folds flat against the forearm at term.

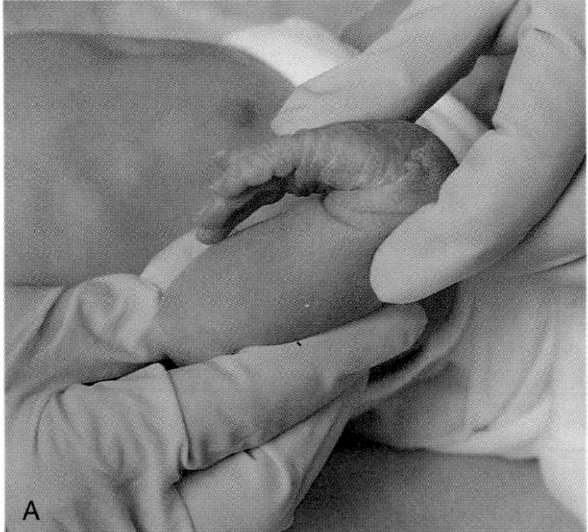

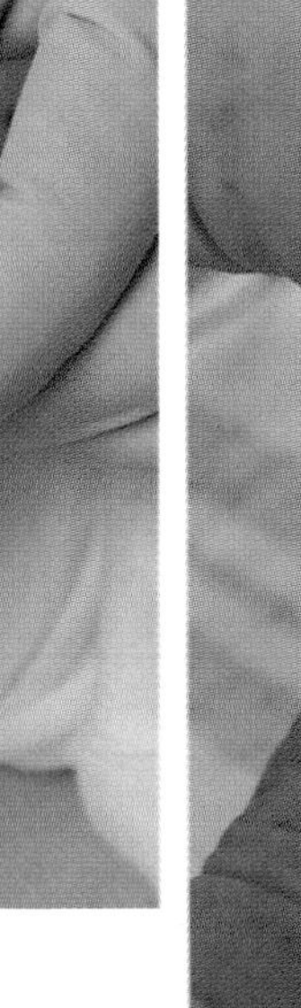

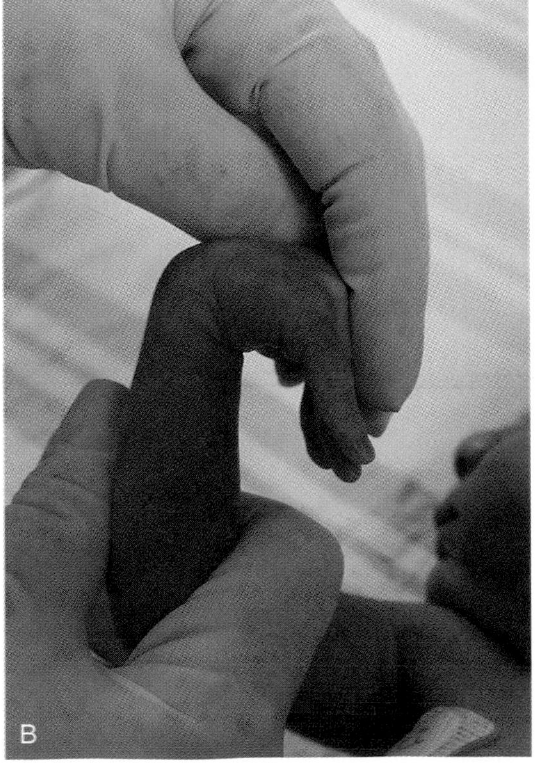

**FIGURE 20–21**

The square window sign is performed on the arm without the identification bracelet. The nurse bends the wrist and measures the angle. A, Infant near full term. B, Preterm infant.

#### ARM RECOIL

In testing for arm recoil, the nurse holds the neonate's arms fully flexed at the elbows for 5 seconds, then pulls the hands straight down to the sides (Fig. 20–22). The hands are quickly released and the degree of flexion as the arms return to their normally flexed position is measured. Preterm infants may not move the arms at all and receive a score of 0. Some-

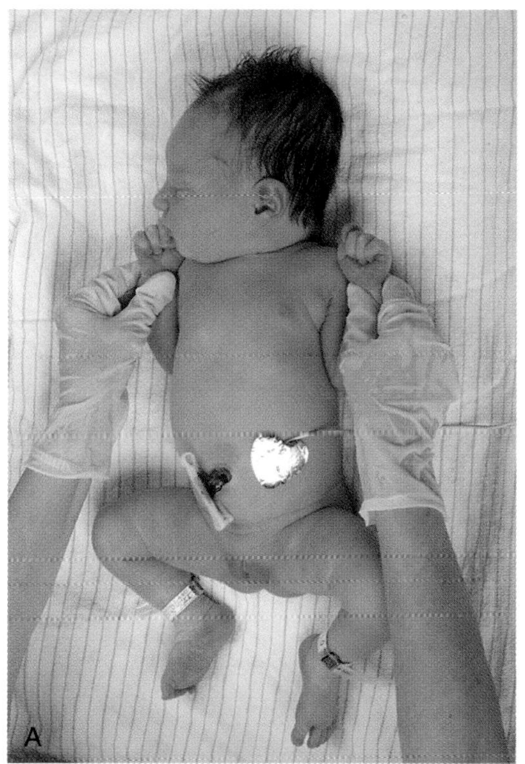


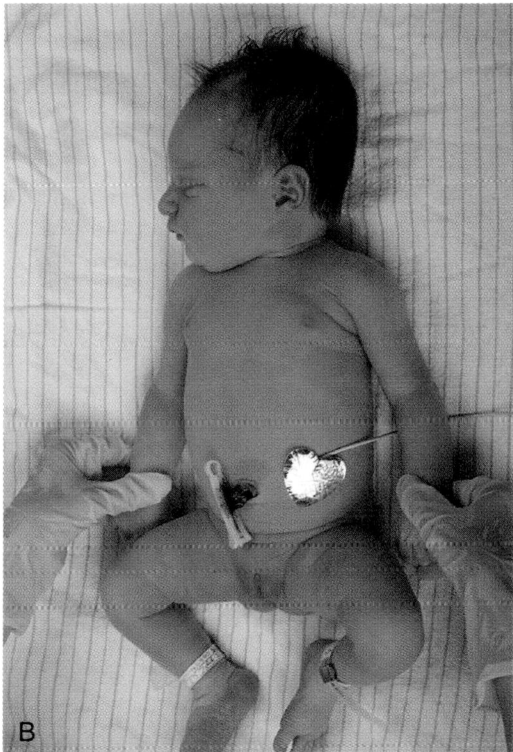


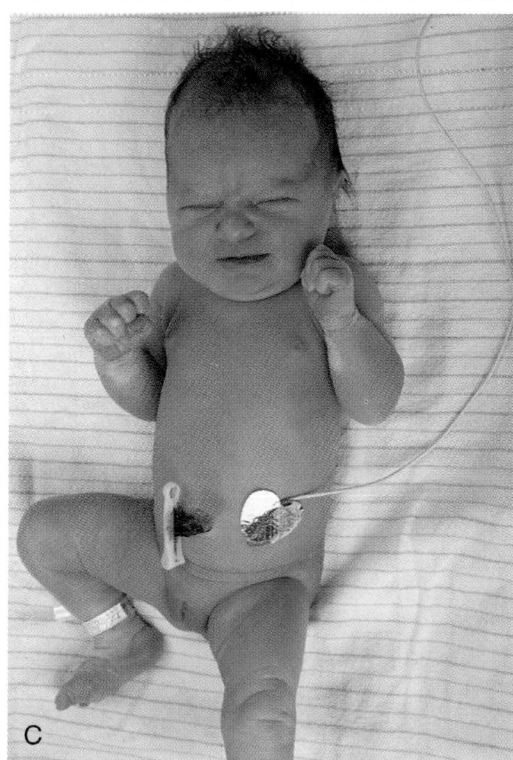


**FIGURE 20–22**

Arm recoil. A, Arms flexed. B, Arms extended. C, Recoil for the full-term infant.

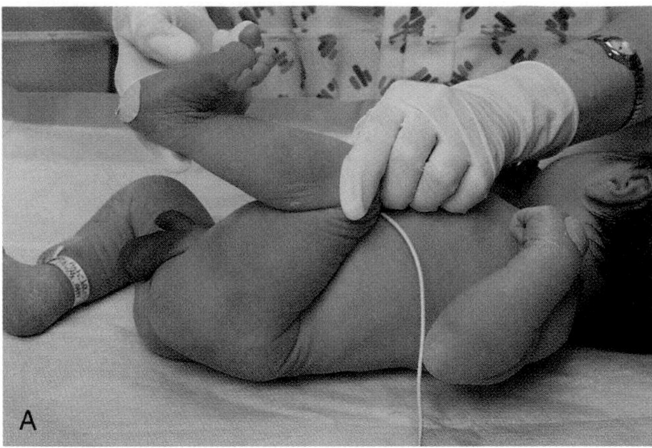


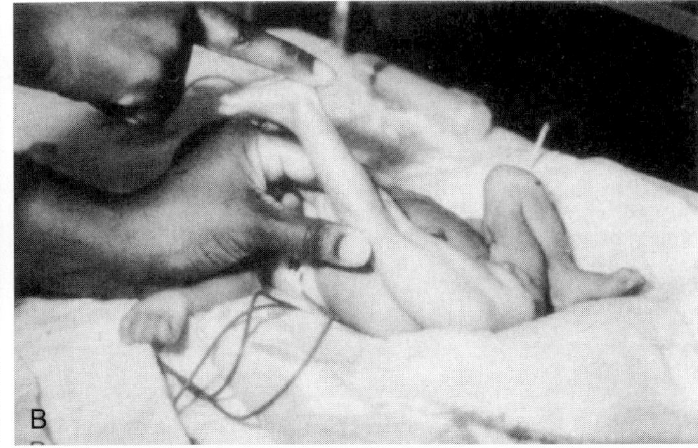


**FIGURE 20–23**

The popliteal angle is measured by flexing the thigh against the abdomen and extending the lower leg to the point of resistance. A, Full-term infant. B, Preterm infant.

what older infants have a sluggish recoil, with only partial return to flexion. If the arms move quickly to an angle of less than 90 degrees at the elbows, the score is 4.

#### POPLITEAL ANGLE

To measure the popliteal angle, the newborn's lower leg is folded against the thigh, with the thigh on the abdomen (Fig. 20–23). The infant's hips must remain flat on the bed. With the thigh still flexed on the abdomen, the lower leg is straightened just until resistance is met. Continued pressure causes the infant to further extend the leg and results in an inaccurate score. The angle at the popliteal space when resistance is first felt is scored, with a range of −1 if the leg can be fully extended to a score of 5 if the angle at the popliteal space is less than 90 degrees.

#### SCARF SIGN

For the scarf sign, the nurse grasps the infant's hand and brings the arm across the body to the opposite side (Fig. 20–24). The shoulder should not be lifted from the surface upon which the infant is lying. The position of the elbow in relation to the midline of the infant's body is noted. The infant with such poor muscle tone that the arm wraps across the body like a scarf with the elbow beyond the edge of the body receives a score of −1. A full score (4) shows that the elbow fails to reach near to midline.

#### HEEL TO EAR

The heel-to-ear assessment is similar to the measurement of the popliteal angle. However, in this case, the nurse grasps the infant's foot and pulls it straight up toward the ears while the hips remain flat on the surface of the bed (Fig. 20–25). When resistance is felt, the position of the foot in relation to the head and the amount of flexion of the leg are compared with the diagrams. The more resistance and flexion, the more mature the infant.

Record the position when resistance is first felt, as the neonate may relax the leg if pressure continues.

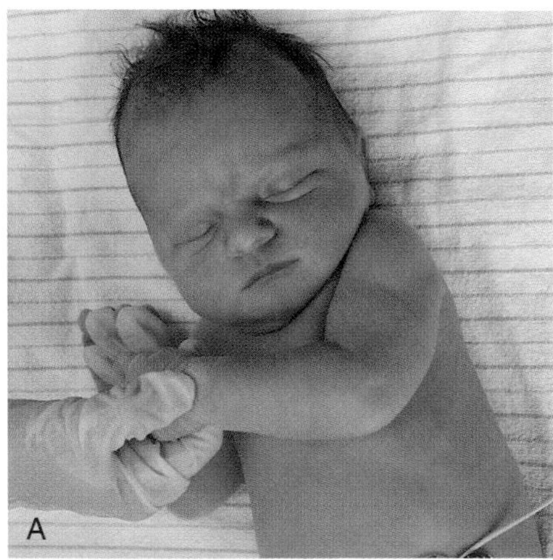


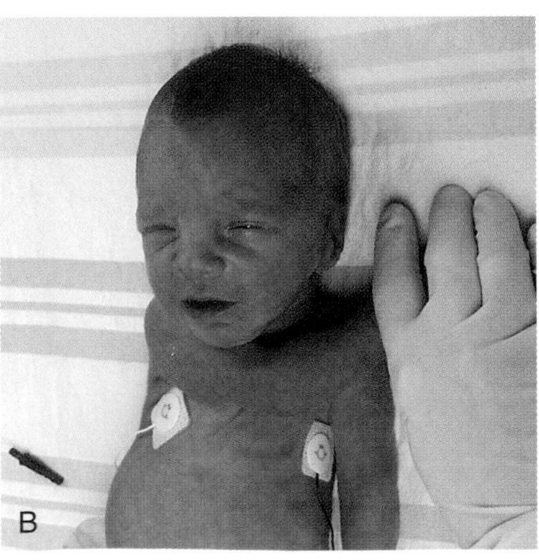


**FIGURE 20–24**

Scarf sign. The nurse determines how far the arm will move across the chest and observes the position of the elbow when resistance is felt. A, Full-term infant. B, Preterm infant. (Note the many visible veins in the preterm infant and the absence of visible veins in the full-term infant.)

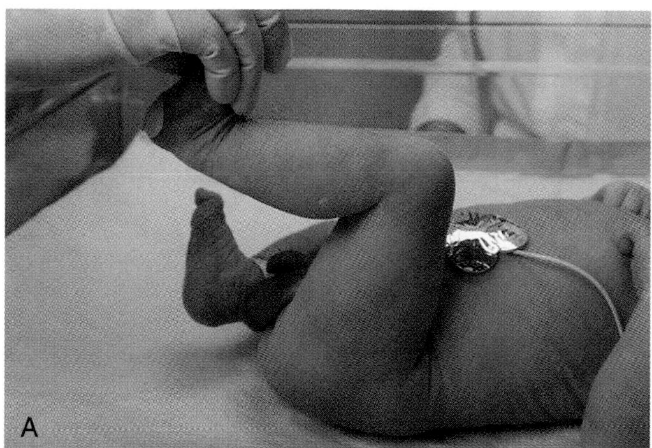


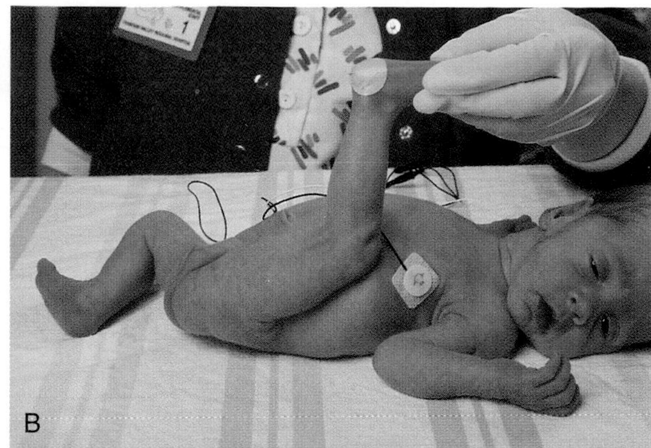


**FIGURE 20–25**

Heel to ear. The nurse grasps the foot and brings it up toward the ear, keeping the hips flat. The score is recorded when resistance is felt. A, Full-term infant. B, Preterm infant.

This assessment may be inaccurate in infants who were in a breech position at delivery because they may lie with the legs extended toward the head. It may be necessary to omit this part of the examination until later or to estimate the score temporarily.

## Physical Characteristics

### SKIN

The skin is assessed for color, visibility of veins, and peeling and cracking. The very preterm infant's skin is almost transparent because it is thin and has little subcutaneous fat beneath the surface. The skin is red, sticky, and fragile, with veins that are easily visible. In the mature newborn, the skin color is paler and few veins are visible, usually over the chest and abdomen (see Fig. 20–24). At term, vernix is present only in the creases.

The full-term infant exhibits some peeling and cracking of the skin, especially around areas with creases, such as the ankles and feet. The postmature infant has deeply cracked skin that appears as dry and thick as leather. Peeling becomes even more apparent during the hours after birth as the skin loses moisture (Fig. 20–26).

### LANUGO

Lanugo appears at 20 weeks of gestation and increases in amount until 28 to 30 weeks (see Fig. 20–13). At that time, it begins to disappear until little remains at term. A small amount may remain over the upper back and shoulders, over the ears, or on the sides of the forehead. Newborns with dark coloring may have more lanugo (which is dark and more easily noticed) than infants with fair skin and very light hair even though they are the same gestational age. The infant receives a score based on the amount of lanugo present.

### PLANTAR SURFACE

Plantar creases begin to appear at 32 weeks of gestation (Fig. 20–27). Although the creases are only red lines near the toes at first, they gradually spread down toward the heel and become deeper. At 37 weeks, creases cover the anterior two thirds of the sole. By 40 weeks, the entire sole is covered with deep creases. The plantar creases must be assessed during the early hours after birth because, as the infant's skin begins to dry, the creases appear more prominent. For the very preterm infant, the length of

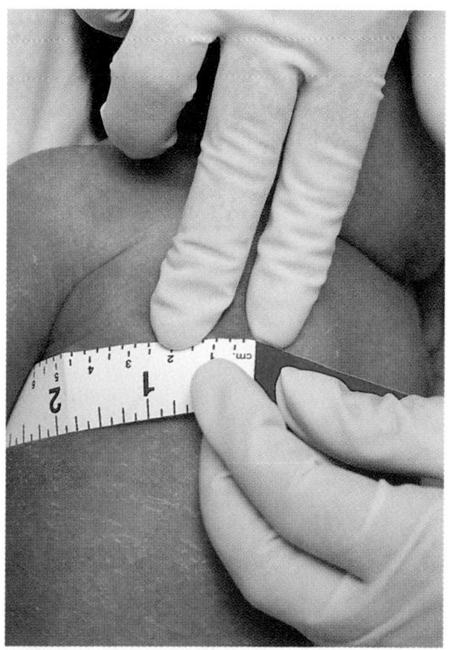

**FIGURE 20–26**

The nurse places a finger on either side of the breast bud tissue and measures the size. In the full-term infant, breast tissue is raised and the nipple is easily distinguished from surrounding skin. (Note the peeling skin.)

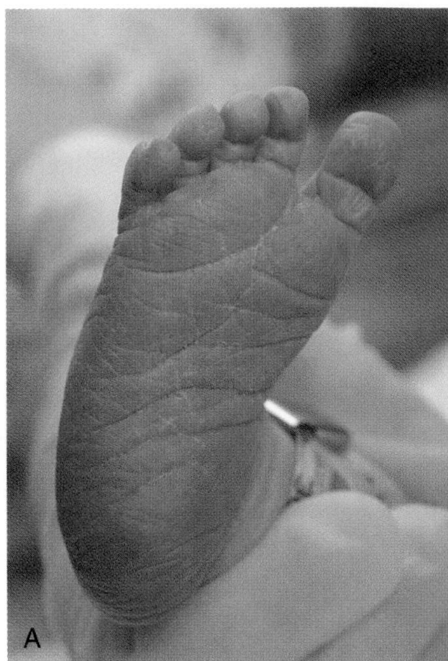


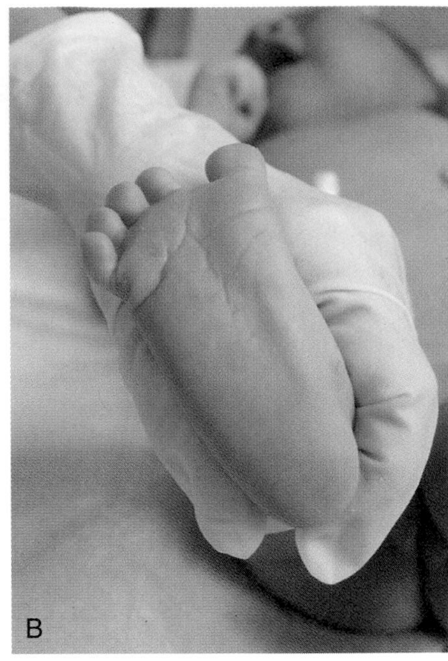


**FIGURE 20–27**

Plantar creases begin to develop at the base of the toes and extend to the heel. A, The postterm infant has deep creases. B, The preterm infant has few creases on the entire foot.

the foot is measured to help determine gestational age.

#### BREASTS

The nipples, areolae, and subcutaneous fat pads (or breast buds) are assessed and scored. In very preterm infants, the structures are not visible. Gradually they grow larger, and the areolae become raised above the chest wall. The fat pads or buds enlarge until they are approximately 1 cm at term. To determine their size, the nurse places a finger on each side and measures the diameter (see Fig. 20–26). Use of the thumb and forefinger may cause excess tissue to be drawn together, resulting in an inaccurate score.

#### EYES AND EARS

In the very preterm infant, the eyelids are fused. They open at 26 to 28 weeks. At about 33 to 34 weeks of gestation, the upper pinnae, which have been flat, begin to curve over. The incurving continues around the ear until it reaches near the earlobe

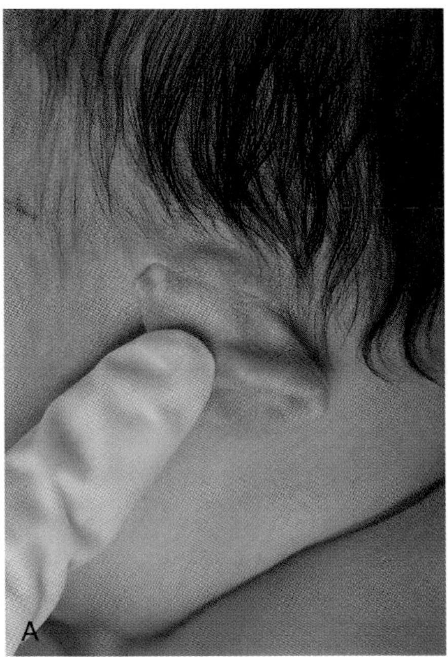


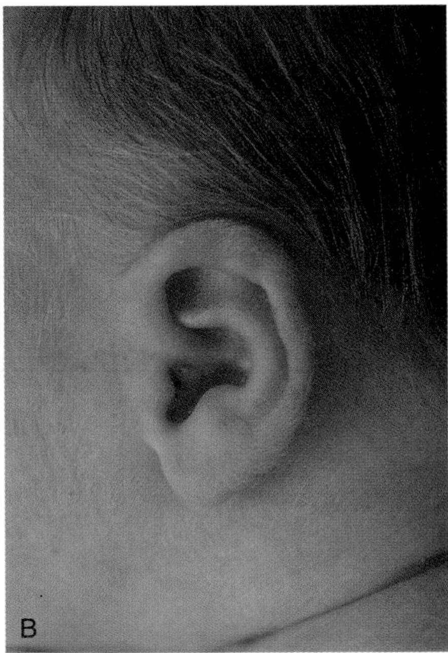


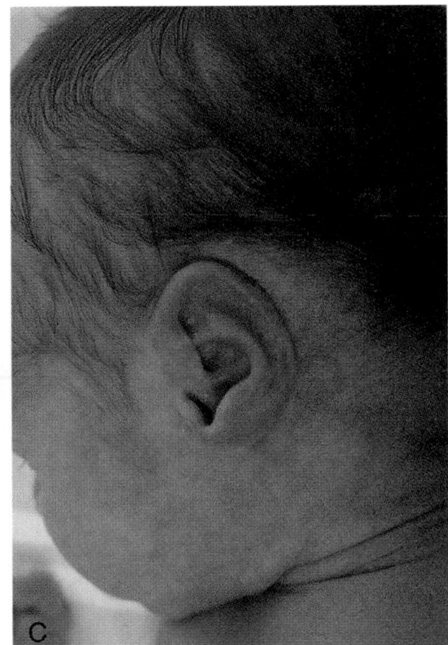


**FIGURE 20–28**

Ear maturation. A, The nurse folds the ears and notes how quickly they return to position. B, Ears in the full-term infant are well formed and have instant recoil. C, In the preterm infant, ears show less curving of the pinna and recoil slowly or not at all.

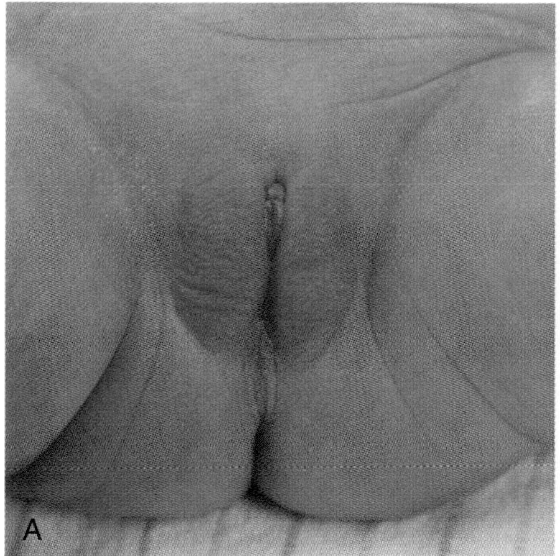


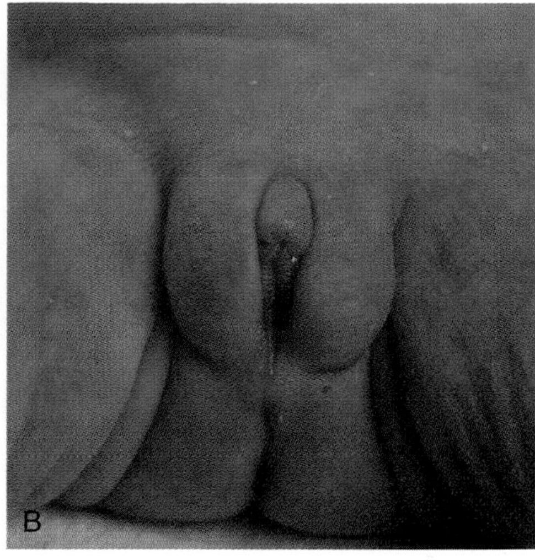


**FIGURE 20–29**

Female genitals. As the female matures, the labia majora cover the labia minora and clitoris completely; in the preterm infant, these structures are not covered. A, Near-term infant. B, Preterm infant.

at 39 to 40 weeks. The amount of cartilage present in the ears is a more accurate guide to gestational age than the curving of the pinnae because of individual differences in ear shape. As cartilage is deposited in the pinnae, the ears become stiff and stand away from the head.

In assessing the ear, the incurving and thickness of each pinna are rated (Fig. 20–28). The ear is folded longitudinally and horizontally to assess the resistance and how fast the ear returns to its original state. In infants less than 32 weeks of gestational age, the ear has little cartilage to keep it stiff. When folded, it remains folded over or returns slowly. In the term neonate, the ear springs back to its original position immediately.

### GENITALS

In the female infant, the relationship in size of the clitoris, labia minora, and labia majora is noted (Fig. 20–29). In the preterm infant, the labia majora are small and separated, whereas the clitoris and labia minora are large by comparison. As the infant nears term, the labia majora enlarge until the clitoris and labia minora are completely covered. Because the size of the labia majora is affected by the amount of fat deposited, the infant who is malnourished in utero may have genitalia with an immature appearance.

In the male infant, the location of the testes and the rugae on the scrotum are assessed (Fig. 20–30).

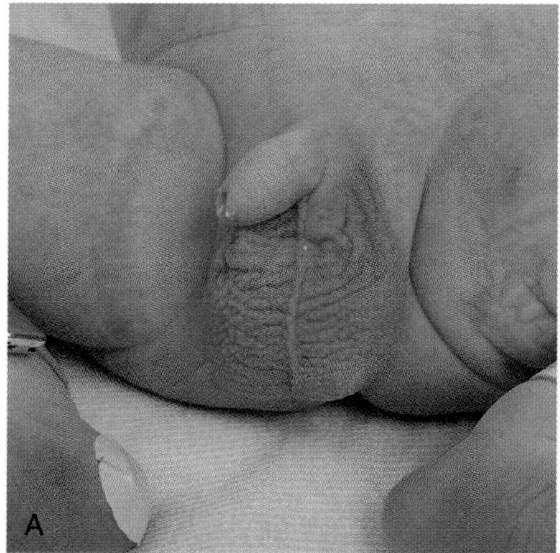


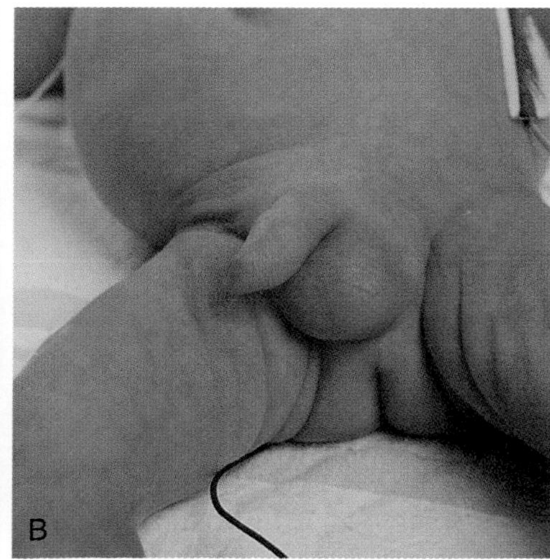


**FIGURE 20–30**

Male genitals. A, The full-term infant has a pendulous scrotum with deep rugae. B, In the preterm infant, the testes may not be descended and rugae are few.

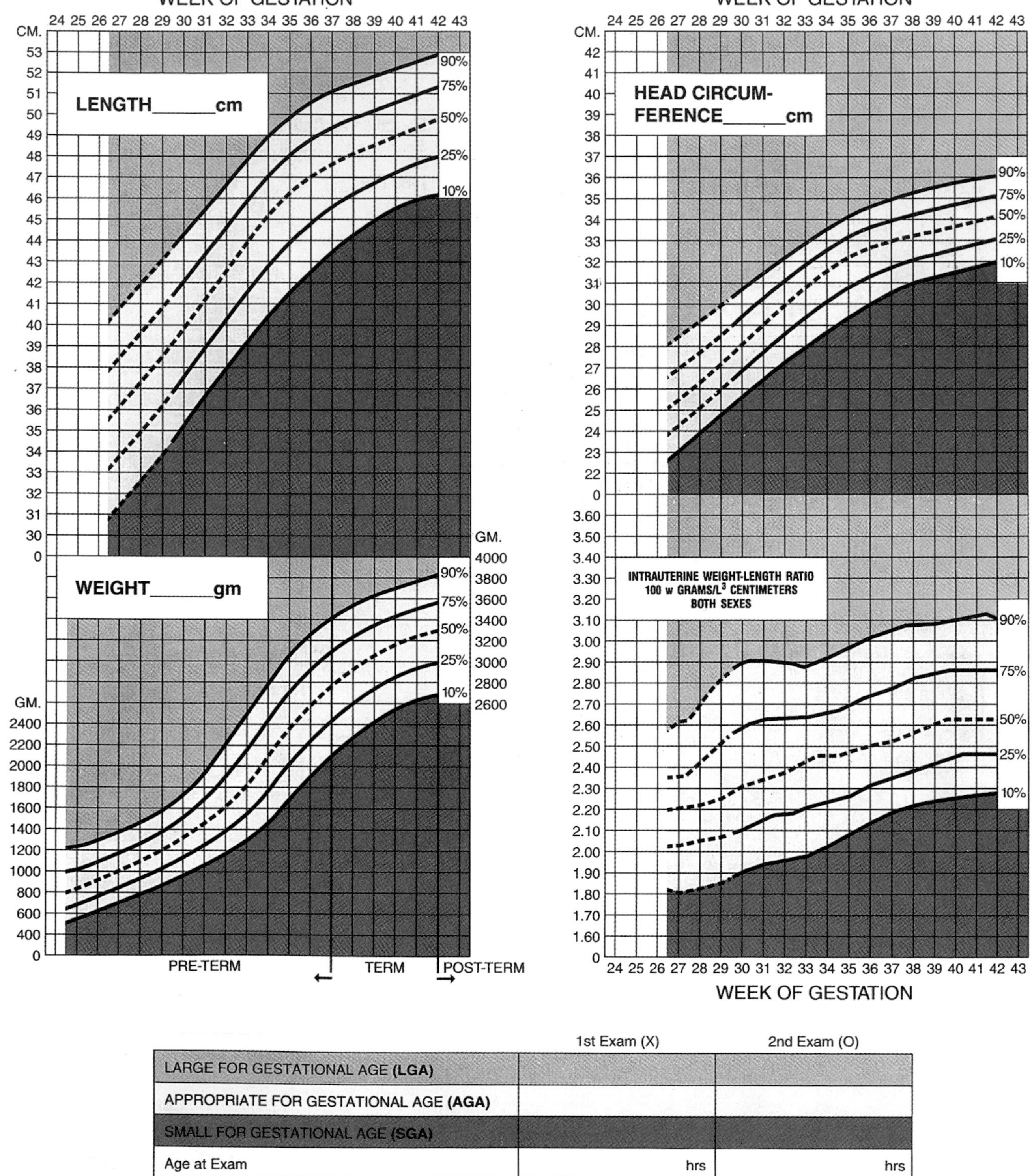


| | 1st Exam (X) | 2nd Exam (O) |
|---|---|---|
| LARGE FOR GESTATIONAL AGE **(LGA)** | | |
| APPROPRIATE FOR GESTATIONAL AGE **(AGA)** | | |
| SMALL FOR GESTATIONAL AGE **(SGA)** | | |
| Age at Exam | hrs | hrs |
| Signature of Examiner | M.D. | M.D. |

**FIGURE 20–31**

Intrauterine growth grids. (Courtesy of Bristol-Myers Company, Evansville, Indiana. Adapted from Lubchenko, L.C., Hansman, C, & Boyd, E. [1966]. *Pediatrics*, 37,403. Adapted by permission of Pediatrics, Vol. 37, p. 403, 1966; and from Battaglia, F.C., & Lubchenko, L.C. [1967]. *Journal of Pediatrics*, 71, 159.)

The testes originate in the abdominal cavity but move down into the inguinal canal at 30 weeks of gestation. By 37 weeks, they are located high in the scrotal sac, and they are generally completely descended by term. Rugae form on the surface of the scrotum beginning at about 36 weeks and cover the sac by 40 weeks. Once the testes are completely down into the scrotum, it appears large and pendulous.

### Scoring

As each part of the assessment is performed, the infant's response is matched with the diagrams and explanations on the assessment tool. The total score is compared with the corresponding gestational age. Although slight differences in the scores may be obtained by different examiners, a difference of 2.5 points is necessary to change the gestational age by 1 week. Therefore, slight differences in the scores of different examiners are not likely to cause significant differences in the outcome of the examination.

### Gestational Age and Infant Size

The appropriateness of the neonate's size for gestational age is determined by plotting the gestational age, weight, length, and head circumference on a graph of intrauterine development (Fig. 20–31). This score determines how well the infant has grown for the amount of time spent in the uterus. An infant may be small, large, or appropriate for gestational age. The infant who is appropriate for gestational age falls between the 10th and the 90th percentile on the graph. The large-for-gestational age (LGA) infant is above the 90th percentile, whereas the small-for-gestational age (SGA) infant is below the 10th percentile.

Although people sometimes think that the SGA infant is born before term, the preterm infant can be appropriate, SGA, or LGA. Similarly, the LGA infant can be born before term, at term, or beyond term. For example, an infant born at 28 weeks of gestation may have measurements that correspond to the 92nd percentile on the intrauterine growth curve chart. The infant would be LGA even though preterm. An infant judged to be 43 weeks' gestational age may have measurements that correspond to the seventh percentile on the growth curve. The infant would be SGA.

### Further Assessments

When an infant's gestational age or measurements fall outside the range expected, the nurse monitors for complications. Specific complications are common to the preterm, postterm, SGA, and LGA infant. For example, pregnancy complications may cause an SGA infant from a poorly functioning placenta. These infants are more prone to hypoglycemia as well as thermoregulation and respiratory problems.

The most common causes of an LGA infant are diabetes in the mother and very large parents. The nurse monitors these infants especially carefully for hypoglycemia and birth injuries because of the difficulty of the large infant passing through the birth canal.

## Assessment of Behavior

Assessment of the infant's behavior helps determine intactness of the central nervous system and provides information about ability to respond to caretaking activities. Because behavior differs at various times after birth, it is important for the nurse to be aware of the periods of reactivity and the six different states of behavior so that nursing care can be adapted appropriately.

### Periods of Reactivity

During the first and second periods of reactivity (see Chap. 19, p. 503), newborns may have elevated pulse and respiratory rates, low temperatures, and excessive respiratory secretions. It is important to observe infants carefully during this time, but assessment can usually be done unobtrusively so that parents can continue to enjoy their newborn. During the sleep period between the first and second periods of reactivity, newborns cannot be awakened easily and are not interested in feeding. Infants in the sleep phase have relaxed muscle tone that may affect the score on a gestational age assessment.

### Behavioral Changes

Nurses assess the infant's behavior and alert the physician of abnormalities. Assessment includes the six different behavioral states: deep sleep, active sleep, drowsy, quiet alert, active alert, and crying. Movement between states should be smooth and not abrupt. The Brazelton neonatal behavioral assessment scale is often used when detailed knowledge about the infant is needed. In addition to assessing behavioral states, the scale analyzes other aspects of the newborn's behavior, such as orientation, habituation, self-consoling behaviors, social behaviors, and the appropriateness of the amount of time in each of these activities.

#### ORIENTATION

The nurse notes the infant's orientation (ability to pay attention) to interesting visual or auditory stimuli. It is most prominent during the quiet alert state. Infants focus their eyes and turn their heads toward a stimulus in an attempt to prolong contact with it.

Preterm or ill neonates have less ability to orient to stimuli. Attempts to stimulate these newborns may result in overfatigue.

#### HABITUATION

The infant's response to a visual, auditory, or tactile stimulus is an important assessment. Generally, the first response of a healthy newborn to an interesting stimulus, such as a brightly colored object or a bell, is a period of alertness. If the stimulus is disturbing, like a bright light flashed in the eyes or a pinprick to the foot, the infant startles and attempts to escape by averting the eyes or pulling the foot away.

Infants gradually stop responding to continued noxious stimuli. This allows them to ignore the stimuli and save energy for physiologic needs. Newborns may go into a dull drowsy state or fall into a deep sleep. Those who seem unresponsive in a bright, noisy nursery may be in a state of habituation. The preterm infant or one with damage to the central nervous system may not be able to habituate.

#### SELF-CONSOLING ACTIVITIES

Normal newborns are able to console themselves for short periods of time. Self-consoling activities include attempting to bring their hands to the mouth, sucking on their fists, and watching objects in the environment. Infants who are ill, preterm, or exposed to drugs prenatally have less ability to console themselves.

#### PARENTS' RESPONSE

The parents' growing ability to respond to the infant's behavioral cues should be noted. The nurse can point out the infant's behavioral changes to facilitate bonding and help the parents learn how to interpret the infant's cues. The methods the parent's use to meet the infant's needs during different behavior states are also noted.

### CHECK YOUR READING

11. When should the first voiding occur? How often do infants void?
12. What is the nurse's responsibility regarding marks on the newborn's skin?
13. Why is the gestational age assessment important?
14. How do the periods of reactivity affect nursing care?

## SUMMARY CONCEPTS

- Nurses assess newborns immediately after birth to detect serious abnormalities. If no problems are detected with a quick assessment, a more comprehensive examination is performed.
- Molding of the head is normal during birth and may cause the head to appear misshapen. There may be caput succedaneum (localized swelling from pressure against the cervix) or a cephalhematoma (bleeding between the periosteum and the bone).
- Measurements are an important way to learn about growth before birth. Abnormal measurements alert the nurse that complications may occur.
- Assessment of cardiorespiratory status includes history, airway, color, heart sounds, pulses, and blood pressure.
- Axillary temperatures are preferred over rectal temperatures because they are safer and provide accurate measurement.
- Hypoglycemia can cause damage to the brain. Early signs of hypoglycemia include jitteriness, poor muscle tone, respiratory distress, perspiration, low temperature, and poor suck.
- In performing heel sticks for blood glucose, the nurse must choose the site carefully to avoid damage to the bone, nerves, or blood vessels of the heel.
- Reflexes are an indication of the health of the central nervous system. Asymmetry or retention of reflexes beyond the time when they should disappear is abnormal.
- The initial feeding provides information about the neonate's ability to coordinate sucking, swallowing, and breathing and tolerance to feeding.
- Newborns usually pass the first stool within 24 hours of birth. Feeding and taking a rectal temperature may stimulate stool passage. Absence of stool for 48 hours may signify an obstruction.
- The newborn's first void occurs within 24 to 48 hours. Infants void two to six times the first two days and five to 25 times daily thereafter.
- Marks on the skin should be documented, including location, size, color, elevation, and texture. Explain marks to parents, and offer emotional support if they are upset.
- The gestational age assessment provides an estimate of the infant's age from conception. It alerts the nurse to possible complications of age and development.
- During the first and second periods of reactivity, the infant may have a low temperature, elevated pulse and respirations, and excessive respiratory secretions. Between these periods, the infant is in a deep sleep with relaxed muscle tone and no interest in feeding.

### References and Readings

American Academy of Pediatrics, Committee on Fetus and Newborn. (1993). Routine evaluation of blood pressure, hematocrit, and glucose in newborns. *Pediatrics*, 92(3), 474–476.

American Academy of Pediatrics and American College of Obstetricians and Gynecologists (AAP). (1992). *Guidelines for perinatal care* (3rd ed.). Elk Grove, Ill.: American Academy of Pediatrics.

Anand, S.K. (1991). Hypertension. In H.W. Taeusch, R.A.

Ballard, & M.E. Avery (Eds.), *Schaffer's diseases of the newborn* (6th ed.). Philadelphia: W.B. Saunders.

Avery, G.B., Fletcher, M.A., & MacDonald, M.G. (Eds). (1994). *Neonatology: Pathophysiology and management of the newborn* (4th ed.). Philadelphia: J.B. Lippincott.

Association of Women's Health, Obstetric, and Neonatal Nurses (AWHONN). (1996). *Physiologic assessment of the healthy newborn*. Washington, D.C.: Author.

Ballard, J.L., Khoury, J.C., Wedig, K., Wang, L., Eilers-Walsman, B.L., & Lipp, R. (1991). New Ballard score, expanded to include extremely premature infants. *Journal of Pediatrics*, 19(3), 417–423.

Behrman, R.E., Kliegman, R.M., & Arvin, A.M. (1996). *Nelson textbook of pediatrics* (15th ed.). Philadelphia: W.B. Saunders.

Bell, E.F., & Oh, W. (1994). Fluid and electrolyte management. In G.B. Avery, M.A. Fletcher, & M.G. Macdonald (Eds.), *Neonatology: Pathophysiology and management of the newborn* (4th ed.). Philadelphia: J.B. Lippincott.

Berkowitz, C.D. (1996). *Pediatrics: A primary care approach*. Philadelphia: W.B. Saunders.

Blackburn, S.T., & Loper, D.L. (1992). *Maternal, fetal, and neonatal physiology: A clinical perspective*. Philadelphia: W.B. Saunders.

Blackburn, S.T., & VandenBerg, K.A. (1993). Assessment and management of neonatal neurobehavioral development. In C. Kenner, A. Brueggemeyer, & L.P. Gunderson (Eds.), *Comprehensive neonatal nursing, a physiologic perspective*. Philadelphia: W.B. Saunders.

Blake, W.W., & Murray, J.A. (1993). Heat balance. In G.B. Merenstein & S.L. Gardner (Eds.), *Handbook of neonatal intensive care*. St. Louis: C.V. Mosby.

Brazelton, T.B. (1994). Behavioral competence. In G.B. Avery, M.A. Fletcher, & M.G. Macdonald (Eds.), *Neonatology: Pathophysiology and management of the newborn* (4th ed.). Philadelphia: J.B. Lippincott.

de Steuben, C. (1992). Breastfeeding and jaundice: A review. *Journal of Nurse-Midwifery*, 37(Suppl. 2), 59–66.

Dodd, V. (1996). Gestational age assessment. *Neonatal Network*, 15(1), 27–36.

Dubowitz, L., & Dubowitz, V. (1977). *Gestational age of the newborn*. Reading, Mass.: Addison-Wesley.

Fletcher, M.A. (1994). Physical assessment and classification. In G.B. Avery, M.A. Fletcher, & M.G. Macdonald (Eds.), *Neonatology: Pathophysiology and management of the newborn* (4th ed.). Philadelphia: J.B. Lippincott.

Glenn, L.H. (1993). Biological and behavioral characteristics. In S. Mattson & J.E. Smith, NAACOG *core curriculum for maternal-newborn nursing*. Philadelphia: W.B. Saunders.

Gomella, T.L., Cunningham, M.D., & Eyal, F.G. (Eds.) (1994). *Neonatology* (3rd ed.). Norwalk, Conn.: Appleton & Lange.

Hagedorn, M.I., Gardner, S.L., & Abman, S.H. (1993). Respiratory diseases. In G.B. Merenstein & S.L. Gardner (Eds.), *Handbook of neonatal intensive care* (2nd ed.). St. Louis: C.V. Mosby.

Kenner, C., Brueggemeyer, A., & Gunderson, L.P. (1993). *Comprehensive neonatal nursing, a physiologic perspective*. Philadelphia: W.B. Saunders.

Lepley, C.J., Gardner, S.L., & Lubchenco, L.O. (1993). Initial nursery care. In G.B. Merenstein & S.L. Gardner (Eds.), *Handbook of neonatal intensive care*. St. Louis: C.V. Mosby.

Mattson, S., & Smith, J.E. (1993). NAACOG *core curriculum for maternal-newborn nursing*. Philadelphia: W.B. Saunders.

Miklos, A.B., & Creehan, P.A. (1996). Newborn physical assessment. In K.R. Simpson & P.A. Creehan (Eds.), AWHONN's *perinatal nursing*. Philadelphia: Lippincott-Raven.

Nicholson, J.F., & Pesce, M.A. (1996). Laboratory medicine and reference tables. In R.E. Behrman, R.M. Kliegman, & A.M. Arvin. *Nelson textbook of pediatrics* (15th ed.). Philadelphia: W.B. Saunders.

Philip, A. (1996). *Neonatology, a practical guide* (4th ed.). Philadelphia: W.B. Saunders.

Smith, J.B., Ley, S.J., Curley, M.A.Q., Elixson, E.M., & Dodds, K.M. (1996). Tissue perfusion. In M.A.Q. Curley, J.B. Smith, & P.A. Moloney-Harmon, *Critical care of infants and children*. Philadelphia: W.B. Saunders.

Tappero, E.P., & Honeyfield, M.E. (Eds.). (1993). *Physical assessment of the newborn*. Petaluma, Calif. NICU INK.

Vargo, L. (1993). Cardiovascular assessment of the newborn. In E.P. Tappero & M.E. Honeyfield (Eds.), *Physical assessment of the newborn*. Petaluma, Calif.: NICU INK.

Wong, D.L. (1995). *Nursing care of infants and children* (5th ed.). St. Louis: C.V. Mosby.

# 21

# Care of the Normal Newborn

**OBJECTIVES**

1. Describe the purpose and use of routine prophylactic medications for the normal newborn.
2. Explain the nurse's responsibility in cardiorespiratory and thermoregulatory assessments and care.
3. Describe collaborative interventions for hypoglycemia.
4. Discuss prevention and parent teaching for jaundice.
5. Explain the risks and benefits of circumcision.
6. Describe the care of circumcised and uncircumcised male infants.
7. Describe ongoing nursing assessments and care of the newborn.
8. Describe methods of protecting newborns by proper identification.
9. Explain how nurses can help prevent infant abductions.
10. Describe methods of preventing infections in newborns.
11. Discuss important considerations in parent teaching.
12. Explain the importance of newborn screening tests.

The role of the nurse in ongoing assessments and care of the newborn is to help the newborn and parents have a successful transition after birth. To do this the nurse identifies changes in the condition of newborns as they adapt to life outside the uterus, keeps infants safe, and teaches parents how to provide care.

## Clinical Pathways

One way to assist parents and infants to reach the goal of successful transition after childbirth is the use of clinical pathways, introduced in Chapter 1. These guides are developed by birth facilities to see that all the necessary tasks involved in helping infants and mothers prepare for discharge are accomplished in the time available. They are also used to see that mothers and infants meet the criteria for discharge. Figure 21–1 provides one example of a clinical pathway for newborns. Pathways are individualized by each institution based on protocols to meet the needs of their clients.

## Early Care

Early care after birth involves assessment, the assignment of Apgar scores, and stabilization of the infant as necessary. Immediate care is discussed on page 332, and infant resuscitation is discussed on page 849. Once the infant is stable, prophylactic medications are given.

Two prophylactic medications are administered to the infant soon after birth. They are vitamin K, to prevent hemorrhagic disease of the newborn, and erythromycin, to prevent ophthalmia neonatorum.

### Administering Vitamin K

Vitamin K is given to the neonate within the first hour after birth (Procedure 21–1 and Drug Guide: Vitamin $K_1$ [Phytonadione]). Although vitamin K is available in oral form, current recommendations are that it be given intramuscularly (AAP, 1993). Because infants cannot synthesize vitamin K in the intestines without bacterial flora, they are deficient in clotting factors. One dose of vitamin K prevents bleeding problems until the infant is able to produce it on his or her own.

### Providing Eye Treatment

All infants receive prophylactic treatment to prevent ophthalmia neonatorum in case the mother is infected with gonorrhea or *Chlamydia*. Currently, the most common medication for eye prophylaxis is erythromycin (Fig. 21–2 and Drug Guide: Erythromycin Ophthalmic Ointment).

Some infants develop a mild inflammation a few hours after prophylactic treatment. However, any discharge from the eyes, especially if it is purulent, should alert the nurse to the possibility of infection. Drainage should be removed with sterile saline and cotton. If the mother is infected, the infant needs additional antibiotics because routine prophylactic treatment may not completely prevent infection.

Because the ointment may temporarily blur the infant's vision, parents may wish to delay treatment for a short time during initial bonding. It may be delayed for as long as an hour after birth without adverse effects.

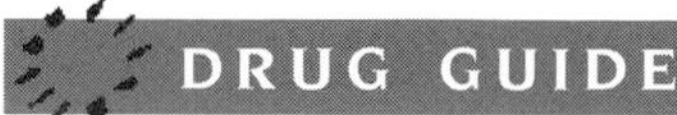


## VITAMIN $K_1$ (Phytonadione)

***Classification:*** Fat-soluble vitamin

***Other Names:*** AquaMEPHYTON, Konakion

***Action:*** Promotes the formation of Factors II (prothrombin), VII, IX, and X by the liver for clotting. Provides vitamin K, which is not synthesized in the intestines for the first 5 to 8 days after birth because the newborn lacks intestinal flora necessary for vitamin K production.

***Indication:*** Prevention or treatment of hemorrhagic disease of the newborn.

***Neonatal Dosage and Route:*** 0.5 to 1 mg (0.25 to 0.5 ml) given once intramuscularly within 1 hour of birth for prophylaxis. (The lower dose may be used for small infants weighing less than 2500 g.) May be repeated or higher doses used if the mother took oral anticoagulants or anticonvulsants during pregnancy. May be repeated if the infant shows bleeding tendencies.

***Absorption:*** Readily absorbed after intramuscular injection. Effective within 1 to 2 hours.

***Adverse Reactions:*** Pain and edema at site of administration. Hemolysis or hyperbilirubinemia, especially in a preterm infant or when large doses are used.

***Nursing Considerations:*** Protect the drug from light until just before administration, as it decomposes and loses potency on exposure to light. Incompatible with other drugs. Observe all infants for signs of vitamin K deficiency: ecchymoses or bleeding from any site.

## Application of Nursing Process: Cardiorespiratory Status

In the early newborn period, problems of transition may include temporary problems in cardiorespiratory status. If identified and managed promptly, most resolve within a short time.

*Text continued on page 556*

**YORK HOSPITAL**
YORK, PENNSYLVANIA
**CLINICAL PATHWAY**

**NEWBORN**

| CLINICAL PATH DAY | | EXPECTED PATIENT/ FAMILY OUTCOMES | MULTIDISCIPLINARY ASSESSMENT | TESTS | CONSULT |
|---|---|---|---|---|---|
| Immediate Newborn Care | Date & Time | ☐ Apgar score >7 at 5 min. [4]<br>☐ Maintains axillary temp of 36.5C to 37.2C while in radiant warmer or in double blankets [1]<br>☐ Physiologic parameters WNL [4}<br>☐ Demonstrates proper latch when breastfeeding [2] | ☐ Apgar score 1 & 5 min.<br>☐ Transitional newborn assessment q 30 min.<br>☐ Suck reflex | ☐ Hypoglycemia protocol when indicated | ☐ ____________ |
| Newborn Admission | Date & Time | ☐ Maintains axillary temp of 36.5C to 37.2C while in radiant warmer or in double blankets [1]<br>☐ Physiologic parameters WNL [4]<br>☐ Tolerates initial feeding [2]<br>☐ Mother's blood type O/Rh-<br>☐ ____________ | ☐ Weight<br>☐ V/S q 30 min x 4<br>☐ Multisystem admission assessment<br>☐ Suck reflex<br>☐ ____________ | ☐ Hypoglycemia protocol when indicated<br>☐ ____________ | ☐ ____________<br>☐ ____________ |
| Day of Birth | Date | N D E<br>☐☐☐ Maintains axillary temp of 36.5C to 37.2C independent of external heat source [1]<br>☐☐☐ Parents/family verbalize understanding of safety & security measures [6]<br>☐☐☐ Physiologic parameters WNL [4]<br>☐☐☐ Parent(s)/family & infant demonstrate attachment behaviors [3]<br>☐☐☐ Feeding [2]<br>☐☐☐ Latch score is 7 or greater for breastfed newborn [2]<br>☐☐☐ No jaundice [4]<br>☐☐☐ Infant seen by physician within 12 hours [6] | N D E<br>☐☐☐ Temp, apical pulse, neuro, cardiac, resp., GI, GU, integ. q shift<br>☐☐☐ Parent/infant attachment<br>☐☐☐ Positioning and LATCH score of breastfed newborn<br>☐☐☐ Freq. and amount of bottlefeeding<br>☐☐☐ ____________ | N D E<br>☐☐☐ Hypoglycemia protocol when indicated<br>☐☐☐ ____________ | N D E<br>☐☐☐ ____________<br>☐ Social service consult if indicated |

| NAME | INITIALS | NAME | INITIALS |
|---|---|---|---|
| | | | |
| | | | |

8035 (4/96)

**FIGURE 21-1**

An example of a clinical pathway for the newborn from birth through the second day and discharge. This form is printed on both sides, and is used by all caregivers to plan and document care. (Courtesy of Women and Children Services of the York Health System, York, Pennsylvania. Modified with permission.)

**DOCUMENTATION CODES**
Initial = Meets Standard
★ = Exception on pathway identified
C = Chronic problems
N/A = Not applicable

**PATIENT/FAMILY PROBLEMS**
1. Thermoregulation
2. Nutrition
3. Parent-Infant attachment
4. Potential alteration in newborn metabolism
5. Risk for infection
6. Infant safety
7. ______
8. ______

| TREATMENTS | MEDS | NUTR. | EDUC & DC PLANNING |
|---|---|---|---|
| ☐ Clamp cord<br>☐ Dry newborn<br>☐ Radiant warmer or double blanket while being held until temp stable<br>☐ ID bands | ☐ Neonatal eye prophylaxis & Aquamephyton<br>☐ HBIG if indicated | ☐ Determine if bottlefeeding or breastfeeding<br>☐ Assist with initial breastfeeding | ☐ Initiate safety & security measures with parents/family<br>☐ Teach breastfeeding mother proper latch |
| ☐ Cord care<br>☐ Admission bath | ☐ ______ | Initial feeding:<br>☐ ______ | |
| N D E<br>☐☐☐ Cord care<br>☐☐☐ Circumcision care when indicated<br>☐☐☐ ______ | N D E<br>☐☐☐ ______ | N D E<br>☐☐☐ Breast/bottle feed on demand (breast: q 2–3 hrs, bottle: q 3–4 hrs) | N D E<br>☐☐☐ Reinforce safety and security measures w/ parents/family<br>☐☐☐ Observe & reinforce proper latch and instruct breastfeeding mother/family in alternative positioning<br>☐☐☐ Give and review new pamphlets:<br>-Message to mothers<br>-Newborn screening<br>-Car seat<br>-Health insurance for newborns<br>-Preparing formula<br>-Breastfeeding, A Guide for Success |

| NAME | INITIALS | NAME | INITIALS |
|---|---|---|---|
| | | | |
| | | | |

**FIGURE 21–1** *Continued*

*Illustration continued on following page*

| CLINICAL PATH DAY | | EXPECTED PATIENT/ FAMILY OUTCOMES | MULTIDISCIPLINARY ASSESSMENT | TESTS | CONSULT |
|---|---|---|---|---|---|
| Day 1 | Date | N D E<br>Maintains axillary temp of 36.5C to 37.2C independent of external heat source [1]<br>Parent(s)/family & newborn demonstrate attachment behaviors [3]<br>Physiologic parameters WNL [4]<br>Feeding [2]<br>LATCH score 7 or greater for breastfed newborn [2]<br>No jaundice [4]<br>No signs of infection [5]<br>__________ | N D E<br>Temp, apical pulse, cardiac, resp., neuro, GI, GU, integ. q 8 hr.<br>N/A N/A Weight<br>Parent(s)/family & infant attachment behaviors<br>LATCH score of breastfed newborn<br>Frequency & amt. of bottle feeding<br>__________ | N D E<br>__________ | N D E<br>Referral made to lactation consultant for LATCH score <7<br>__________ |
| Day 2 | Date | Maintains axillary temp of 36.5C to 37.2C independent of external heat source [1]<br>Parent(s)/family & newborn demonstrate attachment behaviors [3]<br>Physiologic parameters WNL [4]<br>Feeding [2]<br>LATCH score 7 or greater for breastfed newborn [2]<br>No jaundice [4]<br>No signs of infection [5]<br>__________ | Temp, apical pulse, cardiac, resp., neuro, GI, GU, integ. q 8 hr.<br>N/A N/A Weight<br>Parent(s)/family & infant attachment behaviors<br>LATCH score of breastfed newborn<br>Frequency & amt. of bottle feeding<br>__________ | __________ | Referral made to lactation consultant for LATCH score <7<br>__________ |
| Discharge | Date | Maintains axillary temp of 36.5C to 37.2C independent of external heat source [1]<br>Parent(s)/family & newborn demonstrate attachment behaviors and appropriate care of newborn [3]<br>Physiologic parameters WNL [4]<br>Circumcision w/o bleeding [5]<br>Voided at least x 1 [4]<br>Stooled at least x 1 [4]<br>Feeding [2]<br>LATCH score 7 or greater for breastfed newborn [2]<br>Parent(s)/family verbalize newborn D/C instruction [6]<br>No jaundice [4]<br>Physician aware of Coombs results<br>Discharge Day 2<br>No signs of infection | Temp, apical pulse, cardiac, resp., neuro, GI, GU, integ. q 8 hr.<br>Discharge weight<br>Parent(s)/family & infant attachment behaviors<br>LATCH score of breastfed newborn<br>Frequency & amt. of bottle feeding<br>__________ | Newborn screening tests prior to D/C<br>__________ | Referral made to lactation consultant for LATCH score <7<br>__________ |

| NAME | INITIALS | NAME | INITIALS |
|---|---|---|---|
| | | | |
| | | | |

NOTE: EACH PATIENT REQUIRES AN INDIVIDUAL ASSESSMENT & TREATMENT PLAN. THIS CLINICAL PATH IS A RECOMMENDATION FOR THE AVERAGE PATIENT WHICH REQUIRES MODIFICATION WHEN NECESSARY BY THE PROFESSIONAL STAFF.

**FIGURE 21-1** *Continued*

| TREATMENTS | MEDS | NUTR. | EDUC & DC PLANNING |
|---|---|---|---|
| N D E<br>N/A N/A Cord care<br>Circumcision care when indicated<br>________ | N D E<br>________ | N D E<br>Breast/bottle feed on demand (breast: q 2–3 hrs, bottle: q 3–4 hrs) | N D E<br>Observe return demonst. of breast-feeding mother's use of<br>-alternative positioning<br>-infant's suck, swallow<br>Observe parent(s) providing appropriate newborn care; reinforce.<br>________ |
| N/A N/A Cord care<br>Circumcision care when indicated<br>________ | ________ | Breast/bottle feed on demand (breast: q 2–3 hrs, bottle: q 3–4 hrs) | Observe return demonst. of breast-feeding mother's use of<br>-alternative positioning<br>-infant's suck, swallow<br>Observe parent(s) providing appropriate newborn care; reinforce.<br>________ |
| Cord care<br>Circumcision care when indicated<br>Cord clamp removed prior to D/C<br>________ | Hepatitis B vaccine per order<br>________ | NPO for circumcision when indicated<br>Breast/bottle feed on demand (breast: q 2–3 hrs, bottle: q 3–4 hrs) | Review D/C instructions with parent(s)/family<br>Discuss plan for follow-up care<br>D/C to mother's care |

| NAME | INITIALS | NAME | INITIALS |
|---|---|---|---|
| | | | |
| | | | |

**FIGURE 21–1** *Continued*

## Procedure 21-1

# Administering Intramuscular Injections to Newborns

**PURPOSE:** To place medication in the muscle without injury.

1. **Prepare medication for injection. Use a 1-ml syringe with a 5/8-inch 25-gauge needle. If the medication is in a glass ampule, use a filter needle to draw it up. Remove the filter needle and replace the original sterile needle to give the injection.** *A small needle reaches the newborn's muscle but avoids the possibility of striking the bone. Use of a filter needle prevents particles of glass from being drawn into the syringe.*

2. **Put on gloves.** *Protects the nurse from contamination with blood.*

3. **Locate the correct site. Intramuscular medication for an infant is given in the vastus lateralis muscle or, if necessary, the rectus femoris muscle. Divide the area between the greater trochanter of the femur and the knee into thirds. Give the injection in the middle third of the muscle, lateral to the midline of the anterior thigh.** *The large vastus lateralis muscle is located away from the sciatic nerve, femoral artery, and femoral vein. The rectus femoris muscle is located nearer to these structures and poses more of a danger.* (**Note:** *The dorsogluteal muscle is never used until a child has been walking for at least a year. These muscles are poorly developed and dangerously near the sciatic nerve.*)

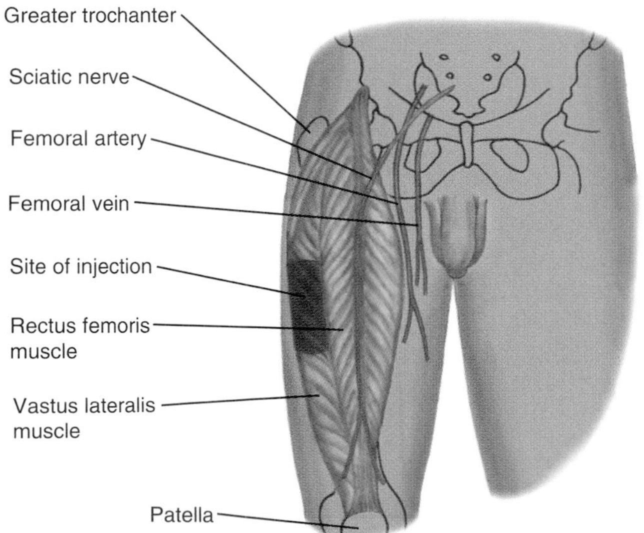


4. **Cleanse the area with an alcohol wipe.** *Removes organisms and prevents infection. (If the area is covered with thick vernix caseosa and/or blood, wash the area first.)*

5. **Stabilize the leg firmly while grasping the thigh between the thumb and fingers.** *Prevents sudden movement by the infant and possible injury.*

6. **Insert the needle at a 90-degree angle.** *Places the medication into the muscle rather than the subcutaneous tissue.*

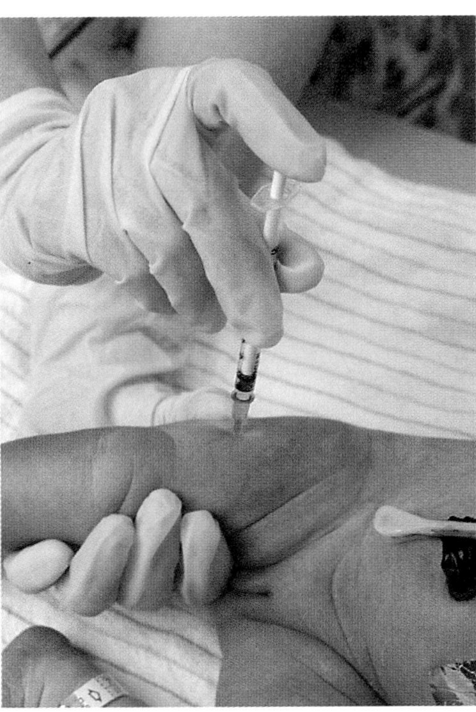

7. **Aspirate and inject the medication slowly if there is no blood return. If blood returns, withdraw the needle. Discard the medication and syringe and prepare new medication.** *Blood return on aspiration indicates that the needle is in a blood vessel. Slow injection reduces discomfort.*

8. **Withdraw the needle quickly and massage the site with alcohol wipe.** *Both increase comfort. Massage helps absorption of medication.*

## Assessment

Assess the newborn for signs of difficult transition to newborn life. Note the rate and character of the heart rate, respirations, and breath sounds. Look for signs of respiratory distress, including tachypnea, retractions, flaring of the nares, pallor or cyanosis, grunting, seesaw respirations, and asymmetry. Check pulses and blood pressure.

## Analysis

Fluid from the lungs must be removed by absorption or drainage from the respiratory passages after birth.

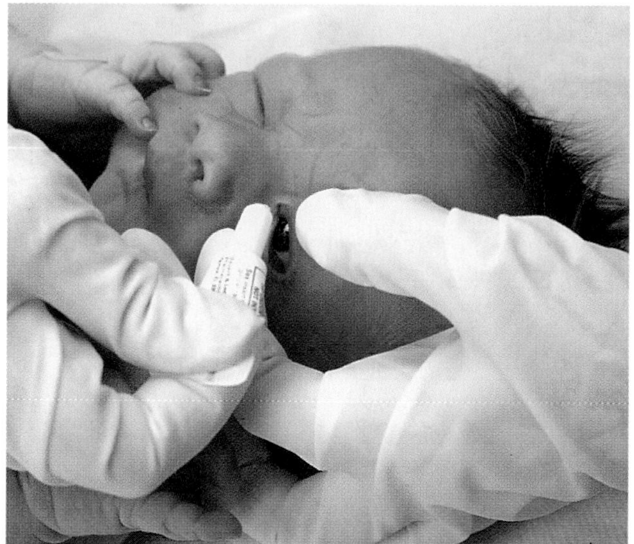

**FIGURE 21–2**

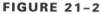

Administration of ophthalmic ointment. The nurse gently cleans the eyes of blood or vernix using sterile saline. Then, placing a finger and thumb near the edge of each lid, the nurse gently presses against the periorbital ridges to open the eyes, avoiding pressing on the eye itself. A ribbon of ointment is squeezed into each conjunctival sac.

This does not happen immediately and may cause a temporary problem during the early hours after birth. One of the most common nursing diagnoses for the newborn is Ineffective Airway Clearance related to excessive secretions in the respiratory passages.

## Planning

The goals for this nursing diagnosis are that the newborn do the following:

- Maintain a patent airway with a respiratory rate within the normal range of 30 to 60 breaths per minute.
- Show no signs of respiratory distress.

## Interventions

### POSITIONING THE INFANT

Position the infant with the head slightly lower than the extremities to aid in draining fluid from the respiratory passages immediately after birth. Use this position briefly whenever the infant is having difficulty clearing the airways, such as during regurgitation. Do not leave the infant in a head-dependent position longer than necessary because pressure from the intestines may interfere with movement of the diaphragm.

### SUCTIONING SECRETIONS

Use the bulb syringe frequently to suction secretions as they drain into the infant's mouth or nose (Procedure 21–2). Suction the mouth first because the infant may gasp when the nose is suctioned, and aspiration could occur if mucus or fluid is in the mouth. Then gently suction the nose, taking care to avoid trauma to the delicate mucous membranes. (Trauma could cause edema and occlude the passages.) Keep the bulb syringe in the crib near the infant's head, where it is available if needed quickly. Teach both parents how to use the bulb syringe correctly. Send the syringe home with the infant so that the parents can use it if the infant experiences a problem.

If mechanical suctioning is necessary to remove deeper secretions, choose a small catheter to avoid damaging the tissues of the respiratory tract. Suction for no more than 5 seconds at a time using minimal negative pressure to avoid trauma, laryngospasm, and bradycardia.

### PROVIDING CONTINUING CARE

Continue monitoring the infant for problems throughout the stay at the birth facility. By the time of the second period of reactivity, the infant may be alone with the mother without constant attendance by the nurse. Although nurses know that regurgita-

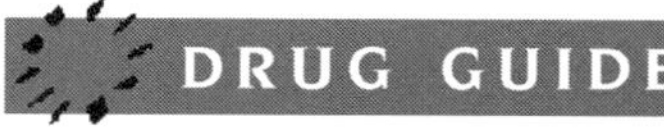

DRUG GUIDE

## ERYTHROMYCIN OPHTHALMIC OINTMENT

***Classification:*** Antibiotic

***Action:*** Inhibits cell wall replication in bacteria

***Indications:*** Prophylaxis against the organisms *Neisseria gonorrhoeae* and *Chlamydia trachomatis*. Prevents ophthalmia neonatorum in infants of mothers infected with gonorrhea and conjunctivitis in infants of mothers infected with *Chlamydia*. Prophylaxis against gonorrhea is required by law for all infants, whether or not the mother is known to be infected.

***Neonatal Dosage and Route:*** A "ribbon" of 0.5 percent erythromycin ointment, 0.5 to 1 cm (0.25 to 0.5 inch) long, is applied to the lower conjunctival sac of each eye within 1 hour after birth. May also be used in drop form.

***Adverse Reaction:*** Irritation may result in chemical conjunctivitis, lasting 24 to 48 hours. Ointment may cause temporary blurred vision.

***Nursing Considerations:*** Cleanse the infant's eyes before application, as needed. Hold the tube in a horizontal rather than a vertical position to prevent injury to the eye from sudden movement. Administer from the inner canthus to the outer canthus. Do not touch the tip of the tube to any part of the eye, as this may spread infectious material from one eye to the other. Do not rinse. Ointment may be wiped from outer eye after 1 minute. Observe for irritation. Use a new tube for each infant to prevent spread of infection. Other medications used for prevention of gonorrhea include tetracycline and silver nitrate solution.

## Nursing Care Plan 21–1
# The Normal Newborn

**ASSESSMENT:** Nicholas, a full-term newborn, was delivered after 18 hours of normal labor. He weighs 7 pounds, 8 ounces and is 20 inches long. His parents, Vicki and Peter, are happy and excited about their first baby. Nicholas receives Apgar scores of 8 at 1 minute and 9 at 5 minutes. During the initial assessment, Nicholas has an excessive amount of mucus. His respiratory rate is 62, apical pulse is 156, and breath sounds are slightly moist. He has mild substernal retractions. His color is pink with acrocyanosis.

### Critical Thinking

Should the nurse worry about Nicholas, based on the assessment above? What other signs would indicate a serious problem?

**ANSWER**

The infant's condition is not unusual immediately after birth. The nurse should be concerned if Nicholas develops central cyanosis, flaring of the nares, grunting, or further increases in pulse and respiratory rate or if signs do not improve during the first hour or two after birth.

**NURSING DIAGNOSIS:** Risk for Ineffective Airway Clearance related to excessive secretions in airways

**GOALS/EXPECTED OUTCOMES**

1. Nicholas will maintain a patent airway and have no signs of respiratory distress throughout birth facility stay as demonstrated by respiratory rate of 30 to 60 breaths per minute, clear breath sounds, and no cyanosis, retractions, flaring, or grunting.
2. Before discharge, Vicki and Peter will demonstrate correct use of the bulb syringe and verbalize when it should be used.

| INTERVENTION | RATIONALE |
|---|---|
| 1. Place Nicholas in a side-lying position with his head slightly lower than the rest of his body just until drainage has occurred. | 1. A head-down position uses gravity to facilitate drainage of secretions from the airways. |
| 2. Use a bulb syringe to suction the mouth. If the nose also requires suctioning, suction it after suctioning the mouth. | 2. Suctioning removes secretions. Suctioning the mouth first prevents aspiration of oral secretions should Nicholas gasp when his nose is suctioned. |
| 3. Change the infant's position frequently. | 3. Position changes promote expansion and drainage of all parts of the lungs. |
| 4. Demonstrate and explain use of the bulb syringe to Vicki and Peter. Assess their ability and make suggestions as needed during a return demonstration. | 4. Demonstration and return demonstration help ensure that parents learn correct techniques. |
| 5. Continue to observe Nicholas for signs of respiratory distress. Count pulse and respirations every 30 minutes until they have been stable for 2 hours. Once they are stable, assess vital signs every 8 hours, or according to birth facility procedure. Increase frequency of assessment if there is any sign of abnormality. Continue to assess for other signs of ineffective airway clearance and respiratory difficulty, such as cyanosis, retractions, flaring, and grunting. | 5. Monitoring should be based on history of excessive mucus, ability to cope with mucus, and other signs of respiratory difficulty and changes in the infant's condition. |

**EVALUATION**

Nicholas maintains a patent airway throughout his birth facility stay. His breath sounds are clear within 3 hours of birth, and his respiratory rate stays within normal limits. He has no signs of respiratory difficulty. Vicki and Peter use the bulb syringe to suction Nicholas appropriately.

**ASSESSMENT:** Nicholas's axillary temperature ranges from 36.2 to 36.8°C (97.2 to 98.2°F). When he has less problem with mucus, Peter and Vicki are anxious to hold him. As they admire their infant, they frequently unwrap him and leave him uncovered. When reminded about the need to keep Nicholas warm, Peter states, "It seems hot in here to me. Will he get too warm with so many blankets?"

## Nursing Care Plan 21–1 *Continued*

# The Normal Newborn

**NURSING DIAGNOSIS:** Risk for Ineffective Thermoregulation related to parental lack of knowledge of newborn thermoregulation abilities and needs

**GOALS/EXPECTED OUTCOMES**

Nicholas will maintain a temperature within the normal range of 36.5 to 37.5°C (97.7 to 99.5°F) axillary throughout his birth facility stay.

Peter and Vicki will verbalize and practice methods of preventing heat loss for their son by the end of the first day.

| INTERVENTION | RATIONALE |
|---|---|
| 1. Explain the reasons why newborns have problems with thermoregulation. | 1. When parents understand the reasons behind precautions given them, they are more likely to practice them. |
| 2. Teach Vicki and Peter to dry Nicholas promptly whenever he is wet, such as during bathing and when changing wet diapers or clothing. | 2. Heat loss from evaporation occurs when the infant's skin is wet. |
| 3. Instruct them to keep the infant's crib away from cold walls, windows, or drafts from air conditioners and open doors or windows. | 3. Heat loss by radiation and convection occurs from exposure to cold objects or air drafts. |
| 4. Point out commonly used objects that may be cold when they touch Nicholas. Explain the effect of this contact, and suggest methods to warm them prior to use. | 4. Heat can be gained or lost by conduction. |
| 5. Assess the infant's axillary temperature every 30 minutes until it has been stable for 2 hours, or according to birth facility procedure and the infant's response. Report Nicholas's progress to Vicki and Peter. | 5. Continued assessment shows response to interventions. Keeping the parents aware of the infant's progress involves them in his care. |
| 6. Check blood sugar according to birth facility routine, especially if Nicholas is jittery or lethargic. Feed him if blood sugar is at or below 45 mg/dl by screening test. Help Vicki to breastfeed him if she wishes, or use formula. | 6. Nonshivering thermogenesis results in stores of glycogen being used. Infants may show tremors or lethargy as a result of hypoglycemia. Feeding provides calories for heat production. |
| 7. Monitor for tachypnea or other signs of respiratory distress. Suction and apply oxygen if needed. | 7. Nonshivering thermogenesis requires use of large amounts of oxygen, increases work of the respiratory system, and may lead to hypoxia. |
| 8. If Nicholas is slow to warm or has repeated episodes of low temperature, place him back under the radiant warmer. Alert the physician or nurse practitioner if the problem continues. | 8. Radiant heat warms infants and can be adjusted according to their needs. Temperature instability is one sign of infection in newborns. The health care provider may order further tests or transfer to an incubator for continued low temperature. |
| 9. When Nicholas is ready to go into an open crib, warm his clothes before dressing him. Place two warmed blankets, wrapped separately, around him. After he is swaddled, place one or two blankets over him. | 9. Warming clothing and blankets keeps Nicholas warm by conduction. Wrapping blankets separately traps air between layers, which acts as an insulating agent. |
| 10. Remove extra blankets according to the infant's temperature. | 10. Overheating increases oxygen and glucose consumption. |
| 11. Apply a stockinette or insulated hat to the infants' head. | 11. Covering the head decreases heat loss from this large surface area. |
| 12. After transfer to an open crib, monitor the infant's temperature every 30 to 60 minutes until it is stable. | 12. Continued monitoring provides prompt identification of problems infants may have in adjusting to changes in environmental temperature. |
| 13. Teach Vicki and Peter how to take their son's axillary temperature at home. | 13. Teaching increases parents' competence in infant care. |

*Nursing Care Plan continued on following page*

## Nursing Care Plan 21–1 *Continued*
## The Normal Newborn

**EVALUATION**

Nicholas's axillary temperature at 3 hours after delivery is 37°C (98.6°F). He has no further problems with temperature instability during his birth facility stay. Vicki and Peter are conscientious in using correct measures to keep Nicholas warm.

**ADDITIONAL NURSING DIAGNOSES TO CONSIDER**

Risk for Altered Parenting
Risk for Infection
Health Seeking Behaviors

tion, gagging, and episodes of cyanosis are normal during the first and second periods of reactivity, these may be very frightening to the mother. Teach the appropriate responses to the behaviors common to this phase. Remind the mother to use the bulb syringe and to call for help if needed. Check frequently with the mother to see if the infant is having difficulty. Assess her ability to use the bulb syringe and her comfort with its use.

### Evaluation

The normal newborn has little difficulty clearing the airway after the first few hours of life. Goals are met if

- The respiratory rate is between 30 and 60 breaths per minute.
- The infant shows no signs of respiratory distress.

## Procedure 21–2
## Using a Bulb Syringe

**PURPOSE:** To provide an open airway by removing secretions or regurgitated feeding from the infant's mouth and nose.

1. **Position the infant's head to the side, or pick up the infant and hold with the head lower than the rest of the body.** *Allows for drainage of mucus from the mouth to prevent aspiration.*
2. **Compress the bulb before inserting it into the infant's mouth.** *Removes the air from the syringe so that it suctions. (Do not compress the bulb while it is in the infant's mouth, or secretions in the bulb will be expelled back into the mouth.)*
3. **Insert the bulb into the side of the infant's mouth. Do not insert it straight to the back of the throat.** *A vagal response could be stimulated, with bradycardia or even apnea resulting. The infant might gag as well.*
4. **Release the bulb slowly while it is in the mouth. Remove and empty it by compressing several times before using again.** *Release the bulb to draw secretions from the infant's mouth into the bulb. Empty it to prepare it for use again.*
5. **Suction the nose if necessary *after* the mouth is cleared.** *Infants often gasp when the nares are suctioned and might aspirate secretions in the mouth if the mouth is not cleared out first.*
6. **Suction the nose carefully and gently.** *Trauma could cause edema to the delicate tissues and lead to obstruction. Infants are obligate nose breathers and have respiratory difficulty if the nasal passages are blocked.*

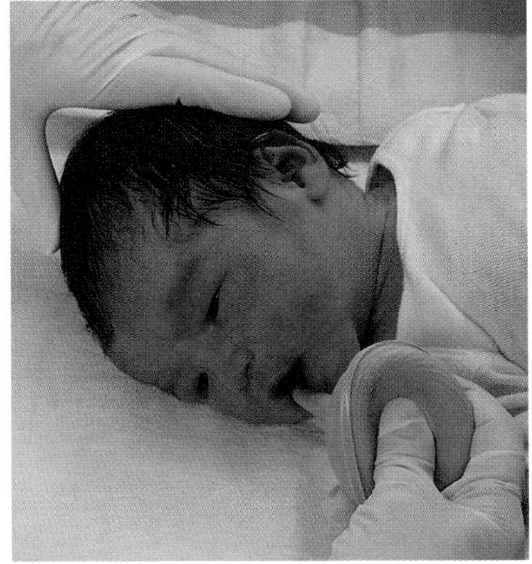

## Application of Nursing Process: Thermoregulation

Any neonate may have difficulty with thermoregulation. The nurse can identify problems and intervene to prevent complications related to this vital function.

### Assessment

Assess the newborn's temperature shortly after birth and then according to agency policy. Generally the temperature is assessed every half hour until it has been stable for 2 hours. It is checked again at 4 hours and then once a shift (every 8 hours). Assess the newborn more often if the temperature is abnormal.

### Analysis

Newborns often have temporary difficulty maintaining a stable temperature. Therefore, an appropriate nursing diagnosis is Risk for Ineffective Thermoregulation related to immature compensation for changes in environmental temperature.

### Planning

The goal for this diagnosis is that the infant will maintain body temperature within the normal ranges:

- Axillary, 36.5 to 37.5°C (97.7 to 99.5°F)
- Rectal, 36.5 to 37.6°C (97.7 to 99.7°F)

### Interventions

#### PREVENTING HEAT LOSS

**Preparing the Environment Before Birth.** Begin preventive measures before the infant is born. Prepare a neutral thermal environment with a radiant warmer to use during initial assessments. This ensures that the infant's metabolic rate does not have to increase and that excess oxygen and glucose are not necessary to maintain body temperature. Check the radiant warmer to be sure it is functioning properly before the delivery. Turn it on early enough that the bed is ready and warm for the newborn. Set the servocontrol between 36.0 and 36.5°C (96.8 and 97.7°F). This regulates the amount of heat produced by the warmer to maintain the infant's skin temperature at the normal level.

**Providing Immediate Care.** Immediately after birth, place the infant on the mother's abdomen or under the radiant warmer to counteract the cool temperature of the delivery room. Dry the wet infant quickly with warm towels to prevent heat loss by evaporation. Pay particular attention to drying the hair because the head is a large surface area and hair that remains damp increases heat loss. Remove towels or blankets as soon as they become wet, and replace them with dry, warmed linens. Cover the infant's head with a cap when the infant is not under a radiant warmer.

If the infant is moved from the mother's abdomen to a radiant warmer, attach a skin probe to the abdomen. The probe allows the warmer to monitor and display the infant's temperature continuously. Check the apparatus frequently to be certain it is working properly and that the infant's skin temperature is increasing as expected.

**Providing Ongoing Prevention.** Warm anything that comes in contact with the infant to avoid conduction of heat away from the body. Pad cool surfaces such as scales before placing infants on them. Warm stethoscopes and clothing before using them on the infant. Before touching the infant, run warm water over your hands if they are cold.

To prevent heat loss by radiation, position the newborn's crib or incubator away from walls or windows that are part of the outside of the building. It is easy to overlook this source of heat loss when the objects and air around the infant seem warm, but infants may lose heat to objects not in close contact with them. Keep this in mind when positioning cribs in mothers' rooms, which are often short of space. Place the crib at the end of the mother's bed or between the beds (in a two-bed room) rather than next to the windows. Avoid areas where there is a draft. Keep traffic low around radiant warmers, as movement increases air currents.

When assessing or caring for newborns, avoid exposing more of their bodies than necessary. Remove clothing and blankets only from the areas being assessed. Keep the upper part of the infant covered when changing diapers. Wrap them in blankets, and use a stockinette or insulated hat to prevent heat loss from the large surface area of the head.

#### RESTORING THERMOREGULATION

Infants who have attained a normal temperature may have a decrease later. When this happens, institute nursing measures to assist thermoregulation immediately. If the axillary temperature is low, some nurses check the rectal temperature to determine core temperature. However, do not wait for the rectal temperature to drop. The process of nonshivering thermogenesis begins in the infant before the core temperature becomes abnormal. Core temperature changes indicate that the infant's thermoregulatory resources are exhausted.

First look for obvious causes for the infant's low temperature. Perhaps the infant is unwrapped or is wearing wet diapers or clothing. The mother's room

## CRITICAL THINKING EXERCISE

You are caring for Nancy Belinsky and her son, Andy, who have both been doing well since Andy was born early this morning. As you enter the room after lunch, Nancy says, "Andy's hands and feet are so cold! But I've heard that all babies have cold hands and feet. Are they always so shaky, too?"

**Q:**
1. What are the nursing priorities in this situation?
2. What expanded assessments are necessary?
3. What interventions are necessary?
4. How will you respond to Nancy?

**A:**
1. Determine whether Andy is showing signs of hypothermia, hypoglycemia, or both. Reassure and teach Nancy as assessments and interventions are completed.
2. While taking the infant's temperature, assess for skin temperature, jitteriness, and general behavior. Check the blood glucose level if indicated.
3. If the baby's temperature is slightly low, intervene by changing any wet linens, double wrapping, and applying a hat. Recheck temperature in 30 minutes. If it is still low, place Andy under a radiant warmer. Feed Andy if the blood glucose level is low. Notify the physician if Andy continues to have difficulty maintaining temperature. (See Nursing Care Plan 21–1 for other interventions.)
4. Praise Nancy for being so observant of her son. If Andy's temperature is normal and he is not jittery, discuss the fact that peripheral circulation is sluggish in newborns and that their hands and feet tend to be cool. If "shakiness" is the Moro reflex or normal newborn behavior, discuss the reflex and the immaturity of the central nervous system. Show Nancy how to wrap Andy so that he stays warm and the Moro reflex is not elicited. Discuss methods of temperature control, and be sure that Nancy knows how to read a thermometer. Explain all interventions.

may be cold, or the crib may be placed near the air conditioner. These causes can easily be corrected.

A slight drop in temperature may require only the addition of extra clothing. Put a shirt on the baby upside down by placing the baby's legs in the sleeves for added warmth. Use two blankets, each wrapped separately around the infant, to increase insulation of heat by trapping air between the layers. Place another blanket over the infant in the crib, and be sure that a hat is on his or her head. Place linens in a warmer prior to use if added warmth is desired.

A greater drop in temperature requires additional measures. Place the infant under a radiant warmer for a short time. For an infant with a markedly decreased temperature, set the temperature control on the warmer to warm the infant slowly. Too rapid warming can cause complications, including apnea.

#### PERFORMING EXPANDED ASSESSMENTS

Expanded assessments are necessary whenever temperature is decreased in a newborn. Assess the respiratory rate because nonshivering thermogenesis increases the need for oxygen. Observe for signs of respiratory distress brought on by the additional oxygen requirement.

Because the cold infant uses more glucose to produce heat, test the blood glucose level when the temperature is abnormal. A reading of 45 mg/dl or lower by screening tests requires feeding. Have the mother breastfeed or use warmed formula. Heating the formula helps warm the infant.

Infants who do not respond to these simple measures need additional treatment. Notify the physician or nurse practitioner, and keep the infant in an incubator in the nursery for close observation until the temperature stabilizes. Observe for signs of infection, because low temperature is a common sign of infection.

### Evaluation

When a temperature within the normal range has been maintained for several hours, the infant can be considered stable in thermoregulation. Assess the infant's temperature according to agency routine, generally every 4 to 8 hours unless further problems develop.

## CHECK YOUR READING

1. Why are prophylactic medications given to all newborns?
2. How can nurses prevent heat loss in newborns?

# Application of Nursing Process: Hepatic Function

The major early assessments and care of the hepatic system are related to blood glucose levels and bilirubin conjugation.

## Blood Glucose

### Assessment

Assess all infants for risk factors and signs of hypoglycemia (see Signs of Hypoglycemia, Chapter 20, p. 525). Perform screening tests for blood glucose according to signs exhibited and agency policy.

### Analysis

For infants who have glucose levels of 40 mg/dl by laboratory analysis or 45 mg/dl by screening tests, the collaborative problem Potential complication: Hypoglycemia is appropriate.

### Planning

Client-centered goals for hypoglycemia are inappropriate because this problem requires collaboration between the nurse and the physician. Planning revolves around the nurse's role in the following:

- Monitoring for signs of hypoglycemia.
- Notifying the physician about signs of hypoglycemia or following routine orders left by the physician for infants with hypoglycemia.
- Intervening to minimize hypoglycemia.

### Interventions

#### MAINTAINING SAFE GLUCOSE LEVELS

If glucose is not constantly available to the brain, permanent damage may occur. To prevent this, follow agency policy and physician orders regarding feeding infants with low glucose levels. A common practice is to feed the newborn if the glucose screening test shows a level of 45 mg/dl or less to prevent further depletion of glucose. (Screening tests are less accurate than laboratory analysis, and intervening at a higher level treats the problem before hypoglycemia becomes severe.) If this is the infant's first feeding, provide breast milk or formula. Some agencies give glucose water for the first feeding, but this is not recommended. Glucose water raises the blood glucose, but insulin production also increases, causing a drop in blood glucose again. Milk provides a longer-lasting supply of glucose because of the other nutrients included.

Assist the breastfeeding mother with the first feeding. If she is unable to nurse the infant immediately (because of pain or exhaustion from delivery), feed the infant formula and help her breastfeed at the next feeding. Assist formula-feeding mothers to give the bottle.

#### REPEATING GLUCOSE TESTS

Closely observe newborns who have shown signs of hypoglycemia until glucose levels are stable. A schedule for retesting is routine in many agencies. An example of such a routine is a second screening 1 hour after the first test, and another screening every 2 hours for the next 6 hours. If the test results are normal at that time, further testing is unnecessary unless new indications of hypoglycemia develop.

Keep the physician or nurse practitioner aware of the newborn's status. If the blood glucose does not remain at an adequate level, other causative factors are investigated. The infant may be transferred to a nursery for more intensive treatment, including intravenous feedings, until blood glucose is regulated with oral feedings.

#### PROVIDING OTHER CARE

Watch for signs of other complications. If infants do not have enough glucose, they may experience a drop in temperature that could lead to respiratory distress as oxygen is used for nonshivering thermogenesis. Explain the situation to parents. They will be distressed over the multiple heel sticks their infant must endure. Explain the importance of maintaining adequate blood glucose levels and why the tests and frequent feedings are necessary. Encourage parents to feed the newborn as instructed so that enough glucose is available to meet the infant's needs. Discuss the routine for blood testing and when the infant will no longer require it.

### Evaluation

In evaluating collaborative interventions for hypoglycemia, note the presence or absence of continued signs of hypoglycemia and compare blood glucose screening with normal values. The blood glucose should remain above 45 mg/dl on screening or 40 mg/dl on laboratory analysis.

## Bilirubin

Because elevated bilirubin levels are common in newborns, be alert to situations that require intervention. Infants who need treatment for hyperbilirubinemia in the birth facility are discussed in Chapter 30, p. 852, in more detail. Preventive aspects are discussed here.

### Assessment

Assess for jaundice by blanching the infant's skin on the nose or sternum. Determine how far down the body the jaundice extends. When serum bilirubin tests are ordered, compare the results with what is expected for the infant's age and previous results.

### Analysis

When infants are discharged within 24 hours of birth, hyperbilirubinemia may not occur until after they are at home. It is important to teach parents appropriately so that infants with jaundice receive proper treatment. A nursing diagnosis for this situation is Risk for Injury related to lack of parental knowledge about hyperbilirubinemia.

### Planning

The goals/outcomes for this diagnosis are the following:

- Infants with jaundice will be identified early in the birth facility or at home.
- Parents will identify infants with jaundice when at home.
- Parents will identify methods of preventing or reducing jaundice when at home.

### Interventions

During assessment and care of newborns, be aware of which infants are at increased risk for hyperbilirubinemia (see Table 20–2, p. 527). By using extra vigilance in caring for infants at higher risk, nurses can detect jaundice earlier and take measures to decrease it.

Explain to parents the importance of adequate feedings to stimulate passage of stools and help prevent high levels of bilirubin in the infant. When a newborn is feeding poorly, determine the reasons for jaundice and intervene appropriately. Help mothers wake sleepy infants to feed, spend extra time with an infant with a poor suck, or teach the mother the appropriate amount to feed at each feeding. Encourage breastfeeding mothers to nurse within 2 hours after birth and every 2 to 3 hours thereafter. Avoid giving water to jaundiced infants, as water does not stimulate stool excretion.

Explain the significance of the color change in the skin and why blood testing is necessary. Answer parents' questions, especially if their infant needs phototherapy (see Nursing Care Plan 30–1, p. 855).

Before discharge, instruct parents about how to check for jaundice at home and to contact their care provider if they think they see it. Tell them to call the physician if the infant is not eating every 3 to 4 hours, voiding 6 to 10 times a day, and producing stools appropriately (at least once daily for formula-fed infants, at least three stools daily for breastfed infants).

Continue to check the infant for jaundice during the early home or clinic visits. Use a transcutaneous bilirubinometer (jaundice meter), if available, to verify the level of bilirubin. The meter is placed on the infant's skin to measure the intensity of the skin color, which is correlated with bilirubin levels (Ruchala et al., 1996). Reinforce teaching about identification of jaundice and importance of feedings and stooling. Answer questions parents may have developed since discharge from the birth facility.

If an infant develops true breast milk jaundice at 4 to 7 days after birth, explain it to the parents. The mother who must discontinue breastfeeding for a day or two will be very concerned. Reassure her that her milk is adequate and not harmful to the infant. Help her maintain her milk supply by using a manual or electric breast pump during the time the infant is taking formula.

### Evaluation

With proper nursing observation and parent teaching, infants with hyperbilirubinemia are identified early to allow for appropriate treatment and prevention of injury.

**CHECK YOUR READING**

3. What should the nurse do for infants with signs of hypoglycemia?
4. What are some interventions for preventing jaundice in newborns?

## Circumcision

Circumcision is the most common surgical procedure of the neonate. It is the removal of the prepuce (foreskin), a fold of skin that covers the glans penis. Although it can be retracted easily for cleaning in the older child, the prepuce is not usually fully retractable until age 3 or older. The prepuce should never be forcibly retracted in any infant because trauma and adhesions can result.

Until 1988, the American Academy of Pediatrics' (AAP) position was that circumcision of newborns as a routine procedure had no medical indications. In 1989, the AAP issued a more neutral statement that "newborn circumcision has potential medical benefits and advantages as well as disadvantages and risks" (AAP, 1989).

### Reasons for Choosing Circumcision

Circumcision may reduce urinary tract infections, which occur in approximately 1 percent of uncircumcised infants (Roberts, 1996). Inflammation of the glans or prepuce and cancer of the penis, although uncommon, occur more frequently in uncircumcised males. A large study showed that uncircumcised men were more likely to have syphilis and gonorrhea, but circumcised men were more likely to have genital warts (Cook et al., 1994).

Some parents choose circumcision for religious, cultural, or social reasons. Jewish parents may have their infants circumcised on the eighth day after birth as part of a special ceremony. Muslim culture also includes circumcision. Some parents want their son to look like his circumcised father or peers. Others feel circumcision is an expected part of newborn care, and some do not realize that they have a choice in the matter.

Parents may be concerned that when older, the child might develop phimosis, a tightening of the prepuce that prevents its retraction and requires circumcision. Although the number of such cases is very small, surgery after the newborn period involves hospitalization and anesthesia and can be psychologically disturbing to the young child.

Lack of knowledge about the care of the prepuce leads to some circumcisions. Poor hygiene may increase the risk of infections and other problems. Teaching the proper care of the uncircumcised penis to the parents and child can prevent surgery and complications related to inadequate cleanliness.

### Reasons for Rejecting Circumcision

Reasons why parents decide against circumcision are varied. It is uncommon in many countries and less often practiced by families from Asian, Latino, and Native American cultures. Some believe that although a few conditions are seen more often in uncircumcised males, the total incidence is too low to make the pain and risk of surgery necessary for every infant. Others believe that having the infant circumcised to look like the father or peers is cosmetic surgery and unnecessary. They especially object to subjecting their sons to the pain during and after the surgery.

Parents may be concerned about removing the prepuce, which serves to protect the glans. When unprotected by the prepuce, the glans is more prone to irritation from constant exposure to urine and rubbing against diapers. Many believe that circumcision decreases sexual pleasure later in life because the glans becomes less sensitive.

Complications are unusual but most often include hemorrhage and infection (Kaplan, 1994). Other complications include the removal of too much or too little of the prepuce, stenosis or fistulas of the urethra, adhesions, necrosis, or other damage to the glans.

Only healthy newborns should undergo circumcision. The preterm or sick infant should not be circumcised until he is healthy enough to tolerate the procedure. Infants with blood dyscrasias may have excessive bleeding if circumcised. For the repair of anatomic abnormalities of the penis, such as hypospadias or epispadias, an intact prepuce may be needed for use in plastic surgery.

### Pain Relief

Circumcision is often performed without anesthesia. Although at one time it was commonly thought that newborns do not feel pain, it is now known that the fetus is able to perceive pain by the third trimester. During circumcision, newborns show changes in vital signs, oxygen saturation levels, and responses by the adrenals, indicating that they feel pain. Infants may show irritability, more frequent crying, and changes in eating and sleeping behavior during the first day after the procedure. Later in infancy, circumcised boys may show more pain responses than uncircumcised boys when undergoing painful procedures such as vaccinations (Taddio et al., 1995).

Injection of the dorsal penile nerves or the area around the foreskin with an anesthetic such as lidocaine is a safe method to eliminate pain during circumcision. Complications are uncommon but include hematomas, local skin necrosis, and absorption of the medication into the blood stream. Anesthetic cream applied before the procedure may also be used but is less effective and requires a longer waiting period before it is effective.

Nonpharmacologic pain relief methods include pacifiers, soothing music, recordings of intrauterine sounds, and talking softly to the infant. All have shown some success in reducing an infant's pain responses to circumcision. The effect of these measures is distraction from rather than actual elimination of pain.

### Methods

The Gomco (Yellen) clamp (Fig. 21–3) and the Plastibell (Fig. 21–4) are two commonly used devices for performing circumcisions. In each method, the prepuce is first separated from the glans with a probe and incised to expose the glans. A Mogan clamp may also be used for circumcisions, especially for ritual circumcisions for Jewish families.

### Nursing Considerations

Circumcision is a somewhat controversial procedure. Parents may ask for information when they are making a decision about circumcision. If they decide to have it performed, they need information about caring for the infant after the procedure.

#### ASSISTING IN DECISION MAKING

Ideally, parents decide about circumcision early in pregnancy on the basis of careful consideration of the risks and benefits. However, this is not always the case. Some parents are not well informed about circumcision. The physician is responsible for explaining the risks and benefits to the parents, but the nurse may be called on to answer questions or clarify misconceptions that the parents may have.

Nurses must be certain that their own biases about circumcision do not interfere with their ability to give objective information to parents. Once the

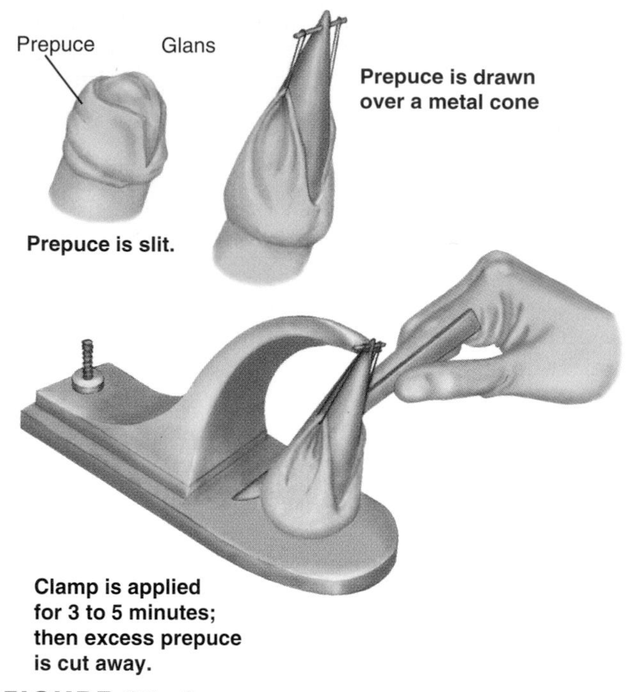
Prepuce
Glans
Prepuce is drawn over a metal cone
Prepuce is slit.
Clamp is applied for 3 to 5 minutes; then excess prepuce is cut away.

**FIGURE 21-3**

Circumcision using the Gomco (Yellen) clamp. The physician pulls the prepuce over a cone-shaped device that rests against the glans. A clamp is placed around the cone and prepuce and is tightened to provide enough pressure to crush the blood vessels. This prevents bleeding when the prepuce is removed after 3 to 5 minutes.

parents come to a decision, the nurse should support it. Although nurses generally teach parents of circumcised infants how to care for the penis, they may not think about providing teaching for parents who decide against circumcision. They should include care of the intact penis in the teaching plan for these parents.

#### PREPARING FOR THE PROCEDURE AND PROVIDING CARE DURING CIRCUMCISION

As with any surgical procedure, informed consent is necessary from the parents before a circumcision is performed. The nurse sees that the consent has been signed and should inform the physician of any problems that might impair the infant's ability to withstand circumcision. The infant should be at least 12 hours old so that he has recovered from the stress of birth.

The nurse gathers equipment and supplies before the procedure. To prevent regurgitation, the infant may not be fed for 2 to 4 hours before the procedure. Because he is restrained in a supine position, regurgitation may cause aspiration. A bulb syringe should be placed nearby in case suction is necessary.

When the physician and equipment are ready, the infant is placed on a circumcision board. This is a plastic holder that is molded to fit the infant's body and has restraints for his arms and legs (Fig. 21–5). A blanket is placed under the infant and only the diaper is removed. A drape provides warmth and maintains sterility. A heat lamp or radiant warmer helps prevent cold stress.

The nurse should comfort the infant during the procedure, especially if no anesthesia is used. A pacifier, talking to the infant, or soft music or tapes of intrauterine sounds may help distract the infant from pain.

#### PROVIDING POSTPROCEDURE CARE

The infant should be removed from the restraints immediately after the circumcision is completed. If a Gomco clamp was used, the nurse squeezes petroleum jelly or antibiotic ointment over the circumcision site to prevent the diaper from sticking to it. A 2 × 2 inch piece of gauze may be placed over the area. Petroleum jelly should not be used with a Plastibell. The infant should be comforted and returned to his mother, who may be anxious about her son.

The nurse watches carefully for signs of complications following the circumcision. The wound is checked frequently for bleeding during the first few hours after the procedure. If the infant is to be discharged after the circumcision, he should be observed for at least 1 hour before release.

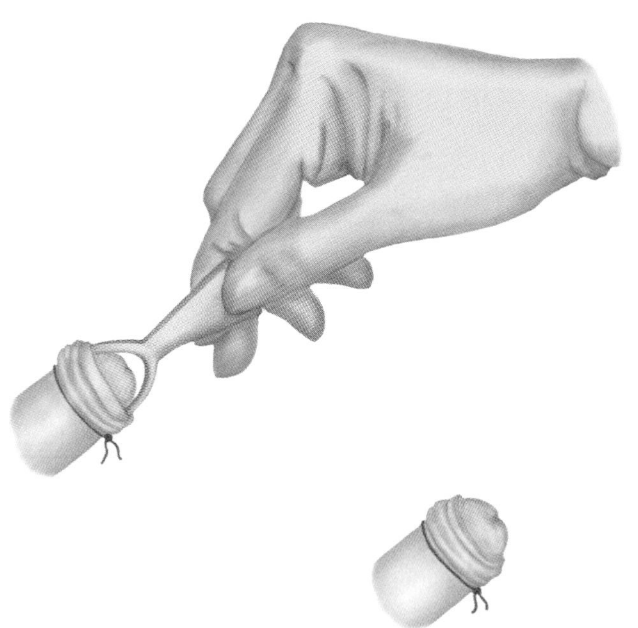

**FIGURE 21-4**

Circumcision using the Plastibell. The physician places the Plastibell, a plastic ring, over the glans, draws the prepuce over it, and ties a suture around the prepuce and Plastibell. This prevents bleeding when the excess prepuce is removed. The handle is removed, leaving only the ring in place over the glans. The Plastibell falls off in 5 to 8 days.

## Parents Want to Know

### Caring for the Uncircumcised Penis

Wash your son's penis daily and when soiled diapers are changed. There is no need to retract the foreskin because it is still attached to the glans, or end of the penis. It will gradually separate from the glans, but it may take 3 or more years for complete separation to occur.

Occasionally, you can gently pull back on the foreskin to see how much separation has occurred. However, *never* force the foreskin to retract. This is painful and may cause bleeding, infections, and adhesions.

As your son gets older and takes over his own care, teach him to wash the area during his daily bath. He should wash under the foreskin by gently pulling it back only as far as it retracts easily. This should become a daily routine, like washing his arms or legs.

If excessive bleeding occurs, steady pressure is applied to the penis with sterile gauze. The physician is notified if bleeding continues. A small amount of blood loss may be significant in an infant, who has a small total blood volume. The physician may apply Gelfoam sponge or suture the small blood vessels.

Noting the first urination after circumcision is important because edema could cause an obstruction. If the infant goes home before voiding, the mother is instructed to call the physician if there is no urinary output within 6 to 8 hours.

#### TEACHING PARENTS

Because circumcision is often performed on the day of discharge, the parents take over care of the site. Each time the site is checked for bleeding, the nurse should show the parents the amount of blood on the diaper to help them understand how much to expect. The normal yellowish exudate that forms over the site should be described and differentiated from purulent drainage. Signs of complications should be discussed fully.

### CHECK YOUR READING

5. What are the reasons parents decide for or against circumcision?
6. What information do parents need about care of the intact and circumcised penis?

## Daily Assessments and Care

Keys to Clinical Practice: Components of Daily Care provides a summary of daily nursing activities in meeting newborn needs (see Appendix D, p. 986). Certain areas are discussed more fully here.

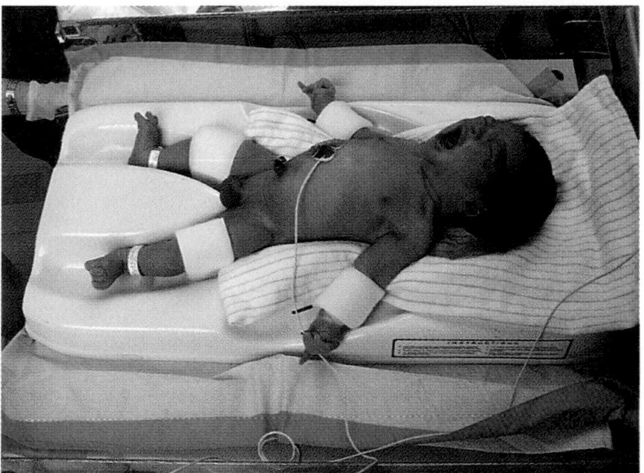

**FIGURE 21–5**

The infant is placed on the circumcision board just before the procedure is begun.

## Ongoing Assessments and Care

A complete assessment is necessary every 8 hours according to the birth facility's routine, but the nurse should be alert at all times for signs of change in the newborn's condition. Vital signs are assessed once every 8 hours, or more often if they are abnormal. The infant is weighed once daily and weight loss or gain noted.

### Providing Skin Care

The skin should be assessed for new marks or changes in old ones. Marks on the scalp may not be obvious if covered by abundant hair. To assess skin turgor, the nurse pinches up a small area of skin over the chest or abdomen and notes how quickly it returns to its normal position. The return should be immediate in the normal newborn, with no "tenting." Skin that remains "tented" is an indication of dehydration.

## Critical to Remember

### SIGNS OF COMPLICATIONS AFTER CIRCUMCISION

- Bleeding more than a few drops with first diaper changes
- Failure to urinate
- Signs of infection: fever or low temperature, purulent or foul-smelling drainage
- Displacement of the Plastibell
- Scarring (after healing)

### Parents Want to Know
## How to Care for the Circumcision Site

Observe the circumcision site at each diaper change. Note the amount of bleeding. Call the physician if there are more than a few drops of blood with diaper changes during the first day or any bleeding thereafter.

Continue to apply petroleum jelly to the penis with each diaper change for the first 24 to 48 hours. If a Plastibell was used, petroleum jelly should not be applied.

Keeping the circumcision site clean is important for healing. Squeeze warm water from a clean washcloth over the penis to wash it. Fasten the diaper loosely to prevent rubbing or pressure on the incision site.

Expect a yellow crust to form over the circumcision site. This is a normal part of healing and should not be removed. Watch for signs of infection such as fever or drainage that smells bad or has pus in it. *Call your physician if you suspect any abnormalities.* If a Plastibell was used, the plastic rim will fall off in 5 to 8 days. If it does not fall off by that time, notify your physician. The circumcision site should be fully healed in approximately 10 days.

## Bathing

The infant receives a bath to remove blood and excessive vernix as soon after birth as the temperature is stable. Early bathing decreases exposure to maternal blood and possible blood-borne organisms on the infant's skin. In one study, infants were bathed as soon as the rectal temperature reached 36.5°C (97.7°F), approximately 1 hour after birth. They had no significant drop in temperature compared with infants bathed at 4 hours after birth (Penny-MacGillivray, 1996).

While shampooing the hair, the nurse combs through it to remove dried blood. The infant must be returned to the radiant warmer quickly and dried well to minimize heat loss. Combing the hair out hastens drying.

The nurse wears gloves during all contact with the infant until the bath is completed because of the blood on the infant's skin from birth. After the bath, gloves are necessary only when contact with body fluids will occur.

After the initial bath, the infant may not receive another full bath during the birth facility stay. However, the skin is cleansed at diaper changes and to remove regurgitated milk. Only clear water or a mild soap solution should be used according to agency policy.

## Providing Cord Care

The cord should be checked for bleeding or oozing during the early hours after birth. The cord clamp must be securely fastened with no skin caught in it. Purulent drainage or redness or edema at the base indicates infection. The cord begins to dry shortly after birth. It becomes brownish black within 2 to 3 days and falls off within approximately 10 to 14 days.

The cord may be treated with a bactericidal substance such as triple dye solution, an antibiotic ointment, or alcohol. Parents should continue to clean the cord with alcohol at least three times a day at home until the cord falls off. They are taught to fold the diaper below the cord to keep it dry and free from contamination by urine.

The cord clamp is removed about 24 hours after birth if the end of the cord is dry (Fig. 21–6). The

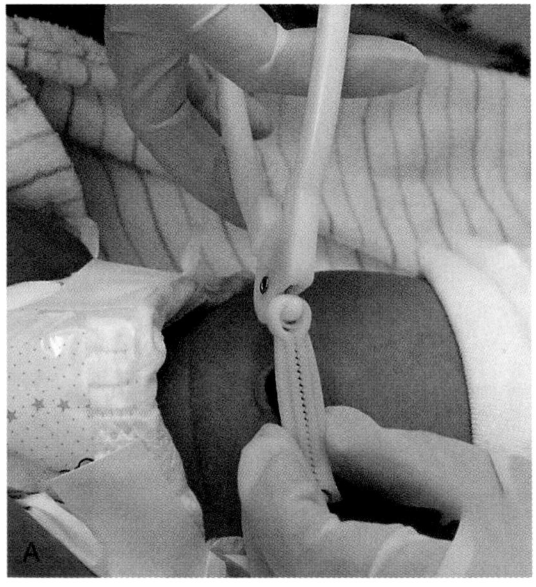


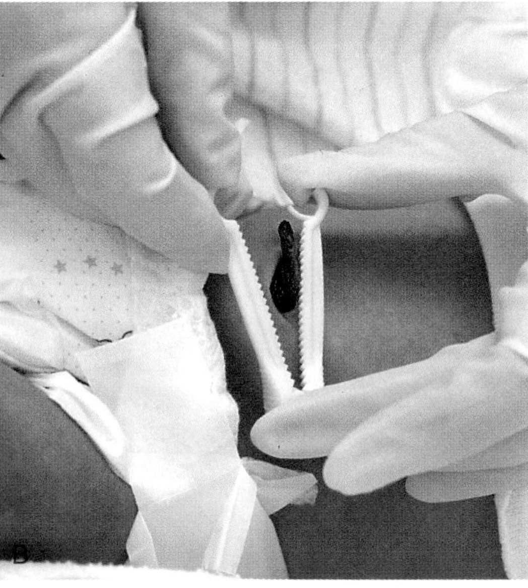


**FIGURE 21–6**

The cord clamp is removed when the end of the cord is dry and crisp. The clamp is cut (A) and separated (B).

base of the cord is still moist, but there is no danger of bleeding if the end is dry and crisp. If the neonate is discharged before the cord is dry enough for the clamp to be removed, it may be tied. In some birth facilities, the nurse removes the clamp during the home visit.

## Cleansing the Diaper Area

Because contact with body fluids is likely while changing diapers, it is important to wear clean gloves. Meconium is very thick and sticky and can be difficult to remove from the skin. Plain water or special soap solutions may be used for cleaning the diaper area. Petroleum jelly or other skin preparations are sometimes used to make cleaning meconium stools easier and to prevent skin irritation.

## Assisting with Feedings

Ensure that the infant is eating well and that the parents understand their chosen feeding method. Assign a LATCH score to breastfeeding mothers and infants, and look for changes in the score (see Chapter 22, p. 589).

Position infants on the side after feedings to promote emptying of the stomach. This allows regurgitated fluid to run out of the mouth and decreases chances of aspiration. Because the lower end of the stomach is on the right side, turning the infant to the right allows gravity to help empty the stomach more quickly. The head of the bed may be elevated for a short time after the feeding. This helps keep stomach contents from flowing into the esophagus through the relaxed cardiac sphincter.

## Protecting the Infant

Safeguarding the infant is a major role of the nurse. Primary ways nurses protect newborns are by (1) ensuring that infants always go to the correct parents, (2) taking precautions to prevent infant abductions, and (3) preventing or recognizing early signs of infection.

### IDENTIFYING THE INFANT

A method to identify newborns is instituted at birth, before mothers and infants are separated, to ensure that the wrong infant is never given to a mother. This type of mistake could result in interference with bonding, lack of confidence in the reliability of the staff, and lawsuits.

The most common method of identifying infants is the use of identification bands, which are placed on the mother, the infant, and the father or other support person. Information on each band is identical and includes a number that is imprinted on the plastic band. The imprinted number is used to identify the mother and the infant every time the infant is brought to the mother after a period of separation, however brief (Procedure 21–3 and Fig. 21–7).

Other methods of identifying infants include taking footprints of the infant and a fingerprint of the mother. The infant is photographed, and a notation of birthmarks or other distinguishing features is made on the nurses' notes.

### PREVENTING INFANT ABDUCTION

An unfortunate but essential role of the nurse is protection of the infant against infant abduction (kidnapping). In 1994, 14 newborns were abducted from health care facilities (AWHONN, 1995). Precautions include teaching parents how to recognize birth facility personnel, whether by a picture identification badge or by other means. Written and verbal information, including a picture of the special identification badge worn by staff, should be given to parents. Parents must be cautioned never to give their infant

---

**Procedure 21–3**

## Identifying Infants

**PURPOSE:** To ensure that each infant is *always* given to the correct mother.

1. **Identify infants and mothers (or fathers) with identification bands whenever reuniting them, even after a brief separation.** *Ensures that the infant is always given to the correct mother.*
2. **When taking an infant into the mother's room, unwrap the blankets enough to expose the identification band on the infant's wrist or ankle. Do *not* rely on memory of the number.** *Allows visualization of the band to check the numbers.*
3. **Explain the identification procedure and its purpose to the mother. Show her the imprinted identification number on her band and the matching number on the infant's bands.** *Ensures the mother's understanding and cooperation.*
4. **Look at the number on the infant's band and ask the mother to read off the identification number on her band. Do *not* reverse the process by reading the infant's number to the mother.** *If the numbers are read to a mother who does not understand the process, she might indicate that the numbers are correct when they are not.*
5. **An alternative procedure is for the nurse to compare the infant's and the mother's bands visually.** *If the mother does not speak English or might have difficulty with the process, the nurse can be sure that the infant is identified correctly.*
6. **If the infant is to be released to a support person wearing an identification band, follow the same identification procedure.** *Ensures that the infant is given to the correct support person.*

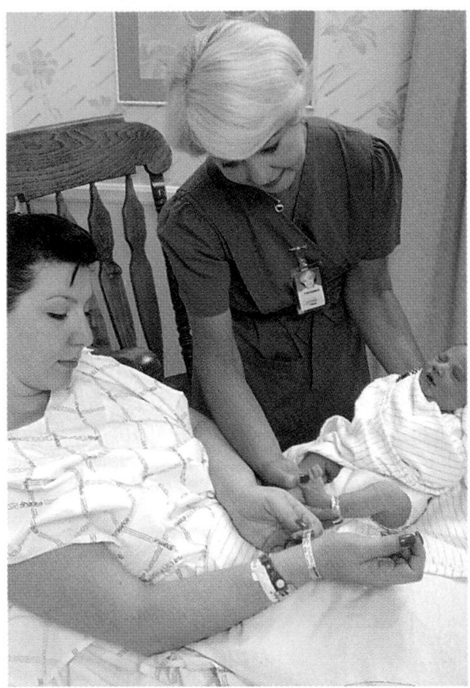

**FIGURE 21–7**

The nurse checks the infant's identification band with the mother's band.

to anyone who does not have proper identification (Table 21–1).

Staff who are working temporarily on the unit must have a special means of identification that is recognized by parents and other staff. Temporary identification badges are assigned and monitored each shift so that none can be removed from the premises without alerting the staff.

In some agencies, an electronic device is attached to each infant's wrist, ankle, or clothing. The maternity unit exits are wired so that an alarm is triggered when the device is near.

Entrances to the maternity unit should be in areas where staff can watch those entering and leaving. Unit doors may be locked at all times. Entrance requires knocking on the door or use of a card-key or a code on the lock (Fig. 21–8). Visitors to maternity units may be required to check in with security guards and wear special visitor identification tags.

Remote exits are often locked and equipped with video cameras and alarms. Staff must respond quickly whenever a door alarm sounds. Although alarms are usually triggered accidentally, it is always possible that a kidnapper is using a remote exit for a quick getaway.

Newborns are usually abducted by women who are familiar with the birth facility and its routines. They are often married and living near the birth facility. They usually visit several times to learn the routines so that they can impersonate birth facility staff to gain access to a newborn. They often know the layout of the facility and the locations of exits well. The abductor usually impersonates a member of the staff. The woman may have had a previous pregnancy loss or has been unable to have a child of her own. She may want an infant to solidify a relationship with her boyfriend. Although the woman plans the kidnapping, she waits for an appropriate opportunity to take any infant.

### PREVENTING INFECTION

Because the newborn has a limited ability to respond to infection, prevention is of utmost importance throughout the birth facility stay and constitutes a major part of parent teaching.

A number of nursing actions are designed to prevent infection. At the beginning of their shift, nurses

**TABLE 21–1 PRECAUTIONS TO PREVENT INFANT ABDUCTIONS**

1. All personnel must wear appropriate identification at all times. No one without appropriate identification should handle or transport infants.
2. Enlist parents' help in preventing kidnapping. Teach them to allow only hospital staff with proper identification to take their infants from them.
3. Teach parents and staff to transport infants only in their cribs and never by carrying them. Question anyone walking in the hallway carrying an infant.
4. Question anyone with a newborn near an exit or in an unusual part of the facility.
5. Be suspicious of anyone who does not seem to be visiting a specific mother or who asks detailed questions about nursery or discharge routines.
6. Be suspicious of unknown people carrying large bags or packages that could contain an infant.
7. Respond immediately when an alarm sounds signaling that a remote entrance has been opened or an infant has been taken into an unauthorized area.
8. Never leave infants unattended at any time. Teach parents that infants must be observed at all times. Suggest that they send the infant to the nursery if they or a family member cannot watch the infant.
9. Take infants to mothers one at a time. This avoids having an infant in a crib waiting outside in the hall while the nurse is in a room with another mother. Never leave an infant in the hall unsupervised.
10. When infants are left in mothers' rooms, place them away from the doorways.
11. If entrances to the maternity unit or nurseries are equipped with locks that open to codes, protect the code from others.
12. Identification bracelets are often given to mothers' support persons so that they can come to the nursery to get the infant. When a parent or family member comes to the nursery to take an infant, always match the infant and adult identification bracelet numbers. Never give an infant to anyone without an identification bracelet or other proper identification.
13. Alert hospital security when any suspicious activity occurs.

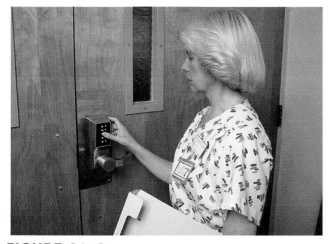

**FIGURE 21-8**

The nurse uses a code to open the door to the nursery.

in many agencies perform a scrub of their hands and arms. Throughout the day, hand washing is important before and after touching any infant. It is essential not to handle one neonate and then go to another without again washing one's hands. An infection that develops in one infant could quickly spread to others if these precautions are not taken.

The nurse should encourage parents and visitors to wash their hands before handling infants. Parents should be instructed to discourage visitors with colds or other infections from coming in contact with the mother or newborn at the birth facility or during the early days at home.

Each infant's supplies should be kept separate from those used for other infants to avoid cross-contamination. Supplies in drawers or cupboards of the crib unit belonging to one infant should be used only for that infant because they are likely to be touched by the nurse while giving care. Using them for another neonate could result in the transfer of infectious organisms.

When the mother has an infection, the physician or nurse practitioner decides whether it is safe for the newborn to remain with her. Although mothers and infants may well share the same organisms, if a mother is acutely ill, her infant may need to stay in the nursery until the mother is no longer contagious and feels able to perform infant care.

Some birth facilities have a policy governing when separation of mother and newborn is necessary. Often the degree of the mother's fever is one of the determining factors. The separation of mother and infant should be as short as possible, of course, to promote attachment.

Nurses must be vigilant for signs of infection during assessment and care of the infant. These signs are often different from those of the older infant or child and may be very subtle (see Signs of Infection, Chapter 30, p. 860). Instead of a fever, there may be a decrease in temperature. The infant may feed poorly or be lethargic. Periods of apnea sometimes occur without obvious cause. Any change in behavior that is unexplained should be recorded and investigated. The same holds true, of course, for the more obvious signs of infection such as drainage from the eyes, cord, or circumcision site (sepsis is discussed in Chapter 30, p. 857).

**CHECK YOUR READING**

7. How can the nurse prevent a parent from getting the wrong baby?
8. How can infant abductions be prevented?
9. What is the most important method of preventing infection in newborns?

## Application of Nursing Process: Parents' Knowledge of Newborn Care

Teaching is particularly important because most mothers go home from the birth facility very early after birth. New mothers often feel unprepared, physically and emotionally, to take over full care of a newborn and themselves. In addition, their ability to learn may be impaired by the stress of labor and birth. One study (Eidelman et al., 1993) found that women 1 day after childbirth were less able to remember information than women during pregnancy. New fathers also had trouble with memory tests. Therefore, finding creative teaching methods is especially important. The nurse must use every contact with the parents as an opportunity for further teaching.

### Assessment

Assess parents' changing learning needs throughout the birth facility stay. Consider the mother's and infant's physical conditions and any special concerns that the mother may have. Review the principles of teaching discussed in Chapter 2 for special considerations when planning teaching sessions.

Determine learning needs for experienced mothers. They may be unaware of information that has changed since the birth of the last infant. For example, mothers who have always placed their infants in the prone position for sleep need to know that this position is no longer recommended because it may be associated with sudden infant death syndrome. Mothers should be taught to use the side or back position (AAP, 1992). Differences in physical requirements or even in temperament between siblings cause concern. Parents may need information about helping other children adjust to the newborn.

Assess the father's learning needs and his plans for involvement with infant care. Whether or not the father participates in care of the infant may depend on cultural beliefs about his role. In some cultures, the father participates very little in the care of the young infant. He may become more involved as the children get older. In other families, fathers actively participate in child care, even during the birth facility stay. They often have many questions and are very eager to learn about care of their infant.

## Analysis

A nursing diagnosis that is appropriate for the family with learning needs is Health Seeking Behaviors related to the desire for information about infant care.

## Planning

The primary goals for the diagnosis of Health Seeking Behaviors are that the parents will do the following:

- Identify their own information needs and seek assistance from nurses to meet those needs.
- Correctly demonstrate infant care before discharge.
- Express confidence in their ability to meet their infant's needs.

## Interventions

### DETERMINING WHO TEACHES

In many agencies, the same nurse is responsible for care of both mother and infant. This may be called couplet care. The extended contact between the nurse and the mother increases the nurse's understanding of the mother's learning needs. There is more time for teaching as additional learning needs become apparent.

If the mother and infant are cared for by separate nurses, be certain that all learning needs are met. Traditionally, postpartum nurses taught mothers how to care for themselves, and nursery nurses taught them how to care for their newborn. However, nurses from both areas must be able to teach about both subjects to ensure that all the concerns of mothers are addressed. Many facilities use a checklist to ensure that all important topics are covered with every parent.

### SETTING PRIORITIES

Because of the short time available for teaching, it is important to set priorities in determining what to teach. After assessing the parent's individual learning needs, make a teaching plan. Use a topic list to help them point out major concerns regarding infant care. This ensures that precious teaching time is spent most effectively. Begin by discussing their most pressing concerns. This enhances further learning by decreasing their anxiety so that they can concentrate on the information. Then, as time allows, go on to other subjects.

### USING VARIOUS TEACHING METHODS

Use a variety of teaching methods to increase effectiveness, make the subject more interesting, and increase retention of the material. Use verbal and written methods, as well as demonstrations. Ask the parents to return each demonstration of care skills. It is helpful to the parents to see skills performed correctly and then practice under supervision while the nurse gives suggestions and makes corrections as needed.

Discuss information with the mother alone or with her family members, roommate, or a group of mothers. Some women learn better with one-to-one teaching, whereas others benefit from watching and listening to others. Group teaching allows nurses to make more efficient use of time.

Use audiovisual materials, including pamphlets, baby magazines, films or videos, and television programs. Highlight the most important areas in written material, watch the videos with her, and clarify information as necessary. This helps reinforce the learning.

Explain the rationale for each point made during teaching sessions. Understanding the reasons behind the actions increases the likelihood that parents will follow the nurse's instructions.

### MODELING BEHAVIOR

Modeling by the nurse is an important teaching tool. Mothers watch closely when nurses handle infants. The nurse demonstrates mothering behavior by the way the infant is held and care is given and by talking to the infant. This is particularly important for the mother with no experience in child care.

### TEACHING INTERMITTENTLY

Plan teaching in small segments that are interspersed with the care of the infant. Check the parents' understanding frequently. Encourage them to take over until they are performing all of the infant's routine care.

### INCLUDING THE FATHER

Identify fathers who would like to participate in care of their infants but hesitate because of lack of experience. Offer them the same teaching given the inexperienced mother. Give praise liberally when

## Parents Want to Know

## Techniques for Infant Care

*This guide is written in language that the nurse might use when teaching parents about infant care. Adapt the subjects to meet the needs of individual parents.*

**Handling the Infant**

*Head Support*

An infant's head is the heaviest part of the body and makes up one fourth of the total body length. Infants are unable to support their head when held in an upright position. Place your hand behind the baby's head whenever you hold him or her to help support the head. Babies' muscles become strong enough to support the head after the first few months of life.

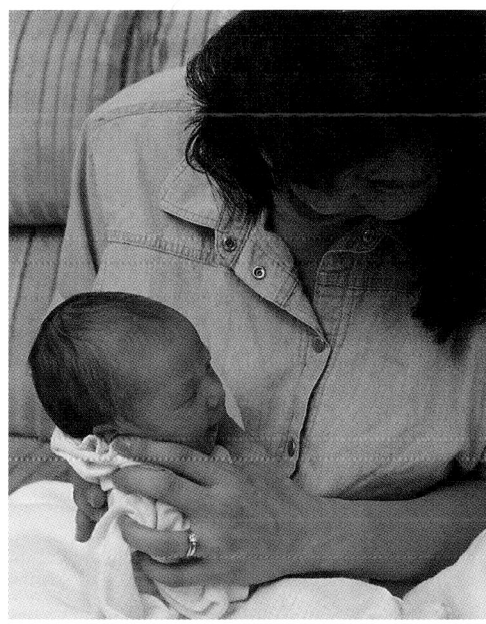

*Positions*

Most mothers hold the infant in the cradle position. In the "football" position, the baby's head is supported in the palm of the hand and the body is held along the arm and supported against your side. This position allows one hand to be free when washing the baby's hair or breastfeeding.

The shoulder hold is good for burping the baby. Or sit the baby on your lap and support the head and chest with one hand while gently patting or rubbing the infant's back with the other hand. This allows you to see the baby's face in case of "spit ups."

Always place your baby on the back or side for sleep. This position is recommended by the American Academy of Pediatrics for all infants. It is thought to help prevent sudden infant death syndrome (SIDS), the sudden unexplained death of an infant. Use a rolled blanket behind the back to help the baby stay in place on the side. The baby should sleep on a firm mattress.

*Wrapping*

Young infants seem more secure when wrapped firmly in a blanket, which may feel like the small space of the uterus. Fussy babies often respond well to swaddling. To swaddle the infant, turn down one corner of a blanket and position the baby's head over the edge. Fold one side of the blanket over the body and arm. Bring the lower corner up and fold it over the chest. Then bring the other side around the infant and tuck it underneath.

**Normal Body Processes**

*Breathing*

Newborns normally breathe about 30 to 60 times a minute. Their breathing is irregular and may vary from loud to very soft. Sometimes breathing is so quiet that mothers wake babies to be sure that they actually are breathing. Sneezing is usually a normal response to lint from new baby clothes rather than a sign of a cold.

*Using a Bulb Syringe*

Use the bulb syringe when the infant has excessive mucus in the mouth or nose or spits up milk. Squeeze the bulb before you insert it into the mouth and aim it to the side of the mouth rather than to the back. Extra mucus is common in the first days of life but is usually not a problem thereafter unless a cold develops. Clean the bulb as necessary with soap and water. Rinse and dry well before using again. *Call your physician if the baby's skin becomes blue or if the baby stops breathing for more than 15 seconds, has difficulty breathing, or has yellow or green drainage from the nose.*

*Temperature*

Newborns have difficulty regulating their temperature. If they become cold, they need more calories and more oxygen than when they are warm enough. A drop in body temperature can be dangerous for them. Dress your baby as you would like to be dressed. Add a light receiving blanket over the young infant, except in very hot weather.

*Using a Thermometer*

Check your baby's temperature during illness. It is best to take the temperature under the infant's arm to prevent injury to the rectum. Place the thermometer under the arm so that the bulb does not protrude behind the arm. Hold the arm firmly over the thermometer and read it at 5 minutes. If you do not know how to read a glass thermometer, a nurse will teach you. *Call your physician if the baby has a temperature higher than 100°F or lower than 97.7°F.*

*Urine Output*

Your baby will have at least 2 to 6 wet diapers a day during the first day or two and 6 to 10 wet diapers a day thereafter. Counting the number of wet diapers helps you know if the baby is getting enough milk. *Call your baby's doctor if the baby has no wet diapers for more than 12 hours.*

*Stool Output*

Formula-fed infants pass one to several stools each day that are pale yellow to light brown and formed. Breastfed infants pass very soft, seedy stools that have a sweet-sour odor and are mustard yellow. They should have at least 3 stools a day. Babies may appear constipated when they turn red and seem to strain when passing a stool. However, constipated infants pass dry stools, and there may be small, hard pieces. There are usually fewer stools per day than is average. If the movement is soft, you do not need to worry if the baby seems to strain.

*Parents Want to Know continued on following page*

## Parents Want to Know *Continued*

## Techniques for Infant Care

*Diarrhea*

Babies with diarrhea pass an increased number of stools, and the color and consistency change. Because the contents move through the intestines more quickly than normal, the color is greener and the stools are more liquid than usual. There may be a water ring—an area in the diaper where the liquid has absorbed, sometimes around an area of more solid stool. *Call your physician for further instructions if the infant passes more than two diarrhea stools.*

*Skin Care*

A number of normal marks occur on the newborn's skin. One is a rash called erythema toxicum that resembles small insect bites. Another is small whiteheads called milia. These are normal and disappear without treatment. Do not squeeze them or they may become infected and last longer.

Newborns have very dry, peeling skin because they were surrounded by water for 9 months and the outer layers of the skin were not shed. After peeling, the baby has soft skin. It is not necessary to use lotions or creams, as they may cause irritation.

*Cord*

Use a cotton swab dipped in alcohol to clean the cord and the crevices at the base of the cord about three times a day. This does not hurt the baby, as there are no nerves in the cord. *Notify your physician if you see bleeding or signs of infection, such as redness, drainage, or a foul odor.*

Keep the cord dry by folding the diaper below it so that it is not wet by urine. The cord generally falls off in about 10 to 14 days. It may bleed a few drops when it detaches. Do not start tub baths until the cord is off and the area is well healed.

*Diaper Area*

Clean the diaper area with each diaper change. For girls, separate the labia (folds) and remove all stool. For boys, wash under the scrotum to help prevent rashes. If the diaper area becomes red, change the diaper more often. Leaving the diaper off to expose the area to air is also helpful. If an ointment is needed, petroleum jelly or a barrier-type ointment may be used. *If redness persists, ask your baby's doctor for suggestions.*

*Bathing*

Give your baby a sponge bath until the cord and circumcision areas are healed. At that time, tub baths can begin. Because infants are washed as needed after regurgitation and with diaper changes, it is not necessary to give them a bath every day. Fathers often enjoy giving the infant a bath and make this their special time with the baby.

*Sponge Baths*

Before the bath, gather all the supplies. You need a container or sink for the warm water, washcloth, towel, baby shampoo, alcohol, cotton or cotton-tipped swabs, and clean clothes. Soap is not necessary for the young infant, but if it is used, it should be gentle and nonalkaline to protect the natural acids of the infant's skin.

Give the bath in a room that is warm and free of drafts. Bathe the baby on a surface that is comfortable and safe. If you use a counter, pad it with blankets or towels.

*Never leave the infant alone on an unprotected surface, even for a minute.* Keep one hand on the infant at all times to prevent falls. Taking the phone off the hook during the bath prevents distractions. If you must leave the room, take the baby along or place him or her in the crib.

Keep the baby warm by uncovering only the area you are washing. Wash and dry the baby's body, one part at a time, to prevent chilling. Start by washing the face with clean water. Use a separate clean area of the washcloth to wipe each eye. Use a washcloth to clean in and around the ears, where regurgitated milk may accumulate. Do not use cotton-tipped swabs in the infant's ears or nose, as injury may occur if the baby moves suddenly. Clean the diaper area last, using the principle of "clean to least clean." For baby girls, wipe the diaper area from front to back. This avoids infections that may occur if stool gets into the vagina or urethra.

To clean the neck folds, put one hand under the baby's shoulders and lift slightly. This causes the head to drop back enough that the creases in the neck can be washed.

Shampoo the head while holding the baby in a football position. Although the fontanelle or "soft spot" may seem delicate, it is covered with a tough membrane. It is not injured by washing. You may see pulse movements in the fontanelle, but this is normal. Dry the hair well to prevent heat loss.

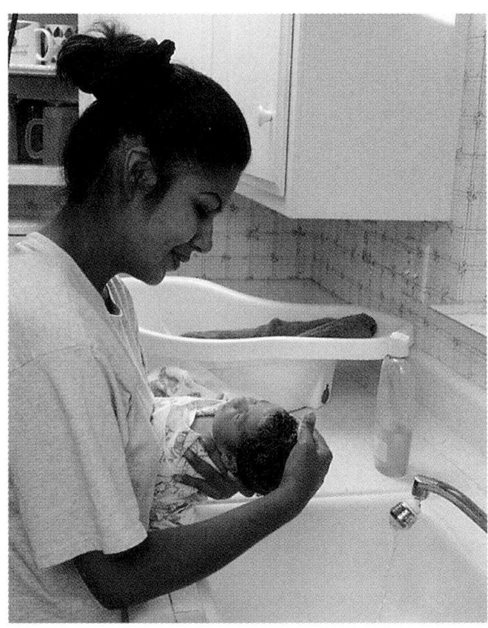

*Tub Bath*

For a tub bath, use a small plastic tub or a clean sink. Pad the bottom with a towel or foam pad to make it more comfortable and prevent the infant from slipping. Place about 3 inches of warm water in the tub. Wash the face and hair before placing the baby in the tub. Keeping the baby dressed until after the hair is washed helps prevent chilling.

It may be easier, at first, to lather your hands with soap and water and then lather the infant's body. Then immerse the baby in the tub for rinsing. It is not unusual for young

## Parents Want to Know *Continued*

### Techniques for Infant Care

infants to be frightened when they are first put in water. Talk to your baby softly and calmly while holding him or her securely to help the baby adjust to this new experience.

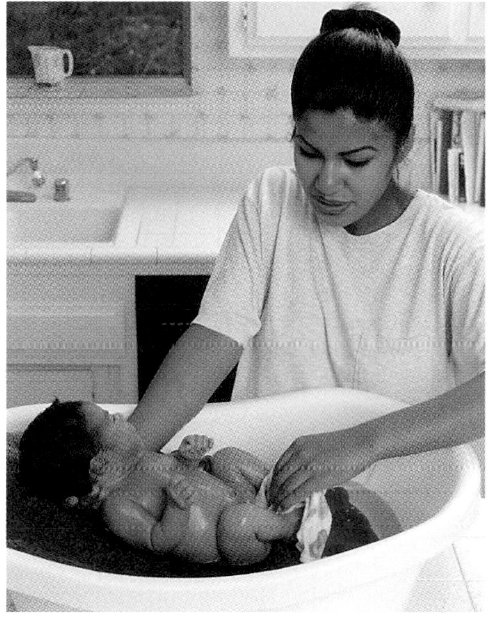

**Feeding**

*Breastfeeding, Formula Feeding* (see Chapter 22, Infant Feeding)

Hold a bottle so that the nipple is filled with milk to prevent the infant from swallowing air. Gently rubbing the palate with the nipple encourages the infant to begin sucking. However, excessive movement of the nipple in the baby's mouth is distracting to the baby.

Burp the baby once midway during the feeding, using the shoulder or the sitting position. After feeding, always place the baby on his or her side with a rolled blanket behind the back to prevent choking if the baby spits up.

**Behavior**

Knowing infants' different behavioral states helps you learn about your baby's individual characteristics.

***Sleep Phases.*** During quiet sleep, the infant sleeps soundly with quiet breathing and little movement. Your baby will not be disturbed by noises from appliances or other children at this time. In active sleep, the baby moves or fusses while still asleep. If your baby sleeps in your room, you may have difficulty sleeping because of the baby's noises and movements. During the drowsy state, the baby is beginning to wake but may go back to sleep if not disturbed. However, if it is time for feeding or other activities, talk softly to help the baby awaken.

***Awake Phases.*** The quiet alert state is the one that parents enjoy most because the infant seems so intent on studying the objects and people nearby. This is a good time for infant stimulation and "play time." Parents soon learn to recognize the active alert or "fussy" phase in their infants. The infant may be signaling hunger or discomfort from wet and cold diapers. If you do not intervene, the baby soon moves to the crying state. If the baby cries too long, he or she may not respond at first to care activities. A few minutes of rocking and holding close may be necessary before the infant settles down.

*Socialization*

Infants are social beings who enjoy contact with people. They hear voices in the uterus and respond with interest when their mothers talk to them after birth. The baby should be part of the life of the family. Use an infant seat or an infant carrier to keep the baby near you and the rest of the family. Infants enjoy watching the human face. Hold your baby close and talk to him or her to provide social stimulation.

*Stimulation*

***Sounds.*** Play music of different types to provide auditory stimulation. Infants prefer music that is not too loud. Music boxes, tapes, or a radio can provide a variety of sound.

***Sights.*** Because babies focus their eyes best at a distance of 7 to 12 inches, items such as mobiles should be placed within this range. Infants especially like black-and-white geometric figures. They enjoy bright colors very early but are not particularly interested in pastels.

***Variety.*** Place the baby in an infant seat in the kitchen while you prepare meals to stimulate the senses of sight, hearing, and smell. An infant carrier pack provides the stimulation of motion as well.

***Timing.*** Stimulation is best used during the baby's quiet alert state. Do not try to use stimulation techniques with a fussy infant because it can cause overstimulation. This causes the baby to be irritable and have difficulty going to sleep.

---

mothers and fathers practice their new infant care skills. This increases their confidence and skill.

#### DOCUMENTING TEACHING

All teaching performed and the parent's abilities to carry out infant care should be documented. This documentation helps other nurses to know what teaching has been completed and what is still needed. It also provides legal proof that teaching was completed before discharge.

#### PROVIDING FOR FOLLOW-UP CARE

Provide information about unmet learning needs to the home or clinic nurse who will see the mother and infant, especially if they are discharged at 24 hours or less after birth. Reinforcement can then be provided at a time when the mother's memory has improved after the stress of birth.

Provide as much information as possible in written form. The parents can then refer to areas where they have concerns. Also provide telephone numbers that they can call for further help. Offer written information in the parents' primary language, if possible. Even if they speak English, they may prefer to read in their own language.

Remind parents about when the infant should be seen for follow-up care. Suggest that they call for an appointment well in advance of that time so that the infant can receive care on time.

#### INCORPORATING CULTURAL CONSIDERATIONS

Take the family's cultural beliefs about child care into consideration when teaching. For example, some Southeast Asian and Latino women are hesitant to breastfeed in the birth facility and wish to wait until the milk comes in when they are home. Asian parents may be uneasy when caregivers are too complimentary about the baby or casually touch the infant's head. However, Latino parents may prefer that a person who compliments the infant touch the infant's face or head to ward off the "evil eye."

Teaching should include family members who will be caring for the infant. This may vary according to the culture and whether the traditional caregiver is available. In addition to the father of the infant, the woman's mother is often the major support person. However, in the Korean culture, the husband's mother is the primary caregiver for the infant and the mother in the early weeks to allow the mother to recover from the birth. If the mother will not be the primary infant caregiver, she may appear uninterested in the nurse's teachings. Asking the parents who will be helping them care for the baby helps determine family members to be included in the teaching.

### Evaluation

Ongoing evaluation of parents' learning is necessary throughout the birth facility stay and during the follow-up home, clinic, or office visits. Determine whether they can demonstrate important aspects of infant care safely and correctly. As they learn more caregiving skills, their confidence should increase as well.

## Immunization

Hepatitis B is a growing problem in the United States. Immunization for this disease is now included with other routine childhood vaccinations. The series of injections for hepatitis B is begun at birth in many facilities.

Infants of mothers with acute or chronic hepatitis B infection (HBsAg positive) may become infected from exposure to the mother's blood at birth. Infants infected at birth have a very high chance of becoming chronically infected. Chronic infection may cause later cancer or other serious liver damage.

These infants should receive both the vaccine and hepatitis B immune globulin (HBIG). The immune globulin provides passive immunity to hepatitis to protect infants until they develop their own antibodies and should be given within 12 hours of birth. The vaccine promotes antibody formation to protect infants from further exposure to the disease.

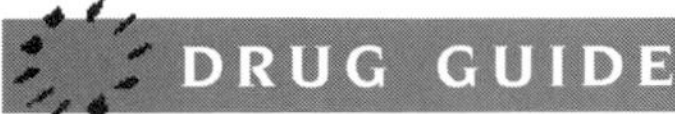


### HEPATITIS B VACCINE

***Classification:*** Vaccine

***Other Names:*** Engerix-B, Recombivax HB

***Action:*** Immunization against hepatitis B infection

***Indications:*** Prevention of hepatitis B in exposed and unexposed infants

***Neonatal Dosage and Route:*** Recombivax HB: 5 μg (0.5 ml) to infant of infected mother, 2.5 μg (0.25 ml) if mother not infected

Engerix-B: 10 μg (0.5 ml) (whether or not mother is infected)

For infants of uninfected mothers the vaccine is given at birth, 1 to 2 months, and 6 to 18 months. An alternate schedule is birth to 2 months, 1 to 4 months, and 6 to 18 months.

For infants of infected mothers the vaccine is given at birth and at 1 and 6 months. If immune globulin is also given at birth because the mother is infected, it should be at a different site than the vaccine.

Give intramuscularly in the anterolateral thigh.

***Absorption:*** Well absorbed from muscle

***Contraindications:*** Hypersensitivity to yeast

***Adverse Reactions:*** Pain or redness at site. Fever

***Nursing Considerations:*** Shake solution before preparing. Give vaccine within 12 hours of birth to infants of infected mothers. Bathe infants before the injection to remove blood and prevent contamination of the injection site with maternal blood on the infant's skin. Obtain parental consent before administering.

## Newborn Screening Tests

Most states require that certain screening tests be performed on the blood of all newborns before discharge from the birth facility. These tests are performed to detect conditions that result from inborn errors of metabolism or other genetic conditions. Without early treatment, the disorders may cause mental retardation or other serious problems. The tests are easy and inexpensive. More thorough testing is necessary to confirm any abnormal test results. Although each state determines which conditions must be tested, those most commonly included are phenylketonuria (PKU), hypothyroidism, galactosemia, and hemoglobinopathies.

Screening tests require a blood sample taken from the infant's heel and are usually performed shortly before discharge. Parents may have questions about the purpose of the tests that the nurse will need to answer. Nurses often refer to the tests as "PKU tests," but they should call them screening tests to emphasize that a number of conditions are included in the tests.

When infants are discharged early, they may have the screening tests performed within the first 24 hours of life. However, the tests are less sensitive at that time. These infants should have repeat tests within 1 to 2 weeks of age so that disorders are not missed because of early testing (AAP, 1992). These tests can be performed at a home, clinic, or office visit.

### Phenylketonuria

Phenylketonuria is a condition in which the infant cannot metabolize the amino acid phenylalanine, which is common in protein foods such as milk. Although some phenylalanine is essential to growth, accumulations of it can result in severe mental retardation. If treatment is begun in the first 2 months of life, retardation can be prevented. Phenylketonuria is treated with a special low-phenylalanine diet, in which the amount of the amino acid is carefully regulated.

### Hypothyroidism

One in 3600 to 1 in 5000 newborns has hypothyroidism (U.S. Public Health Service, 1995). In this condition, the thyroid does not produce enough of the hormone thyroxine. Thyroid hormones affect the entire body, and the symptoms in an untreated infant include respiratory, feeding, and growth problems as well as irreversible brain damage. Early and consistent treatment with thyroid hormones allows normal growth and development of full intellect.

### Galactosemia

Absence of the enzyme necessary for the conversion of the milk sugar galactose to glucose causes galactosemia. The condition results in damage to the liver, brain, and eyes and eventually causes death. Treatment includes elimination of milk from the diet.

### Hemoglobinopathies

Hemoglobinopathies include sickle cell anemia, thalassemia, and other diseases. The diseases are most often found in infants of African, Mediterranean, Asian, or South and Central American background. In sickle cell anemia, erythrocytes may become sickle shaped, resulting in obstruction of blood vessels and erythrocyte destruction. The other hemoglobinopathies cause chronic anemias, sepsis, and other serious conditions.

### Other Conditions

Screening may also be performed for maple syrup urine disease, homocystinuria, and other conditions. Knowing which conditions are included in testing allows the nurse to include appropriate information in parent teaching.

**✓ CHECK YOUR READING**

10. What are some important considerations in planning parent teaching?
11. What immunization may be performed at the birth facility and why?
12. Why is it important to perform screening tests on infants as close to discharge as possible? When is retesting important?

## Discharge and Newborn Follow-up Care

### Discharge

Early discharge may be considered for term newborns who are appropriate for gestational age and have normal physical examination results. Infants who are discharged early should have vital signs within normal limits, have fed successfully, and show that they are making the transition from fetal to neonatal life without difficulty. The mother should show adequate knowledge, ability, and confidence to provide adequate care of the newborn (AAP, 1995).

Although state and federal legislation has been passed to allow women and infants to stay in the birth facility for 48 hours after vaginal birth and 96 hours after cesarean birth, some women choose to go home earlier. The time of discharge varies according to the mother and newborn's needs and wishes and the primary caregivers' assessment of their conditions.

### Follow-up Care

Follow-up care after discharge from the birth facility is very important. The American Academy of Pediatrics recommends that follow-up by a health care professional be provided to all newborns who go home from the birth facility less than 48 hours after birth. This should occur within 48 hours of discharge and can be provided in the home, clinic, or office (AAP, 1995).

Follow-up care can be provided in a number of ways. One or more home visits by a nurse are offered as a part of the maternity package in many birth facilities. In other areas, families return to the birth facility, a clinic, or the pediatrician's office to have the newborn checked.

Some birth facilities have "hot lines" or "warm lines" that mothers can call when they have questions about care of their infants or themselves. In many facilities, nurses call mothers during the first few days after discharge to assess the adjustment and health of the mother and baby, clarify information given before discharge, and answer questions. If problems are identified, appropriate referrals are made. This method is less expensive than home visits but does not allow the nurse to perform assessments in person. It may be combined with home visits used only for high-risk families. Follow-up care for newborns is discussed further in Chapter 23, p. 615.

## SUMMARY CONCEPTS

- Prophylaxis against hemorrhagic disease of the newborn and ophthalmia neonatorum are necessary shortly after birth. It is provided by an injection of vitamin K and use of erythromycin ophthalmic ointment.
- Newborns may need help in clearing the airway. Positioning, suction, and close observation may be necessary.
- Nurses can prevent heat loss in newborns by keeping them dry and covered, avoiding contact between them and cold objects or surfaces, and keeping them away from drafts and outside windows and walls.
- The nurse must identify actual or potential hypoglycemia and intervene appropriately.
- Important interventions for jaundice are to monitor for its occurrence, to be sure that the infant is feeding well, and to explain the condition to the parents.
- Potential benefits of circumcision may include decreased incidence of urinary tract infections and inflammation of the glans, prepuce, or meatus. Other reasons for circumcision include religious dictates, parent preference, and lack of knowledge about care of the foreskin. Potential risks of circumcision include hemorrhage, infection, over-removal, urethral stenosis or fistula, adhesions, and damage to the glans.
- Parents with uncircumcised sons should be taught not to retract the foreskin until it becomes separate from the glans later in childhood.
- Parents of circumcised infants should be taught signs of complications and how to care for the area.
- The nurse must prevent mistaken identification of infants by checking the mother and infant identification bands whenever they have been separated.
- Parents and nurses must work together to prevent infant abductions. Parents must know how to identify hospital staff. Nurses should be alert for suspicious behavior.
- Infection can best be prevented by scrupulous hand washing by staff and all who come in contact with newborns.
- Every nursing contact with parents should be used as an opportunity to teach.
- Screening tests are commonly performed to rule out PKU, hypothyroidism, galactosemia, and hemoglobinopathies.

### References and Readings

American Academy of Pediatrics (AAP). (1989). Report of the AAP task force on circumcision. *Pediatrics*, 84(4), 388–391.

American Academy of Pediatrics (AAP). (1993). Controversies concerning vitamin K and the newborn. *Pediatrics*, 91(5), 1001–1003.

American Academy of Pediatrics (AAP). (1995). Hospital stay for healthy term newborns. *Pediatrics*, 96(4), 788–789.

American Academy of Pediatrics (AAP), American College of Obstetricians and Gynecologists (ACDG). (1992). *Guidelines for perinatal care* (3rd ed). Washington, D.C.: Author.

American Academy of Pediatrics, Committee on Genetics. (1992). Issues in newborn screening. *Pediatrics* 89(2), 345–349.

American Academy of Pediatrics, Task Force on Infant Positioning and SIDS. (1992). Positioning and SIDS. *Pediatrics*, 89(6) 1120–1126.

Avery, G.B., Fletcher, M.A., & MacDonald, M.G. (Eds.) (1994). *Neonatology: Pathophysiology and management of the newborn* (4th ed.). Philadelphia: J.B. Lippincott.

Association of Women's Health, Obstetric, and Neonatal Nurses (AWHONN). (1994). Neonatal circumcision. Washington, D.C.: Author.

Association of Women's Health, Obstetric, and Neonatal Nurses (AWHONN). (1995). New data on infant abductions released. AWHONN *Voice*, 3(3), 11.

Association of Women's Health, Obstetric, and Neonatal Nurses (AWHONN). (1996). Physiologic assessment of the healthy newborn. Washington, D.C.: Author.

Association of Women's Health, Obstetric, and Neonatal Nurses (AWHONN) and National Center for Missing and Exploited Children. (1993). For healthcare professionals: Guidelines on preventing infant abductions: Washington, D.C.: AWHONN.

Barnes, L.P. (1995). Using the telephone in patient and family teaching. *American Journal of Maternal-Child Nursing*, 20(6), 341.

Beachy, P., & Deacon, J. (1992). Preventing neonatal kidnapping. *Journal of Obstetric, Gynecologic, and Neonatal Nursing*, 21(1), 12–16.

Choi, E.C. (1995). A contrast of mothering behaviors in women from Korea and the United States. *Journal of Obstetric, Gynecologic, and Neonatal Nursing*, 24(4), 363–369.

Cook, L.S., Koutsky, L.A., & Holmes, K.K. (1994). Circumcision and sexually transmitted diseases. *American Journal of Public Health*, 84(2), 197–201.

Crawford, N.G., & Pruss, A.M. (1993). Preventing neonatal hepatitis B infection during the perinatal period. *Journal of Obstetric, Gynecologic, and Neonatal Nursing*, 22(6), 491–497.

D'Avanzo, C.E. (1992). Bridging the cultural gap with Southeast Asians. MCN: *American Journal of Maternal-Child Nursing*, 17(4), 204–208.

Eidelman, A.I., Hoffman, N.W., & Kaitz, M. (1993). Cognitive deficits in women after childbirth. *Obstetrics and Gynecology*, 81(5), 764–767.

Faucher, M.A., & Jackson, G. (1992). Pharmaceutical preparations: A review of drugs commonly used during the neonatal period. *Journal of Nurse-Midwifery*, 37(2), 74S–86S.

Freitag-Koontz, M.J. (1997). Prevention of hepatitis B and C transmission during pregnancy and the first year of life. *Journal of Perinatal and Neonatal Nursing*, 10(2), 40–55.

Fuentes-Afflick, E. (1996). Circumcision. In H.W. Taeusch, R.O. Christiansen, & E.S. Buescher, *Pediatric and neonatal tests and procedures*. Philadelphia: W.B. Saunders.

Kaplan, G.W. (1994). Structural abnormalities of the genitourinary system. In G.B. Avery, M.A. Fletcher, & M.G. Macdonald (Eds.), *Neonatology: Pathophysiology and management of the newborn* (4th ed.). Philadelphia: J.B. Lippincott.

Lerner, H. (1993). Sleep position of infants: Applying research to practice. *American Journal of Maternal-Child Nursing*, 18(5), 275–277.

Mattson, S. (1995). Culturally sensitive perinatal care for Southeast Asians. *Journal of Obstetric, Gynecologic, and Neonatal Nursing*, 24(4), 335–341.

Mattson, S., & Smith, J.E. (1993). NAACOG *core curriculum for maternal-newborn nursing*. Philadelphia: W.B. Saunders.

McGregor, L.A. (1994). Short, shorter, shortest: Improving the hospital stay for mothers and newborns. *American Journal of Maternal-Child Nursing*, 19(2), 91–96.

McGregor, L.A. (1996). Short, shorter, shortest: Continuing to improve the hospital stay for mothers and newborns. *American Journal of Maternal-Child Nursing*, 21(4), 191–196.

Penny-MacGillivray, T. (1996). A newborn's first bath: When? *Journal of Obstetric, Gynecologic, and Neonatal Nursing*, 25(6), 481–487.

Philip, A. (1996). *Neonatology, a practical guide* (4th ed.). Philadelphia: W.B. Saunders.

Rabinowitz, R., & Hulbert, W.C. (1995). Newborn circumcision should not be performed without anesthesia. *Birth*, 22(1) 45–46.

Rabun, J.B., & Lincoln, J. (1994). Preventing infant abductions from health care facilities. *Neonatal Network*, 13(8), 61–63.

Roberts, J.A. (1996). Neonatal circumcision: An end to the controversy? *Southern Medical Journal*, 89(2), 167–171.

Ruchala, P., Seibold, L., & Stremsterfer, K. (1996). Validating assessment of neonatal jaundice with transcutaneous bilirubin measurement. *Neonatal Network*, 15(4), 33–37.

Schneiderman, J.U. (1996). Postpartum nursing for Korean mothers. *American Journal of Maternal-Child Nursing*, 21(3), 155–158.

Simpson, K.R., & Creehan, P.A. (Eds. 1996). AWHONN's *perinatal nursing*. Philadelphia: Lippincott-Raven.

Sinai, L.N., Kim, S.C., Casey, R., & Pinto-Martin, J.A. (1995). Phenylketonuria screening: Effect of early newborn discharge. *Pediatrics*, 96(4), 605–608.

Snellman, L.W., & Stang, H.J. (1995). Prospective evaluation of complications of dorsal penile nerve block for neonatal circumcision. *Pediatrics*, 95(5), 705–708.

Taddio, A., Goldbach, M., Ipp, M., Stevens, B., & Koren, G. (1995). Effect of neonatal circumcision pain responses during vaccination in boys. *Lancet*, 345(Feb. 4), 292–293.

U.S. Public Health Service (1995). Put prevention into practice: Newborn screening. *Journal of the American Academy of Nurse Practitioners*, 7(10), 513–517.

# 22

# Infant Feeding

**OBJECTIVES**

1. Identify the nutritional and fluid needs of the infant.
2. Compare the composition of breast milk with that of formula.
3. Explain important factors in choosing a method of infant feeding.
4. Explain the physiology of lactation.
5. Describe nursing management of initial and continued breastfeeding.
6. Describe nursing assessments and interventions for common problems in breastfeeding.
7. Describe nursing assessments and interventions in formula feeding.

**DEFINITIONS**

**colostrum** *Breast fluid secreted during pregnancy and the first 2 to 3 days following childbirth.*

**engorgement** *Swelling of the breasts resulting from feedings that are delayed, too short, or not frequent enough.*

**foremilk** *First breast milk received in a feeding.*

**hindmilk** *Breast milk received near the end of a feeding; contains higher fat content than foremilk.*

**latch-on** *Attachment of the infant to the breast.*

**let-down reflex** *See milk-ejection reflex.*

**mastitis** *Inflammation of the breast, usually caused by stasis of milk in the ducts or by infection.*

**mature milk** *Breast milk that appears after the first 2 weeks of lactation.*

**milk-ejection reflex** *Release of milk from the alveoli into the ducts; also known as the let-down reflex.*

**non-nutritive sucking** *Sucking during which no milk flow is obtained.*

**nutritive suckling or sucking** *Steady rhythmic suckling at the breast or sucking at a bottle to obtain milk.*

**oxytocin** *Hormone produced by the posterior pituitary gland that stimulates uterine contractions and the milk-ejection reflex; also prepared synthetically.*

**prolactin** *Anterior pituitary hormone that promotes growth of breast tissue and stimulates production of milk.*

**suckling** *Giving or taking nourishment from the breast. Sometimes used interchangeably with sucking, which refers only to drawing into the mouth with a partial vacuum, as with a bottle or pacifier.*

**transitional milk** *Breast milk that appears between secretion of colostrum and mature milk.*

Infant feeding is an important part of parenting, and a woman may derive much of her satisfaction as a mother from her perception of success with feeding. Helping her as she chooses a feeding method and learns to feel comfortable using it are important nursing contributions that require knowledge of the infant's nutritional needs and the techniques to meet those needs.

## Nutritional Needs of the Newborn

### Calories

The full-term newborn needs 110 to 120 kcal/kg (50 to 55 kcal/pound) of body weight each day. The infant must consume sufficient calories to meet energy needs, prevent use of body stores, and provide for growth. The diet should contain enough carbohydrate and fat that dietary proteins are not used for energy, as this would decrease protein available for growth.

Breast milk and formulas used for the normal newborn contain 20 kcal/ounce. The average newborn weighing 3.4 kg (7.5 pounds) requires approximately 19 to 21 ounces of breast milk or formula each day to meet caloric requirements. This is 45 to 75 ml (1.5 to 2.5 ounces) at each feeding for infants who breastfeed every 2 to 3 hours. Formula-fed infants who feed every 3 to 4 hours need 75 to 105 ml (2.5 to 3.5 ounces) at each feeding.

During the early days after birth, many infants lose 5 to 10 percent of their birth weight. This is due to normal loss of extracellular water and the fact that they often consume fewer calories than needed. Newborns may fall asleep before feeding adequately or sleep through feeding times in the early days. The stomach capacity at birth is only about 6 ml/kg (Blackburn & Loper, 1992), making it difficult to meet caloric needs. Capacity increases rapidly so that many infants take 2 to 3 ounces by the end of the first week. Infants usually regain the lost weight by age 10 days. This information should be explained to parents.

### Nutrients

The calories needed by the newborn are provided by carbohydrates, proteins, and fat in breast milk or formula. Full-term neonates digest simple carbohydrates and proteins well. Fats are less well digested because of the lack of pancreatic lipase in the newborn. Vitamins and minerals are provided by both breast milk and formula.

### Water

The newborn needs much larger amounts of fluid in relationship to size than does the adult because infants lose water more easily from the skin, kidneys, and intestines. As a result, they must take in fluids equal to 10 to 15 percent of their body weight each day, whereas adults need only 2 to 4 percent of their body weight daily (Behrman et al., 1996). The normal newborn needs approximately 100 to 150 ml/kg (45 to 68 ml/pound) a day after the first 2 days of life (DeMarini et al., 1993). Breast milk or formula supplies the infant's fluid needs. Additional water is unnecessary.

**Critical to Remember**

**Daily Calorie and Fluid Needs of the Newborn**

Calories: 110 to 120 kcal/kg (50 to 55 kcal/lb)
Fluid: 100 to 150 ml/kg (after first 2 days of life)

## Breast Milk and Formula Composition

### Breast Milk

Breast milk is species-specific for human infants and offers many advantages over formula. The nutrients in breast milk are proportioned appropriately for the neonate and change to meet the newborn's changing needs. Breast milk provides protection against infection and is easily digested. Table 22–1 compares breast milk, cow's milk, and modified cow's milk formulas according to the recommended nutrient intake for infants.

#### CHANGES IN COMPOSITION

The composition of breast milk changes in three phases: colostrum, transitional milk, and mature milk, which vary in makeup to meet the newborn's changing nutritional needs.

**Colostrum.** The major secretion of the breasts during the first week of lactation is colostrum—a thick, yellow substance. Colostrum is higher in protein, fat-soluble vitamins, and minerals than mature milk but lower in calories, fat, and lactose. It is rich in immunoglobulins, especially secretory IgA, which helps protect the infant's gastrointestinal tract from infection. Colostrum helps establish the normal flora in the intestines, and its laxative effect speeds the passage of meconium.

**Transitional Milk.** Transitional milk appears by 7 to 10 days after lactation begins as the milk changes from colostrum to mature milk. Immunoglobulins and proteins decrease while lactose, fat, and calories in-

**TABLE 22-1 COMPARISON OF RECOMMENDED DIETARY ALLOWANCES WITH INFANT MILKS PER DECILITER**

| Nutrient | Recommended Dietary Allowances Infants to 6 Months | Mature Human Milk | Cow's Milk | Modified Cow's Milk Formulas |
|---|---|---|---|---|
| Kilocalories | * | 73 | 63 | 68 |
| Protein (g) | 13 | 1 | 3.3 | 1.5 |
| Fat (g) | | 4.5 | 3.3 | 3.6 |
| Vitamin A (IU) | 1238 | 190–240 | 310 | 203 |
| Vitamin D (IU) | 300 | 2.2 | 4.2 | 41 |
| Vitamin C (mg) | 30 | 4.3–5 | 0.8 | 5.4 |
| Thiamin (mg) | 0.3 | 0.14 | 0.04 | 0.06 |
| Riboflavin (mg) | 0.4 | 0.37 | 0.17 | 1.01 |
| Niacin (mg) | 5 | 0.15–0.18 | 0.08 | 0.7 |
| Calcium (mg) | 400 | 33 | 121 | 51 |
| Phosphorus (mg) | 300 | 15 | 95 | 39 |
| Iron (mg) | 6 | 0.02 | 0.04 | 0.12 |
| Sodium (mg) | 120 | 16 | 50 | 22 |

*Recommendation for kilocalories is based on infant's weight: 110–120 kcal/kg.
*Source:* Data from Institute of Medicine, National Academy of Sciences, Food and Nutrition Board (1991). *Nutrition during lactation.* Washington, D.C.: National Academy Press; Mahan, L.K., & Escott-Stump, S (Eds.). (1996). *Krause's food, nutrition, and diet therapy* (9th ed). Philadelphia: W.B. Saunders; Merenstein, G.B., & Gardner, S.L. (1989). *Handbook of neonatal intensive care* (2nd ed.). St. Louis: C.V. Mosby.

crease. The vitamin content is approximately the same as that of mature milk.

**Mature Milk.** After the first 2 weeks of lactation, mature milk replaces transitional milk. Because breast milk is bluish and not as thick as colostrum, some mothers think their milk is not "rich" enough for the infant. Nurses should explain the normal appearance of breast milk. Mature milk contains approximately 20 kcal/ounce and nutrients sufficient to meet the infant's needs. In general, discussions of breast milk and its contents refer to mature milk unless otherwise stated.

### NUTRIENTS

Although unmodified cow's milk is not given to infants in developed countries, it forms the base for most infant formulas. Comparing human milk with cow's milk demonstrates the adaptations that are necessary to produce infant formulas.

**Protein.** The concentrations of amino acids in breast milk are suited to the infant's needs and ability to metabolize them. Breast milk contains a high level of taurine, which is important for bile conjugation and brain development. Tyrosine and phenylalanine are low in breast milk to correspond to the infant's low level of enzymes to digest them. The proteins produce a lower solute load for the infant's immature kidneys than the proteins in cow's milk.

Casein and whey are the proteins in milk. Casein forms a large, insoluble curd that is harder to digest than the curd from whey, which is very soft. Breast milk is more easily digested because it has a higher ratio of whey to casein than cow's milk. The larger proportion of casein in cow's milk results in a curd that takes longer to digest and is less completely digested. Commercial formulas are adapted to increase the amount of whey so that the curd is more digestible.

The body's immune system recognizes and may react to the protein in cow's milk, making it one of the most common allergens. Allergies develop in approximately 3 to 5 percent of infants fed cow's milk formulas (Adams, 1992). Because breast milk is made for the human infant, it does not cause allergies (Lawrence, 1994). Long-term follow-up studies have shown a significant decrease in allergic conditions when infants are breastfed exclusively for at least 1 month (Saarinen & Kajosaari, 1995) This is of particular importance when there is a family history of allergies.

**Carbohydrate.** Lactose is the carbohydrate in breast milk. Its higher level in breast milk may improve absorption of calcium (Lawrence, 1994). Lactose also promotes growth of the normal bacterial flora in the intestines.

**Fat.** Thirty to 55 percent of the calories in breast milk are from fat. The fat composition of human milk differs greatly from that of cow's milk. The majority is in the form of triglycerides, with higher amounts of several essential fatty acids. Cholesterol is also higher in breast milk than in cow's milk. The high level of cholesterol may aid in the development of the central nervous system. The fat in breast milk is more easily digested by the newborn than that in cow's milk.

The amount of fat in breast milk varies during the feeding and according to the time of day. More fat is present in the hindmilk, the milk produced at the end of the feeding. Hindmilk produces satiety and helps the infant gain weight. Fat is lowest in the early morning and is increased during the middle-of-the-day feedings (Riordan, 1993a).

**Vitamins.** The vitamin content varies between human and cow's milk as well. Vitamin C must be added to commercial formulas to match the levels in human milk, which meet the infant's needs if the mother has an adequate intake. Vitamin D may be inadequate and need supplementation if the mother's diet is poor and she or the infant is not exposed to the sun. The infant of a vegan mother may need supplementation with vitamin $B_{12}$.

**Minerals.** Although iron in breast milk is lower than in formula, approximately 49 percent is absorbed, compared with only 4 percent of that in iron-fortified formula (Lawrence, 1994). The increased absorption may be due to the higher lactose and vitamin C content in breast milk. The infant who is breastfed exclusively maintains iron stores for the first 6 months of life. However, the addition of formula or other foods may decrease the absorption of iron, making supplementation necessary.

Sodium, calcium, and phosphorus are higher in cow's milk than in human milk. This could cause an excessively high renal solute load if formula is not diluted properly. The amount of fluoride in breast milk is not influenced by the mother's diet. Fluoride supplements may be given to ensure adequate intake.

#### ENZYMES

Breast milk contains enzymes that aid in digestion. Pancreatic amylase, necessary to digest carbohydrates, is low in the newborn, but the enzyme is present in breast milk. Breast milk also contains lipase to increase fat digestion.

**CHECK YOUR READING**

1. Why do some newborns lose weight after birth?
2. What are the differences between colostrum, transitional milk, and mature breast milk?
3. How does breast milk compare to commercial formulas?

#### INFECTION-PREVENTING COMPONENTS

Other factors present in human milk help prevent infection in the newborn. *Bifidus factor* promotes the growth of *Lactobacillus bifidus*, an important part of the intestinal flora that helps produce an acid environment in the gastrointestinal tract. This protects the infant against infection from common intestinal pathogens.

*Leukocytes* present in breast milk also help protect against infection. Macrophages are most abundant and secrete lysozyme and lactoferrin. *Lysozyme* is a bacteriolytic enzyme that acts against gram-positive and enteric bacteria. *Lactoferrin* is a protein that binds iron in iron-dependent bacteria, such as *Staphylococcus* and *Escherichia coli*, preventing their growth. It also acts against *Candida albicans*. Giving infants supplementary iron may interfere with the effectiveness of lactoferrin.

*Immunoglobulins* are present in highest amounts in colostrum but are present throughout lactation. Higher levels occur when the infant is born prematurely. Lymphocytes in the milk produce secretory IgA, which helps prevent viral or bacterial invasion of the intestinal mucosa, resulting in fewer intestinal infections in breastfed than in formula-fed infants. This protection is especially important because the infant does not produce adequate amounts of IgA in the intestinal tract until 6 to 12 weeks of age. IgA also helps prevent respiratory infections and prevents absorption of foreign molecules that might precipitate development of allergies. Infants who are breastfed, even partially, have a significantly decreased incidence not only of respiratory and gastrointestinal infections, but of ear infections and hospitalization as well (Beaudry et al., 1995).

#### EFFECT OF MATERNAL DIET

Although the fatty acid content of breast milk is influenced by the mother's diet, malnourished mothers have about the same proportions of protein, carbohydrates, and most minerals as those who are well nourished. However, levels of vitamins in breast milk are affected by the mother's intake and stores. It is important that breastfeeding women eat a well-balanced diet to maintain their own health and energy levels. (Nutrition for the lactating mother is discussed in Chapter 9, p. 213.)

## Formulas

Commercial formulas are produced to replace or supplement breast milk. Manufacturers adapt commercial formulas to correspond to the components in breast milk as much as possible, although an exact match is not possible. A variety of formulas that differ in price and ingredients is available.

#### COW'S MILK

Modified cow's milk is the source of approximately 80 percent of commercial formulas. Manufacturers specifically formulate it for infants by reducing protein to decrease renal solute load. Saturated fat is removed and replaced with vegetable fats. Vitamins and other nutrients are added to simulate the contents of breast milk. Examples of formulas are Similac and Enfamil. These formulas are also available with added iron.

#### FORMULAS FOR ALLERGIC INFANTS

Infants who have formula intolerance or allergies or come from families in which allergies are prevalent are given soy or protein hydrolysate formulas. Soy milk is derived from the protein of soybeans and supplemented with amino acids. It is also used for infants who are unable to tolerate lactose. Examples of soy formulas are ProSobee and Isomil.

Many infants with cow's milk allergy are also allergic to soy formulas. Protein hydrolysate formulas, such as Nutramigen, are more universally tolerated by infants with allergies. The protein in these cow's milk–based formulas is treated so that they are hypoallergenic. The formulas are also used for infants with fat malabsorption.

#### SPECIAL FORMULAS

Some formulas are designed to meet the needs of infants with special problems. The preterm infant may require a more concentrated formula with more calories in less liquid, such as Enfamil Premature and Similac Special Care. Specific nutrients are added for the preterm infant's higher requirements in a more easily digestible form. Human milk fortifiers, such as Similac Natural Care, can be added to human milk to adapt it to the needs of preterm infants. Formulas such as Pregestimil are produced for infants with gastrointestinal problems. Lactofree formula is modified for infants who do not tolerate lactose. Lofenalac is low in the amino acid phenylalanine and is given to infants with phenylketonuria (PKU), who are deficient in the enzyme to digest phenylalanine found in standard formulas.

## Considerations in Choosing a Feeding Method

Many women decide on a feeding method well ahead of birth. Some may not have questions about which method is best for them until late in their pregnancy. Nurses can help mothers decide on a method and gain confidence in feeding their infants. In fact, being advised during the prenatal period to breastfeed was the most important predictor of whether Mexican-American and non-Hispanic white women in one study breastfed their newborns (Balcazar et al., 1995). Although many woman who receive Women, Infants, and Children (WIC) assistance do not choose to breastfeed, those who receive breastfeeding advice from WIC staff are more likely to choose that method of feeding their infants (Schwartz et al., 1995).

It is very important for nurses to be sensitive to mothers' feelings about feeding. Although nurses should encourage breastfeeding as the best method of feeding in most circumstances, they should be supportive of the mother's chosen method once the decision is made. The early days of parenting are a very vulnerable time for new mothers, who may feel that their feeding ability reflects on their mothering ability. The nurse's teaching and encouragement about the chosen feeding method increase their self-confidence.

### Breastfeeding

Breastfeeding offers many advantages, which are summarized in Table 22–2. Although breastfeeding was once the major method of feeding, many factors have decreased the incidence of breastfeeding. The advent of refrigeration, the development of commercial formulas, and the increased incidence of maternal employment have led to an increase in the number of mothers choosing formula feeding. In addition, advertisements by formula companies and formula gift packs given to mothers at discharge, which may imply an expectation that nursing mothers will need formula, have aided the move away from breastfeeding.

It has been increasingly recognized, however, that formula feeding can never fully equal breastfeeding in terms of providing for the infant's optimal growth

**TABLE 22–2 BENEFITS OF BREASTFEEDING**

**For the Infant**

- No allergic reaction to breast milk
- Immunologic properties help prevent infections. May have fewer respiratory, ear, and gastrointestinal infections and less risk for hospitalization
- Composition meets infant's specific nutritional needs
- Nutritional and immunologic properties change according to infant's needs
- Breast milk easily digested
- Protein, fat, and carbohydrate in most suitable proportions
- No possibility of improper (and potentially dangerous) dilution
- Breast milk unlikely to be contaminated, not affected by water supply
- Less likely to result in overfeeding
- Unlikely to have constipation

**For the Mother**

- Oxytocin release enhances involution of uterus
- She is more likely to rest while feeding
- She is likely to eat balanced diet that improves healing
- May help with postpartum weight loss
- Frequent, close contact may enhance bonding
- Convenient: always available, no bottles to prepare, no formula to buy or heat
- Economical: eliminates cost of formula and bottles
- Traveling easier: no bottles to prepare, carry, refrigerate, or warm

and development. Both the American Academy of Pediatrics and the U.S. Surgeon General recommend breastfeeding. A goal set by the U.S. Department of Health and Human Services (USDHHS) for the year 2000 is for 75 percent of all new mothers to breastfeed at the time of birth facility discharge and for at least 50 percent to continue breastfeeding for 5 to 6 months. This is based on the 1988 figures of only 54 percent of mothers breastfeeding at discharge from the birth facility and only 21 percent still breastfeeding at 5 to 6 months (USDHHS, 1991). Although slight progress has been made, the goal is not near to being met at this time. In 1995, 59.7 percent of mothers were breastfeeding at the time of discharge and 21.6 percent were still breastfeeding at 6 months (Ross Products Division, 1995).

In an effort to promote breastfeeding, the United Nations Children's Fund (UNICEF) and the World Health Organization (WHO) are advocating that birth facilities become certified as baby-friendly hospitals, where policies are initiated to actively encourage breastfeeding. Guidelines to becoming certified as a baby-friendly hospital emphasize education of staff and parents about breastfeeding, early initiation of breastfeeding, demand feedings, avoidance of formula and pacifiers, and rooming in.

## Formula Feeding

Mothers choose formula feeding for many reasons. Some mothers are embarrassed by breastfeeding, seeing the breast only in a sexual context. Many mothers have little experience with family or friends who have had positive breastfeeding experiences. Some women feel a need to maintain a strict feeding schedule and are uneasy not knowing exactly how much milk the infant will take at each feeding. A mother who has many other commitments may feel that formula feeding would meet her needs best. Some women may require medications that enter breast milk and are harmful to the infant. A frequent reason that mothers choose formula feeding instead of breastfeeding may be a lack of adequate knowledge about the two methods.

## Combination Feeding

Some parents prefer a combination of breastfeeding and bottle feeding. It is best to delay this until lactation has been well established at 3 to 4 weeks, if possible. Either breast milk or formula may be given in the bottle. The mother may give a bottle each day or only occasionally, such as when a baby sitter is with the infant. This allows the mother to be away from the infant for longer periods of time, yet allows the closeness with the infant that many mothers enjoy, as well as the physical advantages of breastfeeding, to continue.

## Factors Influencing Choice

Many factors influence a woman's choice of feeding method. These factors must be considered when educating women about their choices.

### CULTURE

Cultural influences may dictate decisions about how a mother feeds her infant. For example, many Mormon women believe that breastfeeding is an important part of motherhood. Muslim women often breastfeed for the first 2 years. Some immigrants from countries where breastfeeding is the norm may breastfeed for shorter durations or not at all because they lack the support system they had in their own country. In addition, formula feeding may be seen as a symbol of the new way of life. It may be considered a way to help infants grow larger and be stronger (Riordan, 1993b). For example, Cambodian women rarely bottle fed infants before coming to the United States but rarely breastfeed infants born in the United States. However, their style of bottle feeding mimics breastfeeding methods used previously in that infants have unlimited access to formula and are weaned late (Rasbridge & Kulig, 1995).

In one study, 58 percent of Hmong women who had previously given birth in Laos or Thailand breastfed there, but almost all chose to formula feed when they gave birth in the United States (Jambunathan & Stewart, 1995). Ethiopian women often breastfeed for more than a year in their home country but may breastfeed for much shorter periods when they come to the United States (Meftuh et al., 1991). Nurses should be particularly watchful for ways to help mothers from other cultures who might wish to breastfeed but fail to do so because of lack of support.

In some Asian and Latino cultures, mothers give their infants formula while in the birth facility and do not begin to breastfeed until at home. This may be due to modesty and embarrassment about nursing in front of others in the birth facility, as well as lack of understanding about the value of colostrum. Some may believe that breastfeeding before the milk comes in may drain heat and fluids from the mother (Mattson, 1995). Women in some cultures believe that colostrum may be "spoiled" because it has been in the breasts for a long time. They may manually express colostrum and discard it before they begin to breastfeed the infant.

Some mothers may be amenable to nursing the infant with help while in the birth facility, especially if the antibody and laxative properties of colostrum are explained. Breastfeeding involves a learning process for both mother and infant, and this is best started where assistance is available. Nurses can help women learn by offering to help them "practice" breastfeeding at least a few times before discharge. This helps build their confidence and allows for early identification and correction of problems. If the mother is firm in her desire to wait until discharge to begin breastfeeding, nurses can support her by teaching her what she will need to know when she goes home. Cultural values about feeding, as about other areas of health care, must be respected.

#### EMPLOYMENT

The need to return to employment soon after birth may cause concern about feeding methods. The mother may choose formula from the beginning, plan a short period of breastfeeding before weaning the infant to formula, or use a combination of breastfeeding and bottle feeding. Nurses provide information about options, breastfeeding and working, using breast pumps (see p. 605), and storage of breast milk. Pamphlets and books for the working breastfeeding mother are particularly helpful.

#### SUPPORT FROM OTHERS

Family members and friends may also share in the decision-making process. The woman's own mother and the baby's father are often most important in helping her make a decision. The mother with little support or with active discouragement from her family will probably have a difficult time nursing. Involvement of the father in feedings is important in some families and may be thought possible only if he can give a bottle regularly. Nurses can suggest other ways that fathers can participate in infant care, such as holding and rocking. Educating family members about the advantages of breastfeeding and how to deal with problems may lead to their encouragement of the breastfeeding mother.

The support the mother receives from the nursing staff plays a significant part in whether she feels comfortable with the feeding method she chooses. Those who do not feel confident in their ability to breastfeed before they leave the birth facility are less likely to continue breastfeeding if they encounter difficulties at home.

#### OTHER FACTORS

Other factors may also influence a woman's decision. Her knowledge and past experience with infant feeding are important. Very young mothers are less likely to breastfeed. More women with higher education and social class breastfeed than mothers with less education or low incomes. White mothers breastfeed more often than black or Latino women. The time when the decision is made is also important. Many mothers choose their feeding methods before pregnancy and the majority by the end of pregnancy. An early decision to breastfeed often leads to a longer duration of breastfeeding (Losch et al., 1995).

#### ✓ CHECK YOUR READING

4. What factors does breast milk contain that help prevent infection?
5. What types of commercial formulas are available?
6. What factors influence a woman's choice of feeding method?

## Normal Breastfeeding

To be most helpful to lactating mothers, the nurse must have a good understanding of the physiology of lactation. The anatomy and physiology of the breast are discussed in Chapter 4 (p. 68), and breast changes occurring in pregnancy are discussed in full in Chapter 7 (p. 124) (see Figs. 4–8 and 7–3).

### Breast Changes During Pregnancy

Breast changes begin early in pregnancy with development of the ducts, lobules, and alveoli in response to the hormones estrogen, progesterone, placental lactogen, prolactin, and chorionic gonadotropin. The breasts begin to secrete colostrum by the second trimester, and women who give birth after the 16th week of gestation produce colostrum (Lawrence, 1994). During pregnancy, the anterior pituitary secretes high levels of prolactin, the hormone that causes the breasts to produce milk. However, milk production is prevented by estrogen, progesterone, and placental lactogen, which inhibit breast response to prolactin.

### Milk Production

Milk is produced in the alveoli of the breasts through a complex process by which materials are removed from the mother's blood stream and reformulated into breast milk. Thus, amino acids, glucose, lipids, enzymes, leukocytes, and other materials are used to manufacture the various proteins, carbohydrates, fats, and other substances needed to nourish and protect the infant. Most milk is synthesized when the infant is suckling, although a small amount is made between feedings and stored for the next feeding (Lawrence, 1994).

The milk is ejected from the secretory cells of the alveoli into the alveolar lumen by contraction of the myoepithelial cells. From there, it travels into the lactiferous ducts, which lead from the alveoli to the nipple. The ducts widen in the area of the areola to become the lactiferous sinuses (or ampullae), which the infant compresses during nursing to eject a stream of milk through pores in the nipple.

## Hormonal Changes at Birth

### PROLACTIN

Separation of the placenta and suckling of the infant are responsible for initiation of lactation. Loss of progesterone, estrogen, and placental lactogen from the placenta results in increasing levels and effectiveness of prolactin and brings about milk production. The tactile stimulation of suckling and the removal of colostrum or milk causes continued increased levels of prolactin.

### OXYTOCIN

Oxytocin, from the posterior pituitary, increases in response to nipple stimulation. Oxytocin causes the milk-ejection reflex, commonly known as the let-down reflex. The resulting contraction of myoepithelial cells around the alveoli releases milk into the ducts, making it available to the infant.

When mothers see, hear, or think about their infants, they often have an increase in oxytocin level, bringing about a let-down of milk. Pain or lack of relaxation can inhibit oxytocin release. Assisting the mother to a comfortable position and relieving her pain helps the let-down reflex occur more quickly. Oxytocin is also responsible for the uterine contractions mothers may feel at the beginning of nursing sessions; these contractions hasten involution of the uterus (Fig. 22–1).

## Continued Milk Production

The amount of milk produced depends primarily on adequate stimulation of the breast and removal of the milk by suckling or a breast pump, which causes production of prolactin. This "supply and demand" effect continues throughout lactation. That is, increased demand with more frequent and longer nursing results in more milk available for the infant.

If milk (or colostrum) is not removed from the breasts, the alveoli become very distended. Pressure on the blood vessels reduces blood flow and prevents prolactin from reaching the secretory cells. Lack of nipple stimulation causes release of prolactin inhibiting factor by the hypothalamus, and milk production gradually ceases. The milk in the ducts is absorbed, the alveoli become smaller, and the cells return to a resting state.

## Preparation of Breasts for Breastfeeding

Little preparation is needed during pregnancy for breastfeeding. The mother should avoid soap on her nipples to prevent removal of the natural protective oils from the Montgomery tubercles of the breasts. The use of creams, nipple rolling, pulling, and rubbing to "toughen" nipples does not necessarily de-

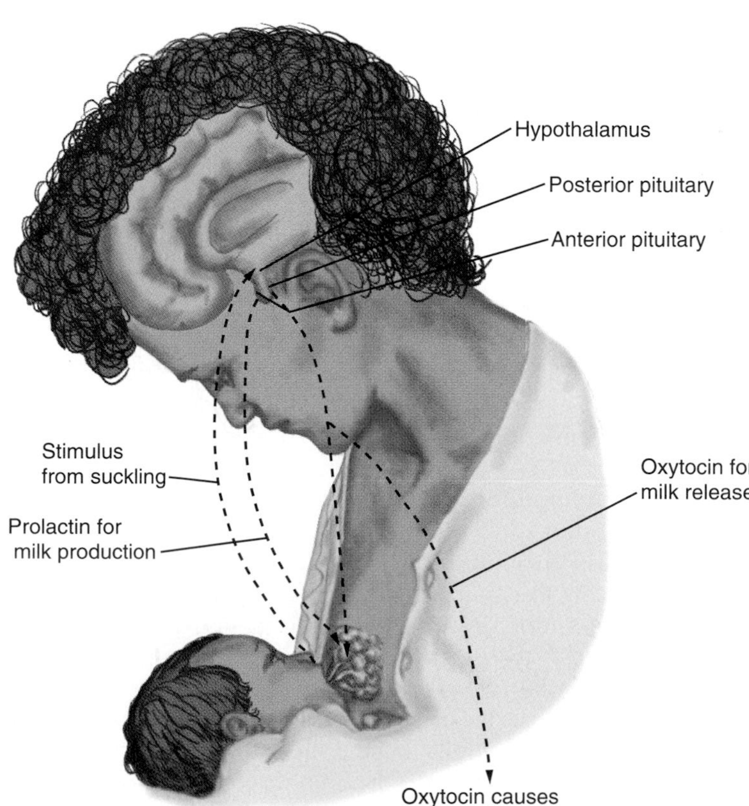


**FIGURE 22–1**

Effect of prolactin and oxytocin on milk production. When the infant begins to suckle at the breast, nerve impulses travel to the hypothalamus, which causes the anterior pituitary to secrete prolactin to increase milk production. Suckling also causes the posterior pituitary to secrete oxytocin, producing the let-down reflex, which releases milk from the breast. Oxytocin also causes the uterus to contract, which aids in involution.

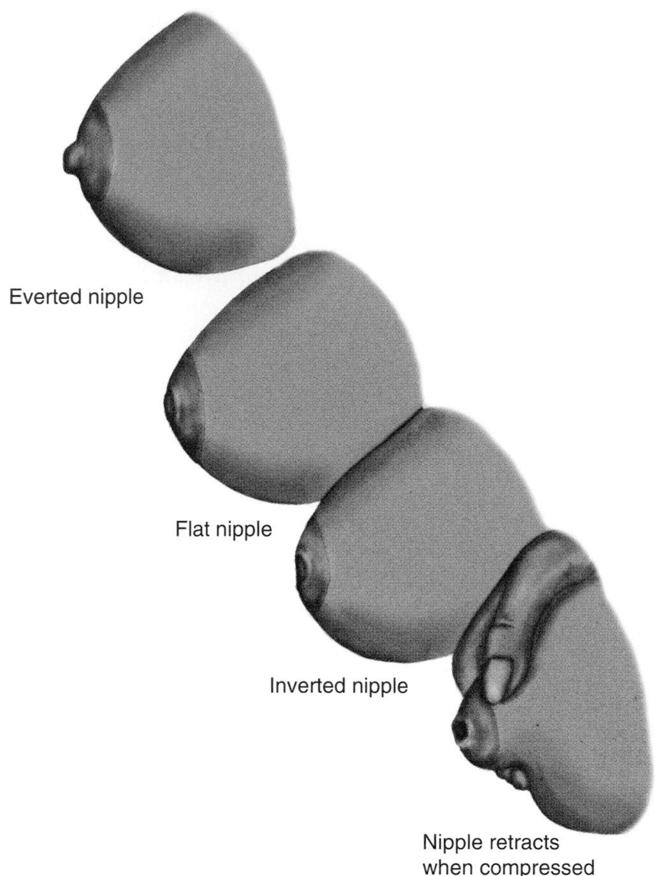


**FIGURE 22–2**

Normal everted nipple and other types of nipples that may cause the infant difficulty in latching-on. Nipples shown after stimulation.

crease nipple pain after birth and may cause irritation or uterine contractions from release of oxytocin. In addition, some women feel that extensive nipple preparation is too much trouble or distasteful and may decide not to breastfeed if they believe that this preparation is necessary.

The breasts should be assessed during pregnancy to identify flat or inverted nipples (Fig. 22–2). Normally, the nipples protrude. Flat nipples appear soft, like the areola, and do not stand erect unless stimulated by rolling them between the fingers. Nipples may also be inverted, or drawn into the breast tissue. Both conditions make it difficult for infants to draw the nipples into the mouth. Some nipples appear normal but draw inward when the areola is compressed in the infant's mouth. Compressing the areola between the thumb and the forefinger determines whether the nipple projects normally or becomes inverted.

Women with flat or inverted nipples sometimes use breast shells during the last weeks of pregnancy and after birth. The shells (also called breast cups) are worn in the bra with the opening over the nipple. They exert slight pressure against the areola and help the nipples protrude. Some shells are solid and milk may collect in them. Warn the mother not to give this milk to the infant because bacteria multiply rapidly in it. Pumping the breasts for a few minutes before beginning nursing also helps bring the nipples out. Exercises for inverted nipples are not recommended during pregnancy because they may cause uterine contractions.

**CHECK YOUR READING**

7. What is the effect of suckling on the let-down reflex and milk production?
8. How does the principle of "supply and demand" apply to breastfeeding?
9. What preparation of the breasts is needed during pregnancy?

## Application of Nursing Process: Breastfeeding

### Assessment

Assess both the mother and the infant during the breastfeeding process. Various scoring tools have been developed for assessing breastfeeding, but none is completely satisfactory. One method used is the LATCH scoring tool, shown in Table 22–3.

#### MATERNAL ASSESSMENT

Assess the condition of the breasts and nipples and the mother's knowledge about breastfeeding to determine her needs for assistance.

**Breasts and Nipples.** Examine the breasts and nipples during pregnancy so that problems that might interfere with feeding can be corrected. If this assessment did not occur before birth, examine the breasts and nipples before the initial feeding. Assess the protrusion of the nipples to identify flat or inverted nipples.

Ongoing assessments include identification of breast fullness and breast engorgement. Fullness is the swelling of the breasts that may occur early in lactation as a result of increased blood and lymph circulation. It may progress to engorgement if feedings are delayed, too short, or not frequent enough. Palpate the breasts to see if they are soft, filling, or engorged. Soft breasts feel like a cheek. If milk is beginning to come in, the breasts may be slightly firmer, which is charted as "filling." Engorged breasts are hard and tender, with taut, shiny skin. Note any redness, tenderness, or lumps within the breasts.

**TABLE 22-3 THE LATCH SCORING TOOL**

| | 0 | 1 | 2 |
|---|---|---|---|
| L<br>Latch | Too sleepy or reluctant<br>No latch achieved | Repeated attempts necessary<br>Must hold nipple in infant's mouth<br>Must stimulate infant to suck | Grasps breast<br>Tongue down<br>Lips flanged<br>Rhythmic sucking |
| A<br>Audible swallowing | None | A few with stimulation | Spontaneous and intermittent <24 hr old<br>Spontaneous and frequent >24 hr old |
| T<br>Type of nipple | Inverted | Flat | Everted (after stimulation) |
| C<br>Comfort (breast/ nipple) | Engorged<br>Cracked, bleeding, large blisters, or bruises<br>Severe discomfort | Filling<br>Reddened/small blisters or bruises<br>Mild to moderate discomfort | Soft<br>Nontender |
| H<br>Hold (positioning) | Full assist (staff holds infant at breast) | Minimal assist (e.g., elevate head of bed; place pillows for support)<br>Teach one side; mother does other<br>Staff holds and then mother takes over | No assist from staff<br>Mother able to position or hold infant |

The nurse can use the LATCH scoring system to assess and document need for assistance with breastfeeding. Each assessment area is scored 0 to 2. Modified from Jensen, D., Wallace, S., & Kelsay, P. (1994). LATCH: A breastfeeding charting system and documentation tool. *Journal of Obstetric, Gynecologic, and Neonatal Nursing,* 23(1), 27–32.

Assess the nipples, which may be red, bruised, blistered, fissured, or bleeding. Ask about tenderness of the nipples and when it occurs. Evaluate the breastfeeding techniques of the mother having problems with her nipples.

**Knowledge.** Assess the mother's knowledge of breastfeeding techniques. The mother breastfeeding for the first time may have many questions and may need substantial guidance during her first attempts. Although the mother who has nursed before may have a better understanding of breastfeeding, she may have questions or have forgotten some aspects. Current information about breastfeeding may have been unavailable when she breastfed her last infant.

#### INFANT FEEDING BEHAVIORS

Assess an infant's readiness for feeding before initiating a breastfeeding session. The infant should be awake and hungry. Trying to feed an infant in a deep sleep period is frustrating to both mother and infant. On the other hand, waiting too long to start the feeding can cause an infant to be too upset to feed well. Sucking on the hands, rooting when the cheek or side of the mouth is touched, smacking of the lips, and slight fussiness are signs that an infant is ready for feeding.

### Analysis

Women with and without experience often need information to have a successful breastfeeding experience. Therefore, a common nursing diagnosis for the breastfeeding mother is Risk for Ineffective Breastfeeding related to lack of knowledge of breastfeeding techniques.

### Planning

The goals and expected outcomes for this nursing diagnosis are the following:

- The infant will breastfeed using nutritive suckling for an average of at least 15 minutes total per feeding before discharge.
- The mother will demonstrate breastfeeding techniques as taught before discharge.
- The mother will verbalize satisfaction and confidence with the breastfeeding process before discharge.

### Interventions

Interventions are centered on teaching that nurses should provide to all inexperienced breastfeeding mothers. These techniques should be adapted as

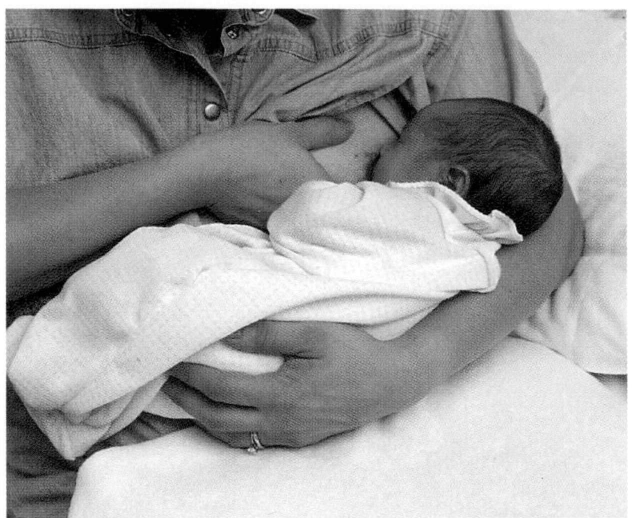

**FIGURE 22-3**

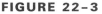

For the cradle hold, the mother positions the infant's head at or near the antecubital space and level with her nipple with her arm supporting the infant's body. Her other hand is free to hold the breast. Once the infant is positioned, pillows or blankets can be used to support the mother's arm, which may tire from holding the baby.

appropriate for mothers who have some knowledge of breastfeeding but need review or clarification. Interventions used for the first feeding session are summarized in Keys to Clinical Practice: Assisting the Inexperienced Breastfeeding Mother (see Appendix D, p. 989).

#### ASSISTING WITH THE FIRST FEEDING

The first feeding should take place within the first 1 to 2 hours after birth if both mother and infant are stable. Ideally, it occurs immediately after birth, when infants are in an alert state and many begin to nurse at once. Others may nuzzle, lick, or suck intermittently at the breast, all of which stimulate production of prolactin necessary for lactation. Feeding at this time also helps establish early bonding. It may be very gratifying to a mother to see her infant nurse right after birth.

Help the mother move to her side or into Fowler's position. Show her how to hold the breast and explain proper positioning of the infant. This is a short session, and teaching should be repeated at the next feeding for reinforcement. Observe the infant's response to the feeding and watch for signs, such as cyanosis or choking, that may indicate the presence of problems that need to be referred to the primary caregiver.

Women who are fatigued or uncomfortable after birth may prefer to wait until later to nurse. Breastfeeding should be initiated as soon as possible once the mother's needs for rest and comfort measures have been met. Whenever it occurs, the first feeding is a time for assessment of the mother's knowledge and technique. Teaching at this time helps prevent problems later.

#### TEACHING FEEDING TECHNIQUES

Teach the new mother many feeding techniques.

##### POSITION OF THE MOTHER AND INFANT

Both the mother and the infant must be positioned properly for optimal breastfeeding. Make the mother as comfortable as possible before she begins to nurse. Pain or an awkward position may interfere with the let-down reflex and cause her to tire. Prevent interruptions and provide privacy so she can concentrate on learning techniques.

The cradle and football holds and the side-lying position are most commonly used (Figs. 22–3 to 22–5). The cross-cradle hold is helpful for the very small infant. The infant's head is held in the hand opposite the breast used for feeding, with the mother's arm supporting the infant's body across her lap. The other hand holds the breast. This position provides more support for a small infant and allows the mother to see the infant's mouth on the breast.

Use pillows behind the mother's back to protect an abdominal incision or to increase her comfort. Arrange folded blankets or pillows to elevate the

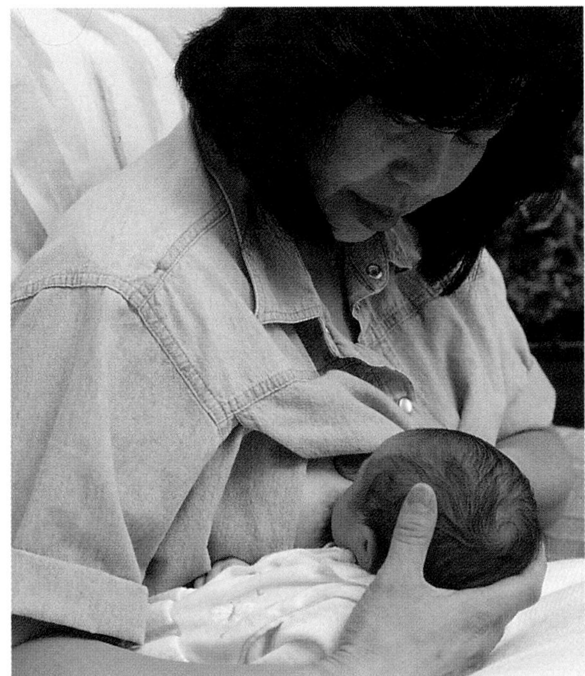

**FIGURE 22-4**

For the football hold, the mother supports the infant's head in her hand, with the infant's body resting on pillows alongside her hip. This method allows the mother to see the position of the infant's mouth on the breast, helps her control the infant's head, and is especially helpful for mothers with heavy breasts. This hold also avoids pressure against an abdominal incision.

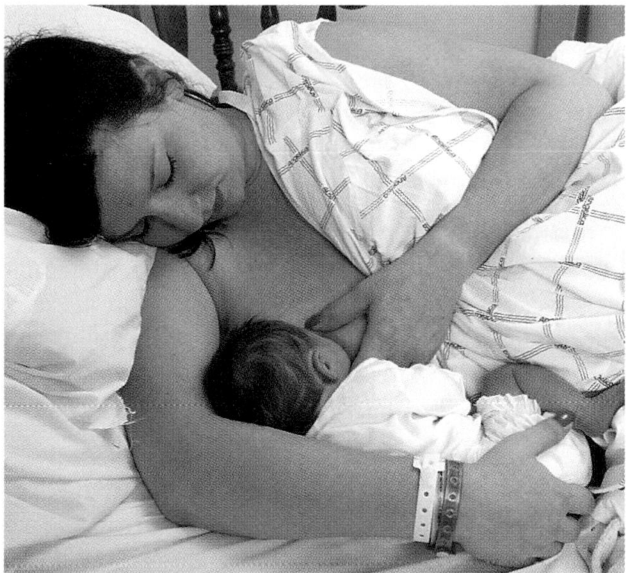

**FIGURE 22–5**

The side-lying position avoids pressure on episiotomy or abdominal incisions and allows the mother to rest while feeding. She lies on her side, with her lower arm supporting her head or placed around the infant. A pillow behind her back and between her legs provides comfort. Her upper hand and arm are used to position the infant on his or her side at nipple level and hold the breast. When the infant's mouth opens to nurse, the mother leans slightly forward or draws the infant to her to insert the nipple into the mouth.

infant to the level of the nipple and prevent pulling and tension on the nipple, which would cause it to become sore. The infant's head and body should directly face the breast with the infant's nose and chin lightly touching the breast. If the infant must turn the head to reach the breast, swallowing is difficult. The neck should be flexed because hyperextension also makes swallowing difficult. The infant body should be aligned so that the ear, shoulder, and hips are on a straight line.

#### POSITION OF THE MOTHER'S HANDS

The mother's hand position is also important. In the C position, the mother holds her breast with her thumb on top and the fingers against the chest wall and supporting the underside of the breast (Fig. 22–6). Be sure that her fingers are behind the areola and her thumb does not press on the breast enough to make the nipple tip upward, or the infant will suck improperly and the nipple may become sore.

In the "scissors hold" the woman uses her forefinger and middle finger to support the breast. This hold increases the risk that her fingers will slip down the wet areola and interfere with the placement of the infant's mouth. Therefore, encourage women to use the C position instead. However, if the mother prefers the scissors position, show her how to place her hands correctly with the fingers well back on the breast.

Although mothers worry about the infant's ability to breathe while nursing, it is unnecessary to indent the breast tissue near the infant's nostrils. This might cause improper positioning of the nipple in the infant's mouth, interfere with the grasp of the nipple, or interfere with milk flow. Unless the mother's breasts are very heavy and the infant buries the nose in the tissue, breathing is not occluded. Lifting the infant's hips to a slightly more horizontal position or bringing them closer to the mother is usually sufficient if there appears to be a problem.

#### LATCH-ON TECHNIQUES

Teach the mother techniques to help the infant latch on to the breast. The infant should be awake and hungry. The mother can talk and cuddle to help a sleepy infant awaken and calm an upset infant.

**Eliciting Latch-on.** After positioning the infant to face the breast, the mother holds her breast so that the nipple brushes against the center of the infant's lower lip. A hungry infant usually opens the mouth as soon as anything comes near it, but some need up to a minute of stroking the area around the mouth. The breast should not be inserted until the infant's mouth is opened wide, or the infant will compress the end of the nipple, causing pain and trauma and little milk flow. When the mouth opens wide, the mother should quickly bring the infant close to her so that the infant can latch on to the areola.

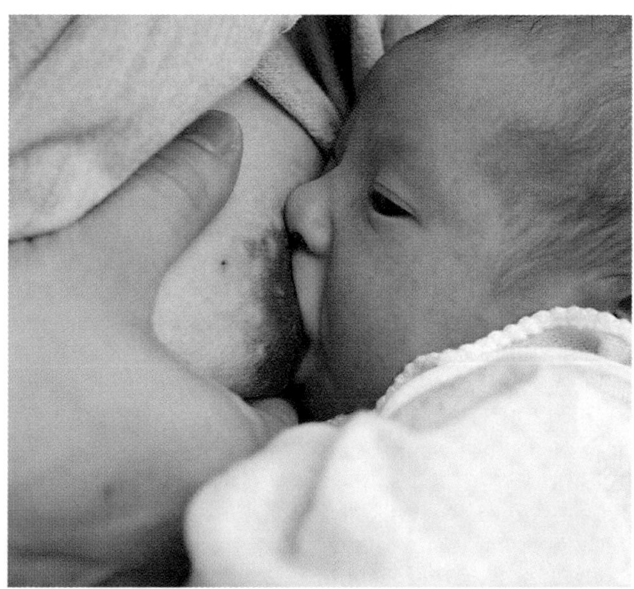

**FIGURE 22–6**

C position of hand on breast. The hand is positioned so the thumb is on top of the breast while the fingers support the breast from below. Note the flaring of the infant's lips.

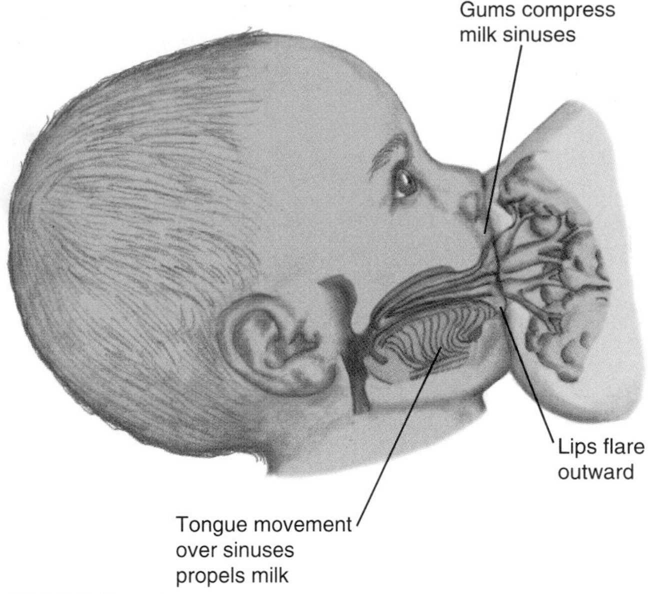
Gums compress milk sinuses
Lips flare outward
Tongue movement over sinuses propels milk

**FIGURE 22–7**

Position of infant's mouth while suckling. When the nipple and areola are properly positioned in the infant's mouth, the gums compress the milk sinuses behind the areola. The tongue is between the lower gum and the breast. The tongue moves over the sinuses like a peristaltic wave to bring the milk forward into the infant's mouth. The infant's lips are flared outward.

**Position of the Mouth.** Assess the position of the infant's mouth on the breast (Fig. 22–7). As much of the areola as possible should be in the infant's mouth to allow the nipple to be drawn toward the back of the mouth. This prevents the infant from sucking on the nipple only, which leads to sore nipples and insufficient milk production. The infant's lips should be about 1 to 1.5 inches from the base of the nipple (Lawrence, 1994). This positions the gums over the milk sinuses just behind the areola and causes milk to be released into the infant's mouth each time the gums compress them.

Assess the position of the infant's tongue by gently pulling down on the lower lip. The tongue should be under the breast and over the top of the lower gums. The lips should be flared outward. Be sure that the lower lip is not turned in, as a friction burn on the lower nipple results.

SUCKLING PATTERN

Observe the infant's suckling pattern. During nutritive suckling, the infant sucks with smooth, continuous movements with only occasional pauses to rest. Each suck may be followed by a swallow, or there may be two or three sucks before the swallow. Nonnutritive sucking often occurs when the infant is falling asleep. There may be a fluttery or choppy motion of the jaw that is not accompanied by the sound of swallowing. The mother should remove the infant from the breast when this occurs because her nipples may become sore. If she thinks that the infant should feed longer, she can try burping and waking the infant before resuming the feeding.

Explain the milk-ejection reflex to the mother. Many mothers learn to recognize a feeling of tingling in the nipples as the let-down occurs. The reflex occurs several times throughout the feeding. She sees the infant begin to swallow more rapidly each time a new let-down brings more rapid expulsion of milk.

**Mothers often wonder whether or not their infants are actually receiving milk from the breast. Call their attention to the sound of swallowing when it occurs. A soft "ka" or "ah" sound indicates that the infant is swallowing colostrum or milk. The infant swallows a number of times in succession and then has a period of no swallowing until another let-down of milk occurs.**

Short pauses are normal during nursing. Caution mothers not to jiggle the breast in the infant's mouth in an effort to start the suckling again. This may cause the infant to lose the grasp on the nipple and areola, resulting in "chewing" on the nipple and soreness. If necessary, she should take the infant off the breast to awaken him or her, then start again.

REMOVAL FROM THE BREAST

Teach the mother to remove the infant from the breast for burping midway in the feeding and whenever suckling becomes non-nutritive. Show her how to avoid trauma to the breast by inserting her finger into the corner of the infant's mouth between the gums to break the suction. She should then remove the breast quickly before the infant begins to suck again. Another method is to indent the breast tissue with a finger near the infant's mouth and remove the infant when the suction is released.

FREQUENCY OF FEEDINGS

Mothers are often concerned about how often they should feed. Because breast milk moves through the stomach within 1.5 to 2 hours, infants usually feed every 2 to 3 hours. Frequent feedings are especially important in the early days after birth, while lactation is being established and stomach capacity is small. Explaining that the hormone prolactin, which is responsible for milk production, is released in increased amounts while the infant is suckling helps mothers understand the relationship of frequent feeding to milk supply.

Infants who are fed frequently during the daytime often sleep longer during the night. However, during the early weeks of life, the infant should usually not be allowed to sleep beyond 5 hours at a time. Long periods between feedings increase the likelihood of breast engorgement. The resulting decreased stimulation of prolactin may reduce milk supply. Generally, the mother should nurse 8 to 12 times in each 24-hour period.

Some infants cluster their feedings and vary the length of feeding and time between each feeding. Several feedings close together (sometimes called "cluster feedings") may be followed by a longer interval between feedings (Mulford, 1995). Strict scheduling of infant feedings is unnecessary and leads to frustration for both mother and infant. A mother should take her cues from her infant.

#### LENGTH OF FEEDINGS

Although early feedings were once limited to only a few minutes per breast in an attempt to prevent sore nipples, improper positioning, rather than time at breast, is the usual cause of nipple trauma. When feedings are too short, the infant may receive little or no colostrum or milk. It may take as long as 5 minutes for the milk-ejection (let-down) reflex to occur during the early days after birth.

Generally mothers can allow the infant to set the length of feedings. The infant should suckle vigorously for a period of time. When choppy non-nutritive suckling without the sound of swallowing occurs, the mother should burp the infant and complete the feeding at the other breast. When the infant is satisfied, the suckling pattern changes and the infant may fall asleep.

Mothers who are uneasy without a specific length of time for feedings can be instructed to start with feedings lasting approximately 10 minutes on each side, or longer if the infant continues to nurse vigorously. The feeding should continue on the second breast until the infant falls asleep or begins non-nutritive suckling, generally about 10 to 15 minutes. Although variations in the length of feedings occur, early feedings should last no less than a total of 15 minutes on the average (Riordan & Auerbach, 1993). Feeding time increases as needed by the infant over the next few days. Instruct the mother that longer feedings do not cause nipple tenderness.

Inform the mother about the differences between foremilk, the watery first milk that quenches the infant's thirst, and hindmilk, which is richer in fat, more satisfying, and leads to weight gain. Feeding for too short a time prevents the infant from getting the hindmilk and decreases weight gain. Although the infant may go to sleep for a brief time, hunger causes early awakening. The frustration of having a fussy infant who "always wants to eat" may lead some mothers to discontinue breastfeeding.

Switching back and forth between breasts several times during a feeding increases the amount of foremilk the infant receives but decreases the amount of hindmilk. Therefore the mother should continue feeding on the first side as long as the infant nurses vigorously before burping and continuing on the other breast.

#### PREVENTING PROBLEMS

Check on the woman often as she feeds her infant so that she can ask questions as they occur to her. Continue to assess her feeding techniques throughout the initial feeding and periodically during subsequent feedings. If the mother is taking medications that might make her sleepy, stay nearby to ensure that the infant is safe at all times.

Once women leave the birth facility, they often have no one to advise them about breastfeeding. Help prevent problems by intensive teaching during the short birth facility stay. Include suggestions on how to improve positioning and techniques and common problems and their solutions. Allow ample time to answer questions. Some facilities hold classes for groups of women during the birth facility stay. If the birth facility provides follow-up telephone calls or home visits, explain the service.

Give the mother breastfeeding pamphlets, and review them with her before discharge. Breastfeeding videos provide another means of providing education. (Before using pamphlets or videos, review them to be sure that the information is correct and they contain no advertisements for formula.)

One of the major reasons mothers give for early weaning to formula is their perception of an insufficient milk supply. Therefore, give the mother suggestions for assessing whether the infant is receiving enough milk. Although mothers are not usually encouraged to weigh normal infants at home because it focuses too much attention on weight gain, the physician or nurse practitioner assesses weight gain at well-baby check-ups. After the initial weight loss following birth, infants generally gain approximately 15 to 30 g (0.5 to 1 ounce) each day during the early months of life. Weight gain generally begins by the fifth day of life.

The mother's general health may affect her continuation of breastfeeding. For example, one study shows than women who have hemoglobin levels below 10 g/dl are more likely to feel that they have insufficient milk (Henly et al., 1995). Therefore, advise the woman to take prescribed iron, eat foods high in iron content, and get adequate rest.

If the mother needs to increase her milk supply, suggest that she feed more often and use a breast pump after feedings to increase milk production. Assess for common causes of decreased milk supply,

## Mothers Want to Know
### Is My Baby Getting Enough Milk?

Your baby is probably getting enough milk if

- You hear the baby swallow frequently during feedings. It sounds like a soft "ka" or "ah" sound.
- You see nutritive suckling, a smooth series of sucking and swallowing with occasional rest periods. This is different from short, choppy sucks that occur when the baby is falling asleep and not getting milk. After rest periods, you may feel a tingling of your nipples as a new let-down reflex occurs. This is followed by more nutritive suckling as the infant swallows the increased milk available.
- Your breast is getting softer during the feeding. (However, your breasts do not have to be hard [engorged] for you to have enough milk for the baby.)
- You can see milk in the baby's mouth or dripping from your breast occasionally.
- You feed your baby 8 to 12 times every 24 hours. You produce more milk when you nurse more often. (Keep track, at first, by writing down the time you start each feeding. Once breastfeeding is well established, it is not necessary to keep close track of the time—your baby lets you know when it is time for feedings.)
- Your baby has at least two to six wet diapers a day for the first 2 days after birth and at least six to eight wet diapers a day by the fifth day. Disposable diapers are very absorbent, and it is sometimes hard to tell if they are wet. If you are unsure, place a tissue or cotton ball inside the diaper to show even small amounts of urine. Urine should be light, not dark, yellow in color.
- Your baby passes at least three bowel movements daily during the first month and often more. The bowel movements are yellow in color by the end of the first week.
- Your baby seems satisfied after feedings. Babies remain quietly awake or go to sleep for at least an hour after most feedings. (An occasional fussy time is not unusual and does not mean that the baby is not getting enough to eat.)
- Your baby has gained weight at the first well-baby checkup.

such as formula use, inadequate rest or diet, smoking, and use of caffeine, alcohol, or some medications. Intervene appropriately if any common causes are found.

### Evaluation

Evaluation of interventions should be continued throughout the birth facility stay. Before discharge, the infant should be feeding well at each breast. The woman should demonstrate the feeding techniques that she has learned and should voice satisfaction with breastfeeding and confidence in her ability. Satisfaction and confidence are major determinants of whether she continues breastfeeding once she is home.

**CHECK YOUR READING**

10. How can the nurse help the mother establish breastfeeding during the initial feeding sessions?
11. What should the nurse teach the mother about frequency and length of feedings?

## Common Breastfeeding Concerns

Many women experience breastfeeding problems that nurses can help them solve. Problems may be divided into those originating with the infant and those involving the mother. Because mothers may be discharged from the birth facility before problems arise, nurses should teach them how to prevent and treat common problems (see Nursing Care Plan 22–1).

Guidance for breastfeeding problems can be continued at home by referring the mother to lactation specialists or organizations such as La Leche League, a support group that gives ongoing assistance to breastfeeding mothers. La Leche League chapters are available in most communities and are listed in the telephone book. Support groups may also be provided by the birth facility.

Some birth facilities provide one or two home visits for new mothers by a nurse who can assess both the mother's and the infant's progress and intervene appropriately. These visits are especially important for mothers who have had any difficulty establishing breastfeeding during the birth facility stay. "Warm lines" may also be available for mothers to call their birth facility and talk to a nurse about breastfeeding problems. Women with more serious breastfeeding problems need referral to a lactation consultant, a professional educated to deal with more complex situations. Assistance helps prevent infant readmission for dehydration and hyperbilirubinemia.

### Infant Problems

Infant problems generally involve a sleepy infant, problems with suckling, and difficulties related to complications of the infant such as jaundice and prematurity. Crying and fussiness are common problems during the first weeks after birth for all infants and are discussed in Chapter 23 (p. 621).

#### SLEEPY INFANT

During the first few days after birth, infants often sleep longer than expected or fall asleep at the

## Mothers Want to Know

### Solutions to Common Breastfeeding Problems

**Problem:** *Infant is sleepy at feeding time or falls asleep shortly after beginning feeding.*

**Prevention**

- Gently awaken your baby at feeding time. Talk, gently move the infant's arms and legs, and play with the infant for a short time before beginning the feeding.
- Unwrap the baby's blankets and change the diaper. Swaddling infants by wrapping them tightly with blankets is a calming technique that often helps them sleep. Leave the blanket off as you begin the feeding. Your body and a blanket draped over both of you after your baby begins to nurse will provide adequate warmth.

**Solutions**

If your baby goes to sleep during the feeding and has fed less than 5 minutes, try the following:

- Rub the baby's hair or cheeks gently, stroke around his or her mouth, or shift the baby's position slightly to see if the infant will wake up.
- Remove the baby from the breast and rub his or her back to bring up bubbles of air that may cause a sensation of stomach fullness. Rubbing the back also stimulates the central nervous system and awakens the baby.
- Express a few drops of colostrum onto the nipple. The baby tastes the colostrum as soon as the nipple is offered and often begins renewed suckling.
- Wash the baby's face with a lukewarm washcloth to help the infant wake up.

If your baby cannot be aroused with a few of the above gentle techniques, a longer sleep period may be needed. Let the infant sleep another half hour, then begin again. Watch for movement of the eyes even though the eyelids are closed and small twitches of the face muscles. These signs indicate that the baby is in a lighter phase of sleep and can be awakened more easily.

**Problem:** *Infant who has taken bottles pushes the nipple out of the mouth and sucks poorly during breastfeeding. Infant has become confused about how to suck from the breast.*

**Prevention**

- Avoid all bottles and pacifiers unless absolutely necessary. If they are necessary, stop as soon as possible.
- Do not give the baby formula during the night. Although the extra sleep is nice, it is seldom worth it if the infant develops later feeding difficulties.
- Avoid giving formula at the end of a breastfeeding session, as it is unnecessary for healthy newborns. It may cause the infant's stomach to become distended, may result in more "spitting up," and may cause the infant to wait longer before nursing again. This decreases milk production.

**Solution**

- Stop all bottle feeding and pacifier use so that the baby gets used to suckling from the breast instead of the bottle. Nurse more often to stimulate milk and help the baby learn what to do.

**Problem:** *Infant sucks on the end of the nipple or fails to open his or her mouth widely enough.*

**Prevention**

- Be sure that the baby has the nipple at the back of the mouth and 1 to 1.5 inches of the areola in the mouth.
- Do not insert the breast into the infant's mouth until the infant opens his or her mouth wide.
- Pull down gently on the infant's chin to help the infant open the mouth if necessary.

**Solutions**

- Stop the feeding and start again if you see dimples in the infant's cheeks or hear "smacking" or clicking sounds. Short, choppy movement of the jaw means that the infant is going to sleep or has finished feeding.
- If you believe that the infant should nurse longer, awaken the infant and begin again.

**Problem:** *Breasts are hard and tender from engorgement.*

**Prevention**

- Breastfeed the infant every 2 to 3 hours day and night. Do not give a bottle during the night, as this increases the risk of engorgement. Waiting even 4 hours between feedings may increase the risk of engorgement, but frequent breastfeeding can often prevent it.

**Solutions**

- Apply cold packs to the breasts between feedings to reduce edema and pain. Make inexpensive cold packs from clean rubber gloves or plastic bags filled with crushed ice, or frozen washcloths. Cover with a washcloth before applying to the skin.
- Before feedings, apply heat with compresses or a shower to stimulate milk flow. Moisten disposable diapers with warm water and apply over each breast. Fasten the tabs to keep the diapers in place and prevent dripping.
- Massage the breasts before and during feedings to stimulate the let-down reflex so that the baby can nurse more easily. Massaging the breasts in the shower provides comfort and helps prepare for feeding.
- If the breasts are very hard and your baby cannot latch on, express a little milk by hand or with a breast pump. As soon as the areola is soft, begin to feed.
- Feed more often—every 1.5 to 2 hours.
- Wear a well-fitting bra for support day and night.
- Take prescribed pain medication to help you feel more comfortable.

**Problem:** *Nipples are sore and may be cracked, blistered, or bleeding.*

**Prevention**

- Position the baby at the breast with enough of the areola in the mouth that the nipple is not compressed between the baby's gums during nursing.
- Avoid engorgement by nursing frequently. Express enough milk to soften the areola if engorgement occurs.
- Do not use soap on the nipples because it removes the protective oils and causes drying.
- If you use breast pads for leaking milk, remove them when they become wet to prevent irritation of the skin. Avoid pads with plastic linings that retain moisture. Cut a cotton diaper or handkerchief into squares and use as inexpensive, washable substitutes for commercial breast pads.

*Mothers Want to Know continued on following page*

## Mothers Want to Know *Continued*

### Solutions to Common Breastfeeding Problems

- Breast creams are unnecessary and may cause sensitivity and irritation. If you are allergic to wool, you may be allergic to lanolin. Use only USP modified lanolin. Creams that have to be removed before each feeding may increase soreness.

**Solutions**

- Begin each feeding with the least sore side first. The hungry baby nurses more vigorously at first, which may be painful. The let-down reflex is started, causing milk to flow more quickly on the second breast.
- Do not use nipple shields (latex nipples that fit over your own nipples). They decrease milk flow so that the baby does not get enough milk and milk production is decreased.
- Vary the position of the infant during nursing. The area of the nipple directly in line with the infant's nose and chin is most stressed during the feeding.
- Apply colostrum or breast milk to the nipples after feedings, as it has healing properties. Or try warm water or warm, wet tea bag compresses to the nipples.
- Expose the nipples to air between feedings by lowering the flaps of your nursing bra. Use a hair dryer held 6 to 8 inches from the breast to apply heat and dry the nipples.
- If you have burning, itching, or stabbing pain throughout your breast, look in the baby's mouth for the white patches of thrush, a yeast infection that can infect the nipples. Call the health care provider for medication to treat both you and your baby.

**Problem:** *Flat or inverted nipples that the baby has difficulty drawing into his or her mouth.*

**Prevention**

None. Can be treated during pregnancy or after birth with breast shells.

**Solutions**

- Wear breast shells in your bra for flat or inverted nipples to help make the nipples protrude.
- Just before beginning breastfeeding, roll the nipple between your thumb and forefinger to help it protrude.
- Use a breast pump just before feedings to draw out inverted nipples. Put the baby to your breast immediately after the pump causes the nipple to become erect. Once the infant gets the nipple in his or her mouth, the normal suckling process usually causes the nipple to stay erect.

breast after feeding for only a short time. They may be tired from the birth process and may not recognize or respond appropriately to hunger. When infants fall asleep before they have fed adequately, they often wake up again within an hour, only to repeat the process. The mother should be informed that this common situation does not reflect on her ability or her breast milk.

The nurse should show mothers how to arouse sleepy infants for breastfeeding. If infants start the feeding fully awake, they are more likely to stay awake to finish the feeding. Pointing out the various behavioral states to the mother helps her develop a greater understanding of her infant and recognize when attempts to feed will be most successful.

When infants fall asleep during feedings, the nurse should evaluate whether the infant has fed adequately, should be awakened to feed longer, or should be fed again sooner than usual. Emphasizing that wake-up techniques should be gentle is important. Using excessively irritating techniques might cause the infant to associate them with feeding and be unwilling to breastfeed. Infants who continue to be excessively sleepy or to nurse poorly need further evaluation. Poor feeding may be an early sign of a complication such as sepsis (see Chapter 30, p. 857).

#### NIPPLE CONFUSION

Nipple confusion (or nipple preference) may occur when an infant who has received bottle feedings confuses the tongue movements necessary for bottle feeding with the suckling of breastfeeding. The infant may refuse to breastfeed or may use tongue movements that push the breast out of the mouth. Some infants develop a preference for the bottle, from which milk flows freely without effort.

A comparison of sucking during bottle feeding and suckling during breastfeeding aids in understanding.

## Critical to Remember

### INFANT SIGNS OF BREASTFEEDING PROBLEMS

- Falling asleep after feeding less than 5 minutes
- Refusal to breastfeed
- Tongue thrusting
- Smacking or clicking sounds
- Dimpling of cheeks
- Failure to open mouth wide at latch-on
- Lower lip turned in
- Short, choppy motions of jaw
- No audible swallowing
- Use of formula

## Nursing Care Plan 22–1

# Breastfeeding for the First Time

**ASSESSMENT:** Melinda Barber plans to breastfeed her first infant, David, but tells the nurse that she is afraid she won't be successful. She asks many questions and appears unsure during her first feeding attempts.

**NURSING DIAGNOSIS:** Risk for Ineffective Breastfeeding related to lack of understanding of breastfeeding techniques

**GOALS/EXPECTED OUTCOMES**

1. David will feed with nutritive suckling for at least 15 minutes per feeding within 24 hours.
2. Melinda will demonstrate correct breastfeeding techniques, including positioning and latch-on, before discharge.
3. Melinda will verbalize satisfaction and confidence with the breastfeeding process before discharge and at the first postpartum home visit.

| INTERVENTION | RATIONALE |
|---|---|
| 1. Assess Melinda's knowledge about breastfeeding techniques. Determine her special concerns. | 1. Teaching should start with and build on the mother's basic knowledge and focus on her perceived needs. |
| 2. Demonstrate cradle and football holds, side-lying position, and use of pillows for support. Help Melinda try out each one. Place David on his side, facing the breast at nipple level. | 2. Knowledge about a variety of positions to use increases the mother's confidence. |
| 3. Demonstrate C position of hand—hand cupped around breast with thumb and fingers behind areola. | 3. Position allows infant to take enough of the nipple and areola into mouth without interference from mother's fingers, reduces trauma to the nipple, and provides support to the breast to keep it in place. |
| 4. Elicit latch-on by rubbing the nipple against the center of David's lower lip and inserting it when he opens his mouth wide. | 4. Rubbing the lip stimulates the infant to open the mouth. Waiting for a wide-open mouth allows insertion of the nipple and areola and prevents the infant from compressing only the nipple and causing trauma. |
| 5. Assess the position of mouth, suck, and swallow. | 5. Proper positioning prevents trauma to the nipple and ensures that the infant is able to compress the milk sinuses. |
| 6. Demonstrate removal of the infant from the breast. | 6. Breaking suction before removal prevents trauma to the nipple. |
| 7. Answer Melinda's questions about the frequency and length of feedings. Ask her if she has other questions. | 7. Eliciting questions gives the mother the information that she needs for continued successful nursing. |
| 8. Instruct Melinda to begin each feeding with the breast where the infant finished the last feeding. Suggest that she place a safety pin on her bra strap to help her remember which side to use first. | 8. Even stimulation and emptying of each breast increase production of milk. |
| 9. Observe Melinda and David at intervals throughout the first feeding session and periodically during subsequent sessions. | 9. Periodic reassessment helps determine if techniques are performed correctly, identifies problems, and allows the nurse to correct misconceptions and answer questions. |
| 10. Instruct Melinda to feed David every 2 to 3 hours. | 10. Frequent feeding provides adequate nourishment and stimulates milk production. |
| 11. Explain how to tell if the infant is receiving enough milk. Include infant behaviors that indicate satisfaction with feedings, how to assess swallowing, the characteristics of breast milk, and the principles of supply and demand in breastfeeding. | 11. A frequent reason for discontinuation of breastfeeding is the mother's perception of inadequate milk supply. Teaching the mother how to assess the infant's intake of milk may help prevent early weaning to formula. |
| 12. Offer praise as Melinda learns about breastfeeding techniques. | 12. Praise helps the mother feel more confident in her abilities and helps prolong the breastfeeding process. |

*Nursing Care Plan continued on following page*

## Nursing Care Plan 22–1 *Continued*
# Breastfeeding for the First Time

**Critical Thinking**

What other interventions might be necessary if Melinda had flat nipples?

**ANSWER**

Reassure Melinda that she can breastfeed even if her nipples are flat. Teach her to roll her nipples just before David latches on to begin feeding.

**EVALUATION**

Melinda and David seem satisfied with feedings that consist of approximately 10 to 15 minutes of nutritive suckling per side. Melinda verbalizes confidence and demonstrates correct positioning and latch-on techniques. Breastfeeding is going well at the postpartum home visit.

Infants must push their tongue over the latex nipple of a bottle to slow the flow of milk and prevent choking (Fig. 22–8). This can be demonstrated by noting the steady drip of milk when a bottle is held upside down. In bottle feeding, the infant's lips are relaxed because there is no need to hold the nipple in place. If the infant uses the same thrusting tongue motion and relaxed lips while nursing, the breast may be pushed out of the mouth.

Ultrasound studies have shown that the mouth is used differently during breastfeeding. Suction is necessary to hold the nipple in place near the back of the throat. The tongue cups around the nipple and areola with the tip over the lower gum. With each compression of the lower jaw over the milk sinuses behind the areola, the tongue presses against the breast like a peristaltic wave, causing the milk to move forward from the sinuses and into the infant's mouth for swallowing.

Nurses should discourage use of formula in normal breastfeeding infants. It reduces breastfeeding time and decreases production of prolactin and, therefore, milk supply. Formula takes longer to digest, and the infant is not hungry again for about 4 hours. This further limits breast stimulation and milk supply and may lead to engorgement. Women who avoid using bottles during the first month are more likely to continue breastfeeding over 6 months (Piper & Parks, 1996).

### SUCKLING PROBLEMS

Suckling problems may occur when the nipple is poorly positioned in the mouth. Dimpling of the cheeks and smacking or clicking sounds may indicate that the infant needs more of the areola in the mouth and is sucking on the nipple only. Some infants do not open their mouth widely and suck on the end of the nipple. Short, choppy motions of the jaw signal non-nutritive suckling.

Suckling can be assessed by inserting a gloved finger into the infant's mouth. The peristaltic motion of the tongue should be felt as the infant sucks. The infant who is thrusting the tongue may have become confused by use of latex nipples, which should be avoided until the problem is resolved. If the infant tends to place the tongue on top of the nipple, placing a finger in the mouth and pressing the infant's tongue down just before latch-on may be effective. More complicated suckling problems may require assistance from a lactation educator or consultant.

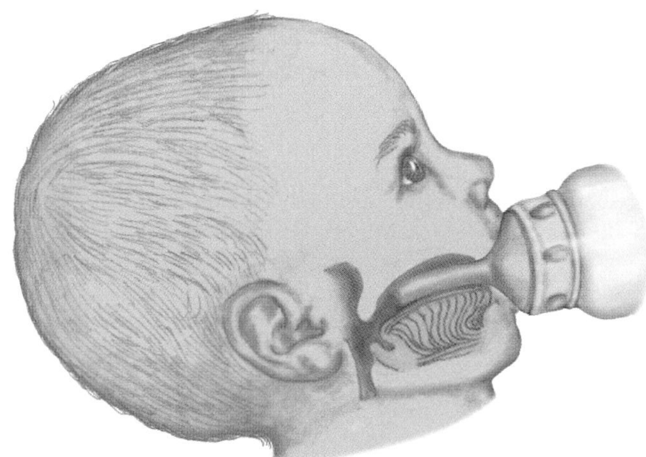
Tongue thrusts forward
to control milk flow

**FIGURE 22–8**

During bottle feeding, infants must thrust the tongue forward to slow the rapid flow of milk.

**CHECK YOUR READING**

12. What wake-up techniques should the nurse teach the mother of a sleepy infant?
13. How does sucking from a bottle differ from suckling from the breast?

### INFANT COMPLICATIONS

Infant complications may be minor and cause minimal interference with breastfeeding. However, the very preterm or ill infant may be unable to breastfeed for a long period of time.

#### JAUNDICE

Jaundice (hyperbilirubinemia) need not interfere with breastfeeding. Even when infants receive phototherapy, they can usually be removed from the lights for feedings. Concern over adequate intake may be more prevalent in caring for the infant with jaundice. Insensible water loss from the skin is increased as a result of the heat and lights used in treatment and could lead to dehydration. Decreased intestinal motility from insufficient milk intake allows reabsorption of bilirubin through the intestinal wall into the blood stream, increasing the work of the immature liver. Therefore, frequent and adequate feedings are important. Jaundice is discussed in detail in Chapters 19 (p. 498) and 30 (p. 852).

Infants receiving phototherapy should not be given extra water because it may decrease the intake of breast milk. Because albumin is necessary to bind bilirubin, frequent breastfeeding is necessary to provide adequate intake of protein and stimulate production of milk. In addition, breastfeeding increases the number of stools and aids in excretion of bilirubin.

#### PREMATURITY

If the preterm infant is unable to breastfeed immediately after birth, the mother needs encouragement and instruction on how to use a breast pump to establish and maintain her milk supply. Breast milk offers immunologic and nutritional benefits and is adapted to preterm needs. It may help prevent necrotizing enterocolitis, a serious complication of preterm infants. It also helps the mother feel she is providing care for her infant even if she cannot take the infant home with her. The woman can pump her milk and take it to the nursery for the infant's feedings. The nurse should provide sterile containers for the woman to take home and instruct her in special nursery requirements. Feeding the preterm infant is discussed in detail in Chapter 29, p. 824.

Some preterm infants or those with breastfeeding problems respond well to the use of supplementary feeding devices. These consist of a container of milk with a small plastic feeding tube that is attached to the breast. When the infant begins to breastfeed, milk flows from the container as well as the breast, increasing the infant's intake and motivation to continue suckling. As the infant gains weight and feeding ability increases, use of the device is gradually decreased until it can be discontinued completely.

#### ILLNESS AND CONGENITAL DEFECTS

Illness in the infant and congenital defects such as a cleft palate may cause breastfeeding problems. Parents of these infants need the same type of assistance as parents with preterm infants. The focus is on helping the mother maintain lactation until she is able to nurse the infant. Referral to support groups can be particularly helpful. Some groups focus on particular congenital defects, and others focus on breastfeeding infants with special problems.

## Maternal Concerns

The most frequent breastfeeding problems of the mother involve problems of the breasts or nipples. The mother who is ill needs special help to continue breastfeeding. Other common concerns include feeding after multiple birth, working, and weaning.

### COMMON BREAST PROBLEMS

Engorgement, nipple trauma, flat or inverted nipples, plugged ducts, and mastitis are common problems involving the breasts.

#### ENGORGEMENT

Many women have a temporary swelling or fullness of the breasts in response to increased blood flow when the milk begins to "come in" or change from colostrum to transitional breast milk. This does not usually occur until the third day after birth but may begin earlier in women who have nursed previously. The fullness does not interfere with breastfeeding.

Engorgement, which is likely to occur if breastfeeding is delayed or infrequent, is different from the temporary fullness of early milk production. Engorged breasts are edematous, hard, and tender, making feeding or even movement painful. The areola may become so hard that the infant cannot compress it for nursing. An engorged areola causes the nipple to become flat, making it more difficult for the infant to draw it into the back of the mouth. In addition to the discomfort engorgement causes the mother, the condition may lead to nipple trauma, mastitis, and even the discontinuation of breastfeeding.

Nurses can help prevent engorgement by assisting women to begin breastfeeding early and to feed frequently and for adequate lengths of time. The nurse

## Nursing Care Plan 22–2
# Breastfeeding an Infant Who Has Complications

**ASSESSMENT:** Ruth James' son John develops respiratory complications at birth and is admitted to the neonatal intensive care unit. Ruth had looked forward to breastfeeding her infant, but John will probably not be able to feed at the breast for a few days. Although Ruth understands the situation, she sounds disappointed and discouraged about whether or not she will be able to breastfeed at all. She states that she will probably have to use formula after John is better because "it will be too late to start breastfeeding."

**NURSING DIAGNOSIS:** Interrupted Breastfeeding related to separation from infant secondary to illness

**GOALS/EXPECTED OUTCOMES**

Ruth will do the following:

1. Verbalize the importance of breastfeeding her infant and her desire to maintain lactation.
2. Pump her breasts as taught.
3. Breastfeed John successfully when it becomes possible.

| INTERVENTION | RATIONALE |
|---|---|
| 1. Explore Ruth's perception of the problem and her understanding of the cause for separation and the effect on breastfeeding. | 1. Discussion of the problem identifies misconceptions and determines the type of teaching and support that are required. |
| 2. Use therapeutic communication techniques to help Ruth express her feelings of disappointment with the unexpected change in plans. | 2. Helping the mother express her feelings and accepting them helps her cope with the situation. |
| 3. Explain to Ruth how valuable breast milk is for her infant and that she can use a breast pump to maintain lactation until John is able to breastfeed. | 3. Reinforcing the value of breastfeeding and offering encouragement increase the chance of success. |
| 4. Teach Ruth to use a breast pump and store her milk. Instruct her to pump her breasts for 15 to 20 minutes every 3 hours during the day and at least once at night. | 4. Frequent use of a breast pump helps establish lactation by causing release of prolactin and oxytocin so that milk is produced and released from the breasts. |
| 5. Feed John breast milk if possible, whether by bottle or gavage. Teach Ruth how to store her milk and how to prepare it for use for her infant. | 5. Breast milk has properties that are especially valuable for the sick infant. |
| 6. Arrange for Ruth to spend as much time with John as possible. Accompany her during the early visits and when she begins to breastfeed to answer her questions and provide support. | 6. Bonding occurs more easily if a mother is able to be with her baby. Accompanying a mother during visits with her infant allows the nurse an opportunity to offer support, encouragement, and teaching as needed. |
| 7. Offer praise and realistic encouragement frequently. | 7. A mother needs reinforcement of her abilities to increase self-esteem as a mother. Encouragement must be suited to actual circumstances. |

**EVALUATION**

Ruth verbalizes her determination to provide breast milk for John. She maintains lactation and brings breast milk at each visit. At 5 days of age, John is ready to begin breastfeeding. Ruth is very patient in helping John learn to breastfeed with the nurses' help. John is able to nurse well at each feeding by discharge.

should encourage them to breastfeed at night, unless there are extenuating circumstances, so that the breasts are emptied regularly. The use of water and formula should be discouraged.

The nurse should teach women with engorgement about application of cold and heat, massage, and breastfeeding techniques. Cold is used between feedings to reduce edema and pain. Heat applied just before feedings increases vasodilation and milk flow. Massage of the breasts causes release of oxytocin and increases the speed of milk release. This decreases the length of time the infant nurses on

## Critical to Remember

### MATERNAL SIGNS OF BREASTFEEDING PROBLEMS

- Hard, tender breasts
- Painful, red, cracked, blistered, or bleeding nipples
- Flat or inverted nipples
- Localized edema or pain in either breast
- Fever, generalized aching, or malaise

painful breasts (Fig. 22–9). Cabbage leaves are sometimes applied to the breasts for short periods of time to provide relief from engorgement (Lawrence, 1994).

If the areola is too engorged for the infant to compress it, the nurse should help the mother express milk by hand or with a breast pump to soften the areola. Nurses should always wear gloves if there is a possibility they will come in contact with colostrum or breast milk, as for any other body fluid.

Mothers with engorgement may need medication for discomfort so that they can relax while breastfeeding. Medications safe for use during breastfeeding may be ordered by the physician. Medicating the mother 15 to 30 minutes before she feeds decreases her pain, and she finishes nursing before peak amounts reach the blood stream and enter the milk being produced. A well-fitting bra should be worn both day and night to help support the breasts.

#### NIPPLE TRAUMA

Nipple pain is common during breastfeeding. Pain for a minute or less may occur during early breastfeeding at the beginning of feedings as the infant stretches the tissue. Nipple trauma causes more sustained pain. Nipple pain tends to be greatest on the third or fourth day after birth and then improve.

Traumatized nipples appear red, cracked, blistered, or bleeding (Fig. 22–10). Minor nipple trauma can be treated by independent nursing interventions. Redness of breast tissue, purulent drainage, and fever indicate mastitis or breast abscess and require antibiotic treatment (see Chapter 28, p. 800).

**Prevention.** Nipple trauma can often be prevented by teaching the mother proper positioning, latch-on techniques, and avoidance of common

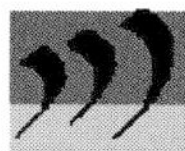

## THERAPEUTIC COMMUNICATION

### Anxiety About Breastfeeding

Jenny Lavelle gave birth to her second baby, Robin, by cesarean. She tells her nurse, Teresa Hernandez, that she breastfed her first infant for a week and then switched to bottle feeding because she didn't have enough milk. Robin is a sleepy baby but does nurse at times. Jenny's breasts are engorged, and her nipples are sore.

**Jenny:** I really wanted to nurse Robin, but I don't know if it's worth the effort. My breasts hurt, and I don't know if he's getting enough milk. I probably should just use the bottle again.

**Teresa:** You sound really discouraged!

*Reflecting the feelings expressed*

**Jenny:** When I couldn't nurse my daughter, I was so disappointed. I had this "Mother Earth" view of the kind of mother I was going to be. But "Mother Earth's" baby wouldn't stop crying, so I went to the bottle.

**Teresa:** That must have been hard for you!

*Reflecting the feelings expressed*

**Jenny:** It was awful, and now it looks like I'm going to fail again. Robin won't nurse half the time, and I'm going home this afternoon.

**Teresa:** Sounds like you're worried about what's going to happen at home.

*Seeking clarification of mother's concerns*

**Jenny:** What if he won't nurse at home? I feel so stupid! This is my second baby!

**Teresa:** You feel you shouldn't have problems breastfeeding when it's your second baby.

*Paraphrasing and clarifying*

**Jenny:** That's right.

**Teresa:** You know, people think breastfeeding is an automatic process, but it isn't always easy. Mothers and babies both have to learn the process, and that takes time and a lot of patience. Robin's hungry now—would you like to try again? I'll stay with you and answer your questions.

*Offering realistic encouragement and assistance in techniques*

**Jenny:** That would be great! Maybe I'll get the hang of this yet!

*By allowing Jenny to express her feelings of discouragement and disappointment before beginning to teach, the nurse learns how important breastfeeding is to Jenny and how best to go about teaching her. Jenny feels accepted even though she feels she should know more because she is a second-time mother.*

## Nursing Care Plan 22–3

# Engorged Breasts and Painful Nipples

**ASSESSMENT:** Sally Portner says during a feeding, 'I'm going to give a bottle for the next few feedings. I'm too sore to nurse anymore today." Her breasts are engorged, warm, and tender. Her son, Grady, has difficulty grasping Sally's nipple and areola to feed. Her nipples are everted but red. There are no blisters, fissures, or bleeding. Sally says she has been breastfeeding for 3 minutes per side every 4 to 4 1/2 hours. She holds Grady lying on his back with his hips and legs lower than the rest of his body during feedings. A few swallowing sounds are heard during nursing.

### Critical Thinking

Evaluate the information above and assign a LATCH score that can be used in planning care for Sally and Grady. (See Table 22–3.)

**ANSWER**

The LATCH score is 6. One point is given for latch, audible swallowing, comfort, and hold. Two points are given for type of nipple. The focus of teaching will be on improving the areas where only one point is assigned.

**NURSING DIAGNOSIS:** Impaired Skin Integrity related to incorrect positioning and engorgement

### GOALS/EXPECTED OUTCOMES

Sally will do the following:

1. Demonstrate correct positioning within 1 day.
2. Describe prevention and treatment of engorgement and sore nipples within 1 day.
3. Have no engorgement or redness of the nipples within 2 days.

| INTERVENTION | RATIONALE |
|---|---|
| 1. Apply warm compresses (such as clean wet disposable diapers) to Sally's breasts before feeding. | 1. Heat dilates blood vessels and milk ducts, encourages the let-down reflex, and relieves pain. |
| 2. Offer Sally ordered medication approximately 30 minutes before feedings. Be sure that the medication ordered is safe for the infant. | 2. Medication relieves pain that could interfere with the let-down reflex, yet only minimal amounts reach breast milk within the feeding time. |
| 3. Demonstrate gentle massage of the breasts before feedings. | 3. Massage causes release of oxytocin, resulting in the let-down reflex. The infant gets milk more quickly, reducing nonproductive time on a painful breast. |
| 4. Demonstrate hand expression or use of a breast pump if necessary to soften the areola enough so that Grady can grasp it to suckle. | 4. If the areola is hard, the infant compresses the nipple rather than the milk sinuses because the nipple is not deep enough in the mouth. This causes nipple trauma, inadequate emptying, and decreased milk production. |
| 5. Demonstrate correct positioning of the infant. Place Grady on his side so that he faces the nipple with his abdomen against Sally. | 5. If the infant must turn his head to feed, it interferes with swallowing and causes traction on the nipple. |
| 6. Have Sally begin the feeding on the less sore side. | 6. The let-down reflex occurs in both breasts at once. Vigorous suckling on the sore side before let-down increases nipple trauma. |
| 7. Assess Grady's mouth position by gently pulling down the lower lip to see that his tongue covers the lower gum. If the lower lip is turned in, gently pull it out so that the lips flare. Assess the position of the nipple. | 7. The tongue cushions the lower gum compression of the areola. A turned-in lower lip causes a friction rub on the nipple and areola. If the lips are 1 to 1.5 inches from the base of the nipple, the nipple should be at the back of infant's mouth. |
| 8. Instruct Sally to wear a well-fitting bra both day and night. | 8. A bra provides support to painful breasts. |
| 9. Prevent further engorgement by teaching Sally to feed Grady every 2 to 3 hours during the day and at least every 4 hours at night. She should feed an average of at least 15 minutes per feeding. | 9. Frequent feedings empty the breasts, prevent stasis, stimulate milk production, and reduce the risk of mastitis. Adequate length allows time for the let-down reflex, which may be delayed at first, to occur. |

## Nursing Care Plan 22–3 *Continued*
## Engorged Breasts and Painful Nipples

| INTERVENTION | RATIONALE |
|---|---|
| 10. Suggest that Sally use a variety of positions for feeding and demonstrate each. | 10. Changing the area of stress on the nipple allows healing of the sore area. |
| 11. Teach Sally to apply warm water compresses or colostrum to the nipples after feedings. Instruct her to leave the flaps of her nursing bra down between feedings. | 11. Warm water compresses are soothing. Colostrum has lysozymes and other healing properties. Increased air circulation promotes healing. |
| 12. Teach Sally to avoid creams that must be removed before nursing or to which she may have allergies. If she uses breast pads, suggest that she change them frequently. Tell her to avoid soap on her nipples. | 12. Cream removal, allergies, and wet pads increase irritation. Prolonged exposure to wet pads can cause maceration and breakdown of skin. Soap removes protective oils from nipples. |

**Critical Thinking**

Should Sally use a bottle for the next few feedings?

**ANSWER**

If Sally skips feedings, her engorgement will increase. Grady will not be ready to feed again for 3 to 4 hours after taking formula, increasing the time between breastfeedings. The lack of suckling and engorgement decrease milk production. Using the above interventions, Sally should be able to breastfeed with less discomfort and prevent further problems.

EVALUATION

Sally breastfeeds Grady every 2 to 3 hours for approximately 10 minutes per side during the day and at least every 4 hours at night. She demonstrates correct positioning at every feeding and can describe causes and care for sore nipples. When she is seen by the home visit nurse on the day after discharge, her engorgement, nipple redness, and tenderness have resolved. Sally verbalizes methods she will use to prevent further engorgement.

causes of nipple trauma. Exposure to soaps, prolonged moisture, or irritating creams may cause sore nipples. Some inflammation and skin changes of the nipple may result from suction during normal sucking (Ziemer & Pigeon, 1993). Prevention may not be entirely possible.

**Care.** Teaching includes increasing air flow to the nipples, feeding with the less inflamed side first, and varying positions for feeding to rotate strain on the nipples. Unfortunately, studies have not shown that any one comfort measure is significantly more effective than others in treating painful nipples. More research is needed in this area.

Warm water compresses or warm, wet tea bags applied to the nipples have often been found to have some effectiveness in reducing pain. Application of breast milk to the nipples after feedings is effective for some women. It is thought to help prevent infection and aid in healing because of the presence of lysozymes in the milk. Ointments are no more effective than other treatments. Women who plan to use lanolin should use only USP modified lanolin that has no pesticides and is hypoallergenic. Many creams have to be removed before feeding and may further irritate sore nipples.

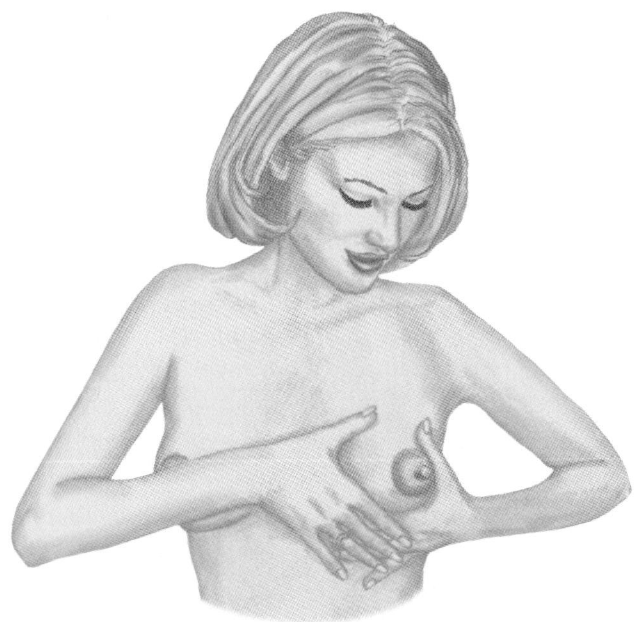

**FIGURE 22–9**
To massage the breasts, the mother places her hands against the chest wall with her fingers encircling the breasts. She gently slides her hands forward until the fingers overlap. The position of the hands is rotated to cover all breast tissue.

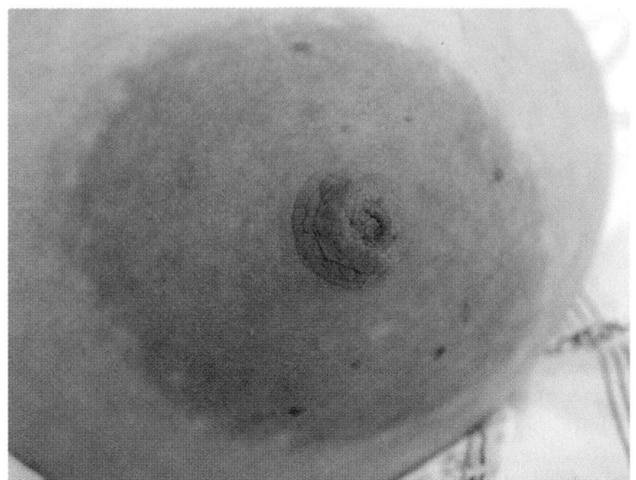

**FIGURE 22–10**
Note the cracked area on this nipple.

Mothers with vaginal candidiasis may transmit it to the infant during birth. If oral infection with *Candida albicans* (thrush) develops in the infant, the mother's nipples may become infected. The infant may or may not have visible white patches in the mouth. The woman has burning, itching, or stabbing pain throughout the breast. The health care provider should be notified, and both mother and infant are usually treated with nystatin.

Women should be cautioned against using nipple shields—latex nipples with wide bases that are placed over a mother's own nipple to decrease pain during feedings. The shields interfere with adequate emptying of the breast and markedly reduce the amount of milk the infant receives.

#### FLAT AND INVERTED NIPPLES

Nipple abnormalities should be treated during pregnancy, if possible, but interventions can begin after birth if necessary. Use of breast shells can be taught at this time. Nipple rolling just before feeding helps flat nipples become more erect so that the infant can grasp them more readily (Fig. 22–11). A breast pump may help draw out inverted nipples.

### CHECK YOUR READING

14. How can the nurse help the mother who has engorged breasts?
15. How should the nurse advise the mother with sore nipples?

#### PLUGGED DUCTS

Although the exact cause of occlusion of a lactiferous duct is unknown, engorgement, missed feedings, or a constricting bra may be involved. Localized edema and tenderness are present, and a hard area may be palpated. There may be a tiny white area on the nipple. Massage of the area followed by heat and continued breastfeeding using varied positions cause the duct to open. A plugged duct may progress to mastitis if not treated promptly. Mastitis involves localized pain accompanied by fever, generalized aching, and malaise. The mother with mastitis is discussed in Chapter 28, p. 800.

### ILLNESS IN THE MOTHER

When the mother is ill, breastfeeding may have to be postponed temporarily because of the mother's condition or the drugs she receives. However, abrupt weaning may lead to mastitis as well as maternal depression from decreased prolactin, which has been associated with feelings of well-being (Lawrence, 1994). Another factor in depression may be the mother's emotional reaction to having to stop her chosen method of feeding. The nurse should explain the mother's condition to her and her family and help them explore appropriate options, including use of a breast pump until she resumes breastfeeding.

#### CONDITIONS IN WHICH BREASTFEEDING SHOULD BE AVOIDED

Some situations occur in which breastfeeding is contraindicated, such as a mother's serious illness that can be transmitted to the infant. Examples are active tuberculosis, hepatitis B or C, and human im-

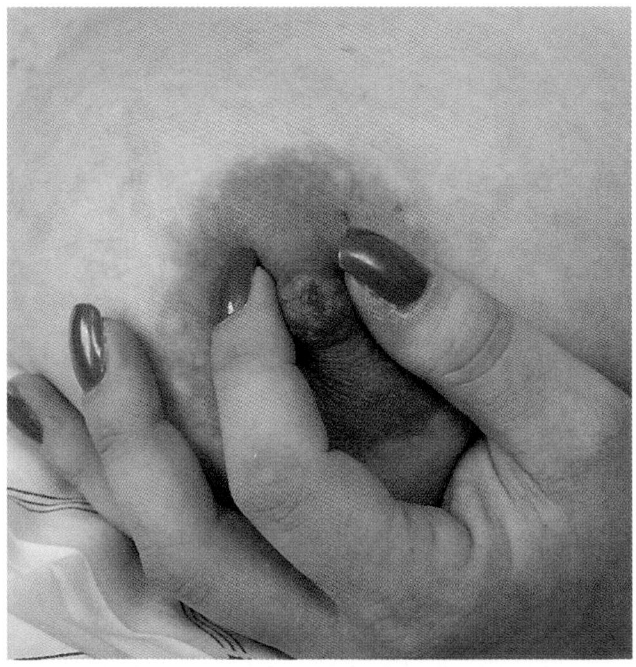

**FIGURE 22–11**
Rolling helps flat nipples become erect in preparation for latch-on.

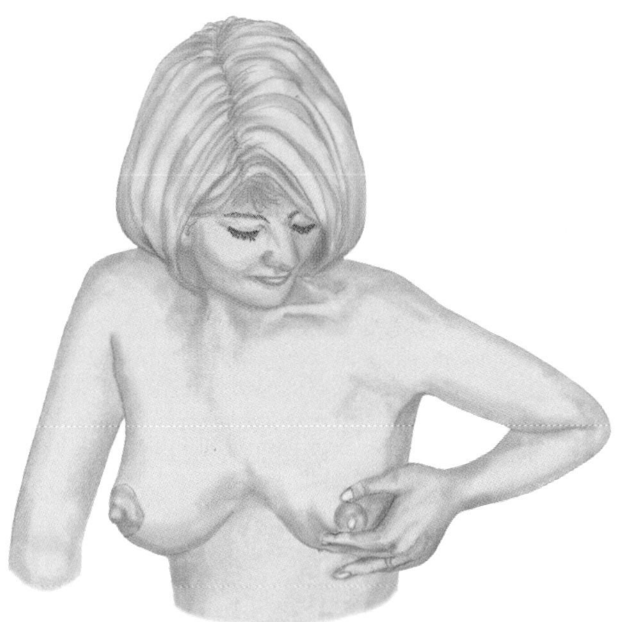

**FIGURE 22-12**

To express milk from the breast, the mother places her hand just behind the areola, with the thumb on top and the fingers supporting the breast. The tissue is pressed back against the chest wall, then the fingers and thumb are brought together and toward the nipple. This compresses the milk sinuses and causes milk to flow. The action is repeated to simulate the suckling of the infant. Moving the hands around the areola allows compression of all sinuses and complete removal of milk from the breast. Compression should be gentle to avoid trauma.

munodeficiency virus (HIV) infection. Conditions such as cancer may become worse owing to hormonal changes of lactation. Maternal drug abuse is also a contraindication.

DRUG TRANSFER TO BREAST MILK

Most medications taken by the mother cross into the breast milk to some degree. Some interfere with milk production. Therefore, both prescription and over-the-counter drugs should be approved by a physician. Another drug can often be substituted for one that affects the infant. Scheduling medication to be given after feedings decreases the amount that passes into the milk. If a mother must take a drug that will be harmful to her infant, she should pump her breasts while she is taking the medication. Once the drug clears her blood stream, she may resume breastfeeding (see Appendix C for more information about drug effects during breastfeeding).

### MILK EXPRESSION

When there is a need for milk expression, the nurse helps the mother use hand expression (Fig. 22–12) or a breast pump (Fig. 22–13). Hand expression can be done without other equipment but is not as effective as a breast pump. Hand expression or manual pumps are useful for the mother who wants to save breast milk for another feeding or whose areola is so engorged that the infant cannot grasp it.

The mother who needs to pump her milk for a prolonged period may prefer using a battery-operated or electric breast pump. Battery-operated pumps are small, portable, and relatively inexpensive. Large electric pumps can often be rented for home use. They are more efficient than hand or battery pumps and are indicated when the mother must pump to maintain her milk supply for a long period of time. Some pumps can be used on both

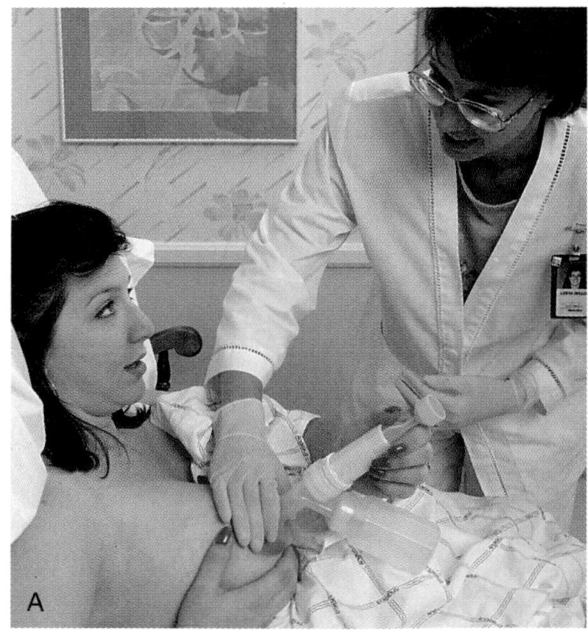

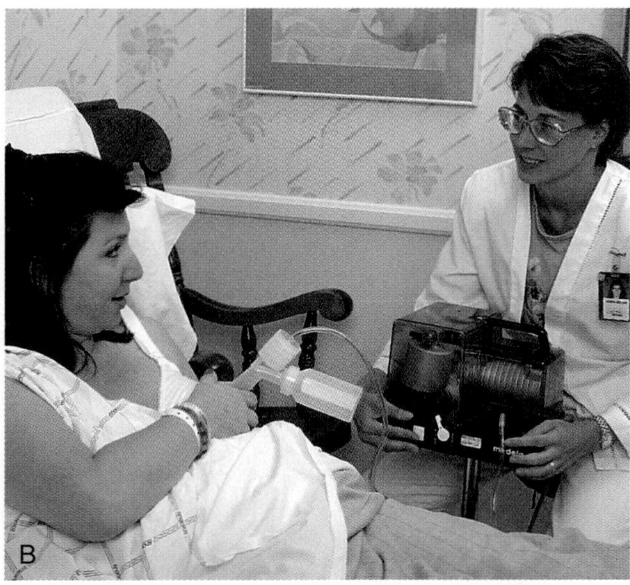

**FIGURE 22-13**

The nurse demonstrates methods of pumping breast milk. A, Manual breast pump. B, Electric breast pump.

breasts at once, which saves time and increases production.

Use of the breast pump should begin within the first 24 hours after birth for the woman who cannot breastfeed her infant. She should pump her breasts approximately every 3 hours during the day and at least once at night when prolactin levels are elevated. Sessions should last approximately 15 to 20 minutes. A total of eight or more sessions in each 24 hours is best to maintain milk supply.

Use of massage and heat before pumping helps initiate the flow of milk. Massage of each quadrant of the breast during pumping may increase the volume of milk obtained at each session. The amount of suction should be set at a low level in the beginning and gradually increased, if necessary. Too much negative pressure traumatizes the breast. If the woman needs to increase her milk supply, pumping more often rather than for longer periods of time is more effective.

### BREASTFEEDING AFTER MULTIPLE BIRTHS

Mothers who have multiple births may have many concerns about their ability to breastfeed more than one infant. They need help and support from nurses and family members.

### HOME CARE

Many infants have not breastfed well by the time of discharge from the birth facility. Problems with engorgement and sore nipples are more likely to occur after discharge. Facilities often provide home visits by nurses who check the mother and baby for problems, including feeding difficulties. A visit within 1 to 2 days after discharge is ideal and may increase the length of time the mother breastfeeds (Serafino-Cross & Donovan, 1992). A home visit allows assessment of the breastfeeding process in the mother's own surroundings. The nurse can observe a feeding session and offer suggestions. The mother can ask

## Mothers Want to Know

## Breastfeeding After the Birth of More Than One Infant

**Ensuring Adequate Milk Production**

Mothers often wonder whether they can produce enough milk to feed more than one infant. Because the amount of milk produced depends on the amount of suckling the breasts receive, providing enough milk should not be a problem. It is important that you nurse frequently, every 2 to 3 hours, to build up the milk supply. You may decide to have each infant nurse on the same breast at each feeding or to alternate breasts for each baby. Production of milk may be more evenly stimulated if you alternate breasts, especially if one infant has a weaker suck.

**Using a Breast Pump**

If your infants are not ready for breastfeeding, use a breast pump to build up your milk supply and provide milk for them until they are ready to breastfeed. Use the pump every 2 to 3 hours while you are awake and at least once during the night. Pump for 15 to 20 minutes at each session. Work up to at least 8 pumping sessions daily. Pumps that can be used on both breasts at the same time decrease the time spent pumping and increase the production of milk. If one baby is ready to breastfeed before the other(s), nurse the baby and pump your breasts after each feeding to stimulate enough milk production to meet the needs of all infants. An alternative is to nurse the infant on one breast and use a breast pump on the other at the same time.

**Feeding Simultaneously or Individually**

You can feed each baby individually or feed two infants at once. Simultaneous nursing shortens feeding times, but both infants must be awake at once. You need help positioning the infants at first. Individual feeding can be done without help and on each infant's own schedule, but a larger portion of your day will be spent feeding.

**Positioning Infants for Simultaneous Feeding**

Use a variety of positions for breastfeeding two infants at once. Place pillows under both infants to bring them to the right height and to keep them in place. Use pillows under your arms and behind your back so that you are comfortable.

***Football* Hold:** Place each infant's head on your lap and support each infant's body with pillows alongside your body. Support each infant's head in your hand and bring the infants to the nipples.

***Football and Cradle* Hold:** Place one infant in a cradle position on pillows across your lap. Place the other in a football position with the body supported on pillows alongside you. Once the infants are in position, help one and then the other to latch on to the breast.

***Criss-cross* Hold:** Place pillows on your lap and hold each baby in the cradle position. The infants' legs criss-cross over each other.

**Keeping Track**

Keep track of when and for how long each baby eats, especially if you feed them individually. Record the number of wet diapers and bowel movements each infant has each day. Six to eight wet diapers and at least three bowel movements usually show adequate intake.

**Care for Yourself**

All new mothers need to eat well and get enough rest. This is especially true for mothers who have had a multiple birth. Ask for help from family and friends. Pamper yourself as much as possible, and leave care of the house and cooking to others if you can. Your major responsibility during this time should be to care for yourself and your new babies!

questions that she did not get answered during her birth facility stay (Fig. 22–14).

Some facilities provide outpatient clinics as an alternative to the home visit. The mother and infant return to the agency for assessment and education by a nurse. The care provided is similar to that received during a home visit. The nurse can see more mothers in a shorter period of time, although the home situation cannot be assessed as well. Access to a nurse by telephone is also an important way of helping women with questions about breastfeeding. (See Chapter 23 for more information about home care.)

#### EMPLOYMENT

Mothers who plan to return to work soon after birth may have many questions about managing breastfeeding and employment. Working and breastfeeding can be combined very well. Although some advance planning is necessary, many mothers feel that continuing the nursing relationship is well worth the effort.

Although some mothers remain at home for 6 weeks or more after birth, others must return to work earlier. Milk supply can be well established by frequent breastfeeding during the time at home. A week or two before she returns to work, the mother can begin using a breast pump once or twice a day to practice pumping her breasts and to build up a small supply of frozen breast milk. This avoids the stress of having to learn the technique or worry about having enough milk while adjusting to the work situation again.

Milk should be stored in rigid polypropylene plastic containers, as antibodies in the milk adhere to glass. The rigid plastic containers maintain the stability of the milk components and are easier to use than plastic bottle liners, which spill easily. The milk can be kept in a refrigerator for 48 hours, a refrigerator freezer for a month, or a deep freeze at 0°F for 6 months. Leukocytes are destroyed by freezing, but most of the other immunologic properties are preserved. Breast milk should be thawed in a refrigerator or by holding the container under running water rather than by heating it. It should not be refrozen or heated in a microwave. Refrigerated milk should be used as much as possible so that the leukocytes are available for the infant.

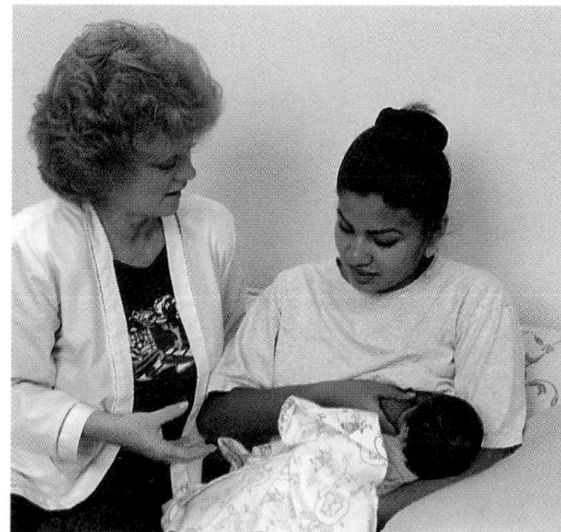

**FIGURE 22–14**

The nurse offers suggestions on hand position during the home visit.

Most working mothers use a battery-operated or electric pump once or twice a day during lunch or coffee breaks. The woman needs to find a place at her work where she can pump her milk in privacy. The milk should be refrigerated or placed in an insulated container with ice and can be used for the next day's feeding. Breastfeeding just before leaving for work and again as soon as the mother returns home keeps the time between feedings at a minimum. The infant is breastfed frequently throughout the evening hours and on weekends to continue to build up the milk supply.

Some mothers choose to use formula during work hours but to breastfeed when at home. They should prepare for this by gradually eliminating the feedings that occur during work hours and substituting a bottle. Although the total milk supply is diminished, breastfeeding can continue in the mornings and evenings.

#### WEANING

Weaning is a concern for many mothers. Because they are often subjected to pressure and opinions offered by family and friends about weaning, mothers benefit from the fact-based information that nurses can offer.

There is no one "right" time to wean the infant. Mothers choose to wean their infants for a variety of reasons. The woman who wants to breastfeed for a short time but does not wish to continue when she returns to work may wean early. Another pregnancy requires a decision of whether to wean or to continue breastfeeding. As infants mature, they show less interest in breastfeeding and increased ability to use a cup. If the mother becomes ill, she may have to stop breastfeeding.

The nurse should provide information so that women can make informed decisions about weaning and should support the woman once her decision is made. Explaining that even a short period of breastfeeding offers her infant many advantages is reassuring. Mothers may need help in planning a gradual weaning process, if it is possible. This allows them to avoid engorgement and infants can get used to a bottle or cup over a period of time. (Introduction of solids is discussed in Chapter 23, p. 629.)

## Mothers Want to Know
### How to Wean from Breastfeeding

**Deciding When to Wean**

Only you can make the decision about when to wean your baby. Breastfeeding has many benefits, and you can continue to breastfeed as long as you are comfortable. However, you may decide at any time that weaning is appropriate for you and your baby. Look at all the reasons for continuing nursing or beginning weaning and then decide.

**How to Proceed**

Gradual weaning is best for both you and your baby. Abrupt weaning can lead to engorgement and mastitis for you and can upset your baby. You both need to get used to this change slowly.

- Eliminate one feeding at a time. Replace it with a bottle for the young infant who needs to continue sucking. Infants generally do not drink as much from a cup as they do from a bottle. They may need a bottle to get enough milk to meet their nutritional requirements. The older infant who has learned to use a cup may not need a bottle at all. Use formula instead of cow's milk until the infant is at least 1 year old, as it is more suited to an infant's needs.
- Wait several days before eliminating another feeding. This allows time for your milk production to adjust and for the baby to accept the changes.
- Omit daytime feedings first. Start with the feeding at which the baby seems least interested, probably during the day when the baby is busy with play.
- Eliminate the baby's favorite feedings last. Many infants are particularly fond of morning and bedtime feedings. Mothers often continue the bedtime feeding for some time, even though the infant is completely weaned during the day. This often helps the baby settle down for the night.
- Expect your infant to want to nurse again when tired, ill, or hurt during the weaning process. This is sometimes called "comfort nursing." A few minutes of nursing may be all that is necessary to comfort the baby.

## CHECK YOUR READING

16. What types of care may be available after discharge for the breastfeeding mother?
17. What teaching should be included for the mother who plans to work and breastfeed?

# Formula Feeding

Although formula feeding may require less knowledge and skill than breastfeeding, the inexperienced mother often has many questions and may need assistance in learning to use formula correctly. Although breastfeeding is preferable, once the mother has made the choice to use formula the nurse should support her decision.

# Application of Nursing Process: Formula Feeding

## Assessment

Assess both the mother and the infant during the feeding process.

### MOTHER'S KNOWLEDGE

Assess the mother's knowledge of bottle feeding. Ask her if she has fed an infant before and if she has questions. Observe her technique during the initial and subsequent feedings. Note how she holds the infant and the bottle, assess her burping technique, and identify areas in which she seems unsure. Determine whether she knows how to prepare formula when she goes home.

### INFANT FEEDING BEHAVIORS

Hungry infants show the same behaviors whether breastfeeding or formula feeding. They may fuss or cry, suck on their hands, and root for the nipple. Waiting until the infant is frantic may result in a feeding taken too fast, with excess swallowing of air or choking. Assess how the infant sucks during the feeding to identify sucking problems.

## Analysis

Because improper formula preparation and feeding techniques could harm the infant, an appropriate nursing diagnosis for the mother using formula feeding is Risk for Altered Health Maintenance related to lack of understanding of formula preparation and feeding techniques.

## Planning

The mother will do the following:

- Demonstrate correct techniques in holding the infant and bottle during feedings.
- Describe how to prepare formula and the frequency of feedings.

## Interventions

### TEACHING ABOUT FORMULA

The mother must learn what type of formula she is to use and how to prepare it. Improper preparation can cause problems for the infant. Infection may occur if the milk or water used for preparation is contaminated. Improper dilution of the formula may cause undernutrition or imbalances of sodium, which can be dangerous to the infant.

### TYPES OF FORMULA

Many types of formula are available, and the physician or nurse practitioner prescribes the type of formula the mother is to use. If milk allergies are prevalent in the family, a soy-based or protein hydrolysate formula may be chosen from the start. Formula may be purchased in three different forms.

**Ready-to-Use.** This formula is available in bottles to which a nipple is added or in cans to be poured directly into a bottle. Although expensive, it is practical when there is difficulty mixing the formula or the water supply is in question. An open can should be refrigerated and used within 24 hours.

**Concentrated Liquid.** This type must be diluted before use. Be sure that the mother understands the directions for dilution. Equal parts of concentrated liquid formula and water are mixed together in a bottle to provide the amount desired for each feeding.

**Powdered.** Powdered formula is more economical and is particularly useful when a breastfeeding mother plans to give an occasional bottle of formula. Usually one scoop of powder is added to each 2 ounces of warm water in a bottle. Formula should be well mixed to dissolve the powder and make the solution uniform.

### EQUIPMENT

Many different types of bottles and nipples are available. Bottles may be glass or plastic, or a plastic liner that fits into a rigid container is used. The liners are designed to prevent swallowing of air from within the bottle. However, the infant still swallows some air around the nipple. Some nipples are designed to simulate the human nipple to promote jaw development. Selection of type of bottles and nipples depends on individual preference.

### PREPARATION

Discuss preparation of formula with the mother. She can prepare a single bottle or a 24-hour supply. If the water supply is safe, sterilization is not necessary. Bottles and nipples can be washed in hot, sudsy water, rinsed well, and allowed to air dry. Bottles may be washed in a dishwasher, but nipples tend to deteriorate quickly unless washed by hand. The top of the can and a can opener are washed just before opening the can. The formula and water are poured into the bottles, which are then capped. Be sure that the mother understands that the proportion of water and liquid or powdered formula must be adhered to exactly to prevent illness in the infant.

When safety of the water supply is questionable, sterilization, by aseptic or terminal method, is required. In both methods, all equipment is washed and rinsed well before beginning. In the aseptic method, equipment needed for the procedure is boiled for 5 minutes in a sterilizer or deep pan. Water for diluting the formula is boiled separately. The bottles are then assembled, using sterilized tongs to avoid contamination by the hands. The formula and boiled water are added, and the bottles are capped and refrigerated until needed.

In the terminal sterilization method, the formula is prepared in the bottles, which are loosely capped. The bottles are then placed in the sterilizer or pan of water, where they are boiled for 25 minutes. After the bottles cool, the caps are tightened and the bottles refrigerated.

## EXPLAINING FEEDING TECHNIQUES

The method for bottle feeding is similar to that for breastfeeding.

**Positioning.** The infant should be positioned in a semi-upright position such as the cradle hold. This allows the mother to hold the infant close in a face-to-face position. The bottle is held so that the nipple is kept full of formula to prevent excessive swallowing of air (Fig. 22–15).

**Burping.** The infant should be burped or "bubbled" after every half ounce for the first few days. The infant is gradually able to take more milk before burping. Show the mother how to place the infant over her shoulder or in a sitting position with the head supported while she pats and rubs the infant's back. After the feeding, the infant should always be placed on the side and propped with a rolled blanket. This helps prevent aspiration should more bubbles of air come up with formula.

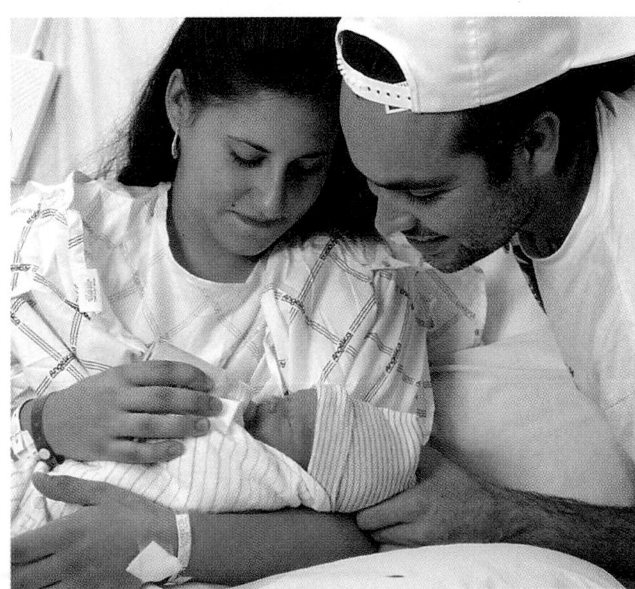

**FIGURE 22–15**

This mother holds her infant close during bottle feeding. The bottle is positioned so the nipple is filled with milk at all times. The father offers encouragement.

**Frequency.** The infant should be fed every 3 to 4 hours. Teach the mother to avoid rigid scheduling and to take her cues from the infant.

**Amount.** The appropriate amount for each feeding is a frequent concern of inexperienced mothers. The bottle-fed infant takes only 0.5 to 1 ounce per feeding during the first day of life but gradually increases to 2 to 3 ounces per feeding by the third day. Again, it is important for the mother to adapt to her infant's needs. An infant who is satisfied often goes to sleep.

**Cautions.** Caution the mother not to prop the bottle. Propping increases the likelihood of choking if regurgitation occurs and eliminates the holding and cuddling that should accompany feeding. Some mothers put an infant to bed with a bottle propped. This not only increases the danger of aspiration but allows milk to stay in the mouth for prolonged periods. The milk may pool in the mouth, promoting growth of bacteria and leading to cavities once the teeth are in. Ear infections are also more common in infants who sleep with a bottle.

The mother should not try to coax the infant to finish the bottle at each feeding. This could result in regurgitation and excessive weight gain. She should not save formula from one feeding to the next because of the danger of rapid growth of bacteria in warm milk. Any formula not used within an hour should be discarded.

Formula should not be heated in a microwave oven because the heating is uneven and may result in some parts of the liquid being very hot even when the outside of the bottle feels only warm. Formula can be heated by placing it in a container of hot water until it is warm. The mother should test the formula temperature by allowing a few drops from the bottle to fall on her inner arm.

**Infant Variations.** Infants vary in their feeding preferences. Some infants drink from the bottle reluctantly. Although formula is usually given at room temperature, some infants take heated formula better. The mother of a sleepy infant needs to use the same wake-up techniques discussed for the breastfeeding mother.

Soft nipples may be helpful for the infant with a weak suck or small mouth. Angling the tip of the nipple so that it rubs the palate triggers the suck reflex in most infants. Placing a finger under the chin for support may help some infants to suck better. It often takes patience and persistence to find the most effective techniques.

## Evaluation

The mother should be able to do the following:

- Demonstrate correct positioning of the infant and the bottle during feedings.
- Explain preparation of formula, the amount the infant should take, and the feeding techniques to be used.

### ✓ CHECK YOUR READING

18. What questions might a mother have about formula feeding?

## SUMMARY CONCEPTS

- The newborn may lose weight in the first few days after birth as a result of insufficient intake and normal loss of extracellular fluid.
- Colostrum is rich in protein, vitamins, minerals, and immunoglobulins. Transitional milk appears between colostrum and mature milk. Mature milk is present after the first 2 weeks of lactation.
- Breast milk has nutrients in proportions that the newborn requires and in an easily digested form. The majority of commercial formulas are cow's milk adapted to simulate human milk.
- Breast milk contains factors that help establish the normal intestinal flora and prevent infection. These include *bifidus* factor, leukocytes, lysozymes, and immunoglobulins.
- A variety of commercial formulas are available. They include modified cow's milk formula, soy-based or protein hydrolysate formulas, and formulas for preterm infants or those with special problems.
- Factors that influence the mother's choice of feeding method include knowledge about each method, support from family and friends, cultural influences, and employment.
- Suckling at the breast causes the mother's posterior pituitary to release oxytocin, which triggers the let-down reflex. It also causes the anterior pituitary to release prolactin, which increases milk production.
- The principle of "supply and demand" applies to breastfeeding. Milk production increases when the infant feeds frequently. When breastfeeding ceases, prolactin is decreased and eventually the alveoli of the breasts atrophy and stop producing milk.
- Flat and inverted nipples should be identified during pregnancy. Creams and methods to toughen the nipples are not necessary.
- The nurse can help the mother establish breastfeeding by initiating early feeding, assisting her to position the infant at the breast, and showing her how to position her hands. The nurse should teach the mother how to help the infant latch on to the breast, assess the position of the mouth on the breast, and remove the infant from the breast.

- The mother should feed the infant 8 to 12 times each day for an average of at least 15 minutes per feeding, nursing until the infant is satisfied at the second breast.
- Wake-up techniques for sleepy infants include unwrapping the blankets, talking to the infant, changing the diaper, rubbing the infant's back, and expressing colostrum onto the breast.
- When infants suck from a bottle, they must push the tongue against the nipple to slow the flow of milk. When they suckle at the breast, they position the nipple far into the mouth so that the gums compress the areola as the tongue moves over the milk sinuses in a wave-like motion.
- The nurse can help the woman with engorged breasts by encouraging her to nurse frequently, apply heat and cold, and massage and express milk to soften the areola if necessary.
- The nurse should help the mother with sore nipples to check the positioning of the infant at the breast. The mother should vary the position of the infant at the breast, apply breast milk, warm water compresses, or warm, wet tea bags to the nipples, and expose the nipples to air.
- Teaching for the mother who plans to work and breastfeed includes expression of breast milk by hand or pump and proper storage of the milk.
- Mothers who use formula need information about the types of formula available, how to prepare them correctly, and feeding techniques.

### References and Readings


Adams, E.J. (1997). Nutritional care in food allergy and food intolerance. In L.K. Mahan & S. Escott-Stump (Eds.), *Krause's food, nutrition, and diet therapy* (9th ed.). Philadelphia: W.B. Saunders.

American Academy of Pediatrics and American College of Obstetricians and Gynecologists. (1992). *Guidelines for perinatal care* (3rd ed.). Elk Grove Village, Ill.: American Academy of Pediatrics.

Auerbach, K.D. (1993). Maternal employment and breastfeeding. In J. Riordan & K.C. Auerbach (Eds.), *Breastfeeding and human lactation*. Boston: Jones & Bartlett.

Auerbach, K.D., & Walker, M. (1994). When the mother of a premature infant uses a breast pump: What every NICU nurse needs to know. *Neonatal Network*, 13(4), 23–29.

Balcazar, H., Trier, C.M., & Cobas, J.A. (1995). What predicts breastfeeding intention in Mexican-American and non-Hispanic white women? Evidence from a national survey. *Birth*, 22(2), 74–80.

Beaudry, M., Dufour, R., & Marcoux, S. (1995). Relation between infant feeding and infections during the first six months of life. *Journal of Pediatrics*, 126(2), 191–197.

Behrman, R.E., Kliegman, R.M., Arvin, A.M., & Nelson, W.E. (Eds.). (1996). *Nelson Textbook of Pediatrics* (15th ed.). Philadelphia: W.B. Saunders.

Blackburn, S.T., & Loper, D.L. (1992). *Maternal, fetal, and neonatal physiology: A clinical perspective*. Philadelphia: W.B. Saunders.

Bronner, Y.L., & Paige, D.M. (1992). Current concepts in infant nutrition. *Journal of Nurse-Midwifery*, 37(Suppl. 2), 43S–58S.

Buchko, G.L., Pugh, L.C., Bishop, B.A., Cochran, J.F., Smith, L.R., & Lerew, D.J. (1994). Comfort measures in breastfeeding primiparous women. *Journal of Obstetric, Gynecologic, and Neonatal Nursing*, 23(1), 46–51.

Buescher, E.S. (1995). Host defense mechanisms of human milk and their relations to enteric infections and necrotizing enterocolitis. *Clinics in Perinatology*, 21(2), 247–262.

Darby, M.K., & Loughead, J.L. (1996). Neonatal nutritional requirements and formula composition: A review. *Journal of Obstetric, Gynecologic, and Neonatal Nursing*, 25(3), 209–217.

D'Avanzo, C.E. (1992). Bridging the cultural gap with Southeast Asians. *MCN: American Journal of Maternal-Child Nursing*, 17(4), 204–208.

DeMarini, S., Tsang, R.C., & Rath, L.L. (1993). Fluids, electrolytes, vitamins, and trace minerals: Basis of ingestion, digestion, elimination, and metabolism. In C. Kenner, A. Brueggemeyer, & L.P. Gunderson (Eds.), *Comprehensive neonatal nursing, a physiologic perspective*. Philadelphia: W.B. Saunders.

Dungy, C.I., Christensen-Szalanski, J., Losch, M., & Russell, D. (1992). Effect of discharge samples on duration of breast-feeding. *Pediatrics*, 90(2), 233–237.

Furman, L. (1995). A developmental approach to weaning. *MCN: American Journal of Maternal-Child Nursing*, 20(6), 322–325.

Gigliotti, E. (1995). When women decide not to breastfeed. *MCN: American Journal of Maternal-Child Nursing*, 20(6), 315–321.

Harris, M.K.B. (1993). Breastfeeding. In S. Mattson & J.E. Smith (Eds.), *NAACOG core curriculum for maternal-newborn nursing*. Philadelphia: W.B. Saunders.

Henly, S.J., Anderson, C.M., Avery, M.D., Hills-Bonczyk, S.G., Potter, S., & Duckett, L.J. (1995). Anemia and insufficient milk in first-time mothers. *Birth*, 22(2), 87–92.

Huggins, K. (1995). *The nursing mother's companion* (3rd ed.). Boston: Harvard Common Press.

Hughes, V., & Owen, J. (1993). Is breastfeeding possible after breast surgery? *MCN: American Journal of Maternal-Child Nursing*, 18(4), 213–217.

Hutchinson, M.K., & Baqi-Azia, M. (1994). Nursing care of the childbearing Muslim family. *Journal of Obstetric, Gynecologic and Neonatal Nursing*, 23(9), 767–771.

Institute of Medicine, National Academy of Sciences, Food and Nutrition Board. (1989). *Recommended dietary allowances* (19th ed.). Washington, D.C.: National Academy Press.

Institute of Medicine, National Academy of Sciences, Food and Nutrition Board. (1991). *Nutrition during lactation*. Washington, D.C.: National Academy Press.

Isabella, P.H., & Isabella, R.A. (1994). Correlates of successful breastfeeding: A study of social and personal factors. *Journal of Human Lactation*, 10(4), 257–264.

Jacobi, A.M., & Levin, M. (1997). Promotion and support of breastfeeding. In B. Worthington-Roberts & S.R. Williams (Eds.), *Nutrition in pregnancy and lactation* (6th ed.). St. Louis: Times Mirror/Mosby.

Jambunathan, J., & Stewart, S. (1995). Hmong women in Wisconsin: What are their concerns in pregnancy and childbirth? *Birth*, 22(4), 204–210.

Jensen, D., Wallace, S., & Kelsay, P. (1994). LATCH: A breastfeeding charting system and documentation tool. *Journal of Obstetric, Gynecologic, and Neonatal Nursing*, 23(1), 27–32.

Kovach, A.C. (1996). An assessment tool for evaluating hospital breastfeeding policies and practices. *Journal of Human Lactation*, 12(1), 41–45.

Lavergne, N.A. (1997). Does application of tea bags to sore nipples while breastfeeding provide effective relief? *Journal of Obstetric, Gynecologic, and Neonatal Nursing*, 26(1), 53–58.

Lawrence, P.B. (1994). Breast milk: Best source of nutrition for term and preterm infants. *Pediatric Clinics of North America*, 41(5), 925–941.

Lawrence, R.A. (1994). *Breastfeeding: A guide for the medical profession* (4th ed.). St. Louis: C.V. Mosby.

Lawrence, R.A. (1995). The clinician's role in teaching proper infant feeding techniques. *Journal of Pediatrics*, 126(6), S112–117.

Losch, M., Dungy, C.I., Russell, D., & Dusdieker, L.B. (1995). Impact of attitudes on maternal decisions regarding infant feeding. *Journal of Pediatrics*, 126(4), 507–514.

Mahlmeister, L. (1996). Breastfeeding [letter]. *Journal of Obstetric, Gynecologic, and Neonatal Nursing*, 25(1), 15.

Mattson, S. (1995). Culturally sensitive perinatal care for southeast Asians. *Journal of Obstetric, Gynecologic, and Neonatal Nursing*, 24(41), 335–341.

Meftuh, A.B., Tapsoba, L.P., & Lamounier, J.A. (1991). Breastfeeding practices in Ethiopian women in southern California. *Indian Journal of Pediatrics*, 58(3), 349–356.

Moore, K., & Chute, G. (1996). Newborn nutrition. In D.R. Simpson & P.A. Creehan (Eds.), *AWHONN's perinatal nursing*. Philadelphia: J.B. Lippincott.

Mulford, C. (1995). Swimming upstream: Breastfeeding care in a nonbreastfeeding culture. *Journal of Obstetric, Gynecologic, and Neonatal Nursing*, 24(5), 464–474.

Neuhouser, M.L.S. (1996). Nutrition during pregnancy and lactation. In L.K. Mahan & S. Escott-Stump (Eds.), *Krause's food, nutrition, and diet therapy* (9th ed.). Philadelphia: W.B. Saunders.

Nurses' Association of The American College of Obstetricians and Gynecologists (NAACOG). (1991). *OGN nursing practice resource: Facilitating breastfeeding*. Washington, D.C.: Author.

Nurses' Association of the American College of Obstetricians and Gynecologists (NAACOG) Executive Board. (1992). NAACOG position statement. Issue: Breastfeeding. *NAACOG Newsletter*, 19(1), 8.

Orlando, S. (1995). The immunologic significance of breast milk. *Journal of Obstetric, Gynecologic, and Neonatal Nursing*, 24(7), 678–683.

Pascale, J.A., Brittian, L., Lenfestey, C.C., & Jarrett-Pulliam, C. (1996). Breastfeeding, dehydration, and shorter maternity stays. *Neonatal Network*, 15(7), 37–43.

Piper, S., & Parks, P. (1996). Predicting the duration of lactation: Evidence from a national survey. *Birth*, 23(1), 7–12.

Pipes, P.L. (1996). Nutrition in infancy. In L.K. Mahan & S. Escott-Stump (Eds.), *Krause's food, nutrition, and diet therapy* (9th ed.). Philadelphia: W.B. Saunders.

Powers, N.G., Naylor, A.J., & Wester, R.A. (1994). Hospital policies: Crucial to breastfeeding success. *Seminars in Perinatology*, 18(6), 517–524.

Pugh, L.C., Buchko, B.L., Bishop, B.A., Cochran, J.F., Smith, L.R., & Lerew, D.J. (1996). A comparison of topical agents to relieve nipple pain and enhance breastfeeding. *Birth*, 23(2), 88–93.

Rasbridge, L.A., & Kulig, J.C. (1995). Infant feeding among Cambodian refugees. *MCN: American Journal of Maternal-Child Nursing*, 20(4), 213–218.

Righard, L., & Alade, M.O. (1992). Sucking technique and its effect on success of breastfeeding. *Birth*, 19(4), 16–20.

Riordan, J. (1993a). The biologic specificity of breastmilk. In J. Riordan & K.C. Auerbach (Eds.), *Breastfeeding and human lactation*. Boston: Jones & Bartlett.

Riordan, J. (1993b). The cultural context of breastfeeding. In J. Riordan & K.C. Auerbach (Eds.), *Breastfeeding and human lactation*. Boston: Jones & Bartlett.

Riordan, J., & Auerbach, K.C. (Eds.). (1993). *Breastfeeding and human lactation*. Boston: Jones & Bartlett.

Riordan, J.M., & Koehn, M. (1997). Reliability and validity testing of three breastfeeding assessment tools. *Journal of Obstetric, Gynecologic, and Neonatal Nursing*, 26(2), 181–187.

Ross Products Division. (1995). *Updated breastfeeding trend 1987–1995. Mothers' survey*. Columbus, Ohio: Ross Products Division, Abbott Laboratories.

Saadeh, R., & Akre, J. (1996). Ten steps to successful breastfeeding: A summary of the rationale and scientific evidence. *Birth*, 23(3), 154–160.

Saarinen, U.M., & Kajosaari, M. (1995). Breastfeeding as prophylaxis against atopic disease: Prospective follow-up study until 17 years old. *Lancet*, 346, 1065–1069.

Schwartz, J.B., Popkin, B.M., Tognetti, J., & Zohoori, N. (1995). Does WIC participation improve breast-feeding practices? *American Journal of Public Health*, 85(5), 729–731.

Serafino-Cross, P., & Donovan, P.R. (1992). Effectiveness of professional breastfeeding home-support. *Journal of Nutrition Education* 24(3), 117–122.

Timbo, B., Altekruse, S., Headrick, M., & Klontz, K. (1996). Breastfeeding among black mothers: Evidence supporting the need for prenatal intervention. *Journal of the Society of Pediatric Nurses*, 1(1), 35–40.

U.S. Department of Health and Human Services (USDHHS). (1991). *Healthy children 2000*. Washington, D.C.: Author.

Walker, M. (1997). Breastfeeding the sleepy baby. *Journal of Human Lactation*, 13(2), 151–153.

Williamson, M.T., & Murti, P.K. (1996). Effects of storage, time, temperature, and composition of containers on biologic components of human milk. *Journal of Human Lactation*, 12(1), 31–35.

Wong, D.L. (1995). *Whaley & Wong's nursing care of infants and children* (5th ed.). St. Louis: C.V. Mosby.

Worthington-Roberts, B. (1997). Human milk composition and infant growth and development. In B. Worthington-Roberts & S.R. Williams (Eds.), *Nutrition in pregnancy and lactation* (6th ed.). St. Louis: Times Mirror/Mosby.

Worthington-Roberts, B. (1997). Lactation: Basic considerations. In B. Worthington-Roberts & S.R. Williams (Eds.), *Nutrition in pregnancy and lactation* (6th ed.). St. Louis: Times Mirror/Mosby.

Ziemer, M.M., & Pigeon, J.G. (1993). Skin changes and pain in the nipple during the first week of lactation. *Journal of Obstetric, Gynecologic, and Neonatal Nursing*, 22(3), 247–256.

# 23

# Home Care of the Infant

**OBJECTIVES**

1. Explain why nurses need knowledge about care of the infant during the early weeks after birth.
2. Describe postdischarge nursing care included in home visits, clinic visits, and telephone follow-up.
3. Explain the safety features of infant equipment that parents must consider.
4. Explain methods of resolving common problems involving infant crying and sleep patterns during the early weeks of parenting.
5. Answer common questions that parents might have about care of the young infant.
6. Describe the normal changes in growth and development of the infant during the first 12 weeks of life.
7. Explain the purpose and importance of well-baby checkups and immunizations for infants.
8. List signs that indicate illness in the infant.
9. Discuss current knowledge about sudden infant death syndrome.

**DEFINITIONS**

**extrusion reflex** *Automatic nervous system response that causes an infant to push anything solid out of the mouth.*

**miliaria (prickly heat)** *Rash caused by heat.*

**reflux** *A condition in which stomach contents enter the esophagus and may be aspirated into the lungs.*

**seborrheic dermatitis (cradle cap)** *Yellowish, crusty area of the scalp.*

**sudden infant death syndrome (SIDS)** *Sudden death of an infant that is unexplained by autopsy, examination of the scene of death, or history.*

Nurses are often called on to answer parents' questions about care of infants during the early weeks. This is especially important when the birth facility stay is short and nurses give follow-up care in the home or clinic. This chapter provides information to help nurses assist parents in adjusting to their new role and providing care for the infant during the first 12 weeks of life. The focus is on teaching about infants beyond the usual birth facility discharge teaching, which is included in Chapter 21. Detailed information about ill or older infants can be found in pediatric textbooks.

## Information for New Parents

### Needs

The early weeks after birth are often very stressful for new parents. This is particularly true for the first birth but also applies to families with other children. The mother is tired from the pregnancy and birth, both parents may be anxious about their new role, and the newborn may be awake much of the night or behave in other unexpected ways. Parents have many questions not only about the newborn but also about adjustment to parenthood and ongoing care of the infant. The need for information and support varies according to the experience, age, and individual concerns of parents.

### Sources of Information

In the birth facility, parents often receive more information about care of the newborn than they can absorb in the very short time available. New mothers may have physical needs and anxieties that interfere with their ability to learn. Women have been found to have more difficulty remembering information given them on the first day after birth than at other times (Eidelman et al., 1993). This may leave parents inadequately prepared to deal with the multiple demands of early parenting.

In the past, the extended family was the usual source of support and information for new parents. Today, family members are frequently widely separated, and parents must rely on friends, health care personnel, child care classes, books, and magazines. Friends can be important sources of support and information, but their knowledge may be incorrect or outdated. For example, they may not have accurate information about breastfeeding and the latest recommendations for immunizations. Nurses are ideal sources of assistance in these situations.

## Care After Discharge

The American Academy of Pediatrics and the American College of Obstetricians and Gynecologists recommend that women and their infants stay in the birth facility for 48 hours after vaginal birth and 96 hours after cesarean birth. The optimal time of discharge should be based on the individual needs of the woman and her infant. Those who are discharged earlier should have follow-up care within 48 hours after discharge (AAP & ACOG, 1992; AAP, 1995).

Although longer stays have been legislated, women may choose to go home before 48 hours after a vaginal birth. Early follow-up is essential for these families. Various programs have been instituted to provide after-discharge care. They may include nursing contact with the family in the home and clinic and by telephone. Some birth facilities offer a package of services. For example, one program includes perinatal classes, two home visits by nurses, 24-hour

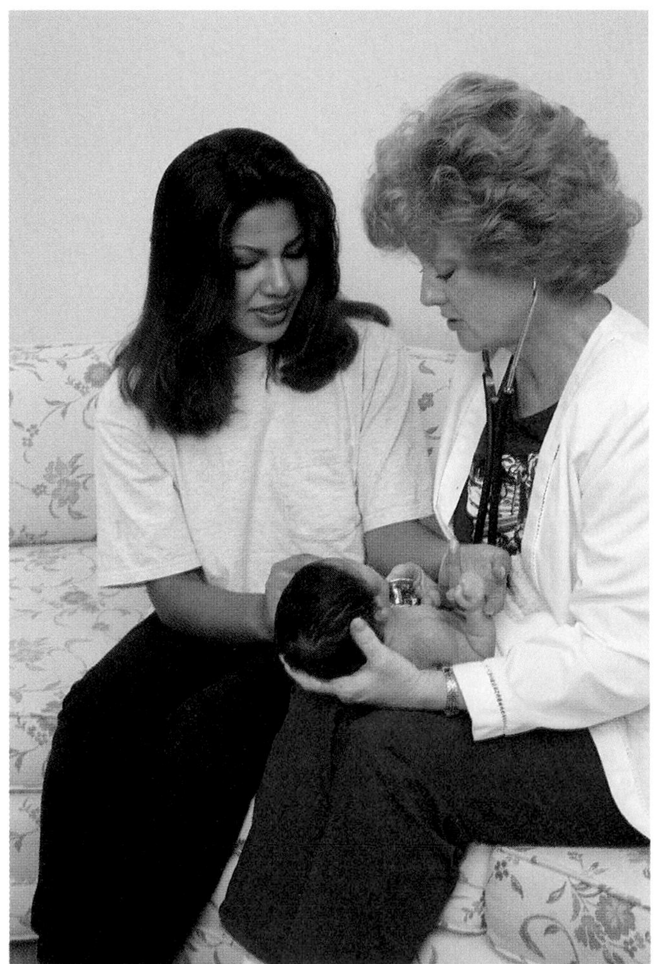

**FIGURE 23–1**

During the home visit, the nurse performs a complete assessment of the infant. Here she is checking the apical pulse and listening to breath sounds.

telephone access, and availability of a home health aide for 16 hours (Mendler et al., 1996). Other programs are less inclusive and may contain only one or two components. These programs have been very successful. One study of a comprehensive program for visits and phone access showed a 99 percent client satisfaction rate as well as a decrease in infant hospital readmissions (Williams & Cooper, 1996).

## Home Visits

The home visit is ideally scheduled during the first 24 to 48 hours after discharge. This timing allows early assessment and intervention for problems in nutrition, jaundice, newborn adaptation, and maternal-infant interaction. Visits usually are 60 to 90 minutes to allow enough time for assessment and teaching. Nurses may visit low-risk mothers and infants (Figs. 23–1 to 23–4) or may follow high-risk infants after discharge from the neonatal intensive care nursery.

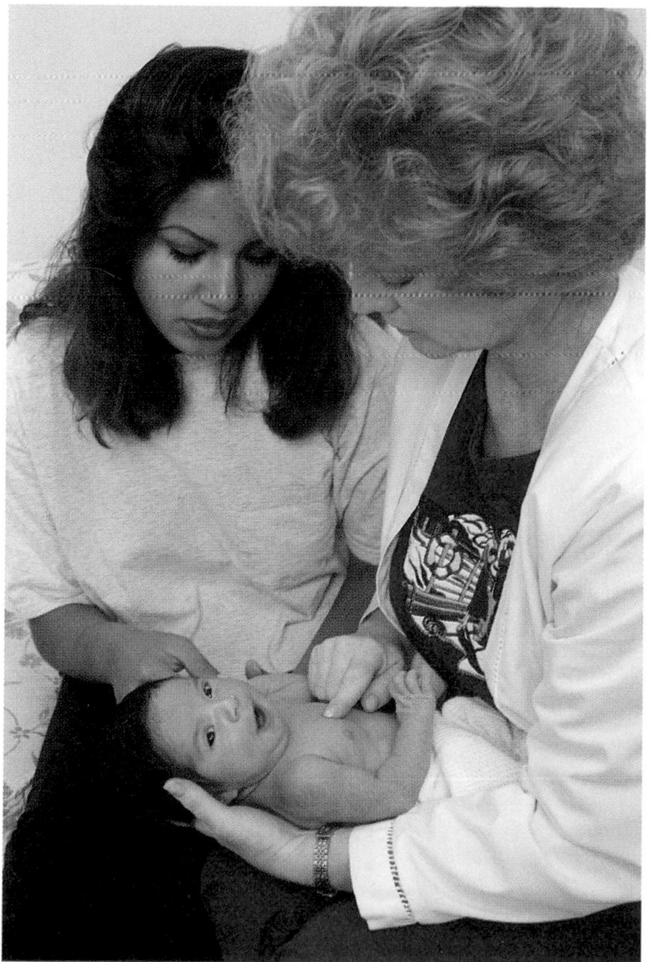

**FIGURE 23–2**

Jaundice is especially of concern when infants are discharged early after birth. The nurse shows the mother how to blanch the skin to check for jaundice and discusses what the mother should do if she sees it.

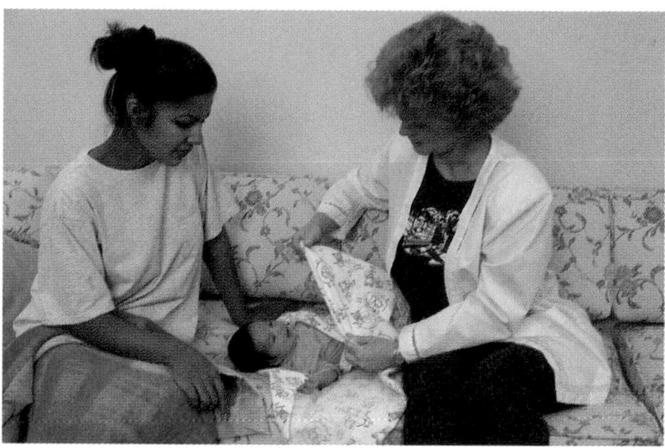

**FIGURE 23–3**

The nurse discusses thermoregulation with the mother and demonstrates swaddling.

### VISITS TO LOW-RISK FAMILIES

During the home visit, the nurse performs a physical examination of the mother and infant. Family adaptation to the addition of a new member and the adequacy of the mother's support system are assessed. The nurse reinforces and continues the teaching about self- and infant care that was begun at the birth facility, and parents have an opportunity to ask questions. A feeding session should be assessed, especially if the mother is breastfeeding. Blood may be obtained for metabolic screening if the infant went home too early for reliable testing in the birth facility. See the summary of components of the home visit in the Clinical Pathway for the Normal Newborn Home Visit (Fig. 23–5). Home care services for mothers are discussed in Chapter 17.

Home visits provide reassurance for parents and may increase a woman's confidence and competence

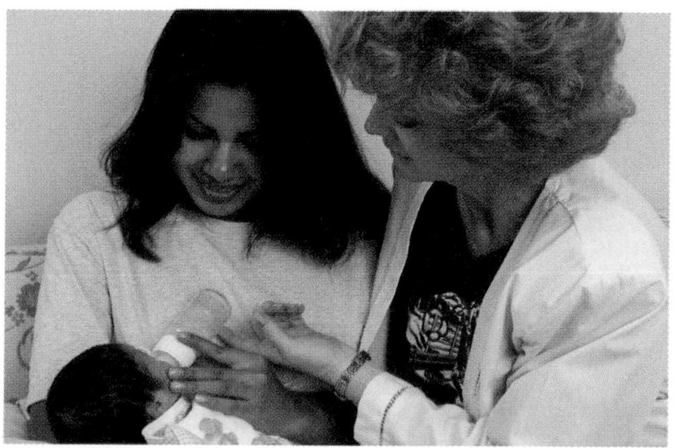

**FIGURE 23–4**

The nurse observes a feeding during the visit to assess feeding techniques and provide a chance for parents to ask questions about feeding concerns. This is a good time to assess parent-infant interaction. The infant is weighed to help determine adequacy of intake.

| EXPECTED NEWBORN/FAMILY OUTCOMES | ASSESSMENTS | INTERVENTIONS | RESPONSE |
|---|---|---|---|
| Physical assessment: The newborn assessment is within normal limits. | Vital signs, weight<br><br>Respiratory status (color, retractions, etc.)<br><br>Skin (rash, jaundice, cord, circumcision)<br><br>Fontanelles<br><br>Activity, sleep, behavior, crying<br><br>Elimination (number of voids and stools in 24 hours) | Complete systematic assessment. | Outcomes met.<br><br>Outcome not met (requires further documentation). |
| Nutrition: Infant's intake is adequate. LATCH score is over 7 if infant breastfed. (See Chapter 22, p. 589.) | Infant's and mother's behaviors during a feeding | Discuss frequency, length of feedings, and amount (in oz. or time at breast). Discuss breastfeeding or other problems. Provide written educational materials. | Outcome met.<br><br>Outcome not met (requires further documentation).<br><br>Referral made |
| Caregiving: Parents correctly describe infant characteristics and needs and demonstrate care. | Parent's knowledge and performance of infant care | Teach and clarify as necessary. Provide written educational materials. | Outcome met.<br><br>Outcome not met (requires further documentation). |
| Infant/family relationships: The family demonstrates attachment behaviors. | Interaction of parents and family members with infant | Discuss emotional adjustment of all family members, sibling rivalry, postpartum blues. Provide written educational materials. | Outcome met.<br><br>Outcome not met (requires further documentation). |
| Support system: Parents have an adequate support system. | Interaction of family members, sources of support within and outside the immediate family | Discuss availability and need for support, resources. Provide written educational materials. | Outcome met.<br><br>Outcome not met (requires further documentation).<br><br>Referral made. |
| Environment: The home is safe and has adequate facilities and baby equipment and supplies are safe. | Safety and potential hazards in the home; availability of heat, electricity, telephone, sanitation, sleeping arrangements | Provide written educational materials. | Outcome met.<br><br>Outcome not met (requires further documentation). |
| Need for care: The parents understand need for well baby care. They recognize signs of infant illness and how to get help. | Knowledge about well baby checkups and immunizations, signs of illness, how to take a temperature, where to get care | Discuss areas in which there is need; demonstrate temperature taking. Provide written educational materials. | Outcome met.<br><br>Outcome not met (requires further documentation). |

**FIGURE 23–5**

An example of a clinical pathway for a home visit by a nurse to the family of a normal newborn.

| EXPECTED NEWBORN/FAMILY OUTCOMES | ASSESSMENTS | INTERVENTIONS | RESPONSE |
|---|---|---|---|
| Other care: Metabolic screening or other care is received, as ordered. | Need for specimen collection or other care | Collect blood specimens for newborn metabolic screening; give other care (phototherapy, etc.) as ordered. Provide written educational materials. | Outcome met.<br><br>Outcome not met (requires further documentation). |
| Referrals: Parents receive necessary referrals. | Need for referrals | Refer to physician, lactation consultant, WIC, community resources, etc. Provide written educational materials. | Outcome met (document to whom referral made).<br><br>Outcome not met (requires further documentation). |

**FIGURE 23–5** *Continued*

in caring for herself and her infant. Early return to her own environment, coupled with the knowledge that she can receive needed assistance from nurses, helps the woman to feel more in control of her experience (Hall & Carty, 1993).

Home visits are especially valuable in recognizing jaundice and intervening before bilirubin levels become dangerously high. When jaundice is found, the nurse can discuss the implications and draw blood for testing bilirubin levels. Appropriate care is discussed, as necessary, including hydration and phototherapy (see Parents Want to Know: Home Care for the Infant Receiving Phototherapy, Chapter 30, p. 854).

Feeding is a subject about which mothers often have questions, especially when they are breastfeeding. Breastfeeding problems were found in one study in almost a third of infants (Williams & Cooper, 1996). When the nurse observes a feeding and helps a woman deal with problems, the infant's intake may increase. Increased intake helps to prevent dehydration and possible hospital readmission. It also leads to increased excretion of bilirubin, which may prevent a need for phototherapy at home or in the hospital.

### VISITS TO FAMILIES WITH HIGH-RISK INFANTS

High-risk infants (discussed in Chapters 29 and 30) often need special care after discharge. Parents may be very anxious about taking over care of an infant who has had a prolonged hospitalization. Many hospitals have programs that enable parents to take over their infant's care gradually before discharge.

A nurse may visit the home before the infant's discharge to help the family plan for accommodating the equipment and the type of care the infant needs. The home is checked for the availability of electricity, heat, and a telephone. The nurse makes sure that the family has notified its utility companies if they have a technology-dependent infant to ensure that no disruption of services occurs.

After the infant is discharged, nursing visits can help the family maintain the infant's health and decrease the need for rehospitalization. Components of each visit vary according to the infant's needs. The nurse provides assessment of the infant and the parents' caregiving ability, as well as necessary teaching and nursing.

Medically fragile infants may require home treatment with mechanical ventilation, oxygen therapy, or apnea monitors. Parents may have to perform such nursing skills as tracheostomy care, tube feedings, suctioning, and care of intravenous sites. Mothers often have concerns about feeding the infant, which may be very different from feeding a normal full-term infant. Follow-up telephone calls from nurses between visits help families adapt to the needs of these infants and may also decrease the need for rehospitalization.

The home health nurse may be part of an interdisciplinary team of health care providers working with families in the home. The nurse may help coordinate care by different professionals. Some infants are eligible for home health aides who provide direct care in the home. The aide is supervised by a nurse.

Infants with complications often need more frequent visits to the pediatrician or nurse practitioner or are rehospitalized during the early months after birth. Common problems include respiratory illness, infections (gastroenteritis, sepsis, urinary tract infections, otitis media), and need for surgery. These parents need more information on preventive measures and care of the infant with acute illness.

Although parents' greatest concerns involve the infant's health, other problems may exist as well. Finding a baby sitter who is qualified to care for an infant on oxygen or who might need cardiopulmonary resuscitation may be difficult. Siblings often have difficulty adjusting to the needs of the infant and may resent the diversion of the parents' attention. The nurse can make suggestions and put the parents in touch with parent groups that offer practical help in caring for a high-risk infant.

#### GENERAL CONSIDERATIONS IN HOME VISITS

The nurse making a home visit is a guest of the family and must adapt nursing care usually given in the birth facility to the home setting. The needs of other family members may make care in the home quite different from care given in the hospital. For example, the examination of the infant may need to wait for a short time while the mother meets the needs of her other small children.

Careful planning before the visit is essential to make the most of the limited time available. A telephone call allows the nurse to schedule the visit at a time convenient for the family and obtain directions to the home. It is important to set priorities very carefully based on the needs identified by the nurse and the family, especially when only one visit is planned. After the home visit, the nurse may schedule additional visits or provide the family with a telephone number where they may receive further help if needed.

Communication skills are particularly important when the setting is the home and the client is the family. The nurse must develop rapport with family members quickly and work with them to meet shared goals for the visit. A brief social interaction may be beneficial at the beginning of the visit to develop a trusting relationship. The purpose of the visit should be explained and the family's expectations and desires discussed. Open-ended questions and therapeutic communication techniques help the nurse identify and address the family's needs. It is important to make suggestions in a positive manner.

The nurse should be aware of any cultural practices affecting the family's view of care. For example, many Asians find direct eye contact, pointing a finger, or showing the bottom of the shoe offensive. In patriarchal cultures, the father is the head of the family, and teaching should be performed through him. The elder members of the family may also play a large role in determining what health care is essential. In some cultures, the mother-in-law is a very important influence in the care of the mother and infant.

Documentation of the visit is essential. The results of the assessments, teaching, nursing care, referrals, and plans for follow-up should be recorded. Copies of the record are usually sent to the primary caregiver.

## Outpatient Visits

Outpatient visits may be provided by the birth facility in clinics managed by nurses. Mothers and infants are seen by a nurse within the first 48 to 72 hours after discharge. The charge is often included in the maternity care package. Assessment and care are essentially the same as those provided for home visits. The advantage of outpatient visits is that the nurse does not have to travel to the home and can see more clients each day, thereby reducing the cost of the service. The disadvantage is that the nurse does not have the opportunity to assess the home setting and the family interaction there. Clinic visits usually last 30 to 45 minutes. Clinic appointments may be made during the discharge procedure from the birth facility.

In some areas nurses take a van to various neighborhoods to provide nursing care. This allows clients with transportation problems easy access to care. Nurses in the van carry out the same assessment and care of the mother and infant that is provided during clinic visits. Care may begin in the prenatal period and extend through the postpartum period.

## Telephone Counseling

Telephone counseling can occur during follow-up calls to discharged clients or when parents call "warm lines" for help with problems or questions. Telephone calls have the advantage of being much less expensive than home or clinic visits. The major disadvantage is that the nurse cannot perform an in-person assessment of the mother, baby, or home environment and must rely on the caller to present an accurate picture of the situation.

#### FOLLOW-UP CALLS

Follow-up calls are placed by nurses in the first few days after discharge. The nurse asks a series of questions to assess the physical condition of the mother and infant and to identify any needs or problems. All mothers may receive calls or only those considered at risk for problems. In some facilities, the nurse who cared for the woman makes the calls. In others, certain nurses are assigned to make all calls. The nurse may schedule another call or a home visit, if available, or refer the woman to her primary care provider if problems are discovered.

#### WARM LINES

Warm lines, also called help lines, provide parents with an opportunity to ask a nurse the questions that often arise after the reality of parenting has been faced. They are used for situations that cause parents concern but are not emergencies. The service should be available 24 hours each day to best meet the needs of the callers. Parents often call about infant feeding, breastfeeding concerns, and basic care of the mother and infant. Calls last about 15 to 20 minutes. The nurse answers the caller's questions and assesses for other problems. The nurse may call back later to see if the situation has resolved.

#### TELEPHONE TECHNIQUES

It is important that nurses caring for clients by telephone understand telephone counseling techniques. They need special training in telephone communication and triage. Open-ended questions such as, "How have you been getting along since you left the hospital?" or "Have there been situations where you weren't sure what to do?" help the mother describe any problems in her own terms.

Telephone triage involves determining whether a serious problem exists and what needs to be done about it. The nurse should help the mother (or caller) describe the major concerns, which may not be those discussed first. "What worries you most?" may help focus on the most important problems. Although most problems discussed are concerns about normal infants, the nurse must be alert for "red flags" that signal serious situations needing immediate referral.

The nurse should determine if the parents know where and when to obtain more care if the problem is not resolved. They should be told approximately how long it is appropriate to wait before calling the primary care provider or telephone warm line if the situation does not improve. Nurses often call parents back to check on the progress of the problem.

### Critical to Remember

#### RED FLAGS OF TELEPHONE TRIAGE

- An emergency situation (e.g., respiratory difficulty, bleeding). Tell the parent to call 911 or take the infant to a hospital emergency department immediately. Call back in 5 minutes to see that parents did seek help.
- Illness (fever, dehydration, change in feeding or behavior, unusual rashes)
- Severe feeding problems (Infant may become dehydrated, jaundiced, or fail to thrive.)
- Problem has been present for longer than usual or usual remedies are ineffective (e.g., prolonged crying or sleeping, rash is spreading).
- Parent's affect seems inappropriate for situation (extremely emotional with apparently minor situation or unconcerned when situation could be serious).

*Note*: Callers should be referred to the primary health care provider or the hospital emergency room, if necessary, when a serious problem may be present. It is always better to be overcautious and refer parents to the primary care provider early rather than to miss a serious situation.

#### GUIDELINES AND DOCUMENTATION

When nurses are giving care by telephone, it is important that they have written protocols and policies that provide guidelines for care. This helps ensure that all who perform this service provide clients with similar information. A list of common questions can be compiled to help nurses obtain appropriate information when parents call about a problem.

Parents should always be told when and how to seek more care if problems are not resolved. If the infant appears ill, referral to the pediatrician or hospital emergency department is most appropriate. The nurse's judgment, based on education, expertise, and experience, is the most important factor in how helpful the service is to clients.

All calls should be documented so that accurate, legal records are available for future reference. The nurse may use a check-off form or a simple written description of the call. Documentation should include identifying information for the caller, including address and phone number. The reason for the call, problems described, advice given, and any referrals should also be recorded. In some agencies, all calls are audiotaped. A copy of the information is sent to the primary caregiver to provide continuity of care.

### CHECK YOUR READING

1. Where do parents obtain information about caring for their infant during the early weeks after birth?
2. What are some ways in which nurses offer follow-up services to new parents?

## Infant Equipment

Many parents have questions about choosing infant equipment. Ideally, they have obtained most of the equipment before the infant is born, but nurses may receive questions in the weeks after the birth. Although nurses should never recommend specific brand names of equipment, their guidance about features and safety is very helpful.

### Safety Considerations

Parents, especially those of limited means, need to understand that few, if any, pieces of equipment are absolutely essential for newborns. Infants sleep in padded dresser drawers and canopied cribs with equal comfort. Safety is the most important consideration.

New equipment sold in the United States is generally safe because manufacturers are required to follow certain governmental standards for safety.

However, hand-me-down equipment may have been produced before newer requirements were in effect. Older equipment should be checked carefully to be certain that all parts are strong and working properly. See Table 23–1 for a summary of safety considerations.

## Car Seats

It is never safe for an adult to carry an infant while riding in a car. A sudden stop or accident could cause the infant to be hurled against the dash board or crushed by the adult, who would be thrown forward by the force of the impact. In the United States and Canada, laws require restraint of infants and young children in car seats when they are riding in automobiles. Generally, laws require that special seats be used for children under 4 years or 40 pounds. Discharge teaching should include information about state car seat laws. In some birth facilities, car seat rentals or loans are available.

**TABLE 23-1 SAFETY CONSIDERATIONS FOR INFANT EQUIPMENT**

**Cribs**

Crib slats must be no more than 2⅜ inches apart so that the infant's head cannot become wedged between them. Remove corner posts that extend more than 1/16 inch above the end panel to prevent strangulation if clothing catches on them. Plastic teething guards should be firmly attached to side rails.

Bumper pads prevent the infant from hitting against the side rails. They should fit well around the entire crib and must be anchored to keep them in place so that infants cannot get caught between the side rail and the bumper.

The crib mattress should fit snugly, with less than an inch between the mattress and the sides of the crib so that the infant cannot become wedged in that space. The mattress should be firm. There should be no soft pillows in the crib that would increase the risk of suffocation.

Crib toys or mobiles should be firmly attached, with no straps or strings in the infant's reach. Mobiles should be removed when the infant can reach them.

Cribs should be placed away from hanging cords of blinds or drapes, which could become wrapped around an active infant.

**Other Equipment**

Paint used to refurbish infant equipment should be marked lead-free and safe for children's equipment to prevent lead poisoning.

All parts should function properly: crib side rails must be secure, highchair trays must stay firmly in place, latches must remain fastened, etc. The frame and basic construction of all equipment should be sturdy.

All moving parts should be examined carefully to see whether little fingers could get caught or whether the infant could trigger a catch that would cause the equipment to become unsafe.

Safety straps for infant seats, swings, changing tables, high chairs, or other equipment in which the infant should be secured to prevent falling must be in good condition. Straps should fit around the infant but not be long enough that the infant could become entangled.

Automatic swings should have legs that are stable, without a tendency to tip over. Note how difficult it is to put the infant into the swing and to remove the infant from the swing safely.

All toys should be examined carefully for parts that can be moved and swallowed.

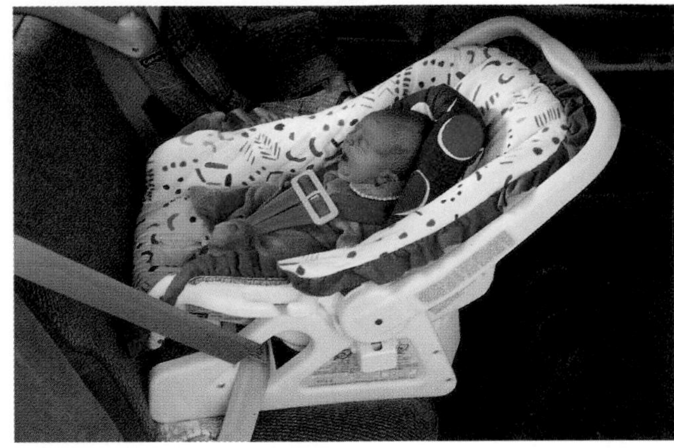

**FIGURE 23-6**

A car seat for an infant under 20 pounds should face the rear of the car. Note the clip that holds the straps together for a snug fit.

The many different car seats available may be confusing to parents. Some car seats are designed for infants younger than 1 year and weighing up to 20 pounds. Others are convertible and meet the needs of both newborns and young children. Seats for newborns face the rear of the car and recline at a 45-degree angle. Those for older children face forward and allow the child to sit up or recline.

Parents should examine the harness restraint carefully before buying a car seat. Three-point harnesses are used in infant-only seats (Fig. 23–6). In convertible seats, a five-point harness is safest for very young infants. The harness should firmly restrain the infant yet be quick and easy to fasten. All car seats should be secured by the automobile seat belt so that there is no chance that the infant could be hurled forward on impact.

In most cars, car seats are safest when they are placed in the center back seat of the car. They should never be placed in the front passenger seat in a car with air bags, which can kill or injure the infant when they inflate. Very small infants may need special adaptations because of their size. Blankets placed at the head, along the sides, and between the legs may improve the fit. They should not be placed under the infant. Special seats or beds designed specifically for preterm or low-birth-weight infants are also available.

**TABLE 23–2 SAFETY CONSIDERATIONS FOR INFANT CAR SEATS**

1. Use only car seats that are approved for use in automobiles. Seats designed for use in the home do not provide adequate protection in a car.
2. Use car seats that are appropriate for the infant's age and size. Place the seat in the center of the back seat of the car, never where there is an air bag.
3. Follow the manufacturer's directions for fastening the seat in the car and the infant in the car seat. Recheck the restraint straps each time the seat is used.
4. Be certain that the straps are tight enough to prevent the infant from getting out of the restraints or turning over in the seat. Infants who turn over can suffocate in the padding of the seat.
5. Check to see that the infant cannot become caught with the straps tightly around the neck.
6. Use car seats only in an automobile. Do not place them on a soft surface, such as a bed, where they might turn over and suffocate the infant. Do not place them on surfaces from which they might fall, such as grocery carts.
7. Never leave infants alone in a car, even for a few minutes. They could be kidnapped or injured in an accident involving the car even though it is parked. Cars quickly become very warm, and the infant could become dangerously overheated.

Many parents use their car seats improperly. An incorrectly fastened harness may not restrain the infant in an accident and could cause damage, such as laceration of the liver. If the automobile seat belt is not routed through the correct area of the car seat, the seat may tip or become a flying missile during an accident. Car seats should be used only in cars and only according to manufacturer's directions. Safety considerations for car seat use are summarized in Table 23–2.

**CHECK YOUR READING**

3. What advice can the nurse offer about safety features of equipment used for infants?
4. What should the nurse teach parents about buying and using a car seat?

# Early Problems

## Infant Crying

Crying is a major parental concern during the early weeks after birth. Infants cry for periods totaling about 60 to 90 minutes a day during the first 3 weeks of life; then crying time increases to 2 to 4 hours a day by 6 weeks and gradually decreases by age 3 months (Wong, 1995). Crying is most frustrating to parents when they cannot find a cause for it. Infants cry for many reasons, including hunger, discomfort, fatigue, overstimulation, and boredom. Sometimes no specific cause can be determined.

When the cause for crying is not obvious, some parents are afraid that responding may spoil the infant. This concern may increase if the infant stops crying when picked up. However, changing the infant's position may help gas move in the intestines, relieve tired muscles, or distract the infant by changing the scenery, bringing about a temporary cessation of crying.

Infants cannot signal that they have unmet needs in any other way but crying and are not spoiled by parents meeting their needs. In fact, it is essential that their needs be met in a consistent, warm, prompt manner for the development of trust to occur. Infants of parents who intervene appropriately for crying are less likely to cry excessively as they get older.

Some families develop creative methods for dealing with crying infants. Others benefit from a nurse's suggestions about appropriate techniques to use.

When parents have searched for causes of crying and tried a variety of comfort measures to no avail, the infant may need to "cry it out" alone. Some infants have a need to discharge excess tension by crying for a period of time before going to sleep. Although this is difficult for parents, leaving the infant safely in the crib for 10 to 15 minutes or so may be enough to allow the infant to fall asleep.

Some parents find that setting a timer is helpful. At the end of the period allowed, they can quietly check to be sure that the infant is all right. Changing the diaper or holding the infant for a few minutes before putting the infant back to bed may be all that is necessary. Talking softly to provide reassurance and patting the infant's back without picking the infant up may be effective. Occasionally, the process may need to be repeated before the infant drifts off to sleep.

## Colic

### DESCRIPTION

Colic is characterized by irritable crying for no obvious reason, usually for 3 hours or more a day. It usually occurs during the late afternoon or early evening and lasts 3 to 4 hours or longer. It occurs in 10 to 20 percent of all infants (Grover, 1996), beginning in the first 3 weeks of life. Although it usually ends about 3 months after birth, some infants continue to have colic until 6 months of age. The infant is in good health, eats well, and gains weight appropriately, despite the daily crying episodes.

Infants with colic cry as though in pain, draw their knees onto the abdomen, and may pass flatus. The

## Parents Want to Know

## Methods to Relieve Crying in Infants

### Treating Common Causes

***Hunger***: Try feeding the infant if it has been more than 1½ hours since the last feeding. A bubble of air may have caused a feeling of fullness too soon during the last feeding. The infant may be experiencing a "growth spurt" and need more frequent feedings for a day or two to provide necessary nutrients for rapid growth.

***Air Bubbles***: Fussy infants may need more frequent burping during and after feedings than other infants. Try burping during crying spells because the infant may swallow air.

***Diapers***: Although most infants do not mind wet or soiled diapers, they may become cold or their skin may be irritated when diapers are not changed frequently enough.

***Clothing***: Check the infant's clothing for anything that could cause discomfort. Be sure that pins are closed, that there are no irritating seams or neck tags, and that elastic on sleeves is not too tight.

***Warmth***: Be sure that the infant is warm enough, yet not too warm. The abdomen should feel warm even if the hands and feet are cool. Dress the infant as an adult would want to be dressed, but add a receiving blanket. Infants who are overdressed rarely perspire but often cry because of their discomfort.

***Overstimulation***: Too many visitors handling the infant or too much noise and commotion in the household may be overstimulating. A quiet environment, rocking, or just being left to work off excess tension alone in the crib may be necessary for the infant.

### Quieting Techniques

***Rocking***: The gentle motion of rocking, reminiscent of intrauterine life, is often soothing for infants.

***Automatic Swings***: Swings may be battery-operated or wind-up. Check the noise level on wind-up swings to be sure that winding does not wake the infant going off to sleep. Very small infants may need padding with blankets for safety and comfort.

***Walking, Jiggling, Swaying***: Sometimes newborns prefer a particular style of motion. Rocking sideways with the infant held in an upright position is helpful for some infants, whereas others prefer vertical rocking. Taking a walk outside may provide distraction from new sights and sounds.

***Swaddling***: Wrap the infant snugly. This is comforting because infants are used to restricted activity in the uterus. Swaddling is especially helpful during the first few weeks after birth.

***Stroller or Buggy Rides***: The motion of a stroller or buggy may be soothing to some infants. The ride can be in or outside the house. A parent can move a stroller back and forth with one foot while doing chores or eating meals. The stroller should allow the infant to lie down rather than sit. Padding may increase comfort.

***Car Rides***: Some infants go to sleep in a moving car. A short ride around the block may put the infant to sleep. The infant may stay asleep when carried into the house.

***Music***: The sound of a parent singing may be reassuring to the infant. Some newborns respond well to a music box, radio, or tape of music. Music with a steady beat or classical music may be particularly effective. Music should be played softly.

***White Noise***: Background noise sometimes puts infants to sleep by diffusing other noises. A radio set on low, a clock ticking, or the sound of a dishwasher, dryer, or even a vacuum cleaner may be effective. Tapes of sounds heard in utero are available and work best if introduced in the first week of life.

***Heat***: A well-covered warm water bottle placed against the infant's abdomen may be soothing. (Take care not to burn the infant's skin). A blanket warmed in the clothes dryer for a few minutes serves the same purpose. Placing the newborn in an infant seat on top of a dishwasher or clothes dryer provides heat and background noise. Be sure that the infant is well secured, of course. Do not use a heating pad.

***Bathing***: Although older infants love baths, very young infants may not yet have reached that stage. However, giving a bath may be a distraction for both parent and infant, and the infant may sleep afterward.

***Water***: Infants who have been crying may be thirsty. Although extra water is not necessary, some mothers like to give it on occasion. It may help bring up bubbles of air that the infant has swallowed while crying. The breastfed infant's thirst can be alleviated by nursing.

***Infant Carriers or Packs***: Front carriers are designed for the young infant and may be especially helpful during crying episodes. A parent's warm body, soothing voice, and gentle swaying motion can often put an infant to sleep. At the same time, the parent can move around and accomplish other tasks. Backpacks should be used only for older infants who are able to support the head alone.

***Pacifiers***: Parents may find pacifiers useful for an irritable infant. The infant may be comforted by sucking even though not hungry.

***Position Changes***: Try varying the infant's position.

- Laying the infant prone across a parent's lap (or over a warmed blanket) may help expel gas.
- Try the "colic holds" (see Fig. 23–7). They may help the infant pass gas. Placing the infant in a supine position and flexing the knees on the abdomen may also help.

***Mother's Diet***: Breastfeeding mothers should review their diet. Some infants react when the mother's diet includes cow's milk, orange juice, foods in the cabbage family, onion, or chocolate. Others react to highly acidic or spicy foods. Caffeine passes into breast milk and can cause wakefulness and irritability. Omit the suspected food for 5 to 7 days; then try it again and watch for irritability after the next feedings to identify the cause of the crying.

***Massage***: Gentle massage may be soothing for some infants. Massage of the abdomen may help infants with colic.

***Smoking***: Ask anyone in the home who smokes to do so away from the infant, preferably outside.

crying is intense and may last until the infant falls asleep exhausted. Persistent crying may interfere with the mother-infant relationship (Keefe et al., 1996). Because it causes so much parental distress and may be a factor in parenting disorders or child abuse, it is important that nurses provide support to parents of colicky infants.

Although many theories have been investigated, the cause of colic remains unknown. Allergies, feeding techniques, parental tension, and exposure to smoking have all been considered. Colic may be due to immaturity of the gastrointestinal tract or nervous system or to a combination of factors.

#### INTERVENTIONS

Nursing interventions include using therapeutic communication to help parents express their frustrations and teaching techniques for coping with the problem. Parents should be encouraged to talk about their feelings and should be reassured that colic does not indicate poor parenting. They often feel inadequate about their failure to manage the problem and guilty if their frustration develops into anger. The nurse should explain that it is not abnormal to feel ambivalent or even angry with the infant. Taking time away from infant care to rest and recoup energy needed to deal with the demands of a crying infant is essential. Parents can leave the infant with a baby sitter for short periods or take turns consoling the infant to provide breaks from the crying.

The techniques listed in Parents Want to Know: Methods to Relieve Crying in Infants may alleviate crying from colic temporarily, but generally none gives prolonged relief. The colic holds may be particularly effective for some infants (Fig. 23–7). Changing from a cow's milk formula to a protein hydrolysate formula may help the infant with allergies. Breastfeeding mothers whose diet includes cow's milk, orange juice, the cabbage family, onions, or chocolate should try eliminating these foods for 5 to 7 days to see if improvement occurs.

A quiet environment, calm approach, and fairly regular schedule may help some infants with colic. Parents should be assured that spoiling does not result from responding to the infant's cries. In severe cases, the infant may be given an antiflatulent, sedative, antispasmodic, or antihistamine for a short time.

**CHECK YOUR READING**

5. Why should parents respond to crying without fear of spoiling the infant?
6. How can nurses help parents of crying infants?

## THERAPEUTIC COMMUNICATION

### Coping with Crying

Shannon Gray tells the nurse, Mark Winston, about her daughter, Marina, who has been having crying spells every night lasting 4 hours or longer. Shannon looks tired and worried. Marina, age 4 weeks, eats well, shows good weight gain, and is developing appropriately for her age.

**Shannon:** It seems like I can't do anything at night anymore, except try to stop Marina's crying.

**Mark:** You spend a lot of time trying to find ways to comfort her.

*Paraphrasing to encourage the mother to continue*

**Shannon:** I've tried everything! I rock her, walk with her, feed and change her. We go for car rides and put her in her swing, but nothing works for long. She just starts crying again.

**Mark:** It's so frustrating when nothing seems to work!

*Reflecting mother's feelings shows that the nurse is trying to understand them.*

**Shannon:** Sometimes I wonder why I ever wanted to have a baby. I never thought it would be like this. Isn't that an awful thing to say! But it's true! (sounds defiant).

**Mark:** Being a mother is so much harder than you expected that sometimes you aren't sure you made the right choice.

*Reflects the content of what the mother said to help her focus. Shows acceptance.*

**Shannon:** But I really do love her. I just don't know how to help her. I must be a terrible mother (becomes teary).

**Mark:** Parents often feel guilty when they can't find a way to help an upset baby. And yet, we really don't know all the reasons why babies cry. You've tried very hard to help Marina. Maybe we can work together to think of some other techniques to use.

*Gives reassurance that what the mother is feeling is normal, then offers information and further help.*

**Shannon:** I'd love that. Marina really is a good baby when she isn't crying so much. And it worries me to have her so unhappy. What else can I do for her?

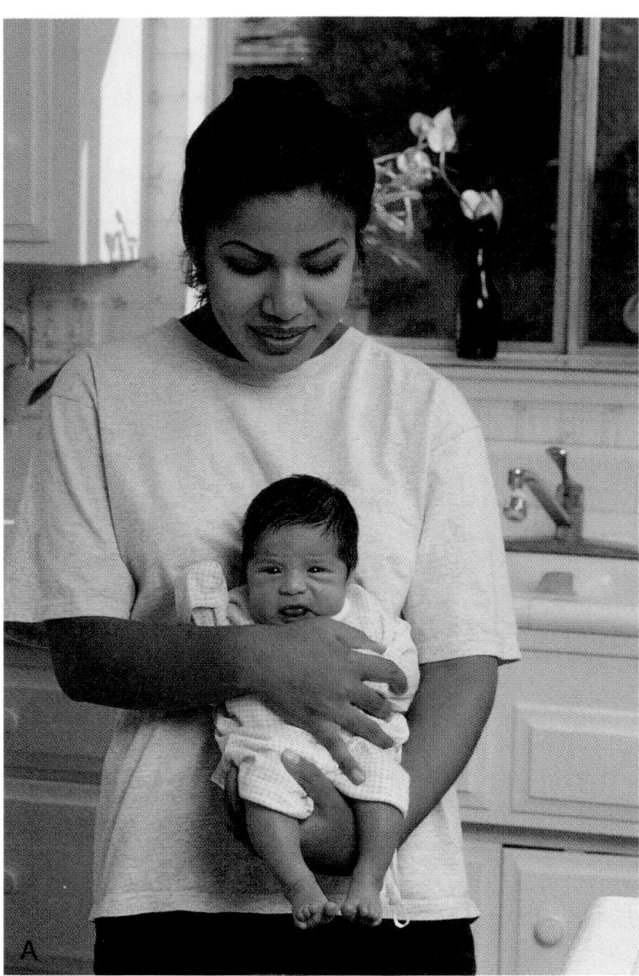

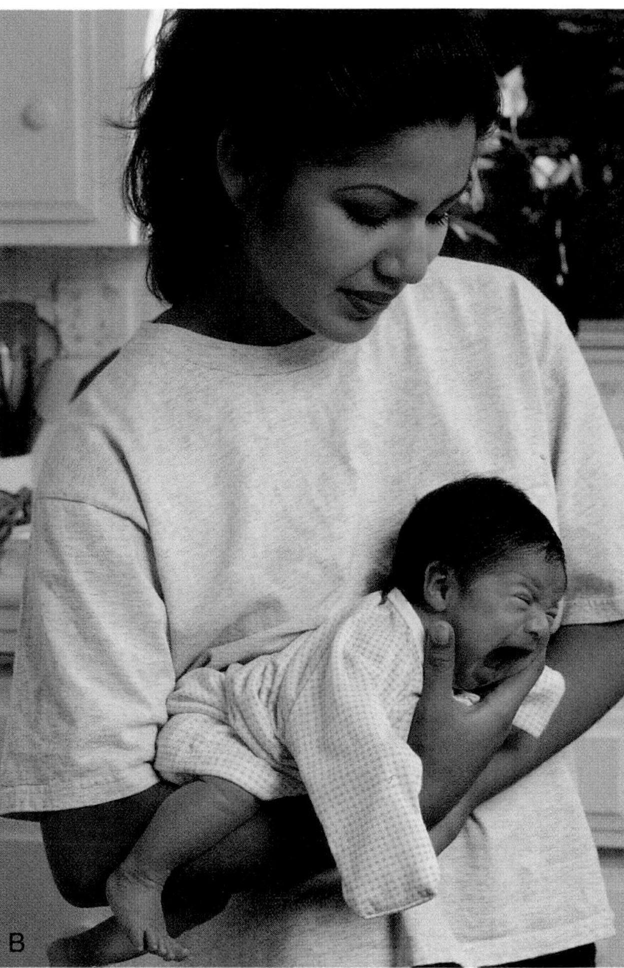

**FIGURE 23-7**

Positions for holding an infant with colic. A, The mother holds the infant facing forward. One hand creates slight pressure against the abdomen, while the other flexes the legs. This position may help the infant expel flatus. B, The prone hold is also effective for some infants. The mother holds the infant in a horizontal position along her arm.

## Sleep

### PARENTS

During the early months after birth, parents often wonder whether they will ever get a full night's sleep again. Because they are so often up during the night, they should try to make up lost sleep at other times. If the mother has not returned to work, she can sleep during the day when the infant naps. If she is working, parents can alternate responsibility for night or early morning feedings. When mothers are breastfeeding, fathers can change the diaper, bring the infant to the mother for night feedings, and then settle the infant back in bed when the feeding is finished. This allows the mother more time to sleep and shares the middle-of-the-night care.

### INFANT SLEEP PATTERNS

Infants spend less time than adults in deep sleep. They have a larger percentage of lighter rapid eye movement (REM) sleep. During this type of sleep, they make noises loud enough to wake parents in the same room, and they move about as if awakening. Going to them at this time is likely to wake them, but they may return to deep sleep if left alone.

Infants should be positioned on the side or back for sleep. The nurse should explain to parents that the prone position has been associated with sudden infant death syndrome (SIDS). No pillows or soft stuffed animals should be allowed in the crib, as they could cause suffocation. Some infants sleep better in an enclosed space and may scoot themselves into a corner of a large crib. The nurse should suggest to parents that they use rolled blankets around the infant to provide a "nest," which feels more like the circumscribed area of the uterus.

### SLEEPING THROUGH THE NIGHT

Parents are often confused about when infants should sleep through the night. Newborns should not be expected to sleep through the night because

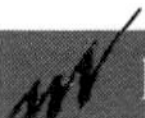

**Parents Want to Know**

### How to Help Infants Sleep Through the Night

- Allow the infant to cry for a few minutes before responding. The infant may not be completely awake and often returns to sleep if undisturbed.
- Keep night feedings for feeding only. Avoid unnecessary activity, or the infant may learn to think of this as a playtime.
- Use a soft light that provides only the amount of light essential for care.
- Give night feedings in the infant's room to further avoid stimulation.
- Keep sounds subdued. Soft music or humming may help the infant return to sleep, but talking should be kept to a minimum.
- Keep night feedings short, and put the infant back to bed immediately.
- Change diapers in the middle of the feeding to avoid awakening the infant after feeding.
- As the infant nears the age when sleeping through the night is more likely, try patting him or her on the back instead of feeding. Offer water instead of milk.
- Allow the infant to fall asleep at bedtime on his or her own instead of always rocking or feeding the infant. This may help the infant go back to sleep alone after awakening in the night.

they are neurologically unable to do so during the early weeks of life. By 12 weeks of age, many infants sleep at least 5 hours at night. Sleep lasting for 9 to 11 hours may begin by 12 to 16 weeks of age (Wong, 1995).

Once infants establish longer sleep patterns, they often awaken at night again when they are teething or ill. Therefore, parents can expect to be awakened frequently during the early years. Parents should be taught methods of helping infants achieve longer sleep periods at night.

## Concerns of Working Mothers

Although it has been traditional for women who work to have at least 6 weeks of maternity leave, this is not always possible. Some women must return to work as early as 3 weeks after childbirth. Working mothers have a number of problems that are different from those of mothers who have a longer time at home. They must find adequate child care, identify methods of managing the household, and try to find enough time and energy to meet the needs of the infant, other family members, and themselves (see Chapter 18, pp. 467–469).

It is important that working mothers not become so involved in their many responsibilities that they have little time for their own needs. Some mothers regularly schedule time for themselves and for family activities. Many working mothers find that the time they can spend with their infant is particularly precious.

## Concerns of Adoptive Parents

Although adoptive parents have not experienced pregnancy and childbirth, they must make adjustments similar to those of biologic parents. In some adoptive situations, the parents meet the biologic mother during pregnancy and may even be with her during birth. In others, parents receive a call after months of waiting telling them that their new infant is ready for them. In either case, the lives of the parents abruptly change.

**CRITICAL THINKING EXERCISE**

Mary and John Reynolds received their adoptive daughter, Ashley 3 days ago. They bring the 6-day-old infant to the pediatrician's office and discuss their concerns with the nurse. They received basic discharge teaching at the hospital where Ashley was born but have many questions about Infant care. The last two nights Ashley slept very little, and both parents are exhausted, "We've waited so long to get Ashley," Mary says, "but I'm beginning to wonder if she's all right and if I'll be a good mother."

**Q:**
1. What are the priorities in this situation?
2. What information should the nurse include in teaching these parents?
3. How should the nurse deal with Ashley's night wakefulness?
4. How should the nurse support Mary and John?

**A:**
1. The major priorities are to support the parents in their new role and to determine if Ashley is progressing normally.
2. Information should be based on the parent's concerns. Explain normal characteristics and behaviors of the newborn. Determine if Mary and John need more information about basic infant care, such as feeding, sleeping, cord care, and signs of illness. Provide frequent opportunities for them to ask questions.
3. Obtain more information about Ashley's sleep patterns. Discuss normal sleep in newborns and methods of helping infants sleep. Offer suggestions for methods of dealing with crying. Help Mary and John work out a plan for sharing the burdens as well as the joys of parenthood.
4. Use therapeutic communication techniques to allow Mary and John to express their feelings adequately. If Ashley appears to be progressing normally, emphasize that she is doing well. Point out that the problems they are encountering are quite common for both biologic and adoptive parents.

In some agencies, adoptive parents receive the same teaching given to other parents. However, their ability to absorb information may be impaired by the excitement of the situation. Although adoptive mothers have not been pregnant or undergone childbirth, they are still very tired from the loss of sleep and sudden changes that they experience. This may be a surprise and very worrisome to some. They have many questions that nurses can answer.

Nurses must offer the same support to adoptive parents that they do to biologic parents. Parents need information about infant care and parenting techniques. They also need reassurance and emotional support as they go through this happy but exhausting change in their lives.

## Common Questions and Concerns

Parents often ask nurses or others questions about infant care. Some of the most common concerns are summarized here.

### Dressing and Warmth

A room temperature of about 70°F is warm enough for the infant. The infant should be dressed as the parents would like to be dressed, with a receiving blanket added. The abdomen should be checked to see if the infant is warm enough. The hands and feet are slightly cooler than the rest of the body but should not be mottled or blue. The infant's head should be kept warm because many thermal skin sensors are located in the scalp. A hat is appropriate if the infant is outside when it is cold or windy.

### Stool Patterns

Formula-fed infants generally pass at least one stool each day, whereas breastfed infants may pass a stool after every feeding or, occasionally in the older infant, only one every 2 to 3 days. Infants may get red in the face and appear to be straining when having a bowel movement, but this is normal behavior and does not indicate constipation. Stools that are dry, hard, and marble-like indicate constipation.

Watery stools indicate diarrhea. A watery stool is absorbed into the diaper with little or no solid material left at the surface. A "water ring" remains on the diaper, showing where the liquid was absorbed. Diarrhea stools occur more frequently than the infant's normal stools and are greenish from bile moving quickly through the intestines. Diarrhea can be serious because life-threatening dehydration develops quickly. Infants should be taken to the pediatrician or nurse practitioner for treatment.

### Smoking

Many mothers quit smoking before or during pregnancy but may not realize that not exposing infants to smoke is just as important after birth as before. Infants exposed to smoke from parents' cigarettes are more likely to develop frequent respiratory problems (Wong, 1995). Smoking is a risk factor in SIDS. Smoke absorption by infants occurs even when smoking is done in another room. Parents who continue to smoke should do so outside the house and away from the infant.

### Eyes

Parents can wipe away small amounts of mucus that accumulate in the corner of the eyes with a damp, clean washcloth. A large amount of mucus, redness, or excessive tearing indicates an infection or a blocked lacrimal duct. The infant should be seen by the pediatrician or nurse practitioner.

Transient strabismus, or crossing of the eyes, can be frightening to parents. The nurse should reassure them that this is normal for infants for the first few months, until they gain control of the small muscles of the eye. It does not indicate that the infant will have later problems.

### Baths

Giving sponge and tub baths is discussed in Chapter 21 (p. 574), as is care of the cord (p. 574) and the circumcision site (p. 568). It is not necessary for parents to give a bath every day if the infant is washed well at diaper changes and when milk is regurgitated. Bathing should be a time for infant stimulation and parent-infant interaction. It can be done at any time of the day that is convenient for parents.

### Nails

Nails should be cut straight across with either blunt-ended scissors or clippers. The edges can be carefully smoothed with an emery board. Mothers should not attempt to cut nails too short, as this increases the danger of cutting the infant's fingertip. Some mothers prefer to cut nails while the infant is sleeping. Others have someone else hold the hand steady while the mother cuts the nails. Nails grow rapidly and may need trimming twice a week.

### Sucking Needs

Parents often have questions about pacifiers and thumb or finger sucking. Nurses should explain that all infants have an urge to suck, although the amount of sucking needed varies with individual infants. Some seem satisfied by feedings, but others suck their hands or a pacifier even when not hungry.

Parents may be concerned that sucking a pacifier or thumb will cause the teeth to become maloccluded. The nurse should reassure them that intermittent sucking that does not continue beyond age 4 years does not result in changes to the teeth (Wong, 1995). If sucking continues after the permanent teeth erupt, malocclusion is more likely. Trying to stop an infant from sucking is difficult and may cause emotional problems if it becomes a major focus.

Some infants increase non-nutritive sucking because the time they spend sucking during feedings is too short. Using bottle nipples with small holes and replacing the nipples every couple of months before they get soft increase the amount of sucking that feedings provide. Breastfed infants should be allowed to continue sucking at the breast long enough to meet basic sucking needs. A short time of sucking after the infant is finished feeding generally satisfies sucking needs and increases production of milk.

When infants use a pacifier, parents should be instructed to examine it often to see if it is in good condition. If the nipple is cracked, torn, or sticky or can be pulled away from the shield, it should be discarded. Pacifiers should be replaced every month or two because they may come apart as they deteriorate and cause aspiration of parts.

Pacifiers should be kept clean by frequent washing, and parents should buy several so that one is always clean when needed. Pacifiers should never be placed on a string around the infant's neck. The string could become tangled tightly around the neck and cause strangulation. Clips with a short band to attach pacifiers to the infant's clothing without danger are available.

Some parents find that an advantage to a pacifier is that the infant gives it up more quickly than a thumb or finger because it is not so easily accessible. Parents who resort to the pacifier as the first response when the infant is fussy are likely to reinforce its use and increase dependence on it. Pacifiers used only after other causes of distress are ruled out may be given up sooner. Because the need for non-nutritive sucking begins to diminish between 4 and 6 months of age, pacifier use may begin to decrease at that time with parents' help.

## Teething

There is much individual variation in the time frame for tooth eruption. The first tooth may appear as early as 3 months or as late as 13 months of age. Generally the two lower central incisors come through the gums at about 6 to 8 months. The average age for eruption of all deciduous teeth is 2 ½ years.

The actual time when teeth erupt has no relationship to the infant's development in other areas. Parents may think that teething has begun when the infant is about 3 months of age, when the normal increased production of saliva causes drooling. Infants must learn to swallow the extra saliva without drooling.

Some infants show signs of teething for weeks before the first tooth comes through the gums. These signs include excessive salivation, biting, irritability, slight fever, and decreased feedings. Many infants who were sleeping through the night begin to wake again as a result of teething discomfort. Some infants have looser stools, and diaper rash may develop. A rash around the mouth may result from drooling. The infant's gums may look red and swollen over the area where the tooth will erupt.

Instruct parents that high fevers or other signs of illness are not normal symptoms of teething. Infants may be more susceptible to illness at the time of teething because of poor eating and sleeping. In addition, teething begins at about the time many of the antibodies received in utero are disappearing.

Some teething infants like to bite on hard objects such as teething rings. Some rings can be frozen to soothe inflammation of the gums. Over-the-counter local anesthetics or analgesics, such as acetaminophen, are safe in small amounts for teething discomfort. Alcoholic beverages should never be rubbed on the gums because infants swallow the alcohol.

## Common Rashes

### DIAPER RASH

Diaper rash occurs as a result of prolonged exposure of skin to wetness combined with a chemical reaction between the urine and fecal enzymes that increases skin sensitivity to irritation. About half of all infants have diaper rash at some time, and 5 percent have severe rashes (Wong, 1995). A rash is more likely to develop when infants begin to sleep for longer periods and the time between diaper changes increases. Other causes include incomplete rinsing of home-laundered diapers and sensitivity to commercial disposable washcloths or components of paper diapers.

Treatment of diaper rash centers on keeping the diaper area clean and dry. The nurse should instruct the parents to change diapers as soon as they are wet or soiled. They should gently wash the perineum with mild soap and warm water, avoiding excessive washing. Plastic coverings should be avoided, as they prevent air flow to the diapered area and keep it damp. Removing the diapers and exposing the perineum to warm air help healing. Superabsorbent disposable diapers draw the wetness away from the skin and may provide relief.

Applying a thin layer of creams such as those with zinc oxide may speed healing and help prevent further outbreaks. The nurse should tell parents not to apply the ointments too thickly, as they may be difficult to remove. Ointments contaminated with fecal matter may accumulate in the skin folds and hold bacteria. Low-potency corticosteroid preparations may be necessary for severe cases.

If the rash becomes severe or pustules or crusted areas develop, infection has set in. The infant should be taken to a pediatrician or nurse practitioner for treatment. *Candida albicans* or *Staphylococcus* is a common cause of infections. Antibiotic creams may be necessary for infections.

#### MILIARIA (PRICKLY HEAT)

Although most common during hot weather, miliaria or prickly heat develops in infants who are too warmly dressed in any weather. This rash is due to occlusion and inflammation of the sweat (eccrine) glands. It has a red base with papules or vesicles in the center.

Treatment is cooling the infant by removing excess clothing or by giving a soothing lukewarm bath. The condition clears quickly with removal of the cause, and ointments or other skin preparations should be avoided. The nurse should discuss the appropriate amount of clothing with parents when infants develop prickly heat.

#### SEBORRHEIC DERMATITIS (CRADLE CAP)

Cradle cap is a chronic inflammation of the scalp or other areas of the skin characterized by yellow, scaly, oily lesions. It sometimes results when parents do not wash over the anterior fontanelle carefully for fear that they will hurt the infant.

Treatment is application of oil or shampoo to the area to help the lesions soften, then removal with a comb before shampooing the head. The nurse should teach parents how to shampoo the scalp and explain that they will not damage the fontanelle by normal gentle shampooing. The scalp should be rinsed well to remove all soap, which may cause irritation if it remains.

**✓ CHECK YOUR READING**

7. What are common signs of teething?
8. How can parents prevent or treat diaper rash?

## Nutrition During the Early Weeks

Infant feeding is discussed in detail in Chapter 22. The discussion here addresses only the most frequent early concerns parents have about feeding.

### Formula Feeding

Mothers using formula may be unsure about how much to feed the infant during the early weeks after birth. Although infants take about 1 ounce at a time during the first day or two of life, this rapidly increases to 2 or 3 ounces per feeding in the first 2 weeks. By 12 weeks they usually drink 5 to 6 ounces every 3 to 4 hours. Considerable variation is seen between infants, and mothers should be encouraged to adapt to their own infant's needs.

Formula-fed infants generally eat every 3 to 4 hours. However, a mother should be taught not to set a strict timetable but to feed her infant when signs of hunger are present. Fussiness or crying, rooting, sucking on hands, and eagerly taking the bottle indicate that the infant is hungry.

Mothers should not urge infants to drink all of the formula if they do not seem interested. Infants vary, as adults do, in the amount taken at each meal. Encouraging the infant to complete all feedings places undue emphasis on the feeding and may lead to later feeding problems or obesity.

### Breastfeeding

The mother of the breastfed infant should also avoid strict schedules but should know that her infant will want to feed more often than if formula-fed, about every 2 to 3 hours. Generally, feedings should last at least 15 minutes initially (see Chapter 22). As nursing becomes well established, mothers often feed approximately 15 minutes on the first side and then continue on the second side as long as the infant is interested. The feeding should be ended when the infant falls asleep or after a short period of nonnutritive suckling.

The total time for each breastfeeding session varies with individual infants and from feeding to feeding. The time may be as short as 20 minutes or as long as 40 minutes. As infants become older, they become more efficient at nursing and obtain all the milk they need in a shorter period of time.

### Water

Both formula and breast milk contain enough water for infants who are eating well. There is no need to give additional water. Some mothers give water to formula-fed infants who are fussy and do not respond to other interventions. Sips of water can also be given to infants with hiccups. However, hiccups go away shortly, with or without water.

Infants should not be given water with sugar added. Sugar only adds empty calories and accustoms them to the sweet taste. Honey should never be used for young infants because of the risk of botulism.

### Regurgitation

Infants often regurgitate ("spit up") because they may eat more than their stomach can easily hold and because their normally relaxed cardiac sphincter allows the stomach contents to flow into the esophagus easily. "Wet burps" result when air is trapped under stomach contents. As the air is expelled, a small amount of milk comes with it.

The nurse should teach parents to differentiate normal spitting up from vomiting, which is a sign of illness. Regurgitation may occur frequently, but usually only a small amount at a time. Vomiting may involve the entire feeding and it is expelled forcefully. Parents should always seek treatment for the infant with projectile vomiting, in which the vomitus is expelled with such force that it travels some distance. This is a sign of pyloric stenosis, which may require surgery.

If an infant has very frequent regurgitation, parents can elevate the head of the bed or use an infant seat after feedings to help air rise and to decrease regurgitation. Turning the infant to the side promotes drainage of regurgitated fluids and prevents aspiration.

Some infants swallow excessive air because they eat very rapidly. Nurses should instruct parents to feed infants before they get too hungry and to stop often for burping. Switching breasts every 5 minutes with a burp in between helps some nursing infants. If the hole in a bottle nipple is too small, an infant may swallow air around the nipple. Enlarging the nipple hole slightly with a hot needle may prevent this.

Some infants experience reflux due to the flow of liquids across a dilated lower esophageal sphincter. These infants may have vomiting, and aspiration pneumonia develops in as many as one third of afflicted infants (Behrman et al., 1996). The infant who has excessive regurgitation or vomiting should be referred for follow-up with the pediatrician or nurse practitioner.

### Introduction of Solid Foods

Infants do not need solid foods until 4 to 6 months of age. Some mothers introduce solids earlier in the hope that the infant will sleep longer at night. This is seldom successful, as the infant receives no more calories from the small amounts of solids taken than from milk. In addition, early introduction of solids may cause other problems. Foods given before the infant is ready may precipitate allergies or cause intestinal upsets because they are incompletely digested. When infants start solids, they drink less milk, thus replacing a food that meets their nutrient needs well with a food that is poorly digested.

The extrusion reflex, in which infants push the tongue out against anything that touches it, continues until approximately 4 months of age. This makes feeding a younger infant difficult, as the infant pushes almost all of every spoonful out of the mouth. The nurse should explain the problems involved with early introduction of solid foods and encourage parents to wait until the infant is physiologically ready, at 4 to 6 months of age. The concerns that made the parents consider changing the feeding routine should also be discussed.

### Weaning

Some mothers decide to wean the infant from the breast to the bottle during the first 12 weeks after birth. Information about weaning is included in Chapter 22, p. 607.

**CHECK YOUR READING**

9. How much should infants eat during the early weeks after birth?
10. Why should solid foods be avoided until the infant is 4 to 6 months old?

## Growth and Development

### Anticipatory Guidance

Parents often have questions about normal patterns of growth and stages of development. Nurses should provide parents with anticipatory guidance about these areas to help them develop realistic expectations about infants' abilities at various ages. It can also help prepare parents for changes they must make to keep the infant's environment safe, especially during the second half of the first year of life, when the infant begins to explore the house alone.

### Growth and Developmental Milestones

A brief summary of the changes that can be expected during the infant's first 12 weeks is included here. More in-depth information is included in pediatrics textbooks. The nurse should emphasize to parents that guidelines are only averages, that the range of normal is often broad, and that individual differences are expected.

During the first 6 months of life, growth proceeds at a very predictable rate in normal infants. The weight lost after birth is usually regained by 10 days of age. Each month, the average infant gains 680 g (1.5 pounds), grows 2.5 cm (1 inch), and has an increase in head circumference of 1.5 cm (0.5 inch) (Wong, 1995). The posterior fontanelle closes by 2 to

3 months and the anterior fontanelle closes by 12 to 18 months of age. Tears appear 2 to 4 weeks after birth.

The Moro, grasp, tonic neck, and rooting reflexes are especially noticed by parents. The nurse should point out that their gradual disappearance helps prepare the infant to learn new skills, such as voluntary grasping or turning over, which are impossible if the reflexes continue. The infant gradually develops more control of the heavy head and has little bobbing or head lag by the end of the third month of life.

Infants are social beings. They stare at objects of interest within a range of 8 to 9 inches as newborns and learn to follow objects by turning the head a full 180 degrees during the first 12 weeks of life. A social smile begins as early as 3 to 5 weeks and is well developed by 6 to 8 weeks. Infants make vowel sounds (cooing) by 2 months and begin some consonant sounds (babbling) and may even squeal with delight at 3 months.

### Accident Prevention

Knowing what infants can do helps prevent accidents. In the first 3 months after birth, they are totally helpless. Although they can communicate their needs through crying, someone must be available at all times to care for them. Parents must be taught the dangers of leaving the infant on any unprotected surface even for seconds. In a very short time, an infant can wiggle from the middle to the edge of a double bed and fall. Crib sides should be raised whenever the infant is in bed. Cribs should be positioned away from hanging cords of blinds or drapes, as these could become wrapped around an active infant and cause strangulation.

Parents should keep one hand on an infant lying on an unprotected surface if they must turn away. Infants should never be left for an instant in even an inch of water because of the danger of drowning. Parents should take the telephone off the hook and ignore the doorbell when bathing the infant, or take the infant out of the water and with them if they must leave the room.

After infants learn to grasp objects with increasing accuracy, parents must be certain that nothing is in the infant's reach that could be swallowed or otherwise cause harm. Help parents to think ahead to the time when the infant will be crawling and walking and make plans for how they will "child proof" their home.

## Well-Baby Care

### Well-Baby Checkups

Well-baby checkups are an opportunity for the pediatrician or nurse practitioner to assess the infant's growth and development, answer questions about feeding and infant care, observe for abnormalities, and give immunizations. These checkups may be provided by a private practitioner or in a well-baby clinic, where examinations and immunizations are free or are provided at reduced cost. Infants are usually taken to their first well-baby checkup at 2 to 4 weeks of age. They generally receive well-baby checkups at 2, 4, 6, 9, and 12 months of age.

Well-baby checkups are a good time for mothers to learn about what is normal for their infants in terms of growth and behaviors. Anticipatory guidance is a major part of well-baby visits. Many mothers are reassured to find that such problems as wakefulness at night or changes in feeding habits are normal. Safety is discussed as the parents learn about skills infants will soon learn that might place them in danger.

**TABLE 23-3 RECOMMENDED IMMUNIZATION SCHEDULE**

| Immunization | Age for Original Immunization | Age for Booster |
|---|---|---|
| DTaP or DTP (diphtheria, tetanus, pertussis)[1,2] | 2, 4, 6 months | 12–18 months, 4–6 yr |
| Hib (*Haemophilus influenzae* type B) | 2, 4, 6 months or 2, 4 months[3] | 12–15 months |
| Oral polio | 2, 4 months | 6–18 months 4–6 yr |
| *or* | | |
| Injectable polio vaccine | 2, 4 months | 12–18 months 4–6 yr |
| *or* | | |
| Injectable polio vaccine | 2, 4 months | |
| *and* | | |
| Oral polio vaccine | | 12–18 months 4–6 yr |
| MMR (measles, mumps, rubella) | 12–15 months | 4–6 yr or 11–12 yr |
| HBV (hepatitis B) | Birth–2 months, 1–4 months, 6–18 months[4] | |
| Varicella-zoster virus vaccine | 12–18 months | |
| Tuberculin skin test (not an immunization but a test) | 12–15 months | Every 1–2 yr |

From Advisory Committee on Immunization Practices, the American Academy of Pediatrics and the American Academy of Family Physicians and Centers for Disease Control and Prevention (1997) data.

[1] May be combined with Hib into one vaccine.

[2] Diphtheria and tetanus toxoid and acellular pertussis vaccine combination (DTaP) is the preferred vaccine for all doses.

[3] The time of immunization for Hib depends on the vaccine used.

[4] Infants who have been exposed to hepatitis B should receive the first injection at birth with hepatitis immune gobulin at a different site.

### Immunizations

Nurses often receive questions about the need for immunizations for uncommon diseases, such as diphtheria, that parents have never seen. Parents may consider a condition such as chickenpox to be a harmless childhood illness. They may be reluctant to have their infants undergo painful procedures when they do not understand the need for them.

The nurse must explain to parents the importance of immunizations. In the United States, national health objectives for the year 2000 include full immunization of at least 90 percent of children by age 2 years. Although most children are immunized by school age, those under 2 years have much lower rates. When immunization rates decline, the occurrence of communicable diseases begins to rise, as happened in the late 1980s, when a resurgence of measles occurred in many U.S. communities. The same may happen with other diseases that are preventable with immunization.

The nurse should briefly describe each of the conditions for which infants receive immunizations to help parents understand that the conditions can cause serious illness and even death. Discuss the age at which each immunization is given and when boosters are needed (Table 23–3).

Common reactions to immunizations should also be discussed with the parents. For example, infants may develop a fever and local tenderness after administration of vaccines. Many care providers suggest that infants receive acetaminophen at the time of the vaccine to decrease the reaction and increase comfort.

**CHECK YOUR READING**

11. How can parents make use of knowledge about infant development to prevent accidents in the first 12 weeks of life?
12. What is the importance of well-baby checkups?
13. Why are immunizations important?

## Illness

Parents have many questions about illness in the infant. They are concerned about recognizing an illness and when to call the pediatrician or nurse practitioner.

### Recognizing Signs

Parents may need help in recognizing signs of illness in infants (Table 23–4). The nurse should explain that any time the infant appears sick or parents believe that something is wrong with the infant, they should call the pediatrician or nurse practitioner. Office staff are usually educated to help parents determine if the infant is sick enough to be seen.

**TABLE 23–4 COMMON SIGNS OF ILLNESS IN INFANTS**

Fever above 100°F axillary
Vomiting all of a feeding more than once or twice in a day
Watery stools or significant increase in number of stools over what is normal for the infant
Blisters, sores, or rashes that are unusual for the infant
Unusual changes in behavior: listlessness or sleeping much more than usual, irritability or crying much more than usual
Coughing, frequent sneezing, runny nose. (*Note*: Occasional sneezing may be due to lint from new clothes or blankets.)
Pulling or rubbing at the ear, drainage from the ear

### Calling the Pediatrician or Nurse Practitioner

When calling the pediatrician or nurse practitioner about an illness, parents should prepare by writing down the information about the illness to avoid forgetting something. They should have the name and telephone number of a pharmacy available in case a prescription drug is needed, and they should be ready to write down instructions (Table 23–5).

Office staff are usually able to answer questions on the telephone about common concerns and simple illnesses. They can help determine if an infant should be brought into the office, but parents should be assertive in asking for an appointment if they believe that one is needed. They have a more complete picture of the infant's condition than can be given over the telephone. If there is a real emergency, the parents should say so immediately so that the staff can act accordingly. Parents can expect the pediatrician or nurse practitioner to return calls about acute illness as soon as possible and those about other concerns near the end of the day.

### Knowing When to Seek Immediate Help

Parents should take the infant to the pediatrician or to an emergency room if signs of dyspnea are present. An infant from birth to 3 months of age should not have a sustained respiratory rate above 60 breaths per minute. If retractions, cyanosis, or extreme pallor is present, parents should get immediate help. If respiratory difficulty occurs suddenly in an infant who is well, the infant may have aspirated a feeding or small object. Parents should call paramedics. Nurses should encourage all parents to take classes in cardiopulmonary resuscitation.

**TABLE 23-5 CALLING THE PEDIATRICIAN OR NURSE PRACTITIONER**

Write down pertinent information before calling. Have your pharmacy name and telephone number handy and a pen and paper to write down instructions.

1. Give the infant's name and age first.
2. Describe the illness or problem.
   a. When did it start?
   b. How often does it occur? (Reporting the number of times the infant vomits or passes a stool gives the pediatrician or nurse practitioner a better idea of the problem.)
   c. How does this compare with the infant's normal patterns?
   d. What does it look like? Describe the rash; describe the color and consistency of the stools.
3. Describe any fever.
   a. How high is it?
   b. Was it taken by axillary or rectal method?
   c. How long has the fever been present?
   d. Has it been higher than it is now?
4. Describe other signs of illness.
   a. Are there changes in eating behavior?
   b. Have sleep patterns changed?
5. Describe the infant's behavior.
   a. Does the infant seem sick?
   b. Is the infant irritable, lethargic, acting differently from normal?
6. Describe what has been done so far to treat the condition and the results.
7. Discuss other relevant information.
   a. Is there a similar illness in family members?
   b. Was the infant treated recently for a similar or different illness?
   c. Does the infant take any other medications?

If an infant's respiratory rate is below 30, parents should stimulate the infant and see if the respirations increase and stay within the normal range of 30 to 60 breaths per minute. If the respiratory rate continues to be below normal, the infant should be seen by a pediatrician or nurse practitioner.

Parents should call the pediatrician if the infant is hard to arouse and keep awake. The infant could be semi-comatose and showing signs of central nervous system disease such as meningitis or encephalitis.

## Learning About Sudden Infant Death Syndrome

Sudden infant death syndrome is the abrupt death of an infant that is unexplained by autopsy, examination of the scene of death, or history. In the United States, more than 3200 SIDS deaths occur each year. It is the third leading cause of death between birth and 1 year of age (Guyer et al., 1996).

Sudden infant death syndrome occurs in apparently healthy infants during sleep, more often in males and during cold weather. It peaks between 2 to 4 months of age. In the United States, Native Americans and African-Americans have the highest rates of SIDS. The lowest rates occur in Asians and Latinos (Hoffman & Hillman, 1992). The reasons for these differences are not known.

Although there have been many studies, the cause of SIDS remains unknown. Maternal smoking, young maternal age, prematurity, low birth weight, low socioeconomic status, infections, maternal drug abuse, and cardiorespiratory and neurologic abnormalities are some of the factors that have been associated with SIDS. It occurs more often in siblings of SIDS victims and preterm infants but is less frequent in breastfed and first-born infants (Hoffman & Hillman, 1992).

An association has been found between SIDS and infants sleeping in the prone position. The prone position may increase the risk of upper airway obstruction, rebreathing expired air, and hyperthermia. Therefore, current recommendations are that a healthy infant be placed on the side or back for sleep. It may be necessary to place a premature infant with respiratory disease or an infant with reflux in the prone position to promote drainage or improve oxygenation. Parents should consult their caregiver about what is best for their infant (AAP, 1992).

Nurses should teach parents about proper positioning of their infants for sleep. Rates of SIDS have dropped as much as 50 percent in countries that have advocated the supine or side-lying position for sleep (Willinger, 1995). A large drop in deaths from SIDS has occurred in the United States since 1992, when the change in position was recommended (Guyer et al., 1996). Therapeutic communication techniques may assist parents concerned about SIDS to talk about their fears. They may need reassurance that the chance that any one infant will experience SIDS is small.

**✓ CHECK YOUR READING**

14. When should immediate help be sought for an infant?
15. What should nurses teach parents about SIDS?

## SUMMARY CONCEPTS

- New parents have a need for information about care of the infant and the mother during the early weeks after birth. Because of shorter hospital stays and decline of the extended family, the traditional sources from which to obtain this information are limited. Nurses assist parents during this time by home or clinic visits and telephone calls.

- Home visits may be provided to low-risk families or those with high-risk infants. For normal infants, the nurse provides assessment for the development of problems such as jaundice and teaching to ensure a successful transition of the infant and mother. For high-risk infants, nurses provide care and teaching adapted to the infant's special needs.
- Careful planning, good communication skills, and knowledge of cultural practices are necessary during home visits.
- Clinic visits include the same assessment and teaching as home visits but do not allow the nurse to assess the home. However, they are more cost-effective.
- Nursing care may also be given by telephone with calls after discharge from the birth facility. These are less expensive but do not allow the nurse to assess the client or home environment in person. However, they are useful for screening and teaching about common concerns.
- All equipment, particularly older, used articles, should be checked by parents for safety. Car seats must be chosen according to the size of the infant and must be used correctly to maintain safety.
- Crying is a major source of concern for parents. They should be reassured that infants are not spoiled by prompt attention to their needs. Nurses can help parents determine the cause and appropriate techniques for dealing with a crying infant. The nurse should use therapeutic communication techniques to help parents deal with negative feelings.
- Colic, crying lasting 3 to 4 hours, usually occurs in the afternoon or evening and often disappears after 3 months. The cause is unknown, and infants with colic grow and develop appropriately.
- Infants may sleep 5 or more hours at night beginning about 12 weeks. By that time they are more mature neurologically and do not need night feedings.
- Common signs of teething include drooling, irritability, decreased appetite and sleep, rash, loose stools, and red and swollen gums. High fever or other signs of illness are not due to teething.
- Diaper rash can be avoided by keeping the area clean and dry and avoiding plastic pants and products to which infants seem sensitive. If rash occurs, exposing the area to air and applying creams sparingly help.
- Both breastfed and formula-fed infants vary in amounts taken at each feeding but average about 1 ounce per feeding initially and 5 to 6 ounces per feeding at 12 weeks of age. Both breast milk and formula contain enough water to meet the infant's needs.
- Solid foods cannot be completely digested until the infant is 4 to 6 months old, and they may cause allergies, gastric upsets, and decreased intake of needed nutrients from milk in a younger infant.
- Well-baby checkups are important for assessment of growth and development, guidance, and immunizations. Immunizations safeguard infants and communities from spread of communicable diseases.
- Parents should learn signs of illness in the infant and when immediate medical care is necessary. When calling the pediatrician or nurse practitioner, parents should think through the information before calling to be sure that all important facts are discussed. They should seek immediate medical attention when infants have difficulty breathing, show cyanosis, or are difficult to arouse from sleep.
- The nurse should teach parents about current knowledge about SIDS and the fact that the cause remains unknown. The nurse should provide reassurance and support using therapeutic communication techniques to help parents with their fears. Parents should be taught not to place the infant in a prone position for sleep.

### References and Readings


American Academy of Pediatrics (AAP). (1995). Hospital stay for healthy term newborns. *Pediatrics, 96*(4), 788–789.

American Academy of Pediatrics (AAP) and American College of Obstetricians and Gynecologists (ACOG). (1992). *Guidelines for perinatal care* (3rd ed.). Elk Grove, Ill.: Author.

American Academy of Pediatrics (AAP) Task Force on Infant Positioning and SIDS. (1992). Positioning and SIDS. *Pediatrics, 89*(6), 1120–1126.

Association of Women's Health, Obstetric, and Neonatal Nurses. (1994). *Didactic content and clinical skills verification for professional nurse providers of perinatal home care*. Washington, D.C.: Author.

Barnes, L.P. (1995). Using the telephone in patient and family teaching. MCN: *American Journal of Maternal-Child Nursing, 20*(6), 341.

Behrman, R.E., Kliegman, R.M., & Arvin, A.M. (Eds.). (1996). *Nelson textbook of pediatrics* (15th ed.). Philadelphia: W.B. Saunders.

Bellig, L.L. (1995). Immunization and the prevention of childhood diseases. *Journal of Obstetric, Gynecologic, and Neonatal Nursing, 24*(7), 669–677.

Berkowitz, C.D. (1996). SIDS and apnea. In C.D. Berkowitz, *Pediatrics: A primary care approach*. Philadelphia: W.B. Saunders.

Blakewell-Sachs, S., & Porth, S. (1995). Discharge planning and home care of the technology-dependent infant. *Journal of Obstetric, Gynecologic, and Neonatal Nursing, 24*(1), 77–83.

Christian, A. (1996). Clinical nurse specialists: Creating new programs for neonatal home care. *Journal of Perinatal and Neonatal Nursing, 10*(1), 54–63.

Dahlberg, N.L.F., & Koloroutis, M. (1994). Hospital-based perinatal home-care program. *Journal of Obstetric, Gynecologic, and Neonatal Nursing, 23*(8), 682–686.

Eidelman, A.I., Hoffman, N.W., & Kaitz, M. (1993). Cognitive deficits in women after childbirth. *Obstetrics and Gynecology, 81*(5), 764–767.

Evans, C.J. (1995). Postpartum home care in the United States. *Journal of Obstetric, Gynecologic, and Neonatal Nursing, 24*(2), 180–186.

Grover, G. (1996). Crying and colic. In C.D. Berkowitz, *Pediatrics: A primary care approach*. Philadelphia: W.B. Saunders.

Guyer, B., Strobino, D.M., Ventura, S.J., MacDorman, M., &

Martin, J.A. (1996). Annual summary of vital statistics—1995, *Pediatrics*, 98(6), 1007–1019.

Hall, W.A., & Carty, E.M. (1993). Managing the early discharge experience: Taking control. *Journal of Advanced Nursing*, 18, 574–582.

Hoffman, H.J., & Hillman, L.S. (1992). Epidemiology of the sudden infant death syndrome: Maternal, neonatal, and postneonatal risk factors. *Clinics in Perinatology*, 19(4), 717–737.

Jones, L.C., Maestri, B.O., & McCoy, K. (1993). Why parents use the warm line. MCN: *American Journal of Maternal-Child Nursing*, 18(5), 258–263.

Keefe, M.R., Kotzer, A.M., Froese-Fretz, A., & Curtin, M. (1996). A longitudinal comparison of irritable and nonirritable infants. *Nursing Research*, 45(1), 4–9.

Keppler, A.B. (1995). Postpartum care center: Follow-up care in a hospital based clinic. *Journal of Obstetric, Gynecologic, and Neonatal Nursing*, 24(1), 17–21.

Lowe, M., Millea, D., & Simpson, K.R. (1996). Discharge planning. In K.R. Simpson & P.A. Creehan (Eds.), AWHONN's *perinatal nursing*. Philadelphia: J.B. Lippincott.

Lust, K.D., Brown, J.E., & Thomas, W. (1996). Maternal intake of cruciferous vegetables and other foods and colic symptoms in exclusively breastfed infants. *Journal of the American Dietetic Association*, 96(1), 46–48.

Mendler, V.M., Scallen, D.J., Kovtun, L.A., Balesky, J., & Lewis, C. (1996). The conception, birth, and infancy of an early discharge program. MCN: *American Journal of Maternal-Child Nursing*, 21(5), 241–246.

Miller, M.A., Sutter, R.W., Strebel, P.M., & Hadler, S.C. (1996). Cost effectiveness of incorporating inactivated poliovirus vaccine into the routine childhood immunization schedule. *Journal of the American Medical Association*, 276(12), 967–971.

Pascale, J.A., Brittian, L., Lenfestey, C.C., & Jarrett-Pulliam, C. (1996). Breastfeeding, dehydration, and shorter maternity stays. *Neonatal Network*, 15(7), 37–43.

Selekman, J. (1994). The guidelines for immunizations have changed again! *Pediatric Nursing*, 20(4), 376–378.

Selekman, J. (1995). Children in the community. In C.M. Smith & F.A. Maurer, *Community health practice: Theory and practice*. Philadelphia: W.B. Saunders.

Simpson, K.R., Seibold, L., & Stremsterfer, K. (1996). Perinatal homecare services. In K.R. Simpson & P.A. Creehan (Eds.), AWHONN's *perinatal nursing*. Philadelphia: J.B. Lippincott.

Smith, C.M. (1995). The home visit: Opening doors for family health. In C.M. Smith & F.A. Maurer, *Community health practice: Theory and practice*. Philadelphia: W.B. Saunders.

Stock, C.M. (1995). Standardization of telephone triage: Is it time? *Journal of Nursing Law*, 2(2), 10–25.

U.S. Department of Health and Human Services, Public Health Service. (1995). *Healthy people 2000: Midcourse review and 1995 revisions*. Washington, D.C.: Author.

Valaitis, R., Tuff, K., & Swanson, L. (1996). Meeting parents' postpartal needs with a telephone information line. MCN: *American Journal of Maternal-Child Nursing*, 21(2), 90–95.

Vessey, I.A., & Ritchie, S.R. (1993). The who, what, and why of pediatric immunization. RN, 56(9), 42–48.

Weekly, S.J., & Neumann, M.L. (1997). Speaking up for baby: The case for individualized neonatal discharge plans. AWHONN's *Lifelines*, 1(1), 24–29.

Weinberg, S.H. (1994). An alternative to meet the needs of early discharge: The Tender Beginnings postpartum visit. MCN: *American Journal of Maternal-Child Nursing*, 19(6), 339–342.

Williams, L.R., & Cooper, M.K. (1996). A new paradigm for postpartum care. *Journal of Obstetric, Gynecologic, and Neonatal Nursing*, 25(9), 745–749.

Willinger, M. (1995). SIDS prevention. *Pediatric Annals*, 24(7), 358–364.

Wong, D.L. (1995). *Whaley & Wong's nursing care of infants and children* (5th ed.). St. Louis: C.V. Mosby.

# Part V

# Families at Risk During the Childbearing Period

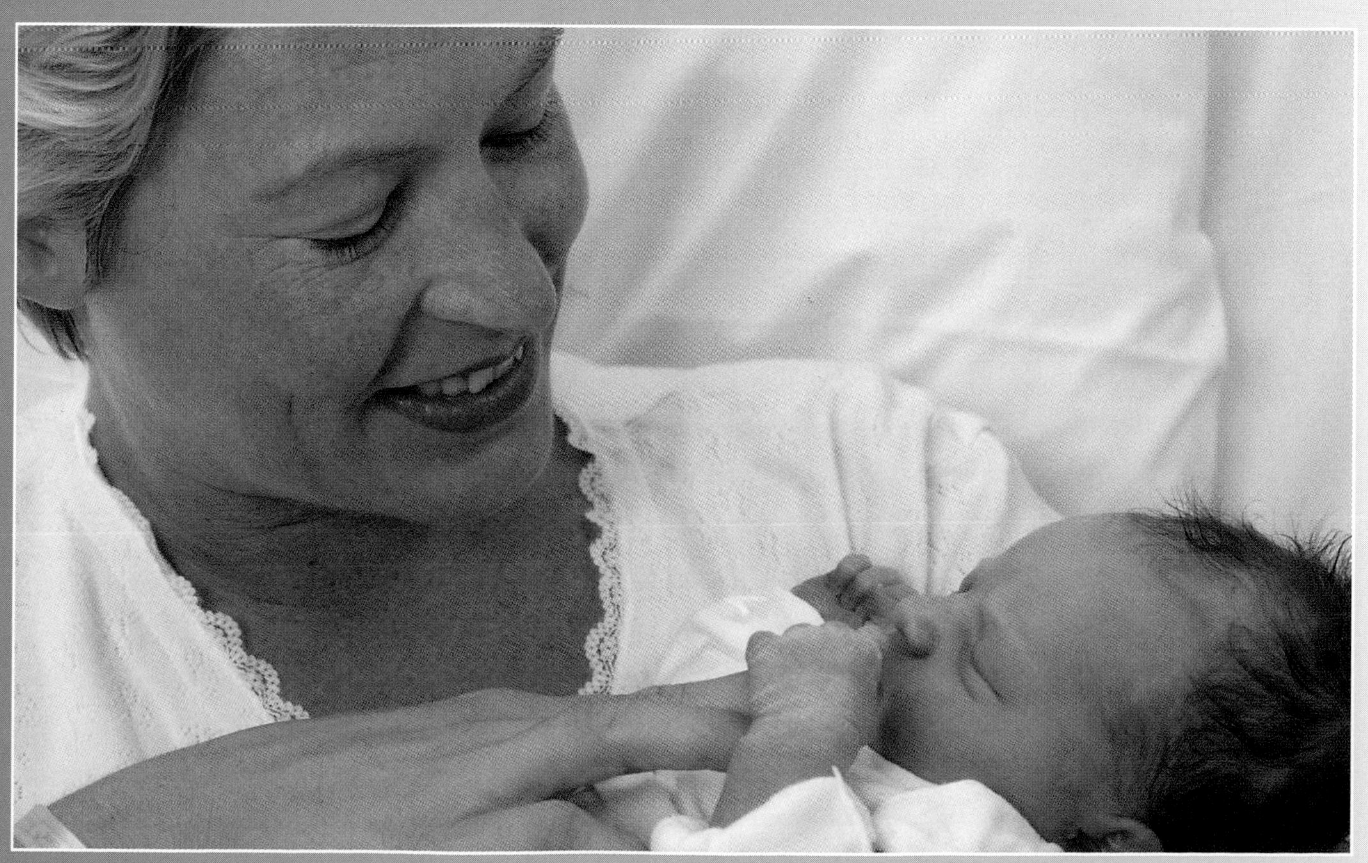

# 24

# The Childbearing Family with Special Needs

**OBJECTIVES**

1. Discuss the incidence and identify the factors that contribute to teenage pregnancy.
2. Identify the effects of pregnancy on the adolescent mother, her infant, and family.
3. Describe the role of the nurse in the prevention and management of teenage pregnancy.
4. Relate the major implications of delayed childbearing in terms of maternal and fetal health.
5. Describe the effects of substance abuse on the mother and the infant, and identify nursing interventions to reduce or minimize the effects in the antepartum, intrapartum, and postpartum periods.
6. Discuss parental responses when an infant is born with congenital anomalies, and identify nursing interventions to assist the parents.
7. Describe parental responses to pregnancy loss, and identify nursing interventions to assist parents through the grieving process.
8. Examine the role of the nurse when the mother relinquishes the infant for adoption.
9. Identify the factors that promote violence against women, and describe the role of the nurse in terms of assessment, prevention, and interventions.

**DEFINITIONS**

**abstinence syndrome** *A group of symptoms that occur when a person who is addicted to a specific drug withdraws or abstains from taking that drug.*

**addiction** *Physical or psychological dependence on a substance such as alcohol, tobacco, or drugs, either legal or illicit.*

**alcoholism** *A chronic, progressive, and potentially fatal disease characterized by tolerance for and physical dependency on alcohol or by pathologic organ changes due to alcohol abuse, or both.*

**amphetamines** *Central nervous system stimulants that create a perception of pleasure that is unrelated to external stimuli.*

**crack** *A highly addictive form of cocaine that has been processed to be smoked.*

**egocentrism** *Interest centered on the self rather than on the needs of others.*

**fetal alcohol syndrome** *A group of physical and mental disorders of the offspring associated with maternal use of alcohol during pregnancy.*

**methadone** *A synthetic compound with opiate properties. Used as an oral substitute for heroin and morphine in the opiate-addicted person.*

**neonatal abstinence syndrome** *A cluster of physical signs exhibited by the newborn who was exposed in utero to maternal use of substances such as cocaine or heroin. See also Abstinence syndrome.*

**opiate** *Any narcotic containing opium or a derivative of opium.*

**prune-belly syndrome** *An absence of abdominal muscles that results in a flabby, distended, and creased abdomen that may occur in the infant exposed to cocaine in utero.*

**withdrawal syndrome** *See Abstinence syndrome.*

All families must make major changes as they adapt to pregnancy and childbirth. For some families, however, the changes are particularly difficult. Those families with special needs include adolescent parents, parents who delayed childbirth, and families that have problems with substance abuse. In addition, many couples need assistance to cope with the birth of an infant with congenital abnormalities or with the unexpected loss of a pregnancy or neonate. Finally, many families exist in an atmosphere of continual violence and require multidisciplinary assistance to protect the safety of the mother and children. Perinatal nurses can make a difference in the lives of these families, particularly in the lives of infants born into them.

# Adolescent Pregnancy

## Incidence

The pregnancy rate for teenagers in the United States is higher than in any other developed country. Eleven percent (110 per 1000) of all infants are born to women under 19 years of age (ACOG, 1996). It is estimated that 1.2 million pregnancies occur in teenaged girls each year. The majority of these are unplanned and unwanted. Moreover, adolescents who become pregnant are likely to become pregnant again within 2 years (Fig. 24–1).

## Factors Associated with Teenage Pregnancy

The high level of sexual activity among adolescents and the low incidence of contraceptive use are directly related to the incidence of teenage pregnancies in the United States. Of all students in grades 9 through 12, more than half are sexually active and use contraceptives sporadically. Approximately three fourths of those report having used some form of contraception, such as birth control pills, condoms, or withdrawal, some of the time (Centers for Disease Control, 1992).

Moreover, many adolescents fail to understand their vulnerability to pregnancy as a result of their sexual activity. Many subscribe to the "personal fable" that because they are unique they are immune to pregnancy. Others risk pregnancy and parenthood as a means of gaining a love relationship. Still others see it as a means to gain independence. Other factors that contribute to teenage pregnancy are listed in Table 24–1.

## National Health Goals

Teenage pregnancies result in numerous personal, social, and financial problems. As a result of these problems the U.S. Department of Health and Human Services (1995) established goals for the year 2000. A partial list of the goals is as follows:

- To reduce the rate of pregnancies among females aged 15 to 17 from 71.1 to no more than 50 per 1000 adolescents
- To reduce the incidence of unintended pregnancies from 56 percent to no more than 30 percent

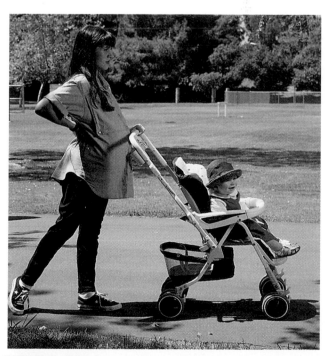

**FIGURE 24–1**

Pregnant adolescent. Thirty-eight percent of teenaged girls who become pregnant will be pregnant again within 24 months.

**TABLE 24–1 FACTORS CONTRIBUTING TO TEENAGE PREGNANCY**

| |
|---|
| Lack of accurate information about how to use contraceptives |
| Limited access to contraceptive devices |
| Fear of reporting sexual activity to parents |
| Ambivalence toward sexuality; intercourse not "planned" |
| Feelings of invulnerability |
| Peer pressure to begin sexual activity |
| Low self-esteem and consequent inability to set limits on sexual activity |
| Means to attain love or to escape present situation |
| Lack of appropriate role models |
| Low level of education correlated with incorrect use of contraceptives |

- To reduce the proportion of adolescents age 15 and younger who have engaged in sexual intercourse from 27 to 15 percent and to reduce the proportion in those aged 17 years and younger from 50 percent to no more than 40 percent.

There is a great deal of controversy about how to achieve the national health goals. The controversy centers on the debate over who should provide sex education. Some believe that families should provide all information about sex and contraceptives to their children. These families are convinced that providing sex education in schools gives tacit approval to sexual activity among teenagers. Conversely, many families advocate early continuing sex education in the public schools. Within this context, information about prevention of pregnancy and sexually transmissible diseases (STDs), including exposure to the human immunodeficiency virus (HIV), is presented on an ongoing basis. Many believe public schools should combine this information with other aspects of teenage sexuality, such as personal adjustments, interpersonal associations, and the establishment of values.

## Sex Education

When sex education is allowed by the community, most educators emphasize that two major strategies should be employed. First, teenagers should be helped to understand how to set limits on sexual activity. Second, they must be instructed in effective measures to prevent pregnancy and STDs.

Learning how to set limits on sexual behavior is particularly important for younger teenagers, who may be pressured to become sexually active before they have developed the maturity to deal responsibly with intercourse, contraception, or unplanned pregnancy. They need advice about how to handle pressure so they can postpone sexual intercourse until they are emotionally and physically ready. In clinical practice, adolescent females often say they wish they had been taught how to say "not now," "not yet," and "not you."

When providing sex education, nurses must keep in mind that adolescent males and females mature at different rates and it may be desirable to form segregated groups until the teenagers indicate that they would feel comfortable in a combined group. It is also important for nurses to use simple but correct language such as uterus, testicles, penis, and vagina. Once the meanings of the terms are understood, most teenagers prefer to use them in their discussions.

For complete information about appropriate contraceptive methods, see Chapter 31.

## Options When Pregnancy Occurs

An adolescent who becomes pregnant must choose one of three options: (1) to terminate the pregnancy, (2) to continue the pregnancy and place the infant for adoption, or (3) to continue the pregnancy and keep the infant. Almost 40 percent (411,000) of all pregnancies among teenagers in the United States are terminated by abortion each year; however, termination of pregnancy is not an acceptable alternative for many families. Moreover, many teenagers do not acknowledge the pregnancy until late in the second trimester, when abortion is complicated.

Few teenagers choose to continue the pregnancy and place the infant for adoption. Those who do may have complicated feelings of grief, relief that a "bad" experience is over, and anger at parents who were unwilling to provide assistance and thus made adoption the only realistic option. However, the autonomous decision to relinquish the child "for the child's good" may be an important step toward maturity.

The choice of abortion or adoption leaves the adolescent with no tangible evidence of her pregnancy and with mixed messages from society regarding her decision. Unlike the teenager who decides to keep her infant, these adolescents receive less assistance about how to deal with their experience. They need help in understanding that their decision to terminate the pregnancy or to place the infant for adoption is an acknowledgment of a significant event, and they need assistance in dealing with their feelings. See the text on relinquishment by adoption, p. 664, for additional information.

## Socioeconomic Implications

The financial cost of teenage pregnancy in the United States is estimated to be almost $17 billion per year. This figure includes funds for Aid to Families with Dependent Children (AFDC), Medicaid, food stamps, direct payment to care providers, and administrative costs (March of Dimes, 1992). Teenaged mothers are more likely than older mothers to be nonwhite, poor, less well educated, and unmarried. Moreover, teenaged mothers are more likely to have larger families at an earlier age, resulting in more children to feed and clothe on an already inadequate income.

Although the financial cost of teenage pregnancy is enormous, the cost in human terms is often tragic. The developmental tasks of adolescence, such as achieving independence from parents and establishing a lifestyle that is personally satisfying, are interrupted (Table 24–2). Educational goals are often curtailed, which limits employment opportunities and results in reliance on the welfare system. Children born into this situation do not escape unscathed. They show a higher incidence of impaired intellectual functioning and poor school adjustment. The negative cycle is often repeated: a large percentage of teenaged parents were children of teenaged parents. As a result, children of adolescent parents are often among the poorest people in the United States.

## Implications for Maternal Health

Pregnancy presents significant problems for the health of adolescent females. They are at increased risk for (1) pregnancy-induced hypertension and (2) anemia and nutritional deficiencies. (Cunningham et al., 1997). Moreover, the maternal mortality rate is higher for adolescents when compared with that of older women.

The high incidence of STDs among pregnant teenagers is another concern. It is estimated that 86 percent of all STDs occur between the ages of 15 and 24 years (Centers for Disease Control, 1992). Gonorrhea and chlamydial infection are particularly prevalent during these years.

The reason for the high incidence of complications among teenagers is unclear. It may be due to delayed prenatal care rather than to age. Some pregnant adolescents do not start prenatal care until the third trimester, and others receive none at all. Early prenatal care that includes counseling about nutritional needs and close observation of the client for the onset of pregnancy-induced hypertension can reduce the high rate of fetal and maternal complications that occur when the expectant mother is very young.

## Implications for Fetal-Neonatal Health

An infant born to a teenaged mother is at higher risk for two major complications: prematurity and low birth weight (<2500 g). This is particularly true when the mother is between 13 and 17 years (Fraser et al., 1995). Low-birth-weight infants have increased incidence of morbidity, and they are more likely to die within the first month of life than infants born at the expected weight.

The cause of low birth weight may be intrauterine growth restriction, which means that the fetus does not grow as expected. This may be due to a variety of causes, such as poor placental perfusion, which occurs during pregnancy-induced hypertension, or the underdeveloped vasculature of the uterus in young primigravidas. When placental perfusion is decreased, the newborn may have a low birth weight even if the pregnancy goes to term because there has been inadequate transport of nutrients and oxygen to the placenta throughout the pregnancy.

Prematurity is also a major cause of low-birth-weight infants. When the infant is born before 38 weeks of gestation, it is likely to weigh less than 2500 g, and in this case the newborn has the added risks associated with immature organs. Respiratory distress syndrome, which occurs as a result of immature lungs, is the leading cause of prolonged hospitalization and neonatal death. Other neonatal conditions that add to the high incidence of morbidity and mortality are birth trauma, congenital anomalies, and perinatal infections.

## The Teenaged Expectant Father

Many adolescent mothers become pregnant by men who are not teenagers but are in their early to mid 20s. These men may accept responsibility for the child, or they may become "phantom fathers," which means that they are absent and rarely involved in parenting the child.

Almost all teenaged expectant fathers indicate that they are not ready for fatherhood, and this attitude does not diminish as the pregnancy progresses. Many are depressed as they grapple with the conflicting roles of adolescence and fatherhood. Although some express interest in learning about childbirth and child care, those who do not want to be fathers are less likely to be supportive. Some do not wish to interact with the infant, leaving the pregnant girl to seek support elsewhere.

A disproportionate number of teenaged expectant fathers are from environments of poverty and lack job skills or educational preparation. Many need job training before they are able to earn enough money to contribute to the support of their children.

## Impact on Parenting

Research indicates that adolescent mothers are at risk to become nonnurturing parents (Thompson et al., 1995). Whether this is due to adolescence per se, the higher incidence of premature births, the lower

**TABLE 24-2 IMPACT OF PREGNANCY ON THE DEVELOPMENTAL TASKS OF ADOLESCENCE**

| Developmental Task* | Impact of Pregnancy | Nursing Considerations |
|---|---|---|
| **Achievement of a Stable Identity:** how the person sees him/herself and how the person perceives that others see and accept him/her; peer group approval provides confirmation and is a major component of identity development. | The ability to adapt and respond to stress is a good indicator of identity development, and adolescents who become pregnant before a stable identity is developed may not be able to accept the responsibilities of parenthood and to plan for the future. | Explore the availability of a school-based mothers' program that will provide the peer support that is so important. Emphasize the importance of prenatal classes and the effect of prenatal care on the pregnancy. Encourage both parents to attend parenting classes and describe the expected growth and development of infants. Focus on the infant's need to develop trust and on the parenting behaviors that promote this. For instance, prompt, gentle, consistent responses to infant signals. |
| **Achievement of Comfort with Body Image:** requires internalization of mature body size, contour, and function. | The adolescent must learn to deal with body changes of pregnancy (increasing size, contour, increased pigmentation, and striae) before she has learned to accept the body changes associated with puberty. May deny pregnancy or severely restrict calories to prevent gaining weight. May be disgusted with the physical changes of pregnancy that make her look different from her peers. | Allow time for the teenager to verbalize her feelings about the body changes of pregnancy. Emphasize that dieting is harmful to the infant and will not stop the changes in body size and contour. Provide exercises that will help her regain her figure after the birth of the infant. |
| **Acceptance of Sexual Role and Identity:** requires internalization of strong sexual urges and achievement of intimacy with others. | The adolescent may need to achieve an intimate relationship with another and to form an exclusive relationship before ready. The pregnant teenager will also need to cope with changes in relationships with friends. She often has difficulty seeing herself as a sexual being or as a mother. | Allow the teenager to express her feelings about sexuality and about motherhood. Initiate classes designed specifically for adolescents and encourage all teenage expectant mothers to join a group with similar interests (childbirth education classes, parenting classes, or special groups that require nutrition counseling). This will help her deal with the changing relationship she has with her peers in school and move toward a mothering role. |
| **Development of a Personal Value System:** able to consider the rights and feelings of others. | Pregnancy occurs before the adolescent is able to move from following rules to considering the rights and feelings of others and developing ethical standards. May experience conflict when they must adjust to the responsibilities of premature motherhood. | Initiate a discussion of teenager's feelings of conflict about her role as mother versus her role as student. Explore her views about motherhood: How does she expect it to change her life? What are her future plans? Present options and assist her to explore her goals. |
| **Preparation for Vocation or Career:** completing educational or vocational goals; youths living in poverty may not have the means or encouragement to accomplish this. | Pregnancy often interrupts school for both parents; this may be a major frustration or it may result in permanent withdrawal from school and limited access to jobs that pay more than the minimum wage. | Discuss the importance of continued education and elicit teenager's feelings and plans to accomplish this. Determine the amount and availability of support from her parents. Refer her to social services for needed assistance. |
| **Achievement of Independence from Parents:** competent in social environment and able to function without parental guidance. | Must adjust to the need for continued financial assistance and dependence on parents at a time when achieving independence is a major priority. | Assist teenager to verbalize her feelings about continued dependence on parents. Discuss the reality of the situation—for instance, that she needs financial support and help with the care of the infant. Determine if she will continue to live at home and the reaction of her parents to the pregnancy. How much support will they provide? What are the conditions for her remaining at her parents' home with the infant? |

* From Mercer, R.T. (1990). *Parents at risk.* New York: Springer.

socioeconomic status, or the particular home environment is difficult to determine. However, teenaged mothers tend to be more insensitive to infant cues. They display fewer instances of mutual gazing, verbal interaction, and touching than do older mothers. Clinical observations of parent-child interaction in adolescent mothers indicate inappropriate parental behaviors, such as pinching, poking, or picking at the infant, although these behaviors are rare in older mothers.

Moreover, adolescent parents may have little understanding of the expected growth and development of infants. They may expect too much too soon from their child. For instance, they may expect that the infant will sleep through the night, smile, or be toilet trained before it is possible for infants to do these things.

It also appears that family functioning decreases as the infant of the adolescent mother grows. The period of time immediately after the infant is brought home has been termed a honeymoon phase. That phase seems to pass as time elapses and child care difficulties arise (Records, 1994). When family support begins to deteriorate, the teenaged mother is likely to experience a great deal of stress.

The ability to deal with stress plays an important part in mothering skills. Young adolescents have immature coping mechanisms, and they may be unable to separate the stress of other life events from the stress that occurs when the infant cries and cannot be consoled. They may respond with immature or punitive measures toward the infant when the source of stress is other factors, such as social isolation or inadequate financial resources.

**CHECK YOUR READING**

1. How does pregnancy affect the developmental tasks of adolescence?
2. What are the major problems associated with teenage pregnancy in terms of maternal and fetal health?
3. How does teenage parenting differ from that of older parents?

## Application of Nursing Process: The Pregnant Teenager

### Assessment

#### PHYSICAL ASSESSMENT

Assessment of pregnant teenagers is similar to that of older women in many respects. At the initial visit, obtain a thorough health and family history to determine whether there are conditions, such as diabetes or infectious diseases, that increase the risk for the mother and fetus. Monitor closely for signs of iron-deficiency anemia or pregnancy-induced hypertension. If STDs are diagnosed, elicit information about sexual partners so that therapeutic management can be initiated. Attempt to identify lifestyle behaviors, such as poor nutrition, smoking, or alcohol or drug use, that could harm the mother or fetus.

**Teenagers are sometimes defensive and inconsistent in their responses. Because they may not volunteer information about nutrition, exercise, and the use of alcohol or other drugs, the nurse needs to press for details. The teenager's statement "I eat okay, and I am pretty active" requires follow-up questions worded to obtain specific information: "What did you eat yesterday? Begin with when you first got up." "What activities do you enjoy most?"**

Structure the interview so that questions can be interspersed in a more general conversation that explores the teenager's likes and concerns. For example, a question such as, "So, you are a member of the choir, will you be able to continue with that after the baby is born?" may establish rapport and help determine whether the teenager is making plans for the future.

#### KNOWLEDGE OF INFANT NEEDS

Assess knowledge of infant needs and parenting skills. How does the teenager plan to feed the infant? What will she do when the infant cries? How will she know when the infant is ill and should be taken to a pediatrician? Does she know how much the infant should sleep? What plans have been made to provide for the hygiene and safety needs of the infant?

#### COGNITIVE DEVELOPMENT

Determine the teenager's cognitive development and ability to absorb health counseling. The three most important areas of cognitive development are the following:

1. *Egocentrism,* which involves the ability to defer personal satisfaction to respond to the needs of the infant: "What would you do if the baby were sick?" "How would you make the baby better?"
2. *Present-future orientation,* which involves the ability to make long-term plans: "What are your plans for finishing high school?" "What will you and the infant need in the first year of the infant's life?"
3. *Abstract thinking,* which involves identifying cause and effect: "Why is it important to keep clinic appointments?" "Why should condoms be used during sexual intercourse?"

#### FAMILY ASSESSMENT

Begin assessment of the family unit by determining the degree of participation by the father of the infant. Some may plan to marry the expectant mother; others deny responsibility for the pregnancy; still others do not plan to marry the expectant mother but plan to participate in the pregnancy and rearing of the child.

It is important to assess the adolescent without the presence of her parents, yet it is also crucial to determine the availability and amount of family support. Will the pregnant teenager continue to live with her parents? How do her parents feel about the pregnancy? How will they incorporate the mother and her infant into the family?

Families generally respond in one of three ways:

1. A family member (often the adolescent's mother) assumes the mothering role, which the teenager may abdicate willingly.
2. All care and responsibilities are left to the adolescent mother, although shelter and food are provided.
3. The family shares care and responsibilities, which allows the teenager to grow in the mothering role while completing the developmental tasks of adolescence.

The pregnant teenager's mother is particularly important when assessing the family. How does she feel about becoming a grandmother? Many women feel embarrassed and disgraced. She may feel that she has "failed" as a mother, or she may resent the new cycle of child care in which the pregnancy involves her. Is communication with her daughter open? Is she aware of the difficult role conflict (as adolescent and mother) that her daughter will experience? If the family is unable or unwilling to provide care for an adolescent with an infant, what other social support can be located?

### Analysis

Many adolescents wait until the second or third trimester to seek prenatal care because they either do not realize that they are pregnant or continue to deny that they are pregnant. Moreover, many teenagers have little information about the physiologic demands that pregnancy imposes on their bodies, such as the increased need for nutrients. As a result, they may have a pattern of sporadic prenatal care and missed appointments (Nursing Care Plan 24–1). One of the most relevant nursing diagnoses is Risk for Altered Health Maintenance related to lack of knowledge of measures to promote health during pregnancy and increased family stress.

### Planning

For the nursing diagnosis Risk for Altered Health Maintenance, the most appropriate goals or outcomes are the following:

- The expectant mother will keep scheduled prenatal appointments and actively participate in recommended group classes.
- She will communicate concerns and seek knowledge of measures that promote her health and the health of the fetus throughout the pregnancy.
- She will express knowledge of infant needs and the expected pattern of infant growth and development before the end of the third trimester.
- The family will verbalize emotions and concerns and maintain functional support of the expectant mother and her infant.

### Interventions

#### ELIMINATING BARRIERS TO HEALTH CARE

The two major barriers to health care are (1) scheduling conflicts and (2) negative attitudes of health care workers. Determine the most convenient location and time for appointments. It may be necessary to help the adolescent locate the clinic closest to her and to provide information about public transportation to that location. Moreover, appointments must be available when the girl (and her partner, if he wishes) are not in school. Some clinics are open in the evening or on Saturday; however, this is not always the case, and alternative plans may have to be made.

Pregnant women of all ages state that the attitude of health care workers can discourage attendance at prenatal clinics. Some health care workers, including nurses, physicians, and social workers, are described as rude, insensitive, patronizing, judgmental, hostile, and condescending. This attitude is particularly unfortunate because it discourages families that would benefit most from early, consistent prenatal care.

Nurses can be instrumental in finding ways to overcome these negative attitudes and thus encourage pregnant women, including teenagers, to return to prenatal clinics for needed follow-up care. Recommended strategies are to do the following:

- Identify pervasive attitudes of the health care team.
- Acknowledge that frustration, stress, and staff burnout are common when health care workers attempt to provide care for families with multiple problems.
- Recognize that many health care workers who are parents of teenagers may feel vulnerable and fear-

# Nursing Care Plan 24–1
# Adolescent's Responses to Pregnancy and Birth

**ASSESSMENT:** Ann Killian, a 16-year-old white female, presented at the neighborhood health clinic during the 20th week of her pregnancy. She lives with her mother and father and a younger sister. Her father works full time in a food processing plant. Her mother works part time as a gardener's helper. Ann remains in school but verbalizes concern about how she looks and feels: "How much bigger am I going to get?" "Why is my face so blotchy?" "My feet swell and it looks gross."

**NURSING DIAGNOSIS:** Body Image Disturbance related to perceived negative effects of pregnancy as evidenced by verbalized concern about appearance

**GOALS/EXPECTED OUTCOMES**

Ann will do the following:

1. Verbalize her feelings about pregnancy and her perception of self during each antepartum visit.
2. Make decisions about times for follow-up appointments by end of current visit.
3. Make two positive statements about herself during next antepartum visit.

| INTERVENTION | RATIONALE |
|---|---|
| 1. Allow time at each prenatal visit for Ann to express concerns about weight gain and other physiologic changes of pregnancy, such as hyperpigmentation and stretch marks. | 1. The adolescent is often ashamed and uncomfortable with her pregnant body. She feels more comfortable if she is allowed to share these feelings and be reassured that they are a normal part of pregnancy. |
| 2. Initiate interaction about body changes by asking open-ended questions such as "How do you feel about needing to wear maternity clothes?" | 2. Adolescents are often intimidated by health care professionals and may think that their own feelings are not important enough to discuss. |
| 3. Provide anticipatory guidance about expected changes during pregnancy; for example, the pattern of weight gain during pregnancy and the rate of weight loss following childbirth. | 3. Most adolescents do not know what to expect during pregnancy, and their fears are often unexpressed. Anticipatory guidance reduces fear and provides information about expected changes. |
| 4. Explain the reason for changes that are most troublesome at each prenatal visit (weight gain, hyperpigmentation, stretch marks, breast changes). | 4. It is often helpful for the adolescent to know that some changes are temporary and that increasing weight indicates that the fetus is growing and developing. This often becomes a source of pride for the young teenager as well as for the older woman. |
| 5. Involve Ann in scheduling follow-up prenatal appointments and other activities related to the birth of the infant (classes, plans for childbirth). | 5. Participation in decision making promotes a positive sense of self. |
| 6. Promote positive self-image by praising grooming, posture, and responsible behavior such as keeping prenatal appointments and folllowing recommendations: "You have never missed an appointment, and your baby is growing so well." | 6. Positive reinforcement is particularly important to help the adolescent meet the developmental tasks of developing a sense of identity and self-worth. |

**EVALUATION**

The plan of care can be considered successful if Ann verbalizes her concerns about how she looks and feels about herself, makes positive statements about herself, and participates in planning future appointments.

**ASSESSMENT:** Ann reveals that her father has said that she has "shamed the family," and she is worried that her friends will reject her when they learn that she is pregnant. Ann states that she will have to "drop out of everything." She confides, in a trembling voice, that she feels guilty for "putting her family through this."

**NURSING DIAGNOSIS:** Anxiety related to feelings of rejection by family and friends as manifested by statements indicating uncertainty about future support for self and infant

**GOALS/EXPECTED OUTCOMES**

Ann will do the following:

1. Identify at least two new measures to cope with anxiety by end of current antepartum visit.
2. Demonstrate ability to implement these measures during subsequent antepartum visits.

*Nursing Care Plan continued on following page*

## Nursing Care Plan 24–1 *Continued*

# Adolescent's Responses to Pregnancy and Birth

| INTERVENTION | RATIONALE |
|---|---|
| 1. Help Ann identify what she can do to overcome anxiety about rejection of family and friends before next prenatal appointment.<br>a. Role play how Ann can initiate a conversation with friends to discuss activities that they can continue to share.<br>b. Suggest that she request a family meeting and acknowledge to them how she feels (guilty for the unhappiness that she is causing them and fearful that they will not assist her through the pregnancy and birth).<br>c. Recommend that she share her feelings with the father of the infant if she continues to see him. | 1. Planning how to approach family and friends reduces anxiety.<br>a. Acceptance by peer group and participation in peer group activities are primary concerns of the adolescent, and a change in the status within the group is a threat to self-concept that precipitates acute anxiety.<br>b. Although adolescents strive for independence, family values continue to be a significant influence. Rejection by the family at this time would leave her vulnerable to stress with which it is beyond her ability to cope.<br>c. Expectant fathers may be a source of emotional and financial support. |
| 2. Encourage Ann to discuss her economic needs as well as her plans for continuing school when the infant is born. | 2. Beginning to develop plans for the future provides some sense of control over the situation and increases feelings of competency. |
| 3. Assist Ann in locating and joining the school-aged mothers' program if available through her school. | 3. This peer group (teenagers who are either mothers or expectant mothers) often replaces the pregnant teenager's previous peer group. The shared concerns and activities provide an opportunity for growth. |

### EVALUATION

The plan of care can be considered successful if Ann identifies and follows up on suggested measures that may reduce her anxiety and if she begins to make future plans.

**ASSESSMENT:** Ann has given birth to a 6 pound, 3 ounce girl at 38 weeks' gestation. She had a difficult labor and received continuous epidural anesthesia. She has decided not to breastfeed because she plans to go back to school as soon as possible. Ann will live at home, and her mother has agreed to care for the infant while Ann is in school. Ann is very concerned about caring for the newborn. She seems unsure how to respond when the infant cries and handles her only during feedings.

**NURSING DIAGNOSIS:** Risk for Altered Parenting related to knowledge deficit of infant needs and lack of confidence in ability to care for infant, as evidenced by uncertain responses to infant

### GOALS/EXPECTED OUTCOMES

Ann will do the following:

1. Demonstrate basic infant care (cord care, bathing, burping, feeding, swaddling) by discharge.
2. Verbalize infant needs for gentle, prompt response to crying.
3. Demonstrate attachment behaviors (eye contact, gazing, holding, verbal stimulation, and positive comments about infant) before discharge.

| INTERVENTION | RATIONALE |
|---|---|
| 1. Demonstrate infant care on first postpartum day, and obtain a return demonstration on second postpartum day before discharge. (For a complete description of infant care, see Chapters 21 and 23.) | 1. Confidence is increased by returning the demonstration of infant care. |
| 2. Role play for Ann how to respond when the infant cries, and emphasize the importance of promptness and gentleness. | 2. Observing how nurses respond to the infant increases the likelihood that adolescents will respond in the same manner. Trust develops when needs are met consistently in a prompt and gentle manner. |

## Nursing Care Plan 24–1 *Continued*

## Adolescent's Responses to Pregnancy and Birth

| INTERVENTION | RATIONALE |
| --- | --- |
| 3. Emphasize the importance of touch and verbal stimulation, and point out the reciprocal bonding behaviors that the infant exhibits (see p. 464). | 3. Many teenaged parents do not provide adequate tactile and verbal stimulation for their infants, which may result in the infant's decreased ability to learn and respond to the environment. The infant has a repertoire of behaviors that stimulates mutual attachment between parent and child. |
| 4. Include the grandmother and the father of the infant in as many demonstrations as possible. | 4. When all primary caregivers are included, family cohesiveness and consistency of care are enhanced. |
| 5. Instruct Ann in early growth and development of the infant (how often infants need to eat, how much they sleep, what to do when they cry). | 5. Some teenaged parents expect "too much, too soon" from infants and become frustrated when the infant does not respond as expected. In addition, anticipatory guidance may reduce some of the stress that many new parents experience. |

**EVALUATION**

Demonstration of basic care, prompt and gentle response to infant crying, and verbalization of the expected growth and development of infants indicate that the plan of care was implemented successfully.

**ADDITIONAL NURSING DIAGNOSES TO CONSIDER**

Risk for Altered Family Processes
Risk for Altered Health Maintenance
Risk for Altered Growth and Development

ful about their own children and project these feelings onto clients.

- Allocate time for staff development, planning programs, and stress reduction.
- Find ways to obtain increased assistance from clerical and support personnel.
- Initiate a scheduling plan that allows health care workers to see the same families whenever possible so that a caring relationship can be established.

### APPLYING TEACHING/LEARNING PRINCIPLES

Because peers are important to adolescents, they benefit from participating in small groups with common concerns. Specific needs that might be addressed are the benefits of prenatal care or education to eliminate unhealthful habits such as smoking, drug use, or alcohol consumption. As pregnancy progresses, needs and group focus change. For example, how to prepare for labor and delivery and how to care for an infant become the priorities.

Repetition is an important method of teaching and clarifying misconceptions. Remember that "telling is not teaching," so allow ample time for questions and discussions. Although teenagers do not read or benefit from printed materials to the same degree that older parents do, many learn well from audiovisual aids. Numerous well-made videos and slide presentations deal with all aspects of prenatal and infant care. Time spent waiting for clinic appointments can be used to view videos that reinforce information.

Above all, remember the importance of nonverbal communication. Maintain an open, friendly posture, and convey empathy by using attending behaviors such as eye contact, frequent nodding, and leaning toward the speaker. As with all expectant families, avoid closed posture (arms folded across the chest), finger pointing, and lack of attention to the person speaking. It is particularly important to avoid sounding like a parent. Avoid using the word "should" or "ought," offering unwanted advice, or making decisions for the teenagers. Table 24–3 summarizes additional recommended methods for teaching adolescents.

### COUNSELING

Allow time to counsel teenagers about their specific problems, such as nutrition, stress reduction, and infant care.

**Nutrition.** Nutrition counseling is one of the most effective means of reducing the incidence of low-

**TABLE 24-3 RECOMMENDED METHODS FOR TEACHING PREGNANT ADOLESCENTS**

Identify and correct barriers to prenatal care
Communicate with kindness and respect
Form small groups with like concerns
Allow ample time for clarification and discussion
Use audiovisual materials
Provide information in appropriate language
Convey empathetic concern by nonverbal communication skills
Include other family members when appropriate

birth-weight infants. Tailor information to the individual adolescent's likes and peer group habits. She often needs instruction in how to make the most nutritious selection from fast-food menus and how to select and plan for healthy snacks when she is away from home.

Referrals to food stamp providers, the special supplemental food program for Women, Infants, and Children (WIC), surplus food distributors, food banks, and food preparation equipment may be necessary because many teenagers have limited access to food and lack the ability to store or prepare food. Nutrition education must be socially and culturally appropriate. (For additional information about the nutritional needs of adolescents and how to help them make good choices, see Chapter 9.)

**Stress Reduction.** Stress is an important factor in perinatal outcome, and teenagers are vulnerable to many sources of stress. Stress may be related to basic needs such as food, shelter, and health care. Fear of labor and delivery and fear of being single, alone, and unsupported all create stress. Perhaps a major source of stress for teenagers occurs when they attempt to meet the developmental tasks of adolescence while working on the developmental tasks of pregnancy (overcoming ambivalence, attaining the role of parent). (See Chapter 8 for additional information about the developmental tasks of pregnancy.)

A variety of measures may be used to reduce stress, depending on the teenager's age, situation, and available support. Adolescents with chronic life stress may require the concentrated efforts of a social worker to achieve stabilization. The pregnant teenager often experiences stress because she has not told her parents or the father of the infant about the pregnancy. It may be helpful to explore her reluctance to do this and to role play the encounter so that she can work out a plan for breaking the news. If appropriate, encourage her to tell the prospective father so that he can work out his role. If the girl is very young or if the pregnancy occurred as a result of rape or incest, social service and law enforcement agencies must become involved to provide protection and assistance.

**Infant Care.** The priorities for teaching gradually change from maternal to infant needs, with particular emphasis on normal growth and development. For example, to reduce the worry that many mothers feel when the newborn trembles or startles in response to loud noises, demonstrate reflexes and explain that the diffuse and uncoordinated motor responses are normal. Explain that development proceeds from the head downward. This helps the young mother understand that the infant must learn to sit before walking and must walk before toilet training is possible.

Explain and demonstrate infant cues (using behaviors of the infants in videos or in the group as examples) in terms of gaze, vocalization, facial expression, body position, and limb movement. Describe how infants use these behaviors to "talk" without words and how parents can use the same behaviors to respond to their infants. Demonstrate how mothers (and fathers) can adjust their position, distance, face, voice, and touch to correspond to their infant's cues. Emphasize that eye contact, holding, cuddling, and verbal stimulation are important for the child's development.

Because adolescents tend to have a more rigid and punitive approach to child care, emphasize to them that infants develop a sense of *trust* when their needs are met promptly and gently. Moreover, their future development depends on attaining a sense of trust during infancy. Emphasize that crying does not indicate that the infant is spoiled but simply that the infant has a need. Perhaps the need is for food, warmth, or comfort and love.

### PROMOTING FAMILY SUPPORT

The pregnant teenager needs encouragement to include her family in her decision making and problem solving. The involvement of her mother, older sister, or other close relative is particularly important in terms of future plans. Topics that should be discussed include who will care for the infant, whether the teenager will return to school, and what financial assistance is available from the family and from the father of the infant. However, if the family has multiple problems that include substance abuse or domestic violence, it may be inappropriate to involve them; the teenager should be encouraged to communicate instead with a family friend or other trusted adult.

### PROVIDING REFERRALS

Nurses who are knowledgeable about national and community resources for pregnant adolescents can make referrals to the closest and most convenient locations. These include well baby clinics offered by the Public Health Service, programs for school-aged mothers offered by many high schools, AFDC offered by state social service agencies, and WIC. Church and community organizations may also provide needed assistance. When incest or rape is suspected, law enforcement agencies must be notified.

### Evaluation

Nursing care has been effective if the pregnant adolescent keeps clinic appointments and participates actively in her plan of care, as demonstrated by asking questions, sharing concerns, and adhering to the recommended program of care. Demonstrating knowledge of the infant's needs as well as the infant's expected pattern of growth and development by the end of the pregnancy increases the teenager's confidence in her ability to provide a nurturing environment. Family support is often available, but if it is not, nurses must often make referrals to agencies that can provide assistance.

**✓ CHECK YOUR READING**

4. What methods are effective for teaching pregnant teenagers?
5. What should prospective teenaged parents be taught about infant growth and development? Why?

## Delayed Pregnancy

An increasing number of women become pregnant relatively late in their reproductive life. Such pregnancies are often the result of contraceptive techniques that provide women with freedom to time the birth of their first child. Furthermore, advances in reproductive medicine increase the chance for infertile women to have a child. Economic motives have also been suggested. For instance, some women may delay childbearing to pursue a career or to establish financial security.

Although a 35-year-old woman can hardly be considered elderly, she is often referred to as an "elderly primigravida" or "older mother"; however, the term *mature primigravida* is preferred by some.

### Maternal and Fetal Implications

When the mature woman decides to conceive, she may experience a delay in becoming pregnant. This is particularly true after the age of 35 years because of the normal aging of the ovaries and the increased incidence in reproductive tract disorders. For instance, pelvic inflammatory disease can cause pelvic and tubal adhesions that interfere with fertilization and implantation.

Once the mature woman conceives, she is at increased risk for complications associated with pregnancy. The risks may be considered in three categories: genetic, preexisting medical conditions, and obstetric complications. The increased risk of fetal chromosomal abnormalities with advancing maternal age is well documented. Trisomy 21 (Down syndrome) is the most common example. The likelihood of a 20-year-old woman having an affected child is approximately 1 in 1400, compared with a 1 in 100 risk for a 40-year-old woman (Cunningham et al., 1997). The use of chorionic villus sampling or amniocentesis permits detection of some chromosomal abnormalities, and legalized abortion allows the woman to terminate the pregnancy if that is an option she would consider.

The most common examples of *preexisting diseases* that increase maternal or fetal jeopardy are hypertension and diabetes mellitus. Uterine myomas (fibroids) occur with greater frequency in women older than 35 years and may be associated with postpartum hemorrhage. The older primigravida is also at increased risk for *obstetric complications*, such as multiple gestation, preterm labor, dysfunctional labor, and cesarean birth. Moreover, the risk of a small-for-gestational age infant increases with maternal age.

### Advantages of Delayed Childbirth

Unlike adolescents, for whom pregnancy may be unplanned and unwanted, women older than 35 years of age seldom make the decision to have a child without careful thought. These women come to the parenting role with a range of personal resources: psychosocial maturity, self-confidence, and a sense of control over their lives (Fig. 24–2). They demonstrate a high level of empathy and flexibility in child-rearing attitudes.

In addition, mature primigravidas are capable of solving complex problems and are often adept at maintaining interpersonal relationships. Because they are more likely to be financially secure, they can afford excellent care for their infants. They are experienced at setting priorities and developing plans. Moreover, they are usually able to manage stress and will independently seek support and assistance.

### Disadvantages of Delayed Childbirth

Mature primiparas need more time to recover from childbirth, and they have less energy than their younger counterparts. They may find child care an exhausting experience for the first few weeks. This is particularly true if they had a cesarean birth

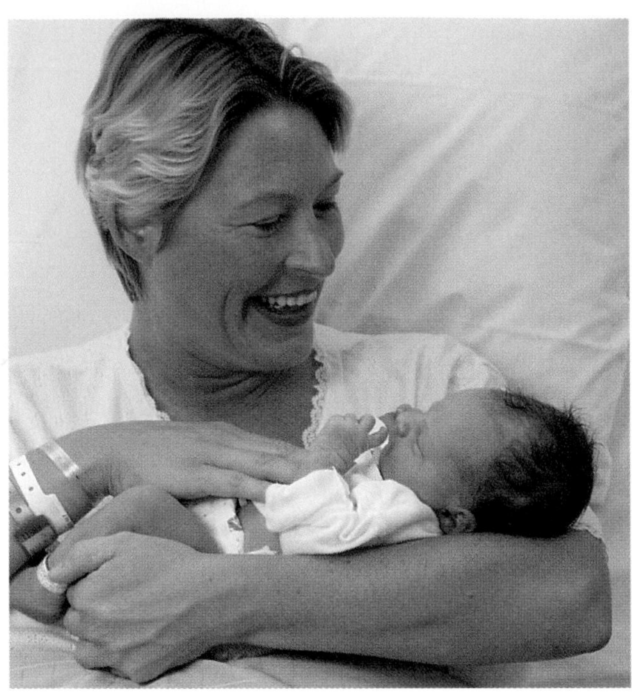

**FIGURE 24-2**

Older primigravidas bring maturity and problem-solving skills to the maternal role, but they are at somewhat increased risk for physiologic problems related to pregnancy and birth.

or other complications of pregnancy, such as excessive bleeding.

Mature primiparas may lack peer support. Many of their friends have teenaged children and do not relate to the concerns of a new mother. Younger mothers have some of the same concerns, but they often do not share the perspective of older mothers.

Family support may also be lacking for the older woman. Her parents are usually in their 60s or 70s and may not be able to assist with child care to the extent that younger grandparents can.

## Nursing Considerations

### REINFORCING AND CLARIFYING INFORMATION

Because the fetus of a mature primigravida is at increased risk for chromosomal anomalies, the woman will be informed about diagnostic tests that are available. Only physicians, certified nurse-midwives, and professionals with special preparation in genetics should provide genetic counseling. All nurses, however, must be prepared to reinforce and clarify the information that has been provided. The tests most often recommended are alpha-fetoprotein screening, chorionic villus sampling, amniocentesis, and ultrasonography. (See Chapter 10.)

The family's beliefs and attitudes about abortion often determine whether to have the recommended tests. The woman who would not consider abortion regardless of the condition of the fetus may refuse diagnostic studies. Nurses must respect the decision and acknowledge that it may have been a difficult one to make.

### FACILITATING EXPRESSION OF EMOTIONS

Several days may pass between performance of diagnostic studies and when results of the tests are known. This is a particularly difficult time for many expectant parents, and nurses often assist the couple to express their concerns and emotions.

**A broad statement such as "Many couples find it difficult to wait for the results" will often elicit free expression of how they feel. Follow-up questions such as "What concerns you most?" may reveal worry about the procedure itself or about the possible effects of the procedure on the fetus. Simply acknowledging that it is a stressful time helps the couple to cope with their emotions.**

### PROVIDING PARENTING INFORMATION

Nurses often help the mature primipara prepare for effective parenting. This may begin by pointing out her individual strengths and advantages. These often include financial security, a stable relationship, and personal maturity. However, the older mother may have unique needs. She often has less energy than younger mothers and must learn to conserve it, particularly during the early weeks following childbirth. Anticipatory guidance about measures that will help conserve energy following childbirth is very useful. Such measures may include meal planning and setting realistic housekeeping goals. In addition, many older mothers need to mobilize all available support so that they can reserve their energy for care of the infant.

During the first weeks following childbirth, the mother may experience feelings of social isolation, particularly if her friends have children who are a great deal older. If she is accustomed to a great deal of mental stimulation, she may miss this while staying at home. If she elects to return to work, she is likely to experience guilt and grief because she must leave her infant. (See Chapter 18 for a discussion of this problem.)

First-time mothers older than age 35 are especially receptive to prenatal classes. These include classes in childbirth education, preparation for cesarean birth, breastfeeding, and early parenting. When teaching infant care following childbirth, the nurse should allow time for demonstrations and return demonstrations so that the expectant parents feel comfortable with routine care. Older couples are particularly interested in learning how the infant grows and develops and what they can do to provide nurturing care for the infant. They generally comprehend printed materials that can be used to reinforce teaching.

**✔ CHECK YOUR READING**

6. What special resources do mature primigravidas often have?
7. Why is it important to offer prenatal testing (alpha-fetoprotein, chorionic villus sampling, amniocentesis) to the mature primigravida?
8. What is the nurse's role in genetic counseling?
9. What anticipatory guidance should the nurse provide the older mother for the first weeks at home following childbirth?

## Substance Abuse

The use of legal substances, such as alcohol and tobacco, as well as illicit drugs, such as cocaine and marijuana, increases the risk of medical complications in the mother and poor birth outcomes in the infant. The problem of substance abuse is not new. However, since the advent of the highly addictive crack cocaine and its popularity among women of reproductive age, the problem of substance abuse in pregnancy has expanded dramatically.

### Incidence

The problem of trying to determine the incidence of drug use is compounded by the fact the use of one drug is often associated with the use of other drugs. The American College of Obstetricians and Gynecologists (1994) reports that, based on current studies, 10 percent represents a reasonable *minimal* estimate of the prevalence of positive toxicology screening in pregnant women nationwide. Although tobacco, alcohol, and marijuana are the most commonly abused drugs, the use of cocaine has had a major impact on health care for pregnant women and their offspring. Prevalence studies for the use of cocaine vary widely; however, 6.1 percent of high school seniors admit to trying it (U.S. Department of Health and Human Services, 1994). An estimated 9000 babies are born to heroin addicts each year in the United States (U.S. Department of Health and Human Services, 1992).

It is estimated that more than 2.25 million women in the United States are problem drinkers. Smoking is also prevalent; 20 to 30 percent of women of childbearing age in the United States smoke cigarettes despite overwhelming evidence of the adverse effects of smoking on pregnancy outcomes.

### Maternal and Fetal Effects

When the pregnant woman takes a substance, by drinking, smoking, snorting, or injecting it, the fetus receives the same substance. The fetus experiences the same systemic effects as the expectant mother but often more severely. For instance, cocaine raises the blood pressure of the woman and the fetus and puts both at risk for intracranial bleeding. A drug that causes intoxication in the woman causes it for prolonged periods of time in the fetus. This is because the fetus is unable to metabolize drugs as efficiently as the expectant mother and will experience the effects long after they have abated in the woman. Therefore, substances taken by the woman can have great impact on the fetus and can interfere with normal fetal development and health. For a summary of the maternal, fetal, and neonatal effects of commonly abused substances, see Table 24–4.

#### TOBACCO

The active ingredients of cigarette smoke are nicotine, tar, and harmful gases, such as carbon monoxide and cyanide. Nicotine, which causes vasoconstriction, transfers readily across the placenta and reduces placental blood circulation. This contributes to fetal hypoxia and increased incidence of fetal death. Carbon monoxide inactivates fetal and maternal hemoglobin and further reduces the amount of oxygen delivered to the fetus. Indirect effects of cigarette smoking include decreased maternal appetite, which results in inadequate intake of calories as well as added difficulties in absorbing nutrients such as calcium and vitamins A, B, and C.

Neonatal consequences of smoking tobacco during pregnancy are low birth weight and prematurity. On average, infants exposed to tobacco in utero weigh 100 g to 320 g less than normal at birth (Lambers & Clark, 1996). Infants born to women who smoke are symmetrically smaller in all areas, including head circumference (Bell & Lau, 1995). Smoking during pregnancy is also associated with delayed neurologic and intellectual development of children. Examples of related problems include hyperactivity, shorter attention span, and lower reading and spelling scores during the primary grades.

#### ALCOHOL

Researchers are unsure how alcohol causes damage to the fetus. However, it is known that alcohol passes easily through the placental barrier, and concentrations found in the fetus are believed to be at least as high as those found in the mother. During the first trimester, alcohol is believed to affect cell membranes and alter the organization of tissue.

**TABLE 24-4 MATERNAL AND FETAL OR NEONATAL EFFECTS OF COMMONLY ABUSED SUBSTANCES**

| Substance | Maternal Effects | Fetal or Neonatal Effects |
|---|---|---|
| Caffeine (coffee, tea, cola, chocolate, cold remedies, analgesics) | Stimulates CNS and cardiac function, causes vasoconstriction and mild diuresis, half-life triples during pregnancy | Crosses placental barrier and stimulates fetus; teratogenic effects are undocumented |
| Tobacco | Decreased placental perfusion, anemia, PROM, preterm labor, spontaneous abortion | Prematurity, LBW, fetal demise, developmental delays, increased incidence of SIDS, pneumonia |
| Alcohol (beer, wine, mixed drinks, after-dinner drinks) | Spontaneous abortion | Fetal demise, IUGR, FAS (facial and cranial anomalies, developmental delay, mental retardation, short attention span), fetal alcohol effects (milder form of FAS) |
| Narcotics (heroin, methadone, morphine) | Spontaneous abortion, PROM, preterm labor, increased incidence of STDs, HIV exposure, hepatitis, malnutrition | IUGR, perinatal asphyxia, intellectual impairment, neonatal abstinence syndrome, neonatal infections, neonatal death (SIDS, child abuse and neglect) |
| Sedatives (barbiturates, tranquilizers) | Lethargy, drowsiness, CNS depression | Neonatal abstinence syndrome, seizures, delayed lung maturity, possible teratogenic effects |
| Cocaine ("crack") | Hyperarousal state, generalized vasoconstriction, hypertension, increased spontaneous abortion, abruptio placentae, preterm labor, cardiovascular complications (stroke, heart attack), seizures, increased STDs | Stillbirth, prematurity, IUGR, irritability, decreased ability to interact with environmental stimuli, poor feeding reflexes, nausea, vomiting, diarrhea, decreased intellectual development; distended, flabby, creased abdomen (prune-belly syndrome) due to absence of abdominal muscles |
| Amphetamines ("speed" or "ice" when processed in crystals to smoke) | Malnutrition, tachycardia, withdrawal symptoms (lethargy, depression) | Increased risk for cardiac anomalies and cleft palate, IUGR, withdrawal symptoms |
| Marijuana ("grass" or "pot") | Often used with other drugs: alcohol, cocaine, tobacco; increased incidence of anemia and inadequate weight gain | Unclear, more study needed, believed related to prematurity, IUGR, neonatal tremors, sensitivity to light |

*Abbreviations*: CNS, central nervous system; PROM, premature rupture of membranes; LBW, low birth weight; SIDS, sudden infant death syndrome; IUGR, intrauterine growth restriction; FAS, fetal alcohol syndrome; STDs, sexually transmissible diseases; HIV, human immunodeficiency virus.

Throughout pregnancy, alcohol interferes with the metabolism of carbohydrates, lipids, and proteins and thus retards cell growth and division. The central nervous system is probably most vulnerable during the third trimester, a time of rapid brain growth.

The teratogenic effects of alcohol have been known for many years. Fetal alcohol syndrome (FAS), first described almost 30 years ago, is the most serious condition related to drinking during pregnancy. This syndrome is characterized by three clinical features: (1) prenatal and postnatal growth restriction, (2) central nervous system impairment, and (3) a recognizable combination of facial features. Common facial anomalies associated with FAS include short palpebral fissures (the openings between the eyelids), flat midface, indistinct philtrum (median groove on the external surface of the upper lip), and a thin upper lip (Fig. 24–3). Growth restriction is noted in length, weight, and head circumference. Manifestations of central nervous system impairment include mental retardation, high activity level, short attention span, and poor short-term memory. Although the range is broad, the average intelligence quotient (IQ) of individuals with FAS is about 70 (Hankin & Sokol, 1995).

A second term—*fetal alcohol effects* (FAE)—is now being used to describe infants who exhibit mild or partial manifestations of FAS, such as low birth weight, developmental delay that may not be obvious for 1 to 2 years, and hyperactivity.

Not all fetuses exposed to alcohol in utero develop FAS. However, no safe level of alcohol consumption during pregnancy has been established,

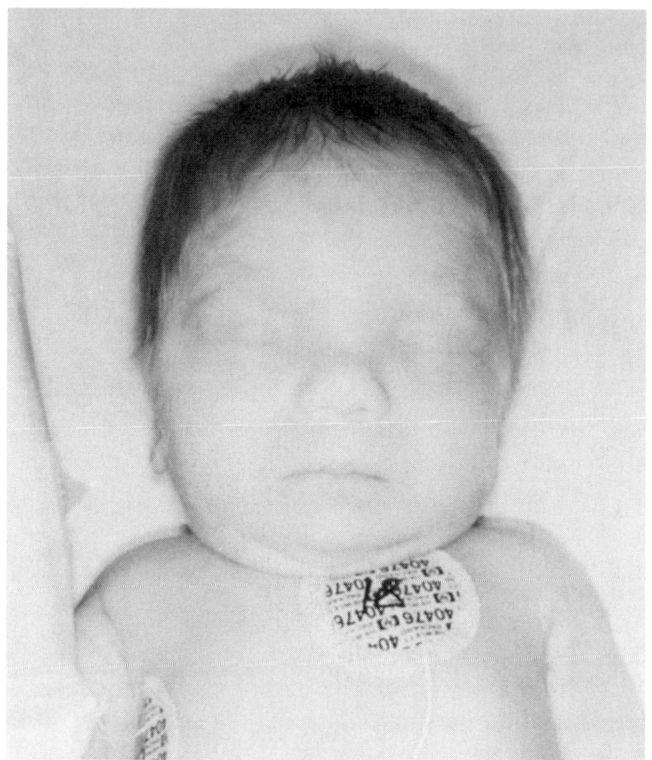

**FIGURE 24-3**

Infant with fetal alcohol syndrome. Subtle indicators that are present are flat midface, indistinct philtrum, and low-set ears. (Courtesy of Trish Beachy, M.S., R.N., Perinatal Program Coordinator. University of Colorado Health Sciences, Denver.)

and it is *recommended that women abstain from drinking alcohol throughout their pregnancies.*

### COCAINE

**How Cocaine Works.** Cocaine is a powerful, short-acting stimulant of the central nervous system. Chemically, cocaine works by blocking the presynaptic reuptake of the neurotransmitters norepinephrine and dopamine, producing an excess of these substances at nerve terminals. The excess of neurotransmitters acts on the cerebral cortex to produce a hyperarousal state that results in euphoria, physical excitement, reduced fatigue, and a heightened sense of well-being and power. Anorexia, hyperglycemia, hyperthermia, and tachypnea are among the array of side effects of cocaine use.

When the initial euphoria wears off, a period of irritability, fatigue, lethargy, depression, and impatience occurs, which elicits a strong desire for additional cocaine so that the initial feelings can be recaptured.

Physical effects of cocaine use are related to cardiovascular stimulation and vasoconstriction. The heart rate, systolic blood pressure, and demand for oxygen all increase. Complications of generalized vasoconstriction include myocardial ischemia, myocardial infarction, or cardiac arrhythmias. In addition, cocaine has been associated with stroke, subarachnoid hemorrhage, and temporal lobe seizures.

**Maternal and Fetal Effects.** Identifying a clear-cut, cause-and-effect relationship between cocaine use and perinatal morbidity is difficult. This is because many women who use cocaine have a lifestyle that includes the use of additional drugs, such as alcohol, tranquilizers, or marijuana, to "come down" from the superarousal state that cocaine produces. In addition, women who abuse cocaine are less likely to seek prenatal care or to eat a diet that contains adequate nutrition. Moreover, sex is often exchanged for drugs, which places the woman at increased risk for STDs.

Cocaine directly stimulates uterine contractions, and one of the most common problems attributed to cocaine use in the pregnant woman is premature delivery (Bell & Lau, 1995). There is also increased incidence of spontaneous abortion and abruptio placentae because of the cocaine-induced vasoconstriction of placental vessels. Additional complications include premature rupture of membranes, precipitous delivery, and stillbirths.

Cocaine crosses the placental barrier and causes the same physical stress on the fetus as on the expectant mother. Moreover, clearance of the drug takes a prolonged period of time in the fetus. Fetal effects have been documented extensively and include tachycardia, decreased beat-to-beat variability of the fetal heart rate baseline, fetal overactivity, and intrauterine growth restriction.

**Neonatal Effects.** Clinical symptoms observed in neonates exposed to cocaine in utero include tremors, tachycardia, marked irritability, muscular rigidity, hypertension, and exaggerated startle reflex. These infants are difficult to console and exhibit an inability to respond to voices or environmental stimuli. They are often poor feeders and have frequent episodes of diarrhea.

The behavioral and developmental characteristics of cocaine-exposed infants may become lifelong disabilities, including both short-term and long-term learning problems, slower intellectual development, and delayed language and motor development. These infants may continue to be irritable and have limited interaction with people and objects in their environment.

### MARIJUANA

The active constituent of marijuana is delta-9-tetrahydrocannabinol (THC), which crosses the placenta and accumulates in the fetus. Although marijuana is one of the most commonly used drugs, very little research has been conducted on the effects of marijuana on the pregnant woman or fetus. One reason is that marijuana is often paired with other drugs such as cocaine and alcohol, making it difficult to determine the effects that are solely the result of marijuana use.

There appears to be an increased incidence in maternal anemia and inadequate maternal weight gain with repeated use of marijuana. Clinically, the neonate may exhibit hyperirritability, tremors, and unusual sensitivity to light. Long-term effects of marijuana on the development of the child deserve much more study before they can be ruled out or confirmed.

#### HEROIN

Heroin is an illegal opiate derived from morphine that produces severe physical addiction. Like all opiates, heroin is a central nervous system depressant that soothes and lulls. It produces a feeling of mental dullness, drowsiness, and finally stupor ("on the nod"). Addiction may be said to exist when discontinuance causes withdrawal symptoms (abstinence syndrome) that are quickly relieved by a dose of the drug.

Heroin use during pregnancy has been studied extensively, and the effects on the pregnant woman, the fetus, and the newborn have been described repeatedly. Women who abuse heroin have poor general health with multiple medical problems associated with their drug abuse and addicted lifestyle. Heroin is an appetite suppressant that also interferes with absorption of nutrients that are ingested, and many women start pregnancy malnourished and anemic. Additional problems include a high incidence of STDs such as gonorrhea, syphilis, and herpes. In addition, infections such as hepatitis and exposure to HIV occur frequently as a result of sharing unclean needles.

**Fetal Effects.** The fetus suffers both direct and indirect effects of heroin use by the expectant mother. The street supply of heroin is usually not steady, and direct effects on the fetus are due to frequent episodes of maternal overdose alternating with periods of withdrawal from the drug. This exposes the fetus to intermittent episodes of hypoxia in utero, which increases the risk of prematurity, growth restriction, and stillbirth. Indirect effects are due to maternal malnutrition and fetal exposure to STDs.

**Neonatal Effects.** Infants born to mothers who are addicted to opiates, including heroin, methadone, meperidine, or morphine, exhibit a neonatal abstinence (withdrawal) syndrome. This syndrome affects all body systems; however, the most consistent symptoms described are neurologic: tremors, jitteriness, restlessness, and, on occasion, seizures. Other manifestations include hypertonicity and prolonged continuous crying.

Additional symptoms of newborn abstinence syndrome include poorly coordinated sucking and swallowing reflexes, vomiting, and diarrhea, which may result in dehydration and failure to gain weight normally. Long-term developmental and learning problems are common. Moreover, the lifestyle of parents who are substance abusers is strongly associated with child neglect and abuse, which are major causes of infant death in this population.

Management of withdrawal syndrome is usually the most immediate problem in the newborn period. Initial management is more general than specific. Decreased environmental stimulation, swaddling, and small frequent feedings may be helpful. Caretakers often become frustrated because the infant's body is stiff and extended, and the newborn does not respond to cuddling or soothing behaviors that usually console a crying infant. Some infants are comforted when they are snugly swaddled with their hands brought to midline. These infants cannot tolerate simultaneous visual and tactile stimulation. They are consoled more easily if positioned with their face away from the caregiver and if rocking movements are vertical rather than horizontal. See Figure 24–4.

## Diagnosis and Management of Substance Abuse

In addition to toxicology screening, the pregnant woman who uses illicit drugs must be tested throughout pregnancy for STDs, hepatitis, and exposure to HIV. Physicians also use all available methods to assess the fetus. These methods include ultrasonography, nonstress tests, and biophysical profiles to help pinpoint problems. Nurses monitor weight gain and provide guidance in nutrition at each opportunity to prevent maternal anemia and inadequate weight gain.

Therapeutic management depends on the type of drug used. In the case of opiates, such as heroin, withdrawal during pregnancy has been associated with significant fetal stress and even fetal death due to the effects of abstinence syndrome. One approach to treatment of the pregnant woman who uses heroin is to place her on an alternative drug such as methadone. Methadone is useful because it can be taken orally and is long-acting; therefore, the woman is able to maintain fairly consistent blood levels, in contrast to the use of heroin, which is short-acting and results in wide swings in blood level that can have severe adverse effects on the fetus.

Treatment for a great deal of substance abuse is aimed at establishing abstinence and preventing relapse. It is often helpful to combine education, individual and group therapy sessions, and peer support groups (Narcotics Anonymous, Alcoholics Anonymous, or Cocaine Anonymous). All members of the health care team must acknowledge that women have extremely positive memories associated with cocaine

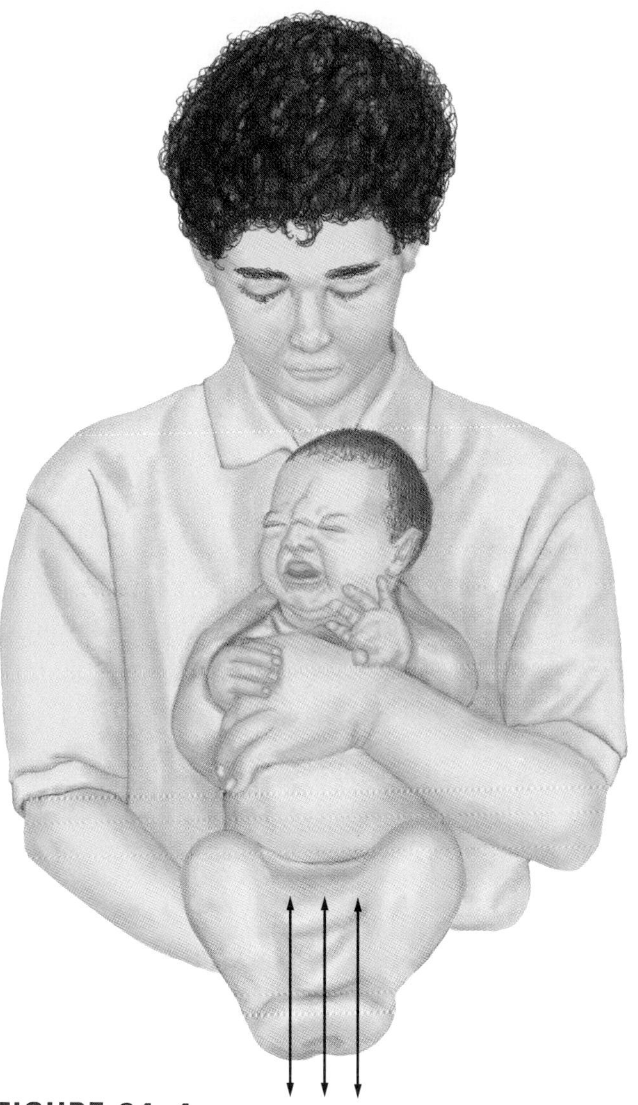

**FIGURE 24-4**

Consoling behaviors for a drug-exposed infant. Note that the infant is swaddled with the hands positioned in the midline, facing away from the caregiver to reduce simultaneous stimuli, and that the caregiver uses vertical rocking.

use, and thus relapse is common. Written contracts that focus on abstinence for one day at a time are often used to help the patient who has relapsed and experiences severe feelings of guilt and self-blame.

Most women are referred for additional treatment for substance abuse during pregnancy. The treatment may be conducted in outpatient clinics; however, residential treatment may provide the optimal setting for needed support.

**CHECK YOUR READING**

10. How does smoking affect the fetus? What are the long-term effects on the child?
11. How does FAS compare with FAE in terms of severity and physical effects?
12. What are the long-term effects of maternal cocaine use on the child?
13. How does neonatal abstinence syndrome affect the caregiver?

# Application of Nursing Process: Maternal Substance Abuse

## Antepartum Period

### Assessment

Multiple drug abuse appears to be the most common substance abuse problem among women, and all women must be screened at the first prenatal visit for nicotine, alcohol, and other drugs. *Because substance abuse occurs in all populations, the nurse must not make assumptions based on class, race, or economic status.*

Certain behaviors are strongly associated with substance abuse: seeking prenatal care late in the pregnancy, failing to keep appointments, and following recommended regimens inconsistently. Physical appearance offers additional clues. Poor grooming, inadequate weight gain, or a pattern of weight gain that does not correspond to the stated gestational age may be signs of a lifestyle that includes substance abuse. Intravenous drug users may have fresh needle punctures, thrombosed veins, or signs of cellulitis.

Defensive or hostile behaviors may be overt signs of substance abuse. Women who use drugs have low self-esteem, and they are dealing with conflicting issues: the physical or psychological need for the substance, the need to deny that the substance is harming the fetus, guilt that they may be responsible for harming the fetus, and, finally, fear that they will be prosecuted for use of illegal drugs. Moreover, many women with substance abuse problems face the discrimination and resentment of health care profes-

**Critical to Remember**

**BEHAVIORS ASSOCIATED WITH SUBSTANCE ABUSE**

- Seeking prenatal care late in pregnancy
- Failure to keep prenatal appointments
- Inconsistent follow-through with recommended care
- Poor grooming, inadequate weight gain
- Needle punctures, thrombosed veins, cellulitis
- Defensive or hostile reactions
- Anger or apathy regarding pregnancy

sionals who direct their frustration at the woman rather than at the problem.

Given the powerful deterrents to self-disclosure, extensive history taking provides the best opportunity to determine current and past substance use. The nurse taking the health history must exhibit patience, empathy, and tolerance and must use a blend of approaches that reinforce concern for the woman and her infant.

#### MEDICAL HISTORY

Determine whether the woman has medical conditions that are prevalent among women who use drugs, such as depression, seizures, hepatitis, pneumonia, cellulitis, STDs, hypertension, or suicide attempts. Current problems may include insomnia, panic attacks, exhaustion, or heart palpitations.

#### OBSTETRIC HISTORY

Evaluate for past and current complications of pregnancy. Spontaneous abortions, premature deliveries, abruptio placentae, and stillbirths are associated with substance abuse, although they also occur in the population that has never used drugs. Current complications may include STDs, vaginal bleeding, and an inactive or hyperactive fetus. Fundal height may be inconsistent with gestational age, suggesting intrauterine growth restriction.

Investigate emotional responses, such as anger or apathy, regarding the pregnancy. These feelings are particularly significant during the latter half of the pregnancy, when one would expect the normal feelings of ambivalence to be resolved. Negative feelings toward the pregnancy may interfere with prenatal compliance with follow-up care.

#### HISTORY OF SUBSTANCE ABUSE

Obtaining an accurate history of substance abuse is difficult and depends in large part on the way the health care worker approaches the woman. A sincere, nonjudgmental, empathetic approach promotes an open exchange of information.

Investigate all forms of drug use, including cigarettes, over-the-counter drugs, prescribed medications, and alcohol, as well as illicit drugs such as cocaine, marijuana, and heroin. Examine patterns of drug use, which can range from occasional recreational use to weekly binges to daily dependence on a particular drug or group of drugs. Suggestions for interviewing are shown in Table 24–5.

Urine toxicology screening is used to validate drug use. This is particularly important when the woman denies current use but presents with a group of symptoms that suggest that she is using one or more drugs.

**TABLE 24–5 TECHNIQUES FOR INTERVIEWING A WOMAN ABOUT SUBSTANCE ABUSE**

To determine whether the woman abuses substances:

Express an accepting and nonjudgmental attitude.

Explain why it is important to know about substance abuse: "We need to know about anything that might affect you or your baby during the pregnancy."

Acknowledge that women may be reluctant to disclose information: "I know it's difficult to talk to us about this, but we need to know so that we can give you and your baby the best care possible."

Begin with questions about over-the-counter or prescription drugs and lead up to use of tobacco, alcohol, and, finally, illicit drugs.

Demonstrate knowledge of types and forms of drugs commonly used in the community: "Do you see much cocaine in your neighborhood?" "Do you have friends who are using crack?"

When substance abuse is acknowledged, the important points in the drug history are the following:

- The type of drug used
- The amount of drug used
- The frequency of use

The nurse can ask specific questions:

How often have you taken over-the-counter medications?

What drugs did you take last month? Were they prescribed?

How many cigarettes do you smoke on a daily basis? Are there times when you smoke more?

How many times a week do you drink alcoholic beverages (beer, wine, mixed drinks)? How many in a day? Are there times when you have more drinks?

How often did you use cocaine before becoming pregnant? How often do you use it now? Do you snort? Smoke crack? Shoot cocaine? How many lines or rocks do you use? How long do you stay high?

### Analysis

Data collected during the interview and during the physical examination are analyzed to formulate nursing diagnoses. Some women acknowledge the use of harmful substances but have a lack of knowledge of their effects. Other women acknowledge the use of drugs and are aware of their harmful effects but are unable to stop using the substances. A nursing diagnosis that addresses both these factors is Risk for Altered Health Maintenance related to lack of knowledge of the effects of substance abuse on self and fetus and inability to manage stress without the use of drugs.

### Planning

Realistic goals for this diagnosis are that the woman will do the following:

- Identify harmful effects of substance on self and infant.

- Verbalize feelings related to continued use of harmful substances.
- Identify personal strengths and accept support offered by the health care delivery system to stop using drugs.

## Interventions

Effective interventions for substance abuse require the combined efforts of nurses, physicians, social workers, law enforcement, and numerous community and federal agencies. Nurses must be aware that progress is slow and frustrating. Keep in mind that the major priority is to protect the fetus and the expectant mother from the harmful effects of drugs.

### EXAMINING ATTITUDES

When working with substance-abusing pregnant women, nurses must identify and acknowledge their own feelings and prejudices. One of the most common emotions expressed by nurses is anger at the woman who not only is engaging in self-destructive behavior but also may be inflicting harm on an innocent victim. Nurses may find it difficult to maintain feelings of empathy, concern, or helpfulness without becoming judgmental or even unknowingly punitive to the pregnant woman. Nurses may also feel helpless, incompetent, and discouraged when the pregnant woman continues to abuse drugs despite the best efforts of the health care team.

Inservice education, professional consultation, and peer support are all avenues to follow when working with pregnant women who abuse drugs. These processes can allow opportunities for discussion, sharing of feelings, problems, and particularly troublesome treatment issues.

### PREVENTING SUBSTANCE ABUSE

The key to any preventive strategy is to provide accurate information in terms that the client can easily understand. Use posters, diagrams, pamphlets, and other visual aids to describe the effects of alcohol, tobacco, cocaine, and heroin on the fetus. The visual aids should be posted in high schools, colleges, supermarkets, shopping centers, and other areas where women of childbearing age will be exposed to them.

Focus on the benefits of remaining drug free. These benefits include a decrease in maternal and neonatal complications. For example, the effects of smoking tobacco are potentially dose-related and cumulative, and nurses need to encourage and support cessation at any point during pregnancy.

### PROVIDING FOLLOW-UP CARE

At each antepartum visit, consider the current status of substance use, social service needs, education needs, and compliance with treatment referrals. In particular, address current drug use because women may change their pattern of drug use during pregnancy. For instance, they may stop using cocaine but increase their use of marijuana or alcohol.

Verify compliance with recommended treatment regimens, such as antepartum clinics and chemical-dependence referral programs. Coordinate care among various service providers, such as group therapy and prenatal classes. Establish communication with all agencies that provide care, and facilitate communication that helps the woman with a chaotic lifestyle meet treatment objectives.

Provide continuing prenatal education classes that include the anatomy and physiology of pregnancy and consequences of prenatal substance abuse. Describe how the newborn benefits when the mother abstains from using drugs, including tobacco and alcohol. Praise any attempts at abstinence and encourage the expectant mother to try again if she relapses.

### COMMUNICATING WITH THE WOMAN

If possible, allow time to get acquainted with the expectant mother. This often involves asking questions about various aspects of her life to obtain a better picture of what other stressors may be contributing to the pattern of substance abuse. Additional stressors may include inadequate housing, economic predicaments, family discord, and emotional or physical illness.

Continue to exercise patience because a hurried or impatient nurse may lose the trust of the expectant mother. Be honest at all times while displaying a nonjudgmental attitude as well as genuine interest and concern. This is especially important when the woman relapses into substance-abusing patterns. Allow her to express guilt, and reassure her that abstinence is possible and that she must simply begin again.

### HELPING THE WOMAN IDENTIFY STRENGTHS

Assist the substance-abusing pregnant woman in identifying personal strengths because she generally has a poor self-image. Acknowledge her actions when she abstains from the use of drugs or alcohol for even a short time. Praise for maintaining an adequate weight gain and attending prenatal classes may increase self-esteem and compliance with the recommended regimen of care.

## Evaluation

Interventions have been successful if the expectant mother does the following:

- Identifies the harmful effects of substance abuse on herself and on the fetus.

- Verbalizes feelings engendered by continued use of substances that adversely affect her or the fetus.
- Identifies personal strengths and accepts support from the health care team to stop using drugs.

## Intrapartum Period

### Assessment

#### COCAINE

Nurses who work in labor and delivery units must become skilled at identifying drug-induced signs and symptoms. Behaviors associated with frequent or recent use of crack cocaine pose the greatest problems. These include profuse sweating, high blood pressure, and irregular respirations, combined with a lethargic response to labor and lack of interest in the necessary interventions. Additional signs include dilated pupils, increased body temperature, and sudden onset of severely painful contractions. Fetal signs often include tachycardia and excessive fetal activity.

Emotional signs of recent cocaine use may include angry, caustic, or abusive reactions to those attempting to provide care. Emotional lability and paranoia are signs of cocaine intoxication.

#### HEROIN

Typically, the pregnant woman addicted to heroin comes to the labor and delivery unit intoxicated from a recent drug administration. When the effects of the drug begin to wear off, withdrawal symptoms may be observed. These include yawning, diaphoresis, rhinorrhea, restlessness, and excessive tearing of the eyes.

### Analysis

One of the most relevant nursing diagnoses during the intrapartal period is Risk for Injury related to physiologic and psychological effects of recent drug use.

### Planning

The major goal for this nursing diagnosis is that the woman and the fetus will remain free from injury during labor and childbirth.

### Interventions

#### PREVENTING INJURY

When a laboring woman has recently used a substance such as cocaine, her life and the life of the fetus depend heavily on the nurse, who must intervene to meet the needs for safety, oxygen, and comfort.

**Critical to Remember**

**SIGNS AND SYMPTOMS OF RECENT COCAINE USE**

- Diaphoresis, high blood pressure, irregular respirations
- Dilated pupils, increased body temperature
- Sudden onset of severely painful contractions
- Fetal tachycardia, excessive fetal activity
- Angry, caustic, abusive reactions and paranoia

**Admitting Procedure.** Two nurses may be needed to admit the woman into the labor unit and to persuade her to assume a safe position. One nurse helps the woman assume the position, initiates electronic fetal monitoring, and begins administration of oxygen, as needed. The other nurse acts as communicator.

Because the woman who has recently used a drug such as cocaine often has difficulty following directions, she should hear only one voice telling her what to do. The second nurse states firmly what is happening and exactly what the woman must do: "Lie on your left side." "This helps us watch how the baby is doing." "This gives you more oxygen." This nurse maintains eye contact with the woman while giving her instructions.

**Setting Limits.** It is critical to realize the importance of setting limits to protect the safety of the mother and the fetus. For instance, the mother cannot smoke. The nurse may say, "It must be difficult not to smoke, but there is real danger to you and to all of us if you do smoke when oxygen is flowing." When the mother is in active labor or after the membranes are ruptured, she must remain in bed even though this may cause her to be agitated. The nurse may say, "I know it is hard to stay in bed, but we can't take good care of the baby when you walk." If it is safe for the woman to walk, the nurse must set limits about where she can walk (in the labor room, not to the cafeteria).

**Initiating Seizure Precautions.** The laboring woman who recently used cocaine is at risk for hypertensive crisis and must be protected from injury in case of seizures. Seizure precautions are as follows:

- Keep the bed in a low, locked position.
- Pad side rails and keep them up at all times.
- Make sure suction equipment functions properly to prevent aspiration.
- Reduce environmental stimuli (lights, noise) as much as possible.

#### MAINTAINING EFFECTIVE COMMUNICATION

Establishing a therapeutic pattern of communication is one of the primary methods of providing care for the patient who has recently used cocaine. Avoid confrontation; instead, acknowledge feelings: "I know you hurt, and I know how frightened you are. I will do everything I can to make you comfortable." When the woman is abusive, be careful not to take the abuse personally or react in a nontherapeutic manner. On the other hand, acknowledge the impact of abusive behavior: "I know this is so difficult for you, and I'm doing my best to take care of you. I feel sad and hurt when you talk to me like that."

Examine your own feelings when women are abusive and acknowledge when anger is getting in the way of providing care. Another nurse may need to assume care of the woman for a time to allow some relief from unrelenting abusive comments.

#### PROVIDING PAIN CONTROL

Pain control for women who are substance abusers poses a difficult problem because it is often impossible to determine the type or combination of drugs that were used before admission. If the woman has used heroin, drugs such as morphine, hydromorphone, and meperidine must be used with caution. Avoid some drugs, such as butorphanol, because they may cause acute withdrawal symptoms in the woman and the fetus. Comfort measures may require nonpharmacologic nursing interventions, such as sacral pressure, back rubs, a cool cloth on the head, and continual support and encouragement. If medications can be administered safely, do not withhold them under the false assumption that their use will contribute to addiction.

#### PREVENTING HEROIN WITHDRAWAL

To prevent or stabilize heroin withdrawal during labor, administer methadone intramuscularly if the woman is nauseated or vomiting. Give methadone to the woman who usually receives methadone at chemical-dependence centers if she did not receive her daily dose. If signs of withdrawal are present, do not order narcotic agonists-antagonists, such as butorphanol (Stadol), because they may cause acute abstinence syndrome in the woman and fetus.

### Evaluation

Both the expectant mother and the fetus may have experienced harmful effects of drugs throughout pregnancy. However, the interventions for this nursing diagnosis can be considered effective if neither the woman nor the fetus sustains additional injury during labor and childbirth.

## Postpartum Period

### Assessment

In the postpartum unit, be aware of the signs of recent drug use and abstinence syndrome and continue to assess the vital signs and level of consciousness of the mother. Observe the mother-infant interaction so that bonding and attachment can be promoted (see Chapter 18). Observe the infant for signs of drug exposure or abstinence syndrome. Obtain a urine sample for toxicology on the newborn as soon after birth as possible. In addition, become aware of visitors who indicate a willingness to provide assistance when the mother and infant are discharged.

### Analysis

Nurses are particularly concerned about discharging an infant to a mother who is known to use drugs. The most worrisome nursing diagnosis is Risk for Altered Parenting related to lack of knowledge of infant needs and inadequate family support.

### Planning

Goals for this nursing diagnosis are the following:

- The mother (and at least one family member) will demonstrate effective feeding and appropriate consoling behaviors before discharge.
- The mother will verbalize plans to obtain the support of family members who are available to provide assistance before discharge.
- The infant will receive appropriate care from the mother, a family member, or an alternative care provider.

### Interventions

#### PROMOTING EFFECTIVE PARENTING

Child neglect, child abuse, and failure to respond to infant signals and cues are associated with alcohol and drug abuse. Begin anticipatory guidance early in the pregnancy and repeat it frequently. Provide information about the growth and development of infants, how much sleep they need, how often they need to eat, and when they can be expected to sleep through the night.

Parents of a drug-exposed infant need to know that they may experience feelings of rejection, frustration, and even hostility. These feelings are likely to occur when the infant stiffens while being held, cries after being fed, or looks away. Parents must also know that drug-exposed infants are easily stressed because of the decreased stability of their central nervous system. They display stress in a vari-

## Parents Want to Know

### Measures to Prevent Frantic Crying in a Drug-Exposed Infant

- Swaddle the infant with the hands brought to the midline and secured (see Fig. 24–4).
- Provide a pacifier.
- Keep the infant's back toward you and support the head while flexing the knees. Slowly and smoothly rock in a vertical motion.
- Coo softly and gently.
- Place the infant over your shoulder and gently stroke the back.
- Keep the room fairly dark because some infants are particularly sensitive to light.
- Avoid simultaneous auditory and visual stimuli.
- Curtail stimulation if infant shows signs of stress (yawning, sneezing, jerky movements, or spitting up).

ety of ways, such as yawning, sneezing, hiccoughing, furrowing their brow, wearing a worried look, grunting, gagging, and averting their gaze.

Because of their hyperexcitable nervous systems, most infants born to women who used cocaine or other drugs during pregnancy have very low thresholds for overstimulation. When they are unwrapped or handled excessively, they often change color, begin thrashing about, and quickly escalate to frantic crying.

Emphasize that the infant needs gentle handling and that crying does not mean that the infant is spoiled but, rather, indicates a need. Teach parents that infants need physical contact and soft verbal stimulation; however, visual and auditory stimulation should not be presented simultaneously to these infants.

#### PROVIDING ASSISTANCE WITH FEEDING

Infants exposed to drugs prenatally often have uncoordinated sucking and swallowing reflexes, and parents need instruction in how to get the infant to feed. Demonstrate measures that help, such as the following:

- Holding the infant in a semisitting position with the arms forward in slight trunk flexion
- Keeping the infant's chin tucked downward; drug-exposed infants often push the head back, which causes an abnormal swallowing pattern
- Supporting the infant's chin or chin and cheeks with the hand if the infant has trouble sucking. Figure 29–6 (p. 828) illustrates correct positioning.

#### MOBILIZING A SUPPORT SYSTEM

Assist the mother to establish a support system that is knowledgeable and reliable because infants who experienced prenatal drug exposure are difficult to care for. Often the grandmother, a neighbor, or a friend will agree to stand by during times when the mother senses that she is about to lose control. It is most beneficial if the support person commits to providing care at a specified time so that the mother does not have to wait for assistance until she feels out of control.

#### ADDRESSING LEGAL IMPLICATIONS

The urine of the mother is tested for metabolites of drugs. The urine, meconium, or hair of the newborn is also tested. If metabolites of drugs are found in either the mother or the infant, legal implications of illicit drug use must be addressed. In many areas, the infant is removed from the mother's care and the mother must complete a program of drug rehabilitation before she gains access to the infant. Notify the social service department so that plans can be made to place the infant in a foster home or with alternative caregivers until long-term care can be obtained for the mother.

### Evaluation

Interventions are effective if the mother and at least one family member demonstrate how to feed and console the infant before discharge and if adequate family support is identified. If family support is unavailable, an alternative caregiver is found to provide nurturing care for the infant.

#### CHECK YOUR READING

14. What prenatal behaviors indicate substance abuse?
15. What signs and symptoms indicate recent cocaine use?
16. How does nursing care differ during the intrapartum period when the woman has recently taken cocaine?
17. How can nurses promote positive parenting of drug-exposed infants?

## Birth of an Infant with Congenital Anomalies

Even when everything goes according to plan, childbirth is a time of stress for parents. Their anxiety about the condition of the infant is obvious as they carefully trace the features and count the fingers and toes of their newborn. When the infant is not perfect but is born with anomalies, the parents are often overwhelmed with feelings of shock and grief. Because nurses are with the parents more than other members of the perinatal team, they have an opportunity to help the family adjust and to cope with their feelings.

## Factors Influencing Emotional Responses of Parents

### TIMING AND MANNER OF BEING TOLD

It was common practice at one time to remove the infant born with congenital anomalies from the delivery area before parents could see him or her. Parents were told about the anomalies at a later time, often after the physician had prepared them for disturbing news. This practice changed, however, when it was realized that parents experienced less stress if they were told at once and were permitted to hold the newborn if the physical status of the infant allowed (Fig. 24–5).

The manner of presenting information changed as well. Physicians and nurses became aware of the importance of helping the parents accept and bond with the newborn. Many now present the infant to the parents in a very sensitive manner, as the following incident illustrates.

A baby girl was delivered with a major irreparable anomaly: the right arm below the elbow was missing entirely. While the placenta was still intact and the cord attached, the physician placed the infant on the mother's abdomen and said, "Oh, we have a very special baby." As mother and father stroked the infant, the physician pointed out how healthy and beautiful the child was and allowed time for the parents to hold their child.

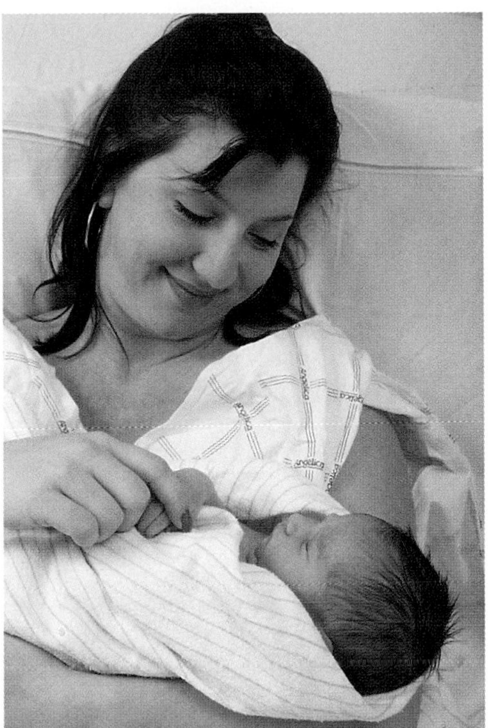

**FIGURE 24–5**

Touching and cuddling between parents and the infant with a congenital anomaly foster attachment and help resolve the grieving process.

### PRIOR KNOWLEDGE OF THE DEFECT

In this age of sophisticated prenatal examinations, the parents may be aware of the existence of a congenital anomaly before the infant is born. These parents may not experience the shock and disbelief that parents who are unprepared experience. This should not be interpreted to mean that they do not experience grief but rather that they have completed some of the early stages of grieving before the birth.

One young couple was aware from the 18th week of gestation that the fetus had hydrocephalus and protrusion of brain tissue from the skull. The mother elected to carry the fetus to term so that the infant would have "every chance at life." When the infant died within minutes after birth, the parents calmly held their child and called the infant by the name that they had selected several weeks previously. The only overt signs of grief were silent tears and a request to see their minister.

### TYPE OF DEFECT

Although any defect in a newborn produces feelings of extreme concern and anxiety, certain defects are associated with long-term parenting problems. It is particularly difficult for the family and the community to accept an infant with facial or genital anomalies. The face is visible to everyone, and parents are fearful about whether the child will be accepted. If the defect is cleft lip and palate, the parents are extremely concerned about surgical repair. Common questions are: "When can it be done?" "Will the child look normal?" "Will the child sound normal?" "Will the scars be obvious?" Parents are often anxious about how grandparents and siblings will accept the child. With time and support, families often work out unique methods to help the family develop strong feelings of attachment.

One young father, profoundly disturbed about the birth of a daughter with a cleft lip and palate and extremely concerned about how his 6-year-old daughter would respond to the infant, took control of the situation. He carefully presented the infant to her sister and pointed out that the baby was small and had special problems; she would need the love of her big sister to overcome them. The 6 year old held the infant and promised to help care for her. After a long talk, the older child, with the help of a nurse, fashioned a sign that was placed in the infant's crib. The sign said, "Hello, my name is Rachel. As you can see, I have a problem, but I am going to be fine."

Gender is at the core of a person's identity, and any defect of the genitals, however slight or correctable, arouses deep concern in both parents. Some anomalies, such as hypospadias (opening of the urethra on the underside of the penis), are repaired in early childhood. Other genital anomalies, such as ambiguous genitalia when assignment of gender is in doubt, cause extreme concern in the family and affect such basic things as what to name the infant, how to dress the infant, and how to respond to questions about the infant's sex.

#### IRREPARABLE DEFECT

Although the initial impact of any defect is profound disappointment and concern, when the defect is irreparable, the parents have no time limit to their endeavors. Eventually, they must grapple with the knowledge that the infant will have a lifelong handicap. Examples of irreparable defects include Down syndrome, microcephaly, and amelia (absence of an entire extremity).

## Grief and Mourning

*Grief* describes the emotional response to loss. *Mourning* is the process of going through the phases of grief until one can accept and resolve the loss. Birth of an infant with an anomaly evokes a grief response, and the family must mourn the loss of the perfect infant they fantasized during pregnancy. Early emotions include denial, anger, and guilt. Denial and disbelief are the initial reactions of most parents to the birth of an infant with a congenital defect. "This can't be true." "How could this happen?" Anger is often a pervasive response, and it may take the form of fault-finding or resentment. Anger may be directed toward the family, the medical personnel, or the self, but it is seldom directed toward the infant. Guilt may be expressed as a question of responsibility for the defect: "I shouldn't have taken that trip while I was pregnant." Other emotions include fear, which may be expressed as concern about what must be done in the immediate or distant future (surgical procedures, complicated health care, the infant's potential for a normal life). Sadness and depression, manifested by crying, withdrawal from relationships, lack of energy, inability to sleep, and decreased appetite, may precede acceptance and resolution. Gradually, often after a prolonged time, the feelings of sadness abate and the family is able to accept and resolve their grief.

#### ✓ CHECK YOUR READING

18. When should parents be told that the infant has anomalies?
19. What types of defects affect parenting most?
20. How can the reaction of parents to birth anomalies be described?

## Nursing Considerations

#### ASSISTING WITH THE GRIEVING PROCESS

Parents must grieve the loss of the perfect infant that they expected before they can form an attachment with this newborn. It is helpful if nurses remain with the parents through the initial phase of shock and disbelief and maintain an atmosphere that encourages them to express their feelings. One way to do this is to listen carefully to what the parents say and to respond by reflecting the content and feelings that they express. For example, the mother of an infant girl with cleft palate says, "How could this happen? I should have gone to the doctor earlier." A helpful response might be, "Actually, we don't know what causes cleft palate, but let's talk about how you are feeling." This offers reassurance but keeps the interaction open to explore the underlying feelings of guilt that the mother may be expressing.

Nurses must recognize that grief responses vary with individuals. Moreover, cultural and religious beliefs affect the expression of grief. Some groups express grief openly by crying, becoming angry, or seeking comfort from a support group. Other cultures (such as Chinese, Japanese, or Native Americans) do not. They may appear stoic and not reveal the depths of their grief. In some cultures (such as Latino), it is acceptable for women, but not for men, to grieve publicly.

#### PROMOTING BONDING AND ATTACHMENT

A priority nursing intervention is to promote bonding and attachment, which may be disrupted when parents who expected a perfect infant give birth to an infant with an abnormality. The process often begins when the nurse communicates acceptance of the infant.

**To do this the nurse handles the newborn gently and presents the infant as something precious. Parents are particularly sensitive to facial expressions of shock or distress. Many nurses emphasize the normal aspects of the infant's body: "She is so alert and she has the most beautiful eyes." Touching and cuddling are essential to caring. Perhaps it is most important to help the parents hold their infant as soon as possible.**

#### PROVIDING ACCURATE INFORMATION

Nurses who work in perinatal settings are responsible for becoming informed about follow-up treatment and timing of surgical procedures so that they can clarify and reinforce information provided by the physician. This involves discussing the plan of care with the physician as well as researching the nursing care that will be required. Parents develop trust in the health care team when consistent information is presented clearly and explained fully.

It may be wise to designate a primary nurse or team to work with the family throughout the hospital stay. Be prepared to repeat information frequently because it may be difficult for the grieving parents to retain it.

#### FACILITATING COMMUNICATION

Nurses are sometimes fearful of being asked questions that they are unable to answer, or they fear that they will say the wrong thing.

**The most helpful course of action is to answer questions as honestly as possible. If unsure of information, say so: "I am not sure about that, but I will find someone with more experience than I have to answer." In addition to answers, parents need kindness, support, and genuine concern.**

It is crucial that family members communicate with one another as well as with the health professionals. Fathers should be included in all discussions, demonstrations, and care of the infant. Information and empathy should be offered consistently to both parents. Without this, the father cannot be expected to support his partner, explain the infant's condition to relatives and friends, or begin to deal with his own shock and sadness.

#### PLANNING FOR DISCHARGE

Often the parents need to learn the special feeding, holding, and positioning techniques that their infant needs; for example, how to feed an infant with cleft palate or how to hold and position the infant with meningocele (protrusion of meninges through a defect in the bony spine). Early participation in infant care fosters feelings of attachment and responsibility for the infant.

Anticipatory guidance may help prevent problems in the family when the infant is discharged to home care. Sibling reaction and behavior depend on their age and ability to understand the needs of the infant. Young children, who are often jealous of the attention and care that the infant requires, may regress to infantile behaviors, such as bed wetting or thumb sucking. Parents should be reminded that this indicates a need for attention rather than naughtiness.

Although grandparents can be a great source of strength and support, they may also have difficulty adjusting to the infant with an abnormality. When appropriate, or if the parents indicate their willingness, include grandparents when teaching special care that the infant will need.

#### PROVIDING REFERRALS

Finally, nurses often initiate referrals to national and community resources. Besides a referral to the social worker in the hospital, parents may also benefit from information about the National Easter Seal Society for Crippled Children, the March of Dimes Birth Defects Foundation, or the crippled children's services of the public health department. In addition, organizations such as the Shriners provide funds for the care of children. Support groups vary from community to community, and perinatal nurses may wish to make a list of the names, addresses, and telephone numbers of these organizations.

**CHECK YOUR READING**

21. How do nurses promote bonding and attachment in families with an infant with congenital anomalies?
22. What should discharge planning for the family of an infant with congenital anomalies include?

## Pregnancy Loss

Perinatal death can occur at any time. Early spontaneous abortion, fetal demise during the latter half of pregnancy, stillbirth, or neonatal death when the infant survives for a few days or weeks can be equally devastating for the parents who experience profound sadness and grief.

Parents experiencing perinatal death often feel alone in their grief, because many people do not consider perinatal loss to be on the same level as the loss of an older child or adult. Moreover, friends and family members are often hesitant to discuss the loss for fear of saying the wrong thing.

Fathers often feel a need to appear strong so that they can support their partners. As a result, fathers often hold back their own feelings of grief and pain and are sometimes perceived as needing less support than the mother.

### Early Pregnancy Loss

Early pregnancy loss, either because of spontaneous abortion or ectopic pregnancy, may precipitate intense grief by the parents. However, many people, even health professionals, minimize the grief that occurs at this time. Comments such as "You shouldn't have any problems getting pregnant again" discount the feelings of mothers and fathers.

When ectopic pregnancy is the reason for the loss, the woman has to deal with the loss of the pregnancy as well as with the possible loss of one fallopian tube. Health care workers mean well when they say, "You still have one fallopian tube left; you'll get pregnant again," but this does not acknowledge to the mother that a child has been lost.

### Concurrent Death and Survival in Multifetal Pregnancy

Parents experience conflicting and complex feelings of joy and grief when one or more infants in a multifetal pregnancy survive and one or more infants in the same gestation die. Contrary to common belief, parents do not grieve less for the dead infant because of the joy that they experience in the living child. They experience an acute sense of loss despite having an infant, and they grieve no less for the infant who did not survive.

For parents experiencing both survival and death of an infant, the grieving process may be more complicated. They may have fears about the health of the surviving infant, especially if the infant is preterm or ill. They may be unable to grieve for the dead child because of their concerns and responsibilities for the surviving child. They may also experience problems with attachment to the surviving infant because of grieving. Moreover, they may receive less support than parents who lost the only child in a single gestation.

Parents who experience the death of one infant and the survival of another need the same interventions as those offered for couples who lose the only child in a single gestation. These interventions include allowing the parents to hold the dead infant and gathering mementos. In addition, nurses must be prepared to confirm the cause of death, if known, and the health status of the surviving infant.

## Application of Nursing Process: Pregnancy Loss

### Assessment

Nursing assessment of the family that has experienced the loss of a fetus or infant requires a great deal of sensitivity. In the case of infant death, collect as much information as possible before meeting with the woman and her family for the first time so that hurtful mistakes can be avoided. Knowing the child's sex, weight, length, and gestational age and whether any abnormalities were noted will help the nurse communicate effectively.

Many perinatal units design a sticker to place on the door, chart, and Kardex so that all staff who come into contact with the family, including auxiliary, housekeeping, laboratory, and radiology personnel, will be alerted that the infant has not survived. Designs include a flower, a teardrop, or a rainbow. This visual symbol diminishes the chance that an uninformed person will make inadvertent comments that cause the family pain.

**Nurses are often unsure how to interact with a family that has experienced the loss of an infant. It is helpful for the nurse to acknowledge the situation and to clarify her or his role at once: "I am Bette Turner. I will be your nurse for the next 8 hours. I am so sorry for your loss. Let me know if there is any way I can be of help." This is not an appropriate time for self-disclosure or for false reassurance. Keep the focus on the family's response and their ability to support one another.**

Initial grief responses, such as crying and expressions of anger, often occur during the woman's stay in the birth facility. Nurses who provide home care or who make follow-up telephone calls must be aware of subtle cues of grief, such as sighing, excessive sleeping, apathy, poor hygiene, or loss of appetite. This is especially important when assessing members of cultural groups that do not display grief publicly.

Evaluate also the availability of a support system that includes family members or clergy. It may be necessary to ask whether a spiritual adviser would offer comfort. Many religions emphasize the acceptance of God's will and the immortality of the soul, and hearing these beliefs affirmed may help the family cope with the grief that they are experiencing. Some fathers focus all their energy on supporting the mother and may not acknowledge their own grief. As a result, they may not receive the support they need.

### Analysis

The most obvious nursing diagnosis for any women who experiences perinatal death is Grieving related to newborn (or fetal) death.

### Planning

Grief reactions are unique to each person, and it is inappropriate to assign a time frame in which parents will acknowledge or share their grief. Goals for this diagnosis are that the parents will do the following:

- Acknowledge their grief and express the meaning of the loss.
- Share their grief with significant others.

## Interventions

### ACKNOWLEDGING THE INFANT

For many years, it was believed that when an infant was stillborn or died shortly after birth the less parents knew of the infant the less they would grieve. The infant was often whisked away so that the parents never saw their newborn. Relatives often disposed of the clothes and the bassinet of the expected infant before the mother returned home, and the parents were left with very few memories of the birth or the infant.

The response to perinatal death changed as nurses discovered that the most helpful interventions for grieving parents were those that acknowledged the rights of the baby. These include the right

- To be recognized as a person who was born and died
- To be named
- To be seen, touched, and held by the family
- To have life-ending acknowledged
- To be put to rest with dignity (Primeau & Lamb, 1995)

**Presenting the Infant to the Parents.** How the infant is presented to the parents is extremely important because these are the memories that they will retain. If necessary, wash the infant and apply baby lotion or powder. Wrap the infant in a soft, warm blanket. If possible, bring parents and infant together while the infant is still warm and soft. It may be necessary to keep the infant in a warmed incubator if some time elapses before the parents have contact with the infant. If this is not possible, tell the parents that the skin may feel cool. Allow parents to keep the infant as long as they wish, and make them feel free to unwrap the infant if they wish.

Many nurses are concerned about how to present the stillborn infant with severe deformities. Explain the defect briefly and gently. Wrap the infant to expose the most normal aspect. Use diapers to cover genital defects, and use booties and mittens to cover abnormalities of the hands and feet. However, it is not advisable to try to hide the defects completely. Allow parents to progress at their own speed in inspecting the infant. Clinical experience shows that many parents never unwrap the infant but instead quietly discuss positive features of the infant: "He has my father's eyes." "Look at the long fingers."

In one case, a stillborn infant had a severely deformed head and face. The nurse wrapped the infant loosely and draped a corner of the blanket over the part of the face that was most affected before giving the infant to the father and mother to hold. Neither parent lifted the blanket, although they did reach under the blanket to hold the infant's hands and feet.

Allow as much privacy and time as the parents and other family members need to be together. Avoid prying, and remain sensitive to cues that members of the family want to talk or prefer not to. It is not necessary to keep up a flow of conversation. A sympathetic smile, a gentle touch of the hand, and a promise to return in a specific time and returning at that time are equally important. It is all right to ask, "Do you want to talk?" Then listening quietly and reflecting the mother or father's feelings are all that is required.

**Preparing a Memory Packet.** The death of a newborn is a loss that must be mourned by the parents, and mourning requires memories. In this climate, nurses have explored measures that help the family create memories of the infant so that the existence of the child is confirmed and the parents can complete the grieving process.

Most parents treasure a memory packet that includes a photograph; footprints; a birth bracelet with the date and time of birth; the crib card with the infant's name, weight, and length; and, if possible, a lock of hair. Some parents and grandparents want pictures taken of themselves with the infant. The memory packet should be kept on file if the parents do not wish to take it home; they may change their minds later.

### PROVIDING REFERRALS

Parents may find that friends and relatives expect them to recover quickly from perinatal loss and are unable to understand their continued grief. The greatest help often comes from contact with persons who have experienced similar loss, and a variety of support groups have been formed. These include Resolve Through Sharing, AMEND (Aiding a Mother Experiencing Neonatal Death), SHARE (Source of Help in Airing and Resolving Experiences), and HAND (Helping After Neonatal Death).

## Evaluation

Nursing care has been successful if the parents acknowledge their feelings of loss and grief and communicate them to significant others.

**✓ CHECK YOUR READING**

23. How should the stillborn infant be presented to the parents? Why?
24. What are the "rights of the baby"?
25. What is a memory packet, and what should it include?

## Relinquishment by Adoption

Some women carry the pregnancy to term and then relinquish the newborn to the care of another family for adoption. The decision to place the infant for adoption is a painful one that can produce long-lasting feelings of ambivalence. On the one hand, the expectant mother may be satisfied that the infant is going into a stable home in which a child is wanted and will receive excellent care; on the other hand, the social pressures against giving up one's child are often intense.

The process of adoption is relatively simple for the expectant mother. Each state and many organized churches have an adoption agency. In addition, private adoptions are becoming more common, although the legality of these adoptions may be called into question in some states. In private adoptions, an attorney acts as the intermediary between the expectant woman and the couple wanting to adopt the infant. The adoptive family usually agrees to pay the medical expenses of the woman, and sometimes a supportive relationship is established between the expectant mother and the adoptive family. Some adoptive mothers want to experience as much of the birth as possible and elect to act as coach or support person during the birth.

Nurses are sometimes unsure of how to communicate with the woman who is relinquishing her infant. First, the nursing staff who come into contact with the woman must be informed of her decision to place the infant for adoption. This prevents inadvertent comments that could cause distress. Second, nurses must remember that adoption is *an act of love, not one of abandonment*, as the woman relinquishes the newborn to a family that is better able to provide financial and emotional support.

Nurses must also be prepared to respect any special wishes that the mother may have about the birth. For instance, most birth mothers want to know all about the infant—how big he or she is, how healthy, how beautiful. They may want to see and hold the newborn. Some wish to name the infant or to give it a gift. Many take photographs or save mementos such as the birth bracelet or the crib card. Such actions provide memories of the infant and help the mother through the grieving process that may accompany relinquishment of the child.

**The nurse should try to establish rapport and a trusting relationship with the mother. The first step in this process is to acknowledge the situation at the initial contact with the woman: "Hello, my name is Denise, and I will be your nurse today. I understand the adoptive family is coming this morning. What can I do to help you get ready for that?" This is much more helpful than providing postpartum care without reference to an event that is of utmost concern to the mother. It also provides a broad opening for her to express feelings that may include strong attachment and love for the infant, ambivalence about her decision, and profound sadness.**

Therapeutic communication techniques, such as reflecting, paraphrasing, and summarizing, are useful to help the mother explore her feelings. Be careful not to offer advice, and remain nonjudgmental.

Nurses also teach adoptive families how to care for the newborn and what to expect in terms of growth and development. This requires that adequate time and a place that is private be provided. This family benefits from all the teaching that is provided for new parents. They may be anxious, and demonstrations as well as return demonstrations are appropriate.

**✓ CHECK YOUR READING**

26. What is meant by the phrase "adoption is an act of love"?
27. What are the nurse's responsibilities to the adoptive parents?

## Violence Against Women

Physical abuse may start or become worse during pregnancy; it has been recognized as a risk to the health of both mothers and infants. Battering of women by their male partners affects an estimated 3 to 4 million women each year (Harris, 1993). The incidence during pregnancy is reported to be 16 percent (1 in 6) (McFarlane et al., 1996a). It is higher among pregnant teenagers, with 20 percent (one in five) reporting physical abuse within the past year (Parker et al., 1993). Physical abuse is recurrent, with 60 percent of abused women reporting two or more episodes of violence. Although all ethnic groups report similar rates of abuse, major ethnic differences exist, with white women experiencing more frequent and more severe abuse (McFarlane et al., 1996a).

Physical abuse may involve threats, slapping, or pushing. It may also escalate to punching, kicking, and beating that results in internal injury or to wounds from weapons. It may end in death. Sexual abuse, including rape, is often part of physical abuse, with almost half the abused women reporting being forced into sex by their male partner.

Women who were physically abused during pregnancy describe relentless abuse. Physical violence occurs within the context of continuous mental abuse, threats, and coercion. Women go through a process of shame, loss of self-respect, diminished ability to cope as a free adult, and a distancing between self and sources of help and support (Smith et al., 1995). Moreover, physical abuse of the mother may be an indication of what life holds for the unborn child. The majority of men who batter the woman also batter the children, and some women who are battered will physically abuse their children.

## Factors That Promote Violence

Family violence occurs in cultures in which the roles of males and females are gender-based and little value is placed on the woman's role. Men hold power, and women are viewed as less worthy of respect than men. In these cultures, strength and aggression, the ability to "show her who is boss," are considered attractive and desirable in males.

In many cultures, women are treated as if they have less power than men. They earn less than men in the job market, and they are often victimized by marriage. For example, women who hold full-time jobs continue to carry the major responsibilities for housekeeping and child care. They often remain in unhealthy relationships because they are financially dependent on the man. If they divorce, most women become single parents with a standard of living much lower than that of their former husbands.

Stereotyping males as powerful and females as weak and without value has a profound effect on the self-esteem of women. Many women internalize the messages and come to believe that they are less worthy than their partner and that they are the cause of their own punishment. They accept the message from society that when women are battered or raped "they got what they deserved." Furthermore, American culture accepts and condones violence. Movies, television, and sports such as football, hockey, and boxing glorify aggression, physical strength, and the ability to hurt and dominate the opponent.

Alcohol is often stated as a cause of violence against women; however, chemical dependence and domestic violence are two separate problems. Chemical dependence is a disease of addiction; abuse is a learned behavior that can be unlearned. However, violence may become more severe or bizarre when alcohol or drugs are involved. See Table 24–6 for a summary of the myths and realities of violence against women.

**TABLE 24–6 MYTHS AND REALITIES OF VIOLENCE AGAINST WOMEN**

| Myths | Realities |
|---|---|
| The battered woman syndrome affects only a small percentage of the population. | Battering is the single major cause of injury to women; 3–4 million women are battered each year by their partners. |
| Battering of women occurs only in lower socioeconomic classes and in minority groups. | Violence occurs in families from all social, economic, educational, racial, and religious backgrounds. |
| The problem is really "spouse abuse," couples who assault each other. | 95 percent of serious assaults are male against female; violence against women is about control and power. |
| Alcohol and drugs cause abusive behavior. | Substance abuse and violence against women are two separate problems: substance abuse is a disease, violence is a learned behavior; it can be unlearned. |
| The abuser is "out of control." | He is not out of control; he is making a decision, because he chooses who, when, and where he abuses. |
| The woman "got what she deserved." | No one deserves to be beaten. No one has the right to beat another person. Violent behavior is the responsibility of the violent person. |
| Women "like" it or they would leave. | Women are threatened with severe punishment or death if they attempt to leave; many have no resources and are isolated, and they and their children are dependent on the abuser. |
| Couples counseling is a good recommendation for abusive relationships. | Couples counseling is not only ineffective for the couple; it can be dangerous for the abused woman. |

## Characteristics of the Abuser

Physical abuse concerns power, and it is only one of many tactics that abusive men use to control their partners. Other tactics include isolation, intimidation, and threats. Extreme jealousy and possessiveness are typical of the abuser. An abusive male often attempts to control every aspect of the woman's life, including where she goes, to whom she speaks, and what she wears. He controls access to money and transportation and may force the woman to account for every moment spent away from him.

The abusive male often has a low tolerance for frustration and poor impulse control. He does not perceive his violent behavior as a problem and often denies responsibility for the violence by blaming the woman. Most abusive men come from homes in which they witnessed the abuse of their mothers or were themselves abused as children. Although many abusive men have alcohol problems, many also batter their partners when they are sober.

## Cycle of Violence

Violence occurs in a cycle that consists of three phases: (1) a tension-building phase, (2) a battering incident, and (3) a "honeymoon phase." Being aware of behaviors that accompany each phase will enable the nurse to counsel the woman. Figure 24–6 depicts these behaviors.

## Effects of Battering During Pregnancy

Abuse during pregnancy is correlated with health problems for the mother and the infant. Women battered during pregnancy are more likely to have multiple injury sites, particularly of the abdomen as well as the face and breasts. Abused women tend to enter prenatal care late in the pregnancy, with up to one fourth starting prenatal care in the third trimester. They are at increased risk for low maternal weight gain and anemia, and a higher percentage report the use of alcohol and illicit drugs (McFarlane et al., 1996b). Pregnant women in battering relationships face an increased risk of prematurity and bearing low-birth-weight infants.

## Nurse's Role in Prevention

Nurses can do a great deal to prevent physical abuse. First, they must examine their beliefs to determine whether they accept the prevailing attitude that blames the victim: "Why was she wearing that?" "She shouldn't have flirted with someone else." "Why does she stay with him?"

Second, nurses can consciously practice in ways that empower women and make it clear that the woman owns her body. Once the woman is clear about ownership of her body, she has the right to decide how it should be treated. Nurses must use language that indicates that the woman is an active partner in her care: "You understand your body: what do you think?" "How did your body respond when you tried that?"

During examinations, nurses can introduce aspects of care that increase the woman's control over the situation. For example, make sure that the woman meets the physician or nurse practitioner who is to examine her while seated and clothed rather than while unclothed and in a lithotomy position. Nurses can place the examination table so that the woman's head, and not her genitalia, meets the examiner's eye when he or she enters the room. When the woman is positioned for the examination, the table can be raised 45 degrees so that she has an oppor-

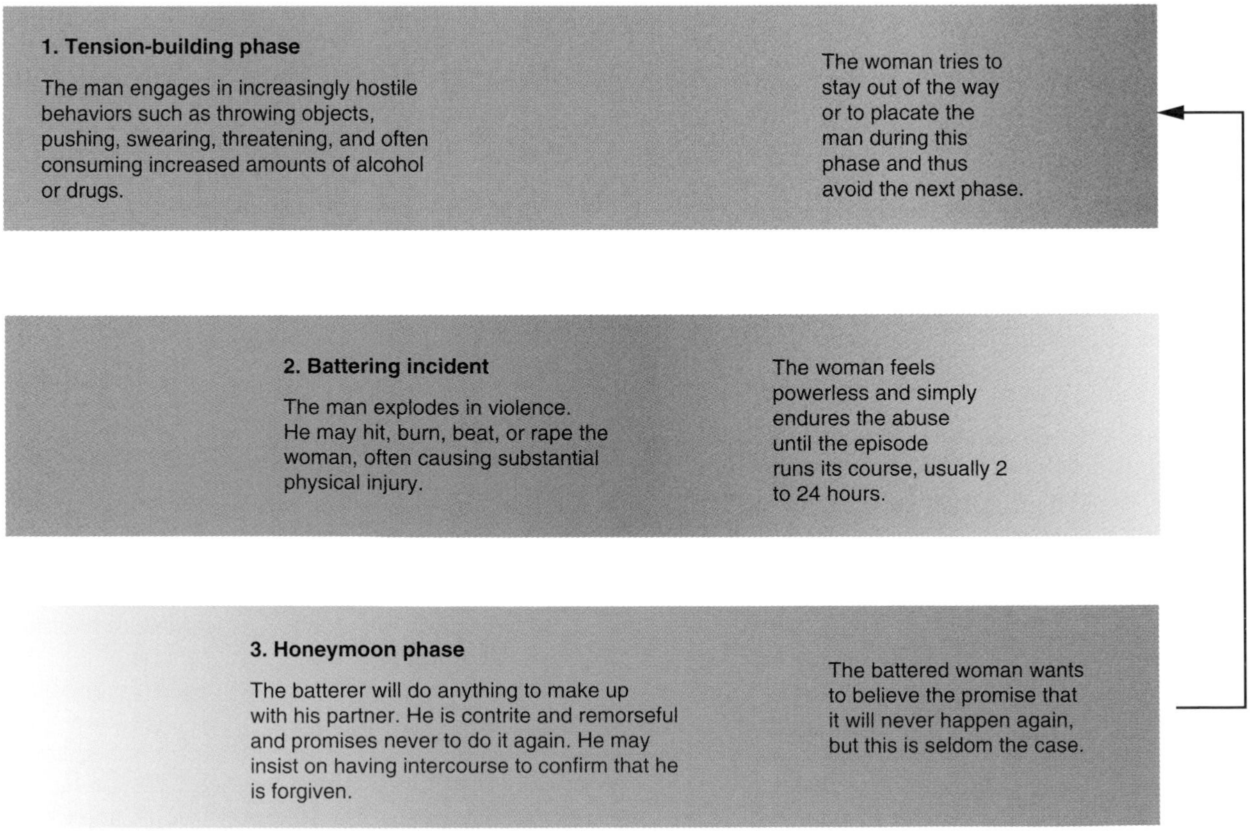

**1. Tension-building phase**

The man engages in increasingly hostile behaviors such as throwing objects, pushing, swearing, threatening, and often consuming increased amounts of alcohol or drugs.

The woman tries to stay out of the way or to placate the man during this phase and thus avoid the next phase.

**2. Battering incident**

The man explodes in violence. He may hit, burn, beat, or rape the woman, often causing substantial physical injury.

The woman feels powerless and simply endures the abuse until the episode runs its course, usually 2 to 24 hours.

**3. Honeymoon phase**

The batterer will do anything to make up with his partner. He is contrite and remorseful and promises never to do it again. He may insist on having intercourse to confirm that he is forgiven.

The battered woman wants to believe the promise that it will never happen again, but this is seldom the case.

**FIGURE 24–6**

Types of behaviors that are evident in each step of the cycle of violence.

tunity to make eye contact with the examiner. Many nurses now provide the woman with a mirror so that she can view the examination and be fully informed about her body parts.

School nurses are in an excellent position to influence how teenagers define gender roles: "Real men don't beat up women." "Girls don't have to put up with verbal or physical abuse from anyone." "Use a condom; it's not cool to give someone you love sexually transmissible diseases or an unwanted pregnancy."

Nurses should be familiar with national resources that are designed to provide health care workers with technical assistance, training materials, posters, bibliographies, and relevant articles. These include the following:

- National Domestic Violence Health Resource Center
  1–800–313–1310
- National Clearinghouse for the Defense of Battered Women
  1–215–351–0010
- National Coalition Against Domestic Violence
  1–303–839–1852
- National Domestic Violence Resource Center
  1–800–537–2238

**CHECK YOUR READING**

28. What is the effect of pregnancy on battering behavior?
29. How can nurses alter their practice to help prevent violence against women?

## Application of Nursing Process: The Battered Woman

### Assessment

It is not an exaggeration to state that there are battered women in every prenatal clinic and in every obstetrician's or nurse-midwife's office. Unfortunately, few women identify themselves as such, and many remain unrecognized. Because of the prevalence of physical abuse during pregnancy, it is recommended that all women be screened for physical abuse.

Nurses are often unsure of how to approach the issue of suspected abuse. Women often seek care and are assessed in the "honeymoon phase" of the violence cycle. It is during this phase that the man is often overly solicitous (hovering husband syndrome) and eager to explain any injuries that the woman exhibits. *Introducing the subject of violence in the presence of the man who may be responsible for it places the woman in*

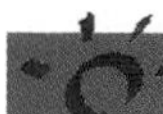

**CRITICAL THINKING EXERCISE**

Joan Piszarek, a 28-year-old primigravida, is admitted to the labor, delivery, and recovery unit in active labor. The right side of her face is swollen, there is evidence of old bruises that look like fingerprints on her upper arms, and there is a large bruised area on her abdomen. She is accompanied by her husband, who is very solicitous. He verbalizes concern about her labor status and remains close beside her at all times. Joan appears lethargic and avoids eye contact with the nurse who is admitting her. She states that she fainted at home and hurt herself when she fell against the bathtub. The nurse accepts the explanation and asks no further questions.

**Q:** 1. What assumptions has the nurse made?
2. What should make the nurse examine her conclusion that the injuries resulted from falling?

When the relief nurse arrives, she waits for time alone with Joan and asks, "Did you get these injuries from being hit?" Joan appears extremely anxious and says, "Don't say anything; he got so mad when I was late getting home from shopping. It was my fault."

**Q:** 3. Why did the nurse wait for time alone before asking questions?
4. How should the nurse respond? What bias must she guard against?
5. How can Joan be protected?

**A:**

1. The nurse assumed that the husband's solicitous behavior indicated concern for his wife. Instead it may have been a "hovering husband syndrome" that occurs in the honeymoon phase of the cycle of violence.
2. Facial injury, signs of previous bruising that resemble "grab marks," and abdominal bruising. Joan's story of falling and hurting herself is not congruent with the location of abdominal injury and injuries on her arms. Joan's lethargy and avoidance of eye contact also suggest that she is afraid.
3. The nurse should not question Joan's explanation of the injury in the presence of the husband because this can increase the danger of escalating violence when the mother and infant are discharged.
4. The nurse should respond, "No one deserves to be hurt; it's not your fault. How can I help you?" Nurses must examine their own thinking to be certain that they do not accept a common bias that physical abuse is deserved by the victim.
5. Joan needs information about how to protect herself and the coming infant from future harm. However, this is not the appropriate time to give her this information. The nurse must inform the physician and the postpartum staff of the problem, and she must make the necessary referrals to the hospital's social service department for follow-up contact with the staff that intercedes for women who are admitted to the emergency department for injuries sustained during an episode of battering.

## Critical to Remember

### CUES INDICATING VIOLENCE AGAINST WOMEN

*Nonverbal*: Facial grimacing, slow and unsteady gait, vomiting, abdominal tenderness, absence of facial response
*Injuries*: Welts, bruises, swelling, lacerations, burns, vaginal or rectal bleeding; evidence of old or new fractures of the nose, face, ribs, or arms
*Vague somatic complaints*: Anxiety, depression, panic attacks, sleeplessness, anorexia
*Discrepancy between history and type of injuries*: Wounds do not match woman's story, multiple bruises in various stages of healing, bruising on the arms (which she may have raised to protect herself), old, untreated wounds

---

*danger; it is absolutely essential to separate the woman from the man for the interview.*

When a private, secure place has been found, reassure the woman that her privacy will be protected and that confidentiality will be absolute. Ask questions directly. If there is trauma, appropriate questions are, "Did someone hurt you?" "Did you receive these injuries from being hit?" The abused woman often appears hesitant, embarrassed, or evasive. She may be unable to look the nurse in the eye and appears guilty, ashamed, jumpy, or frightened.

Evaluate and document all signs of injury, both past and present. This includes areas of welts, bruising, swelling, lacerations, burns, and scars. Injuries are most commonly noted on the face, breasts, abdomen, and genitalia. Many women have new or old fractures. These are usually fractures of the face, nose, ribs, or arms. If there has been sexual abuse, a gynecologic examination is necessary because there is often trauma to the labia, vagina, or cervix. The types of forced sex may include vaginal intercourse, anal intercourse, and insertion of objects into the vagina and anus. Vaginal or rectal bleeding or trauma must be documented according to hospital protocol.

Be particularly alert for nonverbal cues that indicate that abuse has occurred. Facial grimacing or a slow, unsteady gait may indicate pain. Vomiting or abdominal tenderness may indicate internal injury. A flat affect, that is, absence of facial response, is indicative of women who mentally withdraw from the situation to protect themselves from the horror and humiliation they experience during an abusive episode. Keep in mind that the woman may fear for her life because abusive episodes tend to escalate. Open-ended questions help prompt full disclosure and the expression of feelings.

## Analysis

Nursing diagnosis depends on the data collected during the assessment. However, the most meaningful diagnosis for perinatal nurses to make may be Fear related to possibility of severe injury to self and/or children during unpredictable cycle of violence.

## Planning

The abused woman may have difficulty developing a long-term plan of care without a great deal of specialized assistance. She is often unwilling to leave the abusive situation, and nurses often must focus on working with the woman to plan short-term goals that will protect her from future injury.

For realistic short-term goals, the woman will do the following:

- Acknowledge the physical assaults.
- Develop a specific plan of action to implement when the abusive cycle begins.
- Identify community resources that provide protection for her and her children.

## Interventions

### DEVELOPING A PERSONAL SAFETY PLAN

Help the woman make concrete plans to protect her safety and the safety of all children in the home. For example, if the woman insists on returning to the shared home, describe the cycle of behavior that culminates in physical abuse and instruct her in factors that precipitate a violent episode. These include the use of alcohol or other drugs and behaviors that indicate that the level of frustration and anger is increasing. Additional plans will be needed to do the following:

- Locate the nearest shelter or safe house and make specific plans to go there once the cycle of violence begins.
- Identify the safest, quickest routes out of the home.
- Obtain extra keys to the car. Keep them and some necessities packed and hidden until needed.
- Devise a code word, and prearrange with someone to call the police when the word is used.
- Memorize the telephone number of the shelter or hotline because time is often a crucial element in the decision to leave.
- Review the safety plan frequently because leaving the batterer is one of the most dangerous times.

### AFFIRMING SHE IS NOT TO BLAME

The abused woman often believes that she is responsible for the abuse. Let her know that no one deserves to be hit for any reason. The one who hit her is the person responsible; she did not provoke it, and she did not cause it. Nurses are often responsible for teaching basic family processes, such as the following:

- Violence is not normal.
- Violence is usually repeated and usually escalates.
- Battering is against the law.
- Battered women have alternatives.

#### PROVIDING REFERRALS

When contact with the battered woman is short-term, acknowledge that many interventions are outside the scope of nursing practice. As a result, be prepared to refer the family to community agencies that are available to the victim. These include the local police department, legal services, community shelters, counseling services, and social service agencies.

It is essential to accept the decisions of the battered woman and acknowledge that she is on her own timetable. She may not contact the police, go to a shelter, or take any actions at the time that they are recommended. Therefore, listening to her, believing her, and providing information about resources may be the only help the nurse can provide.

Do not become negative or pass judgment on the partner of an abused woman. She is often tied to the man by both economic and emotional bonds and may become defensive if her partner is criticized. Tell her that resources are available for her partner but that it is necessary for him to admit abuse and seek assistance before help can be offered. To initiate referrals for the partner before he asks for help will increase the danger to the woman if her partner feels that he has been betrayed.

### Evaluation

The plan of care can be judged successful if the woman does the following:

- Acknowledges violent episodes in the home
- Makes concrete plans to protect herself and her children from future injury
- Uses the community resources available to her

#### CHECK YOUR READING

30. What are the major cues that indicate that a woman has been physically abused?
31. How can nurses intervene to help women protect their safety if they choose to remain in a home situation with a partner who physically abuses them?

## SUMMARY CONCEPTS

- Teenage pregnancy is a major health problem in the United States that requires that adolescents receive accurate information not only about contraceptives but also about how to set limits on sexual behavior.
- Pregnancy imposes serious physiologic risks for the adolescent and the fetus that result in a higher incidence of pregnancy-induced hypertension, anemia, and nutritional deficiencies for the expectant mother as well as prematurity and low birth weight for the infant.
- Teenage pregnancy interrupts the developmental tasks of adolescence and may result in childbirth before the parents are capable of providing a nurturing home for the infant without a great deal of assistance.
- The mature primigravida often has financial and emotional resources that younger women do not have; however, she may experience anxiety about recommended antepartum testing and her ability to parent effectively.
- Multidrug substance abuse is a widespread problem that can have devastating fetal and neonatal effects that may persist and become long-term developmental problems for the child.
- The lifestyle associated with illicit drug abuse includes inadequate nutrition, inadequate prenatal care, and increased incidence of STDs and necessitates interdisciplinary interventions to prevent injury to the expectant mother and to the fetus.
- The birth of an infant with congenital anomalies produces strong emotions of shock and grief in the family and calls for a sensitive response from the health care team to help the family grieve for the loss of the perfect or "fantasy" infant and to form an attachment to the newborn.
- Pregnancy loss at any stage of pregnancy produces grief that must be acknowledged and expressed before it can be resolved. Nurses realize that mourning requires memories, and they intervene to arrange unlimited contact between the family and the stillborn infant and to gather a memento packet for the family.
- Nursing care for the mother who is placing her infant for adoption is based on the knowledge that relinquishment (adoption) is an act of love, not abandonment.
- Multiple factors are associated with violence against women, which is deliberate, severe, and generally repeated in a predictable cycle that often causes severe physical harm (or death) to the woman.
- All perinatal nurses come into contact with abused women who require assistance to protect themselves and their children from serious injury.

#### References and Readings

American College of Obstetricians and Gynecologists (ACOG). (1996). *Guidelines for women's health care*. Washington, D.C.: Author.

American College of Obstetricians and Gynecologists (ACOG). (1994). Substance Abuse in Pregnancy. ACOG *technical bulletin* No. 195. Washington, D.C.: Author.

Barnet, B., Duggan, A.K., Wilson, M.D., & Joffe, A. (1995). Association between postpartum substance abuse and depressive symptoms, stress, and social support in adolescent mothers. *Pediatrics,* 96(4), 659–666.

Bell, G.L., & Lau, K. (1995). Perinatal and neonatal issues of substance abuse. *Pediatric Clinics of North America,* 42(2), 261–279.

Bloom, K.C. (1995). The development of attachment behaviors in pregnant adolescents. *Nursing Research,* 44(5), 284–289.

Byrne, M.W., & Lerner, H.M. (1992). Communicating with addicted women in labor. MCN: *American Journal of Maternal Child Nursing,* 17(1), 22–26.

Censullo, M. (1994). Strategy for promoting greater responsiveness in adolescent parent/infant relationships: Report of a pilot study. *Journal of Pediatric Nursing,* 9(5), 326–332.

Centers for Disease Control. (1992). Sexual behavior among high school students. *Morbidity and Mortality Weekly Report,* 40(51 and 52), 885–888.

Chazotte, C., Youchah, J., & Freda, M.C. (1995). Cocaine use during pregnancy and low birth weight: The impact of prenatal care and drug treatment. *Seminars in Perinatology,* 19(4), 293–299.

Chez, R.A., & Jones, R.F. (1995). The battered woman. *American Journal of Obstetrics and Gynecology,* 173(3), 677–679.

Chiriboga, C. (1993). Fetal effects. *Neurologic Clinics,* 11(3), 707–729.

Christian, A. (1995). Home care of the battered pregnant woman: One battered woman's pregnancy. *Journal of Obstetric, Gynecologic, and Neonatal Nursing,* 24(9), 836–842.

Cornelius, M.D., Taylor, P.M., Geva, D., & Day, N.L. (1995). Prenatal tobacco and marijuana use among adolescents: Effects on offspring, gestational age, growth, and morphology. *Pediatrics* 95(5), 738–743.

Cunningham, P.G., MacDonald, P.C., Gant, N.F., Leveno, K.J., Gilstrap, L.C., Hankins, G.D.U., et al. (1997). *Williams obstetrics* (20th ed.). Stamford, Conn. Appleton & Lange.

Dicker, M., & Leighton, E.A. (1994). Trends in the U.S. prevalence of drug-using parturient women and drug-affected newborns, 1979–1990. *American Journal of Public Health,* 84(9), 1433–1438.

Fraser, A.M., Brockert, J.E., & Ward, R.H. (1995). Association of young maternal age with adverse reproductive outcomes. *New England Journal of Medicine,* 332(17), 1113–1117.

Fretts, R.C., Schmittdiel, J., McLean, F.H., Usher, R.H., & Goldman, M.B. (1995). Increased maternal age and the risk of fetal death. *New England Journal of Medicine,* 333(15), 953–957.

Hadley, S.M., Short, L.M., Lezin, N., & Zook, E. (1995). Womankind: An innovative model of health care response to domestic abuse. *Women's Health Issues,* 5(4), 189–198.

Hankin, J.R., & Sokol, R.J. (1995). Identification and care of problems associated with alcohol ingestion in pregnancy. *Seminars in Perinatology,* 19(4), 286–291.

Harris, L., & Associates, Inc. (1993). *The Commonwealth Fund survey of women's health.* New York: The Commonwealth Fund.

Jecker, N.S. (1993). Privacy beliefs and the violent family: Extending the ethical argument for physician intervention. *Journal of the American Medical Association,* 269(6), 776–780.

Laken, M.P., & Hutchins, E. (1996). *Recruitment and retention of substance-using pregnant and parenting women: Lessons learned.* Arlington, VA.: National Center for Education in Maternal and Child Health.

Lambers, D.S., & Clark, K.E. (1996). The maternal and fetal physiologic effects of nicotine. *Seminars in Perinatology,* 20(2), 115–126.

Landry, S.H., & Whitney, J.A. (1996). The impact of prenatal cocaine exposure: Studies of the developing infant. *Seminars in Perinatology,* 20(2), 99–106.

Lee, R.V. (1995). Drug Abuse. In G.N. Burrow & T.F. Ferris (Eds.), *Medical complications during pregnancy* (4th ed., pp. 579–596). Philadelphia: W.B. Saunders.

March of Dimes (1992a). Adolescent pregnancy. Series 4. Nursing issues for the 21st Century. Module 2.

March of Dimes. (1992b). Prevention of battering during pregnancy [pamphlet].

McFarlane, J., Parker, B., & Soeken, K. (1996a). Abuse during pregnancy: Associations with maternal health and infant birth weight. *Nursing Research,* 45(1), 37–42.

McFarlane, J., Parker, B., & Soeken, K. (1996b). Physical abuse, smoking, and substance use during pregnancy: Prevalence, interrelationships, and effects on birth weight. *Journal of Obstetric, Gynecology, and Neonatal Nursing,* 25(4), 313–320.

Mercer, R.T. (1990). *Parents at risk.* New York: Springer.

O'Reilly-Green, C., & Cohen, W.R. (1993). Pregnancy in women aged 40 and older. *Obstetrics and Gynecology Clinics of North America,* 20(2), 313–331.

Parker, B., McFarlane, J., Soeken, K., Torres, S., & Campbell, D. (1993). Physical and emotional abuse in pregnancy: A comparison of adult and teenage women. *Nursing Research,* 42(3), 173–178.

Poland, L.M., & Hutchins E. (1995). *Building and sustaining systems of care for substance-using women and their infants: Lessons learned.* Arlington, Va.: National Center for Education in Maternal and Child Health.

Primeau, M.R., & Lamb, J.M. (1995). When a baby dies: Rights of the baby and parents. *Journal of Obstetric, Gynecologic, and Neonatal Nursing,* 24(3), 206–208.

Primeau, M.R., & Recht, C.K. (1994). Professional bereavement photographs: One aspect of a perinatal bereavement program. *Journal of Obstetric, Gynecologic, and Neonatal Nursing,* 23(1), 22–25.

Prysak, M., Lorenz, R.P., & Kisly, A. (1995). Pregnancy outcome in nulliparous women 35 years and older. *Obstetrics and Gynecology,* 85(1), 65–70.

Records, K.A. (1994). Adolescent mothers: Caregiving, approval, and family functioning. *Journal of Obstetric, Gynecologic, and Neonatal Nursing,* 23(9), 792–797.

Roye, C.F., & Balk, S.J. (1996). Evaluation of an intergenerational program for pregnant and parenting adolescents. *Maternal-Child Nursing Journal,* 24(1), 32–40.

Smith, P.H., Tessaro, I., & Earp, J.A. (1995). Women's experiences with battering: A conceptualization from qualitative research. *Women's Health Issues,* 5(4), 173–182.

Thompson, P.J., Powell, M.J., Patterson, R.J., & Ellerbee, S.M. (1995). Adolescent parenting: Outcomes and maternal perceptions. *Journal of Obstetric, Gynecologic, and Neonatal Nursing,* 24(8), 713–717.

U.S. Department of Health and Human Services. (1992). *National household survey of drug abuse.* Washington, D.C.: Author.

U.S. Department of Health and Human Services. (1994). *National household survey of drug abuse.* Washington, D.C.: Author.

U.S. Department of Health and Human Services. (1995). *Healthy people 2000: Midcourse review and 1995 revisions.* Washington, D.C.: Author.

Warrick, L., Christianson, J.B., Walruff, J., & Cook, P.C. (1993). Educational outcomes in teenage pregnancy and parenting programs: Results from a demonstration. *Family Planning Perspective,* 25(4), 148–155.

# 25

# Complications of Pregnancy

**OBJECTIVES**

1. Describe the hemorrhagic conditions of early pregnancy, including spontaneous abortion, ectopic pregnancy, and hydatidiform mole.
2. Explain disorders of the placenta, such as placenta previa and abruptio placentae, that result in hemorrhagic conditions of late pregnancy.
3. Discuss the effects and management of hyperemesis gravidarum.
4. Describe the development and management of hypertensive disorders of pregnancy.
5. Compare Rh and ABO incompatibility in terms of etiology, fetal and neonatal complications, and management.

**DEFINITIONS**

**abortion** *A pregnancy that ends before 20 weeks' gestation, either spontaneously or electively. Miscarriage is a lay term for a spontaneous abortion.*

**abruptio placentae** *Premature separation of a normally implanted placenta.*

**antiphospholipid antibodies** *Autoimmune antibodies directed against phospholipids in cell membranes; associated with recurrent spontaneous abortion, fetal loss, and severe pregnancy-induced hypertension.*

**bicornuate (bicornate)** *Malformed uterus having two horns.*

**cerclage** *Encircling of the cervix with suture to prevent recurrent spontaneous abortion caused by early cervical dilation.*

**culdocentesis** *Needle puncture through the upper posterior vaginal wall (cul-de-sac of Douglas) to aspirate blood or fluid from the pelvic cavity.*

**dilation and curettage (D&C)** *Stretching the cervical os to permit suctioning or scraping of the walls of the uterus. The procedure is performed in abortion, to obtain samples of uterine lining tissue for laboratory examination, and during the postpartum period to remove retained fragments of placenta.*

**dilation and evacuation (D&E)** *Wide cervical dilation followed by mechanical destruction and removal of fetal parts from the uterus. Following complete removal of the fetus, a vacuum curet is used to remove the placenta and remaining products of conception.*

**eclampsia** *Convulsive form of pregnancy-induced hypertension.*

**ectopic pregnancy** *Implantation of a fertilized ovum in any area other than the uterus; the most common site is the fallopian tube.*

**erythroblastosis fetalis** *Agglutination and hemolysis of fetal erythrocytes due to incompatibility between maternal and fetal blood. In most cases, the fetus is Rh-positive and the mother is Rh-negative.*

**gestational trophoblastic disease** *A spectrum of diseases that includes benign hydatidiform mole and gestational trophoblastic tumors, such as invasive moles and choriocarcinoma.*

**hydatidiform mole** *Abnormal pregnancy resulting from proliferation of chorionic villi that give rise to multiple cysts and rapid growth of the uterus.*

**hypovolemic shock** *Acute peripheral circulatory failure due to loss of circulating blood volume.*

**kernicterus** *Staining of brain tissue caused by accumulation of unconjugated bilirubin in the brain. Also called bilirubin encephalopathy.*

**laparoscopy** *Insertion of an illuminated tube into the abdominal cavity to visualize contents, locate bleeding, and perform surgical procedures.*

**linear salpingostomy** *Incision along the length of a fallopian tube to remove an ectopic pregnancy and preserve the tube.*

**maceration** *Discoloration and softening of tissues and eventual disintegration of a fetus that is retained in the uterus after its death.*

**perinatologist** *A physician who specializes in the care of the mother, fetus, and infant during the perinatal period (from the 20th week of pregnancy to 4 weeks following childbirth).*

**pre-eclampsia** *A hypertensive disorder induced by pregnancy that usually includes a triad of signs and symptoms: hypertension, edema, and proteinuria.*

**salpingectomy** *Surgical removal of a fallopian tube.*

**toxemia** *A term occasionally used to denote pregnancy-induced hypertension, pre-eclampsia, and eclampsia.*

**vacuum curettage (vacuum aspiration)** *Removal of the uterine contents by application of a vacuum through a hollow curet or cannula introduced into the uterus.*

**vasoconstriction** *Narrowing of the lumen of blood vessels.*

Although childbearing is a normal process, numerous maternal and fetal adaptations must occur in an orderly sequence. If problems develop in these physiologic processes, complications may arise that threaten the well-being of the expectant mother or the fetus, or both. Family physicians or nurse-midwives may be responsible for co-managing women with complications of pregnancy; however, these women are often referred to an obstetrician or a perinatologist or to a perinatal center for management.

Nurses who work at the primary care site or at the perinatal center frequently fill the role of case manager or coordinator of services provided for the woman. Often the nurse is the only consistent provider involved in the woman's care and therefore is the person on whom the woman counts to guide her through the system.

Conditions that complicate pregnancy are divided into two broad categories: (1) those that are related to pregnancy and are not seen at other times and (2) those that could occur at any time but when they occur concurrently with pregnancy may complicate its course. Concurrent conditions that affect pregnancy are considered in Chapter 26.

The most common pregnancy-related complications are hemorrhagic conditions that occur in early pregnancy, hemorrhagic complications of the placenta in late pregnancy, hyperemesis gravidarum, hypertensive disorders of pregnancy, and blood incompatibilities.

# Hemorrhagic Conditions of Early Pregnancy

The three most common causes of hemorrhage during the first half of pregnancy are abortion, ectopic pregnancy, and hydatidiform mole.

## Abortion

Abortion is the loss of pregnancy before the fetus is viable, that is, capable of living outside the uterus. The medical consensus today is that a fetus of less than 20 weeks' gestation or one weighing less than 500 g is not viable; termination of pregnancy before this time is considered to be an abortion. Abortion may be either spontaneous or induced. Lay people often use the term *miscarriage* to denote an abortion that has occurred spontaneously as opposed to one that has been induced. Abortion is the accepted medical term for either, and this point should be clarified in discussions with women to avoid misinterpretation or confusion. Induced abortion is described in Chapter 33.

### SPONTANEOUS ABORTION

Spontaneous abortion is defined as termination of pregnancy without action taken by the woman or any other person.

INCIDENCE AND ETIOLOGY

Determining the exact incidence of spontaneous abortion is difficult because unrecognized losses occur in early pregnancy. However, it is believed that 15 percent of all recognized pregnancies end in spontaneous abortion (Glass & Golbus, 1994). Most spontaneous abortions occur in the first 12 weeks of pregnancy, with the rate declining rapidly thereafter.

The causes of spontaneous abortion are varied; however, the most common cause is genetic abnormalities that are incompatible with life or that would result in gross deformity of the fetus. Spontaneous abortion due to genetic abnormalities may reflect nature's way of extinguishing imperfect embryos. Additional causes include maternal infections such as syphilis, listeriosis, toxoplasmosis, brucellosis, rubella, and cytomegalic inclusion disease. There is inconclusive evidence that genital herpes and *Chlamydia trachomatis* also increase the risk of abortion. (See Chapter 26 for additional information about maternal infections.) Maternal endocrine disorders such as hypothyroidism and abnormalities of the reproductive organs have also been implicated. In addition, immune factors such as antiphospholipid antibodies are currently being investigated.

Spontaneous abortion is divided into six subgroups: threatened, inevitable, incomplete, complete, missed, and recurrent. Figure 25–1 illustrates threatened, inevitable, and incomplete abortion.

THREATENED ABORTION

**Clinical Manifestations.** The first symptom of threatened abortion is vaginal bleeding, which is rather common during pregnancy. Up to 25 percent of all women experience "spotting" or bleeding in early pregnancy. About half of these pregnancies will end in spontaneous abortion, whereas the remainder will progress to term (Cunningham et al., 1997).

Vaginal bleeding may be followed by rhythmic uterine cramping, persistent backache, or feelings of pelvic pressure. These symptoms increase the chance that the threatened abortion will progress to inevitable abortion.

**Therapeutic Management.** Bleeding in the first half of pregnancy must always be considered a threatened abortion, and women should be advised to notify their physician or nurse-midwife whenever vaginal bleeding is noted. When vaginal bleeding is reported, the nurse obtains a detailed history that includes length of gestation and the onset, duration,

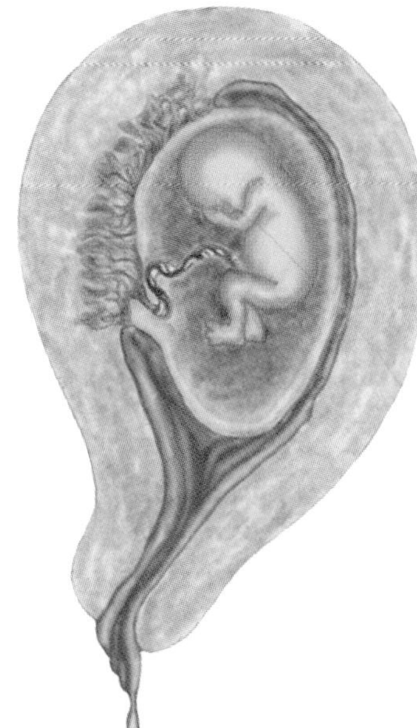
Threatened abortion
Vaginal bleeding occurs.

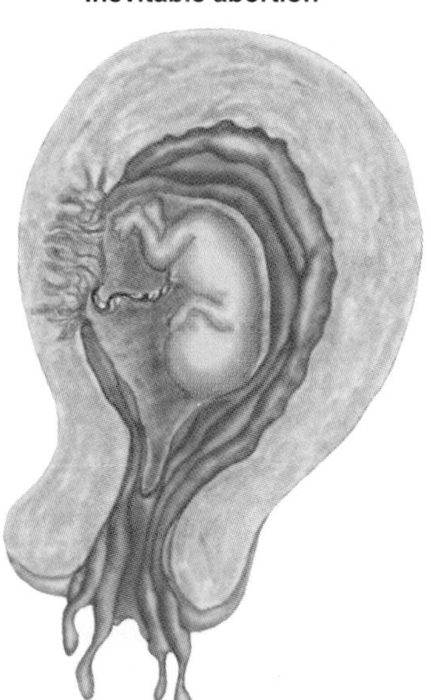
Inevitable abortion
Membranes rupture and cervix dilates.

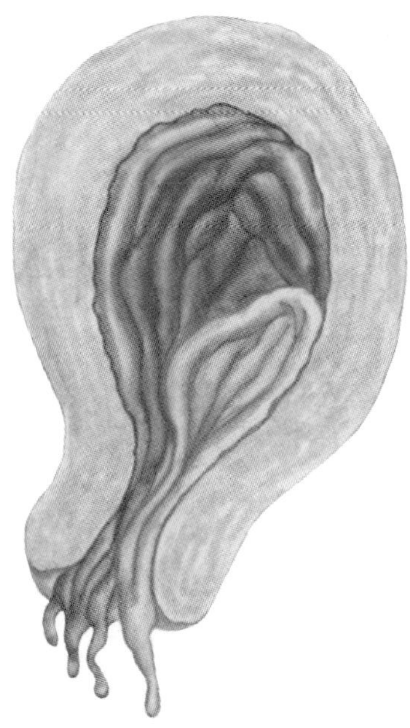
Incomplete abortion
Some products of conception have been expelled, but some remain.

**FIGURE 25–1**

Three types of spontaneous abortion.

and amount of vaginal bleeding. Any accompanying discomfort, such as cramping, backache, or sharp abdominal pain is also evaluated.

Ultrasound examination is often performed to determine whether the fetus is present and, if so, whether it is alive. Although bedrest may be recommended after each bleeding episode, many physicians now believe that there is no valid basis for advising bedrest (Enkin et al., 1995). Therefore, the preference of individual women should be the deciding factor in whether they rest in bed. Some women may wish to rest, and they should be encouraged to do whatever feels best for them.

The woman is advised to curtail sexual activity until bleeding has ceased and for 2 weeks following the last evidence of bleeding, or as recommended by the physician or nurse-midwife. The woman is instructed to count the number of perineal pads used and to note the quantity and color of blood on the pads. She should also look for evidence of passage of tissue.

Bleeding episodes are frightening, and psychological support is very important. The woman often wonders whether her actions may have contributed to the situation and is anxious about her own condition and that of the fetus. The nurse should offer accurate information and avoid false reassurance, because the woman may lose her pregnancy despite every precaution.

#### INEVITABLE ABORTION

**Clinical Manifestations.** Abortion is usually inevitable (that is, it cannot be stopped) when there is rupture of the membranes and dilation of the cervix. Rupture of membranes is generally experienced as a sudden gush of fluid from the vagina followed by uterine contractions and bleeding. If complete evacuation of the products of conception does not occur spontaneously, excessive bleeding or infection can occur.

**Therapeutic Management.** Initial treatment of inevitable abortion involves allowing a natural evacuation of the uterine contents. Vacuum curettage is used to evacuate the uterus if the natural process is ineffective. If the pregnancy is more advanced or if bleeding is excessive, a dilation and curettage (D&C) while the woman is under anesthesia is carried out by the physician.

#### INCOMPLETE ABORTION

**Clinical Manifestations.** Incomplete abortion occurs when some but not all products of conception are expelled from the uterus. The major symptoms are uterine bleeding and severe abdominal cramping. The cervix is open and there is passage of fetal and placental tissue.

**Therapeutic Management.** The retained tissue prevents the uterus from contracting firmly, thus allowing profuse bleeding from uterine blood vessels. Initial treatment should be focused on stabilizing the woman from a cardiovascular standpoint. A blood specimen is drawn for crossmatching and blood typing, and an intravenous line is inserted for fluid replacement. When the woman's condition is stable, a D&C is usually performed to remove the remaining tissue. This procedure may be followed by intravenous administration of oxytocin (Pitocin) or intramuscular administration of methylergonovine (Methergine) to contract the uterus and control bleeding.

A D&C may not be performed if the pregnancy has advanced beyond 14 weeks because of the danger of excessive bleeding. In this case, oxytocin or prostaglandin is administered to stimulate uterine contractions until all products of conception (fetus, membranes, placenta, and amniotic fluid) are expelled.

#### COMPLETE ABORTION

**Clinical Manifestations.** Complete abortion occurs when all products of conception are expelled from the uterus. After passage of all products of conception, uterine contractions and bleeding abate and the cervix closes. The uterus feels smaller than the length of gestation would suggest. The symptoms of pregnancy are no longer present, and the pregnancy test becomes negative.

**Therapeutic Management.** Once complete abortion is confirmed, no additional intervention is required unless excessive bleeding or infection develops. The woman should be advised to rest and to watch for further bleeding, pain, or fever. She should schedule a follow-up visit with her health care provider.

#### MISSED ABORTION

**Clinical Manifestations.** Missed abortion occurs when the fetus dies during the first half of pregnancy but is retained in the uterus. When the fetus dies, the early signs of pregnancy (nausea, breast tenderness, urinary frequency) disappear. Moreover, the uterus not only stops growing but also decreases in size, reflecting the absorption of amniotic fluid and maceration of the fetus.

**Therapeutic Management.** The first step is to confirm death of the fetus by real-time ultrasound examination, which provides reliable information by the sixth week of pregnancy. In addition, serial pregnancy tests should indicate a decline in placental hormone production. Once fetal demise is confirmed, the usual management is to wait 3 to 5 weeks for spontaneous abortion, which occurs in 93 percent of cases (Hayashi & Castillo, 1993). Waiting for the spontaneous expulsion of the pregnancy may be a trying time for the woman, particularly if it takes weeks.

Two major complications of missed abortion are infection and disseminated intravascular coagulation (DIC). If there are signs of uterine infection, such as elevation in temperature, vaginal discharge with a foul odor, or abdominal pain, evacuation of the uterus will be delayed until antibiotic therapy is initiated.

**Disseminated Intravascular Coagulation.** A life-threatening defect in coagulation, DIC may occur if the fetus is retained for a prolonged period. This defect is also associated with abruptio placentae and with pregnancy-induced hypertension. With DIC, anticoagulation and procoagulation factors are activated simultaneously. DIC develops when the clotting factor thromboplastin is released into the maternal blood stream as a result of placental bleeding and consequent clot formation. The circulating thromboplastin activates widespread clotting in small vessels throughout the body. This process consumes or "uses up" other clotting factors such as fibrinogen and platelets. The condition is further complicated by activation of the fibrinolytic system to lyse, or destroy, clots. The net result is a simultaneous decrease in clotting factors and increase in circulating anticoagulants that leaves the circulating blood unable to clot. This allows profuse bleeding to occur from any vulnerable area, such as intravenous sites, incisions, or the gums or nose, as well as from expected sites such as the site of placental attachment during the postpartum period.

Laboratory studies are helpful in establishing a diagnosis. Fibrinogen and platelets are usually decreased, prothrombin and partial thromboplastin time may be prolonged, fibrin degradation products, the most sensitive measurement, are increased.

The priority in treatment of DIC is delivery of the fetus and placenta so that the production of thromboplastin, which is fueling the process, is stopped. In addition, blood replacement products, such as whole blood, packed red blood cells, and cryoprecipitate, are administered to maintain the circulating volume and to transport oxygen to body cells.

### RECURRENT SPONTANEOUS ABORTION

**Clinical Manifestations.** Recurrent spontaneous abortion is sometimes referred to as "habitual" abortion; the current definition is three or more consecutive spontaneous abortions. The primary causes of recurrent abortion are believed to be genetic or chromosomal abnormalities and anomalies of the reproductive tract, such as bicornuate uterus or incompetent cervix. Additional causes include an inadequate luteal phase in which there is insufficient secretion of progesterone and immunologic factors that involve increased sharing of human leukocyte antigens by the sperm and ovum of the man and woman who conceived. The theory is that, because of this sharing, the woman's immunologic system is not stimulated to produce blocking antibodies that protect the embryo from maternal immune cells or other damaging antibodies. Systemic diseases such as lupus erythematosus and diabetes mellitus have been implicated in recurrent abortions. Reproductive infections and some sexually transmissible diseases discussed in Chapter 26 are also associated with recurrent abortions.

**Therapeutic Management.** The first step in management of recurrent spontaneous abortion is a thorough examination of the cervix to determine whether anatomic defects are the cause. If the cervix is normal, the woman is usually referred for genetic screening to determine the presence of genetic factors that would increase the possibility of recurrent abortions.

Additional therapeutic management of recurrent pregnancy loss depends on the cause. For instance, treatment may involve assisting the woman to develop a regimen to maintain normal blood glucose if diabetes mellitus is a factor; administration of appropriate antibiotics is necessary if the cause is infection.

Recurrent spontaneous abortion may be due to cervical incompetence, an anatomic defect that results in painless dilation of the cervix in the second trimester. In this instance, the cervix may be sutured to keep it from opening. The most common procedures are cerclage, McDonald's procedure, or Shirodkar's procedure. These three procedures vary according to the type and placement of the sutures. Sutures are sometimes removed near term in preparation for vaginal delivery; however, they may be left in place if a cesarean birth is planned. Prophylactic antibiotics may be necessary if the woman is judged to be at high risk for infection.

### NURSING CONSIDERATIONS

Nurses must consider the psychological needs of the family experiencing spontaneous abortion. Vaginal bleeding is frightening, and waiting and watching is often difficult, although it may be the only treatment recommended. Moreover, many families feel an acute sense of loss and grief with spontaneous abortion. Grief often includes feelings of guilt that may be expressed in terms of wondering if the woman could have done something to prevent the loss. It is very helpful if nurses emphasize that abortions usually occur as the result of factors or abnormalities that could not be avoided.

Anger, disappointment, and sadness are commonly experienced emotions, although the intensity of the feelings may vary. For many couples the fetus has not yet taken on specific physical characteristics, but they grieve for their fantasies of the unseen, unborn child. The couple may want to express their feelings of sadness but may feel that family, friends, and often health personnel are uncomfortable or unable to provide emotional support after early pregnancy loss.

It is important to recognize the meaning of the loss to each individual family. To do this, nurses must listen carefully to what the couple says and observe how they behave. Nurses must attempt to convey unconditional acceptance of the feelings expressed or demonstrated. The couple should be permitted to remain together as much as possible. Providing information and simple brief explanations of what has occurred and what will be done facilitates the family's ability to grieve.

It is helpful for the family to realize that grief may last from 6 months to a year, or even longer. Family support, knowledge of the grief process, spiritual counselors, and the support of other bereaved couples may provide needed assistance during this time. Chapter 24 provides additional information about pregnancy loss and grief.

**CHECK YOUR READING**

1. What are the signs of threatened abortion, and how do they differ from those of inevitable abortion?
2. What is DIC?
3. What are the major causes of recurrent spontaneous abortion?
4. How can nurses intervene for the grief families experience as a result of early pregnancy loss?

## Ectopic Pregnancy

The term *ectopic pregnancy* refers to implantation of a fertilized ovum in an area outside the uterine cavity. Although implantation can occur in the abdomen or in the cervix, almost 92 percent of ectopic pregnancies are in the fallopian tube (Jehle et al., 1994). Figure 25–2 illustrates common sites of implantation.

Ectopic pregnancy has been called "a disaster of reproduction" for two reasons:

- It remains a leading cause of maternal death from hemorrhage.
- It sharply reduces the woman's chance of subsequent pregnancies because of damage or destruction of a fallopian tube.

### INCIDENCE AND ETIOLOGY

The incidence of ectopic pregnancy has increased dramatically throughout the world in the last 20 years. In the United States, the rate has more than quadrupled, to 14 in every 1000 reported pregnancies. The highest rate is seen in nonwhite women older than 35 years (Cunningham et al., 1997). The rapid increase in incidence is attributed to the growing number of women of childbearing age who experience scarring of the fallopian tubes because of pelvic infection, inflammation, or surgery. Pelvic infection is often due to *Chlamydia* or *Neisseria gonorrhoeae*. Failed tubal ligation and a history of previous ectopic pregnancy also increase the risk for an ectopic pregnancy that implants in the fallopian tube.

In addition, the use of contraception that prevents

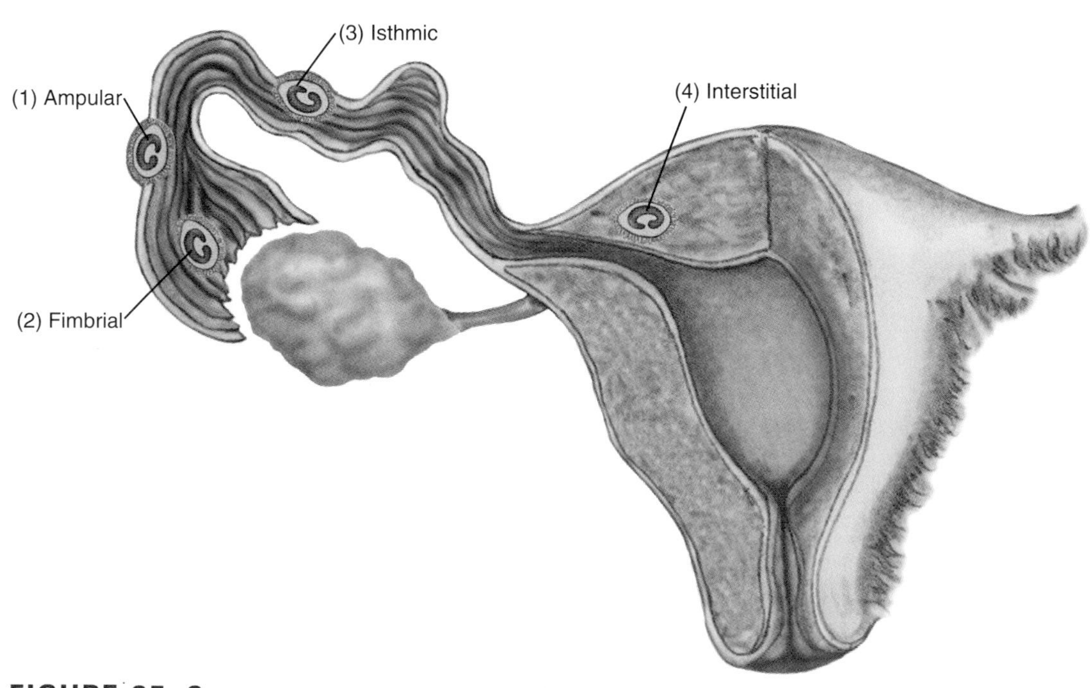


**FIGURE 25–2**

Sites of ectopic pregnancy. Numbers indicate the order of prevalence.

intrauterine pregnancy, such as intrauterine contraceptive devices or low-dose progesterone agents, is associated with increased risk of extrauterine (ectopic) pregnancy (Cunningham et al., 1997). Whether this is due to latent infection or some other mechanism is unknown.

Additional causes of ectopic pregnancy are delayed or premature ovulation, with the tendency of the fertilized ovum to implant before arrival in the uterus, and altered tubal motility in response to changes in estrogen and progesterone levels. Multiple induced abortions are associated with increased risk of tubal pregnancy, possibly because of salpingitis (infection of the fallopian tube) that has occurred following induced abortion. Table 25–1 summarizes the major risk factors for ectopic pregnancy.

Regardless of the cause of ectopic pregnancy, the effect is that transport of the fertilized ovum through the fallopian tube is hampered.

#### CLINICAL MANIFESTATIONS

The classic signs of ectopic pregnancy are the following:

- Missed menstrual period
- Abdominal pain
- Vaginal "spotting"

More subtle signs and symptoms depend on the site of implantation. If implantation occurs in the distal end of the fallopian tube, which is able to accommodate the growing embryo for longer periods of time, the woman may at first exhibit the usual early signs of pregnancy and consider herself to be normally pregnant. Several weeks into the pregnancy, intermittent abdominal pain and small amounts of vaginal bleeding occur that initially could be mistaken for threatened abortion.

If implantation has occurred in the proximal end of the fallopian tube, rupture of the tube may occur within 2 to 3 weeks of the missed period. Symptoms include sudden, severe pain in one of the lower quadrants of the abdomen as the tube tears open and the embryo is expelled into the pelvic cavity, often with profuse hemorrhage. Radiating pain in the shoulder may indicate bleeding into the abdomen caused by phrenic nerve irritation (Jehle et al., 1994). Hypovolemic shock is a major concern because systemic signs of shock may be rapid and extensive without obvious bleeding.

**TABLE 25–1 RISK FACTORS FOR ECTOPIC PREGNANCY**

History of sexually transmissible diseases (gonorrhea, chlamydial infection)
History of pelvic inflammatory disease
History of previous ectopic pregnancies
Failed tubal ligation
Intrauterine device
Multiple induced abortions
Maternal age older than 35 years

#### DIAGNOSIS

The combined use of transvaginal ultrasound examination (described in Chapter 10) and determination of the beta subunit of human chorionic gonadotropin ($\beta$-hCG) are helpful in early detection of ectopic pregnancy. An abnormal pregnancy is suspected if $\beta$-hCG is present but at lower levels than expected. If a gestational sac cannot be visualized when $\beta$-hCG is present, a diagnosis of ectopic pregnancy may be made with great accuracy. Visualization of an intrauterine pregnancy, however, does not absolutely rule out an ectopic pregnancy. It is possible for a woman to have an intrauterine pregnancy and concurrently to have an ectopic pregnancy.

The use of sensitive pregnancy tests and high-resolution ultrasound has largely eliminated invasive tests for ectopic pregnancy. A culdocentesis may be performed when ultrasound is not readily available or when the patient is unstable from a cardiovascular standpoint and rapid surgical intervention is necessary to prevent hypovolemic shock (Jehle et al., 1994). In this procedure, an aspiration needle is inserted through the posterior vaginal wall into the cul-de-sac of Douglas (located between the rectum and the uterus). Aspiration of blood from the cul-de-sac indicates bleeding from rupture of a fallopian tube. Laparoscopy (examination of the peritoneal cavity by means of a laparoscope) may be necessary to diagnose ectopic pregnancy. A characteristic bluish swelling within the tube is the most common finding.

#### THERAPEUTIC MANAGEMENT

Management of tubal pregnancy depends on whether the tube is intact or ruptured. Medical management may be possible if the tube is unruptured. The chemotherapeutic agent methotrexate (a folic acid antagonist that interferes with cell reproduction) is currently recommended as a means of inhibiting cell division in the developing embryo. The primary impetus for medical management is preserving the tube and improving the chance of future fertility.

Surgical management of a tubal pregnancy that is unruptured may involve a linear salpingostomy to salvage the tube (Fig. 25–3). Linear salpingostomy may also be attempted if the tube is ruptured but damage to the tube is minimal. Salvaging the tube is particularly important to women who are concerned about future fertility.

When ectopic pregnancy results in rupture of the fallopian tube, the goal of therapeutic management

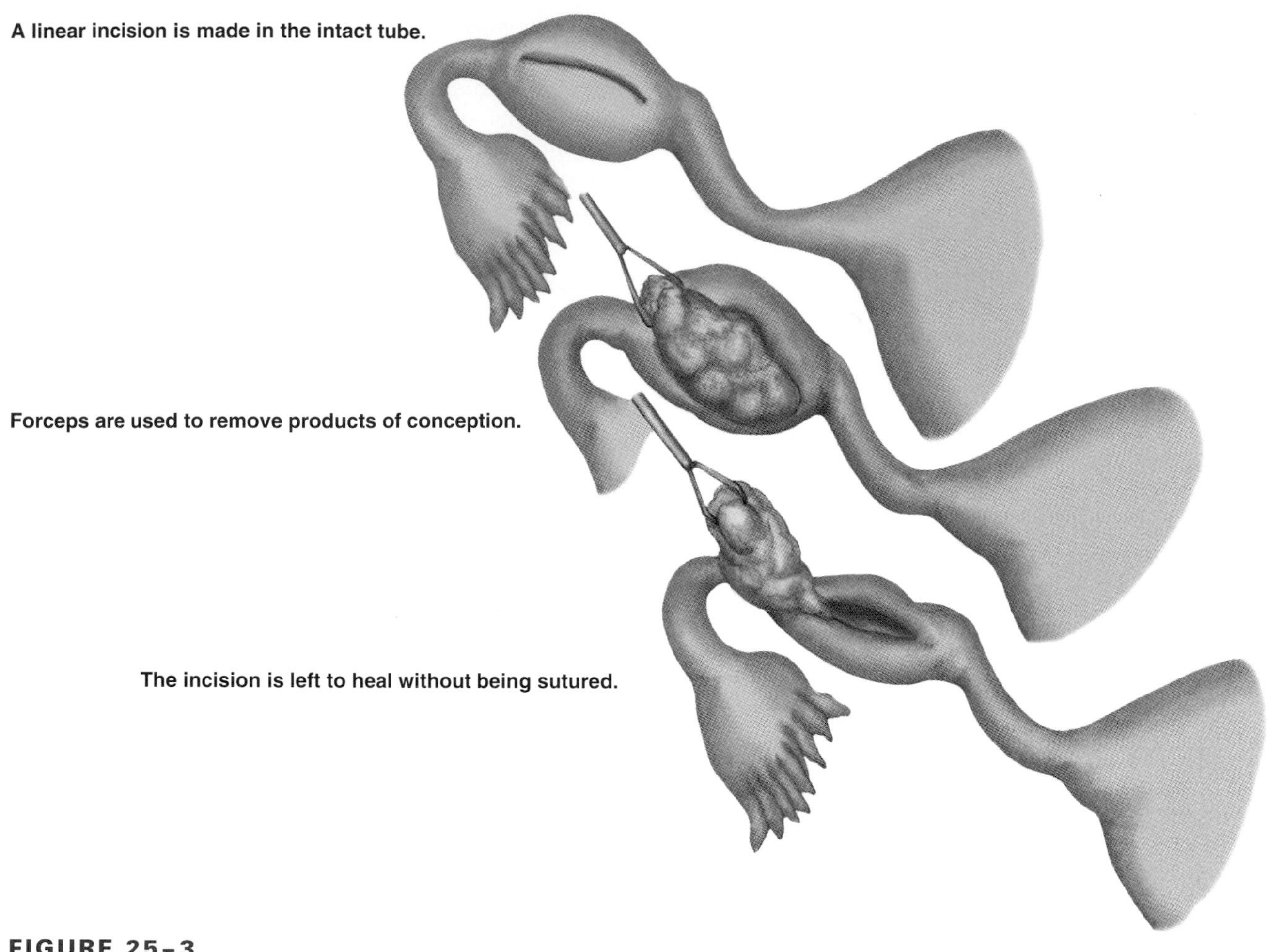
A linear incision is made in the intact tube.
Forceps are used to remove products of conception.
The incision is left to heal without being sutured.

FIGURE 25–3

Linear salpingostomy.

is to control the bleeding and prevent hypovolemic shock. When the woman's cardiovascular status is stable, a salpingectomy is performed to remove the affected tube and to ligate bleeding vessels. Future pregnancies can still occur when only one tube is present; however, the probability of pregnancy declines.

#### NURSING CONSIDERATIONS

Nursing care is focused on preventing or identifying hypovolemic shock, controlling pain, and providing psychological support for the woman who experiences an ectopic pregnancy. Nurses monitor the woman for decreasing hematocrit levels and pain that would indicate a ruptured ectopic pregnancy. Nurses administer analgesics and evaluate their effectiveness so that pain can be controlled.

If methotrexate is used, the nurse must explain adverse side effects, such as nausea and vomiting, and the importance of communicating any physical changes to the health care team. The woman must also be instructed to refrain from drinking alcohol, which decreases effectiveness, ingesting vitamins that contain folic acid, and having sexual intercourse until hCG is not detectable. If the treatment is successful, this hormone disappears from plasma within 2 to 4 weeks (Cunningham et al., 1997). Moreover, the importance of keeping follow-up appointments should be emphasized.

The woman and her family will need psychological support to resolve intense emotions that may include anger, grief, guilt, and self-blame. The woman may also be anxious about her ability to become pregnant in the future, and it may be necessary for nurses to clarify the physician's explanation and to use therapeutic communication techniques that assist the woman to deal with her anxiety.

### Gestational Trophoblastic Disease (Hydatidiform Mole)

Hydatidiform mole is a form of gestational trophoblastic disease that occurs when the trophoblasts (peripheral cells that attach the fertilized ovum to the uterine wall) develop abnormally. As a result of the abnormal growth, the placenta, but not the fetal part of the pregnancy, develops. The condition is characterized by proliferation and edema of the chorionic villi. The fluid-filled villi form grape-like clusters that may grow large enough to fill the uterus to the size of an advanced pregnancy (Fig. 25–4).

### INCIDENCE AND ETIOLOGY

In the United States and Europe, the incidence of hydatidiform mole is 1 in every 1000 pregnancies (Cunningham et al., 1997). Age is also a factor, with the frequency of molar pregnancies highest at both ends of the reproductive life. The incidence is 10 times greater in women older than 45 years (Cunningham et al., 1997). Women who have had one molar pregnancy are at increased risk to have another. About 10 to 20 percent of complete moles advance to invasive, potentially metastatic choriocarcinoma (Kohorn, 1994).

Although there are variations, *complete mole* is believed to occur when the ovum is fertilized by a sperm that duplicates its own chromosomes while the chromosomes of the ovum are inactivated. In a *partial mole*, the maternal contribution is usually present but the paternal contribution is double, and thus the karyotype is triploid (69,XXY or 69,XYY).

### CLINICAL MANIFESTATIONS

The most common signs and symptoms of molar pregnancy include the following:

- Elevated levels of hCG.
- Vaginal bleeding, which varies from dark-brown spotting to profuse hemorrhage.
- A uterus that is larger than one would expect based on the duration of the pregnancy. For instance, at 10 weeks of gestation, the uterus may be palpated midway between the symphysis and the umbilicus, which is consistent with a pregnancy of 16 weeks.
- Failure to detect fetal heart activity even with sensitive instruments.
- Excessive nausea and vomiting (hyperemesis gravidarum), which may be related to excessive hCG from the proliferating trophoblasts.
- Early development of pregnancy-induced hypertension, which is rarely diagnosed before 24 weeks in an otherwise normal pregnancy.

### DIAGNOSIS

Ultrasound examination allows a differential diagnosis to be made between two types of molar pregnancies: (1) a partial mole that includes some fetal tissue and membranes and (2) a complete mole that is composed only of enlarged villi and contains no fetal tissue or membranes.

### THERAPEUTIC MANAGEMENT

Medical management includes two phases: (1) immediate evacuation of the mole and (2) continuous follow-up of the woman to detect any malignant changes of the remaining trophoblastic tissue. Before evacuation, chest radiography, computed tomography, or magnetic resonance imaging may be per-

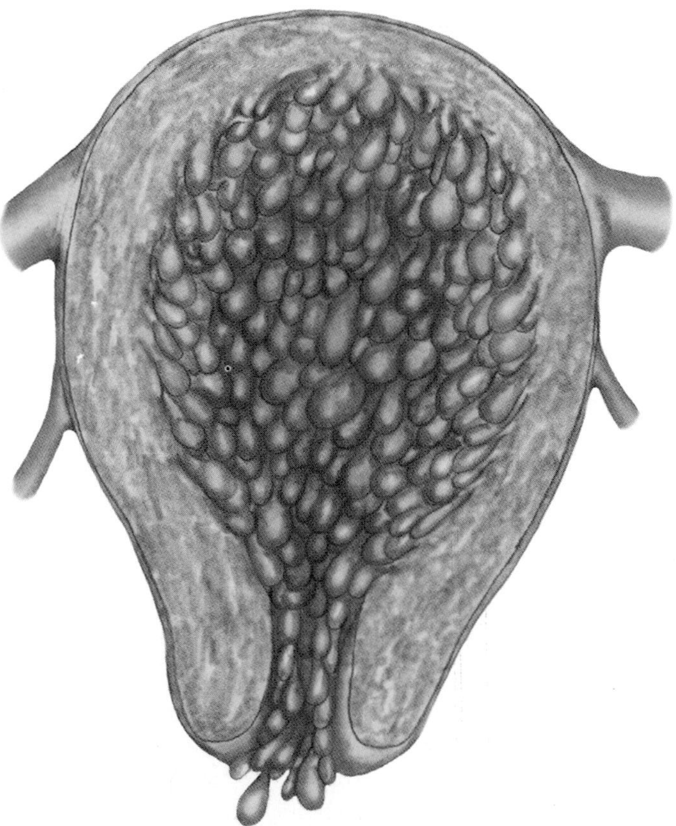

**FIGURE 25–4**
Hydatidiform mole.

formed to detect metastatic disease. A complete blood count, laboratory assessment of clotting factors, and blood typing and crossmatching are also necessary in case a transfusion is needed.

Most often, vacuum aspiration is used to extract the mole. After tissue has been removed, intravenous oxytocin can be used to contract the uterus. It is important to avoid uterine stimulation with oxytocin before evacuation. Uterine contractions can cause trophoblastic tissue to be engulfed by the large venous sinusoids in the uterus, resulting in pulmonary embolus (Berman & Disaia, 1994). Curettage follows the evacuation, and the tissue obtained is sent for careful laboratory evaluation. This is extremely important because, although a hydatidiform mole is usually a benign process, choriocarcinoma is sometimes a complication.

Follow-up is critical to detect any changes suggestive of trophoblastic malignancy. Follow-up protocol involves evaluation of serum chorionic gonadotropin levels every 1 to 2 weeks until normal pre-pregnancy levels are attained. The test is repeated every 1 to 2 months for a year. Pregnancy must be avoided during the 1 year follow-up because it would obscure the evidence of choriocarcinoma. Affected women should also be advised that oral contraceptives are safe to use but that intrauterine devices may cause irregular bleeding and should not be used.

#### NURSING CONSIDERATIONS

Women who have had a hydatidiform mole experience many of the same emotions as those who have had any other type of pregnancy loss. In addition, they may be anxious about follow-up evaluations and the need to delay pregnancy for at least a year.

### ✓ CHECK YOUR READING

5. Why is ectopic pregnancy called a "disaster of reproduction"?
6. Why is the incidence of ectopic pregnancy increasing in the United States? How is it treated?
7. What is a hydatidiform mole, and why are two phases of treatment necessary?

## Application of Nursing Process: Hemorrhagic Conditions of Early Pregnancy

Regardless of the cause of antepartum bleeding, nurses play a vital role in its management. Nurses are responsible for monitoring the condition of the pregnant woman and for collaborating with the physician to provide treatment.

### Assessment

Confirmation of pregnancy and length of gestation are important initial data to obtain. Physical assessment focuses on determining the amount of bleeding and the description, location, and severity of pain. Estimate the amount of vaginal bleeding by examining linen and peripads. If necessary, make a more accurate estimation by weighing the linen and peripads (1 g weight equals 1 ml volume).

**When asking a woman how much blood she lost at home, ask her to compare the amount lost with a common measure such as a tablespoon or a cup. Ask also how long the bleeding episode lasted and what has been done to control the bleeding.**

Bleeding may be accompanied by pain. Uterine cramping usually accompanies spontaneous abortion; deep, severe pelvic pain is associated with ectopic pregnancy. Remember that in ruptured ectopic pregnancy, bleeding may be concealed and pain is the only symptom.

Assess the woman's vital signs to determine her cardiovascular status. Check laboratory values for hemoglobin and hematocrit and report abnormal values to the health care provider. Determine the Rh factor so that all women who are Rh-negative can receive $Rh_0(D)$ immune globulin. Additional information about $Rh_0(D)$ immune globulin appears in the discussion of Rh incompatibility (p. 703).

Moreover, because abortion may be associated with infections, assess the woman for fever, malaise, and prolonged or malodorous vaginal discharge.

Determine the family's knowledge of needed follow-up care and how to prevent complications such as infection.

### Analysis

Nursing diagnoses are, of course, based on information obtained during assessment. A variety of complications and nursing diagnoses are possible. These include the possibility of Hypovolemic Shock (see p. 688) and Risk for Infection. A more complete diagnosis might be Knowledge Deficit of diagnostic and therapeutic procedures, signs and symptoms of infection, dietary measures to prevent infection, and recommended follow-up care.

### Planning

Goals for this nursing diagnosis are that the woman will do the following:

- Verbalize understanding of diagnostic and therapeutic procedures.

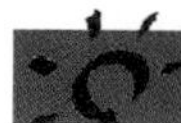

## CRITICAL THINKING EXERCISE

All women who have experienced prenatal bleeding and invasive procedures are at increased risk for infection.

**Q:** What common assumptions do nurses make about those who are at risk for developing infections?

**A:** Nurses often assume that patients know how to use a thermometer and that they know the signs of infection. Moreover, many nurses assume that patients realize the connection between blood loss and the tendency to develop infection. As a result, nurses may not emphasize the need for a diet that is high in nutrients that increase hemoglobin and hematocrit.

- Verbalize signs of infection that should be reported to the health care provider.
- Develop a plan for obtaining follow-up care.

### Interventions

#### PROVIDING INFORMATION ABOUT TESTS AND PROCEDURES

Women and their families experience less anxiety if they understand what is happening. Explain necessary diagnostic procedures, such as transvaginal or transabdominal ultrasonography (see Chapter 10). Include the purpose of the tests, how long they will take, and whether the procedures cause discomfort. If surgical intervention is necessary, explain anesthesia or analgesia that may be administered. Briefly describe the reasons for blood tests such as hCG, hemoglobin, or hematocrit. Explain that diagnostic and therapeutic measures are performed quickly at times to prevent excessive bleeding.

#### TEACHING MEASURES TO PREVENT INFECTION

The risk for infection is greatest during the first 72 hours following spontaneous abortion or operative procedures; however, most women are discharged within a few hours. Ensure that the woman knows how to use a thermometer, and instruct her to take her temperature every 8 hours for the first 3 days at home.

Personal hygiene should include careful hand washing before and after changing perineal pads and daily showers. Perineal pads instead of tampons should be used until bleeding has subsided. The woman should consult with the health care provider before sexual intercourse is resumed.

#### PROVIDING DIETARY INFORMATION

Nutrition and adequate fluid intake play a vital role in maintaining the body's defense against infection, and the nurse must promote adequate diet. The woman who is at risk for infection needs foods that are high in iron to increase hemoglobin and hematocrit values. These foods include liver, red meat, spinach, egg yolks, carrots, and raisins. In addition, she needs foods that are high in vitamin C, which increases the utilization of iron (Mahan & Escott-Stump, 1996). These foods include citrus fruits, broccoli, strawberries, cantaloupe, cabbage, and green peppers. Adequate fluid intake (2500 ml per day) helps prevent dehydration after bleeding episodes and maintains digestive processes.

Iron supplementation is also frequently prescribed, and the woman may require information on how to lessen the gastrointestinal upsets that many people experience when iron is administered. Less gastric upset is experienced when iron is taken with meals, and a diet that is high in fiber and fluid helps to reduce constipation that is an associated problem for many.

#### TEACHING SIGNS OF INFECTION TO REPORT

Instruct the woman to seek medical help if her temperature goes above 37.8°C (100°F). She should also report additional signs of infection, such as vaginal discharge with foul odor, pelvic tenderness, or general malaise, to the health care provider so that treatment can be initiated.

#### RECOMMENDING FOLLOW-UP CARE

A variety of follow-up procedures such as repeat ultrasonic examinations or serum hCG levels may be necessary. Genetic testing and counseling may be advisable. The couple who experiences recurrent abortions may become involved in complex investigations of immunologic or genetic abnormalities. Moreover, all couples who have had a pregnancy loss should be seen and counseled.

At this time, answer questions that the couple has about the cause of pregnancy loss and the chances of reproductive success. Acknowledge their grief, which often manifests as anger. Many women have guilt feelings that must be recognized. They often need repeated reassurance that the loss was not due to anything they did or to anything they neglected.

### Evaluation

Interventions are judged successful if the family does the following:

- Verbalizes comprehension of diagnostic and therapeutic procedures.
- Verbalizes hygienic and dietary measures that reduce the risk of infection.
- Verbalizes signs of infection that should be reported to a health care professional.
- Develops and complies with a follow-up plan of care.

## CRITICAL THINKING EXERCISE

Alice Starkey, a 24-year-old primigravida, experienced an incomplete abortion at 12 weeks' gestation. When she was admitted to the hospital, intravenous fluids were administered and blood was taken for blood grouping and cross-matching. General anesthesia was administered, and a D&C was performed to remove retained placental tissue. When bleeding subsided, Alice was discharged to go home. Helen Clabo, the nurse providing discharge instructions, comments to Alice, "These things happen for the best, and you are so lucky it happened early." "You can have other children."

**Q:**

1. What assumptions has Helen made? How do these affect Alice?
2. Is the comment that Alice can have other children comforting? Why not?
3. What responses from the nurse would be most helpful for Alice?

**A:**

1. Many people wrongly assume that early pregnancy loss does not produce the grieving that accompanies loss at a later stage. Telling Alice that she is lucky ignores her feelings and invalidates the grief she feels.
2. The nurse also mistakenly assumes that there is little cause for grief over the loss of this one if later children are possible. However, there is a unique relationship between Alice and this fetus. Alice may experience an emotional upheaval when this special relationship comes to an abrupt end.
3. It would be beneficial if Helen examined her assumptions before having the interaction with Alice. She might then allow Alice to express her feelings and acknowledge the grief that she is feeling.

# Hemorrhagic Conditions of Late Pregnancy

After 20 weeks of pregnancy, the two major causes of hemorrhage are the disorders of the placenta called placenta previa and abruptio placentae. Abruptio placentae may be further complicated by DIC.

## Placenta Previa

Placenta previa is defined as implantation of the placenta in the lower uterine segment. As a result, it is closer to the cervical os than the presenting part (usually the head) of the fetus. The three classifications of placenta previa (total, partial, and marginal) depend on how much of the cervical os is covered by the placenta (Fig. 25–5).

Marginal or low-lying placentas (implanted in the lower uterine segment but not extending to the cervical os) that are found on early ultrasound examinations frequently "move" upward and away from the internal cervical os as the pregnancy develops. Follow-up ultrasonography is performed to locate the placenta and to determine whether the problem of marginal or low-lying placenta resolves during the last weeks of pregnancy.

### INCIDENCE AND ETIOLOGY

In the United States, the incidence of placenta previa averages 1 in 200 to 250 pregnancies. It is much more common in multiparas, in women who have had a cesarean birth, and in women who have had multiple early pregnancy terminations. The groups at highest risk are those who have had previous placenta previa and those who have had multiple prior cesarean births (Green, 1994).

Marginal

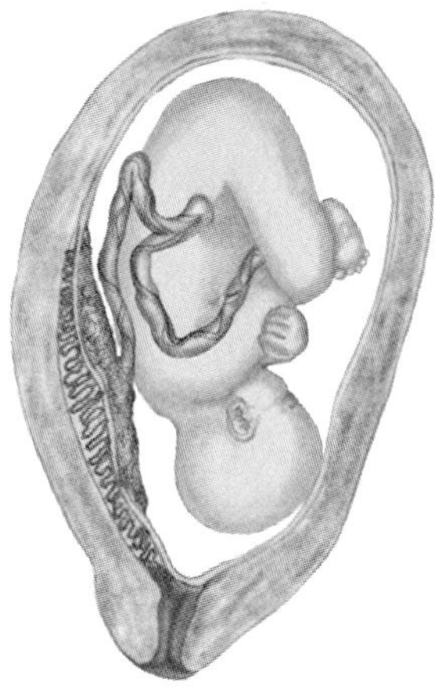

Placenta barely extends to cervical os.

Partial

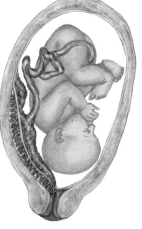

Placenta partially covers cervical os.

Total

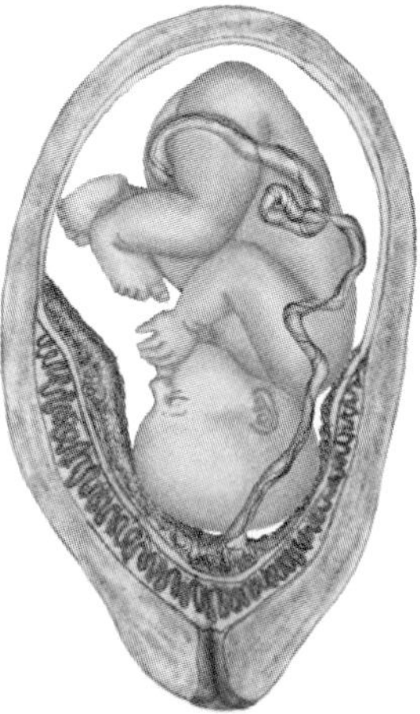

Placenta completely covers cervical os.

**FIGURE 25–5**

The three classifications of placenta previa.

### CLINICAL MANIFESTATIONS

The classic sign of placenta previa is the sudden onset of painless uterine bleeding in the latter half of pregnancy; however, many cases of placenta previa are diagnosed by ultrasound examination before the onset of bleeding. Bleeding occurs when the placental villi are torn from the uterine wall, resulting in hemorrhage from the uterine vessels. Bleeding is painless because it is not occurring in a closed cavity and does not cause pressure on adjacent tissue; it may be scanty or profuse, and it may cease spontaneously, only to recur later.

Bleeding may not occur until labor starts, when cervical changes disrupt placental attachment. The admitting nurse may be unsure whether the bleeding is heavy "bloody show" or a sign of a placenta previa.

*If there is any doubt, the nurse never performs a vaginal examination or takes any action that would stimulate uterine activity.* Digital examination of the cervical os when a placenta previa is present can cause additional placental separation or tear the placenta itself, causing severe hemorrhage and extreme risk to the fetus. Until the location and position of the placenta are verified by ultrasonography, no manual examinations should be performed, and administration of oxytocin should be postponed to prevent strong contractions that could result in sudden placental separation and rapid hemorrhage.

### THERAPEUTIC MANAGEMENT

When the diagnosis of placenta previa is confirmed, medical interventions are based on the condition of the expectant mother and fetus. The woman is evaluated carefully to determine the amount of hemorrhage, and electronic fetal monitoring is initiated to determine the condition of the fetus.

Options for management include conservative management if the mother's cardiovascular status is stable and the fetus is immature and without signs of distress. Conservative management may take place in the home or in the hospital.

**Home Care.** When the mother's condition permits, home care may be initiated. Criteria for home care include the following:

- No evidence of active bleeding.
- No evidence of signs and symptoms of preterm labor.
- Home is no more than 15 to 20 minutes from the hospital.
- Emergency support systems are in place for immediate transport to the hospital (Simpson, 1992).

Nurses are often responsible for helping the family develop a plan of care that includes strict bedrest, the presence of a responsible adult at all times, and ready transportation to the hospital. Nurses must teach the mother and the family what to monitor and emphasize the importance of (1) assessing vaginal discharge or bleeding after each urination or bowel movement or more often as needed, (2) counting fetal movement daily, (3) assessing uterine activity daily, and (4) curtailing sexual intercourse to prevent disruption of the placenta. Nurses are often responsible for making daily phone contact for assessments of uterine activity (cramping, regular or sporadic contractions), bleeding, fetal activity, and adherence to the prescribed treatment plan. In addition, they make regular home visits for comprehensive maternal-fetal assessments, including nonstress tests. The family is instructed to report at once whether fetal movements decrease or uterine contractions or vaginal bleeding occurs.

Nurses are also responsible for providing specific, accurate information about the condition of the fetus. For example, parents are reassured when they hear that the fetal heart rate is within the expected range and daily "kick counts" indicate the fetus is not in distress. Moreover, it may be necessary for nurses to help the family understand the physician's plan of care. For instance, they may explain why a cesarean birth is necessary when the placenta extends over the cervical os.

**Inpatient Care.** Women with placenta previa are admitted to the antepartum unit if they do not meet the criteria for home care or if they require constant assessment and care. When the expectant mother is confined to the hospital, nursing assessments are focused on determining whether she experiences bleeding episodes or signs of preterm labor. Periodic electronic fetal monitoring is necessary to determine whether there are changes in fetal heart activity that indicate fetal distress. A significant change in fetal heart activity, an episode of vaginal bleeding, or signs of preterm labor should be reported immediately to the physician.

At times conservative management is not an option. For instance, delivery is scheduled if the fetus is older than 36 weeks' gestation and the lungs are mature. Immediate delivery may be necessary regardless of fetal immaturity if bleeding is excessive, the woman demonstrates signs of hypovolemia, or there are signs of fetal compromise.

If cesarean birth becomes necessary, nurses must prepare the expectant mother for surgery. Preparation includes inserting an indwelling urinary catheter, confirming that appropriate preoperative permission forms are signed, validating that blood typing and crossmatching have been done, and starting intravenous fluids as directed by the physician.

The preoperative procedures are often performed quickly, and the family may become anxious and concerned about the condition of the fetus and the expectant mother. Nurses must use whatever time is available to keep the family informed.

**During the rapid preparations for surgery, the nurse can reassure both the woman and the family by briefly describing the necessary preparations: "I'm sorry we have to rush, but we need to start the IV in case she needs extra fluids." "Do you have questions I might answer as we prepare for the cesarean?"**

## Abruptio Placentae

Separation of a normally implanted placenta before the fetus is delivered (called abruptio placentae, placental abruption, or premature separation of the placenta) occurs when there is bleeding and formation of a hematoma (clot) on the maternal side of the placenta. As the clot expands, further separation occurs. Hemorrhage may be apparent (vaginal bleeding) or concealed. The severity of the complication depends on the amount of bleeding and the size of the hematoma. If there is continued bleeding, the hematoma expands and obliterates intervillous spaces. Moreover, fetal vessels will be disrupted as placental separation occurs, and there is fetal as well as maternal bleeding.

Abruptio placentae is a dangerous condition for both the pregnant woman and the fetus. The major danger for the woman is hemorrhage and consequent hypovolemic shock and clotting abnormalities (see disseminated intravascular coagulation, p. 675). The major dangers for the fetus are anoxia, excessive blood loss, and delivery before the fetus is mature enough to survive.

### INCIDENCE AND ETIOLOGY

Published incidence of abruptio placentae varies widely; however, it probably averages about 1 in 200 deliveries. Placental abruption extensive enough to cause the death of the fetus has declined to about 1 in 830 deliveries (Cunningham et al., 1997).

The cause is unknown; however, several factors that increase the risk have been identified. The risk factors include maternal hypertension, maternal cigarette smoking, multigravida status, short umbilical cord, abdominal trauma, and history of previous premature separation of the placenta. Maternal use of cocaine, which causes vasoconstriction in the endometrial arteries, is one of the leading causes of abruptio placentae.

### CLINICAL MANIFESTATIONS

The four classic signs and symptoms of abruptio placentae are the following:

- Vaginal bleeding
- Abdominal pain
- Uterine hyperactivity with poor relaxation between contractions
- Uterine tenderness

Additional signs include back pain, fetal distress, signs of hypovolemic shock, and fetal death.

Cases of abruptio placentae are divided into two main types: (1) those in which hemorrhage is concealed and (2) those in which hemorrhage is apparent. In either type, the placental abruption may be complete or partial. Concealed hemorrhage occurs when there is bleeding behind the placenta but the margins remain intact, causing formation of a hematoma. The hemorrhage is apparent when bleeding separates or dissects the membranes from the endometrium and blood flows out through the vagina. Figure 25–6 illustrates abruptio placentae with external and concealed bleeding. Appar-

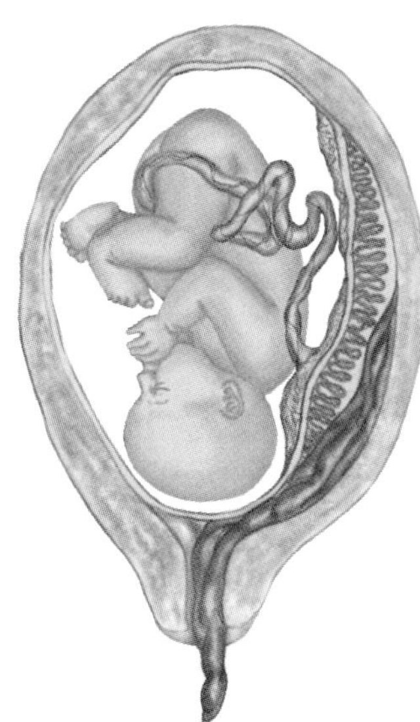


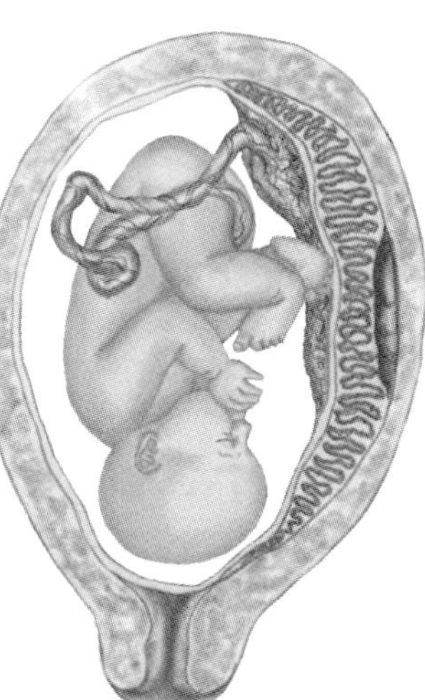


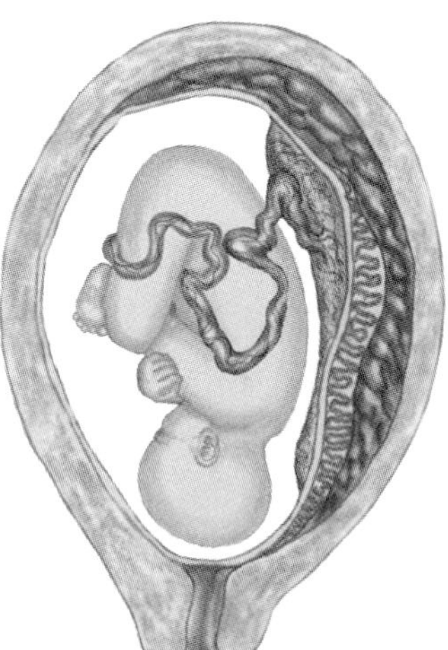


**FIGURE 25–6**

Types of abruptio placentae.

ent bleeding does not indicate the actual amount of blood lost, and signs of shock (tachycardia, hypotension, pale color, and cold, clammy skin) may be present when there is little or no external bleeding.

Abdominal pain is also related to the type of separation. It may be sudden and severe when there is bleeding into the myometrium (uterine muscle) or intermittent and difficult to distinguish from labor contractions. The abdomen may become exceedingly firm (board-like) and tender, making palpation of the fetus difficult. Ultrasound examination is helpful to rule out placenta previa as the cause of bleeding, but it cannot be used to diagnose abruptio placentae because the separation and bleeding may not be obvious on ultrasonography.

#### THERAPEUTIC MANAGEMENT

Any woman who exhibits signs of abruptio placentae should be hospitalized and evaluated at once. Evaluation focuses on the condition of the fetus and the cardiovascular status of the expectant mother. If the condition is mild and the fetus is immature and shows no signs of distress, conservative management may be initiated. This includes bedrest and may include administration of tocolytic medications to decrease uterine activity (Green, 1994). Conservative management is rare, however, owing to the great risks of fetal death and maternal hemorrhage associated with abruptio placentae.

Immediate delivery of the fetus is necessary if there are signs of fetal compromise or if the expectant mother exhibits signs of excessive bleeding, either obvious or concealed. Intensive monitoring of both the woman and the fetus is essential because rapid deterioration of either can occur. Blood products for replacement should be available, and two large-bore intravenous lines should be secured for replacement of fluid and blood.

#### NURSING CONSIDERATIONS

Abruptio placentae is extremely frightening for the woman. She experiences severe pain and is aware of the danger to herself and to the fetus. She must be carefully assessed for signs of concealed hemorrhage.

If immediate cesarean delivery is necessary, the woman may feel powerless as the health care team hurriedly prepares her for surgery. If it is at all possible in the time available, nurses must explain anticipated procedures to the woman and her family to reduce their feelings of fear and anxiety.

Excessive bleeding and fetal hypoxia are always major concerns with abruptio placentae, and nurses are responsible for continuous monitoring of both the expectant mother and the fetus so that problems can be detected early before the condition of the woman or the fetus deteriorates.

**Critical to Remember**

**SIGNS OF CONCEALED HEMORRHAGE**

- Increase in fundal height
- Hard, board-like abdomen
- High uterine base tone on electronic monitoring strip
- Persistent abdominal pain
- Systemic signs of early hemorrhage (tachycardia, falling blood pressure, restlessness)
- Persistent late deceleration in fetal heart rate or decreasing baseline variability
- Vaginal bleeding may be slight or absent

**CHECK YOUR READING**

8. What are the signs and symptoms of placenta previa? How is it managed in the home?
9. What are the signs and symptoms of abruptio placentae?
10. What are the major dangers to the expectant mother and the fetus during the placental abruption?

## Application of Nursing Process: Hemorrhagic Conditions of Late Pregnancy

### Assessment

For hemorrhagic conditions of late pregnancy, some nursing assessments should be performed immediately and others can be deferred until initial measures have been taken to stabilize the cardiovascular status of the woman. The priority nursing assessments are the following:

- *Amount and nature of bleeding.* Time of onset, estimated blood loss before admission to hospital, and description of tissue or clots passed. Peripads and linen savers should be saved so that blood loss can be estimated accurately.
- *Pain.* Type (constant, intermittent, sharp, dull, severe), onset (sudden, gradual), and location (generalized over abdomen, localized). Is the uterus tender to gentle palpation?
- *Maternal vital signs.* Within normal limits, deviation from baseline.
- *Condition of the fetus.* Application of an electronic monitor to determine fetal heart rate, baseline variability, and fetal response to uterine activity

(late decelerations or loss of baseline variability are of particular concern).

- *Uterine contractions*. Application of a monitor to determine uterine resting tone and frequency and duration of contractions. A uterus that does not relax between contractions and frequent, long contractions are associated with abruptio placentae.
- *Obstetric history*. Gravida, para, previous abortions, preterm infants, previous pregnancy outcomes.
- *Length of gestation*. Date of last menstrual period, fundal height, correlation of fundal height with estimated gestation. *If there is bleeding into the myometrium, the fundus enlarges rapidly as bleeding progresses.* Some nurses use a piece of tape to mark the top of the fundus at a given time and then observe and report increasing fundal size, which indicates that bleeding into uterine muscles is occurring.
- *Laboratory data*. Hemoglobin, hematocrit, clotting factors, blood type, partial thromboplastin time, and clotting time. Laboratory data are obtained to prepare for transfusions should they become necessary and to determine whether signs of DIC are developing.

Despite the emphasis on physical assessment, the emotional response of the expectant mother and her partner must also be addressed. They will most likely be anxious, fearful, confused, and overwhelmed by the activity. They may have very little knowledge of expected medical management and may not realize that the fetus will need to be delivered as quickly as possible and that a surgical procedure is necessary. Moreover, they may fear for the life of the woman and the fetus.

### Analysis

Nursing diagnoses vary, depending on the cause and severity of the bleeding. The most commonly used nursing diagnoses for antepartum bleeding appear in Nursing Care Plan 25–1. The most dangerous potential complication is *hypovolemic shock*, which jeopardizes the life of the mother as well as the fetus.

## Nursing Care Plan 25–1
## Antepartum Bleeding

ASSESSMENT: Beth Dixon, a 28-year-old gravida 2, para 1, is admitted to the antepartum unit following an episode of vaginal bleeding that has been diagnosed as being due to total placenta previa. Vital signs are stable, and fetal heart rate is 140 beats per minute with no signs of distress. The gestational age is estimated to be 34 weeks. Beth and her husband, Bob, appear anxious about the condition of the fetus and the plan of care. Beth is particularly worried about her 5-year-old son who is at home with a neighbor.

NURSING DIAGNOSIS: Anxiety related to unknown effects of bleeding and lack of knowledge of predicted course of management

**Critical Thinking**

Although this diagnosis is correct, what are priority nursing actions for Beth? Why?

**ANSWER**

To monitor the condition of the fetus and to observe Beth for vaginal bleeding or change in vital signs. These priorities are based on a hierarchy of needs; physiologic needs and the need for safety must be ensured before psychological needs are addressed.

GOALS/EXPECTED OUTCOMES

1. The couple will verbalize expected routines and projected management by the end of the first day following admission.
2. The couple will relate less anxiety following teaching.

| INTERVENTION | RATIONALE |
|---|---|
| 1. Remain with the couple and acknowledge the emotions that they exhibit: "I know this is unexpected, and you must have many questions; perhaps I can answer some of them." | 1. The nurse's presence and empathetic understanding are potent therapeutic tools to prepare the family to cope with the unexpected situation. |
| 2. Determine the couple's level of understanding of the situation and the projected management: "Tell me what you've been told to expect." | 2. Allows the nurse to reinforce the physician's explanations and to notify the physician if additional explanations are necessary. |

## Nursing Care Plan 25–1 *Continued*

# Antepartum Bleeding

| INTERVENTION | RATIONALE |
|---|---|
| 3. Provide the couple with factual information about projected management.<br>a. Explain that Beth will need to remain in the hospital so that her condition and the condition of the fetus can be watched closely.<br>b. Explain why a cesarean birth is necessary this time even though she delivered vaginally before.<br>c. Provide information about hospital routines (meals, visiting hours) and monitoring techniques that will be used (electronic fetal monitoring, nonstress tests). | 3. Patient education has proved to be an effective measure for preventing and reducing anxiety. |
| 4. Allow Beth and her family to participate in the routine as much as possible. This may mean scheduling procedures around times when Tom and their son can visit. | 4. Many women feel a sense of powerlessness when they are confined to bed and a course of treatment is prescribed without consultation. |

### EVALUATION

The interventions are judged to be successful if the couple demonstrates knowledge of the projected management and why it is necessary and verbalizes reduced anxiety.

**ASSESSMENT:** Although Beth has no more episodes of vaginal bleeding, she cries frequently. She tells the nurse, "I miss my son so much. He just started kindergarten and he is so shy. I feel useless and he really needs me now. It's hard on Bob, too; he has to do everything."

**NURSING DIAGNOSIS:** Situational Low Self-Esteem related to temporary inability to provide care for family

### GOALS/EXPECTED OUTCOMES

Beth will do the following:

1. Identify positive aspects of self during hospitalization.
2. Identify ways of providing comfort and affection for her son during the hospital stay.

| INTERVENTION | RATIONALE |
|---|---|
| 1. Encourage Beth to express her concerns about the need for hospitalization: "What bothers you most about being away from home?" | 1. Major concerns may not be identified or may be misunderstood unless the woman clarifies them. |
| 2. After acknowledging feelings, encourage examination of the need for hospitalization and its consequences: it provides time for the fetus to mature. | 2. Identifies positive aspects of the situation and her important role. |
| 3. Explore reality of Beth's self-appraisal ("I feel useless") by assisting her to investigate ways to provide nurturing care for her son while she is hospitalized:<br>a. Keep in close touch by telephone (wake-up, good-night, and after-school calls).<br>b. Make small handmade items such as book marks.<br>c. Explain in simple, nonfrightening terms why she must stay in the hospital.<br>d. Offer reassurances of continued love. | 3. Daily involvement in the life of the child helps reduce feelings of isolation and failure to meet obligations to her family. |
| 4. Assist Beth to involve her son in plans for the newborn. He might benefit from sibling classes or playtime with the mother that involves caring for dolls. | 4. Provides goals for combined family interaction that increase feeling of self-worth. |

### EVALUATION

Beth is able to make positive comments about the importance of bedrest to the health of the fetus, and she initiates numerous activities that permit her to continue close, comforting contact with her child during the period of hospitalization.

### ADDITIONAL NURSING DIAGNOSES TO CONSIDER

Risk for Altered Family Processes
Diversional Activity Deficit
Fear

## Planning

The nurse cannot independently manage hypovolemic shock but must confer with physicians for medical orders for treatment. Planning should reflect the nurse's responsibility to do the following:

- Monitor for signs of hypovolemic shock.
- Consult with the physician if signs of hypovolemic shock are observed.
- Perform actions to minimize the effects of hypovolemic shock.

## Interventions

### MONITORING FOR SIGNS OF HYPOVOLEMIC SHOCK

Assess for any sign of developing hypovolemic shock. The body attempts to compensate for decreased blood volume and to maintain oxygenation of essential organs by increasing the rate and effort of the heart and lungs and by shunting blood from less essential organs, such as the skin and the extremities, to more essential organs, such as the brain and the kidneys. This compensatory mechanism results in the early signs and symptoms of hypovolemic shock:

- Tachycardia, diminished peripheral pulses
- Normal or slightly decreased blood pressure
- Increased respiratory rate
- Cool, pale skin and mucous membranes

The compensatory mechanism fails if hypovolemic shock progresses and there is insufficient blood to perfuse the brain, heart, and kidneys. Later signs of hypovolemic shock include the following:

- Falling blood pressure
- Pallor, skin becomes cold and clammy
- Urine output less than 30 ml per hour
- Restlessness, agitation, decreased mentation

**Critical to Remember**

**SIGNS AND SYMPTOMS OF IMPENDING HYPOVOLEMIC SHOCK**

- Increased pulse rate, falling blood pressure, increased respiratory rate
- Weak, diminished, or "thready" peripheral pulses
- Cool, moist skin, pallor, or cyanosis (late sign)
- Decreased urinary output (<30 ml/hr)
- Decreased hemoglobin, hematocrit levels
- Change in mental status (restlessness, agitation, difficulty concentrating)

### MONITORING THE FETUS

If possible, initiate continuous electronic fetal monitoring so that signs of fetal distress, such as decreasing baseline variability or late deceleration, can be seen (see Chapter 14). If fetal distress is noted, contact the physician at once because the fetus sometimes experiences distress before maternal signs of hemorrhage or hypovolemia are obvious.

### PROMOTING TISSUE OXYGENATION

To promote oxygenation of tissues:

- Place the woman in a lateral position, with the head of the bed flat to increase cardiac return and thus to increase circulation and oxygenation of the placenta and other vital organs.
- Restrict maternal movements and activity to decrease the tissue demand for oxygen.
- Provide simple explanations, reassurance, and emotional support to the woman to help reduce anxiety, which increases the metabolic demand for oxygen.

### COLLABORATING WITH THE PHYSICIAN FOR FLUID REPLACEMENT

To replace fluids:

- Obtain an order for blood typing and crossmatching so that whole blood is available for replacement if necessary.
- Insert intravenous lines according to hospital protocol; usually two lines that use large-bore catheters are recommended so that whole blood can be administered if necessary.
- Administer fluids for replacement as directed by the physician to maintain a urinary output of at least 30 ml per hour.

### PREPARING THE WOMAN FOR SURGERY

It may be necessary to prepare the woman quickly for cesarean delivery. The nurse is responsible for the following:

- Surgical preparation and insertion of an indwelling urinary catheter.
- Validating that preoperative permits have been correctly signed.
- Validating that appropriate laboratory work has been done.
- Administering nonparticulate antacid or other medications as ordered by the anesthesiologist.
- Remaining with the woman and providing information and reassurance to the family (this is particularly important because the hurried activity and unusual procedures provoke fear and anxiety in the family).
- Assessing bleeding from the vagina as well as from any surgical sites or puncture wounds (epidural or

intravenous sites) so that uncontrolled bleeding or bleeding from unexpected sites, which may indicate DIC, can be reported to the physician for immediate, aggressive medical management.

#### PROVIDING EMOTIONAL SUPPORT

Once the safety of the woman and the fetus is ensured, nursing interventions are aimed at promoting comfort and providing emotional support. Explain what is causing the discomfort, and reassure the woman that pain relief measures will be initiated as soon as possible without causing harm to the fetus. Although it is unwise to offer false reassurance about the condition of the fetus, remain with the woman and provide accurate and timely information. Find time to explain what is going on to the woman and her family. They can feel overwhelmed by all the activity and the sense of haste.

### Evaluation

Although client-centered goals are not developed for collaborative problems, the nurse collects and compares data with established norms and judges whether the data are within normal limits. For hypovolemic shock, the maternal vital signs remain within normal limits and the fetal heart demonstrates no signs of compromise, such as late decelerations or decreasing baseline variability.

## Hyperemesis Gravidarum

Hyperemesis gravidarum is a condition of persistent, uncontrollable vomiting that begins in the first weeks of pregnancy and may continue throughout pregnancy. Unlike so-called morning sickness, which is self-limiting and causes no serious complications, hyperemesis gravidarum can have serious consequences. It can lead to severe weight loss, dehydration, and electrolyte imbalance (both sodium and potassium are lost from gastric fluids). Thiamine, retinol-binding protein, vitamin $B_{12}$, and chloride are also decreased (van Stuijvenberg et al., 1995). Metabolic alkalosis may develop because large amounts of hydrochloric acid are lost in the vomitus.

### Etiology

Although the cause of hyperemesis gravidarum is not known, some demographic factors have been studied. It is more common among unmarried white women and during first pregnancies. Other theories include endocrine or allergic origins. Elevated hormone levels, such as estrogen and hCG, are considered a possible cause as is thyroid dysfunction. Psychological factors, such as ambivalence toward the pregnancy, and family-related stress may also play causal roles.

### Therapeutic Management

Treatment often occurs in the home, where the woman attempts to control the nausea by the palliative methods that are used for morning sickness (see Chapter 7). In addition, some physicians prescribe vitamins, such as pyridoxine (vitamin $B_6$), that may provide some relief. The use of antiemetic medications is controversial because reported fetal anomalies associated with them have been widely circulated. A daily vitamin and mineral supplement may be recommended.

If palliative methods are unsuccessful and weight loss or electrolyte imbalance persists, intravenous fluid and electrolyte replacement or total parenteral nutrition may be necessary.

### Nursing Considerations

Because management frequently occurs in the home, nurses are often responsible for assessing and intervening for the woman with hyperemesis gravidarum. Physical assessment begins with determining the intake and output. Intake includes intravenous fluids and parenteral nutrition, as well as oral nutrition, which is allowed once vomiting is controlled. Output includes the amount and character of emesis and urinary output. As a rule of thumb, the normal urinary output is about 1 ml per kg (2.2 pounds) per hour. A record of bowel elimination also provides significant information about oral nutrition.

Samples of blood are taken frequently so laboratory data can be evaluated. Elevated levels of hemoglobin and hematocrit may occur as a result of inability to retain fluid, which results in hemoconcentration. Moreover, concentrations of sodium, potassium, and chloride may be reduced, resulting in hypokalemia and alkalosis.

The woman should be weighed frequently and her urine tested for ketones. Weight loss and the presence of ketones in the urine suggest that fat stores and protein are being metabolized to meet energy needs.

Signs of dehydration include decreased fluid intake ($<$2000 ml/day), decreased urinary output, increased specific gravity of urine ($>$1.025), dry skin or dry mucous membranes, and nonelastic skin turgor.

Nursing interventions focus on reducing nausea and vomiting, maintaining nutrition and fluid balance, and providing emotional support.

#### REDUCING NAUSEA AND VOMITING

When food is offered to the woman, portions should be small so that the amount does not appear overwhelming. Food should be attractively presented, and foods with strong odors should be eliminated from the diet because nausea is often associated with food smells. Low-fat foods and easily digested carbohydrates, such as fruit, breads, cereals, rice, and pasta, provide important nutrients and help prevent low blood sugar, which can cause nausea. Soups and other liquids should be taken between meals, so as not to overly distend the stomach and trigger vomiting. Sitting upright after meals reduces the frequency of gastric reflux.

#### MAINTAINING NUTRITION AND FLUID BALANCE

Women with nausea and vomiting should eat every 2 to 3 hours. Salting food helps replace chloride lost when hydrochloric acid is vomited. Potassium- and magnesium-rich foods should be encouraged because these nutrients are likely to be depleted and magnesium deficiency can exacerbate nausea.

Intravenous fluids and total parenteral nutrition are administered as directed by the physician. Small oral feedings of clear liquids are started when nausea and vomiting begin to subside. When oral fluids are tolerated, parenteral nutrition is gradually discontinued. Any inability to tolerate oral feedings or continued episodes of vomiting should be reported to the physician so that continued parenteral fluids and nutrition can be prescribed.

#### PROVIDING EMOTIONAL SUPPORT

The woman with hyperemesis gravidarum needs the opportunity to express how it feels to be pregnant and to live with ever-present nausea.

There is often a curious lack of sympathy and support for these women, however. The underlying reason for this is obscure; it may be because one reported cause has been termed psychogenic. Whatever the cause, nurses must use critical thinking to examine their own beliefs and biases so that they can provide comfort and support. It may be necessary to have case conferences or inservice educational programs to overcome preset beliefs and to establish a level of care that meets the needs of the woman.

### ✓ CHECK YOUR READING

11. How do "morning sickness" and hyperemesis gravidarum compare in terms of onset, duration, and effect on the client?
12. What are the goals in therapeutic management of hyperemesis gravidarum?
13. Why is critical thinking particularly important in the care of the woman with hyperemesis gravidarum?

## Hypertensive Disorders of Pregnancy

### Hypertension in Pregnancy

Terminology used to describe hypertension in pregnancy is nonuniform and confusing. Several overlapping terms are commonly applied to different clinical manifestations of the same disease process. However, in clinical practice two distinct entities are commonly encountered: chronic hypertension and pregnancy-induced hypertension (PIH). Furthermore, these two conditions can coexist. In fact, the risk of developing PIH is higher in women with underlying hypertension.

### Pregnancy-Induced Hypertension

Pregnancy-induced hypertension is a multiorgan disease process that may involve more than elevated blood pressure. It develops as a consequence of pregnancy and regresses in the postpartum period. Several clinical subsets have been given distinct labels, depending on end-organ effects (Table 25–2). In clinical practice, the terms PIH and pre-eclampsia are often used interchangeably.

### Pre-eclampsia

Pre-eclampsia is a condition in which hypertension develops during the last half of pregnancy in a woman who previously had normal blood pressure. In addition to hypertension, renal involvement leads to proteinuria. Many women also experience generalized edema; however, pre-eclampsia may be diagnosed without edema being present. The only known

**TABLE 25–2 CLASSIFICATION OF HYPERTENSIVE DISORDERS OF PREGNANCY**

| | |
|---|---|
| Pregnancy-induced hypertension | Development of hypertension (BP >140/90) during second half of pregnancy in previously normotensive woman |
| Pre-eclampsia | Renal involvement leads to proteinuria |
| Eclampsia | Central nervous system involvement leads to seizures |
| HELLP | Clinical picture dominated by hematologic and hepatic signs and symptoms |
| Chronic hypertension | Elevation of blood pressure before 20 weeks' gestation |

Adapted from American College of Obstetrics and Gynecology. (1996). Hypertension in pregnancy. *Technical Bulletin* No. 219. Washington, D.C.: ©ACOG, January 1996.

cure is delivery of the fetus. If the fetus is immature, however, this may not be practical. Although the disease cannot be cured, maternal and fetal morbidity can be minimized if detected early and managed carefully.

### INCIDENCE AND RISK FACTORS

Pre-eclampsia is relatively common. Seven percent of all pregnancies that progress to the second trimester are affected (Magann & Martin, 1995). It is a major cause of perinatal death, and it is often associated with intrauterine fetal growth restriction (also known as intrauterine growth retardation).

Although the cause of pre-eclampsia is not understood, several factors are known to increase a woman's risk that the condition will develop. For example, it is most likely to occur in a first pregnancy, in a woman older than 40 years of age, in African-Americans, and in those with chronic hypertension or renal disease. A family history of PIH also increases the risk. Although low socioeconomic status and young maternal age have traditionally been identified as risk factors, the actual independent contribution of these factors to the risk for PIH is questionable (ACOG, 1996).

Less well-known risk factors include both genetic and immunologic factors. The presence of the angiotensinogen gene T235 greatly increases the woman's sensitivity to angiotensin, a powerful vasoconstrictor that could lead to hypertension. Antiphospholipid syndrome (APS) is also strongly associated with the development of PIH. This syndrome is due to the development of antiphospholipid antibodies (aPL). These antibodies are directed against phospholipids that are widely distributed in cell membranes. The clinical picture of APS includes thrombosis, recurrent fetal loss, intrauterine fetal growth restriction, and the presence of aPL. Not everyone with PIH has aPL, but women who have them and become pregnant are at increased risk to develop PIH (Scott & Branch, 1994). Table 25–3 summarizes risk factors for the development of PIH.

### PATHOPHYSIOLOGY

Pre-eclampsia is due to generalized vasospasm. The underlying cause of the vasospasm remains a mystery; however, some of the physiologic processes are known. In normal pregnancy, there is a significant increase in vascular volume as well as increased cardiac output. Despite these factors, blood pressure does not rise in normal pregnancy. This is probably because pregnant women develop resistance to the effects of vasoconstrictors, such as angiotensin II. Moreover, there is a decrease in peripheral vascular resistance due to the effects of certain vasodilators, such as prostacyclin ($PGI_2$), prostaglandin E (PGE), and endothelium-derived relaxing factor (EDRF).

In pre-eclampsia, however, peripheral vascular resistance increases because of sensitivity of some women to angiotensin II and a decrease in vasodilators. For instance, there is an increase in the ratio of thromboxane ($TXA_2$) to $PGI_2$. Thromboxane, produced by kidney and trophoblastic tissue, causes vasoconstriction and platelet aggregation (clumping). Prostacyclin, produced by placental tissue and endothelial cells, causes vasodilation and inhibits platelet aggregation.

Vasospasm decreases the diameter of blood vessels, which results in endothelial cell damage and decreased EDRF. Vasoconstriction also results in impeded blood flow and elevated blood pressure. As a result, circulation to all body organs, including the kidneys, liver, brain, and placenta, is decreased. The following changes are most significant:

- Decreased renal perfusion causes a decline in glomerular filtration rate; consequently, blood urea nitrogen, creatinine, and uric acid levels begin to rise.

  Reduced blood flow to the kidneys also results in glomerular damage. This allows protein to leak across the glomerular membrane, which is usually impermeable to large protein molecules. Loss of protein reduces colloid osmotic pressure and allows fluid to shift to interstitial spaces. This may result in edema and relative hypovolemia, which causes increased viscosity of the blood and a rise in hematocrit. In response to hypovolemia, additional angiotensin II and aldosterone are secreted to trigger the retention of both sodium and water. The pathologic processes spiral: additional angio-

**TABLE 25–3 RISK FACTORS FOR PREGNANCY-INDUCED HYPERTENSION (PIH)**

First pregnancy
Age >40 years
African-American
Family history of PIH
Chronic hypertension
Chronic renal disease
Antiphospholipid syndrome
Diabetes mellitus
Twin gestation
Angiotensin gene T235
Low socioeconomic status and young maternal age are traditional risk factors; the actual independent contribution of these factors to the risk of pregnancy-induced hypertension is questionable.

From American College of Obstetrics and Gynecology. (1996) Hypertension in pregnancy. *Technical Bulletin* No. 219. Washington, D.C.: ©ACOG, January 1996.

tensin II results in further vasospasm and hypertension; aldosterone increases fluid retention, and edema is worsened.

- Decreased circulation to the liver leads to impaired liver function as well as to hepatic edema and subcapsular hemorrhage, which can result in hemorrhagic necrosis. This is manifested by elevation of liver enzymes in maternal serum.
- Vasoconstriction of cerebral vessels leads to pressure-induced rupture of thin-walled capillaries, resulting in small cerebral hemorrhages. Symptoms of arterial vasospasm include headache and visual disturbances, such as blurred vision and "spots" before the eyes, as well as hyperreflexia.
- Decreased colloid oncotic pressure can lead to pulmonary capillary leak that results in pulmonary edema. Dyspnea is the primary symptom.
- Decreased placental circulation has serious consequences. Placental ischemia results in infarctions that increase the risk of abruptio placentae and DIC. In addition, when maternal blood flow through the placenta is decreased, the fetus is likely to experience intrauterine growth restriction and persistent fetal hypoxemia, which can result in fetal acidosis, mental retardation, or death. Figure 25–7 summarizes the pathologic processes of pre-eclampsia.

### PREVENTIVE MEASURES

**Prenatal Care.** Proper prenatal care with attention to pattern of weight gain as well as careful monitoring of blood pressure and urinary protein may minimize maternal and fetal morbidity and mortality.

**Low-Dose Aspirin.** In recent years, low doses of aspirin (60 to 80 mg daily) have been administered to women at high risk for developing pre-eclampsia. Low-dose aspirin helps to prevent injury to endothelial cells that line the blood vessels. This reduces the aggregation of platelets and allows increased production of EDRF. In addition, aspirin suppresses synthesis of $TXA_2$, the vasoconstrictor described earlier. However, aspirin is not recommended for PIH prophylaxis in women with normal blood pressure who are not at risk to develop PIH (ACOG, 1996).

**Calcium Supplementation.** Some evidence suggests that women who receive calcium supplementa-

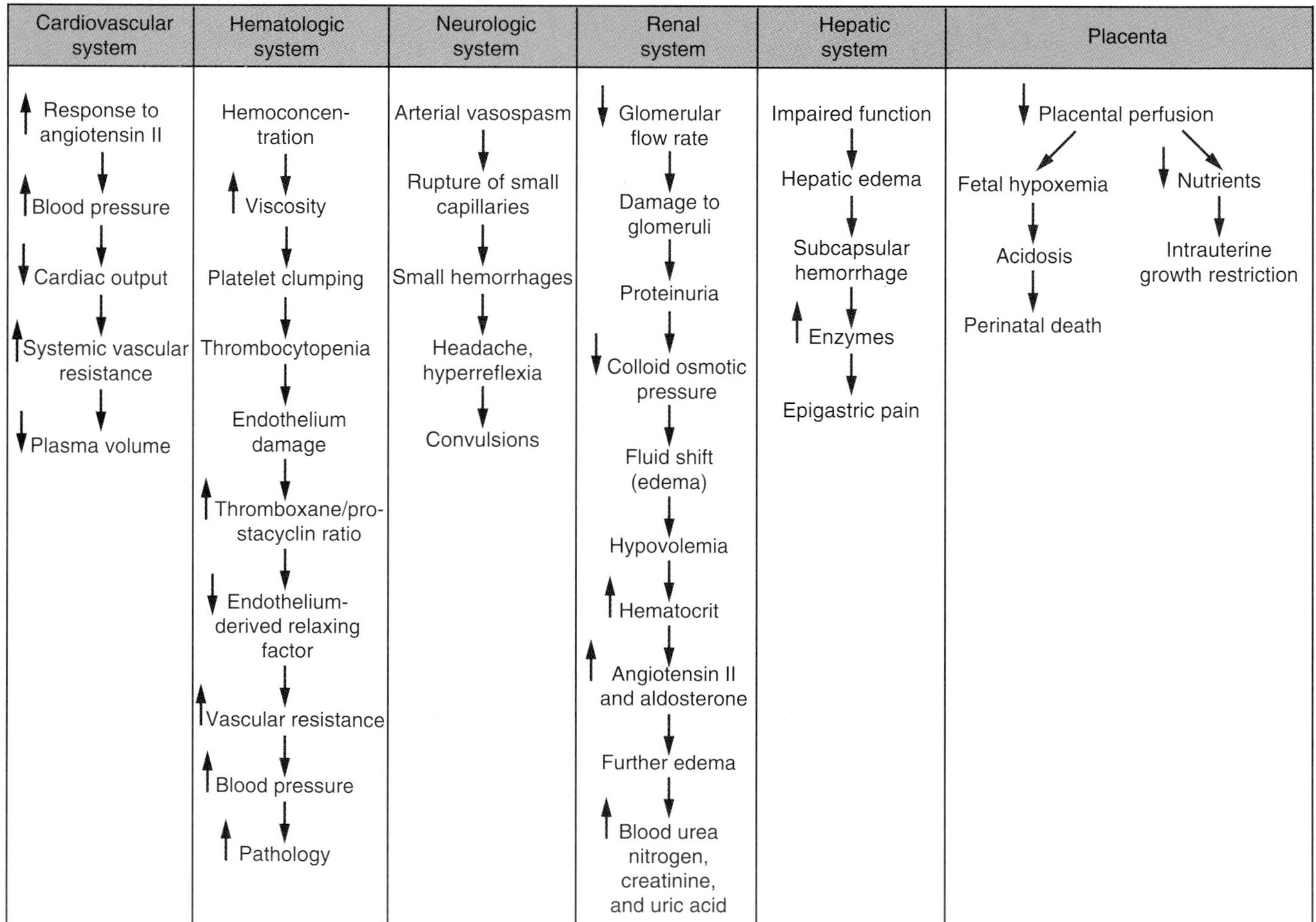


**FIGURE 25–7**

The pathologic processes of pre-eclampsia.

tion are less sensitive to the pressor effects of angiotensin II and have a lower overall incidence of hypertension (Ferris, 1995).

### CLINICAL MANIFESTATIONS OF PRE-ECLAMPSIA

**Classic Signs.** Hypertension, generalized edema, and proteinuria are the three classic signs of pre-eclampsia. The first indication of pre-eclampsia is usually hypertension; however, the first sign that the pregnant woman may notice is a rapid weight gain, which is due to fluid retention and consequent generalized edema. Edema is obvious not only in the lower legs, as is common in pregnancy, but also in the hands and face (Fig. 25–8). However, edema may not be present in all women who develop pre-eclampsia.

Hypertension is defined as sustained blood pressure equal to or above 140/90. Earlier data suggested that an increase of 30 mmHg systolic or 15 mmHg diastolic from baseline was also of diagnostic value; however, this concept is no longer considered valid (ACOG, 1996).

Because of the potential errors associated with determination of blood pressure, blood pressure should be taken in the sitting position with the arm supported in a horizontal position at heart level. Outpatient and inpatient departments should use the same position. There continues to be controversy about whether Korotkoff's fourth phase (muffling) or the fifth Korotkoff sound (disappearance) correlates better with true diastolic pressure. Most clinicians use the fifth phase, although it is 5 to 10 mmHg lower than the fourth phase (Knuppel & Drukker, 1993). Some clinicians record both the fourth and the fifth phases.

Proteinuria usually develops later than hypertension and edema, and the combination of proteinuria and hypertension increases the possibility of fetal jeopardy. A clean-catch specimen is needed to prevent contamination of the specimen by vaginal secretions.

**Additional Signs.** Careful assessment may reveal additional signs of pre-eclampsia. For instance, when the retina is examined, vascular constriction and narrowing of the small arteries are obvious in most women with pre-eclampsia. The vasoconstriction that can be seen in the retina is occurring throughout the body. If deep tendon reflexes are elicited, they may be very brisk (hyperreflexia). This suggests cerebral irritability secondary to decreased circulation and edema.

**Symptoms.** Pre-eclampsia is particularly dangerous for the expectant mother and fetus for two reasons: (1) it develops and progresses rapidly and (2) the early signs are not noticed by the woman. By the time she experiences symptoms, the disease has often progressed to an advanced state and valuable treatment time has been lost.

Certain symptoms, such as continuous headache, drowsiness, or mental confusion, indicate poor cerebral perfusion and may be precursors of convulsions. Visual disturbances, such as blurred or double vision or spots before the eyes, indicate arterial spasms and edema in the retina. Numbness or tingling of

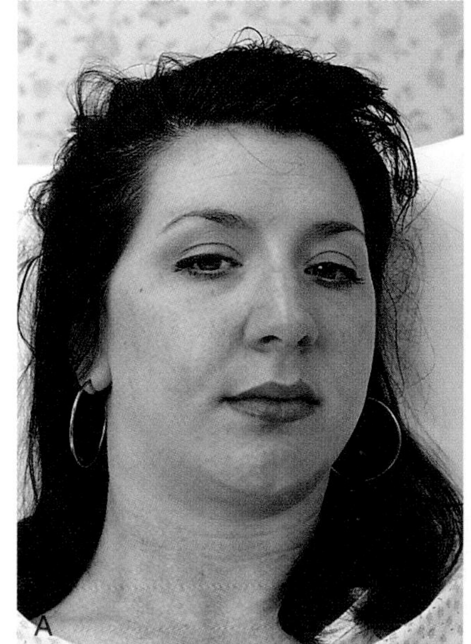


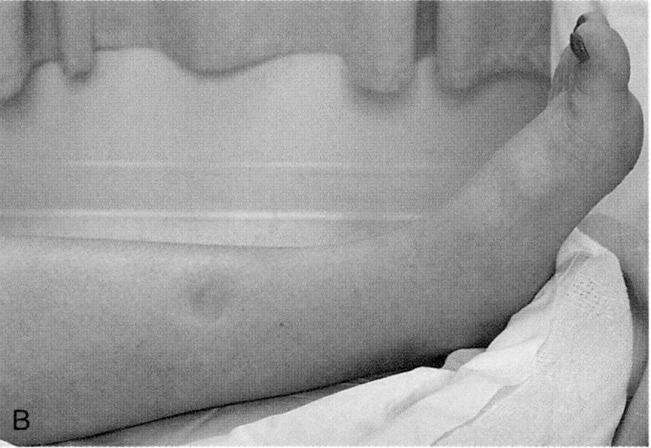


**FIGURE 25–8**

Generalized edema is a classic sign of pre-eclampsia. A, Facial edema may be subtle. B, Pitting edema of the lower leg.

the hands or feet occurs when nerves are compressed by retained fluid. Some symptoms, such as epigastric pain or "upset stomach," are particularly ominous because they indicate distention of the hepatic capsule and often warn that a convulsion is imminent. Decreased urinary output indicates poor perfusion of the kidneys and may precede acute renal failure.

### THERAPEUTIC MANAGEMENT OF MILD PRE-ECLAMPSIA

Pre-eclampsia continues to be categorized as either mild or severe, depending on the frequency and intensity of presenting signs and symptoms. However, because the disease may progress rapidly, an apparently mild condition can become severe in a very short time. Pre-eclampsia is considered mild when the diastolic blood pressure does not exceed 100 mmHg; proteinuria is no more than 500 mg/day (trace to 1+), and symptoms, such as headache, visual disturbances, or abdominal pain, are absent (Ferris, 1995). In addition, signs of kidney or liver involvement are absent, and the fetus demonstrates normal growth.

#### HOME CARE

Management in the home may be possible for selected women if the condition is mild. Criteria for home management varies with primary health care providers and home care agencies. In general the woman must be in stable condition with no evidence of worsening maternal or fetal status. Moreover, the woman and her family must be willing to adhere to a prescribed treatment plan that usually includes the following:

- Activity restriction
- Fetal movement counting
- Blood pressure monitoring
- Daily weights
- Frequent urinalysis
- Uterine activity monitoring
- Medication administration
- Documentation (Simpson, 1992; Grohar, 1994)

**Maternal Restrictions.** Bedrest is prescribed with bathroom privileges only. The expectant mother is instructed to rest in the left lateral position as much as possible. This position decreases pressure on the vena cava, thereby increasing cardiac return and circulatory volume and thus improving perfusion of vital organs. Increased renal perfusion decreases angiotensin II levels, promotes diuresis, and lowers the blood pressure. The woman is advised to remain quiet and calm. This may involve restricting visitors or telephone calls that cause agitation.

**Fetal Activity.** While home management is in effect, the expectant mother is asked to keep a record of fetal movements, commonly called a "kick count" (see Chapter 10). She should report a decrease in movements or if no movement is felt during a 4-hour period.

**Blood Pressure.** The family must be taught to use electronic blood pressure equipment. Blood pressure should be checked two to four times per day in the same arm and in the same position.

**Weight.** The woman should weigh herself at the same time each day, usually in the morning, preferably on the same scale.

**Urinalysis.** Urine dipstick for protein, using first voided midstream specimen, should be performed daily.

Most protocols allow a regular diet that does not restrict salt or fluids. Most also require daily contact with a home care nurse for assessment of signs and symptoms, review of blood pressure, urinalysis, fetal movement, weight, activity level, and adherence to treatment plan. Indications of disease progression or fetal deterioration require admission to the hospital.

Additional fetal surveillance is often recommended and may include serial sonography, weekly nonstress testing, and a contraction stress test or biophysical profile if the nonstress test indicates there is fetal compromise.

### THERAPEUTIC MANAGEMENT OF SEVERE PRE-ECLAMPSIA

The disease is considered severe when blood pressure is higher than 160/110 mmHg, proteinuria is higher than 5 gm in 24 hours (3+ or more), and there is oliguria (500 ml or less in 24 hours). If symptoms occur that were absent in the mild form of the disease, or if laboratory findings indicate liver involvement (elevated enzymes or hyperbilirubinemia) or kidney damage (elevated creatinine), the disease is judged to be severe (ACOG, 1996). Table 25–4 compares mild and severe pre-eclampsia.

**TABLE 25–4 MILD VERSUS SEVERE PRE-ECLAMPSIA**

| | Mild | Severe |
|---|---|---|
| Systolic BP | <160 | >160 |
| Diastolic BP | <100 | >110 |
| Proteinuria | Trace | >5 g/24 hr |
| Creatinine | Normal | Elevated |
| Thrombocytopenia | Absent | Present |
| Oliguria | Absent | <500 ml/24 hr |
| Liver enzyme elevation | Minimal | Marked |
| Fetal growth restriction | Absent | Present |
| Headache, visual disturbances, abdominal pain | Absent | Present |

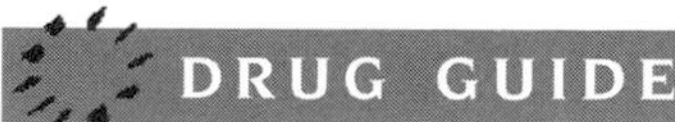
DRUG GUIDE

## HYDRALAZINE

***Classification:*** Antihypertensive.

***Action:*** Relaxes arterial smooth muscle to reduce blood pressure.

***Indications:*** Used in pre-eclampsia when blood pressure is elevated to a degree that might be associated with intracranial bleeding.

***Dosage and Route:*** For obstetric use, 10 to 50 mg is administered intramuscularly. Following a test dose to determine hypotensive effects, 5 to 10 mg may be administered by intravenous bolus infusion as often as every 20 minutes if necessary (ACOG, 1996).

***Absorption:*** Well absorbed from intramuscular sites. Widely distributed, crosses the placenta; enters breast milk in minimal concentrations.

***Excretion:*** Metabolized and excreted by the liver.

***Contraindications and Precautions:*** Contraindicated in coronary artery disease, cerebrovascular disease, and hypersensitivity to hydralazine. Used cautiously in obstetrics because safety during pregnancy and lactation has not been established.

***Adverse Reactions:*** Headache, dizziness, drowsiness, hypotension that can interfere with uterine blood flow, epigastric pain, which may be confused with worsening pre-eclampsia.

***Nursing Implications:*** Obstetric clients are hospitalized before initiation of hypertensive medications. Blood pressure and pulse must be monitored every 2 to 3 minutes for 30 minutes after initial dosage and periodically throughout the course of therapy. Therapy is repeated only when diastolic pressure exceeds limits set by physician or facility protocol (usually >110 mmHg).

**Antepartum Management.** Goals of management are to prevent convulsions and to maintain the pregnancy until it is safe to deliver the fetus. Home care is not appropriate if pre-eclampsia becomes severe. The woman will be hospitalized for constant assessment and management.

**Bedrest.** As during home management, the hospitalized woman is kept on bedrest and her environment is kept quiet. External stimuli (lights, noise) that might precipitate a convulsion should be reduced.

**Antihypertensive Medications.** Blood pressure control does not improve fetal oxygenation, and thus the use of antihypertensives is usually reserved for severe hypertension when there is the possibility of intracranial bleeding (Roberts, 1994). Various antihypertensive agents such as hydralazine may be used (ACOG, 1996). Other antihypertensive medications, such as nifedipine (a calcium channel blocker) or labetalol (a $\beta$-adrenergic blocker), may be administered in some cases (Ferris, 1995).

**Anticonvulsant Medications.** In the United States, magnesium sulfate ($MgSO_4$) is the drug of choice to prevent convulsions; however, phenytoin (Dilantin, Diphenylan) is occasionally used. Magnesium acts as a central nervous system depressant by blocking neuromuscular transmission and decreasing the amount of acetylcholine liberated. Magnesium is not an antihypertensive medication, but it relaxes smooth muscle and thus reduces vasoconstriction. Decreased vasoconstriction promotes circulation to the vital organs of the expectant mother and increases placental circulation. Increased circulation to the maternal kidneys leads to diuresis, as interstitial fluid is shifted into the vascular compartment and excreted.

Magnesium is generally administered by intravenous infusion, which allows for immediate onset of action and does not cause the discomfort associated with intramuscular administration. Intravenous magnesium is administered via a secondary ("piggyback") line so that the medication can be discontinued at any time while the primary line remains open and functional.

One of the major advantages of magnesium is that it can be used to prevent convulsions without harming the fetus or neonate. Fetal magnesium levels are nearly identical with those of the expectant mother. As a result, there may be decreased fetal heart rate variability on fetal monitor tracing. However, there is no cumulative effect because the fetal kidneys excrete magnesium effectively (Roberts, 1994).

Significant adverse reactions and side effects are associated with parenteral administration of magnesium. The most important is central nervous system depression, including depression of the respiratory center. Magnesium is excreted solely by the kidneys, and administration of parenteral magnesium depends on kidneys that function effectively.

**Intrapartum Management.** Most seizures occur during labor and the postpartum period (Roberts, 1994), so these are the times when continued assessment and therapy are most important. During labor, the fetus and the expectant mother must be monitored continuously to detect signs of imminent convulsions. The woman should be kept in a lateral position to promote circulation through the placenta, and efforts should be focused on controlling pain that may cause agitation and precipitate seizures.

Induction of labor by intravenous oxytocin is often planned once the fetus is mature. Oxytocin to stimulate uterine contractions and magnesium sulfate to prevent convulsions are often administered simultaneously during labor. Infusion pumps should be used to ensure that the medications are administered at the prescribed rate, and equipment and intravenous lines should be checked carefully for correct placement and function.

Narcotic analgesics or epidural anesthesia may be

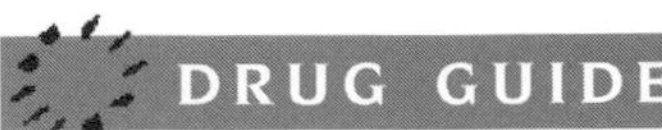

## MAGNESIUM SULFATE

***Classification:*** Miscellaneous anticonvulsant.

***Action:*** Decreases acetylcholine released by motor nerve impulses, thereby blocking neuromuscular transmission. Depresses the central nervous system to act as an anticonvulsant; also decreases frequency and intensity of uterine contractions. Produces flushing and sweating due to decreased peripheral blood pressure.

***Indications:*** Prevention and control of seizures in severe pre-eclampsia. Prevention of uterine contractions in preterm labor.

***Dosage and Route:*** Magnesium sulfate is generally administered parenterally. An intravenous loading bolus (4 g over 20 minutes) is given and followed by continuous infusion (2 to 3 g/hour) via a controlled infusion device (ACOG, 1996). Therapeutic range for magnesium is generally considered to be 4 to 8 mg/dl (ACOG, 1996).

***Absorption:*** Immediate onset following intravenous administration. Duration of action is 3 to 4 hours.

***Excretion:*** Excreted by the kidneys.

***Contraindications and Precautions:*** Contraindicated in persons with myocardial damage, heart block, myasthenia gravis, or impaired renal function.

***Adverse Reactions:*** Result from magnesium overdose and include flushing, sweating, hypotension, depressed deep tendon reflexes, and central nervous system depression, including respiratory depression.

***Nursing Implications:*** Monitor blood pressure closely during administration. Assess client for respiratory rate above 12 per minute, presence of deep tendon reflexes, and urinary output greater than 30 ml per hour before administering magnesium. Place resuscitation equipment (suction, oxygen) in the room. Keep calcium gluconate, which acts as an antidote to magnesium, in the room along with syringes and needles.

administered to provide comfort and to reduce painful stimuli that could precipitate a convulsion.

Continuous fetal electronic monitoring is necessary to determine any change in fetal heart activity that could indicate fetal hypoxia. Oxygen is administered to the expectant mother if fetal compromise is noted.

A pediatrician, neonatologist, or neonatal nurse practitioner must be available to care for the newborn at birth.

**Postpartum Management.** Following birth, careful assessment of the mother's blood loss and signs of shock are essential because the hypovolemia caused by pre-eclampsia may be aggravated by blood loss during the delivery. Assessments for signs and symptoms of pre-eclampsia must be continued for at least 48 hours, and magnesium may be continued to prevent seizures.

Signs that the woman is recovering from pre-eclampsia are as follows:

- Urinary output of 4 to 6 liters per day, which causes a rapid reduction in edema and rapid weight loss
- Decreased protein in the urine
- Return of blood pressure to normal, usually within 2 weeks

### THERAPEUTIC MANAGEMENT OF ECLAMPSIA

Eclampsia is marked by convulsions that typically begin with twitching about the mouth. The body then becomes rigid in a state of tonic muscular contractions that last 15 to 20 seconds. Suddenly the facial muscles and then all body muscles alternatively contract and relax in rapid succession. This clonic phase of the convulsion may last about 1 minute. Respiration is halted during the convulsion because the diaphragm tends to remain fixed. Breathing usually resumes shortly after the convulsion and is most often rapid and deep (Usta & Sibai, 1995).

Magnesium may be given intravenously to control the convulsions. Sedatives such as phenobarbital or diazepam are used only if magnesium fails to bring the seizures under control. Sedatives should not be given if birth is expected within an hour or two because of their depressant effects on the fetus.

Pulmonary edema, circulatory or renal failure, and cerebral hemorrhage are complications that may occur with eclampsia. The woman's lungs should be auscultated frequently, and furosemide (Lasix) may be administered if pulmonary edema develops. Digitalis may be needed to strengthen contraction of the heart if circulatory failure results. Urine output should be assessed hourly; if output drops below 30 ml per hour, renal failure should be suspected.

The woman should be monitored carefully for ruptured membranes, signs of labor, or abruptio placentae because eclampsia stimulates uterine irritability. While the woman is comatose, she should be kept on her side to prevent aspiration and to improve placental circulation. The side rails should be kept up to prevent a fall and possible injury. When vital signs have stabilized, delivery of the fetus should be considered.

Aspiration is a leading cause of maternal morbidity following an eclamptic seizure. After initial stabilization, the nurse should anticipate orders for chest radiographs and possibly arterial blood gases to rule out the possibility of aspiration.

**CHECK YOUR READING**

14. What are the effects of vasospasm on the fetus?
15. What are the signs and symptoms of pre-eclampsia? Why is bedrest recommended for management?
16. What is the effect of vasospasm on the brain?

17. What are the effects of magnesium sulfate, including the primary adverse effect?
18. What are the major complications of eclampsia?

## Application of Nursing Process: Pre-eclampsia

### Assessment

Nursing assessment is one of the most important components of successful management of pre-eclampsia. Careful assessment is the only way to determine whether the condition is responding to medical management or whether the disease is worsening. Many hospitals assign nurses to women on a one-to-one basis or admit the woman to the antepartum intensive care unit.

Weigh the woman on admission and daily after that. Check vital signs, and auscultate the chest for moist breath sounds that indicate pulmonary edema. Assess the location and severity of edema at least every 4 hours. Table 25–5 provides a useful method for describing edema. Insert an indwelling catheter and measure urinary output hourly. Check the urine for protein every 4 hours. Apply an external electronic monitor to determine whether there are changes in fetal heart rate or variability.

Check brachial and patellar reflexes for hyperreflexia that may indicate increasing cerebral irritability. Determine whether clonus is present by dorsiflexing the woman's foot sharply while her knee is held in a flexed position. Normally, no clonus is present; however, if oscillations or "jerking" motions occur as the foot drops, clonus is present and should be reported to the physician. Procedure 25–1 illustrates how to assess and rate deep tendon reflexes.

**TABLE 25–5 ASSESSMENT OF EDEMA**

| | |
|---|---|
| Minimal edema of lower extremities: | +1 |
| Marked edema of lower extremities: | +2 |
| Edema of lower extremities, face, hands, and sacral area: | +3 |
| Generalized massive edema that includes ascites (accumulation of fluid in peritoneal cavity): | +4 |

Question the woman carefully about symptoms she may be experiencing, such as headache, visual disturbances, epigastric pain, or increased edema.

**An open-ended question such as "How do you feel?" may not be adequate, and detailed questions should follow if the woman states that she feels "fine." Ask targeted questions, such as "Do you have a headache? Describe it for me." "Do you have any pain in the abdomen? Show me where it is and describe it." "Do you see spots before your eyes? Flashes of light? Double vision?" "Is your vision blurred?" "I see you have removed your rings. Did you do that because your hands were swollen? When did that happen?"**

#### ASSESSMENTS FOR MAGNESIUM TOXICITY

Adverse side effects of magnesium include central nervous system depression that includes depression of the respiratory center. As a result, nursing assessments should focus on these areas. Determine respiratory rate hourly. Assess the woman's level of consciousness (alert, drowsy, confused, oriented). Hypotonic reflexes indicate central nervous system depression. Table 25–6 summarizes nursing assessments and their implications.

**TABLE 25–6 NURSING ASSESSMENTS FOR PRE-ECLAMPSIA AND MAGNESIUM TOXICITY**

| Assessment | Implications |
|---|---|
| Daily weight | Provides estimate of fluid retention |
| Blood pressure | To determine response to treatment |
| Respiratory rate | Drug therapy ($MgSO_4$) causes respiratory depression, and drug should be held if respiratory rate is $<12$/min |
| Breath sounds | To detect onset of pulmonary edema |
| Deep tendon reflexes | Hyperreflexia indicates increased cerebral edema; hyporeflexia indicates magnesium excess |
| Edema | For estimation of interstitial fluid |
| Urinary output | More than 30 ml/hr indicates adequate perfusion of the kidneys |
| Level of consciousness | Drowsiness, dulled sensorium indicate therapeutic effects of magnesium; nonresponsive behavior or muscle weakness indicates magnesium excess |
| Headache, epigastric pain, visual problems | Indicate increasing severity of condition and development of eclampsia |
| Fetal heart rate and baseline variability | Rate should be between 110 and 160; decreasing baseline variability may be due to magnesium or to continuous fetal hypoxemia and fetal distress |
| Laboratory data | Elevated serum creatinine, elevated liver enzymes, or decreased platelets (thrombocytopenia) are significant signs of increasing severity of disease; serum magnesium levels should be in therapeutic range designated by physician |

Procedure 25–1

## Assessing Deep Tendon Reflexes

**PURPOSE:** To determine whether there are exaggerated reflexes (hyperreflexia) or diminished reflexes (hyporeflexia).

Assess both the brachial and the patellar reflex, plus clonus. Equipment: reflex hammer.

1. **To assess the brachial reflex, support the woman's arm and instruct her to let it go totally limp while it is being held.** *This position partially relaxes and partially flexes the person's arm.*

2. **Place your thumb over the woman's tendon, as illustrated, and strike the thumb with the small end of the reflex hammer. The normal rsponse is slight flexion of the forearm.** *The tendon response can be felt as well as seen when the tendon is tapped.*

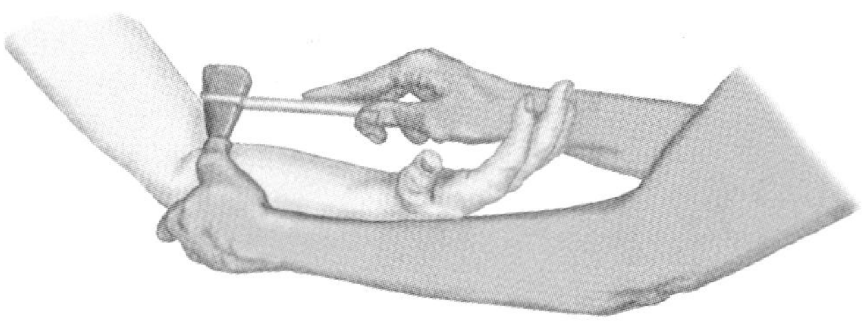

3. **The patellar reflex can be assessed in two positions, sitting or lying. When the woman is sitting, allow her lower legs to dangle freely to flex the knee and stretch the tendons. Strike the tendon with the reflex hammer just below the patella.** *Determines deep tendon reflexes in the lower extremities when the person is sitting.*

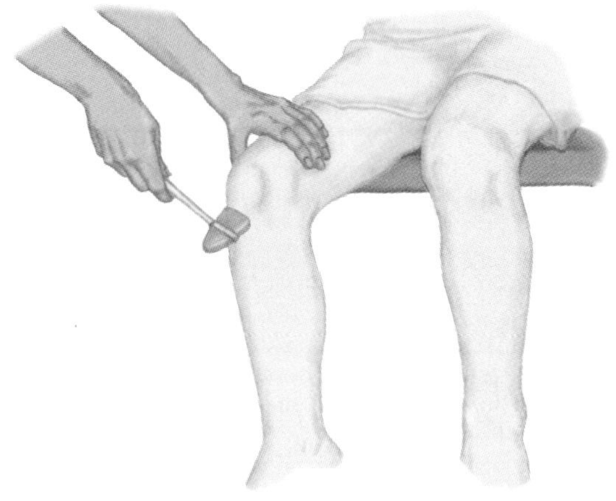

4. **When the woman is in the supine position, the weight of her leg must be supported to flex the knee and stretch the tendons. Strike the partially stretched tendons just below the patella. Extension of the leg is the expected response.** *It is necessary to support the leg because an adequate response requires that the limb be relaxed and the tendon partially stretched.*

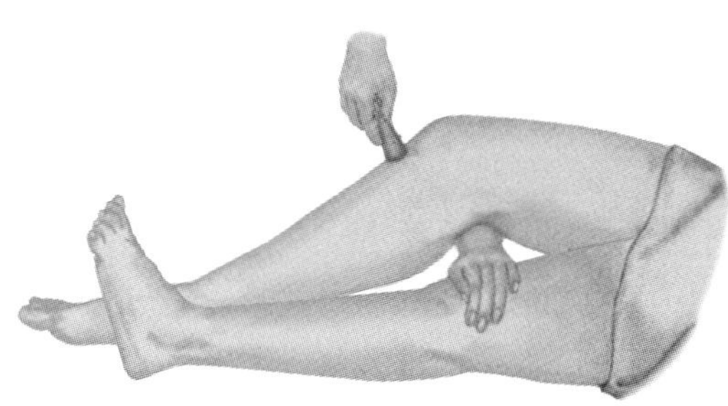

5. **Clonus should be tested, particularly when the reflexes are hyperactive. The woman's lower leg should be supported, as illustrated, and the foot sharply dorsiflexed. Hold the stretch. With a normal response, no movement will be felt. When clonus is present, rapid rhythmic jerking motions of the foot are obvious.** *Dorsiflexion stretches the tendon, and rapid rhythmic contractions indicate hyperreflexia.*

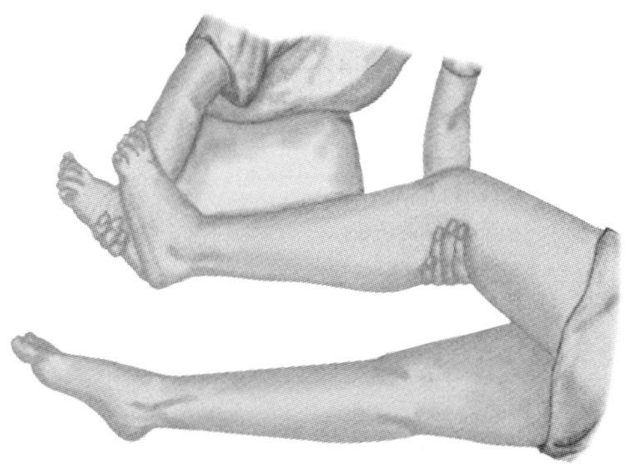

DEEP TENDON RATING SCALE

0 = Reflex absent
+1 = Reflex present, hypoactive
+2 = Normal reflex
+3 = Hyperactive reflex
+4 = Hyperactive reflex with clonus present

#### PSYCHOSOCIAL ASSESSMENT

The development of pre-eclampsia places a great deal of stress on the childbearing family. The woman may be on bedrest or hospitalized for some time. This creates anxiety about the condition of the fetus as well as that of the expectant mother. Moreover, many families do not understand the seriousness of the disease; after all, the woman feels well for some time after its onset.

Investigate how the family will function while the expectant mother is hospitalized. Determine how the woman is adapting to the "sick role" and the necessity of being dependent on others instead of functioning in her primary role. Ask how much support is available and who is willing to participate. Finally, determine the major concerns of the family.

### Analysis

Analysis of the data collected can lead to both nursing diagnoses (see Nursing Care Plan 25–2) and collaborative problems or potential complications. Potential complications necessitate that nurses monitor to detect onset or changes in status. Both physician-prescribed and nurse-prescribed interventions are used to minimize the complication. Potential complications for the woman with pre-eclampsia are eclamptic seizures and magnesium toxicity.

### Planning

Client-centered goals are inappropriate for the potential complications of eclamptic seizures and magnesium toxicity because the nurse cannot independently manage these conditions but must confer with physicans for medical orders for treatment. For seizures, planning should reflect the nurse's responsibility to do the following:

- Monitor for signs of impending seizures
- Consult with the physician if signs of impending seizures are observed
- Perform actions that will minimize the risk of seizures occurring and prevent injury if seizures do occur

For magnesium toxicity:

- Monitor for signs of magnesium toxicity
- Consult with the physician if signs of magnesium toxicity are observed
- Perform actions that will minimize the possibility of magnesium toxicity

### Interventions

#### INTERVENTIONS FOR SEIZURES

##### MONITORING FOR SIGNS OF IMPENDING SEIZURES

Signs of impending seizures include the following:

- Hyperreflexia or the presence of clonus, or both
- Increasing signs of cerebral irritability (headache, visual disturbances)
- Epigastric pain

None of these signs is an absolutely reliable predictor of imminent seizure. Nurses must be alert for subtle changes and prepared for seizures in all women with pre-eclampsia.

##### INITIATING PREVENTIVE MEASURES

In the presence of cerebral irritability, seizures may be precipitated by excessive visual or auditory stimuli. Nurses should reduce external stimuli by doing the following:

- Admitting the woman to a private room in the quietest section of the unit and keeping the door to the room closed
- Padding the door to reduce noise when the door must be opened and closed
- Keeping lights low and noise to a minimum; this may include blocking incoming telephone calls
- Grouping nursing assessments and care to allow the woman long periods of undisturbed quiet
- Moving carefully and calmly around the room and avoiding bumping into the bed or startling the woman
- Collaborating with the woman and her family to restrict visitors

##### PREVENTING SEIZURE-RELATED INJURY

The bed's side rails should be padded and the bed kept in the lowest position with the wheels locked to prevent trauma should the woman hit the side rails or fall from the bed during a convulsion.

Oxygen and suction equipment should be assembled and ready to use to prevent aspiration and to provide oxygen as necessary. Check equipment at the beginning of each shift because there will not be time to set up equipment if convulsions occur.

A pre-eclampsia tray, sometimes called a "toxemia tray," should be in the room. It should contain a medium plastic airway, an Ambu bag with mask, an ophthalmoscope, a tourniquet, a reflex hammer, syringes and needles. Medications that should be in the PIH tray include magnesium sulfate, sodium bicarbonate, heparin sodium, epinephrine, phenytoin, and calcium gluconate.

## Nursing Care Plan 25–2

# Pre-eclampsia

**ASSESSMENT:** Julie Frost, a 16-year-old primigravida, is seen in the prenatal clinic at 30 weeks of gestation. Her blood pressure is 136/90, and there is some edema of the lower legs and trace proteinuria. Although the signs are minimal, she is referred to home care and given instructions about home care regimen for pregnancy-induced hypertension. This includes bedrest; frequent monitoring of blood pressure, weight, and urine; and how to do fetal "kick counts." She is told that she must return to the clinic in a week. Julie states that she feels fine and doesn't want to miss school. She says that she doesn't see the reason for bedrest.

**NURSING DIAGNOSIS:** Impaired Adjustment related to lack of knowledge of health status and the need for a change in lifestyle

**GOALS/EXPECTED OUTCOMES**

Julie will do the following:

1. Verbalize the benefits of the recommended regimen by the end of the first prenatal appointment.
2. Comply with the recommended care for the next week.
3. Keep prenatal appointments.

| INTERVENTION | RATIONALE |
|---|---|
| 1. Initiate an interaction that allows Julie to verbalize her feelings about the recommended regimen: "What concerns you most about missing school?" Acknowledging her feelings as important: "It must be difficult to think of falling behind in your schoolwork." "It isn't any fun to miss all the afterschool activities." | 1. When feelings are identified and acknowledged as important, anxiety decreases and teaching and learning can begin. |
| 2. Identify family support that will permit compliance with the recommended regimen of bedrest and home care. | 2. Compliance with the regimen is impossible without family assistance that includes assistance with activities of daily living and necessary assessments. |
| 3. Describe in general terms the physiologic processes that are occurring and their effect on her and the fetus: "The small blood vessels in your body may be narrowed so they don't carry enough blood to your vital organs or to the baby." "Staying in bed on your left side helps the blood to move to all parts of your body and to carry oxygen to the baby." | 3. Expectant mothers are highly motivated to comply with a therapeutic management that will benefit the fetus, and knowledge of how the planned program provides the fetus with oxygen improves the possibility of compliance with bedrest and frequent assessments. |
| 4. Explain that she may feel well even when the condition worsens and that she must be observed for painless symptoms daily at home and frequently at the clinic. | 4. Hypertension and proteinuria are not noticed by the expectant mother. Edema is considered normal by many clients, and they may not identify edema above the waist as more significant than dependent edema. |
| 5. Instruct Julie to call the clinic if she notices headache, double vision, or spots before her eyes. | 5. These signs indicate rapid progression of the disease and that additional management is needed. |
| 6. Collaborate with Julie to arrange for contact with her boyfriend or selected friends and to arrange for ongoing homebound classes. | 6. Such an agreement will allow a schedule to be developed that provides peer support but that allows for prolonged periods of quiet. Homebound classes alleviate the concern that she is falling behind with schoolwork, and related anxiety will decrease. |

**EVALUATION**

Despite maintaining the recommended regimen of bedrest with the help of her mother and sister, Julie's symptoms escalated with a rise in blood pressure and a rapid gain in weight, indicating generalized edema.

**ASSESSMENT:** Julie is admitted to the hospital at 32 weeks of gestation with blood pressure 160/110, heart rate 92, and respirations 22. There is 2+ proteinuria and marked edema of the hands and face. Electronic fetal monitoring is initiated. Fetal heart rate is 136 with adequate variability. She is started on a continuous intravenous infusion of magnesium sulfate ($MgSO_4$), seizure precautions are initiated, and environmental stimuli are carefully reduced. Julie is agitated and verbalizes concern that the procedures are going to hurt her or the fetus. She frequently asks, "How sick am I?" "Is the baby going to be okay?" Her hands are perspiring, and they shake when she reaches for a tissue.

**NURSING DIAGNOSIS:** Anxiety related to hospitalization and concern about her health and the health of the fetus

## Nursing Care Plan 25–2 *Continued*

# Pre-eclampsia

### GOALS/EXPECTED OUTCOMES

Julie will do the following:

1. Verbalize her concerns and describe the benefits of the treatment while her family is present.
2. Manifest less anxiety (agitation, physiologic signs such as tremors, tachycardia, and perspiration).

| INTERVENTION | RATIONALE |
|---|---|
| 1. Initiate measures to reduce anxiety.<br>a. Provide positive reassurance that a solution to anxiety can be found: "I can see you are really worried, and I will try to answer all your questions."<br>b. Allow her to cry, get angry, or express any feeling that is present.<br>c. Encourage a discussion of feelings: "Tell me more about how you feel."<br>d. Reflect observations: "I see you wringing your hands; do you want to talk about it?"<br>e. Convey empathy and positive regard; use nonverbal behavior, including touch, when appropriate. | 1. Anxiety is an ominous feeling of tension resulting from a physical or emotional threat to the self. It is a global, often unnamed, sense of doom, a feeling of helplessness, isolation, and insecurity. Anxiety needs to be ventilated and then addressed by conveying that the person is not alone and that they will be protected. |
| 2. Provide information about hospital routines and procedures when anxiety is diminished enough for learning to take place.<br>a. Be very specific about procedures, such as fetal monitoring, assessment of deep tendon reflexes, and vital signs. Explain what they are for, who will do them, and how long they will be maintained.<br>b. Focus on Julie's present concerns; she is not able to be future-oriented at this time.<br>c. Speak slowly and calmly, give very short directions, and do not ask Julie to make decisions: "Turn on your side." "Breathe slowly."<br>d. Allow a friend or family member to remain with Julie and instruct the person on the necessity for a low-stimulus environment. | 2. Knowledge of the procedures that will be performed and the purpose of the procedures provides a sense of control that reduces anxiety. Perception is somewhat narrowed when anxiety is high; therefore, short, brief instructions are easier for the anxious person to understand than long explanations. |

### EVALUATION

Julie discusses her feelings with the nurse and with her sister. She feels in control of anxiety as manifested by a decrease in signs of agitation and physiologic signs (tachycardia, tachypnea) and by the ability to use relaxation techniques.

### POTENTIAL COMPLICATIONS TO CONSIDER

Magnesium toxicity
Seizures

### Critical Thinking

1. What two potential complications cause the greatest concern for nurses who care for Julie?
2. Why do nurses not develop goals for these problems?
3. What are the nurses' responsibilities for these complications?

### ANSWER

1. The most common complications that cause the greatest concern are magnesium toxicity and seizures.
2. These are collaborative problems that require interventions from the entire health care team. The nurse does not develop goals because she cannot independently manage magnesium toxicity or seizures.
3. The nurse must monitor for signs of these conditions, administer prescribed medications, observe and report Julie's response to the medications, and collaborate with the physicians to lessen the chance that these complications will occur.

PROTECTING THE WOMAN AND FETUS DURING A CONVULSION

Nurses must protect the woman and the fetus during a convulsion. The nurse's primary responsibilities are the following:

- Remain with the woman and press the emergency bell for assistance.
- If there is time, attempt to turn the woman on her side when the tonic phase begins. A Sims position permits greater circulation through the placenta, and it may also help prevent aspiration.
- Note the time and sequence of the convulsion. Eclampsia is marked by a tonic-clonic convulsion that may be preceded by facial twitching that lasts for a few seconds. A tonic contraction of the entire body is followed by the clonic phase, which may last about a minute.
- Insert an airway following the convulsion, and suction the woman's mouth and nose to prevent aspiration; administer oxygen by mask to increase oxygenation of the placenta and all maternal body organs.
- Notify the physician as soon as possible that a convulsion has occurred. This is an obstetric emergency that is associated with cerebral hemorrhage, premature separation of the placenta, severe fetal hypoxia, and death.
- Administer medications and prepare for additional medical interventions as directed by the physician.

PROVIDING INFORMATION AND SUPPORT FOR THE FAMILY

Explain to the family what has happened, but do not minimize the seriousness of the situation. A convulsion is very frightening for anyone who witnesses it, and the family is often reassured when the nurse explains that the convulsion lasts for only a few minutes and that the woman will probably not be conscious for some time. Acknowledge that the convulsion indicates worsening of the condition and that it will be necessary for the physician to determine future management, which may include delivery of the infant as soon as possible.

#### INTERVENTIONS FOR MAGNESIUM TOXICITY

MONITORING FOR SIGNS OF MAGNESIUM TOXICITY

Magnesium excess depresses the entire central nervous system, including the brain stem, which controls respirations and cardiac function, and the cerebrum, which controls memory, mental processes, and speech. Carbon dioxide accumulates if the respiratory rate is reduced, leading to respiratory acidosis and further central nervous system depression, which could culminate in respiratory arrest.

Signs of magnesium toxicity include the following:

- Respiratory rate under 12 breaths per minute
- Absence of deep tendon reflexes
- Sweating, flushing
- Altered sensorium (confused, lethargic, slurring of speech, drowsiness, disorientation)
- Hypotension
- Serum magnesium above the therapeutic range of 4 to 8 mg per dl (ACOG, 1996)

RESPONDING TO SIGNS OF MAGNESIUM TOXICITY

Discontinue magnesium if the respiratory rate is below 12 breaths per minute or if deep tendon reflexes are absent. These are signs of magnesium toxicity, and administration of additional magnesium will make the condition worse. Notify the physician of the woman's condition so that additional orders can be received. Magnesium is excreted by the kidneys, and if the urinary output falls below 30 ml per hour, the physician should be notified before magnesium is administered.

Calcium gluconate is the antidote for magnesium sulfate, because it effectively antagonizes the effects of magnesium at the neuromuscular junction, and it should be readily available whenever magnesium is administered. Magnesium toxicity can be reversed by intravenous administration of 1 g (10 ml of 10 percent) calcium gluconate over 2 minutes (ACOG, 1996).

### Evaluation

Collect and compare data with established norms and then judge whether the data are within normal limits. For seizures, interventions are judged to be successful if

- Deep tendon reflexes remain within normal limits (+1 to +3).
- Clonus is absent.
- The woman is free of visual disturbances, headache, and epigastric pain.
- The woman remains free of seizures or free of injury if a seizure occurs.

For magnesium toxicity, determine whether respiratory rates remain above 12 breaths per minute, deep tendon reflexes are present, and maternal plasma levels of magnesium do not exceed the therapeutic dose.

**CHECK YOUR READING**

19. What nursing assessments should be made for the woman with pre-eclampsia? Why?
20. What measures may be initiated to prevent or manage convulsions?

21. How can injury during convulsion be prevented?
22. What are the signs of magnesium toxicity? How should it be managed?

## Hemolysis, Elevated Liver Enzymes, and Low Platelets Syndrome

The acronym HELLP (hemolysis, elevated liver enzymes, low platelets) is used to identify a potentially life-threatening variation of pre-eclampsia. Hemolysis is believed to occur as a result of the fragmentation and distortion of erythrocytes during passage through small damaged blood vessels. Elevated liver enzymes occur when hepatic blood flow is obstructed by fibrin deposits. Hyperbilirubinemia and jaundice may also be observed as a result of liver impairment. Low platelets are due to vascular damage resulting from vasospasm; platelets aggregate at sites of damage, resulting in thrombocytopenia.

The prominent symptom of HELLP syndrome is pain in the right upper quadrant, the lower chest, or epigastric area. There may also be tenderness due to liver distention. Additional signs include nausea, vomiting, and severe edema. Laboratory data include irregular, damaged red blood cells, progressive anemia, thrombocytopenia, and elevated liver enzymes (Fallon & Riely, 1995).

It is important to avoid traumatizing the liver by abdominal palpation and to use care in transporting the woman. A sudden increase in intra-abdominal pressure could lead to rupture of the subcapsular hemotoma, which is most likely to occur during convulsions (Usta & Sibai, 1995).

Management of women with HELLP syndrome should be in a setting with full intensive care facilities. Treatment includes magnesium sulfate and hydralazine, followed by cesarean delivery if the fetus is mature (Fagan, 1994). Once delivered, most mothers will have an uneventful recovery. Platelet count generally returns to normal within 7 days (Fallon & Riely, 1995).

## Chronic Hypertension

A diagnosis of chronic hypertension is made whenever there is evidence that hypertension preceded pregnancy, or when a woman is hypertensive before 20 weeks' gestation. Chronic hypertension is seen most often in older women, in those who are obese, and in those with diabetes. Heredity, which includes racial factors, plays a role in the development of chronic hypertension, which is common in African-Americans (Cunningham et al., 1997).

Pregnancy aggravates hypertension. The most common hazard faced by women with chronic hypertension is the development of pre-eclampsia. The diagnosis is made on the basis of a rise in blood pressure, sustained proteinuria, and generalized edema (Roberts, 1994). Treatment of superimposed pre-eclampsia often requires hospitalization and measures to prevent the development of eclampsia.

A high-protein diet with adequate but not excessive salt is recommended, and the woman is advised to weigh herself every 3 days to detect abnormal weight gain. Antihypertensive medication should be continued if already in use. If not in use, antihypertensive medication should be initiated once the diastolic pressure is consistently higher than 90 mmHg (Ferris, 1995). The choice of antihypertensive medication is of great concern because of the possible teratogenic effects of these medications. Methyldopa (Aldomet) is one of the most commonly prescribed antihypertensives during pregnancy, and long-term follow-up evaluations of children whose mothers took methyldopa indicate no signs of teratogenic effects (Roberts, 1994).

**CHECK YOUR READING**

23. What does the acronym HELLP stand for? What are the prominent signs and symptoms of this syndrome? Why should the liver not be palpated?
24. Compare pre-eclampsia with chronic hypertension in terms of onset and treatment.

## Incompatibility Between Maternal and Fetal Blood

### Rh Incompatibility

Rhesus (Rh) factor incompatibility during pregnancy is possible only when two specific circumstances coexist: (1) the expectant mother is Rh-negative and (2) the fetus is Rh-positive. For such a circumstance to occur, the father of the fetus must be Rh-positive. Rh incompatibility is basically a problem that affects the fetus; it causes no harm to the expectant mother.

Rh-negative blood is a recessive trait; therefore, a person must inherit the same gene from both parents to be Rh-negative. Approximately 15 percent of the white population in the United States is Rh-negative. The incidence is lower in the African-American and Asian populations.

#### PATHOPHYSIOLOGY

People who are Rh-positive have the Rh antigen on their red blood cells, whereas people who are

Rh-negative do not have the antigen. When blood from a person who is Rh-positive enters the blood stream of a person who is Rh-negative, the body reacts as it would to any foreign substance: it develops antibodies to destroy the invading antigen. To destroy the Rh antigen, which exists as part of the red blood cell, the entire red blood cell must be destroyed.

Theoretically, there is no mixing of fetal and maternal blood during pregnancy. In reality, small placental accidents may occur that allow a drop or two of fetal blood to enter the maternal circulation and initiate the production of antibodies to destroy the Rh-positive blood. Sensitization can also occur during a spontaneous or elective abortion or during antepartal procedures such as amniocentesis and chorionic villus sampling. Figure 25–9 illustrates the process of maternal sensitization.

Most exposure of maternal blood to fetal blood occurs during the third stage of labor, when there may be active exchange of fetal and maternal blood from damaged placental vessels. In this case, the woman's first child is not affected because antibodies are formed following the birth of the infant. Subsequent Rh-positive fetuses may be affected, however, unless the mother receives $Rh_0(D)$ immune globulin (RhoGAM) to prevent antibody formation after the birth of each Rh-positive infant.

## Critical to Remember

### TREATMENT FOR Rh-NEGATIVE WOMEN

All unsensitized Rh-negative women should receive $Rh_0(D)$ immune globulin (RhoGAM) following abortion, ectopic pregnancy, chorionic villus sampling, amniocentesis, or birth of an Rh-positive infant. RhoGAM prevents the development of Rh antibodies that would result in destruction of fetal erythrocytes in subsequent pregnancies.

### FETAL AND NEONATAL IMPLICATIONS

If antibodies to the Rh factor are present in the expectant mother's blood, they cross the placental barrier and cause massive destruction of fetal red blood cells. The fetus becomes deficient in red blood cells, which are needed to transport oxygen to fetal tissue. As fetal red blood cells are destroyed, fetal bilirubin levels increase (icterus gravis), which

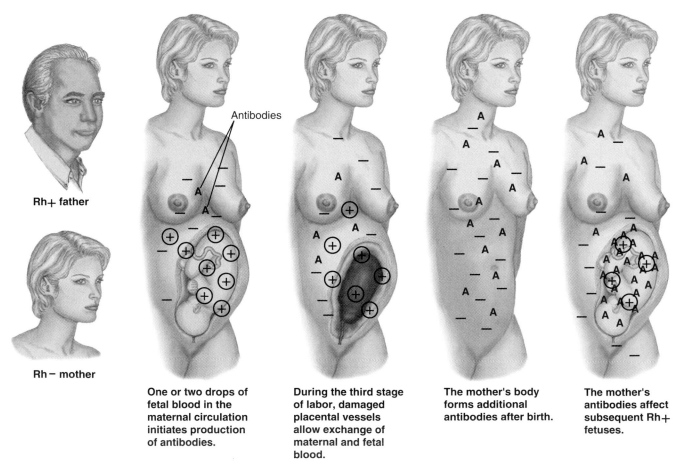

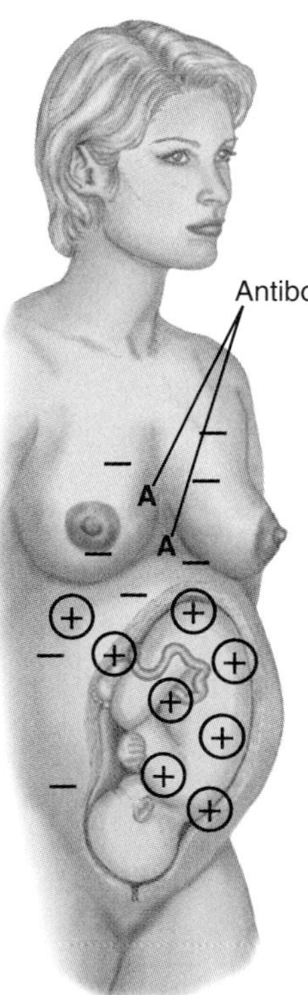


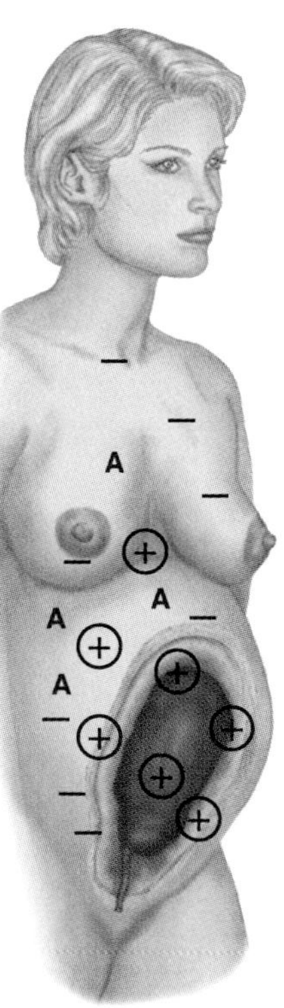


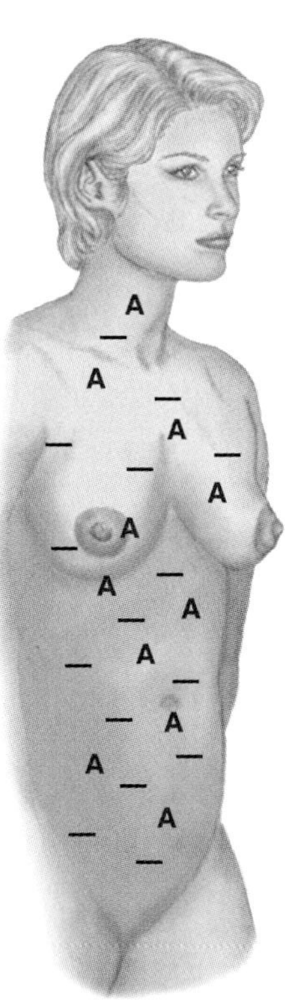


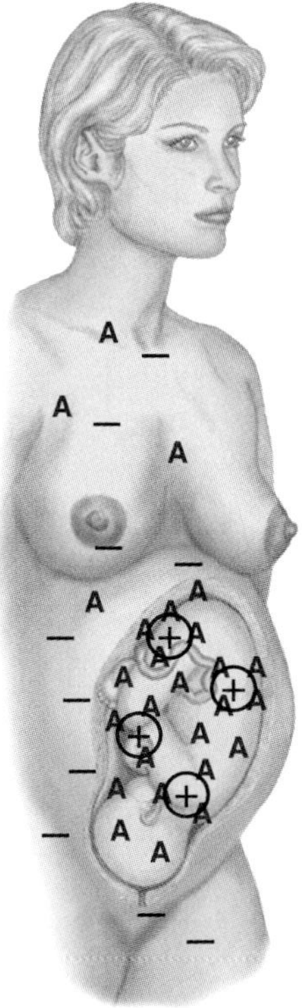


Rh+ father

Rh− mother

The mother's body forms additional antibodies after birth.

**FIGURE 25–9**

The process of maternal sensitization to the Rh factor.

can lead to severe neurologic disease (kernicterus). This hemolytic process results in rapid production of erythroblasts (immature red blood cells), which cannot carry oxygen. The entire syndrome is termed erythroblastosis fetalis. The fetus becomes so anemic that generalized fetal edema (hydrops fetalis) results and can terminate in fetal congestive heart failure.

Management of the infant born with erythroblastosis fetalis is discussed in Chapter 30.

#### PRENATAL ASSESSMENT AND MANAGEMENT

All pregnant women should have a blood test to determine blood type and Rh factor at the initial prenatal visit. Rh-negative women should have an antibody titer (indirect Coombs' test) to determine whether they are sensitized (have developed antibodies) as a result of previous exposure to Rh-positive blood. If the indirect Coombs' test is negative, it is repeated at 28 weeks of gestation to identify cases of subsequent sensitization. A negative indirect Coombs' test result accurately identifies the fetus as not at risk for hemolytic disease of the newborn.

An $Rh_0(D)$ immune globulin (such as RhoGAM), is administered to the unsensitized, Rh-negative woman at 28 weeks of gestation as a preventive measure. RhoGAM is a commercial preparation of passive antibodies against Rh factor. It effectively prevents the formation of active antibodies if there is accidental transport of fetal Rh-positive blood into the circulation of an Rh-negative mother during the remainder of the pregnancy.

If the indirect Coombs' test result is positive, that is, if it indicates maternal sensitization and the presence of antibodies, it is repeated at frequent intervals throughout the pregnancy to determine whether the antibody titer is rising. An increase in titer indicates that the process is continuing and that the fetus will be in jeopardy.

Amniocentesis may be performed to evaluate change in the optical density ($\Delta$OD) of amniotic fluid. This reflects the amount of bilirubin (residue of red blood cell destruction) that is present in the amniotic fluid. If the fluid optical density remains low, it may indicate that the fetus is Rh-positive but in no jeopardy or, more likely, that the fetus is Rh-negative. If the optical density is elevated, indicating fetal jeopardy in a hostile environment, intrauterine transfusion may be planned. If the fetal age is more than 32 weeks, early delivery may provide the best opportunity for survival.

Ultrasound examination is also used to evaluate the condition of the fetus. Generalized fetal edema, ascites, enlarged heart, or hydramnios indicates serious fetal compromise. Figure 25–10 summarizes assessments.

#### POSTPARTUM MANAGEMENT

If the mother is Rh-negative, umbilical cord blood is taken at delivery to determine blood type, Rh factor, and antibody titer (direct Coombs' test) of the newborn. Rh-negative, unsensitized mothers who give birth to Rh-positive infants are given an intra-

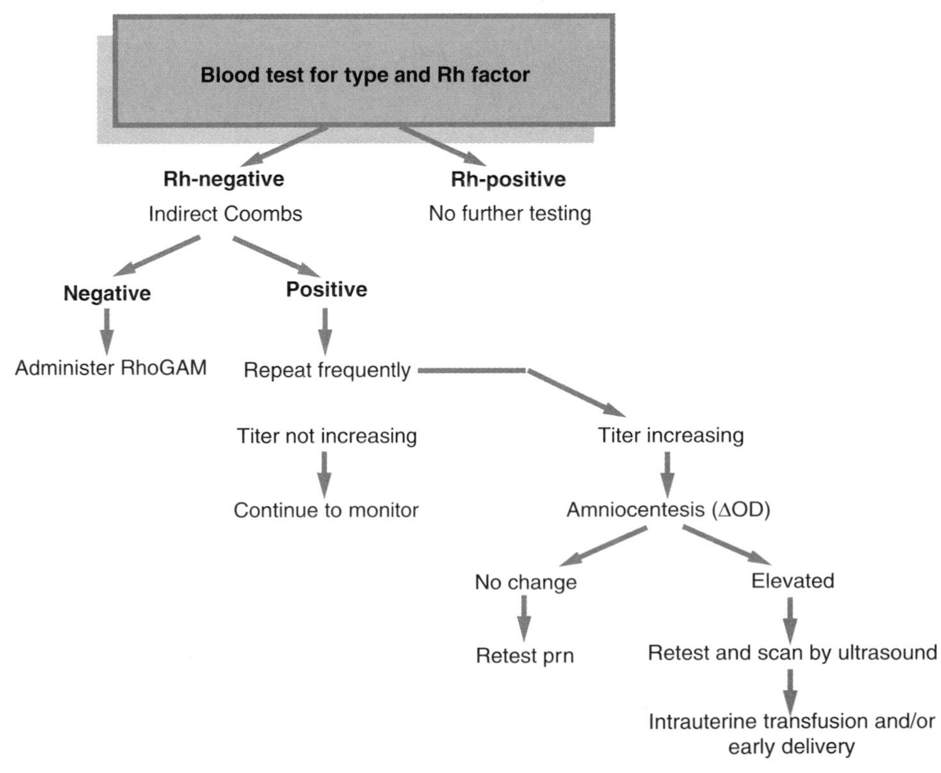


**FIGURE 25–10**

Sequence of assessments for Rh sensitization. prn, as needed; $\Delta$OD, change in optical density of bilirubin.

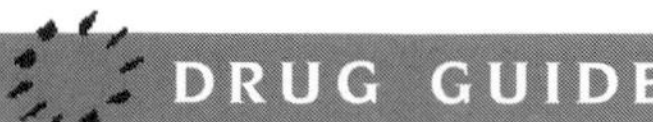

## Rh$_0$(D) IMMUNE GLOBULIN (RhoGAM, HypRhoD, Gamulin Rh)

***Classification:*** Concentrated immunoglobulins directed toward the red blood cell antigen Rh$_0$(D).

***Action:*** Prevents production of anti-Rh$_0$(D) antibodies in Rh-negative women who have been exposed to Rh-positive blood by suppressing the immune reaction of the Rh-negative woman to the antigen in Rh-positive blood. Prevents antibody response and subsequently prevents hemolytic disease of the newborn in future pregnancies of women who have conceived an Rh-positive fetus.

***Indications:*** Administered to Rh-negative women who have been exposed to Rh-positive blood by

1. Delivering an Rh-positive infant.
2. Aborting an Rh-positive fetus.
3. Having chorionic villus sampling, amniocentesis, or intra-abdominal trauma while carrying an Rh-positive fetus.
4. Following accidental transfusion of Rh-positive blood to an Rh-negative woman.

***Dosage and Route:*** One standard dose administered intramuscularly

1. At 28 weeks of pregnancy and within 72 hours of delivery.
2. Within 72 hours following termination of a pregnancy of 13 weeks or more of gestation.

One *microdose* within 72 hours following the termination of a pregnancy of less than 13 weeks' gestation.

Dose is calculated based on the volume of blood erroneously administered in transfusion accidents.

***Absorption:*** Well absorbed from intramuscular sites.

***Excretion:*** Metabolism and excretion unknown.

***Contraindications and Precautions:*** Women who are Rh-positive or women previously sensitized to Rh$_0$(D) should not receive Rh$_0$(D) immune globulin. Used cautiously for women with previous hypersensitivity reactions to immune globulins.

***Adverse Reactions:*** Local pain at intramuscular site, fever, or both.

***Nursing Implications:*** Type and crossmatch of mother's blood and cord blood of the newborn must be performed to determine the need for the medication. The mother must be Rh-negative and negative for Rh antibodies; the newborn must be Rh-positive. If there is doubt regarding the fetus' blood type following termination of pregnancy, the medication should be administered. The drug is administered to the mother, not the infant. The deltoid muscle is recommended for intramuscular administration.

---

muscular injection of RhoGAM within 72 hours following delivery. If RhoGAM is given to the mother in the first 72 hours following delivery of an Rh-positive infant, any Rh antigens present are destroyed, and therefore the mother forms no natural antibodies.

If the infant is Rh-negative, there is no possibility of antibody formation and RhoGAM is not necessary. As stated previously, RhoGAM is also administered following abortion, chorionic villus sampling, and amniocentesis when fetal-to-maternal transfusion is possible, and at 28 weeks of gestation if the mother is Rh-negative and unsensitized.

Nurses must be prepared to reassure the expectant parents that the medical management is generally effective and to answer questions that are commonly asked.

Families are often very concerned about the fetus, and nurses must be sensitive to cues and signals that indicate that the family is anxious and must be able to offer honest reassurance. This is especially important if the expectant mother is sensitized and fetal testing is necessary throughout pregnancy.

During labor, the nurse is often responsible for reminding the physician that cord blood is needed to determine the blood type and Rh factor of the newborn. During the postpartum period, nurses are responsible for follow-up to determine whether RhoGAM is necessary and for administering the injection within the prescribed time.

### ABO Incompatibility

ABO incompatibility occurs when the expectant mother is blood type O and the fetus is blood type A, B or AB. Type A, B, and AB blood contains a protein component (antigen) that is not present in type O blood.

### Parents Want to Know About Rh Incompatibility

*What does it mean to be Rh-negative?*

Those who are Rh-negative lack a substance that is present in the red blood cells of those who are Rh-positive.

*How can the expectant mother be Rh-negative and the fetus be Rh-positive?*

The fetus can inherit the Rh-positive factor from the father.

*What does sensitization mean?*

Sensitization means that the expectant mother has been exposed to Rh-positive blood and has developed antibodies against the Rh factor.

*Do the antibodies harm the expectant mother?*

No, because she does not have the Rh factor.

*Do Rh-positive men always father Rh-positive children?*

No. Rh-positive men who have an Rh-positive gene and an Rh-negative gene can father Rh-negative children.

*Why is RhoGAM necessary during pregnancy and following childbirth?*

RhoGAM prevents the development of Rh antibodies, which might be harmful to subsequent fetuses.

*Why will the next fetus be jeopardized if RhoGAM is not administered?*

If RhoGAM is not administered when the fetus is Rh-positive, the expectant mother may develop antibodies that cross the placental barrier and affect the next Rh-positive fetus.

People with type O blood develop anti-A or anti-B antibodies naturally as a result of exposure to antigens in the foods that they eat or to infection by gram-negative bacteria. As a result, some women with blood type O have developed high serum anti-A and anti-B antibody titers before pregnancy. The antibodies may be either IgG or IgM. When the woman becomes pregnant, the IgG antibodies cross the placental barrier and cause hemolysis of fetal red blood cells. Although the first fetus can be affected, ABO incompatibility is less severe than Rh incompatibility because the primary antibodies of the ABO system are IgM, which do not cross the placenta.

No specific prenatal care is needed; however, the nurse must be aware of the possibility of ABO incompatibility. During the delivery, cord blood is taken to determine the blood type of the newborn and the antibody titer (direct Coombs' test). The newborn is carefully screened for jaundice, which indicates hyperbilirubinemia. See Chapter 30 for medical and nursing management of hyperbilirubinemia in newborns.

**CHECK YOUR READING**

25. Why do unsensitized Rh-negative expectant mothers receive RhoGAM during pregnancy and following an abortion, amniocentesis, and childbirth?
26. What are the effects on the fetus of maternal Rh sensitization?
27. Why is the first fetus sometimes affected if there is ABO incompatibility? Why are the effects of ABO incompatibility milder than Rh-sensitization?

## SUMMARY CONCEPTS

- Spontaneous abortion is one of the leading causes of pregnancy loss. Treatment is aimed at preventing complications, such as hypovolemic shock and infection, and providing emotional support for grieving, which accompanies any pregnancy loss.
- The incidence of ectopic pregnancy is increasing in the United States as a result of pelvic inflammation associated with sexually transmissible diseases. The goals of therapeutic management are to prevent severe hemorrhage and to preserve the fallopian tube so that future fertility is retained.
- Management of hydatidiform mole involves two phases: (1) evacuation of the molar pregnancy and (2) continuous follow-up for 1 year to detect malignant changes in the remaining trophoblastic tissue.
- Disorders of the placenta (placenta previa and abruptio placentae) are responsible for hemorrhagic conditions of the last half of pregnancy. Either condition may result in maternal hemorrhage and fetal or maternal death.
- Disseminated intravascular coagulation is a life-threatening complication of missed abortion, abruptio placentae, and pre-eclampsia, in which procoagulation and anticoagulation factors are simultaneously activated.
- The cause of hyperemesis gravidarum remains obscure, but the goals of management are to prevent dehydration, malnutrition, and electrolyte imbalance. Emotional support is a most important therapy and a responsibility of nurses.
- Hypertensive disorders of pregnancy may include pregnancy-induced hypertension, pre-eclampsia, eclampsia, or preexisting (chronic) hypertension. The underlying process is generalized vasospasm, which decreases circulation to all organs of the body, including the placenta. Major maternal organs affected include the liver, kidneys, and brain.
- Treatment of pre-eclampsia includes bedrest, reduction of environmental stimuli, and administration of anticonvulsants.
- Magnesium sulfate, an anticonvulsant used to prevent pre-eclampsia from progressing to eclamptic convulsions, is associated with adverse effects, the most serious being central nervous system depression, which includes depression of the respiratory center.
- Nurses monitor the woman with pre-eclampsia to determine the effectiveness of medical therapy and to identify signs that the condition is worsening, such as increasing hyperreflexia. Nurses also control external stimuli and initiate measures to protect her in case of eclamptic seizures.
- Nurses also monitor the woman with pre-eclampsia for signs of magnesium toxicity, which include decreased respiratory effort and hyporeflexia.
- Women who have chronic hypertension are at increased risk for pre-eclampsia and should be monitored closely for proteinuria or generalized edema. Antihypertensive medication should be continued or initiated if diastolic blood pressure is consistently higher than 90 mmHg.
- Rh incompatibility can occur when an Rh-negative woman conceives a child who is Rh-positive. As a result of exposure to the Rh-positive antigen, maternal antibodies may develop that cause hemolysis of fetal Rh-positive red blood cells in subsequent pregnancies.
- Administration of RhoGam prevents production of anti-Rh antibodies, thus preventing destruction of Rh-positive red blood cells in subsequent pregnancies.
- ABO incompatibility usually occurs when the mother has type O blood and naturally occurring anti-A and anti-B antibodies, which cause hemolysis if the fetus' blood is not type O. ABO incompatibility may result in hyperbilirubinemia of the infant, but it usually presents no serious threat to the health of the child.

### References and Readings

American College of Obstetricians and Gynecologists (ACOG) (1996). Hypertension in pregnancy. *Technical Bulletin* 219. Washington, D.C.: Author.

Arias, F. (1994). Third-trimester bleeding. In F.P. Zuspan & E.J. Quilligan (Eds.), *Current therapy in obstetrics and gynecology* (4th ed.). Philadelphia: W.B. Saunders.

Berman, M.L., & DiSaia, P.J. (1994). Pelvic malignancies, gestational trophoblastic neoplasia, and nonpelvic malignancies. In R.K. Creasy & R. Resnik (Eds.), *Maternal-fetal medicine: Principles and practice* (3rd ed., pp. 1112–1134). Philadelphia: W.B. Saunders.

Bernstein, J. (1995). Ectopic pregnancy: A nursing approach to excess risk among minority women. *Journal of Obstetric, Gynecologic, and Neonatal Nursing*, 24(9), 803–809.

Bowman, J.M. (1994). Hemolytic disease (erythroblastosis fetalis). In R.K. Creasy & R. Resnik (Eds.), *Maternal-fetal medicine: Principles and practice* (3rd ed., pp. 711–743). Philadelphia: W.B. Saunders.

Carpenito, L.J. (1996). *Nursing diagnosis: Application to clinical practice* (6th ed.). Philadelphia: J.B. Lippincott.

Cunningham, F.G., MacDonald, P.C., Gant, N.F., Leveno, K.J., & Gilstrap, L.C., Hankins, G.D.V., et al. (1997). *Williams obstetrics* (20th ed.). Norwalk, Conn.: Appleton & Lange.

Enkin, M., Keirse, M.J., Renfrew, M., & Neilson, J. (1995). *A guide to effective care in pregnancy and childbirth* (2nd. ed.). Oxford and New York: Oxford University Press.

Fagan, E.A. (1994). Diseases of liver, biliary system, and pancreas. In R.K. Creasy & R. Resnik (Eds.), *Maternal-fetal medicine: Principles and practice* (3rd ed., pp. 1040–1061). Philadelphia: W.B. Saunders.

Fallon, K.J., & Riely, C.A. (1995). Liver diseases. In G.N. Burrow & T.F. Ferris (Eds.), *Medical complications during pregnancy* (4th ed., pp. 307–342). Philadelphia: W.B. Saunders.

Ferris, T.F. (1995). Hypertension and pre-eclampsia. In G.N. Burrow & T.F. Ferris (Eds.), *Medical complications during pregnancy* (4th ed., pp. 1–28). Philadelphia: W.B. Saunders.

Glass, R.H., & Golbus, M.S. (1994). Recurrent abortion. In R.K. Creasy & R. Resnik (Eds.), *Maternal-fetal medicine: Principles and practice* (3rd ed., pp. 445–452). Philadelphia: W.B. Saunders.

Green, J.R. (1994). Placenta previa and abruptio placentae. In R.K. Creasy & R. Resnik (Eds.), *Maternal-fetal medicine: Principles and practice* (3rd ed., pp. 602–619). Philadelphia: W.B. Saunders.

Grohar, J. (1994). Nursing protocols for antepartum home care. *Journal of Obstetric, Gynecologic, and Neonatal Nursing*, 23(8), 687–694.

Hayashi, R.H., & Castillo, M.S. (1993). Bleeding in pregnancy. In R.A. Knuppel & J.E. Drukker (Eds.), *High-risk pregnancy: A team approach* (2nd ed., pp. 539–560). Philadelphia: W.B. Saunders.

Hewell, S.W., & Hammer, R.H. (1997). Antiphospholipid antibodies: A threat throughout pregnancy. *Journal of Obstetric, Gynecologic, and Neonatal Nursing*, 26(2), 162–168.

Jehle, D., Krause, R., & Braen, G.R. (1994). Ectopic pregnancy. *Emergency Medicine Clinics of North America*, 12(1), 55–72.

Knuppel, R.A., & Drukker, J.E. (1993). Hypertension in pregnancy. In R.A. Knuppel & J.E. Drukker (Eds.), *High-risk pregnancy: A team approach* (2nd ed., pp. 468–575). Philadelphia: W.B. Saunders.

Kohorn, E.I. (1994). Hydatidiform mole. In F.P. Zuspan & E.J. Quilligan (Eds.), *Current therapy in obstetrics and gynecology* (4th ed., pp. 180–184). Philadelphia: W.B. Saunders.

Lucas, L.S., & Jordan, E.T. (1997). Phenytoin as an alternative treatment for pre-eclampsia. *Journal of Obstetric, Gynecologic, and Neonatal Nursing*, 26(3), 263–269.

Magann, E.F., & Martin, J.N. (1995). Complicated postpartum preeclampsia-eclampsia. *Obstetrics and Gynecology Clinics of North America*, 22(2), 337–357.

Mahan, I.K., & Escott-Stump, S. (1996). *Krause's food, nutrition, and diet therapy* (9th ed.). Philadelphia: W.B. Saunders.

Maiolatesi, C.R., & Peddicord, K. (1996). Methotrexate for nonsurgical treatment of ectopic pregnancy: Nursing implications. *Journal of Obstetric, Gynecologic, and Neonatal Nursing*, 25(3), 205–208.

Nathan, L., & Huddleston, J.F. (1995). Acute abdominal pain in pregnancy. *Obstetrics and Gynecology Clinics of North America*, 22(1), 55–68.

Newman, V., Fullerton, J.T., & Anderson, P.O. (1993). Clinical advances in the management of severe nausea and vomiting during pregnancy. *Journal of Obstetric, Gynecologic, and Neonatal Nursing*, 22(6), 483–490.

O'Brien, B., & Zhou, Q. (1995). Variables related to nausea and vomiting during pregnancy. *Birth*, 22(2), 95–100.

Probst, B.D. (1994). Hypertensive disorders of pregnancy. *Emergency Medicine Clinics of North America*, 12(1), 73–89.

Richardson, P. (1994). Body experience differences of women with pregnancy-induced hypertension. *Maternal-Child Nursing Journal*, 22(4), 121–133.

Roberts, J.M. (1994). Pregnancy-related hypertension. In R.K. Creasy & R. Resnik (Eds.), *Maternal-fetal medicine: Principles and practice* (3rd ed., pp. 804–843). Philadelphia: W.B. Saunders.

Rosevear, S. (1994). Bleeding in early pregnancy. In. D.K. James, P.J. Steer, C.P. Weiner, & B. Gonik (Eds.), *High-risk pregnancy: Management options* (pp. 75–117). Philadelphia: W.B. Saunders.

Scott, J.R., & Branch, D.W. (1994). Immunologic disorders. In R.K. Creasy & R. Resnik (Eds.), *Maternal-fetal medicine: Principles and practice* (3rd ed., pp. 467–481). Philadelphia: W.B. Saunders.

Simpson, K.R. (1992). *Protocols for homecare management of high-risk pregnancies.* St. Louis: Healthy Homecomings, Inc.

Thompson, W.B. (1994). Therapeutic abortion. In F.P. Zuspan & E.J. Quilligan (Eds.), *Current therapy in obstetrics and gynecology* (4th ed., pp. 310–313). Philadelphia: W.B. Saunders.

Urbanski, T.K., Higgins, P.G., Murray, M.L., & Joffe, G. (1996). Caring for a woman with a hydatidiform mole and coexisting pregnancy. *American Journal of Maternal Child Nursing*, 21(2), 85–89.

Usta, I.M., & Sibai, B.M. (1995). Emergent management of puerperal eclampsia. *Obstetrics and Gynecology Clinics of North America*, 22(2), 315–335.

van Stuijvenberg, M.E., Schabort, I., Labadarios, D., & Nel, J.T. (1995). The nutritional status and treatment of patients with hyperemesis gravidarum. *American Journal of Obstetrics and Gynecology*, 172(5), 1585–1591.

Yero, T., Mayer, J., Parsons, A., & Maroulis, G. (1995). A prospective of unruptured ectopic pregnancies treated by tubal injection with hyperosmolar glucose. *Obstetrics and Gynecology*, 85(2), 265–268.

# 26

# Concurrent Disorders During Pregnancy

**OBJECTIVES**

1. Describe the effects of pregnancy on fuel metabolism.
2. Discuss the effects and management of preexisting diabetes mellitus during pregnancy.
3. Explain the effects and management of gestational diabetes mellitus.
4. Describe the major effects of pregnancy on the woman who has heart disease, and identify the goals of therapy.
5. Explain the maternal and fetal effects of specific anemias and the required management during pregnancy.
6. Identify the effects, management, and nursing considerations of specific preexisting conditions; such as lupus erythematosus, rheumatoid arthritis, and epilepsy.
7. Identify the major causes of trauma during pregnancy and describe therapeutic management.
8. Discuss the maternal, fetal, and neonatal effects of the most common infections that may occur during pregnancy.

**DEFINITIONS**

**acquired immunodeficiency syndrome (AIDS)** *Syndrome caused by the human immunodeficiency virus* (HIV), *resulting in loss of defense against malignancies and opportunistic infections.*

**cardiac decompensation** *Failure of the heart to maintain adequate circulation to the tissues. See also congestive heart failure.*

**caudal regressive syndrome** *A severe malformation that results when the sacrum, lumbar spine, and lower extremities fail to develop.*

**congenital anomaly** *Abnormal intrauterine development of an organ or structure.*

**congestive heart failure** *Condition resulting from failure of the heart to maintain adequate circulation; characterized by weakness, dyspnea, and edema in body parts that are lower than the heart.*

**diabetes mellitus** *A disorder of carbohydrate metabolism caused by a relative or complete lack of insulin secretion. Characterized by glycosuria (glucose in the urine) and hyperglycemia.*

**diabetogenic** *Condition, such as pregnancy, that produces the effects of diabetes mellitus.*

**dystocia** *Difficult or prolonged labor; often associated with abnormal uterine activity and cephalopelvic disproportion.*

**gestational diabetes** *Impaired glucose tolerance that is induced by pregnancy and diagnosed during pregnancy. Usually disappears after childbirth.*

**gluconeogenesis** *Formation of glycogen by the liver from noncarbohydrate sources, such as amino or fatty acids.*

**human immunodeficiency virus (HIV)** *A retrovirus that results in the development of AIDS.*

**hydramnios** *Excess volume of amniotic fluid (more than 2000 ml at term). Also called polyhydramnios.*

**ketosis** *Accumulation of ketone bodies (metabolic products) in the blood; frequently associated with acidosis.*

**lipogenic** *Substance, such as insulin, that stimulates the production of fat.*

**macrosomia** *Unusually large fetal size; infant birth weight more than 4000 g.*

**Marfan's syndrome** *A hereditary condition that involves weakness in connective tissue, bones, and muscles; the vascular system is affected, particularly the aorta.*

**neonatologist** *A physician who specializes in the care of newborn infants (from birth until the 29th day of life).*

**osmotic diuresis** *Secretion and passage of large amounts of urine as a result of increased osmotic pressure that can result from hyperglycemia.*

**perinatologist** *A physician who specializes in the care of the mother, the fetus, and the infant during the perinatal period (from the 20th week of pregnancy to 4 weeks after childbirth).*

**polydipsia** *Excessive thirst.*

**polyphagia** *Excessive ingestion of food.*

**polyuria** *Excessive excretion of urine.*

**seroconversion** *Change in a blood test result from negative to positive, indicating the development of antibodies in response to infection or immunization.*

Pregnancy affects the care of women with a medical condition in two ways. First, pregnancy may alter the course of the disease. Second, the disease or its treatment may have unwanted effects on the pregnancy. As a result, the usual antepartum care must be adapted to include increased surveillance of the mother and the fetus. Moreover, some disorders that are mild or even subclinical in the pregnant woman can produce massive damage to the fetus. This chapter describes the most common disorders that can cause significant fetal jeopardy.

# Diabetes Mellitus

## Pathophysiology

### ETIOLOGY

Diabetes mellitus is a complex disorder of carbohydrate metabolism caused primarily by a partial or complete lack of insulin secretion by the beta cells of the pancreas. Some cells, such as those in skeletal and cardiac muscles and in adipose tissue, rely on insulin to carry glucose across the cell membranes. Without insulin, glucose accumulates in the blood, resulting in hyperglycemia. The body attempts to dilute the glucose load by any means possible. The first strategy is to increase thirst (polydipsia), one of the classic symptoms of diabetes mellitus. Next, fluid from the intracellular spaces is drawn into the vascular bed, resulting in dehydration at the cellular level but fluid volume excess in the vascular compartment. The kidneys attempt to excrete large volumes of this fluid plus the heavy solute load of glucose (osmotic diuresis). This excretion produces the second symptom of diabetes, polyuria, as well as glycosuria (glucose in the urine). Without glucose, the cells starve, so that there is weight loss even though the person ingests excessive amounts of food (polyphagia).

Because the body is unable to metabolize glucose, it begins to metabolize protein and fat to meet energy needs. Metabolism of protein produces a negative nitrogen balance, and the metabolism of fat results in the buildup of ketone bodies (such as acetone, acetoacetic acid, or $\beta$-hydroxybutyric acid) or ketosis (accumulation of acids in the body).

If the disease is not well controlled, serious complications may occur. Hypoglycemia or hyperglycemia can result if the amount of insulin does not match the diet. Moreover, fluctuating periods of hyperglycemia and hypoglycemia damage small blood vessels throughout the body. This damage can cause serious impairment, especially in the kidneys, eyes, and heart.

### EFFECT OF PREGNANCY ON FUEL METABOLISM

To comprehend the relationship of diabetes mellitus and pregnancy, it is necessary to understand how pregnancy and diabetes alter the metabolism of food.

**Early Pregnancy.** Metabolic changes can be divided into those that occur early in pregnancy (from 1 to 20 weeks) and those that occur late in pregnancy (from 20 to 40 weeks). During early pregnancy, maternal metabolic rates and energy needs change little. During this time, however, insulin release in response to serum glucose levels accelerates. As a result, significant hypoglycemia may occur, particularly in women who experience the nausea, vomiting, and anorexia that often occur during the first weeks of pregnancy.

In an uncomplicated pregnancy, the availability of glucose and insulin, a lipogenic substance, favors the development and storage of fat during the first half of pregnancy. Accumulation of fat prepares the mother for the rise in energy use by the growing fetus during the second half of pregnancy.

**Late Pregnancy.** During the second half of pregnancy when fetal growth accelerates, placental hormones rise sharply. These hormones, particularly estrogen, progesterone, and human placental lactogen, create *resistance to insulin* in maternal cells. This resistance allows an abundant supply of glucose to be available for the fetus. However, the hormones have a diabetogenic effect in that they may leave the woman with insufficient insulin and episodes of hyperglycemia.

For many women, insulin resistance is not a problem; the pancreas responds by simply increasing the production of insulin. If the pancreas is unable to respond, however, the woman will experience fluctuating periods of hyperglycemia.

During late pregnancy, there is continuous withdrawal by the fetus of nutrients, such as glucose and amino acids, from maternal blood. The result is an earlier-than-normal switch from carbohydrate metabolism to gluconeogenesis (formation of glycogen from noncarbohydrate sources such as proteins and fat). Because the fetus uses many of the amino acids, the process becomes predominantly one of fat utilization. This process produces high levels of free fatty acids that further inhibit the uptake and oxidation of glucose and, thus, preserves glucose for use by the central nervous system and the fetus. These metabolic changes are similar to those occurring during "accelerated starvation," when fat is metabolized to meet many of the body's energy needs.

**TABLE 26–1 CLASSIFICATION OF DIABETES MELLITUS**

**TYPE I—INSULIN DEPENDENT**

Onset in childhood or young adulthood; no insulin produced; prone to ketosis.

**TYPE II—NON–INSULIN DEPENDENT**

Usual onset after 40 years; associated with obesity; usually sufficient insulin produced to prevent ketosis.

**TYPE III—GESTATIONAL**

Onset of glucose intolerance first diagnosed during pregnancy; exogenous insulin may or may not be needed.

From National Institute of Diabetes and Digestive and Kidney Diseases. (1994). *Insulin-dependent diabetes.* NIH Publication No. 95-2098. Washington, D.C.: Author.

## Classification

Diabetes is classified as type I (insulin dependent) or type II (non–insulin dependent) according to whether the client requires the administration of insulin to prevent ketoacidosis. The onset of glucose intolerance during pregnancy is termed *gestational diabetes* (Table 26–1).

At one time the classification of diabetes during pregnancy considered the age of onset and the duration of diabetes as well as the presence of maternal complications (Table 26–2). Improvements in fetal

**TABLE 26–2 CLASSIFICATION OF DIABETES COMPLICATING PREGNANCY**

**Pre-gestational Diabetes**

| Class | Age of Onset | | Duration (yr) | Vascular Disease | Therapy |
|---|---|---|---|---|---|
| A | Any | | Any | None | A-1 Diet only |
| B | >20 | *or* | <10 | None | Insulin |
| C | 10–19 | *or* | 10–19 | None | Insulin |
| D | <10 | | >20 | Benign retinopathy | Insulin |
| F | Any | | Any | Nephropathy | Insulin |
| R | Any | | Any | Proliferative retinopathy | Insulin |
| H | Any | | Any | Heart disease | Insulin |

**Gestational Diabetes**

| Class | Fasting Plasma Glucose | Postprandial Plasma Glucose |
|---|---|---|
| A-1 | <105 mg/dl | <120 mg/dl |
| A-2 | >105 mg/dl | >120 mg/dl |

From American College of Obstetrics and Gynecology. (1986). ACOG *Technical Bulletin* No. 92. Washington, D.C.: Author.

assessment, neonatal care, and metabolic management of the pregnant woman made the classification less helpful than in the past (ACOG, 1994).

## Incidence

The pregnant woman may have preexisting diabetes (type I or type II) or she may develop gestational diabetes mellitus (type III) during the course of the pregnancy. Diabetes mellitus is a common medical condition complicating pregnancy. One of every 200 pregnant women has preexisting diabetes. Five of every 200 pregnant women will develop gestational diabetes (Reece, 1996).

## Preexisting Diabetes Mellitus

### MATERNAL EFFECTS

The course of pregnancy for women with diabetes mellitus has improved greatly as a result of new treatments and more effective methods of fetal surveillance. However, the incidence of complications that affect the mother and fetus remains higher than that experienced by the general population.

Diabetes adversely affects pregnant women in several ways. The risk of pregnancy-induced hypertension is four times greater than in the normal population even if there is no evidence of vascular or renal complications (Cunningham et al., 1997). The development of ketoacidosis is a threat to women with insulin-dependent diabetes and is most often precipitated by infection or missed insulin doses. Moreover, ketoacidosis may develop during pregnancy at lower thresholds of hyperglycemia than those seen in nonpregnant individuals. Untreated ketoacidosis can progress to fetal and maternal death. Urinary tract infections are more common, possibly because of spilling of glucose into the urine, which provides a nutrient-rich medium for bacterial growth. Other effects include hydramnios, which may result from fetal hyperglycemia and consequent fetal diuresis, and premature rupture of membranes, which may be caused by overdistention of the uterus by hydramnios or a large fetus. Problems that arise during labor and childbirth because the fetus is frequently large (more than 4000 g) include a difficult labor, shoulder dystocia (delayed or difficult birth of fetal shoulders after the head is born), and consequent injury to the birth canal. Large fetal size also increases the likelihood that a cesarean birth will be necessary and increases the risk of postpartum hemorrhage.

During the first trimester, when major fetal organ development is occurring, the effects of the abnormal metabolic environment, such as hypoglycemia, hyperglycemia, and ketosis, may also lead to increased incidence of spontaneous abortion or major fetal malformations.

### FETAL EFFECTS

Fetal and neonatal effects of pre-existing diabetes depend on the timing and severity of maternal hyperglycemia and the degree of vascular impairment that has occurred.

**Congenital Malformation.** The most common major congenital malformations associated with preexisting diabetes are neural tube defects, caudal regression syndrome, and cardiac defects. Major malformations have been reported in 4 to 11 percent of infants born to mothers with type I diabetes compared with only 1.2 to 2.1 percent in infants of nondiabetic mothers (Healy et al., 1995). The incidence correlates directly with the degree of maternal hyperglycemia during the first trimester. Fewer malformations occur if the woman is able to maintain a normal blood glucose level before conception and throughout early pregnancy.

**Variations in Fetal Size.** Fetal growth is related to maternal vascular integrity. In women without vascular impairment, glucose and oxygen are easily transported to the fetus; if the woman is hyperglycemic, so is the fetus. Although maternal insulin does not cross the placental barrier, the fetus produces insulin by the 10th week of gestation. Fetal *macrosomia* results when elevated levels of blood glucose stimulate excessive production of fetal insulin, which acts as a powerful growth hormone. This is a major neonatal effect (birth weight more than 4000 g), with consequent increase in cesarean birth or birth injury from shoulder dystocia.

Conversely, if there is vascular impairment, placental perfusion may be decreased. Vascular impairment may be caused by complications of the diabetes or to vasoconstriction that occurs in pregnancy-induced hypertension, a common complication for the woman with diabetes. When placental perfusion is impaired, the supply of glucose as well as oxygen will be decreased. As a result, the infant is likely to be small-for-gestational age. This condition is frequently called *intrauterine growth restriction* (IUGR).

### NEONATAL EFFECTS

The four major neonatal complications of preexisting diabetes are hypoglycemia, hypocalcemia, hyperbilirubinemia, and respiratory distress syndrome.

**Hypoglycemia.** The neonate is at higher risk for hypoglycemia because fetal insulin production was accelerated during pregnancy to metabolize excessive glucose received from the expectant mother. The constant stimulation of hyperglycemia leads to hyperplasia and hypertrophy of the islets of Langerhans in the pancreas. At birth, when the maternal glucose supply is withdrawn, the level of neonatal insulin exceeds the available glucose and hypoglycemia develops rapidly.

**Hypocalcemia.** During the last half of pregnancy, large amounts of calcium are transported across the placenta from the mother to the fetus. At the time of birth, this transfer is abruptly stopped, leading to a dramatic decrease in total and ionized calcium. Hypocalcemia, defined as 7 mg/dl or less, most often occurs between 24 and 36 hours after birth (Tyrala, 1996). It is associated with preterm birth, birth trauma, and perinatal asphyxia, all common problems of the infant born to a mother with diabetes mellitus.

**Hyperbilirubinemia.** The fetus who experiences recurrent hypoxia compensates by production of additional erythrocytes to carry oxygen supplied by the mother. After birth, the excess in erythrocytes is broken down, releasing large amounts of bilirubin into the neonate's circulation.

**Respiratory Distress Syndrome.** Fetal hyperinsulinemia retards cortisol production, which is necessary for synthesis of surfactant (lipoproteins that prevent collapse of alveoli), and the inadequate production of surfactant increases the risk that the newborn will experience respiratory distress syndrome. (See Chapter 29 for additional information about neonatal complications.)

The occurrence of maternal and fetal-neonatal complications can be greatly diminished by maintaining normal blood glucose levels. The objective of the team providing treatment is to devise a plan that allows the woman to maintain a level as close to normal as possible (Nursing Care Plan 26–1).

### MATERNAL ASSESSMENT

Whenever a pregnant woman with preexisting diabetes initiates prenatal care, a thorough evaluation of her health status must be completed. This evaluation includes history, physical examination, and laboratory tests.

**History.** A detailed history should include the onset and management of the diabetic condition. How long has she had the disease? How does she maintain normal blood glucose? Is she familiar with how to monitor blood glucose and administer insulin? The degree of glycemic control before pregnancy is of particular interest. Effective management depends on her adherence to a plan of care. Therefore, her knowledge of how diabetes affects pregnancy and how pregnancy affects diabetes must be determined. The support person's knowledge also must be assessed, and specific learning needs should be identified. In addition, the woman's emotional status should be assessed to determine how she is coping with pregnancy superimposed on preexisting diabetes.

All women with diabetes should be seen by a qualified nurse-educator for an individualized assessment to ensure that they can monitor blood glucose accurately. A variety of battery-powered portable blood glucose reflectance meters are currently available for home use. Accurate readings depend on performing the test correctly and as often as recommended by the health care team. In addition to home monitoring of blood glucose, the nurse must observe the woman's skill in mixing and administering insulin.

**Physical Examination.** In addition to routine prenatal examination (see Chapter 7), specific efforts should be made to assess the effects of diabetes. A baseline electrocardiogram (ECG) should be obtained to determine cardiovascular status. Evaluation for retinopathy should be performed, with referral to an ophthalmologist if necessary. The woman's weight and blood pressure must be monitored carefully because of the increased risk for the development of pregnancy-induced hypertension. Fundal height should be measured, noting any abnormal increase in size that may indicate macrosomia or hydramnios, which may occur as a result of diuresis by the hyperglycemic fetus.

**Laboratory Tests.** In addition to routine prenatal laboratory examinations (see Chapter 7), baseline renal function should be assessed with a 24-hour urine collection for total protein excretion and creatinine clearance. The urine should be checked at each prenatal visit for possible urinary tract infections that are common in women with diabetes. Urine should also be checked for the presence of glucose and ketones. Thyroid function tests should be performed because of the risk for coexisting thyroid disease.

Glycemic control should be evaluated on the basis of *glycosylated hemoglobin*. With prolonged hyperglycemia, a percentage of hemoglobin will remain saturated with glucose for the life of the red blood cell. The glycosylated hemoglobin assay (HbA1c) is an accurate measurement of the average glucose concentrations during the preceding 4 to 8 weeks (Homko & Khandelwal, 1996). Unlike other tests that reflect the amount of glucose in the plasma at that moment, the HbA1c is not affected by recent intake or restriction of food.

### FETAL SURVEILLANCE

Because of the increased risk for congenital anomalies, fetal surveillance should begin early for women with preexisting diabetes mellitus. Maternal serum alpha-fetoprotein should be offered at approximately 16 weeks' gestation to screen for neural tube defects, which increase by as much as 20-fold in offspring of mothers with diabetes (Reece et al., 1996). A detailed ultrasonographic evaluation of the fetus should

## Nursing Care Plan 26–1

# Pregnancy and Diabetes Mellitus

**ASSESSMENT:** Kathy Ringold is a 24-year-old primigravida of 9 weeks' gestation who was diagnosed with type I diabetes mellitus 6 years ago. She has been on a daily regimen of insulin and is comfortable with insulin administration and blood glucose monitoring. She is experiencing daily nausea and vomiting. Kathy states that she is concerned because she is not eating as much as before becoming pregnant. She also reveals that she had sometimes "binged" on food before becoming pregnant and didn't always monitor blood glucose as often as directed. She does not see why her blood glucose has to be watched so carefully.

**NURSING DIAGNOSIS:** Risk for Altered Health Maintenance related to knowledge deficit of the effects of pregnancy on diabetes control

**GOALS/EXPECTED OUTCOMES**

Kathy will do the following:

1. Describe predicted changes in insulin needs throughout pregnancy.
2. Follow prescribed schedule of blood glucose monitoring, insulin administration, diet, and exercise.
3. Describe the importance of frequent fetal surveillance and follow the prescribed schedule.

| INTERVENTION | RATIONALE |
|---|---|
| 1. Reduce barriers to learning<br>a. Allow Kathy to express emotions and concerns before teaching.<br>b. Examine her beliefs and past experiences related to diabetes.<br>c. Assess readiness to learn, based on interest, attention, and participation in scheduled learning sessions. | 1. Motivation and readiness to learn are essential for permanent learning to occur. She will learn only if she sees the value of the information. |
| 2. Instruct Kathy about the predicted changes in insulin needs during pregnancy.<br>a. Explain the importance of blood glucose testing; Kathy will need less insulin because of the nausea and vomiting occurring in the first trimester.<br>b. Emphasize that later (during the second and third trimesters) she will probably require more insulin because of the effects of the placental hormones.<br>c. Describe the importance of following the prescribed diet and exercise regimen to maintain normal blood glucose. | 2. Behaviors change when learning occurs. Understanding how insulin needs change throughout pregnancy, labor, and the postpartum period increases the likelihood that Kathy will follow the recommended regimen. |
| 3. Inform Kathy about specific fetal surveillance techniques recommended during pregnancy (serial nonstress tests, contraction stress tests, biophysical profiles), and explain the importance of the tests. | 3. Some frequently ordered tests are time-consuming and expensive. The woman is more likely to comply if she understands the importance of monitoring the fetal condition at frequent intervals. |
| 4. Allow time for Kathy to focus on her feelings and concerns at each teaching session; offer praise and encouragement for her adherence to the prescribed regimen. | 4. Motivation to comply with the regimen is strengthened by praise and the awareness that the woman's feelings are important. |
| 5. Explain in simple, positive terms the advantages to the fetus of maintaining a normal maternal blood glucose level. These advantages include an optimal pattern of growth, the increased likelihood that the baby will be born near term, and fewer complications associated with prematurity. | 5. Understanding that the fetus benefits when maternal glucose levels are normal reduces anxiety and increases the likelihood that the mother will comply with recommended treatment. |
| 6. Review the recommended plan for diet and exercise during pregnancy, and determine whether Kathy knows the importance of these factors in her care. | 6. Maintenance of normal blood glucose depends on coordinating the amount of food, insulin, and exercise. If any of these factors is altered, the others must also be altered to prevent hypoglycemia or hyperglycemia. |

## Nursing Care Plan 26–1 *Continued*
## Pregnancy and Diabetes Mellitus

**EVALUATION**

Kathy verbalizes her understanding of changing insulin needs and the importance of glucose monitoring. She states that she feels in better control of the diabetes and plans to comply with the recommended schedule of fetal surveillance, diet, and exercise.

**ASSESSMENT:** At 32 weeks' gestation, Kathy's blood glucose is consistently above the desired level and daily nonstress tests are prescribed. The tests are reactive, indicating no present fetal compromise; however, Kathy verbalizes anxiety about the condition of the fetus and asks when it will be safe for the baby to be born.

**NURSING DIAGNOSIS:** Anxiety related to perceived threat to the health of the fetus and lack of knowledge about the timing of the delivery

**GOALS/EXPECTED OUTCOMES**

Kathy will do the following:

1. Relate her perception of the condition of the fetus and the significance of the reactive nonstress test as the tests are performed.
2. Describe her concerns about timing of the delivery at the conclusion of the next nonstress test.

| INTERVENTION | RATIONALE |
|---|---|
| 1. Ask Kathy to describe her concern about the fetus, and clarify her feelings. | 1. Her concerns must be identified and clarified so that misconceptions do not occur. For example, Kathy may begin to be anxious about labor and delivery or she may worry that the elevated blood glucose level poses an immediate threat to the baby. |
| 2. Explain that a reactive nonstress test indicates that the fetal heart rate accelerates whenever the fetus moves; this is a good sign that the fetus is not in immediate jeopardy. | 2. Reassurance that the fetus is not in jeopardy and that the daily tests will detect early signs if a problem develops reduces anxiety about the fetal condition. |
| 3. Ask Kathy how she feels about the labor and delivery; determine whether she is taking childbirth education classes and whether she has selected her coach. | 3. It is normal for women to become concerned about the birth process and how they will cope with labor during the last few weeks of pregnancy. Medical professionals sometimes neglect the need for normal pregnancy care for women with high-risk pregnancies. |
| 4. Assist her in investigating a childbirth education class if she has not done so previously, and suggest that she and her coach begin classes. | 4. Knowledge learned at childbirth classes may reduce the anxiety about the birth processes. |
| 5. Acknowledge that the prospect of labor and delivery causes many women some anxiety even when the condition of the infant is not in question. | 5. Knowledge that her feelings are common to most women may provide some relief from anxiety. |

**EVALUATION**

Kathy has been reassured by explanations regarding the reactive nonstress test, but is concerned about how she will do in labor. She initiates plans to attend a childbirth education class with her sister as the coach.

**ADDITIONAL NURSING DIAGNOSES TO CONSIDER**

Risk for Altered Family Processes
Risk for Altered Parenting
Risk for Injury

be recommended at 18 weeks, and an assessment of fetal cardiac structure by echocardiography should be done at 20 weeks (Gabbe & Landon, 1994).

During the third trimester, fetal surveillance includes maternal assessment of fetal movement ("kick counts"), nonstress tests, contraction stress tests, and biophysical profiles. Doppler velocimetry may be recommended if vascular complications exist or if hypertension develops. See Chapter 10 for a complete description of fetal diagnostic procedures.

### THERAPEUTIC MANAGEMENT

The goals of therapeutic management for a pregnant woman with diabetes are to (1) maintain normal blood glucose levels, (2) give birth to a healthy baby, and (3) avoid accelerated impairment of blood vessels and other major organs. The improved outcome for women with diabetes mellitus is the result of the advent of the *team approach to management* and the widespread use of home glucose monitoring (Rotondo & Coustan, 1993).

Members of the team include a diabetologist, who assists in regulation of maternal blood glucose; a perinatologist, who monitors the mother and fetus and determines the optimal time for birth; a dietitian, who provides a balanced meal plan; and a nurse, who provides ongoing education and support. The team is completed by a neonatologist, who will care for the newborn, as well as the family physician and the pediatrician, who will provide ongoing care for the infant and mother.

**Preconception Care.** Ideally, the team approach should begin before conception. Both prospective parents should participate in care sessions to learn more about the following issues:

- Establishing the optimal time for pregnancy on the basis of maintenance of normal maternal blood glucose levels so that the risk of major fetal malformations can be reduced.
- Evaluating the degree of maternal vascular complications.
- Providing information about the importance of maintaining normal blood glucose levels throughout the pregnancy; this is particularly important if excellent control has not been accomplished before conception.
- Providing instruction, if necessary, in the use of home glucose monitoring techniques.

**Diet.** The average daily intake for the pregnant woman with diabetes ranges from 2200 to 2400 calories per day. Approximately 45 percent of the calories should be from carbohydrates, 20 percent from protein, and 35 percent from fat (Gabbe & Landon, 1994). Caloric intake should be distributed between three meals and two to four snacks. Women who are restricted in activity or who gain excessive weight may require fewer calories.

**Self-Monitoring of Blood Glucose.** Women with preexisting diabetes mellitus should monitor blood glucose four to six times a day (Rotondo & Coustan, 1993). In addition to regular monitoring, they should also perform a glucose test whenever they have symptoms of hypoglycemia. They should record all test results on a log sheet for review by the health care provider at each visit.

**Insulin Therapy.** The need to maintain rigorous control of the maternal metabolism during pregnancy necessitates more frequent doses of insulin than usual. Most treatment regimens rely on three daily injections, with a combination of short-acting (regular) insulin and intermediate-acting (NPH) insulin given before breakfast, regular insulin before dinner, and NPH insulin at bedtime. Some regimens call for long-acting (Ultralente) insulin to be given once or twice daily, supplemented by regular insulin before meals (Moore, 1994).

Because insulin needs change throughout pregnancy owing to the effect of the placental hormones, insulin coverage will need to be adjusted as pregnancy progresses.

***First Trimester.*** Insulin needs generally decline during the first trimester because the secretion of placental hormones that are antagonistic to insulin remain low during this time. The woman also may experience nausea, vomiting, and anorexia, resulting in decreased intake of food, and thus require less insulin. Moreover, the fetus receives its share of glucose, and this reduces maternal plasma glucose levels and decreases the need for maternal insulin.

***Second and Third Trimesters.*** Insulin needs increase markedly during the second and third trimesters when placental hormones, which initiate maternal resistance to the effects of insulin, reach their peak. In addition, the nausea of early pregnancy usually resolves and the diet includes 300 additional calories per day, which is necessary to meet the increased metabolic demands of pregnancy.

***During Labor.*** Insulin needs during labor are based on the blood glucose level. The vigorous muscular exertion and lack of oral intake should decrease the amount of insulin needed. However, intravenous glucose is sometimes given, making it necessary to administer insulin. The only accurate way to determine insulin needs is to evaluate blood

#### Critical to Remember

**SIGNS AND SYMPTOMS OF MATERNAL HYPOGLYCEMIA**

- Shakiness (tremors)
- Sweating
- Pallor; cold clammy skin
- Disorientation; irritability
- Headache
- Hunger
- Blurred vision

glucose levels hourly during labor (Rotondo & Coustan, 1993). If insulin is needed, regular insulin may be added to the intravenous solution and infused at a rate to maintain normal levels. Tight glucose control during labor is needed to reduce the severity of neonatal hypoglycemia.

***Postpartum.*** Insulin needs should decline rapidly after delivery of the placenta and the abrupt cessation of placental hormones. Blood glucose levels should be monitored at least four times daily, however, so that the insulin dose can be adjusted to meet individual needs.

**Timing of Delivery.** If possible, the pregnancy should be allowed to progress to term so that the fetal lungs have a chance to mature and so that the risk of neonatal respiratory distress syndrome can be reduced. However, if there is evidence of fetal compromise, such as nonreactive nonstress tests or late decelerations on a contraction stress test, an amniocentesis may be performed to evaluate the ratio of lecithin to sphingomyelin. If the ratio is at least 2:1 and the phospholipid phosphatidylglycerol is present, the lungs are judged to be mature and early delivery may be planned (Moore, 1994).

## Type III (Gestational) Diabetes Mellitus

### RISK FACTORS

Gestational diabetes is a carbohydrate intolerance of variable severity that develops or is first recognized during pregnancy. Diagnosis begins with a history that identifies whether the woman is at risk to develop gestational diabetes. Factors known to increase the risk include the following:

- Obesity (>90 kg or 198 pounds)
- Chronic hypertension
- Maternal age older than 25 years
- Family history of diabetes
- Previous birth of a large infant (>4000 g)
- Previous birth of an infant with unexplained congenital anomalies
- Previous unexplained fetal demise
- Gestational diabetes in previous pregnancy

Patients with any of these factors should be screened for gestational diabetes at the first prenatal visit (Moore, 1994).

### SCREENING

**Glucose Challenge Test.** The American Diabetes Association (1993) recommends that *all* pregnant women who have not been identified with glucose intolerance earlier in pregnancy be screened with a 50-g 1-hour glucose challenge test (GCT) between 24 and 28 weeks of pregnancy. This is a convenient test because it can be done at a regular clinic visit. The woman does not need to fast, and the test does not follow a meal. The woman should ingest 50 g of oral glucose solution; 1 hour later a blood sample should be taken. If blood glucose is equal to or above 140 mg/dl, a 3-hour oral glucose tolerance test (OGTT) should be recommended (ACOG, 1994).

**Oral Glucose Tolerance Test.** The OGTT is diagnostic for diabetes mellitus. Although it is the gold standard for diagnosing diabetes, it is a more complicated test and requires the woman's participation. She must eat a high-carbohydrate diet for 2 days before the scheduled test and fast from midnight on the day of the test. After a fasting plasma glucose level is obtained, the woman should ingest 100 g of oral glucose solution. Plasma glucose levels should be obtained at 1, 2, and 3 hours. Gestational diabetes is the diagnosis if the fasting blood glucose is abnormal or if two or more of the following values are found (ACOG, 1994):

- Fasting, greater than 105 mg/dl
- 1 hour, greater than 190 mg/dl
- 2 hours, greater than 165 mg/dl
- 3 hours, greater than 145 mg/dl

### MATERNAL, FETAL, AND NEONATAL EFFECTS

With a few important exceptions, the effects of gestational diabetes are similar to those associated with preexisting diabetes. The exceptions are that gestational diabetes is not associated with an increased risk for ketoacidosis or spontaneous abortion. Because gestational diabetes develops after the first trimester, which is the critical period of major fetal organ development (organogenesis), it is not usually associated with an increase in major congenital malformations. Nevertheless, gestational diabetes, characterized by maternal hyperglycemia during the third trimester, is associated with increased neonatal morbidity and mortality. The major fetal complications are macrosomia, leading to birth injuries or making cesarean birth necessary, and neonatal hypoglycemia. Other problems, such as hypocalcemia, hyperbilirubinemia, and respiratory distress may also occur. Table 26–3 summarizes maternal, fetal, and neonatal effects of diabetes mellitus and their probable causes.

### THERAPEUTIC MANAGEMENT

**Diet.** Nutritional counseling is the mainstay of therapy for women with gestational diabetes mellitus. The diet should provide the calories and nutrients needed for maternal and fetal health, result in euglycemia, and prevent ketosis due to inadequate carbohydrate intake. Although the diet must be individualized, in general an intake of 2200 to 2400 calories per day is recommended. Complex carbohydrates from foods high in soluble fiber should pro-

**TABLE 26–3 MAJOR EFFECTS OF DIABETES MELLITUS ON PREGNANCY**

| Increased Maternal Risks | Probable Cause |
|---|---|
| Pregnancy-induced hypertension | Unknown but increased even without renal or vascular impairment |
| Urinary tract infections | Increased bacterial growth in nutrient-rich urine |
| Hydramnios | Fetal diuresis caused by hyperglycemia |
| Ketoacidosis | Uncontrolled hyperglycemia |
| Preterm labor and premature rupture of membranes | Overdistention of uterus caused by hydramnios and fetal macrosomia |
| Difficult labor, injury to birth canal, cesarean birth, and postpartum hemorrhage | Fetal macrosomia and overdistention of uterus |
| **Increased Fetal and Neonatal Risks** | **Probable Cause** |
| Perinatal death | Poor placental perfusion because of maternal vascular impairment |
| Congenital anomalies | Maternal hyperglycemia in the first trimester |
| Macrosomia (>4000 g) | Fetal hyperglycemia stimulates production of insulin |
| Birth injury | Large fetal size |
| IUGR | Maternal vascular impairment |
| Polycythemia | Fetal hypoxemia |
| Hyperbilirubinemia | Breakdown of excessive red blood cells after birth |
| Hypoglycemia | Neonatal hyperinsulinemia after birth when maternal glucose is no longer available |
| Hypocalcemia | Transfer of calcium abruptly stopped at birth |
| Respiratory distress syndrome | Inadequate production of pulmonary surfactant |

vide 50 to 60 percent of total calories. Simple sugars found in concentrated sweets should be eliminated from the diet. Protein sources should supply 10 to 20 percent, with the remaining 25 to 30 percent coming from fat (Gabbe & Landon, 1994). Calories should be divided among three meals and at least two snacks.

**Exercise.** Exercise can play a significant role in managing blood glucose levels in women who develop gestational diabetes and in women with type II diabetes who become pregnant. A contracting skeletal muscle increases its glucose uptake and helps regulate the capacity for glucose transport. Moderate exercise for active women and regular activity for sedentary women show promise for normalizing blood glucose levels (Artal, 1996). Prescribing exercise, however, requires knowledge of a pregnant woman's physical capacity, anatomy, and physiologic alterations. The exercise regimen should be recommended by a physician who takes into account each patient's risk factors and risks to the fetus.

**Glucose-Level Monitoring.** Blood glucose levels should be evaluated to determine if glucose levels are normal. The most common methods are *fasting blood sugar* (no food for the previous 4 hours) and *postprandial blood sugar* (2 hours after a meal). The American College of Obstetrics and Gynecology (1994) recommends that fasting blood glucose be maintained below 105 mg/dl and that postprandial levels be less than 120 mg/dl. Insulin is recommended if levels repeatedly exceed these thresholds (Landon & Gabbe, 1994).

**Fetal Surveillance.** Women with diet-controlled gestational diabetes who maintain normal fasting and postprandial glucose values are at low risk for fetal death (Landon & Gabbe, 1996). However, maternal assessment of fetal activity or "kick counts" are often initiated during the last trimester. In addition, antepartum fetal testing is usually initiated if (1) the mother requires insulin, (2) hypertension develops, or (3) there is a history of previous stillbirth. The most common fetal surveillance techniques of the third trimester include fetal movement counts (kick counts), the nonstress test, amniotic fluid index, and biophysical profile (see Chapter 10).

#### NURSING CONSIDERATIONS

The care of a pregnant woman with diabetes mellitus focuses primarily on maintaining normal blood glucose. As stated earlier, this maintenance involves a rather rigid schedule of controlling the diet, testing blood glucose, administering insulin, and monitoring the fetus. Some women respond calmly to the intense medical supervision; others respond with anxiety, fear, denial, or anger and feel inadequate or unable to control the diabetes to the degree expected by the health care team. These feelings may not be shared spontaneously, but they may affect the woman's ability to achieve the desired outcomes. Also, nurses should remember to provide for normal pregnancy care in addition to monitoring the pregnant woman's diabetes.

**Increasing Effective Communication.** A woman often does not volunteer information about her feelings and concerns, especially if she has negative feelings about her care. Moreover, the woman and the nurse may both be unaware of the misunderstandings or conflicts regarding the plan of care. Nurses must ask specifically about the feelings and concerns the woman and her family have about the pregnancy. Broad opening questions, such as "What are your major concerns?" and "How do you feel about the plan of care?" are helpful. These should be followed with more specific questions, such as

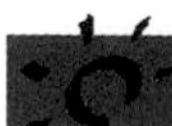

## CRITICAL THINKING EXERCISE

Marcia Mahoney, a 28-year-old primigravida, is diagnosed with gestational diabetes in her 30th week of pregnancy. The health care team provides her with a diet and exercise regimen and tells her that she will need weekly tests to monitor her condition and that of the fetus. Although Marcia accepts the information without comment, she does not keep the next scheduled appointment.

**Q:**
1. What assumptions has the health care team made?
2. What could the team have done to ensure Marcia's compliance with the recommendations?

**A:**
1. The team may have assumed that Marcia knew the maternal and fetal effects of gestational diabetes and the importance of following the plan of care.
2. The team could have explained the reasons for the recommended plan and allowed adequate time to answer all questions. It is particularly important to emphasize why it is necessary to monitor the condition of the fetus, because mothers are usually motivated to do whatever they can to ensure the health of the fetus.

Marcia is located and agrees to return to the clinic for follow-up care. She states she does not "see what all the fuss is about." She understands she may have a large baby, but states that her mother had a 10-pound baby who did just fine. She wonders if the weekly tests are necessary and if they could harm the baby.

**Q:**
1. How can the nurse respond to Marcia's comments about having a large baby without frightening her?
2. How can the nurse explain the necessity for weekly nonstress tests?

**A:**
1. The nurse should acknowledge Marcia's belief. "I realize that we haven't made our concerns clear to you. Let me explain why it is important for you and for your baby to be watched carefully during these last weeks." The nurse must then provide clear, simple explanations and allow time to answer questions.
2. The nurse must acknowledge that weekly tests are time-consuming but that they provide valuable information about the well-being of the baby. Usually the information is reassuring, but additional tests can be performed if there are questions.

"How do you feel about the fetal testing?" and "What would you like to change about the diet?" The woman's comments can provide valuable information about her emotional response to the care plan. One woman remarked, "I can tell you one thing, I don't feel like a person; I feel like an incubator, a faulty incubator." Another woman, who had a difficult time achieving the desired blood glucose level, said: "I feel as if my whole life has been taken over by diabetes. I'm tired of feeling like a sick person."

The nurse must be an active listener and allow time for the woman and her family to express concerns and feelings. The nurse must convey acceptance of feelings that are expressed whether they are negative or positive. Many women are reassured to hear that their feelings of stress or anger are normal and to know that the health care team understands those feelings. Sharing of emotions will help her prevent or diminish unnecessary guilt, anxiety, or frustration and thus promote positive feelings about her ability to participate successfully in her plan of care.

Most women benefit from praise when diabetic control is well maintained; they feel competent and trusted by the health care team and are motivated to continue their efforts.

**Providing Opportunities for Control.** Allowing the woman to make as many decisions as possible increases her sense of being in control. For instance, she can select foods from the exchange list that provide the necessary nutrients but still allow her some choice. She may also develop a regular schedule of exercise and sleep that helps to keep the blood glucose level under control. Nurses should allow as much flexibility as possible when scheduling stressful events, such as fetal monitoring tests and amniocentesis.

Some women resent being "treated as though ill" even though their diabetic control is excellent. These women may be capable of making more decisions regarding their care during pregnancy, but they need the support of an understanding team to do this.

**Providing Normal Pregnancy Care.** Some women express a need for normal pregnancy care that is sometimes ignored because of the focus on preventing complications that might occur as a result of diabetes. Women with diabetes also experience the discomforts that nondiabetic women experience during pregnancy, such as morning sickness, fatigue, backache, and difficulty sleeping. The nurse caring for women with diabetes should provide education and counseling regarding normal pregnancy discomforts. Also, because women with diabetes are concerned about how they will manage during labor and delivery, nurses should offer childbirth preparation classes and discuss with them the experiences that are common to all pregnant women.

## CHECK YOUR READING

1. What effects do the hormones of pregnancy have on maternal glucose metabolism?
2. What are the maternal effects of type I diabetes mellitus? What are possible fetal and neonatal effects?

3. What is the importance of glycosylated hemoglobin in monitoring diabetes mellitus?
4. How do insulin needs vary from the first trimester through the postpartum period?
5. How does gestational diabetes compare with type I diabetes mellitus in terms of onset and treatment?
6. What is the difference between a glucose challenge test and a glucose tolerance test?
7. How do the maternal, fetal, and neonatal effects of gestational diabetes differ from those of preexisting diabetes?

## Application of Nursing Process: The Pregnant Woman with Diabetes Mellitus

### Assessment

Determine how well the woman understands the prescribed management and how the family plans to carry out the recommended regimen. She may be newly diagnosed and may have no experience in the necessary skills and procedures. On the other hand, she may be skilled in monitoring glucose and administering insulin but may have no knowledge of the effects that diabetes has on the pregnancy nor of the effects of pregnancy on diabetes.

To determine whether her techniques are accurate, ask the expectant mother to demonstrate how she monitors blood glucose and observe how she mixes and injects insulins. Verify that she and her family are aware of the need to select appropriate sites and injection techniques that prevent insulin leakage.

Although diet is prescribed by a dietitian, it is necessary to assess how well the family understands the diet. Determine whether there are special problems with food preferences or availability of recommended foods. It may be necessary to review the exchange list and ask the woman how she plans to substitute and exchange foods.

Identify the woman's knowledge of potential complications, such as hypoglycemia and hyperglycemia, so that she and her family can be provided with pertinent information.

Determine her knowledge of fetal surveillance techniques and her response to the need for frequent tests. Some women are highly motivated to continue the treatment regimen when test results indicate the fetus is thriving. Other women dread the tests and are puzzled by the need for such frequent testing.

### Analysis

One of the most common nursing diagnoses is Risk for Altered Health Maintenance related to knowledge deficit of specific measures to maintain normal blood glucose levels; signs, symptoms, and management of hypoglycemia and hyperglycemia; and recommended fetal surveillance procedures.

### Planning

Expected outcomes for this nursing diagnosis are that the woman (and her family) will do the following:

- Demonstrate competence in home glucose monitoring and administration of insulin before home management is initiated.
- Describe a plan for meeting dietary recommendations.
- Identify signs and symptoms of hypoglycemia and hyperglycemia and the necessary management required in each.
- Verbalize knowledge of fetal surveillance procedures and keep scheduled appointments for testing.

### Interventions

Although management of diabetes mellitus during pregnancy is a team effort, the nurse's major responsibility is to provide accurate information about the recommended therapeutic regimen and to offer consistent support for the woman's efforts to comply with the recommendations. It may be necessary to demonstrate specific skills that the client and her family must master and to review and reinforce information that comes from other members of the health care team.

#### TEACHING SELF-CARE SKILLS

Demonstration and return demonstration are the most effective ways to teach and evaluate psychomotor skills. The woman (and her family) must learn to mix and inject insulin and to obtain a small sample of blood to test for glucose. Both of these procedures are invasive and cause mild discomfort; this may make the woman reluctant to start. Acknowledge these feelings before teaching begins.

**Home Blood Glucose Monitoring.** The blood glucose level is monitored several times a day, and the patient must be comfortable with the procedure. Spring devices, available for sticking the finger, make the procedure easier and less painful. Recommend that the expectant mother use the side of the finger, which is less sensitive than the tip. Teach her to cleanse the area with warm water before obtaining a sample to prevent infection. Each home monitoring kit contains specific instructions for timing and washing or blotting the blood from the reagent strip, and these directions must be followed exactly to obtain an accurate reading.

**Insulin Administration.** Two types of insulin are usually prescribed: intermediate-acting and short-acting (regular) insulin. Teach the expectant mother the difference in onset, peak, and duration of each type of insulin. She also needs to learn how to mix the two insulins in the same syringe.

Insulin is administered subcutaneously. Common sites include the upper thighs, abdomen, and upper arms. Aseptic technique is recommended to prevent infection.

Because the pregnant woman is injecting insulin frequently, emphasize these precautions:

- To prevent hypoglycemia, a meal should be taken 30 minutes after insulin is injected.
- Unless the woman is very thin, insulin should be injected at a 90-degree angle so the tip of the needle reaches the fatty tissue layer.
- The needle should be inserted quickly to minimize discomfort.
- The tissue pinch, if used, is released after inserting the needle and before injecting insulin because pressure from the pinch can promote insulin leakage from the subcutaneous tissue.
- It is not necessary to aspirate when injecting into subcutaneous tissue.
- Insulin is injected slowly (over 2 to 4 seconds) to allow tissue expansion and to minimize pressure, which can cause insulin leakage.
- The needle is withdrawn quickly to minimize the formation of a track, which might permit insulin to leak out.

Emphasize the importance of administering the correct dose at the correct time. Teach the woman and her family the function of insulin and the importance of following the directions of her physician in regard to coordinating meals with the administration of insulin.

**Continuous Subcutaneous Insulin Infusion.** Many women use continuous subcutaneous insulin infusion and wish to continue with this method during pregnancy. The use of programmable insulin infusion pumps allows tailoring of insulin administration to the woman's individual lifestyle. Prompt emergency counseling and assistance must be available 24 hours a day to deal with unexpected problems such as pump malfunction.

### TEACHING DIETARY MANAGEMENT

Although a dietitian prescribes the recommended diet, the nurse must be aware of the general requirements and must be sensitive to the expectant mother's dietary habits and preferences. There is often a need to review and clarify how the exchange lists are used to plan meals and snacks. Encourage the patient to avoid simple sugars (candy, cake, cookies), which raise the blood glucose levels quickly, and to include foods high in fiber, which are believed to help reduce glucose levels.

Finances are often a problem, and it may be necessary to help the woman select foods that are high in nutrients but low in cost. Animal protein is especially expensive, and alternative sources of protein (beans, peas, corn, grains) can be substituted to meet some of the protein needs.

Allow the expectant mother to verbalize her frustrations or problems with the diet, and collaborate with the dietitian if she has a particular problem.

### RECOGNIZING AND CORRECTING HYPOGLYCEMIA AND HYPERGLYCEMIA

Every woman and her family must be aware of the signs and symptoms that indicate abnormal blood glucose levels. Hypoglycemia and hyperglycemia pose a threat to mother and fetus if they are not identified and corrected quickly.

**Hypoglycemia.** Treat hypoglycemia at once to prevent damage to the brain, which is dependent on glucose (see p. 716). If the woman is able to swallow, have her drink 8 ounces of milk and eat two crackers. Repeat the snack in 15 minutes if symptoms persist or her blood glucose level is between 40 and 80 mg. She, and another family member, should be taught that sucrose or unrefined sugar should not be ingested during hypoglycemic episodes. They can result in high levels of blood glucose that disturb glycemic control for many hours (Moore, 1994).

Teach family members how to inject glucagon in the event that the woman cannot swallow or retain food. Notify the physician at once. Intravenous glucose will be administered if she is hospitalized. If untreated, hypoglycemia can progress to convulsions and death.

To prevent episodes of hypoglycemia, instruct the woman to have meals at a fixed time each day and to plan snacks at 10 A.M., 3 P.M., and at bedtime. Suggest that she carry a container of milk and some dry crackers whenever possible.

**Hyperglycemia.** Because infection is the most common cause of hyperglycemia, pregnant women must be instructed to notify the physician whenever they have an infection of any type.

If untreated, hyperglycemia can lead to ketoacidosis, coma, and maternal and fetal death. If signs and symptoms occur, notify the physician at once so that treatment can be initiated. Hospitalization is often necessary for monitoring blood glucose levels and intravenous administration of insulin.

## Critical to Remember

### SIGNS AND SYMPTOMS OF MATERNAL HYPERGLYCEMIA

- Fatigue
- Flushed, hot skin
- Dry mouth; excessive thirst
- Frequent urination
- Rapid, deep respirations; odor of acetone on the breath
- Drowsiness; headache
- Depressed reflexes

#### EXPLAINING PROCEDURES, TESTS, AND PLAN OF CARE

Explain the schedule and the reasons for frequent checkups and tests that are necessary. Encourage the woman and her family to ask questions if any part of the schedule is confusing. This is particularly important for women who are aware that their prenatal care differs significantly from that of their friends who do not have diabetes. Knowing that the tests provide information about the condition of mother and fetus reduces frustration and anxiety. Specifically, pregnant women and their families need to know why weekly (or daily) nonstress tests are necessary. Inform them why it is necessary to perform contraction stress tests or a biophysical profile. Women may be especially concerned if they think that the test results have changed because the condition of the fetus is deteriorating. They need to know that their diabetic care will require more of their time and effort than it did before pregnancy but that this care greatly improves the likelihood that they will have healthy infants.

### Evaluation

After procedures, tests, and plan of care have been explained, the family should be evaluated to ensure that

- The expectant mother and one family member can demonstrate competence in blood glucose monitoring and administration of insulin.
- The family can describe a plan for meeting dietary requirements.
- The woman and her family can list the signs and symptoms of hypoglycemia and hyperglycemia.
- The woman and her family can describe the initial management of these conditions.
- The woman can verbalize knowledge of the reason for fetal surveillance procedures and can keep appointments for tests.

## Heart Disease

Alterations in cardiovascular function are necessary in every pregnancy to meet additional maternal metabolic demands and to meet the needs of the fetus. Plasma volume, venous return, and cardiac output all increase. Heart rate and stroke volume, the components of cardiac output, increase during pregnancy. The heart rate gradually rises above the baseline during the third trimester; however, increases in stroke volume are primarily responsible for the overall rise in cardiac output during early pregnancy.

A normal heart can adapt to the changes so that pregnancy and birth are tolerated without difficulty. If there is preexisting or underlying heart disease, however, the changes can impose an additional burden on an already compromised heart, and cardiac decompensation and congestive heart failure can result.

### Incidence and Classification

Heart disease complicates about 1 percent of pregnancies (Cunningham et al., 1997). Pregnancy may unmask a previously asymptomatic heart condition, or it may aggravate known heart disease.

The two major categories of heart disease are rheumatic heart disease and congenital heart disease. Although rheumatic fever is uncommon in the United States, it is prevalent in less-developed countries. It is still the most common heart disease encountered in pregnancy (McAnulty et al., 1995). The incidence of pregnancy complicated by congenital heart disease is increasing because more women with congenital heart disease now survive to reproductive age. A third category, mitral valve prolapse, is a benign condition that usually does not complicate pregnancy.

#### RHEUMATIC HEART DISEASE

There has been a remarkable decline in rheumatic heart disease in North America and western Europe as a result of early treatment of streptococcal pharyngitis (strep throat), which often precedes the onset of rheumatic fever. Even one bout of rheumatic fever may cause scarring of the valves in the heart. This results in narrowing (stenosis) of the openings between the chambers of the heart.

The mitral valve is the most common site of stenosis. Mitral stenosis obstructs free flow of blood from the left atrium to the left ventricle. The left atrium becomes dilated. As a result, pressure in the left atrium, the pulmonary veins, and pulmonary capillaries is chronically elevated. This elevation may lead to pulmonary hypertension, pulmonary edema, or congestive heart failure. The first warnings of heart failure include persistent rales at the base of the lungs, dyspnea on exertion, cough, and hemoptysis. Progressive edema and tachycardia are additional signs of heart failure.

### CONGENITAL HEART DISEASE

Congenital heart defects can be grouped into those that cause a left-to-right shunt and those that result in a right-to-left shunt. Those defects that produce left-to-right shunting include atrial and ventricular septal defects and patent ductus arteriosus. On the other hand, right-to-left shunting occurs when there is a cyanotic heart defect, such as tetralogy of Fallot. Right-to-left shunting may also occur through a septal defect or patent ductus arteriosus when pulmonary vascular resistance exceeds peripheral vascular resistance and pulmonary hypertension (Eisenmenger syndrome) occurs.

#### LEFT-TO-RIGHT SHUNT

**Atrial Septal Defect.** Atrial septal defect is often first discovered in women of childbearing age because symptoms are absent or vague. This defect produces a left-to-right shunt because pressure in the left side of the heart is higher than it is in the right side. Pregnancy is well tolerated by patients with an uncomplicated atrial septal defect, and no specific treatment is recommended (McAnulty et al., 1995). Bacterial endocarditis is rare, and prophylactic antibiotics are not required. Atrial septal defects are not associated with heart failure; therefore, digitalis, diuretics, and extreme limitation of intravenous infusions are not warranted (Monga & Creasy, 1994). Left-to-right shunting, however, may increase the chance of pulmonary hypertension because the additional blood that moves to the right side of the heart is transported to the lungs via the pulmonary artery.

**Ventricular Septal Defect.** Although ventricular septal defects are more common than atrial septal defects at birth, they are usually detected and corrected before childbearing age. Most women with ventricular septal defects who become pregnant are asymptomatic, but occasionally fatigue or symptoms of pulmonary congestion occur.

Pregnancy is well tolerated with small to moderate left-to-right shunts (Cunningham et al., 1997). However, pregnancy occasionally precipitates heart failure or an arrhythmia, either of which is managed as in non-pregnant patients. Bacterial endocarditis is common with unrepaired defects, and antibacterial prophylaxis is recommended.

**Patent Ductus Arteriosus.** The communicating shunt between the pulmonary artery and aorta is usually discovered and treated in childhood. If untreated, the physiologic effects are related to size. If small, this lesion, like septal defects, may be well tolerated during pregnancy unless complicated by pulmonary hypertension. The patent ductus arteriosus tends to become infected, so antibiotic prophylaxis is recommended, particularly at the time of labor.

#### RIGHT-TO-LEFT SHUNT

**Tetralogy of Fallot.** The primary cause of right-to-left shunting is tetralogy of Fallot, a combination of four defects (ventricular septal defect, pulmonary valve stenosis, right ventricular hypertrophy, and rightward displacement of the aorta). Untreated patients with tetralogy of Fallot have obvious symptoms of heart disease that include (1) cyanosis; (2) clubbing of the fingers, indicating proliferation of capillaries to transport blood to the extremities; and (3) inability to tolerate activity.

Women who have undergone repair, and in whom cyanosis did not reappear, may do well during pregnancy. With uncorrected tetralogy of Fallot, maternal mortality approaches 10 percent (Cunningham et al., 1997).

**Eisenmenger Syndrome.** Eisenmenger syndrome develops when pulmonary resistance exceeds systemic resistance and a right-to-left shunt develops in a patient with a previous left-to-right shunt. In this case, pregnancy is a dangerous undertaking and should be avoided (McAnulty et al., 1995).

### MITRAL VALVE PROLAPSE

Mitral valve prolapse is one of the most common cardiac conditions among the general population. The incidence among otherwise normal young women is 5 percent (Cunningham et al., 1997). Although the condition appears to be inherited, mitral valve prolapse is associated with a variety of other cardiac disorders, such as atrial septal defects and *Marfan's syndrome*.

The leaflets of the mitral valve prolapse into the left atrium during ventricular contraction. Mitral valve prolapse is considered a benign condition, and most women with mitral valve prolapse are asymptomatic. Some women experience arrhythmias or chest pain; however, most women with mitral valve prolapse tolerate pregnancy well. The condition is considered by some to be a significant risk factor for bacterial endocarditis, and some physicians administer prophylactic antibiotics before and during labor and delivery. If arrhythmia or chest pain occurs, $\beta$-blockers, such as propranolol hydrochloride (Inderal), are administered to prevent stimulation of myocardial, vascular, and pulmonary receptor sites.

### PERIPARTUM AND POSTPARTUM CARDIOMYOPATHY

Cardiomyopathy in the peripartum or postpartum period is a rare condition that is exclusively associated with pregnancy. Women with this condition have no underlying heart disease, but symptoms of cardiac decompensation appear during the last weeks of pregnancy or 2 to 20 weeks post partum. The symptoms are those of congestive heart failure: dyspnea, edema, weakness, chest pain, and heart palpitations. The condition is treated with digitalis, diuretics, sodium restriction, and prolonged bedrest. Peripartum cardiomyopathy tends to recur with subsequent pregnancies, and prognosis for future pregnancies is related to heart size. Future pregnancies are definitely contraindicated if the heart remains enlarged after the initial episode.

## Diagnosis and Classification

Early recognition of underlying heart disease is essential, and careful assessment for specific signs and symptoms of heart disease is part of every initial prenatal visit. Signs and symptoms include dyspnea, syncope (fainting) with exertion, hemoptysis, paroxysmal nocturnal dyspnea, and chest pain with exertion. Additional signs that confirm the diagnosis are (1) diastolic, presystolic, or continuous heart murmur; (2) cardiac enlargement; (3) a loud, harsh systolic murmur associated with a thrill; or (4) serious arrhythmias (Shabetai, 1994).

Diagnosis of heart disease may be made from clinical signs and symptoms and physical examination. It is often confirmed by chest radiograph, electrocardiography, or echocardiography.

Once the diagnosis is made, the severity of the disease can be determined by the client's ability to endure physical activity. A clinical classification based on the effect of exercise on the heart has been developed by the New York Heart Association (Table 26–4).

**TABLE 26–4 NEW YORK HEART ASSOCIATION FUNCTIONAL CLASSIFICATION OF HEART DISEASE**

**CLASS I**

Uncompromised. No limitation of physical activity. Asymptomatic with ordinary activity.

**CLASS II**

Slightly compromised, requiring slight limitation of physical activity. Comfortable at rest, but ordinary physical activity causes fatigue, dyspnea, palpitations, or anginal pain.

**CLASS III**

Marked limitation of physical activity. Comfortable at rest, but less than ordinary activity causes excessive fatigue, palpitation, dyspnea, or anginal pain. Markedly compromised.

**CLASS IV**

Inability to perform any physical activity without discomfort. Symptoms of cardiac insufficiency even at rest.

In general, maternal and fetal risks for class I and II disease are small but are greatly increased with class III and IV.

## Therapeutic Management

### CLASS I AND CLASS II HEART DISEASE

All pregnant women with heart disease should do the following:

- Limit physical activity so that cardiac demand does not exceed the functional capacity of the heart. In other words, the woman should remain free of symptoms of cardiac stress, such as dyspnea, chest pain, or tachycardia.
- Avoid excessive weight gain, which places further demands on the heart. A diet adequate in protein, calories, and sodium is necessary; however, a low-sodium diet prevents excessive expansion of blood volume (McAnulty et al., 1995).
- Prevent anemia, which decreases the oxygen-carrying capacity of the blood and results in a compensatory increase in heart rate. Most anemia is prevented by administration of iron and folic acid.
- Prevent infection; this may include administration of prophylactic antibiotics.
- Undergo careful assessment for the development of congestive heart failure, pulmonary edema, or cardiac arrhythmias.

### CLASS III AND CLASS IV HEART DISEASE

The primary goal of management is to prevent cardiac decompensation and the development of congestive heart failure. Moreover, every effort is also made to protect the fetus from hypoxia and IUGR which can occur if placental perfusion is inadequate.

### DRUG THERAPY

**Anticoagulants.** During pregnancy, clotting factors normally increase and thrombolytic activity decreases. These changes may predispose the pregnant woman to thrombus formation. Superimposed cardiac problems, such as mitral valve stenosis, may necessitate anticoagulant therapy during pregnancy. Warfarin is associated with fetal malformations and should be restricted throughout pregnancy. Heparin, which does not cross the placental barrier, is an effective alternative. Heparin should be administered subcutaneously to decrease the likelihood of maternal and placental bleeding. Careful monitoring of partial thromboplastin time, activated partial thromboplastin time, and platelets is essential to achieve effective anticoagulation.

**Antiarrhythmics.** When medication to control arrhythmias is necessary during pregnancy, the effect on the fetus must be considered. Digoxin, quinidine, and procainamide are not harmful to the fetus, and despite early concerns, $\beta$-blocker therapy is not associated with adverse fetal outcomes (McAnulty et al., 1995).

**Anti-infectives.** Anti-infectious agents, such as ampicillin and gentamicin, may be administered as prophylaxis against bacterial endocarditis.

**Diuretics.** When congestive heart failure is uncontrolled by restriction of activity and sodium intake, diuretics should be instituted, with careful monitoring of electrolytes and water balance. Experience is greatest with thiazides and furosemide; neither has an apparent direct detrimental effect on the fetus (McAnulty et al., 1995).

#### INTRAPARTUM MANAGEMENT

Every effort is made to minimize the effects of labor on the cardiovascular system. For example, with every contraction, 300 to 500 ml of blood is shifted from the uterus and placenta into the central circulation. This extra fluid causes a sharp rise in cardiac workload. Therefore, careful management of intravenous fluid administration is essential to prevent fluid overload. The woman should also be positioned on her side, with the head and shoulders elevated. Oxygen is administered to increase the oxygen-carrying capacity of the blood. Sedation and epidural anesthesia are recommended early in labor to reduce discomfort. The environment is kept as quiet and calm as possible to decrease anxiety, which can cause tachycardia.

The fetus is electronically monitored, and signs of fetal distress as well as maternal signs of cardiac decompensation (tachycardia, rapid respirations, moist rales, exhaustion) should be reported immediately to the physician.

A vaginal delivery produces less trauma and is recommended for a woman with heart disease unless there are indications for cesarean birth. Outlet forceps are often used to shorten the second stage of labor.

The fourth stage of labor is associated with special risks. After delivery of the placenta, about 500 ml of blood is added to the intravascular volume. To minimize the risks of overloading the circulation, the woman's legs are kept level with the body by avoiding the use of stirrups or by lowering them during the third stage of labor. Moreover, the uterus should not be massaged to expedite separation of the placenta. Careful assessment for signs of circulatory overload, such as bounding pulse, distended neck and peripheral veins, and moist rales in the lungs, is performed during the third and fourth stages of labor.

#### POSTPARTUM MANAGEMENT

Women who have shown no evidence of distress during pregnancy, labor, or childbirth may still decompensate during the postpartum period. They must be observed closely for signs of infection, hemorrhage, or thromboembolism. These conditions can act together to precipitate postpartum heart failure in women with underlying heart disease.

If there is no evidence of cardiac compromise during labor and the early postpartum period, breastfeeding is usually not contraindicated.

## Application of Nursing Process: The Pregnant Woman with Heart Disease

### Assessment

Begin with a review of the woman's medical record to determine the functional classification assigned (see Table 26–4). Assess the woman at each prenatal appointment to determine how pregnancy affects the functional capacity of the heart.

- Take vital signs, and compare them with preconception levels; note any changes since the last prenatal appointment.
- Assess the level of fatigue and any changes in fatigue since the last prenatal appointment; this is especially important when fluid volume peaks and the chance of cardiac decompensation is greatest (18 to 32 weeks' gestation).
- Observe for signs or symptoms of congestive heart failure.

**Critical to Remember**

**SIGNS AND SYMPTOMS OF CONGESTIVE HEART FAILURE**

- Cough (frequent, productive, hemoptysis)
- Progressive dyspnea with exertion
- Orthopnea
- Pitting edema of legs and feet or generalized edema of face, hands, or sacral area
- Palpitations of heart
- Progressive fatigue or syncope with exertion
- Moist rales in lower lobes, indicating pulmonary edema

- Note additional factors that may increase the workload of the heart (anemia, infections, anxiety, lack of adequate support to manage the activities of daily living).
- Weigh the client, and compare the desired pattern of weight gain with the actual one to detect excessive weight gain or fluid retention.
- Assess the woman's knowledge of the prescribed regimen of care and her ability to comply with it.

## Analysis

The pregnant woman with a cardiac defect may be unable to tolerate activity to the same degree as before pregnancy because of the stress imposed on the cardiovascular system. Arriving at the nursing diagnosis Activity Intolerance related to insufficient knowledge of measures that reduce cardiac stress is a priority.

## Planning

Goals and outcomes are as follows:

- The woman (and her family) will identify factors that increase cardiac workload.
- They will describe measures that promote adaptation to activity restrictions.

## Interventions

Prenatal nursing care focuses on teaching the woman and her family how the disease may affect their lives. This teaching may include specific instructions about factors that increase the workload of the heart and measures that promote adaptation to restrictions in activity.

### TEACHING ABOUT INCREASED CARDIAC WORKLOAD

**Excessive Weight Gain and Anemia.** Excessive weight gain and anemia increase the workload of the heart and should be avoided. A well-balanced diet that contains approximately 2200 calories is recommended, with adequate high-quality protein.

Emphasize the importance of taking iron and folic acid supplements to prevent anemia and thus reduce the risk of tachycardia.

**Exertion.** Instruct the woman to modify approaches to activities to regulate energy expenditures and to reduce cardiac workload. For example, she might take rest periods during the day and for an hour after meals. She can sit rather than stand, if possible, when performing activities. She should rest every few minutes when performing an activity that increases the heart rate to allow the heart time to recover. Emphasize that she should stop an activity if she experiences dyspnea, chest pain, or tachycardia.

**Exposure.** Instruct the woman to avoid unnecessary exposure to environmental extremes. She should dress warmly during cold weather and create a barrier to cold temperatures by wearing layers of clothing. She must become aware that exertion in hot, humid weather or during extreme cold weather places additional demands on the heart and should be avoided.

**Emotional Stress.** Help the woman to identify areas of stress in her life, if applicable, and explain the effects of emotional stress on the cardiovascular system (increased blood pressure, heart rate, and respiratory rate). Discuss various methods for stress management, such as meditation, progressive relaxation of muscles, and biofeedback. Teach that cigarette smoking and use of illicit drugs, such as cocaine and amphetamines, greatly increase stress on the heart.

### HELPING THE FAMILY ACCEPT RESTRICTIONS ON ACTIVITY

Assist family members to accept the need for activity restriction. The amount of activity that can be tolerated depends on the severity of the disease; however, all women with heart disease require 8 to 10 hours of sleep each night, with a period of morning and afternoon rest. For some women, complete bedrest (with bathroom privileges only) is necessary during the last half of pregnancy, and this may create special problems for the family. Nurses often help family members plan how to meet their needs while the expectant mother remains on bedrest. See Chapter 27 and the Nursing Care Plan for Preterm Labor (p. 767) for additional interventions when a prolonged period of bedrest is required.

### PROVIDING CARE POST PARTUM

After childbirth, the mother may be unable to assume care of the newborn; however, every effort should be made to promote contact between the mother and baby. Many nurses assess the baby and perform the necessary newborn care at the bedside, and then allow the mother ample time to hold the infant. The father and other family members should be included in the care of the infant whenever possible.

Breastfeeding may not be recommended because of the demands on the mother's energy. However, she should be allowed to feed the infant, whenever possible, to promote maternal-infant attachment. Consult with physicians, and make referrals as necessary for follow-up care, which may include home care by a nurse or nursing assistant. Be certain that the family understands the signs and symptoms of cardiac complications and when to notify the physician that problems have developed.

### Evaluation

The ability to identify the factors that increase cardiac workload offers reassurance that the family will initiate measures that promote adaptation to restricted activity.

**✓ CHECK YOUR READING**

8. How do the cardiovascular changes of pregnancy affect the condition of the woman who has a cardiac defect?
9. What are the two major categories of heart disease? What is the functional classification of heart disease?
10. What are the primary goals for management of heart disease in terms of diet, activity, and weight gain?
11. Why must the administration of fluids be monitored closely during labor?
12. Why is the fourth stage of labor particularly dangerous for the woman with heart disease?

## Anemias

Anemia is a condition in which there is a decline in circulating red blood cell mass that reduces the capacity to carry oxygen to the vital organs of the mother or fetus. During pregnancy and the puerperium, anemia is defined as a hemoglobin concentration of less than 10.5 to 11.0 g/dl (Laros, 1994).

Anemia is one of the most common problems of pregnancy. It is estimated that between 20 to 60 percent of prenatal patients will be found to be anemic at some time during their pregnancy (Laros, 1994). The incidence varies according to geographic location and socioeconomic group. Anemia may be caused by a variety of factors, including nutrition, hemolysis, or blood loss. The most common types of anemia observed during pregnancy include iron-deficiency anemia, folic acid–deficiency anemia, sickle cell anemia, and thalassemia.

### Iron-Deficiency Anemia

The total iron requirement for a typical pregnancy with a single fetus is approximately 1000 mg. Unfortunately, most women do not have iron stores that equal this amount. Furthermore, it is difficult to meet pregnancy needs by diet alone, although iron is present in many foods. The primary sources are meat, fish, chicken, liver, and green leafy vegetables.

#### MATERNAL EFFECTS

Signs and symptoms of iron-deficiency anemia include pallor, fatigue, lethargy, and headache. Clinical findings may also include inflammations of the lips and tongue. Pica (consuming nonfood substances such as clay, dirt, ice, or starch) is also a sign of iron-deficiency anemia (Laros, 1994). Laboratory findings for severe anemia include red blood cells that are *microcytic* (small) and *hypochromic* (pale). The plasma iron and serum ferritin are low, whereas the total iron-binding capacity is higher than normal.

#### FETAL AND NEONATAL EFFECTS

The effects of maternal iron-deficiency anemia on the fetus and neonate are unclear. In general, even with significant maternal iron deficiency, the fetus will receive adequate stores at a cost to the mother. If the mother is severely anemic, the fetus may have reduced red cell volume, hemoglobin, and iron stores.

#### THERAPEUTIC MANAGEMENT

Iron replacement is easily achieved in most patients with administration of ferrous sulfate, gluconate, or fumarate tablets. The daily dose should equal about 200 mg of *elemental iron*. Many women experience less gastrointestinal discomfort if iron is taken with meals. Therapy is often continued for about 3 months after the anemia has been corrected. Parenteral therapy may be necessary if the woman cannot take oral preparations.

### Folic Acid–Deficiency (Megaloblastic) Anemia

Folic acid, which functions as a coenzyme in the synthesis of deoxyribonucleic acid (DNA), is essential for cell duplication and for fetal and placental growth. It is also an essential nutrient for the formation of red blood cells.

#### MATERNAL EFFECTS

Maternal needs for folic acid double during pregnancy in response to the demand for greater production of erythrocytes and for fetal and placental growth. A deficiency in folic acid results in a reduction in the rate of DNA synthesis and mitotic activity of individual cells, resulting in the presence of *large, immature erythrocytes* (*megaloblasts*). Folate deficiency is the primary cause of megaloblastic anemia during pregnancy.

Non-nutritional factors that contribute to folic acid deficiency include hemolytic anemias with increased red blood cell turnover; some medications, such as phenytoin (Dilantin); and malabsorption entities. Folic acid deficiency is often present in association with iron-deficiency anemia.

#### FETAL AND NEONATAL EFFECTS

Folate deficiency is associated with increased risk of spontaneous abortion, abruptio placentae, and fetal anomalies. There is particular interest in the relation between folic acid–deficiency anemia and an increase in neural tube defects.

#### THERAPEUTIC MANAGEMENT

The recommended daily allowance for folic acid doubles during pregnancy, and some women have difficulty ingesting the amount needed even though it does occur widely in foods. The best sources of folic acid are liver, kidney beans, lima beans, and fresh dark-green leafy vegetables (see Table 9–5). Folic acid is often destroyed in cooking. As a result of the increased demands for this vitamin during pregnancy, folate supplementation has become a standard component of care (see Chapter 9).

### Sickle Cell Anemia

Sickle cell anemia is an autosomal recessive genetic disorder. It occurs when the gene for the production of S hemoglobin is inherited from both parents. The defect in the hemoglobin causes erythrocytes to be shaped like a sickle, or crescent. Because of their distorted shape, the erythrocytes have difficulty passing through small arteries and capillaries and tend to clump together and occlude the blood vessel.

The disease is characterized by chronic anemia, increased susceptibility to infection, and periodic episodes of obstruction of blood vessels by the abnormally shaped erythrocytes. Sickle cell anemia occurs most often in people of African-American or Mediterranean ancestry. The incidence is one in 2000 persons in African-Americans (Nuwayhid & Khalife, 1992).

#### MATERNAL EFFECTS

Pregnancy may exacerbate sickle cell anemia and bring on *sickle cell crisis*. This broad term includes several different conditions, particularly temporary cessation of bone marrow function, hemolytic crisis with massive erythrocyte destruction resulting in jaundice, and severe pain caused by infarctions located in the joints and all the major organs. In addition, expectant mothers with sickle cell anemia are prone to pyelonephritis, bone infection, and heart disease.

#### FETAL AND NEONATAL EFFECTS

The fetus is prone to serious complications, including prematurity and IUGR. The incidence of fetal death is particularly high in the presence of sickle cell crisis.

#### THERAPEUTIC MANAGEMENT

Women with sickle cell disease should seek early prenatal care and should be informed of the maternal and fetal risks associated with the pregnancy. Frequent evaluations of hemoglobin, complete blood count, serum iron, total iron-binding capacity, and serum folate are necessary to determine the degree of anemia and iron and folic acid stores.

Fetal surveillance studies (ultrasonography, nonstress tests, biophysical profiles) are necessary to assess fetal growth and development and placental function.

The goal of nursing management is to help the pregnant woman maintain a healthy status and avoid hospitalization. Women must be encouraged to keep all prenatal care appointments, usually every other week. Topics in prenatal education include the need (1) to maintain adequate hydration to prevent sickling; (2) for adequate nutrition to meet metabolic needs; (3) for folic acid supplementation for erythrocyte production; (4) for rest periods throughout the day as well as good hygiene practices and the avoidance of persons with infectious illnesses; and (5) for prompt treatment for fever or other signs of infection.

Nurses must be alert for signs of sickle cell crisis. The most common indications are pain in the abdomen, chest, vertebrae, joints, or extremities; pallor; and signs of cardiac failure. Nurses must also provide comfort measures, such as repositioning, good skin care, assisting with ambulation and movement in bed, and assisting the woman to splint the abdomen with a pillow when she must cough or breathe deeply.

Intrapartum care focuses on preventing the development of sickle cell crisis. Oxygen is administered continuously, and fluids should be administered to prevent dehydration because *hypoxemia and dehydration as well as exertion, infection, and acidosis stimulate the sickling process.*

### Thalassemia

Like sickle-cell anemia, thalassemia is a genetic disorder that involves the abnormal synthesis of $\alpha$ or $\beta$ chains of hemoglobin. This leads to alterations in the red blood cell membrane and decreased life span of red blood cells. Thalassemia is named and classified by the type of chain that is inadequately produced. $\beta$-Thalassemia is most frequently encountered in the United States. $\beta$-Thalassemia minor refers to the heterozygous form that results from the inheritance of one abnormal gene from either parent. $\beta$-Thalassemia major is the term used to refer to inheritance of the gene from both parents (homozygous form). Females with *$\beta$-thalassemia major* (*Cooley's anemia*) usually die in childhood or adolescence. Those who survive are often sterile (Cunningham et al., 1997). $\beta$-Thalassemia is most often found in those of Mediterrean or Asian (particularly Chinese) origin.

#### MATERNAL EFFECTS

Women with β-thalassemia minor are often mildly anemic but healthy otherwise. Laboratory values normally associated with β-thalassemia minor indicate a mild hypochromic and microcytic anemia. This can lead to the diagnosis of iron-deficiency anemia and iron supplementation therapy. This treatment is potentially dangerous because β-thalassemia is associated with increased iron absorption and storage and a susceptibility to iron overload (Blackburn & Loper, 1992).

#### FETAL AND NEONATAL EFFECTS

There is controversy regarding whether this disorder is associated with increased fetal or neonatal morbidity. There appears to be no increase in prematurity, low-birth-weight infants, or abnormal size for gestation. The fetus may inherit the serious problem of β-thalassemia major.

#### THERAPEUTIC MANAGEMENT

There is no specific therapy for β-thalassemia minor during pregnancy. Most often the outcomes for the mother and fetus are satisfactory (Cunningham et al., 1997). Infections, which depress production of red blood cells and accelerate erythrocyte destruction, should be identified and treated promptly.

#### CHECK YOUR READING

13. Why is supplemental iron needed by almost all women who are pregnant?
14. What are the neonatal effects of iron-deficiency anemia?
15. What are the fetal and neonatal effects of folic acid deficiency?
16. What are the maternal effects of sickle cell anemia?
17. How is sickle cell anemia treated during pregnancy?
18. Why is iron supplementation often not recommended for women with thalassemia?

## Medical Conditions

Women with a preexisting medical condition should be aware of the effect that pregnancy will have on the condition as well as the impact the medical condition will have on pregnancy outcome. Some of the conditions that complicate pregnancy are discussed in this section.

### Immune-Complex Diseases

#### SYSTEMIC LUPUS ERYTHEMATOSUS

Systemic lupus erythematosus (SLE) is a chronic, inflammatory, autoimmune disease that can affect any organ or system in the body. Although the cause is unknown, there appears to be an imbalance between immune response and tolerance of specific antigens in which the body produces antibodies to its own cells and tissue. Signs and symptoms result from inflammation of multiple organ systems, especially the joints, skin, kidneys, and nervous system. The most common symptoms are joint pain, photosensitivity, and a "butterfly rash" on the face.

The disease tends to affect young women, but it may occur in any age group. The incidence is believed to be approximately one per 1000 persons. It is more common in African-Americans and persons of Latin descent.

Although women with SLE can have a normal pregnancy and give birth to a normal baby, the pregnancy must be treated as high risk. There is an increased incidence of abortion and fetal death during the first trimester. Moreover, almost half of all deliveries will be premature because of complications such as pre-eclampsia (Kuper & Failla, 1994).

Because pregnancy can exacerbate SLE, the woman must be carefully observed during pregnancy for signs that the disease has worsened. Renal complications pose a special risk. Women with a history of kidney problems should be advised to seek the advice of a physician before becoming pregnant.

#### ANTIPHOSPHOLIPID SYNDROME

Antiphospholipid syndrome is a recently described autoimmune condition characterized by the production of antiphospholipid antibodies combined with certain clinical features. The most specific clinical features include thrombosis, decreased platelets, and pregnancy loss. An unusually high rate of pre-eclampsia has been noted in patients with antiphospholipid syndrome. Pre-eclampsia contributes to the high rate of preterm births with this condition.

Although the syndrome occurs most often in women with other underlying autoimmune diseases, such as SLE, it is also diagnosed in women with no other recognizable autoimmune disease.

Women with antiphospholipid syndrome should be informed of the potential maternal and obstetric problems, including a possible risk of stroke. They should be assessed for evidence of anemia, thrombocytopenia, and underlying renal disease. Some physicians believe that treatment with heparin may be warranted on the basis of increased risk for thrombosis; however, this is controversial. Combinations of low-dose aspirin and subcutaneous heparin are sometimes recommended.

#### RHEUMATOID ARTHRITIS

Rheumatoid arthritis is a chronic inflammatory disease that usually affects the synovial (hinged) joints. Although the cause is unknown, an autoimmune mechanism is suspected. It is strongly associated with rheumatoid factor, an autoantibody that is present in 80 to 90 percent of patients with inflammatory rheumatoid arthritis (de Swiet, 1994). It occurs in 1 to 2 percent of the population and affects females two to three times more frequently than males (Gladman & Urowitz, 1995).

There is often marked improvement in symptoms of rheumatoid arthritis during pregnancy. The exact reason is unclear, but improvement is reported to parallel the rise in pregnancy-specific protein, which suppresses inflammatory reactions. Hormonal factors have also been suggested. For instance, increased levels of cortisol as well as estrogen and progesterone may be beneficial in suppressing the immune response. Unfortunately, most women relapse within 6 weeks to 6 months post partum.

In contrast to SLE, there appears to be no increased risk of abortion in women with rheumatoid arthritis. Moreover, there have been no reports of particular obstetric problems unless there is significant deterioration in the hips or cervical spine (Gladman & Urowitz, 1995).

## Neurologic Disorders

### EPILEPSY

Convulsive seizures are the most common form of epilepsy, which is a recurrent disorder of cerebral function. Epilepsy occurs in 0.3 to 0.6 percent of pregnant women (Blackburn & Loper, 1992).

The effect of pregnancy on the course of epilepsy is variable and unpredictable. The frequency of seizures may increase, decrease, or remain the same. In general, the longer the woman has been seizure-free before pregnancy, the less likely she is to develop seizures during pregnancy. Women with epilepsy have a higher than normal incidence of stillbirth and may have a higher incidence of preterm labor. Maternal bleeding may occur as a result of a deficiency of clotting factors associated with anticonvulsant drugs such as diphenylhydantoin (Dilantin) or phenobarbital. Anticonvulsant drugs also compete with folate for absorption, which may result in folate deficiency.

A major concern is the teratogenic effects of anticonvulsant drugs. A specific syndrome, known as *fetal hydantoin syndrome*, which includes craniofacial abnormalities, limb reduction defects, growth restriction, mental retardation, and cardiac anomalies, has been described. Other anticonvulsants, such as trimethadione, paramethadione, and carbamazepine are also associated with malformation syndromes. The teratogenic effects of phenobarbital are difficult to assess because it is often combined with other drugs.

Health professionals should recommend that the pregnant woman consult a neurologist before conception. The goal of treatment is to prevent grand mal seizures and also to reduce the effects of anticonvulsant medications. The family must be made aware of the risks involved when anticonvulsant drugs must be used. They also should realize that treatment cannot be stopped during pregnancy unless the woman has been seizure-free for a prolonged time. Grand mal seizures result in fetal hypoxia and acidosis and thus pose a serious problem for the fetus.

### BELL'S PALSY

Bell's palsy is a sudden unilateral neuropathy of the seventh cranial (facial) nerve that causes facial paralysis with weakness of the forehead and lower face. It is thought to be caused by a virus. It is three times more common during pregnancy and generally occurs in the third trimester. Although the reason for the increase during pregnancy is unknown, one theory suggests that estrogen-induced edema puts pressure on the facial nerve, making the pregnant woman more vulnerable to the disease. Pregnancy does not affect recovery rate, and nearly 90 percent of women will recover function within a few weeks to months (Aminoff, 1994).

The face feels stiff and pulled to one side. It may be difficult or impossible to close the eye on the affected side. There may be difficulty with eating or with fine facial movements. There may also be a disturbance in the ability to taste.

Treatment is controversial; however, many physicians prescribe steroids within the first few days. Supportive care may include patching the eye and applying ointment or eye drops to prevent dryness or injury to the exposed cornea. Facial massage may be helpful, and the woman should be cautioned to chew carefully. Psychological support is necessary to assist the woman and her family deal with anxiety that they naturally feel when there is sudden paralysis of the face. They must be reassured that the condition is usually temporary. Table 26–5 describes the maternal, fetal, and neonatal effects and relevant nursing considerations of additional conditions.

**CHECK YOUR READING**

19. What are the maternal and fetal effects of SLE?
20. How does pregnancy affect rheumatoid arthritis?
21. What is the major concern about administering anticonvulsant drugs for the woman with epilepsy?
22. What is the recommended supportive care for those with Bell's palsy?

**TABLE 26–5 INFREQUENT CONDITIONS AND THEIR EFFECT ON PREGNANCY**

| Condition | Maternal-Fetal Effects | Nursing Considerations |
|---|---|---|
| **Appendicitis** | | |
| Inflammation of the appendix. The most common nongynecologic surgical emergency during pregnancy. | Difficult to diagnose during pregnancy. Early symptoms mimic common conditions of pregnancy. Ultrasonography may help rule out other diagnoses. | When there is a reasonable doubt that the patient has appendicitis, the appendix should be removed to prevent rupture and consequent complications. |
| **Asthma** | | |
| An obstructive lung disease, caused by airway inflammation. Characterized by dyspnea, cough, wheezing. Course in pregnancy is variable. | No significant increase in prematurity or spontaneous abortion. Medications used are well tolerated in pregnancy and appear to be safe for the fetus. | Early use of anti-inflammatory agents such as inhaled corticosteroids may prevent severe attacks. Outpatient use of $\beta$-agonists often controls mild asthma. |
| **Glucose-6-Phosphate Dehydrogenase Deficiency** | | |
| Female-linked genetic disorder that predisposes to lysis of red blood cells when exposed to oxidizing drugs (salicylates, acetaminophen, phenacetin, and some sulfa drugs). | Not affected by pregnancy unless complicated by anemia. Iron and folic acid supplementation recommended. | Advise patient of risks and suggest she consult with her health care provider for recommended list of drugs for minor discomforts. |
| **Hyperthyroidism** | | |
| An overactive, enlarged thyroid gland that is difficult to diagnose and manage during pregnancy because the normal changes of pregnancy increase the metabolic rate and mimic hyperthyroidism. Graves' disease is the most common cause during pregnancy. | Increased incidence of pregnancy-induced hypertension and postpartum hemorrhage if not well controlled during pregnancy. Treatment is complicated by the presence of the fetus, which may be jeopardized by surgery or antithyroid medications. Propylthiouracil has limited placental transfer and is widely used during pregnancy to control thyroid function. | Be aware of the major signs that should be reported. These include a resting pulse rate greater than 100/min, loss of weight or failure to gain weight in spite of normal intake of food, heat intolerance, and abnormal protrusion of the eyes (exophthalmos). |
| **Hypothyroidism** | | |
| Characterized by inadequate thyroid secretion; confirmed by an elevated level of thyroid-stimulating hormone and low levels of triiodothyronine and thyroxine. | If the expectant mother is untreated, there is an increased risk of neonatal goiter and congenital hypothyroidism; severity of symptoms depend on time of onset and severity of the deprivation. | Suspect neonatal hypothyroidism when the infant is large-for-gestational age, with respiratory and feeding difficulties, rough dry skin, and an umbilical hernia. |
| **Maternal Phenylketonuria (PKU)** | | |
| Inherited single-gene recessive anomaly leading to an inability to metabolize the amino acid phenylalanine, resulting in high serum levels of phenylalanine. Irreparable mental retardation occurs if the pregnant woman is not treated early with a diet that provides adequate protein but restricts phenylalanine. | The woman must be on a low-phenylalanine diet before conception and pregnancy. If not, there is an increased fetal risk of microcephaly, mental retardation, heart defects, and intrauterine growth restriction. | Advise women that the child will either be a carrier of the gene or will inherit the disease, depending on the presence of the gene in the father of the child. Treatment at a PKU center is recommended. |

## Trauma in Pregnancy

### Blunt Force Injuries

Automobile accidents cause most cases of blunt force injuries to the pregnant woman. Maternal deaths are most often caused by head injury or intra-abdominal hemorrhage, which may follow sudden premature separation of the placenta or rupture of the uterus. Pelvic fracture is also a commonly reported injury in automobile accidents or as a result of falls.

During the first trimester, the fetus is protected from external forces by the bony pelvis, the amniotic fluid, and soft tissue surrounding the pelvis. Later in pregnancy, the fetal compartment extends beyond the bony pelvis, and as a result the fetus is more vulnerable to blunt force injury. Fetal injury may include skull fracture and intracranial hemorrhage. Moreover, disruption of uteroplacental blood flow because of premature separation of the placenta can result in fetal anoxia.

Use of seat belt restraints improves maternal and fetal outcomes in automobile accidents significantly. Current recommendations are that the pregnant woman wear three-point restraint seat belts during automobile travel (Gonik, 1994).

### Penetrating Injuries

Gunshot and knife wounds are the most common penetrating injuries and may be associated with aggravated assaults or suicide attempts. Mortality rates from penetrating wounds in the pregnant woman are less than those in non-pregnant women because the uterus acts as a shield for the abdominal structure (Gonik, 1994). The fetus fares less well, with high injury and mortality rates.

### Therapeutic Management

Initial management of trauma in pregnancy is similar to that in the non-pregnant state. Primary goals are evaluation and stabilization of maternal injuries. Basic rules are applied to resuscitation, including establishing ventilation and arrest of hemorrhage. During attempted resuscitation, however, prolonged supine positioning should be avoided so that compression of the large blood vessels can be minimized. Lateral displacement of the uterus can be accomplished by placing a wedge along the right side of the woman. Moreover, the need for large amounts of fluid replacement should be anticipated. After resuscitation, evaluation is continued for fractures, bleeding sites, and internal injuries. Exploratory abdominal surgery may be necessary to identify and control internal bleeding. The uterus and fetus must also be evaluated for injuries.

Electronic fetal monitoring may reflect the condition of the mother as well as that of the fetus. For example, although the mother is stable, electronic monitoring may detect signs of premature separation of the placenta, such as uterine contractions, fetal tachycardia, and late decelerations.

The necessity for cesarean delivery of a live fetus depends on several factors, including the age of the fetus and the fetal condition as well as the extent of uterine injury. Because placental abruption usually develops soon after trauma, electronic monitoring is begun as soon as the maternal condition is stabilized. It is continued as long as there are signs of uterine contractions, vaginal bleeding, uterine tenderness, or ruptured membranes.

## Infections During Pregnancy

The acronym TORCH is sometimes used to denote a group of diseases that can cross the placenta and cause permanent physical or mental disability in the neonate. TORCH stands for Toxoplasmosis, Other diseases such as syphilis, Rubella, Cytomegalic inclusion disease, and Herpes genitalis. Although the acronym is helpful in recalling the diseases, it does not include all infections that can cause harm to the fetus. In this section, infections are divided into those caused by viruses and those caused by other organisms. Table 26–6 presents nursing considerations of sexually transmissible diseases and vaginal infections. Table 26–7 summarizes urinary tract infections and their effect on pregnancy (see also Chapter 33).

### Viral Infections

Although viral infections are mild or even asymptomatic in adults, they are of great concern during pregnancy because fetal or neonatal consequences can be catastrophic. Maternal infection with cytomegalovirus, rubella, varicella-zoster virus, herpes simplex, hepatitis B, and human immunodeficiency virus (HIV) have the greatest potential for harming the fetus or neonate.

#### CYTOMEGALOVIRUS

Cytomegalovirus, a member of the herpesvirus group, is widespread and eventually infects most humans. Cytomegalovirus has been isolated from urine, saliva, blood, cervical mucus, semen, breast milk, and stool. Transmission may occur from contamination of any of these bodily fluids. The highest rate of infection occurs between the ages of 15 and 35 years; thus, the possibility of cytomegalovirus infection occurring during pregnancy is high.

## TABLE 26–6 SEXUALLY TRANSMISSIBLE DISEASES AND VAGINAL INFECTIONS: THEIR IMPACT ON PREGNANCY

| Maternal, Fetal, and Neonatal Effects | Nursing Considerations |
|---|---|
| **Sexually Transmissible Diseases** | |
| ***Syphilis* (*Causative Organism: Spirochete* Treponema pallidum)** | |
| If untreated, the infection may be passed across the placenta to the fetus and result in spontaneous abortion, a stillborn infant, premature labor and birth, or congenital syphilis. Major signs of congenital syphilis are enlarged liver and spleen, skin lesions, rashes, osteitis, pneumonia, and hepatitis. | Penicillin is the only treatment that will cure the disease without harming the fetus. Women who are allergic are desensitized and then treated (Martens, 1994). |
| ***Gonorrhea* (*Causative Organism: Bacterium* Neisseria gonorrhoeae)** | |
| Not transmitted via the placenta; vertical transmission from mother to newborn during birth may cause ophthalmia neonatorium. Endocervicitis and weakness of the fetal membranes increase the risk of premature rupture of membranes and preterm labor. | Ceftriaxone or cefixime with erythromycin are now recommended for penicillin-resistant organisms. The partner must also be treated to prevent reinfection. All infants are treated with an ophthalmic antibiotic at birth to prevent serious eye infections (CDC, 1993). |
| ***Chlamydial Infection* (*Causative Organism: Bacterium* Chlamydia trachomatis)** | |
| The fetus may be infected during birth and suffer neonatal conjunctivitis or pneumonitis, which manifests within 4 to 6 weeks. Conjunctivitis is prevented by erythromycin ophthalmic ointment. Chlamydia may also be responsible for premature rupture of membranes, premature labor, and chorioamnionitis. | Education is particularly important because chlamydia is the most common sexually transmissible disease in the United States, and infection is usually asymptomatic. Both partners should be treated to prevent recurrent infection. As with all sexually transmitted diseases, the use of condoms decreases the risk of infection. Erythromycin is the recommended treatment (CDC, 1993). |
| ***Trichomoniasis* (*Causative Organism: Protozoan* Trichomonas vaginalis)** | |
| Not transmitted across the placental barrier; the organism cannot survive in the infantile, nonestrogenized vagina. Associated with premature rupture of membranes and postpartum endometritis. | Metronidazole (Flagyl) can only be used safely during the second and third trimesters because of teratogenity. Clotrimazole may provide relief of symptoms during first trimester (Martens, 1994). |
| ***Condyloma Acuminatum* (*Causative Organism: Human Papillomavirus*)** | |
| Transmission of condyloma acuminatum, also called veneral warts, may occur during vaginal birth and is associated with the development of epithelial tumors of the mucous membranes of the larynx in children. Pregnancy can cause proliferation of lesions, which are associated with cervical dysplasia and cancer. | Podophyllin is contraindicated as treatment during pregnancy because of the possible teratogenic effects. Applications of trichloracetic acid or cryotherapy is recommended instead (Youngkin, 1995). |
| **Vaginal Infections** | |
| ***Candidiasis* (*Causative Organism: Yeast* Candida albicans)** | |
| Oral candidiasis (thrush) may develop in newborns if infection is present at birth. Thrush is treated with application of nystatin (Mycostatin) over the surfaces of the oral cavity four times a day for several days. Characteristic "cottage cheese" vaginal discharge with vulvar pruritus, burning, and dyspareunia. Vulva may be red, tender, and edematous. | Candidiasis (previously called *Monilia*) is a persistent problem for many women during pregnancy. Effective treatment may be obtained with miconazole nitrate (Monistat) or clotrimazole (Gyne-Lotrimin), both available over the counter. |
| ***Bacterial Vaginosis* (*Causative Organism:* Gardnerella vaginalis*)** | |
| No known fetal effects; may be associated with postpartum endometritis. Marked by a major shift in vaginal flora from the normal predominance of lactobacilli to a predominance of anerobic bacteria. Causes profuse, malodorous, "fishy" vaginal discharge, itching, and burning. | The causative organism is sensitive to metronidazole, which may be used during the second and third trimesters without concern about teratogenic effect (Lee, 1995). |

*Formerly called nonspecific vaginitis or *Gardnerella* vaginitis.

**TABLE 26–7 URINARY TRACT INFECTIONS AND THEIR EFFECT ON PREGNANCY**

| Maternal, Fetal, and Neonatal Effects | Nursing Considerations |
|---|---|
| **Asymptomatic Bacteriuria (Causative Organisms: *Escherichia coli, Klebsiella, Proteus*)** | |
| Ascending bacteria can result in cystitis or pyelonephritis in later pregnancy if condition remains untreated. | Defined as recovery of the same pathogen from two consecutive urine samples of 100,000 colony-forming units per milliliter of urine. Diagnosed by midstream, clean-catch specimen. Treated with oral sulfonamides or ampicillin in early pregnancy; sulfonamides displace bilirubin from albumin in fetal circulation in late pregnancy and can result in neonatal jaundice. |
| **Cystitis (Causative Organisms: E. *coli, Klebsiella, Proteus*)** | |
| Emphasize importance of reporting signs of urinary tract infection. Stress the importance of taking all the medication prescribed even if the symptoms abate. Provide information about hygiene measures. | Signs and symptoms include dysuria, frequency, urgency, and suprapubic tenderness. Ascending infection may lead to pyelonephritis. |
| **Acute Pyelonephritis (Causative Organisms: E. *coli, Klebsiella, Proteus*)** | |
| Increased risk of preterm labor and premature delivery. Maternal complications include septic shock and adult respiratory distress syndrome. | Inform women with asymptomatic bacteriuria or cystitis of signs and symptoms, such as sudden onset of fever, chills, flank pain or tenderness, nausea, and vomiting so that treatment can begin promptly. May be hospitalized for intravenous administration of antibiotics. |

After primary infection, the virus becomes latent, but like other herpesvirus infections, there may be periodic reactivation and shedding of the virus. The best way to establish the presence of cytomegalovirus is by isolating the virus (Gibbs & Sweet, 1994). However, most infections are asymptomatic, so they may not be suspected or diagnosed.

**Fetal and Neonatal Effects.** Two percent of all live neonates are infected with the virus; about 90 percent of these are asymptomatic and appear normal (Collins et al., 1995). The most serious complications of those affected are deafness, mental retardation, seizures, blindness, and dental abnormalities. Some of these conditions may not be obvious for several months or even years.

**Therapeutic Management.** No effective therapy is currently available for the treatment of congenital infection. Antiviral agents, such as adenosine arabinoside, have been used for severe infections; however, these drugs are toxic and only temporarily suppress shedding of the virus (Collins et al., 1995). In those instances in which a primary infection is diagnosed during the first 20 weeks of gestation, a therapeutic termination of the pregnancy may be considered.

### RUBELLA

Rubella is caused by a virus that is transmitted from person to person by droplets or through direct contact with articles contaminated with nasopharyngeal secretions. Rubella is a mild disease; fever, general malaise, and a characteristic maculopapular rash that begins on the face and migrates over the body are the major symptoms. Although the overall incidence has declined since rubella vaccine became available, up to 20 percent of the adults in the United States remain susceptible (Collins et al., 1995).

**Fetal and Neonatal Effects.** Rubella remains a serious concern because the virus crosses the placental barrier and can infect the fetus. The greatest risk to the fetus occurs during the first trimester, when fetal organs are developing. If maternal infection occurs during this time, approximately one third of these cases will result in spontaneous abortions and the surviving fetuses may be seriously compromised. Deafness, mental retardation, cataracts, cardiac defects, IUGR, and microcephaly are the most common fetal complications. Moreover, infants who are born to mothers who had rubella during pregnancy shed the virus for many months and thus pose a threat to other infants as well as to susceptible adults who come in contact with them.

**Therapeutic Management.** Prevention is the only effective protection for the fetus. Women who are immune do not become infected, so it is critical to determine the immune status of all women of childbearing age. A serologic test, hemagglutination inhibition, determines rubella titers. A titer of 1:8 or greater provides evidence of immunity. Women who are not immune should be vaccinated before they become pregnant, and they should be advised not to become pregnant for 3 months after vaccination because there is a possible risk to the fetus from the live-virus vaccine. Many women are vaccinated during the postpartum period so that they will be immune before becoming pregnant again. In some facilities, women of childbearing age must read and sign a document indicating that they understand the risks to the fetus if they become pregnant before 3 months.

### VARICELLA-ZOSTER VIRUS

Varicella infection (chickenpox) is caused by varicella-zoster virus, a herpesvirus that is transmitted by direct contact or via the respiratory tract. The varicella virus can become latent in nerve ganglia. When the virus is reactivated, herpes zoster (shingles) results. Potential maternal complications of acute varicella infection may include preterm labor, encephalitis, and varicella pneumonia, which is the most serious complication associated with varicella-zoster virus.

**Fetal and Neonatal Effects.** Fetal and neonatal effects depend on the time of maternal infection. If the infection occurred during the first trimester, the fetus may be at risk for congenital varicella syndrome; clinical findings include limb hypoplasia, cutaneous scars, chorioretinitis, cataracts, microcephaly, and symmetric IUGR (Gibbs & Sweet, 1994). In later pregnancy, transplacental passage of maternal antibodies usually protects the fetus. If the fetus is exposed to the virus in utero and is born before the development of maternal antibodies, however, the infant is at risk for development of life-threatening neonatal varicella infection.

**Therapeutic Management.** Immune testing may be recommended for pregnant women who are presumed to be susceptible. Varicella-zoster immune globulin should be administered to women who have been exposed and are susceptible (Rouse et al., 1996). Those infected with chickenpox during pregnancy should be instructed to report pulmonary symptoms immediately. Hospitalization, fetal surveillance, full respiratory support, and hemodynamic monitoring should be available for women diagnosed with varicella pneumonia.

For infants born to mothers with varicella, authorities recommend immunization with varicella-zoster immune globulin within 72 hours of birth. Women and infants with varicella are highly contagious and should be placed in strict isolation. Only staff members known to be immune to varicella should come in contact with these clients.

### HERPESVIRUS SEROTYPES 1 AND 2

Genital herpes is one of the most common sexually transmissible diseases. It may be caused by herpesvirus serotype 1 or serotype 2; however, 90 percent of the episodes of genital herpes are caused by type 2. Infection occurs as a result of direct contact of the skin or mucous membrane with an active lesion. Lesions form at the site of contact and begin as a group of painful papules that progress rapidly to become vesicles, shallow ulcers, pustules, and crusts. The woman sheds the virus until the lesions are completely healed. The virus then migrates along the sensory nerves to reside in the sensory ganglion, and the disease enters a latent phase. It can be reactivated later as a recurrent infection.

*Vertical* transmission (from mother to infant) generally occurs in two ways: (1) after rupture of membranes, when the virus ascends from active lesions; and (2) during birth, when the fetus comes into contact with infectious genital secretions.

Diagnosis is usually based on clinical signs and symptoms; however, definitive diagnosis involves isolation of the virus from a lesion. (See Chapter 33 for implications of herpes genitalis in nonpregnant women.)

**Fetal and Neonatal Effects.** Complications of pregnancy from a recurrent infection are rare. However, if primary infection occurs during the first 20 weeks, there is an increase in the rate of spontaneous abortions, IUGR, and preterm labor (Martens, 1994). Neonatal herpes infection is the major perinatal problem. The incidence of neonatal herpes in the United States is about one in 7500 births (Martens, 1994). Symptoms usually appear within 2 to 3 days of birth, and the disease progresses rapidly. The mortality rate for infants with disseminated herpes infection is approximately 60 percent, with as many as 50 percent of the surviving infants suffering severe neurologic complications (Ricci, 1992).

**Therapeutic Management.** There is no known cure for herpes infection, although antiviral chemotherapy (acyclovir) is prescribed in non-pregnant women to reduce symptoms and shorten the duration of the lesions. Acyclovir is sometimes administered in pregnancy; however, it is in pregnancy risk category C according to the U.S. Food and Drug Administration and should be used with caution. See Appendix C: Effects of Drug Use During Pregnancy and Breastfeeding.

For women with a history of genital herpes, vaginal delivery is allowed if there are no genital lesions at the time of labor. For women with active lesions, either recurrent or primary, at the time of labor, cesarean birth is often recommended. After delivery, isolation of the mother from her infant is not necessary as long as direct contact with lesions is avoided and mothers are instructed in careful hand washing techniques. Mothers may breastfeed if there are no lesions on the breasts.

The infant is observed carefully for signs of infection, including temperature instability, lethargy, poor sucking reflex, jaundice, seizures, and herpetic lesions.

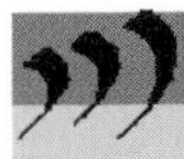

## THERAPEUTIC COMMUNICATION
### Concern About Confidentiality

Mary Smith, who had a cesarean delivery because of an active herpes lesion, appears anxious and uncomfortable during the morning assessment by nurse Eileen Sinclair.

**Mary:** Why does everyone wear gloves whenever they come near me?
**Eileen:** You wonder why we wear gloves when we care for you?

*Reflecting content*

**Mary:** Well, it bothers me that you think I am so contagious.
**Eileen:** You think we wear gloves because you have a herpes outbreak and that upsets you?

*Clarifying content and feeling*

**Mary:** Yes, why else would it be necessary?
**Eileen:** We wear gloves when we care for all patients, whenever there is a chance that we will come into contact with body fluids. I'm sorry you thought it was only because of the herpes.

*Providing information and conveying empathy*

**Mary:** I'm just so touchy about having my family find out I have herpes.
**Eileen:** You don't want your family to know why you had a cesarean?

*Clarifying and reflecting feelings*

**Mary:** Yes, I'm so embarrassed. I wish they didn't have to know.
**Eileen:** They will know only if you tell them. We do everything possible to protect your privacy. I'd like to come back in a few minutes and we can talk more about how you feel.

*Offering reassurance about Mary's privacy and giving her the option to express her feelings more completely at a later time*

Expectant mothers need information about effective ways to deal with the emotional as well as the physical effects of herpes. Many women are concerned about privacy and do not want family members to know why cesarean birth is necessary. Such women must be assured that their wishes will be respected. Many women need an opportunity to discuss their feelings of shame, anger, or anxiety about the disease.

#### PARVOVIRUS B19

Erythema infectiosum, also called *fifth disease*, caused by human parvovirus B19, is an acute, communicable disease that is characterized by a highly distinctive rash. The rash starts on the face with a "slapped-cheeks" appearance, followed by a generalized maculopapular rash. Other symptoms include fever, malaise, and joint pain. Erythema infectiosum is more common among children and often occurs in community epidemics. The prognosis is usually excellent. However, if the disease occurs in pregnancy, there are potential fetal and neonatal effects. Parvovirus titers can be drawn if exposure during pregnancy is suspected.

**Fetal and Neonatal Effects.** When infection occurs during pregnancy, fetal death can result, usually from failure of fetal red blood cell production, followed by severe fetal anemia, hydrops (generalized edema), and heart failure. The mother should be assessed for elevated levels of alpha-fetoprotein, which may be a marker for hydrops. Serial ultrasonography can also be performed to detect hydrops. At delivery, the umbilical cord blood should be examined for virus or IgM antibody, which reveals whether or not the virus has crossed the placenta and infected the fetus. If this has occurred, the infant is examined for any defect and is followed up for several years to exclude the possibility of delayed complications.

**Therapeutic Management.** There is no specific treatment. Starch baths may help reduce pruritus, and analgesics may be necessary to relieve mild joint pain.

#### HEPATITIS B

Hepatitis B, formerly known as serum hepatitis, is caused by a virus that is transmitted via blood, saliva, vaginal secretions, semen, or breast milk and across the placental barrier. The disease is prevalent in certain population groups, such as Asians, Native Americans, Eskimos, Southeast Asian immigrants, and intravenous drug users. Symptoms may include vomiting, abdominal pain, jaundice, fever, rash, and painful joints. Fortunately, most infected adolescents and adults recover within 6 months and acquire long-lasting immunity.

**Fetal and Neonatal Effects.** There is an increased incidence of prematurity, low birth weight, and neonatal death when the mother has hepatitis B infection during pregnancy. Infants born to mothers who have hepatitis B during pregnancy or who are chronic carriers of hepatitis B surface antigen (HBsAg) are at risk for the development of acute infection at birth. Newborns as well as children infected with hepatitis B virus before the age of 5 years will become chronic carriers of the virus.

**Therapeutic Management.** Hepatitis B is completely preventable. Simple hygiene measures such as safe sex and standard precautions with body fluids are easy ways to begin. However, pre-exposure and postexposure prophylaxes are more effective. Highly effective hepatitis B vaccines have been available for more than a decade in the United States. A series of three intramuscular injections given during a 6- to 12-month period produces a protective antibody response for most infants, children, and adults.

All pregnant women should be screened for HBsAg. Women at high risk for hepatitis should be rescreened in the third trimester if the initial screen is negative. Household members and sexual contacts should be tested and offered vaccination if they are susceptible. No specific treatment exists for hepatitis. Recommended supportive treatment includes bedrest and a high-protein, low-fat diet.

Infection of the newborn whose mother is known to be HBsAg positive can usually be prevented by administration of hepatitis B immune globulin (HBIG, Hep-B-Gammagee), followed by hepatitis B vaccine (Heptavax B) soon after birth. *The newborn must be carefully bathed before any injections are given to prevent infections from skin surface contamination.* The vaccine should be repeated at 1 month and 6 months of age.

Infants born to mothers who were not screened for HBsAg should receive the vaccine soon after birth. If the mother is found to be HBsAg positive, HBIG should be administered as well as the second and third doses of vaccine.

Breastfeeding is considered safe as long as the newborn has been vaccinated. Vaccination is recommended for any population at risk; this includes nurses who frequently come into contact with blood.

### HUMAN IMMUNODEFICIENCY VIRUS

Acquired immunodeficiency syndrome (AIDS) is caused by a retrovirus known as HIV. Transmission of HIV infection is predominantly through three modes: (1) sexual exposure to genital secretions of an infected person, (2) parenteral exposure to infected blood or tissue, and (3) perinatal exposure of an infant to an infected mother. The virus must enter the recipient's blood stream to produce infection.

In the past, the populations at highest risk for HIV exposure included homosexual and bisexual men, intravenous drug users (who often share contaminated needles), and inhabitants of West Africa and Haiti. However, since the mid 1980s, heterosexual transmission has rapidly become the major mode of spread throughout the world (Chin, 1994). The receptive partner in sexual intercourse, whether it be anal or vaginal intercourse, has a greater likelihood of acquiring an HIV infection than the insertive partner. Thus, although there is a greater probability that infected men will transmit the virus, there is no doubt that transmission occurs in both directions. The incidence is increasing rapidly among young, disadvantaged African-Americans and Latinos. There are approximately 1 million persons in the United States infected with HIV. Of this number, at least 80,000 are women of childbearing age (Minkoff, 1994).

**Pathophysiology.** Like other retroviruses, HIV can integrate its viral genetic makeup into the genetic makeup of the cell when infecting it. This results in an abnormal cell, one that cannot perform its functions properly. At the same time, this cell replicates and produces more viruses that invade more cells. The disease worsens as more and more cells cease to function, and at the same time, a greater number of viruses are produced. The principal mechanism whereby HIV leads to immunodeficiency is via its effect on helper (CD4) lymphocytes. These cells play a key role in organizing the body's immune response.

As the number of CD4 cells declines, the immune response becomes inadequate and opportunistic infections are able to overwhelm the person who is HIV positive. A CD4 count of less than 200 cells/mm$^3$ confirms the diagnosis of AIDS.

The clinical course of HIV infection follows fairly predictable stages:

1. There is an early, or acute, stage that occurs several weeks after HIV exposure. Flu-like symptoms may develop and last a few weeks. Antibodies to HIV (seroconversion) generally appear within a few months, but occasionally delays of more than a year have been reported.
2. A middle, or asymptomatic, period of minor or no clinical problems follows. This period is characterized by continuous low-level viral replication and CD4 cell loss. The latent period from infection to AIDS is approximately 11 years (Minkoff, 1994).
3. A transitional period of symptomatic disease follows.
4. A late or crisis period of symptomatic disease lasts months or years.

During stages 1 and 2, the infected person is said to be HIV positive; during stages 3 and 4, the immune system no longer offers adequate protection, and opportunistic diseases occur. The person is then said to have AIDS.

**Fetal and Neonatal Effects.** Although techniques for diagnosis are not standardized, an infant born to an HIV-positive mother has a 20 to 40 percent risk for developing the disease (Chin, 1994). Characteristically, the newborn is asymptomatic at birth, but signs and symptoms usually become obvious during the first year of life. The most common early signs are enlargement of the liver and spleen, lymphadenopathy, failure to thrive, persistent thrush, and ex-

## Critical to Remember

### FACTS ABOUT HIV

- After initial exposure, there is a period of from 3 to 12 months before seroconversion; the person is considered infectious during this time.
- There is a long period of time (often years) from seroconversion to development of AIDS; persons must be considered infectious during this time.
- As of now, AIDS will eventually develop in all those who are HIV-positive.
- There is no cure for AIDS; however, certain medications slow replication of the virus and delay onset of opportunistic diseases. Effects of these medications on the fetus are not completely understood.
- Human immunodeficiency virus is transmitted by sexual contact with an infected person, by contact with infected body fluids, and through the placenta from mother to fetus.

tensive seborrheic dermatitis (cradle cap). Unlike adults, infants frequently experience chronic bacterial infections, such as meningitis, pneumonia, osteomyelitis, septic arthritis, and septicemia.

Infants infected with HIV progress to AIDS more rapidly than adults. Approximately 80 percent will die as a result of AIDS within 5 years (Chin, 1994).

**Prevention.** Prevention remains the only way to control HIV infection. Sexual transmission can be avoided by several methods. Abstinence would render a person safe from all sexually transmissible diseases, including HIV; however, for many people sexual expression adds to the quality of life, and many are not willing to practice total abstinence. Transmission of HIV can also be prevented if infected persons do not have intercourse with susceptible persons. If intercourse does occur, barrier methods, such as latex condoms in conjunction with spermicidal jellies containing nonoxynol 9, have been demonstrated to be effective. A rubber dam or plastic wrap (condom) offers protection from transmission through cunnilingus or fellatio (oral sex).

Intravenous drug users who refuse rehabilitative treatment must be taught to wash the equipment with water, soap, and bleach before each use to prevent transmission of the virus from one person to another via a soiled needle.

**Medical Management.** Although HIV was thought to be universally fatal, several medications have proven to be beneficial. Zidovudine (previously called azidothymidine [AZT]) is thought to inhibit replication of the virus and thus to prolong the mother's life. Currently, zidovudine is recommended for pregnant women who are HIV positive to reduce vertical transmission of the virus (CDC, 1994). Didanosine is used to treat symptomatic HIV infection in those who cannot tolerate zidovudine. Recently, protease inhibitors were found to reduce the amount of virus in the blood and prolong the life of those with HIV infection. Saquinavir (Invirase) is the first protease inhibitor approved by the Food and Drug Administration in the United States.

*Pneumocystis carinii* pneumonia is the most common serious HIV-related infection in children. The drug of choice for prophylaxis is trimethoprim-sulfamethoxazole (co-trimoxazole). Aerosolized pentamidine is also recommended for adults and children older than 5 years.

**Nursing Considerations.** Learning of HIV infection during pregnancy can have a devastating and immobilizing effect on the entire family. A nursing diagnosis of Anticipatory Grieving related to multiple losses that include probable loss of her life and possible death of the infant should be considered. Crisis intervention may be necessary initially to help the family cope.

Nurses must frequently determine what the family perceives as the most pressing needs and worries. Some of the most common fears are loss of control, loss of support and love, social isolation, and loss of privacy. The nurse's response may involve finding ways for the woman to retain control while she is physically able and to assist her in selecting those in her family who will provide continued love and emotional support. Above all, it is necessary to reassure the woman that her right to privacy will not be violated.

Nurses can help the woman maintain the highest level of wellness possible. Adequate, high-quality nutrition decreases the risk of opportunistic infections and promotes vitality. A daily regimen should include sufficient rest and activity. It is important to avoid large crowds, travel to areas with poor sanitation, or exposure to infected individuals. Meticulous skin care is essential, especially during recurrent herpes infections.

The woman will need to know that breastfeeding is contraindicated but that she can provide all other care for her infant. She will almost certainly experience a great deal of anxiety about whether the infant will be HIV positive. Nurses need to respond honestly that testing will be required but that many infants do not get the virus. Moreover, nurses must reinforce information about medication, such as zidovudine, that may slow the progression of the disease and decrease the incidence of vertical transmission.

### CHECK YOUR READING

23. What are the fetal and neonatal effects of cytomegalovirus infection?
24. Why is rubella infection most dangerous in the first trimester?

25. How can rubella be prevented?
26. How are infants born to mothers with varicella treated?
27. How does vertical transmission of the herpes virus occur?
28. What are the fetal and neonatal effects of parvovirus B19 infection?
29. How is hepatitis B virus transmitted? How are newborns treated?
30. How can HIV infection be prevented?
31. What is the medical management for HIV infection?

## Nonviral Infections

### TOXOPLASMOSIS

Toxoplasmosis is a protozoal infection caused by *Toxoplasma gondii.* Infection is transmitted through organisms in raw or undercooked meat, through contact with infected cat feces, or across the placental barrier to the fetus if the expectant mother acquires the infection during pregnancy.

Toxoplasmosis is often subclinical; the woman may experience a few days of fatigue, muscle pains, and swollen glands but may be unaware of the disease. If the infection is suspected, diagnosis can be confirmed by positive serologic test results, which include indirect fluorescent antibody tests for IgG and IgM.

**Fetal and Neonatal Effects.** Although toxoplasmosis may go unnoticed in the pregnant woman, it may cause abortion or result in the birth of a liveborn infant with the disease. About 50 percent of infants born to mothers who were infected during pregnancy acquire congenital toxoplasmosis. Affected infants may be asymptomatic at birth or may have low birth weight, enlarged liver and spleen, jaundice, and anemia. Complications, usually chorioretinitis, or signs of neurologic damage may develop several years later.

**Therapeutic Management.** All pregnant women should be advised to do the following:

- Cook meat thoroughly, particularly pork, beef, and lamb.
- Avoid touching mucous membranes of the mouth or eyes while handling raw meat.
- Wash all kitchen surfaces that come into contact with uncooked meat.
- Wash the hands thoroughly after handling raw meat.
- Avoid uncooked eggs and unpasteurized milk.
- Wash fruits and vegetables before consumption.
- Avoid contact with materials that are possibly contaminated with cat feces (cat litter boxes, sandboxes, or garden soil).

Toxoplasmosis is usually self-limiting, and treatment for mothers is controversial in the United States. Some physicians recommend a combination of pyrimethamine, sulfadiazine, and folinic acid. All authorities agree, however, that this combination should be administered to symptomatic infants with congenital toxoplasmosis (Gibbs & Sweet, 1994). The most serious consequences occur if the disease is contracted during the first 20 weeks of pregnancy, so abortion may be presented as an option for the parents to consider.

### GROUP B STREPTOCOCCUS INFECTION

Group B streptococcus (GBS) is a leading cause of life-threatening perinatal infections in the United States. The gram-positive bacterium colonizes the rectum, vagina, cervix, and urethra of pregnant and non-pregnant women. Approximately 10 to 30 percent of pregnant women are colonized with GBS in the vaginal or rectal area (CDC, 1996). Often, these women are asymptomatic, although symptomatic maternal infections can occur. These infections include urinary tract infection, chorioamnionitis, and endometritis. Most women respond quickly to antimicrobial therapy; however, potentially fatal complications, such as meningitis, fascitis, or intra-abdominal abscess can occur.

**Fetal and Neonatal Effects.** Early-onset GBS disease occurs within 7 days of birth and accounts for approximately 80 percent of all GBS disease in newborns (ACOG, 1996). In these newborns, the mortality rate ranges from 5 to 20 percent (ACOG, 1996, CDC, 1996). Sepsis, pneumonia, or meningitis are the primary infections. Late-onset disease occurs after the first week of life, and meningitis is the most common clinical manifestation. Permanent neurologic consequences may be seen in 15 to 30 percent of those who survive meningeal infections. See Chapter 30 for additional information about manifestations and recommended management of neonatal sepsis.

**Therapeutic Management.** Health care providers have difficulty identifying women who are asymptomatic GBS carriers during pregnancy because the duration of carrier status is unpredictable. Prenatal screening cultures may not identify the woman who will be a GBS carrier at the time of membrane rupture or onset of labor (CDC, 1996). Optimal identification of the GBS carrier depends on culture timing and technique. Cultures should be obtained from the rectum and vagina (not the cervix) between 35 and 37 weeks' gestation, and if GBS is present the woman should be offered intrapartum penicillin to prevent neonatal infection (CDC, 1996).

The Centers for Disease Control and Prevention (1996) also recommends that intrapartum penicillin be administered in specific high-risk situations:

- Previous infant with GBS disease
- The presence of GBS in urine during this pregnancy
- Birth before 37 weeks' gestation

- Maternal fever during labor
- Membranes ruptured 18 or more hours before childbirth

### TUBERCULOSIS

Tuberculosis results from infection by *Mycobacterium tuberculosis*. It is transmitted by aerosolized droplets of liquid containing the bacterium, which are inhaled by a noninfected individual and taken into the lung. Initially, most individuals are asymptomatic. Women obtaining prenatal care should be screened for tuberculosis. This screening involves an intradermal injection of mycobacterial protein (purified protein derivative). If the reaction is positive, the woman's abdomen should be protected by a lead shield while a radiograph is taken of her chest. Diagnosis is confirmed by isolating and identifying the bacterium in the sputum.

Symptomatic patients have general malaise, fatigue, loss of appetite, weight loss, and fever. These symptoms occur in the late afternoon and evening and are accompanied by night sweats. As the disease progresses, a chronic cough develops and a mucopurulent sputum is produced.

Tuberculosis is associated with poverty, malnutrition, and HIV infection. Worldwide, it is responsible for more deaths than any other communicable disease. Moreover, the incidence is increasing in inner city areas and among homeless persons. It is also prevalent among immigrants from Southeast Asia and Central and South America.

**Fetal and Neonatal Effects.** Although perinatal infection is rare, it may be acquired as a result of the fetus swallowing infected amniotic fluid. Diagnosis is made by finding the bacilli in gastric aspirate of the neonate or in placental tissue. Signs of congenital tuberculosis include failure to thrive, lethargy, respiratory distress, fever, and enlargement of the spleen, liver, and lymph nodes. If the mother remains untreated, the newborn is at high risk for acquiring tuberculosis by inhalation of infectious respiratory droplets from the mother.

**Therapeutic Management.** Treatment of tuberculosis is based on two principles. First, more than one drug must be used to prevent growth of resistant organisms. Second, treatment must continue for a prolonged period of time. The preferred treatment for pregnant women is isoniazid plus rifampin every day for a total of 9 months. Ethambutol is added initially if drug resistance is suspected (Weinberger & Weiss, 1995). Pyridoxine (vitamin $B_6$) is often administered with isoniazid to prevent fetal neurotoxicity.

Management of the infant born to a mother with tuberculosis involves preventing the disease or treating early infection. Prevention focuses on teaching family members how the disease is transmitted so they can protect the infant from airborne organisms. The infant should be skin tested at birth and may be started on preventive isoniazid therapy. Skin testing should be repeated at 3 months, and isoniazid may be stopped if the skin test result remains negative. If the skin test result converts to positive, a full course of isoniazid should be given.

**CHECK YOUR READING**

32. How can toxoplasmosis be prevented?
33. What are the risk factors for colonization of the newborn with GBS during the intrapartum period? How is colonization prevented?
34. How is tuberculosis treated in the mother? How is it diagnosed and treated in the newborn?

## Application of Nursing Process: The Pregnant Woman with Tuberculosis

### Assessment

Question each pregnant woman about signs or symptoms of tuberculosis. These include fever, night sweats, fatigue, weight loss, and cough. Ask if the cough is productive and if the sputum is purulent. Administer and read a purified protein derivative skin test as directed. Examine factors that increase the risk of tuberculosis, such as poverty, homelessness, recent immigration from an area that has a high incidence of tuberculosis, and HIV infection. Determine whether a family member or close friend has a history of tuberculosis.

If a woman has tuberculosis, determine how much knowledge she has about the disease. For example, does she know how the disease is transmitted, how important it is to complete the prescribed course of medications, and major side effects of medications?

### Analysis

The woman with tuberculosis must adhere to a prolonged treatment regimen that has significant side effects. The most relevant nursing diagnosis for this woman might be Ineffective Individual Management of Therapeutic Regimen related to lack of knowledge of disease process and expected course of treatment.

### Planning

Outcome statements for this nursing diagnosis are that the woman will do the following:

- Verbalize information about the mode of transmission of tuberculosis, the importance of medications, and possible side effects of antituberculosis medications.

- Adhere to the treatment plan as directed by the physician.

## Interventions

**PROVIDING INFORMATION**

1. Teach how tuberculosis is transmitted to decrease the chance of transmission:
   - Isolating infants from infected persons is essential.
   - Covering the mouth when coughing, sneezing, or laughing helps prevent bacteria from entering the air.
   - Washing the hands carefully after any contact with body substances or soiled tissues decreases exposure of others.
2. Furnish reassuring information about pregnancy and tuberculosis:
   - Tuberculosis does not usually affect the type of delivery (forceps, vaginal, or cesarean) or the birth weight of newborns.
   - Congenital tuberculosis of the newborn is rare.
   - There are no adverse fetal effects to skin testing.
   - Antituberculosis medications are in pregnancy risk category C (see Appendix C).
   - Tuberculosis may be cured or arrested if medication is taken as prescribed.
3. Instruct about correct administration of medications:
   - Take medication at the same time each day.
   - Take medication on an empty stomach (1 hour before or 2 hours after a meal).
   - Do not skip medications or double up on missed doses.
   - Avoid the use of alcohol, which increases the risk of liver toxicity.
   - Avoid antacids containing aluminum because they impair absorption of isoniazid and rifampin.
4. Educate about expected or potential side effects:
   - Oral contraceptives are less effective when a woman is taking rifampin.
   - Body fluids, such as urine or saliva, may become a characteristic red-orange when taking rifampin.
   - Nausea, heartburn, diarrhea, and flatulence are fairly common side effects. Rifampin may cause drowsiness.
   - Symptoms of hepatitis (jaundice, anorexia, excessive fatigue) should be reported to the physician.
5. Teach the necessity of continuing medication although symptoms have disappeared.
6. Emphasize the importance of keeping follow-up appointments.

**PROVIDING SUPPORT**

Respiratory isolation may be necessary, and a new mother may be separated from her newborn. The nursing staff must provide emotional support and counseling so the mother can deal with the anxiety and frustration she may feel at not being allowed to care for the infant. Language barriers and cultural implications should also be addressed. A referral to social services may be needed to arrange temporary care of the newborn outside the home until the infant and mother have received adequate treatment.

## Evaluation

Goals or outcomes are met if the mother does the following:

- Demonstrates knowledge of the mode of transmission.
- Verbalizes the importance of taking medications as prescribed.
- Adheres to the treatment regimen as directed.

## SUMMARY CONCEPTS

- During early pregnancy, the release of insulin accelerates, which may result in episodes of hypoglycemia. Moreover, the availability of glucose and insulin favors the development and storage of fat that the mother will need later.
- Placental hormones, which reach their peak during the second and third trimesters, create resistance to insulin in maternal cells and precipitate changes in insulin needs throughout pregnancy.
- Diabetes is classified according to onset and to whether the woman requires the administration of insulin to prevent ketoacidosis.
- Type I diabetes mellitus adversely affects the mother in a variety of ways. The risk of pregnancy-induced hypertension, urinary tract infections, and ketosis are examples.
- Because maternal hyperglycemia during the first trimester increases the risk for congenital anomalies in the fetus, a major goal of management is to establish normal blood glucose levels before pregnancy occurs.
- Fetal growth depends on the condition of maternal blood vessels; if there is no vascular impairment, placental perfusion is adequate and the infant is likely to be large (macrosomia). If there is vascular impairment, placental perfusion may be compromised and the fetus may experience IUGR.
- In addition to congenital anomalies, the infant of a diabetic mother is at increased risk for hypoglycemia, hypocalcemia, hyperbilirubinemia, and respiratory distress syndrome.

- Maternal effects of gestational diabetes include increased risks for urinary tract infections, hydramnios, premature rupture of membranes, and the development of pregnancy-induced hypertension.
- Gestational diabetes is responsible for two major complications for the fetus or neonate: fetal macrosomia and neonatal hypoglycemia.
- Gestational diabetes can usually be treated by diet and exercise; however, insulin may be administered if blood glucose remains high.
- Cardiovascular changes that occur in normal pregnancy impose an additional burden that may result in cardiac decompensation if the expectant mother has preexisting heart disease.
- The primary goal of management of the pregnant woman with heart disease is to prevent the development of congestive heart failure by restricting activity, limiting weight gain, and preventing anemia and infection, so that cardiac demand does not exceed cardiac reserves.
- Intrapartum and postpartum management of heart disease focuses on preventing fluid overload, which can cause a sharp rise in cardiac effort.
- Iron supplementation is necessary during pregnancy because most women do not have sufficient iron stores to meet the demands of pregnancy.
- Folic acid deficiency is associated with increased risk of spontaneous abortion, abruptio placentae, and fetal anomalies, such as neural tube defects. A folic acid supplement may be necessary to prevent maternal and fetal effects.
- Sickle cell anemia is exacerbated by pregnancy, and a primary goal is to prevent sickle cell crisis during pregnancy.
- Laboratory values for thalassemia are similar to those of iron deficiency; however, administration of iron is risky because increased iron absorption and storage makes the woman susceptible to iron overload.
- Although women with SLE can have a normal pregnancy and give birth to a normal newborn, the pregnancy must be treated as high risk because of the increased incidence of abortion, fetal death during the first trimester, and possible exacerbation of the disease.
- Antiphospholipid syndrome (an autoimmune disorder) is a cluster of clinical entities that includes increased risk for thrombosis, fetal loss, and the presence of antiphospholipid antibodies.
- There is often marked improvement in rheumatoid arthritis during pregnancy, possibly as a result of pregnancy-specific hormone and hormonal factors. However, most women relapse soon after childbirth.
- Management of epilepsy is complicated because of the teratogenic effects of anticonvulsant medications.
- Although Bell's palsy is usually temporary, the woman experiences anxiety. Supportive care and emotional support are essential.
- Automobile accidents are the major cause of blunt force trauma that may result in premature separation of the placenta, hemorrhage, fractures, and internal injuries. Penetrating injuries caused by knife or gunshot wounds are particularly dangerous for the fetus.
- Treatment of trauma during pregnancy is similar to that in a non-pregnant state. Cardiopulmonary resuscitation and controlling bleeding are the priorities. Evaluation of the mother for internal injuries may necessitate surgical exploration. Careful evaluation of the uterus and fetus are also essential.
- Viral infections that occur during pregnancy can be transmitted to the fetus in two ways: across the placental barrier or by exposure to organisms during birth. Although they are mild or even subclinical in the mother, viral infections can have serious effects for the fetus.
- The health care team is responsible for teaching how infectious diseases can be prevented and that early treatment may also reduce fetal and neonatal exposure to infections.
- Human immunodeficiency virus is a retrovirus that invades the CD4 subset of lymphocytes and destroys them, producing AIDS, which allows opportunistic infections to overwhelm the immune system.
- Pregnant women who are HIV-positive or who are at risk for HIV-positive status experience anxiety, fear, and grief as they contemplate the losses they will experience as a result of the disease. Nurses must provide emotional support, information, and counseling, which will help the woman cope with her emotions and retain control of her care for as long as possible.
- Nonviral infections such as toxoplasmosis, GBS infection, and tuberculosis can be prevented or treated.

### References and Readings


American College of Obstetricians and Gynecologists. (1991). *Fetal macrosomia*. ACOG Technical Bulletin No. 159. Washington, D.C.: Author.

American College of Obstetricians and Gynecologists. (1994). *Diabetes and pregnancy*. ACOG Technical Bulletin No. 200. Washington, D.C.: Author.

American College of Obstetricians and Gynecologists. (1996). *Committee Opinion: Prevention of early-onset group B streptococcal disease in newborns* (pp. 173). Washington, D.C.: Author.

American Diabetes Association. (1993). Position statement: Gestational diabetes. *Diabetes Care*, Suppl. 2, 5.

Aminoff, M.J. (1994). Neurologic disorders. In R.K. Creasy & R. Resnik (Eds.), *Maternal-fetal medicine: Principles and practice* (3rd ed., pp. 1071–1100). Philadelphia: W.B. Saunders.

Artal, P. (1996). Exercise: An alternative therapy for gestational diabetes. *The Physician and Sports Medicine*, 24(3), 54–66.

Bevier, W.C., Jovanovic-Peterson, L., & Peterson, C.M. (1995). Pancreatic disorders of pregnancy: Diagnosis, management, and outcome of gestational diabetes. *Endocrinology and Metabolism Clinics of North America*, 24(1), 103–138.

Blackburn, S.T., & Loper, D.L. (1992). *Maternal, fetal, and neonatal physiology*. Philadelphia: W.B. Saunders.

Boden, G. (1996). Fuel metabolism in pregnancy and in gestational diabetes mellitus. *Obstetrics and Gynecology Clinics of North America*, 23(1), 1–10.

Buchanan, T.A., & Coustan, D.R. (1995). Diabetes mellitus. In G.N. Burrow & T.F. Ferris (Eds.). *Medical complications during pregnancy* (4th ed., pp. 29–61). Philadelphia: W.B. Saunders.

Centers for Disease Control and Prevention. (1993). Sexually transmitted diseases treatment guidelines. *Morbidity and Mortality Weekly Report* 42 (RR-14), 1–73.

Centers for Disease Control and Prevention. (1996). Recommendations of the U.S. Public Health Service Task Force on the use of zidovudine to reduce perinatal transmission of human immunodeficiency virus. *Morbidity and Mortality Weekly Report* 43(No. RR-11), 81–84.

Centers for Disease Control and Prevention. (1996). Prevention of perinatal group B streptococcal disease: A public health prospective. *Morbidity and Mortality Weekly Report* 45(No. RR-7), 1–24.

Chin, J. (1994). The growing impact of the HIV/AIDS pandemic on children born to HIV-infected women. *Clinics in Perinatology*, 21(1), 1–14.

Collins, T.M., Saltzman, R.L., & Jordan, M.C. (1995). Viral infections. In G.N. Burrow & T.F. Ferris (Eds.), *Medical complications during pregnancy* (4th ed., pp. 381–403). Philadelphia: W.B. Saunders.

Coustan, D.R. (1996). Screening and testing for gestational diabetes mellitus. *Obstetrics and Gynecology Clinics of North America*, 23(1), 125–136.

Cunningham, F.G., MacDonald, P.C., Gant, N.F., Levend, K.J., Gilstrap, L.C., Hankins, G.D.V., et al. (1997). *Williams obstetrics* (20th ed.). Norwalk, Conn: Appleton & Lange.

de Swiet, M. (1994). Rheumatologic and connective tissue disorders. In R.K. Creasy & R. Resnik (Eds.), *Maternal-newborn medicine: Principles and practice* (3rd ed., pp. 1062–1070). Philadelphia: W.B. Saunders.

Dinsmoor, M.J. (1994). HIV infection and pregnancy. *Clinics in Perinatology*, 21(1), 85–95.

Doshier, S. (1995). What happens to the offspring of diabetic pregnancies? *American Journal of Maternal-Child Nursing*, 20(1), 25–28.

Duffy, T.P. (1995). Hematologic aspects of pregnancy. In G.N. Burrow & T.F. Ferris (Eds.), *Medical complications during pregnancy* (4th ed., pp. 62–82). Philadelphia: W.B. Saunders.

Finch, C.M. (1995). Human parvovirus B19 in pregnancy. *Journal of Obstetric, Gynecologic, and Neonatal Nursing*, 24(6), 495–498.

Freeman, S.B. (1995). Common genitourinary infections. *Journal of Obstetric, Gynecologic, and Neonatal Nursing*, 24(8), 735–741.

Frenkel, L.D., & Gaur, S. (1994). Perinatal HIV infection and AIDS. *Clinics in Perinatology*, 21(1), 95–108.

Gabbe, S.G., & Landon, M.B. (1994). Diabetes mellitus in pregnancy. In F.P. Zuspan & E.J. Quilligan (Eds.), *Current therapies in Obstetrics and gynecology* (4th ed., pp. 235–241). Philadelphia: W.B. Saunders.

Gibbs, R.S., & Sweet, R.L. (1994). Clinical disorders. In R.K. Creasy & R. Resnik (Eds.), *Maternal-fetal medicine* (3rd ed., pp. 639–703). Philadelphia: W.B. Saunders.

Gladman, D.D., & Urowitz, M.B. (1995). Rheumatic disease in pregnancy. In G.N. Burrow & T.F. Ferris (Eds.), *Medical complications during pregnancy* (4th ed., pp. 501–529). Philadelphia: W.B. Saunders.

Gonik, B. (1994). Intensive care monitoring of the critically ill pregnant patient. In R.K. Creasy & R. Resnik (Eds.), *Maternal-fetal medicine: Principles and practice* (3rd ed., pp. 865–890). Philadelphia: W.B. Saunders.

Graves, C.R., & Boehm, F.H. (1994). Diabetes mellitus. *Infertility and Reproductive Medicine Clinics of North America*, 5(4), 671–684.

Healy, K., Jovanovic-Peterson, L., & Peterson, C.M. (1995). Pancreatic disorders of pregnancy. *Endocrinology and Metabolism Clinics of North America*, 24(1), 73–101.

Homko, C.J., & Khandelwal, M. (1996). Glucose monitoring and insulin therapy during pregnancy. *Obstetrics and Gynecology Clinics of North America*, 23(1), 47–74.

Kuper, B.C., & Failla, S. (1994). Shedding new light on lupus. *American Journal of Nursing*, 94(10), 26–32.

Landon, M.B., & Gabbe, S.G. (1994). Controversies in gestational diabetes. *Infertility and Reproductive Medicine Clinics of North America*, 5(4), 685–697.

Landon, M.B., & Gabbe, S.G. (1996). Fetal surveillance and timing of delivery in pregnancy complicated by diabetes mellitus. *Obstetrics and Gynecology Clinics of North America*, 23(1), 109–124.

Langer, O., & Hod, M. (1996). Management of gestational diabetes mellitus. *Obstetrics and Gynecology Clinics of North America*, 23(1), 137–160.

Laros, R.K. (1994). Maternal hematologic disorders. In R.K. Creasy & R. Resnik (Eds.), *Maternal-fetal medicine: Principles and practice* (3rd ed., pp. 905–933). Philadelphia: W.B. Saunders.

Larrabee, K., & Cowan, M. (1995). Clinical nursing management of sickle cell disease and trait during pregnancy. *Journal of Perinatal Neonatal Nursing*, 9(2), 29–41.

Lee, R.V. (1995). Sexually transmitted infections. In G.N. Borrow & T.F. Ferris (Eds.), *Medical complications during pregnancy* (4th ed., pp. 404–438). Philadelphia: W.B. Saunders.

Lewis, R., O'Brien, J. M., Ray, D.T., & Sibai, B.M. (1995). The impact of initiating a human immunodeficiency virus screening program in an urban obstetric population. *American Journal of Obstetrics and Gynecology*, 173(4), 1329–1333.

Lindberg, C.E. (1995). Perinatal transmission of HIV: How to counsel women. *American Journal of Maternal Child Nursing*, 20(4), 207–212.

Martens, K.A. (1994). Sexually transmitted and genital tract infections during pregnancy. *Emergency Medicine Clinics of North America*, 12(1), 91–113.

McAnulty, J.H., Metcalfe, J., & Ueland, K. (1995). Cardiovascular disease. In G.N. Burrow & T.F. Ferris (Eds.), *Medical complications during pregnancy* (4th ed., pp. 123–154). Philadelphia: W.B. Saunders.

Mercer, B.M., Ramsey, R.D., & Sibai, B.M. (1995). Prenatal screening for group B streptococcus. *American Journal of Obstetrics and Gynecology*, 173(3, Pt. 1), 842–846.

Minkoff, H.L. (1994). Human immunodeficiency virus. In R.K. Creasy & R. Resnik (Eds.), *Maternal-fetal medicine: Principles and practice* (3rd ed., pp. 704–710). Philadelphia: W.B. Saunders.

Monga, M. & Creasy, R.K. (1994). Cardiovascular and renal adaptation to pregnancy. In R.K. Creasy & R. Resnik (Eds.), *Maternal-fetal medicine: Principles and practice*. (3rd ed., pp 758–767). Philadelphia: W.B. Saunders.

Montgomery, K.S. (1996). Caring for the pregnant woman with sickle cell disease. *American Journal of Maternal-Child Nursing*, 21(5), 224–228.

Moore, T.R. (1994). Diabetes and pregnancy. In R.K. Creasy & R. Resnik (Eds.). *Maternal-fetal medicine: Principles and practice* (3rd ed., pp. 934–978). Philadelphia: W.B. Saunders.

Munro, C.L. (1995). The impact of recent advances in microbiology and immunology on perinatal and women's health care. *Journal of Obstetric, Gynecologic, and Neonatal Nursing*, 24(6), 525–531.

National Institute of Diabetes and Digestive and Kidney Diseases. (1994). *Insulin dependent diabetes.* NIH Publication No. 95-2098. Washington, D.C.: Author.

Nuwayhid, B., & Khalife, S. (1992). Medical complications of pregnancy. In N.F. Hacker & J.G. Moore (Eds.), *Essentials of obstetrics and gynecology* (2nd ed., pp. 197–222). Philadelphia: W.B. Saunders.

Reece, E.A. (1996). Preface. *Obstetrics and Gynecology Clinics of North America,* 23(1), xi–xii.

Reece, E.A., & Eriksson, U.J. (1996). The pathogenesis of diabetes-associated congenital malformations. *Obstetrics and Gynecology Clinics of North America,* 23(1), 29–46.

Reece, E.A., Homko, C.J., & Hagay, Z. (1996). Prenatal diagnosis and prevention of diabetic embryopathy. *Obstetrics and Gynecology Clinics of North America,* 23(1), 11–28.

Rotondo, L., & Coustan, D.R. (1993). Diabetes mellitus in pregnancy. In R.A. Knuppel & J.E. Drukker (Eds.), *High-risk pregnancy: A team approach* (2nd ed., pp. 518–538). Philadelphia: W.B. Saunders.

Rouse, D.J., Gardner, M., Allen, S.J., & Goldenberg, R.L. (1996). Management of presumed susceptible varicella (chicken pox)-exposed gravida: A cost-effectiveness/cost-benefit analysis. *Obstetrics and Gynecology,* 87(6), 932–936.

Shabetai, R. (1994). Cardiac diseases. In R.K. Creasy & R. Resnik (Eds.), *Maternal-fetal medicine: Principles and practice.* (3rd ed., pp. 768–791). Philadelphia: W.B. Saunders.

Shermer, R.H. (1995). Group B streptococcus during the perinatal period. *Journal of Obstetric, Gynecologic, and Neonatal Nursing,* 24(6), 562–566.

Simpkins, S.M., Hench, C.P., & Bhatia, G. (1996). Management of the obstetric patient with tuberculosis. *Journal of Obstetric, Gynecologic, and Neonatal Nursing,* 25(4), 305–312.

Tyrala, E.E. (1996). The infant of the diabetic mother. *Obstetrics and Gynecology Clinics of North America,* 23(1), 221–241.

Weinberger, S.E., & Weiss, S.T. (1995). Pulmonary disease. In G.N. Burrow & T.F. Ferris (Eds.), *Medical complications during pregnancy* (4th ed., pp. 439–483). Philadelphia: W.B. Saunders.

Youngkin, E.Q. (1995). Sexually transmitted diseases: Current and emerging concerns. *Journal of Obstetric, Gynecologic, and Neonatal Nursing,* 24(8), 743–758.

# 27

# Intrapartum Complications

## OBJECTIVES

1. Explain abnormalities that may result in dysfunctional labor.
2. Describe maternal and fetal risks associated with premature rupture of the membranes.
3. Analyze factors that increase a woman's risk for preterm labor.
4. Explain maternal and fetal problems that may occur if pregnancy persists beyond 42 weeks.
5. Describe common intrapartum emergencies.
6. Explain therapeutic management of each intrapartum complication.
7. Apply the nursing process to care of women with intrapartum complications and to their families.

## DEFINITIONS

**abruptio placentae** *Premature separation of a normally implanted placenta.*

**amniotic fluid embolism** *An embolism in which amniotic fluid with its particulate matter is drawn into the pregnant woman's circulation, lodging in her lungs.*

**cephalopelvic disproportion (CPD).** *Fetal head size that is too large to fit through the maternal pelvis at birth. Also called fetopelvic disproportion.*

**chorioamnionitis** *Inflammation of the amniotic sac (fetal membranes); usually caused by bacterial or viral infection. Also called amnionitis.*

**dystocia** *Difficult or prolonged labor; often associated with abnormal uterine activity and cephalopelvic disproportion.*

**hydramnios** *Excessive volume of amniotic fluid (more than 2000 ml at term). Also called polyhydramnios.*

**hypertonic labor dysfunction** *Ineffective labor characterized by erratic and poorly coordinated contractions. Uterine resting tone is higher than normal.*

**hypotonic labor dysfunction** *Ineffective labor characterized by weak, infrequent, and brief but coordinated uterine contractions. Uterine resting tone is normal.*

**macrosomia** *Unusually large fetal size; infant birth weight more than 4000 g.*

**multifetal pregnancy** *A pregnancy in which the woman is carrying two or more fetuses. Also called multiple gestation.*

**occult prolapse** *See Prolapsed cord.*

**oligohydramnios** *Abnormally small volume of amniotic fluid (less than 500 ml at term).*

**placenta accreta** *A placenta that is abnormally adherent to the uterine muscle. If the condition is more advanced, it is called placenta increta (the placenta extends into the uterine muscle) or placenta percreta (the placenta extends through the uterine muscle).*

**placenta previa** *Abnormal implantation of the placenta in the lower uterus, at or very near the cervical os.*

**precipitate birth** *A birth that occurs without a trained attendant present.*

**precipitate labor** *An intense, unusually short labor (less than 3 hours).*

**preterm labor** *Onset of labor after 20 weeks and before the beginning of the 38th week of gestation.*

**prolapsed cord** *Displacement of the umbilical cord in front of or beside the fetal presenting part. An occult prolapse is one that is suspected on the basis of fetal heart rate patterns; the umbilical cord cannot be palpated or seen.*

**shoulder dystocia** *Delayed or difficult birth of the fetal shoulders after the head is born.*

**tocolytic** *A drug that inhibits uterine contractions.*

**uterine inversion** *Turning of the uterus inside out after birth of the fetus.*

**uterine resting tone** *Degree of uterine muscle tension when the woman is not in labor or during the interval between labor contactions.*

**uterine rupture** *A tear in the wall of the uterus.*

For most women, birth is a normal process free of major complications. However, complications sometimes make childbearing hazardous for the woman or her baby. The nurse's challenge is to identify the complications promptly and to provide effective care for these mothers while nurturing the entire family at this significant time in their life.

The complications addressed in this chapter are often interrelated. For example, a dysfunctional labor is likely to be prolonged, and the woman is more vulnerable to infection and psychological distress. Also, women who have complications are more likely to need interventions such as cesarean birth. The nurse should provide nursing care that relates to all problems experienced by the woman.

## Dysfunctional Labor

Normal labor is characterized by progress. Dysfunctional labor is one that does not result in normal progress of cervical effacement, dilation, and fetal descent. *Dystocia* is a general term that describes any difficult labor or birth. A dysfunctional labor may result from problems with the powers of labor, the passenger, the passage, the psyche, or a combination of these. Dysfunctional labor is often prolonged but may be unusually short and intense.

An operative birth (vacuum extractor– or forceps-assisted or cesarean) may be needed if dysfunctional labor does not resolve or if fetal or maternal compromise occurs. These signs include persistent nonreassuring fetal heart rate (FHR) patterns (see p. 356), fetal acidosis, and meconium passage. Maternal exhaustion or infection may occur, especially with long labors. However, nursing measures that enhance progress and maternal comfort and promote fetal well-being are discussed in this chapter.

### Problems of the Powers

The powers of labor may not be adequate to expel the fetus because of ineffective contractions or ineffective maternal pushing efforts.

#### INEFFECTIVE CONTRACTIONS

Effective uterine activity is characterized by coordinated contractions that are strong and numerous enough to propel the fetus past the resistance of the woman's bony pelvis and soft tissues. It is not possible to say how frequent, long, or strong labor contractions must be. One woman's labor may progress with contractions that would be inadequate for another woman. Possible causes of ineffective contractions include the following:

- Maternal fatigue
- Maternal inactivity
- Fluid and electrolyte imbalance
- Hypoglycemia
- Excessive analgesia or anesthesia
- Maternal catecholamines secreted in response to stress or pain
- Disproportion between the maternal pelvis and the fetal presenting part
- Uterine overdistention, such as with multiple gestation or hydramnios

Two patterns of ineffective uterine contractions are hypotonic and hypertonic dysfunction. Hypotonic dysfunction is more common than hypertonic. Characteristics and management of each are different, but the result—poor labor progress—is the same if they persist (Table 27–1).

**Hypotonic Dysfunction.** Hypotonic contractions are coordinated but are too weak to be effective. They are infrequent and brief and can be easily indented with fingertip pressure at the peak.

Hypotonic dysfunction usually occurs during the active phase of labor, when progress normally quickens. This is usually when the woman has reached at least 4 cm of cervical dilation. Uterine overdistention is associated with hypotonic dysfunction because the stretched uterine muscle contracts poorly.

The woman may be fairly comfortable because her contractions are weak. However, she is often frustrated because labor slows down at a time when she expects quicker progress. Persistent hypotonic dysfunction is fatiguing for the mother. Fetal hypoxia is not usually seen with hypotonic labor.

**TABLE 27–1 PATTERNS OF LABOR DYSFUNCTION**

| Hypotonic Dysfunction | Hypertonic Dysfunction |
|---|---|
| **Contractions** | |
| Coordinated, but weak<br>Become less frequent and shorter in duration<br>Easily indented at peak<br>Woman may have minimal discomfort because the contractions are weak. | Uncoordinated, irregular<br>Short and poor intensity, but painful and cramp-like |
| **Uterine Resting Tone** | |
| Not elevated | Higher than normal. Important to distinguish from abruptio placentae, which has similar characteristics (p. 684). |
| **Phase of Labor** | |
| Active. Typically occurs after 4 cm dilation<br>More common than hypertonic dysfunction | Latent. Usually occurs before 4 cm dilation<br>Less common than hypotonic dysfunction |
| **Therapeutic Management** | |
| Amniotomy (may increase the risk of infection)<br>Oxytocin augmentation<br>Cesarean birth if no progress | Correct cause if it can be identified.<br>Sedation<br>Hydration<br>Tocolytics to reduce high uterine tone and promote placental perfusion |
| **Nursing Care** | |
| Interventions related to amniotomy and oxytocin augmentation<br>Encourage position changes. An abdominal binder may help direct the fetus toward the mother's pelvis if her abdominal wall is very lax.<br>Ambulation if no contraindication and if acceptable to the woman<br>Emotional support: Allow her to ventilate feelings of discouragement. Explain measures taken to increase effectiveness of contractions. Include her partner/family in emotional support measures as they may have anxiety that will heighten the woman's anxiety. | Promote uterine blood flow: side-lying position<br>Promote rest, general comfort, and relaxation<br>Pain relief<br>Emotional support: Accept the reality of the woman's pain and frustration.<br>Reassure her that she is not being childish. Explain reason for measures to break abnormal labor patterns and their expected results. Allow her to ventilate her feelings during and after labor. Include partner/family (see hypotonic labor). |

Management depends on the cause. Many women respond to simple measures. Providing intravenous or oral fluids corrects maternal fluid and electrolyte imbalances or hypoglycemia. Maternal position changes, particularly upright positions, favor fetal descent and promote effective contractions. The woman who moves about actively typically has better labor progress and is more comfortable than one who remains in one position.

The nurse should use therapeutic communication to help the woman identify anxieties or beliefs about labor and its progress. Helping her to get her anxieties in the open is the first step to managing them effectively so that the stress response does not slow her labor. For example, the nurse might ask, "What do you think is making your labor slow?"

Some women need measures such as amniotomy or oxytocin infusion to promote labor progress. The birth attendant evaluates the woman's labor to confirm that she is having hypotonic active labor rather than a long latent phase of labor. The latent phase of labor occurs within the first 3 cm of cervical dilation. The maternal pelvis and fetal presentation and position are assessed to identify abnormalities.

Amniotomy or oxytocin augmentation may be used to stimulate a labor that slows after it is established. The risks of amniotomy are umbilical cord prolapse, infection, and abruptio placentae. Reduced placental perfusion due to excessive uterine contractions is the most common risk of oxytocin labor augmentation.

**Hypertonic Dysfunction.** Hypertonic dysfunction of labor is less common than hypotonic. Contractions are uncoordinated and are erratic in their frequency, duration, and intensity. The contractions are painful but ineffective. Hypertonic dysfunction usually occurs during the latent phase of labor.

Although each contraction varies in its intensity, the uterine resting tone between contractions is high, reducing uterine blood flow. This ischemia decreases fetal oxygen supply and causes the woman to have almost constant cramping pain. Because high resting tone and constant pain are also seen in abruptio placentae, this complication should be considered as well.

The mother becomes very tired because of nearly constant discomfort. She may lose confidence in her ability to give birth and to cope with labor. She often thinks, "If it hurts this much so early, I must be a real baby." Frustration and anxiety further reduce her pain tolerance and interfere with the normal processes of labor. The nurse should accept her frustration and discomfort. It is important not to equate cervical dilation with the amount of pain a woman "should" experience.

Management of hypertonic labor depends on the cause. Relief of pain is the primary intervention to promote a normal labor pattern. Warm showers or baths promote relaxation and rest, often allowing a normal labor pattern to ensue. Systemic analgesics or occasionally epidural analgesia may be required to achieve this purpose.

Oxytocin is not usually given because it can intensify the already high uterine resting tone. However, very low doses of oxytocin are sometimes given to promote coordinated uterine contractions. Tocolytic drugs may be ordered to reduce uterine resting tone and improve placental blood flow.

#### INEFFECTIVE MATERNAL PUSHING

A reflex urge to push with contractions usually occurs as the fetal presenting part reaches the pelvic floor during second-stage labor. However, ineffective pushing may result from the following:

- Use of incorrect pushing techniques or inappropriate pushing positions
- Fear of injury because of pain and tearing sensations felt by the mother when she pushes
- Decreased or absent urge to push
- Maternal exhaustion
- Analgesia or anesthesia that suppresses the woman's urge to push
- Psychological unreadiness to "let go" of her baby

Management focuses on correcting causes contributing to ineffective pushing. If maternal and fetal vital signs are normal, there is no maximum allowable duration for the second stage. Each woman is evaluated individually by her birth attendant to determine whether labor should be ended with an operative delivery or can continue safely. For most women, this occurs after about 2 to 3 hours of *vigorous* pushing efforts that do not result in fetal descent to the pelvic floor.

Nursing care to promote effective pushing helps the mother make each effort more productive. Upright positions such as squatting add the force of gravity to her efforts. Semi-sitting, side-lying, and pushing while sitting on the toilet are other options (see Chapter 13).

The woman who fears injury because of the sensations she feels when she pushes may respond to accurate information about the process of fetal descent. If she understands that sensations of tearing often accompany fetal descent but that her tissues can expand to accommodate the baby, she may be more willing to push with contractions. Warm perineal compresses and massage increase perineal distensibility and reduce the chance of tearing.

A reduced urge to push may occur when epidural block analgesia is given. Most epidural blocks for labor use a mixture of a local anesthetic agent (one of the *-caine* drugs) and an epidural opioid analgesic to provide pain control without the major loss of sensation that is likely if local anesthetic is used alone. However, if a woman cannot feel the urge to push or cannot feel it strongly, she can be coached to push as each contraction begins.

The woman who is exhausted may push more effectively if she is encouraged to rest and to push only when she feels the urge, or she may push with every other contraction. Giving oral or intravenous fluids, as ordered, provides energy for the strenuous work of second-stage labor. Reassuring her about fetal well-being and the fact that she has no deadline to meet helps her work with her body's efforts most effectively. This reassurance also helps the woman who may be emotionally readying herself to "let go" of her fetus in exchange for a newborn as she labors.

### Problems with the Passenger

Fetal problems associated with dysfunctional labor are those related to the following:

- Fetal size
- Fetal presentation or position
- Multifetal pregnancy
- Fetal anomalies

These variations may cause mechanical problems and contribute to ineffective contractions.

#### FETAL SIZE

**Macrosomia.** The macrosomic infant weighs more than 4000 g (8.8 pounds) at birth. The head may be so large that it cannot mold enough to adapt to the pelvis. Even if the head makes it through the pelvis, the shoulders may be too large to pass. In addition, distention of the uterus by the large fetus reduces the strength of contractions both during and after birth.

Size is relative, however. The woman with a small pelvis or one that is abnormally shaped may not be able to deliver an average-sized or small infant. The woman with a large pelvis may easily give birth to an infant heavier than 4000 g.

**Shoulder Dystocia.** Delayed or difficult birth of the shoulders may occur as they become impacted above the maternal symphysis pubis. As soon as the head is born, it retracts against the perineum, much like a turtle's head drawing into its shell ("turtle sign"). Shoulder dystocia is more likely with a large fetus or with a maternal pelvis that is small relative to fetal size.

Shoulder dystocia is an urgent situation because the umbilical cord is easily compressed between the fetal body and the maternal pelvis. Although the infant's head is out of the vaginal canal, the chest is compressed, preventing respirations. Any of several methods may be used to quickly relieve the impacted fetal shoulders (Fig. 27–1). The infant's clavi-

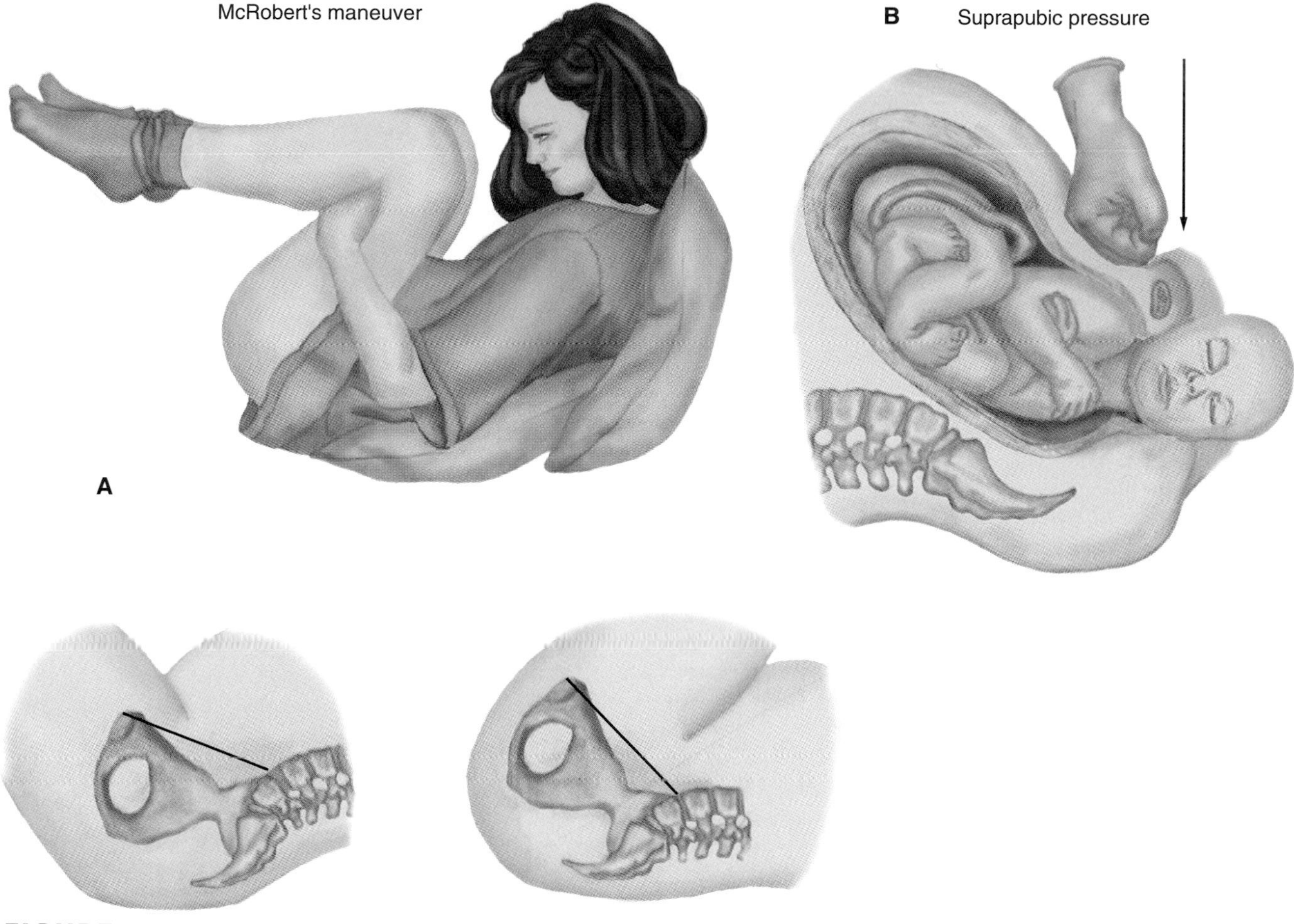


**FIGURE 27–1**

Methods that may be used to relieve shoulder dystocia. A, McRobert's maneuver. The woman flexes her thighs sharply against her abdomen, which straightens the pelvic curve somewhat. A supported squat has a similar effect and adds gravity to her pushing efforts. B, Suprapubic pressure by an assistant pushes the fetal anterior shoulder downward to displace it from above the mother's symphysis pubis. Fundal pressure should not be used, as it will push the anterior shoulder even more firmly against the mother's symphysis.

cles should be checked for crepitus, deformity, or bruising, each of which suggests fracture.

### ABNORMAL FETAL PRESENTATION OR POSITION

An unfavorable fetal presentation or position may interfere with cervical dilation or fetal descent.

**Rotation Abnormalities.** Persistence of the fetus in the occiput posterior (OP) or occiput transverse (OT) position can contribute to dysfunctional labor. These positions prevent the mechanisms of labor (cardinal movements) from occurring normally. Most fetuses that begin labor in an occiput posterior position rotate spontaneously to an occiput anterior position, promoting normal extension and expulsion of the head. The fetus may not rotate, or it may partly rotate and remain in an occiput transverse position. Although many women cannot readily deliver their fetus in the occiput posterior position, the woman with a large pelvis compared with the fetal size may be able to do so.

Labor is usually longer and more uncomfortable when the fetus remains in the occiput posterior or occiput transverse position. Intense back or leg pain that is poorly relieved with analgesia makes it difficult for the woman to cope with labor. "Back labor" aptly describes the sensations a woman feels when her fetus is in an occiput posterior position.

Maternal position changes promote fetal head rotation to an occiput anterior position and descent (see Fig. 13–4, p. 322). Examples are as follows:

- Hands and knees. Rocking the pelvis back and forth while on hands and knees encourages rotation.
- Side-lying (on her left side if the fetus is in a right occiput posterior position and on her right side for a left occiput posterior position)
- The lunge (Simkin, 1995), in which the mother places one foot on a chair with her foot and knee pointed to that side. She lunges sideways repeatedly during a contraction for 5 seconds at a time.

## CRITICAL THINKING EXERCISE

A woman having her first baby has been in labor for several hours. Her nurse-midwife performs a vaginal examination and says that the cervix is 6 cm dilated and completely effaced, with the fetus in right occiput posterior position. The mother is having persistent back pain that worsens during contractions.

**Q:** How should the nurse interpret this information? Should the nurse take any specific action based on the nurse-midwife's examination?

**A:** When the fetus is in one of the occiput posterior positions, back pain is usually persistent because the fetal head presses on the mother's sacrum with each contraction, often called "back labor." Additionally, the fetal head has to rotate internally through a wider arc to ultimately reach an occiput anterior position for birth; this process prolongs labor in most women.

The nurse should take actions to make the woman more comfortable and to promote rotation of the fetal head to an occiput anterior position. The nurse should encourage the woman to change positions regularly. Positions that cause her uterus to fall forward reduce pressure on her sacrum and straighten the pelvic curve somewhat to encourage fetal rotation. Examples of these are leaning forward while sitting, kneeling, standing, and a hands-and-knees position. Lunging toward her right side provides slightly more room on that side of her pelvis. If she wants to lie in bed, a left side-lying position favors fetal rotation toward an occiput anterior position. Consult with the nurse-midwife if the woman wants analgesia or anesthesia.

It can also be done in a kneeling position. The nurse or her partner must secure the chair and help her balance.

- Squatting (for second-stage labor)
- Sitting, kneeling, or standing while leaning forward

Upright maternal positions promote descent, which is usually accompanied by fetal head rotation. The first two maternal positions promote rotation because the mother's abdomen is dependent in relation to her spine. The convex surface of the fetal back tends to rotate toward the convex anterior uterus, similar to nesting two spoons together (Fig. 27–2). Moreover, these positions decrease the mother's discomfort by reducing fetal head pressure on her sacrum. A side-lying position has a similar effect, although not quite as pronounced.

The lunge widens the side of the pelvis toward which the woman lunges. If the fetal position is known, she lunges toward the side where the occiput is located (Fig. 27–3). If the fetal position is not known, the woman can lunge toward the side that gives her greater comfort.

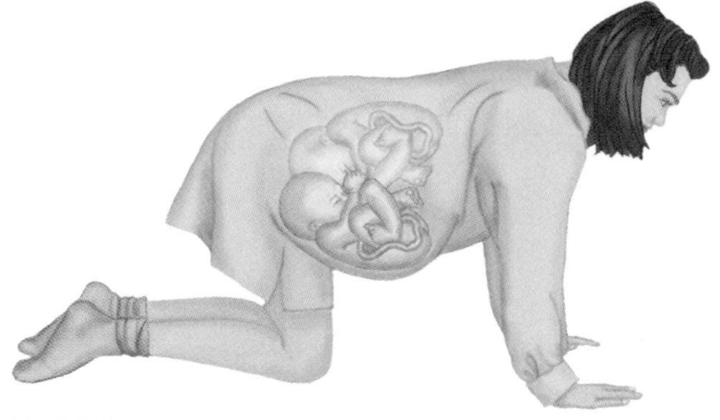

**FIGURE 27–2**

A "hands and knees" position helps the fetus rotate from a left occiput posterior (LOP) position to an occiput anterior position.

All variations of the squatting position aid rotation and fetal descent by straightening the pelvic curve and by enlarging the pelvic outlet. They also add gravity to the force of maternal pushing.

If spontaneous rotation does not occur, the physician may assist rotation and descent of the head with forceps. The vacuum extractor cannot usually be applied to the fetal head when it remains in an

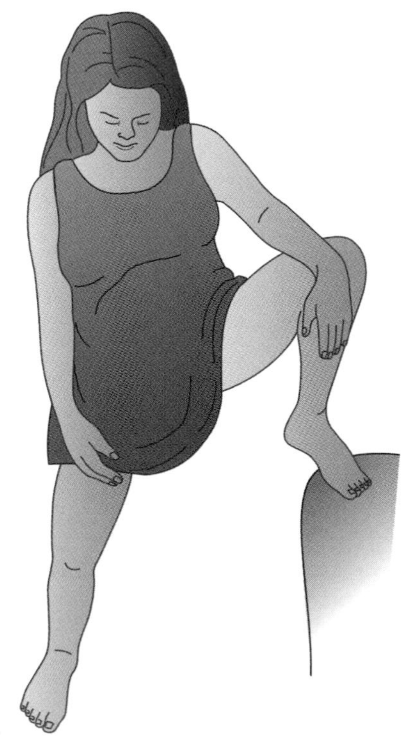

**FIGURE 27–3**

The "lunge" to one side promotes rotation of the fetal occiput from a posterior position to an anterior one.

occiput posterior position. However, a vacuum extractor may be used for minor degrees of malrotation because the fetal head tends to rotate as downward traction is applied and it descends. Cesarean birth may be needed if forceps use is not successful.

**Deflexion Abnormalities.** The poorly flexed fetal head presents a larger diameter to the pelvis than if flexed with the chin on the chest (see Fig. 12–8, p. 277). In the *vertex presentation*, the head diameter is smallest; in the *military* and *brow presentations*, the head diameter is larger. In the *face presentation*, the head diameter is similar to that of the vertex presentation, but the maternal pelvis can be traversed only if the fetal chin (mentum) is anterior.

**Breech Presentation.** Cervical dilation and effacement are often slower when the fetus is in a breech presentation because the buttocks or feet do not form a smooth, round dilating wedge like the head. The greatest fetal risk is that the head—the largest fetal part—is last to be born. By the time the lower body is born, the umbilical cord is well into the pelvis and may be compressed. The shoulders, arms, and head must be delivered quickly so that the infant can breathe.

A breech presentation is common well before term, but only 3 to 4 percent of term fetuses remain in this presentation. Adverse outcomes for infants that remain in a breech presentation may relate to causes other than their mode of birth:

- Fetal injury with a difficult vaginal birth
- Prolapsed umbilical cord
- Low birth weight due to preterm gestation, multifetal pregnancy, or intrauterine growth restriction
- Fetal anomalies, such as hydrocephalus
- Complications secondary to placenta previa or cesarean birth

*External version* may be attempted to change the fetus in a breech presentation or transverse lie to a cephalic presentation (see p. 404). If the fetus remains in the abnormal presentation, cesarean birth is usually performed to avoid complications of a difficult vaginal birth. Birth for the nulliparous woman with a fetus in a breech presentation is almost al-

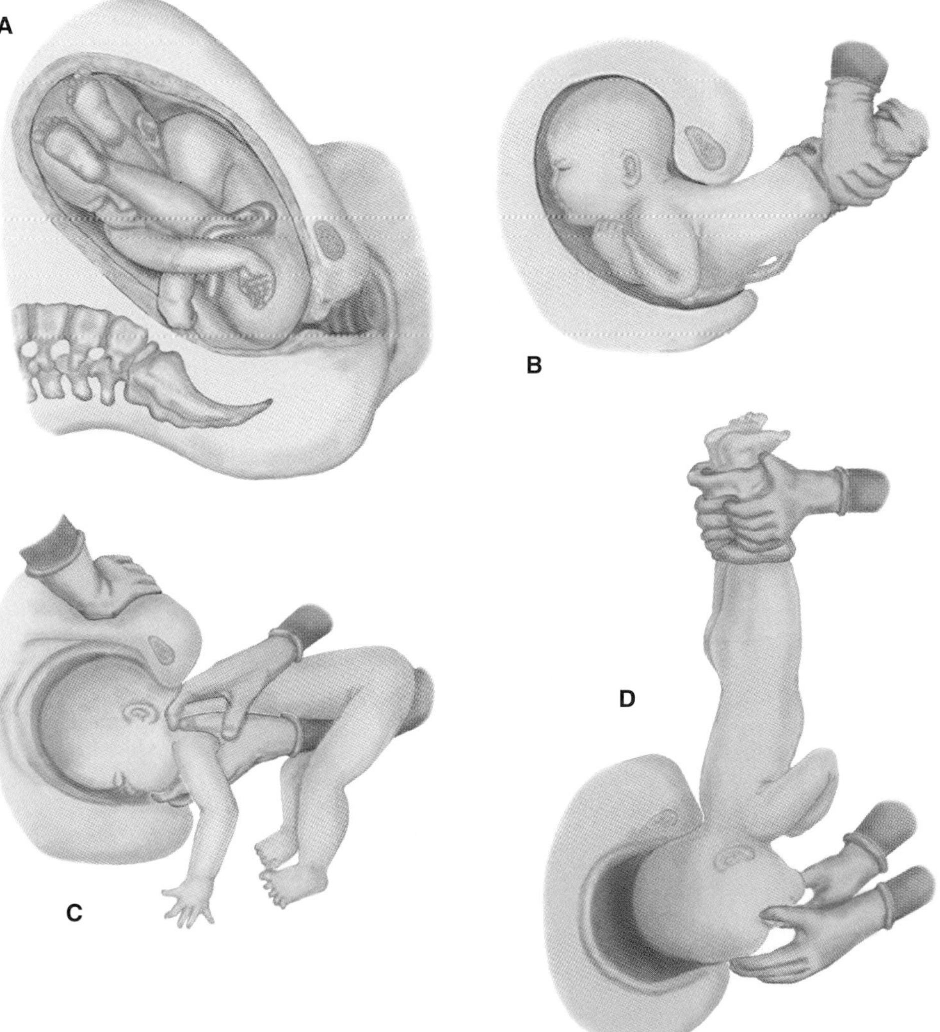


**FIGURE 27–4**

Sequence for vaginal birth in a frank breech presentation. A, Descent and internal rotation of the fetal body. B, Internal rotation complete; extension of the fetal back as the trunk slips under the symphysis pubis. The birth attendant uses a towel for traction when grasping the fetal legs. C, After the birth of the shoulders, the attendant maintains flexion of the fetal head by using the fingers of the left hand to apply pressure to the lower face; the fetal body straddles the attendant's left arm. An assistant provides suprapubic pressure to help keep the fetal head well flexed. D, After the fetal head is brought under the symphysis pubis, an assistant grasps the fetal legs with a towel for traction while the attendant delivers the face and head over the mother's perineum.

ways cesarean. The fetus remaining in a transverse lie is delivered by cesarean.

The physician may recommend that vaginal birth be attempted when the fetus is in a breech presentation if

- The maternal pelvis is of normal size and shape
- The estimated fetal weight is less than 3600 g (8 pounds)
- Other complications, such as placenta previa and prolapsed cord, are not present

Because some women are admitted in advanced labor with the fetus in a breech presentation, birth attendants and intrapartum nurses must be prepared to care for the woman having either a planned or an unexpected vaginal breech birth. Figure 27–4 illustrates the mechanisms of vaginal birth for an infant in a breech presentation.

### MULTIFETAL PREGNANCY

Multifetal pregnancy may result in dysfunctional labor because of uterine overdistention, which contributes to hypotonic dysfunction, and abnormal presentation of one or both fetuses (Fig. 27–5). In addition, the potential for fetal hypoxia during labor is greater because the mother must supply oxygen and nutrients to more than one fetus. She is also at greater risk for postpartum hemorrhage resulting from uterine atony because of uterine overdistention.

Because of these problems, birth for a woman with a multifetal pregnancy is often cesarean. If three or more fetuses are involved, the birth is almost always cesarean. Some women having twins may have a safe vaginal birth. The physician considers fetal presentations, maternal pelvic size, and presence of other complications, such as pregnancy-induced hypertension.

During labor, each twin's FHR is monitored separately. When in bed, the woman should remain in a lateral position to promote adequate placental blood flow. After vaginal birth of the first twin, assessment of the second twin's FHR continues until birth. The nurse observes for signs of hypotonic dysfunction throughout labor.

Whether the birth is vaginal or cesarean, the intrapartum staff must be prepared for the care and possible resuscitation of multiple infants. Cord clamps, bulb syringes, radiant warmers, and resuscitation equipment must be prepared for each infant. One or more neonatal nurses, a neonatal nurse-practitioner, a pediatrician, or a neonatologist should be available to care for each infant. One nurse should be free to care for the mother.

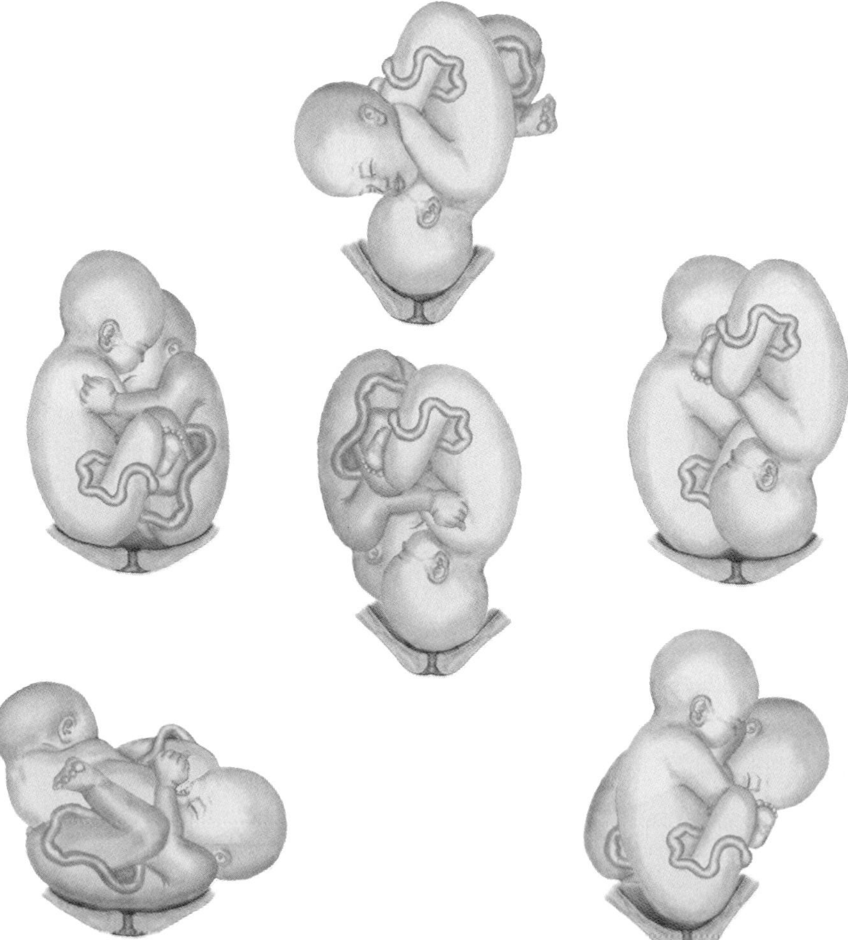

**FIGURE 27–5**

Twins can present in any combination.

### FETAL ANOMALIES

Fetal anomalies, such as hydrocephalus, or a large fetal tumor may prevent normal descent of the fetus. Abnormal presentations, such as breech or transverse lie, are also associated with fetal anomalies. These abnormalities may be discovered by ultrasound examination before labor. A cesarean birth is scheduled if vaginal birth is not possible or if it is inadvisable.

### CHECK YOUR READING

1. How does hypotonic labor dysfunction differ from hypertonic labor in terms of the most common labor phase when it becomes evident? Uterine contractions? Presence of pain? Therapeutic management?
2. How can maternal position changes favor rotation of the fetus from an occiput transverse or occiput posterior position to an occiput anterior position?
3. Why does a cesarean birth not eliminate all adverse outcomes for infants in a breech presentation?
4. How does preparation for the birth of twins (vaginally or cesarean) differ from preparation for a single infant's birth?

## Problems of the Passage

Dysfunctional labor may occur because of variations in the maternal bony pelvis or because of soft tissue problems that inhibit fetal descent.

### PELVIS

A small (contracted) or abnormally shaped pelvis may retard labor and obstruct fetal passage. The woman may experience poor contractions, slow dilation, slow fetal descent, and a long labor. The danger of uterine rupture is greater with thinning of the lower uterine segment, especially if contractions remain strong.

There are four basic pelvic shapes, each with different implications for labor and birth (Fig. 27–6).

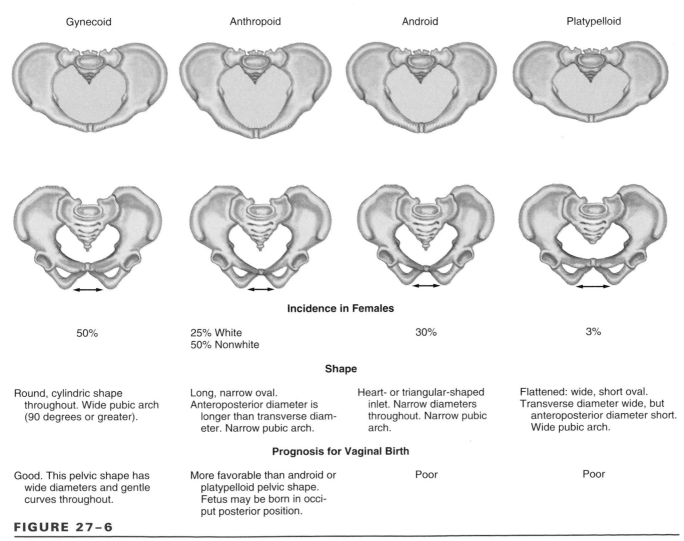

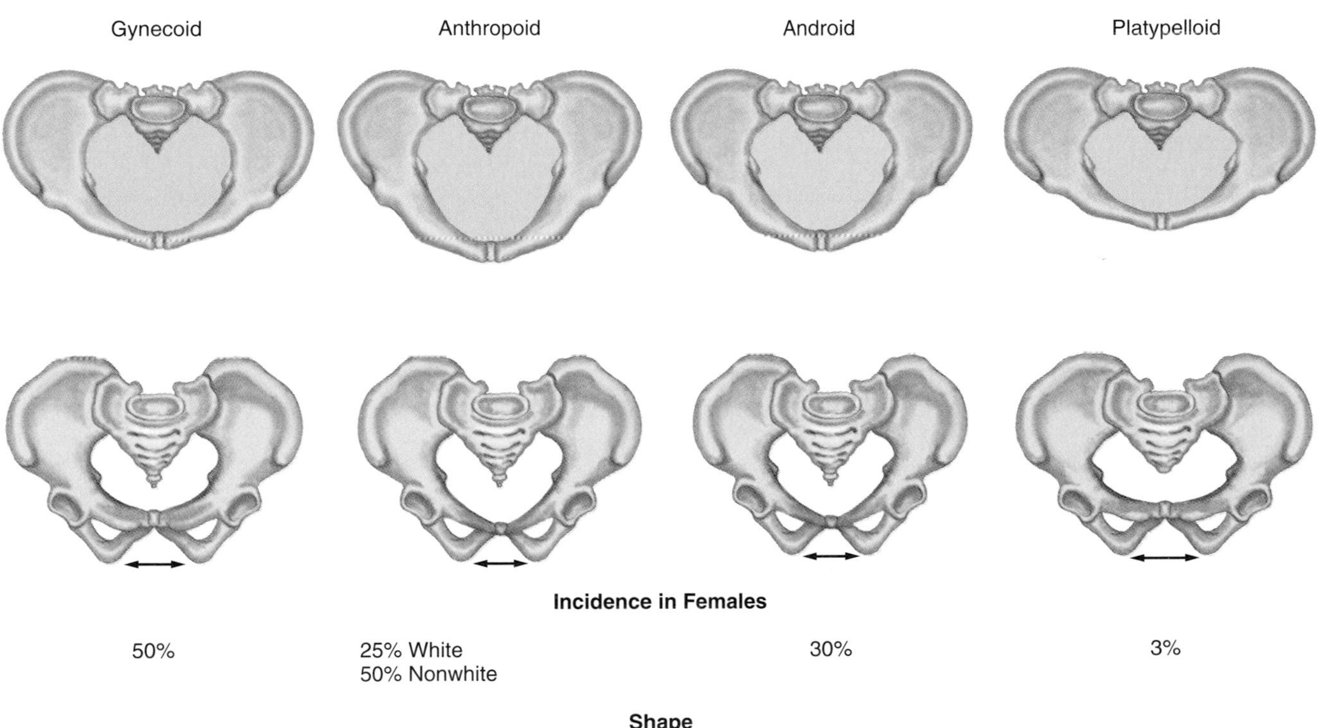


| | Gynecoid | Anthropoid | Android | Platypelloid |
|---|---|---|---|---|
| **Incidence in Females** | 50% | 25% White<br>50% Nonwhite | 30% | 3% |
| **Shape** | Round, cylindric shape throughout. Wide pubic arch (90 degrees or greater). | Long, narrow oval. Anteroposterior diameter is longer than transverse diameter. Narrow pubic arch. | Heart- or triangular-shaped inlet. Narrow diameters throughout. Narrow pubic arch. | Flattened: wide, short oval. Transverse diameter wide, but anteroposterior diameter short. Wide pubic arch. |
| **Prognosis for Vaginal Birth** | Good. This pelvic shape has wide diameters and gentle curves throughout. | More favorable than android or platypelloid pelvic shape. Fetus may be born in occiput posterior position. | Poor | Poor |

**FIGURE 27–6**

Pelvic shapes.

Most women do not have a pure pelvic shape but have mixed characteristics from two or more types.

#### MATERNAL SOFT TISSUE OBSTRUCTIONS

During labor, a full bladder is a common soft tissue obstruction. Bladder distention reduces available space in the pelvis and intensifies maternal discomfort. The woman should be assessed for bladder distention regularly and encouraged to void every 1 to 2 hours. Catheterization may be needed if she cannot urinate.

Less common obstructions are pelvic tumors such as benign uterine fibroids (myomas), cysts, and septa that form a wall within the uterus, cervix, or vagina.

### Problems of the Psyche

Labor is a stressful event for most women. However, a perceived threat caused by pain, fear, nonsupport, or one's personal situation can result in excessive maternal stress and interfere with normal labor progress. The woman's perception of stress—more than the actual existence of a threat—is important.

The body responds to stress, preparing itself for fight or flight. However, responses to excessive or prolonged stress interfere with labor in several ways:

- Increased glucose consumption reduces the energy supply available to the contracting uterus.
- Secretion of catecholamines (epinephrine and norepinephrine) by the adrenal glands stimulates uterine beta-receptors, which inhibit uterine contractions (an action similar to that of tocolytic drugs, such as terbutaline).
- Adrenal secretion of catecholamines diverts blood supply from the uterus and placenta to skeletal muscle.
- Labor contractions and maternal pushing efforts are less effective because these powers are working against the resistance of tense abdominal and pelvic muscles.
- Pain perception is increased and pain tolerance is decreased, which further increase maternal anxiety and stress.

Helping the woman relax helps her body work more effectively with the forces of labor and promotes normal progress. General nursing measures involve the following:

- Establishing a trusting relationship with the woman and her family
- Making the environment comfortable by adjusting temperature and light
- Promoting physical comfort, such as cleanliness
- Providing accurate information
- Implementing nonpharmacologic and pharmacologic pain management

Chapters 13 and 15 describe specific methods to encourage relaxation and promote comfort.

**CHECK YOUR READING**

5. Why should the nurse observe the laboring woman's bladder frequently?
6. Why is psychological support during labor important for effective physiologic function?

### Abnormal Labor Duration

An unusually long or short labor may result in maternal, fetal, or neonatal problems.

#### PROLONGED LABOR

Prolonged labor is a type of dysfunctional labor that results from problems with any of the factors in the birth process. After the woman reaches the active phase of labor, cervical dilation should proceed at a minimum rate of 1.2 cm per hour in the nullipara and 1.5 cm per hour in the parous woman. Descent of the fetal presenting part is expected to occur at a minimum rate of 1.0 cm per hour in the nullipara and 2.0 cm per hour in the parous woman (ACOG, 1995b). If all previous births were by cesarean before much cervical dilation occurred, the criteria that apply to a nullipara may be applied.

Potential maternal and fetal problems in prolonged labor include the following:

- Maternal infection, intrapartum or postpartum
- Neonatal infection, which may be severe or fatal
- Maternal exhaustion
- Higher levels of anxiety and fear during a subsequent labor

Maternal and neonatal infections are more likely if the membranes have been ruptured for a prolonged time because organisms ascend from the vagina. The mother is more likely to have an intrapartum or a postpartum infection, or both.

Nursing measures for the woman who has prolonged labor include promotion of comfort, conservation of energy, emotional support, position changes that favor normal progress, and assessments for infection. Nursing care for the fetus includes observation for signs of intrauterine infection and for compromised fetal oxygenation (see Chapter 14).

#### PRECIPITATE LABOR

Precipitate labor is one in which birth occurs within 3 hours of its onset. Often there is an abrupt onset of intense contractions rather than the more gradual increase in frequency, duration, and intensity that typify most labors.

Precipitate labor is not the same as a precipitate birth. A precipitate birth occurs after a labor of any length, in or out of the hospital or birth center, when a trained attendant is not present to assist. However, a woman in precipitate labor may also have a precipitate birth. The nurse should simply wear gloves while supporting the baby as it emerges. The mother's legs should not be locked or the fetal head held back to delay birth. Such actions can result in fetal hypoxia or other injury.

If the maternal pelvis is adequate and the soft tissues yield easily to fetal descent, little maternal injury is likely. However, if the soft tissues are firm and resist stretching, trauma (uterine rupture, cervical lacerations, hematoma) of the vagina or vulva may occur.

The fetus may suffer direct trauma, such as intracranial hemorrhage or nerve damage, during a precipitate labor. The fetus may become hypoxic because intense contractions with a short relaxation period reduce time available for gas exchange in the placenta. Fetal bradycardia and late decelerations are probable electronic fetal monitor patterns if this occurs.

Priority nursing care of the woman in precipitate labor includes promotion of fetal oxygenation and maternal comfort. The woman should remain in a side-lying position to enhance placental blood flow and reduce the effects of aortocaval compression. An added benefit of the side-lying position is to slow the rapid fetal descent and minimize perineal tears. Additional measures to enhance fetal oxygenation include administering oxygen to the mother and maintaining adequate blood volume with nonadditive intravenous (IV) fluids. If oxytocin is being used, it should be stopped. A tocolytic drug may be ordered.

Promoting comfort is difficult in a precipitate labor because intense contractions give the woman little time to prepare and to use coping skills, such as breathing techniques. Pharmacologic measures (opioid analgesia or regional block) may not be useful because rapid labor progression does not allow time for them to become effective. Also, possible newborn respiratory depression must be considered when opioids are given near birth. The nurse helps the woman focus on techniques to cope with pain one contraction at a time. The nurse must remain with her, both to provide support and to assist with an emergency birth if it occurs.

**CHECK YOUR READING**

7. During the active phase of labor, what is the minimum dilation and fetal descent rate expected for a nulliparous woman? For the parous woman?
8. What is the priority nursing care for a woman in prolonged labor?
9. What are the maternal and fetal risks when labor is unusually short?

## Application of Nursing Process: Dysfunctional Labor

Several nursing diagnoses and collaborative problems may be appropriate in dysfunctional labor. The potential complication of fetal compromise should be part of all intrapartum management (see Chapter 14). Pain management is especially important to women in dysfunctional labor because they may find that their coping skills are inadequate. Anxiety or fear is often higher with abnormal labor, which limits the woman's ability to cope with pain. Maternal or newborn injury may become apparent after the birth.

In addition to these problems, nursing care is directed toward two other nursing diagnoses: possible intrauterine infection and maternal exhaustion.

## Intrauterine Infection

### Assessment

Infection can occur with both normal and dysfunctional labors. Assess the FHR and maternal vital signs for evidence of infection:

- Fetal tachycardia (>160 beats per minute [BPM] for a term fetus), often the first sign of intrauterine infection
- Maternal temperature; assess every 2 to 4 hours in normal labor and every 2 hours after membranes rupture; assess hourly if elevated (38°C, or 100.4°F) or if other signs of infection are present.
- Maternal pulse, respirations, and blood pressure at least hourly to identify tachycardia or tachypnea, which often accompany temperature elevation.

Assess amniotic fluid for normal clear color and mild odor. Yellow or cloudy fluid or fluid with a foul or strong odor suggests infection. The strong odor may be noted before birth or afterward on the infant's skin.

### Analysis

For the woman without signs of infection but with risk factors, the nursing diagnosis selected is Risk for Infection related to presence of favorable conditions (specify) for development.

### Planning

Goals relate to detecting onset of infection:

- Maternal temperature will remain below 38°C (100.4°F).
- The FHR will remain near the baseline and below 160 BPM.
- The amniotic fluid will remain clear and without a foul or strong odor.

### Interventions

#### REDUCING THE RISK FOR INFECTION

Nurses should wash their hands before and after each contact with the woman and her infant to reduce transmission of organisms. Use gloves and other protective wear to prevent contact with potentially infectious secretions before and after birth.

Limit vaginal examinations to reduce transmission of vaginal organisms into the uterine cavity, and maintain aseptic technique during essential vaginal examinations. The intrapartum nurse learns to estimate a woman's progress with few vaginal examinations. For example, there may be increased bloody show and heightened anxiety when the cervix is about 6 cm dilated; she may become irritable and lose control at about 8 cm dilation.

Keep underpads as dry as possible to reduce the moist, warm environment that favors bacterial growth. Periodically clean excess secretions from the vaginal area in a front-to-back motion to limit fecal contamination and promote the mother's comfort.

#### IDENTIFYING INFECTION

Assess the woman and fetus for signs of infection. Increase frequency of assessments if labor is prolonged. If signs of infection are noted, report them to the birth attendant for definitive treatment. Note the time at which the membranes ruptured to identify prolonged rupture, which adds to the risk for infection.

The birth attendant may collect specimens from the uterine cavity or placenta for culture to identify infectious organisms and determine antibiotic sensitivity. Both aerobic and anaerobic culture specimens may be collected in containers specifically made for these two types of organisms. Follow directions on the container for proper handling and prevention of contamination with extraneous organisms, which would result in inaccurate results. Transport specimens to the laboratory promptly because living organisms are required for culture and sensitivity study.

Inform the newborn nursery staff if signs of infection are noted or if increased maternal risk factors exist. Specimens of infant secretions also may be obtained for testing.

The infant is often given prophylactic antibiotics to prevent neonatal sepsis (see p. 858). If results of infant cultures indicate that no infection is present, the antibiotic is usually discontinued. Culture and sensitivity testing may reveal an infection and indicate that a different antibiotic would be more effective.

**Critical to Remember**

**SIGNS ASSOCIATED WITH INTRAPARTUM INFECTION**

- Fetal tachycardia (more than 160 beats per minute)
- Maternal fever (38°C or 100.4°F)
- Foul or strong-smelling amniotic fluid
- Cloudy or yellow appearance to amniotic fluid

### Evaluation

If the goals are achieved,

- The woman's temperature will remain below 38°C (100.4°F).
- The amniotic fluid will have normal characteristics.
- Fetal tachycardia, either sudden or gradual in onset, will be absent.

Even if the woman has no signs of intrapartum infection, she remains at higher risk for postpartum infection and should be observed for signs and symptoms of infection.

## Maternal Exhaustion

### Assessment

Many women begin labor with a sleep deficit because of fetal movement, frequent urination, and shortness of breath associated with advanced pregnancy. As labor drags on, the mother's reserves are further depleted.

Assess the mother for signs and symptoms of exhaustion:

- Verbal expression of tiredness, fatigue, or exhaustion
- Verbal expression of frustration with a prolonged, unproductive labor ("I can't go on any longer. Why doesn't the doctor just take the baby?")
- Ineffectiveness or inability to use coping techniques (such as patterned breathing) that she previously used effectively
- Changes in her pulse, respiration, and blood pressure (increased or decreased)

### Analysis

The intense energy demands of a dysfunctional labor may exceed a woman's physical and psychological ability to meet them. For this reason, Activity Intolerance related to depletion of maternal energy reserves is an appropriate nursing diagnosis.

### Planning

Contractions must continue for labor to progress. Two realistic goals are that the woman will do the following:

- Rest between contractions with her muscles relaxed.
- Use coping skills, such as breathing and relaxation techniques.

### Interventions

#### CONSERVING MATERNAL ENERGY

Reduce factors that interfere with the woman's ability to relax. Lower the light level, and turn off overhead lights. Reduce noise by closing the door or masking it with soft music or other comforting sounds. Maintain a comfortable maternal temperature with blankets or a fan. If there is no contraindication, a warm shower or bath is soothing.

Position the woman to encourage comfort, promote fetal descent, and enhance fetal oxygenation. Support her with pillows to reduce muscle strain and added fatigue. Help her change positions regularly (about every 30 to 60 minutes) to reduce muscle tension from constant pressure.

A soothing back rub may reduce muscle tension, which increases fatigue. Firm sacral pressure or assuming some of the positions discussed with fetal occiput posterior positions may reduce back pain.

Maintain the intravenous fluids at the rate ordered to provide fluid, electrolytes, and sometimes glucose. Assess intake and output to identify dehydration, which may accompany prolonged labor. Dehydration may also cause maternal fever. If there is no contraindication, provide juice, lollipops, Popsicles, or other clear liquids, as ordered by the physician or nurse-midwife, to moisten the woman's mouth and replenish her energy.

#### PROMOTING COPING SKILLS

When position changes or medical therapy is used to enhance labor, explain their purpose and expected benefits. Encourage the woman to visualize her baby passing downward smoothly through her pelvis as a result of her efforts. Provide her with mental images that allow her to "see" herself giving birth.

Generous praise and encouragement of the woman's use of skills, such as breathing techniques, motivate her to continue them even when she is discouraged. As with any laboring woman, tell her when she is making progress. Tell her that fetal heart rates and patterns are reassuring if this is true. Knowing that her efforts are having the desired results and that her fetus is doing well gives the woman courage to continue.

### Evaluation

Goals are met if the woman does the following:

- Rests and relaxes between contractions. If she is unable to relax, discuss analgesia options with her. Inability to relax between contractions is associated with pain beyond the woman's tolerance.
- Continues to demonstrate adequate use of learned skills to cope with labor.

In addition, solicit the woman's perceptions of her ability to relax and cope with labor.

## Premature Rupture of the Membranes

Rupture of the amniotic sac before onset of true labor, regardless of length of gestation, is called *premature rupture of the membranes* (PROM). A similar term, *preterm premature rupture of the membranes* (PPROM), describes ruptured membranes earlier than the end of the 37th week of gestation, with or without contractions. PPROM is strongly associated with preterm labor and birth.

### Etiology

Several conditions are associated with PROM, but the exact cause often remains unclear. Possible causes are as follows:

- Infections of the vagina or cervix, such as gonorrhea, group B streptococcal infection, and *Gardnerella vaginalis* infection
- Chorioamnionitis
- Incompetent cervix
- Fetal abnormalities or malpresentation
- Hydramnios
- Amniotic sac with a weak structure
- Recent sexual intercourse
- Nutritional deficiencies

### Complications

Both mother and newborn are at risk for infection during the intrapartum and postpartum periods. Chorioamnionitis can be both a cause and a result of PROM. The mother is at higher risk for postpartum infection, and the newborn is vulnerable to neonatal sepsis.

If chorioamnionitis does not precede PROM, it is more likely to occur if a long time elapses between membrane rupture and birth because vaginal organisms can readily enter the uterus. The exact time at which infection occurs cannot be predicted, but the risk is known to be greatly increased after 24 hours have elapsed. However, infection may occur after just a few hours of ruptured membranes.

If preterm birth occurs, the infant is more likely to have respiratory distress syndrome (RDS) and complications related to prematurity. The hazards of prematurity are greatest before 34 weeks' gestation.

Other infant complications result from the loss of the amniotic fluid cushion (oligohydramnios). Umbilical cord compression, reduced lung volume, and deformities resulting from compression may occur.

### Therapeutic Management

Management of PROM depends on the gestation and whether there is evidence of infection or other fetal or maternal compromise. For a woman at term, PROM may herald the imminent onset of true labor. Usually, the cervix is soft with some dilation and effacement. The fetal head is at or near zero (0) station. If the woman is not at term or if her cervix is not soft and favorable for labor, therapeutic management is more complex. The risk of infection or preterm birth is weighed against the hazards of labor induction by oxytocin or cesarean birth.

#### DETERMINING TRUE MEMBRANE RUPTURE

The first step is to determine whether the membranes are truly ruptured. Urinary incontinence, increased vaginal discharge, or loss of the mucus plug can make a woman think that her membranes have ruptured when they have not. A vaginal examination is avoided, particularly if the gestation is preterm and there is no evidence of labor. Instead, the physician or nurse-midwife performs a sterile speculum examination to look for a pool of fluid near the cervix and estimate cervical dilation and effacement. A Nitrazine or fern test may be done on the fluid to verify that the liquid is amniotic fluid. Tests to assess fetal lung maturity and identify infection are often done as well.

#### GESTATION NEAR TERM

If the woman is at or near term and her cervix is soft, induction may be done if labor does not begin spontaneously. Walking may help stimulate contractions. If the cervix is not favorable and no infection is present, induction may be delayed 24 hours, or sometimes longer, to allow cervical softening. If induction is unsuccessful or if infection develops, a cesarean birth may be necessary. However, the nurse should remember that cesarean birth also increases the risk for postpartum infection.

#### PRETERM GESTATION

If the gestation is preterm, the physician weighs the risks of maternal-fetal infection against the infant's risk for complications of prematurity. The cervix is usually not favorable for induction far from term. The physician considers factors such as gestational age, amount of amniotic fluid remaining, and fetal lung maturity.

### Nursing Considerations

The woman may remain hospitalized until birth, or she may return home after a few days of hospital observation. If she is hospitalized, the nurse observes for signs of infection. Preparation for home management includes teaching the woman to do the following:

- Avoid sexual intercourse, orgasm, or insertion of anything into the vagina, which increases the risk for infection caused by ascending organisms and can stimulate contractions.
- Avoid breast stimulation if the gestation is preterm because it can cause release of oxytocin from the posterior pituitary and thus stimulate contractions.
- Take her temperature at least four times a day, reporting any temperature above 37.8°C (100°F).
- Maintain any activity restrictions recommended.
- Note uterine contractions.

See care of the woman with preterm labor for additional care if her membranes are ruptured before term.

**✓ CHECK YOUR READING**

10. How does PROM differ from PPROM?
11. What is the relationship of infection to PROM?
12. What is the usual therapeutic management of PROM if the woman is at or near term?
13. What factors does the physician consider if the woman with PROM is not near term gestation?

## Preterm Labor

Preterm labor begins after the 20th week but before the end of the 37th week of pregnancy. The physical risks to the mother are no greater than labor at term unless there are other complications, such as infection. However, preterm labor may result in the birth of an infant who is ill equipped for extrauterine life.

### Associated Factors

Just as all of the causes of labor's onset at term are not known, the causes of preterm labor are not fully known either. Several factors are associated with preterm labor:

- Medical conditions
- Present and past obstetric conditions
- Social and environmental factors
- Demographic factors such as race and age (Table 27–2)

However, many women who have preterm labor and birth have none of these risk factors.

## Signs and Symptoms

Signs and symptoms of early preterm labor are more subtle than those of labor at term and often occur in normal pregnancies as well. The woman may be only vaguely aware that something seems different, or she may not detect that anything is amiss. Only when preterm labor reaches the active phase is it likely to have characteristics typical of term labor. Symptoms vary among women, but common ones are as follows:

- Uterine contractions that may or may not be painful; the woman may not feel contractions at all
- A sensation that the baby is frequently "balling up"
- Cramps similar to menstrual cramps
- Constant low backache
- Sensation of pelvic pressure or a feeling that the baby is pushing down
- Pain, discomfort, or pressure in the vulva or thighs
- Change or increase in vaginal discharge (increased, watery, bloody)
- Abdominal cramps with or without diarrhea
- A sense of "just feeling bad" or "coming down with something"

## Preventing Preterm Birth

### COMMUNITY EDUCATION

Preterm birth can impose substantial physical, emotional, and financial burdens on the child, the family, and society. Nurses play an important role in preventing preterm birth. Ideally, strategies begin before conception, with community education. Programs often include teaching about the following:

- Duration of normal pregnancy
- Consequences of preterm birth
- Role of early and regular prenatal care in preventing preterm birth
- Conditions that increase risk for preterm birth

Women who are aware of the consequences of preterm birth may be more likely to take action to prevent it. If they recognize that they have risk factors, they may seek prenatal care earlier in gestation than they otherwise might.

### DURING PREGNANCY

During pregnancy, measures to prevent preterm birth include the following:

- Reducing barriers and improving access to early prenatal care for all women
- Assessing for risk factors to permit changes in those that can be changed
- Promoting adequate nutrition
- Educating women and their partners about the subtle signs and symptoms of preterm labor and how they differ from normal pregnancy changes
- Empowering women and their partners to take an active approach in seeking care if they have signs and symptoms of preterm labor

**TABLE 27–2 MATERNAL RISK FACTORS FOR PRETERM LABOR**

| Medical History | Obstetric History | Present Pregnancy | Lifestyle and Demographics |
|---|---|---|---|
| Uterine or cervical anomalies | Previous preterm birth | Uterine distention (such as multifetal pregnancy or hydramnios) | Little or no prenatal care |
| Diethylstilbestrol (DES) exposure as a fetus | Previous preterm labor | Abdominal surgery during pregnancy | Poor nutrition |
| History of cone biopsy | Previous first trimester abortions (>2) | Uterine irritability | Age under 18 or over 40 |
| Low weight for height | Previous second trimester abortion | Uterine bleeding | Low education level |
| Chronic illness (such as cardiac, renal, hypertension) | History of previous pregnancy losses (2 or more) | Dehydration | Low socioeconomic status |
| | Incompetent cervix | Infection | Smoking >10 cigarettes daily |
| | | Anemia | Nonwhite |
| | | Incompetent cervix | Chronic physical or psychological stress |
| | | Pre-eclampsia | Substance abuse |
| | | Preterm premature rupture of membranes (PPROM) | |
| | | Fetal or placental abnormalities | |

**Improving Access to Care.** Improving access to prenatal care must be customized for the community. What works in one area may be inappropriate for another. Difficult access is a serious problem for women who rely on public clinics for their care. Long waits, fragmented care, language barriers, and insensitivity of caregivers may discourage women from obtaining care. Expanding the number of caregivers by using nurses with advanced education, such as certified nurse-midwives and nurse practitioners, can reduce waits for care significantly. Nurses can help coordinate various aspects of care to limit the number of different appointments a woman needs to obtain complete care.

**Identifying Risk Factors.** Women who have risk factors for preterm birth can benefit from programs to reduce the risk and identify preterm labor early. These women benefit from care such as more frequent prenatal care appointments, reinforcement of the symptoms of preterm labor, telephone contacts, and assessments of fetal growth and health.

Some risk factors can be reduced or eliminated if the woman changes her lifestyle. Although it may have been difficult for them, many women have stopped smoking or using drugs to benefit their baby. A woman may need to rest more or to stop working, and this may be difficult or impossible for many. Nurses can work with the woman to help reduce her risks as much as possible by helping her identify sources of support.

Infections of the urinary and reproductive tracts are associated with PPROM and preterm labor. Screening for abnormal microorganisms in the urine, vagina, or cervix identifies women who may benefit from antibiotic therapy.

**Promoting Adequate Nutrition.** An adequate maternal diet contributes positively to the length of gestation and the infant's weight. Every pregnant woman should be offered culturally sensitive diet counseling. The Women, Infants, and Children (WIC) program is available to supplement the diet of some low-income women. Anemia can be corrected with appropriate supplements.

**Educating Women and Their Partners About Preterm Labor.** *All pregnant women and their partners should be taught about symptoms of preterm labor because most preterm births occur in women who have no identified risk factors.* Language barriers can be reduced by using fluent interpreters and printed materials in the woman's primary language. Diagrams should supplement the words of any language because some women have limited reading skills. Jones and Collins (1996) recommend that written materials have a reading level no higher than sixth grade.

The vague signs and symptoms of early preterm labor should be reinforced regularly. The woman should be taught how to respond if she detects them. Typical responses to signs and symptoms of preterm labor include the following:

- Drinking three glasses of water to counteract dehydration that stimulates uterine contractions
- Emptying the bladder because a full bladder can stimulate uterine contractions
- Lying down, usually on the left side, to promote uterine blood flow
- Palpating contractions for 1 hour
- Notifying the birth attendant if more than four contractions occur during 1 hour

The nurse should verify the woman's understanding by seeking feedback, such as having her restate the signs and symptoms of preterm labor and the appropriate responses to them.

**Empowering Women and Their Partners.** Delaying birth when preterm labor occurs depends critically on identifying it early. Women should be encouraged to seek treatment promptly if they suspect preterm labor. They should be encouraged to communicate their concerns when they arrive at the clinic or hospital. Otherwise, they may wait for hours to be seen in a public facility. It is equally important not to make the woman feel foolish if she reports signs and symptoms but is not in labor. Otherwise, she may not seek care for recurrent episodes when she truly is in labor; the opportunity to delay preterm birth may be lost.

**The nurse might suggest this approach to a woman seeking care for possible preterm labor: "I'm not due for 8 more weeks, but I think I may be in labor. I need to be seen right away, or I might have a premature baby."**

## Therapeutic Management

Management focuses on identifying preterm labor early, delaying birth, and accelerating fetal lung maturity if preterm birth is likely.

### IDENTIFYING PRETERM LABOR

The reason to identify preterm labor early is to delay birth, thus promoting further fetal maturation.

**Frequent Prenatal Visits.** Women at risk for preterm labor have more frequent prenatal visits and are checked for signs and symptoms of preterm labor and their ability to follow therapy to prevent it. Gentle cervical examinations or ultrasound examinations identify painless effacement or dilation that often precedes onset of labor. Infections can be identified and treated promptly before they result in rupture of the membranes or labor.

**Fetal Fibronectin.** Fetal fibronectin is a protein in the amniotic fluid and fetal membranes. It is also found in vaginal secretions until about 22 weeks' gestation and again at or near term. If infection or other processes compromise fetal membrane integrity, fetal fibronectin appears in vaginal secretions at a time when it is not expected to be present (Escher-Davis, 1996). It is evaluated by testing secretions obtained from the posterior cul-de-sac with a swab.

Because of the vague qualities of early preterm labor, assessment for fetal fibronectin can help the birth attendant decide on the best course of management. For example, if the woman in suspected preterm labor has a positive fetal fibronectin test, she may be treated more aggressively with tocolytics or transported to a facility where neonatal intensive care is available rather than being treated conservatively.

**Home Uterine Activity Monitoring.** Home uterine activity monitoring detects uterine activity that the woman may not perceive. A vital part of this service is 24-hour phone availability of perinatal nurses to (1) evaluate uterine activity patterns, (2) determine signs and symptoms that are present, (3) reinforce signs and symptoms to report, and (4) notify the physician of significant signs or symptoms.

Studies of the benefits of home uterine activity monitoring have shown mixed results. Increased uterine activity often occurs about 24 hours before preterm birth occurs. Although the home monitor can detect these contractions, it is not clear whether the actual preterm *birth* incidence is reduced enough to justify its use in all women at risk (ACOG, 1995c). Further study is needed to clarify what role this technology should have in the prevention of preterm birth.

Monitoring is usually done twice a day for 60 minutes, or any time the woman detects symptoms. Information is transmitted by phone to a central site, where a nurse evaluates it. The nurse contacts the woman and asks her about signs or symptoms of preterm labor. Depending on the uterine activity data, the woman's report, and the physician's orders, the nurse instructs the woman to monitor at the next scheduled time or remonitor after emptying her bladder and drinking water. The nurse informs the physician of any uterine activity that exceeds a prescribed limit and discusses the physician's recommendation with the mother.

### STOPPING PRETERM LABOR

Once diagnosis of preterm labor is made, management focuses on stopping the uterine activity before it reaches the point of no return, usually after 3 cm dilation. If preterm delivery is inevitable, therapy is directed toward reducing the infant's risk for respiratory distress.

#### INITIAL MEASURES

Before attempting to halt preterm labor, the physician determines whether any maternal or fetal conditions contraindicate continuing the pregnancy. Examples of these conditions are pregnancy-induced hypertension, maternal hypovolemia, chorioamnionitis, and fetal compromise.

Initial measures to stop preterm labor may include identifying and treating infections, restricting activity, and hydrating the woman.

**Identifying and Treating Infections.** Infection has a strong association with preterm birth, as it does with premature rupture of the membranes. Blood studies identify infection and other conditions, such as anemia, that are also associated with preterm labor or that affect its management. Common studies include a complete blood count with differential white blood cell analysis, C-reactive protein, electrolytes, and glucose and creatinine levels (Iams, 1994).

Urinary tract infections are often associated with preterm labor and reduce the effectiveness of methods to stop it. A catheterized urine specimen is usually obtained for analysis and for culture and sensitivity testing.

Cultures of vaginal and cervical secretions may identify infection in the lower reproductive tract, which permits better management of the preterm labor. Amniocentesis may be done if chorioamnionitis is suspected.

The value of treating overt infections is clear. However, the value of giving antibiotics prophylactically to women who are simply *at risk* for infection is less clear. Several studies have demonstrated prolonged gestation when antibiotics were given in addition to tocolytic therapy. More study is needed to determine the exact role of antibiotics in preterm birth prevention (ACOG, 1995c).

**Restricting Activity.** Bed rest, usually on the left side, increases placental blood flow and reduces fetal pressure on the cervix. However, bedrest has not been shown to lengthen pregnancy significantly and is associated with serious maternal side effects (Burke & Poole, 1996; Maloni, 1996). Physical side effects include cardiovascular deconditioning, muscle and calcium loss, and weight loss (or failure to gain normally). Other side effects may include depression, anxiety, and sleep changes. Because of significant maternal problems with no clear benefit to the infant, lengthy bedrest is less often prescribed for women who are at risk for preterm labor. Or activity restrictions may be modified, such as resting in a semi-Fowler's position or partial bedrest. Alternating sides from left to right reduces discomfort of constant side-lying.

Most women have difficulty maintaining activity restrictions such as bedrest. Reasons include the need to care for their children, not feeling sick, household demands, lack of support, need to work, and discomfort of bedrest (Josten et al., 1995). Additionally, this study found that the pregnancy outcomes were similar for women who did and did not comply with bedrest.

**Hydrating the Woman.** Intravenous fluids are often prescribed for the woman hospitalized for possible preterm labor and may delay need for tocolytic drugs. The posterior pituitary gland responds to dehydration by secreting antidiuretic hormone, and oxytocin along with it. However, benefits of intravenous hydration are unclear if the woman is not dehydrated. The American College of Obstetricians and Gynecologists (1995c) recommends use of hypotonic fluids to reduce the risk of pulmonary edema that may occur if tocolytic therapy is needed.

#### TOCOLYTICS

One problem related to treatment of preterm labor is that no consensus exists on what findings diagnose it. If the physician waits until the woman is clearly in preterm labor, preventing preterm birth may be impossible. Tocolysis is less likely to be effective if the cervix is 3 cm or more dilated. However, tocolytic drugs have significant side effects, and physicians do not want to treat a nonexistent disorder. Iams (1994) suggests that these criteria be met before starting tocolytic therapy:

- Gestational age is 20 to 37 weeks.
- If the cervix is less than 80% effaced (longer than about 0.4 cm) and less than 2 cm dilated at admission, cervical change (effacement and/or dilation) must occur to start a tocolytic drug.
- If the cervix is more than 80% effaced (shorter than about 0.4 cm) or more than 2 cm dilated at admission, a tocolytic drug may be started if contractions are present (four per 20 minutes or eight per 60 minutes) despite bed rest in a lateral position and hydration with intravenous fluids.

Tocolysis is most likely to be ordered if preterm labor occurs before the 34th week of gestation because the infant's risk for respiratory and other complications of prematurity is high if born at that time. The benefit of tocolysis is less clear if labor begins between 34 and 37 weeks because infants of older gestation usually have less severe complications. Tocolytic drugs do not typically *prevent* preterm birth but may *delay* it. This delay may provide time to allow use of corticosteroids to accelerate fetal lung maturity or to transfer the woman to a facility having a neonatal intensive care unit.

Most tocolytic drugs are used primarily for conditions other than preterm labor and therefore have effects on body systems other than the reproductive. The lowest possible dose that inhibits contractions is used. Four types of drugs are used for tocolysis: (1) β-adrenergics, (2) magnesium sulfate, (3) prostaglandin synthesis inhibitors, and (4) calcium antagonists. Table 27–3 summarizes doses and routes of administration for each of these drugs.

A new drug, atosiban, which opposes the action of oxytocin, is being researched. The early trials on this drug suggest that it offers a delay until birth similar to that of other tocolytic drugs. Its side effects have been minimal. If further study confirms the beneficial effects of atosiban, it offers another drug to counteract preterm labor.

**TABLE 27–3 DRUGS USED IN PRETERM LABOR**

| Drug/Purpose | Common Doses* | Side or Adverse Effects |
|---|---|---|
| β-Adrenergics (tocolysis) | | |
| Ritodrine | IV: Start at 0.05 mg/min (50 μg/min). Increase by 0.05 mg/min until labor stops or significant side effects develop. Maximum dose is 0.35 mg/min (350 μg/min).<br>Hold rate for 60 min after contractions stop, then decrease by 0.05 mg/min (50 μg/min) increments until lowest effective dose is reached. Hold this dose for 12 hr.<br>*Oral*: Give first oral dose before discontinuing IV ritodrine. 10 mg q 2 hr or 20 mg q 4 hr for 24–48 hr. Maximum daily oral dose: 120 mg/day. | Side effects are dose-related and more prominent during increases in the infusion rate than during maintenance therapy.<br>Cardiovascular: maternal and fetal tachycardia. Wide pulse pressure<br>Pulmonary: Shortness of breath, chest pain<br>Gastrointestinal: Nausea, vomiting, diarrhea, ileus<br>Tremors, jitteriness, restlessness, feeling of apprehension<br>Metabolic alterations: hyperglycemia; hypokalemia<br>Pulmonary edema (more likely if the woman receives corticosteroids at the same time) |

**TABLE 27-3 DRUGS USED IN PRETERM LABOR** *Continued*

| Drug/Purpose | Common Doses* | Side or Adverse Effects |
|---|---|---|
| Terbutaline | See Drug Guide: Terbutaline (p. 764)<br>IV: Begin at 0.0025 mg/min (2.5 μg/min). Increase by 0.0025 mg/min (2.5 μg/min) at 20-min intervals until contractions stop (maximum of 0.02 mg/min [20 μg/min]) or significant side effects develop. Maintain dose for at least 1 hr; then reduce rate at 20-min intervals to reach lowest effective dose. Continue maintenance dose for 12 hr after contractions stop before changing route of administration.<br>*Subcutaneous* (SC) (most common parenteral route): 0.25 mg (250 μg) every 1–3 hr. Continuous pump may be used for SC administration.<br>*Oral*: 2.5–5 mg every 2–4 hr. | Cardiovascular: Maternal and fetal tachycardia, palpitations, cardiac arrhythmias, chest pain, wide pulse pressure<br>Respiratory: Dyspnea, chest discomfort<br>Central nervous system: Tremors, restlessness, weakness, dizziness, headache<br>Metabolic: Hyperglycemia, hypokalemia<br>Gastrointestinal: Nausea, vomiting, reduced bowel motility<br>Skin: Flushing, diaphoresis<br>Infection at injection site (subcutaneous terbutaline pump) |
| Magnesium sulfate (tocolysis) | IV: Loading dose: 4–6 g; continue at 2–4 g/hr<br>Higher doses can usually be given than for pre-eclampsia because these women usually have normal renal function. | Side and adverse effects are dose-related, occurring at higher serum levels.<br>Depression of deep tendon reflexes<br>Respiratory depression<br>Cardiac arrest (usually at serum levels above 12/mg/dl)<br>Less serious side effects include: Lethargy, weakness, visual blurring, headache, sensation of heat, nausea, vomiting, constipation<br>Fetal-neonatal effects: Reduced FHR variability. Hypotonia |
| Indomethacin (tocolysis) | *Oral or rectal*: 25–50 mg every 6 hr for 48 hr. Discontinue if birth is imminent or likely to occur within 24 hr. 48 hr is a common maximum time for administration. | Gastrointestinal: Epigastric pain, gastrointestinal bleeding<br>Fetus: May have constriction of the ductus arteriosus and decreased urine output. Decreased urine output is associated with oligohydramnios, which may result in cord compression. Adverse fetal effects usually resolve within a day after treatment is stopped. |
| Nifedipine (tocolysis) | *Oral*: 30 mg initially; 20 mg 4 hr later | Maternal flushing<br>Transient maternal tachycardia<br>Maternal hypotension |
| Corticosteroids (accelerating fetal lung maturation)<br>* Betamethasone<br>* Dexamethasone | See Drug Guide: Betamethasone and Dexamethasone (p. 766)<br>*Betamethasone*: 12 mg IM for two doses, 24 hr apart<br>*Dexamethasone*: 6 mg IM q 12 hr for four doses<br>Greatest fetal benefits if at least 24 hr elapse between first dose and birth | Concurrent administration with beta-adrenergics and corticosteroids has been associated with development of pulmonary edema.<br>May worsen conditions such as diabetes and hypertension and may delay wound healing. |

* Doses and frequency of administration are common, but protocols do vary.

**β-Adrenergic Drugs.** Ritodrine (Yutopar) is the only β-adrenergic currently approved by the U.S. Food and Drug Administration (FDA) for tocolysis, although terbutaline (Brethine) is the more widely used drug in this class.

The main side effects involve the cardiorespiratory system. Maternal and fetal tachycardia are common; other side effects include decreased blood pressure, wide pulse pressure, arrhythmias, myocardial ischemia, chest pain, and pulmonary edema. Metabolic changes include hyperglycemia and hypokalemia. Tremors and restlessness are also side effects. See the Drug Guide below for nursing care related to terbutaline tocolysis.

$\beta$-Adrenergics may be given by the intravenous, subcutaneous, or oral route. Ritodrine is typically begun intravenously; terbutaline is often started subcutaneously. After the preterm contractions are stopped, the dose is gradually reduced to the lowest one that is effective and is maintained at that level for 12 hours. Oral therapy begins 30 minutes before the intravenous dose is stopped to maintain consistent blood levels of the drug. Oral therapy continues for another 24 to 48 hours (Boyle, 1995) or may continue until 35 to 37 weeks of gestation (ACOG, 1995c). Glucose tolerance may decrease if terbutaline therapy lasts longer than 1 week, so the woman is often screened for gestational diabetes (see Chapter 25).

Subcutaneous terbutaline may be given with a continuous, low-dose infusion pump at home or in the hospital. No clear evidence supports the benefit of this administration method over other methods, however (ACOG, 1995c).

Propranolol should be available to reverse adverse effects of $\beta$-adrenergic drugs.

**Magnesium Sulfate.** Magnesium sulfate is used in management of pregnancy-induced hypertension to prevent seizures (see the Drug Guide on p. 696). Because of its added effect of quieting uterine activity, it is often used to inhibit preterm labor. Magnesium sulfate therapy has a well-established record of safety during pregnancy. The woman who cannot tolerate other drugs or for whom other drugs are ineffective may benefit from magnesium sulfate tocolysis.

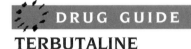

Magnesium sulfate for tocolysis is given intra-

DRUG GUIDE

## TERBUTALINE

***Classification:*** Beta-adrenergic agent

***Action:*** Stimulates beta-adrenergic receptors of the sympathetic nervous system. Action primarily results in bronchodilation and inhibition of uterine muscle activity. Increases pulse rate and widens pulse pressure.

***Indications:*** Stop preterm labor. Reduce or stop hypertonic labor contractions, whether natural or stimulated.

**Dosage and Route**

1. *Intravenous* (IV) *infusion.* Begin at 0.0025 mg/minute (2.5 $\mu$g/minute). Increase by 0.0025 mg/minute (2.5 $\mu$g/minute) at 20-minute intervals until contractions stop (maximum of 0.02 mg/minute [20 $\mu$g/minute]). Maintain this dose for at least 1 hour; then reduce the rate at 20-minute intervals to reach minimum maintenance dose. Continue maintenance dose for 12 hours after contractions stop before changing route of administration.
2. *Subcutaneous* (SC) (most common parenteral route). 0.25 mg (250 $\mu$g) every 1 to 3 hours
3. *Oral.* 2.5 to 5 mg every 2 to 4 hours

When changing from intravenous therapy to oral therapy, give oral dose 30 minutes before discontinuing intravenous infusion.

**Absorption**

1. *Intravenous.* Prompt; duration about 2 hours
2. *Subcutaneous.* 6 to 15 minutes; duration 1.5 to 4 hours
3. *Oral.* 1 to 2 hours; duration 4 to 8 hours

***Excretion:*** Metabolized in the liver. Excreted in urine.

***Contraindications:*** Hypersensitivity. Contraindicated before 20 weeks' gestation and if continuing the pregnancy is hazardous to the mother or fetus, as in fetal distress, hemorrhage, chorioamnionitis, and intrauterine fetal death. Contraindicated in conditions that may be adversely affected by $\beta$-adrenergic agents (uncontrolled diabetes, hyperthyroidism, bronchial asthma treated with other beta-mimetic agents or steroids, cardiac dysrhythmias, hypovolemia, and uncontrolled hypertension).

***Precautions:*** Terbutaline is not approved by the U.S. Food and Drug Administration for inhibiting uterine activity, although it is widely used for this purpose based on extensive clinical experience. It is most effective if begun as soon as a diagnosis of preterm labor is made.

**Adverse Reactions**

1. *Cardiovascular:* Maternal and fetal tachycardia, palpitations, cardiac arrhythmias, chest pain, wide pulse pressure
2. *Respiratory:* Dyspnea, chest discomfort
3. *Central nervous system:* Tremors, restlessness, weakness, dizziness, headache
4. *Metabolic:* Hypokalemia, hyperglycemia
5. *Gastrointestinal:* Nausea, vomiting, reduced bowel motility
6. *Skin:* Flushing, diaphoresis

***Nursing Considerations:*** Diagnostic studies that may be ordered related to terbutaline therapy: electrocardiogram, blood glucose, electrolytes, urinalysis. Explain common side effects that are usually well tolerated, such as palpitations, tremors, restlessness, weakness, headache. Assess FHR, usually with continuous electronic fetal monitoring, recording rate and patterns every 15 minutes during IV dose increases. Assess maternal pulse, respirations, and blood pressure by same schedule as for FHR. Maintain adequate IV or oral hydration. Encourage the woman to empty her bladder every 2 hours. Notify the physician for significant or unacceptable side effects (maternal heart rate above 110/BPM, respirations above 24/minute, systolic blood pressure lower than 90 mmHg, FHR above 160/BPM, chest pain, dyspnea). Report continuing or recurrent uterine activity. Teach signs and symptoms of recurrent preterm labor and follow-up medical care after discharge.

venously using a similar protocol to that for pregnancy-induced hypertension. The criteria needed to continue magnesium sulfate therapy include the following:

- Urine output of at least 30 ml per hour
- Presence of deep tendon reflexes
- Respirations of at least 12 per minute

In addition, the nurse should check heart and lung sounds with hourly vital signs because excessive fluid and electrolyte imbalances can lead to pulmonary edema or cardiac dysrhythmias. Bowel sounds are checked when therapy begins and every 4 to 8 hours because the smooth muscle in the intestinal tract may be relaxed just as the uterus is relaxed. Serum magnesium level measurements are often ordered.

The magnesium sulfate infusion continues for 12 to 24 hours, when it is gradually reduced. The woman is often shifted to oral terbutaline to maintain tocolysis when the magnesium sulfate is discontinued.

Calcium gluconate, 10 percent, should be available to reverse magnesium toxicity and prevent respiratory arrest if serum levels become high. Excess serum levels of magnesium are less likely when the drug is given for preterm labor because the woman's renal function is usually normal. However, the nurse must remain alert for this complication of magnesium sulfate therapy.

**Prostaglandin Synthesis Inhibitors.** Because prostaglandins stimulate uterine contractions, drugs may be used to inhibit their synthesis. Indomethacin is the drug in this class that is most often used for tocolysis.

Constriction of the fetal ductus arteriosus may occur, particularly if the drug is given after 34 weeks' gestation. Indomethacin temporarily impairs fetal renal function, which reduces the volume of amniotic fluid. Its effect in reducing the amount of amniotic fluid also makes indomethacin useful for normalizing the volume if hydramnios is present.

Indomethacin can alter neutrophil and platelet function, particularly in the fetus. This effect may lead to sepsis, intracranial hemorrhage, necrotizing enterocolitis, or renal dysfunction (Gordon & Samuels, 1995). These adverse effects are more likely to occur if indomethacin is given for more than 48 hours, or if less than 24 hours elapse between the last dose and birth. Therefore, indomethacin is not usually given if birth within 24 hours is likely, and the length of therapy is often limited to a maximum of 48 hours.

The nurse should observe the woman for side effects such as nausea, vomiting, and rash. Because indomethacin can prolong bleeding time, the nurse observes for abnormal bleeding, such as prolonged bleeding from injections and bruising with no apparent cause. The antipyretic effect of indomethacin can mask infection because fever may not be present. Checking the height of the fundus at the beginning of therapy and daily thereafter helps identify reduced amniotic fluid. Fetal movements may slow and fetal heart accelerations with fetal movements may decrease if the fetal condition deteriorates.

**Calcium Antagonists.** Nifedipine (Procardia) is a calcium channel blocker usually given for problems such as hypertension. Calcium is essential for muscle contraction in smooth muscles such as the uterus, so blocking calcium reduces the muscular contraction. Flushing of the skin, headache, and a transient increase in the maternal and fetal heart rates are common side effects. Because nifedipine is a vasodilator, the woman may have postural hypotension.

The nurse should observe for side effects of nifedipine and report a maternal pulse greater than 110. The woman should be assisted when sitting or standing and should do so gradually to reduce the effects of postural hypotension.

#### ACCELERATING FETAL LUNG MATURITY

The physician may order corticosteroids to speed fetal lung maturation if preterm birth seems inevitable. Steroid therapy may reduce the incidence and severity of RDS in the preterm infant. Evidence also suggests that steroids given before preterm birth reduce mortality and decrease the incidence of intraventricular hemorrhage and necrotizing enterocolitis. Betamethasone and dexamethasone are common drugs for this purpose.

Corticosteroids are indicated if the woman is between 24 and 34 weeks' gestation because of the high incidence of RDS at this age. For greatest benefit in reducing RDS, birth must occur no sooner than 24 hours after beginning the drug but within 7 days. Evidence shows that birth within 24 hours offers some benefits to the infant, so steroids are recommended unless birth is imminent. Although the National Institutes of Health concluded that steroids are beneficial for women with ruptured membranes between 24 and 32 weeks, the American College of Obstetricians and Gynecologists (1995c) recommends further study of this issue. Repeat steroid doses may be given if birth does not occur within 7 days (up to 34 weeks of gestation), although further study is needed to determine if repeat dosing is safe and effective.

The nurse should observe for and teach the woman signs of pulmonary edema because corticosteroids can cause sodium retention with accompanying fluid retention. The nurse assesses lung sounds with other vital signs. The woman is taught to

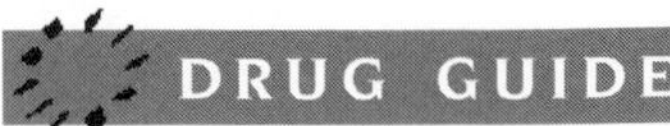

## BETAMETHASONE DEXAMETHASONE

***Classification:*** Corticosteroids

***Indications:*** Acceleration of fetal lung maturity to reduce the incidence and severity of respiratory distress syndrome. Studies suggest that antenatal steroids can also reduce the incidence of intraventricular hemorrhage and necrotizing enterocolitis in the preterm infant. Greatest benefits accrue if at least 24 hours elapse between the initial dose and birth of the preterm infant, but the drug is indicated if birth is not actually imminent.

***Dosage and Route:*** *Betamethasone*: 12 mg IM for two doses, 24 hours apart
*Dexamethasone*: 6 mg IM every 12 hours for four doses

The doses may be repeated if birth has not occurred within 7 days.

***Absorption:*** Rapid and complete after IM administration

***Excretion:*** Metabolized in the liver. Excreted in urine.

***Contraindications:*** Active infection, such as chorioamnionitis, is a relative contraindication, although further study is needed. The National Institutes of Health recommend use of corticosteroids for the woman who has preterm rupture of the membranes (24 to 32 weeks' gestation), but the American College of Obstetricians and Gynecologists has not yet endorsed this recommendation.

***Precautions:*** Possible infection. Pregnancies complicated by diabetes.

***Adverse Reactions:*** Few, owing to the short-term use of the drug. Pulmonary edema is possible secondary to sodium and fluid retention.

***Nursing Considerations:*** Explain the potential benefits of corticosteroid administration to the preterm neonate. Explain that the drug cannot prevent or lessen the severity of all complications of prematurity. If the woman is diabetic, explain that more frequent blood glucose determinations are common because these levels are often slightly higher. Assess lung sounds. Report chest pain or heaviness or dyspnea.

report any chest pain or heaviness or any difficulty breathing.

### CHECK YOUR READING

14. What symptoms of preterm labor should be taught to women at risk?
15. Why is it important to identify preterm labor early?
16. What four drugs may be used to stop preterm labor contractions?
17. What is the purpose of giving corticosteroids to a woman who is in preterm labor at 27 weeks' gestation? Why is it important that birth be delayed at least 24 hours?

# Application of Nursing Process: Preterm Labor

Nursing care for the woman experiencing preterm labor often includes interventions related to tocolytic, corticosteroid, or antibiotic drug therapy. If labor cannot be halted, care is similar to that for other laboring women, with additional care to prepare for a preterm infant's needs at birth. Support for anticipatory grieving may be needed if the infant is very immature and is expected to die.

Care for the family when an extremely preterm infant (20 to 25 weeks' gestation) is expected to be born can be heavily laden with ethical and legal issues. For example, if labor cannot be halted, should fetal monitoring be used if fetal survival is unlikely? If no intervention is done for a nonreassuring pattern, it can distress parents and caregivers alike. On the other hand, knowledge of the fetal response to labor helps the neonatologist make better decisions about how to treat the infant. In addition, ultrasound estimates of gestational age have considerable variation at this time. A fetus presumed to be 24 weeks of gestation before birth may be assessed to be 26 weeks after birth and thus suited to more aggressive treatment than was planned.

Much of the general nursing care for a woman having preterm labor also applies to women experiencing other types of high-risk pregnancies. Women may need multiple hospitalizations, and these may occur in the middle of the night, disrupting sleep and family routines. These women often have some activity restriction and may have to stop working. Therefore, this section focuses on the family's psychosocial concerns, management of home care, and the woman's boredom.

## Psychosocial Concerns

### Assessment

The entire family is affected by stressors associated with a complicated pregnancy. Assess how the woman and her family usually cope with crisis situations and how they are coping with this one. Identify their greatest concerns to prioritize care. For example, the nurse might say, "This development in your pregnancy must have been a shock. How are you handling things? What concerns you the most right now?"

The woman or her family may have physical, emotional, and cognitive impairments because of the unexpected problems. Physical signs of emotional distress, such as tremulousness, palpitations, and restlessness, are also side effects of β-adrenergic drugs. The woman may express fear, helplessness, or disbelief. She may be irritable and tearful. Her ability to concentrate may be impaired at a time when she needs to absorb new information.

Her partner often feels at loose ends. He struggles to keep the household running if she must be inactive. Young children pick up on their parents' anxiety and may misbehave or regress.

The family may be under financial strain. The woman must often curtail or stop working. If she does not have sick time or other benefits, the family sustains an abrupt drop in income at a time when medical expenses are mounting.

Overlaid on the sudden change in lifestyle is the family's concern for fetal well-being. A woman may feel pulled in opposite directions by the needs of all her children—those already born and the fetus she is trying to mature. She may be concerned about the effects of drug therapy on the fetus and on her own body.

### Analysis

The unexpected development of complications during pregnancy can prevent a woman and her family from using their normal coping mechanisms. Therefore, the nursing diagnosis selected is Anxiety related to uncertain outcome of the pregnancy, disruption of family relationships, and financial concerns.

### Planning

The outcome of any pregnancy is never certain, and this is especially true when the pregnancy is a high-risk one for any reason. Goals focus on the family's ability to cope with the crisis of preterm labor. An appropriate goal is: The family will identify methods to cope with the temporary disruption in their lives.

### Interventions

#### PROVIDING INFORMATION

Knowledge decreases anxiety and fear related to the unknown. Include appropriate family members so that they are more likely to be supportive. Determine what the woman knows about preterm birth and about the specific therapy that is recommended. Determine what information the parents need about problems that a preterm infant may face. Use this opportunity to correct misinformation and reinforce accurate information.

## Nursing Care Plan 27–1
## Preterm Labor

**ASSESSMENT:** Rhonda Ellis is a 28-year-old gravida IV, para III. Her first child was born at 40 weeks of gestation, the second at 28 weeks, and the third at 32 weeks. Her oldest child is a second grader, the second is 4 years old, and the youngest is 18 months old. She is having her regular prenatal appointment today at 12 weeks of gestation. Her pregnancy has progressed normally, with normal weight gain. Rhonda tells the nurse she and her husband, Carl, are anxious to avoid having another premature baby.

**NURSING DIAGNOSIS:** Health Seeking Behaviors related to Rhonda's expressed desire for a full-term pregnancy

**GOALS/EXPECTED OUTCOMES**

At the end of teaching, Rhonda will restate the following:

1. Actions that may prevent preterm labor.
2. Signs and symptoms that suggest early preterm labor.
3. What to do if she has symptoms of preterm labor.

| INTERVENTION | RATIONALE |
|---|---|
| 1. Ask Rhonda what she already knows about preterm labor related to her previous experience. For example,<br>a. How long pregnancy should last for the baby to have minimal problems.<br>b. How serious she believes preterm labor and birth are and her beliefs about the causes of preterm labor.<br>c. How likely preterm labor is to recur.<br>d. Whether preterm labor can be detected and stopped.<br>e. What measures she used to try to stop it previously and their effectiveness. | 1. Knowledge is best retained if it is related to something the learner already knows and if the learner is motivated to learn. Relating it to the woman's previous experience with preterm labor and birth helps identify her individual perceptions of and beliefs about her situation. |

Nursing Care Plan continued on following page

## Nursing Care Plan 27–1 *Continued*

# Preterm Labor

**INTERVENTION**

2. Discuss methods to prevent preterm labor that are appropriate for Rhonda's present situation. Examples are to
   a. Avoid physically or psychologically stressful activities.
   b. Plan several rest periods during the day.
   c. Eat a well-balanced diet so that she gains about 1 pound per week.
   d. Drink eight large glasses of fluid each day, excluding caffeine-containing beverages.
   e. Avoid excessive breast stimulation during sexual activity or bathing.
   f. If preterm contractions do occur, sexual activity should stop.

**RATIONALE**

2. Rhonda is in a high-risk group because she has already had two preterm infants. Prevention focuses on usual health-promoting activities, with preparation for other restrictions that may be needed.
   a. Physical or psychological stress increases the risk for preterm labor. Rhonda has three young children, including two preschoolers.
   b. Rest promotes uterine blood flow and relieves some of the stress of everyday life.
   c. A high-quality diet and adequate weight gain have a positive effect on pregnancy outcomes. Low prepregnancy weight and inadequate weight gain are associated with preterm labor and birth.
   d. Dehydration causes the pituitary to secrete antidiuretic hormone. Oxytocin, a stimulant of uterine activity, may be released along with it. Adequate hydration reduces the risk for urinary tract infection.
   e. Breast stimulation may cause release of oxytocin from the posterior pituitary.
   f. Sexual activity can cause orgasm and semen contains prostaglandins, both of which may stimulate contractions.

---

**INTERVENTION**

3. Ask Rhonda how labor started in her other preterm births and how these differed from her term birth. Explain that she should promptly go to the hospital if she has any of these signs and symptoms of preterm labor:
   a. Uterine contractions, painful or painless. These may feel like the baby is "balling up"
   b. Cramping similar to menstrual cramps
   c. A constant backache
   d. A sensation of pelvic pressure or thigh pain
   e. A change or increase in vaginal discharge
   f. Abdominal or intestinal cramps, with or without diarrhea
   g. A sense of "feeling bad" or that something is not quite right

**RATIONALE**

3. Symptoms of early preterm labor are often vague and not as obvious as signs of early term labor. If preterm labor is considered as a possible cause for the symptoms, a woman is more likely to seek early therapy to halt it.

---

**INTERVENTION**

4. Teach Rhonda signs of a urinary tract infection:
   a. Fever (either low or high)
   b. Burning or pain on urination
   c. Unusual urinary frequency
   d. Flank pain
   e. Strong-smelling or cloudy urine

**RATIONALE**

4. Urinary tract infection is associated with preterm labor. Treatment of the infection improves effectiveness of other measures to halt preterm labor and birth.

**EVALUATION**

Rhonda already knows about the need for rest but acknowledges that this is difficult with small children. She tries to eat a well-balancd diet but is often rushed during meals because of the demands of her family. She dislikes water and prefers colas but says she will try to drink more water and fewer caffeinated drinks. Rhonda discusses several early symptoms of preterm labor, including those she had with her other pregnancies. She says she will come to the hospital right away if she suspects preterm labor.

**ASSESSMENT:** Rhonda has mild cramping and pelvic pressure at 28 weeks and comes to the hospital right away. The physician does a speculum examination of her cervix and finds that it is dilated 1 to 2 cm and is beginning to efface. She responds to intravenous magnesium sulfate to stop her contractions. The physician also orders betamethasone, 12 mg, IM for two doses, 24 hours apart. After her contractions stop, Rhonda is started on oral terbutaline to maintain tocolysis and will be discharged home in 48 hours if no recurrent symptoms develop.

## *Nursing Care Plan 27–1 Continued*
# *Preterm Labor*

**Critical Thinking**

What should you tell Rhonda about each of these drugs?

**Answer**

Explain that magnesium sulfate is eliminated by the kidneys, so you will be measuring her urine output to be sure it is adequate. Tell her that you will be checking her reflexes and vital signs to identify toxicity if it develops. Serum magnesium levels are often assessed as well.

Because Rhonda's fetus is likely to have significant respiratory and other problems if born at this early gestation, explain that the use of corticosteroids, such as betamethasone, help speed fetal lung maturity.

Tell Rhonda that she will notice a faster heart rate when taking terbutaline. Tell her that the drug tends to increase her glucose level and reduce her potassium level, so checks of these substances may be done if she needs long-term terbutaline therapy.

The physician recommends that she remain on modified bed rest in a semi-Fowler position for much of the day. She may be up for meals, showering, and use of the restroom. She says she is worried about how she will care for her three children. Her mother-in-law lives nearby but works part-time.

**NURSING DIAGNOSIS:** Impaired Home Maintenance Management related to activity restrictions and family demands

**GOAL/EXPECTED OUTCOME**

By hospital discharge, Rhonda will relate ways that she can maintain prescribed activity restrictions.

| INTERVENTION | RATIONALE |
|---|---|
| 1. Assess what support systems are available and financially feasible to help Rhonda with child care and transportation, such as daycare, mother's day out programs at churches, family, and friends. | 1. Responsibilities for other children may impede a woman's ability to maintain activity limits. Coordination among several resources helps provide all-day coverage for child care. |
| 2. Encourage Rhonda to temporarily lower her standards for home management:<br>a. Eat nourishing take-out or fast food.<br>b. Prioritize household tasks that must be done.<br>c. Let her children do tasks that are within their abilities.<br>d. Make lists of tasks that need to be done for different people who will be available to help her. | 2. Many usual roles must be reallocated during this time. Having alternative arrangements increases the chance that the woman can maintain therapy. |
| 3. Encourage Rhonda to accept help from others. Remind her that this situation is temporary and that she may be able to help someone else at another time. | 3. If a woman feels that she can help others at another time, she may be more willing to accept help when she needs it. |

**EVALUATION**

Rhonda identifies three friends in addition to her mother-in-law who may be able to help with child care. She says she cannot afford to continue sending her children to their daycare center if she is not working. She feels that if her children are cared for, her husband can handle her home management needs.

**ASSESSMENT:** At 31 weeks' gestation, Rhonda again experiences preterm labor and goes to the hospital. Her cervix is dilated 2 to 3 cm and is 75 percent effaced (about 0.5 cm long). Her contractions occur every 6 to 7 minutes, lasting about 20 to 30 seconds each. The physician again orders a magnesium sulfate infusion and betamethasone injections. The physician explains that preterm birth may be delayed but will probably occur within the next 24 to 48 hours. Rhonda begins crying, and says, "I did what I was supposed to do and now I'm still going to have another preemie! It will be weeks before I can be a real mother!"

**NURSING DIAGNOSIS:** Rhonda will probably lose the experience of a term birth that she has been hoping for and working toward. The nursing diagnosis chosen is Anticipatory Grieving related to loss of expected birth experience.

**GOAL/EXPECTED OUTCOME**

Rhonda will express her feelings about the loss of her expected birth at term.

*Nursing Care Plan continued on following page*

## Nursing Care Plan 27–1 *Continued*
# *Preterm Labor*

| INTERVENTION | RATIONALE |
|---|---|
| 1. Sit down and spend time with Rhonda. Use therapeutic communication to encourage her to express her feelings. | 1. Unhurried time allows expression of feelings, which is the first step in dealing with the anticipated loss. |
| 2. When she has expressed her frustration about this development in her pregnancy, explain that much remains unknown about why labor begins, whether at term, preterm, or postterm. | 2. If a woman knows that professionals do not have all the answers but must make recommendations based on what is known or appears to work for an individual woman, she may be more accepting of the inevitability of preterm birth. |
| 3. Explain that Rhonda's efforts have paid off because she has gained 3 valuable weeks of gestation for her baby. | 3. Knowing that her self-care has benefits, although not the hoped-for term birth, reduces the sense of failure that she may feel. |

**EVALUATION**

Rhonda cries and expresses her frustration about the developments in her pregnancy. She says that she knew she was more likely to have another preterm infant but hoped that this time would be different. As the day goes by, Rhonda gradually begins expressing feelings that she did do something positive for this baby. She begins making specific plans to deal with the probable preterm birth.

**ADDITIONAL NURSING DIAGNOSES TO CONSIDER**

Altered Family Processes
Altered Health Maintenance
Ineffective Individual or Family Coping

Initially, the woman for whom activity restriction is prescribed may be highly motivated to maintain the recommended level of activity. However, because she usually feels well, she may begin to feel lazy and unproductive. Continue to explain how limiting her activity benefits her baby and to affirm that she is indeed doing an important job.

#### PROMOTING EXPRESSION OF CONCERNS

Encourage the woman and her family to express their concerns. Begin by exploring common concerns of women with problem pregnancies. For example, say, "Most women are worried when they have to stop working. How has this affected your family?" An open question gives them a chance to ventilate their feelings so that they can take the next step: identifying constructive methods to cope with the situation. Collaboration with a social worker may identify financial or other community resources available.

#### TEACHING WHAT MAY OCCUR DURING A PRETERM BIRTH

Because preterm birth may occur despite all interventions, a pregnant woman and her partner should be prepared for that possibility. If the hospital has a neonatal intensive care unit, a nurse often visits the parents to explain what might occur if their baby is born early. One or both parents tour the unit to see the equipment and care the infants receive there. A tour of the intensive care nursery may motivate the woman to maintain the recommended therapy to prevent preterm birth.

In hospitals with neonatal intensive care units, one or more neonatal nurses, a neonatal nurse-practitioner, a neonatologist or a combination of these is present at birth to care for the infant. The woman who has planned to give birth in a hospital without a neonatal intensive care unit may be transferred to a facility with this type of unit before the birth to allow immediate care and stabilization of her newborn. The infant may also be transferred after birth if there is no time to transfer the woman before birth or if the infant has more problems than were anticipated. Hospitalization of the mother or infant, or both, at a distant location adds to the stress on the family.

### Evaluation

The goal for this nursing diagnosis is achieved if the woman and her family can identify constructive methods to deal with their anxiety. If a high-risk pregnancy situation is prolonged or if the family has difficulty adapting constructively to the situation, a nursing diagnosis of Altered Family Processes may be more appropriate.

## Management of Home Care

### Assessment

Part of the care of women who have high-risk pregnancies, including a risk for preterm birth, often occurs in their home. Many daily household activities are probably managed by the woman. When she is disabled, even briefly, the usual roles of family members are disrupted.

Determine the level of activity prescribed by the physician and identify the role of each family member. A good way to do this is to have the woman describe a usual day before she had any limitations. Determine the number and ages of children in the home.

Evaluate the home itself, either by visual inspection or by questioning the family. Does the home have more than one level or, if it is an apartment, is it upstairs or downstairs? Determine if a telephone is available for emergency contact.

Evaluate the family's resources and their willingness to use them. Ask whether family members and friends in the area are available to help. Explore local support groups, such as churches or mother-to-mother networks, that the family might contact for assistance. Determine whether insurance covers assistance such as homemaker services.

### Analysis

The diagnosis chosen is Impaired Home Maintenance Management related to change in usual roles and responsibilities.

### Planning

Two goals are appropriate for this nursing diagnosis:

- *Short-term*: The family will identify methods for management of daily household routines.
- *Long-term*: The woman will be able to maintain the prescribed level of activity and drug therapy.

### Interventions

The pregnancy threatened by preterm labor or other complications is a self-limiting situation, making temporary adjustments somewhat easier. Needed changes in home routines may be brief but sometimes extend over several weeks.

#### CARING FOR CHILDREN

The woman who has children has different concerns than the woman who does not. Knowledge of growth and development helps the nurse identify the most appropriate way to ensure adequate care for the children and strengthen family relationships.

Toddlers and preschoolers rarely understand why their mother does not play with them as usual. If they are already in daycare, this may continue if the family can afford it. They may live with a relative or friend temporarily. Toddlers may feel that their parents have abandoned them if they are sent away, although this may be the only realistic solution if no one besides the mother is available to supervise them.

School-aged children usually understand the situation better and are often quite helpful. They may assist with care of other children, but they should not be put into the role of an adult. They may resent responsibility that is excessive for their age.

Adolescents may welcome the trust their parents have in them, but they also may resent the intrusion on independent activities with their peers. Teenagers who drive can be very helpful in taking younger siblings to school and other activities. They may be enlisted for grocery shopping and meal preparation. If resentment flares, the parents and nurse can remind teenagers that the situation is temporary and that they are valuable contributors to the health of the new baby.

#### MAINTAINING THE HOUSEHOLD

The first step to home maintenance during this time may be for the woman to lower her standards of housekeeping. Things may not be as clean or organized as she would like. The partner may take over many household tasks, but these compete with his responsibilities outside the home.

Advise the woman to have a list of tasks ready when friends and family ask, "Can I do anything to help?" If they offer to bring a meal or do laundry, encourage her to accept. Remind her that people who offer to help mean it and that she may be able to return the favor to someone else. Homemaker services may be an option to help the family deal with the woman's temporary disability.

Transportation of school-aged children may be a concern. If no family or friends are available, the school nurse or Parent-Teacher Association (PTA) may help find someone willing to take the children to school each day.

### Evaluation

Goals are met under the following conditions:

- The short-term goal is met if the family can identify how to manage minimum household care.
- The long-term goal is met if she can maintain the prescribed therapy.

# Boredom

## Assessment

If activity is to be restricted, determine what skills the woman has for coping with boredom. Although the benefit of bedrest in prolonging gestation is questionable, there is often at least some reduction in activity prescribed. At first, a prescription for rest may sound wonderful, but after a short while it can become trying.

Ask about a usual day to identify activities that are still appropriate within the restrictions prescribed. Ask about hobbies, present and past. What type of leisure activities does the woman enjoy? Which activities are available or possible? Does she have good alternative places to maintain rest and still give her a change of scenery?

Assess her personality. Is she calm and composed, taking whatever comes with serenity? Or does she need to be busy most of the time? No matter how motivated, the woman who finds inactivity tiresome will find even limited activity restriction difficult to maintain.

## Analysis

The nursing diagnosis is Diversional Activity Deficit related to lack of knowledge about alternative activities.

## Planning

Two goals are appropriate for this nursing diagnosis. The woman will do the following:

- Identify activities that are appropriate for her level of activity restriction.
- Pursue (with help of others) activities to relieve boredom.

## Interventions

### IDENTIFYING APPROPRIATE ACTIVITIES

Determine the woman's understanding about needed activity restrictions to identify misunderstandings and reinforce correct information. Help her identify which usual activities are permitted and which ones should not be done and why. If she understands the rationale, she may be more willing to comply with restrictions.

Some women continue work activities, such as paperwork or phone calls, that can be accomplished while at rest. Workplace deadlines can increase stress, even if she works at home. However, the feeling of usefulness gained by such activities may be beneficial because she is willing to maintain activity restrictions. Moreover, work-related activities can help reduce some of the family's financial concerns.

Suggest activities to help women keep busy and productive. These may include household activities that can be done at rest, volunteering for activities such as phone calls, and leisure activities, such as puzzles, games, and hand needlework. Help her identify someone who can obtain the necessary supplies for her. This might be a good time to reactivate an old (quiet) hobby.

The woman can participate in some activities with her children while she is in bed. She can read to them and play board or card games. Encourage her to help the children with their homework and stimulate their development with thought-provoking discussions.

### CHANGING THE PHYSICAL SURROUNDINGS

Encourage the woman to identify at least two areas where she can maintain her prescribed rest. This gives her a change of scene and helps her feel more a part of the family activities. Each area should include pillows, blankets, and a clipboard with writing materials. An adjustable ironing board can provide a movable table for her things, and a shoe bag helps keep supplies organized and at hand. Ideally, the telephone is within reach or is cordless and she has a television with a remote control unit.

## Evaluation

The first goal is short term and may be met when activity restrictions are first instituted if the woman can accurately discriminate between appropriate and inappropriate activities. The second goal is met over time if she actually pursues only appropriate activities.

# Prolonged Pregnancy

A prolonged pregnancy is one that lasts longer than 42 weeks. Many apparent cases of prolonged pregnancy may be only miscalculation of the estimated date of delivery (EDD) because the woman has had irregular menstrual periods or has forgotten the date of her last normal one. Late prenatal care limits the use of clinical methods such as ultrasonography, which might otherwise be used to pinpoint her EDD.

## Complications

The main physical risk in prolonged pregnancy is to the fetus or newborn. Insufficiency of the placental function secondary to aging and infarction reduces transfer of oxygen and nutrients to the fetus and removal of waste. Because the fetus with placental insufficiency has less reserve to tolerate uterine contractions, signs of fetal compromise, such as late decelerations and decreased variability, may develop during labor. In addition, reduced amniotic fluid volume (oligohydramnios) that often accompanies placental insufficiency can result in umbilical cord compression. Meconium in the amniotic fluid may cause respiratory distress in the newborn if it is aspirated before or during birth. The infant may be growth-restricted and may appear to have lost weight.

Many postterm fetuses do not suffer from placental insufficiency and may continue growing. The woman and fetus then may have complications related to dysfunctional labor, inadequate postpartum uterine contraction to control bleeding, and injury if the birth is traumatic.

Psychologically, the woman often feels as if her pregnancy will never end. She may fear induction of labor, a possible cesarean birth, and problems with her baby. The added fatigue imposed by prolonged pregnancy diminishes her resources for tolerating the added stress and anxiety.

### Therapeutic Management

Therapeutic management begins with determination of the true gestation with the greatest accuracy possible. If a woman did not have early prenatal care, several markers used to pinpoint gestation, such as ultrasonography, fundal height measurements, dates of quickening, and first auscultation of the fetal heart tones with a nonamplified fetoscope, may be lost. Also, the woman may have forgotten her last menstrual period date.

Another factor in management decisions is whether the fetus is thriving in the uterus. If antepartum tests, such as a biophysical profile, indicate that the fetus is doing well, the birth attendant can take a more conservative approach than if the fetus is suffering from reduced placental function.

If the gestation appears to be truly postterm and there is no fetal urgency to deliver quickly, management depends on whether the cervix is favorable for induction of labor. If the cervix is favorable for induction, that is usually begun. If the cervix is not favorable, the physician may take a "wait and see" approach, repeating fetal surveillance tests as needed. Or the woman may have a cervical ripening procedure (see Chapter 16) to make the cervix more favorable for induction.

### Nursing Considerations

Nursing care for the woman with a prolonged pregnancy is tied to the management chosen. The nurse's role may include the following:

- Teaching about procedures, such as antepartum testing or induction of labor
- Support for her psychological and physical fatigue
- Nursing care related to specific procedures, such as induction of labor

## Intrapartum Emergencies

### Placental Abnormalities

Women with placental abnormalities (see p. 682) may experience hemorrhage during the antepartum or intrapartum period. Placenta previa is sometimes associated with an abnormally adherent placenta (placenta accreta). Placenta accreta may cause immediate or delayed hemorrhage immediately after birth because the placenta does not separate cleanly, often leaving small fragments that prevent full uterine contraction. More extreme degrees of abnormal adherence occur when the placenta penetrates the uterine muscle itself (placenta increta) or even all the way through the uterus (placenta percreta). All or only part of the placenta may be involved. A hysterectomy is often required if a large portion of the placenta is abnormally adherent.

### Prolapsed Umbilical Cord

A prolapsed umbilical cord slips downward after the membranes rupture, subjecting it to compression between the fetus and pelvis (Fig. 27–7). It may slip down immediately with the fluid gush or long after the membranes rupture. Interruption in blood flow through the cord interferes with fetal oxygenation and is potentially fatal.

#### CAUSES

Prolapse of the umbilical cord is more likely when the fit is poor between the fetal presenting part and the maternal pelvis. When the fit is good, the fetus fills up the pelvis, leaving little room for the cord to slip down. Although prolapse of the cord is possible during any labor, it is more likely if these conditions are present:

- A fetus that remains at a high station
- A very small fetus
- Breech presentations (the footling breech is more likely to be complicated by a prolapsed cord because the feet and legs are small and do not fill the pelvis well)
- Transverse lie
- Hydramnios (often associated with abnormal presentations; also, the unusually large amount of fluid exerts more pressure to push the cord out)

#### SIGNS OF PROLAPSE

Prolapse may be complete, with the cord visible at the vaginal opening. A prolapsed cord may not be

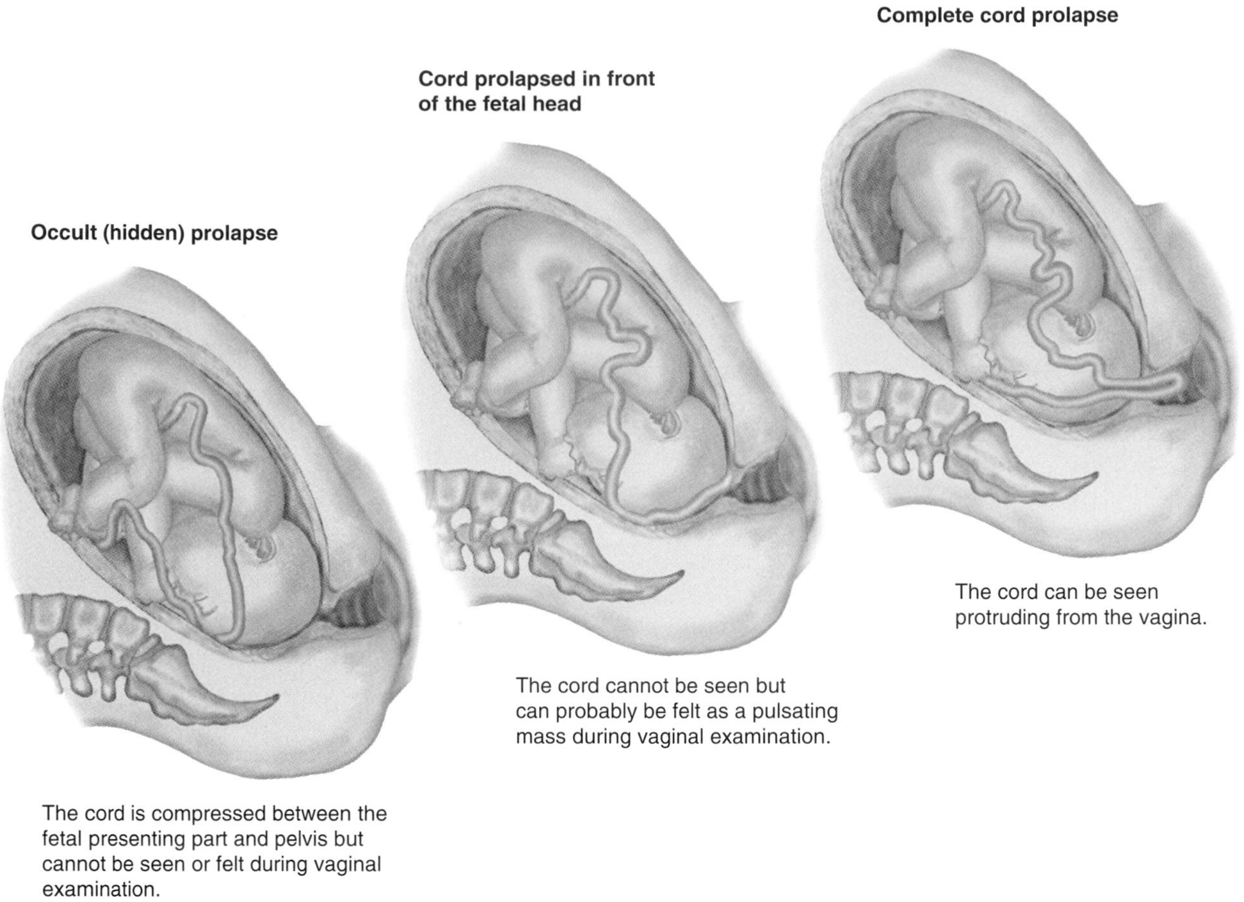

Occult (hidden) prolapse

The cord is compressed between the fetal presenting part and pelvis but cannot be seen or felt during vaginal examination.

Cord prolapsed in front of the fetal head

The cord cannot be seen but can probably be felt as a pulsating mass during vaginal examination.

Complete cord prolapse

The cord can be seen protruding from the vagina.

**FIGURE 27–7**

Variations of prolapsed umbilical cord.

visible but may be palpated on vaginal examination as it pulsates synchronously with the fetal heart. An occult prolapse of the cord is one in which the cord slips alongside the fetal head or shoulders. The prolapse cannot be palpated or seen but is suspected because of changes in the FHR, such as bradycardia or variable decelerations.

### THERAPEUTIC MANAGEMENT

Medical and nursing management often overlap, as they do in many emergency situations. Either the nurse or the birth attendant may be the first to discover umbilical cord prolapse. Birth is almost always cesarean unless vaginal delivery can be accomplished more quickly and less traumatically.

When cord prolapse occurs, the priority is to relieve pressure on the cord to restore blood flow through it until delivery. None of these interventions should delay the promptest possible delivery. Push the call light to summon help. Others should call the physician and prepare for birth. Notify the neonatal nurses and pediatrician and prepare for possible neonatal resuscitation.

Prompt actions are taken to relieve cord compression and increase fetal oxygenation:

1. Position the woman's hips higher than her head to shift the fetal presenting part toward her diaphragm. Any of these methods (Fig. 27–8) may be used:
   a. Knee-chest position
   b. Trendelenburg position
   c. Hips elevated with pillows, with side-lying position maintained
2. With a gloved hand, push the fetal presenting part upward. Maintain this position until the

## Critical to Remember

**FACTORS THAT INCREASE A WOMAN'S RISK FOR A PROLAPSED UMBILICAL CORD**

Ruptured membranes *and*

- The fetal presenting part at a high station
- A fetus that poorly fits the pelvic inlet because of small size or abnormal presentation
- Excessive volume of amniotic fluid (hydramnios)

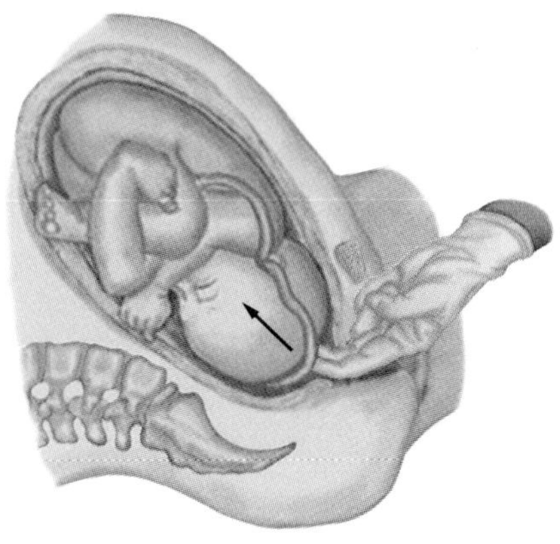

A gloved hand in the vagina pushes the fetus upward and off the cord.


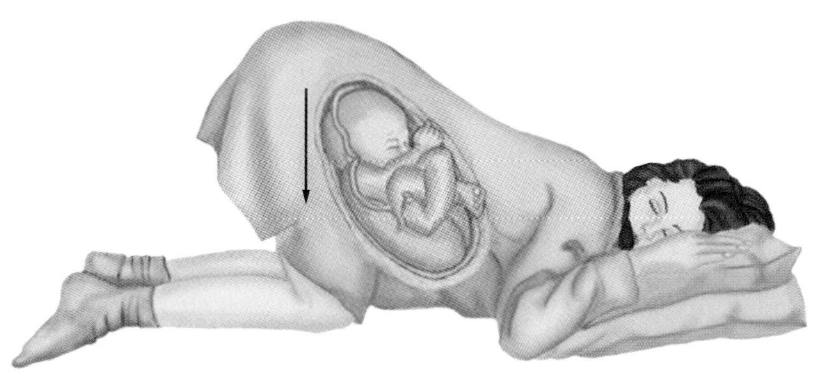

Knee-chest position uses gravity to shift the fetus out of the pelvis. The woman's thighs should be at right angles to the bed and her chest flat on the bed.


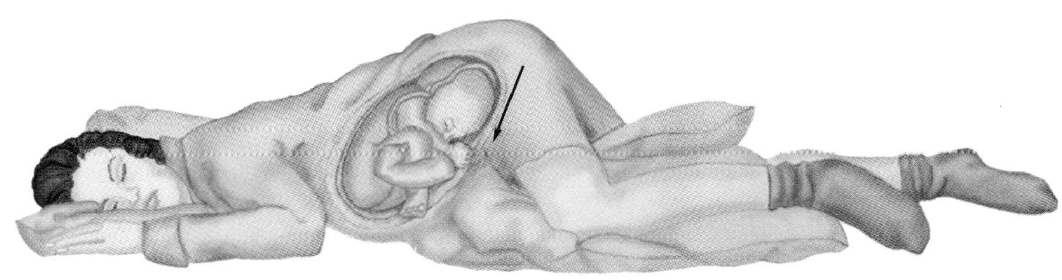

The woman's hips are elevated with two pillows; this is often combined with the Trendelenburg (head down) position.


**FIGURE 27–8**

Measures that may be used to relieve pressure on a prolapsed umbilical cord until delivery can take place.

physician orders it stopped, which may not be until a cesarean incision is made.

Give oxygen at 8 to 10 liters per minute by face mask to increase maternal blood oxygen saturation, making more available for the fetus.

Other actions may enhance fetal oxygenation, but prompt delivery is the priority and often no time remains for these measures. A tocolytic drug, such as terbutaline, may be ordered to inhibit contractions, increasing placental blood flow and reducing intermittent pressure of the fetus against the pelvis and cord. Warm saline-moistened towels retard cooling and drying of the cord. If the cord is protruding from the vagina, no attempt should be made to replace it because to do so could traumatize it and further reduce blood flow through it.

Prognosis for the woman is good because the only additional risks are those associated with cesarean birth. Prognosis for the infant depends on how long and how severely blood flow through the cord has been impaired. With prompt recognition and corrective actions, the infant usually does well.

#### NURSING CONSIDERATIONS

In addition to prompt corrective actions, the nurse must consider the woman's anxiety. The nurse must remain calm during this time and acknowledge the woman's anxiety. Explanations must be simple because anxiety interferes with the woman's ability to comprehend them. Her partner and family should be included as much as possible.

### Uterine Rupture

Sometimes a tear in the wall of the uterus occurs because the uterus cannot withstand the pressure against it (Fig. 27–9). There are three variations of uterine rupture:

**Complete rupture** a direct communication between the uterine and peritoneal cavities.

**Incomplete rupture** rupture into the peritoneum covering the uterus or into the broad ligament but not into the peritoneal cavity.

**Dehiscence** a partial separation of an old uterine scar. There may be little or no bleeding. There

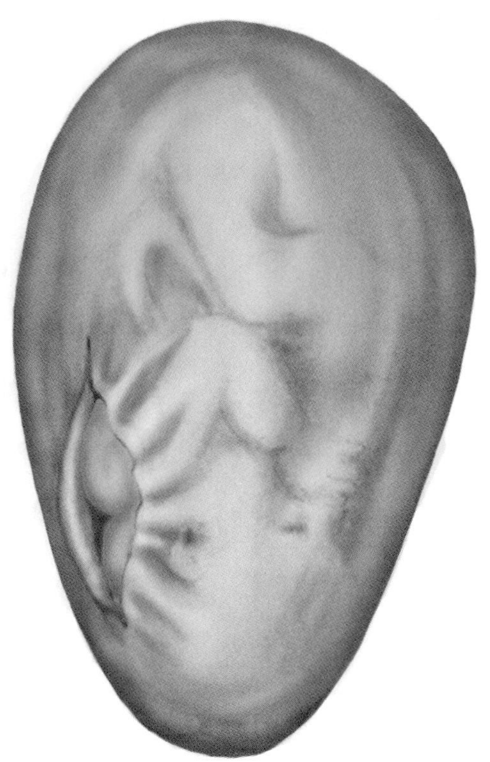

**FIGURE 27-9**

Uterine rupture in the lower uterine segment.

may be no signs or symptoms, and the rupture ("window") may be found incidentally during a subsequent cesarean birth or other abdominal surgery.

### CAUSES

Although uterine rupture is rare, dehiscence is not unusual. Uterine rupture is associated with previous uterine surgery, such as cesarean birth or surgery to remove fibroids. The risk for rupture in a woman who has had a prior cesarean birth depends on the type of uterine incision. The risk for rupture is greater in women with a classic incision (vertical into the upper uterine segment) than in women with a low transverse incision. For this reason, vaginal birth after cesarean is not recommended for women who have had a previous classic cesarean birth.

Rupture of the unscarred uterus is more likely for women of high parity with a thin uterine wall, women sustaining blunt abdominal trauma, and women having intense contractions, especially if fetopelvic disproportion is present. Excessively strong contractions (hypertonic) may cause the intrauterine pressure to exceed the tensile strength of the uterine wall. If the fetus cannot be expelled downward through the pelvis, contractions may push it through the lower uterine segment. Intense contractions are more likely to occur when oxytocin is administered for induction or augmentation of labor, but they also may occur spontaneously.

### SIGNS AND SYMPTOMS

Dehiscence does not have symptoms initially and may not interfere with labor or vaginal delivery if the area is small. However, labor progress may stop because the open area prevents efficient expulsion of the fetus. Intrauterine pressures may have little change during contractions. A larger area of dehiscence may cause abdominal pain that persists despite analgesia.

Manifestations of uterine rupture vary with the degree of rupture and may mimic other complications. Possible signs and symptoms of uterine rupture are as follows:

- Abdominal pain and tenderness. The pain may not be severe; it may occur suddenly at the peak of a contraction. The woman may describe a feeling that something "ripped."
- Chest pain, pain between the scapulae, or pain on inspiration. Pain occurs because of the irritation of blood below the woman's diaphragm.
- Hypovolemic shock caused by hemorrhage: falling blood pressure, tachycardia, tachypnea, pallor, cool and clammy skin, anxiety. Signs of shock may not occur until after birth.
- Signs associated with impaired fetal oxygenation, such as late decelerations, reduced variability, tachycardia, and bradycardia.
- Absent fetal heart tones with a large disruption of the placenta.
- Cessation of uterine contractions.
- Palpation of the fetus outside the uterus (usually occurs only with a large, complete rupture). The fetus is likely to be dead.

If the rupture is incomplete, blood loss is slower and signs of shock, chest pain, or intrascapular pain may be delayed. Complete rupture results in massive blood loss. Signs of shock and pain develop quickly. External bleeding may not be impressive, because most of the blood is lost into the peritoneal cavity.

### THERAPEUTIC MANAGEMENT

Initial management is to stabilize the woman and fetus and to perform cesarean delivery. If the rupture is small and the woman wants other children, it may be repaired. A woman with a large uterine rupture requires hysterectomy. Blood is replaced if needed.

### NURSING CONSIDERATIONS

The nurse must be aware of women who are at increased risk for uterine rupture and must stay alert for the signs and symptoms. Administer oxytocin cautiously to reduce the likelihood of excessive contractions. The nurse must keep in mind that hypertonic contractions can occur in either a stimulated or an unstimulated labor. Notify the birth attendant if hypertonic contractions occur. A tocolytic drug may be ordered to reduce the intensity of hypertonic contractions.

Uterine rupture may not be detected before birth. If postpartum bleeding is excessive and the fundus is firm, injury to the birth canal, including uterine rupture, is possible. Bleeding may be concealed if the ruptured area bleeds into the broad ligament. In this case, signs of hypovolemic shock are likely to develop quickly.

## Uterine Inversion

An inversion occurs when the uterus completely or partly turns inside out, usually during the third stage of labor. Such an event is uncommon but potentially fatal.

### CAUSES

Often no single cause is identified. Predisposing factors are as follows.

- Pulling on the umbilical cord before the placenta detaches from the uterine wall
- Fundal pressure during birth
- Fundal pressure on an incompletely contracted uterus after birth
- Increased intra-abdominal pressure
- An abnormally adherent placenta
- Congenital weakness of the uterine wall
- Fundal placenta implantation

### SIGNS AND SYMPTOMS

The birth attendant notes that the uterus is either absent from the abdomen or a depression in the fundal area is present. The interior of the uterus may be seen through the cervix or protruding into the vagina. Massive hemorrhage, shock, and pain quickly become evident. The woman has severe pelvic pain.

### MANAGEMENT

Quick action by nursing and medical personnel is required to reduce maternal morbidity and mortality. The physician tries to replace the uterus through the vagina into a normal position. If that is not possible, laparotomy with replacement is done. Hysterectomy may be required.

Two intravenous lines are established to allow rapid fluid and blood replacement. General anesthesia or a tocolytic drug is often needed to relax the uterus enough to replace it. After the uterus is replaced, oxytocin is given to contract the uterus and control blood loss. *Oxytocin is not given until the uterus is repositioned to avoid trapping the inverted fundus in the cervix.*

### NURSING CONSIDERATIONS

Nursing care during the emergency supplements that of other staff members. Postpartum nursing care is directed toward observing and maintaining maternal blood volume and correcting shock. The woman may be transferred to the intensive care unit.

Assess the uterine fundus for firmness, height, and deviation from the midline. Assess vital signs every 15 minutes or more frequently until stable, then according to recovery room routine. Observe for tachycardia and a falling blood pressure, which are associated with shock. A cardiac monitor identifies dysrhythmias, which may occur with shock. Invasive hemodynamic monitoring is common.

An indwelling catheter is often inserted to observe fluid balance and to keep the bladder empty so that the uterus can contract well. Assess the catheter for patency, and record intake and output. Urine output should be at least 30 ml per hour. A fall in urine output may indicate hypovolemia or an obstructed catheter.

The woman is allowed nothing by mouth until her condition is stable. She can usually receive fluids and progress to solid foods quickly because uterine inversion does not usually recur. However, it may recur in a future pregnancy if conditions favor its development.

## Amniotic Fluid Embolism

Amniotic fluid embolism occurs when amniotic fluid is drawn into the maternal circulation and carried to the woman's lungs. Fetal particulate matter (skin cells, vernix, hair, meconium) in the fluid obstructs pulmonary vessels. Abrupt respiratory distress, heart failure, and circulatory collapse occur. Disseminated intravascular coagulation (see p. 675) is likely because thromboplastin-rich amniotic fluid interferes with normal blood clotting. This infrequent disorder is often fatal. Survivors may have neurologic deficits.

Amniotic fluid embolism is more likely when the labor is very strong. High intrauterine pressure forces amniotic fluid into open uterine or cervical veins. Meconium that often accompanies a stressed fetus in such a labor adds to the particulate matter forced into the woman's circulation and increases the likelihood of death from this embolism.

Therapeutic management of amniotic fluid embolism is primarily medical and includes the following:

- Cardiopulmonary resuscitation
- Oxygen with mechanical ventilation
- Blood transfusion
- Correction of coagulation deficits with platelets or fibrinogen

**✓ CHECK YOUR READING**

18. What are three risks to the fetus or neonate when pregnancy lasts longer than 42 weeks?

19. What is the immediate management if prolapse of the umbilical cord occurs?
20. How can oxytocin-stimulated contractions increase the risk for uterine rupture?
21. What are the primary complications of a uterine inversion? How are they managed?
22. Under what circumstances does a woman have an increased risk for amniotic fluid embolism?

## Trauma

Most trauma during pregnancy occurs because of accidents, assault, or suicide. Battering is a significant cause of maternal-fetal trauma during pregnancy. (The social and emotional issues of battering are addressed in Chapter 24.) Trauma may be blunt, such as that sustained in an automobile accident, or penetrating, such as gunshot and knife wounds. Burns and electrical injuries also may occur.

Although fetal injury may not be fatal, later neurologic deficits are sometimes found. Direct fetal trauma, such as skull fracture or intracranial hemorrhage, may occur from pelvic fracture, penetrating wounds, or blunt trauma. Indirect causes of fetal injury or death include abruptio placentae and disruption of the placental blood flow secondary to maternal hypovolemia or uterine rupture. The most common cause of fetal death is death of the mother.

Anatomic and physiologic changes of pregnancy make trauma care unique. During early pregnancy, the uterus is surrounded by the pelvis and is well protected from direct damage. As the uterus grows, it protrudes and becomes a large target for trauma. At the same time, it acts as a shield for other maternal organs such as the kidneys, often protecting them from direct trauma.

Normal alterations of pregnancy can affect the maternal and fetal outcomes after traumatic injury and can affect interpretation of diagnostic studies that may be done. Pregnant women have greater blood volume than non-pregnant women, which gives them a cushion against blood loss. However, the fetus may suffer if the woman hemorrhages because maternal blood is diverted from the placenta. This can lead to fetal hypoxia, acidosis, and death of the fetus.

Maternal fibrinogen levels are higher during pregnancy (300 to 600 mg/dl). A decrease to lower levels is associated with abruptio placentae and may indicate that disseminated intravascular coagulation is developing.

### MANAGEMENT

Care of the pregnant trauma victim first focuses on injuries that threaten her life. Management of the fetus depends on whether the fetus is living and on the gestational age. The fetus may be delivered by cesarean birth if it is mature enough to survive and if the maternal or fetal condition is likely to be improved by prompt delivery. The fetus that is dead or too immature to survive is not usually delivered unless birth can improve the outcome for the mother.

### NURSING CONSIDERATIONS

Nursing care of the pregnant trauma victim also focuses first on maternal, then fetal stabilization. A wedge is placed under one side to prevent supine hypotension and further hemodynamic instability and to improve placental blood flow. Vital signs are taken as needed, based on her condition. Vital signs and urine output (at least 30 ml per hour) provide information about the adequacy of her blood volume. Bloody urine suggests bladder or renal damage. Other nursing care is directed toward care of her specific injuries and implementation of medical care.

Signs suggesting abruptio placentae (vaginal bleeding with uterine pain and tenderness) should be reported because this complication may occur with abdominal trauma. The uterine height may also increase as the uterus fills with blood.

Once the woman's condition is stable, nursing care intensifies for the fetus. External monitoring is appropriate if the fetus has reached a viable gestational age. Preterm labor may occur but may not be recognized if the woman is unconscious or if pain from injuries overshadows discomfort from contractions. Recurrent restlessness or moaning may accompany contractions. The nurse should palpate the woman's uterus for contractions periodically because they may not be evident on the fetal monitoring strip.

**CHECK YOUR READING**

23. What is the primary focus of medical and nursing care of the pregnant trauma victim?
24. What are common causes of fetal injury and death when a pregnant woman suffers trauma?
25. What are important nursing considerations for each kind of intrapartum emergency: Prolapsed umbilical cord? Uterine rupture? Uterine inversion? Amniotic fluid embolism? Trauma?

## Application of Nursing Process: Intrapartum Emergencies

Nursing care of the woman with an intrapartum emergency overlaps with care in other situations discussed elsewhere. Much of the nursing care is collaborative and supports medical management. Parents may suffer loss if the fetus dies or if the mother loses her ability to bear future children, as may occur with uterine rupture. One problem that is expected in any emergency situation is the emotional distress of the woman and her family.

## Assessment

When an emergency occurs, simply because of its suddenness, the woman and her family have little time to absorb what has happened. In umbilical cord prolapse, for example, labor has often been uneventful up to that point. Suddenly, nurses place the woman in a strange position, apply oxygen, and pull her toward the operating room.

Under such circumstances, the woman and her family have a very narrow focus. They are obviously apprehensive and may lose control. The woman or her partner may be immobilized by fear. Reactions are similar for other emergency situations.

## Analysis

The nursing diagnosis is Anxiety related to sudden development of complications. This diagnosis is expected to differ from the anxiety associated with preterm labor because the onset is acute; the anxiety also may lessen more quickly because the emergency is sometimes resolved quickly.

## Planning

The focus of a goal is very narrow in an emergency situation. Two appropriate goals, during and after the emergency, are that the woman and her family will do the following:

- Indicate an understanding of emergency procedures.
- Express their feelings about the complication.

## Interventions

Although there is little time for discussion, explain honestly and simply what is occurring. Tell the woman what is happening and why to reduce fear and anxiety of the unknown. Include her partner and family if appropriate. Provide continued reassurance and support to the woman because her partner must often be excluded from the emergency or operating room when an emergency occurs.

The infant born in an emergency situation may need resuscitation or other supportive measures. Nurses and a neonatal nurse-practitioner or pediatrician from the neonatal intensive care unit, if there is one, are usually present at the birth to attend the infant. Explain to the family who the other professionals are and what their roles are. If possible, explain what is being done to care for the baby.

After the emergency, give the woman and her family a chance to ask questions. The ability to absorb new knowledge during periods of severe anxiety is very limited. Adequate explanations afterward help them understand and assimilate the experience.

**Although the nurse is usually anxious in an emergency situation too, it is important to keep a calm attitude. The woman and her family quickly pick up on the staff's anxiety, and consequently theirs escalates. Remain with the woman to reduce fears of abandonment. If possible, hold her hand. Speak in a low, calm voice.**

## Evaluation

Evaluation of the goals is probably impossible until the emergency is over and the woman's physical condition stabilizes. Goals for this nursing diagnosis are achieved if the woman and her family do the following:

- Indicate that they understand the problem and the rationale for emergency procedures.
- Express, over several days, their feelings about what has occurred.

## SUMMARY CONCEPTS

- Dysfunctional labor may occur because of abnormalities in the powers, the passenger, the passage, or the psyche. Combinations of abnormalities are common.
- Nursing care in dysfunctional labor focuses on prevention or prompt identification and action to correct additional complications: fetal hypoxia, infection, injury to the mother or fetus, and postpartum hemorrhage.
- Premature rupture of the membranes is associated with infection as both a cause and an effect.
- The early indications of preterm labor are often vague. Prompt identification of preterm labor enables the most effective therapy to delay preterm birth.
- Nursing care for the woman at risk for a very early preterm birth focuses on helping her delay birth long enough to provide time for fetal lung maturation with corticosteroids, allow transfer to a facility that has neonatal intensive care, or reach a gestation at which the infant's problems with immaturity are minimal.
- The main risk in prolonged pregnancy is reduced placental function. This may compromise the fetus during labor and may result in meconium aspiration in the neonate. Dysfunctional labor may occur as a fetus continues growing during the prolonged pregnancy.
- The key intervention for umbilical cord prolapse is to relieve pressure on it and to expedite delivery.
- Be aware of women at risk for uterine rupture, and observe for signs and symptoms: signs of shock, abdominal pain, a sense of tearing, chest pain,

pain between the scapulae, abnormal FHR patterns, cessation of contractions, and palpation of the fetus outside the uterus.
- Uterine inversion is often accompanied by massive blood loss and shock. Recovery care promotes uterine contraction and maintenance of adequate circulating volume.
- Amniotic fluid embolism is more likely to occur when labor is intense and the membranes have ruptured.
- Medical and nursing care of the pregnant trauma victim focuses on stabilization of the mother first. Management of the fetus depends on gestational age and whether the fetus is alive. Abruptio placentae and uterine rupture are obstetric complications that may occur with direct abdominal trauma.

### References and Readings


Abbott, J.T. (1995). Emergency management of the obstetric patient. In G.N. Burrow & T.F. Ferris (Eds.), *Medical complications during pregnancy* (4th ed., pp. 249–263). Philadelphia: W.B. Saunders.

American College of Obstetricians and Gynecologists (ACOG). (1995a). *Technical bulletin no. 196: Operative vaginal delivery*. Washington, D.C.: Author.

American College of Obstetricians and Gynecologists (ACOG). (1995b). *Technical bulletin no. 218: Dystocia and the augmentation of labor*. Washington, D.C.: Author.

American College of Obstetricians and Gynecologists (ACOG). (1995c). *Technical bulletin no. 206: Preterm labor*. Washington, D.C.: Author.

Asrat, T., & Quilligan, E.J. (1994). Postterm pregnancy. In F.P. Zuspan & E.J. Quilligan (Eds.), *Current therapy in obstetrics and gynecology* (4th ed., pp. 275–277). Philadelphia: W.B. Saunders.

Bachman, J., & Kendrick, J.M. (1996). Childbirth. In K.R. Simpson and P.A. Creehan (Eds.), AWHONN's *perinatal nursing* (pp. 151–186). Philadelphia: J.B. Lippincott.

Biancuzzo, M. (1993). Six myths of maternal posture during labor. MCN: *American Journal of Maternal-Child Nursing*, 18(5), 264–269.

Blackburn, S.T., & Loper, D.L. (1992). *Maternal, fetal, and neonatal physiology: A clinical perspective*. Philadelphia: W.B. Saunders.

Bowes, W.A. (1994). Clinical aspects of normal and abnormal labor. In R.K. Creasy & R. Resnick (Eds.), *Maternal-fetal medicine: Principles and practice* (3rd ed., pp. 527–557). Philadelphia: W.B. Saunders.

Boyle, J.G. (1995). Beta-adrenergic agonists. *Clinical Obstetrics and Gynecology*, 38(4), 688–696.

Burke, M.E., & Poole, J. (1996). Common perinatal complications. In K.R. Simpson & P.A. Creehan (Eds.), AWHONN's *perinatal nursing* (pp. 109–148). Philadelphia: J.B. Lippincott.

Creasy, R.K. (1994). Preterm labor and delivery. In R.K. Creasy & R. Resnick (Eds.), *Maternal-fetal medicine: Principles and practice* (3rd ed., pp. 494–523). Philadelphia: W.B. Saunders.

Creatsas, G.C., Charalambidis, V.M., Zagotzidou, E., & Aravantinos, D.I. (1995). Untreated cervical infections, chorioamnionitis and prematurity. *International Journal of Obstetrics and Gynecology*, 49, 1–7.

Crowther, C.A. (1995). Commentary: Bed rest for women with pregnancy problems: Evidence for efficacy is lacking. *Birth*, 22(1), 13–14.

Cunningham, F.G., MacDonald, P.C., Gant, N.F., Leveno, K.J., Gilstrap, L.C., Hankins, G.D.V., et al. (1997). *Williams obstetrics* (20th ed.). Norwalk, Conn.: Appleton & Lange.

Curet, L.B. (1994). Dysfunctional labor. In F.P. Zuspan & E.J. Quilligan (Eds.), *Current therapy in obstetrics and gynecology* (4th ed., pp. 243–245). Philadelphia: W.B. Saunders.

de Veciana, M., Porto, M., Major, C.A., & Barke, J.I. (1995). Tocolysis in advanced preterm labor: Impact on neonatal outcome. *American Journal of Perinatology*, 12(4), 294–298.

Devoe, L.D., Youssef, A.E., Croom, C.S., & Watson, J. (1994). Can fetal biophysical observations anticipate outcome in preterm labor or preterm rupture of membranes? *Obstetrics and Gynecology*, 84(3), 432–438.

Escher-Davis, L. (1996). Fetal fibronectin: A biochemical marker for preterm labor. AWHONN *Voice*, 4(3), 1, 6–7.

Freda, M.C. (1995). Arrest, trial, and failure. *Journal of Obstetric, Gynecologic, and Neonatal Nursing*, 24(5), 393–394.

Gardner, M.O., & Goldenberg, R.I. (1995). The clinical use of antenatal corticosteroids. *Clinical Obstetrics and Gynecology*, 38(4), 746–754.

Garite, T.J. (1994). Premature rupture of the membranes. In R.K. Creasy & R. Resnick (Eds.), *Maternal-fetal medicine: Principles and practice* (3rd ed., pp. 625–638). Philadelphia: W.B. Saunders.

Goodwin, T.M., Valenzuela, G., Silver, H., Hayashi, R., Creasy, G., & Lane, R. (1996). Treatment of preterm labor with the oxytocin antagonist atosiban. *American Journal of Perinatology*, 13(3), 143–146.

Gordon, M.C., & Iams, J.D. (1995). Magnesium sulfate. *Clinical Obstetrics and Gynecology*, 38(4), 706–712.

Gordon, M.C., & Samuels, P. (1995). Indomethacin. *Clinical Obstetrics and Gynecology*, 38(4), 697–705.

Griese, M.E., & Prickett, S.A. (1993). Nursing management of umbilical cord prolapse. *Journal of Obstetric, Gynecologic, and Neonatal Nursing*, 25(3), 257–264.

Gupton, A., & Heaman, M. (1994). Learning needs of hospitalized women at risk for preterm birth. *Applied Nursing Research*, 7(3), 118–124.

Hall, S.P. (1997). The nurse's role in the identification of risks and treatment of shoulder dystocia. *Journal of Obstetric, Gynecologic, and Neonatal Nursing*, 26(1), 25–32.

Hannah, M.E. (1996). Tocolytics: More good than harm, or is it the reverse? *Birth*, 23(1), 41–43.

Hodnett, E. (1996). Nursing support of the laboring woman. *Journal of Obstetric, Gynecologic, and Neonatal Nursing*, 22(4), 311–315.

Huzel, P.A., & Remsburg-Bell, E.A. (1995). Fetal complications related to minor maternal trauma. *Journal of Obstetric, Gynecologic, and Neonatal Nursing*, 25(2), 121–124.

Iams, J.D. (1994). Prevention and management of preterm birth. In F.P. Zuspan & E.J. Quilligan (Eds.), *Current therapy in obstetrics and gynecology* (4th ed., pp. 283–287). Philadelphia: W.B. Saunders.

Iams, J.D. (1996). The role of tocolysis in the prevention of preterm birth. *Birth*, 23(1), 40–41.

Iams, J.D., Johnson, F.F., & Parker, M. (1994). A prospective evaluation of the signs and symptoms of preterm labor. *Obstetrics and Gynecology*, 84(2), 227–230.

Joffe, G.M., Symonds, R., Alverson, D., & Childton, L. (1995). The effect of a comprehensive prematurity prevention program on the number of admissions to the neonatal intensive care unit. *Journal of Perinatology*, 15(4), 305–309.

Jones, D.P., & Collins, B.A. (1996). The nursing management of women experiencing preterm labor: Clinical guidelines and why they are needed. *Journal of Obstetric, Gynecologic, and Neonatal Nursing*, 25(7), 569–592.

Josten, L.E., Savik, K., Mullett, S.E., Campbell, R., & Vincent, P. (1995). Bed rest compliance for women with pregnancy problems. *Birth*, 22(1), 1–12.

Kosasa, T.S., Busse, R., Wahl, N., Hirata, G., & Nakayama, R.T. (1994). Long-term tocolysis with combined intravenous terbutaline and magnesium sulfate: A 10-year study of 1000 patients. *Obstetrics and Gynecology*, 84(3), 369–373.

Lewis, R., & Mercer, B.M. (1995). Adjunctive care of preterm labor: The use of antibiotics. *Clinical Obstetrics and Gynecology*, 38(4), 755–770.

Luke, B., Mamelle, N., Keith, L., et al. (1995). The association between occupational factors and preterm birth: A United States nurses' study. *American Journal of Obstetrics and Gynecology*, 173(3), Part I, 849–862.

MacLennan, A.H. (1994). Multiple gestation: Clinical characteristics and management. In R.K. Creasy & R. Resnick (Eds.), *Maternal-fetal medicine: Principles and practice* (3rd ed., pp. 589–601). Philadelphia: W.B. Saunders.

Maloni, J.A. (1996). Bed rest and high-risk pregnancy: Differentiating the effects of diagnosis, setting, and treatment. *Nursing Clinics of North America*, 31(2), 313–325.

McCain, G.C., & Deatrick, J.T. (1994). The experience of high-risk pregnancy. *Journal of Obstetric, Gynecologic, and Neonatal Nursing*, 23(5), 421.

McFarland, M., Hod, J., Piper, J.M., Xenakis, E.M-J., & Langer, O. (1995). Are labor abnormalities more common in shoulder dystocia? *American Journal of Obstetrics and Gynecology*, 175(4), 1212–1214.

McGregor, J.A., French, J.I., Parker, R., et al. (1995). Prevention of premature birth by screening and treatment for common genital tract infections: Results of a prospective controlled evaluation. *American Journal of Obstetrics and Gynecology*, 173(1), 158–167.

Morrison, J.C. (1994). Premature rupture of the membranes. In F.P. Zuspan & E.J. Quilligan (Eds.), *Current therapy in obstetrics and gynecology* (4th ed., pp. 281–283). Philadelphia: W.B. Saunders.

Nelson, L.H., Anderson, R.L., O'Shea, T.M., & Swain, M. (1994). Expectant management of preterm premature rupture of the membranes. *American Journal of Obstetrics and Gynecology*, 171(2), 352–358.

Poole, G.V., Martin, J.N., Perry, K.G., Griswold, J.A., Lambert, C.J., & Rhodes, R.S. (1996). Trauma in pregnancy: The role of interpersonal violence. *American Journal of Obstetrics and Gynecology*, 174(6), 1873–1876.

Potter, J. (1996). Controversies in preventing and managing preterm labor. (Cassette recording no. T6). New Orleans: MCN Convention.

Ray, D., & Dyson, D. (1995). Calcium channel blockers. *Clinical Obstetrics and Gynecology*, 38(4), 713–721.

Reedy, N.J. (1994). Crises in the delivery room: Recognition and response. Dallas, Tex.: MCN Convention.

Resnik, R. (1994). Post-term pregnancy. In R.K. Creasy & R. Resnick (Eds.), *Maternal-fetal medicine: Principles and practice* (3rd ed., pp. 521–526). Philadelphia: W.B. Saunders.

Sanmire, H.F. (1996). Roundtable discussion: What is the role of tocolytic therapy in preterm birth? *Birth*, 23(1), 38–39.

Sauve, R.S. (1996). Tocolytics: The neonatal perspective. *Birth*, 23(1), 43–45.

Schroeder, C.A. (1996). Women's experience of bed rest in high-risk pregnancy. *Image: Journal of Nursing Scholarship*, 28(3), 253–258.

Simkin, P. (1995). Reducing pain and enhancing progress in labor: A guide to nonpharmacologic methods for maternity caregivers. *Birth*, 22(3), 161–171.

Sisson, M.C. (1997). Preventing preterm labor: Is terbutaline our best option? *Lifelines*, 1(2), 42–46.

U.S. Preventive Services Task Force (1993). Home uterine activity monitoring for preterm labor. *Journal of the American Medical Association*, 270(3), 371–376.

Wapner, R.J., Cotton, D.B., Artal, R., Librizzi, R.J., & Ross, M.G. (1995). A randomized multicenter trial assessing a home uterine activity monitoring device used in the absence of daily nursing contact. *American Journal of Obstetrics and Gynecology*, 172(3), 1026–1034.

Wright, L.L., Horbar, J.D., Gunkel, H., et al. (1995). Evidence from multicenter networks on the current use and effectiveness of antenatal corticosteroids in low birth weight infants. *American Journal of Obstetrics and Gynecology*, 173(4), 263–269.

# 28

# Postpartum Maternal Complications

**OBJECTIVES**

1. Describe postpartum hemorrhage in terms of predisposing factors, causes, clinical signs, and therapeutic management.
2. Explain major causes, clinical signs, and therapeutic management of subinvolution.
3. Describe three major thromboembolic disorders (superficial venous thrombosis, deep vein thrombosis, pulmonary embolism) in terms of predisposing factors, causes, clinical signs, and therapeutic management.
4. Discuss puerperal infection in terms of location, predisposing factors, causes, signs and symptoms, and therapeutic management.
5. Describe two major affective disorders (postpartum depression and psychosis).
6. Describe the role of the nurse in the management of women who have a postpartum complication.

**DEFINITIONS**

**atony** *Absence or lack of usual muscle tone.*

**dilation and curettage (D&C)** *Stretching of the cervical os to permit suctioning or scraping of the walls of the uterus. The procedure is performed in abortion, to obtain samples of uterine lining tissue for laboratory examination, and during the postpartum period to remove retained fragments of placental.*

**embolus** *A clot, usually part or all of a thrombus, brought by the blood from another vessel and forced into a smaller one, thus obstructing circulation.*

**hematoma** *Localized collection of blood in a space or tissue.*

**hydramnios** *Excess volume of amniotic fluid (more than 2000 ml at term). Also called polyhydramnios.*

**hypovolemia** *Abnormally decreased volume of circulating fluid in the body.*

**hypovolemic shock** *Acute peripheral circulatory failure due to loss of circulating blood volume.*

**placenta accreta** *A placenta that is abnormally adherent to the uterine muscle. If the condition is more advanced, it is called placenta increta (the placenta extends into the uterine muscle) or placenta percreta (the placenta extends through the uterine muscle).*

**psychosis** *Mental state in which a person's ability to recognize reality, communicate, and relate to others is impaired.*

**thrombus** *Collection of blood factors, primarily platelets and fibrin, that may cause vascular obstruction at the point of formation.*

Pregnancy and childbirth are natural functions that most women recover from without complication. However, nurses must be aware of problems that may occur and their effect on the family. The most common physiologic complications are hemorrhage, thromboembolic disorders, and infection. Complications that are psychogenic in origin include postpartum depression and postpartum psychosis.

## Postpartum Hemorrhage

Postpartum hemorrhage is defined as blood loss that exceeds 500 ml after vaginal childbirth or 1000 ml after cesarean birth. Blood loss to this extent in the first 24 hours after childbirth is termed *early postpartum hemorrhage*; such blood loss occurring after 24 hours is called *late postpartum hemorrhage*.

It is difficult to estimate blood loss, especially when bleeding is brisk or when hemorrhage is concealed. Furthermore, blood loss during childbirth is frequently underestimated and constitutes only about half the actual loss (Cunningham et al., 1997). This is important to remember when excessive bleeding occurs later.

Postpartum hemorrhage complicates approximately 5 to 8 percent of deliveries (Druelinger, 1994). Hemorrhage, along with infection and hypertensive disorders, is one of the three leading causes of maternal morbidity and mortality.

### Early Postpartum Hemorrhage

There are two major causes of early postpartum hemorrhage: uterine atony and trauma to the birth canal during labor and delivery. Abnormalities of the third stage of labor, such as placenta accreta (abnormal adherence of the placenta to the uterine wall), and inversion of the uterus are described in Chapter 27.

#### UTERINE ATONY

Up to 90 percent of cases of early hemorrhage are caused by uterine atony (Druelinger, 1994). Atony refers to lack of muscle tone that results in failure of the uterine muscle fibers to contract firmly around blood vessels when the placenta separates. The relaxed muscles allow rapid bleeding from the endometrial arteries at the placental site. Bleeding continues until the uterine muscle fibers contract to stop the flow of blood.

Figure 28–1 illustrates the effect of uterine contraction on the size of the placental site and the amount of bleeding that occurs.

**Predisposing Factors.** Knowledge of factors that increase the risk of uterine atony can be used to anticipate and thus to reduce excessive bleeding. Overdistention of the uterus from any cause (multiple gestation, a large infant, hydramnios) makes it more difficult for the uterus to contract with enough firmness to prevent excessive bleeding. Multiparity results in muscle fibers that have been stretched

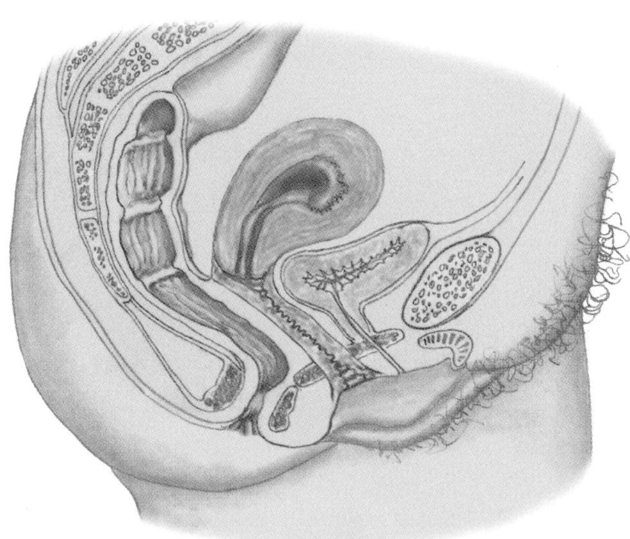

**A Contracted uterus**

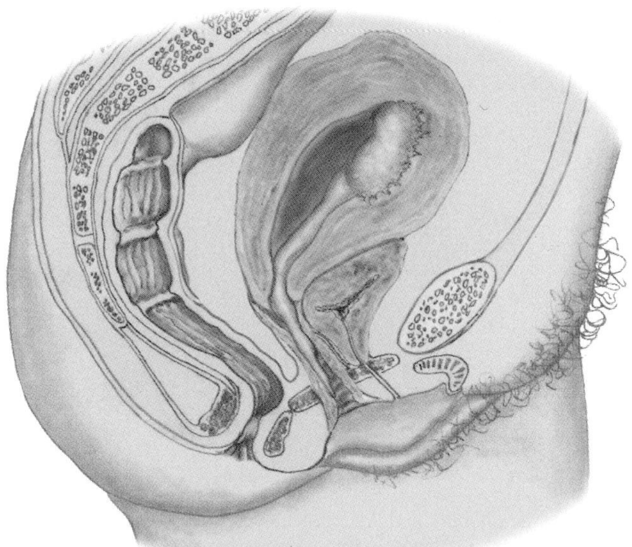

**B Uterine atony**
Uterus remains uncontracted.

**FIGURE 28–1**

A, When the uterus remains contracted, the placental site is smaller, so bleeding is minimal. B, If uterine muscles fail to contract around the endometrial arteries at the placental site, hemorrhage occurs.

**TABLE 28–1 COMMON PREDISPOSING FACTORS FOR POSTPARTUM HEMORRHAGE**

Overdistention of the uterus (multiple gestation, large infant, hydramnios)
Multiparity (>5)
Use of tocolytic drugs
Precipitate labor or delivery
Prolonged labor
Use of forceps or vacuum extractor
Cesarean birth
Manual removal of the placenta
Previous postpartum hemorrhage
General anesthesia
Additional factors:
 Low implantation of placenta
 Administration of magnesium sulfate
 Clotting disorders
 Previous uterine surgery

repeatedly, and these flaccid muscle fibers may not remain contracted after birth. Intrapartum factors include contractions that were barely effective, resulting in *prolonged labor*, or contractions that were excessively vigorous, resulting in *precipitate labor*. Labor that was induced or augmented with oxytocin is more likely to be followed by postdelivery uterine atony and hemorrhage. Retention of a large segment of the placenta does not allow the uterus to contract firmly and can result in uterine atony. Table 28–1 summarizes predisposing factors.

**Clinical Signs.** Major signs of uterine atony are as follows:

- A uterine fundus that is difficult to locate
- A soft or "boggy" feel when the fundus is located
- A uterus that becomes firm as it is massaged, but loses its tone when massage is stopped
- The uterine fundus is located above the expected level, which is at or near the umbilicus
- Excessive lochia

For the first 24 hours after birth, the uterus should feel like a firmly contracted ball roughly the size of a large grapefruit. It should be easily located at about the level of the umbilicus. Lochia should be dark red and moderate in amount. Saturation of more than one peripad per hour is considered excessive, even in the early postpartum period. The nurse must realize that although bleeding may be profuse and dramatic, a constant steady trickle is just as dangerous. (Refer to Chapter 17 for information about how to assess the uterus and lochia).

**Therapeutic Management.** Nurses are with the mother during the hours after childbirth and are responsible for assessments and initial management of

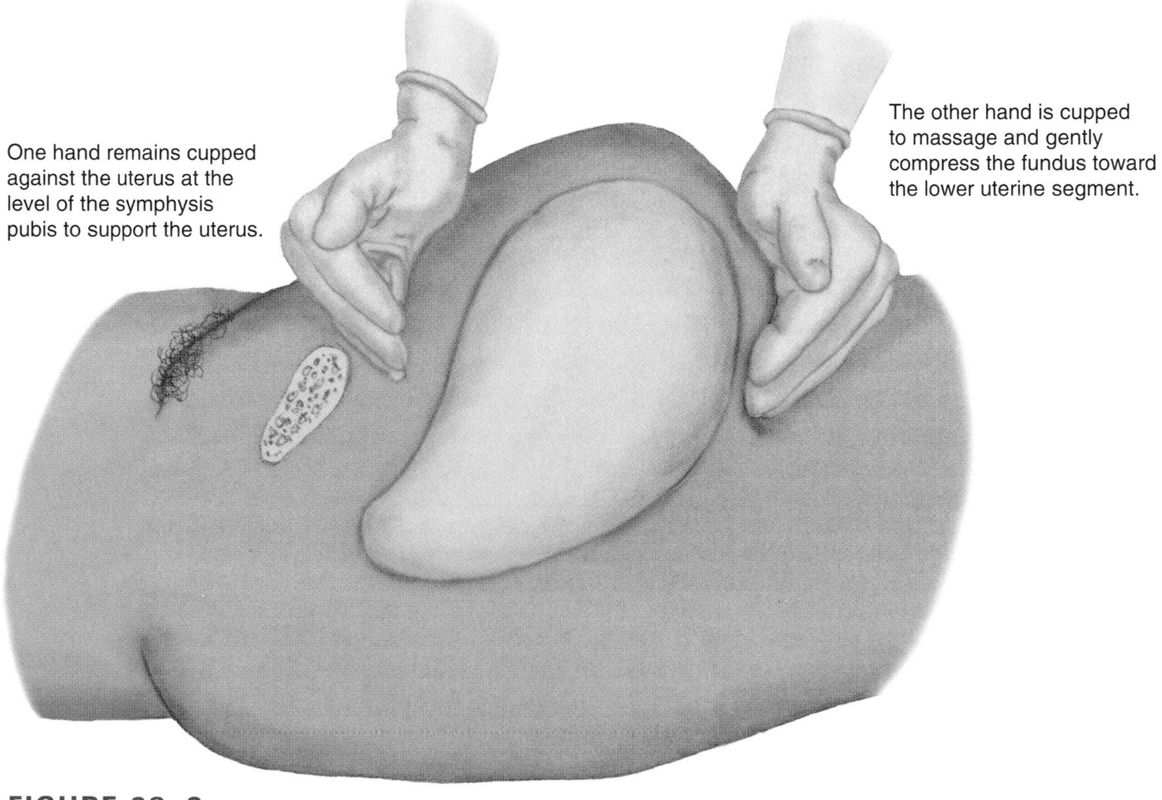
One hand remains cupped against the uterus at the level of the symphysis pubis to support the uterus.
The other hand is cupped to massage and gently compress the fundus toward the lower uterine segment.

**FIGURE 28–2**

Technique for fundal massage.

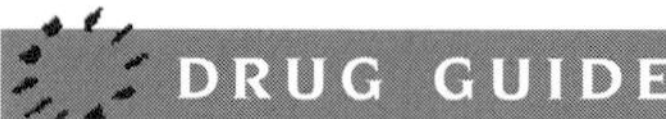

## METHYLERGONOVINE (Methergine)

***Classification:*** Oxytocic.

***Action:*** Directly stimulates contraction of the uterus.

***Indications:*** Used for the prevention and treatment of postpartum or postabortion hemorrhage caused by uterine atony or subinvolution.

***Dosage and Route:*** Usual dosage is 0.2 mg intramuscularly (IM) every 2 to 4 hours for up to five doses. Change to oral route 0.2 mg every 6 to 12 hours for 2 to 7 days.

***Absorption:*** Well absorbed after oral or IM route.

***Excretion:*** Metabolic fate unknown, probably metabolized by the liver.

***Contraindications and Precautions:*** Do not use to induce labor; do not use IM if the mother is hypersensitive to phenol. Contraindicated for hypertensive women, those with severe hepatic or renal disease, and during third stage of labor.

***Adverse Reactions:*** Dizziness, headache, dyspnea, palpitations, hypertension, nausea, and uterine and gastrointestinal cramping.

***Nursing Considerations:*** Before administering medication, check expiration date and monitor blood pressure. Follow facility protocol if medication must be withheld (usually a reading of 136/90). Caution the mother to avoid smoking because nicotine constricts blood vessels. Remind her to report any adverse reactions.

---

uterine atony. If the uterus is not firmly contracted, the first intervention is to massage the fundus until it is firm and to express clots that may have accumulated in the uterus. One hand is placed just above the symphysis pubis to support the lower uterine segment while the fundus is gently but firmly massaged in a circular motion. Clots that may have accumulated in the uterine cavity are expressed by applying firm but gentle pressure on the fundus in the direction of the vagina. *It is critical to not attempt to express clots until the uterus is firmly contracted.* Pushing on an uncontracted uterus could invert the uterus and cause massive hemorrhage. Figure 28–2 illustrates correct hand placement for fundal massage.

If the uterus does not remain contracted as a result of uterine massage, the problem may be a distended bladder. A full bladder lifts and displaces the uterus and prevents effective contraction of the uterine muscles. Nurses should assist the mother to urinate or catheterize her, if necessary, to correct uterine atony caused by bladder distention.

Pharmacologic measures may also be necessary to maintain firm contraction of the uterus. A rapid intravenous infusion of dilute oxytocin (Pitocin) often increases uterine tone and controls bleeding. Twenty units in 1000 ml of lactated Ringer's or normal saline at a rate of 600 ml per hour is often recommended (Cunningham et al., 1997). If the uterus remains atonic and bleeding continues, methylergonovine (Methergine) may be given by intramuscular or intravenous injection (Hauth, 1994; Cunningham et al., 1997). Methylergonovine has the side effect of elevating blood pressure and should not be given to a woman who is hypertensive. Analogues of prostaglandin $F_{2\alpha}$ (carboprost tromethamine) given intramuscularly are sometimes effective in controlling postpartum hemorrhage caused by uterine atony. Table 28–2 summarizes management for early postpartum hemorrhage.

If uterine massage and pharmacologic measures are ineffective in stopping uterine bleeding, the physician or nurse-midwife may use bimanual compression of the uterus to stop the bleeding. In this procedure, one hand is inserted in the vagina and the other compresses the uterus through the abdominal wall (Figure 28–3). It may also be necessary to return the woman to the delivery area to explore the uterine cavity and to remove placental fragments that interfere with uterine contraction.

Hemorrhage requires prompt replacement of intravascular fluid volume. Lactated Ringer's solution and whole blood as well as other plasma extenders may be used. Enough fluid should be given to maintain urine flow of at least 30 ml per hour (Cunningham et al., 1997). The nurse is often responsible for obtaining properly typed and crossmatched blood and for inserting large-bore intravenous lines that are capable of carrying whole blood.

Operative procedures are the last resort. A hysterectomy may be necessary to save the life of

**TABLE 28–2 THERAPEUTIC MANAGEMENT FOR EARLY POSTPARTUM HEMORRHAGE**

| Cause | Treatment |
|---|---|
| Uterine atony | Massage of the fundus, express clots from uterus, assist to empty bladder<br>Pharmacologic measures:<br>Rapid intravenous, infusion of dilute oxytocin (20 units/1000 ml to infuse at 600 ml/h) (Cunningham et al., 1997)<br>Parenteral administration of methylergonovine 0.2 mg or analogues of prostaglandin<br>Intravenous replacement of intravascular fluids and blood<br>Bimanual compression of the uterus<br>Abdominal hysterectomy if other interventions fail to control bleeding |
| Trauma | Locate and repair lacerations and hematomas in the genital tract |
| Retained placental fragments | Oxytocin, methylergonovine, prostaglandins, or curettage if hemorrhage continues; antibiotics if infection suspected |

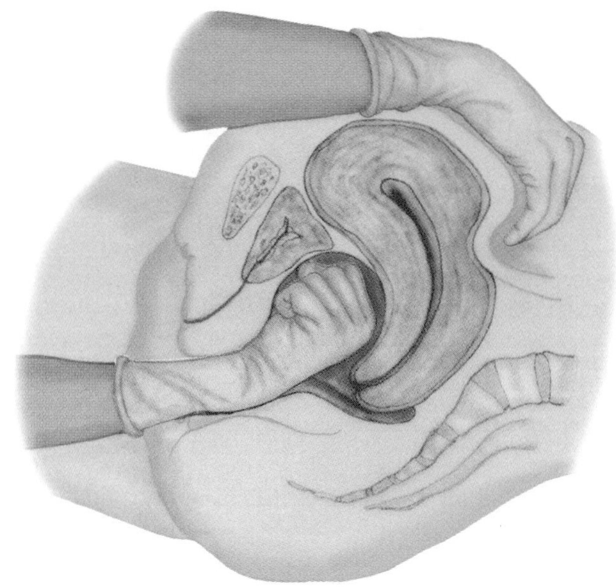

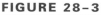

**FIGURE 28-3**

Bimanual compression. One hand is inserted in the vagina, and the other compresses the uterus through the abdominal wall.

a woman with uncontrollable postpartum hemorrhage.

#### TRAUMA

Trauma to the birth canal is the second most common cause of early postpartum hemorrhage. Trauma can include vaginal, cervical, or perineal lacerations as well as hematomas.

**Predisposing Factors.** Many of the same factors that increase the risk of uterine atony also increase the risk of soft tissue trauma during childbirth. For example, trauma to the birth canal is more likely to occur if the infant is large or if labor and delivery occur rapidly. Induction and augmentation of labor increase the risk of tissue trauma, as does the use of assistive devices. (See Chapter 27 for intrapartum complications. See Table 28-1 for a more complete list of predisposing factors.)

**Lacerations.** The perineum, vagina, cervix, or the area around the urethral meatus are the most common sites for lacerations. Cervical lacerations occur frequently when the cervix dilates rapidly during the first stage of labor. Lacerations of the vagina, perineum, and periurethral area usually occur during the second stage of labor, when the fetal head descends rapidly or when assistive devices, such as forceps or a vacuum extractor, are used to assist in delivery of the fetal head.

*Lacerations of the birth canal should always be suspected if excessive uterine bleeding continues when the fundus is contracted firmly and is at the expected location.* Bleeding from lacerations of the genital tract is often bright red, in contrast to the darker red color of lochia.

**Hematomas.** Hematomas occur when there is bleeding into loose connective tissue while overlying tissue remains intact. Hematomas develop as a result of injury to soft tissue in spontaneous deliveries as well as in deliveries in which forceps or vacuum extractors are used. Hematomas may be found in vulvar, vaginal, or retroperitoneal areas.

Visible vulvar hematomas appear as a discolored bulging mass that is caused by rapid bleeding into soft tissue. Hematomas produce deep, severe, unrelieved pain and feelings of pressure. Formation of a hematoma should also be suspected if the mother demonstrates systemic signs of concealed blood loss, such as falling blood pressure or tachycardia, when the fundus is firm and lochia is within normal limits. Figure 28-4 illustrates a vulvar hematoma.

**Therapeutic Management.** When postpartum hemorrhage is caused by trauma of the birth canal, surgical repair is often necessary. It is difficult to visualize lacerations of the vagina or cervix, and it is necessary to return the mother to the delivery area, where surgical lights are available. She is placed in a lithotomy position and carefully draped. Surgical asepsis is required while the laceration is being visualized and repaired.

Small hematomas usually reabsorb naturally; however, large hematomas may require incision, evacuation of the clots, and location of the bleeding vessel so that it can be ligated. (See Table 28-2 for a summary of therapeutic management for early postpartum hemorrhage.)

## Late Postpartum Hemorrhage

The most common causes of late postpartum hemorrhage are subinvolution (delayed return of the uterus

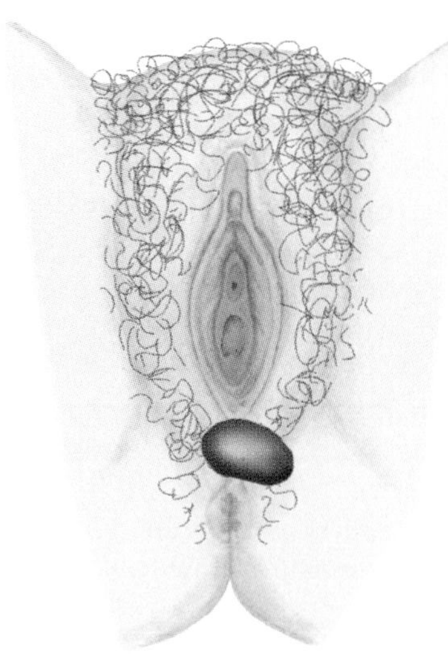

**FIGURE 28-4**

A vulvar hematoma is caused by rapid bleeding into soft tissue, and it causes severe pain and feelings of pressure.

to its prepregnant size and consistency) and fragments of placenta that remain attached to the myometrium when the placenta is delivered. Clots form around the retained fragments, and excessive bleeding can occur when the clots slough, several days after delivery.

Late postpartum hemorrhage caused by retained placental fragments is generally preventable. The placenta should be carefully inspected by the nurse-midwife or physician to determine if it is intact. If a portion of the placenta is missing, the health care provider can explore the uterus, locate the missing fragments, and remove them soon after delivery of the placenta.

Late postpartum hemorrhage, which typically occurs without warning after the woman is discharged from the birth facility, can be dangerous for the unsuspecting mother. Families must be taught how to assess the fundus and the normal duration of lochia. Moreover, they must be instructed to notify their health care provider if bleeding persists or becomes unusually heavy.

#### PREDISPOSING FACTORS

Attempts to deliver the placenta before it separates from the uterine wall, manual removal of the placenta, and placenta accreta are the primary predisposing factors for retention of placental fragments.

#### THERAPEUTIC MANAGEMENT

Initial treatment for late postpartum hemorrhage is directed toward control of the excessive bleeding. Oxytocin, methylergonovine, or prostaglandins are the most commonly used pharmacologic measures. Placental fragments are often dislodged and swept out of the uterus by the bleeding, and if the bleeding subsides when oxytocin is administered, no other treatment is necessary. Sonography can exclude placental fragments as the cause of delayed postpartum hemorrhage (Cunningham et al., 1997). If bleeding continues or recurs, curettage may be carried out. This treatment should be performed only when other treatment has failed, because curettage may cause trauma and additional bleeding. Broad-spectrum antibiotics may also be given if postpartum infection is suspected because of uterine tenderness, foul-smelling lochia, or fever.

## Application of Nursing Process: Excessive Bleeding

### Assessment

The initial postpartum assessment includes a chart review to determine whether there are factors such as prolonged labor or birth of a large infant that increase the risk for the woman to bleed excessively (see Table 28–1).

#### UTERINE ATONY

Priority assessments for uterine atony include the fundus, bladder, lochia, vital signs, skin temperature, and color. Assess the consistency and the location of the uterine fundus. The fundus should be firmly contracted, at or near the level of the umbilicus, and midline. If the uterus is not firmly contracted, the fundus feels soft (boggy) and bleeding from the placental site is rapid and continuous. If the fundus is above the level of the umbilicus and displaced, a full bladder may be the cause of excessive bleeding. A full bladder lifts the uterus and impedes contraction, which allows excessive bleeding. The accumulation of clots also expands the uterus, making contraction difficult and resulting in continued bleeding. See Procedure 17–1 (p. 441) for complete information about assessing the fundus.

It is difficult to estimate the volume of lochia by visual examination of peripads. More accurate information is obtained by weighing peripads and bed liners before and after use and subtracting the difference. One gram (weight) equals 1 ml (volume). When inspecting for blood loss, always ask the woman to turn on her side to be certain that large amounts of blood are not pooling undetected underneath her. Although bleeding may be profuse and dramatic, a constant, steady trickle may lead to significant blood loss that becomes increasingly life-threatening.

Measure vital signs at least every 15 minutes to detect trends, such as tachycardia or a decrease in pulse pressure, that may reveal a deteriorating status in a woman with significant blood loss. Remember that initially the body compensates for excessive bleeding by constricting the blood vessels and shunting blood to vital organs. As a result, vital signs may remain normal although the woman is becoming hypovolemic. (See p. 790 for a discussion of hypovolemic shock.)

The skin should be warm and dry; mucous membranes of the lips and mouth should be pink; and there should be prompt capillary return when the nails are blanched. These signs confirm that there is adequate circulating volume to perfuse the peripheral tissue.

#### TRAUMA

If the fundus is firm but bleeding is excessive, the cause may be lacerations of the cervix or birth canal. Inspect the perineum to determine whether a laceration is visible in that area. Lacerations of the cervix or vagina are not visible, but bleeding in the presence of a contracted uterus is suggestive of a lacera-

**TABLE 28–3 NURSING ASSESSMENTS FOR POSTPARTUM HEMORRHAGE**

| Assessments | Abnormal Signs/Symptoms | Nursing Implications |
|---|---|---|
| Chart review | Presence of predisposing factors | More frequent evaluations. |
| Fundus | Soft, boggy, displaced | Massage, express clots, assist to empty bladder, notify primary health care provider if measures are ineffective. |
| Lochia | Excessive bleeding (saturation of more than 1 pad/hr, steady trickle or profuse flow) | Assess for trauma, save and weigh pads and bed liner so estimation of blood loss will be more accurate. Notify physician or nurse-midwife. |
| Vital signs | Tachycardia, decreasing pulse pressure | Signs of excessive blood loss should be reported. |
| Comfort level | Severe pelvic or rectal pain | Signs of hematoma, usually perineal or vaginal; examine vulva for masses or discoloration. |
| Skin | Cool, damp, pale | Signs of hypovolemia, vigilant assessment and management by entire health care team is necessary. |

tion; this sign warrants examination of the vaginal walls and the cervix by the health care provider.

Assess comfort level. If the mother complains of deep, severe pelvic or rectal pain or if vital signs or skin changes suggest hemorrhage but excessive bleeding is not obvious, the cause may be concealed bleeding and the formation of a hematoma. Examine the vulva for bulging masses or discoloration of the skin. However, a hematoma may be developing in the vagina or in the retroperitoneal area and will not be obvious when the vulva is examined. Table 28–3 summarizes assessments, abnormal signs and symptoms, and nursing implications.

## Analysis

Certain signs and symptoms, such as uterine atony that does not respond to massage, excessive lochia, pelvic or rectal pain, or changes in vital signs may be the earliest signs of postpartum hemorrhage. Postpartum Hemorrhage is a potential complication that requires the efforts of the health care team to control the hemorrhage and to prevent further complications, such as hypovolemic shock.

## Planning

Client-centered goals are inappropriate for this potential complication because the nurse cannot manage postpartum hemorrhage independently but must confer with the physicians or nurse-midwives for medical orders to treat the condition. Planning should reflect the nurse's responsibility to do the following:

- Monitor for signs of postpartum hemorrhage.
- Consult with the health care provider if signs of postpartum hemorrhage are observed.
- Perform actions that will minimize postpartum hemorrhage and prevent hypovolemic shock.

## Interventions

### PREVENTING HEMORRHAGE

Every nurse should be aware of factors that put the new mother at risk for postpartum hemorrhage. This knowledge alerts the nurse to be particularly vigilant in monitoring these women so that excessive bleeding can be anticipated and minimized.

When predisposing factors are present, initiate frequent assessments. Many hospitals and birth centers have a standard of care that calls for assessments every 15 minutes during the first hour after delivery, every 30 minutes for the next 2 hours, and hourly for the next 4 hours. However, this may not be adequate for the woman at known risk for postpartum hemorrhage because bleeding occurs rapidly. A delay in assessment may result in a great deal of blood loss.

### COLLABORATING WITH THE HEALTH CARE PROVIDER

Notify the physician or nurse-midwife when excessive bleeding is suspected. In addition, initiate actions, such as uterine massage, to control bleeding. In some hospitals or birth centers, protocols permit nurses to initiate specific laboratory studies, such as

**Critical to Remember**

**EARLY SIGNS OF POSTPARTUM HEMORRHAGE**

- An uncontracted uterus
- Large gush or slow, steady trickle of blood from the vagina
- Saturation of more than one peripad per hour
- Severe, unrelieved perineal or rectal pain
- Tachycardia

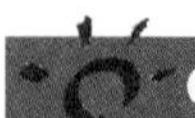

## CRITICAL THINKING EXERCISE

Dolores Navarra, a 26-year-old multipara, is admitted to the postpartum unit after rapid labor and the birth of her fourth infant 2 hours ago. The baby weighed 4000 g (8 pounds, 12 ounces). At the initial assessment, Dolores' fundus is firm, at the level of the umbilicus. Lochia is heavy, with occasional small clots expressed. Vital signs are unchanged from prenatal norms.

**Q:** 1. What are the "red flags" that suggest a potential problem or complication? What actions should the nurse take as a result?

**A:** Some data (multiparity, birth of large infant, rapid labor and delivery) in her history indicate that she is at risk for postpartal hemorrhage. The nurse will increase the frequency of her assessments of the fundus, lochia, vital signs, and skin temperature and color.

**Q:** 2. The nurse observes that the fundus is soft and that lochia is excessive. What are the priority interventions? Why?

**A:** Massage the fundus, express clots that may have accumulated in the uterus. Massage often stimulates uterine contractions that compress torn myometrial blood vessels and stop excessive bleeding. Continued assessment of the fundus and lochia are imperative.

**Q:** 3. Within an hour, the fundus becomes "boggy" again and is located 3 cm above the umbilicus and displaced to the right. What is the priority nursing action? Why?

**A:** Assist Dolores to void, because a distended bladder lifts the uterus, making contraction more difficult and resulting in excessive bleeding.

**Q:** 4. Dolores voids 500 ml; however, the fundus is difficult to locate and lochia is excessive. What is the next nursing action? Why?

**A:** Notify the physician, the nurse-midwife, or both because excessive bleeding requires the combined efforts of primary health care providers and nurses to prevent postpartum hemorrhage.

hemoglobin and hematocrit levels and typing and crossmatching of blood, so that blood is available should transfusions be necessary. Many protocols also allow the nurse to start intravenous fluids while the health care provider is being informed of the mother's condition. These actions do not substitute for notifying the health care provider, but they do allow nurses to make initial interventions quickly.

Maintain the woman on bedrest to increase venous return and maintain cardiac output. Trendelenburg's position may interfere with cardiac function and is not advised. Continue the assessments described earlier, call for assistance, and save all pads, linen savers, and linen so that an accurate estimation of blood loss can be made. Assistance is necessary because one nurse must continue to massage the uncontracted uterus and perform and record assessments while the other notifies the health care provider of the mother's condition.

When the health care provider is notified, the time and content of each communication must be documented. For example, "On 2/1/98 at 1300 hours (1 P.M.), Dr. X was notified of difficulty maintaining uterine contraction and continued excessive bleeding. Requested Dr. X to see client. Orders for 1000 ml of normal saline with 20 units of oxytocin to infuse at 120 gtts (drops)/minute received."

Administer medications and fluids ordered by the health care provider, and evaluate their effect. For example, add the prescribed amount of oxytocin to the intravenous solution and infuse the solution at the prescribed rate. Evaluate the effect of the medication on the uterus, and relay this information to the health care provider. Physicians and nurse-midwives depend on the nurse for accurate information, and they base medical management on information relayed by the nurse.

If measures fail to control bleeding, notify the health care provider so that additional procedures can be initiated. These may include preparation for operative intervention (surgical prep, consent signed for operative procedure, or confirmation that blood replacement is available).

### PROVIDING SUPPORT FOR THE FAMILY

The unusual activity of the hospital staff may make the mother and her family anxious. Be alert to their nonverbal cues, and when they appear frightened, acknowledge their feelings. Moreover, keeping them informed is one of the most effective ways of reducing anxiety.

Acknowledge the anxiety, and provide simple appropriate explanations of the activity. "I know all this activity must be frightening; she is bleeding a little more than we would like, and we are doing several things at once."

### Evaluation

Although client-centered goals are not developed for potential complications (collaborative problems), the nurse collects and compares data with established norms and judges whether the data are within normal limits. For postpartum bleeding:

- The fundus remains firm.
- Lochia is moderate.
- Vital signs remain near predelivery levels.

## Hypovolemic Shock

The pregnant woman can tolerate blood loss that approaches the volume of blood added during pregnancy (approximately 1.5 liters) (Knuppel & Hatangadi, 1995). When more than this reserve is lost, hypovolemic shock can ensue. Hypovolemia endangers vital organs by depriving them of oxygen. The brain, heart, and kidneys are especially vulnerable to hypoxia and may suffer damage in a brief period.

### How the Body Compensates for Hypovolemia

Nurses must remember that recognition of hypovolemic shock may be delayed because the body activates compensatory mechanisms that mask the severity of the problem. For example, carotid and aortic baroreceptors are stimulated to constrict peripheral blood vessels. This shunts blood to the central circulation and away from less essential organs, such as the skin and extremities. This causes the skin to become pale and cold but maintains cardiac output and perfusion of vital organs.

In addition, the adrenal glands release catecholamines, which compensate for decreased blood volume by promoting vasoconstriction in nonessential organs, increasing the heart rate, and raising the blood pressure. As a result, blood pressure remains normal initially, although a decrease in pulse pressure may be noted. The tachycardia that develops is an early sign of compensation for excessive blood loss.

### Pathophysiology of Hypovolemic Shock

As shock worsens, the compensatory mechanisms fail and physiologic insults spiral. Inadequate organ perfusion and decreased cellular oxygen for metabolism result in a buildup of lactic acid and the development of metabolic acidosis. Decreased serum pH (acidosis) results in vasodilation, which further increases bleeding. In this instance, the effects of hemorrhage now become additional causes of further blood loss.

Eventually, circulating volume becomes insufficient to perfuse cardiac and brain tissue; cellular death occurs as a result of anoxia, and the mother dies.

### Clinical Signs and Symptoms

Tachycardia is one of the earliest signs of hypovolemic shock, and even gradual increases in the pulse rate should be noted. A decrease in blood pressure and narrowing of pulse pressure (difference between systolic and diastolic blood pressure) occurs when the circulating volume of blood is sufficiently decreased. The respiratory rate increases as the woman becomes more anxious and as she attempts to take in more oxygen to overcome the need created when hemoglobin is inadequate to transport oxygen to all organs.

Skin changes also provide early cues. Increased catecholamine levels initiate vasoconstriction in the skin, and the skin becomes pale and cool to the touch. As hemorrhage worsens, the skin changes become more obvious; pallor increases, and the skin temperature changes from warm and dry to cold and clammy.

As shock progresses, changes also occur in the central nervous system. The mother becomes anxious, then confused, and finally lethargic when blood loss totals 30 to 40 percent of the total blood volume. Urine output also progressively decreases from more than 30 ml per hour in early shock to less than 5 ml per hour when more than 40 percent of the blood is lost.

### Therapeutic Management

The goals of therapy are to control bleeding and to prevent hypovolemic shock from becoming irreversible. Assessment and intervention goals include those described for postpartum hemorrhage. In addition, a second intravenous line should be inserted with a large-bore (16-gauge) catheter that is capable of carrying whole blood. Sufficient fluid volume is infused to produce a urinary output of at least 30 ml per hour. At the same time, every effort is made by the health care team to locate the source of bleeding and to stop the loss of blood. Interventions may include uterine packing; ligation of uterine, ovarian, or hypogastric artery, or hysterectomy.

### Nursing Considerations

One person should be assigned to evaluate and record every 3 to 5 minutes vital signs, location and consistency of the fundus, amount of lochia, skin temperature and color, and capillary return. Nurses collaborate with the physician or nurse-midwife to provide initial care. Many facilities also have protocols that allow nurses to initiate specific procedures.

If not already done, blood should be drawn for hemoglobin, hematocrit, clotting studies, and type and crossmatch. In addition, a pulse oximeter should be applied to determine oxygen saturation of the blood. A urinary catheter should be inserted so that hourly urinary output can be measured; the indwelling catheter is also necessary if a surgical procedure to control the hemorrhage is required. Oxygen may be needed to increase the saturation of fewer red blood cells. It should be administered by tight face mask at 6 liters per minute or as directed by the health care provider.

Nurses are also responsible for administering fluids, whole blood, and medications as directed and for reporting on their effectiveness. Moreover, nurses must make every effort to provide information and emotional support for the woman and her family.

### Home Care

Nurses involved in home care or who work in nurse-managed postpartum clinics must be aware that women who have postpartum hemorrhage are subject to a variety of complications. In general, they are exhausted, and it may take weeks for them to feel well again. Anemia often results, and a course of iron therapy may be prescribed to restore hemoglobin level. Activity may be restricted until strength returns. Some women need extra assistance with housework and care of the new infant. Exhaustion may interfere with bonding and attachment. Moreover, extensive blood loss increases the risk of postpartum infection, and the woman and her family must be taught to observe for specific signs and symptoms.

**CHECK YOUR READING**

1. Why does the nurse examine the mother's prenatal record as well as her labor and delivery record?
2. Why is a mother who has given birth to twins at increased risk for postpartum hemorrhage?
3. Can the nurse be positive that bleeding is controlled when the fundus is firm and the lochia is moderate? Why or why not?
4. How is uterine atony treated?
5. How are hematomas treated?
6. Why is it sometimes difficult to recognize that the woman is becoming hypovolemic?

## Subinvolution of the Uterus

Subinvolution refers to a slower-than-expected return of the uterus to its prepregnancy size after childbirth. Normally, the uterus descends at the rate of about 1 cm or one fingerbreadth per day. By 2 weeks, it is no longer palpable above the symphysis pubis. The endometrial lining has sloughed off as part of lochia, and the site of placental attachment is well healed by 6 weeks after childbirth if involution progresses as expected.

The most common causes of subinvolution are retained placental fragments and pelvic infection. Signs of subinvolution include prolonged lochial discharge, irregular or excessive uterine bleeding, and sometimes profuse hemorrhage (Cunningham et al., 1997). Pelvic pain or feelings of pelvic heaviness, backache, fatigue, and persistent malaise are reported by many women. On bimanual examination, the uterus feels larger and softer than normal for the particular period of the puerperium.

### Therapeutic Management

Treatment is tailored to correct the cause of subinvolution. Oral methylergonovine maleate (Methergine), 0.2 mg every 3 to 4 hours for 24 to 48 hours, provides long, sustained contraction of the uterus. Infection responds to antimicrobial therapy.

### Nursing Considerations

In most cases, subinvolution is not obvious until the mother has returned home after childbirth. For this reason, nurses must teach the mother and her family how to assess for the condition and how to recognize its occurrence.

The nurse should demonstrate how to locate and palpate the fundus and how to estimate fundal height in relation to the umbilicus. The nurse should request return demonstrations until the mother is confident of her skill. The uterus should become smaller each day (by approximately one fingerbreadth). The nurse also explains the progressive changes from lochia rubra, to lochia serosa, and then to lochia alba (see Chapter 17).

The mother is instructed to report any deviation from the expected pattern or duration of lochia. A foul odor often indicates uterine infection, for which treatment must be sought. Additional signs must be reported to the physician or midwife, such as pelvic or fundal pain, backache, or feelings of pelvic pressure or fullness.

**CHECK YOUR READING**

7. What are the major signs of subinvolution?
8. What is the nurse's primary responsibility in the management of subinvolution?

## Thromboembolic Disorders

The three most common thromboembolic disorders encountered during pregnancy and the postpartum period are superficial venous thrombosis, deep venous thrombosis, and pulmonary embolism. Superficial venous thrombosis generally involves the saphenous venous system and is confined to the lower leg. Deep venous thrombosis can involve veins from the foot to the iliofemoral region. It is a major concern because it predisposes to pulmonary embolism. Pulmonary embolism is a dangerous and potentially fatal complication that occurs when the pulmonary artery is obstructed by a blood clot that was swept into circulation from a vein. Figure 28–5 illustrates the venous system of the leg.

### Incidence and Etiology

The incidence of thromboembolic disease in pregnancy and the puerperium is five times higher than that in non-pregnant women of a similar age. Thromboembolic disease remains a major cause of maternal death in the United States. Although the incidence has remained fairly constant during pregnancy, there has been a decrease in the frequency of deep venous thrombosis and pulmonary embolism in the puerperium. This is a result of early ambulation after childbirth. Ambulation prevents stasis of blood in the legs and decreases the likelihood of thrombus formation.

A *thrombus* is a collection of blood factors, primarily platelets and fibrin, on a vessel wall. Thrombi can form whenever the flow of blood is impeded. Once started, the thrombus can enlarge with successive layering of platelets, fibrin, and blood cells as the blood flows past the clot. Thrombus formation is often associated with an inflammatory process in the vessel wall, which is termed *thrombophlebitis*.

The three major causes of thrombosis are venous stasis, hypercoagulable blood, and injury to the intima (the innermost layer) of the blood vessel. At least two of these conditions, venous stasis and hypercoagulable blood, are present in all pregnancies.

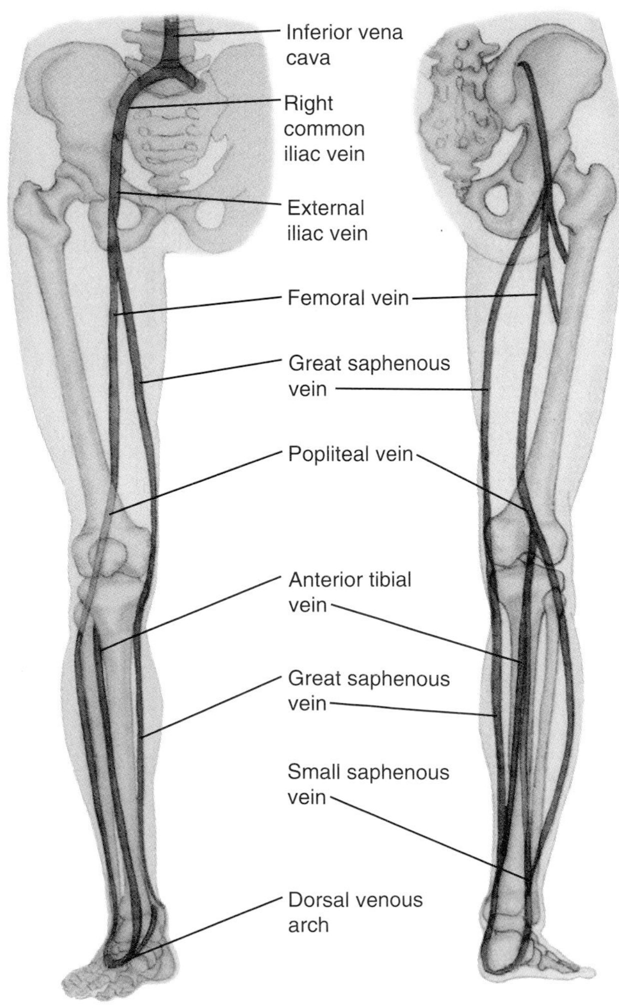


**FIGURE 28–5**

The venous system of the leg is affected when deep venous thrombosis occurs.

#### VENOUS STASIS

Pregnancy is characterized by an increase in venous stasis in the lower extremities and pelvis as a result of compression of the large vessels by the enlarging uterus. Stasis is most pronounced when the pregnant woman stands for prolonged periods of time. Stasis of blood in the lower extremities during pregnancy results in dilated vessels and the potential for continued pooling of blood postpartum. Relative inactivity during pregnancy also leads to venous pooling and stasis of blood in the lower extremities.

Prolonged time in stirrups for delivery and repair of the episiotomy may also promote venous stasis and increase the risk of thrombus formation.

#### HYPERCOAGULATION

Pregnancy is also characterized by changes in the coagulation and fibrinolytic systems that persist in the postpartum period. During pregnancy, the levels of most coagulation factors (particularly fibrinogen and factors III, X, and VIII) are elevated. In addition, there is also a suppression of the fibrinolytic system (plasminogen activator and antithrombin III), which causes clots to disintegrate (lyse). The net result is that factors that promote clot formation are increased to prevent maternal hemorrhage and factors that prevent clot formation are decreased, resulting in a higher risk for thrombus formation during pregnancy and the postpartum period.

#### BLOOD VESSEL INJURY

Injury to the intima of the blood vessel probably plays no role in initiation of thrombosis in pregnancy, except for the possibility of injury during cesarean births, which could conceivably trigger a pelvic vein thrombosis. Thrombosis is three times more likely to occur if the birth was cesarean (Ingardia & Pitcher, 1993).

#### ADDITIONAL PREDISPOSING FACTORS

Certain factors create additional risk for some women. These factors include varicose veins, obesity, a history of thrombophlebitis, and smoking. Women older than 35 years or who have had more than three pregnancies and, as stated earlier, women who had a cesarean birth, are also at increased risk (Table 28–4).

### Superficial Venous Thrombosis

#### CLINICAL SIGNS AND SYMPTOMS

Thrombosis of superficial veins is usually accompanied by signs and symptoms of inflammation and can be diagnosed by clinical signs and symptoms. In most people superficial thrombophlebitis is limited to the calf area. Signs and symptoms include swelling of the involved extremity as well as redness, tenderness, and warmth. It may be possible to palpate the enlarged, hardened vein. Patients sometimes experience pain when they walk.

#### THERAPEUTIC MANAGEMENT

Superficial venous thrombosis is often seen in association with varicose veins. Thrombosis that is limited to the superficial veins of the saphenous system is treated with analgesics, rest, and elastic support. Elevation of the lower extremity to improve venous return may also be recommended. Warm packs may be applied to the affected area to promote healing. There is no need for anticoagulants or anti-inflammatory agents unless the condition persists. After 5 to 7 days of bedrest and when symptoms disappear, the woman may ambulate gradually. She should avoid standing for long periods of time and continue to wear support hose to help prevent venous stasis and a subsequent episode of superficial thrombosis. There is little chance of pulmonary embolism if thrombosis occurs and remains in the superficial veins of the lower leg.

**TABLE 28–4 FACTORS THAT INCREASE THE RISK OF THROMBOSIS**

Inactivity
Obesity
Cesarean birth
Smoking
History of previous thrombosis
Varicose veins
Diabetes mellitus
Prolonged time in stirrups in second stage of labor
Maternal age older than 35 yr
Parity greater than 3

### Deep Venous Thrombosis

Deep venous thrombosis is much more difficult to diagnose on the basis of clinical manifestations because signs and symptoms are often absent or diffuse. If they are present, they are caused by an inflammatory process and obstruction of venous return; calf swelling, erythema, heat and tenderness, and pedal edema are the most common signs.

It is a common belief that a positive Homans' sign (presence of pain behind the knee when the foot is dorsiflexed) is an indicator of deep venous thrombosis in postpartum women. However, Homans' sign has proved to be of little value in the diagnosis because pain may also be caused by a strained muscle or contusion. Contusions may be common during the early postpartum period as a result of inappropriate contact between the calf and delivery bed stirrups (Cunningham et al., 1997). Reflex arterial spasms may cause the leg to become pale and cool to the touch with decreased peripheral pulses. At one time, this condition was called *milk-leg*.

Additional symptoms may include pain on ambulation, chills, general malaise, and stiffness of the affected leg.

#### DIAGNOSIS

Noninvasive tests to diagnose deep venous thrombosis include duplex Doppler scanning of the deep veins of the upper legs to detect alterations in blood flow. Impedance plethysmography measures changes in venous blood volume and flow. Venography is an accurate method for diagnosing deep venous thrombosis; however, there are significant risks associated with the use of the radiographic dye that is used. These include pain, anaphylaxis, and radiation exposure (Clarke-Pearson, 1994).

#### THERAPEUTIC MANAGEMENT

**Preventing Thrombus Formation.** The mother should ambulate frequently and as early as possible to prevent thrombus formation. If she is unable to ambulate, range of motion and gentle leg exercises, such as flexing and straightening the knee and raising one leg at a time, should begin within 8 hours after childbirth. In addition, the mother should avoid using pillows or the knee gatch to prevent sharp flexion at the knees and pressure on the popliteal space and consequent pooling of blood in the lower extremities.

Nurses should obtain an order for antiemboli stockings for mothers with varicose veins or a history of thrombosis or for those who had a cesarean birth. The stockings should be applied before the mother

**Women Want to Know**

**How Do I Prevent Thrombosis?**

*Methods to improve peripheral circulation will help prevent the occurrence of thrombophlebitis:*

- Improve your circulation with regular schedule of activity, preferably walking.
- Avoid prolonged standing or sitting in one position.
- When sitting, elevate your legs and avoid crossing them. This will increase the return of venous blood from the legs.
- Maintain a fluid intake of at least 2500 ml (approximately 2½ quarts) to prevent dehydration and consequent sluggish circulation.
- Stop smoking. Not only is smoking a risk factor for thrombosis, but it can cause respiratory problems in you and your newborn.

rises in the morning to prevent venous congestion, which begins as soon as she gets up. It is important that she understand the correct way to put on the antiemboli stockings; improperly applied stockings can roll or bunch and may cause slower venous return from the legs, possibly worsening the condition.

Stirrups should be padded during childbirth to prevent prolonged pressure against the popliteal angle during the second stage of labor. It may also be possible to decrease the time in stirrups to no more than 1 hour.

Before discharge from the birth facility, the mother should be taught about lifestyle changes that can improve peripheral circulation.

**Initial Treatment.** Initial treatment of deep venous thrombosis consists of the following:

- Bedrest, with the affected leg elevated to decrease interstitial swelling and to promote venous return from that leg.
- Gradual ambulation, which is allowed when symptoms have abated and with permission of the health care provider.
- Anticoagulant therapy, which usually begins with continuous infusion of intravenous heparin to prevent extension of the thrombus by delaying the clotting time of the blood. Activated partial thromboplastin time should be monitored and the heparin dose should be adjusted to maintain a therapeutic level of 1.5 to 2.5 times control (Laros, 1994).
- Analgesics, as necessary, to control pain.
- Antibiotic therapy, if necessary, to prevent or control infection.

**Subsequent Treatment.** The long-term management of deep venous thrombosis depends on whether the woman is pregnant or in the postpartum period. After several days of treatment with heparin, the postpartum woman is started on warfarin (Coumadin), which is often continued for 3 to 6 months (Vaccaro, 1994). The usual anticoagulating dose of warfarin is 10 to 15 mg daily until a therapeutic level is reached. Prothrombin time and the international normalized ratio are used to monitor coagulation time when warfarin is used. The international normalized ratio corrects for variations in the potency of the thromboplastins used by different laboratories. An appropriate ratio for treatment of deep venous thrombosis is 2.0 to 3.0 (Laros, 1994).

Warfarin is contraindicated during pregnancy because of teratogenic effects and the increased risk of fetal hemorrhage. Therefore, pregnant women are given heparin, which is administered subcutaneously (Clarke-Pearson, 1994). After symptoms have completely abated, well-fitting elastic stockings should be applied, and gradual ambulation may begin while heparin is continued (Clarke-Pearson, 1994).

## Application of Nursing Process: The Mother with Deep Venous Thrombosis

### Assessment

Assessment focuses on determining the status of the venous thrombosis. Palpate pedal pulses to determine whether they are absent, diminished, or easily palpable and equally strong on both sides. Inspect the affected leg for *unusual* warmth or redness, which indicates inflammation, or for unusual coolness or cyanosis, which indicates venous obstruction. Compare the affected and unaffected leg for size and color. Sometimes the nurse measures the legs and compares the circumference to obtain an accurate estimation of the edema that may be present in the affected leg.

Determine the degree of discomfort present. Pain is caused by tissue hypoxia, and increasing pain indicates progressive obstruction.

Evaluate the laboratory reports of clotting studies to monitor circulating heparin levels. In addition to activated partial thromboplastin time, whole-blood partial thromboplastin time and platelets may be evaluated when heparin is used. Thrombocytopenia is a concern when heparin is administered for a prolonged time (Laros, 1994). As stated previously, prothrombin time and international normalized ratio are evaluated when the anticoagulant for the postpartum woman is changed to warfarin.

## Analysis

The treatment of deep venous thrombosis includes the administration of anticoagulants for a prolonged time. As a result, Hemorrhage secondary to anticoagulation therapy is one of the most troubling potential complications.

## Planning

Client-centered goals are inappropriate for potential complications because the nurse cannot independently manage them. The nurse must confer with physicians for medical orders to treat the condition. Planning should reflect the nurse's responsibility to do the following:

- Monitor for signs of hemorrhage.
- Consult with the physician if signs of hemorrhage are observed.
- Perform actions that will minimize the risk of hemorrhage.

## Interventions

### MONITORING FOR SIGNS OF BLEEDING

At least twice a day, visually inspect the mother for the appearance of bruising or petechiae. Instruct her to report the appearance of any bleeding: bloody nose, blood in urine, bleeding gums, or increased vaginal bleeding.

Be alert to signs of hemorrhage, such as tachycardia, falling blood pressure, or other signs of shock that may indicate internal bleeding.

Unless frank hemorrhage is present, the usual treatment for excessive anticoagulation is temporary discontinuance of the anticogulant. However, keep *protamine sulfate*, the antidote for heparin, available. The antidote for warfarin is vitamin K.

### EXPLAINING CONTINUED THERAPY

Instruct the woman in measures to prevent excessive anticoagulation. Carefully explain the treatment regimen, including the schedule of medication and possible side effects, such as unexplained fever, unusual fatigue, or sore throat (signs of agranulocytosis or diminished number of neutrophils). Assist her to devise a method for remembering to take the medication as directed, for example, marking a calendar each time the drug is taken. Caution her not to "double up" if a dose is missed. If necessary, teach her and another family member how to inject heparin.

Emphasize the importance of keeping the health care provider informed about any medications the mother takes, because oral anticoagulants are associated with many clinically significant drug interactions. Caution the woman that common over-the-counter medications, such as aspirin and nonsteroidal anti-inflammatory drugs, increase the risk of hemorrhage. Also emphasize the importance of reporting unusual bleeding.

Suggest that the mother use a soft toothbrush and floss her teeth gently to prevent bleeding from the gums. She should postpone dental appointments until the therapy is completed. Recommend a depilatory to remove unwanted hair; this is safer than a razor during anticoagulant therapy.

Caution the new mother against going barefoot, about the importance of avoiding activities that may cause injury, and against the use of alcohol, which inhibits the metabolism of oral anticoagulants.

### HELPING THE FAMILY ADAPT TO HOME CARE

In addition to the assessments, physical care, and teaching described above, nurses must often help the family adapt to home care. The first step may be to assess family structure and function to determine how prepared the family is to cope with the mother's illness. How many children are in the family? What are their ages? Who is usually the primary caregiver? Are family members available to provide care while the mother is confined to bed or on limited activity? Who helps the family in times of need?

Note interactions between the mother and the newborn as well as between the father and the newborn. If the father is not present, determine who else will be available to support the mother during the subsequent weeks.

It may be necessary to help the family develop a plan of care that includes temporary assistance by members of the extended family. Although the health of the mother is of primary importance, care must be taken that the attachment process between her and the infant progresses normally.

## Evaluation

Although client-centered goals are not developed for potential complications, the nurse collects and compares data with established norms and judges whether the data are within normal limits:

- The woman receiving anticoagulant therapy maintains ordered therapeutic levels.
- The mother demonstrates no signs of unusual bleeding or other side effects of the medication.

## Pulmonary Embolism

### PATHOPHYSIOLOGY

Pulmonary embolism is a rare but dreaded complication of deep venous thrombosis. It occurs when fragments of a blood clot dislodge and are carried to the pulmonary artery or one of its branches. The embolus occludes the vessel and obstructs the flow of blood into the lungs, either entirely or partially. If pulmonary circulation is severely compromised, death may occur within a few minutes. If the embolus is small, adequate pulmonary circulation may be maintained until treatment can be initiated.

#### CLINICAL SIGNS AND SYMPTOMS

Clinical signs and symptoms depend on how much the flow of blood is obstructed. Sudden, sharp chest pain; tachycardia; syncope; tachypnea; pulmonary rales; cough; and hemoptysis are the most common signs. Arterial blood gas determinations show decreased partial pressure of oxygen, and chest radiography reveals areas of atelectasis and pleural effusion.

#### THERAPEUTIC MANAGEMENT

Treatment of pulmonary embolism is aimed at dissolving the clot and maintaining pulmonary circulation. Heparin therapy is initiated and may be continued for many months to prevent further emboli. Oxygen is used to decrease hypoxia, and narcotic analgesics are used to reduce pain and apprehension. The woman is kept at bedrest, with the head of the bed slightly elevated to reduce dyspnea. Intensive care, support of ventilation, and other supportive measures depend on her pulmonary status. Pulse oximetry should be initiated and arterial blood gases should be evaluated. Emergency medications, such as dopamine, may be used to support falling blood pressure. Thrombolytic drugs, such as streptokinase or urokinase, may be used for massive pulmonary emboli. Embolectomy (surgical removal of the embolus) may be attempted if there is no time to allow the clot to dissolve.

#### NURSING CONSIDERATIONS

**Monitor for Signs.** When caring for a woman with deep venous thrombosis, nurses must be aware of the danger of pulmonary embolism and focus the assessment for early signs and symptoms. This includes frequent assessment of respiratory rate and auscultation of breath sounds. Abnormalities, such as diminished or unequal breath sounds, or coughing should be reported immediately to the health care provider. Additional signs that require immediate attention include air hunger, dyspnea, tachycardia, pallor, or cyanosis.

**Facilitate Oxygenation.** Oxygen should be administered at 8 to 10 liters by tight face mask (Simpson & Creehan, 1996). The nurse should remain with the mother to allay fear and apprehension. The head of the bed should be raised to facilitate breathing, and the woman should be kept warm. Narcotic analgesics, such as morphine, may be used to relieve pain.

**Seek Assistance.** The woman's condition is precarious until the clot is lysed or until it adheres to the pulmonary artery wall and is reabsorbed. The primary nurse should call for assistance to initiate interventions. These include intravenous administration of heparin, continuous assessment of vital signs, and administration of emergency drugs that may be needed. The woman who has pulmonary embolism requires critical-care nursing skills and is usually transferred to an intensive care unit.

#### ✓ CHECK YOUR READING

9. Why is the risk of thrombus formation increased in pregnancy and in the postpartum period?
10. What are the signs and symptoms of superficial venous thrombosis?
11. How does the long-term treatment for deep venous thrombosis differ for the pregnant woman from that of the woman who is in the postpartum period?
12. Why is strict bedrest prescribed for the woman with deep venous thrombosis?
13. What additional nursing assessments are necessary when the mother is receiving anticoagulation medication?
14. In addition to assessment, physical care, and teaching, what are the home care nurse's responsibilities?

## Puerperal Infection

*Puerperal infection* is a term used to describe bacterial infections after childbirth. It occurs in 2 to 5 percent of all women who have had vaginal births and in 15 to 20 percent of those who have had cesarean births (Savoia, 1995). Until the advent of antibiotics, puerperal infection resulting in death was not uncommon. Even today, it is one of the three leading causes of maternal deaths.

The most common postpartum infections are metritis, wound infections, urinary tract infections, mastitis, and septic pelvic thrombophlebitis.

### Definition

The definition of puerperal infection, according to the Joint Committee on Maternal Welfare, is a fever of 38°C (100.4°F) or higher after the first 24 hours following childbirth, occurring on at least 2 days during the first 10 days. Although a slight elevation of temperature may occur during the first 24 hours because of dehydration or the exertion of labor, any mother with fever should be assessed for other signs of infection.

## Effect of Normal Anatomy and Physiology on Infection

To understand the seriousness of infection of the reproductive tract, it is important to consider the anatomy of the region. Every part of the reproductive tract is connected to every other part, and organisms can move from the vagina, through the cervix, into the uterus, up the fallopian tubes, and out the tubes to infect the ovaries and the peritoneal cavity. Moreover, the entire reproductive tract is particularly well supplied with blood vessels during pregnancy and after childbirth. Bacteria that invade or are picked up by the blood vessels or lymphatics can carry the infection to the rest of the body, which can result in life-threatening septicemia.

The normal physiologic changes of childbirth increase the risk of infection. During labor, the acidity of the vagina is reduced by the amniotic fluid, blood, and lochia, which are alkaline. An alkaline environment encourages growth of bacteria.

Necrosis of the endometrial lining and the presence of lochia provide a favorable environment for the growth of anaerobic bacteria. Many small lacerations, some microscopic in size, occur in the endometrium, cervix, and vagina during birth and allow bacteria to enter the tissue. Although the uterine interior is not sterile until 3 to 4 weeks after delivery, infection does not develop in most women. This is partly because of the presence of granulocytes in the lochia and endometrium that prevent infection. Scrupulous aseptic technique during labor and birth and careful hand washing during the postpartum period are also major preventive factors.

## Other Risk Factors

In addition to the normal physiologic changes of the puerperium, other factors may predispose a woman to infection (Table 28–5). A cesarean birth, a major predisposing factor, increases the risk five to 30 times above that for vaginal delivery (Gibbs & Sweet, 1994). This is because of the trauma to the tissue that occurs in surgery; the incision, which provides an entrance for bacteria; the possibility of contamination during surgery; and the presence of foreign bodies such as sutures. In addition, women who must have a surgical delivery because of a problem that develops during labor may have other risk factors, such as prolonged labor, that raise the chances of infection. Colonization of the vagina with virulent organisms, such as group B streptococcus, *Chlamydia trachomatis*, *Mycoplasma hominis*, and *Gardnerella vaginalis*, also predisposes to the development of infection after childbirth.

Any trauma to maternal tissues increases the haz-

**TABLE 28–5 RISK FACTORS FOR PUERPERAL INFECTION**

| Risk Factor | Reason |
|---|---|
| History of previous infections (urinary tract infection, mastitis, thrombophlebitis) | May be more vulnerable to infectious process |
| Colonization of lower genital tract with pathogenic organisms such as group B streptococcus, *Chlamydia trachomatis*, *Staphylococcus aureus*, *Escherichia coli*, and *Gardnerella vaginalis* | Infections usually caused by several microbes that have ascended to the uterus from the lower genital tract |
| Cesarean birth | Increased portals of infection |
| Trauma | Provides entrance for bacteria and makes tissues more susceptible |
| Prolonged rupture of membranes | Removes barrier of amniotic fluid and allows access for organisms to interior of uterus |
| Prolonged labor | Increases number of vaginal examinations; allows time for bacteria to multiply |
| Catheterization | Could introduce organisms into bladder |
| Excessive number of vaginal examinations | Increases chance that organisms from vagina or outside source are carried into the uterus |
| Retained placental fragments | Provide growth medium for bacteria and may interfere with flow of lochia |
| Hemorrhage | Loss of infection-fighting components of blood |
| Poor general health (excessive fatigue, anemia, frequent minor illnesses) | Increases vulnerability to infections and complications of labor |
| Poor nutrition (decreased protein, vitamin C) | Less able to repair tissue and defend against infection |
| Poor hygiene | Excessive exposure to pathogens |
| Medical conditions, such as diabetes mellitus | Decreases ability to defend against infections of any kind |
| Low socioeconomic status | More likely to have poor nutrition and inadequate prenatal care |

ard of infection. Trauma may occur with rapid delivery, birth of a large infant, use of forceps or a vacuum extractor, or the need for manual delivery of the placenta as well as lacerations and episiotomies. Catheterization during labor increases the chance of introduction of organisms into the bladder and adds to the trauma of the urinary tract that occurs during normal childbirth.

When there is prolonged rupture of membranes during labor, organisms from the vagina are more likely to ascend into the uterine cavity. This is especially true if more than 24 hours pass before delivery. A long labor or many vaginal examinations during labor increase the danger of infection. Each vaginal examination increases the possibility of contamination from gloves or from organisms in the vagina being pushed through the open cervix. If part of the placenta remains inside the uterus after delivery, the tissue becomes necrotic and provides a good place for bacteria to grow.

Additional factors include postpartum hemorrhage, which causes loss of some of the infection-fighting components of the blood, such as leukocytes, and leaves the mother in a weakened condition. Prenatal conditions (poor nutrition, anemia) interfere with the mother's ability to resist infection. Lack of knowledge of hygiene or lack of access to facilities that permit adequate hygiene increases the risk of postpartum infection.

## Specific Infections

### METRITIS

Infections of the uterus have been called endometritis, endomyometritis, and endoparametritis. The preferred term is *metritis with pelvic cellulitis* because infection involves the decidua, myometrium, and parametrial tissues (Cunningham et al., 1997).

**Etiology.** Metritis is usually caused by organisms that are normal inhabitants of the vagina and cervix. More than one organism is responsible for most infections. Organisms most often involved include gram-negative coliform bacteria, such as *Escherichia coli*, *Bacteroides*, *Staphylococcus*, and anaerobic nonhemolytic *Streptococcus*. Although group A hemolytic streptococcal infections were once the source of epidemics of puerperal infections (then known as "childbed fever"), improved routine care has made it uncommon today. Group B streptococcus is involved in as many as 30 percent of metritis cases today. This organism is also the major cause of sepsis in the newborn.

**Clinical Signs and Symptoms.** The mother with severe metritis looks sick. She presents a different picture from the typical happy new mother. The major signs and symptoms of metritis are fever, chills, malaise, lethargy, anorexia, abdominal pain and cramping, uterine tenderness, and purulent, foul-smelling lochia. Additional signs include tachycardia and subinvolution. In most cases, the signs and symptoms occur within the first 2 to 7 days (Gibbs & Sweet, 1994). Not all women have all these symptoms. When the causative organisms are group A or group B streptococci, the woman may exhibit no signs except fever.

Laboratory data may confirm the diagnosis. The results of a complete blood count may show an elevation of leukocytes. However, leukocytes are normally elevated to 20,000 or as high as 30,000 during labor and for a short time afterward. Elevations in the upper ranges of normal should cause suspicion.

Specimens may be taken from the blood, endocervix, and uterine cavity for cultures. A catheterized urine specimen should also be obtained. The antibiotic sensitivity from these cultures may be used to determine the appropriate second-line antibiotic therapy in case the broad-spectrum therapy is unsuccessful in halting the infection.

**Therapeutic Management.** Intravenous administration of antibiotics is the initial treatment for metritis. The goal of this therapy is to confine the infectious process to the uterus and to prevent spread of the infection throughout the body. Broad-spectrum antibiotics, such as ampicillin and cephalosporins, are rapidly effective for mild to moderate infection after vaginal birth. Response to antibiotics after cesarean birth is less dramatic, and a combination of clindamycin plus gentamicin may be necessary (Gibbs & Sweet, 1994).

Improvement in clinical signs usually follows within 48 to 72 hours. If the symptoms persist, additional investigation is needed to determine the cause and precise location. Oral antibiotics may be used after completion of an intravenous course of treatment. Some physicians give prophylactic antibiotics intravenously, orally, or both for any woman who is having a cesarean birth or who is particularly at risk for infection. Other drugs include antipyretics for fever and oxytocics, such as methylergonovine, to increase drainage of lochia and promote involution.

**Complications.** If the infection spreads outside the uterine cavity, there may be infection of the fallopian tubes (*salpingitis*) or the ovaries (*oophoritis*), which could result in sterility. *Peritonitis* (inflammation of the membrane lining the walls of the abdominal and pelvic cavities) may occur and lead to formation of a pelvic abscess. In addition, the risk of pelvic thrombophlebitis is increased when pathogenic bacteria enter the blood stream during episodes of metritis. Figure 28–6 illustrates complications of metritis.

Signs and symptoms that the infection is spreading (or extending) may be similar to those of metritis, but more severe. Fever and abdominal pain will be particularly pronounced. Peritonitis may result in

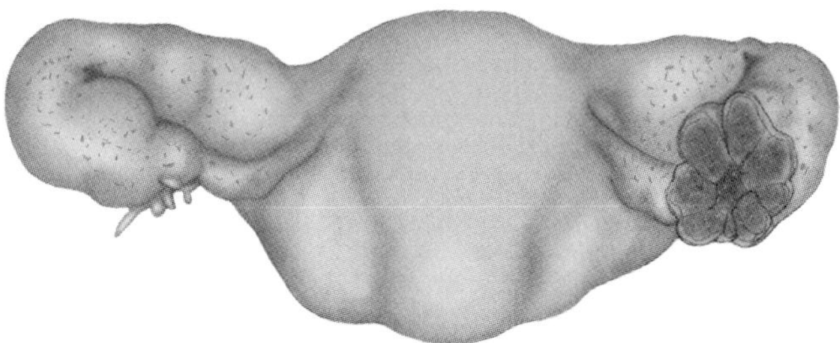

**Salpingitis:** Infection in fallopian tubes causes them to become enlarged, hyperemic, and tender.

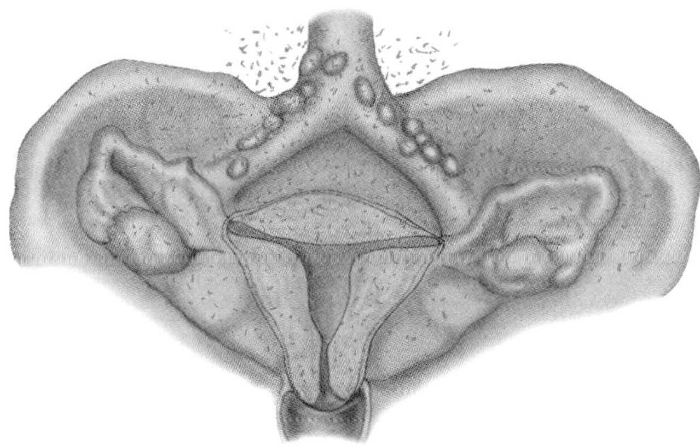

**Peritonitis:** Infection spreads through the lymphatics to the peritoneum; a pelvic abscess may form.

**FIGURE 28–6**

Areas of spread of uterine infection.

paralytic ileus and a distended, board-like abdomen with absent bowel sounds.

**Nursing Considerations.** The mother with metritis should be placed in a Fowler's position to promote drainage of lochia. She may be medicated as needed for abdominal pain or cramping, which may be severe. The nurse should give the medications as directed and observe the mother for signs of improvement or new symptoms, such as nausea and vomiting, abdominal distention, absent bowel sounds, and severe abdominal pain. Comfort measures include warm blankets, cool compresses, sponge baths, perineal care, cold or warm drinks, or use of a heating pad.

Teaching incorporates signs and symptoms of worsening condition, side effects of therapy, and the importance of adhering to the treatment plan and follow-up care. If the woman must be isolated from her infant, a nursing diagnosis of Risk for Altered Parenting related to separation from infant should be considered. If the mother is breastfeeding, she will need help to pump her breasts to establish and maintain lactation. If she is not isolated from the infant, a nursing diagnosis Risk for Infection related to knowledge deficit of preventive measures is appropriate. In that instance, she can be instructed in methods to prevent the spread of infection to her infant.

#### WOUND INFECTION

Wound infections are common types of puerperal infection because any break in the skin or mucous membrane provides a portal for bacteria. The most common sites are the perineum, where episiotomies and lacerations are common (Figure 28–7); the vagina; and cesarean surgical incisions.

**Clinical Signs and Symptoms.** Signs of wound infection are edema, warmth, redness, tenderness, and pain. The edges of the wound may pull apart, and there may be seropurulent drainage from the wound. If the wound remains untreated, generalized signs of infection, such as fever and malaise, may develop as well.

As with other puerperal infections, cultures may reveal mixed aerobic and anaerobic bacteria. The most common pathogens of abdominal wounds are group A streptococcus or *Clostridium* (Gibbs & Sweet, 1994). Lower genital tract wounds usually are colonized with organisms typically found in that area and include *E. coli*, *Proteus*, and *Bacteroides* species.

**Therapeutic Management.** The physician or nurse-midwife may decide to remove some sutures to open the area and allow for drainage. Packing, such as iodoform gauze, may be placed in the open lesion to keep it open and to facilitate drainage. Broad-spectrum antibiotics will be ordered until a report of the antibiotic-sensitive organism is returned. Analgesics are often necessary, and warm compresses or sitz baths may be used to provide

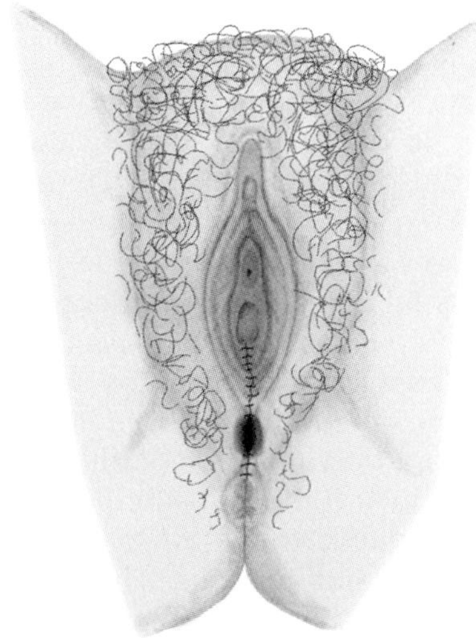

**FIGURE 28–7**

Any break in the skin, such as the episiotomy site, provides a portal of entry for bacteria and can result in localized infection.

comfort and to promote healing by increasing circulation to the area.

**Nursing Considerations.** Wound infections are painful and annoying to the mother out of proportion to their size. Perineal infections cause discomfort during many activities, such as walking, sitting, or defecating, and are particularly troublesome because they are not expected by the new mother.

Wound infections may require readmittance to the hospital or home health care visits. The woman requires reassurance and supportive care. Comfort measures might include sitz baths, warm compresses, and frequent perineal care. The woman is taught to wipe from front to back and to change perineal pads frequently. Good hand washing techniques are emphasized. Adequate fluid intake and diet are important. Activity may be modified depending on the site, severity, and treatment of the wound infection.

The infant is not routinely isolated from the mother with a wound infection, but she must be advised how to protect her infant from contact with contaminated articles. Anticipatory guidance should include teaching side effects of medication, signs of worsening condition, and any self-care measures that will be needed.

### URINARY TRACT INFECTIONS

**Etiology.** Postpartum urinary tract infections occur in approximately 2 to 4 percent of women. Trauma during birth and stasis of urine after birth contribute to the development of urinary tract infections. During childbirth, the bladder and urethra are traumatized by the pressure from the descending fetus. Insertion of a catheter, with its risk of infection, occurs at least once during many labors. After birth, the bladder and urethra are hypotonic, with stasis of urine and urinary retention common problems. Moreover, there may be residual urine and reflux of urine during voiding.

Women who had bacteria in the urine during pregnancy are at increased risk. Urinary tract infections are usually caused by coliform bacteria, such as *E. coli*.

**Clinical Signs and Symptoms.** Symptoms typically begin on the first or second postpartum day. They include dysuria (a burning pain on urination), urgency, and frequency of urination. A low-grade fever is sometimes the only symptom. In some women, an upper urinary tract infection, such as pyelonephritis, may develop the third or fourth day, with chills, spiking fever, costovertebral angle tenderness, flank pain, and nausea and vomiting. This infection of the kidney pelvis may result in permanent damage to the kidney if not promptly treated.

**Therapeutic Management.** With the exception of pyelonephritis, most urinary tract infections can be treated on an outpatient basis. If the mother is breastfeeding, the most commonly prescribed medication is ampicillin, which can be taken safely during pregnancy and lactation (Hodgson et al., 1995). Sulfonamides, nitrofurantoin, or cephalosporin should be used cautiously during lactation.

Pyelonephritis warrants intravenous hydration and intravenous administration of broad-spectrum antibiotics until the causative organism and its sensitivity are known; the antibiotic therapy can then be adjusted.

**Nursing Considerations.** The woman with a urinary tract infection must be instructed to take the medication for the entire time it is prescribed and not stop when symptoms abate. In addition, she must drink at least 3000 ml of fluid each day to help dilute the bacterial count and flush the infection from the bladder. Acidification of the urine inhibits multiplication of bacteria, and drinks that acidify urine, such as apricot, plum, prune, or cranberry juices, are frequently recommended. Carbonated drinks should be avoided because they increase urine alkalinity.

Teaching should also include measures to prevent urinary tract infections, such as proper perineal care, increasing fluid intake, and urinating frequently.

### MASTITIS

Mastitis, an infection of the lactating breast, occurs most often during the second and third weeks after birth, although it may develop at any time during breastfeeding (Lawrence, 1994). It is more common in mothers nursing for the first time and usually affects only one breast.

**Etiology.** Mastitis is generally caused by S. *aureus*, although E. *coli* may also be involved. The bacteria are most often carried on the hands of the mother or birth center staff; however, the mouth of the newborn is also an important source. The organism may enter through an injured area of the nipple, such as a crack or blister, although there may be only redness or no obvious signs of injury. Soreness of a nipple may result in insufficient emptying of the breast resulting from pain during breastfeeding. Engorgement and stasis of milk frequently precede mastitis. This may happen when a feeding is skipped, when the infant begins to sleep through the night, or when breastfeeding is suddenly stopped. Constriction of the breasts from a bra that is is too tight may interfere with emptying of all the ducts and may lead to infection. The mother who is fatigued or stressed or who has other health problems that might lower her immune system is also at increased risk for mastitis.

**Clinical Signs and Symptoms.** At first, the mother may think that she has the flu because of fatigue and aching muscles. Symptoms progress to include fever of 38.4°C (101.1°F) or higher, chills, malaise, and headache. Mastitis is characterized by a localized area of redness and inflammation. Although

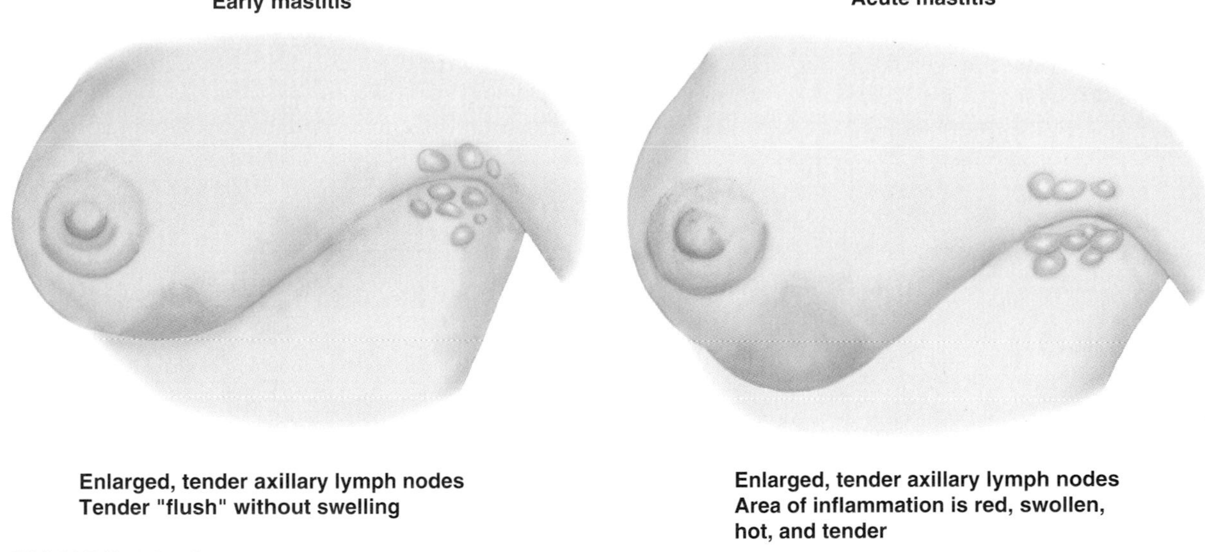


**FIGURE 28–8**

Mastitis is an infection that usually occurs 2 to 3 weeks after birth in the breast of a woman who breastfeeds.

rare, purulent drainage may be present. Untreated mastitis may progress to breast abscess. Figure 28–8 illustrates mastitis.

**Therapeutic Management.** Antibiotic therapy and continued decompression of the breast by breastfeeding or breast pump constitute the first line of treatment. With early antibiotic treatment, mastitis usually resolves within 24 to 48 hours and abscess formation is unusual. Supportive measures include ice packs, breast support, and analgesics (Gibbs & Sweet, 1994). In most cases, the mother can continue to breastfeed from both breasts; however, if the affected breast is too sore, she can pump the breast gently. Regular emptying of the breast is important in preventing abscess formation. If an abscess forms and ruptures into the ducts of the breasts, breastfeeding should be discontinued and a mechanical pump used to empty the breast. Milk obtained should be discarded.

**Nursing Considerations.** Because mastitis rarely occurs before discharge from the birth facility, the nurse must concentrate on providing adequate information for the family. Measures to prevent the development of mastitis include correct positioning of the infant and avoiding trauma to the nipples and milk stasis. The mother should breastfeed every 2 to 3 hours. She should avoid formula supplements and nipple shields, and she should change nursing pads when they are wet. She should also avoid continuous pressure on the breasts from tight bras or infant carriers. Chapter 22 provides complete information about necessary teaching for mothers who plan to breastfeed and those who do not.

Once mastitis occurs, nursing measures are aimed at increasing comfort and helping the mother maintain lactation. Moist heat promotes comfort and increases circulation. A shower or hot packs should be used before feeding or emptying the breasts. One way to apply heat to the breast is to use a disposable diaper moistened with hot water. The thickness helps to retain heat, and the plastic cover prevents dripping.

The breast should be completely emptied at each feeding to prevent stasis of milk, which can result in an abscess. If the mother is too sore to breastfeed on the affected side or if she is taking antibiotics that are contraindicated during lactation, she should be instructed in how to empty the breasts by expressing the milk or using a mechanical pump. Breastfeeding or pumping every 1½ to 2 hours makes the mother more comfortable and prevents stasis. Starting the feeding on the unaffected side causes the milk-ejection reflex to occur in the painful breast and make the process more efficient. Massage over the affected area before and during the feeding helps to ensure complete emptying. The mother should stay in bed during the acute phase of her illness. Her fluid intake should be at least 3000 ml per day. Analgesics may be required to relieve discomfort.

The mother with mastitis is likely to be very discouraged. Some mothers decide to stop breastfeeding because of the discomfort involved. The nursing diagnosis Interrupted Breast Feeding related to discomfort, infectious process, or effects of therapy, may be appropriate. Weaning during an episode of mastitis may increase engorgement and stasis, leading to abscess formation or recurrent infection. The mother may need much encouragement, and she will need help in arranging care for other children or with other responsibilities so that she can remain in bed.

### SEPTIC PELVIC THROMBOPHLEBITIS

Septic pelvic thrombophlebitis is the least common of the puerperal infections. It usually is not seen until 2 to 4 days after childbirth. It occurs when infection spreads along the venous system and thrombophlebitis develops. It occurs more often in women with wound infection. It usually involves the ovarian, uterine, or hypogastric veins.

**Clinical Signs and Symptoms.** The primary symptom is pain in the groin, abdomen, or flank. There may be fever, tachycardia, gastrointestinal distress, and decreased bowel sounds. Laboratory data may be used to exclude other diagnoses and usually include complete blood count with differential, blood chemistries, coagulation studies, and cultures.

**Therapeutic Management.** Readmittance to the hospital is usually necessary. Primary treatment includes anticoagulation therapy with intravenous heparin and intravenous antibiotics. Supportive care is similar to that for deep venous thrombosis and includes monitoring for safe levels of anticoagulation therapy and for signs and symptoms of pulmonary embolism.

## Application of Nursing Process: Infection

### Assessment

Although all women are observed for indications of infection as part of routine nursing assessments, the nurse must practice increased vigilance for mothers who are at increased risk of infection.

## Nursing Care Plan 28–1
## Postpartum Infection

ASSESSMENT: Lisa Pyle, a thin, pale, 16-year-old primipara, is admitted to the postpartum unit after a cesarean birth. Her membranes were ruptured for 14 hours, and she was in labor for 16 hours before the birth. She was catheterized twice during labor and now has an indwelling catheter.

**Critical Thinking**

What data indicate that Lisa is at increased risk for infection? What additional data should be obtained?

**ANSWER**

Factors that increase the risk for infection include a cesarean birth and rupture of membranes several hours before the surgery was performed increase the risks for metritis. Catheterization increases the risk for urinary tract infection. Additional data that should be obtained include estimated blood loss and prenatal conditions such as anemia.

NURSING DIAGNOSIS: Risk for Infection related to presence of favorable conditions for infections

GOALS/EXPECTED OUTCOMES

Lisa will do the following:

1. Remain free of signs of infection during the postpartum period.
2. Verbalize methods of prevention of infection and signs that infection may be present.

| INTERVENTION | RATIONALE |
|---|---|
| 1. Assess vital signs every 4 hours. | 1. Temperature above 38°C (100.4°F) or tachycardia suggests an infectious process and should be reported. |
| 2. Observe the surgical incision for redness, tenderness, or edema every 4 hours; note odor of lochia at each assessment; determine whether Lisa experiences frequency, urgency, or pain with urination when the catheter is removed. | 2. Redness, pain, or swelling of the incision suggests wound infection; foul odor of lochia suggests endometrial infection; frequency, urgency, or painful urination may indicate urinary tract infection. |
| 3. Instruct Lisa in hygienic practices to prevent infection:<br>a. Careful hand washing before and after perineal care<br>b. Perineal cleansing after elimination<br>c. Changing peripads frequently<br>d. Wiping the perineum from front to back | 3. a. Hand washing is the most important defense against infection and its spread.<br>b. Perineal cleansing helps prevent growth of bacteria.<br>c. Frequent pad changes remove accumulated lochia, which provides an excellent culture for bacteria.<br>d. Wiping from front to back prevents fecal contamination of the vagina. |

## Nursing Care Plan 28–1 *Continued*
# Postpartum Infection

| INTERVENTION | RATIONALE |
| --- | --- |
| 4. Initiate measures to reduce the risk of urinary tract infection.<br>a. Provide fluids of Lisa's choice when she is able to take them, and emphasize the importance of drinking at least 2500 ml per day.<br>b. Monitor bladder distention to prevent overfilling; teach Lisa the importance of emptying her bladder every 2 to 3 hours during the first days after childbirth.<br>c. Use methods to promote bladder emptying, such as running water in the shower or sink, running warm water over the perineum, and providing pain medication as needed. | 4. Adequate hydration and frequent emptying of the bladder help prevent stasis of urine, which increases the risk of urinary tract infection; relief of pain may allow the mother to relax enough to void. |
| 5. Offer and encourage Lisa to eat well-balanced meals when she progresses to a regular diet. Emphasize the importance of a diet high in protein and vitamin C. | 5. Adequate protein and vitamin C are necessary for healing damaged tissues. |

**EVALUATION**

Interventions have been successful if Lisa remains free of the signs and symptoms of infection throughout her hospital stay and if she verbalizes measures that reduce the risk of infection when she is discharged from the hospital.

**ADDITIONAL NURSING DIAGNOSES TO CONSIDER**

Activity Intolerance
Pain
Fatigue
Risk for Altered Parenting

Pay particular attention to signs that may be expected in infection, such as fever; tachycardia; pain; or unusual amount, color, or odor of lochia. Generalized symptoms of malaise and muscle aching may also be significant. Examine all wounds each shift for the presence of signs of localized infection, such as redness, edema, tenderness, discharge, or pulling apart of incisions or sutured lacerations. Particularly note whether the mother experiences difficulty emptying her bladder or discomfort related to urination.

Assess the mother's knowledge of hygiene practices that prevent infections, such as proper hand washing, perineal care, and handling of perineal pads. Evaluate her knowledge of breastfeeding and any problems that might result in breast engorgement and stasis of milk in the ducts. Assess the nipples for signs of injury that might provide a portal of entry for organisms.

### Analysis

Because all women are at risk for infection after childbirth, most facilities have developed standards of practice that protect postpartum women from infection and individual nursing care plans are usually not necessary. However, when predisposing factors increase the likelihood of infection, routine assessments and care may need to be modified and pre-

## Critical to Remember
### SIGNS AND SYMPTOMS OF POSTPARTUM INFECTION

- Fever, chills
- Pain or redness of wounds
- Purulent wound drainage or wound edges not approximated
- Tachycardia
- Uterine subinvolution
- Abnormal duration of lochia, foul odor
- Elevated white blood cell count
- Frequency or urgency or urination, dysuria, or hematuria
- Suprapubic pain
- Localized area of warmth, redness, or tenderness in the breasts
- Body aches, general malaise

ventive measures intensified. In this case, the most relevant nursing diagnosis is Risk for Infection related to the presence of significant risk factors.

## Planning

Goals for this nursing diagnosis are as follows. The mother will do the following:

- Remain free of signs of infection during the postpartum period.
- Verbalize methods to prevent infection and signs of infection that should be reported immediately.

## Interventions

### PREVENTING INFECTION

**Promoting Hygiene.** Nursing responsibilities for the woman at risk for puerperal infection focus on prevention of initial infection. Preventive measures include aseptic technique for all invasive procedures and meticulous attention to hand washing. Hand washing is important not only for the nursing staff but also for the mother. She should wash her hands before and after changing pads or touching the perineum. Instruct her on care of the perineum and episiotomy site (see Chapter 17), making sure that she can demonstrate cleansing methods before she is discharged.

**Preventing Urinary Stasis.** An adequate supply of fluids (at least 2500 to 3000 ml/day) is important for preventing stasis of urine. Encourage the woman to empty her bladder at least every 2 to 3 hours during the day. Measure the first two voidings after delivery or removal of an indwelling catheter, and assess the bladder and fundus to be certain the bladder is empty. Instruct her to report any signs of urinary tract infection immediately so that early treatment can be obtained. Use appropriate measures to promote bladder emptying if she has difficulty. Drinking hot fluids, such as tea, helps some mothers to void. Running water or having the mother blow bubbles in a glass of water uses the sound of water to stimulate the urge to urinate. Pouring warm water over the perineum or having the mother void in a sitz bath or shower may help relax the urinary sphincter. Administration of analgesics may help her relax enough to urinate.

**Teaching Breastfeeding Techniques.** Mothers often need assistance in establishing an effective pattern of breastfeeding that results in complete emptying of the breasts at each feeding and that reduces the risk of nipple trauma (see Chapter 22).

**Providing Information.** Advise mothers to obtain adequate rest and sufficient food of high nutritive value to replenish their energy and prevent infection. It may be necessary to identify foods high in protein, which is necessary for repair of damaged tissue. Whole-grain breads, cereals, or pasta; cheese; eggs; chicken; fish; and meat are some of the best sources of protein. This is particularly important if the mother is breastfeeding.

Obtaining adequate rest is a problem for many mothers. Nursing interventions focus on helping them plan a schedule that allows them to rest while the infant sleeps and to identify family members or friends who are available to provide support and assistance.

### TEACHING SIGNS AND SYMPTOMS THAT SHOULD BE REPORTED

Because many women are discharged 24 to 48 hours after childbirth, they must be taught signs and symptoms of infection that should be reported to their health care provider. These include fever, chills, dysuria, and redness and tenderness of a wound. Malodorous lochia or discharge from a wound as well as prolonged lochial discharge should also be reported.

## Evaluation

The interventions can be judged to be successful if

- The mother remains free of signs of infection during the puerperium.
- She identifies signs and symptoms that should be reported to the health care provider as soon as possible.

If infection occurs, the problem is no longer amenable to independent nursing actions but becomes a collaborative problem requiring medical and nursing interventions.

### ✓ CHECK YOUR READING

15. Why is the woman who had an assisted birth or cesarean birth at increased risk for postpartum infection?
16. Why do the normal physiologic changes of childbearing make a mother especially susceptible to infection of the reproductive system?
17. Why is metritis more likely to develop in a mother who had prolonged labor? Who gave birth by cesarean?
18. What are the signs and symptoms of metritis? How is it usually treated?
19. What are the most common sites for wound infections?
20. How does the nurse assess for wound infection?
21. What measures can the woman take to decrease the risk of urinary tract infection? How does the treatment for cystitis differ from that of pyelonephritis?
22. How may mastitis be prevented? How is it treated?
23. How does septic pelvic thrombophlebitis usually develop?

## Affective Disorders

Affective (mood) disorders are disturbances in function, affect, or thought processes that can impact the family after childbirth as severely as physiologic problems. However, one of the difficulties in dealing with affective disorders is that there is no consensus on how to define the disorders. Some practitioners view postpartum "blues," postpartum depression, and postpartum psychosis as part of a continuum of the same disorder, with postpartum blues being the mildest form and postpartum psychosis the most severe form. Others view affective disorders as three separate entities.

Postpartum blues is a transient, self-limiting mood disorder that affects 50 to 70 percent of new mothers. It is believed to be related to hormonal fluctuations after childbirth (see Chapter 18). Postpartum depression and postpartum psychosis are more serious disorders that disrupt the family and require intervention to resolve.

### Postpartum Depression

#### INCIDENCE

Depression is the most common affective disorder of the postpartum period. Although the incidence is difficult to determine, it is believed that between 10 and 15 percent of all new mothers are affected (Green & Adams, 1993). Moreover, many investigators believe that postpartum depression is underdiagnosed and underreported.

#### CLINICAL SIGNS AND SYMPTOMS

Postpartum depression is not the normal worries and "blues" that many new mothers experience from time to time. The woman experiencing depression shows less interest in her surroundings and a loss of her usual emotional response toward her family. Even though she cares for the infant in a loving manner, she is unable to feel pleasure or love. She may have intense feelings of unworthiness, guilt, and shame, and she often expresses a sense of loss of self. Generalized fatigue, complaints of ill health, and difficulty in concentrating are also present. She often has little interest in food and experiences sleep disturbances. She often describes panic attacks and relentless obsessive thinking.

Postpartum depression is differentiated from the normal labile emotions of pregnancy and the postpartum period by the number, intensity, and persistence of symptoms. A majority of the symptoms are intensely and consistently present for at least a 2-week period. These are not mood swings but a persistent depressed state.

#### IMPACT ON THE FAMILY

Postpartum depression has an impact on the entire family. It creates strain on each member's usual methods of coping and often causes difficulties in relationships. Stressors tend to be magnified, and, as a result, family members may decrease their interactions with the depressed mother when she needs support the most. Communication is impaired because she gradually withdraws from contact with others. Moreover, the decreased libido commonly associated with depression may also affect the relationship with the significant other.

Depressed mothers interact differently with their infants than do women who are not depressed. They appear tense, are more irritable, and feel less competent as mothers. They may not pick up on their infants' cues or smiles, thus failing to meet the infants needs and to enjoy their positive feedback (Beck, 1995a). Infants of depressed mothers tend to be fussier, more discontent, and make fewer positive facial expressions.

#### PREDICTORS OF POSTPARTUM DEPRESSION

The cause of postpartum depression is unknown; however, factors believed to increase the risk of its occurrence include the following:

- Hormonal fluctuations that follow childbirth
- Medical problems during pregnancy, such as pregnancy-induced hypertension, preexisting diabetes mellitus, or thyroid dysfunction
- History of depression, mental illness, or alcoholism, either in the woman or in her family
- Personality characteristics, such as immaturity and low self-esteem
- Marital dysfunction or difficult relationship with significant other, resulting in lack of support
- Anger at the pregnancy
- Feelings of isolation
- Fatigue, sleep deprivation, financial worries, and birth of an ill infant or an infant with anomalies

#### THERAPEUTIC MANAGEMENT

Depression responds best to a combination of psychotherapy, social support, and medication, such as antidepressants. The woman's partner and immediate family must be included in counseling sessions so they can develop an understanding of what the woman feels and needs.

## Application of Nursing Process: Postpartum Depression

### Assessment

Observe for subjective symptoms, such as apathy, lack of interest or energy, anorexia, or sleeplessness. The mother's verbalizations of failure, sadness, loneliness, anxiety, or vague confusion are also important cues. Objective data, such as crying, poor personal hygiene, or inability to follow directions or to concentrate may be present.

Determine if family support is available as part of each assessment. Single mothers or mothers with an absent or unavailable support system may feel increasingly isolated; this may lead to stress that they are unable to manage. Inappropriate expressions of blame or anger toward the partner and unmet expectations of the baby or the parenting role are sometimes present.

### Analysis

A likely nursing diagnosis, particularly if predisposing factors are present, is Risk for Ineffective Individual Coping related to depression in response to stressors associated with childbirth and parenting.

### Planning

To achieve the goals for this nursing diagnosis, the new mother will do the following:

- Verbalize feelings with the health care provider and significant other throughout the postpartum period.
- Identify strengths and resources that are available during the postpartum period.

### Interventions

#### DEMONSTRATING CARE

Conveying a caring attitude is one nursing strategy to help mothers decrease their emotional distress and to guide them in regaining their well-being during the postpartum period. According to Beck (1995b), caring means that nurses observe carefully and acknowledge that something is wrong. They have enough information to recognize that the woman is depressed. Caring means that nurses share valuable time and that they provide hope by reassuring the woman that this illness can be treated and it will end. It is particularly important for nurses to reinforce that it is an illness and is not the fault of the woman. Additional nursing actions that demonstrate caring include making an effort to provide continuity of care and to make appropriate referrals.

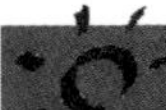

**CRITICAL THINKING EXERCISE**

Aricella Nunez, a 23-year-old multipara, gave birth several days ago to her second baby. It is obvious to the nurse making a telephone follow-up call after discharge that Aricella is crying. She says, "I feel so stupid. I can barely get out of bed in the morning and I am worn out just trying to take care of the kids." The nurse, Sharon Greenspan, responds, "Oh, that is just the 'baby blues.' Just look at those beautiful babies and you will feel better."

**Q:**

1. What assumption has the nurse made?
2. Is her response helpful for Aricella? Why or why not?
3. What would be a more therapeutic response?
4. What additional action should the nurse take?

**A:**

1. The nurse assumes that the feelings Aricella has are transient, self-limiting moods of depression that come and go in the majority of women who give birth. She fails to obtain additional data that may indicate whether Aricella is experiencing postpartum depression that requires additional therapy.
2. Her response is not helpful because it minimizes the feelings Aricella has expressed and it offers no measures for dealing with the feelings.
3. It would be more therapeutic for the nurse to acknowledge the feelings and ask follow-up questions that allow Aricella to express those feelings fully.
4. The nurse must convey her genuine interest and caring. She can do this best by
   a. Indicating that she is aware that something may be wrong
   b. Sharing as much time as Aricella needs to express her feelings
   c. Providing hope by reassuring Aricella that this is not her fault and that it can be cured
   d. Making appropriate referrals that try to provide as much continuity of care as possible

#### PROVIDING ANTICIPATORY GUIDANCE

Some mothers, particularly young mothers, are unprepared for the rapid change in lifestyle that follows the birth of an infant. Initiate a discussion of the changes to present anticipatory guidance about the early weeks at home. Discuss the need for frequent contact with other adults so that the new mother does not become isolated. Emphasize the need for continued communication with the partner or with a close friend who is available to provide support when loneliness or anxiety becomes a problem. Explain the importance of adequate rest and nutrition for maintaining energy and a feeling of health and well-being.

#### HELPING THE MOTHER VERBALIZE FEELINGS

Many women and their families minimize depression because they cannot find the exact cause. Moreover, many in the health care delivery system also trivialize the problem by making comments such as, "You'll get over it; after all, you have a beautiful baby."

Recommend that although some of her feelings may seem "unreasonable" (anger, guilt, shame), she should acknowledge these feelings to herself and insist that others acknowledge them too. It may be helpful to rehearse some of the situations that may occur, such as a fussy baby or being home alone and feeling lonely, as a means to develop perspective and to find solutions before the situation occurs.

#### ENHANCING SENSITIVITY TO INFANT CUES

Plan measures that enhance the depressed mother's sensitivity to infant cues. Music, relaxation therapy, and massage techniques just before mother-infant interactions have been used to alter the depressed mood of the mother at least temporarily and thus increase the mutual response between the mother and infant (Beck, 1995a).

#### DISCUSSING OPTIONS AND RESOURCES

Assist the new mother in identifying those persons who are available to provide support. Suggest that she explain her anticipated needs to those persons before the development of symptoms. In addition, provide her with telephone numbers for support groups in the area.

Additional information and support are supplied by national and international programs:

Depression After Delivery (DAD)
Morrisville, PA 19067
1–800–994–4–PPD
Mothers can obtain the address of the nearest DAD support group.

Postpartum Support International
927 North Kellogg Avenue
Santa Barbara, CA 93111
1–800–967–7636
Provides information and demonstrates that depression is widespread.

Health Science Consortium
201 Silver Cedar Court
Chapel Hill, NC 27514-1517
1–919–942–8731
Markets a video that provides a great deal of support: *Postpartum Depression: You Are Not Alone.*

### Evaluation

The interventions have been successful if

- The mother identifies those stressors in her life that contribute to postpartum depression. Each woman is unique, and the factors will vary from person to person.
- She is able to verbalize her feelings and insist that others acknowledge the feelings and their impact on her. By achieving this goal, she may be able to reduce the severity of the depression. Family and community resources vary, but knowing that she is not alone and that there are support groups is helpful.

## Postpartum Psychosis

Postpartum psychosis is a rare condition that affects about one in 1000 postpartum women. It generally surfaces within 3 weeks of delivery. There are two categories:

1. *Bipolar disorder* is characterized by the occurrence of manic and depressive episodes.
2. *Major depression* is characterized by depression without manic episodes.

Estimates for the risk of relapse for women with bipolar disorder during the postpartum period vary, but range between 20 and 50 percent (Cohen et al., 1995).

Women with bipolar disorder suffer from irritability, hyperactivity, euphoria, and grandiosity. They exhibit little need for sleep and are seldom aware they have a problem. The poor judgment and confusion they experience make self-care and infant care impossible and can create a dangerous, even life-threatening set of conditions for mother and infant. The depressions of the bipolar disorder and major depression are similar and are characterized by tearfulness, preoccupations of guilt, feelings of worthlessness, sleep and appetite disturbances, and an inordinate concern with the baby's health. Delusions about the infant being dead or defective are common.

Assessment and management of postpartum psychosis are beyond the scope of maternity nurses, and mothers who experience these conditions must be referred to specialists for comprehensive therapy.

Hospitalization is usually necessary to treat women with postpartum psychosis, and treatment is aimed toward the particular disorder. Women who have manic symptoms are usually treated with the standard medications (lithium, antidepressants, antipsychotics). Lithium is not recommended during pregnancy; however, it may be resumed in the postpartum period if the mother is not breastfeeding. Women who have depressive symptoms must be assessed for suicidal potential and treated according to the severity of the threat. Antipsychotics and antidepressants are used for treatment, and careful monitoring is required because of the effect of hormonal imbalances on the mother's reaction to the prescribed medication.

**CHECK YOUR READING**

24. What are the symptoms of postpartum depression and how does it differ from postpartum "blues"?
25. How can nurses intervene for postpartum depression?
26. What is the therapeutic management for postpartum psychosis?

## SUMMARY CONCEPTS

- Postpartum hemorrhage can sometimes be anticipated and prevented by careful examination of antepartum and intrapartum factors that predispose to excessive bleeding.
- Overstretching of the muscle fibers during pregnancy or repeated stretching during past pregnancies predispose to uterine atony and excessive uterine bleeding.
- Uterine atony is not the only cause of hemorrhage; soft tissue trauma (lacerations, hematomas) can also cause rapid loss of blood even when the uterus is firmly contracted.
- Initial management of uterine atony focuses on measures to contract the uterus and provide fluid replacement.
- Management of trauma of the reproductive tract involves locating the trauma and repairing it before excessive blood loss occurs.
- Compensatory mechanisms maintain the blood pressure so that vital organs, such as the brain, heart, and kidneys, receive adequate oxygen. When compensatory mechanisms fail, hypovolemic shock follows.
- The process of uterine involution is delayed (subinvolution) when placental fragments are retained or when the inner lining of the uterus is infected (metritis).
- Subinvolution of the uterus develops after the mother has been discharged from the hospital. The nurse teaches the family the process of normal involution and the signs and symptoms that should be reported to the health care provider.
- Venous stasis that occurs during pregnancy, increased levels of coagulation factors, and decreased thrombolytic factors that persist into the postpartum period increase the risk of thrombus formation during the puerperium.
- Treatment for deep venous thrombosis includes anticoagulants, analgesics, and bedrest, with the affected leg elevated to decrease interstitial edema and improve venous return.
- Nurses who administer anticoagulant therapy are responsible for assessing the mother to determine whether her clotting time is within the recommended therapeutic level so that overmedication with anticoagulants does not result in bleeding from unusual sites.
- Pulmonary embolism is a complication of deep venous thrombosis that occurs when a clot is partially or completely dislodged from the vein and carried by the blood to a pulmonary vessel, which may be completely or partially occluded by the clot.
- The risk of infection is increased with childbearing because the anatomy of the reproductive tract provides open access to bacteria from the vagina through the fallopian tubes and out into the peritoneal cavity. Increased blood supply to the pelvis and the alkalinization of the vagina by the amniotic fluid further increase the risk of metritis.
- Any break in the skin or mucous membranes during childbirth provides a portal of entry for pathogenic organisms and increases the risk of puerperal infection. Nurses must assess women with an incision or laceration for signs of localized wound infections.
- Urinary stasis and trauma to the urinary tract increase the risk of postpartum urinary tract infection. Nurses must initiate measures to prevent urinary stasis.
- Nurses must provide information about the importance of completely emptying the breasts at each feeding and about measures to prevent nipple trauma to prevent mastitis.
- Postpartum depression is a disabling affective disorder that affects the entire family. It is often underdiagnosed and underreported. Nurses must help the woman to acknowledge her feelings and assist her in identifying measures that will help her cope with the condition.

### References and Readings


Beck, C.T. (1993). Teetering on the edge: A substantive theory of postpartum depression. *Nursing Research*, 42(1), 42–48.

Beck, C.T. (1995a). The effects of postpartum depression on maternal-infant interaction: A meta-analysis. *Nursing Research*, 44(5), 298–304.

Beck, C.T. (1995b). Perceptions of nurses' caring by mothers experiencing postpartum depression. *Journal of Obstetric, Gynecologic, and Neonatal Nursing*, 24(9), 819–825.

Clark, R.A. (1995). Infections during the postpartum period. *Journal of Obstetric, Gynecologic, and Neonatal Nursing*, 24(6), 542–548.

Clarke-Pearson, D.L. (1994). Venous thromboembolic disease in pregnancy. In F.P. Zuspan & E.J. Quilligan (Eds.), *Current therapy in obstetrics and gynecology* (4th ed., pp. 320–323). Philadelphia: W.B. Saunders.

Cohen, L.S., Sichel, D.A., Robertson, L.M., Heckscher, E., & Rosenbaum, J.F. (1995). Postpartum prophylaxis for women with bipolar disorder. *American Journal of Psychiatry*, 152(11), 1641–1645.

Cunningham, F.G., MacDonald, P.C., Gant, N.F., Leveno, K.J., Gilstrap, L.C., Hankins, G.D.V., et al. (1997). *Williams obstetrics* (20th ed.). Norwalk, Conn.: Appleton & Lange.

Druelinger, L. (1994). Postpartum emergencies. *Emergency Medicine Clinics of North America*, 12(1), 219–237.

Ely, J.W., Rijhsinghani, A., Bowdler, N.C. & Dawson, J.D. (1995). The association between manual removal of the placenta and postpartum endometritis following vaginal delivery. *Obstetrics and Gynecology*, 86(6), 1002–1006.

Gibbs, R.S., & Sweet, R.L. (1994). Clinical disorders. In R.K. Creasy & R. Resnik (Eds.), *Maternal-fetal medicine: Principles and practice* (3rd ed., pp. 639–703). Philadelphia: W.B. Saunders.

Green, S.E., & Adams, W.M. (1993). Chronic psychiatric illness and pregnancy: Nursing implications. *Journal of Perinatal, Neonatal Nursing* 7(3), 7–18.

Hauth, J.C. (1994). Postpartum hemorrhage. In F.P. Zuspan & E.J. Quilligan (Eds.), *Current therapy in obstetrics and gynecology* (4th ed.). Philadelphia: W.B. Saunders.

Hodgson, B.B., Kizior, R.J., & Kingdon, R.T. (1995). *Nurse's Drug Handbook* 1995. Philadelphia: W.B. Saunders.

Ingardia, C.J., & Pitcher, E.F. (1993). Additional medical complications in pregnancy. In R.A. Knuppel & J.E. Drukker (Eds.), *High-risk pregnancy: A team approach* (2nd ed., pp. 597–618). Philadelphia: W.B. Saunders.

Kajs-Wyllie, M. (1994). Venous stroke in the pregnant and postpartum patient. *Journal of Neuroscience Nursing* 26(4), 204–209.

Knuppel, R.A., & Hatangadi, S.B. (1995). Acute hypotension related to hemorrhage in the obstetric patient. *Obstetrics and Gynecology Clinics of North America* 22(1), 111–130.

Laros, R.K. (1994). Thromboembolic disease. In R.K. Creasy & R. Resnik (Eds.), *Maternal-fetal medicine: Principles and practice* (3rd ed., pp. 792–803). Philadelphia: W.B. Saunders.

Lawrence, R.A. (1994). *Breastfeeding: A guide for the medical profession* (4th ed.). St. Louis: C.V. Mosby.

Savoia, M.C. (1995). Bacterial, fungal, and parasitic disease during pregnancy. In G.N. Burrow & T.F. Ferris (Eds.), *Medical complications during pregnancy* (4th ed., pp. 343–380). Philadelphia: W.B. Saunders.

Selig, C. (1996, June). *Clinical guidelines for detection of depression in women's health.* Paper presented at the national AWHONN Conference, Anaheim, CA.

Simpson, K.R., & Creehan, P.A. (1996). AWHONN *perinatal nursing*. Philadelphia: Lippincott-Raven.

Stamp, G.E., Williams, A.S., & Crowther, C.A. (1995). Evaluation of antenatal and postnatal support to overcome postnatal depression: A randomized controlled study. *Birth*, 22(3), 138–143.

Ugarriza, D.N. (1992). Postpartum affective disorders: Incidence and treatment. *Journal of Psychosocial Nursing*, 30(5), 2932.

Vaccaro, P.S. (1994). Thrombophlebitis, venous thrombosis, and pulmonary embolism. In F.P. Zuspan & E.J. Quilligan (Eds.), *Current therapy in obstetrics and gynecology* (4th ed., pp. 427–431). Philadelphia: W.B. Saunders.

# 29

# High-Risk Newborn: Complications Associated with Gestational Age and Development

**OBJECTIVES**

1. List risk factors that may lead to complications of gestational age and development in the newborn.
2. Explain the special problems of the preterm infant.
3. Identify common nursing diagnoses for preterm infants, and explain the nursing care for each.
4. Describe the complications that may result from premature birth.
5. Describe the characteristics and problems of the infant with postmaturity syndrome.
6. Explain the effects of intrauterine growth restriction.
7. Compare the problems of the large-for-gestational age infant with those of the small-for-gestational age infant.

**DEFINITIONS**

**apneic spells** *Cessation of breathing for more than 15 seconds, accompanied by cyanosis or bradycardia.*

**bronchopulmonary dysplasia** *Chronic pulmonary condition in which damage to the infant's lungs requires prolonged dependence on supplemental oxygen.*

**compliance** *Stretchability or elasticity of the lungs and thorax that allows distention without resistance during respirations.*

**containment** *A method of increasing comfort in infants by using swaddling or other methods to keep the extremities in a flexed position near the body.*

**corrected gestational age** *Gestational age that a preterm infant would be if still in utero. May also be called developmental age.*

**enteral feeding** *Nutrients supplied to the gastrointestinal tract orally or by feeding tube.*

**intrauterine growth restriction** *Failure of a fetus to grow as expected for gestational age. May also be called intrauterine growth retardation.*

**large-for-gestational age infant** *An infant whose size is above the 90th percentile for gestational age.*

**low-birth-weight infant** *An infant weighing less than 2500 g at birth.*

**macrosomia** *Unusually large fetal size; infant birth weight more than 4000 g.*

**necrotizing enterocolitis** *A condition of injury, invasion by bacteria, and possible necrosis of the intestines.*

**noncompliance** *Resistance of the lungs and thorax to distention with air during respirations.*

**parenteral nutrition** *Intravenous infusion of all nutrients needed for metabolism and growth.*

**periventricular-intraventricular hemorrhage** *Bleeding into and around the ventricles of the brain.*

**postmaturity syndrome** *Condition in which a postterm infant shows characteristics indicative of poor placental functioning before birth.*

**postterm infant** *An infant born after 42 weeks of gestation.*

**preterm infant** *An infant born before the beginning of the 38th week of gestation. Also called premature infant.*

**pulse oximetry** *Method of determining the level of blood oxygen saturation by sensors attached to the skin.*

**respiratory distress syndrome** *Condition caused by insufficient production of surfactant in the lungs; results in atelectasis (collapse of the lung alveoli), hypoxemia, and hypercapnia.*

**retinopathy of prematurity** *Condition in which interference with blood supply to the retina may cause decreased vision or blindness.*

**small-for-gestational age infant** *An infant whose size is below the 10th percentile for gestational age.*

**transcutaneous oxygen/carbon dioxide monitoring** *Method of continuous noninvasive measurement of oxygen and carbon dioxide levels in the blood by transducers attached to the skin.*

**very-low-birth-weight infant** *An infant weighing 1500 g or less at birth.*

This chapter is designed to provide nurses with knowledge of the gestational complications of newborns, so that nurses will be able to identify and care for the immediate needs of these infants until they are transferred to the neonatal intensive care unit (NICU), provide information and emotional care for parents, and form a basis for further study.

## Care of High-Risk Newborns

Approximately 9 percent of all newborns are sick enough at birth to require intensive care (Behrman et al., 1996). Nurses care for minor illness in the normal newborn nursery, but more serious problems require care in specialized nurseries designed for that purpose. Nurses who work in NICU nurseries have additional education and experience to prepare them for this role.

### Levels of Care

Not every hospital is equipped to provide an NICU. Such hospitals must employ staff members who are specialized clinical experts able to provide complex treatment with expensive technical equipment. Hospitals are categorized according to the level of care they provide. Facilities at each level also provide care for infants with less acute needs as well.

- *Level* I facilities treat normal, low-risk mothers and newborns. They perform immediate resuscitation of infants with respiratory depression, treat physiologic jaundice and preterm infants weighing more than 2000 g, and care for sick newborns until they can be transferred to a level II or III facility.
- *Level* II facilities provide care for infants with moderate- to high-risk problems. They may also serve as "step down" units for infants who no longer need level III care. Infants such as those with mild respiratory distress syndrome or suspected sepsis receive level II care.
- *Level* III facilities, also called tertiary care centers, offer services necessary for extremely high-risk infants. Infants who need prolonged treatment with ventilators or those with symptomatic congenital heart conditions receive level III care (American Academy of Pediatrics and American College of Obstetricians and Gynecologists, 1992) (Fig. 29–1).

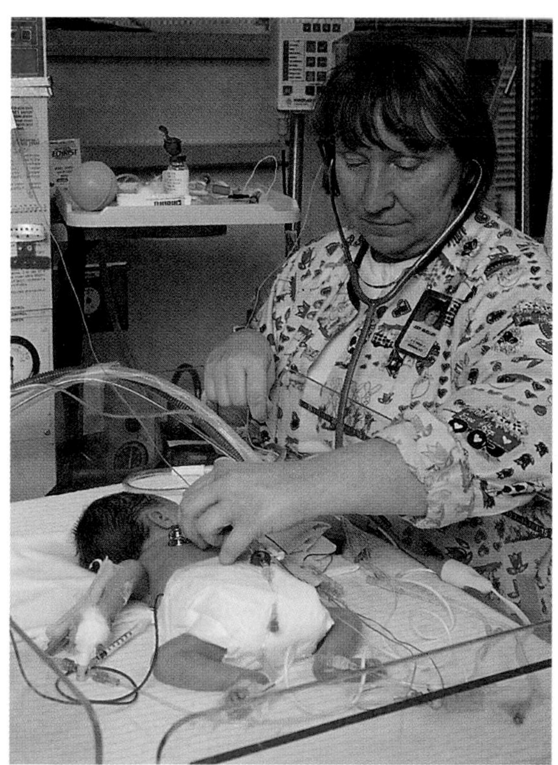

**FIGURE 29–1**

The infant in a neonatal intensive care nursery is cared for by nurses with highly specialized skills.

### Transport

When the birth of an infant with a serious complication is suspected, the woman may be transferred to a tertiary care center before birth. However, not all infants with complications can be identified before birth. Therefore, all maternity nurses must be prepared to give immediate care to the unexpectedly compromised newborn until the infant can be transferred.

A transport ambulance, airplane, or helicopter may take the infant to the new hospital. The team caring for the infant during transit may include specially prepared nurses, nurse practitioners, physicians, and respiratory therapists.

### Multidisciplinary Approach

The care of infants with problems at birth often necessitates collaboration between staff members specialized in many different areas. In the hospital setting on a given day, this care may include nurses, nurse practitioners, physicians with different specialties, respiratory therapists, laboratory personnel, and pharmacists. Care from other professionals, including social workers, physical therapists, feeding specialists, occupational therapists, and infant development experts may begin during the hospital stay and continue after the infant is discharged. Nurses must often coordinate this care and explain or clarify to parents what is being done.

## Preterm Infants

Preterm infants (also called premature infants) are born before the beginning of the 38th week of gestation. A gestational age assessment of preterm infants' size and development may show that they are small, appropriate, or large for the amount of time that they have spent in the uterus. Most preterm infants are appropriate for their gestational age.

The word *preterm* is sometimes confused with the term *low birth weight* (LBW), which refers to infants weighing 2500 g (5 pounds, 8 ounces) or less at birth. *Very-low-birth-weight* (VLBW) infants weigh 1500 g (3 pounds, 5 ounces) or less at birth. Although most of these infants are preterm, others are full-term and have failed to grow normally while in the uterus, a condition called *intrauterine growth restriction* (IUGR).

### Incidence and Etiology

#### SCOPE OF PROBLEM

Advances in technology have resulted in survival at much lower birth weights than ever before. Approximately 95 percent of infants weighing more than 1500 g at birth and 20 percent of infants who weigh 500 to 600 g at birth now survive (Behrman et al., 1996).

Although advances in technology have allowed very small infants to survive, the number of early births is not decreasing. In fact, the preterm birth rate of approximately 7 percent has not changed in recent decades (Whitsett et al., 1994). In terms of medical expense, lost potential, and suffering of infants and their parents, preterm birth is extremely costly.

Care of very preterm infants raises ethical questions concerning the benefit of saving them at great expense versus the risk that they may have permanent, serious disabilities and little chance to live normal lives. The incidence of problems such as blindness, hearing loss, developmental retardation, and cerebral palsy is about 5 to 10 percent in newborns weighing 1000 g to 1500 g but more than 50 percent in those weighing less than 600 g or born before 23 to 24 weeks of gestation (Blackburn, 1995).

#### CAUSES

The exact causes of preterm birth are not known, but all risk factors in pregnancy are potential causes of complications for the newborn as well. Difficulty during pregnancy may lead to preterm birth, and complications during labor or delivery may result in decreased oxygenation of the fetus or trauma during delivery. Multifetal pregnancy may be the cause of early birth. This occurs more often after infertility treatment to achieve pregnancy.

One of the major factors associated with prematurity is low socioeconomic status of the pregnant woman, because many risk factors are often present in low-income women. They are more likely to be malnourished, young, unmarried, and have frequent, closely spaced pregnancies. With little money and inadequate transportation, these women may begin pregnancy in poor health and receive little or no prenatal care. Complications may not be discovered until late in the pregnancy or in labor, when they may be more difficult to treat. Substance abuse may occur more often among (but certainly is not limited to) the poor. All these factors together increase the risk of complications for women and infants who live in poverty.

#### PREVENTION

Prevention of preterm birth is best accomplished by provision of adequate prenatal care for every pregnant woman to identify and treat risk factors as early as possible. Teaching women signs of preterm labor will help them seek care when halting the labor is still a possibility (see Chapter 27, p. 759).

## Characteristics of Preterm Infants

Although the estimated due date is used before delivery to determine whether labor is preterm, the gestational age assessment made after birth is the most accurate method of computing the age of the newborn (p. 538). Characteristics of preterm infants vary by gestational age. For example, the appearance and problems of infants born at 34 weeks' gestation are different from those of infants born at 26 weeks' gestation. However, some characteristics are common to all preterm infants.

### APPEARANCE

Preterm infants appear frail and weak, and they have underdeveloped flexor muscles and muscle tone. Their extremities are limp and offer little or no resistance when moved. Premature newborns typically lie in an extended position (see Fig. 20–20). The head of the normal preterm infant is large in comparison with the rest of the body.

Preterm infants lack subcutaneous fat, which makes their thin skin appear red and almost transparent, with blood vessels clearly visible. The nipples and areola may be barely perceptible, whereas vernix caseosa and lanugo may be abundant. Plantar creases are absent in infants of less than 32 weeks' gestation (see Fig. 20–27).

The pinna of the ear appears flat, lacking the rolled-over look of full-term ears (see Fig. 20–28). When folded, the ears are soft and may remain folded or return slowly to the original position because there is little cartilage. In the female infant, the clitoris and labia minora appear large and are not covered by the small, separated labia majora. The male infant may have undescended testes, with a small, smooth scrotal sac (see Figs. 20–29 and 20–30).

### BEHAVIOR

The behavior of preterm infants differs from that of full-term infants because of the stress of having to adjust to extrauterine life before they are ready. They have little excess energy for maintaining muscle tone. Premature newborns are easily exhausted from noise and routine activities. Their response is varied, including lowered oxygenation levels and behavior changes. The cry is feeble and seldom heard because the infant is too weak to cry.

### CHECK YOUR READING

1. Why are low-income women at increased risk of having preterm infants?
2. How does the appearance of a preterm infant differ from that of a full-term infant?

## Assessment and Care of Common Problems

Because preterm infants are "unfinished" in their growth and development, they are prone to problems that affect all systems and body processes. Some of the most common problems are discussed here. Problems with environmental stress, nutrition, and parenting are discussed in the section on application of nursing process.

### PROBLEMS WITH RESPIRATION

Problems of the respiratory system are a major concern because preterm newborns must go through the same processes as the full-term infant to begin breathing but with less mature lungs. The presence of surfactant in adequate amounts is of primary importance. Surfactant reduces surface tension in the alveoli and prevents their collapse with expiration. Infants born before surfactant production is adequate develop respiratory distress syndrome (p. 837).

**Assessment.** The infant's respiratory status must be observed constantly. The lungs are assessed for adventitious breath sounds or areas of absent breath sounds. The Silverman-Andersen index is a useful tool for evaluating the degree of respiratory distress (Fig. 29–2).

The nurse differentiates periodic breathing from apneic spells. Periodic breathing is the cessation of breathing for 5 to 10 seconds without other changes. Apneic spells generally last more than 15 seconds or are accompanied by cyanosis and bradycardia, or both. They are common in preterm infants, increasing in incidence with lower gestational age. Apnea without an identified cause in a preterm infant is called apnea of prematurity and generally improves as the infant matures. The spells may occur along with periodic breathing, and the infant may require stimulation.

The weak or absent cough reflex and the very small air passages make the preterm infant susceptible to obstruction by mucus. Because they are nose breathers, obstruction of the nasal passages may cause respiratory distress.

The nurse observes the effort required for breathing and the location and severity of retractions. Retractions are particularly noticeable in preterm infants, whose weak chest wall is drawn in with each inspiration. The excessive compliance (elasticity) of the chest cage during retractions may interfere with full expansion of the lungs.

Grunting may be an early sign of respiratory distress syndrome. It closes the glottis and increases the pressure within the alveoli. This keeps the alveoli partially open between breaths and increases the amount of oxygen absorbed.

**Nursing Interventions.** Interventions focus on collaborating with other team members, such as the respiratory therapist, to manage technical equipment and facilitate removal of secretions.

***Working with Respiratory Equipment.*** The infant may need an endotracheal tube and mechanical ventilation. Continuous positive airway pressure may be necessary to keep the alveoli open and improve expansion of the lungs. It can be delivered with nasal prongs or an endotracheal tube. High-frequency ventilation may be used to provide very fast, frequent respirations with less pressure than other methods. Liquid ventilation, the use of oxygenated fluids to ventilate infants at low pressures, is another method that may be used more in the future to decrease lung damage associated with ventilator use.

A hood is often used for infants who are able to breathe alone but who need extra oxygen. The hood is a plastic box-like device that fits over the infant's head. The infant breathes the higher levels of oxygen surrounding the head, and there is no interference with access to the rest of the infant's body for care (Fig. 29–3).

Oxygen may also be given by nasal cannula to the infant who breathes well alone. After discharge, many preterm infants continue to receive oxygen delivered via nasal cannula at home. Oxygen must be humidified to prevent insensible water loss and drying of the delicate mucous membranes. It is warmed to maintain body temperature.

When oxygen is administered, the level of oxygen in the infant's blood must be monitored. Arterial blood may be drawn for testing arterial oxygen levels. Pulse oximetry or transcutaneous monitoring may also be used. They are less invasive and provide continuous information about oxygen partial pressure ($Po_2$) levels through sensors attached to the skin.

The nurse must observe the infant's increasing or decreasing dependence on breathing assistance and need for oxygen. The infant's response to activity that may increase oxygen need, such as handling, feeding, and linen changes, may require changes in settings on equipment to meet the infant's needs.

***Positioning the Infant.*** The infant should be placed in a side-lying or prone position to facilitate drainage of respiratory secretions. The side-lying or prone position allows regurgitated feedings to drain easily from the mouth. The prone position is not recommended for normal newborn infants because it may be associated with increased incidence of sudden infant death syndrome (SIDS). However, in the preterm infant, the prone position allows more efficient use of the respiratory muscles, decreases respiratory effort, and results in better oxygenation and lung compliance (Lefrak-Okikawa & Lund, 1993).

If the infant must be in a supine position, the nurse can elevate the head of the bed and turn the infant's head to the side. Rolled blankets by the head can prevent movement, if necessary. A small roll under the shoulders will straighten the airway. Frequent position changes will help air passages drain and prevent stasis of secretions.

***Suctioning Secretions.*** Suction equipment must be available at all times. The nurse checks equipment at the beginning of each shift to ensure that it is functioning properly. A bulb syringe is less likely to be traumatic than wall suction, but it may not reach mucus deep in the respiratory tract.

The infant is suctioned as mucus becomes apparent. The mouth is always suctioned before the nose to prevent aspiration of fluids if the infant gasps when the nose is suctioned. Suction should always be gentle to avoid traumatizing the delicate mucous membranes. Trauma could cause edema, which could further decrease the size of the air passages and lead to more respiratory difficulty.

***Performing Chest Physiotherapy.*** Chest physiotherapy (postural drainage, percussion, and vibration) and suctioning are used in some hospitals to help keep the airway clear. Postural drainage helps the affected areas of the lung drain into the major bronchi.

Percussion helps loosen secretions and bring them into the bronchi, where they can be removed by suction. The procedure may not be used for the VLBW infant, because the stimulation causes stress and may increase intracranial pressure. When it is a part of the treatment plan for a larger infant, the nurse performs gentle percussion for 30 to 60 seconds at a time with a special rubber instrument, a nipple, or a padded medicine cup. It may be followed with gentle vibration with fingertips or a special mechanical device designed for that purpose. The treatment ends with suction to remove loosened secretions.

Chest physiotherapy should be stopped immediately if lowered blood oxygen levels, bradycardia, or

**FIGURE 29–2**

Assessment of respiratory distress. The Silverman-Andersen index is used to score the infant's degree of respiratory difficulty. The score for individual criteria matches the grade, with a total possible score of 10 indicating severe distress. (Modified from Silverman, W., & Andersen, D. [1956]. A cold clinical trial of effects of water mist on obstructive respiratory signs, death rate and necropsy findings among premature infants. *Pediatrics*, 17, 4.)

| **Grade** | **0** | **1** | **2** |
|---|---|---|---|

CHEST/ABDOMINAL MOVEMENT

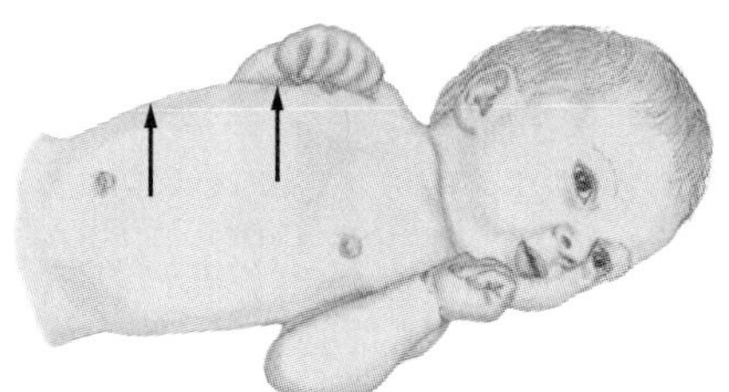

Synchronized respirations

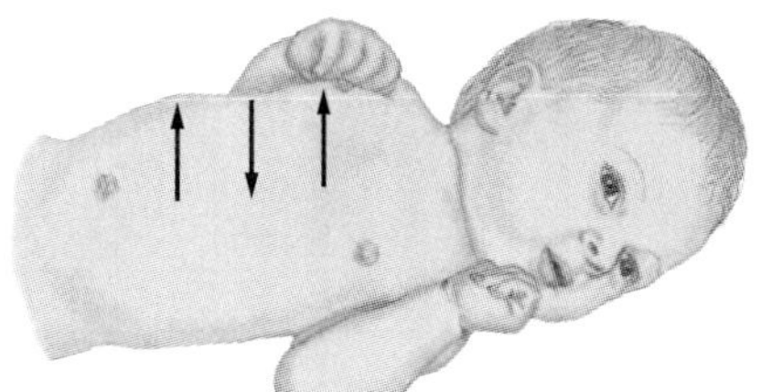

Lag in inspiration

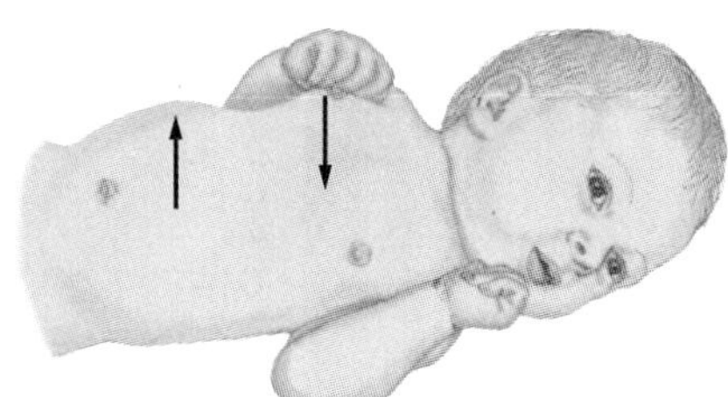

Seesaw respirations

INTERCOSTAL SPACES

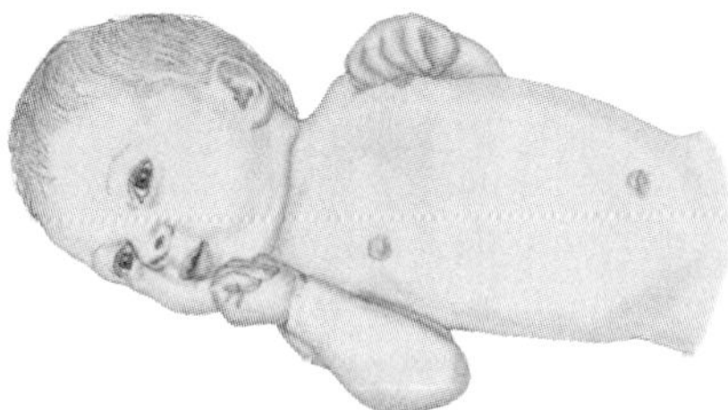

No retraction

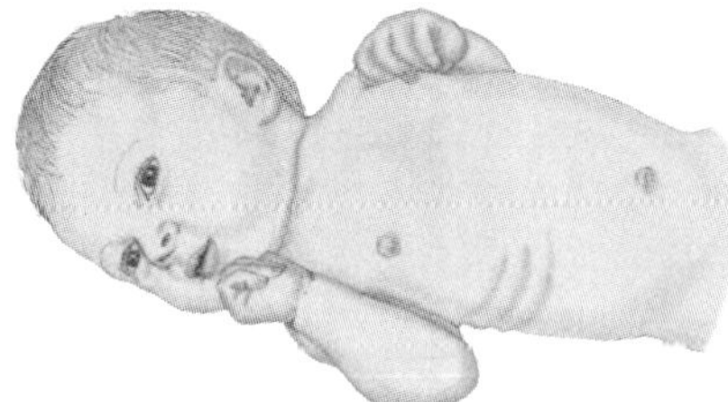

Retraction just visible

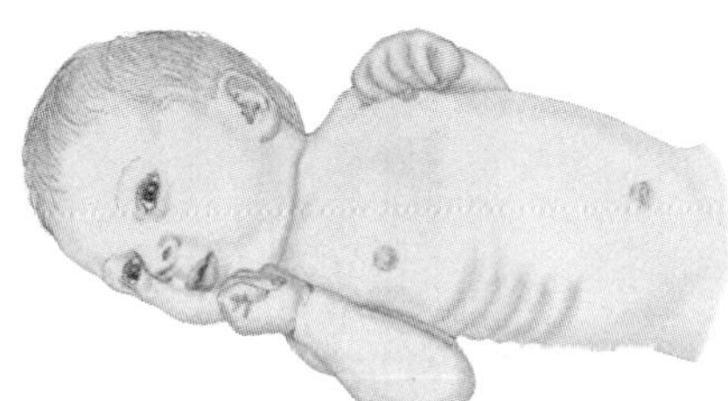

Marked retraction

XIPHOID AREA

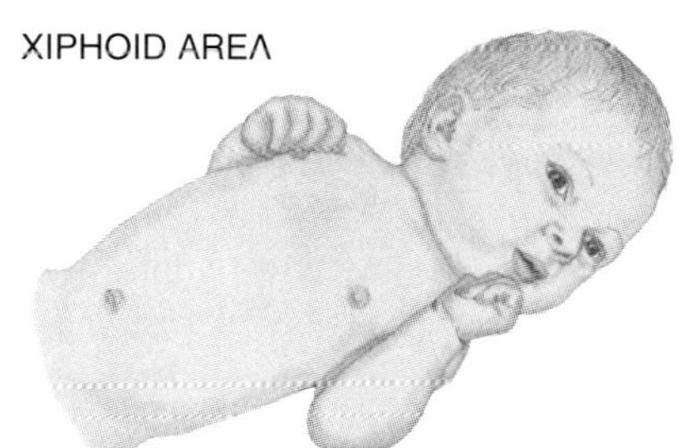

No retraction

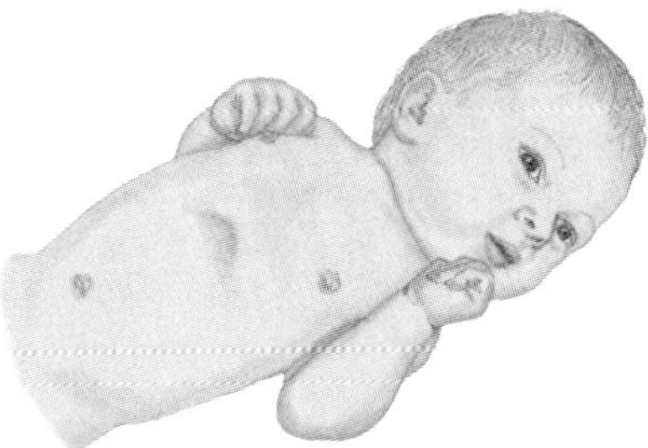

Retraction just visible

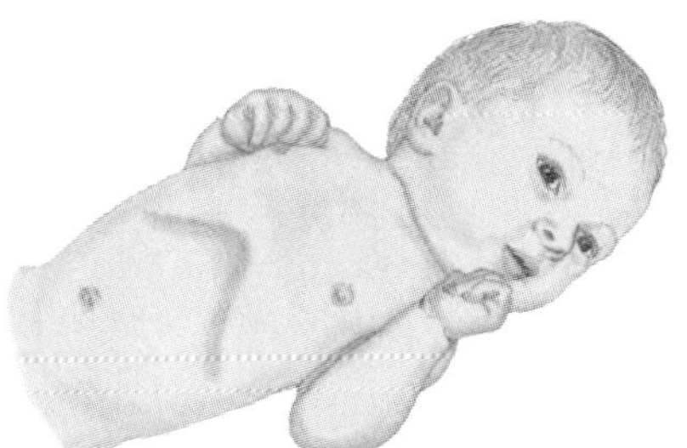

Marked retraction

NARES

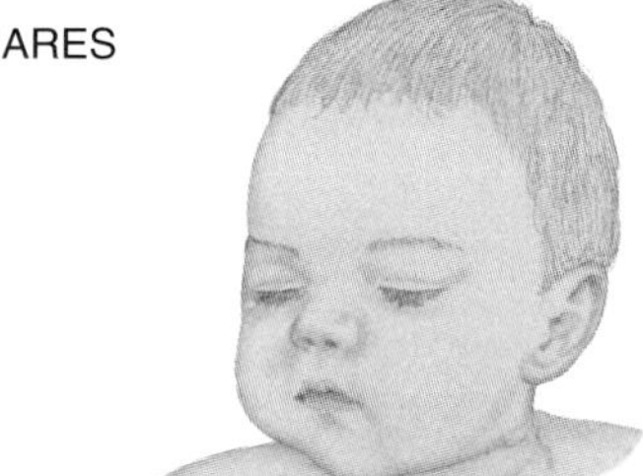

No dilation

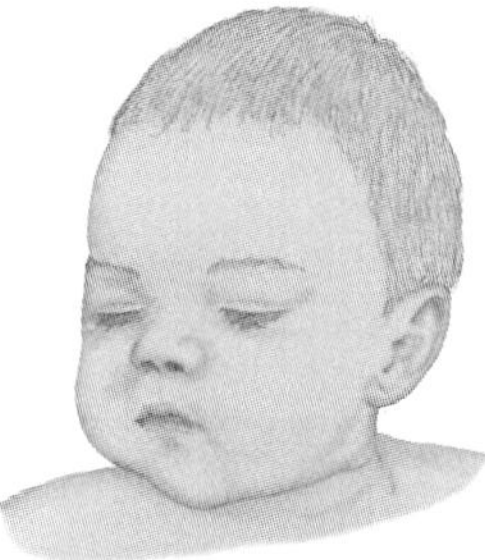

Minimal dilation

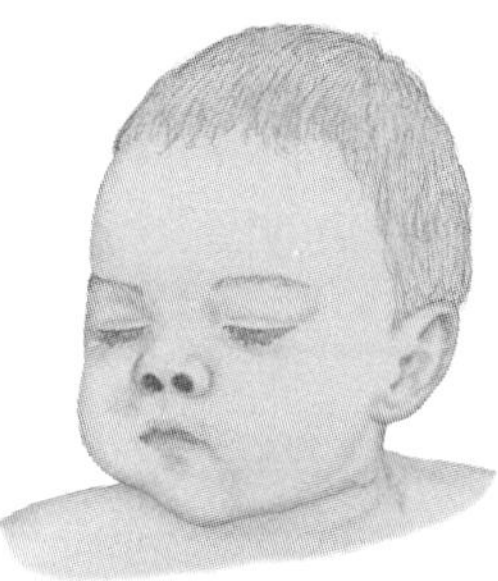

Marked dilation

EXPIRATORY SOUND

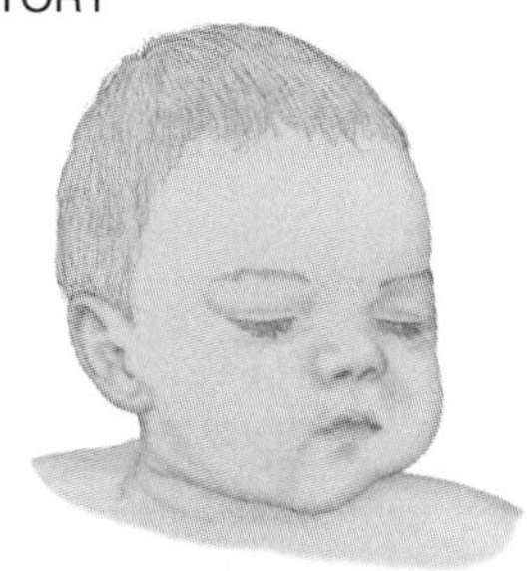

No expiratory grunting

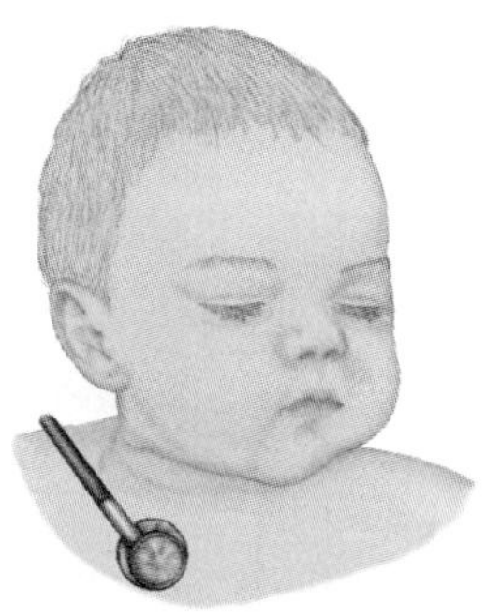

Expiratory grunting audible by stethoscope

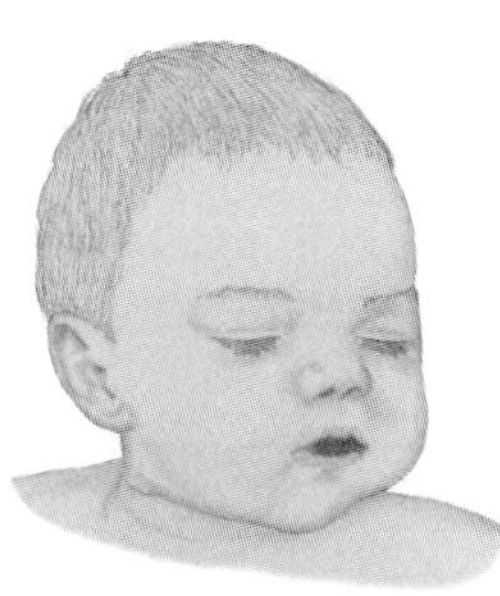

Expiratory grunting audible to unaided ear

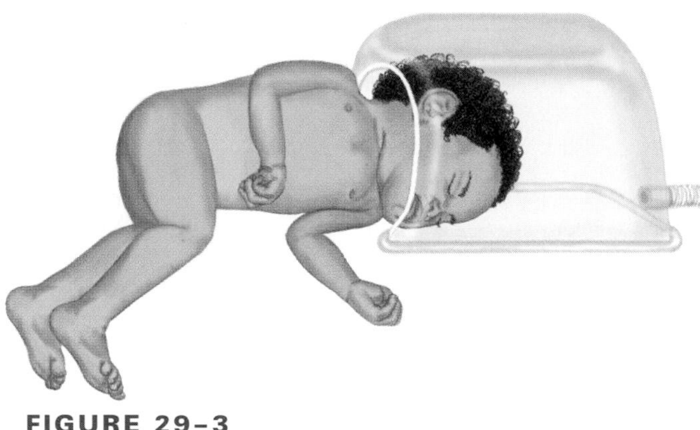

**FIGURE 29–3**

The oxygen hood is one way of delivering oxygen to an infant who can breathe unassisted.

cyanosis occur. Oxygen is increased before, during, or after the treatment, if necessary. The infant should rest after the procedure.

***Maintaining Hydration.*** Adequate hydration is essential to keep secretions thin so that they can be removed by drainage or suction. If infants become dehydrated, secretions will become thick and viscous and could obstruct tiny air passages. Fluid intake should be increased, within the limits of the overall treatment plan, if secretions seem to indicate even minimal dehydration. Small amounts of saline may be administered through endotracheal tubes just before suctioning to thin secretions.

### PROBLEMS WITH THERMOREGULATION

Although heat loss can be a problem for full-term infants, it is even more significant in preterm infants. Because the skin is thin, with blood vessels near the surface, and scant subcutaneous fat is present to serve as insulation, rapid heat loss results. The shorter time in the uterus allows less brown fat to accumulate before birth, impairing the preterm infant's ability to produce heat by nonshivering thermogenesis.

Preterm infants have a large head and more body surface area in proportion to size than full-term infants. Although full-term infants maintain heat by flexion of the extremities, the limp, extended body of preterm newborns exposes a greater surface area to the air for heat loss. The temperature control center of the brain of preterm infants is less mature and may be further impaired by asphyxia.

Full-term newborns increase metabolism to produce heat, but preterm infants are less able to do this. Hypoglycemia and respiratory problems are more likely to develop. This limits the glucose and oxygen available to increase metabolism as a method of heat production. Vasoconstriction, which occurs when body temperature drops, may lead to metabolic acidosis, pulmonary vasoconstriction, interference with production of surfactant, and more respiratory difficulty.

**Assessment.** The infant's temperature is monitored continuously by a skin probe on the infant's abdomen, which is attached to the heat control mechanism of the radiant warmer or incubator. The infant's temperature as shown on the monitor should be recorded at least every hour initially, and every 4 hours when the infant is stable. The nurse should assess the axillary temperature every 4 to 8 hours and compare it with the heat control reading to ensure that the machinery is functioning properly.

The axillary temperature should remain between 36.5° and 37.5°C (97.7° and 99.5°F), and the abdominal skin temperature should be between 36° and 36.5°C (96.8° and 97.7°F). If the infant has accumulated brown fat, a normal axillary temperature when the monitor shows a decreased skin temperature may indicate that brown fat in the axillary space is being used to maintain the infant's core temperature.

Indications of inadequate thermoregulation include poor feeding or intolerance to feedings in an infant who previously had little difficulty, lethargy, irritability, poor muscle tone, cool skin temperature, and mottled skin (Fig. 29–4). Hypoglycemia and respiratory distress may be the first signs that the infant's temperature is low. Because temperature instability may be an early sign of infection, the nurse should assess for other evidence that infection may be present.

**Nursing Interventions.** Maintenance of heat in preterm infants involves the same basic nursing care principles as for the full-term infant (see Chapter 21). However, these principles must be adapted to meet the needs of the preterm infant.

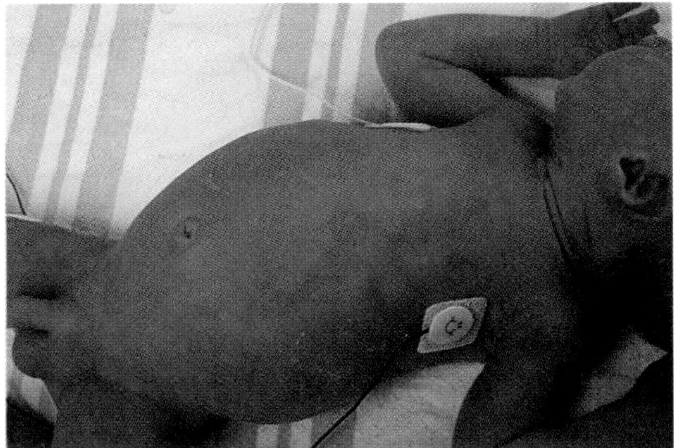

**FIGURE 29–4**

This preterm infant has mildly mottled skin and slight abdominal distention and retractions.

## Critical to Remember

### SIGNS OF INADEQUATE THERMOREGULATION

- Axillary temperature <36.5°C or >37.5°C
- Abdominal skin temperature <36°C or >36.5°C
- Change in feeding behavior
- Lethargy
- Irritability
- Decreased muscle tone
- Cool skin temperature
- Mottled skin
- Signs of hypoglycemia
- Signs of respiratory difficulty

***Maintaining a Neutral Thermal Environment.*** A neutral thermal environment is especially important to prevent need for increased oxygen to maintain body temperature. Radiant warmers or incubators are used until infants can maintain normal body temperature alone. Charts are available that indicate the appropriate temperature setting to maintain a neutral thermal environment according to the infant's size and maturity. Smaller, less mature infants will need more warmth to maintain body heat than larger or older preterm infants because they lose more heat and produce less.

Infants needing many procedures are usually placed under the open radiant warmer to make it easier to see them and work with equipment. However, air currents around an unclothed infant can cause heat loss by convection despite the heat generated by the warmer. Doors near the warmer should be closed and traffic kept to a minimum to further decrease convective heat loss. The infant should receive only warmed oxygen, because thermal receptors in the face are very sensitive to cold. Cold oxygen could quickly lead to cold stress.

Equipment or caregivers should not come between the infant and the heat source, preventing heat from reaching the infant. A transparent plastic blanket over the infant allows heat from the warmer to pass across to the infant and decreases insensible water loss while maintaining visibility of the infant's body parts.

When infants are in an incubator, the nurse should keep portholes and doors closed as much as possible. A significant amount of heat is lost every time the incubator is opened, and it takes time to build up again. On removal from the incubator for procedures or holding, the infant should be placed in heated blankets, and head coverings should be used. The incubator doors should be closed while the infant is out of it to retain heat inside.

Procedures that cannot be performed inside the incubator should be done with infants under a radiant warmer or on a surface padded with warm blankets. A heat lamp provides an alternative source of heat.

Although temperature loss is the most common concern, overheating is also a problem for preterm infants. This may occur when heating devices such as radiant warmers are set too high. This leads to an increase in the metabolic rate, with increased oxygen and glucose needs, and insensible water losses.

**Weaning to an Open Crib.** Preparation of infants for moving to an open crib should begin early. When they are stable, they can be dressed in a shirt, diaper, and hat while in the incubator. This conserves heat and helps them adjust to a different temperature on the face than the rest of the body. Infants who are about 1500 g and gaining approximately 15 to 30 g daily can begin gradual weaning from external heat (Medoff-Cooper, 1994).

Each department has its own protocol for the weaning process. The incubator temperature is usually decreased 1 to 1.5°C each day. It is raised if the infant's temperature falls below 36°C. If the temperature remains stable, the process can continue the next day.

When infants can tolerate the incubator setting at 28°C, they are ready for transfer to an open crib. They should be double-wrapped with warm blankets at first to help insulate body heat. The temperature is assessed at gradually increasing intervals until they are on a routine schedule. A blanket is added for a low temperature, but if the temperature does not rise to normal, infants are returned to the incubator.

Nurses should observe infants carefully during the first few days after transfer to an open crib. Signs that may indicate inadequate thermoregulation include decreased weight gain or poor feeding. When an infant's temperature is lower than normal, complications such as hypoglycemia, respiratory difficulty, and acidosis may occur.

#### PROBLEMS WITH FLUID AND ELECTROLYTE BALANCE

Preterm infants lose fluid very easily. Their thin skin has little protective subcutaneous fat and a greater water content, and it is more permeable than the skin of term infants. The large surface area, in proportion to body weight, and lack of flexion further increase insensible water losses. Radiant warmers and the heat from phototherapy lights cause even more fluid loss through the skin. Radiant warmers heighten insensible water losses enough to result in a 40 to 100 percent increase in fluid needs (Blake & Murray, 1993). Water loss also occurs through the respiratory and gastrointestinal tracts. The rapid respiratory rate and the use of oxygen can increase fluid loss from the lungs. Loose stools will lead to rapid dehydration.

Development of the kidneys is not complete until approximately 35 weeks of gestation. The ability of the kidneys to concentrate or dilute urine is poor before that time, causing a fragile balance between dehydration and overhydration. Although there is variation according to size and gestational age, the fluid needs of preterm infants average 110 to 140 ml/kg per day after the first 2 days of life (Price & Kalhan, 1993). Monitoring intake and output of fluids is important in determining fluid balance. Normal urinary output is 1 to 3 ml/kg per hour.

Regulation of electrolytes by the kidneys is also a problem. Preterm infants need higher intakes of sodium because the kidneys do not reabsorb it well. However, if they receive sodium, they may be unable to increase sodium excretion adequately and are susceptible to sodium and water overload as a result.

**Assessment.** The nurse must be alert for fluid overload or deficit. The infant's intake and output by all routes is carefully calculated. Parenteral, feeding tube, or oral fluids are included when measuring intake. Output from drainage tubes and urine should be measured. A urine output of less than 1 ml/kg per hour may indicate inadequate fluid intake, whereas more than 3 ml/kg per hour is a sign of overhydration (Gomella, 1994). The nurse must also keep track of the amount of blood taken for laboratory tests; the amount can be substantial.

***Urinary Output.*** There are several methods of measuring urinary output. Plastic bags that adhere to the perineum are often not suitable for the preterm infant because they may damage the fragile skin. Weighing diapers is less invasive to the infant. The weight of dry diapers is subtracted from the weight of wet diapers to determine the amount of urine excreted. One gram is equivalent to 1 ml of urine. However, humidification may add moisture to the diaper, and a radiant warmer may cause evaporation of urine on the diaper. When precise measurement is essential, diapers can be fastened instead of placing them open under the infant.

Specific gravity should be checked to determine if urine is more concentrated or dilute than expected. Urine is collected by placing cotton balls at the perineum. The specific gravity should range between 1.005 and 1.015.

***Weight.*** Changes in the infant's weight can give an indication of fluid gain or loss, especially if they are sudden and greater than would be expected from feeding changes. The undressed infant should be weighed daily at the same time each day with the same scale. Very small infants are often placed in a bed that has a scale on it so that they do not have to be disturbed for daily weighing. They may be weighed twice a day to monitor their fluid status more closely.

***Signs of Dehydration or Overhydration.*** The nurse should observe for signs that indicate that the infant has received too little or too much fluid. Early signs of dehydration include decreased urine output and increased specific gravity. Weight loss may exceed that expected for the infant's age and general condition. Dry skin or mucous membranes, sunken anterior fontanelle, and poor tissue turgor are late signs. Changes in the blood include increased sodium, protein, and hematocrit levels resulting from decreased plasma volume.

Signs of overhydration include increased output of urine with a below-normal specific gravity. Edema and weight gain occur from retention of fluids. Bulging fontanelles and decreased blood sodium, protein, and hematocrit levels are also present. Complications of excess fluid may include patent ductus arteriosus and congestive heart failure.

**Nursing Interventions.** The nurse must carefully regulate intravenous fluids and use infusion control devices to help prevent fluid volume overload. Intravenous medications should be diluted in as little fluid as is consistent with safe administration of the

### Critical to Remember

**SIGNS OF FLUID IMBALANCE IN THE NEWBORN**

**Dehydration**

- Urine output $<1$ ml/kg per hr
- Urine specific gravity $>1.015$
- Weight loss greater than expected
- Dry skin and mucous membranes
- Sunken anterior fontanelle
- Poor tissue turgor
- Blood: elevated sodium, protein, and hematocrit levels

**Overhydration**

- Urine output $>3$ ml/kg per hr
- Urine specific gravity $<1.005$
- Edema
- Weight gain greater than expected
- Bulging fontanelles
- Blood: decreased sodium, protein, and hematocrit levels
- Moist breath sounds
- Difficulty breathing

drug and should be included when measuring intake. Starting intravenous lines on infants with poor veins is a lengthy, difficult procedure. Infants must be restrained as necessary to prevent infiltration. Some fluids will cause extensive damage as a result of tissue sloughing if they infiltrate.

#### PROBLEMS WITH INFECTION

The incidence of infection in preterm infants is three to 10 times greater than that in full-term newborns (Behrman et al., 1996). Many preterm infants have one or more episodes of sepsis during their hospital stay. They have several risk factors for infections. The mother may have had an infection that caused labor to begin prematurely, thus exposing the infant to the same infection. The infant may not have been in the uterus long enough to receive adequate passive immunity from the transfer of immunoglobulin G from the mother during the third trimester. In addition, the immune response of a preterm infant is less mature than that of the full-term newborn.

Preterm infants are often exposed to situations that may cause infection. Their skin is fragile, permeable, and easily damaged. Removal of adhesive-based products may strip the epidermal layer of the skin. They are subject to invasive procedures such as insertion of intravenous lines and drawing of blood specimens.

**Assessment.** The nurse should be on the alert for signs of infection at all times (see Chapter 30, p. 860).

**Nursing Interventions.** Nursing care involves scrupulous cleanliness and maintaining the infant's skin integrity.

All precautions in infection control used with the full-term infant apply to the preterm infant. Even the normal flora on the hands of caretakers may cause sepsis. Therefore, parents and staff members should scrub their hands and arms before handling infants. Exposure to family members or staff members who have contagious diseases should be prevented.

The use of adhesives should be restricted to prevent damage to the skin when they are removed. The smallest amount of adhesive possible should be used to stabilize endotracheal tubes and intravenous tubing. Tape that is specially prepared to be less traumatic on removal helps protect the skin. Easily removed pectin-based products are available for skin probes and monitor leads.

The nurse should avoid the use of chemicals that can injure the skin or may be absorbed through it. Adhesives should be removed with water alone or diluted soap instead of chemicals, when possible. If alcohol or other preparations are used on the skin, a sterile water rinse will minimize damage.

Infants and their equipment should be positioned to avoid undue pressure on the skin. Frequent position changes are important, but should be based on the infant's ability to tolerate changes.

#### PROBLEMS WITH PAIN

Infants in the NICU undergo many painful procedures each day. Caregivers once thought that newborns, particularly preterm infants, were neurologically too immature to feel pain. It is now recognized that pain stimuli cause physiologic and behavioral changes in infants. Preterm infants may be even more sensitive to pain than older infants (Stevens et al., 1995). The long-term effects of pain in the neonate are not yet fully understood.

**Assessment.** The nurse must assess the infant for pain level and response to potentially painful stimuli. Physiologic changes include changes in heart rate and respirations, increased blood pressure and intracranial pressure, and decreased oxygen saturation. Hormonal and metabolic changes occur as well. Physiologic changes may be unpredictable and cannot be used alone to assess pain.

Behavioral changes include high-pitched, intense, harsh crying. In infants who are intubated or too weak to cry, a "cry face" is seen, with a crying facial expression without the sound of a cry.

**Nursing Interventions.** Nurses should prepare infants for potentially painful procedures by waking them slowly and gently and using containment. Containment simulates the enclosed space of the uterus and is comforting to infants. It involves keeping the extremities in a flexed position near the body by swaddling, blanket rolls, or the nurse's hands. At least one hand should be near the mouth for sucking.

Comfort measures help the infant cope with short-term, mild pain and reduce agitation. They include non-nutritive sucking, soft talking, restraining the extremities to prevent flailing, and holding and rocking.

### Critical to Remember

#### COMMON SIGNS OF PAIN IN INFANTS

- High-pitched, intense, harsh cry
- "Cry face"
- Eyes squeezed shut
- Mouth open
- Grimacing
- Rigidity or flailing of extremities
- Color changes: red, dusky, pale
- Increased or decreased heart rate
- Increased respirations
- Increased blood pressure
- Decreased oxygen saturation
- Increased intracranial pressure

**LONG BEACH MEMORIAL MEDICAL CENTER**
**MULTIDISCIPLINARY ACTION PLAN**
**Growing Preemie ≤32 Weeks' Gestation at Birth**

| | 32 weeks | 33 weeks | 34 weeks | 35 weeks | 36 weeks | 37 weeks |
|---|---|---|---|---|---|---|
| **DATE** | | | | | | |
| **PATIENT OUTCOMES** | ☐ No AB spells x 24°<br>☐ Gains wt on enteral fdgs<br>☐ Hct >28% | ☐ Parents meet with case manager<br>☐ Temp stable when held<br>☐ Tol up in chair without v/s changes<br>☐ Parents demo use of thermometer and bulb syringe<br>☐ Hct >28% | ☐ Tol nipple feeds x 1/day<br>☐ Hct >28% | ☐ Parents do feeding x 1/day<br>☐ Temp stable in crib<br>☐ Gains wt<br>☐ Hct >28% | ☐ Gains wt<br>☐ Parents return demo med admin<br>☐ Identify signs & symptoms of illness<br>☐ Hct >28% | ☐ Gains wt on 20 cal formula<br>☐ Parents return demo CPR<br>☐ Hct >28%<br>☐ Tol all nipple feeds |
| **VS/CRITICAL ASSESSMENTS** | ☐ V/S q 8 hours<br>☐ HC q day<br>☐ Abd girth AC or q shift<br>☐ Wt q day | ☐ V/S q 8 hours<br>☐ HC q day<br>☐ Abd girth AC or q shift<br>☐ Wt q day | ☐ V/S q 8 hours<br>☐ HC q day<br>☐ Abd girth AC or q shift<br>☐ Wt q day | ☐ V/S q 8 hours<br>☐ HC q day<br>☐ Abd girth AC or q shift<br>☐ Wt q day | ☐ V/S q 8 hours<br>☐ HC q day<br>☐ Abd girth AC or q shift<br>☐ Wt q day | ☐ V/S q 8 hours<br>☐ HC q day<br>☐ Abd girth AC or q shift<br>☐ Wt q day |
| **CONSULTS** | ☐ Ophthalmologist | ☐ OT/PT if not done earlier | | | ☐ OB for circ | |
| **DIAGNOSTIC TESTS** | ☐ Lab tests per protocol<br>☐ Hematest stool q shift<br>☐ Eye Exam (6 wks of age) | ☐ Lab tests per protocol<br>☐ Hematest stool q shift<br>☐ Eye Exam (6 wks of age)<br>☐ Theo/Caffeine levels | ☐ Lab tests per protocol<br>☐ Hematest stool q shift<br>☐ Eye Exam (6 wks of age)<br>☐ Hearing exam | ☐ Lab tests per protocol<br>☐ Hematest stool q shift<br>☐ Eye Exam (6 wks of age)<br>☐ Pneumogram | ☐ Lab tests per protocol<br>☐ Hematest stool q shift<br>☐ Eye Exam (6 wks of age) | ☐ Lab tests per protocol<br>☐ Hematest stool q shift<br>☐ Eye Exam (6 wks of age) |
| **TREATMENT/ INTERVENTION** | ☐ Epogen/Fe if Retic <5% Hct <35%<br>☐ At 1500 gms Protocol to wean to open crib | ☐ Breast fdg eval<br>☐ OT eval | ☐ At 1800 gms wean to open crib | ☐ Check on circ consent | ☐ Circ at 1900 gms<br>☐ OT developmental eval | |



✓ Indicates achievement of outcome/performance or intervention.
• Indicates an unachieved outcome or intervention not performed.
☐ Indicates an intervention that was not applicable.
○ May discontinue after two normal results unless otherwise indicated

**FIGURE 29–5**

An example of a clinical pathway (called a multidisciplinary action plan here) for "growing preemies" (stable preterm infants) at 32 weeks' gestation. (Modified from Long Beach Memorial Medical Center, Long Beach, California.)

**LONG BEACH MEMORIAL MEDICAL CENTER**
**MULTIDISCIPLINARY ACTION PLAN**
**Growing Preemie ≤32 Weeks' Gestation at Birth**

| | 32 weeks | 33 weeks | 34 weeks | 35 weeks | 36 weeks | 37 weeks |
|---|---|---|---|---|---|---|
| **MEDICATIONS** | ☐ Theophylline/Caffeine<br>☐ Reglan/Cisapride<br>☐ MVI | ☐ Theophylline/Caffeine<br>☐ Reglan/Cisapride<br>☐ MVi<br>☐ Fe supplement | ☐ D/C Cisapride/Reglan<br>☐ D/C /Theophylline at 1800 gms if AB free x 2 weeks<br>☐ D/C Caffeine<br>☐ MVI<br>☐ Fe supplement | ☐ MVI<br>☐ Fe Supplement | ☐ MVI<br>☐ Fe Supplement | ☐ MVI<br>☐ Fe Supplement |
| **ACTIVITY** | ☐ Out of isol, Kangaroo care as tol<br>☐ Positioning: Nesting/ head in donut<br>☐ Pacifier for non-nutritive sucking<br>☐ Interaction based on infant cues<br>☐ Up in infant seat x 1hr ac q shift | ☐ Out of isol as tol<br>☐ Positioning: Nesting/ head in donut<br>☐ Pacifier for non-nutritive sucking<br>☐ Interaction based on infant cues<br>☐ Up in infant seat x 1hr ac q shift | ☐ Out of isol as tol<br>☐ Positioning: Nesting/head in donut<br>☐ Pacifier for non-nutritive sucking<br>☐ Interaction based on infant cues<br>☐ Up in infant seat x 1hr ac q shift | ☐ Positioning: Nesting/ head in donut<br>☐ Pacifier for non-nutritive sucking<br>☐ Interaction based on infant cues<br>☐ Up in infant seat x 1hr ac q shift | ☐ Positioning: Nesting/ head in donut<br>☐ Pacifier for non-nutritive sucking<br>☐ Interaction based on infant cues<br>☐ Up in infant seat x 1hr ac q shift | ☐ Positioning: Nesting/ head in donut<br>☐ Pacifier for non-nutritive sucking<br>☐ Interaction based on infant cues<br>☐ Up in infant seat x 1hr ac q shift |
| **NUTRITION** | ☐ 24 cal/oz formula<br>☐ Gavage fdg q 3 hrs | ☐ Nipple x 1/day<br>☐ Gavage other feeds | ☐ Nipple BID<br>☐ Gavage other feeds<br>☐ Parents co nipple feeds x 1/day | ☐ Nipple TID and advance as to<br>☐ Gavage other feeds | ☐ Nipple all feeds<br>☐ 20 cal/oz formula<br>☐ 22 cal/oz at 1800 grams | ☐ Nipple all feeds<br>☐ 20 cal/oz formula |
| **ELIMINATION** | ☐ Wet diaper checks<br>☐ Monitor stooling pattern | ☐ Wet diaper checks<br>☐ Monitor stooling pattern | ☐ Wet diaper checks<br>☐ Monitor stooling pattern | ☐ Wet diaper checks<br>☐ Monitor stooling pattern | ☐ Wet diaper checks<br>☐ Monitor stooling pattern | ☐ Wet diaper checks<br>☐ Monitor stooling pattern |
| **PATIENT/ FAMILY EDUCATION** | ☐ Assess educational needs of parents based on Pt. Ed. Flowsheet<br>☐ Thermometer use<br>☐ Bulb syringe use | ☐ Bath demo<br>☐ Parents identify infant cues | ☐ Baby care class<br>☐ Review: car seat safety & home safety | ☐ CPR class<br>☐ Review signs & symptoms of illness<br>☐ Med admin teaching | ☐ Review D/C instr.<br>☐ Med return demo<br>☐ CPR return demo | |
| **DISCHARGE PLANNING** | ☐ Re-assess funding | ☐ Validate address/phone #<br>☐ Assess home preparedness<br>☐ Parents receive class invitations | ☐ Discuss car seat needs | ☐ WIC referral<br>☐ Peds referral | ☐ Order equipment and supplies<br>☐ Order nursing visits<br>☐ Request letters for priority service from utility services | Parents:<br>☐ Receive equipment & supplies<br>☐ Receive & fill med Rx<br>☐ Receive D/C instructions<br>☐ Receive letters for priority service |
| **BEHAVIORAL** | ☐ Assess infant cues during activity<br>☐ Support self regulatory behaviors | ☐ Assess infant cues during nipple feeds & activity<br>☐ Support self regulatory behaviors | ☐ Assess infant cues during nipple feeds & activity<br>☐ Support self regulatory behaviors | ☐ Assess infant cues during nipple feeds & activity<br>☐ Support self regulatory behaviors | ☐ Assess infant cues during nipple feeds & activity<br>☐ Support self regulatory behaviors | ☐ Assess infant cues during nipple feeds & activity<br>☐ Support self regulatory behaviors |



✓ Indicates achievement of outcome/performance or intervention. • Indicates an unachieved outcome or intervention not performed. ☐ Indicates an intervention that was not applicable. ○ May discontinue after two normal results unless otherwise indicated

**FIGURE 29–5** *Continued*

Measures should be adapted according to infants' responses.

The nurse should discuss the infant's pain with the primary care provider to ensure that medications are available for long-term and more severe pain. Morphine and general anesthesia can be tolerated by preterm infants. The nurse should give ordered medications before painful procedures and when the infant demonstrates pain signs. The nurse should carefully note the infant's response to allow increasing or decreasing dosage as necessary.

**CHECK YOUR READING**

3. What factors contribute to respiratory problems in preterm infants?
4. What nursing responsibilities relate to care of preterm respiratory problems?.
5. How do nurses help infants adjust to the cooler environment of an open crib?
6. How does the nurse keep track of an infant's intake and output?
7. What special problems related to fluid balance, infections, and pain occur in preterm infants?

### Case Management and Clinical Pathways

Preterm infants may remain in the NICU for many days, at a cost of thousands of dollars. Methods to reduce the length of stay to return infants to their parents at home more quickly and to reduce the cost of hospitalization have been explored. One method involves case management and clinical pathways.

The case manager is a nurse who follows infants from admission to discharge to identify or prevent situations that would interfere with progression toward discharge. Clinical pathways are guidelines developed collaboratively by staff members from all disciplines. They list the care infants will need along a time line and the expected outcomes of that care. This allows staff members and parents to know when to expect changes in care. Different pathways are created to meet the needs of different types of infants, such as infants with various complications of prematurity. Figure 29–5 is an example of a clinical pathway used for stable preterm infants.

## Application of Nursing Process: Preterm Infant

Preterm infants commonly have difficulty with stress from the NICU environment and obtaining adequate nutrition. Their parents may have difficulty with bonding.

## Environmentally Caused Stress

Preterm infants are exposed constantly to a bright, loud environment. The sounds of alarms, ventilators, doors, and people create a noise level above that of loud traffic. This stressful environment may be associated with hearing loss, retinopathy of prematurity, and other complications. In addition, stimulation of any kind can cause increased energy expenditure by the preterm infant. Noise and routine nursing interventions are often accompanied by changes in heart rate, oxygen saturation levels, and behavior states.

Although touch is generally thought to be comforting to infants, it is often associated with painful events for preterm infants. During uterine life, the fetus sleeps as much as 80 to 90 percent of the time. However, preterm infants undergo multiple assessments and treatments. These cause frequent interruptions of sleep and may interfere with the development of normal sleep-wake cycles. Energy that must be directed toward coping with an overstimulating and stressful environment may be unavailable for normal growth and development.

### Assessment

Assess the amount of noise to which the infant is exposed. Determine how often interruptions occur and how the infant responds to different types of care.

Assess the infant's ability to tolerate activity and noise. Overstimulation results in changes in oxygenation and behavior. Signs of alteration in oxygenation include pulse and respiratory rate variations from baseline, apnea, rapid color changes and cyanosis, nasal flaring, and drop in oxygen saturation levels.

Behavioral indications of stress include stiffening and extension of the extremities with fisting or splaying (spreading) of the fingers. The infant may appear hyperalert with a worried facial expression or may turn away from eye contact. Coughing, yawning, hiccupping, and regurgitation are also signals that infants are receiving more stimulation than they can tolerate. All signs may be accompanied by increased fatigue.

### Analysis

A nursing diagnosis appropriate for preterm infants having difficulty enduring the multiple stimuli in their environment is Risk for Altered Growth and Development related to stress from an overstimulating environment. Use of this nursing diagnosis can help the nurse plan ways to increase the infant's ability to tolerate interventions.

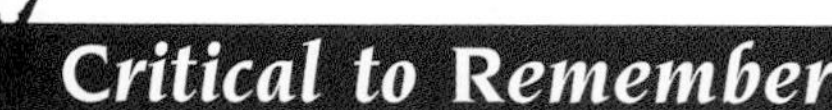

**SIGNS OF OVERSTIMULATION IN PRETERM INFANTS**

**Oxygenation Changes**

- Increase or decrease in pulse and respiratory rate
- Cyanosis, pallor, or mottling
- Flaring nares
- Decreased oxygen saturation levels
- Coughing
- Yawning

**Behavior Changes**

- Stiff, extended arms and legs
- Fisting of the hands or splaying of the fingers
- Alert, worried expression
- Turning away from eye contact
- Hiccupping
- Regurgitation
- Fatigue

## Planning

The goals for this nursing diagnosis are that the infant will do the following:

- Conserve energy for growth and development by showing decreased signs of overstimulation during routine activity.
- Gradually show an ability to withstand more activity before signs of overstimulation occur.

## Interventions

The role of the nurse is to help the infant conserve energy needed for normal body function and growth. Interventions are focused on providing developmentally supportive nursing care that meets the preterm infant's ability to tolerate stimulation. Developmental care keeps stressors in the environment to a minimum based on the infant's physiologic and behavioral responses.

### SCHEDULING CARE

Schedule periods of undisturbed rest throughout the day to allow the infant to recover from treatments. Avoid disturbing rest by arranging routine care to correspond with the infant's awake periods. Group care activities so that several tasks are performed at one time to allow for more rest between interruptions. However, be alert to the infant's signs of stress. Too many activities may be more than the infant can tolerate without rest.

Allow short rest periods within grouped activities or during long or painful procedures if the infant shows signs of overstimulation. Decrease the frequency of taking vital signs and providing other routine care as soon as possible.

The handling involved in routine sponge bathing may cause changes in heart rate and oxygenation saturation levels in small infants (Peters, 1996a). If the procedure causes stress responses in an infant, it should be limited to necessary cleaning to conserve energy.

An important nursing responsibility is managing the infant's care by coordinating activities of different health care workers. For example, many different tests are often needed, and the nurse must see that they are done properly, yet protect the infant from overstimulation.

### REDUCING STIMULI

Keep noise around the infant as low as possible. Place incubators where they are away from traffic and congestion of people. Avoid talking near the incubator. Set volume on alarms on low and respond quickly when they sound. Open and close doors on incubators and cupboards gently. Do not place objects on top of the incubator or use it as a writing surface, because this increases the noise inside.

The lights that are on 24 hours a day in the nursery may interfere with the development of sleep cycles. Position the incubator so that the infant is not facing bright lights, and drape a blanket over one end to decrease light further. Use a dimmer switch to vary the intensity of lights as needed. Place infants in a prone position to help them avoid looking at ceiling lights.

### PROMOTING REST

When possible, schedule "quiet periods," when lights and noise in the unit are kept to a minimum, to promote rest. Scheduled naps when infants are disturbed as little as possible help increase sleep, decrease waking, and lead to longer uninterrupted sleep (Holditch-Davis et al., 1995). They may be associated with decreased periods of apnea and increased weight gain for some infants. A daytime and evening nap and two during the night will help the infant begin to differentiate day and night sleeping patterns.

Contain the infant's arms and legs to promote flexion and reduce energy loss from flailing extremities. Provide a "nest" with rolled blankets placed around the infant for boundaries. Use the prone position to increase quiet sleep periods. In the side or supine position, arrange the infant's arms and legs in a flexed position, with the hands near midline.

### PROMOTING MOTOR DEVELOPMENT

Preterm infants may have musculoskeletal and developmental problems from prolonged immobilization and the effects of gravity on their immature neuromuscular system. Because the extensor muscles mature before the flexor muscles, the infant tends to remain in an extended, "frog-leg" position. Shoulder retraction, abduction of the lower extremities, and lateral flexion of the arms may result. When possible, swaddle the infant with the extremities flexed and the hands positioned near the mouth to allow the infant to suck the hands for comfort. Turn the infant every 2 hours, avoiding the supine position, and use blankets and rolls to maintain flexion.

#### INDIVIDUALIZING CARE

The ability to tolerate stress varies with each individual infant. Adapt general care according to the infant's ability to tolerate it. When possible, the same nurse should care for the infant each day. This allows the nurse to learn the infant's unique behavior and response to stress. Even positive stimuli, such as soft music or soft talking to the infant, can overstimulate the infant. Use it judiciously according to the infant's tolerance level.

Infants often require extra energy to adjust to changes in care. Observe how well they tolerate changes such as moving from assisted to more independent breathing or introduction of new feeding methods. Increase rest periods during these times.

#### MINIMIZING PAIN

Minimizing pain is a part of developmental care to promote rest and conserve energy. Interventions for pain are discussed in the previous section.

#### COMMUNICATING INFANTS' NEEDS

Use the nursing care plan and shift reports to inform other caregivers of techniques that are especially effective for certain infants. Tape notes on the incubator as reminders of needs that are unique to each infant. This also alerts parents to the methods nurses use to help their infant. Explain all techniques to parents.

### Evaluation

As a result of interventions, the infant conserves energy. The infant displays signs of overstimulation less often and an increasing tolerance before signs appear.

**✓ CHECK YOUR READING**

8. What can the nurse do for the infant at risk for overstimulation?

## Nutrition

The need for adequate nutrition in the preterm newborn is especially acute because the infant is born before full accumulation of nutrient stores during the last trimester of pregnancy. Full-term newborns have reservoirs of calcium, iron, and other substances, but these are lacking in preterm infants. Fat stores are minimal or absent, and glucose reserves are used up soon after birth.

Nutrients are needed not only to promote growth but to prevent injury to the brain. Hypoglycemia is a major concern because of the lack of glucose and fat reserves. Low blood glucose develops very quickly and must be prevented or treated quickly because the brain needs a steady supply of glucose.

Preterm infants need to 120 to 150 kcal/kg per day, which is higher than the 110 to 120 kcal/kg per day needed by the full-term newborn. They also need more protein, iron, calcium, and phosphorus.

The gastrointestinal tract of preterm infants does not absorb nutrients as well as that of full-term infants. Although they digest protein fairly well, preterm infants have insufficient bile acids and pancreatic lipase to absorb fat adequately. They have some lactase deficiency but digest glucose and sucrose adequately. Although their smaller stomach capacity limits the volume that they can tolerate at each feeding, preterm infants need more of many nutrients per kg than do full-term infants and require supplementation.

Coordination of sucking and swallowing usually occurs at about 32 to 34 weeks of gestation (Price & Kalhan, 1993). Infants of less than 34 weeks' gestation or weighing under 1600 g generally have difficulty coordinating sucking, swallowing, and breathing. The gag reflex, which helps prevent aspiration, may function poorly. Oral feeding may cause the very weak infant to expend too much oxygen and glucose. When sucking is uncoordinated or takes too much energy, the infant must receive intravenous or gavage feedings.

### Assessment

The focus of assessment in nutrition is on feeding readiness and tolerance. Feedings are often changed according to the nurse's assessment of an infant's adjustment to feedings and signs indicating complications or readiness for change.

#### READINESS FOR NIPPLE FEEDING

Preterm infants are often fed parenterally or by gavage (feeding tube) initially to conserve energy for growth and basic functioning. During feedings, watch for signs that nipple feeding may soon be possible,

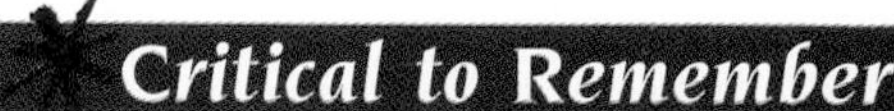

**Critical to Remember**

**SIGNS OF FEEDING READINESS IN AN INFANT**

**Signs of Readiness for Nipple Feedings**

- Rooting
- Sucking on gavage tube, finger, or pacifier
- Able to tolerate holding
- Respiratory rate <60 breaths per minute
- Presence of gag reflex

**Signs of Nonreadiness for Nipple Feedings**

- Respiratory rate >60 breaths per minute
- No rooting or sucking
- Absence of gag reflex
- Excessive gastric residuals

**Adverse Signs During Nipple Feedings**

- Tachycardia
- Bradycardia
- Increased respiratory rate
- Markedly decreased oxygen saturation level
- Apnea
- Coughing
- Gagging
- Falling asleep early in feeding
- Feeding time beyond 25 to 30 minutes

such as rooting, sucking on the gavage tube, a finger, or a pacifier; and an increasing ability to tolerate holding and handling. Note whether the infant gags on the tube or a gloved finger inserted into the mouth. Infants who do not have a gag reflex are more likely to aspirate feedings.

When the infant begins to feed by nipple, assess coordination of suck and swallow and observe for aspiration. Frequent choking, gagging, or cyanosis during feedings may indicate that the infant is unable to coordinate sucking, swallowing, and breathing well enough for nipple feeding. Some infants are so weak that the usual signs of aspiration are minimal or absent.

Assess the respiratory rate before and during feedings. When the respiratory rate is above 60 to 70 breaths per minute before feedings, gavage feed to prevent aspiration. An increased respiratory rate, tachycardia, bradycardia, decreased oxygen saturation levels, or excessive fatigue demonstrates that the effort of nipple feeding requires too much energy and oxygen for the infant.

#### FEEDING TOLERANCE

Assess how well the infant tolerates feedings, whether by feeding tube or nipple. Before beginning a gavage feeding, withdraw the gastric contents to measure the amount left from the previous feeding. This helps determine whether the stomach is emptying and prevents overdistention. A residual of more than 30 percent of the previous feeding indicates that the amount or type of formula may need changing. It may also be an early sign of a complication.

Observe for other signs of intestinal complications. Obtain objective data about abdominal distention by using a tape to measure abdominal girth. Place the tape at the level of the umbilicus, and record the placement on the nursing care plan to ensure consistency. Test stools for reducing substance by dissolving stool in water and mixing with a Clinitest tablet. The presence of reducing substance indicates malabsorption of carbohydrates. Also check for occult blood.

Vomiting or frequent regurgitation may indicate that the feedings are too large. Vomitus containing bile may be a sign of intestinal obstruction and may require surgery. Diarrhea may be caused by rapid advancement of the feeding or intolerance to the type of formula. Report signs of feeding intolerance to the physician or nurse practitioner because they may be early indications of complications, such as ileus, sepsis, obstruction of the gastrointestinal tract, or necrotizing enterocolitis.

### Analysis

When the infant's nutritional needs are met by parenteral methods, the nursing care is mainly collaborative. However, once the infant is able to take formula or to breastfeed, many nursing interventions are involved. They address the nursing diagnosis Risk for Altered Nutrition: Less Than Body Requirements related to uncoordinated suck and swallow and fatigue during feedings.

### Planning

Goals written for an individual infant with this nursing diagnosis take into consideration the specific needs of that infant. The infant will do the following:

- Take in adequate amounts of breast milk or formula to meet nutrient needs for age and weight.
- Gain weight as appropriate for age.

The actual amount of feedings and weight gain will vary according to the infant's gestational age and other conditions. What is appropriate for a particular infant can be discussed with the physician or nurse practitioner.

## Procedure 29-1

# Administering Gavage Feeding

**PURPOSE:** Gavage feeding is used for infants who are unable to take the full feeding by nipple. It may be used alone or along with nipple feedings. Orogastric tubes are often used for intermittent feedings, whereas nasogastric tubes are used for continuous feedings.

1. **Wash hands and gather equipment, including gavage tube of proper size (usually 5 to 8 French, depending on size of the infant), medicine cup or other measured container, and 20-ml syringe. Warm breast milk or formula to room temperature. Check the chart to determine how previous feedings were tolerated. Add fortifier to breast milk if necessary.** *Having all equipment ready helps the procedure go smoothly and avoids disturbing the infant or delaying feedings. Information about previous feedings will help meet the infant's needs.*

2. **If the infant has a tendency to regurgitate when moved after feedings, position him or her on the right side or prone. If parents are present, they may hold the infant in their arms once the tube is inserted or hold the hands if the infant cannot be held.** *Positioning uses gravity to help avoid reflux of milk into the trachea and promotes emptying of the stomach. Feeding is important to parents, and helping increases their sense of involvement.*

3. **Determine the length of catheter to insert by measuring from the infant's mouth or nose to the earlobe and then to the xyphoid process. Mark the tube at the proper point with a piece of tape.** *The measured distance is equal to the distance from the mouth to the stomach.*

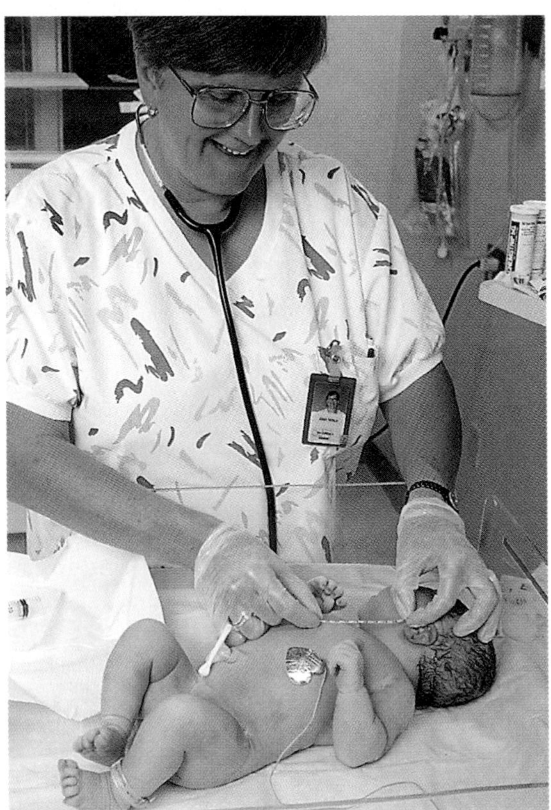

4. **Moisten the tip of the catheter with water, and shake off any excess. While holding the infant's head steady, gently insert the tube through the mouth or nose to the point marked. Remove the tube immediately if persistent coughing, choking, cyanosis, apnea, or bradycardia occurs.** *Moistening the tip provides lubrication. Signs may indicate that the tube is entering the trachea instead of the esophagus. Stimulation of the vagus nerve may cause bradycardia or apnea.*

5. **Check for placement when the tube is first placed, before beginning bolus feedings, and at least once a shift for continuous feedings. Attach a syringe to the tube and insert 0.5 to 1 cc of air through the tube while listening over the stomach with a stethoscope. Gently draw back on the plunger to withdraw the inserted air.** *Hearing air enter the stomach ensures that the catheter is in place. Withdrawing the inserted air provides more room for feeding and helps prevent regurgitation.*

6. **Gently aspirate stomach contents. Move or rotate the tube slightly if the plunger does not withdraw easily.** *Aspirating stomach contents provides further proof that the feeding tube is in the proper place. Use of force could traumatize the stomach lining if the end of the tube is resting against it. Moving the tube may draw it away from the stomach lining.*

7. **Tape the tube in place.** *Taping ensures the tube will remain inserted to the proper length during the procedure.*

8. **Withdraw stomach contents. Observe amount, color, and consistency of the aspirate. During continuous feedings, check the gastric residual every 2 to 4 hours. Do not feed the infant if the aspirate is abnormal. Report abnormal appearance or amount of stomach contents.** *Assessment of stomach contents detects abnormalities. Stomach contents that are red or dark brown may indicate blood. If the aspirate is green with bile or brown with feces, there may be an intestinal obstruction. An excessive amount may mean that the infant is receiving too much or that stomach emptying is delayed. For continuous feedings, residual equal to 2 to 3 hours of volume may be normal if there are no other signs of feeding intolerance.*

9. **Replace the aspirate before beginning feeding. Subtract the amount of gastric residual from the amount of milk to be given.** *Replacement of aspirate prevents loss of electrolytes. Overdistention of the stomach is avoided by subtracting the residual from the feeding to be given.*

10. **Remove the plunger and attach the syringe to the feeding tube. Pour the correct amount of solution into the syringe. If it does not begin to move down the tube, insert the plunger just far enough to get the flow started, then withdraw it. Do not use the plunger to force the contents through the tube. Allow feeding to flow by gravity. Or attach to a feeding pump that will regulate the amount of flow.** *Using the plunger to force the entire feeding may cause damage to the stomach mucosa from too much pressure. A*

## Procedure 29-1 *Continued*

# Administering Gavage Feeding

**PURPOSE:** Gavage feeding is used for infants who are unable to take the full feeding by nipple. It may be used alone or along with nipple feedings. Orogastric tubes are often used for intermittent feedings, whereas nasogastric tubes are used for continuous feedings.

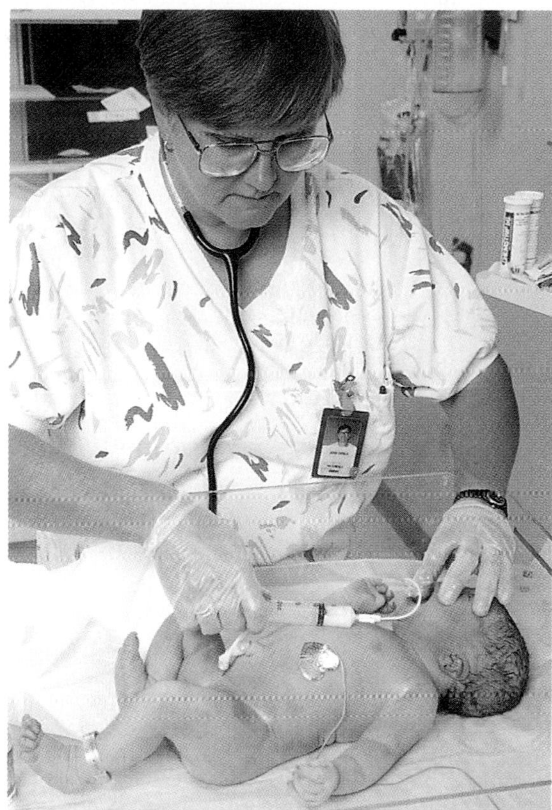

(See step 8)

*gravity flow or regulation of the flow by pump causes less trauma and prevents filling the stomach too fast.*

**11. If using gravity flow, raise or lower the syringe to increase or decrease the rate of flow so that the feeding moves slowly into stomach over 15 to 30 minutes.** *The higher the syringe, the faster the flow of solution and the greater the pressure. Feedings should be given slowly to prevent sudden distention or trauma from pressure.*

**12. For continuous feedings, place no more than a 2- to 4-hour supply of milk in a feeding bag or syringe. Set the pump to deliver the correct rate of flow. Change the equipment every 4 hours or according to hospital policy.** *Limiting the amount and changing equipment prevents excessive growth of bacteria in the milk or tubing. Infusion pumps deliver the feeding at a constant, measured rate.*

**13. Give the infant a pacifier during the feeding.** *Stimulates the sucking reflex, helps prepare the infant for nippling, is comforting, and helps the infant associate sucking with feeding.*

**14. When the catheter is to be withdrawn, pinch the tube and remove quickly.** *Pinching prevents drops of milk from entering the trachea as the tube is removed, and quick removal decreases irritation.*

**15. Burp the infant, and position on the right side or prone, with the head of the bed elevated. If movement tends to cause regurgitation, omit burping. Allow the infant to remain on the right side or prone.** *Air is swallowed around the tube and can cause the infant to regurgitate and aspirate. Position helps prevent reflux of feeding into the esophagus and promotes emptying of the stomach by gravity. If regurgitation occurs, the milk will flow out of the mouth.*

**16. Record time, amount, and characteristics of gastric residual, type and amount of feeding given, and how the infant tolerated it.** *Documentation allows monitoring of infant's ability to tolerate feedings and meet nutritional needs.*

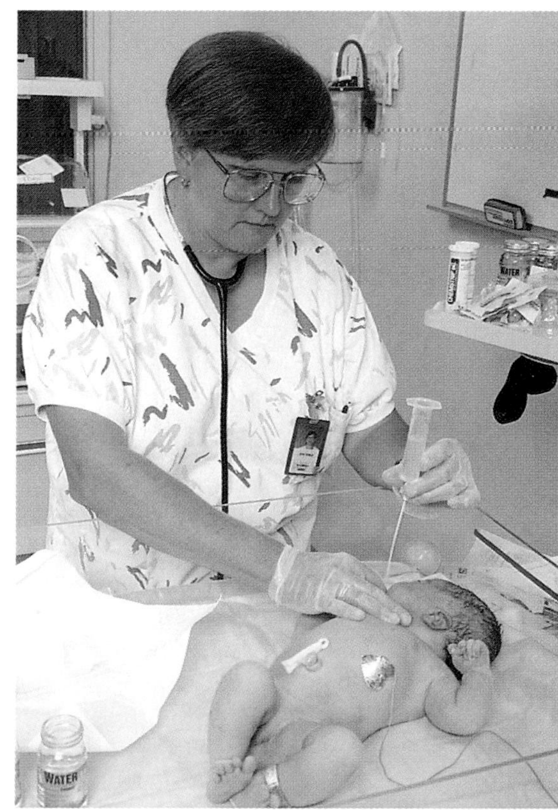


(See step 11)

## Interventions

### ADMINISTERING PARENTERAL FEEDINGS

The nurse manages the administration of parenteral nutrition, which may be necessary for very immature infants. Parenteral nutrition is the intravenous infusion of solutions containing the major nutrients needed for metabolism and growth. It provides calories, amino acids, fatty acids, vitamins, and minerals in amounts adapted to the specific needs of infants.

### ADMINISTERING GAVAGE FEEDINGS

Enteral feedings (feeding into the gastrointestinal tract, orally or by feeding tube) are started as soon as possible because they may help promote intestinal growth and maturity (Townsend et al., 1993). Infants of less than 34 weeks' gestation or weighing less than 1800 g (4 pounds) may need special formulas or fortified breast milk. Special formulas are adapted to meet the need for easily digestible, concentrated nutrients in a smaller volume of fluid. Preterm infants may need 24 or 27 kcal per ounce (instead of 20 kcal/ounce used for the full-term infant) to meet the requirement for 120 to 150 kcal/kg per day. Preterm formulas contain added calcium, phosphorus, and vitamins needed by the preterm infant. Breast milk fortifiers add needed nutrients to breast milk to make it more concentrated.

Gavage feedings are usually started before oral feedings for preterm infants (Procedure 29–1). A small, soft catheter is inserted through the mouth at each feeding for intermittent (bolus) feedings. Or, a nasogastric catheter may be inserted and left in place for a period of time to provide for continuous feedings. Leaving the catheter in place decreases the vagal stimulation that occurs with apnea and bradycardia during multiple insertions, but it may interfere with air flow through the infant's small nasal passages. In addition, bacteria counts in the milk or formula may become too high, and fats tend to adhere to the tubing during continuous feeding.

Gavage feedings are begun in small amounts, with gradual increases as tolerated by the infant. Only a few milliliters of feeding are given at first. Very small feedings may help increase later feeding tolerance (Pereira, 1995). Carefully observe the infant's tolerance at each feeding to determine when the feeding type or amount can be changed.

If the infant is able to suck, use a pacifier during feedings to help associate the comfortable feeling of fullness with sucking. Non-nutritive sucking also helps prepare the infant for nippling, improves weight gain, and decreases oxygen consumption (Estrada & Brennan-Behm, 1992). It may help quiet a fussy infant as well.

### ADMINISTERING ORAL FEEDINGS

Oral feedings are often begun when the infant reaches what would be 32 to 34 weeks' corrected gestational age and weighs at least 1500 g. At this time, most healthy preterm infants are able to coordinate sucking with swallowing and breathing, have a functional gag reflex, and have enough energy to feed orally without compromising oxygenation (Fig. 29–6). The first nipple feedings may be only a few milliliters once a day and completed by gavage. Placing the gavage tube before beginning oral feedings helps prevent regurgitation stimulated by passing the catheter. Gradually increase the amount and frequency of oral feedings until the infant feeds by breast or bottle once a shift, then every second or third feeding, and eventually every feeding.

**Preparing for Feedings.** Provide for maintenance of heat during feeding times. When infants have stable temperature maintenance, wrap them in warm blankets and hold for feedings. If thermoregulation is a problem, use a heat lamp over the infant or feed the infant in the radiant warmer or incubator.

Nipple feedings involve a greater expenditure of energy by the infant than gavage feedings. Allow for a period of rest before and after feedings. Use of a pacifier before feedings helps bring preterm infants

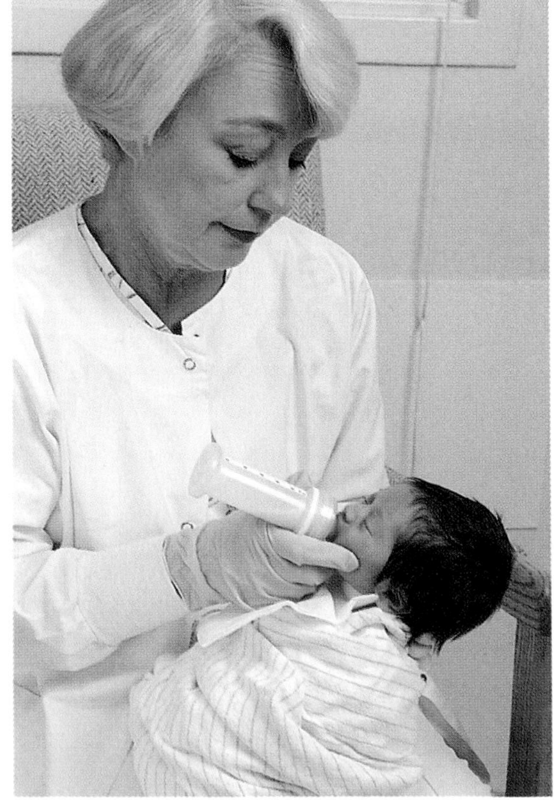

**FIGURE 29–6**

The nurse positions her hands to provide cheek and jaw support for feeding this preterm infant.

to an inactive awake state that enhances oral feeding success (McCain, 1992). Infants may be fed according to a feeding schedule or at times when they demonstrate cues that they are ready.

**Giving Bottle Feedings.** Nursing interventions for bottle feeding the preterm infant are presented in Nursing Care Plan 29–1.

#### FACILITATING BREASTFEEDING

Encourage mothers who would like to breastfeed. Contributing her milk helps the mother feel that she has something important to offer at a time when she may feel there is little she can do to help her baby. The immunologic benefits of breast milk are particularly important to the preterm infant who did not receive passive immunity during fetal life. Nutrients in breast milk are more easily digested, and enzymes, hormones, and growth factors important for the preterm infant are provided. Although milk from mothers of preterm infants is higher in protein, fat, and electrolytes during the early weeks, it may be necessary to add special fortifiers to meet total nutrient needs.

Breast milk may increase feeding tolerance, reduce

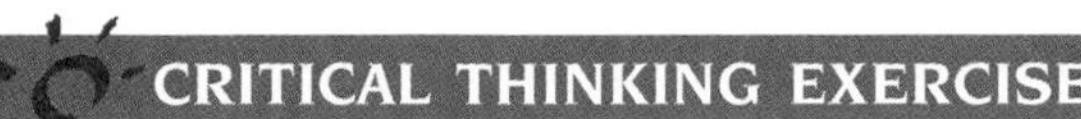


**Q:** What are the major differences between formula feeding a preterm infant and a full-term infant?

**A:** The preterm infant may need a special formula and smaller amounts. The preterm infant will take longer to feed, might need gavage feedings before introduction of a bottle, and would be more prone to complications in feeding. See Nursing Care Plan 29–1 for interventions appropriate for bottle feeding the preterm infant.

## *Nursing Care Plan 29–1*
# *The Preterm Infant*

ASSESSMENT: John was born at 33 weeks' gestation and weighs 1800 g (4 pounds). He breathes on his own with oxygen by hood. John needs many treatments throughout the day. He demonstrates pallor and increased respiratory rate when tired. Noises often cause a drop in oxygen saturation. When held or disturbed for care, John may stiffen and extend his arms with the fingers splayed. He sleeps most of the time when he is undisturbed.

NURSING DIAGNOSIS: Activity Intolerance related to weakness, fatigue, and possible overstimulation

GOALS/EXPECTED OUTCOMES

1. John will not show signs of overstimulation (increased respirations, pallor, decreased oxygen saturation level, stiffening of arms and legs, or splaying of fingers) as a result of normal activity.
2. John will increase tolerance to activity gradually as demonstrated by fewer signs of fatigue or stress.

| INTERVENTION | RATIONALE |
|---|---|
| 1. Arrange to provide routine care to correspond to John's natural awake periods, whenever possible. | 1. Preterm infants need undisturbed sleep to promote growth. |
| 2. Schedule periods of uninterrupted rest, especially before and after energy-draining activities. | 2. Infants tolerate activities best when they begin in a rested state and are allowed to recover from them before other activities are necessary. |
| 3. Experiment with grouping care to determine the number and combination of care activities that John tolerates best. | 3. Flexible nursing care allows individualization to meet the infant's needs. Grouping accomplishes more tasks at once so that longer rest periods are possible between tasks. However, too many activities may cause too much fatigue. |
| 4. Assess carefully to determine what activities bring about signs of overstimulation and fatigue: changes in color, respirations, or pulse; stiff, extended extremities; worried, hyperalert expression. Stop activity and allow short period of rest, if possible. | 4. Careful observation allows the nurse to be sensitive to the infant's ability to tolerate care. |
| 5. Reduce the noise level around John. Avoid talking unnecessarily, open and close doors softly, keep alarm volumes low. | 5. Noise may be overstimulating and result in increased oxygen need. |

*Nursing Care Plan continued on following page*

## Nursing Care Plan 29–1 *Continued*

## The Preterm Infant

| INTERVENTION | RATIONALE |
|---|---|
| 6. Reduce nonessential lighting. Place John's bed facing away from bright lights. Partially cover incubator over John's head to keep out light, but allow visualization of infant. Place John in a prone position. | 6. Continuous lighting interferes with infant's sleep. Reducing light in the infant's face will increase rest. |
| 7. Use blanket rolls to form "boundaries" around John and keep the extremities flexed. | 7. Enclosed space promotes rest and comfort because it is similar to the small space of uterus. Blankets also prevent the infant from hitting the hard walls of the bed. |

**Critical Thinking**

Who else besides the primary nurse needs to know about methods to maintain appropriate stimuli in John's environment? How can this information be made available to other people?

**ANSWER**

Other nurses caring for John, members from other disciplines, and parents so that everyone in contact with him will follow the same plan for developmental care. See interventions below.

| INTERVENTION | RATIONALE |
|---|---|
| 8. Inform everyone working with John about what works best in decreasing fatigue and stimulation for him. Use shift report, the nursing care plan and Kardex, and arrange an interdisciplinary team conference. Ask for suggestions. Tape signs on the bed to provide this information to parents and others. | 8. All caregivers should have information available to help meet the infant's needs consistently. |
| 9. Explain John's needs for rest and low stimulation to parents. Suggest ways that they can interact appropriately to meet John's needs, and point out signs that he is receiving too much stimulation. Ask for their input. | 9. Parents who are informed can care for the infant appropriately and feel that they are members of the team and parenting their child by learning his needs. |

### EVALUATION

John gradually shows increased ability to tolerate progressive activity with fewer episodes of overstimulation. His respirations and oxygen saturation levels remain stable, and he rarely stiffens his arms and legs during activity.

**ASSESSMENT:** John begins to take feedings by nipple supplemented by gavage when he becomes too tired. He has occasional episodes of increased respirations or short cyanotic spells when fed. He sometimes takes only half the feeding before falling asleep and must receive the rest by gavage. John's mother has decided to formula feed.

**NURSING DIAGNOSIS:** Risk for Altered Nutrition: Less Than Body Requirements related to fatigue during feedings

### GOALS/EXPECTED OUTCOMES

John will do the following:

1. Take 216 to 270 kcal per day to meet his needs at a weight of 1800 g.
2. Gain approximately 30 g daily.
3. Complete nipple feedings without signs of excessive fatigue (such as increased respiratory rate or falling asleep during feeding).

| INTERVENTION | RATIONALE |
|---|---|
| 1. Schedule nursing care to provide a rest period before and after nipple feedings. | 1. Nippling consumes a great deal of energy. Rest helps prevent excessive fatigue that might prevent the infant from completing the feeding. |
| 2. Gather equipment. Use a feeding container (such as a Volutrol) on which each milliliter is marked. Place container in warm water to warm milk to room temperature or slightly warmer. Do not use a microwave oven to warm. | 2. Having all equipment ready prevents wasted motion and ensures that infant is fed without interruption. Exact measurement of the amount taken is important to ensure that infants receive required nutrients. Some infants will take slightly warmed milk better. Microwaving provides uneven heating of formula and may cause the infant to be burned. |

## Nursing Care Plan 29–1 *Continued*

# The Preterm Infant

| INTERVENTION | RATIONALE |
|---|---|
| 3. Determine the type of nipple that works best for John. Choose between various sizes and consistencies. | 3. A "preemie" nipple is more pliable than regular nipples and requires less energy for sucking. Some infants need firmer nipples because soft nipples allow milk to flow too fast, cause choking, and interfere with breathing between sucking bursts. Infants with a very small mouth require a smaller nipple. |
| 4. Wrap John in warmed blankets and place a hat on his head. Feed him in the incubator or under warmer if needed. | 4. Hat and blankets help maintain temperature during the time infants are out of the incubator. If infants have difficulty with temperature maintenance, an incubator or warmer provides warmth during feedings. |
| 5. Position John at a 45- to 60-degree angle facing the nurse. Position the head slightly forward and the chin slightly down. Place a finger on each cheek and one under the jaw at the base of the tongue, midway between the chin and the throat. Provide gentle pressure. | 5. This position allows the nurse to observe the infant's suck, response to feeding, and any regurgitation. The finger position increases sucking strength and helps support the tongue. |
| 6. Feed slowly, with frequent stops to burp and allow the infant to stop for rest. | 6. Slow feeding is necessary because of the infant's decreased energy. Preterm infants may swallow more air than full-term infants because sucking is less efficient. They need rest periods during feedings because they have difficulty regulating their breathing while feeding. |
| 7. Observe for coughing, gagging, cyanosis, changes in heart rate or respirations, or apnea. Evaluate the infant's ability to continue. | 7. These signs show difficulty coordinating sucking, swallowing, and breathing and possible aspiration. |
| 8. Assess for signs of overfatigue: falling asleep during feedings, feedings lasting more than 25 to 30 minutes, increased respirations. | 8. Feedings may require more energy than the infant has available. Infants who are overfatigued are more likely to aspirate. |
| 9. Finish feeding by gavage if necessary. | 9. Completing the feeding by gavage conserves energy and prevents aspiration. |
| 10. Position John on the right side or prone, with his head elevated approximately 30 degrees after feeding. | 10. If regurgitation occurs, fluid will run out of the mouth easily so that the infant will not aspirate it. The right-side position and elevation of the head allow gravity to help empty the stomach. |
| 11. Include parents in the feedings. Teach them how to assess the infant's response to feedings. | 11. Feeding allows parents to participate in the infant's care. Their comfort with feedings and learning about the infant's responses will help them prepare for discharge. |

### EVALUATION

John consumes an average of 260 calories and gains an average of 31 g daily. He gradually takes more of his feeding by nipple and rarely needs gavage feeding to finish it. His respiratory rate remains under 60 breaths/minute, and he stays awake for the entire feeding.

### ADDITIONAL NURSING DIAGNOSES TO CONSIDER

Ineffective Thermoregulation
Ineffective Airway Clearance
Altered Family Processes
Risk for Caregiver Role Strain
Risk for Altered Parenting
Risk for Infection
Pain

later allergies, improve retinal function, enhance neurologic development, and help prevent necrotizing enterocolitis (Meier & Brown, 1996). Breastfeeding may be less stressful than bottle feeding for preterm infants. Oxygenation levels are often higher during breastfeeding because the infant can regulate breathing and suckling better than with bottle feeding. In addition, the mother's body temperature helps keep the infant warm.

When the mother plans to breastfeed, she will need help in maintaining lactation until the infant is mature enough for nipple feedings. Teach her how to use a breast pump and give her sterile containers to store her milk. Tell her to place it in a refrigerator or freezer until she brings it to the NICU for the infant. If fortifiers will be added to the milk, explain the higher needs of the preterm infant so the mother does not believe that her milk is inadequate.

Support the mother in her efforts in feeding, which may be difficult at first. Remind her that even full-term infants must learn how to breastfeed. Relaxation needed for feeding is difficult in the busy NICU nursery. Provide as much privacy as possible, using a separate room or screens. Help the mother feel comfortable holding the tiny infant and any attached equipment, such as monitor leads.

Adapt breastfeeding teaching to the needs of a very small infant. Show the mother how to use the cross cradle hold, which is very effective for small infants. She should hold her breast with the hand on the same side and press slightly back and downward behind the areola to make the nipple prominent. The other hand holds the infant's head and brings it to the breast. This allows the mother to see the infant well during latching on and throughout the feeding (Meier & Mangurten, 1993).

Make the same observations of the infant during breastfeeding as during bottle feeding. Signs of fatigue, bradycardia, tachypnea, or apnea may show lack of readiness for breastfeeding. Be sure that the infant stays warm. The mother's body heat will help maintain the infant's temperature during feedings. Kangaroo care (p. 832) can often be combined with breastfeeding.

#### MAKING ONGOING ASSESSMENTS

Continuously assess the infant's responses to all feeding methods. Record the amount of breast milk or formula that the infant takes by gavage or bottle feeding and compare it with the amount needed to meet nutrient needs for the infant's age and weight. Because it is difficult to accurately estimate milk intake, infants may be weighed on an electronic scale before and after breastfeedings. This allows gavage feeding amounts to be calculated based on the infant's oral intake.

Weigh the infant daily at the same time of day with the same scale. Record the length and head circumference each week. Plot measurements on a growth chart for preterm infants to see if changes are within expected ranges. Weight increase not accompanied by increased length may be caused by edema and may be a sign of a complication such as congestive heart failure.

Observe changes in the infant's ability to take feedings. The suck and swallow coordination should gradually improve with maturity and practice. As the infant becomes more mature, less energy should be expended during the feeding sessions. The infant will take the feedings more quickly and show fewer signs of fatigue, such as falling asleep during feedings.

### Evaluation

If the goals have been met, the infant will do the following:

- Consume adequate amounts of formula or breast milk to meet nutrient needs for age and weight.
- Show a pattern of weight gain that is appropriate for his or her age.

**✓CHECK YOUR READING**

9. How does the nurse assess feeding tolerance?
10. How can the nurse help the mother who wants to breastfeed her preterm infant?

## Parenting

The birth of a preterm infant is generally unexpected and always emotionally traumatic to parents. Infants are often hurried away to the NICU shortly after birth. When parents see the infant later attached to an array of machines, they may have difficulty developing a feeling of attachment to a tiny baby who looks so different from what they expected (see section on parental grieving in Chapter 24).

The extended hospitalization of the preterm infant results in separation of the parents from their newborn and disrupts family life. Some parents feel that they play such a small part in the preterm infant's life that the infant almost belongs to the hospital.

Parents need help to understand the infant's condition and what is expected to occur throughout the hospital stay. Parents perceive nurses as being among the most helpful in aiding them to cope with these stresses (Miles et al., 1996). Nurses must evaluate the progress of bonding and assist parents to feel important in caring for their infant.

## Assessment

Assess for signs of parental attachment on the first and subsequent visits to the NICU nursery. Expect parents to be fearful at first but more able to focus on the infant as they get over the initial shock of preterm birth. Assess for common behaviors that show normal progression of attachment. These include talking about the infant in positive terms, pointing out physical characteristics, naming the infant, making eye contact, and calling the infant by name. Parents should ask questions about the infant. When they are able to hold and participate in the care of the infant, observe for gradual increase in comfort and skill. The parents should smile and talk to the infant and verbalize increasing confidence in their caretaking abilities.

Watch for signs that bonding is not occurring as expected. These include failure to perform usual bonding behaviors or a decrease in behaviors that were previously present. Parents who seem as interested in other infants in the NICU as their own or who talk about the infant in an impersonal way may be having difficulty. Note how often the parents make visits or calls to the NICU and changes that may indicate a need for support. Determine if there are other stressors in the parents' lives that may interfere with their ability to visit and attach to the infant.

After the critical period in the early days after birth, healthy preterm infants become more stable. They still require specialized nursing care and hospitalization but gradually need less technologic interventions. They are sometimes called "growers" at this time. This is a time when parent participation in the infant's care should increase in preparation for discharge.

## Analysis

Altered parent-infant attachment is a potential problem for parents of any infant who has a problem at birth. It may occur whenever parents and infants must be separated because of hospitalization during the newborn period. One nursing diagnosis that is appropriate for the parents of preterm infants is Risk for Altered Parenting related to separation of parents from infant and lack of understanding about the preterm infant's condition and characteristics.

## Planning

The goals for this nursing diagnosis are that the parents will do the following:

- Demonstrate bonding behaviors, including visiting frequently and interacting as appropriate for the infant's condition throughout the hospital stay.
- Verbalize understanding of the preterm infant's condition and characteristics within 2 days.
- Express increasing comfort in caring for the infant within 1 week.

### Critical to Remember

**SIGNS THAT BONDING MAY BE DELAYED**

- Using negative terms to describe the infant
- Discussing the infant in impersonal or technical terms
- Failing to give the infant a name or to use the name
- Visiting or calling infrequently or not at all
- Decreasing the number and length of visits
- Showing interest in other infants equal to that in their own infant
- Refusing offers to hold and learn to care for the infant
- Showing a decrease in or lack of eye contact and in time spent talking to or smiling at the infant

## Interventions

### MAKING ADVANCE PREPARATIONS

Preparing for threatening situations such as preterm birth helps parents cope with the actual event. Parents expected to have a preterm birth should visit the NICU nursery before delivery. If the mother is confined to bed, arrange for a nurse from the NICU to visit her so that she feels a link with the nursery and can ask questions. The father or another support person should have a tour of the nursery so that he will know where to go and can discuss the nursery environment with the mother.

### ASSISTING PARENTS AT BIRTH

After the birth, allow the mother to see the newborn in the delivery room, even if only for a few moments, so that she has a realistic idea of the infant's appearance and condition. If possible, allow the father to watch the initial care in the NICU. Explain what is happening and why. This allows him to see the intensive efforts made on behalf of his infant, increases his confidence in the staff, and enables him to give the mother a full description later. Support the father, as well as the mother, by using therapeutic communication techniques during this difficult time.

If the infant must be transported to another facility, it is important to have the transport team visit the mother just before they leave, if possible. This helps the mother feel connected to her infant and to the staff providing care. Leaving photographs with the mother is one way of helping her bond even though the infant is not with her.

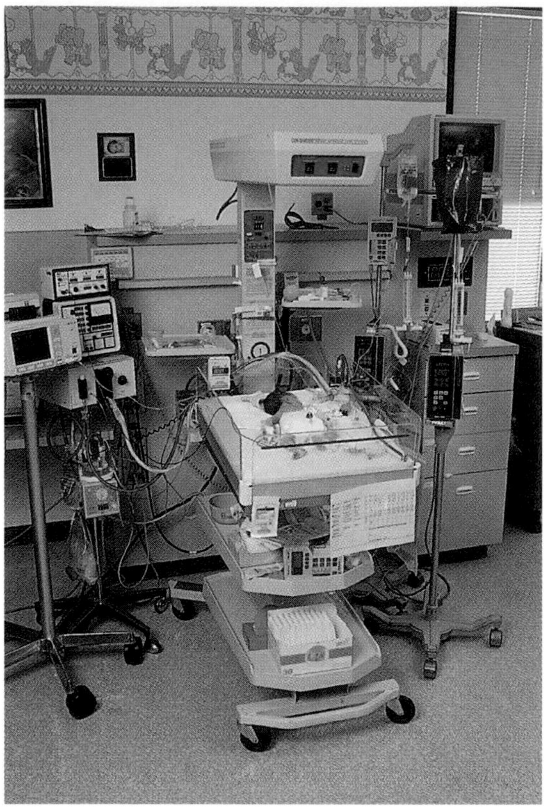

**FIGURE 29–7**

An infant in the neonatal intensive care unit is surrounded by highly technologic equipment. This can be very frightening to parents at first. Preparation of parents before they visit is an important nursing responsibility.

### SUPPORTING PARENTS DURING EARLY VISITS

Take the mother to the NICU nursery as soon as she is able. If she is too sick to be with her infant, bring her photographs. Before parents first visit the infant, prepare them for what they will see by describing the equipment and its purposes, the various attachments to the infant, and the sounds of alarms (Fig. 29–7). Explain how the infant will look and behave. Table 29–1 provides specific steps that the nurse can follow to help parents become familiar with the NICU setting.

At first, stay with the parents during visits. When they are comfortable, allow them time alone with the infant so that they can interact in private. Answer questions and explain changes in the infant's condition and treatment. Use therapeutic communication as the parents cope with their grief, guilt, and emotional turmoil.

Parents should touch the infant as soon as possible because this helps promote the development of attachment. They may be hesitant initially because of fear that they will interfere with equipment. The smaller the infant, the more reluctant parents may be. Show them how to touch in ways appropriate for the infant, such as holding the infant's hand through the portholes of the incubator or stroking the small areas of skin not encumbered by equipment. Some parents may hesitate to touch because they are afraid of becoming attached to an infant whom they may lose. They will need sensitive support from the nurse until they are ready to progress in their relationship with the infant.

### PROVIDING INFORMATION

Explain all nursing care, its purpose, and the expected response. Point out how preterm infants are similar to and different from full-term infants to help parents develop a realistic understanding of the infant's capabilities.

Offer realistic reassurance about the infant's condition. This means emphasizing positive aspects, yet being truthful in all communication with the parents. If they have misconceptions or did not understand a

**TABLE 29–1 INTRODUCING PARENTS TO THE NEONATAL INTENSIVE CARE UNIT SETTING**

**Before Parents Visit the NICU**

Describe the NICU environment. Include the noise of alarms, the busyness of the staff, the number of people and sick infants.

Show parents photographs of the infant. This helps prepare them, but it is not as overwhelming as seeing the infant in person.

Describe the infant. Include the size, the lack of fat, the breathing, the weak cry. Explain that no sound of crying can be heard if the infant is intubated. Include some human aspects: "He's a real fighter" or "She makes the funniest faces during her feedings."

Describe the equipment. Include ventilators, intravenous lines, and monitors. Explain how they look and how they are attached to the infant. Keep the explanations simple, without technical details.

**When Parents Visit the NICU**

Help parents perform scrubbing and gowning procedures while explaining the purpose.

Stay with the parents during their visit. Having a familiar person nearby will help them feel more comfortable while they adjust to this unfamiliar environment.

Introduce them to their infant's nurse. Ask the NICU nurse to explain some of the things being done for the infant.

Provide parents with written information about the NICU so that they can take it home with them to read later. This usually includes visiting hours, calling for updates about the infant, availability of classes on infant care, and support groups.

Tell the parents that they will receive instruction on how to care for their infant in time. Encourage them to visit the infant as much as they are able. Emphasize how important they are to their infant.

Offer realistic encouragement based on the infant's condition.

Provide an opportunity for the parents to express their concerns and feelings and to ask questions.

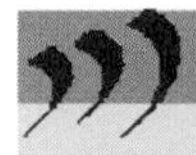

## THERAPEUTIC COMMUNICATION

### Reassuring Parents During Visits to the NICU

Ann Gibson gave birth to a preterm infant, Molly, at 30 weeks' gestation. Ann is visiting the NICU for the first time the day after the birth. The nurse, Lee Wills, has talked to her about what to expect and stays with her during the visit.

**Ann:** Oh, she looks so tiny! I saw her for only a minute after she was born, and I didn't really get a good look. How can she ever survive when she's so small and covered with tubes?

**Lee:** So far, Molly is doing very well. Her vital signs are stable, and she's holding her own. But it is frightening when she looks so small and vulnerable, isn't it?

*Offering realistic reassurance and reflecting Ann's fearful feelings. Using infant's name to promote bonding.*

**Ann:** I stayed in bed like they told me to do. I thought she wouldn't be born so soon if I stayed in bed.

**Lee:** It must have been a shock especially when you tried so hard to prevent it.

*Reflecting feelings and acknowledging that Ann did what she could to prevent early birth.*

**Ann:** Now she's so tiny and so sick! She looks so different from what I expected.

**Lee:** Molly's small, but babies her size grow very quickly. Would you like to touch her?

*Offering realistic reassurance and attempting to bring Ann closer to infant.*

**Ann:** Oh, I might hurt her. Maybe I should wait until she's bigger.

**Lee:** Even tiny babies like to have their mothers stroke their skin and talk to them. She listened to your voice all through your pregnancy, so it is familiar to her. Why don't you hold her hand while I work with her? And I can tell you about all this equipment and what we are doing for Molly.

*Emphasizing the mother's importance, involving her in care being given, and offering information about infant's equipment and care.*

physician's explanations, clarify or ask the physician to go over specific information again. Translate medical terms into words that the parents can understand. Use an interpreter if the parents do not understand English.

Repeat explanations, especially at first. Because of their emotional distress, parents are often unable to fully comprehend or remember what is said to them.

Offer written information in the language of the parents about NICU policies and procedures. Explanations about visiting hours, who can visit, routines for scrubbing, and the role of parents can be reinforced in writing and be available for later reading by parents who are overwhelmed.

#### INSTITUTING KANGAROO CARE

Begin kangaroo care (KC) as soon as possible. Kangaroo care is a method of providing skin-to-skin contact between preterm infants and their parents. Explain the advantages of KC to parents and elicit their participation. This method of care has been found safe for stable infants, even if intubated; provides an opportunity for parents to participate in the infant's care; and increases attachment. The infant, wearing only a diaper and hat, is placed under the mother's clothes between her breasts. Mothers may breastfeed if they wish and the infant is able. Fathers may also participate in KC.

In a study comparing KC with traditional holding (cradle position with the infant wrapped in blankets), infants having KC were able to maintain their temperature better than those without KC. They had stable heart rates and oxygen saturation levels. Mothers generally were pleased with the care and preferred the kangaroo method of holding (Legault & Goulet, 1995).

Kangaroo care provides developmental care so important for the preterm infant and helps with parental attachment. The upright position of the infant against the parent's chest makes breathing easier. The containment of the extremities decreases purposeless movements that use up oxygen and calories. In addition, parents are often gratified when infants fall into a quiet sleep during KC, and feelings of confidence and closeness to the infant are increased (Ludington-Hoe & Swinth, 1996).

#### FACILITATING INTERACTION

Parents may feel rejected by the infant's lack of the response they expect during interactions. Explain to them that infants born at less than 34 weeks of gestation may not be able to cope with socialization. The talking, smiling, and eye contact so effective with full-term infants may be too stimulating for very young or sick preterm infants. Encourage forms of touch and interaction based on the individual infant's capacity. Quiet holding or gentle stroking may be better until the infant is able to tolerate more.

Teach parents signs of overstimulation so that they can adapt their interaction to meet the infant's needs. Discuss methods to avoid too much stimula-

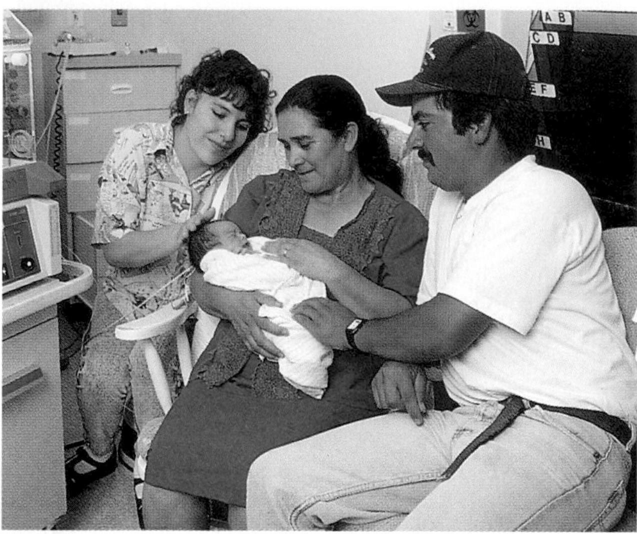

**FIGURE 29–8**

The parents look on while the grandmother holds the infant in the neonatal intensive care unit.

tion and ways to calm the infant. If several types of stimulation (such as rocking, eye contact, and talking) cause signs of overstimulation, suggest they stop one or more activities until the infant has had a period of rest. Show them how to position the infant with the hands near the mouth so the infant can suck on them as a self-comforting measure.

As the infant matures, show parents signs that the infant is ready for more interaction and suggest appropriate types of stimulation. Point out small signs of improvement and even minor strengths. Talk about individual characteristics that make this infant different from all others. The way the infant eats, reacts to sounds, or even how the infant seems to get tangled in the monitor leads may help parents feel closer to their newborn and understand the infant's special characteristics.

Involve the parents in care of the infant as soon as possible (Fig. 29–8). As they become familiar with the NICU nursery setting and the equipment, more involvement will help them to feel a sense of control. At first, plan to change the linens in the incubator or radiant warmer when the parents are there so that they can hold their infant, even if for only a few moments. As the infant's condition improves, parents can develop skill in caring for a tiny infant by changing diapers, feeding, and bathing during the infant's hospitalization.

#### INCREASING PARENTAL DECISION MAKING

Encourage parents to help make large and small decisions about care of the infant. Give them the information they need to take an active part in decisions made about the infant's treatment plan. This will increase their feelings of control over a situation in which many parents feel they have little power.

#### ALLEVIATING CONCERNS

Encourage parents to call the NICU at any time for information about their infant. This helps allay worry when parents wake up at night and wonder how the infant is doing. This is especially beneficial for parents not able to visit the infant because of distance or other reasons.

Parents also need support from others besides nursing staff. Put them in touch with other parents who have had a preterm infant. Talking with those who have faced the same problems can be very comforting. They can compare notes and get down-to-earth suggestions from an experienced parent's point of view.

#### HELPING WITH ONGOING PROBLEMS

Parents are often unprepared for the inconsistent progress infants often make after surviving the risks of the early days. They expect steady progress once the infant can eat and breathe alone. However, complications such as necrotizing enterocolitis can cause major setbacks at this time. Parents need extensive support from the nurse to cope with a new crisis. Use therapeutic communication techniques to help them express and cope with their extreme disappointment. Give information about the infant's changing condition and what to expect in the days ahead.

#### PREPARING FOR DISCHARGE

Because infants go home very early, it is important that the parents understand the expected hospital course. If a clinical pathway is being used for the infant, give them a copy. They can chart the infant's achievement of major milestones in development and changes in care as the infant moves toward discharge. This helps them prepare themselves and their home to provide the special care that their infant may need after discharge.

Teach parents any special procedures that the infant will need after discharge. Begin early to show them how to manage treatments and medications. Observe the parents perform care until they are comfortable and can do it safely. Help them learn what is normal for their infant and how to recognize and respond to abnormal signs. Some hospitals have parents spend a night in a special "parent room," where they take over full 24-hour care of the infant. This provides an opportunity to practice assuming complete care of the infant in an environment where help is available if needed.

Help the parents determine what adaptations they will need to make at home for discharge. Utility companies should be notified if the infant is considered medically fragile. This ensures the family receives priority service in cases of power failure. Ordering special equipment may be necessary before the infant can go home. Home nursing services arrangements should be completed.

Discuss what to expect in care of the infant after discharge. Many infants need feedings every 3 hours, day and night, to help them gain the 20 g to 40 g a day expected (Sifuentes, 1996). Feedings may be time consuming, and parental fatigue resulting from interruptions to their sleep may be more than they expected.

Help parents to have realistic expectations of the infant. For example, they should know that the infant will accomplish developmental tasks, such as crawling and walking, later than full-term infants. Parents should base expectations on the infant's developmental age rather than chronologic age. Developmental age is the chronologic age minus the number of weeks the infant was born early. Many infants catch up to their chronologic age when they are approximately 2.5 years (Sifuentes, 1996).

Assist the parents in planning for integrating the new infant into the family. Meeting the needs of their other children, in addition to the new responsibilities of caring for the preterm infant, is a major source of worry. Listen to their concerns about other children, and encourage siblings to visit, if possible. Caution parents that siblings with infections should not visit the infant who cannot fight off infections well. Help parents explain to the other children what they will see when they visit the infant. Siblings should touch or hold the infant, if possible, to help them bond. Taking photographs of the siblings with the infant will help them remember the visit.

### Evaluation

Goals are met if parents do the following:

- Demonstrate bonding behaviors, including positive verbalization about the infant, frequent visiting, and interacting with the infant as appropriate for the infant's condition.
- Verbalize understanding of the preterm infant's special needs and the treatment given throughout the hospital stay.
- Take an increasingly active role in care of the infant.

**✓ CHECK YOUR READING**

11. How can the nurse help parents be comfortable with their preterm infant?
12. How should the nurse prepare parents for the discharge of their preterm infant?

## Common Complications of Preterm Infants

The preterm infant is at risk for a number of complications that increase as the infant's gestational age and birth weight decrease. Some complications that are common to full-term and preterm infants, such as hyperbilirubinemia and patent ductus arteriosus, are discussed in Chapter 30. Complications most often associated with preterm birth are discussed in this section.

### Respiratory Distress Syndrome

Respiratory distress syndrome (RDS), also called hyaline membrane disease, accounts for 30 percent of all neonatal deaths in the United States (Behrman et al., 1996). The syndrome occurs in half of infants born at 26 to 28 weeks' gestation, but fewer than 20 to 30 percent of those born at 30 to 31 weeks (Whitsett et al., 1994). Respiratory distress syndrome is also seen in birth asphyxia, birth by cesarean, and infants of diabetic mothers because these conditions interfere with surfactant production. However, it is less frequent when chronic fetal stress, such as in heroin addiction, causes the lungs to mature more quickly.

#### PATHOPHYSIOLOGY

Respiratory distress syndrome is caused by insufficient production of surfactant, a phospholipid that lines the alveoli. Surfactant is first produced in the alveoli at 22 weeks of gestation. By 34 to 36 weeks, production of surfactant is usually mature enough to enable the infant to breathe normally outside the uterus (Hagedorn et al., 1993)

Surfactant decreases surface tension to allow the alveoli to remain open when air is exhaled. It must be continuously produced as it is being used. When there is too little surfactant, the alveoli collapse each time the infant exhales. The lungs become noncompliant, or "stiff," and resist expansion. Noncompliant lungs require a much higher negative pressure for the alveoli to open each time the infant inhales. Severe retractions occur with each breath, drawing the weak muscles of the chest wall inward. The resulting pressure on the lungs further interferes with expansion.

As fewer alveoli expand, atelectasis and hypoxia occur. This causes pulmonary vasoconstriction and decreased blood flow to the lungs because of the high resistance within the vessels of the lungs. Persistent pulmonary hypertension can result in a return to fetal circulation patterns, with opening of the ductus arteriosus. Respiratory and metabolic acidosis as well as alveolar necrosis further complicate the condition by interfering with surfactant synthesis.

Surfactant is a composite of a number of different substances. Three of the components are lecithin, sphingomyelin, and phosphatidylglycerol, which can be detected by tests on amniotic fluid. These tests can predict whether the fetal lungs are mature enough so that survival outside of the uterus is possible (see Chapter 10, p. 232). The incidence and severity of RDS may be reduced by giving the mother corticosteroids at least 24 hours before birth.

#### MANIFESTATIONS

Signs of RDS begin during the first hours after birth, often become worse on the next day, and may begin to improve within 72 hours after birth. They include tachypnea, nasal flaring, retractions, and cyanosis. Grunting on expiration is characteristic and signifies physiologic efforts to maintain lung expansion. Breath sounds may be decreased or wet. Acidosis develops as a result of hypoxemia. Chest radiographs shows the "ground glass" appearance of the lungs that is characteristic of RDS. Areas of atelectasis are present.

#### THERAPEUTIC MANAGEMENT

Surfactant replacement therapy is used prophylactically to prevent RDS or as "rescue" treatment once RDS has occurred. It is instilled into the infant's trachea immediately after birth or as soon as signs of RDS become apparent. Improvement in breathing occurs in minutes. Doses are repeated, if necessary. Infants treated with surfactant have higher survival rates and fewer of some complications of RDS, although they may have other complications resulting from their prematurity.

Other treatment is supportive, including mechanical ventilation, correction of the acidosis, intravenous feedings, and care of developing complications.

#### NURSING CONSIDERATIONS

The nurse observes for signs of developing RDS at birth and during the early hours after the delivery. Changes in the infant's condition are constantly assessed. For example, diuresis may occur with improvement in the disease. Changes in ventilator settings may be necessary as the infant's ability to oxygenate increases. Observation for common complications, such as patent ductus arteriosus and bronchopulmonary dysplasia, is important. Other care is similar to general care for the preterm infant.

### Bronchopulmonary Dysplasia

Bronchopulmonary dysplasia (BPD) is a chronic condition occurring in as many as 30 percent of infants treated with mechanical ventilation (Hagedorn et al., 1993), although it may also occur in those without ventilator use. As many as 10 to 15 percent of affected infants do not survive the first year (Davis & Rosenfeld, 1994).

#### PATHOPHYSIOLOGY

Bronchopulmonary dysplasia results from a combination of factors, including oxygen, high pressures of pulmonary ventilation, inflammation, infection, and nutritional factors, that cause damage to the alveoli and lining of the respiratory tract. Inflammation, edema, and airway hyperreactivity lead to thickening of the walls of the alveoli and fibrotic changes. Atelectasis and pneumonia also occur.

#### MANIFESTATIONS

The major sign of BPD is the continued need for oxygen for more than 28 days of life. Infants may need prolonged treatment with mechanical ventilation as well. Characteristic changes in the lungs are seen on chest radiographs.

#### THERAPEUTIC MANAGEMENT

Treatment is supportive, with gradual decreases in the amount of oxygen, bronchodilators, corticosteroids, diuretics, and antibiotics as necessary. The infant may go home on long-term oxygen therapy, and some need frequent rehospitalization for respiratory infections.

Formation of new alveoli, which take the place of those destroyed by BPD, brings about gradual improvement in the condition. The alveoli normally increase in number from 20 to 70 million at birth to as many as 300 to 400 million at 2 to 8 years of age, when the lungs reach adult size (Whitsett et al., 1994). Significant improvement occurs in the first 2 years, but some pulmonary problems may remain. Surfactant replacement therapy has improved survival and led to less severe forms of BPD.

### Periventricular-Intraventricular Hemorrhage

Periventricular-intraventricular hemorrhage (PIVH) occurs in 20 to 30 percent of infants of less than 32 weeks' gestation or weighing less than 1500 g (Minarcik & Beachy, 1993).

#### PATHOPHYSIOLOGY

The condition results from rupture of the fragile blood vessels in the germinal matrix, located around the ventricles of the brain. It is most often associated with hypoxic injury to the vessels, increased blood pressure and cerebral blood flow, and rupture of blood vessels.

Hemorrhage is graded 1 through 4, according to the amount of bleeding. Grade 1 is a very small bleed outside ventricle walls, producing few, if any, clinical changes. Grade 2 hemorrhage extends into the lateral ventricles, and grade 3 distends at least one ventricle. Grade 4 hemorrhage causes ventricular dilation and damage to brain tissue.

Although there are fewer complications and less mortality with grade 1 or 2 hemorrhages, infants with grade 3 and 4 hemorrhages are likely to have neurologic abnormalities and developmental delays. Those with grade 4 hemorrhage have a poor survival rate. The mortality rate for all infants with PIVH ranges from 25 to 50 percent depending on the extent of the hemorrhage and other complications (Blackburn, 1993).

#### MANIFESTATIONS

Signs of PIVH are determined by the severity of the hemorrhage. They may include lethargy, poor muscle tone, deterioration of respiratory status with cyanosis or apnea, drop in hematocrit level, decreased reflexes, full or bulging fontanelle, and seizures. Because some infants show no signs, early and repeated screening by ultrasonography is performed on preterm infants younger than 32 weeks.

#### THERAPEUTIC MANAGEMENT

Treatment is supportive and focuses on maintaining respiratory function and dealing with other complications. Hydrocephalus may develop from blockage of cerebrospinal fluid flow. Lumbar taps or a ventriculoperitoneal shunt may be necessary to drain the fluid.

#### NURSING CONSIDERATIONS

Nursing care includes measurement of the head circumference daily and observation for changes in neurologic status, which may be subtle. Increases in blood pressure from excessive handling or suctioning should be avoided.

### Retinopathy of Prematurity

Retinopathy of prematurity (ROP), or retrolental fibroplasia, may result in visual impairment or blindness in preterm infants. It occurs more often in infants weighing less than 1500 g.

#### PATHOPHYSIOLOGY

Retinopathy of prematurity is caused by damage to immature blood vessels in the retina of the eye. Although the exact cause of the damage is unknown, it is thought to result partly from high arterial blood oxygen levels. It is the level of oxygen in the blood rather than the amount of oxygen the infant receives that is important. Because ROP has developed in some infants who have not received oxygen, other causative factors may also be involved.

The incidence of ROP decreased when accurate monitoring of partial pressure of oxygen in arterial blood ($PaO_2$) levels became available, but it has become more common with the increase in survival of VLBW infants. These infants need higher levels of oxygen to survive, and their less-mature retinas are more prone to the condition.

In ROP, immature blood vessels in the retina of the eye constrict and become permanently occluded. New vessels proliferate, extending throughout the retina and into the vitreous of the eye. Hemorrhages from the fragile vessels may cause scarring, traction on the retina, and retinal detachment.

#### THERAPEUTIC MANAGEMENT

Low-birth-weight infants are screened between 4 and 8 weeks after birth to detect changes of the eye. Cryotherapy and laser surgery have been used to destroy the proliferating blood vessels or to reattach the retina. Many infants have a spontaneous regression with little or no impairment of vision.

### Necrotizing Enterocolitis

Necrotizing enterocolitis (NEC) is a serious condition of the intestinal tract, with a 10 to 50 percent mortality rate (Vanderhoof et al., 1994).

#### PATHOPHYSIOLOGY

Although the exact causes are unknown, the condition may be caused by interference with blood supply to the intestinal mucosa. During asphyxia, blood is diverted from the gastrointestinal tract to the brain, heart, and kidneys. Sepsis, polycythemia, and maternal cocaine use are among other causes of decrease in intestinal blood flow. The resulting ischemia may make the mucosa more susceptible to invasion with bacteria. When infants are fed, bacteria proliferate, and gas-forming organisms may invade the intestinal wall. Eventually, necrosis, perforation, and peritonitis may occur.

#### MANIFESTATIONS

Signs include increased abdominal girth caused by distention, increased gastric residuals, decreased or absent bowel sounds, loops of bowel seen through the abdominal wall, vomiting, signs of infection, and blood in the stools. On radiographs, loops of bowel dilated with air and layers of gas in the intestinal wall are present. Free air in the peritoneum indicates that perforation has occurred.

#### THERAPEUTIC MANAGEMENT

Treatment includes antibiotics, discontinuation of oral feedings, and use of parenteral nutrition to rest the intestines. Surgery may be necessary if there is perforation or continued lack of improvement. The necrotic area is removed, and an ostomy may be performed. Breast milk may have a preventive effect on the development of NEC. Other preventive strategies include corticosteroids given to the mother, slow advancement of feedings, and oral immunoglobulin A (Parker, 1995).

#### NURSING CONSIDERATIONS

Early recognition of signs of NEC is essential to decrease mortality. Because nurses are constantly observing the infant, they are often able to note the early, subtle signs that lead to prompt diagnosis. Noting one or more signs will prompt the nurse to withhold the next feeding and notify the physician.

## Postterm Infants

Postterm infants are those who are born after the 42nd week of gestation. Their longer-than-normal gestation places them at risk for a number of complications.

### Scope of the Problem

Approximately 6 to 12 percent of all pregnancies are considered postterm. Postterm infants have a two to three times higher perinatal mortality rate than infants born at term (Hamilton & Hobel, 1992). The major concern is how well the placenta functions during the last weeks of pregnancy. In 20 to 30 percent of postterm pregnancies, placental function deteriorates, causing interference with oxygen and nutrient supply. This results in hypoxia and malnourishment in the fetus and is called *postmaturity syndrome* or *dysmaturity syndrome*.

However, in most cases, the fetus continues to be well supported by the placenta. Some may grow to more than 4000 g (8 pounds, 13 ounces) and are at risk for birth injuries or the need for cesarean birth because of their size.

### Assessment

Signs of postmaturity syndrome may occur during pregnancy, during labor, or after birth. Diminished fetal growth or oligohydramnios may cause decreased uterine size during the last weeks of pregnancy. When labor begins, poor oxygen reserves may cause fetal distress. The fetus may pass meconium as a result of hypoxia before or during labor, increasing the risk of meconium aspiration at delivery.

At birth, the cord, skin, and nails may be stained, indicating that meconium was present for some time. The hyperalert, wide-eyed, worried look common to these infants is a sign of chronic intrauterine hypoxia. Inadequate oxygen in utero may cause the infant to have polycythemia (Chapter 30, p. 862).

A poorly nourished fetus has wasting and growth restriction. The infant is thin and has loose skin with little subcutaneous fat. The postterm infant has little or no lanugo and vernix caseosa. There is usually abundant hair on the head and long nails. The skin is dry, cracked, and peeling.

### Therapeutic Management

Therapeutic management focuses on prevention and symptomatic treatment. Expectant mothers who are "overdue" are scheduled for tests of placental functioning, and labor is induced if there are signs of placental deterioration. If the fetus cannot tolerate labor, a cesarean birth is necessary. Apgar scores less than 7 are more likely in postterm infants. In cases of asphyxia or meconium aspiration, respiratory support is needed at birth (Chapter 30, pp. 847 and 850).

During the nursery stay, respiratory problems may necessitate continued assessment and care. The infant is prone to hypoglycemia because of poor stores of glycogen at birth. Thermoregulation is a problem because the infant has little subcutaneous fat to act as insulation. Polycythemia makes the infant prone to hyperbilirubinemia.

### Nursing Considerations

The nurse's role is primarily one of prevention of complications, where possible, and monitoring for changes in status. During labor and delivery, the nurse responds appropriately to fetal heart rate decelerations, prepares for and assists in emergency delivery, and cares for respiratory problems at birth.

Signs of postmaturity syndrome in infants are noted during the initial assessment. If there was an error in calculating the mother's due date, the condition will be unexpected. Infants with any indications of postmaturity should be tested for blood glucose level soon after birth and again an hour later. They need early and more frequent feedings to help compensate for the period of poor nutrition in utero.

Temperature regulation may be poor because fat stores have been used for nourishment in utero. The infant may need more time in a radiant warmer or incubator before thermoregulation is stable. Extra blankets, frequent monitoring of temperature, and teaching parents about prevention of cold stress may be necessary throughout the hospital stay.

## Small-for-Gestational Age Infants

Small-for-gestational age (SGA) infants are those who fall below the 10th percentile in size on growth charts. They have had IUGR. It is possible for some infants who do not meet the definition for SGA (below the 10th percentile) to have IUGR and fail to grow to full potential in utero for a variety of reasons. However, SGA and IUGR are often used interchangeably.

Infants who are SGA may be preterm, full-term, or postterm but have failed to grow at the rate expected for the time spent in utero. Approximately one third of all infants who have a low birth weight are full-term but SGA (Behrman et al., 1996).

### Causes

Many risk factors may cause an infant to be SGA. Congenital malformations, chromosomal anomalies, and fetal infections from rubella or cytomegalovirus may cause IUGR. Poor placental function resulting from aging, small size, separation, or malformation may interfere with fetal growth. Illness in the expectant mother, including pregnancy-induced hypertension or severe diabetes, restricts uteroplacental blood flow and decreases fetal growth. Smoking and drug or alcohol abuse also impair fetal growth, as does severe maternal malnutrition.

### Scope of Problem

Intrauterine growth restriction occurs in 3 to 10 percent of all pregnancies, and affected infants have a four to eight times higher perinatal mortality rate than infants who are not growth restricted (Gomella, 1994). Death may occur from asphyxia before or during labor because of poor placental functioning.

Infants who are SGA are subject to many of the same complications as those who are preterm or postterm. The specific complications and their severity depend on the cause and degree of growth restriction. Infants with congenital defects will also have problems at birth that are associated with the anomaly. Drug-exposed infants may have the added complication of drug withdrawal. Problems tend to be greatest in infants who are preterm in addition to being SGA.

Low Apgar scores, meconium aspiration, and polycythemia are increased in the SGA infant as in the postterm infant. Hypoglycemia is common because there is little storage of glycogen in the liver. Although muscle tone enables the SGA infant to maintain better flexion than the preterm infant, SGA infants are prone to inadequate thermoregulation because subcutaneous and brown fat stores have been used to survive in utero. If hypoglycemia develops, there is inadequate glucose for increased metabolism to produce heat, increasing the problem.

### Characteristics

The appearance of the SGA infant varies according to whether the cause of growth restriction began early or late in the pregnancy. This is because growth restriction affects the weight first. If it continues, the length and then the head size will eventually be affected.

- *Symmetric* growth restriction occurs in about 30 percent of cases and involves the entire body (Pittard, 1993). It may be caused by congenital anomalies or exposure to infections or drugs early in pregnancy. Although the infant is small, the body is proportionate and appears normally developed for size. There is a decrease in the total number of cells, and the infant may have long-term complications. These infants are often small throughout their lives.
- *Asymmetric* restriction is caused by complications that begin after the first half of pregnancy, such as pregnancy-induced hypertension. In asymmetric restriction, the head is normal in size but seems large for the rest of the body. The length is normal, but the weight is below that expected for gestational age. The infant appears long and thin. The loose skin has longitudinal thigh creases from loss of subcutaneous fat. The infant has sparse hair, a thin cord, dry skin, and the wide-eyed look associated with intrauterine hypoxia. These infants generally "catch up" in growth if they are adequately nourished after birth.

### Therapeutic Management

Therapeutic management is focused on prevention with good prenatal care to identify and treat problems early. When growth restriction cannot be prevented, ultrasound examination may permit early discovery of the condition so that the infant can be delivered early, if necessary, and preparation can be made for the expected complications at birth. Problems after birth are treated as they occur.

### Nursing Considerations

Because the causes of growth restriction are so varied, care of the SGA infant must be adapted to meet the specific problems that the infant demonstrates. When signs of growth restriction are present, the nurse must observe for complications that commonly accompany it. The general appearance and measurements will give an indication of the type of growth restriction that has occurred. Measurements of the head, chest, length, and weight will be below normal in the infant with symmetric growth restriction. If the restriction is asymmetric, the head circumference and length will be normal and the chest circumference and weight will be low.

The nurse should assess for hypoglycemia, especially in asymmetric growth-restricted infants. The brain of the infant is normal and needs large amounts of glucose, but the liver is small and has inadequate stores of glycogen. Calorie needs will be higher than for a normal infant, making early and more frequent feedings important. Temperature regulation and respiratory support are added nursing concerns. Care is generally similar to that of the preterm or postterm infant, depending on the problems present.

## Large-for-Gestational Age Infants

Large-for-gestational age (LGA) infants are those who are above the 90th percentile on intrauterine growth charts. They may weigh more than 4000 g (8 pounds, 13 ounces) and are usually born at term, although they may be preterm or postterm. The preterm LGA infant may be mistaken for full-term, but has the same problems as other preterm infants.

### Causes

Infants who are LGA may be born to multiparas, large parents, and certain ethnic groups known to have large infants. Diabetes in the mother may also cause increased size (Chapter 30, p. 861), as may erythroblastosis fetalis (Chapter 30, p. 853).

### Scope of the Problem

The LGA infant is more likely to go through a longer labor, have injury during birth, or need a cesarean birth. Shoulder dystocia may occur because the shoulders are too large to fit through the pelvis. Fractures of the clavicle, damage to the brachial plexus or facial nerve, cephalhematoma, and bruising occur more often in these infants than in those of normal size. Congenital heart defects and a higher mortality rate are also more common (Behrman et al., 1996).

### Therapeutic Management

Therapeutic management is based on identification of macrosomia (large size) during pregnancy by measurements of fundal height and ultrasound examination. Delivery problems may lead to use of forceps, vacuum extraction, or cesarean birth. Specific treatment involves identification and treatment of birth injuries and complications as they arise.

### Nursing Considerations

The nurse assists in a difficult delivery or cesarean birth resulting from dystocias when the infant is LGA. After birth, the infant is carefully assessed for injuries or other complications such as hypoglycemia or polycythemia (see pp. 525 and 862). Nursing care is geared to problems presented.

**CHECK YOUR READING**

13. What is the typical appearance of the infant with postmaturity syndrome?
14. What special problems might a postmature infant have?
15. How are symmetric and asymmetric IUGR different?
16. What problems may occur in infants who are LGA?

## SUMMARY CONCEPTS

- Low socioeconomic status increases risk of preterm birth because of possible decreased general health, nutrition, and medical care and lack of economic, social, and emotional support.
- Preterm infants differ in appearance from full-term infants. Some differences include small size, limp posture, red skin, abundant vernix and lanugo, and immature ears and genitals.
- The lungs of preterm infants may lack adequate surfactant, which may cause the lungs to be noncompliant, increasing the amount of energy necessary for breathing and leading to atelectasis.
- Other factors that may increase respiratory problems are poor cough reflex, narrow respiratory passages, and weak muscles.
- Preterm infants should be positioned on the side or prone to increase drainage of respiratory secretions. Prone position decreases breathing effort because respiratory muscles are used efficiently. In the supine position, a small roll should be placed under the shoulders to straighten the airway.
- Preterm infants are prone to cold stress because they have thin skin with blood vessels near the surface, little subcutaneous or brown fat, a large surface area, a limp position, and an immature temperature control center.
- It is important to maintain a neutral thermal environment at all times for infants. The nurse should prevent air drafts, use warmed oxygen, and keep incubator doors and portholes closed. When the infant is taken out of heating devices, he or she should be wrapped in warmed blankets and wear a hat.
- Preterm infants are subject to increased insensible water losses and have difficulty maintaining fluid balance. Their kidneys do not concentrate or dilute urine as well as those of full-term infants. Intake and output must be carefully measured.
- Preterm infants are subject to infections because they lack passive antibodies from the mother, have an immature immune system, have fragile skin, and are subjected to many invasive procedures.
- The nurse must watch carefully for signs of pain and use comfort measures and medications to alleviate it.
- Infants demonstrate that they are receiving too much stimulation by changes in oxygenation and

behavior. The nurse should schedule care to allow rest periods, keep noise to a minimum, and teach parents how to interact with the infant appropriately.

- Preterm infants lack nutrient stores and need more nutrients but do not absorb them well. They lack coordination in sucking and swallowing and fatigue easily.
- Signs indicating that an infant may be ready for nipple feeding include rooting, sucking on a gavage tube or pacifier, presence of gag reflex, and respiratory rate below 60 breaths per minute.
- The nurse can help the mother who wishes to breastfeed her preterm infant by teaching her how to use a breast pump and store her milk until the infant is ready to breastfeed. The nurse can provide privacy, give support and encouragement, explain the infant's behavior, and answer general questions about breastfeeding.
- Nurses can increase parents' comfort with their preterm infant by providing information about the NICU environment, the infant's condition and characteristics, and the equipment and care. Spending time with parents during visits, offering therapeutic communication and realistic encouragement, and involving parents in care of the infant will also help with bonding.
- Preparation for discharge should be started early in the infant's hospital stay. This allows parents to gradually learn about and take on increasing responsibility in the care of the infant until they are comfortable with complete care.
- Common complications of preterm birth are RDS, BPD, PIVH, ROP, and NEC.
- Infants with postmaturity syndrome may appear thin, with loose skin folds, cracked peeling skin, and meconium staining. They appear hyperalert and worried. They may have respiratory difficulties at birth and suffer hypoglycemia and inadequate temperature regulation.
- Infants with IUGR may be SGA at birth. In symmetric growth restriction, the infant is proportionately small; in asymmetric growth restriction, the head and length are normal and the body is thin.
- Large-for-gestational age infants may have birth injuries, such as fractures, nerve damage, or bruising, as a result of their size. They may have hypoglycemia or polycythemia.

### References and Readings

Adcock, E.W., & Consolvo, C.A. (1993). Fluid and electrolyte management. In G.B. Merenstein & S.L. Gardner (Eds.), *Handbook of neonatal intensive care* (3rd ed.). St. Louis: C.V. Mosby.

Affonso, D.D., Hurst, I., Mayberry, L.J., Haller, L., Yost, K., & Lynch, M.E. (1992). Stressors reported by mothers of hospitalized premature infants. *Neonatal Network*, 11(6), 63–70.

American Academy of Pediatrics and American College of Obstetricians and Gynecologists. (1992). *Guidelines for perinatal care* (3rd ed.). Elk Grove Village, Ill.: American Academy of Pediatrics.

Association of Women's Health, Obstetric, and Neonatal Nurses. (1995). *Clinical commentary: Pain in neonates*. Washington, DC: Author.

Behrman, R.E., Kliegman, R.M., & Arvin, A.M. (Eds.). (1996). *Nelson textbook of pediatrics* (15th ed.). Philadelphia: W.B. Saunders.

Bell, E.H., Geyer, J., & Jones, L. (1995). A structured intervention improves breastfeeding success for ill or preterm infants. MCN: *American Journal of Maternal Child Nursing*, 20(6), 309–414.

Bell, R.P., & McGrath, J.M. (1996). Implementing a research-based kangaroo care program in the NICU. *Nursing Clinics of North America*, 31(2), 387–403.

Blackburn, S. (1995). Problems of preterm infants after discharge. *Journal of Obstetric, Gynecologic, and Neonatal Nursing*, 24(1), 43–49.

Blackburn, S.T. (1993). Assessment and management of neurologic dysfunction. In C. Kenner, A. Brueggemeyer, & L.P. Gunderson (Eds.), *Comprehensive neonatal nursing: A physiologic perspective*. Philadelphia: W.B. Saunders.

Blake, W.W., & Murray, J.A. (1993). Heat balance. In G.B. Merenstein & S.L. Gardner (Eds.), *Handbook of neonatal intensive care* (3rd ed.). St. Louis: C.V. Mosby.

Bosque, E.M., Brady, J.P., Affonso, D.D., & Wahlberg, V. (1995). Physiologic measures of kangaroo versus incubator care in a tertiary-level nursery. *Journal of Obstetric, Gynecologic, and Neonatal Nursing*, 24(3), 219–226.

Boyle, K.M., Baker, V.L. & Cassaday, C.J. (1995). Neonatal pulmonary disorders. In S.L. Barnhart & M.P. Czervinske (Eds.), *Perinatal and pediatric respiratory care*. Philadelphia: W.B. Saunders.

Bruno, J.P. (1995). Systematic neonatal assessment and intervention. MCN: *American Journal of Maternal Child Nursing*, 20(1), 21–28.

Corbett, J.V., & Omlin, K.L. (1995). Prenatal and postnatal use of corticosteroids. MCN: *American Journal of Maternal Child Nursing*, 20(6), 346.

Cox, C.A., Wolfson, M.R., & Shaffer, T.H. (1996). Liquid ventilation: A comprehensive overview. *Neonatal Network*, 15(3), 31–43.

Darby, M.K., & Loughead, J.L. (1996). Neonatal nutritional requirements and formula composition: A review. *Journal of Obstetric, Gynecologic, and Neonatal Nursing*, 25(3), 209–217.

Davis, J.M., & Rosenfeld, W.N. (1994). Chronic lung disease. In G.B. Avery, M.A. Fletcher, & M.G. Macdonald (Eds.), *Neonatology, pathophysiology and management of the newborn* (4th ed.). Philadelphia: J.B. Lippincott.

Dodd, V. (1996). Gestational age assessment. *Neonatal Network*, 15(1), 27–36.

Estrada, E.A., & Brennan-Behm, M. (1992). Neonatal nutrition. In P. Beachy & J. Deacon (Eds.), *Core curriculum for neonatal intensive care nursing*. Philadelphia: W.B. Saunders.

Fanaroff, A.A., & Martin, R.J. (1997). *Neonatal-perinatal medicine* (6th ed.). St. Louis: C.V. Mosby.

Gardner, S.L. (1994). Pain and pain relief in the neonate. MCN: *American Journal of Maternal Child Nursing*, 19(2), 85–90.

Gomella, T.L. (Ed.). (1994). *Neonatology: Management, procedures, on-call problems, diseases, drugs* (3rd ed.). Norwalk, Conn.: Appleton & Lange.

Gordon, M., & Montgomery, L.A. (1996). Minimizing epidermal stripping in the very low birth weight infant: Integrating research and practice to affect infant outcome. *Neonatal Network*, 15(1), 37–44.

Hagedorn, M.I., Gardner, S.L., & Abman, S.H. (1993). Respiratory diseases. In G.B. Merenstein & S.L. Gardner (Eds.), *Handbook of neonatal intensive care* (2nd ed.). St. Louis: C.V. Mosby.

Hamilton, L.A., & Hobel, C.J. (1992). Intrauterine growth retardation, intrauterine fetal demise, and postterm pregnancy. In N.F. Hacker & J.G. Moore (Eds.), *Essentials of obstetrics and gynecology* (2nd ed.). Philadelphia: W.B. Saunders.

Haney, C., & Allingham, T.M. (1992). Nursing care of the neonate receiving high-frequency jet ventilation. *Journal of Obstetric, Gynecologic, and Neonatal Nursing,* 21(3), 187–194.

Haut, C., Peddicord, K., & O'Brien, E. (1994). Supporting parental bonding in the NICU: A care plan for nurses. *Neonatal Network,* 13(8), 19–25.

Hicks, M.A. (1995). A systematic approach to neonatal pathophysiology: Understanding respiratory distress syndrome. *Neonatal Network,* 14(1), 29–35.

Higley, A.M., & Miller, M.A. (1996). The development of parenting: Nursing resources. *Journal of Obstetric, Gynecologic, and Neonatal Nursing,* 25(9), 707–713.

Hill, A.S., & Rath, L. (1993). The care and feeding of the low-birth-weight infant. *Journal of Perinatal Neonatal Nursing,* 6(4), 56–68.

Holditch-Davis, D., Barham, L.N., O'Hale, A., & Tucker, B. (1995). Effect of standard rest periods on convalescent preterm infants. *Journal of Obstetric, Gynecologic, and Neonatal Nursing,* 24(5), 424–432.

Kinneer, M.D., & Beachy, P. (1994). Nipple feeding premature infants in the neonatal intensive care unit: Factors and decisions. *Journal of Obstetric, Gynecologic, and Neonatal Nursing,* 23(2), 105–112.

Kirkpatrick, J.M., Alesander, J., & Cain, R.M. (1997). Recovering urine from diapers: Are test results accurate? MCN: *American Journal of Maternal Child Nursing,* 22(2), 96–102.

Klaus, M.H., & Fanaroff, A.A. (Eds.). (1993). *Care of the high-risk neonate* (4th ed.). Philadelphia: W.B. Saunders.

LaGamma, E.F., & Browne, L.E. (1994). Feeding practices for infants weighing less than 1500 g at birth and the pathogenesis of necrotizing enterocolitis. *Clinics in Perinatology: Necrotizing Enterocolitis,* 21(2), 271–306.

Lefrak-Okikawa, L., & Lund, C.H. (1993). Nursing practice in the neonatal intensive care unit. In M.H. Klaus & A.A. Fanaroff (Eds.), *Care of the high-risk neonate.* Philadelphia: W.B. Saunders.

Legault, M., & Goulet, C. (1995). Comparison of kangaroo and traditional methods of removing preterm infants from incubators. *Journal of Obstetric, Gynecologic, and Neonatal Nursing,* 24(6), 501–506.

Ludington-Hoe, S.M., & Swinth, J.Y. (1996). Developmental aspects of kangaroo care. *Journal of Obstetric, Gynecologic, and Neonatal Nursing,* 25(8), 691–703.

Mattson, S., & Smith, J.E. (Eds.). (1992). NAACOG *core curriculum for maternal-newborn nursing.* Philadelphia: W.B. Saunders.

McCain, G.C. (1992). Facilitating inactive awake states in preterm infants: A study of three interventions. *Nursing Research,* 41(3), 157–160.

McGrath, J.M., & Conliffe-Torres, S. (1996). Integrating family-centered developmental assessment and intervention into routine care in the neonatal intensive care unit. *Nursing Clinics of North America,* 31(2), 367–386.

Medoff-Cooper, B. (1994). Transition of the preterm infant to an open crib. *Journal of Obstetric, Gynecologic, and Neonatal Nursing,* 23(4), 329–335.

Medoff-Cooper, B., & Ray, W. (1995). Neonatal sucking behaviors. IMAGE: *Journal of Nursing Scholarship,* 27(3), 195–200.

Meier, P., & Brown, L.P. (1996). State of the science: Breastfeeding for mothers and low birth weight infants. *Nursing Clinics of North America,* 31(2), 351–365.

Meier, P., Engstrom, J.L., Fleming, B.A., Streeter, P.L., & Lawrence, P.B. (1996). Estimating milk intake of hospitalized preterm infants who breastfeed. *Journal of Human Lactation,* 12(1), 21–26.

Meier, P., & Mangurten, H.H. (1993). Breastfeeding the preterm infant. In J. Riordan & K.G. Auerbach (Eds.), *Breastfeeding and human lactation.* Boston: Jones & Bartlett.

Miles, M.S., Carlson, J., & Funk, S.G. (1996). Sources of support reported by mothers and fathers of infants hospitalized in a neonatal intensive care unit. *Neonatal Network,* 15(3), 45–51.

Militello, L., & Lim, L. (1995). Patient assessment skills: Assessing early cues of necrotizing enterocolitis. *Journal of Perinatal Neonatal Nursing,* 9(2), 42–52.

Minarcik, C.J., & Beachy, P. (1993). Neurologic disorders. In G.B. Merenstein & S.L. Gardner (Eds.), *Handbook of neonatal intensive care* (3rd ed.). St. Louis: C.V. Mosby.

Parker, L.A. (1995). Necrotizing enterocolitis. *Neonatal Network,* 14(6), 17–26.

Pereira, G.R. (1995). Nutritional care of the extremely premature infant. *Clinics in Perinatology,* 22(1), 61–75.

Peters, K.L. (1996a). Research update: Dinosaurs in the bath. *Neonatal Network,* 15(1), 71–73.

Peters, K.L. (1996b). Selected physiologic and behavioral responses of the critically ill premature neonate to a routine nursing intervention. *Neonatal Network,* 15(1), 74.

Philip, A. (1996). *Neonatology: A practical guide* (4th ed.). Philadelphia: W.B. Saunders.

Pittard III, W.B. (1993). Classification of the low-birth-weight infant. In M.H. Klaus & A.A. Fanaroff (Eds.), *Care of the high-risk neonate.* Philadelphia: W.B. Saunders.

Price, P.T., & Kalhan, S.C. (1993). Nutrition and selected disorders of the gastrointestinal tract. In M.H. Klaus & A.A. Fanaroff (Eds.), *Care of the high-risk neonate* (4th ed.). Philadelphia: WB Saunders.

Shandor, M., & Holditch-Davis, D. (1997). Parenting the prematurely born child: Pathways of influence. *Seminars in Perinatology,* 21(3) 254–266.

Shellabarger, S.G. (1993). The critical times: Meeting parental communication needs throughout the NICU experience. *Neonatal Network,* 12(2), 39–44.

Short, M.A., Brooks-Brunn, J.A., Reeves, D.S., Yeager, J., & Thorpe, J.A. (1996). The effects of swaddling versus standard positioning on neuromuscular development in very low birth weight infants. *Neonatal Network,* 15(4), 25–31.

Sifuentes, M. (1996). Well child care for preterm infants. In C.D. Berkowitz (Ed.), *Pediatrics: A primary care approach.* Philadelphia: W.B. Saunders.

Simpson, K.R., & Creehan, P.A. (Eds.). (1996). AWHONN's *perinatal nursing.* Philadelphia: Lippincott-Raven.

Stevens, B.J., Johnston, C.C., & Grunau, R.V.E. (1995). Issues of assessment of pain and discomfort in neonates. *Journal of Obstetric, Gynecologic, and Neonatal Nursing,* 24(9), 849–855.

Strauch, C., Brandt, S., & Edwards-Beckett, J. (1993). Implementation of a quiet hour: Effect on noise levels and infant sleep states. *Neonatal Network,* 12(2), 31–35.

Symington, A., Ballantyne, M., & Stevens, B. (1995). Indwelling versus intermittent feeding tubes in premature neonates. *Journal of Obstetric, Gynecologic, and Neonatal Nursing,* 24(4), 321–328.

Thompson, D.G. (1994). Critical pathways in the intensive care and intermediate care nurseries. MCN: *Maternal-Child Nursing Journal,* 19(1), 29–32.

Thompson, D.G., & Maringer, M. (1995). Using case management to improve care delivery in the NICU. MCN: *Maternal-Child Nursing Journal,* 20(5), 257–260.

Townsend, S.F., Johnson, C.B., Hay Jr., W.W. (1993). Enteral nutrition. In G.B. Merenstein & S.L. Gardner (Eds.), *Handbook of neonatal intensive care* (3rd ed.). St. Louis: C.V. Mosby.

Vanderhoof, J.A., Zach, T.L., & Adrian, T.E. (1994). Gastrointestinal disease. In G.B. Avery, M.A. Fletcher, & M.G. Macdonald (Eds.), *Neonatology, pathophysiology and management of the newborn* (4th ed.). Philadelphia: J.B. Lippincott.

Vecchi, C.J., Vasquez, L., Tadin, T., Johnson, P. (1996). Neonatal individualized predictive pathway (NIPP): A discharge planning tool for parents. *Neonatal Network*, 15(4), 7–13.

Whitsett, J.A., Pryhuber, G.S., Rice, W.R., Warner, B.B., & Wert, S.E. (1994). Acute respiratory disorders. In G.B. Avery, M.A. Fletcher, & M.G. Macdonald (Eds.), *Neonatology, pathophysiology and management of the newborn* (4th ed.). Philadelphia: J.B. Lippincott.

Yecco, G.J. (1993). Neurobehavioral development and developmental support of premature infants. *Journal of Perinatal Neonatal Nursing*, 7(1), 56–65.

# 30

# High-Risk Newborn: Acquired and Congenital Conditions

## OBJECTIVES

1. Describe the steps involved in neonatal resuscitation.
2. Explain the common respiratory problems in the newborn.
3. Explain the causes and significance of pathologic jaundice.
4. Describe the nursing care of the infant with pathologic jaundice.
5. Describe causes of neonatal infections and nursing care for infants with infections.
6. Explain the effect of maternal diabetes on the newborn.
7. Describe the effect of maternal substance abuse on the newborn.
8. Describe common congenital anomalies.

## DEFINITIONS

**asphyxia** *Insufficient oxygen and excess carbon dioxide in the blood and tissues.*

**bilirubin encephalopathy** *Brain damage resulting from deposits of unconjugated bilirubin in the brain tissue.*

**erythroblastosis fetalis** *Agglutination and hemolysis of fetal erythrocytes due to incompatibility between the maternal and fetal blood types. In most cases, the fetus is Rh-positive and the mother is Rh-negative.*

**esophageal atresia** *Condition in which the esophagus is separated from the stomach and ends in a blind pouch.*

**gastroschisis** *Protrusion of the intestines through a defect in the abdominal wall. Intestines are not covered by a peritoneal sac or skin.*

**hydrops fetalis** *Heart failure and generalized edema in the fetus secondary to severe anemia resulting from destruction of erythrocytes.*

**kernicterus** *Staining of brain tissue caused by accumulation of unconjugated bilirubin in the brain.*

**meconium aspiration syndrome** *Obstruction and air trapping due to meconium in the infant's lungs, which may cause severe respiratory distress.*

**meningocele** *Protrusion of the meninges through a defect in the vertebrae; a form of neural tube defect.*

**myelomeningocele** *Protrusion of the meninges and spinal cord through a defect in the vertebrae; a form of neural tube defect.*

**neonatal abstinence syndrome** *A cluster of physical signs exhibited by the newborn who was exposed in utero to maternal use of substances such as cocaine or heroin.*

**omphalocele** *Protrusion of the intestines into the base of the umbilical cord. Intestines are covered by a peritoneal sac. May be associated with other anomalies.*

**persistent pulmonary hypertension** *Vasoconstriction of the infant's pulmonary vessels after birth; may result in right-to-left shunting of blood flow through the ductus arteriosus, the foramen ovale, or both.*

**spina bifida** *Defective closure of the bony spine that encloses the spinal cord; a type of neural tube defect.*

**tracheoesophageal fistula** *Abnormal connection between the esophagus and the trachea.*

**transient tachypnea of the newborn** *Condition of rapid respirations due to inadequate absorption of fetal lung fluid.*

In addition to the high-risk conditions related to gestational age discussed in Chapter 29, the newborn at risk may have acquired or congenital complications. Acquired conditions may be associated with prenatal complications or may occur at birth or shortly thereafter.

# Respiratory Complications

Respiratory distress is one of the most common problems of the neonate. It may be caused by asphyxia before or during birth, disease of the respiratory system, or other conditions that affect the infant's ability to breathe. The nurse is responsible for identification and evaluation of respiratory status at birth and throughout the hospital stay. The degree of respiratory distress must be monitored for change, the need for intervention, and the effectiveness of treatment. Use of charts like the Silverman-Andersen index helps evaluate the degree of respiratory distress (Fig. 29–2, p. 814).

## Asphyxia

Asphyxia is a lack of oxygen and increase of carbon dioxide in the blood. It may occur in utero, at birth, or later. Asphyxia may cause the fetus to pass meconium and may lead to reflex gasping, which draws meconium deep into the air passages (see section on meconium aspiration syndrome, p. 850). When asphyxia occurs at birth, it may be a continuation of asphyxia that began in utero, or it may be the result of other factors, such as preterm lungs with insufficient surfactant to function adequately.

Infants may have primary apnea, in which a few gasping breaths at birth are followed by cessation of respirations and a rapid fall in heart rate. Stimulation at this time may be all that is necessary to restart respirations. If asphyxia continues without intervention, gasping respirations may resume weakly until the infant enters a period of secondary apnea. In secondary apnea, the oxygen levels in the blood continue to decrease, the infant loses consciousness, and stimulation is ineffective. Resuscitative measures must be initiated immediately to prevent permanent damage to the brain or death.

Lack of oxygen to the cells leads to anaerobic metabolism and the production of lactic acid. Metabolic acidosis develops when available bicarbonate is no longer able to buffer the accumulating acids. The blood shows a high partial pressure of carbon dioxide in arterial blood ($Paco_2$) and a low partial pressure of oxygen ($Po_2$), pH, and bicarbonate. Vasoconstriction decreases blood flow to all organs except the brain, myocardium, and adrenal glands. The ductus arteriosus and foramen ovale may remain open because of the low oxygen in the blood, high resistance to blood flow through constricted pulmonary vessels, and elevated pressure on the left side of the heart. Thus, even circulating blood remains low in oxygen. Progress toward brain damage and death is rapid unless intervention is prompt.

### INFANTS AT RISK

Whenever there are complications during pregnancy, labor, or birth, the infant may be at risk for asphyxia. In addition, if the expectant mother receives narcotics for analgesia shortly before delivery, the infant may be too depressed at birth to breathe spontaneously. Naloxone (Narcan) is given to these infants (Table 30–1).

**TABLE 30–1 COMMON DOSAGES OF NALOXONE HYDROCHLORIDE (NARCAN)**

Dosage must be calculated based on weight (0.1 mg/kg). The amount for various weights is given below for *two different drug concentrations.*

| Infant's Weight | Total Dose | Drug Concentration *0.4 mg/ml* | Drug Concentration *1.0 mg/ml* |
|---|---|---|---|
| 1 kg (2 lb, 3 oz) | 0.1 mg | 0.25 ml | 0.1 ml |
| 2 kg (4 lb, 7 oz) | 0.2 mg | 0.50 ml | 0.2 ml |
| 3 kg (6 lb, 10 oz) | 0.3 mg | 0.75 ml | 0.3 ml |
| 4 kg (8 lb, 13 oz) | 0.4 mg | 1.00 ml | 0.4 ml |

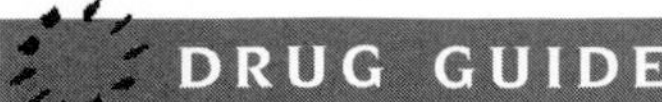


## NALOXONE HYDROCHLORIDE (Narcan)

***Classification:*** Narcotic antagonist.

***Action:*** Reverses central nervous system and respiratory depression caused by narcotics (opiates). Competes with narcotics at receptor sites.

***Indications:*** Severe respiratory depression when the mother has received narcotics within 4 hours of delivery.

***Dosage and Route:*** Available in 0.4 mg/ml and 1 mg/ml. Dosage is 0.1 mg/kg. Given intravenously, intramuscularly, subcutaneously, or into an endotracheal tube. Intravenous and endotracheal routes are preferred during resuscitation.

***Absorption:*** Well absorbed by all routes. Onset of action is 1 to 2 minutes if given intravenously.

***Excretion:*** Metabolized by the liver and excreted by kidneys.

***Contraindications and Precautions:*** Duration of effect is 1 to 4 hours. The dose may need to be repeated because the narcotic may have a longer half life than naloxone. If given to an infant of a mother addicted to drugs, it will cause withdrawal and may cause seizures. Resuscitative measures should be used as necessary.

***Nursing Considerations:*** Note the strength of the medication available when calculating the dose. Prepare the syringe before birth with 1 ml of the drug. After birth, the excess is removed from the syringe, and the amount is given according to the estimate of the infant's weight. Inject rapidly. Monitor for response, and be prepared to give repeated doses if necessary. See Table 30–1 for correct dose for various weights.

### NEONATAL RESUSCITATION

Although asphyxia can sometimes be predicted, it may develop unexpectedly. Therefore, all personnel involved in deliveries should know how to perform resuscitative measures. Courses in neonatal resuscitation are usually required of all staff members working with newborns, and skills are updated annually. Neonatal resuscitation is presented in Procedure 30–1.

Nurses must be prepared for situations in which asphyxia may develop. Equipment should be readily available and functioning properly at all times so that there is no delay in starting resuscitation. Nurses begin resuscitation measures as necessary and assist the physician with intubation, insertion of umbilical vein catheters, and administration of medications. Some nurses are taught to intubate infants in emergency situations.

Once the infant is stabilized, the nurse will assess for further change when the infant is transferred to the regular or intensive care nursery. Infants with asphyxia often have other complications as well. Communication with the parents is a vital nursing function. They will be confused and frightened and will need explanation and realistic reassurance. Parents often need continued support after the crisis to talk about their fears and concerns.

## Transient Tachypnea of the Newborn

Infants who experience transient tachypnea of the newborn (TTN) develop rapid respirations soon after birth. The condition, which resolves within a few days, is also called respiratory distress syndrome, type II. Risk factors include maternal analgesia, bleeding, or diabetes; cesarean birth; and asphyxia. Mild immaturity of surfactant production may also be a factor. Infants may be term or preterm.

### CAUSE

Although the exact cause of TTN is unknown, it is thought to be caused by a delay in absorption of fetal lung fluid by the pulmonary capillaries and the lymph vessels. This causes decreased lung compliance and air trapping and brings about signs similar to respiratory distress syndrome.

### MANIFESTATIONS

In TTN, respirations as high as 150 per minute develop within hours of birth. Retractions, nasal flaring, grunting, and mild cyanosis are also present. Chest radiography shows hyperinflation and presence of fluid in the fissures between the lobes and in the pleural space.

### THERAPEUTIC MANAGEMENT

Treatment is supportive. Usually, moderate amounts of oxygen are sufficient to prevent cyanosis. Intravenous or gavage feeding may be necessary while the respiratory rate is high to prevent aspiration and conserve energy. Because the signs are similar to respiratory distress syndrome and sepsis, the infant is observed for those complications. Antibiotics may be given until sepsis is ruled out.

### NURSING CONSIDERATIONS

The nurse may be the first person to see signs of TTN, especially if they are not apparent at birth. After identifying signs, the nurse notifies the appropriate caregiver and carries out treatment. General nursing care is similar to that of the respiratory care of the preterm infant (see p. 813).

### CHECK YOUR READING

1. What is the result of asphyxia before or during birth?
2. What is the role of the nurse in care of the infant with asphyxia?
3. How is TTN different from respiratory distress syndrome?

## Procedure 30–1

# Performing Resuscitation in Newborns

**PURPOSE:** To ensure adequate oxygenation of the neonate with asphyxia.

1. **Place the infant under a preheated radiant warmer immediately. Dry thoroughly and determine if resuscitation is necessary.** *Prevention of cold stress is important to prevent increased oxygen need.*

2. **Position the infant with the infant's neck only slightly extended, in a "sniffing" position, so that the airway is open. Avoid hyperextension or flexion of the neck. Place a small blanket under the shoulders.** *Proper positioning will help maintain an open airway. Hyperextension or flexion may obstruct the airway.*

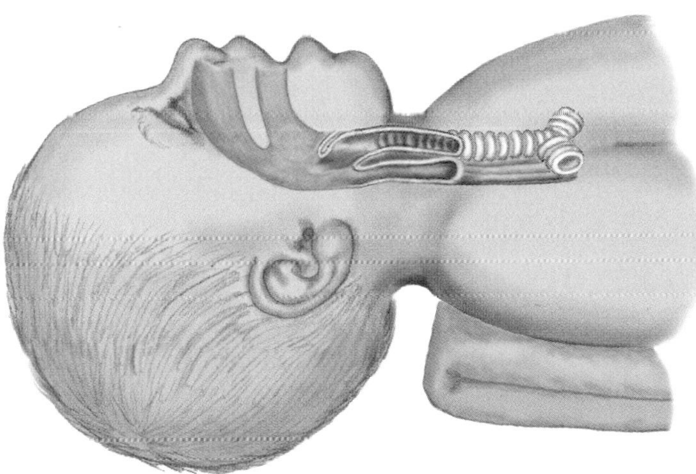

3. **Suction the mouth and then the nose.** *Suctioning removes mucus from the airways. Infants often gasp when the nose is suctioned and may aspirate secretions from the mouth into the lungs.*

4. **Stimulate the infant if necessary. Rub the infant's back or slap the soles of the feet if additional stimulation is needed.** *Spontaneous respirations should begin within the first 30 to 45 seconds after birth. The tactile stimulation of drying the infant and suctioning the mouth and nose may cause spontaneous respirations. If not, additional stimulation may be needed.*

5. **If there is no response after stimulating once or twice, stop and initiate immediate resuscitation. Do not delay resuscitation until the Apgar scores are given. Drying, clearing the airway, and stimulation should take no more than 20 seconds.** *Resuscitation becomes more difficult the longer it is delayed. Immediate resuscitation is necessary to prevent brain damage.*

6. **Begin positive-pressure ventilation with a bag and mask if the infant fails to breathe spontaneously with initial stimulation or the heart rate is less than 100 beats per minute when respirations have begun.** *Positive-pressure ventilation ensures oxygen entry into the lungs.*

7. **Attach the bag to an oxygen source with 100 percent oxygen. Place the mask snugly over the infant's nose and mouth. Squeeze the bag gently to force air into the infant's lungs with a pressure that will deliver 20 to 30 ml of air. If possible, use a bag with a gauge, to show the amount of pressure being used, and a "pop-off" valve, which releases if the pressure is high enough to cause lung damage.** *Great care must be taken to use a pressure that will deliver the 20 to 30 ml of air necessary to inflate the lungs without causing damage from overinflation.*

8. **Observe the rise and fall of the chest during ventilation. If the chest does not move, suction secretions and reposition the head and the mask. Ventilate the infant at a rate of 40 to 60 breaths per minute until the infant is breathing spontaneously and the heart rate is above 100 beats per minute.** *The airway must not be occluded by positioning or secretions.*

9. **Pause after 15 to 30 seconds of ventilation to take a 6-second heart rate. Use a stethoscope or feel the pulsations at the base of the cord. Multiply the rate by 10 to get the heart rate per minute. If the rate is less than 60 beats per minute, or less than 80 beats per minute and not increasing, a second person should begin chest compressions while the first continues to ventilate the infant.** *Adequate ventilation causes improvement of bradycardia in most infants. Evaluation of the infant's status determines whether ventilation can be discontinued or chest compressions must be added for the infant to survive.*

10. **Compress the chest by placing the hands around the infant's chest with the fingers under the back for support and the thumbs over the sternum. Position the**

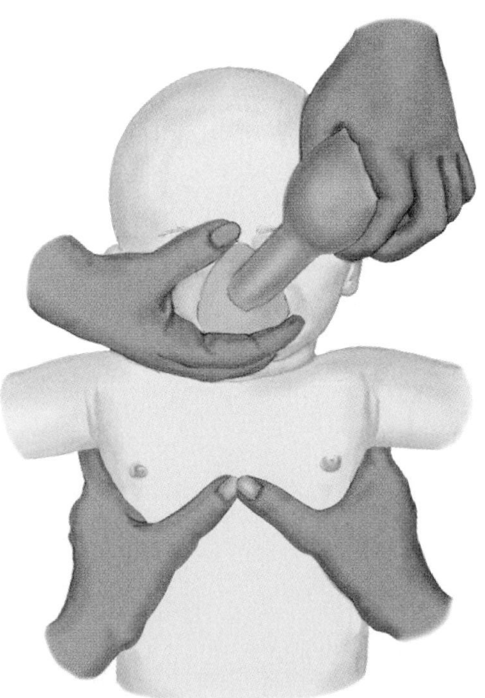

*Procedure 30–1 continued on following page*

Procedure 30–1 *Continued*

## Performing Resuscitation in Newborns

**PURPOSE:** To ensure adequate oxygenation of the neonate with asphyxia.

**thumbs just below the nipple line.** *Fingers under the infant's back provide support. Correct hand position compresses the heart but avoids or minimizes injury to the liver or spleen, fractures of the ribs, or pneumothorax.*

**11. Compress the sternum ½ to ¾ inch, with three compressions followed by one ventilation, for a combined rate of compressions and ventilations of 120 each minute. This is 90 compressions and 30 ventilations each minute. Pause for ½ second after every third compression for ventilation.** *Simultaneous compression and ventilation may interfere with adequate ventilation. The short pause allows air to enter the lungs.*

**12. Stop compressions after 30 seconds to check the heart rate for 6 seconds. If it is above 80 beats per minute, discontinue compressions but continue ventilation until spontaneous breathing begins. If the heart rate is below 80 beats per minute, continue compressions with rechecks of the heart rate periodically.** *Periodic evaluation is necessary to ensure that treatment is appropriate to the infant's status.*

**13. Prepare medications if the heart rate is below 80 after 30 seconds of compression. They may include epinephrine given through an umbilical vein catheter or through an endotracheal tube, volume expanders, and naloxone. A 10 percent dextrose solution may also be given. Sodium bicarbonate is given only after prolonged arrest and only with effective ventilation.** *Epinephrine stimulates the heart. Volume expanders may be used for bleeding. Naloxone counteracts the effects of narcotics given to the mother in labor. Dextrose prevents or treats hypoglycemia. Sodium bicarbonate corrects acidosis after prolonged asphyxia that does not respond to other treatment.*

Data from Bloom, R.S., Cropley, C., & AHA/AAP Neonatal Resuscitation Program Steering Committee. (1994). *Textbook of neonatal resuscitation.* Dallas: American Heart Association and American Academy of Pediatrics.

## Meconium Aspiration Syndrome

Meconium aspiration syndrome occurs most often in postterm infants, who have decreased amniotic fluid and are prone to cord compression. It also occurs in term infants who have suffered intrauterine asphyxia. It is rare before 36 to 38 weeks' gestation. Meconium aspiration syndrome results in obstruction of the airways, pneumonitis, and air trapping. It may lead to persistent pulmonary hypertension of the newborn (Fig. 30–1).

### CAUSES

Although the normal fetus may pass meconium, it is most often seen when hypoxia causes relaxation of the anal sphincter previous to or during labor. Meconium aspiration syndrome develops when meconium enters the lungs during fetal life or at birth. Meconium may be drawn into the lungs if gasping movements occur in utero as a result of asphyxia and acidosis, or the meconium in the upper airways may be pulled deep into the respiratory passages when the infant takes the first breaths after birth.

Obstruction of the airways may be complete or partial. In partial obstruction, air can enter but not escape from the alveoli. During inhalation, the bronchioles expand slightly as air flows into them past the meconium. During exhalation, the passages constrict and meconium blocks the passage of air out of the lungs.

This ball-valve mechanism results in air trapping. The overdistended alveoli may develop an air leak, with escape of air into the pleural cavity (pneumothorax) or mediastinum (pneumomediastinum). In addition, meconium is irritating to lung tissue and causes an inflammatory reaction and chemical pneumonitis. Persistent pulmonary hypertension may result.

Severe meconium aspiration syndrome develops in only a small number of the approximately 4 percent of newborns with meconium below the vocal cords. It most often occurs when the fetal heart rate during labor and delivery indicated asphyxia (Whitsett et al., 1994). The addition of meconium to a lung damaged by asphyxia may increase the severity of the condition. Damage from asphyxia interferes with clearing of lung fluid, surfactant production, and causes pulmonary vasoconstriction that can result in return to fetal circulation.

### MANIFESTATIONS

If meconium in the amniotic fluid is light, respiratory problems usually do not develop. However, thick meconium may cause serious respiratory pathology. Signs of mild to severe respiratory distress are present at birth, with tachypnea, cyanosis, retractions, nasal flaring, grunting, and coarse breath

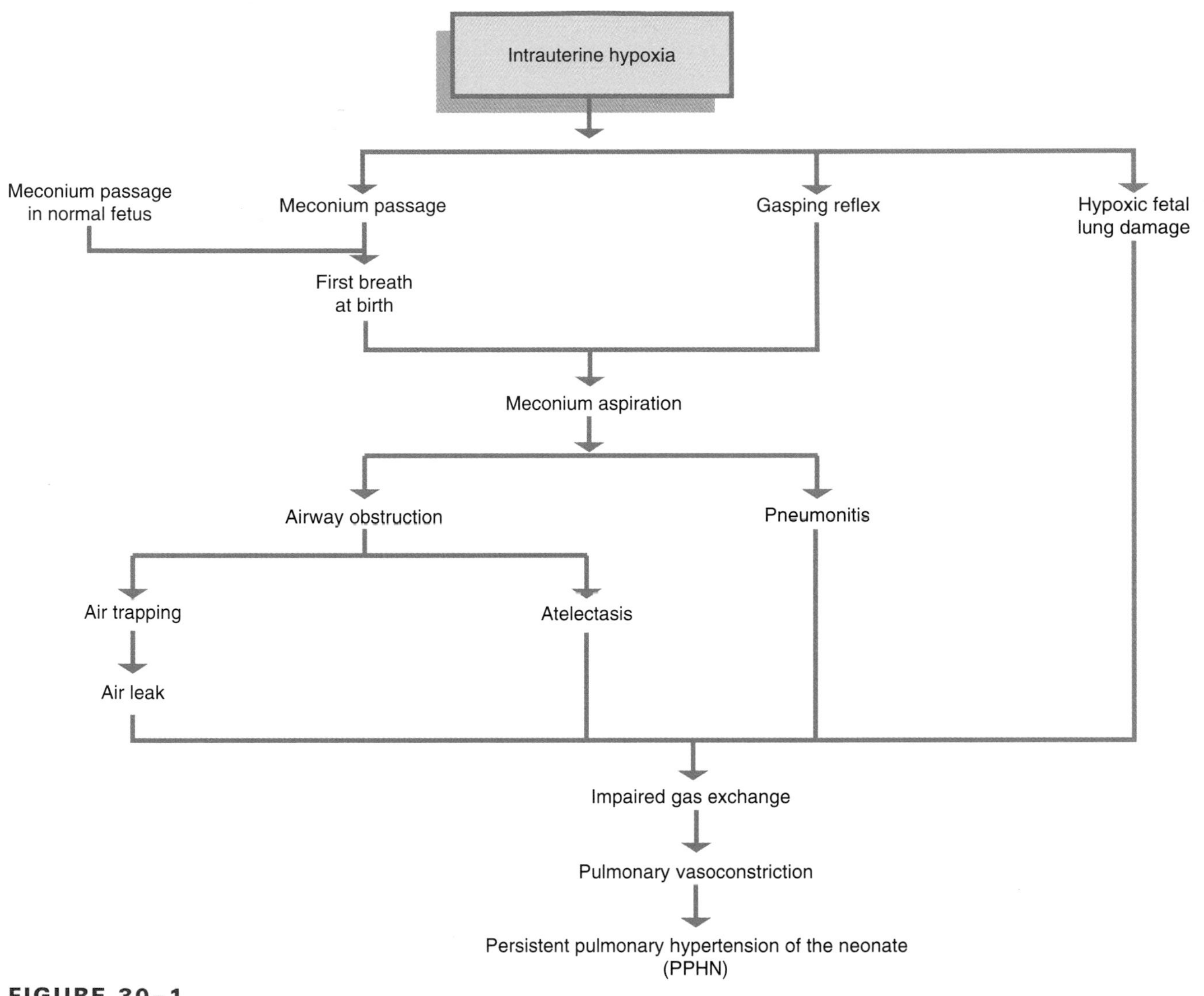


**FIGURE 30–1**

Flow chart showing the effects of meconium aspiration syndrome.

sounds. Radiography shows atelectasis, consolidation, and hyperexpansion from air trapping.

#### THERAPEUTIC MANAGEMENT

At birth, the airway must be cleared, especially if meconium is thick. The infant's mouth and pharynx are suctioned as soon as the head is delivered and before delivery of the rest of the body. This helps prevent drawing the meconium from the upper air passages deep into the lungs during the infant's first breath.

Immediately after birth and before the infant takes the first breath, a laryngoscope is inserted and the trachea suctioned. An endotracheal tube is inserted to allow deep suction of meconium and ventilation, if necessary. If the meconium is thin and the infant is vigorous and showing no respiratory difficulty, intubation may not be necessary.

Infants may only need warmed, humidified oxygen, or extensive respiratory support with a ventilator may be required. High-frequency ventilation may be used. Supportive care to meet the problems presented makes up ongoing management.

Infants with severe meconium aspiration syndrome who do not respond to conventional treatment may benefit from extracorporeal membrane oxygenation (ECMO). This is a method available in some hospitals to oxygenate the blood while bypassing the lungs, much like heart-lung machines used during heart surgery. It allows the infant's lungs to rest temporarily and recover.

#### NURSING CONSIDERATIONS

When meconium is noted in the amniotic fluid during labor, the nurse notifies the primary caregiver of the amount of meconium present so that delivery care can be adapted as necessary. The nurse ensures that equipment is available and functioning and assists with care at delivery. After the infant's birth, nursing care is adapted to the problems presented. Although meconium is sterile, lung damage promotes the growth of bacteria. Infants should be closely observed for infection, which may further complicate the condition.

### Persistent Pulmonary Hypertension of the Newborn

Persistent pulmonary hypertension of the newborn (PPHN) is a condition in which the vascular resistance of the lungs does not decrease after birth and normal changes to neonatal circulation are impaired. For this reason the condition is also called *persistent fetal circulation*.

#### CAUSES

The cause of PPHN may be abnormal lung development, maternal use of nonsteroidal anti-inflammatory agents or aspirin, hypoxia, or it may develop for unknown reasons. It is often associated with hypoxemia and acidosis from conditions such as asphyxia, meconium aspiration, sepsis, or respiratory distress syndrome.

Inadequate oxygenation results in vasoconstriction, instead of the normal dilation, of the pulmonary artery and produces increased resistance in the lungs. It also causes relaxation, instead of constriction, of the ductus arteriosus. The elevated pulmonary vascular resistance causes a rise in pressure on the right side of the heart. This results in a right-to-left shunt of blood through the foramen ovale and patent ductus arteriosus, as occurs during fetal circulation.

#### MANIFESTATIONS

Infants with PPHN are usually term or postterm and develop signs of PPHN within the first 24 hours after birth. Tachypnea, respiratory distress, and progressive cyanosis often become worse with handling. Oxygen saturation and partial pressure of oxygen in arterial blood ($PaO_2$) are decreased. Other signs may result from associated conditions. The mortality rate is high for this condition.

#### THERAPEUTIC MANAGEMENT

Management involves treating the underlying cause of poor oxygenation and relieving pulmonary vasoconstriction. Arterial pH may be increased with respiratory and drug therapy to cause pulmonary vasodilation. High-frequency ventilation, surfactant therapy, and ECMO therapy may all be necessary. Inhalation of nitric oxide, which dilates pulmonary vessels, is being investigated. Nursing care is similar to care of other infants with severe respiratory disease. Because infants become hypoxic with activity and other stimuli, handling and noise are kept to a minimum.

**✓ CHECK YOUR READING**

4. How does meconium get into an infant's respiratory tract? Why is it a problem?
5. What is the role of the nurse when meconium is discovered in amniotic fluid?

## Hyperbilirubinemia (Pathologic Jaundice)

Conjugation of bilirubin and physiologic jaundice are discussed in Chapters 19, p. 498, and 20, p. 525. This discussion focuses on pathologic jaundice. When the bilirubin level reaches 5 to 7 mg/dl, jaundice is visible in the skin (Maisels, 1994). Jaundice is considered pathologic in the following circumstances:

- It appears in the first 24 hours after birth
- The total bilirubin rises above 12 mg/dl in a full-term infant or 10 to 14 mg/dl in a preterm infant, or more than 5 mg/dl in 24 hours
- The direct bilirubin is above 1 mg/dl
- Jaundice continues beyond the second week of life (Behrman et al., 1996)

Pathologic jaundice is a concern because it may lead to kernicterus. In kernicterus, bilirubin deposits cause yellowish staining of the brain, especially the basal ganglia, cerebellum, and hippocampus. It is more likely to occur in infants who have suffered sepsis, hypoxia, or respiratory acidosis, which impairs the blood-brain barrier and allows unconjugated bilirubin to enter the brain. Kernicterus causes bilirubin encephalopathy.

Although bilirubin encephalopathy is rare today because of improved treatment measures, the mortality rate of affected infants is high. Those who survive may suffer from cerebral palsy, mental retardation, hearing loss, or more subtle long-term neurologic and developmental problems. The exact level at which this begins to develop is not known, but it may occur when total bilirubin levels are more than 20 mg/dl in full-term infants and lower levels in preterms or neonates with other complications.

### Causes

The most common cause of pathologic jaundice is hemolytic disease of the newborn caused by incompatibility between the blood of the mother and that of the fetus. The best known cause is Rh incompatibility, in which the Rh-negative mother forms antibodies when Rh-positive blood from the fetus enters her circulation. Antibodies may have developed during a previous pregnancy or after injury, abortion, amniocentesis, or a transfusion of Rh-positive blood. The antibodies cross the placenta and attach to fetal red blood cells and destroy them. This condition is called erythroblastosis fetalis.

Infants with erythroblastosis fetalis are anemic from destruction of red blood cells. However, jaundice usually does not develop until soon after birth because bilirubin crosses the placenta and is excreted by the mother. Severely affected infants may experience hydrops fetalis, a severe anemia that results in heart failure and generalized edema. Use of $Rh_0$(D) immune globulin (RhIG), such as RhoGAM, to prevent the mother from forming antibodies against Rh-positive blood has greatly decreased the incidence of erythroblastosis fetalis. (See Rh Incompatibility, p. 703.)

ABO incompatibility also causes pathologic jaundice. Mothers with type O blood have natural antibodies to type A or B blood. The antibodies cross the placenta and cause hemolysis of fetal red blood cells. However, the destruction is much less severe than with Rh incompatibility and causes milder signs.

Other causes of pathologic jaundice include infection, hypothyroidism, glucuronyl transferase or other enzyme deficiency, polycythemia, and biliary atresia. Any condition that causes destruction of erythrocytes or impairment of the liver may result in pathologic bilirubin levels.

## Therapeutic Management

Therapeutic management is focused on determining the cause of the jaundice, following the course of bilirubin elevation by laboratory work, and treating the condition to prevent the development of kernicterus. The cause is determined by history and diagnostic tests to identify infections or blood abnormalities. During pregnancy, a positive Coombs' test result of the expectant mother's blood shows the presence of antibodies against fetal blood. Amniocentesis may be performed to determine the degree of hyperbilirubinemia.

At birth, a direct Coombs' test is performed on the cord blood. A positive result indicates that antibodies from the mother have attached to the infant's red blood cells. Bilirubin levels are followed closely for changes that indicate that treatment should be initiated or changed.

### PHOTOTHERAPY

The most common treatment of jaundice is phototherapy or "bili" lights. These are special fluorescent lamps placed over the infant at a distance determined by the type of bulb used (usually 12 to 30 inches) (Fig. 30–2). A fiberoptic phototherapy blanket that is placed against the infant's skin is another option. The infant can be swaddled and does not require patches over the eyes when the blanket is used. Double phototherapy lights or a combination of blanket and lights may be used if the bilirubin level is high.

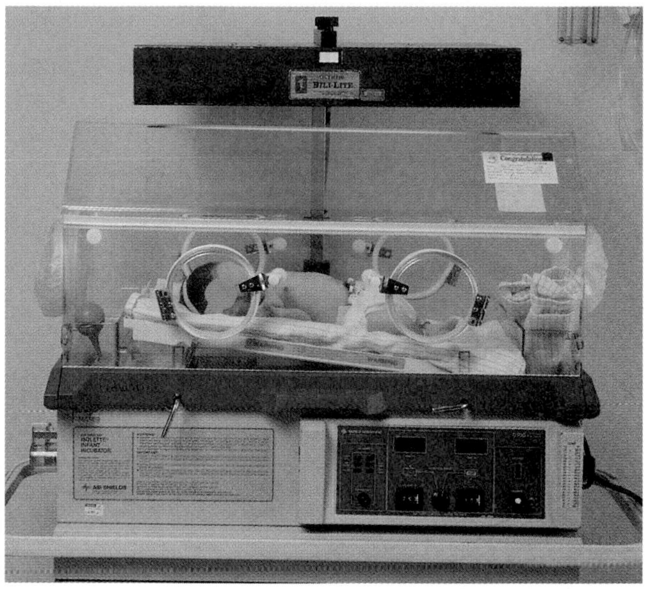

**FIGURE 30–2**

The infant receiving phototherapy is wearing eye patches to protect the eyes and a diaper to protect the gonads.

During phototherapy, bilirubin in the skin absorbs the light and changes into water-soluble products (photobilirubin and lumirubin). These do not require conjugation by the liver and can be excreted in the bile and urine. Because bilirubin encephalopathy develops in preterm infants at lower bilirubin levels than in full-term infants, phototherapy is begun at lower levels for them.

Side effects of phototherapy include frequent loose green stools, resulting from increased bile flow and peristalsis. This causes more rapid excretion of the bilirubin but may be damaging to the skin and result in fluid loss. African-American infants may experience a tanning effect from the light. Bronze baby syndrome, a grayish brown discoloration of the skin, occurs in infants with cholestatic jaundice, in whom liver function and production or flow of bile are impaired. A skin rash similar to erythema toxicum may also occur. The color changes and rash disappear when phototherapy is ended. Some infants experience a temporary lactose intolerance during therapy and need formula without lactose.

Home phototherapy is a way to avoid prolonged hospitalization, separation from parents, and interference with breastfeeding. Parents using phototherapy at home need extensive teaching on how to manage the equipment and the infant's requirements. Home

### Parents Want to Know

## Home Care for the Infant Receiving Phototherapy

- Position the phototherapy or "bili" light at the proper distance from your baby according to the manufacturer's directions. Placing it too close to the infant could result in fever or burns. Placing it too far away will make the treatment ineffective.
- Close the baby's eyes, and place patches over the eyes before placing the infant under the lights. Check at least every hour to see that the patches remain in place. They must cover the eyes but not press on the nose because they can interfere with breathing.
- The infant may be taken out from under the lights for feedings, diaper changes, and other general care but should receive phototherapy for 18 hours every day (or number of hours ordered by the physician). Hold and cuddle your infant during the time that he or she is out of the lights. When the baby is under the lights, you can talk to her or him. The sound of your voice will be comforting.
- If you are using a fiberoptic blanket, keep it next to the baby's skin at all times. Be sure the baby does not roll off the blanket. You may wrap the baby with a receiving blanket over the "bili" blanket and hold the baby for feedings, etc. It is not necessary to cover the infant's eyes if the blanket alone is used.
- Check your baby's temperature under the arm before every feeding. The temperature should remain between 97.7 and 99.5°F. If it is abnormal, see if the heat in the room is too low or high, or if the "bili" light is out of position. Use warm blankets when you remove the baby from the warmth of the light. Call your physician if the baby has a temperature less than 97.7 or above 100°F.
- Change your baby's position about every 2 hours so that the light reaches all areas of the body. Keep diapers on your infant at all times, but no other clothing that would prevent exposure of the skin to the light. You may have to keep the room temperature higher than usual to keep the baby warm.
- Feed your baby every 2 to 3 hours. It is important for the infant to eat well while under the "bili" light because it causes the baby to lose fluid from the skin and have loose stools. This could cause dehydration. The infant needs protein, which helps eliminate the bilirubin that causes the jaundice.
- Keep a list of your baby's wet diapers and stools. The infant should have six to 10 wet diapers a day. If there are fewer, or if the urine appears dark, increase the feedings.
- Call the physician or home care nurse if you have questions about care, if the baby has a fever or appears sick to you, if the mouth seems dry, or if the urine is dark or less than normal.

visits by nurses are important to help ensure the infant is making adequate progress and that the parents understand how to provide care.

#### EXCHANGE TRANSFUSIONS

Exchange transfusions are necessary when phototherapy does not reduce dangerously high bilirubin levels quickly enough. This treatment removes sensitized red blood cells before they break down and release large amounts of unconjugated bilirubin. The transfusion also removes antibodies and unconjugated bilirubin in the blood and corrects severe anemia. If the problem is Rh incompatibility, type O Rh-negative blood, crossmatched against the mother's and infant's blood, is used so that circulating antibodies will not destroy the erythrocytes.

**Procedure.** During the exchange transfusion, 5 to 10 ml portions of blood are removed and replaced with an equal amount of donor blood. Because the donor blood mixes with the infant's blood, it is necessary to administer approximately twice the infant's blood volume. Normal blood volume in a full-term infant is 80 to 85 ml/kg and in a preterm infant, 100 ml/kg. At the end of the transfusion, approximately 85 percent of the infant's red blood cells have been replaced.

The bilirubin level after transfusion is about 45 percent of the pre-exchange level. When the level in the blood decreases, bilirubin from the tissues moves into the plasma. This may increase the blood level to 60 percent or more of the original level (Frank et al., 1993). This rebound elevation of bilirubin may necessitate repeat transfusions, but phototherapy is generally adequate to resolve it.

**Complications.** Many complications may occur during exchange transfusion, including infection, hypervolemia or hypovolemia, cardiac arrhythmias, and air embolism. Hypocalcemia is also a problem because preservatives in the blood lower the infant's blood calcium level. Signs of hypocalcemia include jitteriness, irritability, tachycardia, and electrocardiogram changes. Samples of blood are analyzed before and after the exchange, including a complete blood count, bilirubin and calcium levels, and other tests as needed.

**Role of the Nurse.** The nurse's role during exchange transfusion is to prepare equipment, assess the infant during and after the procedure, and keep accurate records. A cardiac monitor is attached to the infant, and adequate warmth is provided by a radiant heater. The nurse must also clarify any misunderstandings that the parents may have about the treatment and help allay their anxiety.

## Application of Nursing Process: Hyperbilirubinemia

Although collaborative care of the infant with jaundice is an important part of the nurse's role, several nursing diagnoses are appropriate. Risk for Injury associated with bilirubin increases and phototherapy is discussed in this section. The diagnoses Risk for Fluid Volume Deficit and Altered Skin Integrity are discussed in Nursing Care Plan 30–1.

## Nursing Care Plan 30–1

# The Infant with Jaundice

**ASSESSMENT:** Holly, a 2-day-old, full-term infant, is jaundiced secondary to ABO incompatibility and is receiving phototherapy. She weighs 3.2 kg (7 pounds, 1 ounce) and her mucous membranes appear slightly dry. Skin turgor is good with quick recoil, and the anterior fontanelle is flat. Urine appears slightly dark in color. Holly had three loose green stools with no water ring on this shift. She is a sleepy infant who takes formula poorly. Holly's mother, Valerie, had a cesarean birth and appears tired and frustrated with Holly's slow eating behavior.

**NURSING DIAGNOSIS:** Fluid Volume Deficit related to inadequate oral intake to meet needs of increased insensible water loss and frequent loose stools

**GOALS/EXPECTED OUTCOMES**

Holly will do the following:

1. Take at least 320 to 480 ml of fluid per day (100 to 150 ml/kg/day) to meet normal needs
2. Show no signs of dehydration (dry mucous membranes, inelastic skin turgor, sunken fontanelles, inadequate urine output, urine specific gravity >1.020).

| INTERVENTION | RATIONALE |
|---|---|
| 1. Instruct Valerie to feed Holly every 2 to 3 hours. Feed Holly in the nursery at night or when Valerie needs rest, if she prefers. | 1. Adequate intake of formula is necessary to meet the infant's nutrient and fluid needs and ensure excretion of bilirubin in the stools. The mother's need for rest must be met without interfering with the infant's needs. |
| 2. Explain to Valerie why Holly needs frequent feedings | 2. The mother's understanding of the need and the reasons will increase her willingness to work with the infant. |
| 3. Observe Valerie feeding Holly and offer suggestions as needed. Show her how to waken the infant by unwrapping and gentle stimulation. Try warming the formula slightly. Stroke around Holly's mouth, and insert a finger to elicit the suck reflex before feedings. | 3. Observation of feedings may identify problems and interventions that work for this situation. A wide-awake infant is more likely to feed well. Some infants prefer warm milk. Oral exercise may help infant suck effectively. |
| 4. Tell the parents about the need for frequent feeding to provide added fluid, protein, and other nutrients. | 4. Infants under phototherapy have a greater than normal insensible water loss. Adequate albumin is necessary to carry bilirubin to the liver for conjugation. Heightened intestinal motility decreases absorption of nutrients. |
| 5. Avoid offering water or dextrose water. Use formula instead. | 5. Infants who are given water supplements may decrease intake of formula, with its needed nutrients. Protein is especially important to maintain serum albumin. Formula increases motility of intestines and expedites excretion of bilirubin in stools, but water does not have the same effect. |
| 6. If water loss appears excessive, check the specific gravity of the urine and weigh all diapers. Urine output should be 1 to 3 ml/kg/hr. Specific gravity should be 1.001 to 1.020 for full-term infants. | 6. Weighing the diapers and checking specific gravity will identify inadequate output and dehydration early. The diaper weight in grams equals the ml of urine. |
| 7. Use therapeutic communication techniques to help Valerie vent her frustrations. Offer praise for her attempts to feed Holly. | 7. Helping the mother deal with her feelings helps her meet the infant's needs. Feeding difficulties often interfere with the mother's view of herself as a "good" mother. Praise increases her self-concept and sense of adequacy. |

**EVALUATION**

Holly drinks a total of 510 ml (17 ounces) of formula during 24 hours. Valerie is able to wake Holly, who begins to suck more vigorously. Holly's mucous membranes are moist and there are 12 wet diapers during the 24 hours.

**ASSESSMENT:** Holly's diaper area is slightly red and irritated from her frequent loose stools.

**NURSING DIAGNOSIS:** Altered Skin Integrity related to frequent loose stools

*Nursing Care Plan continued on following page*

## Nursing Care Plan 30–1 *Continued*
# The Infant with Jaundice

**GOALS/EXPECTED OUTCOMES**

Skin will return to normal within 2 days without further signs of irritation or breakdown.

| INTERVENTION | RATIONALE |
|---|---|
| 1. Check diapers at least every hour. Cleanse the diaper area with soap and water after each stool. | 1. Extended exposure of the skin to stool and urine may cause skin breakdown. Thorough cleansing removes irritating substances from Holly's skin. |
| 2. Place Holly prone, and expose diaper area to light and air. Place a diaper under Holly (for male infants, use a face mask to cover the scrotum). Expose the entire diaper area to air for short periods when the phototherapy light is off. | 2. Exposure to air dries the area and aids healing. |
| 3. Avoid lotions, powders, ointments, or wipes containing alcohol. | 3. Skin preparations may irritate the skin and increase the risk of burns from the phototherapy lights. |
| 4. Use cloth diapers if paper disposable diapers seem to cause more irritation. | 4. Cloth diapers may be softer on irritated skin than paper diapers. |
| 5. Explain the reason for loose stools and methods of treatment of skin irritation to Valerie. | 5. The mother may need help to understand that the condition is not the result of poor care. She should learn how to care for diaper rash at home. |

**EVALUATION**

Holly's diaper area returns to normal within 1 day.

**ADDITIONAL NURSING DIAGNOSES TO CONSIDER**

Anxiety
Altered Parenting
Ineffective Thermoregulation

## Assessment

Assess the level of jaundice at the initial assessment each shift. Press the skin over a bony prominence, and note the color in the area before the blood returns. Determine the areas of the body affected by the jaundice, and document carefully to use for comparison during future assessment. Jaundice begins at the head and moves down the body as the bilirubin levels rise. Monitor laboratory bilirubin levels for change, especially because visibility of jaundice in the skin may be affected by phototherapy.

Assess for risk factors that might further increase bilirubin levels. Note temperature fluctuations, hypoglycemia, or infection. Determine the infant's oral intake and number of stools as an indication of gastrointestinal motility.

## Analysis

Nurses can do many things to prevent situations that might cause further rises in bilirubin. They must also protect the infant from injury from the light during phototherapy. Therefore, an appropriate nursing diagnosis is Risk for Injury related to preventable causes of further elevation of bilirubin and damage to the eyes or gonads secondary to phototherapy.

## Planning

The goals and expected outcomes for this nursing diagnosis are that the infant will avoid the following:

- Injury resulting from increased bilirubin
- Exposure of the eyes or gonads to phototherapy lights

## Interventions

Interventions are designed to prevent situations that might cause injury to the infant from rising bilirubin levels or effects of treatment.

### MAINTAINING A NEUTRAL THERMAL ENVIRONMENT

Prevent situations, such as cold stress or hypoglycemia, that could result in increased fatty acids in the blood caused by acidosis, thereby decreasing the availability of albumin-binding sites for unconjugated bilirubin. Prevent cold stress at birth and during all care by maintaining the infant in a neutral thermal environment. Use a temperature probe to monitor the temperature, and check the infant's axillary temperature every 2 to 4 hours to identify an early decrease before it becomes a problem. Dress the infant in warmed clothes and blankets when removing him or her from phototherapy lights.

Prevent elevation of the infant's temperature from exposure to the heat of the "bili" lights. Use a skin probe if the infant is in an incubator to maintain the environmental temperature appropriately. Position the lights according to the manufacturer's guidelines to prevent overheating or burning the skin.

#### PROVIDING OPTIMAL NUTRITION

Ensure that the infant receives feedings every 2 to 3 hours, whether by breast or bottle. This prevents hypoglycemia, provides protein to maintain the albumin level in the blood, and promotes gastrointestinal motility and prompt emptying of bilirubin from the bowel. Avoid offering water, if possible, because the infant may take less milk, which is more effective in removing bilirubin from the intestines. If breastfeeding must be supplemented, use formula instead of water.

#### PROTECTING THE EYES

Provide patches to protect the eyes from retinal damage from the phototherapy lights. Close the infant's eyes before placing the patches to avoid abrasions to the cornea. Check the position of the patches at least every hour. Infants often wiggle enough to push the patches above or below the eyes, leaving them exposed. The edges of the patches can dig into the eyes or compress the nose and interfere with breathing. If adhesive is used to fasten patches, check for skin irritation.

#### ENHANCING RESPONSE TO THERAPY

Expose as much skin as possible to the light. Turn the infant frequently to prevent irritation of the skin from lack of position change and to expose the areas evenly. Remove all clothing except a diaper. Use a face mask for a diaper if diapers cover too much skin of very small infants. If the face mask has a metal strip to go over the nose, remove it so that it does not retain heat and burn the infant. Be sure that the testes or ovaries are covered, because there is a possibility that damage to DNA may occur from exposure of the gonads to phototherapy. Turn the light off when changing diapers.

If a fiberoptic blanket is used, check the position of the blanket frequently. Infants sometimes need to be repositioned so that the blanket remains in contact with the skin.

The amount of time that the infant can be removed from phototherapy lights without decreasing the effectiveness is controversial. Generally, short periods of time out of the lights do not decrease effectiveness. The policy in most nurseries is to keep infants under the lights except during feedings. When bilirubin levels are high, some feedings may be given while the infant remains under the lights.

Use a light meter to check the level of irradiance to be sure the apparatus is functioning appropriately.

Observe for other complications. Although bilirubin encephalopathy is rare today, monitor for signs that indicate its presence. These include lethargy, poor muscle tone, decreased or absent Moro reflex, high-pitched cry, opisthotonos, and seizures. Note the presence of rashes or changes in the color of the skin, and inform parents that they are not harmful and will disappear when phototherapy is discontinued.

### Evaluation

- There should be no signs of injury.
- The eyes and gonads will not have been exposed to the phototherapy lights.

**CRITICAL THINKING EXERCISE**

**Q:** Why is it important to remove the patches from the eyes each time the infant is taken from the phototherapy for feeding?

**A:** Patches hide the eye area and an infection might not be noticed immediately. Removal of the patches at feedings allows inspection for signs of infection such as redness, edema, and drainage. Removal also allows a time for visual stimulation for the infant. If parents give the feeding, being able to see the infant's eyes enhances attachment.

**CHECK YOUR READING**

6. When is jaundice considered pathologic?
7. What is the role of the nurse in caring for the infant receiving phototherapy?

## Infection

Neonatal infection is responsible for approximately 30 percent of all neonatal deaths (Lott et al., 1993). The nurse must be constantly alert for this condition.

### Transmission of Infection

Newborns acquire infection in two ways: vertical transmission, which occurs in utero or during birth, and horizontal transmission, which occurs after birth.

Transmission of some organisms, such as cytomegalovirus or *Streptococcus*, may occur either vertically or horizontally.

#### VERTICAL TRANSMISSION

In vertical transmission, the fetus becomes infected by transfer of organisms from the mother across the placenta during pregnancy, by contact with organisms present in the vagina during birth, or by ascending infection after rupture of membranes. Infections that are acquired by vertical transmission include toxoplasmosis, rubella, cytomegalovirus, herpes, and hepatitis. Vertically transmitted infections may cause defects in the fetus and long-term consequences for the newborn and the family. Some of the most common infections and their effects on the neonate are listed in Table 30–2. Some infections are also discussed in Chapter 26, p. 732.

#### HORIZONTAL TRANSMISSION

In horizontal transmission, the infant acquires infection after birth from the mother or other family members, agency staff, or contaminated equipment. A common example is staphylococcal infection.

## Sepsis Neonatorum

Infection that occurs during or after birth may result in sepsis neonatorum, systemic infection with bacteria in the blood stream. Bacterial sepsis occurs in one to eight infants per 1000 live births (Klein & Remington, 1995).

Newborns are particularly susceptible to sepsis because their immune system is immature and they react more slowly to invasion by organisms. They fail to localize infection as well as older children, and this allows infection to spread easily from one organ to another. The blood-brain barrier is less effective in keeping out organisms, and central nervous system infection may occur. Preterm and low-birth-weight infants are especially susceptible to infection.

#### CAUSES

The most common causative agents of neonatal sepsis are group B $\beta$-hemolytic streptococci and *Escherichia coli*. Other common causes include *Staphylococcus epidermidis* (most often in very small preterm infants), *Staphylococcus aureus* (usually hospital acquired), *Haemophilus influenzae*, and *Listeria monocytogenes*. Sepsis may be divided into early onset and late onset, according to when signs of disease begin.

Early-onset sepsis is often caused by complications of labor such as prolonged rupture of membranes, prolonged labor, or chorioamnionitis. It usually begins in the first 24 hours after birth and has a more rapid progression than late-onset sepsis. The mortality rate is 15 to 50 percent (Klein & Marcy, 1995). It often involves the respiratory system or causes meningitis.

Late-onset sepsis generally develops after the first week of life from exposure to organisms during or after birth and usually involves the central nervous system. Mortality rate is 10 to 20 percent (Klein &

**TABLE 30–2 COMMON VERTICAL INFECTIONS IN THE NEWBORN***

| Transmission | Effect on Newborn | Nursing Considerations |
|---|---|---|
| **Viral Infections** | | |
| ***Cytomegalovirus*** | | |
| Transplacental | Most infants asymptomatic at birth. LBW, IUGR, enlarged liver and spleen, jaundice, mental retardation, hearing loss, blindness, epilepsy. May have no signs for months or years. | Most common perinatal infection. A major cause of mental retardation. Diagnosed by urine culture. May shed virus in saliva and urine for months. Antiviral drugs being tested. |
| ***Hepatitis B*** | | |
| Usually during birth through contact with maternal blood. Also transplacental, breast milk. | Asymptomatic at birth. LBW, prematurity. Most become chronic carriers. Risk of later liver cancer. | Wash well to remove all blood before skin is punctured for any reason. After cleaning, administer hepatitis B immune globulin and hepatitis B vaccine to prevent infection. |
| ***Herpes*** | | |
| Usually during birth through infected vagina or ascending infection after rupture of membranes. Transplacental rarely. | Clusters of vesicles, temperature instability, lethargy, poor suck, seizures, encephalitis, jaundice, purpura. Half to two thirds have disseminated infection with death or severe neurologic impairment very high. | Contact precautions. Obtain lesion specimens for culture. Mortality and morbidity rate high even with antiviral drugs. |

**TABLE 30–2 COMMON VERTICAL INFECTIONS IN THE NEWBORN*** *Continued*

| Transmission | Effect on Newborn | Nursing Considerations |
|---|---|---|
| ***Human Immunodeficiency Virus/Acquired Immunodeficiency Syndrome*** | | |
| Transplacental, during birth from infected blood and secretions, from breast milk. Transmission rate in U.S. is 25 to 30%. Transmission less if mother takes antiviral drugs during pregnancy. | Asymptomatic at birth, signs usually apparent at 4 to 12 months. Enlarged liver and spleen, lymphadenopathy, failure to thrive, pneumonia, persistent candida and bacterial infections. | Diagnosed from symptoms or at 6 to 18 months when antibodies from mother gone. Wash early and before skin is punctured to remove blood. Treated with antiviral drugs and prophylaxis against other infections. |
| ***Rubella*** | | |
| Transplacental | Asymptomatic or IUGR, cataracts, cardiac defects, deafness, mental retardation. Damage greatest in first trimester. | Contact precautions. Infant may shed virus for months after birth. Diagnosed by presence of antibody. No treatment. |
| ***Varicella Zoster Virus (Chickenpox)*** | | |
| Transplacental | Skin scarring, limb hypoplasia, eye and brain damage, IUGR, death. Damage greatest before the 20th week of gestation. | Immune globulin for infants of mothers infected just before delivery. Acyclovir. Airborne isolation of infants with lesions. |
| **Other Infections** | | |
| ***Group B β-Streptococcal Infection*** | | |
| During birth or ascending after rupture of membranes | Sudden onset of respiratory distress in infant usually well at birth, pneumonia, shock, meningitis. May have early or late onset. | Early identification essential to prevent death. Treated with IV antibiotics to mother in labor or to infant after birth. |
| ***Gonorrhea*** | | |
| Usually during birth | Conjunctivitis (ophthalmia neonatorum), with red, edematous lids and purulent eye drainage. May result in blindness if untreated. | All infants treated with erythromycin eye ointment or other antibiotic for prevention. Previously treated with silver nitrate. |
| ***Chlamydial Infection*** | | |
| During birth | Conjunctivitis, pneumonia, otitis media. | Erythromycin eye ointment for prevention of conjunctivitis. Infection treated with erythromycin. |
| ***Candidiasis*** | | |
| During birth | White patches in mouth (thrush) that bleed if removed. Rash on perineum. May be systemic. | Administer nystatin drops or cream and teach parents how to administer them. Assess mother for vaginal or breast infection. |
| ***Toxoplasmosis*** | | |
| Transplacental | Asymptomatic, or LBW, thrombocytopenia, enlarged liver and spleen, jaundice, anemia, seizures, microcephaly, hydrocephalus, chorioretinitis. Signs may not develop for years. | Consider in infants with IUGR. Confirmed by serum tests. Treatment: pyrimethamine, sulfadiazine, and folinic acid. |
| ***Syphilis*** | | |
| Transplacental | Asymptomatic or enlarged liver and spleen, jaundice, lymphadenopathy anemia, rhinitis, pink or copper-colored peeling rash, pneumonitis, osteochondritis, CNS involvement. | Diagnosed by blood and cerebrospinal fluid testing. Administer penicillin as ordered. |

*Standard precautions for infection control apply to all patients and are not listed above. They include precautions for contact with blood; all body fluids, secretions, and excretions except sweat; nonintact skin; and mucous membranes. Contact precautions are used when transmission of the disease may occur from direct contact with patient's dry skin or articles in the patient's environment. See Appendix A for more information about infection control.

*Abbreviations*: LBW, low birth weight; IUGR, intrauterine growth restriction; IV, intravenous; CNS, central nervous system.

Marcy, 1995) and serious long-term effects can be frequent.

### THERAPEUTIC MANAGEMENT

Once sepsis has been identified, intravenous antibiotics are given. Intravenous gammaglobulin may also be used in prevention and treatment of sepsis in some preterm infants. Other care is supportive to meet the infant's specific needs.

### NURSING CONSIDERATIONS

#### ASSESSMENT

**Signs of Infection.** In the newborn, signs of infection are not as specific or obvious as those in the older infant or child. Instead, they tend to be subtle and could indicate other conditions. There may be temperature instability, respiratory problems, and changes in feeding habits or behavior. It is often the nurse who notices the early, subtle changes that indicate sepsis. Experienced nurses may have a feeling that the infant is not doing well even before specific signs of infection are present. When this occurs, the nurse expands the assessment and watches carefully for the development of other signs. Early identification and treatment are important because infants can develop septic shock with little warning.

**Testing.** Neonatal sepsis may be confused with other illnesses. For example, group B streptococcal pneumonia has the same symptoms as respiratory distress syndrome at first. Therefore, a variety of tests are ordered.

The nurse is responsible for obtaining or helping to obtain specimens for laboratory analysis and for seeing that other tests ordered by the physician are completed. Specimens of the blood, urine, gastric aspirate, and sometimes the cerebral spinal fluid are obtained for culture to determine areas infected. Although specimens of the nose, throat, cord, and skin surfaces may also be obtained for culture, these are not as reliable in determining the cause of the sepsis because they are contaminated by environmental organisms.

A complete blood count may show decreased neutrophils, increased bands (immature neutrophils), and decreased platelets. Presence of elevated immunoglobulin M levels in cord blood or shortly after birth indicates that infection was acquired in utero, because this immunoglobulin does not cross the placenta. It often indicates transplacental infection. Chest radiography will help differentiate between respiratory distress syndrome and sepsis. Blood glucose levels should be checked, because they may be unstable (high or low) in sepsis.

#### NURSING INTERVENTIONS

**Providing Antibiotics.** Because the signs of sepsis are nonspecific and the disease can be fatal, physicians may order antibiotics before an actual diagnosis is made for infants who are at high risk or who show early signs. Broad-spectrum antibiotics are given intravenously until culture and sensitivity results are available. Continued antibiotic therapy is based on the organisms that are positive on culture. The nurse must be knowledgeable about the specific antibiotics used and possible side effects. Commonly used antibiotics include ampicillin, gentamicin, and cefotaxime (Klein & Macy, 1995).

## Critical to Remember

### SIGNS OF SEPSIS IN THE NEWBORN

**General Signs**

- Temperature instability (usually low)
- Nurse's feeling that infant is not doing well
- Rash

**Respiratory Signs**

- Tachypnea
- Apnea
- Respiratory distress—nasal flaring, retractions, grunting

**Cardiovascular Signs**

- Color changes—cyanosis, pallor, mottling
- Tachycardia
- Hypotension
- Decreased peripheral perfusion

**Gastrointestinal Signs**

- Decreased oral intake
- Vomiting
- Gastric residuals measuring over half of previous feeding
- Diarrhea
- Abdominal distention
- Hypoglycemia or hyperglycemia

**Central Nervous System Signs**

- Decreased muscle tone
- Lethargy
- Irritability
- Bulging fontanelle

**Signs That May Indicate Advanced Infection**

- Jaundice
- Evidence of hemorrhage (petechiae, purpura, pulmonary bleeding)
- Anemia
- Enlarged liver and spleen
- Respiratory failure
- Shock
- Seizures

The nurse starts the intravenous fluids and ensures that medications are administered on time. If more than one antibiotic is ordered, the timing of administration must be coordinated to increase effectiveness. Laboratory analysis of peak and trough levels may be ordered to measure blood levels of the medications at times when they are expected to be at the highest and lowest points. This requires planning with the laboratory so that blood is drawn at the correct time in relation to medication administration. Changes in dosage will be based on results of the laboratory tests. Antibiotics are usually continued for 10 days or longer.

**Providing Other Supportive Care.** Oxygen or other respiratory support is used if needed. The infant may need treatment for shock, hypoglycemia or hyperglycemia, electrolyte imbalances, and problems in temperature regulation. Gavage feeding may be necessary if the infant is unable to take oral feedings.

Infants with sepsis may have additional problems as well. They may be premature or have other transplacentally acquired infections. These may require other intensive nursing care.

**Preventing Spread of Infection.** Transmission of infection to other infants in the nursery must be prevented. This is done by using the same techniques that are used to prevent cross-contamination between normal infants (such as hand washing, separation of supplies, and standard precautions for infection control). They must be conscientiously performed by all who come in contact with the infant. Placing the infant in an incubator provides a physical separation between infected and well infants similar to placing adults in isolation in private rooms. The nurse can observe the infant in an incubator more easily at all times.

**Supporting Parents.** Nurses should support parents of newborns with sepsis, and help them understand their infant's illness and treatment. The infant with sepsis often appears healthy at birth but suddenly becomes critically ill. Parents have feelings of shock, fear, and disappointment when their apparently healthy newborn is suddenly moved to the intensive care nursery. They will benefit from a chance to talk about their feelings with an understanding nurse who can explain the infant's treatment and care. Keeping the parents informed of the infant's changes in condition and involving them in care are essential.

## Infant of a Diabetic Mother

### Scope of Problem

The infant of a diabetic mother faces a number of risks, which depend on the type of diabetes the mother has and how well it is controlled. Infants of mothers with long-term diabetes and vascular changes may be small-for-gestational age because decreased placental blood flow causes intrauterine growth restriction. Hypertension occurs more often in diabetic women and further compromises uteroplacental blood flow. Infants born to women with gestational diabetes or diabetes without vascular changes may be large-for-gestational age, particularly if the diabetes is not well controlled (Fig. 30–3).

When the mother is hyperglycemic, large amounts of amino acids, free fatty acids, and glucose are transferred to the fetus, but maternal insulin is not. This causes hypertrophy of the islet cells of the fetal pancreas. The islet cells produce large amounts of insulin, which acts as a growth hormone. The accelerated protein synthesis and the deposit of fat and glycogen in fetal tissues result in macrosomia. Macrosomic infants are at risk for trauma during birth, including fractures or nerve damage.

Congenital anomalies are 2 to 7.9 times more likely in infants of diabetic mothers (Cordero & Landon, 1993). Caudal regression syndrome and anomalies of the neural tube, heart, and kidney are most common. The incidence of anomalies is less if blood glucose levels remain within normal limits, especially before conception and in the early weeks of gestation, when organs are forming.

Infants of diabetic mothers have a higher risk of respiratory distress syndrome than normal infants

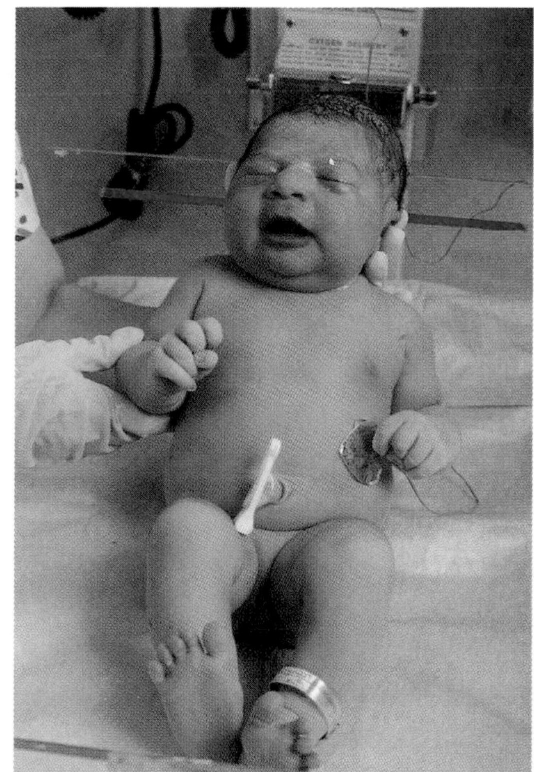

**FIGURE 30-3**
Macrosomia is common in infants of diabetic mothers.

because high levels of insulin interfere with the production of surfactant. Strict control of the diabetes and allowing the pregnancy to progress to full term reduces the incidence of respiratory distress syndrome.

Other complications for which the infant of a diabetic mother is at risk include hypoglycemia after birth, when the maternal supply of glucose ends but the infant's high level of insulin production continues. Hypocalcemia may occur as a result of decreased parathyroid hormone production, especially when the mother's diabetes was poorly controlled.

Polycythemia (hematocrit level above 65 percent) may occur because infants may produce more erythrocytes than normal because of poor oxygenation during fetal life. Organ damage from decreased blood flow, renal vein thrombosis, and necrotizing enterocolitis are possible effects of polycythemia. Polycythemia also results in hyperbilirubinemia as the excessive red blood cells break down after birth.

## Characteristics of Infants of Diabetic Mothers

The small-for-gestational age infant of a diabetic mother is similar to small-for-gestational age infants from other causes, but is more likely to have congenital anomalies. The macrosomic infant of a diabetic mother is different from the large-for-gestational age infant. The infant's size results from fat deposits and hypertrophy of the liver, adrenals, and heart. All organs except the brain are larger than normal. The length and head size are generally within the normal range for gestational age. Other large-for-gestational age infants do not have enlargement of the organs and tend to be long, with large heads to match the rest of the body. Infants of diabetic mothers have a characteristic appearance. The face is round and red, and the body is obese. There is poor muscle tone at rest, but the infant becomes irritable and may have tremors when disturbed.

## Therapeutic Management

Therapeutic management includes controlling the mother's diabetes throughout the pregnancy to decrease complications of the fetus (see Chapter 26). If the infant is large, delivery may be difficult and a cesarean birth may be required. Immediate care of respiratory problems and continued observation for complications determine treatment.

## Nursing Considerations

### ASSESSMENT

Infants of diabetic mothers are assessed for signs of complications, trauma, and congenital anomalies at delivery and during the early hours after birth. Hypoglycemia may be present without observable signs. The blood glucose is screened according to hospital protocol. An example is screening every hour for 4 to 6 hours after birth and every 4 hours until the results are normal (Philip, 1996). Glucose levels of less than 45 mg/dl measured with glucose screening reagent strips should be reported and verified by laboratory analysis.

The most frequent sign of low glucose is jitteriness or tremors. Diaphoresis is uncommon in newborns but may occur with hypoglycemia. Rapid respirations, low temperature, and poor muscle tone are also common (see Chapter 20, p. 525). Because these signs are not specific for hypoglycemia, the nurse must be alert for other complications, particularly if signs continue after feeding.

### NURSING INTERVENTIONS

If hypoglycemia develops, infants must be fed early to correct it. Gavage feeding may be used if the infant does not suck well or if the respirations are high. Some infants need intravenous glucose to maintain balance and prevent damage to the brain.

The nurse must be alert for signs of other complications that occur in infants of diabetic mothers. A check of the hematocrit level will identify polycythemia. These infants must be hydrated adequately to prevent sluggish blood flow and ischemia to vital organs. Monitoring of bilirubin levels is important if jaundice occurs as blood cells break down.

Infants are also at increased risk for low calcium levels. If jitteriness occurs and the glucose levels are normal, the infant may have hypocalcemia.

The nurse must watch for signs of respiratory distress syndrome or other respiratory complications. Cold stress, which would increase the metabolic rate, must be prevented. Increased metabolism uses oxy-

**CRITICAL THINKING EXERCISE**

Although some institutions use 5 or 10 percent dextrose water for the first feeding, it is now more common to use breast milk or formula for low blood glucose.

**Q:** What is the rationale for this?

**A:** Giving infants fluids with high levels of glucose will correct the immediate problem of hypoglycemia, but will stimulate the production of additional insulin. This causes a rebound hypoglycemia. Giving glucose in a form that will be metabolized more slowly provides longer normal glucose levels. If dextrose water is given, it should be followed within an hour by breast milk or formula.

gen and glucose more rapidly and could increase respiratory problems as well as exacerbate hypoglycemia.

Providing support to parents is important. They may not understand why their infant, who appears fat and healthy to them, needs close observation and frequent blood tests. The mother may have had a difficult pregnancy and may feel guilty, even if she followed a program of good diabetic control. Ample opportunity for discussion of feelings as well as information about the care of the infant is important.

### CHECK YOUR READING

8. What is the difference between vertical and horizontal transmission of infection?
9. What is the role of the nurse in caring for the infant with sepsis?
10. What problems occur in infants of diabetic mothers?
11. What are the major nursing responsibilities in caring for infants of diabetic mothers?

## Prenatal Drug Exposure

Substance abuse affects the fetus at any time during pregnancy. Most drugs readily cross the placenta and cause a variety of problems. Abuse during the first 2 months of pregnancy may cause congenital anomalies. Later abuse may interfere with development or functioning of organs already formed. Abuse of more than one substance is common, making it difficult to determine the exact cause of any one effect.

The effects of substance abuse on pregnancy, the fetus, and the neonate are discussed in Chapter 24. This section focuses on nursing care for infants with neonatal abstinence syndrome, the disorder in which neonates demonstrate signs of drug withdrawal.

### Identification of Drug-Exposed Infants

Maternal substance abuse may be identified before an infant is born, but many infants are born to women whose substance use is not known to the health professionals caring for them during labor and delivery. A history of no prenatal care or behaviors during labor and delivery that may indicate substance abuse may raise suspicion. Placental abruption may occur after cocaine use. When there is any cause to suspect drug use, the infant is observed closely for signs of prenatal drug exposure.

Neonatal abstinence syndrome occurs in infants who have suffered prenatal drug exposure sufficient to cause withdrawal signs after birth. It usually begins during the first 48 to 72 hours after birth, depending on the time of the mother's last drug dose. Signs vary according to the drug or combination of drugs, but often include neurologic and gastrointestinal abnormalities. Some infants with prenatal drug exposure show no abnormal signs at all or do not show signs until after the first week.

Infants appear hungry and suck vigorously on their fists but have poor coordination of suck and swallow. Frequent regurgitation, vomiting, and diarrhea are common. Although some behaviors are similar to those of hypoglycemia, the blood glucose level is normal. Infants are restless, and their excessive activity, coupled with poor feeding ability, results in failure to gain weight. Various scoring systems are available to determine the number, frequency, and severity of behaviors that may indicate neonatal abstinence syndrome.

Congenital anomalies and other effects of prenatal drug exposure may be apparent at birth. Many of these infants are small-for-gestational age. They may also be preterm and suffer from related complications. Infants are more likely to have respiratory distress at birth, jaundice, or sudden infant death syndrome. Infants with fetal alcohol syndrome have a characteristic appearance (see Fig. 24–3).

When there is suspicion that exposure may have occurred, a urine specimen is collected from the in-

### Critical to Remember

#### SIGNS OF INTRAUTERINE DRUG EXPOSURE

**Behavioral Signs**

- Irritability
- Jitteriness, tremors
- Muscular rigidity, increased muscle tone
- Restless, excessive activity
- Exaggerated startle reflex
- Prolonged high-pitched cry
- Difficult to console

**Signs Relating to Feeding**

- Uncoordinated sucking and swallowing
- Frequent regurgitation or vomiting
- Diarrhea

**Other Signs**

- Poor sleeping patterns
- Yawning
- Nasal stuffiness, sneezing
- Tachypnea
- Apnea
- Seizures
- Diaphoresis

*Note*: Some infants with prenatal drug exposure will have no abnormal signs at all, or signs may be delayed.

Procedure 30–2

## Applying a Pediatric Urine Collection Bag

**PURPOSE:** To collect a nonsterile urine specimen from an infant.

1. **Wash and dry the genitalia. Apply tincture of benzoin according to hospital policy. Allow to dry until "tacky."** *Removal of gross contaminants prevents contamination of the specimen. The bag adheres to a clean, dry surface best. Tincture of benzoin increases adherence of the bag to the skin.*

2. **Remove the paper covering the posterior adhesive tabs of the bag first. To apply to female infants, stretch the perineum (skin between the rectum and the vagina). Fold the bag in half and apply smoothly over the perineum, extending the tabs to the side. For male infants, place the penis and scrotum (if small) inside the bag and apply the posterior adhesive tabs to the perineum. If the scrotum will not fit in the bag easily, apply the tabs smoothly over the scrotum.** *Covering the perineum with the posterior tabs first helps ensure smooth fit at this area, where leakage of urine may occur in the female infant especially. Care in application prevents losing the specimen.*

3. **Remove the paper covering the anterior adhesive tabs, and apply to cover genitalia. Be sure that there are no wrinkles in the tabs.** *Wrinkles allow openings for urine to leak out of the bag.*

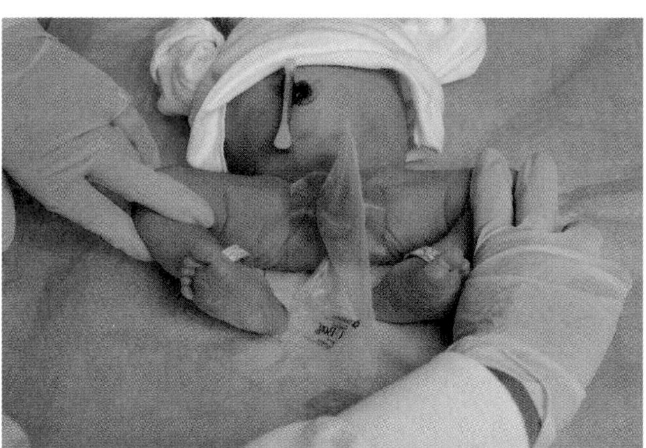

4. **Place the diaper loosely over the bag or cut a slit in the diaper and gently pull the bag through the slit.** *Cutting a slit in the diaper allows visualization of the bag. Placing the diaper too tightly over the bag might pull against the adhesive, causing trauma to the skin and providing an opening through which the specimen is lost.*

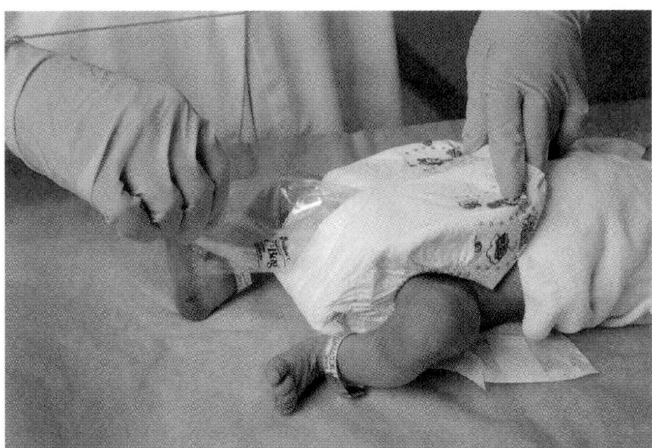

5. **Check the bag for urine frequently. Transfer the urine to a specimen cup by removing the tab over the hole in the bottom or cutting the lower corner and pouring. The specimen can also be aspirated with a syringe.** *Ensures removal of the bag before urine loosens the adhesive. Prepares the specimen to be sent to the laboratory for analysis.*

6. **Clean the genitalia, and observe for irritation.** *Removes urine and adhesive from the skin.*

fant for analysis. Drugs are present in the newborn's urine for various lengths of time after the mother has used them. Some drugs last several days because of the infant's difficulty in excreting them, whereas others disappear very soon. Therefore, it is important to obtain the first urine output from the infant, if possible (Procedure 30–2). Meconium may also be tested for drugs.

### Therapeutic Management

Therapeutic management includes dealing with the complications common to drug-exposed infants during and after birth. Respiratory problems are treated as for other infants. Sedatives may be necessary for severe irritability; drugs commonly used include tincture of opium, tincture of paregoric, phenobarbital, oral morphine, and diazepam (Valium). Use of gavage or intravenous feeding may be required at times because the infant's suck and swallow are uncoordinated. Some infants may need more than the normal caloric requirements because of their excessive activity. Involvement by social services in and out of the hospital is important to deal with the long-term effects of the drugs, placement of the infant after hospitalization, and follow-up of the mother or other caretaker to help provide for the infant's needs.

## Nursing Considerations

The infant who has been exposed to drugs prenatally will need special care to cope with drug withdrawal. Care is focused on feeding, rest, and enhancing parental attachment, if possible. Nursing care is summarized in this section. More detailed interventions are given in Nursing Care Plan 30–2.

### FEEDING

Feeding can be difficult and time consuming. The poor suck and swallow coordination of drug-exposed infants interferes with caloric intake, yet their increased activity increases the calories they need.

**Assessment.** The nurse should assess the infant's ability to coordinate sucking and swallowing. Infants often suck frantically on their fists or a nipple but are unable to coordinate feeding behaviors well. Changes in the frequency and amount of regurgitation or vomiting or the length of time it takes infants to finish feedings should be noted.

**Nursing Interventions.** Distractions during feedings can be prevented by choosing an area of the nursery for feedings where noise and activity are low. Infants should be swaddled to prevent the startling that occurs when drug-exposed infants are handled.

Gavage feedings may be necessary to save the infant's energy and prevent risk of aspiration if the infant is excessively agitated, is unable to suck and swallow adequately, or has rapid respirations. Gastric contents are aspirated before feedings to determine if formula is passing from stomach to intestines between feedings. The amount of gastric aspirate is subtracted from the next feeding.

When oral feedings are begun, infants may need chin and cheek support similar to that used for preterm infants. This helps them suck more efficiently. After feedings, they should be positioned on the

## Nursing Care Plan 30–2
## The Drug-Exposed Infant

Tracy was born at 38 weeks' gestation to Gloria, who was on a methadone maintenance program. However, Tracy tested positive not only for methadone but also for heroin, which Gloria admitted using several times in the days just before she began labor.

ASSESSMENT: Tracy weighs 2240 g (4 pounds, 15 ounces) and is small-for-gestational age. She is jittery, becomes agitated easily, and has a poor suck and swallow. Tracy regurgitates her feedings frequently. She has been fed by gavage but is now taking feedings orally.

NURSING DIAGNOSIS: Altered Nutrition: Less Than Body Requirements related to abnormal coordination of suck and swallow and excessive activity

GOALS/EXPECTED OUTCOMES

1. Tracy will take and retain 246 to 269 kcal daily (110 to 120 kcal/kg/day)
2. Tracy will gain at least ½ ounce each day.

| INTERVENTION | RATIONALE |
|---|---|
| 1. Feed Tracy as soon as she begins to wake at feeding times. | 1. Drug-exposed infants often move from sleeping to an agitated state very quickly. This would make feeding more difficult. |
| 2. Swaddle Tracy with her extremities in a flexed position during feeding. | 2. Infants become more agitated if they are allowed to startle. Swaddling provides a sense of security and prevents excessive movement. |
| 3. Try warming the formula slightly before feeding. | 3. Some infants take warmed formula more readily. |
| 4. Use chin and cheek support during the feedings as needed. | 4. Chin and cheek support increases sucking strength and increases intake. |
| 5. Feed slowly with frequent stops for burping Tracy. If frantic sucking continues when the feeding is stopped, use a pacifier to soothe her. | 5. Frequent burping while keeping the infant calm helps prevent regurgitation. |
| 6. Place Tracy on her right side with her head elevated 30 to 45 degrees after feedings. Keep the environment as nonstimulating as possible after feedings. | 6. Positioning uses gravity to promote gastric emptying and helps prevent aspiration during regurgitation. Quiet surroundings promote sleep and decrease agitation. |

*Nursing Care Plan continued on following page*

## Nursing Care Plan 30–2 *Continued*

# The Drug-Exposed Infant

**EVALUATION**

Tracy's intake averages 250 calories each day. She gains slightly more than ½ ounce daily.

**ASSESSMENT:** Tracy sleeps less than an hour after feedings. When she awakens, her high-pitched cry and agitation begin immediately. She wiggles out of her blankets, and her activity elicits the Moro reflex, which leads to more agitation. She is irritable and does not respond to care taking activities as quickly as other infants.

**NURSING DIAGNOSIS:** Sleep Pattern Disturbance related to agitation from own activity and irritability

**GOALS/EXPECTED OUTCOMES**

Tracy will do the following:

1. Sleep for periods of 2 hours or more after feedings.
2. Decrease crying by at least 1 hour a day within the first week.

| INTERVENTION | RATIONALE |
|---|---|
| 1. Place Tracy's crib in the quietest corner of the nursery. Place a sign nearby to remind others of the need for quiet in that area. For example, "Shh please! Tracy is resting!" | 1. Drug-exposed infants are easily overstimulated by noise and activity. |
| 2. Keep lights turned down as much as possible. Place a blanket over the head end of the crib to help prevent Tracy from looking into lights. | 2. Lowered lighting provides a more restful environment. |
| 3. Keep Tracy tightly swaddled in a flexed position during sleep and feedings. | 3. The drug-exposed infant's own movements can cause startling, awakening, and agitation. |
| 4. Use a pacifier, and position her hands near her mouth. | 4. Non-nutritive sucking may have a calming effect on the infant. Positioning the hands near the mouth allows the infant to self-comfort by sucking. |
| 5. Use a slow vertical rocking motion when Tracy is upset. | 5. Vertical rocking decreases agitation and helps infants to move more smoothly from one behavior state to another. |
| 6. Use a front infant carrier during Tracy's awake periods. | 6. An infant carrier provides the same effect as swaddling. In addition, it provides warmth and a rocking motion from the caretaker's body that may be soothing. |
| 7. Organize nursing care so that Tracy is not disturbed unnecessarily, especially when sleeping. | 7. Once drug-exposed infants are asleep, they should not be disturbed unless necessary because they may have difficulty going back to sleep. |

**EVALUATION**

Tracy gradually lengthens her sleep periods to 2 hours and decreases crying episodes within the first week.

**ASSESSMENT:** Gloria visits Tracy sporadically. She seems hesitant when she comes into the nursery and afraid to touch or care for Tracy. She asks, "Why does she cry so much?" When the nurse helps her hold Tracy, Gloria states, "I don't think she likes me."

**NURSING DIAGNOSIS:** Altered Parenting related to lack of understanding of the infant's characteristics and how to relate to an irritable infant

**GOALS/EXPECTED OUTCOMES**

Gloria will do the following:

1. Visit at least every other day.
2. Participate in Tracy's care by holding and feeding her.
3. Make positive statements about her daughter.

## *Nursing Care Plan 30–2 Continued*

# *The Drug-Exposed Infant*

| INTERVENTION | RATIONALE |
|---|---|
| 1. Show acceptance of Gloria when she comes to visit Tracy. Greet her and provide her with an update on Tracy's progress. | 1. A mother is more likely to visit her infant if she feels accepted by staff. The more she visits, the more she is likely to learn to parent her infant. |
| 2. Assist Gloria to hold and feed Tracy. Explain nursing actions such as placing the crib in a secluded corner and covering the top with a blanket. | 2. Encouraging the mother to participate in care of the infant helps her get to know her infant and how to care for the infant more quickly. |
| 3. Show Gloria how to make Tracy more comfortable. Demonstrate swaddling and rocking and explain the purpose. Show her how to place a rolled blanket around the infant to provide a feeling of security and help promote sleep. | 3. When the mother learns ways to comfort her infant, the positive response from the infant may increase bonding. |
| 4. Explain the behavioral characteristics of infants who are drug-exposed. Explain that Tracy's stiff body posture and failure to "mold" to the mother's body are normal for her. Point out signs that Tracy is overstimulated, such as gaze aversion and increase in irritability. Explain that the high-pitched cry is common. | 4. The mother needs to learn that the infant's behavior is part of the infant's problem, not because of the mother's handling of her. |
| 5. Model ways of interacting with Tracy and calming her when she becomes agitated. Demonstrate holding quietly and point out signs that Tracy is ready to interact. Suggest only one stimulus at a time, such as talking softly without rocking. | 5. The mother learns appropriate interaction when she sees it performed by the nurse. Infants may need short time-outs before they are ready for more stimulation. Decreasing the number of stimuli may be more effective. |
| 6. Point out positive points about Tracy, such as her long eyelashes or delicate fingers. Point out signs that show that Tracy is making progress. | 6. The mother needs help to focus on positive aspects of the infant as well as the problems. |
| 7. Explain the routine care of a newborn. Spread teaching out over Gloria's visits. | 7. The mother needs to learn the usual care of any newborn as well as the infant's special needs. |
| 8. Give praise and encouragement frequently as Gloria works with Tracy. | 8. The mother needs positive reinforcement and help to feel that she is capable of mothering her infant. |
| 9. Use therapeutic communication techniques to help Gloria discuss her feelings as she cares for Tracy. | 9. Mothers often find it frustrating to care for the drug-exposed infant. Helping them vent their feelings may increase their ability to cope with the infant's special needs. |
| 10. Discuss sources of support from family members or friends. Also refer to social services or support groups in the community if Tracy is unaware of them. | 10. Ongoing support is necessary for the woman with addiction problems. Support for the mother will help her care more effectively for her infant. |
| 11. If Gloria will have custody of Tracy, help her begin to make plans for discharge. Discuss ongoing problems and concerns such as sudden infant death syndrome (SIDS). | 11. Preparation for discharge must be made well in advance. Infants will have ongoing problems that will continue in the home setting. Infants exposed to heroin have an increased incidence of SIDS. |

### EVALUATION

Gloria begins to visit more often, coming three to four times a week. She participates in care, begins to talk about her "pretty little girl," and discusses her plans for when she can take Tracy home with her.

### ADDITIONAL NURSING DIAGNOSES TO CONSIDER

Altered Family Processes
Ineffective Individual Coping
Impaired Skin Integrity

right side with the head of the bed elevated 30 to 45 degrees.

#### REST

The excessive activity and poor sleep patterns of drug-exposed neonates interfere with their ability to rest.

**Assessment.** The infant's muscle tone, tremors, and tendency for excessive activity with and without being disturbed should be assessed. The degree of tremors and stimuli that increase or decrease irritability are important. The nurse also keeps track of the number of hours that the infant sleeps after each feeding.

**Nursing Interventions.** Stimulation of the drug-exposed infant should be kept to a minimum, especially at first, when the infant is excessively irritable. Noise and bright lights are reduced as much as possible. The nurse should organize nursing care to reduce handling and disturbances. A calm approach and slow, smooth movements during care help avoid startling the infant.

Swaddling the infant in a flexed position helps prevent startling and agitation. Non-nutritive suckling also helps quiet the infant. Skin abrasions and breakdown from excessive activity or diarrhea may increase discomfort and agitation. They should be prevented if possible and treated promptly if they occur.

#### BONDING

In many areas, infants who test positive for drugs may not be released to the mother until her ability to care for her infant safely has been assessed by social services or a court. She may be required to enter a drug rehabilitation program before she can obtain custody of the infant. After hospital discharge, the infant may receive care in an institution, in a foster home, or by family members approved by the court. However, the mother will most likely gain custody of the infant eventually if she wishes, and attachment to the infant should be encouraged.

**Assessment.** The frequency of her visits and her response to the infant may give an indication of the mother's apparent interest in the infant. Although some substance-abusing mothers are uninterested in their infants, for others the infant provides a reason to attempt to overcome their addiction. Demonstration of bonding behaviors such as calling the infant by name and smiling at the infant should be noted.

**Nursing Interventions.** Because the mother may become the infant's primary caretaker, it is vital that nurses do whatever they can to enhance mother-infant bonding. Helping the mother feel welcome when she visits the infant provides one of the most challenging aspects of nursing care. It is sometimes easy to be judgmental and difficult to be accepting when the mother's behavior has been harmful to her infant. However, a friendly approach will make the mother more likely to visit the infant and to accept teaching from the nurse.

The nurse can promote bonding by encouraging mothers to participate actively in infant care during visits. Including the mother will help her feel that the nurses trust her to care for the infant. This may help increase her determination to go through recovery to regain her newborn.

The mother's participation also provides a chance to assess the mother's infant care skills and areas in which further discussion of the newborn's needs will be helpful. In addition, it gives the nurse an opportunity to demonstrate parenting skills. Many mothers who use drugs have not had good parenting role models and do not know what to do. Frequent positive feedback about the mother's participation is also important.

The mother needs the same teaching given to all new parents, plus special techniques necessary to meet the needs of drug-exposed infants. The nurse should teach her about her newborn's special characteristics and help her take on more of the infant's care as she demonstrates readiness. For example, she will need to learn how to swaddle the infant in a flexed position to prevent excessive startles and tremors (see Fig. 24–4, p. 653, and Parents Want to Know, p. 658).

Signs of overstimulation in drug-exposed infants have some similarities with those for the preterm infant. In addition, these infants cannot tolerate more than brief periods of interaction. They may not make eye contact or they may avert their eyes after 30 to 60 seconds of social interaction. The nurse should teach the mother that the infant responds poorly to everyone so that she does not think that only she is being rejected.

The nurse can provide information and referral to any special programs available to help parents learn special stimulation techniques appropriate for drug-exposed infants. If the mother is unable to care for the newborn, the same interventions can be used to help the person who will take over care of the infant on hospital discharge.

Cocaine, amphetamines, and other drugs pass into breast milk. Trying to breastfeed an infant with poorly developed feeding skills may be too much stress for the mother who is trying to recover from addiction. Therefore, mothers likely to continue drug use after delivery should be discouraged from breastfeeding. However, there are situations in which breastfeeding may be acceptable. If the woman has a strong desire to breastfeed, the nurse should consult the health care provider.

**CHECK YOUR READING**

12. What common problems occur in infants with prenatal exposure to drugs?
13. What special nursing care measures are needed for drug-exposed infants?

## Congenital Anomalies and Congenital Cardiac Defects

Approximately 2 to 3 percent of newborns have major congenital anomalies at birth. These defects are responsible for approximately 20 percent of all neonatal deaths (Lott, 1993). Some infants have more than one anomaly, which may be part of a syndrome or result from separate causes. Although congenital anomalies are generally treated in the pediatrics setting, they are usually identified soon after birth. Common congenital anomalies are noted in Table 30–3. (See a pediatric nursing textbook for more detailed information about care of infants with these conditions.) Congenital cardiac conditions are discussed in this section.

Approximately 1 percent of newborns have congenital heart defects (Daberkow & Washington, 1993). They are a major cause of death in the first year. The exact cause is unknown in most cases, but genetics, teratogens, and viral infections such as rubella are all known to be possible factors. Often, a genetic predisposition is combined with an environmental cause. The heart forms by the sixth week of gesta-

**TABLE 30–3 COMMON CONGENITAL ANOMALIES**

Gastrointestinal Tract

*Cleft Lip and Palate*

These are among the most common congenital anomalies, and they occur together or separately, on one or both sides. *Lip*: minor notching of the lip or all of lip and into floor of nose. *Palate*: only the soft palate or division of entire hard and soft palate. Both genetic and environmental factors are included in cause.

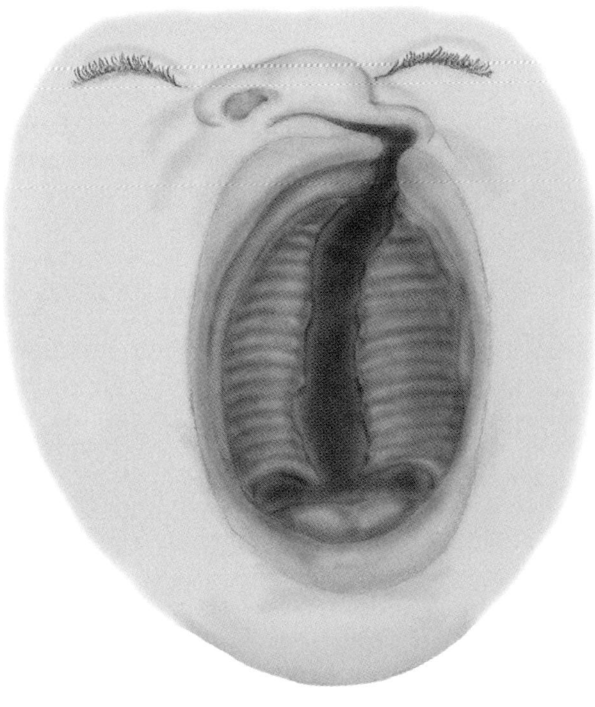

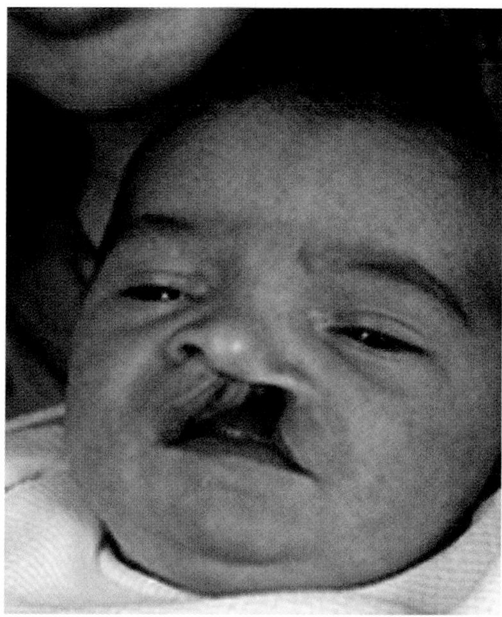

**ASSESSMENT**

Severe clefts are obvious at birth.
Palpate hard and soft palate of all neonates during initial assessment.

**THERAPEUTIC MANAGEMENT**

Lip surgery should be done as soon as possible within the first few days or weeks after birth to enhance appearance and parental bonding.

*Table continued on following page*

## TABLE 30-3 COMMON CONGENITAL ANOMALIES *Continued*

### Gastrointestinal Tract

Palate repair surgery is done in stages, depending on the degree, beginning at about 1 year to minimize speech problems.
Long-term follow-up should be done for orthodontia, speech therapy, and possible hearing problems.

#### NURSING CONSIDERATIONS

Degree of cleft determines approach to feeding.
Experiment to find method that works best for individual infant. Try:

1. Breastfeeding (soft breast tissue fills in the cleft).
2. Soft preemie nipple directed away from a cleft palate.
3. Nipple with enlarged hole.
4. Compressible bottles.
5. Special long nipples that extend beyond cleft.
6. Nipples with extensions to cover cleft.
7. Medicine dropper.
8. Asepto syringe with soft tubing attached.

Feed infant in upright position because milk enters nasal passages through palate, causing increased tendency to aspirate.
Feed slowly with frequent stops to burp, because infant tends to swallow excessive air.
Wash away milk curds with water after feeding.
Help parents deal with disappointment over infant with obvious anomaly. Show before and after pictures of plastic surgery.
Reinforce physician's explanation of plans for surgery.
Teach parents feeding techniques. Have parents observe at first, then take over gradually. Discuss positioning infant upright during feedings and on side after feedings to prevent aspiration.
Prevent infections. Infants are especially susceptible to respiratory and ear infections, which can delay surgery. Ear infections may lead to hearing loss.
Emphasize the need for long-term follow-up. Refer to agencies that help with expense of long-term care and to support groups for help and emotional support from other parents.

#### *Esophageal Atresia and Tracheoesophageal Fistula*

The esophagus is most commonly divided into two unconnected segments (atresia) with a blind pouch at the proximal end. The distal end is connected to the trachea, resulting in tracheoesophageal fistula (TEF). Cause is failure of normal development during the fourth week of pregnancy. Common variations of the condition are shown in the figure.

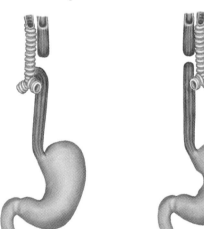

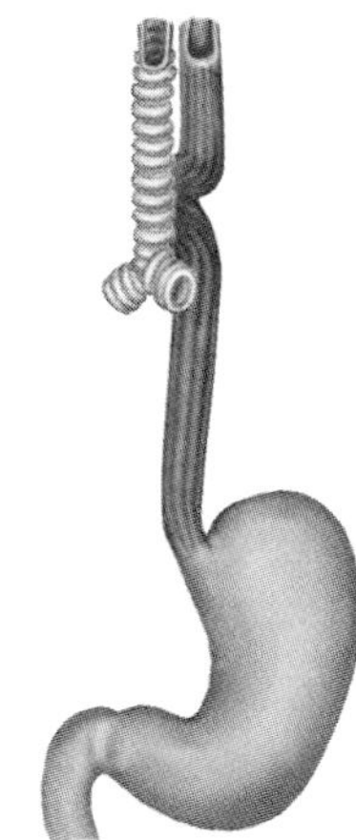

#### ASSESSMENT

Watch for TEF when polyhydramnios occurs, because the excessive fluid may be caused by fetal inability to swallow amniotic fluid.
Other defects (cardiovascular and gastrointestinal most common) occur in 30 to 50%.
Signs vary by type of defect.
Suspect TEF in infant with excessive frothy drooling and more suction needed than usual, when regurgitation occurs from secretions that pool in blind pouch, and when catheter will not pass into stomach.
If upper esophagus connects with trachea, feedings enter lungs and cause immediate coughing, choking, and cyanosis.
If fistula is between distal esophagus and trachea, stomach becomes distended with air from trachea. Gastric secretions aspirate into the lungs, causing severe inflammatory reaction.

#### THERAPEUTIC MANAGEMENT

Diagnosis is confirmed by symptoms and radiography.
Continuous suction should be done to upper pouch and gastrostomy if infant is too unstable for surgery.
Long-term follow-up should be done for esophageal reflux and dilation of strictures that form at surgical site.

#### NURSING CONSIDERATIONS

Observe all infants carefully during first feeding for respiratory difficulty or other signs. A small amount of sterile water is usually given first to prevent aspiration of formula, should TEF be present.
If first feeding is by breast, observe carefully for respiratory difficulty.

## TABLE 30–3 COMMON CONGENITAL ANOMALIES *Continued*

### Gastrointestinal Tract

Prevent aspiration by maintaining in a semi-upright position to prevent reflux of gastric fluids.
Maintain suction equipment.
Care after surgery involves ventilator, chest tubes, intravenous lines, and gastrostomy feedings.

#### *Omphalocele and Gastroschisis*

Both are caused by congenital defects in the abdominal wall. In omphalocele, the intestines protrude into the base of the umbilical cord. Other anomalies often occur with omphalocele.
Gastroschisis is a defect to the side of the abdomen, next to and not involving the cord. The intestines protrude through the defect and float freely in the amniotic fluid.

**ASSESSMENT**

Diagnosis is made by prenatal ultrasound or is obvious at birth.

**THERAPEUTIC MANAGEMENT**

Infant should be intubated at delivery, with gastric tube placed to decrease air in stomach. Gastric suction, parenteral nutrition, and antibiotics should be given.
Surgery should be performed as soon as infant is stable. A Silastic silo (pouch) may be used to replace the intestine gradually over a week.

**NURSING CONSIDERATIONS**

Cover intestines with sterile saline dressings and plastic to prevent drying.
Prevent infection and trauma.

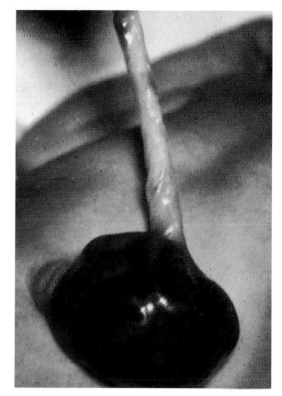

#### *Diaphragmatic Hernia*

The diaphragm fails to fuse during the eighth to 10th weeks of gestation. A large or small part of the abdominal contents moves into the chest cavity, usually on the left side.
If herniation is large enough, the lungs may fail to develop (hypoplastic lungs). When gas fills bowel, further pressure on heart and lungs results.

**ASSESSMENT**

There may be mild to severe respiratory distress at birth, with breath sounds diminished over the affected area, and barrel chest. The heart beat may be displaced to the right.
The abdomen may be scaphoid (concave).
The condition may be diagnosed prenatally by ultrasound.

**THERAPEUTIC MANAGEMENT**

An endotracheal tube is placed for ventilation and a gastric tube for decompression of stomach.
Surgery to replace intestines and repair defect in diaphragm should be done as soon as possible.
Extracorporeal membrane oxygenation (ECMO) may be used.
Fetal surgery has been performed.

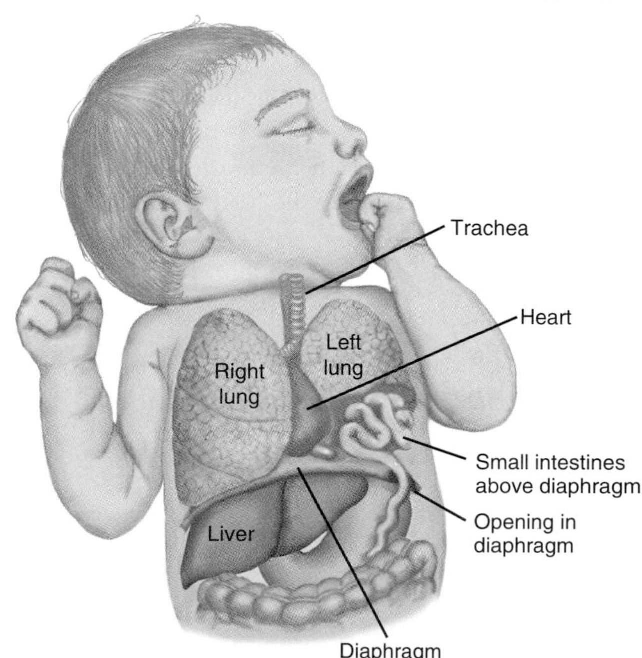


**NURSING CONSIDERATIONS**

Position the infant on the affected side to allow unaffected lung to expand. Elevate the head to decrease pressure on the heart and lungs. Assist with ventilation, and monitor respiratory status. Expect surgery as soon as infant is stable.
Continue to monitor respiratory status after surgery to determine whether lung function will be adequate.

*Table continued on following page*

## TABLE 30-3 COMMON CONGENITAL ANOMALIES *Continued*

### Central Nervous System

***Neural Tube Defects***

Forms of spina bifida are the most common central nervous system defects.

Folic acid supplements in pregnancy may help prevent neural tube defects.

*Spina bifida occulta* is failure of the vertebral arch to close, usually without other anomalies. It is seen by a dimple on the back, which may have a tuft of hair over it.

*Meningocele* is protrusion of meninges through the spina bifida, covered by skin or thin membrane. Because the spinal cord is not involved, there is no paralysis.

*Myelomeningocele* is protrusion of meninges and spinal cord covered with membrane through spina bifida. The degree of paralysis depends on the location of defect. The infant may also have hydrocephalus, or it may develop after surgery.

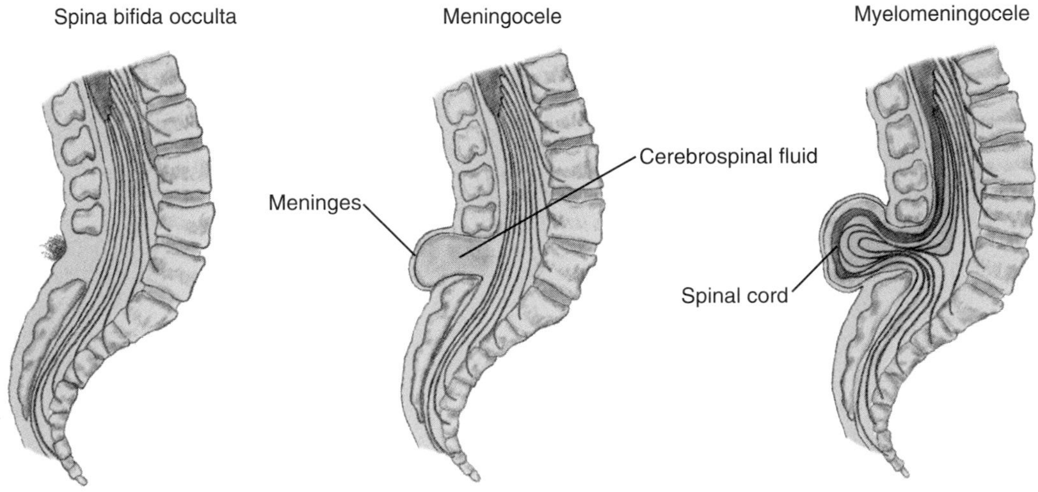


**ASSESSMENT**

Note the position and covering of defect at birth.
Observe movement below the defect to determine degree of paralysis.
Examine for relaxed anus and dribbling of stool and urine.
Check for other anomalies.

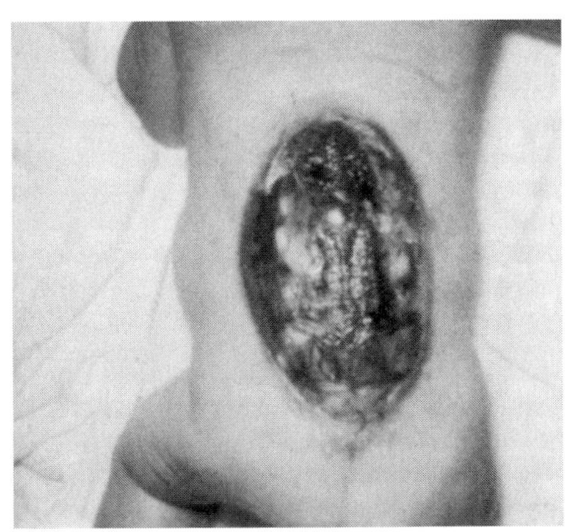

**THERAPEUTIC MANAGEMENT**

Surgery is performed for meningocele and myelomeningocele.
A shunt is placed to divert cerebrospinal fluid if hydrocephalus develops.
Antibiotics are given to prevent infection.
Long-term follow-up should be done, with physical therapy and other care as needed.

**NURSING CONSIDERATIONS**

Apply sterile saline dressing and plastic over the defect covered by membrane to prevent drying.
Handle the infant carefully, and position prone or to side to prevent trauma to sac.
Prevent infection. Keep free of contamination from urine and feces.
Inspect sac for intactness before surgery. Monitor for signs of infection.
Every shift, check for increasing head circumference, bulging fontanelles, separation of sutures, intermittent apnea, and other signs of increased intracranial pressure to identify early hydrocephalus.

***Congenital Hydrocephalus***

This is a problem with absorption or obstruction to flow of cerebral spinal fluid in the ventricles of the brain, causing compression of the brain and enlargement of the head.

**ASSESSMENT**

There is a full or bulging fontanelle or separation of sutures.
The head is enlarged, especially in the frontal area.
The setting-sun sign is apparent (sclera visible above the pupils of the eyes).

**TABLE 30–3 COMMON CONGENITAL ANOMALIES** *Continued*

Central Nervous System

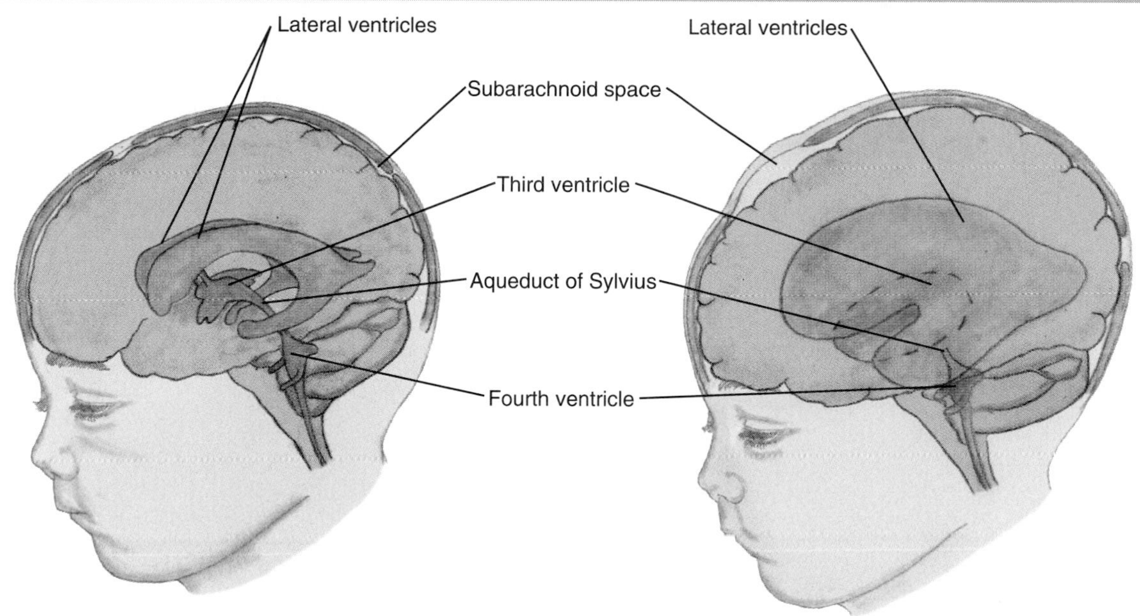


THERAPEUTIC MANAGEMENT

This disorder is corrected surgically, and a shunt is inserted to drain fluid. A ventriculoperitoneal shunt is used most often to drain fluid into the peritoneal cavity.

NURSING CONSIDERATIONS

Measure head circumference daily.
Prevent pressure areas.
Observe for signs of infection.
Teach parents how to care for shunt and observe signs of increased intracranial pressure.

tion, and problems in development during this period may result in anomalies of other structures as well.

## Classification of Cardiac Defects

Cardiac defects are generally categorized according to the pattern of blood flow and whether cyanosis results from the defect. Some of the most common defects are illustrated in Fig. 30–4.

### CYANOTIC DEFECTS

In cyanotic defects, there is a decrease in blood flow to the lungs or mixing of venous and oxygenated blood into the general systemic circulation, or both, decreasing the oxygen carried to the tissues and resulting in cyanosis. This results in a right-to-left shunt where venous blood from the right side of the heart flows through an abnormal opening to the left side of the heart and into the systemic circulation. Although the heart and lungs work harder, adequate oxygenation may be impossible, resulting in hypoxia of the major organs. Infants usually have serious problems from birth. The infant grows poorly, has frequent infections, and is easily fatigued. Heart failure may be an early complication. Transposition of the great vessels is an example of a cyanotic heart defect.

### ACYANOTIC DEFECTS

In acyanotic conditions, there is an obstruction of blood flow from the left side of the heart or a defect that causes increased flow of blood to the lungs. Both increase the work of the heart. In addition, there may be congestion in the lungs that may eventually cause increased resistance of the pulmonary vessels and pulmonary hypertension. Infants are prone to respiratory infections because of the pulmonary congestion and increased work of the heart and lungs. Growth is slowed, and the infant fatigues easily. The heart may fail from overwork. Patent ductus arteriosus is an example of this group.

In some cases, pulmonary resistance increases sufficiently to change the pressures within the heart. This reverses the flow of blood through an abnormal opening and causes mixing of oxygenated and ve-

**A. Ventricular Septal Defect**

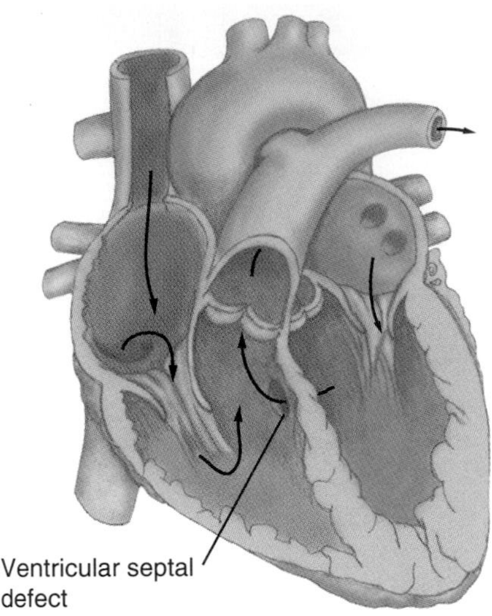


This is the most common type of congenital heart defect. It occurs alone or with other defects. The opening in the septum ranges from the size of a pin to very large. Fifty to 75% of small defects close spontaneously. When the pressure in the left ventricle increases after birth, oxygenated blood is shunted through a large ventricular septal defect into the right ventricle and then recirculated to the lungs (a left-to-right shunt). Increased pulmonary resistance may cause pulmonary hypertension, shunt reversal, heart failure, or a combination of these. Surgery is necessary for a large ventricular septal defect and increasing symptoms.

**B. Patent Ductus Arteriosus**

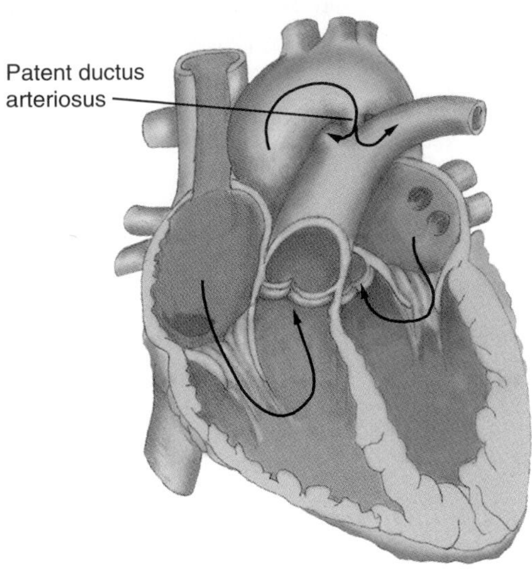


This condition is a failure of the ductus arteriosus to close after birth. Blood flows from the higher pressure of the aorta to the pulmonary artery and the lungs (left-to-right shunt). It is most common in the preterm infant. Prostaglandins cause vasodilation and may interfere with closure of the ductus arteriosus. Indomethacin, a prostaglandin inhibitor, may be effective in causing closure. Symptoms vary from none to early congestive heart failure. Surgical ligation is used when necessary.

**C. Coarctation of the Aorta**

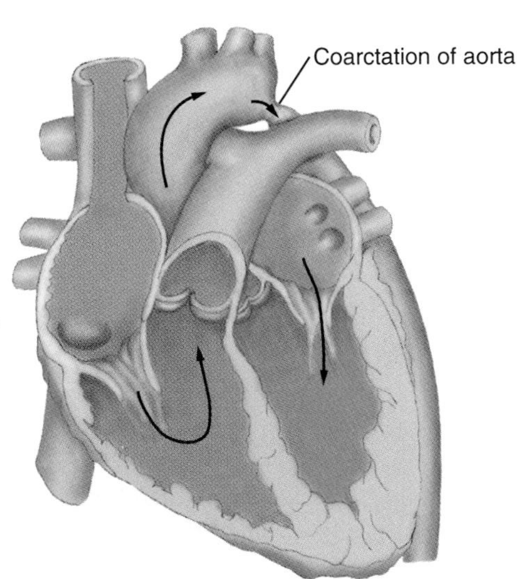


In this condition, blood flow is impeded through a constricted area of the aorta, increasing pressure behind the defect. The constriction may occur before or after the ductus arteriosus. The blood pressure is higher in the upper extremities than in the lower extremities. Carotid, brachial, and radial pulses are bounding, but pulses in the legs are weak or absent. The increased pressure in the left ventricle causes hypertrophy from the added workload. Congestive heart failure may result.

**D. Tetralogy of Fallot**

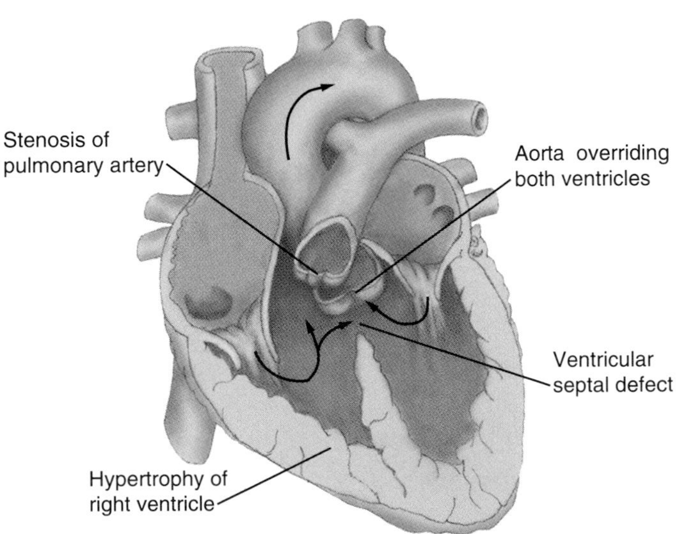


Tetralogy of Fallot has four characteristics: a ventricular septal defect, aorta positioned over the ventricular defect, pulmonary stenosis, and hypertrophy of the right ventricle. Cyanosis occurs when venous blood from the right ventricle flows through the septal defect and into the overriding aorta and blood flow to the lungs is diminished because of the narrowed pulmonary valve. The amount of right-to-left shunting and cyanosis varies according to the degree and position of each defect.

**FIGURE 30-4**

Common congenital heart defects.

**E. Transposition of the Great Arteries**

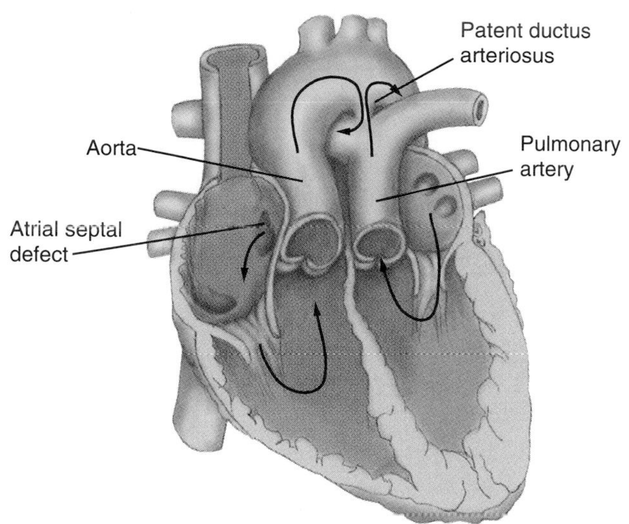


In this condition, the positions of the aorta and the pulmonary artery are reversed. The aorta carries venous blood from the right ventricle back to the general circulation. The pulmonary artery returns oxygenated blood from the left ventricle to the lungs. Unless there is another source for mixing oxygenated and venous blood, the infant cannot survive. A septal defect, open foramen ovale, or patent ductus arteriosus may be present. Prostaglandins may be given to keep the ductus open, and surgical correction is performed.

**FIGURE 30-4** *Continued*

nous blood. Cyanosis then occurs, causing a condition classified as acyanotic to become cyanotic.

The presence of cyanosis depends on the severity and combination of defects and the child's ability to compensate. Some infants with cyanotic heart disease may be pink, and some with acyanotic heart defects may develop cyanosis. Because of this potential change in classification, further classification by blood flow is helpful.

#### DEFECTS WITH INCREASED PULMONARY BLOOD FLOW

Defects with increased pulmonary blood flow are heart defects that allow blood to flow from the higher pressure of the left side of the heart to the right side or from the aorta to the pulmonary artery. This increases blood flow to the lungs and is called a left-to-right shunt. It causes some oxygenated blood to be sent to the lungs instead of to the rest of the body, increasing the work of the right side of the heart. Examples are ventricular septal defects and patent ductus arteriosus.

#### DEFECTS WITH OBSTRUCTION OF BLOOD FLOW

In defects with obstruction of blood flow, there is a decrease in the blood flow through a narrowed vessel or valve. This adds to the work of the heart, causes hypertrophy of the heart or major blood vessels, and may cause heart failure. Coarctation of the aorta fits into this classification.

#### DEFECTS WITH DECREASED PULMONARY BLOOD FLOW

An impairment in the flow of blood from the right side of the heart to the lungs combined with abnormal openings between pulmonary and systemic circulations occur in defects with decreased pulmonary blood flow. An example is tetralogy of Fallot.

#### MIXED DEFECTS

Mixed defects allow survival only if there is a mixing of venous and oxygenated blood in the heart. There is increased blood flow to the lungs and a mixture of venous and oxygenated blood in the systemic circulation. Transposition of the great vessels is a mixed defect.

### Manifestations

Congenital heart defects may present obvious signs at birth, or the indications may not become apparent until later, when changes from fetal to neonatal circulation are completed. Some infants have no difficulty for months or years, whereas others experience early heart failure.

The most common indications of cardiac problems that may be discovered by the nurse on assessment are cyanosis, heart murmurs, and tachycardia and tachypnea.

#### CYANOSIS

Cyanosis is a major sign of cardiac anomaly when there is no respiratory disease. It may be apparent at birth or may develop slowly or suddenly later. If the cyanosis is caused by a right-to-left shunt, giving oxygen will not improve the infant's color. Cyanosis increases with crying, feeding, or other activity. Pal-

***Critical to Remember***

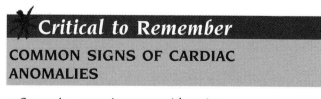

**COMMON SIGNS OF CARDIAC ANOMALIES**

- Cyanosis—may increase with crying
- Pallor
- Murmurs
- Tachycardia
- Tachypnea
- Dyspnea
- Choking spells
- Falling asleep during feedings
- Diaphoresis

lor, mottling, or gray color may be present in infants who do not have cyanosis.

#### HEART MURMURS

Murmurs may be present at birth or develop later. They may sound like clicks, machinery, rumbling, swishing, or other muffled noises. It takes much practice to detect heart murmurs accurately. Although many infants have a temporary murmur until the fetal structures are closed, all abnormal sounds must be referred for follow-up.

#### TACHYCARDIA AND TACHYPNEA

Tachycardia and tachypnea may occur anytime the heart and lungs must work harder to provide sufficient oxygen to the body. Thus, they are present in respiratory conditions as well as in cardiac conditions. They increase in congestive heart failure.

#### FEEDING DIFFICULTIES

Fatigue may interfere with the infant's ability to eat. The infant may feed slowly or fall asleep before the feeding is finished. Although diaphoresis is uncommon in the newborn, it may appear during feedings in the infant with a heart defect.

### Therapeutic Management

Therapeutic management involves diagnosis of the specific defect and supportive and surgical treatment as indicated. Various tests, such as echocardiograms and cardiac catheterizations, confirm the diagnosis. The decision for surgery depends on the status of the infant and whether surgery can be delayed safely. Palliative surgery may be performed to partially correct a defect or to make another defect to allow greater amounts of oxygenated blood to get to the systemic circulation.

Oxygen and drugs such as digitalis, diuretics, potassium supplements, and sedatives may be prescribed. Prostaglandins may be given to prevent the ductus arteriosus from closing in cases in which keeping it open will increase flow of oxygenated blood to the body.

### Nursing Considerations

Nursing care is focused on assessing for changes in condition and reducing the infant's need for oxygen. The need for rest is especially important. Infants with rapid respirations are at risk for aspiration and may need feeding by gavage. Oxygen may be increased during feedings or other exertion, but only enough oxygen to maintain saturation levels adequately should be used. Surgical nursing care may be necessary.

Support of the parents and education about the infant's condition and expected treatment are important. The nurse uses drawings to help parents understand the defect. The parents are taught techniques for accurate administration of medications because the range between the therapeutic and toxic dosage of the drugs is narrow.

**CHECK YOUR READING**

14. How are heart defects classified?

## SUMMARY CONCEPTS

- Asphyxia before or during birth causes apnea, acidosis, pulmonary hypertension, and possible death. Neonatal resuscitation must be initiated immediately.
- Nurses must identify conditions that increase the risk of asphyxia, begin resuscitation promptly, and assist other members of the team during treatment. Continued follow-up of the infant and parental support are important.
- In transient tachypnea of the newborn, respiratory difficulty in full-term or preterm infants is caused by failure of fetal lung fluid to be absorbed completely. It usually resolves spontaneously with supportive care.
- In meconium aspiration syndrome, meconium enters the lungs before birth or during the first breaths after birth. It causes inflammation and blocks air flow.
- The nurse's role in meconium aspiration syndrome is to prepare for care at birth, assist with care, and continue aftercare.
- Pathologic jaundice appears in the first 24 hours of life, rises faster and to higher levels than physiologic jaundice, or both. It may result in damage to the brain from kernicterus.
- The nurse's role in phototherapy includes decreasing situations such as cold stress or hypoglycemia that might further elevate bilirubin levels, seeing that lights are used properly, observing for excessive fluid loss or skin impairment, ensuring adequate oral intake, and teaching parents.
- Infection can be transmitted to neonates vertically (from mother to infant during pregnancy or birth) or horizontally (from family members or agency staff after birth). Infections may have serious consequences.
- The infant of a diabetic mother may have congenital anomalies, may be large- or small-for-gestational age, and may suffer from respiratory distress syndrome, hypoglycemia, hypocalcemia, and polycythemia.
- Nursing responsibilities in caring for infants of diabetic mothers include early identification and follow-up of complications, monitoring blood glucose levels, ensuring early and adequate feedings, and supporting parents.

- Infants with prenatal exposure to drugs may have congenital defects and behavioral and feeding abnormalities. They may have difficulty relating to others and fail to gain weight.
- Nursing care for infants with neonatal abstinence syndrome includes decreasing stimuli from lights, noise, or handling; increasing feeding abilities; and fostering the mother's attachment to and ability to care for her infant.
- In cyanotic heart defects, unoxygenated blood flows into the systemic circulation, producing cyanosis. In acyanotic heart defects, there is impairment of blood flow or flow of oxygenated blood into the pulmonary system. Defects may increase or decrease blood to the lungs.

### References and Readings


American Academy of Pediatrics and American College of Obstetricians and Gynecologists. (1992). *Guidelines for perinatal care* (3rd ed.). Elk Grove Village, Ill.: American Academy of Pediatrics.

American Academy of Pediatrics, Provisional Committee for Quality Improvement and Subcommittee on Hyperbilirubinemia. (1994). Practice parameter: management of hyperbilirubinemia in the healthy term newborn. *Pediatrics*, 94(4), 558–565.

Angeles, D.M. (1992). Pathophysiology and nursing management of persistent pulmonary hypertension of the newborn. MCN: *American Journal of Maternal Child Nursing*, 17(6), 314–332.

Askin, D.F. (1995). Bacterial and fungal infections in the neonate. *Journal of Obstetric, Gynecologic, and Neonatal Nursing*, 24(7), 635–643.

Association of Women's Health, Obstetric, and Neonatal Nurses. (1995). *Clinical commentary: Perinatal group B streptococcal disease.* Washington, D.C.: Author.

Behrman, R.E., Kliegman, R.M., & Arvin, A.M. (Eds.). (1996). *Nelson textbook of pediatrics* (15th ed.). Philadelphia: W.B. Saunders.

Bell, G.L., & Lau, K. (1995). Perinatal and neonatal issues of substance abuse. *Pediatric Clinics of North America*, 42(2), 261–281.

Berkowitz, C.D. (1996). Infants of substance abusing mothers. In C.D. Berkowitz, *Pediatrics: A primary care approach.* Philadelphia: W.B. Saunders.

Blackburn, S. (1995). Hyperbilirubinemia and neonatal jaundice. *Neonatal Network*, 14(7), 15–25.

Bloom, R.S., Cropley, C., & AHA/AAP Neonatal Resuscitation Program Steering Committee. (1994). *Textbook of neonatal resuscitation.* Dallas: American Heart Association and American Academy of Pediatrics.

Boyle, K.M., Baker, V.L., & Cassaday, C.J. (1995). Neonatal pulmonary disorders. In S.L. Barnhart & M.P. Czervinske, (Eds.), *Perinatal and pediatric respiratory care.* Philadelphia: W.B. Saunders.

Composto, R., & Eichelberger, C. (1992). Congenital diaphragmatic hernia: Pathophysiology and nursing care. *Neonatal Network*, 11(6), 57–61.

Cordero, L., & Landon, M.B. (1993). Infant of the diabetic mother. *Clinics in Perinatology*, 20(3), 635–648.

Daberkow, E., & Washington, R.L. (1993). Cardiovascular diseases and surgical interventions. In G.B. Merenstein & S.L. Gardner (Eds.), *Handbook of neonatal intensive care* (3rd ed.). St. Louis: C.V. Mosby.

D'Apolito, K., & McRorie, T.I. (1996). Pharmacologic management of neonatal abstinence syndrome. *Journal of Perinatal and Neonatal Nursing*, 9(4), 70–80.

DeBoer, S.L., & Stephens, D. (1997). Persistent pulmonary hypertension of the newborn: Case study and pathophysiology review. *Neonatal Network*, 16(1), 7–13.

Doshier, S. (1995). What happens to the offspring of diabetic pregnancies? MCN: *American Journal of Maternal Child Nursing*, 20(1), 25–29.

Fanaroff, A.A., & Martin, R.J. (1997). *Neonatal-perinatal medicine* (6th ed.) St. Louis: Mosby–Year Book.

Fanaroff, A.A., Martin, R.J., & Miller, M.J. (1994). Identification and management of high-risk problems in the neonate. In R.K. Creasy & R. Resnik (Eds.), *Maternal-fetal medicine: Principles and practice* (3rd ed.). Philadelphia: W.B. Saunders.

Faro, S., & Pastorek, J.G. (1993). Perinatal infections. In R.A. Knuppel & J.E. Drukker (Eds.), *High-risk pregnancy: A team approach* (2nd ed.). Philadelphia: W.B. Saunders.

Flandermeyer, A.A. (1993). The drug-exposed neonate. In C. Kenner, A. Brueggemeyer, & L.P. Gunderson (Eds.), *Comprehensive neonatal nursing: A physiologic perspective.* Philadelphia: W.B. Saunders.

Franck, L., & Vilardi, J. (1995). Assessment and management of opioid withdrawal in ill neonates. *Neonatal Network*, 14(2), 39–48.

Frank, D.G., Turner, B.S., & Merenstein, G.B. (1993). Jaundice. In G.B. Merenstein & S.L. Gardner (Eds.), *Handbook of neonatal intensive care* (2nd ed.). St. Louis: C.V. Mosby.

Frenkel, L.D., & Gaur, S. (1994). Perinatal HIV infection and AIDS. *Clinics in Perinatology*, 21(1), 95–107.

Hagedorn, M.I., Gardner, S.L., & Abman, S.H. (1993). Respiratory diseases. In G.B. Merenstein & S.L. Gardner (Eds.), *Handbook of neonatal intensive care* (2nd ed.). St. Louis: C.V. Mosby.

Healy, K., Jovanovic-Peterson, L., & Peterson, C.M. (1995). Pancreatic disorders of pregnancy: Pregestational diabetes. *Endocrinology and Metabolism Clinics of North America*, 24(1), 73–101.

Hite, C., & Shannon, M. (1992). Clinical profile of apparently healthy neonates with in utero drug exposure. *Journal of Obstetric, Gynecologic, and Neonatal Nursing*, 21(4), 305–309.

Huffman, D.M., Price, B.K., & Langel, L. (1994). Therapeutic handling techniques for the infant affected by cocaine. *Neonatal Network*, 13(5), 9–13.

Kahn, N.S., & Luten, R.C. (1994). Neonatal resuscitation. *Emergency Medicine Clinics of North America*, 12(1), 239–256.

Kang, J.H., & Shankaran, S. (1995). Double phototherapy with high irradiance compared with single phototherapy in neonates with hyperbilirubinemia. *American Journal of Perinatology*, 12(3), 178–180.

Katz, V.L., & Bowes, W.A. (1992). Meconium aspiration syndrome. Reflections on a murky subject. *American Journal of Obstetrics and Gynecology*, 166(1), 171–183.

Kirsten, D. (1996). Patent ductus arteriosus in the preterm infant. *Neonatal Network*, 15(2), 19–26.

Klaus, M.H., & Kennell, J.H. (1993). Care of the parents. In M.H. Klaus & A.A. Fanaroff (Eds.), *Care of the high-risk neonate.* Philadelphia: W.B. Saunders.

Klein, J.O., & Macy, S.M. (1995). Bacterial sepsis and meningitis. In J.S. Remington & J.O. Klein (Eds.), *Infectious diseases of the fetus & newborn infant* (4th ed.). Philadelphia: W.B. Saunders.

Klein, J.O., & Remington, J.S. (1995). Current concepts of infections of the fetus and newborn infant. In J.S. Remington & J.O. Klein (Eds.), *Infectious diseases of the fetus & newborn infant* (4th ed.). Philadelphia: W.B. Saunders.

Krause, K.D., & Youngner, V.J. (1992). Nursing diagnoses as guidelines in the care of the neonatal ECMO patient.

*Journal of Obstetric, Gynecologic, and Neonatal Nursing*, 21(3), 169–176.

Lefrak-Okikawa, L., & Lund, C.H. (1993). Nursing practice in the neonatal intensive care unit. In M.H. Klaus & A.A. Fanaroff (Eds.), *Care of the high-risk neonate*. Philadelphia: W.B. Saunders.

Lott, J.W. (1993). Fetal development: Environmental influences and critical periods. In C. Kenner, A. Brueggemeyer, & L.P. Gunderson (Eds.), *Comprehensive neonatal nursing: A physiologic perspective*. Philadelphia: W.B. Saunders.

Lott, J.W., & Kenner, C. (1994a). Keeping up with neonatal infection: Designer bugs, Part I. MCN: *American Journal of Maternal Child Nursing*, 19(4), 207–213.

Lott, J.W., & Kenner, C. (1994b). Keeping up with neonatal infection: Designer bugs, Part II. MCN: *American Journal of Maternal Child Nursing*, 19(5), 264–271.

Lott, J.W., Nelson, K., Fahrner, R., & Kenner, C. (1993). Assessment and management of immunologic dysfunction. In C. Kenner, A. Brueggemeyer, & L.P. Gunderson (Eds.), *Comprehensive neonatal nursing: A physiologic perspective*. Philadelphia: W.B. Saunders.

Ludwig, M.A., Marecki, M., Wooldridge, P.J., & Sheman, L.M. (1996). Neonatal nurses' knowledge of and attitudes toward caring for cocaine-exposed infants and their mothers. *Journal of Perinatal Neonatal Nursing*, 9(4), 81–85.

Maisels, M.J. (1994). Jaundice. In G.B. Avery, M.A. Fletcher, & M.G. Macdonald (Eds.), *Neonatology: Pathophysiology and management of the newborn* (4th ed.). Philadelphia: J.B. Lippincott.

Meaux, J.B. (1996). Intravenous immunoglobulin: What nurses need to know. *Journal of Perinatal and Neonatal Nursing*, 9(4), 63–69.

Mosijczuk, A.D., & Ellis-Vaiani, C. (1993). Hematologic diseases. In G.B. Merenstein & S.L. Gardner (Eds.), *Handbook of neonatal intensive care* (2nd ed.). St. Louis: C.V. Mosby.

Mueller, B.U., & Pizzo, P.A. (1995). Acquired immunodeficiency syndrome in the infant. In J.S. Remington & J.O. Klein (Eds.), *Infectious diseases of the fetus and newborn infant* (4th ed.). Philadelphia: W.B. Saunders.

Nash, P. (1996). Common neonatal complications. In K.R. Simpson & P.A. Creehan (Eds.), *AWHONN's perinatal nursing*. Philadelphia: Lippincott-Raven.

O'Donnell, J.P., & Merenstein, G.B. (1993). Infection in the neonate. In G.B. Merenstein & S.L. Gardner (Eds.), *Handbook of neonatal intensive care* (2nd ed.). St. Louis: C.V. Mosby.

Paul, K.E. (1995). Recognition, stabilization, and early management of infants with critical congenital heart disease presenting in the first days of life. *Neonatal Network*, 14(5), 13–20.

Paxton, J.M. (1992). Neonatal infections. In P. Beachy & J. Deacon (Eds.), *Core curriculum for neonatal intensive care nursing*. Philadelphia: W.B. Saunders.

Peng, T.C.C., Gutcher, G.R., & Van Dorsten, J.P. (1996). A selective aggressive approach to the neonate exposed to meconium-stained amniotic fluid. *American Journal Obstetrics and Gynecology*, 175(2), 296–303.

Philip, A. (1996). *Neonatology: A practical guide* (4th ed.). Philadelphia: W.B. Saunders.

Rayburn, W., & Marsden, D. (1993). Medications in pregnancy. In R.A. Knuppel & J.E. Drukker (Ed.), *High-risk pregnancy: A team approach* (2nd ed.). Philadelphia: W.B. Saunders.

Schuman, A.J., & Karush, G. (1992). Fiberoptic vs. conventional home phototherapy for neonatal hyperbilirubinemia. *Clinical Pediatrics*, 31(6), 345–352.

Sham, B. (1992). Perinatal substance abuse. In P. Beachy & J. Deacon (Eds.), *Core curriculum for neonatal intensive care nursing*. Philadelphia: W.B. Saunders.

Shermer, R.H. (1995). Group B streptococcus during the perinatal period. *Journal of Obstetric, Gynecologic, and Neonatal Nursing*, 24(6), 562–566.

Simpson, K.R., & Creehan, P.A. (Eds.). (1996). *AWHONN's perinatal nursing*. Philadelphia: Lippincott-Raven.

Smith, J.B., Baker, A.L., Moynihan, P.J., Lincoln, P., & Kane, P.L. (1996). Cardiovascular critical care problems. In M.A.Q. Curley, J.B. Smith, & P.A. Moloney-Harmon (Eds.), *Critical care nursing of infants and children*. Philadelphia: W.B. Saunders.

Stamos, J.K., & Rowley, A.H. (1995). Timely diagnosis of congenital infections. *Pediatric Clinics of North America*, 41(5), 1017–1033.

Steinhorn, R.H., Millard, L.L., & Morin, F.C. (1995). Persistent pulmonary hypertension of the newborn. *Clinics in Perinatology*, 22(2), 405–428.

Strodtbeck, F. (1995). Viral infections of the newborn. *Journal of Obstetric, Gynecologic, and Neonatal Nursing*, 24(7), 659–667.

Suevo, D.M. (1997). The infant of the diabetic mother. *Neonatal Network*, 16(5), 25–33.

Tan, K.L. (1995). Comparison of the efficacy of fiberoptic and conventional phototherapy for neonatal hyperbilirubinemia. *Journal of Pediatrics*, 125(4), 607–612.

Tyrala, E.E. (1996). The infant of the diabetic mother. *Obstetric Clinics of North America*, 23(1), 221–241.

Whitsett, J.A., Pryhuber, G.S., Rice, W.R., Warner, B.B., & Wert, S.E. (1994). Acute respiratory disorders. In G.B. Avery, M.A. Fletcher, & M.G. Macdonald (Eds.), *Neonatology: Pathophysiology and management of the newborn* (4th ed.). Philadelphia: J.B. Lippincott.

Wiswell, T.E., & Bent, R.C. (1993). Meconium staining and the meconium aspiration syndrome. *Pediatric Clinics of North America*, 40(5), 955–981.

Wolach, B. (1997). Neonatal sepsis: Pathogenesis and supportive therapy. *Seminars in Perinatology*, 21(1), 28–38.

# Part VI

# Other Reproductive Issues

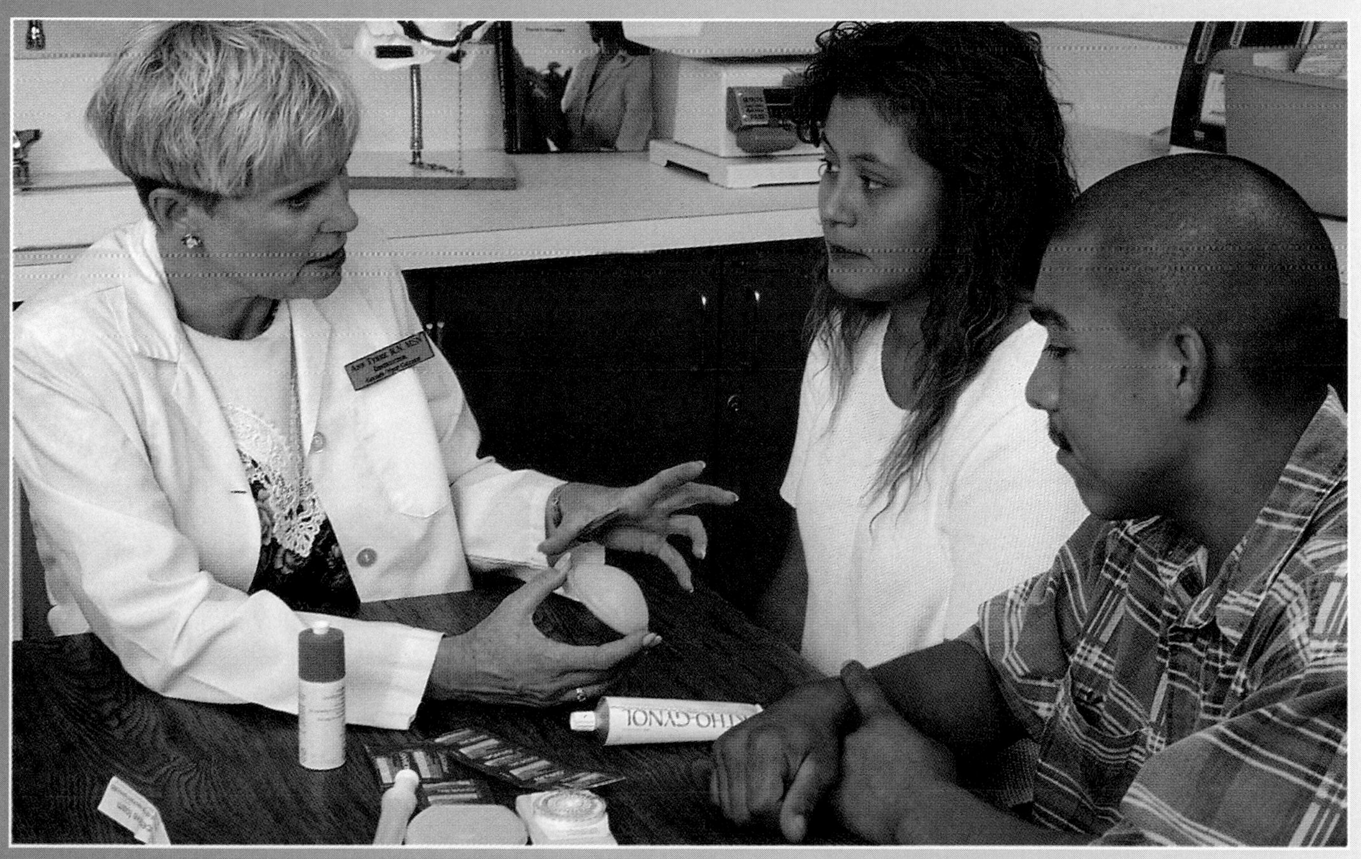

# 31

# Family Planning

## OBJECTIVES

1. Describe the role of the nurse in helping couples choose contraceptive methods.
2. Compare and contrast contraceptive methods in terms of safety, effectiveness, convenience, education needed to use, interference with spontaneity, availability, expense, and preference.
3. Explain why informed consent is important for contraception.
4. Compare and contrast contraceptive needs of adolescent and perimenopausal women.
5. Explain the mechanism of action of each method of family planning available: sterilization, hormonal contraceptives, intrauterine devices, barrier, and natural family planning.

## DEFINITIONS

**basal body temperature** *Body temperature at rest.*

**cervical cap** *A small cup-like device placed over the cervix to prevent sperm from entering, thus preventing pregnancy.*

**coitus** *Sexual union between a male and a female.*

**coitus interruptus** *Withdrawal of the penis from the vagina before ejaculation.*

**condom** *Latex, polyurethane, or natural membrane shield covering the penis or lining the vagina to prevent sperm from entering the cervix or to prevent infection, or both.*

**contraception** *Prevention of pregnancy.*

**diaphragm** *A contraceptive device consisting of a latex dome that covers the cervix and prevents entrance of sperm; must be used with a spermicide to be effective.*

**hormone implant** *Small capsules of progestin inserted subcutaneously to provide contraception.*

**intrauterine device (IUD)** *A mechanical device inserted into the uterus to prevent pregnancy.*

**libido** *Sexual desire.*

**mittelschmerz** *Low abdominal pain that occurs at ovulation.*

**natural family planning** *Method of predicting ovulation based on normal changes in a woman's body.*

**oral contraceptive** *Drug that inhibits ovulation; contains progestins alone or in combination with estrogen.*

**progestin** *Any natural or synthetic form of progesterone.*

**sexually transmissible (or transmitted) disease (STD)** *A disease that is passed to others primarily through sexual contact.*

**spermicide** *A chemical, such as nonoxynol-9, that kills sperm.*

**spinnbarkeit** *Clear, slippery, stretchy quality of cervical mucus during ovulation.*

**tubal ligation** *Occluding the fallopian tubes to prevent passage of ova or sperm, thus preventing pregnancy.*

**vasectomy** *Occluding the vas deferens to prevent passage of sperm, thus preventing pregnancy.*

Family planning involves choosing when to have children. It includes contraception—the prevention of pregnancy—as well as methods to achieve pregnancy. Chapter 32 describes methods used by couples having difficulty attaining pregnancy. This chapter focuses on techniques used to avoid pregnancy.

If both partners are fertile, approximately 90 percent of women will conceive within 1 year if they do not use contraception (Cunningham et al., 1997). Therefore, those who wish to control the timing of pregnancies cannot leave contraception to chance.

Because the majority of contraceptive methods available must be practiced by women, women often choose the type of contraception used. In the United States, more than 90 percent of all women at risk for pregnancy use some method of contraception (Nelson, 1995). During a woman's reproductive lifetime, her needs for contraception change. Most women try a variety of methods before they reach menopause. Because the average woman in the United States bears only two children, she may make contraceptive decisions for more than 30 years.

## Information About Contraception

### Common Sources

Women often obtain information about contraception from friends, relatives, newspapers, and magazines. They seek answers to practical questions about comfort, partners' responses, and problems encountered. However, they may receive incomplete facts or misinformation when their source of information is not a qualified health care professional.

Women frequently turn to nurses in clinics, physicians' offices, birth settings, or even social settings for accurate information about contraception. Some women are more comfortable asking a nurse questions about contraception than a physician, particularly when they are unsure of what technique they desire.

### Role of the Nurse

The nurse's role in family planning is that of counselor and educator. To fulfill this role, nurses need current, correct information about contraceptive methods. More than half of all pregnancies are unintended. This has led to a national goal in the United States to reduce unintended pregnancies from the 1987 baseline of 56 percent to no more than 30 percent (U.S. Department of Health and Human Services, Public Health Service, 1995).

About half of the unintended pregnancies occur in women who are using a contraceptive method but use it incorrectly or have a contraceptive failure. This would occur much less frequently if women had adequate education about their chosen method. The initial teaching that accompanies selection of the contraceptive technique may be insufficient to meet the woman's needs. Reinforcement of teaching and providing an opportunity to ask questions after initial use can help ensure the woman is using her method correctly.

Nurses must feel comfortable discussing contraception and be sensitive to the woman's concerns and feelings. In discussing family planning, the woman's preferences take precedence. Nurses must be careful not to introduce their own biases toward or against specific methods. The nurse's personal experiences and choices regarding contraception are not pertinent. The needs and feelings of the woman and her partner must be the focus of counseling (Fig. 31-1).

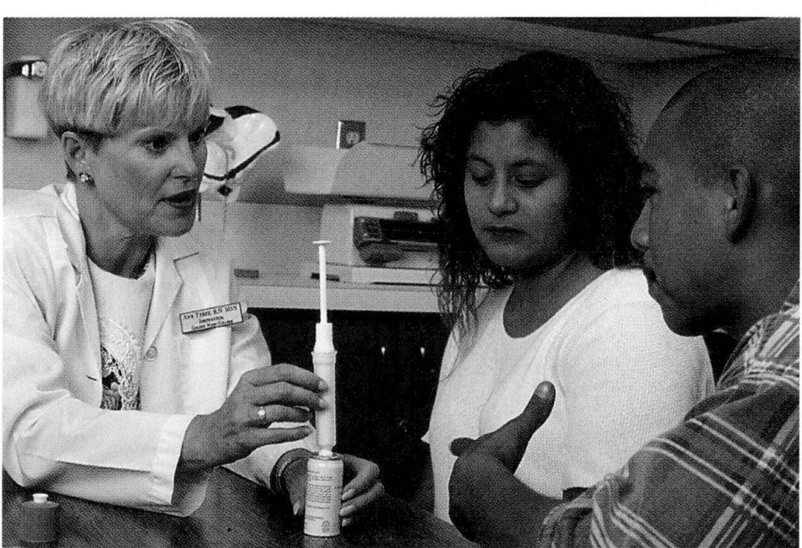

**FIGURE 31-1**

Success of contraception is more likely when both the woman and her partner are involved in discussions. The nurse demonstrates filling a foam applicator.

Nurses working in maternity settings should discuss family planning with every woman after birth to provide an opportunity to clarify misinformation and answer questions. Then the woman will be ready to discuss contraception further with her primary caregiver, if necessary.

## Considerations When Choosing a Contraceptive Method

There is no perfect contraceptive method. Each has advantages and disadvantages (Table 31–1). Women change contraceptive methods as circumstances in their lives change and may try several before finding one that is satisfactory. The rate at which women discontinue the use of their contraceptive method is shown in Table 31–2. The nurse can help women weigh factors involved in choosing a family planning method. Careful consideration of all factors can help women choose methods that best meet their needs and are therefore more likely to prevent pregnancy.

### Safety

The safety of the method is a primary consideration. Although all contraceptives are tested before marketing, medical conditions may make some methods unsafe for certain women. For example, oral contraceptives (OCs) should not be used by women who have had thrombophlebitis or strokes because the hormones used may cause these conditions to recur. The diaphragm and cervical cap are unsafe for women with a history of toxic shock syndrome, a possible complication of these methods.

### Protection from Sexually Transmissible Diseases

There is no contraceptive (other than abstinence) that is 100 percent effective in preventing sexually transmissible diseases (STDs). The risk of exposure to STDs should be considered in counseling women about contraceptive choices. The male condom offers the best protection available. It should be used whenever there is a risk that one partner may have an STD, even when another form of contraception is practiced. Although women are aware of the protection offered by condoms, those reporting use at last intercourse is low (Murphy et al., 1995; Hiltabiddle, 1996). In one large study, 52 percent of the women studied had not used condoms in the last 6 months and only 12 percent reported that they always used condoms (Lauver et al., 1995).

### Effectiveness

The importance of avoiding pregnancy must be considered when choosing a contraceptive method. A woman may wish to put off pregnancy for a time but may not care if pregnancy occurs earlier. Other

**TABLE 31–1 ADVANTAGES AND DISADVANTAGES OF MOST COMMON CONTRACEPTIVE METHODS**

| Method | Advantages | Disadvantages |
|---|---|---|
| Sterilization (tubal ligation and vasectomy) | Ends concern about contraception.<br>Tubal ligation can be performed right after childbirth while still in hospital or as an outpatient at another time.<br>Vasectomy may be performed in physician's office under local anesthesia.<br>Although expensive initially, long-term cost is low. | Does not protect against STDs.<br>Reversal is difficult, expensive, and potentially impossible.<br>Requires surgery with potential complications of all surgeries.<br>Vasectomy requires another contraceptive method until semen is free of sperm. |
| Implant | In place at all times.<br>Unrelated to coitus. | Does not protect against STDs.<br>Expensive initially (although lower overall cost), requires minor surgery to implant and remove.<br>Slightly visible.<br>Side effects may lead to discontinuation if unacceptable. |
| Progestin injections (Depo-Provera) | Unrelated to coitus. | Must be repeated every 3 months. Side effects similar to other progestin contraceptives.<br>Does not protect against STDs. |
| Oral contraceptives | Taken at time unrelated to coitus.<br>See Table 31–3 (Potential Benefits and Risks of Oral Contraceptives). | Must be taken at same time each day.<br>May cause side effects and complications.<br>Does not protect against STDs.<br>See Table 31–3 (Potential Benefits and Risks of Oral Contraceptives). |

**TABLE 31–1 ADVANTAGES AND DISADVANTAGES OF MOST COMMON CONTRACEPTIVE METHODS** *Continued*

| Method | Advantages | Disadvantages |
|---|---|---|
| Intrauterine devices | In place at all times.<br>Low long-term cost. | Does not protect against STDs.<br>High initial cost.<br>Can be expelled without woman's knowledge—must check for strings.<br>Potential side effects or complications—menorrhagia, infection, ectopic pregnancy, abortion, perforation. |
| Barrier | | |
| All methods | Avoids use of systemic hormones.<br>Offers some protection against STDs. | Most coitus related (must be used just before coitus). May interfere with sensation. Some people are sensitive to components of spermicide or latex. |
| Chemical (spermicides) | Quick and easy.<br>No prescription needed.<br>Inexpensive per single use. | Films and suppositories must melt to be effective.<br>Usually effective for only 1 hr.<br>May be messy.<br>New application needed for subsequent intercourse. |
| Condoms | Quick and easy.<br>No prescription needed.<br>Best protection available for STDs, especially if combined with spermicide.<br>Inexpensive per single use.<br>Can be carried discreetly.<br>Vaginal condoms increase women's control over contraceptive use and protection from STDs. | Must be checked for expiration date and holes.<br>Can break or slip off.<br>Can be used only once.<br>Vaginal condom may seem unattractive. |
| Diaphragm | Can be inserted several hours before coitus. | Initially expensive. Requires nurse practitioner, certified nurse-midwife, or physician to fit.<br>Requires education on proper use.<br>Some women have difficulty with correct insertion or removal.<br>Added spermicide necessary for repeat coitus.<br>Possibility of toxic shock.<br>Must be refitted after each birth or weight change of 10 or more pounds.<br>Pressure against bladder may cause infections. |
| Cervical cap | Smaller than diaphragm and may fit women who cannot wear a diaphragm.<br>Requires less spermicide and no additional spermicide for repeated intercourse.<br>No pressure against bladder.<br>Less noticeable than diaphragm.<br>Can remain in place 48 hr. | Sizes are limited.<br>Initially expensive.<br>Requires nurse practitioner or physician to fit.<br>Requires education on proper use.<br>Somewhat more difficult to insert than diaphragm.<br>Can be dislodged during intercourse.<br>Possibility of toxic shock.<br>Must be refitted each year and after birth, abortion, or surgery. |
| Natural family planning | | |
| All methods | Inexpensive.<br>No drugs or hormones.<br>Helps woman learn about her body.<br>Acceptable to most religions.<br>May be used to achieve pregnancy.<br>Can combine with barrier methods to increase effectiveness. | Requires high level of motivation.<br>Extensive education needed.<br>Requires abstinence for large part of each cycle.<br>High risk of pregnancy from error.<br>Many factors may change ovulation time. |

*Abbreviations*: STD, sexually transmissible disease

**TABLE 31-2 CONTRACEPTIVE EFFECTIVENESS, FAILURE, AND DISCONTINUATION RATES**

| Method | Effectiveness Rate: Actual or Typical Use (%) | Failure Rate: Actual or Typical Use (%) | Failure Rate: Ideal or Perfect Use (%) | Discontinuation Rate at 1 Year (%) |
|---|---|---|---|---|
| Sterilization | | | | |
| Tubal ligation | 99.6 | 0.4 | 0.4 | |
| Vasectomy | 99.85 | 0.15 | 0.1 | |
| Hormone implants | 99.91 | 0.09 | 0.09 | 15 |
| Injectable hormones | 99.7 | 0.3 | 0.3 | 30 |
| Oral contraceptives | 97 | 3 | | 28 |
| Combined estrogen/progestin | | | 0.1 | |
| Progestin only | | | 0.5 | |
| Intrauterine devices | | | | |
| Progesterone | 98 | 2 | 1.5 | 19 |
| Copper | 99.2 | 0.8 | 0.6 | 22 |
| Condoms | | | | |
| Male | 88 | 12 | 3 | 37 |
| Female | 79 | 21 | 5 | 44 |
| Diaphragm | 82 | 18 | 6 | 42 |
| Cervical cap | | | | |
| Parous women | 64 | 36 | 26 | 55 |
| Nulliparous women | 82 | 18 | 9 | 42 |
| Spermicides—gel, foam, films, suppositories | 79 | 21 | 6 | 57 |
| Natural family planning | 80 | 20 | | 33 |
| Calendar | | | 9 | |
| Basal body temperature | | | 3 | |
| Symptothermal | | | 2 | |
| Postovulation | | | 1 | |
| Coitus interruptus (withdrawal) | 81 | 19 | 4 | |
| No contraceptive use | 15 | 85 | 85 | |

Percent of women who may be expected to avoid or become pregnant with use of each method from typical and perfect use during the first year. Discontinuation rate is the rate of women who do not wish to become pregnant and stop using a method by the end of 1 year of use. The discontinuation rate often rises with each year of use.
Reprinted and modified with the permission of the Population Council, from James Trussell et al. (1990). Contraceptive failure in the United States: An update. *Studies in Family Planning*, 21(1): 52; and Hatcher, R.A., Trussell, J., Stewart F., et al. (1994). *Contraceptive technology* (16th ed.). New York: Irvington Publishers.

women may be extremely upset about an accidental pregnancy because it would affect their health or have a major impact on their financial stability.

Effectiveness is determined by how often the method fails to prevent pregnancy (see Table 31–2). There are two different types of failure rates:

1. The ideal, perfect, or theoretic failure rate refers to perfect use of the method with every act of intercourse. Failures are due to a problem with the method itself rather than with the use of the method.
2. The typical, actual, or user failure rate is taken from studies of occurrence of pregnancy in real people using the method. Failure is presumably due to incorrect or inconsistent use of the technique. Failures are most often due to not using the method for every act of intercourse.

The difference between the two rates of failure shows how forgiving a method is, that is, how likely pregnancy is to occur if use is occasionally imperfect. The typical failure rate is more meaningful when counseling women and their partners. When comparing different methods, one must use the same method of analysis.

Failure rates are listed as number of pregnancies in 100 women per year. Although a typical failure rate of 12 percent for a method might seem fairly good, it means that 12 of every 100 women using that method experience unintended pregnancies each year. For women who feel that a one in eight yearly risk of pregnancy is too great, a more effective method should be chosen.

Effectiveness varies according to accuracy of use. It drops greatly when the user does not understand how to use the method. The failure rate commonly decreases after the first year of use because experience with the method leads to more accurate use. Methods that are less reliable can sometimes be combined to increase effectiveness, such as using a condom with a spermicide.

The acceptability of the method to the couple

must be balanced against the effectiveness. Surgical sterilization is the most effective method but is unacceptable to couples planning to have children at a later time. Oral contraceptives or intrauterine devices (IUDs) are also highly effective, but some women may dislike the side effects or have religious objections.

## Convenience

Convenience is another important factor. If the woman perceives her contraceptive as difficult to use, time consuming, or too much "bother," she is unlikely to use it consistently unless her level of motivation is very high. The education she receives about the method may affect her perception of its difficulty. Women knowledgeable about the contraceptive technique are less likely to feel that the contraceptive is difficult to use.

Contraceptives that are "messy" may seem inconvenient and unattractive. Spermicide may drip from the vagina and decrease satisfaction for both the woman and the man. Less spermicide may decrease dripping but increase the risk of pregnancy.

## Education Needed

Some methods of contraception involve very little education, whereas others depend on one or more teaching sessions to ensure adequate knowledge. For example, condoms are easy to use and involve less education than some other methods. Natural family planning methods rely on extensive education about body changes that denote ovulation. Women using these methods need rather sophisticated information to practice them successfully.

## Side Effects

Many methods of contraception have side effects that women may dislike. Side effects must be explained clearly in discussing the advantages and disadvantages of each method. When women know what to expect, they are often more willing to tolerate side effects, especially if they know they do not indicate a health risk. This may help them to continue an effective contraceptive method instead of discontinuing it and using no method or one that is less effective.

## Interference with Spontaneity

Coitus-related contraceptive methods, such as spermicides and barrier methods, must be used just before sexual intercourse. They interrupt lovemaking, increasing the chance that the method will not be used. Some couples remedy this by including placement of the contraceptive device, such as a condom or diaphragm, as a part of foreplay. Others prefer methods such as OCs, IUDs, or hormone implants that do not interrupt sexual activity.

## Availability

Condoms and spermicides are readily available without prescriptions. They can be purchased anonymously at any time without a trip to a health care provider. This may be important to an adolescent who wants to hide her sexual activity or to any woman who is embarrassed to discuss contraception with a health care provider.

## Expense

The cost of family planning methods per use can be compared with long-term expense. The price of condoms and spermicides is relatively low, but frequent use makes them expensive over a period of years. Couples may find them economical for occasional sexual intercourse or until they can afford a more expensive method. However they have a higher chance of failure and pregnancy than other, more expensive, methods. The yearly cost of any contraceptive method is less than the cost of a pregnancy.

Methods that depend on periodic visits to a nurse practitioner or physician are more costly than over-the-counter methods. However, the professional counseling given may enhance contraceptive effectiveness. Visits also provide opportunities for health teaching and screening for health problems. In spite of the fact that they require a health practitioner visit, the copper T IUD, implants, and injectable contraceptives are the most cost effective reversible contraceptives available over a 5-year period because they prevent pregnancy so well (Trussel et al., 1995).

Contraceptive information and services are often available at family planning clinics at little or no cost. These clinics provide professional counseling about all contraceptive methods as well as follow-up services. However, women may object to a long wait and the fact that they may see a different health care provider at each visit.

## Preference

The woman makes the final decision about contraceptive method, and it is crucial that she be satisfied with it. Consistent use of any method depends on whether it meets the needs of the woman and her partner. If the woman feels pressured into choosing a method or if the chosen method fails to live up to her expectations, use is likely to be inconsistent. The opinions of the woman's partner and friends may also influence what method she chooses.

Some women are uncomfortable with their bodies and embarrassed by methods that involve touching the vagina. Inserting a diaphragm or cervical cap or performing a daily assessment of cervical mucus may be unacceptable to them.

### Religious and Personal Beliefs

Religious or other personal beliefs also affect the choice of contraceptives. Roman Catholics may not believe in the use of any contraceptives other than natural family planning methods. Some women and their partners are averse to any method linked to abortion, such as postcoital contraception.

### Culture

Culture may also influence the method chosen. In the African-American culture, OCs and female sterilization are most often chosen and male sterilization is rare (Lethbridge, 1995). For some Hispanics, condoms may not be acceptable because they suggest infidelity (Edwards, 1994). Hmong women may report that their husbands do not believe in contraception (Jambunathan & Stewart, 1995).

## Informed Consent

Because some methods have potentially dangerous side effects, it is necessary for the woman to sign an informed consent form to show that she received and understands information about risks and benefits. For example, written consent may be obtained from women choosing surgical sterilization, OCs, hormone implants or injections, and IUDs. Of course, whether or not a formal consent form is used, every woman should receive information about the chosen contraceptive method and its proper use, the risks and benefits, and the alternative methods available.

**✓ CHECK YOUR READING**

1. Why do women usually choose the method of contraception that a couple uses?
2. What is the role of the nurse in helping women with contraceptive choices and use?
3. What are some important considerations in choosing a contraceptive technique?
4. Which contraceptive methods involve an informed consent form?

## Adolescents

Adolescent pregnancy is a major problem. The United States is trying to reduce pregnancies in women aged 15 to 17 to no more than 50 per 1000 adolescents from the 1985 baseline of 71.1 per 1000 in this age group (U.S. Department of Health and Human Services, Public Health Service, 1995). Although the goal may not be met by the target date, the severe impact of pregnancy on the teenager makes finding methods to enhance adolescent contraception use of major importance. (See Chapter 24 for information about adolescent pregnancy.)

### Adolescent Knowledge

Many adolescents have little knowledge about their own anatomy and physiology, including how and when conception occurs. They are likely to learn about contraception from other teenagers, who often pass on incorrect information. Even adolescents who have been pregnant misunderstand contraceptive techniques, and they may become pregnant again because of lack of information about family planning.

#### MISINFORMATION

Misinformation and erroneous beliefs cause adolescents to use ineffective methods of contraception or no method at all. Some teenagers think they cannot become pregnant the first time they have intercourse unless they have an orgasm or have been menstruating a certain length of time. However, pregnancy can result from any intercourse near ovulation. Although many adolescents have anovulatory menstrual cycles during the early months after menarche, they cannot depend on it to prevent pregnancy.

Teenagers may douche (insert a solution into the vagina) after intercourse to prevent pregnancy. However, douching is ineffective because sperm may enter the cervix within 15 seconds after ejaculation (Hatcher et al., 1994). Coitus interruptus (withdrawal) is another unreliable method used by teenagers. It requires more control than most adolescent boys have over timing of ejaculation. Semen spilled near the vagina can enter and cause pregnancy, even without penetration by the penis. In addition, preejaculatory fluid may contain sperm.

#### RISK-TAKING BEHAVIOR

Adolescents are more likely to take risks in sexual activity because they believe that their chances of becoming pregnant are small. They often do not plan intercourse and therefore are not prepared with contraceptives. Their risk-taking behavior may lead to STDs as well as to pregnancy. Schools have helped increase birth control use among adolescents by offering information about family planning and prevention of STDs. Contraceptive services are available on some school campuses, as well.

### Counseling Adolescents

Nurses who counsel adolescents about sexuality must be sensitive to the feelings, concerns, and needs of the teenager. They must be prepared to be accepting of the teenager regardless of personal feelings about adolescent sexuality. For an adolescent to seek information about contraception, she must admit that she is and plans to continue to be sexually active. The teenager may be afraid to ask about contraception because she does not want anyone to know that she is sexually active or she fears that she will be lectured about her behavior. Her need for secrecy may cause her to miss appointments for family planning. The nurse must be adept at determining the adolescent's needs and must reassure her about confidentiality.

Because many teenagers forgo contraception rather than talk to their parents about it, family planning clinics in most states may provide information and supplies to minors without parental permission. Some family planning clinics are designed to meet the special needs of teenagers. For example, because adolescent girls may fear the pelvic examination, clinic staff may wait to perform it until the second visit. During the first visit, the teenager receives information about contraceptive techniques. Taking this extra time to explain different methods helps allay the common concern of adolescents about potential adverse health effects of contraceptives. It also helps the teenager to feel comfortable in the clinic setting.

Because of her youth and possible lack of knowledge about anatomy and physiology, the adolescent often needs more extensive teaching than the older woman. Liberal use of audiovisual materials, such as pictures, anatomic models, and samples of various methods, helps the teenager understand the information more easily. Using a banana and condom or showing her the packet of pills she will be using are important aids.

**Using understandable terminology is especially important when teaching adolescents. The nurse must know street terms for body parts and sexual intercourse, as they may be the only words with which the teenager is familiar.**

Adolescents are most successful when they choose contraceptive methods that are easy to use and that seem unrelated to coitus. Many teenagers choose oral or injectable contraceptives. These methods are safe, seem unrelated to sex, and are not difficult or messy. Long-term OC use has not been found to cause problems in healthy women.

However, adolescent females may be inconsistent in taking pills every day. They are more likely to discontinue any method for minor side effects, such as nausea or spotting. Their concerns should be taken seriously, and attempts should be made to alleviate side effects or they will stop using the method, with pregnancy as a possible result. They should understand all aspects of management of their contraceptive method and when there is need for a back-up method.

Condom use should be encouraged to help prevent STDs, even when using another contraceptive method (Fig. 31–2). In one study, consistent condom use with another method was reported to occur in only 37 percent of young women (Dinerman et al., 1995). Discussing perceived barriers to using condoms will help dispel misconceptions about them. Many young women are uneasy about asking a partner to use a condom. They benefit from learning how to negotiate condom use with a partner. Adolescent males are often more concerned about avoiding pregnancy than about STDs. They may not want to use a condom if they

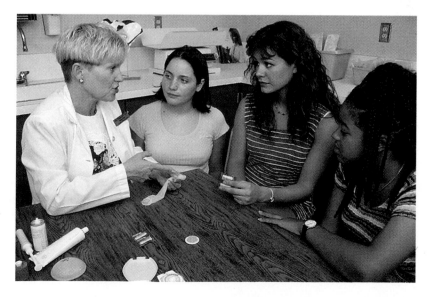

**FIGURE 31–2**

Although many adolescents choose oral contraceptives, the nurse emphasizes the need to use condoms for protection against sexually transmissible diseases. Demonstrating with actual contraceptives increases understanding.

### CRITICAL THINKING EXERCISE

A 15-year-old girl approaches the nurse with questions about contraception. She says she does not want to become pregnant, but her boyfriend does not want to use condoms and she is too embarrassd to go to see a physician for other contraceptive methods.

**Q:** How should the nurse handle the situation?

**A:** Find a private place to talk without interruption. Use therapeutic communication techniques to explore her feelings further. Help her think through how a pregnancy might change her life and how she would feel about those changes. Discuss what happens when a woman is examined during a visit for contraceptive counseling. Explore what she feels would be most embarrassing about seeing a physician. Would a female nurse practitioner, midwife, or physician be more acceptable? Discuss common contraceptive methods and determine her understanding and feelings about them. Also discuss negotiation skills for condom use, because condoms are important for prevention of sexually transmissible diseases as well as pregnancy. Try role playing, with the adolescent acting the role of her partner and the nurse taking the role of the adolescent.

know their partner is using another contraceptive method.

## Perimenopausal Women

Perimenopausal women may continue to ovulate as long as they have regular menstrual periods, and some ovulate even when indications of menopause are present. Pregnancy is rare after age 50, and contraception can be discontinued sooner if menstruation has ceased for at least 2 years (Cunningham et al., 1997). The mature woman who does not smoke and has no other contraindications can use any method of contraception. It is important that she have regular physical examinations to identify any conditions that would necessitate a change in contraceptive method. Many couples who do not plan to have more children choose sterilization. This ends their concerns about contraception permanently.

### CHECK YOUR READING

5. What are some erroneous beliefs about contraception commonly held by adolescents?
6. Why might teenagers be hesitant to seek contraceptive information?
7. How can the nurse increase effectiveness in teaching adolescents about contraception?
8. What considerations are necessary in contraception for perimenopausal women?

## Methods of Contraception

### Sterilization

Sterilization is an extremely popular method of contraception for couples who have completed their families. In the United States, approximately 1 million sterilizations are performed annually and more than 35 percent of women at risk for pregnancy between 14 and 44 years use this method of contraception (Hatcher et al., 1994). Although it is expensive at the time of surgery, it ends all further contraceptive costs. It should always be considered a permanent end to fertility because reversal surgery is difficult, expensive, and usually not covered by insurance. Reversal surgery is not always successful and increases the risk of ectopic pregnancy.

Couples considering sterilization need counseling to ensure that they understand all aspects of the procedure. When surgery is planned for immediately after childbirth, the decision should be made well before labor begins. Future marriage, divorce, or death of a child may cause couples to regret their decision. As with any surgery, informed consent forms are necessary. Complications are those of any surgery, including hemorrhage, infection, and anesthesia complications. Although pregnancy is rare, the risk of failure should be discussed. When pregnancy occurs after tubal ligation, it is more likely to be ectopic.

#### TUBAL LIGATION

Female sterilization is the method of contraception used by approximately 14 million women in the United States (Hatcher et al., 1994). The effectiveness rate is 99.6 percent. The surgery can be performed at any time. It is easiest during the immediate postpartum period, when the fundus is located near the umbilicus and the fallopian tubes are directly below the abdominal wall. For the woman who is not postpartum, the procedure is often performed in an outpatient surgery department. General anesthesia is most common, but regional or local anesthesia may be used.

The procedure can be performed in three ways. A minilaparotomy incision is made near the umbilicus in the postpartum period or just above the symphysis pubis when surgery is not postpartum. The surgeon brings the tubes through the incision, where a piece is removed and the ends are tied.

In the second method, surgery is performed

through a laparoscope inserted through a small incision. The surgeon visualizes the fallopian tubes and blocks them with clips or rings or destroys a portion of the tubes with electrocoagulation. The third method is during other surgery, generally along with cesarean birth, when a woman is sure that she wants the procedure regardless of the outcome of the birth.

#### VASECTOMY

Vasectomy, the male sterilization procedure, is 99.85 percent effective. It involves making a small incision in the scrotum and cutting the vas deferens, which carries sperm from the testes to the penis. After vasectomy, semen no longer contains sperm.

Although performed less frequently than tubal ligation, vasectomy is a very popular method of contraception. It involves lower morbidity rates than tubal ligation, and, because it can be performed in a physician's office under local anesthesia, it is less expensive as well. After surgery, the man applies ice to the area and watches for excessive swelling or bleeding.

The couple should understand that complete sterilization does not occur until all sperm have left the system, which may be a month or more. The man should submit semen specimens for analysis until two specimens show no sperm present.

### Hormonal Contraceptives

Hormonal contraceptives alter the normal hormone fluctuations of the menstrual cycle. They may be given by implant, by injection, or orally.

#### HORMONE IMPLANT

The progestin implant (Norplant System) is the most effective reversible form of contraception available today (99.91 percent). Six flexible capsules about 1.5 inches long (the size of a match) are inserted subcutaneously into the upper inner arm under local anesthetic (Fig. 31–3). This area is used because it is easily accessible and low in fat. The capsules are inserted in a fan-shaped configuration and are only slightly visible. They release progestin continuously at gradually decreasing levels over the 5 years they are effective.

The progestin implant is expensive at the time of insertion, although the long-term cost is relatively low. Medicaid generally covers the cost; insurances often pay all or part. It has been used by approximately 1 million women in the United States and by more than 2.5 million women worldwide (AWHONN, 1995).

**Action.** The action of the hormone implant is similar to that of progestin-only OCs. It inhibits ovulation and development of the endometrium and causes cervical mucus changes that impede penetration by the sperm. The implant provides continuous contraception without estrogens and without effort by the woman. Fertility returns promptly after the capsules are removed.

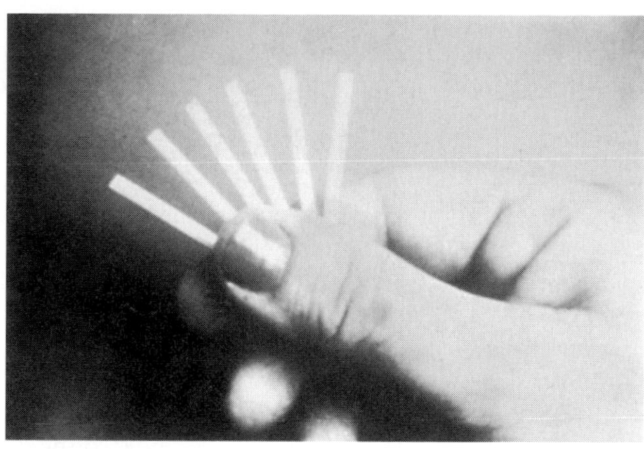

**FIGURE 31–3**

Norplant capsules are inserted under the skin of the upper arm and remain effective for 5 years. (Courtesy of Wyeth-Ayerst Laboratories, Philadelphia, Pennsylvania.)

**Side Effects.** Menstrual changes in up to 80 percent of women are the most common cause for discontinuation of the method (Hatcher et al., 1994). Women may have irregular, midcycle, or prolonged bleeding, which usually decreases by 1 year of use. If necessary, bleeding may be treated with oral estrogen or ibuprofen. Some women have less bleeding than they did before the implants were inserted, or amenorrhea. Other side effects include headaches, weight gain, acne, dizziness, and mood changes. Infection and expulsion of the implants are rare complications. Removal may be difficult if the capsules are deeply implanted. Practitioners must be trained in both insertion and removal.

Women with conditions that would preclude using oral contraceptives generally should not use the implant. It can be inserted after delivery, but breastfeeding women should wait six weeks. It may not be as effective in women weighing more than 150 pounds, as hormone concentration in the blood is less in heavier women.

#### HORMONE INJECTIONS

Depo-Provera, (medroxyprogesterone acetate or DMPA) is an injectable progestin. It prevents ovulation for 14 weeks, although women are advised to repeat doses every 3 months to avoid decreases in hormone levels. It is 99.7 percent effective, convenient, and does not contain estrogen. Action and side effects are similar to those of other progestin contraceptives. Menstrual irregularities are the major reason for discontinuation. Although spotting and breakthrough bleeding are common, amenorrhea occurs in 50 percent of women at 1 year. Weight gain may approximate 4 pounds per year. Other side effects include headaches and hair loss. Women who should not use other hormone contraceptives generally should avoid Depo-Provera as well.

Depo-Provera is given by deep intramuscular injection. The site should not be massaged after injection, as this accelerates absorption. The injection is best given within 5 days of the menstrual period. If given later in the cycle, an additional form of contraception should be used for the rest of the cycle. Women can use Depo-Provera at any age and for any length of time, if they are in good health. For breastfeeding women, it is often started 6 weeks after delivery, when lactation is well established. Fertility returns in approximately 4 to 9 months (AWHONN, 1994).

### ORAL CONTRACEPTIVES

Oral contraceptives are the most widely used contraceptive method in the United States (Hatcher et al., 1994). Combination OCs contain both estrogen and progestin, whereas "minipills" contain only progestin. Both types contain much lower hormone levels than the original OCs, thus decreasing the risk of long-term side effects. Oral contraceptives have a 97 percent typical effectiveness rate.

**Combination.** Estrogen and progestin combinations are the most common OCs and have an action similar to pregnancy in preventing ovulation. The high level of estrogen and progestin prevents the discharge of follicle-stimulating and leuteinizing hormones from the pituitary. This inhibits maturation of the follicle and ovulation. (See Chapter 4 for information about the menstrual cycle.) In addition, the cervical mucus becomes too thick for sperm to penetrate, and the endometrium becomes less hospitable to implantation.

Combination OCs are available in packets of 21 or 28 tablets. With 21-tablet packets, the woman takes one pill daily for 3 weeks, then stops for a week, during which time menses occurs. Packets of 28 tablets include 7 tablets made of an inert substance that the woman takes during the fourth week. This avoids disrupting the everyday routine of taking pills.

Monophasic or multiphasic dosages are available. Monophasic pills have an estrogen and progestin content that remains constant throughout the cycle. With multiphasic pills, the estrogen dose may be constant or increased in the later part of the cycle, whereas the progestin is low at the beginning and is increased later. This helps reduce side effects. Because there may be two or three phases of dose changes, it is important that women take the pills in the proper order.

**Progestin Only.** Oral contraceptives that contain progestin but no estrogen are called minipills. They are useful for women who cannot take estrogen. They are less effective at inhibiting ovulation but cause thickening of the cervical mucus to prevent penetration by sperm and make the endometrial lining unfavorable for implantation. These pills have a lower dose of hormones and may avoid some of the side effects and risk factors associated with estrogen. However, if the woman misses any pills or does not take them at the same time each day, chances of pregnancy increase. Breakthrough bleeding and higher risk of pregnancy have made these OCs less popular than the combination OCs.

**Benefits, Risks, and Cautions.** When choosing oral contraceptives, the balance between the benefits and the risks must be weighed for each individual (Table 31–3). The method has many advantages and can be used by women at any age. Although OCs were once thought unsafe for older women, studies show that women in good health who do not smoke can continue to take OCs until menopause.

**TABLE 31–3 POTENTIAL BENEFITS AND RISKS OF ORAL CONTRACEPTIVES**

| Benefits | Risks* |
|---|---|
| Highly effective contraception. | No protection against sexually transmissible diseases. |
| Reduces ovarian and endometrial cancer by as much as 50%. | May affect carbohydrate metabolism and may worsen diabetes. |
| Protection continues for years after use. Effect on breast and cervical cancer is not yet proven—may increase or decrease risk for breast cancer for certain women. | |
| Regulates menstrual cycles and reduces cramping, menstrual blood loss, and associated anemia. | |
| Decreased incidence of | Increased incidence of |
| Benign breast disease | Deep and superficial vein thrombosis |
| Ovarian cysts | Pulmonary embolism |
| Pelvic inflammatory disease | Myocardial infarction |
| Ectopic pregnancy | Stroke |
| Improves | Hypertension |
| Endometriosis | Migraines |
| Premenstrual syndrome (for some) | Chlamydial infection |
| Dysmenorrhea | Benign liver tumors |
| Fibroids (leiomyomata) | Gallbladder disease |
| | Depression |

* Incidence of many risks is significantly reduced with low-dose oral contraceptives presently used. Avoiding oral contraceptive use in women who smoke or have other risk factors lowers risk for cardiovascular disease significantly.

Smoking increases the incidence of complications for women of all ages. Other risk factors include hypertension, high cholesterol levels, obesity, and diabetes. However, with careful follow-up, diabetic women may use any contraceptive method, if they have no other contraindications (Kjos, 1996).

Although there are risks in using OCs, it is important for women to know that the chances of complications and death during pregnancy and childbirth are greater (Hatcher et al., 1994). Many risks were associated with the higher doses of hormones used in the original OCs but are less of a problem with current OCs. Hazards are decreased by careful screening for risk factors in each woman.

Oral contraceptives provide no protection against STDs and may increase susceptibility to some. Therefore, women should be advised to use a condom and spermicide if their partner may be infected.

**Side Effects.** Approximately 28 percent of women who do not wish to become pregnant discontinue OCs within a year. A major reason is side effects. Most side effects are minor and include signs and symptoms often seen in pregnancy. Decreasing the amount of estrogen helps relieve nausea, headaches, or breast tenderness, whereas increasing the estrogen content prevents breakthrough bleeding. Other side effects include weight gain or loss, fluid retention, amenorrhea, acne, and chloasma. Side effects often decrease after the first few months of use and are less frequent in low dose OCs.

**Teaching.** Education about proper use of OCs greatly increases their effectiveness. Teaching should be extensive when the woman begins to use the hormones. Follow-up is necessary to ensure that her questions and unanticipated problems are resolved. Because the instructions can be complicated, she should have them written clearly and simply in her own language, if she can read. Almost one third of the 3.5 million yearly unintended pregnancies that occur in the United States are due to failure to follow instructions correctly, failure, or discontinuation of OCs (Rosenberg et al., 1995).

The nurse should listen carefully to women's concerns about side effects and help them find methods to relieve them. Accidental pregnancy occurs in almost 25 percent of women who discontinue OCs owing to side effects because they did not use another method of contraception or used a less effective method (Rosenberg, et al., 1995). Women should be instructed that they need a back up contraceptive method readily available should they decide to stop taking their OCs.

***Blood Hormone Levels.*** Because maintaining a constant blood hormone level is important for effectiveness, the woman must take the pills at the same time each day. Many women make them a part of their bedtime routine, whereas others take them with a meal to avoid nausea. Breakthrough bleeding is more likely when there is a significant time variation between doses. Women should use another contraceptive method during the first week of the first cycle until the blood hormones levels are established (Cunningham et al., 1997).

***Missed Doses.*** Instructions for the woman who misses one or more doses should be provided. If a woman misses a period and thinks she may be pregnant because she missed one or more doses, she should stop taking the pills and get a sensitive pregnancy test immediately. It is essential that she use another contraceptive method during this time. Although there is no established association with fetal anomalies, continued use during pregnancy is not advisable.

Another contraceptive method is usually recommended when a dose is missed. The woman should use another method until seven tablets are taken consecutively after the missed dose or for the rest of the cycle if more than one tablet is missed.

***Nutrition.*** Low-estrogen OCs now used do not interfere with nutritional status as those in the past did. Women in good health do not need to take vitamin supplements just because they are taking OCs (Mahan & Escott-Stump, 1996).

***Lactation.*** Combination OCs reduce milk production in lactating women, and very small amounts may be transferred to the milk. Combination forms should be used only after milk production is well established. Progestin-only contraceptives may be a better choice, as they do not affect milk production. Studies to date show no adverse effects on infants breastfed by mothers using OCs (Erwin, 1994).

## Critical to Remember

### CAUTIONS IN USING ORAL CONTRACEPTIVES

Oral contraceptives should not be used by women with a history of any of the following:

- Thrombophlebitis and thromboembolic disorders
- Cerebrovascular or cardiovascular diseases
- Any estrogen-dependent cancer or breast cancer
- Benign or malignant liver tumors

Oral contraceptives should not be used by women who currently have any of the following:

- Any of the above conditions
- Impaired liver function
- Suspected or known pregnancy
- Undiagnosed vaginal bleeding
- Heavy cigarette smoking (more than 15 per day in women older than 35; any use of cigarettes is discouraged and should be evaluated individually)

### Women Want to Know

### What to Do if an Oral Contraceptive Dose Is Missed

The following provides general information about what to do if you miss one or more contraceptive tablets. Talk with your nurse practitioner, nurse-midwife, or physician for specific information suited to your needs.

**One Pill Missed**

Take the pill as soon as you remember it. Take the next pill at the normal time. You will probably not become pregnant after missing one pill, but you may want to use another contraceptive method for 7 days to be sure.

**Two Pills Missed**

Take two pills as soon as you remember. Take two pills the next day also. Taking extra pills 8 to 12 hours apart decreases nausea. *Use another method of contraception until you have been on the pills at least 7 days.*

**Three Pills Missed**

Follow directions of your health care provider who may tell you to throw out the remaining pills and (1) start a new pack immediately or (2) wait for your next period and begin your next pack of pills on the day you usually start them (Sunday or another day as instructed by your health care provider). *Use another method of contraception until you have been on the pills at least 7 days.*

**Inactive Pills Missed Between Days 21 and 28**

Throw away pills missed, and continue to take the rest as scheduled. Contraception will not be affected. Begin a new packet of pills on the same day as usual.

***Other Medications.*** Oral contraceptives may interact with other medications, and the effectiveness of each may be changed. For example, antibiotics, such as ampicillin and tetracycline, and some anticonvulsants decrease the effectiveness of OCs. Therefore, the woman should always tell any health care provider prescribing medications for her what other drugs she is taking.

***Follow-up.*** The woman who takes OCs should have a yearly pelvic examination and a Papanicolaou (Pap) smear, breast examination, and blood pressure measurement. She should report any signs of adverse reaction immediately. Use of the acronym ACHES may help the woman to remember signs that may indicate complications (Table 31–4). Return of fertility usually occurs within 2 to 3 months after the pills are discontinued. A woman should wait until her menstrual cycle is reestablished before conceiving so that she can date the beginning of her pregnancy more accurately.

**Postcoital Emergency Contraception.** Postcoital contraception (often called emergency contraception or the "morning-after pill") is a method to prevent pregnancy after unprotected intercourse. It may be used after contraceptive failure, such as a condom breaking or diaphragm dislodging during intercourse.

**TABLE 31–4 "ACHES"* WARNING SIGNS OF ORAL CONTRACEPTIVE COMPLICATIONS**

| | Warning Sign | Possible Complication |
|---|---|---|
| A | Abdominal pain (severe) | Benign liver tumor, gallbladder disease |
| C | Chest pain, dyspnea, hemoptysis | Pulmonary emboli or myocardial infarction |
| H | Severe headache, weakness or numbness of extremities | Stroke |
| E | Eye problems (visual changes such as blurred or double vision or visual loss, speech disturbance) | Stroke |
| S | Severe leg pain or swelling (calf or thigh) | Deep vein thrombosis |

* The acronym ACHES can be used to help women remember warning signs that may indicate complications when using oral contraceptives. Other signs include jaundice, a breast lump, and depression. The woman should contact her health care provider if any of these signs develop. (Data from Hatcher et al., 1994.)

It may also be used after rape or in other situations when contraceptives were used incorrectly or not at all.

The most common method involves taking a larger than usual dose of an oral contraceptive as soon as possible and not later than 72 hours after unprotected intercourse. A second dose is taken 12 hours after the first. Treatment reduces the risk of pregnancy by 75%. The high hormone levels prevent normal endometrial development and may interfere with fertilization and tubal transport. The treatment is ineffective if pregnancy has already occurred. Antiemetics may be prescribed to treat the side effects of nausea and vomiting.

Combined OC treatment should not be used in women who have contraindications for their use. High doses of progestin-only contraceptives may be preferable for these women. Insertion of the copper T 380A IUD within 5 days of intercourse may also be used and provides 99 percent effectiveness.

## Intrauterine Devices

Intrauterine devices are inserted into the uterus to provide continuous pregnancy prevention. The two types available in the United States, the copper T 380A (ParaGard) and the progestin IUD (Progestasert), are both shaped like the letter T (Fig. 31–4). They are 98 to 99.2 percent effective. Although there was a concern about safety with early models, IUDs are considered very safe at this time. They are often inserted at the 6 weeks postpartum checkup and are safe during lactation. Intrauterine devices are expen-

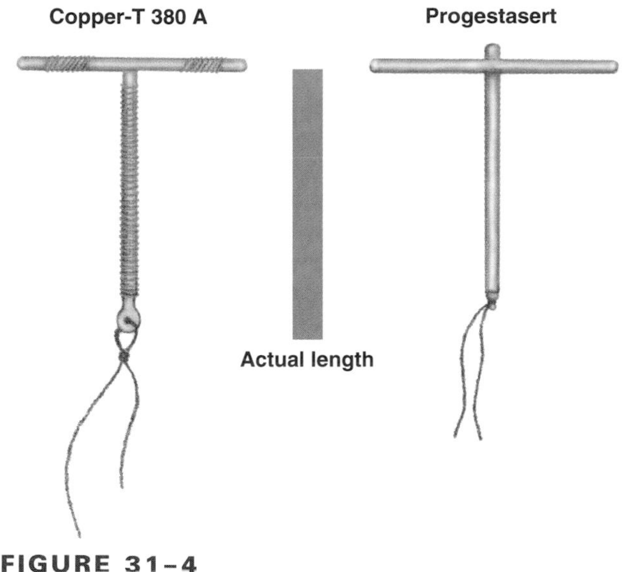


**FIGURE 31-4**

The Copper T 380A (ParaGard) and progestin (Progestasert) intrauterine devices (IUDs). Currently, IUDs are considered a very safe method for preventing pregnancy.

sive at the time of insertion but have a relatively low long-term cost.

#### ACTION

The exact mechanism of action is unknown, but IUDs appear to affect sperm, ova, and the endometrium to prevent fertilization. Sperm are immobilized, and ova move through the fallopian tubes more quickly. The endometrium undergoes a sterile inflammatory response that affects sperm and may prevent implantation. The ParaGard IUD has copper wire wound around it and remains effective for 10 years. Progestin is continuously released from the Progestasert IUD, which must be replaced yearly.

#### SIDE EFFECTS

Side effects include cramping and bleeding with insertion. Menorrhagia (increased bleeding during menstruation) and dysmenorrhea (painful menstruation) are common reasons for removal. They may be more frequent with the copper device. Ibuprofen may relieve cramping, and some women need iron for anemia. Pelvic infections are less common than with the original models. They occur most often in the first few weeks after insertion or are due to STDs. Therefore, only women in mutually monogamous relationships and at low risk for STDs should use IUDs.

Possible complications include expulsion and perforation of the uterus. Women who become pregnant using the IUD are more likely to have ectopic pregnancies, spontaneous abortions, or preterm deliveries. Nulliparous women and those with recent or recurrent pelvic infections, a history of ectopic pregnancy, bleeding disorders, or abnormalities of the uterus should choose another contraceptive method.

#### TEACHING

Teaching the woman about side effects and how to check for the presence of the plastic strings or "tail" extending from the IUD into the vagina is important. The woman should feel for the strings once a week during the first 4 weeks, then monthly after menses, and if she has signs of expulsion (cramping or unexpected bleeding). If the strings are longer or shorter than previously, she should see her health care provider. Signs of infection, such as unusual vaginal discharge, pain or itching, low pelvic pain, and fever, should prompt a call to the physician. Any signs of pregnancy should be reported to rule out ectopic pregnancy and to remove the device if pregnancy occurs. The woman should return yearly for a Pap smear and to check for anemia if menses are heavy.

### Barrier Methods

The barrier methods of contraception involve chemicals or devices that prevent sperm from entering the cervix. The method may kill the sperm or place a temporary partition between the penis and the cervix. All of the barrier methods are coitus-related and may interfere with spontaneity. However, they avoid use of systemic hormones and provide some protection from STDs. Infection with human papillomavirus, an STD, may increase the risk of cervical cancer. Therefore, use of barrier contraceptives may lower the incidence of cervical cancer.

#### CHEMICAL BARRIERS

Chemicals that kill sperm are called *spermicides* and come in many forms. Creams and gels are generally used with mechanical barriers such as the diaphragm or cervical cap. Foams, suppositories, and vaginal film may be used alone. They are inserted into the vagina just before sexual intercourse and are effective for about 1 hour. Vaginal films and suppositories must melt before they become effective, which takes approximately 15 minutes.

Spermicides are readily available without a prescription, are inexpensive per use, and are easy to use. Nonoxynol 9 is used in many products containing spermicide and may provide some protection against chlamydial infection, gonorrhea, genital herpes, trichomoniasis, syphilis, and possibly human immunodeficiency virus (HIV). Spermicides should be used with condoms. They increase lubrication, which decreases the risk of condom breakage.

Women should avoid douching for at least 6 to 8 hours after intercourse and should add more spermicide if coitus is repeated. Sensitivity to the products may cause genital irritation, which could increase susceptibility to HIV infection. Some women and their partners feel that spermicides are messy and interfere with sensation during intercourse. When used alone, spermicides are about 79 percent effective. Effectiveness is increased when spermicides are used with a mechanical barrier method.

#### MECHANICAL BARRIERS

Mechanical barriers are devices placed over the penis or cervix to prevent passage of sperm into the uterus. They include the condom, diaphragm, and cervical cap.

**Male Condom.** Condoms, the only male contraceptive device currently available, are one of the most popular contraceptive methods in the United States. They cover the penis to prevent sperm from entering the vagina. Condoms are most often made of latex and may be coated with spermicide. Some condoms are made from polyurethane or natural membrane. Polyurethane condoms are thinner than latex and can be used by people who are allergic to latex. They may require lubrication to avoid breakage. Natural membrane condoms do not prevent passage of viruses and do not provide protection from STDs caused by viruses. Latex condoms provide the best protection available (other than abstinence) against syphilis, gonorrhea, herpes, chlamydial infection, trichomoniasis, and HIV. For this reason, they should be used during any possible exposure to an STD, even if another contraceptive technique is practiced or if the woman is pregnant.

Condoms are readily available, are inexpensive, and can be carried inconspicuously by the man or the woman. The typical failure rate of 12 percent can be decreased greatly by combining condom use with another method, such as a vaginal spermicide. One large study showed condoms broke at a rate of 1.9 percent and that 2 percent of condoms slipped off during intercourse or withdrawal (Grady & Tanfer, 1994). Reservoir tips and water-based lubricants help prevent breakage. Because condoms must be applied just before intercourse, some couples object to the interference with spontaneity. Others feel that condoms interfere with sensation. People who are allergic to latex should avoid the use of latex condoms, as severe reactions are possible. Condoms may be affected by vaginal medications and should not be used concurrently.

**Female Condom.** The female condom is a polyurethane sheath inserted into the vagina. A flexible ring fits over the cervix like a diaphragm, and another ring extends outside the vagina to partially cover the perineum (Fig. 31–5). Another design is similar to a bikini panty with a pouch that is inserted into the vagina.

The female condom is the first contraceptive device to allow a woman some protection from STDs without relying on the male condom. However, it is less effective, and many women object to it on esthetic grounds. It has a typical failure rate of approximately 21 percent.

**Diaphragm.** The diaphragm is a latex dome surrounded by a spring or coil. The woman places spermicidal cream or gel into the dome and around the rim, then inserts it over the cervix by hand or with a

### Couples Want to Know

### What Is the Proper Way to Use Condoms?

Although condoms are easy to use, proper use increases their effectiveness.

- Condoms are available in a variety of colors, textures, and materials, but those made of latex are most effective. Others may help protect against pregnancy but may not protect against sexually transmissible diseases.

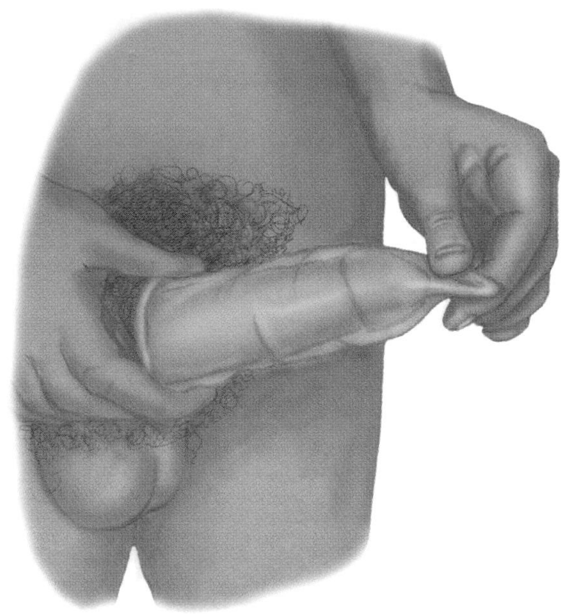

- Check the expiration dates on packages because condoms may deteriorate after 5 years.
- Lubrication may increase comfort for the woman and reduce the risk of breakage. Use a water-soluble lubricant or a spermicide because oil-based products (such as petroleum jelly or baby oil) cause deterioration of the latex.
- Always apply the condom before there is any contact of the penis with the vagina because sperm may be present in pre-ejaculatory fluid.
- Squeeze the air out of the tip of the condom, and leave one-half inch of space at the tip as the condom is rolled onto the erect penis. This allows a place for sperm to collect and helps prevent breakage.
- Withdraw the penis from the vagina before it becomes soft and hold the condom in place so it does not slip off and no semen spills into the vagina.
- Use a new condom each time intercourse is repeated.

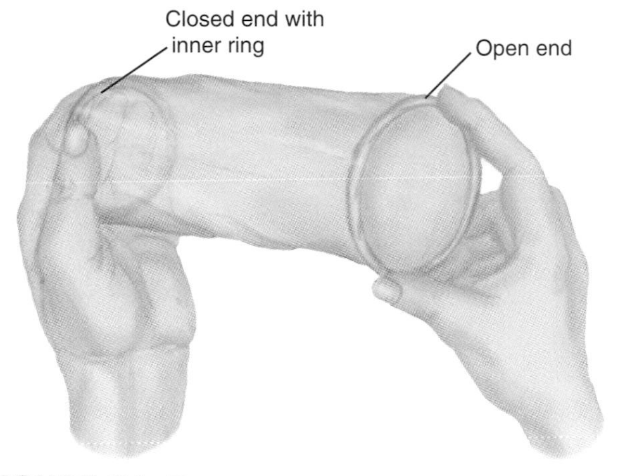


FIGURE 31-5

The female condom. A woman can protect herself from sexually transmissible diseases without relying on use of the male condom.

plastic introducer. When folded, some models arc to form a half-moon shape, which assists in proper placement. Because it covers the cervix, the diaphragm prevents passage of sperm while holding spermicide in place for additional protection. It must be fitted by a nurse practitioner, nurse-midwife, or physician. The woman should be checked for size changes yearly, after a weight gain or loss of more than 10 pounds, and after each pregnancy or abortion. The diaphragm should be replaced every 2 years. The correct size may not be available for all women.

To eliminate interference with spontaneity, some women insert the diaphragm hours in advance when intercourse is possible, although not necessarily planned. Although some women cannot feel the diaphragm once it is in place, others find it noticeable or uncomfortable. Pressure on the urethra may cause irritation and urinary tract infections. Allergies to latex or history of toxic shock syndrome preclude use. The diaphragm may be damaged by some medications used for vaginal candidal infections and should not be used during treatment.

**Cervical Cap.** The cervical cap is similar to the diaphragm but smaller. The flexible latex cup fits over the cervix and remains in place by suction (Fig. 31-6). Women who are difficult to fit with a diaphragm may be able to use the cervical cap. However, cap sizes are limited, and women with cervical abnormalities may not be able to use it. It is 82 percent effective for nulliparous women but only 64 percent effective for women who have already given birth.

Because it is smaller than the diaphragm, the cervical cap is less noticeable and causes no pressure on the bladder. It can remain in place for 48 hours, and more spermicide is not needed if intercourse is repeated. It should not be removed for 6 hours after the last intercourse. Insertion and removal are similar to those for the diaphragm but may be more difficult because the cap is smaller. The nurse should teach the woman to feel her cervix to check placement before and after intercourse because the cap can be dislodged. It should not be used during menses or in women with a history of toxic shock syndrome.

The cap fitting should be checked yearly; after abortion, childbirth, or surgery; or if it dislodges frequently. A Pap smear is required 3 months after the original fitting because some users have had changes indicating cervical neoplasia. If the Pap smear is normal at 3 months, only yearly examinations are necessary.

## Natural Family Planning Methods

Natural family planning methods, also called fertility awareness or periodic abstinence methods, use physiologic cues to predict ovulation and avoid coitus when conditions are favorable for fertilization. They can also help women who wish to become pregnant (see Chapter 32). The ovum may be fertilized for approximately 24 hours, and some sperm may live up to 72 hours in the female genital tract, although most live only 24 hours (Guyton & Hall, 1996). Some research indicates that fertilization is most likely to occur from coitus during the 6 days up to and including ovulation (Wilcox et al., 1995).

Natural family planning helps women learn about how their bodies change throughout the menstrual cycle. It is acceptable to most religious groups and avoids the use of drugs, chemicals, and devices. However, couples must be highly motivated because

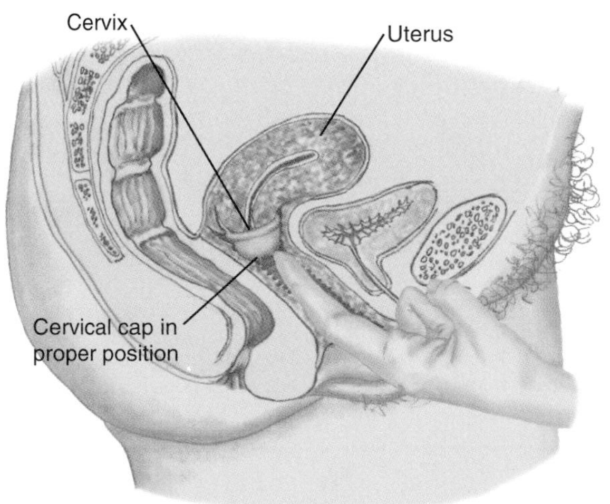


FIGURE 31-6

The cervical cap is inserted much like the diaphragm. The woman should check to be certain that it is placed over the cervix.

## Women Want to Know

### How to Use a Diaphragm

Follow instructions carefully when using your diaphragm. Skill at insertion and removal increases with practice.

- Plan to insert the diaphragm during lovemaking or several hours before. Empty your bladder before insertion.
- Spread about a teaspoon of spermicidal cream or gel inside the dome and around the rim.

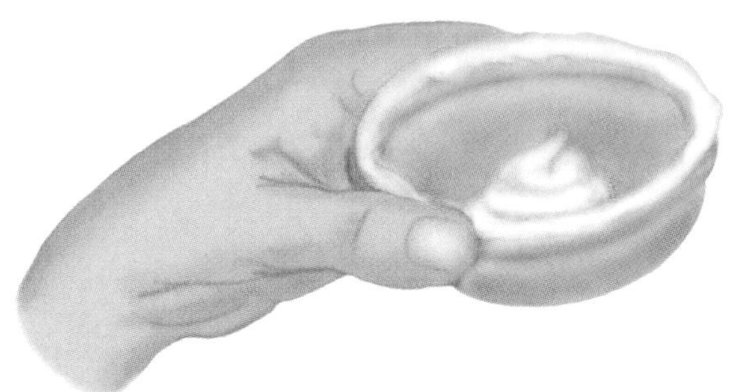

- Fold the diaphragm, and insert it into the vagina with the spermicide toward the cervix. A squatting position or placing one foot on a chair makes insertion and removal easier.

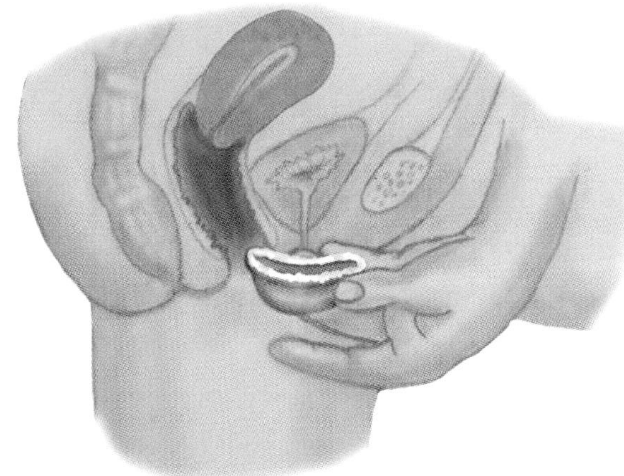

- Be sure that the front rim fits behind your pubic bone and that you can feel the cervix through the center of the diaphragm,

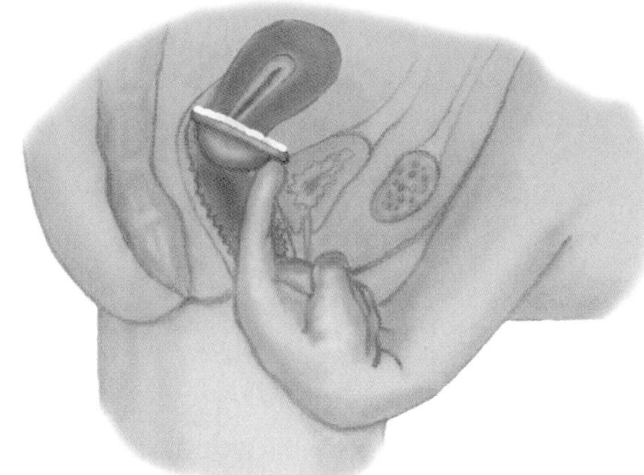

- If more than 6 hours elapse between the insertion and intercourse or if you have intercourse again, insert more spermicide into the vagina without removing the diaphragm. Some women use more spermicide after 2 to 3 hours.
- Leave the diaphragm in place at least 6 hours after the last intercourse, but leave it in place for no more than a total of 24 hours to reduce risk of infection.
- Douching with the diaphragm in place is unnecessary and will lessen the effectiveness.
- To remove the diaphragm, assume a squatting position and bear down. Hook a finger around the front rim to break the suction, and pull down.

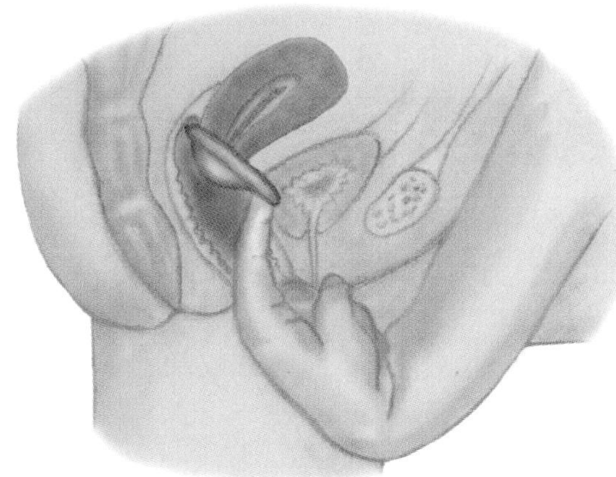

- Wash the diaphragm with mild soap, and dry well after each use. Inspect it occasionally for small holes by holding it up to a light. If you find one, use another contraceptive method and go to your physician, nurse-midwife, or nurse practitioner for a new diaphragm.

they must abstain from intercourse as much as half the menstrual cycle. Natural family planning methods may be very effective if used perfectly. However, the method is very unforgiving and errors in predicting ovulation or intercourse during the forbidden times carry a high risk of pregnancy. Some women use the method to determine when they are fertile and use a barrier contraceptive at that time.

#### CALENDAR

The calendar method is based on the fact that ovulation occurs approximately 14 days before the onset of menses. This allows women with regular cycles to estimate when ovulation will occur. The woman keeps track of the length of her cycles for 6 months to determine the range in cycle length. She subtracts 18 to 20 days from the shortest cycle and 10 days from the longest cycle to predict the time when fertilization is possible. Thus, if her cycles varied from 28 to 32 days, she could be fertile between days 8 and days 22 ($28 - 20 = 8$, $32 - 10 = 22$). The calendar method is unreliable because many factors, such as illness or stress, can affect the time of ovulation.

#### BASAL BODY TEMPERATURE

In the basal body temperature method, the woman charts her oral temperature each morning before getting out of bed or increasing her activity, which would cause her temperature to rise (see Procedure 32–1, p. 909). Her basal body temperature may drop slightly before ovulation and then rise approximately 0.2° to 0.45°C (0.4° to 0.8°F) with ovulation. The temperature remains higher throughout the second half of the cycle because of progesterone. The woman is no longer fertile on the third day after the rise in temperature.

Used alone, this method is not reliable because temperature changes are very small and the rise in temperature indicates that ovulation has already occurred. Intercourse the day before the temperature rise may well result in pregnancy. For some women, the drop that occurs before the rise in temperature may be too small to be noticed. In addition, illness, a sleepless night, or stress could affect the temperature.

#### CERVICAL MUCUS

Also called the Billings or "ovulation" method, the cervical mucus technique is based on changes in cervical mucus due to rising estrogen levels during the follicular phase of the menstrual cycle. The woman assesses the cervical mucus by wiping it from the vaginal orifice with tissue each day. There is no mucus for the first 3 to 4 days after menses, and then thick, sticky mucus begins to appear. As estrogen increases, the mucus changes to clear, slippery, and stretchy, like egg white. This condition is called *spinnbarkeit* (see Procedure 32–1, p. 911). After ovulation, mucus decreases in amount and becomes thick and sticky again.

To prevent pregnancy, couples must avoid intercourse from the time mucus is first present until the evening of the fourth day after the height of slippery mucus. Intercourse during menstruation is forbidden because some women may enter the fertile period before the end of menses. It is allowed only every other day when there is no mucus, because semen interferes with mucus assessment.

#### SYMPTOTHERMAL METHOD

The symptothermal method combines the calendar, basal body temperature, and cervical mucus methods. In addition, other symptoms that occur near ovulation, such as weight gain, abdominal bloating, mittelschmerz (pain on ovulation), or increased libido, are noted. This increases awareness of when ovulation occurs and increases effectiveness.

#### POSTOVULATION METHOD

The postovulation method uses any combination of the natural family planning methods, but intercourse is avoided from the first day of the menstrual cycle until the end of the fertile period. Therefore, abstinence is necessary for more than half the cycle. Although this is the most effective of the natural techniques, it is difficult for many couples to achieve.

#### ✓ CHECK YOUR READING

9. What factors should a couple consider in deciding which method of sterilization to use?
10. What is the mechanism of action of hormonal contraceptives?
11. What education is important for woman choosing an IUD?
12. How do barrier methods of contraception work?
13. What are the advantages and disadvantages of natural family planning methods?

## Least Reliable Methods of Contraception

The following methods of contraception are not considered reliable. However, they are used by women who lack information about their risks and other options or who will not use other methods for medical or personal reasons. The nurse needs to be familiar with these methods to help women understand the risks involved.

#### BREASTFEEDING

Breastfeeding inhibits ovulation because suckling and prolactin interfere with secretion of gonadotropin-releasing hormone and luteinizing hormone. During lactation, the ovarian response to follicle-stimulating hormone and luteinizing hormone may be altered. The frequency, intensity, and duration of suckling are very important in inhibiting ovulation.

Women who breastfeed completely (at least 10 times in 24 hours with no supplementary feedings) may avoid ovulation and resumption of menstrual cycles. However, use of formula or solids decreases the frequency and duration of breastfeeding, increases the length of time between feedings, and reduces night feedings. This may cause ovulation and a return of menses. After the first 3 to 6 months, prolactin levels decrease and the menstrual cycle generally resumes by 6 months. Another method of contraception should be used at this time or before if menses resumes.

#### COITUS INTERRUPTUS

Also called withdrawal, coitus interruptus is the removal of the penis from the vagina before ejaculation. Although it has an effectiveness rate of 81 percent, it requires great control by the man and may be unsatisfying for both partners. Even a man who wishes to use the method may misjudge the timing and withdraw too late. Fluid that escapes from the penis before ejaculation is not felt by the man or woman and may contain sperm. Sperm spilled on the vulva may enter the vagina and cause pregnancy.

## Application of Nursing Process: Choosing a Contraceptive Method

Contraceptive failure often occurs because women lack knowledge of how to use their contraceptive methods correctly or choose methods unsuited to their needs. When contraception fails, the woman is exposed to the physical, psychological, and social consequences of unplanned pregnancy. Lack of understanding may also expose her to unnecessary side effects, possible complications, or STDs.

### Assessment

Because contraception is a very private matter, approach it in a sensitive manner. Perform the assessment in a quiet area where interruptions are unlikely, and keep voices low to increase the woman's comfort. Assure the woman that her confidentiality will be maintained.

#### INTRODUCING THE SUBJECT

In the postpartum setting, introduce the subject by asking the woman if she plans to have more children. Most women indicate a desire to wait a period of time before the next pregnancy. Ask, "What method of family planning are you thinking about using now?" or "How did you feel about the method you used before pregnancy?" These kinds of questions may identify problems that the woman has had with contraception. In other settings, a woman may make some reference to her contraceptive method. The nurse can respond by asking, "How do you like using (name method)?" This shows the nurse is interested if the woman wishes to pursue the topic.

#### DETERMINING THE WOMAN'S UNDERSTANDING

Determine the woman's understanding of her contraceptive technique. For example, ask how she inserts her diaphragm, when and where she adds spermicide, or what time of day she takes her OC. The woman should know how to use her technique effectively and what to do in special circumstances, such as when she misses an OC pill or has difficulty removing her diaphragm. Explore any misinformation, concerns, or problems that she may have in regard to effectiveness, technique, or common side effects of the method.

#### ASSESSING THE WOMAN'S SATISFACTION

Assess the woman's satisfaction with her contraceptive. The length of time that she has used the method is important. Women may be unsure about their method in the early months until they gain comfort from repetitive use. Satisfaction, as well as effectiveness, increases with greater familiarity with the method. Side effects also affect satisfaction. They may be severe enough to cause the woman to consider another method, or they may be relieved by simple techniques. Be sure that what the woman considers simple side effects are not indications of complications that necessitate referral for treatment.

#### DISCUSSING AVAILABLE CHOICES

If the woman is considering a change in contraceptive method, discuss available choices with her. Assess for factors that would help determine the best method for the individual woman. Include past history of medical conditions that might eliminate certain methods, childbearing history, cultural and religious beliefs, and intensity of desire to prevent pregnancy. The woman's ability to understand and follow complicated directions is important as well.

The type of relationship that a couple has is important in terms of contraceptive choice and protection against STDs. If the relationship is mutually monogamous, there is no risk of STDs if neither partner is infected. If either of the couple has more than one partner, protection against STDs with a barrier method is essential, even if the woman uses a contraceptive that is effective against pregnancy.

Frequency of coitus may help determine the best choice of contraception. For occasional sexual intercourse, a barrier method may be most satisfactory. If intercourse is frequent, the woman may desire a method that is always in place, such as an IUD or a hormone implant. Explore her past experience with other methods, what she considers important, and her individual preferences. The woman who wants to avoid hormones that have a systemic effect is not a candidate for OCs or implants. Ask about beliefs and values that might eliminate certain choices.

## Analysis

Lack of knowledge about family planning is common and can lead to physical, psychological, and social complications in a woman's life. A nursing diagnosis that addresses this problem is Risk for Altered Health Maintenance related to lack of understanding about contraceptive methods chosen and available.

## Planning

Outcomes for this diagnosis are that the woman will do the following:

- Correctly describe how to use her contraceptive method, including solving common problems.
- Describe common side effects, indications of complications, and correct follow-up.
- Report that she and her partner are satisfied with their contraceptive method.
- Describe other methods available, and choose one if she desires a different form of contraception.

## Interventions

Interventions involve follow-up of problems that may interfere with the woman's ability to maintain health. Increasing her understanding of contraceptive techniques will be the basis of the teaching plan.

### INCREASING UNDERSTANDING OF THE CHOSEN METHOD

Fill in gaps in the woman's knowledge about how her contraceptive method works, its effectiveness, advantages and disadvantages, common side effects and complications, and when to seek help. Use demonstrations and return demonstrations of how to use the method (such as inserting a cervical cap or checking for IUD strings). Give suggestions for managing side effects and common problems.

### TEACHING ABOUT OTHER METHODS

Provide information about other forms of contraceptives, if the woman wishes. Compare other methods with the one the woman is using. Discuss aspects most important to the individual woman and her lifestyle. If a prescription or fitting is needed, discuss what may happen during the visit.

### PROTECTING AGAINST SEXUALLY TRANSMISSIBLE DISEASES

Address defense against STDs, particularly if the woman is using a method that does not provide protection. Again, this is a delicate subject. A way to approach it might be to say, "The method you are using is very effective against pregnancy but does not protect you against diseases you might catch from a partner. This is important because some diseases, like HIV, can never be cured. Others can cause infections that could prevent you from having children later. If there is any chance that you or your partner might have sex with more than one person or that your partner might have an infection, you should protect yourself by using one of the barrier types of contraception along with the one you are using. Let me explain about those further."

### INCLUDING THE WOMAN'S PARTNER

Invite the woman to include her partner in discussions, if possible. He may influence the woman's choice of contraception and whether she actually uses it and uses it correctly. If the partner understands the proper method of use, he may be more cooperative and this will help to ensure contraceptive success.

## Evaluation

Evaluate the woman's understanding of the correct use of her contraceptive technique. She should describe accurately all aspects of her contraceptive method, including how to solve common problems and when to seek help for side effects or complications. Evaluate continued understanding, compliance with proper use, and satisfaction with the method at later visits. The woman who wishes to change her contraceptive method should describe other contraceptives available and how to use them. She should choose a new method and visit a nurse practitioner, nurse-midwife, or physician, if necessary, for further discussion, examination, fitting, or prescription.

## SUMMARY CONCEPTS

- Women usually choose the contraceptive method a couple uses because they are the ones who must practice most methods and are most affected by contraceptive failure.
- The nurse plays an important role in educating women about contraceptive techniques available and their correct use.
- In choosing the best contraceptive method for an individual woman, safety, protection from STDs, effectiveness, convenience, education needed, side effects, interference with spontaneity, availability, expense, preference, and culture are all important.
- Because some methods have potential for serious complications, an informed consent form may be necessary.
- Adolescents often have erroneous beliefs and incorrect information about contraception that increase their risk of pregnancy and STDs.
- Teenagers may avoid seeking contraceptive information because they are concerned about confi-

dentiality, do not want to admit that they are sexually active, are afraid of pelvic examinations, or fear that contraception will have an adverse effect on their health.

- Adolescents feel more comfortable talking about contraception with a nurse who has an accepting attitude, provides extra time for education, and uses understandable terms and audiovisual materials.
- Contraception is necessary until menstruation has ceased for 2 years. The healthy perimenopausal woman who does not smoke or have contraindications can use any method of contraception safely.
- Sterilization offers permanent contraception. A tubal ligation can be performed soon after birth or at any time. Vasectomy is less expensive and can be performed in an office under local anesthesia. Although surgery to reverse sterilization is possible, it is expensive and not always successful.
- Hormonal contraceptives include OCs, hormone injections, and the progestin implant. They inhibit ovulation and make the cervical mucus unreceptive to sperm. Side effects and complications make these unsuitable for some women.
- Intrauterine devices are very effective and safe in women with no risk of STDs. Women must learn how to check for the device's strings and when to seek medical treatment.
- Barrier methods may be chemical or mechanical. They kill or prevent sperm from entering the cervix and provide some protection against STDs.
- Natural family planning methods involve avoidance of coitus when physiologic cues suggest that ovulation is likely. They help a woman learn about her body, avoid the use of chemicals, are inexpensive, and are acceptable to most religions. However, they involve extensive education and high motivation and have a high risk of pregnancy should error occur.

### References and Readings


American College of Obstetricians and Gynecologists. (1996). Emergency oral contraception. ACOG *Practice Patterns, Number* 2. Washington, D.C.: Author.

Association of Women's Health, Obstetric, and Neonatal Nurses (AWHONN). (1994). Clinical commentary: Medroxyprogesterone acetate for contraceptive use. Washington, D.C.: Author.

AWHONN. (1995). Wyeth-Ayerst offers legal aid to Norplant system prescribers. AWHONN *Voice*, 3(3), 2.

Beckman, L.J., & Harvey, S.M. (1996). Factors affecting the consistent use of barrier methods of contraception. *Obstetrics and Gynecology*, 88(3, suppl.), 65S–71S.

Burkman, R.T. (1994). Contraception and family planning. In A.H. DeCherney & M.L. Pernoll (Eds.), *Current obstetric and gynecologic diagnosis and treatment* (8th ed.). Norwalk, Conn.: Appleton & Lange.

Coker, A.L., Harlap, S., & Fortney, J.A. (1993). Oral contraceptives and reproductive cancers: Weighing the risks and benefits. *Family Planning Perspectives*, 25(1), 17–21.

Cunningham, F.G., MacDonald, P.C., Gant, N.F., Leveno, K.J., Gilstrap, L.C., Hankins, G.D.V., et al. (1997). *Williams obstetrics.* (20th ed.). Norwalk, Conn.: Appleton & Lange.

Dinerman, L.M., Wilson, M.D., Duggan, A.K., & Joffe, A. (1995). Outcomes of adolescents using levonorgestrel implants vs. oral contraceptives or other contraceptive methods. *Arch Pediatric Adolescent Medicine*, 149, 967–972.

Edwards, S.R. (1994). The role of men in contraceptive decision making: Current knowledge and future implications. *Family Planning Perspectives*, 26(2), 77–82.

Erwin, P.C. (1994). To use or not use combined hormonal oral contraceptives during lactation. *Family Planning Perspectives*, 26(1), 26–30+.

Freda, M.C. (1994). Childbearing, reproductive control, aging women, and health care: The projected ethical debates. *Journal of Obstetric, Gynecologic, and Neonatal Nursing*, 23(2), 144–152.

Freda, M.C., Abruzzo-Fogarassy, M., Adams, N.V., Davini, D., DeVore, N., & Merkatz, I.R. (1996). Women's responses to Depo-Provera. MCN: *American Journal of Maternal Child Nursing*, 21(4), 183–186.

Geerling, J.H. (1995). Natural family planning. *American Family Physician*, 52(6), 1749–1756.

Gerchufsky, M. (1995). Updating family planning options. *Advance for Nurse Practitioners*, 3(5), 18–23.

Grady, W.R., & Tanfer, K. (1994). Condom breakage and slippage among men in the United States. *Family Planning Perspectives*, 26(3), 107–112.

Grimes, D.A. (Ed.). (1994). Adolescent pregnancy prevention programs. *The Contraceptive Report*, 5(2), 4–14.

Grimes, D.A. (Ed.). (1995). 30 Years of change: The current perspective on cardiovascular risks and oral contraceptives. *Contraceptive Report*, 6(2), 4–14+.

Gross, T.P., & Schlesselman, J.J. (1994). The estimated effect of oral contraceptive use on the cumulative risk of epithelial ovarian cancer. *Obstetrics and Gynecology*, 83, 419–424.

Guyton, A.C., & Hall, J.E. (1996). *Textbook of medical physiology* (9th ed.). Philadelphia: W.B. Saunders.

Hatasaka, H. (1995). Implantable levonorgestrel contraception: 4 years of experience with Norplant. *Clinical Obstetrics and Gynecology*, 38 (4), 859–871.

Hatcher, R.A., Trussell, J., Stewart, F., et al. (1994). *Contraceptive technology* (16th ed.). New York: Irvington Publishers.

Hesla, J.S., & Murphy, A.A. (1995). The effects of contraceptive agents on the endometrium. *Infertility and Reproductive Medicine Clinics of North America*, 6(2), 379–400.

Hiltabiddle, S.J. (1996). Adolescent condom use, the health belief model, and the prevention of sexually transmitted disease. *Journal of Obstetric, Gynecologic, and Neonatal Nursing*, 25(1), 61–66.

Hinkle, L.T. (1994). Education and counseling for Norplant users. *Journal of Obstetric, Gynecologic, and Neonatal Nursing*, 23(5), 387–301.

Jambunathan, J., & Stewart, S. (1995). Hmong women in Wisconsin: What are their concerns in pregnancy and childbirth? *Birth*, 22(4), 204–210.

Kipersztok, S. (1995). The new progestins. *Infertility and Reproductive Medicine Clinics of North America*, 6(1), 61–75.

Kjos, S. (1996). Contraception in diabetic women. *Obstetrics and Gynecology Clinics of North America*, 23(1), 243–258.

Lande, R.E. (1995). New era for injectables. *Population reports*, Series K, 23(5). Baltimore: Johns Hopkins University, Population Information Program.

Lauver, D., Armstrong, K., Marks, S., & Schwarz, S. (1995). HIV risk status and preventive behaviors among 17,619 women. *Journal of Obstetric, Gynecologic, and Neonatal Nursing*, 24(1), 33–39.

Lethbridge, D.J. (1995). Fertility management in Taiwanese and African-American women. *Journal of Obstetric, Gynecologic, and Neonatal Nursing*, 24(5), 459–463.

Libbus, M.K. (1992). Condoms as primary prevention in sexually active women. MCN: *American Journal of Maternal Child Nursing*, 17(5), 256–260.

Lindberg, C.E. (1997). Emergency contraception: The nurse's role in providing postcoital options. *Journal of Obstetric, Gynecologic, and Neonatal Nursing*, 26(2), 144–152.

Mahan, L.K., & Escott-Stump, S. (1996). *Krause's food, nutrition, and diet therapy* (9th ed.). Philadelphia: W.B. Saunders.

Marquette, C.M., Koonin, L.M., Antarsh, L., Gargiullo, P.M., & Smith, J.C. (1995). Vasectomy in the United States, 1991. *American Journal of Public Health*, 85(5), 644–649.

Moore, R. (1994). *Contemporary studies in women's health: Contraception issues and options for young women*. Fair Lawn, N.J.: MPE Communications, Inc.

Murphy, P., Kirkman, A., & Hale, R.W. (1995). A national survey of women's attitudes toward oral contraception and other forms of birth control. *Women's Health Issues*, 5(2), 94–99.

Nelson, A. (1995). Patient selection key to IUD success. *Contemporary OB/GYN*, 40(10), 49–62.

O'Connell, M.L. (1996). The effect of birth control methods on sexually transmitted disease/HIV risk. *Journal of Obstetric, Gynecologic, and Neonatal Nursing*, 25(6), 476–480.

Potter, L.S. (1996). How effective are contraceptives? The determination and measurement of pregnancy rates. *Obstetrics and Gynecology*, 88(3, suppl.), 113S–123S.

Rosenberg, M.J., Waugh, M.S., & Long, S. (1995). Unintended pregnancies and use, misuse and discontinuation of oral contraceptives. *Journal of Reproductive Medicine*, 40(5), 355–360.

Speroff, L. (1992). The risk of breast cancer associated with oral contraception and hormone replacement therapy. *Women's Health Issues*, 2(2), 63–74.

Still, J.M. (Ed.). (1994). *Contemporary studies in women's health: Issues in contraceptive method selection*. Fair Lawn, N.J.: MPE Communications, Inc.

Tanfer, K. (1994). Knowledge, attitudes and intentions of American women regarding the hormonal implant. *Family Planning Perspectives*, 26(2), 60–65.

Treiman, K., Liskin, L., Kols, A., & Rinehart, W. (1995). IUD's—An update. *Population Reports* (Series B, No. 6). Baltimore: Johns Hopkins University, Population Information Program.

Trussell, J. Ellertson, C., & Stewart, F. (1996). The effectiveness of Yuzpe regimen of emergency contraception. *Family Planning Perspectives*, 28(2), 58–64, 87–88.

Trussell, J., Hatcher, R., Cates, W., Stewart, F.H., & Kost, K. (1990). Contraceptive failure in the United States: An update. *Studies in Family Planning*, 21(1), 51–54.

Trussell, J., Leveque, J.A., Koenig, J.D., London, R., Borden, S., Henneberry, J., LaGuardia, K.D., Stewart, F., Wilson, T.G., Wysocki, S., & Strauss, M. (1995). The economic value of contraception: A comparison of 15 methods. *American Journal of Public Health*, 85(4), 494–503.

Trussell, J., Sturgen, K., Strickler, J., & Dominik, R. (1994). Comparative contraceptive efficacy of the female condom with other barrier methods. *Family Planning Perspectives*, 26(2), 66–72.

U.S. Department of Health and Human Services, Public Health Service. (1995). *Healthy people 2000: Midcourse review and 1995 revisions*. Washington, D.C.: Author.

Wilcox, A.J., Weinberg, C.R., & Baird, D.D. (1995). Timing of sexual intercourse in relation to ovulation. *New England Journal of Medicine*, 333(23), 1517–1521.

# 32

# Infertility

## OBJECTIVES

1. Describe settings in which the nurse may encounter couples who have infertility problems.
2. Explain factors that can impair a couple's ability to conceive.
3. Explain factors that may cause repeated pregnancy losses.
4. Specify evaluations that may be performed when a couple seeks help for their infertility.
5. Explain the use of procedures and treatments that may aid a couple's ability to conceive and carry the fetus to viability.
6. Analyze how infertility can affect a couple and others in their family.
7. Summarize the nurse's role when caring for couples experiencing problems with fertility.

## DEFINITIONS

**anovulatory (or anovular)** *Menstrual cycles occurring without ovulation.*

**azoospermia** *Absence of sperm in semen.*

**climacteric** *Endocrine, body, and psychic changes occurring at the end of a woman's reproductive period. Also informally called menopause.*

**endometriosis** *Presence of endometrial tissue (uterine lining) outside the uterine cavity.*

**ferning (or fern test)** *The microscopic fern-like appearance of dried cervical mucus that is most apparent at the time of ovulation.*

**gametogenesis** *Development and maturation of the sperm and ova.*

**gestational surrogate** *A woman who carries the embryo of an infertile couple and relinquishes the child after birth.*

**impotence** *Inability of a man to achieve or maintain an erection of the penis that is sufficiently rigid to permit successful sexual intercourse.*

**incompetent cervix** *Inability of the cervix to remain closed long enough during pregnancy for the fetus to survive.*

**infertility** *Inability of a couple to conceive after 1 year of regular intercourse (two to three times weekly) without using contraception; also, the involuntary inability to conceive and produce viable offspring when the couple chooses. Primary infertility occurs in a couple who has never conceived; secondary infertility occurs in a couple who has conceived at least once before.*

**oligospermia** *A decreased number of sperm in semen, usually considered to be under 20 million per milliliter.*

**retrograde ejaculation** *Discharge of semen into the bladder rather than from the end of the penis.*

**semen** *Spermatozoa with their nourishing and protective fluid; discharged at ejaculation.*
**spinnbarkheit** *Clear, slippery, stretchy quality of cervical mucus during ovulation.*
**sterility** *Total inability to conceive.*
**surrogate mother** *A fertile woman who is inseminated with the purpose of conceiving and relinquishing a child to an infertile couple.*
**varicocele** *Abnormal dilation or varicosity of veins in the spermatic cord.*

Although infertility care is a specialty, many general practice nurses meet persons who are seeking help for infertility or who have had treatment for it in varied settings. Friends and family members often see the nurse as one who can answer questions and refer them to appropriate resources when they have problems conceiving. Nurses who work in the perioperative area may care for these couples as they have diagnostic or therapeutic surgery. Nurses who work with urology patients often see men who are being evaluated or treated for infertility. In the emergency department, nurses may care for women who are having a spontaneous abortion of a hard-won pregnancy.

Nurses who work in antepartum, intrapartum, and postpartum settings often encounter couples who have a new baby after successful therapy. In addition, parenthood after infertility is not always easy, and nurses who work in pediatric or psychosocial settings may counsel families needing help with parenting and changes in their personal relationships.

## Extent of Infertility

The extent of infertility depends on how the problem is defined. Infertility is not an absolute condition; it is a reduced ability to conceive. Infertility is strictly defined as the inability to conceive after 1 year of unprotected regular sexual intercourse. A more workable definition does not specify a time limit but recognizes that infertility is any involuntary inability to conceive at the time desired. The definition is commonly expanded to include couples who conceive but repeatedly lose a pregnancy (*pregnancy wastage*) before the fetus is old enough to survive. Couples with primary infertility have never conceived. Couples with secondary infertility may have conceived before but are unable to conceive again.

About 15 percent of U.S. couples cannot have a baby when they desire (Edwards & Brody, 1995). Couples who delay childbearing until their mid to late 30s feel pressured by the approaching end of the woman's reproductive years. To older couples, delay in achieving pregnancy or having a living baby is more significant than for young couples, who have more years to pursue pregnancy.

Although the rate of infertility has not increased, more couples are seeking help for impaired conception. Some couples delay childbearing until their mid to late 30s, when a natural decline in fertility begins. Because of advances in diagnosis and treatment, couples who might have accepted childlessness may enter infertility therapy or resume therapy they had abandoned. In addition, some women want to have a child without a male partner and may be served by infertility services.

## Factors Contributing to Infertility

The ability to conceive depends not only on normal reproductive function in each partner but also on a sensitive interaction between the partners. For some couples, identification and treatment of infertility are simple; for other couples, complex evaluation and treatment are required.

The study of infertility underscores the delicacy of the reproductive process. Because some factors contributing to infertility remain unknown, treatment of an identified problem does not always lead to a successful pregnancy. For example, it may be likely that a couple will be infertile because of problems in either or both partners, but the couple nevertheless has several children. About 20 percent of infertile couples have no identified problem, yet some never conceive despite having undergone all available treatments.

### Factors in the Man

The test of a man's fertility is his ability to initiate pregnancy in a fertile woman. Few absolute criteria exist to distinguish normal from abnormal male fertility, although an adequate number of sperm having normal structure and function must be deposited near the woman's cervix. There may be problems with the sperm, with erection or ejaculation, or with the seminal fluid that carries the sperm into the woman's reproductive tract.

#### ABNORMALITIES OF THE SPERM

Many factors can impair the number, structure, or function of sperm. Some conditions are temporary, such as an acute illness; other conditions are perma-

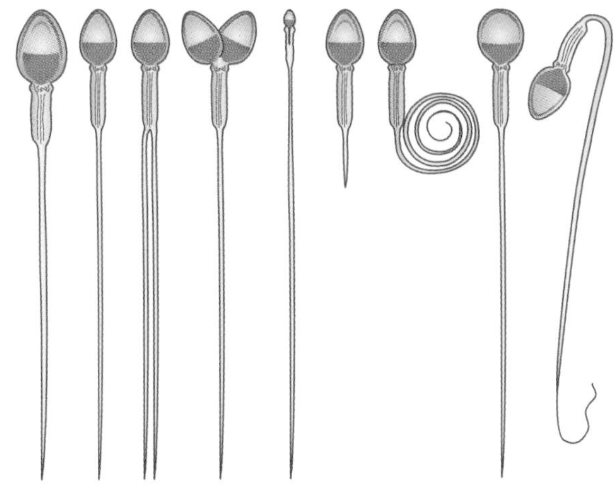

**FIGURE 32–1**

Abnormal infertile sperm compared with a normal sperm on the left. (From Guyton, A.C., & Hall, J.E. [1996]. *Textbook of medical physiology* [9th ed., p. 1008]. Philadelphia: W.B. Saunders.)

nent, such as a genetic disorder. A single finding may be abnormal, or there may be several. Further complicating evaluation of a man's fertility are the normal daily variations in semen.

Evaluation of the semen may reveal that the man has azoospermia or oligospermia. The average number of sperm released at ejaculation is 400 million. Twenty million sperm per milliliter of semen is probably the minimum number adequate for unassisted fertilization.

A sufficient number of normal sperm must move in a purposeful direction to reach the ovum in the fallopian tube. Abnormal sperm structure or movement may reduce fertility, regardless of the actual number of sperm (Fig. 32–1). Inflammatory processes in the man's reproductive organs may cause the sperm to clump, inhibiting their motility and fertilizing ability. Other sperm may look normal yet may be unable to penetrate the ovum.

Many factors can impair the number and function of the sperm, such as the following:

- Abnormal hormonal stimulation of sperm production
- Acute or chronic illness such as mumps, cirrhosis, or renal failure
- Infections of the genital tract
- Anatomic abnormalities, such as a varicocele, or obstruction of the ducts that carry sperm to the penis
- Exposure to toxins, such as lead, pesticides, or other chemicals
- Therapeutic treatments, such as antineoplastic drugs or radiation for cancer
- Excessive alcohol intake
- Use of illicit drugs, such as marijuana or cocaine
- An elevated scrotal temperature resulting from febrile illness or repeated use of saunas or hot tubs
- Immunologic factors, produced by the man against his own sperm (autoantibodies) or by the woman, causing the sperm to clump or be unable to penetrate the ovum

#### ABNORMAL ERECTIONS

Abnormal erections reduce the man's ability to deposit sperm-bearing seminal fluid in the woman's upper vagina. Erections are influenced by both physical and psychological factors. Central nervous system dysfunction, which may be caused by drugs, psychiatric disturbance, or chronic illness, can interfere with erections. Spinal cord disorders and disorders or surgery that affects the autonomic nervous system may also disrupt normal erections. Peripheral vascular disease reduces the amount of blood entering the penis and thus reduces the ability to maintain an erection. Drugs, such as antihypertensives, may reduce the erection or shorten its duration.

#### ABNORMAL EJACULATION

Abnormal ejaculation prevents deposition of the sperm in the ideal place to achieve pregnancy. Retrograde ejaculation is the release of semen backward into the bladder rather than forward through the tip of the penis. Conditions that may cause retrograde ejaculation are diabetes, neurologic disorders, surgery that impairs function of the sympathetic nerves, and drugs such as antihypertensives and psychotropics. Men who have suffered spinal cord injury may retain the ability to ejaculate, depending on the level of cord damage.

Anatomic abnormalities, such as hypospadias (urethral opening on the underside of the penis), may cause deposition of semen near the vaginal outlet rather than near the cervix.

Excessive alcohol intake or use of illicit drugs can adversely affect ejaculation as well as sperm number and function. Ejaculation may be slow, absent, or retrograde when a man takes drugs that affect neurologic coordination of this event. Premature ejaculation is usually related to psychological disorders, such as performance anxiety or unresolved conflicts.

#### ABNORMALITIES OF SEMINAL FLUID

The seminal fluid nourishes, protects, and carries sperm into the vagina until they enter the cervix. Only sperm enter the cervix; the seminal fluid remains in the vagina. Semen coagulates immediately after ejaculation but liquefies within 30 minutes, permitting forward movement of sperm. Seminal fluid that remains thick traps the sperm, impeding their movement into the cervix. The pH of seminal fluid is slightly alkaline to protect the sperm from the acidic secretions of the vagina. Adequate fructose must be present to provide energy for the sperm.

The specific abnormality found in the seminal fluid suggests the cause of the abnormality, such as obstruction or infection in a specific area of the genital tract. Seminal fluid that is abnormal in amount, consistency, or chemical composition suggests obstruction, inflammation, or infection. The presence of large numbers of leukocytes suggests infection.

**CHECK YOUR READING**

1. How is infertility defined? What is the difference between primary and secondary infertility?
2. What are normal characteristics of sperm and of the seminal fluid that carries them into the woman's vagina?
3. What problems in the man can occur with erection? With ejaculation of semen?
4. What can cause abnormalities in the sperm, in ejaculation, or in the seminal fluid?

## Factors in the Woman

A woman's fertility depends on the following:

- Regular production of normal ova
- An open path from her cervix to the fallopian tube to permit fertilization and movement of the embryo into the uterus for implantation
- A uterine endometrium that supports the pregnancy after implantation

See Chapter 4 for a complete discussion of the interrelated factors that contribute to normal female fertility.

### DISORDERS OF OVULATION

Normal ovulation depends on delicately timed and balanced secretions from the hypothalamus and pituitary and an ovarian response to mature and release an ovum. The hypothalamus secretes gonadotropin-releasing hormone (GnRH) beginning at puberty. This hormone, in turn, stimulates the pituitary to release follicle-stimulating hormone (FSH) and luteinizing hormone (LH). Follicle-stimulating hormone stimulates maturation of several follicles in the ovary. As the follicles mature, the ovary secretes estrogen to thicken the endometrium. About 24 to 36 hours before ovulation, there is a marked increase of LH, which stimulates final maturation and release of one ovum from its follicle. The other follicles regress permanently. The collapsed follicle from which the ovum was released, now called a *corpus luteum*, produces progesterone and estrogen, which further prepare the endometrium for implantation and nourishment of the fertilized ovum.

Ovulation can be disrupted by the following:

- A dysfunction in the hypothalamus or pituitary gland that alters the secretion of GnRH, FSH, and LH
- Failure of the ovaries to respond to FSH and LH stimulation, preventing maturation and release of the ovum

Disruption of hormone secretion or of the ovarian response to hormone secretion can be caused by many factors, such as cranial tumors, stress, obesity, anorexia, systemic disease, and abnormalities in the ovaries or other endocrine glands.

A woman does not produce new oocytes after her birth. Her existing oocytes are therefore vulnerable until the end of her reproductive life to cumulative toxic effects from therapeutic drugs, social or abused drugs, and environmental agents. Examples of factors that may impair normal ovulation include cancer chemotherapeutic agents, excessive alcohol intake, and cigarette smoking.

Women with ovulation disorders often have abnormal menses because hormone levels do not permit normal development and shedding of the endometrium. The woman may have absent, scant, or heavy menstrual periods. However, other women may have no menstrual disorders; inability to conceive may be their only complaint.

As a woman approaches the end of her reproductive life, she ovulates and menstruates more erratically. Thus, her fertility naturally declines with age, falling dramatically after 40 years.

### ABNORMALITIES OF THE FALLOPIAN TUBES

At least one open fallopian tube is needed for conception and implantation to occur (Fig. 32–2). Tubal obstruction may occur because of scarring and adhesions following reproductive tract infections. Sexually transmissible diseases, such as chlamydial infection and gonorrhea, are responsible for many cases of infertility owing to tubal obstruction. Prevention or prompt treatment and eradication of pelvic infections can reduce the incidence of fallopian tube damage.

Endometriosis may cause tubal adhesions, painful menstrual periods, and painful intercourse. Small lesions are unlikely to affect tubal function, but large lesions can distort tubal anatomy and lead to infertility.

Tubal obstruction also may occur if adhesions develop after pelvic surgery, ruptured appendix, peritonitis, or ovarian cysts. In addition, the fallopian tubes and other reproductive organs may have congenital anomalies that disrupt normal function.

The conditions that cause obstruction also may interfere with normal motility within the fallopian tube. Poor movement of the fimbriated (distal) end of the

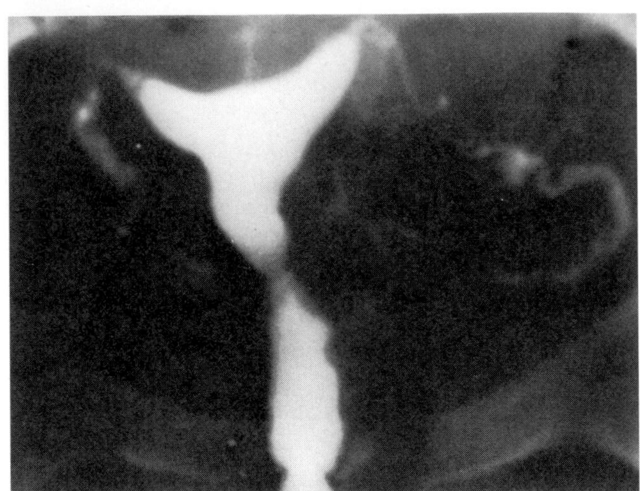

**FIGURE 32-2**

A hysterosalpingogram can determine whether fallopian tubes are patent. When tubes are open, as in this photograph, contrast medium that was injected through the cervix spills out of the fallopian tubes into the peritoneal cavity. (From Hacker, N.F., & Moore, J.G. [1992]. *Essentials of obstetrics and gynecology* [2nd ed., p. 559]. Philadelphia: W.B. Saunders.)

tube may prevent the pickup of the ovum from the ovarian surface after ovulation. Abnormal action of the cilia within the tube prevents normal transport of the ovum toward the uterine cavity.

Depending on the extent and location of the blockage, fallopian tube obstructions can prevent fertilization of the ovum or lead to an ectopic pregnancy. Complete tubal occlusion prevents fertilizing sperm from reaching the ovum, and the woman will be sterile without the use of advanced techniques, such as in vitro fertilization. Partial obstruction may result in a tubal ectopic pregnancy, because sperm can reach the ovum to fertilize it but the embryo cannot reach the uterine cavity to implant.

#### ABNORMALITIES OF THE CERVIX

Estrogen levels from the ovary peak twice during the menstrual cycle—once before ovulation and again about 1 week after ovulation. The first peak occurs about 2 days before ovulation and causes the woman's cervix to dilate slightly and produce a clear, thin, slippery mucus that is similar to egg white in consistency. This mucus facilitates passage of sperm into the uterus and capacitation to ready one sperm for fertilization. Low estrogen levels prevent development of this mucus and are usually associated with anovulation.

Polyps or scarring from past surgical procedures, such as cauterization or conization, may obstruct the woman's cervix. Abnormal cervical mucus caused by estrogen deficiency, surgical destruction of the mucus-secreting glands, and cervical damage secondary to infection or other factors prevent normal capacitation and movement of the sperm into the uterus and fallopian tubes for fertilization.

**CHECK YOUR READING**

5. What factors can result in abnormal ovulation?
6. Why does a woman who has ovulation problems often have abnormal menstrual periods?
7. What are some causes of fallopian tube obstruction?
8. How do abnormalities of cervical mucus contribute to infertility?

## Repeated Pregnancy Loss

Couples who repeatedly lose pregnancies have the same result as those unable to conceive: no living child. Repeated losses may result from abnormalities in the fetus or placenta or from maternal factors.

#### ABNORMALITIES OF THE FETAL CHROMOSOMES

Errors in the fetal chromosomes may result in spontaneous abortion, usually in the first trimester. Chromosome abnormalities often disrupt development severely, and the embryo or fetus cannot survive to live birth.

Most chromosome abnormalities are sporadic, occurring randomly. Others occur because one parent has a balanced chromosome translocation that is passed on to the offspring. The parent with the balanced translocation has a normal total amount of chromosome material; however, when the chromosomes are divided during gametogenesis, the resulting sperm or ovum may receive too much or too little chromosome material. The sperm or ovum also may receive a balanced translocation like the parent, or it may receive a totally normal chromosome complement with no translocation.

#### ABNORMALITIES OF THE CERVIX OR UTERUS

Stenosis or congenital malformations of the cervix or uterine cavity may cause repeated loss of a normal embryo or fetus (Fig. 32-3). These malformations may prevent normal implantation of the fertilized ovum or may prevent normal prenatal growth of the placenta or fetus.

Women who were exposed prenatally to diethylstilbestrol are more likely to have uterine malformations or an incompetent cervix. Cervical or uterine abnormalities also may occur after surgery or trauma from a previous birth. Painless and premature cervical dilation, often early in the second trimester, is characteristic in women with an incompetent cervix. Uterine malformations occur in many forms and may result in early spontaneous abortion or preterm labor.

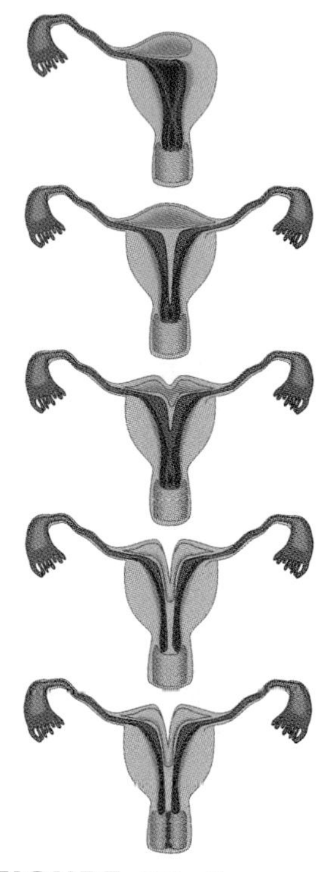


**FIGURE 32-3**

Types of uterine malformations that may cause infertility or repeated pregnancy loss.

Uterine myomas (benign tumors of the uterine muscle) and adhesions inside the uterine cavity may cause repeated fetal losses. These problems can alter the blood supply to the developing fetus or cause uterine irritability that results in preterm labor and birth.

### ENDOCRINE ABNORMALITIES

Inadequate progesterone secretion by the corpus luteum (luteal phase defect) prevents normal implantation and establishment of the placenta. The embryo may not implant, or it may implant poorly. In other cases, the corpus luteum may develop and function properly but the woman's endometrium may not respond to its progesterone secretion.

Hypothyroidism and hyperthyroidism may be associated with the inability to conceive and with recurrent pregnancy loss. Poorly controlled diabetes can result in repeated pregnancy loss as well as many other complications of pregnancy because of its effects on maternal blood glucose levels and the vascular system.

### IMMUNOLOGIC FACTORS

Immunologic factors are implicated in some cases of recurrent pregnancy loss, although not all are established conclusively. The embryo has antigens different from those of the mother and ordinarily would be rejected as any other foreign tissue would be rejected. However, the mother's body normally blocks this rejection response and tolerates the developing baby. Some women's bodies respond inappropriately to the embryo, rejecting it as foreign tissue. These women often have recurrent spontaneous abortions.

Women with autoimmune disease, such as lupus erythematosus, are more likely to experience spontaneous abortion. Pregnancy loss in these women appears related to thrombosis or other damage in placental blood vessels. Women with lupus often have other complications during pregnancy, such as exacerbation of their symptoms, fetal heart block, fetal distress, and stillbirth.

### ENVIRONMENTAL AGENTS

Some environmental agents have a well-established relationship to impairment of fertility and pregnancy loss. Others are believed to be damaging but do not show a conclusive link to pregnancy loss. In addition, the amount of exposure (dose) relates to the pregnancy outcome in most cases. For example, radiation exposure in the form of a chest radiograph is unlikely to have an adverse effect on pregnancy, whereas the larger doses used for cancer therapy might be toxic.

Examples of established toxins are ionizing radiation, alcohol, and isotretinoin (Accutane). Suspected toxins are numerous, for example, cigarette smoke, anesthetic gas, chemicals such as organic solvents or pesticides, and lead and mercury in occupational settings. These agents may be directly toxic to the embryo or fetus, causing its death, or they may interfere with normal placental function that is necessary to sustain the pregnancy.

### INFECTIONS

Infections of the reproductive tract are associated with poor pregnancy outcomes in general, and they may be related to early pregnancy losses as well. These infections are often asymptomatic, making their link to pregnancy loss difficult to establish.

**CHECK YOUR READING**

9. How can anatomic abnormalities of a woman's uterus or cervix cause her to lose a normal pregnancy?
10. What endocrine factors can cause repeated pregnancy loss?
11. What immunologic factors may cause loss of a normal fetus?

## Evaluation of Infertility

When a couple seeks help to conceive, both partners are evaluated in a systematic, timely, and cost-effec-

## Infertile Couples Want to Know

### What Is Infertility Treatment Like?

**General**

- Both members of the couple are evaluated.
- Simpler evaluations and therapies are done before more complex ones are undertaken.
- A complete medical history and physical examination are done for each partner.
- The ages of the partners, particularly the woman's, are considered. Evaluations and therapy may be instituted more quickly if the woman is in her mid 30s or older.
- Costs may be partially covered by insurance; check to see what your insurance covers.
- Difficult decisions may be required at different times during evaluation and treatment, for example, whether to proceed to more complex and expensive tests and therapies, whether to take a break from treatment, or whether to abandon treatment altogether.
- Infertility treatment is often stressful, can occupy many hours per week, and requires a substantial commitment to self-care.
- Infertility remains unexplained in about 20 percent of couples.

**Men**

- Semen analysis is usually the first test. Several semen specimens are obtained over a period of several weeks to obtain the best evaluation.
- Depending on your medical history, physical examination, and semen analysis, other diagnostic tests may be done (hormone assay, an ultrasonogram of your reproductive organs, a biopsy of your testicles, and specialized tests of sperm function).
- Corrective measures may include medications, surgery, and methods to reduce the scrotal temperature.

**Women**

- The first evaluation is usually to determine whether you are ovulating each month. You may be taught to take your basal body temperature each morning and to assess your cervical mucus as the first step. These assessments are often done at the same time as other tests.
- Other evaluations may include a postcoital test to determine how your partner's sperm react in your body, an ultrasound examination, a laparoscopy, and a hysterosalpingogram (x-ray of your uterus and tubes).
- For some tests and therapies, an operative procedure is required (hysteroscopy, laparoscopy, laser surgery, or microsurgery) on either an outpatient or an inpatient basis.
- Typically, infertility evaluations and treatments require more of the woman's time, energy, physical discomfort, and risk than the man's.
- Corrective measures depend on the problem that is identified, for example, medications, surgery, and advanced reproductive techniques, such as in vitro fertilization.

tive manner. Couples are often in a hurry for definitive therapy, but a thorough assessment of their problem is essential for suitable treatment. Some tests, such as semen evaluation, must be repeated sequentially for an accurate picture. The prolonged evaluation process is frustrating to many couples, especially older ones who are anxious for a child before the end of the woman's reproductive years. Another frustration for couples undergoing an infertility work-up is that some diagnostic tests are investigational and their usefulness and normal values are not well established. Other tests are commonly used, but well-accepted normal values have not been established.

Numerous professionals may be involved in evaluation and care of infertile couples: nurses, physicians specializing in reproductive medicine, gynecologists, urologists, microsurgeons, embryologists, and ultrasonographers. In addition, general and specialized laboratory facilities may provide diagnostic services to enhance treatment. Nurses working in infertility clinics often coordinate communication among the many providers and help the couple negotiate the maze of evaluation and treatment.

## History and Physical Examination

A thorough history and physical examination of each partner can help identify the appropriate diagnostic tests and therapy.

### HISTORY

The partners' general health history is reviewed to determine problems that affect their general health as well as their fertility. A reproductive history is also taken and it includes the following:

- The woman's menstrual pattern
- Any pregnancies and their outcomes
- Previous fertility of the man and woman with other partners
- Pattern of intercourse in relation to the woman's menstrual cycles
- Length of time the couple has had unprotected intercourse
- Any home tests the couple has used, such as basal body temperature or over-the-counter ovulation predictor kits

The past medical history, including childhood illnesses and surgery, and a history of exposure to toxins provide clues to the possible cause of infertility. The couple's past and present occupations may identify toxin exposure, stresses, or other adverse influences on reproduction. Investigation of the couple's usual frequency and timing of intercourse may identify the need for a change in practice to promote conception.

### PHYSICAL EXAMINATION

Couples who seek help for infertility are usually healthy. However, a thorough physical examination of each partner may identify endocrine disturbances, cranial tumors, or undiagnosed chronic disease. Examination of the reproductive organs may reveal structural defects, infection, cysts, or other abnormalities. Chromosomal analysis may be performed for couples experiencing repeated pregnancy loss that is not explained by other factors.

## Diagnostic Tests

Each couple's evaluation is individualized, but testing generally proceeds from the simple and less expensive to the more complex and expensive diagnostics. Simple evaluations are done simultaneously, but more complex tests are delayed until the need for them is established. Two methods of identifying ovulation—basal body temperature and assessment of cervical mucus—can be used as contraceptive measures in addition to their use in infertility care (Procedure 32-1).

Five basic tests are common in early infertility evaluation:

- Semen analysis
- Basal body temperature
- Postcoital test

## Procedure 32-1
# Teaching Women Fertility Awareness

**PURPOSE:** To identify whether ovulation occurs and the probable time of ovulation. These techniques can be used in infertility care or as a minimally effective contraceptive method.

### BASAL BODY TEMPERATURE

The basal body temperature (BBT) is designed to detect the slight elevation in temperature that accompanies increased progesterone secretion in response to the luteinizing hormone (LH) surge and ovulation.

**1. Teach the woman the relationship between her BBT and ovulation:**

**a. Explain that the BBT is the lowest, or resting, temperature of the body.**

**b. During the first half of the woman's menstrual cycle, her temperature is lower than during the second half of the cycle.**

**c. The basal temperature often drops slightly just before ovulation. Not all women experience this fall in basal temperature.**

**d. Progesterone is secreted during the second half of the cycle, rising just after ovulation. The BBT rises after the slight drop near ovulation and remains higher during the second half of the cycle.**

**e. The BBT remains high if conception occurs and falls about 2 to 4 days before menstruation if conception does not occur.** *This method of fertility awareness requires careful assessment and record keeping by the woman. She is more likely to have an accurate record if she understands the relationship between her basal temperature and ovulation.*

**2. Explain the occurrences that can interfere with the**

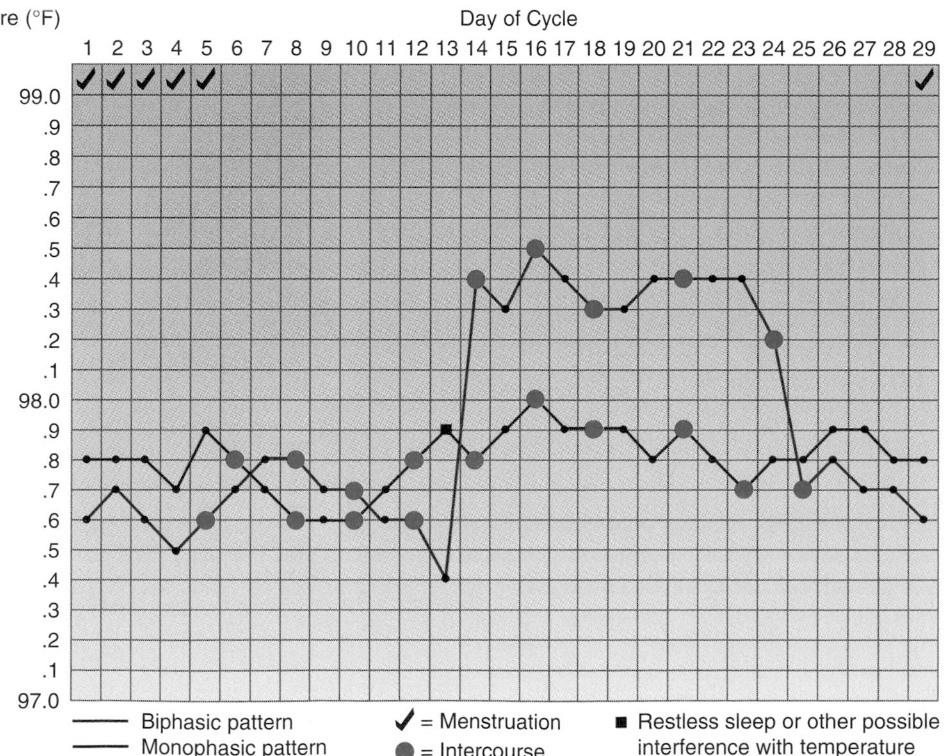


Procedure continued on following page

## Procedure 32–1 *Continued*

# Teaching Women Fertility Awareness

**PURPOSE:** To identify whether ovulation occurs and the probable time of ovulation. These techniques can be used in infertility care or as a minimally effective contraceptive method.

**accuracy of her BBT, for example, illness, restless or inadequate sleep (fewer than six hours), waking later than usual, traveling across time zones (jet lag), alcohol intake the evening before, sleeping under an electric blanket or on a heated water bed, or any activity before taking the temperature.** *Temperature changes are very slight at ovulation; these factors can cause temperature to rise even if ovulation has not occurred.*

3. **Show the woman a glass fever thermometer and a glass basal thermometer. Explain that the range of temperatures on the basal thermometer is smaller (96° to 100°F) and is marked in tenths of a degree. Explain how to read the marks on the thermometer. Electronic basal thermometers are available that digitally display tenths of a degree. These require less time for accurate assessment than glass ones. The woman should read the instructions that come with her specific thermometer.** *Allows the woman to see the differences between a fever thermometer, which may be familiar to her, and a basal thermometer. The temperature rise is very slight (about 0.4°F higher than during the first half of the cycle). A special thermometer is needed to detect the change more accurately. Some women may not know how to read a glass thermometer and should be taught. Reading and following instructions specific for the thermometer increases the accuracy of the assessment.*

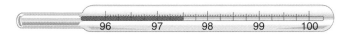

4. **Basal temperatures with glass thermometers can be taken orally, rectally, or vaginally. The woman should use the same site for all readings.** *Body temperatures vary when different sites are used. The basal temperature identifies very small fluctuations, and varying sites may show changes unrelated to ovulation.*

5. **Show the woman the chart for recording her BBT and the symbols for marking relevant events, such as menstrual periods, intercourse, illness, or other occurrences, which may alter her BBT.** *Allows a consistent, more accurate interpretation of temperature fluctuations.*

6. **Teach the woman how to take her basal temperature:**

   a. **If a glass thermometer is used, shake it down the night before.**

   b. **As soon as she awakens, but before any activity, the basal thermometer should be placed under her tongue and remain until the electronic thermometer beeps. A glass thermometer requires up to 10 minutes for an accurate reading if the oral site is used. The thermometer should remain still while it is registering the temperature.**

   c. **Record the reading on the chart provided.** *Any activity before taking the basal temperature, including shaking the thermometer down, can alter the reading enough to cause inaccurate interpretation.*

7. **Encourage the woman to demonstrate taking her temperature and recording the result. Ask her to list events other than ovulation that can alter the BBT.** *Verifies that she has correctly understood the teaching and allows correction of misunderstandings.*

8. **As a method to avoid pregnancy: Explain that for the greatest effectiveness, a woman should avoid intercourse from the onset of the menstrual period through the second day of elevated temperature.** *The most conservative approach requires a long period of abstinence while a viable ovum could be present, because it primarily identifies that ovulation has already occurred. Not all women have a temperature drop at the time of ovulation, and the rise in BBT occurs after ovulation. Also, sperm can remain viable in the woman's reproductive tract for 72 or more hours, although most die within 24 hours. To reduce the time of abstinence, couples using fertility awareness as a method of contraception usually combine methods, such as BBT and the cervical mucus assessment.*

9. **To enhance the chances of conception, the couple should have intercourse when the temperature falls: Emphasize that the BBT primarily identifies that ovulation has already occurred and the adequacy of progesterone**

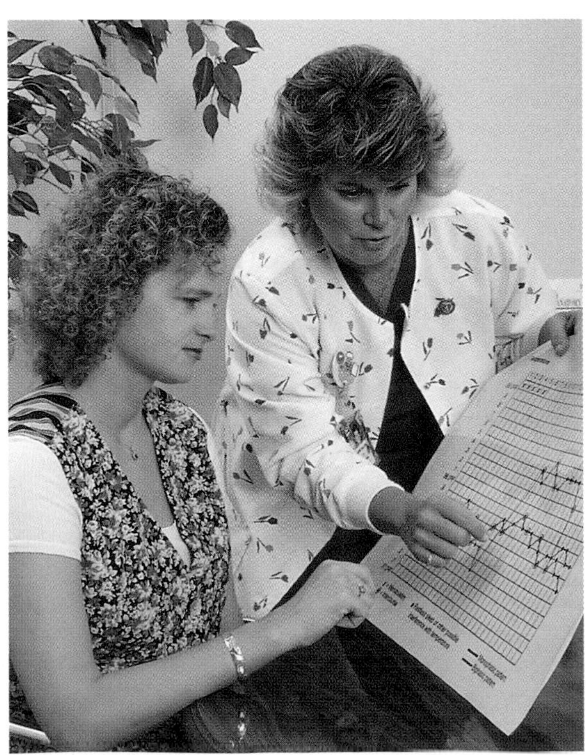

## Procedure 32–1 *Continued*

# Teaching Women Fertility Awareness

**PURPOSE:** To identify whether ovulation occurs and the probable time of ovulation. These techniques can be used in infertility care or as a minimally effective contraceptive method.

**secretion to prepare her endometrium during the second half of her menstrual cycle. The BBT is less effective for timing intercourse to coincide with ovulation because of the short life span of the ovum after ovulation.** *Increases the likelihood that sperm will be available to fertilize the ovum while it is viable. The woman receiving infertility therapy should understand the limitations of the BBT in terms of enhancing conception.*

### CERVICAL MUCUS ASSESSMENT

The cervical mucus normally changes just before ovulation to facilitate survival of the sperm and promote their passage into the woman's uterus.

1. **Teach the woman how her cervical mucus changes throughout the menstrual cycle. Spinnbarkheit describes how much the mucus can be stretched between her fingers or between a microscope slide and coverslip. Before and after ovulation, the cervical mucus is scant, thick, sticky, and opaque. It stretches less than 6 cm. Just before and for 2 to 3 days after ovulation, the cervical mucus is thin, slippery, and clear and is similar to raw egg white. It stretches 6 cm or more. When this ovulatory mucus is present, the woman has probably ovulated and could become pregnant.** *As with the BBT, this method requires careful assessment and record keeping by the woman. She is more likely to perform the assessment and record changes in her cervical mucus accurately if she understands how the changes relate to fertility.*

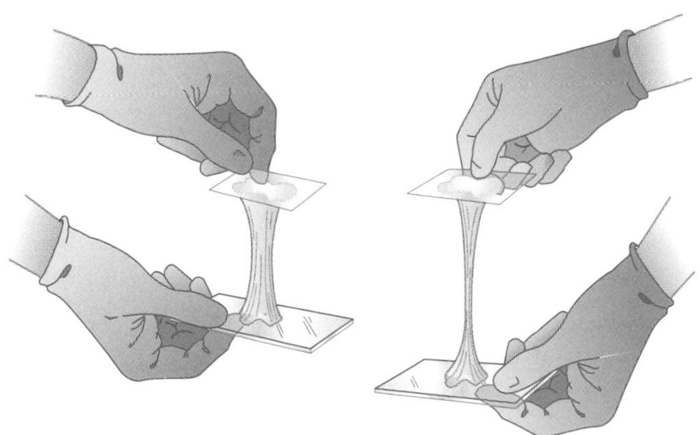

2. **Explain the factors that can interfere with the accuracy of her assessment. The mucus may be thicker if she takes antihistamines. Vaginal infections, contraceptive foams or jellies, sexual arousal, and semen can make the mucus thinner even if ovulation has not occurred. Tell her to record these factors. Factors that interfere with the consistency of the cervical mucus may cause inaccurate identification of the fertile period.**
3. **Demonstrate how to stretch mucus between the thumb and forefinger by using raw egg white. Have the woman return demonstrate the process.** *Provides visual and tactile experiences to enhance learning. Return demonstration allows the nurse to determine whether the woman has misunderstood the teaching.*
4. **Teach the woman to wash her hands before and after assessing her mucus.** *Reduces the chance of introducing infection into the reproductive tract and of transferring infectious organisms from the vagina to other areas.*
5. **Teach the woman to obtain a small mucus sample several times a day from just inside her vagina and to note the following:**
   a. **The general sensation of wetness (around ovulation) or dryness (not near ovulation) on her labia.**
   b. **The appearance and consistency of the mucus: thick, sticky, and whitish or thin, slippery, and clear or watery.**
   c. **The distance the mucus will stretch between her fingers, usually at least 6 cm (2.3 inches) at the time of ovulation.** *Allows the woman to identify cyclic changes in her mucus over the entire duration of her menstrual cycle.*
6. **Have the woman record the day's typical mucus characteristics (often combined with the BBT recording).** *Provides a means of evaluating signs and symptoms associated with ovulation during the entire cycle.*
7. **As a method of contraception, the woman should avoid intercourse from the time the thin, stretchy ovulatory mucus appears until 48 to 72 hours after the mucus returns to its pre-ovulatory characteristics.** *Reduces the chance that sperm are available for fertilization while the ovum is viable.*
8. **As a method to enhance conception, the couple should have intercourse every 2 days during the period of ovulatory mucus (approximately days 12 to 16 if the woman has a 28-day cycle).** *Makes sperm available to fertilize the ovum while it is viable.*

- Hysterosalpingogram
- Endometrial biopsy

Table 32–1 describes diagnostic tests that may be offered to the infertile couple and the nursing care associated with each.

## Therapies to Facilitate Pregnancy

Evaluation of the couple identifies whether therapy might improve their chances to conceive and complete a pregnancy. A variety of procedures may be

**TABLE 32–1 SELECTED DIAGNOSTIC TESTS IN INFERTILITY**

| Test/Purpose | Nursing Implications |
|---|---|
| **Male** | |
| ***Semen Analysis*** | |
| Evaluates structure and function of sperm and composition of seminal fluid.<br>Semen volume: 2.0–6.0 ml<br>pH: 7.2–7.8<br>Sperm concentration: 20 million/ml or more<br>Motility: 50% or more with normal forms<br>Morphology: 60% or more with normal forms<br>Viability: 50% or more live<br>Liquefaction: within 30 min<br>Leukocytes (white blood cells): Fewer than 1 million/ml<br>Fructose: 150–600 mg/dl | Explain purpose of semen analysis: three or more specimens are usually collected over several weeks' time for more accurate analysis.<br>Explain to the man that he should collect the specimen by masturbation after a 2- to 3-day abstinence; semen may be collected in a condom if masturbation is unacceptable.<br>Teach the man to note the time the specimen was obtained so the laboratory can evaluate liquefaction of the semen; the specimen should be transported near the body to maintain warmth and should arrive in the laboratory within 1 hr. |
| ***Endocrine Tests*** | |
| Evaluate function of hypothalamus, pituitary gland, and the response of the testicles.<br>Assays are made to determine testosterone, estradiol, luteinizing hormone (LH), and follicle-stimulating hormone (FSH) levels.<br>Additional tests may be made on the basis of history and physical findings. | Teach the man about the relationship between hypothalamic and pituitary function and sperm formation; LH stimulates testosterone production by Leydig cells of the testes, and FSH stimulates Sertoli cells of the testes to produce sperm. |
| ***Ultrasonography*** | |
| Evaluates structure of prostate gland, seminal vesicles, and ejaculatory ducts by use of a transrectal probe. | Teach the man that ultrasonography uses sound waves to evaluate these structures; no radiation is involved. |
| ***Testicular Biopsy*** | |
| An invasive test for obtaining a sample of testicular tissue; identifies pathology and obstructions. | Explain the purpose of the test; a local anesthetic is used, and there should be little discomfort. |
| ***Sperm Penetration Assay*** | |
| Evaluates fertilizing ability of sperm; assesses ability of sperm to undergo changes that allow penetration of a hamster ovum from which the zona pellucida has been removed. | Explain the purpose of the test; abnormal penetration does not necessarily mean that the sperm cannot fertilize a human ovum. |
| **Female** | |
| ***Ovulation Prediction*** | |
| Uses any of several methods to identify the surge of LH, which precedes ovulation by 24–36 hr; this enables the timing of intercourse to coincide with ovulation and identifies the absence of ovulation. | Explain the purpose of the tests (commercial ovulation predictor kits, basal body temperature, and cervical mucus assessment).<br>Teach the woman to follow the instructions on the commercial product.<br>Teach her how to do the basal body temperature and cervical mucus assessment (see Procedure 32–1). |

used, depending on the couple's initial and ongoing evaluations and on their personal choices. Some therapy is simple, like timing intercourse to coincide with ovulation; other procedures may involve considerable expense, discomfort, or unpleasant side effects. Many couples need a combination of treatments to improve their chances of conception.

Identification of appropriate infertility therapy is not always straightforward. Many factors must be considered, including the couple's history, their medical evaluations, financial resources, age and other time constraints, and religious and cultural values. Generally, simpler treatments are indicated before more complex ones, but the needs of each couple are considered individually. Infertility specialists may proceed more aggressively if the woman is in her mid-30s or older because she has less time before the end of her reproductive years than does the younger woman.

Statistical success rates for various procedures are

**TABLE 32–1 SELECTED DIAGNOSTIC TESTS IN INFERTILITY** *Continued*

| Test/Purpose | Nursing Implications |
|---|---|
| **Female** | |
| ***Ultrasonography*** | |
| Evaluates structure of pelvic organs.<br>Identifies ovarian follicles and release of ova at ovulation.<br>Evaluates for presence of ectopic or multifetal pregnancy. | Teach the woman that ultrasonography uses sound waves to evaluate these structures; no radiation is involved.<br>Explain preparations needed for specific evaluations. |
| ***Post-coital Test*** | |
| Evaluates characteristics of cervical mucus and sperm function within that mucus at time of ovulation. Ultrasonography ensures proper timing for test. | Explain that the test is performed 6 to 12 hours after intercourse; the woman may have to rearrange her personal or work commitments each time this test is done. |
| ***Endocrine Tests*** | |
| Evaluates functions of hypothalamus, pituitary gland, and ovary.<br>Assays are made to determine LH, FSH, estrogen, and progesterone levels.<br>Additional hormone evaluations may be done on the basis of the history and physical findings. | Explain the purpose of each test: FSH and LH stimulate ovulation; estrogen and progesterone prepare uterine endometrium for implantation of a fertilized ovum. Explain the importance of timing within the cycle to provide best information. |
| ***Hysterosalpingogram* (HSG)** | |
| X-ray that uses contrast medium to evaluate the structure and patency of the uterus and fallopian tubes. | The test is performed after the menstrual period during the first half of the cycle to avoid flushing menstrual debris through the tubes into the pelvic cavity and to avoid disrupting a pregnancy that might be in place.<br>Explain the purpose of the test. Contrast medium is injected through the cervix, and x-ray films are made at the same time. |
| ***Endometrial Biopsy*** | |
| An invasive test for obtaining a small sample of endometrial tissue; determines whether endometrium is responding properly to estrogen and progesterone stimulation from ovary. | Explain the purpose of the test.<br>The test is done 2–3 days before the woman expects her menstrual period; some cramping may occur, but it should be relieved with mild analgesics, such as ibuprofen. |
| ***Hysteroscopy and Laparoscopy*** | |
| Examines uterine interior and pelvic organs with an endoscope; general anesthesia is used.<br>Identifies abnormalities (polyps, endometrial adhesions). Some surgical procedures may be done via the endoscope. | Explain the purpose of the test and any procedures that will be done at the same time. The woman takes nothing by mouth and should urinate before the procedure. Carbon dioxide gas, used to separate pelvic organs for better visualization, may cause temporary shoulder pain. |

often difficult for couples to evaluate and vary widely among facilities. Factors that affect a center's success rate for a procedure are numerous. For example, a referral center that accepts only couples with longstanding infertility may have lower success rates than one that accepts couples having fewer problems.

## Medications

Hormones and other medications may be given to either the man or the woman. A medication may be given to improve semen quality, induce ovulation, prepare the uterine endometrium, or support the pregnancy once it is established. Table 32–2 summarizes medications used in infertility therapy.

### Ovulation Induction

Medications to induce ovulation may be prescribed for the woman who does not ovulate or who ovulates erratically. Medications may also be given to provide multiple ova if a woman plans to have in vitro fertilization, gamete intrafallopian transfer, or tubal embryo transfer. Clomiphene citrate is a drug often used to stimulate ovulation. Clomiphene has also been used to stimulate sperm production, although this use is an unlabeled one.

**TABLE 32-2 MEDICATIONS USED FOR INFERTILITY THERAPY**

| Drug | Use |
|---|---|
| Bromocriptine (Parlodel) | Corrects excess prolactin secretion by anterior pituitary, which causes inadequate progesterone production by corpus luteum, thus inhibiting normal implantation of embryo. |
| Clomiphene (Clomid) | Induction of ovulation |
| Chorionic gonadotropin, human (hCG; Pregnyl) | Used with menotropins to stimulate ovulation in the female or sperm formation in the male; stimulates progesterone production by corpus luteum |
| Gonadotropin-releasing hormone (GnRH; Lutrepulse) | Stimulates release of follicle-stimulating hormone (FSH) and luteinizing hormone (LH) from the pituitary gland in men and women who have deficient GnRH secretion by their hypothalamus; FSH and LH, in turn, stimulate ovulation in the female and stimulate testosterone production and spermatogenesis |
| Leuprolide (Lupron) | Reduces endometriosis; adjunct to drug given to stimulate ovulation |
| Menotropins (FSH and LH; Pergonal) | Stimulates ovulation and spermatogenesis (given with hCG) |
| Nafarelin (Synarel) | Reduces endometriosis |
| Progesterone | Promotes implantation of embryo |
| Urofollitropin (Metrodin) | Stimulates ovulation (given in conjunction with hCG) |

Ovulation induction increases the risk of multiple births because several ova may be released and fertilized. Another serious complication is *ovarian hyperstimulation syndrome*, in which there is marked ovarian enlargement, with exudation of fluid into the woman's peritoneal and pleural cavities. Careful adjustment of medication dose and serial ultrasound examinations prevent most cases of high multifetal pregnancy (triplets or more) and ovarian hyperstimulation syndrome.

## Surgical Procedures

In some men, correction of a varicocele improves sperm quality and quantity. Endoscopic procedures may be used to correct obstructions, with minimal invasiveness, in either the man or the woman. The woman may need a laparotomy to relieve pelvic adhesions and obstructions caused by endometriosis, infection, or previous surgical procedures if these cannot be corrected via laparoscopy. Medications may also reduce endometriosis. Laser surgical techniques may be used to reduce adhesions because they are minimally invasive, precise, and less likely to cause formation of new adhesions. For surgical correction of obstructions in the fallopian tubes or tubal structures in the male genital tract, microsurgical techniques are needed because these structures are very narrow.

Transcervical balloon tuboplasty may be used to unblock a woman's fallopian tubes without more invasive procedures, such as laparoscopy or laparotomy. A thin catheter is threaded through the uterus into the fallopian tube, and the balloon is inflated to clear the blockage.

## Therapeutic Insemination

The technique of therapeutic insemination (formerly called "artificial insemination") may use either the partner's semen or that of a donor to overcome a low sperm count. Donor insemination also may be used if the man carries a genetic defect or if a woman wants a biologic child without having a relationship with a male partner. Intrauterine insemination is a variation that allows the sperm to bypass cervical mucus and reduces some immunologic incompatibilities.

Sperm that are to be placed directly in the uterus or the fallopian tube are prepared by washing and spinning the semen in a centrifuge to remove seminal fluid. A technique called *sperm swim-up* uses a suspension to concentrate sperm having the best motility. Although the total number of sperm is lower, the remaining ones (those with normal structure and highest motility) are more likely to fertilize the ovum.

Men who donate semen for therapeutic insemination are screened to reduce the risk of transmitting diseases or genetic defects. They are questioned about their personal and family health history, including genetic disorders or birth defects. Questions about their social habits and personality can disclose high-risk behaviors and also give recipient parents information about traits their child might have. Physical and laboratory examinations are performed to

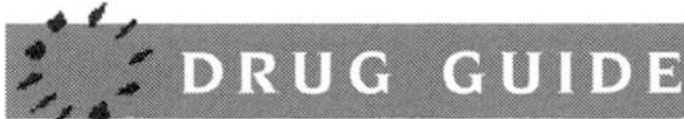

## CLOMIPHENE CITRATE (Clomid)

***Classification*:** Ovarian stimulant.

***Action*:** Stimulates pituitary gland to increase secretion of luteinizing hormone (LH) and follicle-stimulating hormone (FSH). LH and FSH stimulate maturation of the ovarian follicle, ovulation, and development of the corpus luteum.

***Indications*:** Female infertility in which estrogen levels are normal. Treatment of male infertility by increasing sperm production (unlabeled use).

**Dosage and Route**

***Female sterility*:** *First course*: 25–50 mg p.o. daily for 5 days. *Second course*: Same dose if ovulation occurred with first course. If ovulation did not occur, increase dose to 100 mg daily for 5 days. Some women require up to 250 mg daily. An increased dose is not beneficial if ovulation is triggered.

***Male sterility*:** 25 mg p.o. daily for 25 days with a 5 day rest; or 100 mg p.o. every Monday, Wednesday, and Friday.

***Absorption*:** Readily absorbed from the gastrointestinal tract. Time to peak effect is 4 to 10 days after last day of treatment.

***Excretion*;** Excreted in the feces.

***Contraindication and Precautions*:** Pregnancy, liver disease, abnormal bleeding of undetermined origin, ovarian cysts, neoplastic disease. Therapy is ineffective in women with ovarian or pituitary failure.

***Adverse Reactions*:** Ovarian enlargement and symptoms, similar to premenstrual syndrome. Ovarian hyperstimulation. Multiple gestation, if more than one ovum is released. Visual disturbances. Abdominal distention, discomfort, nausea, vomiting. Abnormal uterine bleeding. Breast tenderness. Insomnia, nervousness, headache, depression, fatigue, lightheadedness, dizziness. Hot flashes, increased urination, allergic symptoms, weight gain, reversible alopecia.

***Nursing Considerations*:** Take the history to determine whether the woman has a history of liver dysfunction or abnormal uterine bleeding. Rule out the possibility of pregnancy. Teach the woman to report abdominal distention, pain in the pelvis or abdomen, or visual disturbances. Teach her to avoid tasks requiring mental alertness or coordination because the drug can cause lightheadedness, dizziness, and visual disturbances. Instruct her to stop taking clomiphene and report to the physician if she suspects that she might be pregnant. Teach the woman and her partner that she may notice irritability, mood swings, and other symptoms similar to those in premenstrual syndrome but that these are temporary.

evaluate the man's general health, determine his blood type and Rh factor, and screen for infections such as sexually transmissible diseases or human immunodeficiency virus (HIV). Carrier testing for some genetic defects, such as sickle cell and Tay-Sachs diseases, reduces the risk of passing on these disorders. Donor semen is frozen and held for 6 months before use to reduce the risk of transmitting diseases that may not be apparent at the initial screening.

### Surrogate Parenting

A surrogate mother may enter the picture if the woman is infertile or if she cannot carry a fetus to live birth. The surrogate mother may supply her uterus only (gestational surrogate), with the infertile couple supplying the sperm and ovum. Or she may be inseminated with the male partner's sperm and carry the fetus to birth, thus supplying both her genetic component and the gestational component. Surrogacy is different from therapeutic insemination because it is not anonymous. In addition, the woman who carries the child inevitably forms bonds with the fetus during the months of pregnancy.

Money paid to the surrogate mother can raise issues of baby selling. Could a poor but fertile woman feel compelled to provide her body for a more well-to-do couple? Yet, not compensating a woman for the real physical and emotional risks of this undertaking can be construed as coercive as well.

Custody of the resulting child has been the issue in several court cases involving surrogate mothers. In the *Baby* M case, a woman who was inseminated with the man's sperm refused to relinquish the baby as stated in the contract between the birth mother and the infertile couple. Ultimately, custody was awarded to the man providing the sperm and his spouse, but visitation rights were granted to the surrogate mother.

Custody issues when the birth mother is a gestational surrogate are clearer than when she also donates her ovum to the child. Courts have more often recognized the genetic parents as the legal parents and upheld the contracts between them and the gestational surrogate. Laws vary among states, however. In surrogacy and other advanced techniques, the laws are behind the available technology.

### Advanced Reproductive Techniques

One class of advanced reproductive technologies bypasses many natural obstacles to conception by placing intact gametes together to allow fertilization. This class includes in vitro fertilization (IVF), gamete intrafallopian transfer (GIFT), and tubal embryo transfer (TET). Each of these procedures begins with ovulation induction to permit retrieval of several ova, thus improving the likelihood of a successful pregnancy. Sperm are prepared and concentrated as they are for therapeutic insemination.

Another class of advanced reproductive technologies involves assisting fertilization with microsurgical techniques. These techniques bypass obstacles to fertilization by penetrating the ovum with tiny needles to allow placement of the sperm within the ovum or its surrounding zona pellucida.

Couples who have concerns about a specific genetic defect in their family may be offered preimplantation genetic testing of their embryo. This testing allows them to make informed decisions about whether they wish to actually implant the resulting embryo into the uterus.

### IN VITRO FERTILIZATION

The technique of IVF involves bypassing blocked or absent fallopian tubes. The physician removes the ova by laparoscope or by ultrasound-guided transvaginal retrieval and mixes them with prepared sperm from the woman's partner or a donor. Two days later, up to four embryos are returned to the uterus to increase the likelihood of a successful pregnancy. Additional embryos may be transferred if the woman is older. The woman receives supplemental progesterone to enhance the receptivity of her endometrium to implantation. Excess ova or embryos may be frozen for future attempts at IVF or embryo transfer to the uterus.

In vitro fertilization is not always successful, although the rates vary among infertility centers. Bypassing the obstructions does not necessarily result in pregnancy. Not every ovum is successfully fertilized when this technique is used. Embryos that are transferred to the woman's uterus may not always implant.

### GAMETE INTRAFALLOPIAN TRANSFER

For GIFT to take place, the woman must have at least one patent fallopian tube. The procedure begins in a manner similar to that of IVF, with retrieval of multiple ova and washed sperm. Ova may be retrieved either laparoscopically or transvaginally with ultrasound guidance.

The retrieved ova are drawn into a catheter that also carries prepared sperm. Sperm and up to two ova per tube are injected into each fallopian tube through a laparoscope, in which fertilization may occur (Fig. 32–4). Additional prepared sperm may be injected into the uterus through the cervix to improve the chance of successful fertilization. Progesterone is often given to enhance implantation of any fertilized ova.

### TUBAL EMBRYO TRANSFER

Tubal embryo transfer, also called *zygote intrafallopian transfer* (ZIFT), is a hybrid of IVF and GIFT. The woman's ova are fertilized outside her body, but the resulting fertilized ova are placed in the fallopian tubes and enter the uterus naturally for implantation. The woman must have at least one patent fallopian tube.

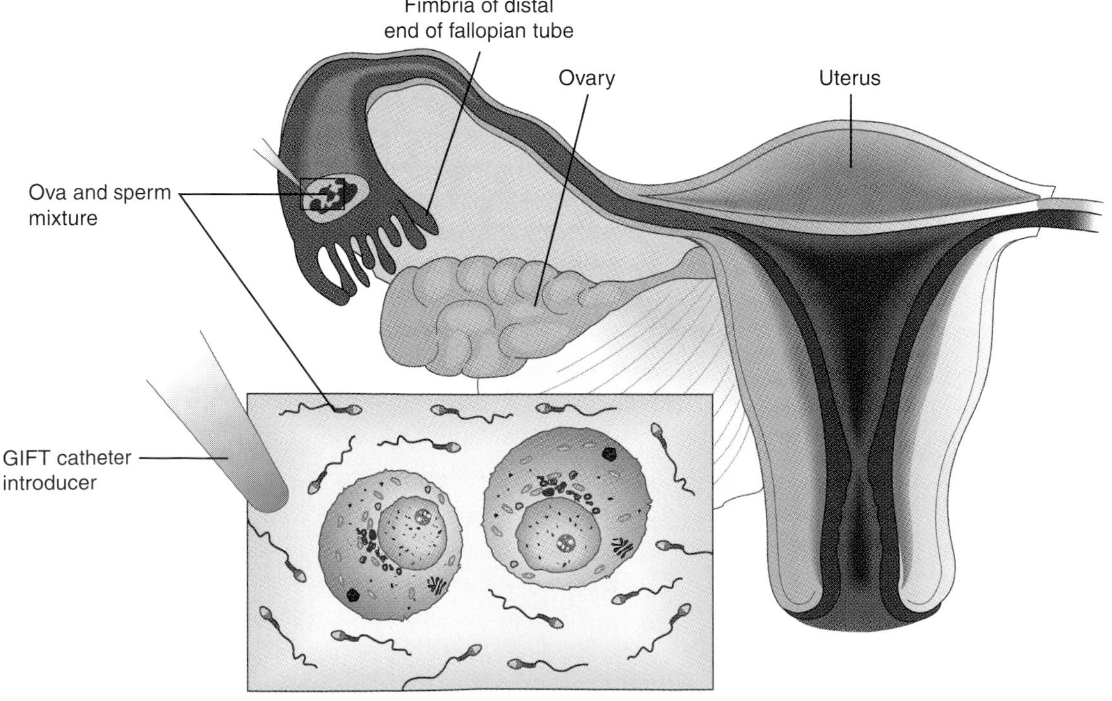


**FIGURE 32–4**

Gamete intrafallopian transfer (GIFT). Multiple ova and washed sperm are injected into the fallopian tube, where fertilization may occur.

### COMPARISON OF IN VITRO FERTILIZATION, GAMETE INTRAFALLOPIAN TRANSFER, AND TUBAL EMBRYO TRANSFER

The primary advantage of GIFT and TET over IVF is that there is a higher pregnancy rate. With IVF or TET, there is evidence of fertilization before placement in the uterus or tubes. The disadvantage of these procedures is that the woman may need to have a laparoscopy to retrieve gametes (IVF) or to place the gametes (GIFT) or fertilized ova (TET) into the fallopian tube. Either GIFT or TET may result in a tubal pregnancy if the embryo cannot reach the uterine cavity to implant.

These reproductive techniques can result in multifetal pregnancy, sometimes more than triplets. Pregnancies of more than twins carry a substantially higher risk to both mother and infants because of preterm labor and birth, placental insufficiency, and a high demand on maternal body systems. Selective reduction in the number of fetuses may be done to give the remaining ones a better chance to progress to a live birth. Such a procedure is, of course, heavily laden with emotional and ethical overtones.

### MICROSURGICALLY ASSISTED FERTILIZATION

Microsurgical techniques, which are related to IVF but are considerably more complex, may help couples for whom straightforward IVF, GIFT, and TET are unlikely to be successful to conceive despite severe male infertility. Only one or a few sperm are required to use these procedures.

One technique involves making small slits in the zona pellucida cells that surround the ovum to allow sperm to access the ovum itself to achieve fertilization. A similar technique injects sperm into the space just under the zona pellucida. Direct injection of a spermatozoon into the cytoplasm of the ovum is called intracytoplasmic sperm injection (ICSI). For these techniques, the retrieval of oocytes and the placement of the resulting conceptus into the uterus are similar to those of IVF.

### BLASTOMERE ANALYSIS

Blastomere analysis is a related technique to genetically analyze the conceptus that results from assisted reproduction. One or two cells from the 4- to 8-cell stage conceptus are withdrawn for analysis. The DNA from the cells is amplified to allow genetic analysis. Because cells are undifferentiated into specialized organ cells at this stage, their loss is quickly made up. If a genetic defect is identified, the couple has the option of not implanting the conceptus.

**CHECK YOUR READING**

12. What elements are included in the history and physical examination for an infertility work-up?
13. What medications may be used to induce ovulation?
14. What screening tests are performed if donor sperm is used for therapeutic insemination or for GIFT?
15. What are the differences in technique among IVF, GIFT, and TET?

## Responses to Infertility

The desire for children is strong in many couples. Even if they delay childbearing, most couples expect to have one or more children before the end of the woman's reproductive years. Couples who chose childlessness earlier may re-evaluate their decision when they are older. If a couple does not achieve pregnancy or produce a living child as expected, the man and woman often experience psychological distress and a threat to their self-images. Either or both partners may feel like failures. Their marital and family relationships may be stressed, and they may withdraw from relationships with others that they previously found satisfying. Every couple is unique, and many reactions depend on the importance attached to having biologic children. The following discussion describes how infertility can alter the lives of those affected.

### Assumption of Fertility

Many couples practice contraception for a number of years before they decide to have a baby. They may want to establish a career and financial security, acquire a comfortable home and lifestyle, or perhaps travel and live freely without the responsibility of a child. They usually assume that they are fertile and must work hard to avoid pregnancy until they are ready.

When they do want a child, they discontinue contraception and assume that pregnancy will occur within a few months at most. They may plan conception so that the baby will be born at a certain time of year (such as not during the hottest weather) or time the birth so that the child is not delayed in starting school.

Either or both partners may experiment with the role of parent as they anticipate pregnancy. They develop a heightened awareness of children and parenting. Being with others who are expecting or who already have children is exciting because they plan to join their ranks shortly. They may discuss issues like full-time parenting by one partner, child care, and future lifestyle changes. The woman often finds that she enjoys shopping in the maternity and children's departments. They may begin acquiring toys and furnishings a child will need. Both partners may develop a fantasy child or a concept of what their baby will be like.

## Growing Awareness of a Problem

As the months pass, the couple gradually becomes concerned about the inability to conceive. If the woman is older, they feel the urgency of the limited time before her reproductive years end. The plan to have a baby at a certain time of year is replaced by the desire for a baby anytime—and soon.

The couple begins to feel uneasy with child-related activities. Now they are not so sure when they will be parents. It begins to hurt when other family members or friends have babies. Events such as baby showers or christenings may become melancholy rather than joyful occasions. They now bypass toy stores and children's departments. Family members and friends who are having children may feel guilty at their good fortune when they are around the couple who cannot conceive.

The potential grandparents may feel that their children are waiting too long to start a family or even that they are selfish. If they are aware that the couple is trying to conceive, they become even more worried as the months pass without the longed-for announcement of a pregnancy. They are twice-saddened by the lack of a grandchild and by the hurt their adult children are enduring.

## Seeking Help for Infertility

Eventually, couples must decide whether to seek help to conceive. They may reach this point after only a few menstrual cycles or, at the opposite extreme, may never seek help. Many factors enter into their decision, such as their age (especially the woman's), how long they have been unable to conceive, how much they want a biologic child, how they regard adoption, and how they feel about a child-free life.

### IDENTIFYING THE IMPORTANCE OF HAVING A BABY

Each partner may place a different priority on having a baby. Conflicts may arise when one partner wants help to conceive sooner than the other. In addition, cultural or religious beliefs influence how each feels about procreation and whether options such as assisted reproductive procedures or adoption are acceptable. How the couple resolves these differences is crucial to the stability of the relationship.

Men and women often differ in their reactions to infertility. Women may want to talk about their feelings and frustrations, but men often internalize their feelings or feel that they must be strong for their partner. The woman may interpret her partner's reluctance to express his feelings and his stoicism as disinterest or lack of concern and care for her.

### SHARING INTIMATE INFORMATION

Although the infertility specialist will limit questions to the necessary ones, evaluation and treatment for infertility require that both partners reveal information about their sexual relationship, such as the frequency and timing of intercourse. This is difficult for those who regard this information as intimate. In addition, infertile couples may feel that the evaluation calls their sexual adequacy into question. They may feel defensive if they perceive a threat to their self-image.

### CONSIDERING FINANCIAL RESOURCES

Financial concerns enter into the couple's decision about whether to seek treatment and how far to carry it. Techniques such as basal body temperature assessment or over-the-counter ovulation predictor kits are inexpensive but have limited usefulness in actually achieving successful pregnancy. Advanced techniques, such as in vitro fertilization, are expensive and may have a low likelihood of success. Health insurance may not cover infertility treatment at all or may not cover all procedures because the problem does not directly threaten the health of either partner. Also, treatments that are investigational are often not covered. The drugs that must be taken to achieve pregnancy can be as expensive as an illegal drug habit. Expense and restricted coverage limit treatment choices for many low-income or middle-income couples. Those who seek and pursue infertility treatment usually have greater financial resources than those who do not.

### COMMITTING TO INVOLVEMENT IN CARE

Infertility evaluation and treatment require a great commitment from the couple in terms of time, energy, and money. Couples can be involved in this process for most or even all of a decade. They participate on a day-to-day basis as they do home assessments, take medications, and keep detailed records. For infertility diagnosis and therapy to be most effective, couples must consider their ability and desire to be directly involved in the process over a long period of time.

## Reactions During Evaluation and Treatment

Couples undergoing infertility evaluation and treatment have different reactions to the process. In addition, their reactions may change as infertility care progresses.

### INFLUENCES ON DECISION MAKING

If their evaluation shows that a treatment or procedure may enable them to conceive, the couple must then decide whether to proceed. The decision-making process begins early and must be repeated during therapy if pregnancy does not occur. A complex array of factors enters into their decisions about beginning and continuing treatment or whether to end their pursuit of pregnancy. Although discussed separately, these factors interact dynamically as the couple makes each decision. The nurse helps them examine each factor and arrive at a decision that is best for them.

**Social, Cultural, and Religious Values.** Some medically appropriate options may not be acceptable to every couple. Surrogate parenting, in vitro fertilization, and therapeutic insemination (especially with donor sperm) are inconsistent with the personal or religious beliefs of many people. If a procedure offers the partners hope for a child but is incompatible with their beliefs, their choices are two: use the technology despite their beliefs or be willing to accept childlessness. Adoption may be a third alternative for some couples if the desire for a biologic child is not absolute. As in other decisions, couples must work out conflicting personal values about what therapy is acceptable.

**Difficulty of Treatment.** The couple must consider how difficult, risky, and uncomfortable therapy will be. The level of difficulty involves physical, psychological, geographic, and time factors. Employment constraints may affect treatment decisions as well.

Several infertility treatments involve invasive procedures or surgery. The person who undergoes the procedure must be the one who ultimately decides whether to do it. That person alone can decide whether the hope of a child is worth the risks and discomfort of the procedure.

Infertility treatment is stressful. Often partners feel or are willing to tolerate different levels of stress. To reduce the stress, they may abandon treatment completely or may take a vacation for a few months from the constant preoccupation with conceiving. Older women nearing or in their 40s often do not feel that they have the luxury of skipping a treatment cycle.

Some couples encounter geographic difficulties if they must travel a long distance for therapy. Time stresses are substantial. The partners, particularly the woman, feel that achieving pregnancy is their new career. One or both partners may spend many hours every week in pursuit of pregnancy.

Employment constraints may be a barrier to infertility therapy because of the time required for treatment. The impact of time is usually greatest on the woman. Time away from work may burden the employer or co-workers. Stopping work may not be an option because the family needs the money and often needs the insurance coverage that comes with employment.

**Probability of Success.** Couples often have a biased interpretation of their statistical probability of success, especially when they begin treatment with a new procedure. For example, if a procedure has a 15 percent likelihood of success with each cycle, they tend to expect that they will be in the successful group rather than in the 85 percent who do not meet with success. As time goes by, however, they must weigh the likelihood of success of any therapy against financial concerns and their own willingness to accept the discomfort and difficulty associated with it.

**Financial Concerns.** Some couples, particularly those with ample resources and a strong desire for a biologic child, pursue expensive treatments and pursue them longer than others of more limited means. They may do so despite a low probability of success. Couples with financial limitations find that they must abandon treatment sooner than they want. Other couples go heavily into debt, adding financial strain to the other stresses of treatment in their quest for a child of their own.

### PSYCHOLOGICAL REACTIONS

A couple's initial reaction to infertility is often one of shock because the partners are usually healthy and often have had no idea that they might have problems conceiving. Their reactions vary according to how easily their infertility is alleviated, their personality and self-image, and the strength of their relationship.

**Guilt.** A partner having the only identified problem might feel that he or she is depriving the other of children. This feeling may be compounded if the "normal" partner has children from another relationship. It may be difficult for this person to understand that not all factors affecting fertility can be detected and that what seems like the problem of only one partner is often a couple problem.

Either partner may feel guilty about past choices that now affect fertility. A woman with adhesions resulting from a sexually transmissible infection may regret her past sexual choices. The man who wanted to delay pregnancy longer than the woman may feel guilty if her age is now affecting her fertility and limiting the length of time she has for achieving conception.

**Isolation.** Infertile couples often feel different from friends and relatives who do not have difficulty conceiving. They may withdraw from these relationships to insulate themselves from painful reminders of their infertility. Some couples develop supportive relationships with others who are also infertile, which somewhat diminishes their sense of isolation.

**Depression.** One or both partners may experience depression as their sense of competence and control over their bodies is challenged, especially if therapy is not successful quickly. They often feel as if they are on a roller coaster of hope alternating with despair when the woman has her menstrual period each month. In an attempt to insulate themselves from disappointment, couples with long-term infertility try not to expect too much with each cycle.

The couple may feel envy at those who conceive easily. They may become judgmental and angry when they see those who seem to "have no business having a baby," such as an adolescent or a poor woman who has several children.

**Stress on the Relationship.** Because infertility can challenge one's identity and self-esteem, the partners may find less satisfaction in their relationship. They may feel unlovable or unappealing to their mate.

The man may find it difficult to perform on demand for semen specimens and postcoital tests, feeling that others will judge his sexual function. The fact that semen samples are best obtained by masturbation is unacceptable to some men. Both partners are stressed when intercourse must be scheduled to coincide with specific evaluations or with ovulation. Intercourse can become a chore more than an expression of love. It may come to be associated with failure rather than fulfillment.

If sperm from an anonymous donor is used for therapeutic insemination or other techniques, the man may feel that his masculinity is further threatened. He does not want to deprive his wife of a child, but he may be ambivalent about use of sperm from a third party. He may have difficulty distinguishing fatherhood as a biologic achievement from fatherhood as a relationship.

The partners find their relationship strained if they disagree on which treatments are appropriate and how long they should be pursued. One partner may want to keep trying "one more month," and the other may want to abandon treatment. If they are considering adoption, their relationship may be strained if they differ on whether to adopt and what kind of child they are willing to accept.

## Outcomes After Infertility Therapy

After infertility therapy, three outcomes are possible. The couple may become parents, either biologically or through adoption. Infertility therapy may be unsuccessful, and the couple must decide whether to pursue adoption. The loss of a pregnancy may result in mixed emotions of grief and optimism.

### Pregnancy Loss After Infertility Therapy

Couples who suffer pregnancy loss after infertility therapy may interpret the experience with mixed feelings of loss and gain. Couples undergoing infertility evaluation and treatment are often aware of a pregnancy much earlier than fertile couples. They want to hope yet expect to be disappointed again. If a spontaneous abortion occurs, they may grieve profoundly for what they achieved and then lost.

Yet, despite their grief about the pregnancy loss, the partners may be encouraged because they have proved that they can achieve a pregnancy. They may feel that if they succeeded once, they can do it again. A spontaneous abortion may give them the courage to continue treatment.

### Parenthood After Infertility Therapy

Couples who achieve conception experience varied emotions. If they have been disappointed many times before, they may hardly believe the good news. They are often thrilled but worry about whether they can complete the pregnancy and take home a baby. Pregnancy after infertility therapy is emotionally tentative for many infertile couples, especially those who have been trying to conceive for a long time or those who have lost a pregnancy. They may distance themselves from the reality of the pregnancy until much later in gestation than would fertile couples. The woman has grown accustomed to sensing and reporting every symptom and may interpret normal physiologic changes of pregnancy as a threat.

The previously infertile couple may find little sympathy from those who do not understand the fear of investing in the pregnancy. Others may be annoyed because they expect the couple to be overjoyed at a successful and apparently normal pregnancy. Outsiders may feel that the partners are self-centered and cannot decide what they want. Other infertile couples, who were previously a source of mutual support, may withdraw from the couple who achieves a pregnancy.

The parents' anxiety may be heightened during labor. They are afraid that something will go wrong at the last moment. Even after the birth of a healthy infant, some parents have difficulty relaxing and enjoying their baby.

These new parents often need much support as they gain experience with their child. Infertile couples who eventually have biologic or adopted children may have unrealistic expectations about parenting. After investing so much financial, physical, and emotional resources in having a child, they may be reluctant to express any unhappiness or frustration over the realities of childrearing.

### Choosing to Adopt

Not every couple who seeks treatment for infertility achieves a "take-home" baby. Some couples discontinue treatment sooner than others, depending on their age and their tolerance for the fatigue, stress, and expense. Some couples investigate adoption early in infertility treatment because advanced age may make them ineligible to adopt through many agencies or because a nonbiologic child is acceptable to them.

Couples who consider adoption must confront their personal preferences, limitations, and even prejudices. As much as they want a child, many couples are not willing to adopt *any* child. Most couples prefer to adopt a newborn or an infant and one of their race. Some prefer an infant but are also willing to adopt an older child, one with special needs, one of a mixed or different race, or a group of siblings. Other couples, for a variety of reasons, will not consider adopting these children.

Some couples fear adopting a child because the woman might become pregnant. Although pregnancy has been the goal for a long time, they may worry that they would love their adopted child differently from their biologic child.

Couples who decide to adopt face further scrutiny of their personal lives. Agencies investigate their home, financial means (which may have been seriously drained), and fitness as parents. Once again, they may feel that their personal competence is questioned.

The couple who decides on adoption may have emotions similar to those who achieve a pregnancy. They may be slow to invest in the process emotionally because they expect disappointment again. In addition, the adopted child often comes to them suddenly and unexpectedly. Although they may have been waiting months for this happy event, they have little time to adjust to the reality that they are becoming parents.

#### ✓ CHECK YOUR READING

16. What factors do couples consider when they are deciding whether to seek help for their infertility?
17. What factors must couples consider when they reach decision points during infertility evaluation and treatment?
18. What are possible psychological reactions to infertility?
19. If the partners become parents, either through birth or adoption, how may they react to parenthood?
20. What are the issues couples must face if they consider adoption?
21. What emotions do couples often experience if they lose a pregnancy after infertility treatment?

## Application of Nursing Process: Care of the Infertile Couple

Nurses may encounter couples facing infertility in many different settings and may identify numerous nursing care needs. Nursing care of the infertile couple is challenging yet can be most satisfying. Regardless of the setting, the nurse often addresses the couple's emotional needs associated with infertility evaluation, treatment, and outcomes of therapy.

### Assessment

In many instances, infertile couples have previously had a positive self-image and feelings of competence about themselves. The diagnosis of infertility shakes their positive view. The nurse should be aware that these feelings may be present, regardless of the practice setting in which the couple is encountered.

Determine at what point the couple is in their infertility treatment. Couples who have just discovered that they may have difficulty conceiving may be shocked, yet optimistic that therapy will result in a baby for them. Couples with longstanding infertility may have a deeper sense of failure and a pessimistic outlook. Listen for remarks that are negative, expressing guilt or helplessness.

Evaluate how infertility has affected the partners' relationship with each other. Are there conflicts or differences in values between the two? Observing their body language, such as eye contact, may provide clues about how similarly or differently they are committed to diagnosis and treatment. Ask them how their relationship has changed. Are they more or less satisfied with their marital relationship than they were before they had problems conceiving?

Ask about support systems. Couples suffering from infertility often withdraw from old relationships yet do not form new supportive ones. Do others who are significant in the partners' lives know that they are trying to conceive? Are family members and friends nearby, and are they supportive? Ask whether they have encountered assumptions by others that infertility is the "fault" of one partner or the other. Are they subjected to questions that invade their privacy, such as "When are you two going to have a baby of your own?"

Elicit information about how the couple's culture

or religion views infertility and the impact of these values on therapy. Are there therapies that are unacceptable to one or both partners? The partners may have differing views that can cause conflict during treatment, and they will need help to work these out.

Determine how the couple is coping with the stresses of treatment. How much has infertility cost them in terms of time, money, and discomfort? Identify the successes and failures they have experienced. Their age, especially the woman's, adds another stressor that they cannot avoid. Older couples may feel that they must try to conceive with every menstrual cycle.

If the woman is pregnant or has given birth recently or if the couple has adopted a child recently, observe for high levels of anxiety in either or both parents. Assess them for negative behaviors and comments, such as reluctance to feel joy or a sense that they will "fail" again.

## Analysis

A nursing diagnosis commonly encountered is Situational Low Self-Esteem related to perception of reproductive inadequacy.

## Planning

Three goals are appropriate for this nursing diagnosis, and they may apply to the man, the woman, or both partners. The person(s) will do the following:

- Express feelings about infertility and its evaluation and treatment.
- Explore ways to increase control within the situation of infertility.
- Identify aspects of self that are positive.

## Interventions

### ASSISTING COMMUNICATION

Therapeutic communication is the primary technique for both assessment and intervention related to this nursing diagnosis. Use a variety of communication techniques, such as active listening and exploration, to encourage the partners to express their feelings honestly. Provide privacy and acceptance of their feelings. Nurses must recognize the validity of the couple's views and emotions, even if they differ from the nurse's own feelings.

Encourage the partners to accept their feelings, both positive and negative. For example, the couple who has finally achieved pregnancy may be living a lie to some extent. The partners may act elated because they believe they should feel happy, yet inside they are cautious and hesitant to become attached to their baby. Explain that feelings are not right or wrong but simply exist. It may be helpful to open the subject of negative feelings (fear of attachment) within a successful situation (pregnancy or birth) to reinforce the normality of their emotions. This technique gives them the opportunity to talk about emotional reactions that they or others feel are inappropriate and might otherwise be reluctant to discuss.

Discuss possible differences in ways the man and the woman communicate. For example, explain that the woman may feel more comfortable than the man in talking about their problem and concerns about treatment. Explain that these differences in communication style can cause misunderstandings because one partner believes that the other does not care as much about their problem. Encourage them to be open with each other for the best mutual support.

### INCREASING THE COUPLE'S SENSE OF CONTROL

Explore how the couple has dealt with stressors in the past and how these techniques might be used to cope with the present crisis. A couple's pattern of dealing with stress in other parts of life is likely to carry over into infertility work-up and treatment and throughout pregnancy and parenthood. Reinforce coping skills that are positive, such as learning more about infertility and the proposed therapy for it.

Couples who experience undue stress may benefit from relaxation techniques, such as visualization and moderate exercise. Frequent strenuous exercise may reduce the woman's ability to ovulate. Although a hot tub is relaxing for many people, it should be avoided because the high temperatures may inhibit spermatogenesis. In addition, the woman could become pregnant with any cycle, and high body temperatures have been associated with fetal anomalies.

Discuss behaviors that enhance the ability to handle stress and that provide a good environment for a pregnancy that might occur. Reinforce healthy choices, such as good nutrition and a balance between exercise and rest. Teach the couple ways to enhance general health if deficiencies are identified.

Explain any procedures and their purpose in language that the couple can understand. Reinforce any medical explanations that may have been given. Encourage questions so that the couple is fully informed. Have the partners restate what was explained to reduce misunderstandings.

Help the couple explore options at each decision point. No one else can decide the best course of action, but the nurse can help identify pros and cons of each choice so that the partners can arrive at a decision appropriate for them. Be nondirective so that the choices are theirs and do not reflect the biases of the nurse or other caregivers.

#### REDUCING ISOLATION

Because couples often distance themselves from friends and family relationships that they find painful, they may have few social supports. Refer them to available support groups to provide emotional outlets, a sense of belonging, and a source of information.

Couples who achieve pregnancy or adopt a child may again find themselves isolated because they are now different from other infertile couples. Encourage them to take the initiative to reestablish ties with relatives and friends, who can be an important source of support during pregnancy and childrearing. Help them to identify ways they can improve communication with these significant others. Remind them that they have undergone significant shifts in self-image that have also affected those around them.

#### PROMOTING A POSITIVE SELF-IMAGE

Because infertility work is often such a dominant factor in their lives, a continuing inability to conceive erodes the partners' perception of themselves. Explore with them other areas of competence and activities that make them feel good about themselves. Reinforce positive attitudes and self-evaluations. Encourage them to maintain activities such as hobbies, sports, or volunteer work. The career of either partner may be a source of stress that needs relief, or it may be an avenue that fosters a positive self-perception.

Some people benefit from self-improvement activities, such as continuing education courses or enhancement of appearance. Encourage these activities if they help the individuals feel better about themselves. If the activity might impair fertility treatments, such as strict dieting, inform the person of this fact as well.

## Evaluation

The goals established are achieved if the individual or both partners does the following:

- Can express their feelings about their situation, usually over a period of time.
- Can explore ways to increase personal control over their lives, as evidenced by expressing feelings of reduced helplessness and dependence.
- Can identify one or more aspects of self perceived as positive and can identify areas of competence.

## SUMMARY CONCEPTS

- Nurses may encounter persons having infertility problems in a variety of settings other than infertility clinics, for example, maternity and gynecology services, urology services, the perioperative area, and the emergency department. Friends and family members also see the nurse as an information resource about infertility care.
- About 20 percent of infertile couples have no identified problem that is explained by current evaluation techniques.
- Because there are many unknown factors in reproduction, identification and correction of problems in one or both partners do not necessarily resolve their infertility.
- A variety of structural and functional abnormalities may contribute to a couple's infertility. The man may have abnormalities of the sperm, the seminal fluid, or with ejaculation. The woman may have ovulation disorders; anatomic problems, such as fallopian tube occlusion; or physiologic disorders, such as hormone imbalances.
- A systematic evaluation of both partners, proceeding from simple to more complex, identifies therapy that is most likely to be successful and cost effective.
- Infertility is a crisis for the couple and often for the extended family. Either or both partners may feel that the inability to conceive represents a personal failure. They may have a variety of psychological reactions.
- Infertile couples must make choices at many points before and during evaluation and therapy. Some major factors that enter into their decisions involve social, cultural, and religious values; difficulty of treatment; probability of success; financial resources; and age, particularly the woman's.
- The possible outcomes after infertility therapy may present new challenges to the couple and their families: unsuccessful therapy and the choice of whether to pursue adoption, pregnancy loss after infertility, and parenthood after infertility.
- Many nursing care needs may be identified as the couple negotiates infertility evaluation and treatment.

#### References and Readings


Bayer, S.R., & DeCherney, A.H. (1994). Cervical factor in infertility. In F.A. Zuspan & E.J. Quilligan (Eds.), *Current therapy in obstetrics and gynecology* 4 (pp. 14–18). Philadelphia: W.B. Saunders.

Blackburn, S.T., & Loper, D.L. (1992). *Maternal, fetal, and neonatal physiology: A clinical perspective*. Philadelphia: W.B. Saunders.

Boxer, A.S. (1996). Images of infertility. *Nurse Practitioner Forum*, 7(2), 60–63.

Edwards, R.G., & Brody, S.A. (1995). *Principles and practices of assisted human reproduction*. Philadelphia: W.B. Saunders.

Friedman, C.I. (1994). Male infertility: Intrauterine insemination. In F.A. Zuspan & E.J. Quilligan (Eds.), *Current therapy in obstetrics and gynecology* 4 (pp. 83–86). Philadelphia: W.B. Saunders.

Garner, C. (1994). Uses of GnRH agonists. *Journal of Obstetric, Gynecologic, and Neonatal Nursing*, 23(7), 563–570.

Grodstein, F., Goldman, M.B., & Cramer, D.W. (1994). Infertility in women and moderate alcohol use. *American Journal of Public Health*, 84(9), 1429–1432.

Guyton, A.C., & Hall, J.E. (1996). *Textbook of medical physiology* (9th ed.). Philadelphia: W.B. Saunders.

Hahn, S.J., Butkowski, C.R., & Capper, L.L. (1994). Ovarian hyperstimulation syndrome: Protocols for nursing care. *Journal of Obstetric, Gynecologic, and Neonatal Nursing*, 23(3), 217–226.

Halman, L.J., Andrews, F.M., & Abbey, A. (1994). Gender differences and perceptions about childbearing among infertile couples. *Journal of Obstetric, Gynecologic, and Neonatal Nursing*, 23(7), 593–600.

Hirsch, A.M., & Hirsch, S.M. (1995). The long-term psychosocial effects of infertility. *Journal of Obstetric, Gynecologic, and Neonatal Nursing*, 24(6), 517–522.

Jirka, J., Schuett, S., & Foxall, M.J. (1996). Loneliness and social support in infertile couples. *Journal of Obstetric, Gynecologic, and Neonatal Nursing*, 25(1), 55–60.

Johnson, C.L. (1996). Regaining self-esteem: Strategies and interventions for the infertile woman. *Journal of Obstetric, Gynecologic, and Neonatal Nursing*, 25(4), 291–295.

Jones, G.S. (1994). Luteal phase defect. In F.A. Zuspan & E.J. Quilligan (Eds.), *Current therapy in obstetrics and gynecology* 4 (pp. 80–83). Philadelphia: W.B. Saunders.

Karch, A.M. (1996). *Lippincott's nursing drug guide* 1996. Philadelphia: J.B. Lippincott.

Kennard, E. (1994). Induction of ovulation. In F.A. Zuspan & E.J. Quilligan (Eds.), *Current therapy in obstetrics and gynecology* 4 (pp. 68–72). Philadelphia: W.B. Saunders.

Keye, W.R., Chang, R.J., Rebar, R.W., & Soules, M.R. (1995). *Infertility: Evaluation and treatment*. Philadelphia: W.B. Saunders.

Mastroianni, L. (1996). Forty years of infertility management—exponential progress and a demanding future. *Nurse Practitioner Forum*, 7(2), 87–91.

Noller, K.L. (1994). In utero DES exposure. In F.A. Zuspan & E.J. Quilligan (Eds.), *Current therapy in obstetrics and gynecology* 4 (pp. 144–146). Philadelphia: W.B. Saunders.

Patrizio, P., & Asch, R.H. (1994a). GIFT procedure. In F.A. Zuspan & E.J. Quilligan (Eds.), *Current therapy in obstetrics and gynecology* 4 (pp. 55–57). Philadelphia: W.B. Saunders.

Patrizio, P., & Asch, R.H. (1994b). Microsurgical epididymal sperm aspiration. In F.A. Zuspan & E.J. Quilligan (Eds.), *Current therapy in obstetrics and gynecology* 4 (pp. 92–94). Philadelphia: W.B. Saunders.

Reshef, E., & Sanfilippo, J.S. (1994). Hysteroscopic evaluation and therapy of mullerian anomalies. In F.A. Zuspan & E.J. Quilligan (Eds.), *Current therapy in obstetrics and gynecology* 4 (pp. 65–69). Philadelphia: W.B. Saunders.

Sandelowski, M. (1994). On infertility. *Journal of Obstetric, Gynecologic, and Neonatal Nursing*, 23(9), 749–752.

Schoener, C.J., & Krysa, L.W. (1996). The comfort and discomfort of infertility. *Journal of Obstetric, Gynecologic, and Neonatal Nursing*, 25(2), 167–172.

Sherrod, R.A. (1992). Helping infertile couples explore the option of adoption. *Journal of Obstetric, Gynecologic, and Neonatal Nursing*, 21(6), 465–470.

Sherrod, R.A. (1995). A male perspective on infertility. *MCN: American Journal of Maternal-Child Nursing*, 20(5), 269–275.

Stansberry, J. (1996). The infertile couple: An overview of pathophysiology and diagnostic evaluation for the primary care clinician. *Nurse Practitioner Forum*, 7(2), 70–86.

Tietz, N.W. (1995). *Clinical guide to laboratory tests* (3rd ed.). Philadelphia: W.B. Saunders.

Timbers, K.A., & Feinberg, R.F. (1996). Recurrent pregnancy loss: A review. *Nurse Practitioner Forum*, 7(2), 64–75.

# 33

# Women's Health Care

**OBJECTIVES**

1. Explain examinations and various screening procedures that are recommended to maintain the health of women.
2. Define four benign disorders of the breast, relate them to expected age of onset, and describe the diagnostic procedures used to rule out cancer of the breast.
3. Describe the incidence, risks, pathophysiology, management, and nursing considerations of malignant tumors of the breast.
4. Discuss the four most common menstrual cycle disorders.
5. Explain nursing considerations for women who experience premenstrual syndrome.
6. Discuss induced abortion in terms of procedures, possible complications, and follow-up care.
7. Describe the physical and psychological changes associated with menopause and the risks versus benefits of hormone replacement therapy.
8. Discuss preventive measures for osteoporosis.
9. Describe the major disorders associated with pelvic relaxation in terms of cause, treatment, and nursing considerations.
10. Discuss the most common benign and malignant disorders of the reproductive tract in terms of signs and symptoms, management, and nursing considerations.
11. Describe care of the woman with an infectious disorder of the reproductive tract, including sexually transmissible diseases, pelvic inflammatory disease, and toxic shock syndrome.

**DEFINITIONS**

**adjuvant therapy** *Additional treatment that increases or enhances the action of the primary treatment.*

**adnexa** *Accessory organs of the uterus, such as the fallopian tubes and ovaries.*

**amenorrhea** *Absence of menstruation. Primary amenorrhea is a delay of the first menstruation. Secondary amenorrhea is cessation of menstruation after its initiation.*

**atrophic vaginitis** *Inflammation that occurs when the vagina becomes dry and fragile, usually as a result of estrogen deficit after menopause.*

**autogenous graft** *Tissue that is moved from one part of the body to another part of the same person's body.*

**axillary tail** *Wedge of tissue extending from the breast into the axilla (also called the tail of Spence).*

**carcinoma in situ** *Malignant neoplasm in surface tissue that has not extended into deeper tissue.*
**climacteric** *Endocrine, body, and psychic changes occurring at the end of a woman's reproductive cycle. Also informally called menopause.*
**colposcopy** *Examination of the vaginal and cervical tissue with a colposcope for magnification of cells.*
**condyloma** *A wart-like growth of the skin seen on the external genitalia, in the vagina, on the cervix, or near the anus; may be caused by human papillomavirus (condyloma acuminatum) or by syphilis (condyloma latum).*
**cryotherapy** *Destruction of tissue using extreme cold.*
**cystocele** *Prolapse of the urinary bladder through the anterior vaginal wall.*
**dysmenorrhea** *Painful menstruation.*
**dyspareunia** *Difficult or painful coitus in women.*
**dysplasia** *Abnormal development of tissue.*
**dysuria** *Painful urination, often associated with urinary tract infection.*
**endometrial hyperplasia** *Excessive proliferation of normal cells of the uterine lining; may be due to administration of estrogen during the postmenopausal period.*
**endometriosis** *Presence of tissue resembling the endometrium outside the uterine cavity.*
**laparoscopy** *Insertion of an illuminated tube into the abdominal cavity to visualize contents, locate bleeding, and perform surgical procedures.*
**laparotomy** *Incision through the abdominal wall to examine the abdominal or pelvic organs.*
**mammogram** *Study of breast tissue using very-low-dose x-ray; primary tool in the diagnosis of breast tumors.*
**menarche** *Onset of menstruation; average age is 12.8 years.*
**menometrorrhagia** *Uterine bleeding that is irregular in frequency and also excessive in amount.*
**menopause** *Permanent cessation of menstruation during the climacteric.*
**menorrhagia** *Excessive bleeding at the time of menstruation in number of days' duration, amount of blood lost, or both.*
**metrorrhagia** *Bleeding from the uterus at any time other than during the menstrual period.*
**osteoporosis** *Increased spaces (porosity) in bone; process greatly accelerates following menopause.*
**peau d'orange** *Dimpled skin condition that resembles an orange; associated with lymphatic edema and often seen over the area of breast cancer.*
**rectocele** *Herniation (protrusion) of the rectum through the posterior vaginal wall.*
**toxic shock syndrome** *Rare, potentially fatal disorder caused by toxin produced by* Staphylococcus aureus*; has been associated with improper use of tampons.*

This chapter focuses on primary and preventive care of women as it relates to routine assessments, screening procedures, and management of specific health concerns. The nurse's role is of particular interest because nurses provide many of the services most valued by women. Some nurses, such as nurse practitioners, provide primary care. Others act as educators and advocates for women. They are responsible for explaining screening and diagnostic procedures and for clarifying options so that women can make informed decisions about care. Finally, nurses have traditionally offered support and comfort to women when they experience disruptions in their health.

## National Health Goals

In 1990 the United States Public Health Service formulated health care objectives for the year 2000 (DHHS, 1995). Some of the major ones relating to women's health are to

1. Reverse the rise in breast cancer deaths from 23.0 per 100,000 women in 1987 to no more than 20.6.
2. Reduce deaths from cancer of the cervix from 2.8 per 100,000 women in 1987 to no more than 1.3.
3. Increase by at least 20 percent the number of women who received a test for cervical cancer within the last 3 years.
4. Reduce the incidence of gonorrhea in women between the ages of 15 and 44 from 501 per 100,000 to 175.
5. Reduce the prevalence of *Chlamydia trachomatis* infections among women under the age of 25 years to no more than 5 percent.
6. Reduce congenital syphilis from an incidence of 91.0 per 100,000 live births to no more than 40.
7. Increase to at least 50 percent the proportion of sexually active women between the ages of 15 and 19 years whose partners used condoms at last sexual experience.

## Health Maintenance

Health maintenance refers to measures that can be taken to prevent or to detect specific diseases. Periodic health examinations, immunizations, and screening procedures are the most commonly recommended measures. Unfortunately, many women do not take advantage of recommended health maintenance procedures. Some seek care only when they have a problem. For others, the only health care they receive comes from a gynecologist or nurse practitioner who conducts a gynecologic examination. Therefore, it is important that those who provide health care for women are familiar with principles of screening and counseling in areas that are not traditionally associated with gynecology, such as assessing risk factors for colon cancer and heart disease.

## Health History

The health history is most important in the determination of risk factors for a variety of conditions. The health history of a well woman may be obtained through individual interviews or a combination of questionnaires, interviews, and previous records.

The focus of a health history depends on the woman's age, but some topics need to be discussed with all women. Table 33–1 provides a summary of information that should be obtained. These topics include dietary intake, physical activity, habits, and sexual practices. When discussing drugs, it is important to include long-term use of prescription and over-the-counter medications.

Family history is essential to assess risk profiles. History on hyperlipidemia, heart disease, osteoporosis, and thyroid disease indicates which screening tests and examinations are needed. A list of family members who had cancer and their ages when it was discovered provides important information about the risk of cancer, particularly breast and colon cancer.

A family history of heart disease is especially important when the woman is postmenopausal because estrogen, which protects against coronary artery disease, decreases after menopause. Therefore, a family history that includes myocardial infarctions increases the risk of coronary artery disease in a postmenopausal woman who does not take estrogen replacement. In this case, a baseline electrocardiogram and periodic laboratory analysis of cholesterol and triglyceride levels may be necessary to identify additional risk factors.

### ✓ CHECK YOUR READING

1. Why is a family history an important part of a health history?
2. What questions should be asked when taking a sexual history?

### TABLE 33–1 HEALTH HISTORY

**Personal History**

Demographic data (name, age, marital status)
Reason for seeking medical care (also termed chief complaint)
Current and past state of health, previous surgeries
Appetite, dietary intake
Exercise pattern
Habits (smoking, use of alcohol, drugs), allergies
Sleep and rest patterns
Patterns of elimination (current or chronic problems)
Degree of stress and stress management techniques

**Sexual History**

Sexually active (one partner, multiple partners, age when first sexually active)
Method of contraception (satisfaction with method, adverse reactions)
Knowledge/practice of measures to protect self from sexually transmissible diseases

**Menstrual History**

Age of menarche
Regularity, duration of menstrual cycle
Menstrual discomfort

**Obstetric History**

Gravida, para, length of gestation, weight of infant at birth
Labor experience and method of delivery

**Family History**

Cardiovascular problems (anemia, hypertension, clotting disorders, stroke, heart attacks)
Cancer (breast, uterine, ovarian, bowel, lung)
Osteoporosis

**Psychosocial History**

Primary language, additional languages spoken or understood
Marital status, employment, occupation, education (relevant to determine financial, social, and emotional support)

## Physical Assessment

A thorough physical examination is necessary to detect general health problems. Blood pressure, temperature, pulse, respirations, and weight are measured at each visit. Height is taken at the initial examination and yearly after that. Loss of height and abnormal curvature of the vertebral column (dorsal kyphosis or scoliosis) are important observations in evaluating osteoporosis in the postmenopausal woman.

The heart is generally auscultated at the initial visit to determine whether rate and rhythm are normal and to detect heart murmurs. The extremities are observed for varicosities or edema, and pedal pulses are palpated. Palpation of the abdomen for tenderness, masses, or distention is an important part of the physical examination.

Additional assessments are necessary if the woman is in a high-risk group. For instance, if she has a family history of diabetes mellitus, a fasting glucose test may be indicated. If she has a history of multiple sexual partners or a sexual partner with multiple contacts, she may require testing for sexually transmissible diseases.

## Preventive Counseling

Physical examination provides an excellent opportunity to counsel women about preventive care. Major preventable problems are obesity, inactivity, and smoking. Approximately one fifth of the women in the United States are obese (ACOG, 1996). Obesity is associated with numerous health problems such as diabetes and hypertension. Inactivity is associated with osteoporosis, elevated levels of cholesterol, and coronary artery disease. Cigarette smoking is on the rise in young women, and smoking increases the risk for a wide variety of diseases, including cardiovascular problems and cancer. Counseling regarding diet should be offered and positive behaviors, such as exercise, should be reinforced. Use of latex condoms provides some protection against transmission of viruses, such as human immunodeficiency virus (HIV) and human papillomavirus (HPV), which is strongly implicated as a risk factor for cervical cancer.

The history or physical examination may indicate other areas for which counseling would be beneficial. These include the dangers of malignant melanoma with repeated exposure to ultraviolet rays of the sun. In addition, the health risks associated with alcohol and other substance abuse may be particularly important for some women.

## Screening Procedures

The value of screening procedures is based on two assumptions: (1) Prevention is better than cure, and (2) early diagnosis allows early treatment while the pathologic process is still reversible.

A variety of screening procedures are recommended for all women, including three screening procedures for early detection of breast cancer as well as vulvar self-examination and screening for cervical cancer.

### BREAST SELF-EXAMINATION

Breast self-examination (BSE) is a supplement to, rather than a substitute for, screening by professional examination and mammography. In many parts of the world, however, BSE is the only realistic means of early cancer detection.

Breast self-examination should be performed monthly by all women after the age of 20 years. Women should perform a BSE about 1 week following the onset of menses, when hormonal influences on the breasts are at a low level. If the woman no longer menstruates, she may choose a day that is easy to remember and perform the test on that day every month. An example is the first day of the month.

### PROFESSIONAL BREAST EXAMINATION

Professional breast examination is similar to BSE; however, professional examiners are more experienced and may detect questionable areas that the woman misses. The examination includes both inspection and palpation. It should be part of every gynecologic examination.

#### INSPECTION

1. While the woman is in an upright position, the examiner inspects the breasts for size, symmetry, color, and skin changes. The nipples and areola are inspected for differences in size and color, unilateral retraction of a nipple, and asymmetric nipple direction, which may indicate an underlying tumor.
2. The woman raises her hands above her head, and the examiner inspects the sides and underneath portions of the breast for asymmetry and differences in color.
3. The woman places her hands on her hips and presses down; this action reveals skin dimpling or masses.

#### PALPATION

1. With the woman in an upright position and while the arm is at the side and relaxed, each axilla is carefully palpated for enlarged or tender lymph nodes.
2. The woman lies in a supine position for palpation of the breasts. A small pillow or folded towel is placed under the shoulder to stretch the tissue and thus flatten the breast. The examiner uses the flat part of the first three fingers to palpate the breast, rotating the fingers against the chest wall. Tissue that extends into the axilla, the so-called tail of Spence, should also be palpated. The procedure is repeated on the opposite side. Normal breast tissue is described as firm, lumpy, nodular, tender, and thickened. Abnormal breast tissue is often likened to a raisin, watermelon seed, or grape. In other words, a discrete mass can be felt and measured. If a suspicious area is found, follow-up by mammography is recommended.
3. The nipples are compressed to detect the presence of discharge. A sample of any discharge should be collected for culture and examination of cells.

## Women Want to Know
### How to Perform Breast Self-Examination

- Lie down. Flatten your right breast by placing a pillow under your right shoulder. If your breasts are large, use your right hand to hold your right breast while you do the examination with your left hand.
- Use the sensitive pads of the middle three fingers on your left hand and a massaging motion to feel for lumps or changes in the breast tissue.
- Press firmly enough to distinguish different breast textures.
- Completely palpate or feel all parts of the breast and chest area. Be sure to examine the breast tissue that extends toward the shoulder. The amount of time required to completely palpate all the breast tissue depends on the size of the breast. Women with small breasts need at least 2 minutes to examine each breast. Larger breasts take longer.

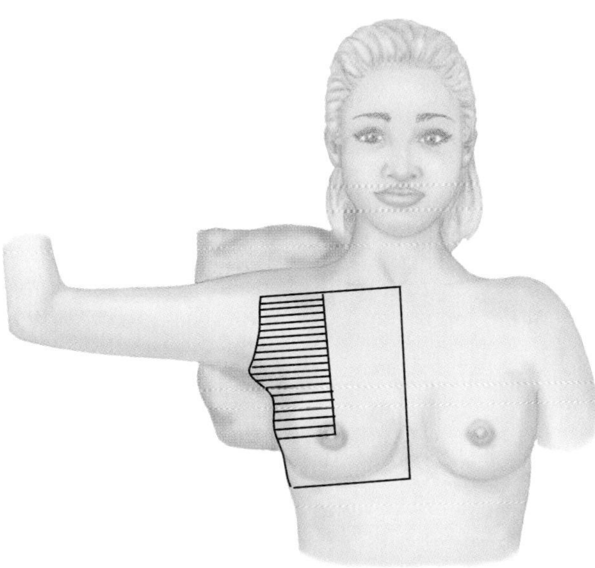

- Use the same routine or pattern to feel every part of the breast tissue. Any of three patterns can help you to make sure you have covered your entire breast: the circular pattern, the vertical strip, and the wedge. Choose the method you find easiest.

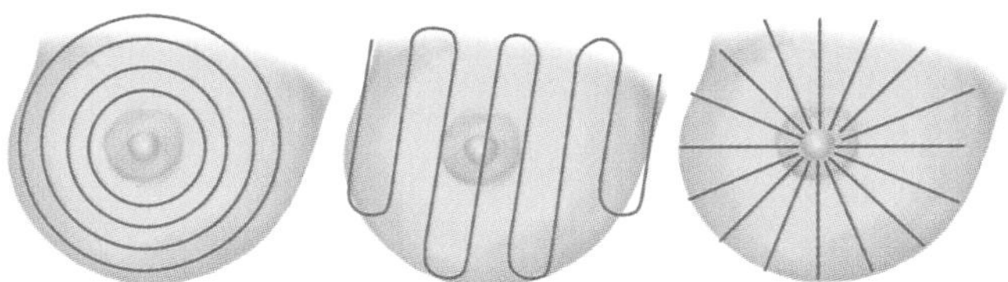

- When you have completely examined your right breast, the left breast should be examined using the same method. Compare what you feel in one breast with the other.
- You may also want to examine your breasts while bathing, when the skin is wet and lumps may be easily palpated.
- You can check your breasts in a mirror by raising your arms and looking for an unusual shape, dimpling of the skin, and any changes in the nipple.

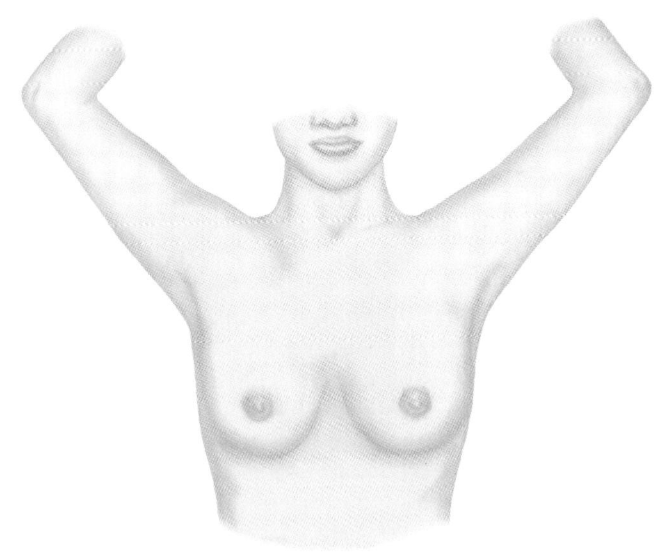

Adapted from the American Cancer Society (1992). *Special touch*. Atlanta: Author.

#### MAMMOGRAPHY

Mammography may be used either to screen for cancer or to assist in the diagnosis of a palpable mass in the breast. At present, mammography is the only screening tool that can detect breast lumps long before they are large enough to be palpated. This allows early diagnosis and treatment and thus increases the chance of long-term survival. The American College of Obstetricians and Gynecologists (1996) continues to recommend that screening mammography be offered routinely every 1 to 2 years to women aged 40 to 49 and annually to women older than 50 years. Women at high risk for breast cancer (see p. 934 for a summary of risk factors) may need earlier or more frequent evaluation.

Despite the known value of mammography, many women have never had a mammogram. Reasons for this include expense, fear that x-ray exposure will cause cancer, fear of pain, and reluctance to hear "bad news."

Nurses provide information and reassurance whenever possible and, in this way, help the woman overcome her objections to the use of this valuable screening tool. Although mammography is relatively expensive, it is often covered by health insurance, and screening mammograms are frequently offered by the community at low cost. It is important to acknowledge that some discomfort occurs when the breast is compressed between two plates while the radiograph is taken. One measure that reduces discomfort is scheduling the mammography following a menstrual period, when the breasts are less tender. Knowledge that the risk of mammography is minimal to nonexistent, because very-low-dose exposure to x-rays is used, may help women to overcome some of their fear.

At one time concern about the safety and reliability of equipment and some questions about the training required for personnel in mammography units were issues. In response to these concerns, the Mammography Quality Standards Act was passed in 1994. This law states that all mammography facilities, including physicians' offices, must be certified by the Food and Drug Administration (FDA). The facilities are responsible for meeting quality standards for film processing, interpretation, and record keeping. Furthermore, mammography units must be monitored closely to ensure appropriate radiation levels and overall operation. Quality assurance programs ensure that positive results are followed up quickly and properly.

## VULVAR SELF-EXAMINATION

Vulvar self-examination should be performed monthly by all women older than 18 and by those younger than 18 who are sexually active. Vulvar self-examination is visual inspection and palpation of the female external genitalia to detect signs of precancerous conditions or infections.

The woman is instructed to sit in a well-lighted area and to use a hand-held mirror to see the external genitalia. She is taught to examine the vulva in a systematic manner, starting at the mons pubis and progressing to the clitoris, labia minora, labia majora, perineum, and anus. Palpation of the vulvar area should accompany visual inspection. New moles, warts or growths of any kind, ulcers, sores, changes in skin color, or areas of inflammation or itching should be reported to the woman's health care provider as soon as possible.

## PELVIC EXAMINATION

Every gynecologic assessment includes a pelvic examination. The woman is advised to schedule the examination between menstrual periods and not to douche or have sexual intercourse for at least 48 hours before the examination. She is also advised not to use vaginal medications, sprays, or deodorants that might interfere with interpretation of cytology specimens that are collected.

Before the examination, the procedure is carefully explained and the woman empties her bladder. Although pelvic examinations are relatively painless, most women dread them and welcome sensitive, considerate support.

The pelvic examination is carried out with the woman in a lithotomy position, with a pillow under her head. If she wishes, she may be placed in a semi-sitting position and offered a hand mirror so that she can observe the external genitalia and the examination. She is carefully draped so that only the parts being examined are exposed.

Necessary equipment to be assembled before the examination begins includes gloves, speculum, slides, cotton swabs, a fixative agent, and a cytobrush and spatula for obtaining material for the Papanicolaou (Pap) smear (see later in this chapter). A stool specimen may be obtained by the examiner during the rectal examination, and a slide for this specimen should also be available.

**External Organs.** The pelvic examination is conducted systematically and gently. The external organs are scrutinized for the degree of development or atrophy of the labia, the distribution of hair, and the character of the hymen. Any cysts, tumors, or inflammation of Bartholin's glands is noted. The urinary meatus and Skene's glands are inspected for purulent discharge. Perineal scarring resulting from childbirth is noted.

**Speculum Examination.** A bivalve speculum of the appropriate size is used to inspect the vagina and cervix. The speculum is warmed with tap water and then gently inserted into the vagina. No other lubrication is used because it interferes with accurate cytology results. The size, shape, and color of the cervix are noted. A sample is taken for the Pap test. In addition, a sample of any unusual discharge is obtained for microscopic examination or culture.

**Bimanual Examination.** The bimanual examination provides information about the uterus, fallopian tubes, and ovaries. The labia are separated, and the gloved, lubricated index finger and middle finger of the examiner's nondominant hand are inserted into the vaginal introitus.

The cervix is palpated for consistency, size, and tenderness to motion. The uterus is evaluated by placing the dominant hand flat on the abdomen with the fingers pressing gently just above the symphysis pubis so that the uterus can be felt between the examining fingers of both hands. The size, configuration, consistency, and motility of the uterus are evaluated (Fig. 33–1).

It is usually impossible to feel the fallopian tubes; however, the ovaries may be palpated between the

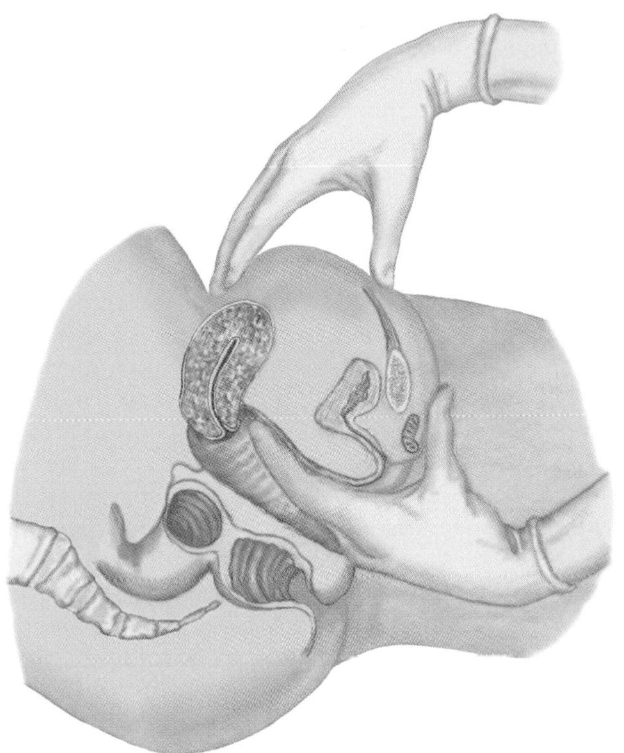

**FIGURE 33–1**

Bimanual palpation provides information about the uterus, fallopian tubes, and ovaries.

fingers of both hands. Because ovaries atrophy following menopause, it is often impossible to palpate the ovaries of a postmenopausal woman.

#### THE PAPANICOLAOU TEST

**Purpose.** It is known that, in virtually all cases, changes occur in cells of the cervix before cervical cancer develops. These changes have variously been called cervical intraepithelial neoplasia, dysplasia, squamous intraepithelial lesions (SIL), and carcinoma in situ. Cervical cytology, or Pap test, is the most useful procedure for detecting precancerous and cancerous cells that may be shed by the cervix. Without question, the Pap test decreases the incidence of cervical cancer and increases the survival rate for those women who develop cervical cancer.

**Procedure.** With the speculum blades open and the cervix in view, samples of the superficial layers of the cervix and endocervix are obtained. Samples are best obtained with a spatula or a cytobrush.

Most lesions develop at the squamocolumnar junction (the border where developing squamous tissue meets the immature columnar epithelium). The cytobrush is most effective in obtaining an adequate specimen from this site, particularly in postmenopausal women, in whom the squamocolumnar junction recedes into the endocervix.

The material is placed on slides that are then either sprayed with or immersed in a fixative solution before being sent to the laboratory for analysis. The FDA recently approved Papnet, an advanced method of computer technology that can greatly increase the detection of abnormalities in Pap smears. The new test automatically detects and displays abnormal cells on a high-resolution color video screen for interpretation and diagnosis. Women can now ask their health care provider to order Papnet testing.

**Classification of Cervical Cytology.** Until recently, a great deal of variation existed in how cervical cytology findings were reported. The Bethesda system was devised to offer standard terminology. It consists of three elements: (1) a statement of specimen adequacy, (2) a general categorization (normal or abnormal), and (3) a descriptive diagnosis regarding abnormal cytology.

The terminology for epithelial cell abnormalities includes the following categories:

1. Atypical squamous cells of undetermined significance
2. Squamous intraepithelial lesion, which is subdivided into (a) low-grade SIL (including cellular changes of HPV) and (b) high-grade SIL (previously categorized as carcinoma in situ).
3. Squamous cell cancer

#### RECTAL EXAMINATION

The anus is inspected for hemorrhoids, inflammation, and lesions. The lubricated index finger is gently inserted, and sphincter tone is noted. A slide may be prepared to test for the presence of occult blood in stool.

Fecal occult blood testing is a useful screening measure for colorectal cancer. Special instructions are necessary to prevent false test results when materials for FOBT are sent home with the woman. She should be instructed to do the following:

- Avoid vitamin C, acetylsalicylic acid, and nonsteroidal anti-inflammatory drugs such as ibuprofen or naproxen for at least 48 hours before collecting the specimen.
- Avoid red meat, turnips, beets, and horseradish for 48 hours before testing.
- Collect a specimen from three consecutive stools.
- Return slides as directed within 4 to 6 days after the specimens are collected.

#### LABORATORY SCREENING TESTS

Additional laboratory tests depend on the history and risk assessment of the woman and might include the following:

- Testing for sexually transmissible diseases, such as chlamydial infection, gonorrhea, syphilis, and HIV.
- Testing for rubella antibodies to determine if the

**TABLE 33–2 SUMMARY OF SCREENING PROCEDURES**

| Procedure | Purpose |
|---|---|
| Breast self-examination | To inspect and palpate the breasts monthly for changes or masses that might indicate breast tumors |
| Professional breast examination | Health care providers may detect masses that the woman might miss. |
| Mammography<br>Every 1–2 yr from 40–49 yr<br>Annually over 50 yr (ACOG, 1996) | To detect breast lumps before they become palpable. Early diagnosis of breast cancer promotes long-term survival. |
| Vulvar self-examination | To detect signs of precancerous conditions or infections |
| Pelvic examination | To inspect and palpate the organs of reproduction for confirmation that no disease exists, or for early detection if disease does exist |
| Papanicolaou test | To detect abnormal cervical cytology as early as possible |
| Rectal examination | To check for hemorrhoids and lesions and to evaluate sphincter control |
| Fecal occult blood test | To determine if there is blood in stool, often an early sign of colon cancer |
| Urinalysis | To screen postmenopausal women; those with diabetes mellitus; history of urinary infections. Almost always performed. |

ADDITIONAL PROCEDURES BASED ON RISK FACTORS

| Procedure | Risk Factors |
|---|---|
| STD testing | History of multiple sexual partners or a partner with multiple contacts, history of STDs |
| HIV testing | Seeking treatment for STDs; IV drug use; sexual partner who is HIV positive or bisexual or injects drugs; recurrent or persistent episodes of STDs such as candidiasis and herpes |
| Lipid profile | History of parent or sibling with high cholesterol or coronary artery disease, diabetes mellitus, or smoking |
| Fasting glucose test | Obesity, history of gestational diabetes, family history of diabetes |
| Thyroid-stimulating hormone | Strong family history of thyroid disease |
| Transvaginal ultrasound examination and/or blood test for CA 125 | Family history of ovarian cancer |
| Colonoscopy | Family history of bowel cancer |

*Abbreviations*: STD, sexually transmissible disease; HIV, human immunodeficiency virus; IV, intravenous.

woman is immune; this is particularly important in the childbearing years.

- Cholesterol testing of women at risk for coronary artery disease. This is particularly important in the postmenopausal period for women who do not have the protection that estrogen offers to prevent coronary artery disease.
- A urinalysis, which is almost always done, to detect signs of infection in the urinary tract.
- A thyroid function test, which may be indicated if the woman exhibits signs of thyroid dysfunction, such as heart palpitations and heat intolerance.
- A serum test for CA 125, a tumor marker that may be elevated with ovarian cancer.
- Transvaginal ultrasonography, which may be recommended for women who are at increased risk for malignant disorders of the reproductive tract (see p. 952).
- A sigmoidoscopy (every 3 to 5 years after the age of 50). A yearly colonoscopy may be recommended if the woman has a family history of colon cancer.

See Table 33–2 for a summary of recommended procedures.

**CHECK YOUR READING**

3. What are the three screening procedures for cancer of the breast?
4. Why is vulvar self-examination recommended?
5. What is a Pap test, and why is it performed?
6. Why is fecal occult blood testing important?
7. What additional screening tests may be recommended for women? Why are these tests recommended?

## Benign Disorders of the Breast

There are four relatively common benign disorders of the breast. The risk for each disorder is related to a specific age.

### Fibroadenoma

Fibroadenomas are the most common benign tumors of the breast, and although they may occur at any age, they are most common during the teenage years and the twenties. Fibroadenomas are composed of both fibrous and glandular tissue. They are felt as firm, hard, freely mobile nodules that may or may not be tender when palpated. Fibroadenomas do not change during the menstrual cycle. They are generally located in the upper, outer quadrant of the breast, and it is not unusual for more than one to be present.

Treatment may involve careful observation for a

few months, or the tumor may be excised and the specimen analyzed to rule out malignancy.

### Fibrocystic Breast Changes

Fibrocystic breast changes, also called mammary dysplasia, are the most common breast disorders during the reproductive years. Fibrosis, or thickening of the normal breast tissue, occurs in the early stages, whereas cysts form in the latter stages and are felt as multiple, smooth, well-delineated nodules.

The most common symptom of fibrocystic changes is pain accompanied by tenderness. The pain is often bilateral and particularly noticeable during the premenstrual phase of the normal cycle. This is believed to be the result of an imbalance in the estrogen-progesterone production. Women with fibrocystic breast changes improve dramatically during pregnancy and lactation because of the large amounts of progesterone produced.

Fibrocystic breast changes are not a disease but represent the way a woman's breasts respond to normal monthly hormonal fluctuation (Isaacs, 1994). Fine-needle aspiration may be performed to study cells in the aspirate. Open biopsy is mandatory if the fluid is bloody or if a residual mass remains following aspiration (Hindle, 1994).

Medical treatment is rare because side effects of the drugs may be more distressing than the breast discomfort. If drugs are administered, they may include progesterone or tamoxifen (an antiestrogen) if an estrogen-progesterone imbalance is suspected to be the cause and if symptoms are severe. Bromocriptine (Parlodel), which inhibits the secretion of prolactin, may relieve breast discomfort. In severe cases, danazol (Danocrine), which suppresses gonadotropins and inhibits estrogen production, may be administered (Fiorica, 1994).

Although controversy exists about whether caffeine contributes to the development of fibrocystic breast changes, some physicians and nurse practitioners recommend limiting consumption of tea, coffee, colas, and chocolate. Some women also benefit from restricting sodium intake to reduce fluid retention the week before menstruation starts, when symptoms are often most acute.

### Ductal Ectasia

Ductal ectasia generally occurs as the woman approaches menopause. It is characterized by dilation of the collecting ducts that become distended and filled with cellular debris. This initiates an inflammatory process resulting in

- A mass that feels firm and irregular
- Enlarged axillary nodes
- Nipple retraction and discharge

These symptoms are similar to those of breast cancer, and accurate diagnosis is vital. Once a surgical biopsy confirms that the condition is benign mammary duct ectasia, no further treatment is necessary.

### Intraductal Papilloma

Intraductal papilloma develops most often just before or during menopause. It occurs when papillomas (small elevations or protuberances) develop in the epithelium of the ducts of the breasts. As the papilloma grows, it causes trauma and erosion within the ducts that result in serous or serosanguinous discharge from the nipple. Treatment consists of excision of the mass and ductal area, plus analysis of nipple discharge to rule out a malignant tumor.

### Diagnosis of Disorders of the Breast

When a lesion or lump is discovered in the breast, the physician must determine if it is benign or malignant. *Ultrasound* examination can be used to differentiate fluid-filled cysts from solid tissue that is potentially malignant. *Needle aspiration biopsy* can be performed to remove fluid from suspected cysts for analysis of the cells. *Surgical biopsy* is performed under these conditions:

- Bloody fluid removed from a cyst on aspiration
- Failure of the mass to disappear completely after fluid aspiration
- Recurrence of the cyst after one or two aspirations
- Solid dominant mass not diagnosed as fibroadenoma
- Bloody nipple discharge
- Nipple ulceration or persistent crusting
- Skin edema and erythema suspicious for inflammatory breast carcinoma
- Suspicious mammography findings (ACOG, 1996)

### Nursing Considerations

It is of primary importance for the nurse to acknowledge the anxiety that all women feel when a breast disorder is discovered. Furthermore, the apprehension continues for most women while they await a final diagnosis. It may be helpful for some women to learn that 90 percent of all breast disorders are benign. For others, the most helpful intervention is to encourage them to express their concerns.

The nurse should explain the diagnostic procedures that are planned, such as ultrasound examination, mammography, needle biopsy, or surgical biopsy. Explanations should include what the procedures entail and how long the woman will have to wait for results to be known.

**CHECK YOUR READING**

8. How are fibrocystic breast changes treated?
9. What three diagnostic procedures are used to determine whether a breast disorder is benign or malignant?

# Malignant Tumors of the Breast

## Incidence

The lifetime risk of developing breast cancer in the United States is one in eight. This reflects the increase in life expectancy of American women and the fact that breast cancer is a disease of older women. The rise in lifetime risk also resulted from the decision to include in the calculations women older than 85 years (Marchant, 1994a). Approximately 182,000 new cases are diagnosed each year, and 46,000 deaths are due to cancer of the breast (American Cancer Society, 1994). Cancer of the breast is second only to lung cancer as a cause of death from cancer among women.

The incidence of breast cancer is approximately five times higher in the United States and northern Europe than in Japan (Prout, 1995). Possible reasons for the high incidence in these areas—high per capita consumption of dietary fat and smoking—are being studied.

## Risk Factors

Although the actual cause of breast cancer remains unknown, several factors are known to increase the risk for the development of breast cancer (Table 33–3). In addition, two genes (BRCA1 and BRCA2), thought to be responsible for the majority of cases of familial breast cancer, have been identified.

Although risk factors are important, it is essential to understand that breast cancer develops in many women who do not fit into any high-risk category. Therefore, it is important that all women, not only those at "high risk," take advantage of the available screening procedures.

**TABLE 33–3 RISK FACTORS FOR BREAST CANCER**

| |
|---|
| Female |
| Age older than 50 yr |
| History of breast cancer |
| Family history (grandmother, mother, sister, aunt) |
| Previous uterine, ovarian, or colon cancer |
| Nulliparity or first pregnancy after 30 yr |
| Early menarche (<12 yr), late menopause (>50 yr) |
| Lifestyle factors: high intake of dietary fat, excessive consumption of alcohol, smoking |

## Pathophysiology

The most common type of breast cancer is infiltrating ductal carcinoma, which originates in the epithelial lining of the mammary ducts. The rate of growth varies, but it is estimated to take 5 to 9 years for the lesion to be large enough to be palpable. As long as the cancer remains in the duct, it is considered to be noninvasive (Silverstein, 1994). When it penetrates the duct into surrounding tissue, it is classified as invasive. Growth occurs in irregular patterns and invades the lymphatic channels, eventually causing lymphatic edema and the dimpling of the skin that resembles an orange peel (peau d'orange).

Cancer cells are carried by the lymph channels to the lymph nodes, and metastasis occurs when the cells are spread by both blood and lymph systems. The most common sites of metastasis are the lungs, liver, and bones.

## Staging

Although confirmation of malignancy is the first step in evaluating the woman with cancer, staging is necessary to understand the severity of the cancer. Staging is generally based on the TNM (tumor, node, metastasis) system used to describe the cancer's anatomic extent. Stages of breast cancer progress from stage 1, indicating a small tumor without lymphatic involvement or metastases, to stage 4, which indicates spread to lymph nodes and metastases to other organs. The stages are often used to determine treatment, and they are useful guides to prognosis. The type of cancer cell, the presence of hormone receptors, and the proliferative rate of the breast cancer cells are also important factors in the rate of recurrence.

## Management

Increasing variations in treatment have evolved over the last decade. There is now less emphasis on very radical procedures, and a combination of surgical excision and adjuvant therapy is often recommended.

### SURGICAL TREATMENT

The surgical procedure depends on the type, stage, and location of the disease. The most common surgeries are the following:

- *Breast conservation treatment,* which involves wide local excision (sometimes called lumpectomy) of the tumor to microscopically clean margins. The excision can be performed without major cosmetic deformity. Some axillary lymph nodes are usually removed to rule out spread of the disease. In most instances radiation therapy is required to complete the treatment.

- *Simple mastectomy*, which is removal of the entire breast. Axillary dissection is omitted, although some lymph nodes may be removed for staging purposes. It is recommended for recurrence after partial mastectomy and for selected cases in which prophylactic removal of the opposite breast is considered. It also performed for elderly women who are poor operative risks and in whom no axillary involvement or distant disease is present (Marchant, 1994a).
- *Modified radical mastectomy*, which involves removal of breast tissue, axillary nodes, and some chest muscles; however, the pectoralis major muscles are preserved. This surgical procedure is recommended when a large primary lesion is found in a relatively small breast, there are contraindications to radiation therapy, or there is evidence of multifocal disease (ACOG, 1996).

#### ADJUVANT THERAPY

Adjuvant therapy is supportive or additional therapy that may be recommended following the surgical procedure. Radiation, chemotherapy, and hormone therapy are adjuvant therapies that are currently recommended. The decision about whether to use adjuvant therapy is based on the woman's age, the stage of the disease, the woman's preference, and the hormone receptor status of the lesion.

Radiation and chemotherapy are known to improve the chance of long-term survival, and one or the other may be recommended following surgical excision of the tumor. Because some tumors are estrogen receptor–positive, meaning that their growth is stimulated by estrogen, estrogen-blocking medications are administered. Tamoxifen is currently the hormone therapy most recommended. Tamoxifen blocks estrogen by binding to estrogen receptors, thereby suppressing tumor growth by reducing the effects of estrogen.

Side effects of tamoxifen vary from woman to woman. The most commonly mentioned side effects are hot flashes, vaginal dryness or increased vaginal discharge, nausea, and anorexia. There is also concern about the recent finding that the risk of endometrial cancer is increased for women taking tamoxifen (Robert, 1994). Laboratory values for cholesterol and triglycerides may also increase. All side effects should be discussed with the woman before tamoxifen is administered so she can weigh the risks versus the benefits and make an informed decision.

#### BREAST RECONSTRUCTION

**Timing.** Breast reconstruction has become an integral part of the treatment of breast cancer, and the timing of reconstruction should be discussed with the woman before surgical treatment. Immediate reconstruction has a psychological appeal. The prospect of having a life-threatening breast cancer and simultaneously facing the loss of a breast may be overwhelming for many women. Conversely, delayed reconstruction may give a woman time to learn about the procedure, to heal from the mastectomy, and to consider the extent of the disease and the side-effects associated with adjuvant therapy.

**Method.** Currently, a variety of methods of breast reconstruction are available. The *tissue expansion method* uses an empty silicone prosthesis fitted with a valve that can be accessed by pericutaneous needle puncture. The bag is filled with saline in small increments to slowly expand the tissue. When the desired volume is attained, the device is removed and the incision is reopened and the expander exchanged for the appropriate implant. In newer models, only the valve must be removed, and the expander serves as the permanent implant (Versaci & Libbey, 1994). This method is the most popular postmastectomy reconstruction in use today. The procedure is more successful than in the past because present-day surgeons often use a skin-sparing technique when performing mastectomies.

*Autogenous grafts* have been successfully used for reconstruction. They are recommended for women who have received radiation therapy. Implants do not do well in such wounds, whereas tissue transfers work well because the flaps carry their own blood supply. The graft is often taken from the abdomen and includes muscle and cutaneous tissue.

**Nipple-Areola Reconstruction.** The nipple can be reconstructed in a variety of ways. Tissue may be taken from the opposite nipple, from skin that covers the prosthesis mound, or from other body tissue. After the nipple has been reconstructed, many surgeons inject pigment into the area to create an areola.

### Psychosocial Consequences of Breast Cancer

The time from discovery to treatment of breast cancer is the most stressful time for many women. Factors that contribute to presurgery distress include a sense of uncertainty, inadequate information, the need to make difficult treatment decisions, and scheduling problems. Treatment usually involves consultations with one or more specialists, including a surgeon, a radiotherapist, a plastic surgeon, and a medical oncologist. Scheduling difficulties arise when women must travel significant distances for treatment. Moreover, conflicting opinions are sometimes expressed by members of the health care team. This results in frustration and confusion for the woman and often leads to additional consultations.

Concerns frequently expressed during treatment for breast cancer include fear of death, uncertainty about the quality of life, changes in body image, the effect on sexuality, and side effects of recommended therapy. For many women, the knowledge that they will lose their hair as a result of chemotherapy creates one of the most difficult situations in therapy.

Breast cancer can have psychological consequences not only for women but also for their husbands, significant others, and other family members. Difficulties reported include sleep disturbances, eating disorders, and problems with work responsibilities. Breast cancer can create strain on the marital relationship, primarily in the areas of sexual relations and communication about matters related to the illness. Women and their partners sometimes differ in regard to how much they want to discuss the illness. Some women have a great need to discuss their diagnosis, treatment, and fears of recurrence. Other women and many men view discussion of such fears as negative thinking that delays adjustment.

### Nursing Considerations

The woman who is diagnosed with breast cancer depends on nurses for emotional support and accurate information. They must allow time for the woman to express her feelings and convey a sense of empathetic understanding by quiet presence, touch, and close attention to the woman's concerns. Many women feel that they have lost control and that their lives have been taken over by cancer and the recommended treatment. Some women are concerned about family relationships, and, as indicated earlier, how their sexual partner will respond. Each woman should be allowed to express her fears and worries. In addition to providing time and demonstrating genuine interest in the woman's concerns, it is important to use communication techniques, such as clarifying, paraphrasing, and reflecting feelings, so that the woman can participate in decisions about her care.

The anxiety that most women experience is reduced when procedures and care are clearly understood. Preoperative teaching is often part of the nurse's responsibility, and husbands and significant others should be included as much as possible in the teaching. Many women are relieved to learn that the hospital stay is short following mastectomy, and they may be relieved by knowing exactly what to expect. For instance, a pressure dressing may be applied over the wound to prevent further bleeding after surgery. Drainage tubes may be attached to portable suction apparatus (Hemovac) to prevent accumulation of fluid under the skin flaps. The incision may appear red and raised for the first few weeks. Lymphedema of the arm on the same side as the mastectomy is possible as a result of blocked lymphatic vessels. Specific exercises such as armlifts and pulley exercises may be necessary.

Discharge teaching focuses on the need for follow-up care and treatment. Some areas of concern include how to minimize the risk of wound infection, side effects of adjuvant therapy, and signs and symptoms that should be reported to the physician. Most women also benefit from information about such groups as Reach to Recovery and Encore, which provide support, information, and guidance following mastectomy.

Using nursing diagnoses to plan and implement care could ensure that care is complete. Relevant diagnoses might include the following:

- Fear of death or pain
- Body image disturbance related to loss of breast and temporary loss of hair during chemotherapy
- Altered family processes related to illness of primary caregiver or lack of information about the course of the disease
- Altered sexuality patterns related to concern about altered body structure

**CHECK YOUR READING**

10. What are the major risk factors for breast cancer?
11. Why is staging for breast cancer important?
12. What is meant by adjuvant therapy, and why is it used?
13. How and when may breasts be reconstructed following mastectomy?
14. What should preoperative teaching include?
15. What should discharge planning emphasize?

## Menstrual Cycle Disorders

The four most common menstrual cycle disorders are absence of menses (amenorrhea), abnormal uterine bleeding, pain associated with the menstrual cycle, and cyclic mood changes, including premenstrual syndrome. Although most of the disorders are benign, all require comprehensive gynecologic assessment. Nurses must be knowledgeable about underlying processes, diagnostic procedures, and expected treatment in order to fulfill the basic core of nursing activities, which include client advocacy, education, and supportive counseling.

### Amenorrhea

Amenorrhea is a symptom that can indicate either normal physiologic processes or pathology in the reproductive system. Amenorrhea before menarche, during pregnancy, during the puerperium and lactation, and following menopause is normal. Amenorrhea at other times is abnormal, and it is called either primary or secondary amenorrhea, depending on when it occurs.

#### PRIMARY AMENORRHEA

The age when primary amenorrhea is diagnosed depends on whether secondary sex characteristics have developed. It is defined as the failure to menstruate by age 16 years in girls who have breast or pubic hair development. On the other hand, it is defined as failure to menstruate by age 14 in girls who have not developed secondary sex characteristics (Brunt, 1995). The most common cause for primary amenorrhea associated with absence of breast or pubic hair development is Turner's syndrome. This syndrome occurs when females have only one normal X chromosome. When the secondary sex characteristics are present, the cause may be incomplete development of the uterus, ovaries, and fallopian tubes. Intrauterine exposure to diethylstilbesterol is associated with abnormal development of the uterus. Other causes may include hormonal imbalances, systemic disease, and hypothalamic-pituitary abnormalities that result in inadequate secretion of gonadotropins. It may also be due to excessive exercise or eating disorders, such as anorexia nervosa and bulemia, that cause a decrease in ovarian hormones.

The condition causes a great deal of concern for the young woman and her family. Amenorrhea is a symptom, not a diagnosis, and they may worry that it indicates a serious disease. Moreover, menstruation is a unique function of women, and absence of menstruation may provoke concerns about femininity and the ability to have children. Concern increases if medical treatment is not successful.

The success of medical management depends on the cause. Counseling for eating disorders, such as anorexia nervosa, and reducing excessive exercise may prove helpful. Hormone therapy may establish normal menses if the cause is hormone imbalance; however, some conditions cannot be successfully treated. For example, if the cause is reproductive tract or congenital anomalies, normal menses and fertility may not be possible, and psychological support becomes the most important therapy.

#### SECONDARY AMENORRHEA

Secondary amenorrhea is the cessation of menstruation for a period of at least three cycles or 6 months in a woman who has established a pattern of menstruation (Ginsburg & Moghissi, 1994). It may be due to a variety of causes, including systemic diseases such as diabetes mellitus, tuberculosis, and hypothyroidism. Hormonal imbalances, strenuous aerobic exercise, poor nutrition, use of oral contraceptives, and ovarian tumors may also be the cause.

Assessment includes a thorough medical and obstetric history, as well as questions about eating habits, history of dieting, and current exercise pattern. Women are also questioned about their uses of drugs, such as oral contraceptives, phenothiazines, and antihypertensives, which can cause secondary amenorrhea.

Medical treatment aims at identifying and correcting the underlying cause. Pregnancy testing is mandatory for any sexually active woman, and medications that are potentially teratogenic must be withheld until pregnancy is ruled out. Hormone replacement therapy, ovulation stimulation, and periodic progesterone withdrawal often result in menstruation.

### Abnormal Uterine Bleeding

Menstruation is considered normal when bleeding occurs every 24 to 35 days and lasts for 2 to 7 days (Weiss, 1995). Abnormal bleeding can be defined as bleeding that occurs with abnormal frequency, lasts an abnormal length of time, or is excessive in amount.

#### ETIOLOGY

The most common causes of abnormal bleeding fall into five basic categories:

1. Pregnancy complications, such as spontaneous abortion
2. Anatomic lesions, either benign or malignant, of the vagina, cervix, or uterus
3. Drug-induced bleeding, such as "breakthrough" bleeding that may occur in women who are on some oral contraceptives, or who have progestin implants, such as Norplant
4. Systemic disorders, such as diabetes mellitus, uterine myomas (fibroids), and hypothyroidism
5. Failure to ovulate (dysfunctional uterine bleeding)

#### MANAGEMENT

Medical treatment for abnormal bleeding depends on the cause. Medications include the use of progestin-estrogen combination oral contraceptives that suppress ovulation and allow a more stable endometrial lining to form. Surgical therapy may include dilation and curettage (D&C) to remove polyps or to diagnose endometrial hyperplasia, which may be treated with progesterone. Hysterectomy is often performed if the uterus is enlarged as a result of fibroids or adenomyosis (benign invasive growth of the endometrium into the muscular layer of the uterus) and if the woman no longer wishes to bear children. Laser ablation is a new procedure that is used to permanently remove the endometrial lining.

Prolonged menorrhagia may result in decreased hemoglobin, and the woman may need treatment for iron-deficiency anemia.

#### NURSING CONSIDERATIONS

Although most nurses (with the exception of nurse practitioners) do not diagnose or treat abnormal bleeding, they are often responsible for encouraging women to seek medical attention promptly when irregular bleeding occurs. Nurses also help the woman keep a record of the bleeding episodes and the amount of blood lost. This involves keeping a calendar and noting any vaginal bleeding (spotting, menses) that occurs, as well as the number of pads and tampons saturated each day.

Nurses are in a unique position to assist the woman to make necessary lifestyle changes. The nurse teaches the importance of adequate nutrition and discourages rigorous dieting. For women who are concerned about amenorrhea, the nurse should explain that, although exercise is beneficial, strenuous workouts or aerobic training can cause amenorrhea. In addition, the nurse teaches methods to reduce stress and promote relaxation. Finally, nurses must provide support for women who fear that irregular bleeding indicates a serious disease, such as cancer. It is unwise to offer false reassurance, but information about diagnostic procedures, such as pelvic examinations, Pap test, and blood tests to detect thyroid function may be helpful.

### ✓ CHECK YOUR READING

16. How does primary amenorrhea differ from secondary amenorrhea in terms of onset, cause, and treatment?
17. What are possible causes of abnormal uterine bleeding, and why should it not be ignored?

## Pain Associated with the Menstrual Cycle

Cyclic pelvic pain must be distinguished from acute pelvic pain. Acute pelvic pain is sudden in onset, and it is not experienced with each menstrual cycle. It may indicate a serious disorder, such as ectopic pregnancy or appendicitis. On the other hand, cyclic pelvic pain occurs repetitively and predictably in a specific phase of the menstrual cycle. The most common causes of cyclic pelvic pain are mittelschmerz, primary dysmenorrhea, and endometriosis.

#### MITTELSCHMERZ

Mittelschmerz ("middle" pain) refers to pelvic pain that occurs midway between menstrual periods, or at the time of ovulation. The pain is due to growth of the dominant follicle within the ovary or rupture of the follicle and subsequent spillage of follicular fluid and blood into the peritoneal space. The pain is fairly sharp and is felt on the right or left side of the pelvis. It generally lasts from a few hours to 2 days, and slight vaginal bleeding may accompany the discomfort. Generally, women do not need medical treatment beyond simple explanation of the discomfort or mild analgesics.

#### PRIMARY DYSMENORRHEA

Primary dysmenorrhea refers to menstrual pain without identified pathology. Commonly called "cramps," primary dysmenorrhea affects at least half of all women and causes 10 percent to miss work or school (Somani, 1995). The pain begins within hours of the onset of menses, and it is spasmodic or colicky in nature. It is felt in the lower abdomen but often radiates to the lower back or down the legs. Primary dysmenorrhea occurs in ovulatory cycles, and it is most common in young nulliparous women.

One of the most confusing aspects of primary dysmenorrhea has been why it is experienced by some, but not all, women. It is now known that some women produce excessive endometrial prostaglandin during the late luteal phase of the menstrual cycle. The prostaglandins (particularly $E_2$ and $F_{2\alpha}$) diffuse into endometrial tissue and cause abnormal uterine muscle contractions, uterine ischemia, and hypoxia. This process accounts for the cramp-like uterine pain, as well as symptoms that often accompany it, such as diarrhea, nausea, and vomiting.

Two recommended treatments of primary dysmenorrhea provide marked relief: oral contraceptives and prostaglandin inhibitors. Oral contraceptives decrease the amount of endometrial growth that occurs during the menstrual cycle and thus reduce the production of endometrial prostaglandin. For women who do not wish to take oral contraceptives, prostaglandin inhibitors also offer relief. The most effective prostaglandin inhibitors include ibuprofen (Motrin, Advil) and naproxen (Naprosyn, Anaprox). To be effective, these must be taken before menses and the onset of cramps.

#### ENDOMETRIOSIS

**Pathophysiology.** Endometriosis is defined as the presence outside the uterus of tissue that resembles the endometrium in both structure and function. The response of this tissue to the stimulation of estrogen and progesterone during the menstrual cycle is identical to that of the endometrium. That is, it grows and proliferates during the follicular and luteal phases of the cycle and then sloughs during menstruation. The menstruation from endometriosis lesions, however, occurs in a closed cavity, which causes pressure and pain on adjacent tissue. In addition, prostaglandins secreted by the endometriosis lesions irritate nerve endings and stimulate uterine contractions that further increase pain. Moreover, cyclic bleeding into the pelvic cavity initiates chronic inflammatory changes that may make conception and implantation difficult. The most common sites of endometriosis lesions are illustrated in Figure 33–2.

Although endometriosis occurs in 5 to 15 percent of all women, the cause remains unknown (Surrey, 1994). One theory is that menstrual discharge contains viable endometrial cells that can attach to sites outside the uterus, where they grow and produce patches of endometrial tissue. It is possible that the endometrial cells are disseminated primarily by retrograde menstruation, that is, reflux of menstrual flow through the fallopian tubes. The cells attach to nearby structures and proliferate, creating spots of endometrial tissue. Also, it has been suggested that endometriosis may represent an autoimmune process that has a genetic basis.

**Signs and Symptoms.** The two major symptoms of endometriosis are pain and infertility. The pain of endometriosis differs from that of primary dysmenorrhea. Endometriosis pain is deep, unilateral or bilateral, and either sharp or dull. It is constant, as opposed to the spasmodic or colicky pain of primary dysmenorrhea. Dyspareunia (painful intercourse) is typical, particularly with deep penetration. Rectal pain is common, especially during defecation. Diarrhea, constipation, and sensations of rectal pressure or urgency are other symptoms of endometriosis. Although the cause of infertility is not completely understood, pelvic adhesions and tubal pathology due to chronic inflammatory changes are certainly contributing factors.

**Management.** Treatment may be either medical or surgical, and the therapy chosen must weigh the need for relief of pain and the desire to maintain fertility against the side effects that accompany many treatment regimens. Because growth of endometriosis depends on the production of ovarian hormones (estrogen and progesterone) during the menstrual cycle, medical therapy is aimed at interrupting the menstrual cycle, thus leaving the woman in a state of "pseudomenopause." As a result, she experiences symptoms associated with estrogen deficit, such as hot flashes and vaginal dryness. Moreover, she is at increased risk for postmenopausal conditions, such as adverse serum lipid changes and osteoporosis (see menopause, p. 943).

Currently, danazol and analogues of gonadotropin-releasing hormone (GnRH) are the drugs of choice. Danazol is an androgen derivative that has been used for many years. The GnRH agonists, such as leuprolide acetate (Lupron) and goserelin acetate (Zoladex), and nafarelin (Synarel), which may be administered by nasal spray, are newer. Both danazol and GnRH agonists interfere with production of gonadotropins (follicle-stimulating hormone and luteinizing hormone) and thus stop the menstrual cycle, creating a "pseudomenopause." Side-effects of danazol include headache, dizziness, irritability, and decreased libido. In addition, danazol often produces masculinizing effects, such as deepening of the voice, facial and body hair, and weight gain. The most common side effects of GnRh drugs are hot flashes, vaginal dryness, decreased libido, and loss of bone mineral density.

Pregnancy also interrupts menstruation, and if the woman wishes to conceive, she may be advised not to delay conception. If pregnancy is not an immediate option, continuous noncyclic oral contraceptives are sometimes recommended, although the effectiveness in treating symptoms of endometriosis is not well documented.

Surgical treatment can take many forms. For the older woman with severe pain who no longer wishes to have children, a hysterectomy with bilateral salpingo-oophorectomy (removal of the uterus, both fallopian tubes, and both ovaries) and excision of all

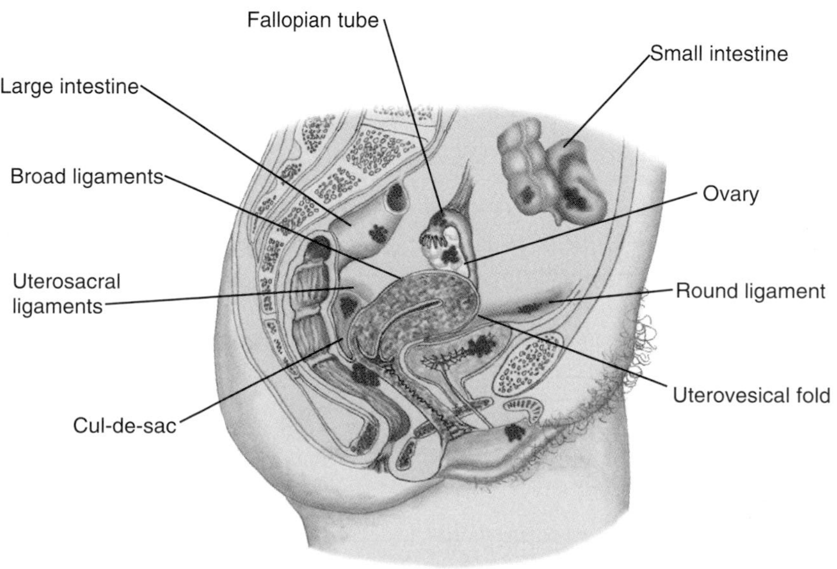


**FIGURE 33–2**

Common sites of endometriosis.

lesions offers the greatest chance for cure. This surgery results in early menopause with permanent estrogen deficit. Postoperative hormone replacement therapy may be recommended if all lesions are removed. More conservative surgery includes laparoscopy for lysis of adhesions and laser vaporization of the lesions of endometriosis.

#### NURSING CONSIDERATIONS

Dysmenorrhea varies from mild "menstrual awareness" to incapacitating pain that affects the quality of life for many days out of each month. Too often the pain is belittled ("It's just cramps"). One of the most important nursing actions is to acknowledge the pain: "I understand this is really uncomfortable, and you are concerned that you have this much pain every month."

Women should be instructed in nonpharmacologic measures to relieve pain, such as frequent rest periods, application of heat to the lower abdomen, moderate exercise, and a well-balanced diet. They may also be advised to schedule stress-provoking situations when they will not coincide with the menstrual period. Nonsteroidal anti-inflammatory drugs provide relief for some women; they should be taken with meals to reduce gastrointestinal irritation. The woman should be counseled to report unusual side effects, such as headache, dizziness, or unusual fluid retention, to the physician or nurse practitioner.

Time must be allowed for the woman to express her concerns about the therapy, and she should be instructed to use a form of contraception other than oral contraceptives when medical therapy, such as GnRH or danazol, is used. Some women benefit from information about measures that promote sleep and relaxation, and, most importantly, from the knowledge that someone is available to provide support and guidance when needed.

#### ✓ CHECK YOUR READING

18. What causes primary dysmenorrhea, and how may it be treated?
19. How does endometriosis cause dysmenorrhea, and how can it be treated?
20. What are the major side effects of danazol? Of the GnRH agonists?

## Premenstrual Syndrome

Although most women experience a variety of physical and emotional changes during the menstrual cycle, the following criteria must met for the condition to be diagnosed as premenstrual syndrome (PMS):

- The signs and symptoms must be cyclic and recur in the luteal phase (after ovulation) of the menstrual cycle.
- The woman should be symptom-free during the follicular phase (before ovulation) of the menstrual cycle, and there must be at least 7 symptom-free days in the cycle.
- Symptoms must be severe enough to have an impact on work, lifestyle, and relationships.
- Diagnosis must be based solely on *prospective* symptom charting by the woman; that is, charting of symptoms as they occur rather than recall of symptoms that occurred in the past (ACOG, 1996).

Several types of PMS diaries are available for symptom charting. Figure 33–3 illustrates one type of calendar or diary on which the woman records the

**Calendar for PMS Symptoms**

| | 1 | 2 | 3 | 4 | 5 | 6 | 7 | 8 | 9 | 10 | 11 | 12 | 13 | 14 | 15 | 16 | 17 | 18 | 19 | 20 | 21 | 22 | 23 | 24 | 25 | 26 | 27 | 28 | 29 | 30 | 31 | 32 |
|---|---|---|---|---|---|---|---|---|---|---|---|---|---|---|---|---|---|---|---|---|---|---|---|---|---|---|---|---|---|---|---|---|
| Menses | M | M | M | M | M | | | | | | | | | | | | | | | | | | | | | | | | | M | | |
| Symptoms | | | | | | | | | | | | | | | | | | | | | | | | | | | | | | | | |
| Depression | | | | | | | | | | | | | | | | | | | | | | | | | | | | | | | | |
| Irritability | | | | | | | | | | | | | | | | | | | | | | | | | | | | | | | | |
| Insomnia | | | | | | | | | | | | | | | | | | | | | | | | | | | | | | | | |
| Bloating | | | | | | | | | | | | | | | | | | | | | | | | | | | | | | | | |
| Headache | | | | | | | | | | | | | | | | | | | | | | | | | | | | | | | | |
| Wt. Increase (lb) | 1 | | | | | | | | | | | | | | | | | | | | | | | 2 | 3 | 4 | 4 | 5 | 4 | | | |
| | | | | | | | | | | | | | | | | | | | | | | | | | | | | | | | | |

Name ____________
Month/year ____________

Severity of symptoms
☐ None
Mild
Moderate
Severe

**FIGURE 33–3**

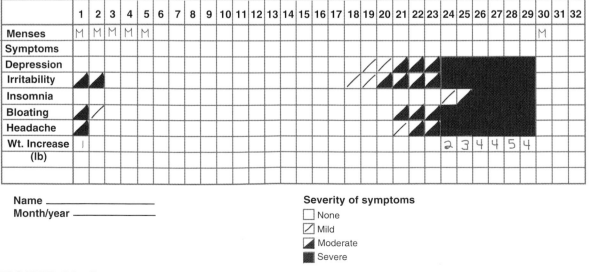

The woman uses a diary to record occurrence and severity of premenstrual symptoms.

**TABLE 33–4 SYMPTOMS OF PREMENSTRUAL SYNDROME (PMS)**

| Physical Symptoms | Behavioral Symptoms |
|---|---|
| Edema | Anxiety |
| Weight gain | Depression |
| Abdominal bloating | Irritability |
| Constipation | Mood swings |
| Hot flashes | Aggressive behavior |
| Breast pain | Increased appetite |
| Headache | Food cravings |
| Acne | Fatigue |
| Rhinitis | Inability to concentrate |
| Heart palpitations | Insomnia |

symptoms that she experiences and the severity of the symptoms.

Numerous symptoms have been ascribed to PMS; however, a relatively small number make up the majority of complaints. They can be divided in behavioral and physical symptoms. Table 33–4 lists those that are most common in approximate order of occurrence.

#### ETIOLOGY

Although the cause of PMS is unknown, several theories or predisposing factors have been put forward. These include the following:

- An imbalance between estrogen and progesterone
- Low levels of $\beta$-endorphins
- Abnormal production of prostaglandins
- Fluid imbalance
- Nutritional deficiency

#### IMPACT ON FAMILY

Premenstrual syndrome puts a consistent strain on family relationships because symptoms recur monthly. The episodes of PMS affect the functioning of the entire family. Clinical descriptions of severe family disruptions include increased family conflict, disrupted communication, and decreased family cohesion. Of particular concern is the group of women who report symptoms of loss of control, child battering, self-injury, and increased accidents.

#### MANAGEMENT

Treatment of PMS is based on the symptom profile of each woman. Mild potassium-sparing diuretics may be prescribed for women with fluid retention and weight gain. Vitamin $B_6$ (pyridoxine), which is an important cofactor in the synthesis of neurotransmitters that influence mood, may be prescribed. Progesterone supplementation is occasionally used, with reported improvement in hot flashes, peripheral edema, and abdominal bloating. Progesterone is less effective therapy for emotional symptoms such as depression and anxiety. Antianxiety medications are usually reserved for severe anxiety that does not respond to other therapy.

Alternative therapy may be helpful for some women. Measures include acupuncture, biofeedback, hypnosis, psychotherapy, and stress management.

#### NURSING CONSIDERATIONS

Many women experience some of the symptoms and diagnose themselves as having PMS. Nurses must discourage this practice because serious systemic disease can be missed if the criteria for diagnosis are ignored. Instead of self-diagnosis, nurses should recommend that the woman consult with her health care provider so that a complete history and physical examination can be performed to rule out other causes.

**Women Want to Know**

**How to Relieve Symptoms of Premenstrual Syndrome**

**Diet**

- Decrease consumption of caffeine (coffee, tea, colas, chocolate), which increases irritability, insomnia, anxiety, and nervousness.
- Avoid simple sugars (cookies, cake, candy) to prevent abnormal elevations of blood glucose followed by a rapid decline and a period of low blood glucose (hypoglycemia).
- Decrease intake of salty foods (chips, pickles) to reduce fluid retention.
- Drink at least 2000 ml (2 quarts) of *water* per day, and do not include other beverages in this total.
- Eat six small meals a day to prevent hypoglycemia; meals should be well balanced, with emphasis on fresh fruits and vegetables, complex carbohydrates, and nonfat milk products.
- Avoid alcohol, which aggravates depression.

**Exercise**

Increase physical exercise to relieve tension and to decrease depression. Aerobic activity, such as jogging or walking, several times a week is recommended.

**Stress Management**

During the time when there are no symptoms of PMS, acknowledge the effect of PMS on daily life and make plans to avoid stressful situations during the premenstrual period when symptoms are acute.

Use guided imagery, conscious relaxation techniques, warm baths, and massage to reduce stress.

**Sleep and Rest**

To reduce fatigue and combat insomnia:

- Adhere to a regular schedule for sleep.
- Drink a glass of milk, which is high in tryptophan and is known to promote sleep, before bedtime.
- Schedule exercise in the morning or early afternoon rather than late afternoon.
- Engage in relaxing activities, such as reading, before bedtime, and avoid excitement at this time.

Once the diagnosis of PMS is confirmed, nurses can educate the family about lifestyle changes that are known to alleviate some symptoms of PMS and decrease the severity of others. Acknowledge that dietary changes are particularly difficult because many women crave salty or sweet foods, which should be restricted. Women also benefit from education about expected cyclic changes. As they learn to predict the pattern of symptoms and gain a sense of control over them, the symptoms often diminish.

Education and support must be expanded to include the family. When the woman exhibits symptoms of PMS, family members often respond by withdrawing or confronting the woman. This increases the woman's feelings of anxiety and vulnerability.

**It is more helpful if the family acknowledges feelings they believe the woman is experiencing. For instance, saying "It must be disturbing to feel so irritable. What can I do to help?" provokes a different emotional response than confronting or blaming comments.**

The family should also be encouraged to express their feelings so that anger and resentment within the family can be diminished.

Nurses must help the woman make concrete arrangements to obtain relief when she feels she is losing control or when she fears that she may harm herself or a child. A neighbor, friend, or family member should be identified to provide immediate relief, without questions or explanations, when the woman feels she is losing control. The telephone number of this important support person should be posted so that it is easily accessible, and the designated person should be called before symptoms are severe.

**✓CHECK YOUR READING**

21. What are the criteria for diagnosing PMS?
22. What are the three most common physical and behavioral symptoms?
23. What lifestyle changes can be made to reduce the symptoms of PMS?

# Induced Abortion

Induced abortion is a voluntary method of terminating a pregnancy. It may be performed to preserve the health of the mother, to prevent the birth of an infant with severe genetic defects, or to end a pregnancy caused by rape or incest. A woman may also choose to terminate a pregnancy for economic or social reasons. Termination of pregnancy for the purpose of safeguarding the health of the mother is termed "therapeutic" abortion. Interruption of the pregnancy at the request of the woman but not for reasons of impaired maternal health or fetal disease is often called "elective" abortion. Therapeutic and elective abortions involve social and ethical implications (see Chapter 3). In 1994, 1,267,415 legal abortions were reported in the United States (DHHS, 1997).

## Methods of Abortion

The technique used to induce abortion depends on the length of gestation. The three most common techniques are vacuum curettage, dilation and evacuation (D&E), and induced labor. Up to 13 weeks' gestation, *vacuum aspiration* or *curettage* is the method of choice. The cervix is dilated gently by inserting a series of tapered metal rods that increase progressively in size. When the cervical canal is open, a plastic cannula is inserted into the uterine cavity. The contents are aspirated with negative pressure within approximately 5 minutes. Many health care providers then gently scrape the uterine cavity with a curet to ensure that the uterus is empty. Cramping may last 20 to 30 minutes after the procedure is completed. Complications may include uterine perforation, hemorrhage, cervical lacerations, and adverse reactions to the anesthetic agent.

RU 486 (mifepristone), a pill that induces early abortion, has been used effectively in France and China for several years. Although it is not licensed for use in the United States, some predict it could be licensed by 1998. RU 486 blocks development of progesterone, which a fertilized ovum needs to implant and develop in the uterus. To end a pregnancy, the woman must take RU 486 within the first 7 weeks of pregnancy (about 3 weeks since a missed menstrual period). The protocol calls for three office or clinic visits, including one for administration of mifepristone, one for the administration of prostaglandin (with 2 to 4 hours of clinical monitoring), and one to verify that the abortion was complete. Abortion generally occurs within 24 hours after administration of prostaglandin.

Other methods that may be available in the future include a combination of methotrexate (a chemotherapeutic agent) and misoprostol, which stimulates uterine contractions.

From 13 to 16 weeks, a *dilation and evacuation* is generally performed. The procedure is similar to vacuum curettage but requires greater cervical dilation and a larger aspirator because the products of conception are larger. The cervix is dilated with laminaria that have been set in place 6 to 24 hours before the procedure. Laminaria are short, rounded pieces of material that are hygroscopic (absorb water). When laminaria are inserted into the cervix, they draw fluid from the cervical canal and expand, causing the cervix to dilate. Cervical dilation occurs slowly and is less traumatic to the cervix. A paracervical block (see Chapter 15) may be administered before the procedure.

After 16 weeks' gestation, *labor induction* can be carried out with several agents that produce uterine contractions or cause fetal death. Laminaria are usually inserted approximately 12 hours before the procedure to begin cervical dilation. Prostaglandin $E_2$, which stimulates contractions, may be given via vaginal suppository or intra-amniotic infusion. Side effects of prostaglandin include nausea, vomiting, and fever.

Prostaglandin may be combined with either hypertonic saline or hypertonic urea. Either may be injected into the amniotic sac. Hypertonic saline carries significant maternal risk for electrolyte imbalance if it accidentally moves into the maternal circulation. These solutions are feticidal, and labor usually starts within 24 hours. Giving oxytocin shortens labor, but second trimester abortion requires overnight hospitalization.

### Nursing Considerations

The nurse's role in caring for women seeking induced abortion is one of providing physical and emotional support and information. History taking and collection of laboratory data depend on the routine of the health care setting in which the nurse is functioning. Counseling and lending emotional support are nursing responsibilities unless a designated counselor performs these services.

Nurses are also responsible for providing information for self-care following an abortion.

> **Women Want to Know**
>
> **Self-Care Measures Following Induced Abortion**
>
> - Normal activities may be resumed, but strenuous work or exercise should be avoided for a few days.
> - Bleeding or cramping may occur for a week or two. If either becomes severe, medical advice should be sought. Light "spotting" may occur for about a month.
> - Sanitary pads rather than tampons should be used for the first week after the abortion to avoid possible infection.
> - Douching should be avoided for at least 1 week to prevent infection.
> - Intercourse should be curtailed for 1 week after the abortion because of the possibility of infection until the uterine lining heals.
> - Birth control measures should be used if sex is resumed before menstruation begins because it is possible to become pregnant during this time. Menstruation usually resumes in 4 to 6 weeks.
> - Temperature should be taken twice a day to detect possible infection; a temperature above 37.8°C (100°F) should be reported to the health care provider.
> - It is important to keep the follow-up appointment in 2 weeks.

## Menopause

Menopause simply means the end of menstruation. However, many people use the term to indicate the array of endocrine, somatic, and psychic changes that occur at the end of the reproductive period. The entire process, frequently called the "change of life," is correctly termed the *climacteric*. Premenopause refers to the early part of the climacteric, before menstruation ceases but after the woman experiences some of the climacteric symptoms, such as irregular menses. Perimenopause includes premenopause, menopause, and at least 1 year after menopause. Postmenopause refers to the phase following menopause, when menstrual periods have ceased altogether.

*Unplanned, or unscheduled, postmenopausal bleeding should always be investigated as soon as possible because it is highly suggestive of endometrial cancer.* Conversely, planned or scheduled postmenopausal bleeding is generally not a cause for concern. It occurs when the woman who takes estrogen and progesterone sequentially stops taking the drugs, usually once a month. This allows the uterine lining to be sloughed and prevents endometrial hyperplasia.

### Age of Menopause

The average age for naturally occurring menopause is 51.5 years in North America (ACOG, 1996). The natural process generally takes place over 3 to 5 years. Menopause can be induced or created artificially, however, at any age. Surgical removal of the ovaries or destruction of the ovaries by radiation creates permanent cessation of ovarian function, including the production of estrogen. The most common reason for performing these procedures is treatment of gynecologic cancer or endometriosis. Young women who experience artificial menopause often have more symptoms associated with menopause than do women who go through the process naturally.

Women can now expect to live another 30 years following menopause. During this period they must deal with physical, psychological, and social changes that often require a re-evaluation of their primary roles and restructuring of personal goals.

### Physiologic Changes

During the normal reproductive cycle, the ovaries respond to gonadotropins (follicle-stimulating hormone and luteinizing hormone) in a predictable pattern: (1) a follicle matures, (2) the ovary secretes estrogen, (3) ovulation occurs, and (4) the corpus luteum produces progesterone. During the premenopausal period, however, the ovaries are less responsive to gonadotropins, and, although increased amounts of follicle-stimulating hormone are secreted, ovulation is sporadic and menstrual periods are irregular. With progressive aging, the ovaries become unresponsive, even to high levels of gonadotropins, and ovulation, menstruation, and the secretion of ovarian hormones (estrogen and progesterone) cease. Lack of estrogen has a significant effect on the health of women during the postmenopausal years.

Estrogen is responsible for the secondary sex characteristics of women; when estrogen levels decline, the organs of reproduction undergo regression. The labia become thin and pale. The vaginal mucosa atrophies, and vaginal tissue loses its lubrication and thus is easily traumatized. Dyspareunia is not uncommon, and bacterial invasion of the epithelium may occur and lead to frequent vaginal infections. This entire process is referred to as atrophic vaginitis. Breasts become smaller, and atrophy of the uterus occurs. However, a concurrent benefit is that uterine myomas (fibroids) and endometriosis lesions also atrophy. Estrogen deficit can also result in atrophic changes in the bladder and urethra that may give rise to loss of urethral tone and frequent atrophic cystitis.

In addition, absence of estrogen is associated with an adverse change in serum lipids. Low-density lipoproteins, which carry cholesterol to blood vessels, increase. High-density lipoproteins, which are known to carry cholesterol to the liver and to protect against the development of coronary artery disease, decrease.

Most menopausal women experience hot flashes or flushes, which are the result of vasomotor instability. The cause of vasomotor instability is not known; however, it is closely associated with increased secretion of gonadotropins. Hot flashes are characterized by a sudden feeling of heat or burning of the skin, followed by perspiration. They occur more frequently during the night, and fatigue due to interrupted sleep is a major problem for some women.

## Psychological Responses

It is easy to understand why menopause is called the "change of life." It is accompanied not only by physical but also by psychological and social changes, and individual responses vary widely. Many women are relieved that their childbearing and childrearing tasks are coming to an end. They look on this as an exciting time, when they can pursue personal development. Other women grieve that the possibility of childbearing is past; this may be particularly true for women who have never had a child.

Menopause makes it necessary for women to come to terms with aging. It may be difficult to accept aging in a society that reveres youth, and many women become extremely concerned with measures that slow the signs of aging. Moreover, many women become grandmothers during the same period, which also confirms aging and requires a major adjustment in how the woman views herself.

Some symptoms do not have a physiologic explanation, but they are no less real to women who experience them. Depression, mood swings, irritability, and agitation are common climacteric complaints. Insomnia and fatigue are frequently mentioned as major problems.

One of the most puzzling aspects of menopause is the wide variation in both physical and psychological symptoms that women experience. For some women, the only changes are mild, infrequent hot flashes and amenorrhea. Other women experience severe, debilitating hot flashes, atrophic vaginitis, and multiple psychological symptoms, such as irritability and prolonged depression.

## Hormone Replacement Therapy

Hormone replacement therapy is considered the treatment of choice for many of the common discomforts of menopause. The type of hormone replacement, either estrogen only or estrogen in combination with progestin, depends on whether or not the woman has had a hysterectomy (removal of the uterus). Estrogen alone is prescribed for women who have had a hysterectomy. Estrogen and progestin are prescribed for women who retain the uterus and are at risk for endometrial hyperplasia if unopposed estrogen is administered.

### BENEFITS

Although hormone replacement therapy is the primary medical treatment for the symptoms of menopause, the risks as well as the benefits of estrogen must be evaluated for each woman. There is ample evidence that estrogen controls hot flashes and alleviates genital atrophy, which is associated with atrophic vaginitis, atrophic cystitis, and urinary incontinence. Either oral or topical estrogen may be administered for atrophic vaginitis.

Estrogen also offers protection from cardiovascular disease, which increases dramatically in postmenopausal women. The cardiovascular benefits of estrogen are believed to be due to its ability to increase high-density lipoprotein, which carries cholesterol to the liver to be excreted, and to decrease low-density lipoprotein, which carries cholesterol from the liver to body cells, including the blood vessels. Progestins have an opposite effect on lipids, but studies have not shown that this effect negates the cardiovascular protection (ACOG, 1996). Estrogen is also known to

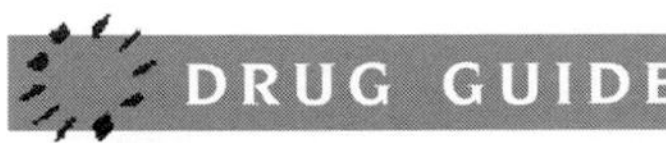

## CONJUGATED ESTROGENS (Estrace, Premarin, Ogen)

***Classification:*** Hormone—estrogen

***Action:*** Increases synthesis of DNA, RNA, and various proteins in responsive tissues. Reduces release of gonadotropin-releasing hormone, thus reducing follicle-stimulating hormone and luteinizing hormone. Promotes normal growth and maintenance of female genital organs, maintaining genitourinary function and vasomotor stability. Restores hormone balance in deficiency states, reduces blood cholesterol, and restores balance of bone resorption. Decreases serum concentration of testosterone.

***Indications:*** Treatment of vasomotor symptoms of menopause, such as hot flashes; prevention of postmenopausal osteoporosis; management of atrophic vaginitis.

***Dosage and Route:*** Dosage for relief of menopausal symptoms and prevention of osteoporosis, 0.6 to 1.25 mg orally. Schedule of administration depends on whether the woman has had a hysterectomy. If she has no uterus, estrogen alone may be administered daily or in a repeating cycle. If the uterus is present, both estrogen and progesterone are administered. Estrogen may be given for 21 days, with progesterone added for the final 10 days. Both medications are then stopped for 7 days. When the medication is stopped, predictable bleeding occurs. An alternative schedule involves the administration of estrogen, 0.625 mg, and progesterone, 2.5 to 5 mg daily. This schedule eliminates episodes of planned bleeding. Vaginal cream applied daily for 21 days, off for 7 days, and then repeated, may be useful for atrophic vaginitis.

***Absorption:*** Well absorbed following oral administration; readily absorbed through skin and mucous membranes.

***Excretion:*** Metabolized largely by the liver; as hepatic recirculation occurs, more absorption occurs from the gastrointestinal tract.

***Contraindications and Precautions:*** Contraindicated in thromboembolic diseases, undiagnosed vaginal bleeding, pregnancy, and lactation. Used cautiously in underlying cardiovascular disease and severe hepatic or renal disease; unopposed use may increase the risk of endometrial carcinoma.

***Adverse Reactions:*** Headache, dizziness, intolerance to contact lenses, nausea, jaundice

***Nursing Considerations:*** Assess blood pressure, pulse, and weight gain periodically throughout therapy; assess frequency and severity of hot flashes. Instruct the woman to report skin changes and to protect skin from excessive exposure to sunlight to prevent hyperpigmentation. Assess for vaginal bleeding, amenorrhea, or changes in menstrual flow, and instruct the woman to report these signs to her health care provider. Caution the woman to avoid use of any medication that has not first been approved by her health care provider.

---

protect against bone loss and the development of osteoporosis, which is described later.

Many women expect more from estrogen than it can deliver. Estrogen does not prevent aging of the skin, and evidence is inconclusive about whether it relieves depression or other psychological symptoms. However, clinical experience suggests that estrogen replacement relieves insomnia, promotes increased energy, and improves the overall quality of life.

### TREATMENT REGIMENS

Three treatment regimens are currently used for hormone replacement therapy. (1) *Cyclic regimen,* in which estrogen is given at specific intervals (such as 25 days per month) with the addition of progestin for the last 10 to 14 days. Many women are unhappy with the monthly "period" that occurs when the hormones are stopped for several days before restarting. (2) *Combined regimen,* in which estrogen and a low dose of progestin are given daily, and planned bleeding is avoided. (3) *Estrogen only,* in which estrogen is given for 25 days per month or daily, without treatment-free intervals or the addition of progestin. This regimen is used for women who have had a hysterectomy.

### RISKS

Administration of unopposed estrogen has been associated with an increased risk of endometrial can-

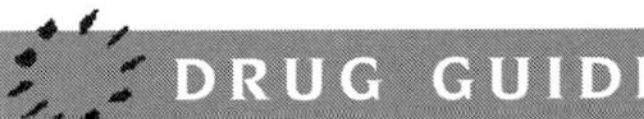

## MEDROXYPROGESTERONE (Provera, Cycrin, Amen)

***Classification:*** Hormone—progestin

***Action:*** A synthetic form of progesterone that transforms the endometrium from a proliferative to a secretory phase and promotes withdrawal bleeding when estrogen is also present. Promotes relaxation of uterine smooth muscle and growth of mammary alveolar tissue.

***Indications:*** Used to reduce the risk of endometrial carcinoma when estrogen is administered to control postmenopausal symptoms or to prevent osteoporosis.

***Dosage and Route:*** For induction of secretory endometrium following estrogen priming, 5 to 10 mg orally for 10 days. Or 2.5 to 5 mg daily with exogenous estrogen to prevent endometrial hyperplasia. Also used for secondary amenorrhea and abnormal uterine bleeding.

***Absorption:*** Unknown; metabolized by the liver

***Excretion:*** Unknown

***Contraindications and Precautions:*** Contraindicated in pregnancy, thromboembolic disease, carcinoma of the breast, and liver disease. Used with caution with cardiovascular disease, seizure disorders, and mental depression.

***Adverse Reactions:*** Depression, thrombophlebitis, edema, weight gain, dizziness, fatigue, headache, insomnia. Fluid retention may complicate other conditions such as asthma, heart disease, and renal disorders.

***Nursing Considerations:*** Assess blood pressure throughout therapy. Monitor weight gain, and emphasize that steady weight gain should be reported to health care provider. Advise women to anticipate withdrawal bleeding 3 to 7 days after discontinuing medication. Emphasize the importance of reporting the following signs and symptoms: visual changes, sudden weakness, headache, leg or calf pain, shortness of breath, jaundice, depression, and skin rash.

cer. To overcome this risk, small doses of progestin are given with estrogen. This eliminates the constant stimulation of the endometrium that occurs when estrogen alone is used. Some data suggest a minimally increased risk of breast cancer for women who used estrogen for more than 10 to 20 years, but the risk is unclear and data are confusing (ACOG, 1996).

Estrogen is contraindicated for some women. Growth of existing breast cancer may be stimulated by estrogen, and women who have had estrogen receptor–positive breast cancer usually do not take estrogen. Estrogen stimulates blood coagulation, and women who have developed a thrombosis should cease estrogen replacement therapy. Because estrogen is metabolized by the liver, it should not be taken by women who have hepatitis or liver disease. Not being able to take estrogen presents a dilemma for some women. Not only is osteoporosis an increased risk, but the atrophic changes of menopause and vasomotor instability remain major problems. When estrogen is contraindicated, women also have increased risk of coronary artery disease because they do not receive the protective effects of increased high-density lipoproteins that estrogen provides. Table 33–5 summarizes contraindications to estrogen replacement therapy.

### Alternative Medications

When hormone replacement therapy is contraindicated, alternative therapy may be prescribed. Clonidine hydrochloride (Catapres, dixarit), an antihypertensive, is sometimes prescribed to decrease the severity and frequency of hot flashes. Bellergal (a combination of phenobarbital, ergotamine tartrate, and belladonna) reduces hot flashes, but it is associated with unwanted side effects such as drowsiness.

### Nursing Considerations

Nursing care focuses on helping women understand the physical changes that occur and the psychological responses that may occur during menopause. Nurses must clarify the individual regimen of hormone replacement therapy as well as the risks and benefits of the therapy. For instance, women should be told that although hormone replacement therapy effectively treats atrophic vaginitis and reduces dyspareunia, it may not overcome the loss of libido that some women experience.

**TABLE 33–5 CONTRAINDICATIONS TO ESTROGEN REPLACEMENT THERAPY**

| |
|---|
| Thromboembolic disease |
| Undiagnosed vaginal bleeding |
| Previous episode of breast cancer or untreated uterine cancer |
| Diabetes mellitus |
| Gallbladder disease |
| Acute or chronic liver disease |

**Women Want to Know About Hormone Replacement Therapy**

- Take the medication with meals to reduce nausea.
- If you miss a dose, take the medication as soon as you remember, but not immediately before the next scheduled dose. *Do not take double doses.*
- Expect withdrawal bleeding (if your uterus is intact) when estrogen and progestin are temporarily discontinued.
- Report unplanned or unanticipated bleeding to your health care provider.
- Stop smoking to reduce the risk of serious thrombotic disorders, such as thrombophlebitis.
- Use sunscreen and protective clothing to prevent increased pigmentation.
- Continue follow-up physical examinations, including blood pressure measurements, Pap tests, and examinations of breasts, abdomen, and pelvis.

If hormone replacement therapy is contraindicated, nurses are often the primary source of information about alternative measures that mitigate symptoms:

- Vitamin E, ginseng, and other herbs can be effective in relieving hot flashes.
- Water-soluble lubricants, such as Lubrin and Replens, provide relief from vaginal dryness and dyspareunia. Oil-based lubricants should not be used because they adhere to the mucous membrane for long periods of time and provide a medium for bacterial growth.
- Kegel exercises increase muscle tone around the vagina and urinary meatus and help counteract the effects of genital atrophy.
- Drinking at least eight glasses of water a day decreases the concentration of urine and reduces bacterial growth, thereby preventing atrophic cystitis.
- Wiping from front to back following urination and defecation reduces the transfer of bacteria from the anus to the urinary meatus and helps prevent cystitis.

### Osteoporosis

Osteoporosis is one of the greatest hazards of the postmenopausal years. It is characterized by decreased bone density, leaving the bones porous, fragile, and susceptible to fractures. The vertebrae, wrists, and hips are the most common sites of fractures. In the United States, 1.3 million fractures occur yearly as a result of osteoporosis. This includes

500,000 vertebral fractures and 250,000 hip fractures in women. Between 12 and 20 percent of the women who suffer hip fracture die as a result of complications, such as pneumonia (Freund, 1995).

#### RISK FACTORS

Small-boned, fair-skinned white women of Northern European extraction and Asian women are at greatest risk for osteoporosis. Other risk factors may include a family history of the disease, early menopause, and a sedentary lifestyle. Women who smoke, drink alcohol, or take corticosteroids, as well as those who consume excessive amounts of caffeine, also have an increased risk for osteoporosis (Freund, 1995). Inadequate lifetime intake of calcium is a major risk factor because it results in failure to achieve peak bone mass.

#### SIGNS AND SYMPTOMS

Osteoporosis has been called the "silent thief" because it takes place gradually throughout the course of many years without any signs or symptoms. The first noticeable signs are loss of height and back pain that occurs when the vertebrae collapse. Later signs include the "dowager's hump," which occurs when the vertebrae can no longer support the upper body in an upright position. Secondary to this, the waistline disappears and the abdomen protrudes because the rib cage moves closer to the pelvis. Depending on the number of fractures, several inches of height may be lost. Figure 33–4 illustrates progressive changes in posture associated with osteoporosis.

Diagnosis of osteoporosis depends on a thorough history, physical examination, and bone mineral analysis. Conventional x-ray is of little help because more than 30 percent of the bone mass must be lost before changes are apparent. Dual-energy x-ray absorptiometry has generally replaced photon absorptiometry. It is highly accurate, fast, and relatively inexpensive. In addition, it involves low exposure to radiation. Computed tomography (CT scan) is accurate but expensive and is not available to all.

#### PREVENTION AND MEDICAL MANAGEMENT

The major goal of treatment is to prevent the development of osteoporosis and to stabilize remaining bone mass. The most effective measures are estrogen replacement, supplemental calcium, and exercise.

**Estrogen Replacement.** Estrogen halts bone loss and reduces the incidence of fractures. It is usually started in the perimenopausal period, and 0.625 mg per day is thought to provide protection from bone loss (ACOG, 1996). When therapy is begun in early menopause, it must be continued for at least 5 to 8 years to protect against the rapid bone loss that occurs during this time (Freund, 1995). Many women continue hormone therapy throughout their lives.

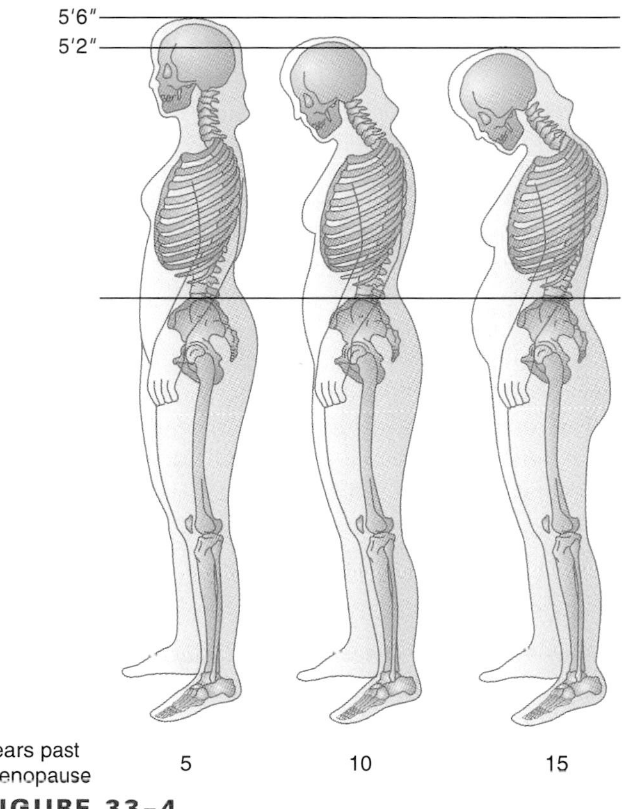


**FIGURE 33–4**

With progression of osteoporosis, the vertebral column collapses, causing loss of height and back pain. "Dowager's hump" is the term used for this curvature of the upper back.

**Calcium.** Although it does not prevent bone loss, other therapies cannot be effective if calcium is deficient. A postmenopausal woman should receive 1500 mg per day of calcium. Because it is difficult to ingest this amount daily, the use of supplements is recommended (ACOG, 1996). Vitamin D is necessary for calcium to be absorbed from the intestine. Supplemental vitamin D, 400 to 800 units, is recommended for many women (Gamble, 1995).

**Exercise.** Weight-bearing exercise has been shown to increase lumbar spine bone mineral density in postmenopausal women. Walking, hiking, stair climbing, and dancing are examples of weight-bearing exercises. High-impact exercises should be avoided because of the risk to fragile vertebrae.

**Alternative Medications.** Calcitonin is recommended for those women who already have low bone densities and for those with high rates of bone turnover. Formerly available only in injection form, calcitonin was approved 1995 by the FDA as a nasal spray (Miacalcin). This medication is indicated for treatment of postmenopausal osteoporosis in women who are 5 years past menopause and demonstrate low bone mass by dual-energy x-ray absorptiometry

(Moore, 1996). Side effects of this medication include nausea, rhinitis (with nasal administration), and arthralgias.

Newer biphosphonates are also potent inhibitors of bone resorption. A new agent of this class, alendronate (Fosamax), was also approved by the FDA in 1995. The most common side effects are nausea, stomach irritation, and abdominal pain. Many of these complaints diminish when women carefully take the medication as directed. Directions include (1) taking first thing on arising in the morning with 6 to 8 ounces of water, (2) remaining upright for at least 30 minutes, and (3) waiting at least 30 minutes before taking food, other fluids, or any other medications (including antacids, calcium supplements, and vitamins). Fluoride and etidronate have been suggested, but questions remain about their long-term effects on bone mass.

#### NURSING CONSIDERATIONS

Nurses often counsel women about lifestyle factors that contribute to bone loss, such as cigarette smoking, excessive alcohol or caffeine intake, and the importance of following the recommended medical regimen. Nurses are also concerned about how to prevent falls and thus reduce the risk of fractures. A major responsibility is to help the woman make her environment as safe as possible. Lighting should be ample, with switches easily accessible. Loose electrical cords should be kept out of the way, and area rugs should have nonskid backing. The bathtub should have nonskid devices, and grab bars near toilets and tubs are advised. Stairways should have handrails, and loose items should be kept out of the walking pathways.

#### NURSING DIAGNOSES

A variety of nursing diagnoses are important for the woman with osteoporosis. Examples include the following:

- Pain related to pressure and inflammation of nerves that exit the vertebral column
- Activity Intolerance related to discomfort and fear of falling
- Body Image Disturbance related to altered posture and functional limitations
- Self-care Deficit (specify) related to physical limitations and depression

#### CHECK YOUR READING

24. Why is menopause often called the "change of life"?
25. How does a deficiency in estrogen affect the reproductive organs?
26. What are the major psychological symptoms associated with menopause?
27. How does hormone replacement affect menopausal and postmenopausal women?
28. Why is osteoporosis called the "silent thief"?
29. How can osteoporosis be prevented?
30. What can nurses do to prevent fractures in women with osteoporosis?

## Pelvic Floor Dysfunction

Pelvic floor dysfunction occurs when muscles, ligaments, and fascia that support the pelvic organs become damaged or weakened. This relaxation of pelvic support allows the pelvic organs to prolapse into, and sometimes out of, the vagina. Pelvic disorders generally occur in the perimenopausal period and may be the delayed result of traumatic childbirth.

### Vaginal Wall Prolapse

The vagina may prolapse at either the anterior or posterior wall. Anterior wall prolapse involves the bladder and urethra and is called cystocele. Prolapse of the posterior wall produces enterocele or rectocele.

#### CYSTOCELE

When the weakened upper anterior wall of the vagina is no longer able to support the weight of urine in the bladder, cystocele develops. The bladder protrudes downward into the vagina, resulting in incomplete emptying of the bladder and consequent cystitis. Urethral displacement, formerly termed *urethrocele*, may occur when the urethra bulges into the lower anterior vaginal wall, producing stress incontinence (Fig. 33–5A).

*Stress incontinence* is the loss of urine that occurs with a sudden increase in intra-abdominal pressure, such as that generated by sneezing, coughing, lifting, or sudden jarring motions. The two most common causes of stress incontinence are damage to the normal supports of the bladder neck and urethra that occurs during pregnancy and childbirth, and tissue atrophy that occurs following menopause.

#### ENTEROCELE

Enterocele refers to prolapse of the upper posterior vaginal wall between the vagina and rectum. This is almost always associated with herniation of the pouch of Douglas (a fold of peritoneum that dips down between the rectum and the uterus) and may contain loops of bowel. Enterocele often accompanies uterine prolapse (Fig. 33–5B).

#### RECTOCELE

Rectocele occurs when the posterior wall of the vagina becomes weakened and thin. Each time the

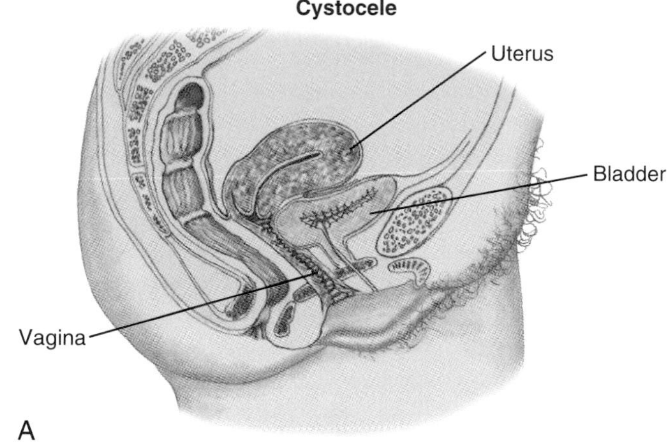


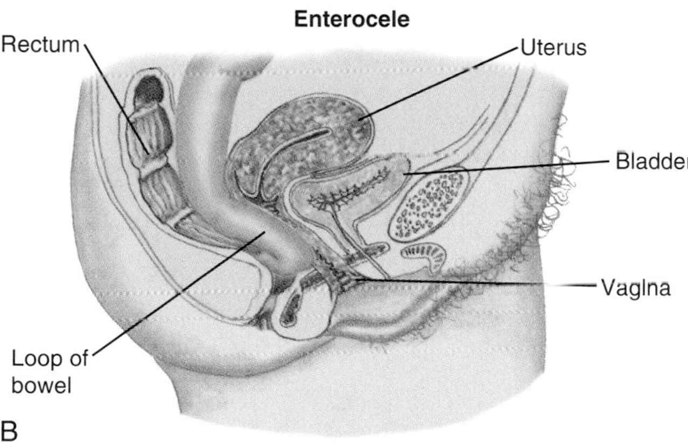


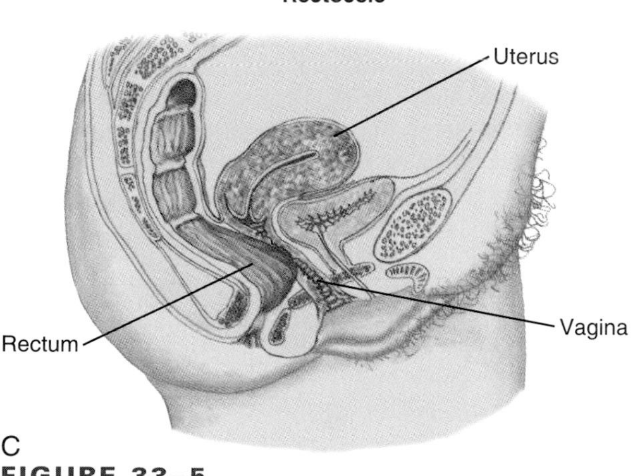


**FIGURE 33-5**

Three types of vaginal wall prolapse. A, Note bulging of bladder into the vagina. B, Note loop of bowel between rectum and uterus. C, Note bulging of rectum into vagina.

woman strains at defecation, feces are pushed against the thinned wall, causing further stretching, until finally the rectum protrudes into the vagina. Many rectoceles are small and produce few symptoms. If the rectocele is large, the patient may have difficulty emptying the rectum. Some women learn to facilitate bowel elimination by applying digital pressure along the posterior vaginal wall to keep the rectocele from protruding during a bowel movement (Fig. 33–5C).

## Uterine Prolapse

Uterine prolapse occurs when the cardinal ligaments, which support the uterus and vagina, are unduly stretched during pregnancy and do not return to normal following childbirth. This allows the uterus to sag backward and downward into the vagina. Uterine prolapse is less common than in the past, largely because of a decrease in traumatic vaginal deliveries. The condition continues to exist, however, particularly when the woman has had many vaginal deliveries or when the infants were large. Figure 33–6 illustrates three degrees of uterine prolapse from first degree, in which the uterus remains in the vagina, to third degree, in which the cervix protrudes through from the vagina.

### SYMPTOMS

Symptoms generally become obvious during the menopausal period. This is because estrogen diminishes at this time, resulting in atrophic changes in the supporting structures.

The most common symptoms of vaginal wall prolapse are feelings of pelvic fullness, a dragging sensation, pelvic pressure, and fatigue. Low backache and a feeling that "everything is falling out" are sometimes described. Symptoms also relate to the structures involved. For instance, urinary frequency, urgency, and urinary incontinence are seen in patients with cystocele. Constipation, flatulence, and difficulty defecating are major symptoms of rectocele. Regardless of the location or structure involved, symptoms become worse after prolonged standing, and they are relieved by lying down.

Symptoms of uterine prolapse are produced by the weight of the descending structures and may

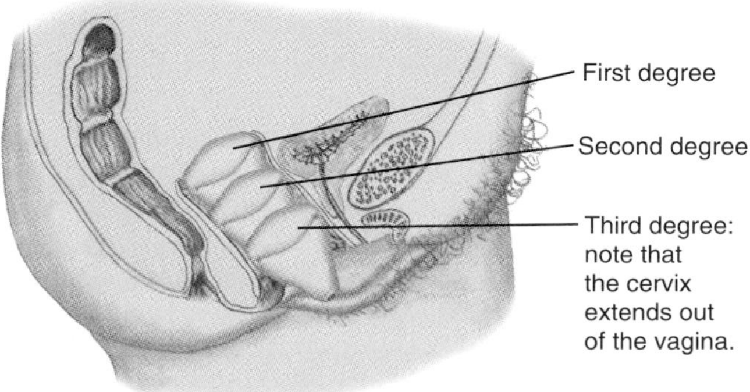


**FIGURE 33-6**

Three degrees of uterine prolapse.

include sensations of pelvic pressure, backache, and fatigue. Cervical ulceration and bleeding occur if the cervix protrudes from the vaginal introitus.

### MANAGEMENT

Treatment of disorders related to pelvic floor dysfunction depends on the woman's age, physical condition, sexual activity, and degree of prolapse. Surgical procedures provide the most satisfactory therapy for women who have significant discomfort. The most common procedures are the anterior and posterior colporrhaphy. The anterior colporrhaphy involves suturing the pubocervical fascia to support the bladder and urethra when a cystocele exists. If a rectocele exists, a posterior colporrhaphy (suturing the fascia and perineal muscles that support the perineum and rectum) is performed.

Surgical treatment for prolapse of the uterus depends on the degree of prolapse. An anterior and posterior colporrhaphy may be effective for a first-degree prolapse. Treatment for more severe prolapse may include vaginal hysterectomy, in which the uterus is removed through the vaginal canal rather than through an abdominal incision. Vaginal hysterectomy may also be combined with anterior and posterior colporrhaphy.

If surgery is contraindicated, a pessary (a device to support pelvic structures) may be inserted into the vagina. The pessary must be inspected and changed frequently by a physician or nurse practitioner to prevent vaginal ulceration or infection. Other devices, such as the Bladder Neck Support Prosthesis, have been found to restore or improve urinary continence in a majority of women (Jenkins et al., 1996).

Medical therapy may include hormone replacement, which is beneficial in reducing the genital atrophy that contributes to pelvic relaxation. Some women have fears about hormone therapy and are reluctant to take it. See p. 944 for information about the risks, benefits, and contraindications of hormone replacement therapy.

### NURSING CONSIDERATIONS

#### PELVIC EXERCISES

Kegel exercises are known to strengthen the pubococcygeal muscle, which surrounds the urethra, vagina, and rectum and is the main support of the pelvic floor. Before teaching Kegel exercise, it is necessary to determine if the woman can contract the pubococcygeal muscle by asking her to sit with her legs apart while she urinates and to squeeze the muscles to stop the stream of urine. If this can be done, the muscle is contracted and it is possible for her to perform the exercise.

Some women mistakenly believe that the Kegel exercise should be performed while urinating, and this idea should be corrected. The stream of urine is stopped only to determine if it is possible for the woman to contract the muscle. Kegel exercises involve conscious contracting and relaxing of the pelvic muscles. Only the pelvic muscles should be used; the abdomen, thighs, and buttocks should NOT tighten. Women should be taught to exhale and keep the mouth open to avoid bearing down when contracting the pelvic muscles. The woman must understand that for muscle tone to be maintained, the exercise must be continued for the rest of her life.

Graduated weight cones may be used as an adjunct to pelvic muscle exercise. Incrementally weighted cones are inserted into the vagina and the woman attempts to hold the weights in place. As the weight of the cones increases, the resistance against which the pelvic muscles contract increases, thereby strengthening the pelvic muscles.

Measures that help reduce the symptoms of pelvic relaxation may also prove helpful. These include lying down with the legs elevated for a few minutes several times a day. Some women are relieved by assuming a knee-chest position for a few minutes. In addition, teaching may include measures to prevent constipation.

#### URINARY INCONTINENCE

Nurses must acknowledge the reluctance many women feel about discussing incontinence and help them overcome these feelings and seek medical intervention.

**Direct questions, such as "Do you have trouble with your bladder?" or "Do you ever unintentionally lose urine?" may encourage women to discuss urine control problems. After the subject is introduced, follow-up questions are asked to determine urinary frequency. For instance, can she sit through a 2-hour movie without emptying her bladder? How many times does she get up to void each night?**

Continence may be enhanced by teaching a number of health promotion activities, such as Kegel exercises and bladder training, which involves adhering to a prescribed schedule for emptying the bladder (Sampselle et al., 1997). Women who cannot execute even a weak pelvic muscle contraction or are unable to implement bladder training may benefit from biofeedback or electrical stimulation provided by a skilled practitioner. Women often benefit from knowing about some of the commercial products that protect the skin and prevent odor. These products are made of material that traps urine and prevents constant contact with the skin.

Women often restrict fluids, believing that this will decrease urinary incontinence. Restricting fluids may actually make the condition worse because the bladder does not fill to its normal capacity. Furthermore, decreased fluid intake can lead to highly concentrated urine that can irritate bladder mucous membranes and increase the urge to void. Alcohol and caffeine can also irritate the bladder and worsen incontinence.

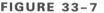

**CHECK YOUR READING**

31. How does cystocele differ from rectocele in terms of location? Symptoms?
32. What causes uterine prolapse, and how is it treated?
33. What are nursing actions to alleviate problems associated with pelvic floor relaxation? Urinary incontinence?

## Disorders of the Reproductive Tract

### Benign Disorders

The most common benign conditions of the reproductive tract include cervical polyps, uterine leiomyomas (fibroids), and ovarian cysts.

#### CERVICAL POLYPS

Polyps are small tumors, usually only a few millimeters in diameter, that are generally on a pedicle (a stem-like structure). They are caused by proliferation of cervical mucosa, and they often cause intermittent vaginal bleeding.

Cervical polyps are surgically removed in an outpatient setting, and the specimen is sent for pathologic examination to rule out the possibility of malignancy.

#### UTERINE LEIOMYOMAS

Leiomyomas, also called fibroids, are one of the most common gynecologic conditions encountered. It has been estimated that one third of all American women older than age 30 have these benign tumors (ACOG, 1996). Although the cause of uterine fibroids is unknown, they develop from smooth muscle cells and are estrogen dependent. As a result, they grow rapidly during the childbearing years but begin to atrophy during menopause, unless growth is stimulated by estrogen replacement therapy. Fibroids may occur throughout the muscular layer of the uterus; Figure 33–7 illustrates the various locations.

Uterine fibroids generally produce no symptoms; however, uterine size is sometimes increased and excessive menstrual bleeding may occur. Excessive bleeding may result in anemia, weakness, and fatigue. Additional symptoms include feelings of pelvic pressure, bloating, and urinary frequency that occurs when the tumor applies pressure on the bladder.

Treatment depends on the size of the fibroids and the symptoms experienced. In the absence of symptoms, treatment may consist of observation only. If abnormal bleeding is a problem, surgical intervention may be necessary. The two most common surgeries are myomectomy or removal of the tumor only, and hysterectomy, which is removal of the uterus. Medical treatment with GnRH may be effective in reducing the size of myomas and lessen the need for surgical removal of the tumor.

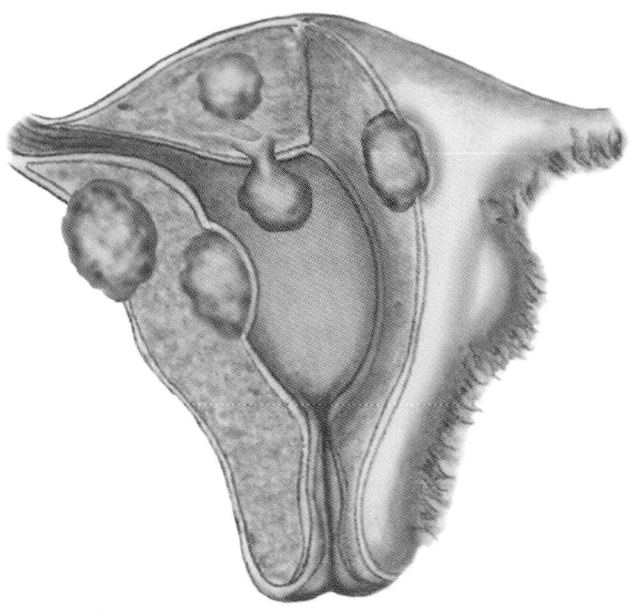

**FIGURE 33–7**

Sites within the uterus where fibroids commonly occur.

#### OVARIAN CYSTS

An ovarian cyst may be either follicular or luteal. If the ovarian follicle fails to rupture during ovulation, a follicular cyst may develop. These cysts are usually asymptomatic, and they generally regress during the subsequent menstrual cycle. A lutein cyst may develop if the corpus luteum becomes cystic and fails to regress. A lutein cyst is more likely to cause pain and some delay in the next menstrual cycle. Occasionally, an ovarian cyst can rupture or twist on its pedicle and become infarcted, causing pelvic pain and tenderness.

Treatment depends on differentiating a cyst from a solid ovarian tumor that may indicate cancer. If the woman is in her childbearing years, when the risk of ovarian cancer is less, the physician may wait until after the next menstrual cycle and examine the woman again. If there is a question about the contents, transvaginal ultrasound examination is useful to determine if it is a fluid-filled cyst or a solid tumor. Laparoscopy may be helpful in ruling out endometriosis, and laparotomy may be necessary to resect the cyst from the ovary for examination by a pathologist.

## Malignant Disorders

The primary sites for cancer in the female reproductive organs are the uterus, ovaries, and cervix. Cancer of the vagina, vulva, and fallopian tubes is relatively uncommon. Although cancer can occur at any age, the incidence increases with age.

### SIGNS AND SYMPTOMS

Cancer of the reproductive organs may not be diagnosed until it is advanced because few symptoms are experienced in the early stages. When symptoms occur, they are often nonspecific and could be caused by infection or other benign conditions. Cancer of the ovaries is particularly difficult to diagnose because the condition may remain "silent" until far advanced, when the chance of long-term survival is greatly reduced.

### RISK FACTORS

Risk factors vary according to the site of the cancer. Risk factors for cervical cancer include a history of sexually transmissible diseases, particularly condyloma acuminatum, or genital warts, caused by HPV. Prolonged use of unopposed estrogen replacement therapy predisposes to overgrowth (hyperplasia) of endometrial tissue and is a significant risk factor for uterine cancer.

Family history is an important risk factor for ovarian cancer. Other factors such as the use of talcum powder and feminine hygiene products that contain talc and the use of fertility drugs have also been implicated; however, their role is inconclusive (Tortolero-Luna et al., 1994). See Table 33–6 for a summary of risk factors for cancer of the reproductive organs.

### DIAGNOSIS

Early diagnosis is strongly associated with long-term survival. A variety of screening and diagnostic procedures are useful in early detection. Screening tests include periodic pelvic examinations, Pap tests, ultrasonography, and serum tests for tumor markers such as CA 125, which may be increased with ovarian or other cancers. Diagnostic procedures include endometrial sampling and colposcopy, which can identify patterns of abnormality near the cervical os, where most cancers of the cervix develop.

### Critical to Remember

**SYMPTOMS THAT MUST ALWAYS BE INVESTIGATED**

- Irregular vaginal bleeding
- Unexplained postmenopausal bleeding
- Unusual vaginal discharge
- Dyspareunia
- Persistent vulvar or vaginal itching
- Elevated or discolored lesions of the vulva
- Persistent abdominal bloating or constipation
- Persistent anorexia or vomiting
- Blood in stools

**TABLE 33–6 RISK FACTORS FOR CANCER OF THE REPRODUCTIVE ORGANS**

**Uterus**

Obesity
Nulliparity
Late menopause
Diabetes mellitus
Hypertension
Gallbladder disease
Breast, colon, or ovarian cancer
Chronic unopposed estrogen stimulation

**Cervix**

First coitus before 20 yr
Multiple sexual partners
Lower socioeconomic status (may be related to infrequent gynecologic examinations)
Race (incidence higher in African-Americans)
History of sexually transmissible diseases (strong link with human papillomavirus)

**Ovaries**

Race (increased in white women)
Menopause >52 yr
Family history of ovarian or uterine cancer
Nulliparity

### MANAGEMENT

Treatment of cancer of the reproductive organs is based on location and extent of the disease as well as the age and desire of the woman to have children. Early treatment of cervical cancer may consist of cryosurgery, destruction of abnormal tissue by laser, loop electrodiathermy excision procedure, or surgical conization of the cervix to remove the affected area. After treatment, a surveillance schedule should be established because there is risk of recurrent SIL after treatment.

Treatment for uterine, ovarian, or advanced cervical cancer usually consists of a total abdominal hysterectomy and bilateral salpingo-oophorectomy and may include adjuvant therapy with radiation or chemotherapy.

**CHECK YOUR READING**

34. What are the symptoms of leiomyomas (uterine fibroids), and how are they treated?
35. Why is ultrasonography used to evaluate ovarian cysts?

36. What signs and symptoms are suggestive of cancer of the reproductive organs and should always be investigated?
37. How may cancer of the cervix be treated?

# Infectious Disorders of the Reproductive Tract

## Sexually Transmissible Diseases

Many diseases can be transmitted through sexual activity. For some diseases, such as syphilis, gonorrhea, and chlamydial infection, sexual activity is almost the only method of transmission. For other diseases, such as candidiasis and trichomoniasis, sexual activity may or may not be the mode of transmission.

### INCIDENCE

Sexually transmissible diseases are epidemic today, with the highest incidence among adolescents and young adults. Furthermore, it is believed that the number of untreated infected individuals with no symptoms is immense. There are many reasons why these diseases remain a major health problem despite advancements in the development of antibiotics. The age of the first sexual experience has been declining steadily, and sexual activity is high among adolescents and young adults. Moreover, multiple sexual partners and inadequate knowledge of transmission and prevention, as well as feelings of invincibility, are common among this age group.

Methods of contraception have a significant impact on the risk of sexually transmissible diseases. Barrier methods, such as condoms, condoms with nonoxynol 9 (spermicide), and female condoms offer the best protection from infection. Diaphragms, cervical caps, and spermicidal foams and jellies do not offer the same protection as condoms, although they can decrease the risk of cervical and upper genital tract infections. When counseling teenagers, nurses must emphasize that oral contraceptives prevent pregnancy, but they do nothing to prevent exposure to sexually transmissible diseases.

Major concerns include the following:

- The vulnerability of women to sexually transmissible diseases
- The resistance of some organisms to antibiotics
- The relationship between HIV infection and other sexually transmissible diseases
- Failure of asymptomatic persons to seek treatment when their sexual partner is infected

See Chapter 26 for the impact of sexually transmissible diseases on pregnancy and the fetus.

### TYPES OF SEXUALLY TRANSMISSIBLE DISEASES

**Candidiasis.** Candidiasis, also known as moniliasis and yeast infection, is the most common form of vaginitis. The cause is believed to be related to a change in vaginal pH that allows accelerated growth of *Candida albicans*, which is a yeast-like fungus that is commonly found in the digestive tract and on the skin. Some conditions, such as pregnancy, diabetes mellitus, oral contraceptive use, and systemic antibiotic therapy, result in changes in vaginal pH and flora that favor accelerated growth of *C. albicans*.

The hallmark presenting symptom for candidiasis is itching. Vulvar and vaginal tissues are inflamed, so burning on urination is also present. Vaginal discharge is white with a typical "cottage cheese" appearance; vaginal and perineal itching is common. Diagnosis is made by identifying the spores of *C. albicans*.

Treatment consists of vaginal application of miconazole nitrate (Monistat), clotrimazole (Gyne-Lotrimin), or nystatin (Mycostatin). These medications are available without prescription; however, women should be advised to seek medical attention with the first infection or if the infection persists or recurs frequently. Recurrent yeast infections that resist treatment are associated with HIV infection.

**Trichomoniasis.** Trichomoniasis is caused by *Trichomonas vaginalis*, an anerobic protozoon that thrives in an alkaline environment. Most infections are believed to be transmitted by sexual contact. The presenting symptoms include a typical vaginal discharge that is thin, malodorous, and greenish-yellow in color. Vulvar itching, edema, and redness may also be present. The diagnosis is made by identifying the organism in a wet-mount preparation.

If the woman is not pregnant, the treatment of choice is metronidazole (Flagyl, Protostat). If the woman is pregnant, clotrimazole (Gyne-Lotrimin) may provide relief of symptoms during the first trimester. Metronidazole may be used during the second and third trimesters. Reinfection may result when the woman's partner is not treated. It is particularly important to emphasize that all sexual partners should be treated and that condoms should be used with a new partner.

**Bacterial Vaginosis.** This infection, previously referred to as nonspecific vaginitis or *Gardnerella* vaginitis, is most often caused by the bacillus *Gardnerella vaginalis*, which inhabits the vagina of healthy women. At times, the organism proliferates or "overgrows" and produces an extremely contagious vaginitis. Cause of the proliferation is not known, although tissue trauma and vaginal intercourse have been identified as contributing factors.

Chief symptoms are a thin grayish-white vaginal discharge that typically exudes a fishy odor. The diagnosis is made by preparing a saline wet mount and identifying characteristic clue cells (epithelial cells with numerous bacilli clinging to their surface).

Treatment for bacterial vaginosis is directed toward re-establishing the balance of flora in the vagina. Metronidazole has been shown to relieve symptoms and to improve vaginal flora. Women should be advised to avoid using alcohol during treatment with metronidazole and for 24 hours thereafter. Clindamycin cream and metronidazole gel are alternative treatments.

**Chlamydial Infection.** The most common sexually transmissible disease in Western countries is caused by the gram-negative bacterium *Chlamydia trachomatis*. The incidence is particularly high in the teenage population. Chlamydial infection is often asymptomatic in women, which makes diagnosis and control of the disease difficult. It should be suspected when the male sexual partner is treated for nongonococcal urethritis and when the culture results for gonorrhea are negative, yet the woman exhibits symptoms similar to those of gonorrhea, such as a yellowish vaginal discharge and painful urination.

Culture is the best method of detection of *C. trachomatis* infection, but it is expensive and time consuming. Rapid detection tests, such as enzyme-linked immunosorbent assay (ELISA) and monoclonal antibody tests, are now commonly used. Unfortunately, both tests may be nonspecific, with false-positive results possible (ACOG, 1996).

Untreated, chlamydial infection ascends from the cervix to involve the fallopian tubes, and it is one of the chief causes of tubal scarring that results in infertility or ectopic pregnancy. The usual treatment is azithromycin, doxycycline hyclate, or tetracycline, and concurrent treatment of all sexual partners is essential to prevent recurrence.

**Gonorrhea.** Gonorrhea is an infection of the genitourinary tract that is caused by the gonococcus *Neisseria gonorrhoeae*. Gonorrhea may be asymptomatic in women; however, when symptoms do occur, they usually include purulent discharge, dysuria, and dyspareunia. Diagnosis is based on a positive culture for the gonococcus. Similar to chlamydial infection, gonorrhea is associated with pelvic inflammatory disease (PID), which increases the risk of tubal scarring and can result in infertility or ectopic pregnancy.

Currently, two factors influence the treatment of gonorrhea: the high numbers of organisms that have become resistant to previously used antibiotics, such as penicillin and tetracycline, and the high frequency of chlamydial infections in persons with gonorrhea. Cefixime or ceftriaxone, in combination with doxycycline, appears to be effective for treatment of all gonococcal infections as well as for treatment of chlamydial infection. If possible, all sexual partners should be treated simultaneously.

**Syphilis.** Syphilis is caused by the spirochete *Treponema pallidum*, and it is divided into primary, secondary, and tertiary stages. The first sign of primary syphilis is a painless chancre that develops on the genitalia, anus, or lips or in the oral cavity. At this time, diagnosis is made by identifying the spirochete on darkfield microscopy in material scraped from the base of the chancre. A serologic test is generally negative in the primary stage. If untreated, the chancre heals in about 6 weeks; the disease is highly infectious at this time.

Although the chancre disappears, the spirochete lives and is carried by the blood to all parts of the body. About 2 months after the initial infection, infected people exhibit symptoms of secondary syphilis, including enlargement of the spleen and liver, headache, anorexia, and a generalized maculopapular skin rash. Skin eruptions, called condylomata lata, may develop on the vulva during this time. Condylomata lata resemble warts; they contain numerous spirochetes and are highly contagious. Serologic tests are generally positive at this time.

If untreated, the disease enters a latent phase that may last for several years. Tertiary syphilis, which follows the latent phase, may involve the heart, blood vessels, and central nervous system. General paralysis and psychosis may result.

In addition to identification of the spirochete in material scraped from a chancre, diagnosis is also made by serology. The usual screening test is the Venereal Disease Research Laboratory (VDRL) serum test, which is based on the presence of antibodies produced in response to the infection. The rapid plasma reagin (RPR) and fluorescent treponemal antibody absorption (FTAABS) tests are more specific and are commonly performed to confirm a positive VDRL.

Treatment of all stages of syphilis is with penicillin. Tetracycline is an alternative if the woman is not pregnant.

**Herpes Genitalis.** Herpes genitalis is a sexually transmissible disease caused by the herpes simplex virus (HSV). Two types of HSV have been identified: type I and type II. HSV II usually causes genital lesions. Transmission occurs through direct contact with an infected person.

Within 2 to 20 days after the primary infection, vesicles (blisters) appear in a characteristic cluster on the vulva, perineum, or perianal area. The initial lesions may cause severe vulvar pain and tenderness as well as dyspareunia. Although they cannot be seen by the woman, the lesions may also occur on the cervix or in the vagina. The vesicles rupture within 1 to 7 days and form ulcers that take an average of 12 days to heal (Bennett, 1994).

At the initial infection, the woman may also experience flu-like symptoms, including fever, general malaise, and enlarged lymph nodes. When symptoms abate, the virus remains dormant in the nerve ganglia and periodically reactivates, particularly in times of stress, fever, and menses. Recurrent episodes are seldom as extensive or painful as the initial episode; however, they are just as contagious. Diagnosis is often based on clinical signs and symptoms and confirmed by viral culture of fluid from the vesicle.

Treatment offers no cure, but acyclovir, an antiviral drug, helps reduce or suppress symptoms, shedding, and recurrent episodes. The safe use of acyclovir in pregnancy has not been established. Women should be advised to abstain from sexual contact while the lesions are present. If it is an initial infection, they should continue to abstain until they become culture-negative, because prolonged viral shedding may occur in such cases.

**Condylomata Acuminata.** Condylomata acuminata, also known as venereal or genital warts, are caused by HPV. The dry wart-like growths may be small and discrete, or they may cluster and resemble cauliflower (Fig. 33–8). Common sites include the vagina, labia, cervix, and perineal area.

Condylomata acuminata are of particular concern because of the increasing evidence of the association of HPV with precursor states of cervical cancer. Colposcopy, examination by a magnifying instrument called the colposcope, is generally recommended to evaluate abnormal cervical tissue and to identify HPV. Women with condylomata acuminata should be advised to have semi-annual or annual Pap tests to detect cervical dysplasia.

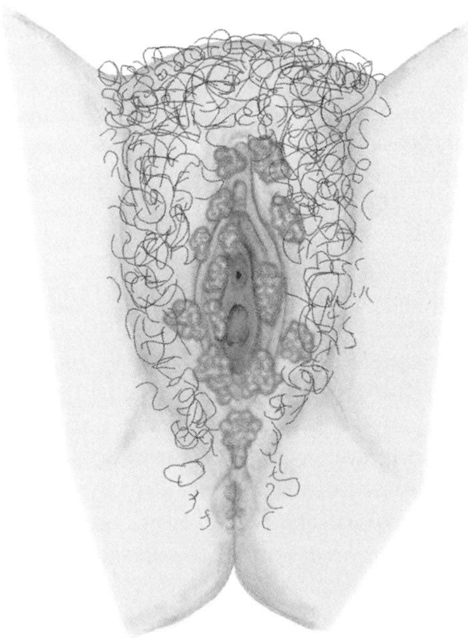

**FIGURE 33–8**

Condylomata acuminata, also called venereal warts, are caused by the human papillomavirus (HPV).

The goal of treatment is to remove the warts, which easily transmit the virus back and forth between sexual partners. Weekly applications of 25 percent trichloroacetic acid is the first line of treatment. Cryotherapy, electrocautery treatment, or laser therapy may be used to remove the warts. Podophyllin is sometimes used as an alternative therapy. It may be applied for 4 hours, and then the area must be carefully washed to prevent damage to surrounding tissue. Interferon, an antineoplastic drug, is sometimes used to treat condylomata acuminata in women older than 18 years of age who have not responded to conventional therapy.

It is important that the woman understands that none of these treatments eradicate the virus and that she may have recurrences. Furthermore, all sexual partners must be treated. Sexual contact should be avoided until all lesions are healed, and the use of condoms is recommended to reduce transmission.

**Acquired Immunodeficiency Syndrome.** Acquired immunodeficiency syndrome (AIDS), caused by HIV, is the most devastating sexually transmissible disease in the world today. Human immunodeficiency virus has been isolated from blood, semen, vaginal secretions, urine, saliva, tears, cerebrospinal fluid, amniotic fluid, and breast milk (McCrone, 1995). The primary modes of transmission are intimate contact with infected bodily secretions, exposure to infected blood and blood products, and perinatal transmission from mother to infant.

The treatment of HIV/AIDS is a rapidly developing and changing field. Although there is currently no cure, new medications show a great deal of promise. In addition to zidovudine and didanosine, which have been used for some time, a new category of drug has been developed. These drugs, known as protease inhibitors, block the working of protease, an enzyme crucial to one step in the reproductive cycle of HIV. They have been found to be effective when used with older drugs that block another enzyme necessary for HIV replication. See Chapter 26 for a complete discussion of HIV and AIDS in pregnant women and neonates.

#### NURSING CONSIDERATIONS

In their role as teachers and counselors, nurses can play a major part in preventing the spread of STDs. To fulfill this role, nurses must be prepared to do the following:

- Teach the signs and symptoms that require medical attention
- Explain diagnostic or screening tests
- Teach preventive measures

## Women Want to Know
## About Sexually Transmissible Diseases

*What are the most common symptoms of sexually transmissible diseases (STDs)?*

- Unexpected nonbloody vaginal discharge (increased amount, unusual color, or odor) or vaginal bleeding
- Vulvar itching or swelling
- Pelvic pain, including painful intercourse, painful urination, and abdominal tenderness
- Skin eruptions or changes (rashes, chancres, warts, painful papules, or vesicles)
- Flu-like symptoms (fever, swollen or painful lymph glands, loss of appetite, nausea or vomiting)
- Presence of symptoms in a sexual partner, even though symptoms are absent in the woman

*What are the common methods of diagnosis?*

- Culture (vaginal discharge, cervix, lesions) to identify organism
- Blood test (serology) to determine if antibodies for specific diseases are present (VDRL or FTAABS test for syphilis, HIV test for human immunodeficiency virus)

*How can STDs be prevented?*

- Limit number of sexual partners.
- Establish monogamous relationship with uninfected partner.
- Use mechanical and chemical barriers (latex condoms in conjunction with nonoxynol 9).
- Remember that one episode of an STD offers no protection from future infection.
- Make sure partner is simultaneously treated to prevent reinfection.

*What are the most important things to know about the treatment?*

- The entire course of medication must be completed even if symptoms subside.
- It is essential to comply with follow-up evaluation as recommended by health care provider.
- Sexual intercourse should be curtailed until free of infection.
- Partner must be examined and treated before sexual intercourse is resumed.
- Importance of reporting side effects of medications, such as skin rashes, difficulty breathing, or headaches.
- Not all STDs can be cured (herpes, AIDS, venereal warts), and treatment is aimed at slowing the disease and preventing complications.

*Are there measures that provide comfort and prevent secondary infections?*

- Keep the vulva clean but avoid strong soaps, creams, and ointments unless prescribed by health care provider.
- Keep the vulva dry; using a hair dryer turned on low is helpful.
- Wear absorbent cotton underwear and avoid pantyhose and tight pants as much as possible.
- Take analgesics (aspirin or acetaminophen) as directed by health care provider.
- Cool or tepid sitz baths may provide relief from itching.
- Wipe vulva from front to back following urination or defecation and then carefully wash hands.

### CHECK YOUR READING

38. What four conditions may change the normal flora and pH of the vagina and result in vaginitis?
39. How does the vaginal discharge of candidiasis differ from that of trichomoniasis?
40. Why are barrier-type contraceptives recommended?
41. How do primary and secondary syphilis differ in terms of signs and symptoms and potential for transmitting the disease?
42. How are condylomata acuminata associated with a precursor state of cervical cancer?

## Pelvic Inflammatory Disease

Pelvic inflammatory disease, infection of the upper genital tract, is a serious health problem in the United States. It is estimated that more than 1 million women seek medical attention for acute pelvic pain, which is the primary symptom of PID. In addition, numerous other women with "silent" sexually transmissible diseases face the risk of chronic pelvic pain, infertility, and ectopic pregnancy, which are common sequelae.

### ETIOLOGY

Although other organisms, such as *Escherichia coli* and gram-positive cocci, may cause PID, the primary infectious organisms are *C. trachomatis* and *N. gonorrhoeae*. These organisms invade the endocervical canal and cause cervicitis. Bacteria ascend and infect the endometrium, fallopian tubes, and pelvic cavity. The chronic inflammatory response is responsible for extensive tubal scarring and peritubal adhesions, which interfere with conception and with transport of the fertilized ovum through the obstructed fallopian tubes.

### SYMPTOMS

Symptoms of PID vary widely. Some women are asymptomatic, whereas others experience pelvic pain, fever, purulent vaginal discharge, nausea, anorexia, and irregular vaginal bleeding. Findings during physical examination may include abdominal or adnexal tenderness, and tenderness of the uterus and cervix when they are moved during bimanual examination (cervical motion tenderness). Laboratory evaluation may reveal a marked leukocytosis and increased sedimentation rate. A urinalysis is needed to rule out urinary tract infection, and cervical cultures for *N. gonorrhoeae* and *C. trachomatis* help to diagnose the disease.

### MANAGEMENT

Women with serious infection, as manifested by fever, abdominal pain, and leukocytosis, may be admitted to a hospital. They are most often treated with intravenous administration of cefoxitin, cefotetan, or clindamycin. Ambulatory treatment is appropriate for some women who are less ill and are able to comply with the recommended regimen.

#### NURSING CONSIDERATIONS

Nurses can play an important role in preventing PID by teaching women how to prevent sexually transmissible diseases in themselves and in their partners. Prevention can be thought of as occurring on two levels: primary and secondary. Primary prevention involves avoiding exposure to these diseases or preventing acquisition of infection during exposure. Primary preventive measures include limiting the number of sexual partners and avoiding intercourse with those who have had multiple partners. Barrier methods (latex condoms with spermicide containing nonoxynol 9, diaphragm with spermicide) used consistently and correctly during all sexual activity help prevent sexually transmissible diseases.

Secondary prevention involves keeping a lower genital tract infection from ascending to the upper genital tract or from being further transmitted within the community. This involves seeking medical attention promptly after having unprotected sex with someone who is suspected of having a sexually transmissible disease and when vaginal discharge or genital lesions are apparent. Moreover, periodic medical assessment is necessary if the woman is not in a mutually monogamous relationship, even if she is asymptomatic. Additional measures include taking medication as prescribed and returning for follow-up evaluation.

### Toxic Shock Syndrome

Although toxic shock syndrome is rare, it is a potentially fatal condition caused by toxin-producing strains of S. *aureus*. The toxin that is produced alters capillary permeability, which allows intravascular fluid to leak from the blood vessels, leading to hypovolemia, hypotension, and shock. The toxin also causes direct tissue damage to organs and precipitates serious defects in coagulation.

If toxin-producing strains of S. *aureus* inhabit the vagina, certain factors increase the risk that the toxin will gain entry into the blood stream. These include the use of high-absorbency tampons during menstruation and barrier methods of contraception (cervical cap or diaphragm), both of which may trap and hold bacteria if left in place for a prolonged time.

Symptoms of toxic shock syndrome include a sudden spiking fever and flu-like symptoms (headache, sore throat, vomiting, diarrhea), hypotension, a generalized rash resembling sunburn, and skin peeling from the palms of the hands and the soles of the feet 1 and 2 weeks after the onset of the illness.

Treatment consists of fluid replacement, administration of vasopressor drugs, and antimicrobial therapy. Corticosteroids may be used to treat skin changes.

Nurses are often responsible for providing information that may help to prevent toxic shock syndrome.

#### TAMPON USE

Nurses should instruct women to do the following:

- Wash the hands thoroughly to remove bacteria before inserting tampons.
- Change tampons at least every 4 hours to prevent excessive bacterial growth on a tampon that is left in place for a longer time.
- Do not use superabsorbent tampons at any time because they may be left in the vagina for a prolonged period, allowing bacteria to proliferate.
- Use pads rather than tampons during hours of sleep, which usually exceeds 6 to 8 hours.

#### DIAPHRAGM USE

Nurses should tell women to do the following:

- Wash hands thoroughly before inserting diaphragm.
- Do not use diaphragm during menstrual periods.
- Remove diaphragm within time recommended by health care provider.

#### ✓ CHECK YOUR READING

43. What organism causes toxic shock syndrome?
44. How can the risk of toxic shock syndrome be reduced?

## SUMMARY CONCEPTS

- Health maintenance refers to examinations and screening procedures that allow early detection of specific conditions, such as breast or cervical cancer, and allow for early treatment that increases the chance of long-term survival.
- A major role of nurses is to explain screening procedures and to encourage women to have them on a regular basis. The most common screening procedures include BSE, professional breast examination, and mammography for breast cancer; vulvar self-examination to detect precancerous conditions or infections; pelvic examination to detect abnormalities of the uterus or ovaries; Pap test for cervical cancer; and screening for fecal occult blood. Additional tests may include transvaginal ultrasonography and CA 125 if the woman is at risk for ovarian cancer.
- Disorders of the breast may be benign, such as fibrocystic changes that occur in relation to the menstrual cycle, or malignant. The discovery of any breast disorder creates anxiety in women, and

nurses must be prepared to explain diagnostic procedures, such as ultrasonography, needle aspiration, and surgical biopsy.

- One in eight women in the United States develops breast cancer; besides gender, the greatest risk factors are advancing age and prior history of breast cancer. Additional factors include family history (grandmother, mother, sister) of breast cancer and previous uterine, ovarian, or colon cancer. Lifestyle factors such as a high intake of dietary fat, smoking, and consumption of alcohol are also suspected to increase risk.
- Management of breast cancer includes surgical removal of the tumor plus varying amounts of surrounding tissue and lymph glands. Adjuvant therapy includes radiation, chemotherapy, and hormone therapy.
- Breast reconstruction is an integral part of the surgical management of breast cancer. Methods include tissue expansion and autogenous grafts.
- Nursing care for women with cancer of the breast focuses on providing emotional support and accurate information.
- Menstrual cycle disorders include amenorrhea, abnormal uterine bleeding, cyclic pelvic pain, and premenstrual syndrome. Some of the disorders, such as premenstrual syndrome, respond to lifestyle alterations such as changes in diet, exercise habits, and stress management.
- Induced abortion may be performed by medical or surgical methods, and each method is associated with social and ethical conflicts.
- Menopause, more correctly termed the climacteric, is a combination of endocrine, somatic, and psychic changes that occur at the end of the reproductive cycle. Women's responses to menopause vary widely; however, following menopause, all women are in a permanent state of estrogen deficit that can result in bone loss (osteoporosis) and increased incidence of coronary artery disease.
- Hormone replacement therapy is commonly prescribed to manage the symptoms of estrogen deficit, such as hot flashes and atrophic vaginitis, and to decrease osteoporosis and cardiovascular disease.
- Estrogen replacement has risks as well as benefits and is contraindicated for women who have thromboembolic disease, undiagnosed vaginal bleeding, previous episodes of breast cancer or untreated uterine cancer, or chronic liver disease. For these women, alternative measures are needed to control the symptoms of menopause.
- Relaxation of pelvic support structures occurs as a delayed result of traumatic childbirth and becomes troublesome when a deficiency in estrogen hastens genital atrophy.
- Although some infections of the reproductive tract are related to a change in the pH or the flora of the vagina, such as candidiasis, the majority are transmitted by sexual contact. The incidence of sexually transmissible diseases is reduced by barrier methods of contraception, particularly the condom, which prevents potentially infected ejaculate from entering the lower genital tract.
- Barrier methods, such as the diaphragm and cervical cap, are less effective than the condom in preventing sexually transmissible diseases; however, they provide some protection for the upper genital tract. Sexually transmissible diseases, including AIDS, are caused by microorganisms, and the best means of protection are abstinence from sexual intercourse or an exclusive sexual relationship with an uninfected person.
- Pelvic inflammatory disease is often a complication of untreated sexually transmissible diseases, particularly chlamydial infection or gonorrhea, which can result in infertility or ectopic pregnancy because of scarring of fallopian tubes resulting from inflammatory processes in the pelvic cavity.
- Toxic shock syndrome is a life-threatening condition resulting from infection with toxin-producing strains of *Staphylococcus aureus*. The infection is believed to be related to use of high-absorbency tampons that trap and hold bacteria in nutrient-rich menstrual blood for an extended time. Tampons should be removed every 4 hours, and other items that trap bacteria, such as cervical caps and diaphragms, should be removed as directed by the health care provider (usually within 6 to 24 hours).

### References and Readings


American Cancer Society. (1988). *Breast self-examination: A new approach*. Atlanta: Author.

American Cancer Society. (1994). *Cancer facts and figures*. Atlanta: Author.

American College of Obstetricians and Gynecologists (ACOG). (1996). *Guidelines for women's health care*. Washington, D.C.: Author.

Bennett, E. (1994). Vaginitis and sexually transmitted diseases. In E. Youngking & M. Davis (Eds.), *Women's health: A primary care clinical guide* (pp. 203–240). Norwalk, Conn.: Appleton & Lange.

Brunt, M.J. (1995). Amenorrhea and oligomenorrhea. In P.L. Carr, K.M. Freund, & S. Somani (Eds.), *The medical care of women* (pp. 168–181). Philadelphia: W.B. Saunders.

Buzby, M. (1996). Viral hepatitis: A sexually transmitted disease? *Nurse Practitioner Forum*, 7(1), 10–15.

Centers for Disease Control. (1992). Sexual behavior among high school students. *Morbidity and Mortality Weekly Report*, 40(5), 885–888.

Creehan, P.A. (1995). Toxic shock syndrome: An opportunity for nursing intervention. *Journal of Obstetric, Gynecologic, and Neonatal Nursing*, 24(6), 557–561.

Dahlbeck, S.W., Donnelly, J.F., & Theriault, R.L. (1995). Differentiating inflammatory breast cancer from acute mastitis. *American Family Physician*, 52(3), 929–934.

Department of Health and Human Services (DHHS). (1995). *Healthy people 2000. Midcourse Review and 1995 Revisions*. Washington, D.C.: U.S. Public Health Service.

Department of Health and Human Services (DHHS). (1997). *Morbidity and Mortality Weekly Report*, 46(SS-4), 37–98.

Donaldson, K., Briggs, J., & McMaster, D. (1994). RU 486: An alternative to surgical abortion. *Journal of Obstetric, Gynecologic, and Neonatal Nursing*, 23(7), 555–559.

Ferreira, N. (1996). Sexually transmitted *Chlamydia trachomatis*. *Nurse Practitioner Fourum*, 7(1), 40–46.

Fiorica, J.V. (1994). Fibrocystic changes. *Obstetrics and Gynecology Clinics of North America*, 21(3), 445–452.

Freeman, S.B. (1995). Common genitourinary infections. *Journal of Obstetric, Gynecologic, and Neonatal Nursing*, 24(8), 735–741.

Freund, K.M. (1995). Osteoporosis. In P.L. Carr, K.M. Freund, & S. Somani (Eds.), *The medical care of women* (pp. 643–651). Philadelphia: W.B. Saunders.

Galsworthy, T.D. (1996). It steals more than bone. *American Journal of Nursing*, 96(6), 27–33.

Gamble, C.L. (1995). Osteoporosis: Drug and nondrug therapies for the patient at risk. *Geriatrics*, 50(8), 39–43.

Ginsburg, K.A., & Moghissi, K. (1994). Secondary amenorrhea. In F.P. Zuspan & E.J. Quilligan (Eds.), *Current therapy in obstetrics and gynecology* (4th ed., pp. 112–116). Philadelphia: W.B. Saunders.

Grady, D., Gebretsadik, T., Ernster, V., & Petitti, D. (1995). Hormone replacement therapy and endometrial cancer risk: A meta-analysis. *Obstetrics and Gynecology*, 85(2), 304–313.

Hautman, M.A. (1996). Changing womanhood: Perimenopause among Filipina-Americans. *Journal of Obstetric, Gynecologic and Neonatal Nursing*, 25(8), 667–672.

Hindle, W.H. (1994). The diagnostic evaluation. *Obstetrics and Gynecology Clinics of North America*, 21(3), 499–518.

Huff, B.C. (1996). Prevention, screening and early detection of gynecologic cancers. *AWHONN Voice*, 4(5), 1–13.

Isaacs, J.H. (1994). Benign tumors of the breast. *Obstetrics and Gynecology Clinics of North America*, 21(3), 487–498.

Jenkins, P., Bernier, F., Davila, G.W., & Harris, L. (1996) Nonsurgical treatment of urinary stress incontinence with the bladder neck support prosthesis; Extended experience. Clinical Research Paper, AWHONN Conference, June 2–6.

Kottmann, L.M. (1995). Pelvic inflammatory disease: Clinical overview. *Journal of Obstetric, Gynecologic, and Neonatal Nursing*, 24(8), 759–767.

Lappe, J.M. (1993). Bone fragility: Assessment of risk and strategies for prevention. *Journal of Obstetric, Gynecologic, and Neonatal Nursing*, 23(3), 260–267.

LeBoeuf, F.J., & Carter, S.G. (1996). Discomforts of the perimenopause. *Journal of Obstetric, Gynecologic, and Neonatal Nursing*, 25(2), 173–180.

Marchant, D.J. (1994a). Contemporary management of breast cancer. *Obstetrics and Gynecology Clinics of North America*, 21(4), 555–560.

Marchant, D.J. (1994b). Risk factors. *Obstetrics and Gynecology Clinics of North America*, 21(4), 561–586.

McCrone, E.L. (1995). Human immunodeficiency virus infection: Epidemiology, risk assessment, and testing. In P.L. Carr, K.M. Freund, & S. Somani (Eds.), *The medical care of women* (pp. 492–500). Philadelphia: W.B. Saunders.

McHahon, S. (1995). Prevention and early detection of cancer in women. *Seminars in Oncology Nursing*, 11(2), 88–102.

McHugh, D.R. (1996). Syphilis: An old disease with modern health concerns. *Nurse Practitioner Forum*, 7(1), 34–39.

Moore, A.A. (1996). Osteoporosis and the older woman. *AWHONN Voice*, 4(5), 1–14.

Moore, A.A., & Noonan, M.D. (1996). A nurse's guide to hormone replacement therapy. *Journal of Obstetric, Gynecologic, and Neonatal Nursing*, 25(1), 24–31.

Newman, R.E., & Nishimoto, P.W. (1996). 1996 human immunodeficiency virus update for the primary care provider. *Nurse Practitioner Forum*, 7(1), 16–22.

Prout, M.N. (1995). Breast cancer: Epidemiology, screening, and prevention. In P.L. Carr, K.M. Freund, & S. Somani (Eds.), *The medical care of women* (pp. 153–160). Philadelphia: W.B. Saunders.

Robert, N.J. (1994). Adjuvant therapy in breast cancer. *Obstetrics and Gynecology Clinics of North America*, 21(4), 693–708.

Sampselle, C.M., Burns, P.A., Dougherty, M.C., Newman, D.K., Thomas, K.K., & Wyman, J.F. (1997). Continence for women. *Journal of Obstetric, Gynecologic, and Neonatal Nursing*, 26(4), 375–385.

Scott, M.A.K. (1996). Reducing the risks: Adolescents and sexually transmitted diseases. *Nurse Practitioner Forum*, 7(1), 23–29.

Silverstein, M.J. (1994). Noninvasive breast cancer: The dilemma of the 1990s. *Obstetrics and Gynecology Clinics of North America*, 21(4), 639–658.

Somani, S. (1995). Evaluation and management of pelvic pain. In P.L. Carr, K.M. Freund, & S. Somani (Eds.), *The medical care of women* (pp. 55–66). Philadelphia: W.B. Saunders.

Surrey, E.S. (1994). Endometriosis and adenomyosis. In F.P. Zuspan & E.J. Quilligan (Eds.), *Current therapies in obstetrics and gynecology* (4th ed., pp. 41–45). Philadelphia: W.B. Saunders.

Tortolero-Luna, G., Mitchell, M.F., & Rhodes-Morris, H.E. (1994). Epidemiology and screening of ovarian cancer. *Obstetrics and Gynecology Clinics of North America*, 21(1), 1–24.

Urso, P., & Jordan, M.L. (1996). Less common dermatological sexually transmitted diseases. *Nurse Practitioner Forum*, 7(1), 30–33.

Versaci, A.D., & Libbey, J.T. (1994). Breast reconstruction following mastectomy. *Obstetrics and Gynecology Clinics of North America*, 21(4), 733–750.

Weiss, R.M. (1995). Abnormal uterine bleeding. In P.L. Carr, K.M. Freund, & S. Somani (Eds.), *The medical care of women* (pp. 113–120). Philadelphia: W.B. Saunders.

Youngkin, E.Q. (1995). Sexually transmitted diseases: Current and emerging concerns. *Journal of Obstetric, Gynecologic, and Neonatal Nursing*, 24(8), 743–758.

# Glossary

**Abortion** A pregnancy that ends before 20 weeks' gestation, either spontaneously or electively. **Miscarriage** is a lay term for a spontaneous abortion.
**Abruptio placentae** Premature separation of a normally implanted placenta.
**Abstinence syndrome** A group of symptoms that occur when a person who is addicted to a specific drug withdraws or abstains from taking that drug.
**Acidosis** A condition resulting from accumulation of acid (hydrogen ions) or depletion of base (bicarbonate). The pH measures acid-base balance.
**Acme** Peak, or period of greatest strength, of a uterine contraction.
**Acquired immunodeficiency syndrome (AIDS)** Syndrome caused by the human immunodeficiency virus (HIV), resulting in loss of defense against malignancies and opportunistic infections.
**Acrocyanosis** Bluish discoloration of the hands and feet due to reduced peripheral circulation.
**Addiction** Physical or psychological dependence on a substance such as alcohol, tobacco, or drugs, either legal or illicit.
**Adjuvant therapy** Additional treatment that increases or enhances the action of the primary treatment.
**Adnexa** Accessory organs of the uterus, such as the fallopian tubes and ovaries.
**Afterpains** Cramping pain following childbirth caused by alternate relaxation and contraction of uterine muscles.
**Agonist** A substance that causes a physiologic effect.
**Alcoholism** A chronic, progressive, and potentially fatal disease characterized by tolerance for and physical dependence on alcohol or by pathologic organ changes due to alcohol abuse, or both.
**Allele** An alternate form of a gene.
**Alpha-fetoprotein (AFP)** Plasma protein produced by the fetus.
**Ambiguity (ambiguous)** Lack of clarity or certainty; having more than one meaning.
**Ambivalence** Simultaneous conflicting emotions, attitudes, ideas, or wishes.
**Amenorrhea** Absence of menstruation. **Primary amenorrhea** is a delay of the first menstruation. **Secondary amenorrhea** is cessation of menstruation after its initiation.
**Amniocentesis** Transabdominal puncture of the amniotic sac to obtain a sample of amniotic fluid that contains fetal cells and biochemical substances for laboratory examination.
**Amnioinfusion** Infusion of lactated Ringer's solution or isotonic saline into the uterine cavity during labor to reduce umbilical cord compression; also done to dilute meconium in amniotic fluid, reducing the risk that the infant will aspirate thick meconium at birth.
**Amnionitis** See **Chorioamnionitis.**
**Amniotic fluid embolism** An embolism in which amniotic fluid with its particulate matter is drawn into the pregnant woman's circulation, lodging in her lungs.
**Amniotomy** Artificial rupture of the amniotic sac (fetal membranes).
**Amphetamines** Central nervous system stimulants that create a perception of pleasure that is unrelated to external stimuli.
**Analgesic** A systemic agent that relieves pain without loss of consciousness.
**Anencephaly** Absence of the cranial vault and all or most of the cerebral hemispheres; a form of neural tube defect.
**Anesthesia** Loss of sensation, especially to pain, with or without loss of consciousness.
**Anesthesiologist** A physician who specializes in administration of anesthesia.
**Anorexia nervosa** Refusal to eat because of a distorted body image and a concern about obesity.
**Anovulatory** (or **Anovular**) Menstrual cycles occurring without ovulation.
**Antagonist** A drug that blocks the action of another drug or of body secretions.
**Antepartum** Term describing the pregnant woman before the onset of labor.
**Antiphospholipid antibodies** Autoimmune antibodies directed against phospholipids in cell membranes; associated with recurrent spontaneous abortion, fetal loss, and severe pregnancy-induced hypertension.
**Apneic spells** Cessation of breathing for more than 15 seconds, accompanied by cyanosis or bradycardia.
**Asphyxia** Insufficient oxygen and excess carbon dioxide in the blood and tissues.
**Aspiration pneumonitis** A chemical injury to the lungs that may occur with regurgitation and aspiration of acidic gastric secretions.
**Assumptions** Beliefs taken for granted without examination.
**Atony** Absence or lack of usual muscle tone.
**Atrophic vaginitis** Inflammation that occurs when the vagina becomes dry and fragile, usually as a result of estrogen deficit after menopause.
**Attachment** Development of strong affectional ties as a result of interaction between an infant and a significant other (mother, father, sibling, caretaker).
**Attenuate** To weaken.
**Attitude** Relationship of fetal body parts to one another.
**Augmentation of labor** Artificial stimulation of uterine contractions that have become ineffective.
**Autogenous graft** Tissue that is moved from one part of the body to another part of the same person's body.
**Autosome** Any of the 22 pairs of **chromosomes** other than the **sex chromosomes.**
**Axillary tail** Wedge of tissue extending from the breast into the axilla (also called the *tail of Spence*).
**Azoospermia** Absence of sperm in semen.
**Baroreceptors** Cells that are sensitive to blood pressure changes.
**Basal body temperature** Body temperature at rest.
**Baseline data** Information that describes the status of the client before treatment begins.
**Bias** A prejudice that sways the mind.
**Bicornuate (Bicornate)** Malformed uterus having two horns.
**Bilirubin** Unusable component of hemolyzed erythrocytes.

**Bilirubin encephalopathy** Brain damage resulting from deposits of unconjugated bilirubin in the brain tissue.
**Bioethics** Rules or principles that govern right conduct, specifically those that relate to health care.
**Biophysical profile (BPP)** Method for evaluating fetal status during the antepartum period based on five variables originating with the fetus: fetal heart rate, breathing movements, gross movements, muscle tone, and amniotic fluid volume.
**Birth defect** An abnormality of structure, function, or body metabolism that often results in a physical or mental handicap, shortens life, or is fatal (according to the March of Dimes Birth Defects Foundation).
**Birth plan** A plan describing a couple's preferences for their birth experience.
**Bloody show** Mixture of cervical mucus and blood from ruptured capillaries in the cervix; often precedes labor and increases with cervical dilation.
**Body image** Subjective image of one's physical appearance and capabilities, derived from own observations and from the evaluation of significant others.
**Bonding** Development of a strong emotional tie of a parent to a newborn; also called *claiming* or *binding-in*.
**Braxton Hicks contractions** Irregular, mild uterine contractions that occur throughout pregnancy; they become stronger in the last trimester.
**Bronchopulmonary dysplasia (BPD)** Chronic pulmonary condition in which damage to the infant's lungs requires prolonged dependence on supplemental oxygen.
**Brown fat** (or **brown adipose tissue**) Highly vascular specialized fat found in the newborn that provides more heat than other fat when metabolized.
**Bulimia** Eating disorder characterized by ingestion of large amounts of food, followed by purging behavior such as induced vomiting or laxative abuse.
**Café au lait spots** Light brown birthmarks.
**Calorie** See **Kilocalorie.**
**Caput succedaneum** Area of edema over the presenting part of the fetus or newborn resulting from pressure against the cervix. Often called simply *caput.*
**Carcinoma in situ** Malignant neoplasm in surface tissue that has not extended into deeper tissue.
**Cardiac decompensation** Failure of the heart to maintain adequate circulation to the tissues. See also **Congestive heart failure.**
**Catabolism** A destructive process that converts living cells into simpler compounds; process involved in **involution** (changes) of the uterus after childbirth.
**Caudal regressive syndrome** A severe malformation that results when the sacrum, lumbar spine, and lower extremities fail to develop.
**Cephalhematoma** Bleeding between the periosteum and skull from pressure during birth. It does not cross suture lines.
**Cephalopelvic disproportion (CPD)** Fetal head size that is too large to fit through the maternal pelvis at birth. Also called *fetopelvic disproportion*.
**Cerclage** Encircling of the cervix with suture to prevent recurrent spontaneous abortion caused by early cervical dilation.
**Cerebrospinal fluid (CSF)** Clear fluid that bathes and cushions the brain and spinal cord.
**Certified nurse-midwife (CNM)** A registered nurse who has completed a nurse-midwifery program approved by the American College of Nurse-Midwives (ACNM) and passed the ACNM National Certification Examination.
**Cervical cap** A small cup-like device placed over the cervix to prevent sperm from entering, thus preventing pregnancy.
**Cesarean birth** Surgical birth of the fetus through an incision in the abdominal wall and uterus.
**Chadwick's sign** Bluish discoloration of the cervix, vagina, and labia during pregnancy as a result of increased vascular congestion.
**Chemoreceptors** Cells that are sensitive to chemical changes in the blood, specifically changes in oxygen and carbon dioxide levels, and in acid-base balance.
**Chignon** Newborn scalp edema created by a vacuum extractor.
**Chloasma** Brownish pigmentation of the face during pregnancy; also called "mask of pregnancy."
**Choanal atresia** Abnormality of the nasal septum that obstructs one or both nasal passages.
**Chorioamnionitis** Inflammation of the amniotic sac (fetal membranes); usually caused by bacterial or viral infection. Also called **amnionitis.**
**Chorionic villus sampling** Transcervical or transabdominal sampling of chorionic villi (projections of the outer fetal membrane) for analysis of fetal cells.
**Chromosomal sex** See **Genetic sex.**
**Chromosome** Thread of DNA (deoxyribonucleic acid) in the cell nucleus that transmits genetic (hereditary) information.
**Cilia** Hair-like processes on the surface of a cell. Cilia beat rhythmically to move a cell or to move fluid or other substances over the cell surface.
**Cleansing breath** A deep breath taken at the beginning and end of each labor contraction.
**Climacteric** Endocrine, body, and psychic changes occurring at the end of a woman's reproductive period. Also informally called **menopause.**
**Coitus** Sexual union between a male and a female.
**Coitus interruptus** Withdrawal of the penis from the vagina before ejaculation.
**Colostrum** Breast fluid secreted during pregnancy and the first 2 to 3 days following childbirth.
**Colposcopy** Examination of the vaginal and cervical tissue with a colposcope for magnification of cells.
**Complete protein food.** Food containing all the essential amino acids.
**Compliance** Stretchability or elasticity of the lungs and thorax that allows distention without resistance during respirations. Also, adherence of the client to a therapeutic plan.
**Conceptus** Cells and membranes resulting from fertilization of the ovum at any stage of prenatal development.
**Condom** Latex, polyurethane, or natural membrane shield covering the penis or lining the vagina to prevent sperm from entering the cervix or to prevent infection, or both.
**Condyloma** A wart-like growth of the skin seen on the external genitalia, in the vagina, on the cervix, or near the anus; may be caused by human papillomavirus (condyloma acuminatum) or by syphilis (condyloma latum).
**Congenital** Present at birth.
**Congenital anomaly** Abnormal intrauterine development of an organ or structure.
**Congestive heart failure** Condition resulting from failure of the heart to maintain adequate circulation; characterized by weakness, dyspnea, and edema in body parts that are lower than the heart.
**Containment** A method of increasing comfort in infants by using swaddling or other methods to keep the extremities in a flexed position near the body.
**Contraception** Prevention of pregnancy.

**Contraction stress test (CST)** Method for evaluating fetal status during the antepartum period by observing response of the fetal heart to the stress of uterine contractions that may induce recurrent episodes of fetal hypoxia.

**Cordocentesis** See **Percutaneous umbilical blood sampling.**

**Corpus luteum** Graafian follicle cells remaining after ovulation that produce estrogen and progesterone.

**Corrected gestational age** Gestational age that a preterm infant would be if still in utero. May also be called *developmental age*.

**Couvade** Pregnancy-related rituals or a cluster of symptoms experienced by some prospective fathers during pregnancy and childbirth.

**Crack** A highly addictive form of cocaine that has been processed to be smoked.

**Cradle cap** See **Seborrheic dermatitis.**

**Craniosynostosis** Premature closure of the sutures of the infant's head.

**Crowning** Appearance of the fetal scalp or presenting part at the vaginal opening.

**Cryotherapy** Destruction of tissue using extreme cold.

**Cryptorchidism** Failure of one or both testes to descend into the scrotum.

**Cul-de-sac** See **Fornix.**

**Culdocentesis** Needle puncture through the upper posterior vaginal wall (cul-de-sac of Douglas) to aspirate blood or fluid from the pelvic cavity.

**Culture** Sum of values, beliefs, and practices of a group of people that are transmitted from one generation to the next.

**Cystocele** Prolapse of the urinary bladder through the anterior vaginal wall.

**Decidua** Name applied to the endometrium during pregnancy; all except the deepest layer is shed after childbirth.

**Decrement** Period of decreasing strength of a uterine contraction.

**Delegated nursing interventions** Physician-prescribed nursing actions that require nursing judgment because nurses are accountable for correct implementation. See also **Independent nursing interventions.**

**Deontologic theory** Ethical theory holding that the right course of action is the one dictated by ethical principles and moral rules.

**Developmental task** A necessary step in growth and maturation that one must complete before additional growth and maturation are possible.

**Diabetes mellitus** A disorder of carbohydrate metabolism caused by a relative or complete lack of insulin secretion. Characterized by *glycosuria* (glucose in the urine) and **hyperglycemia.**

**Diabetogenic** Condition, such as pregnancy, that produces the effects of diabetes mellitus.

**Diagnostic statement** A phrase that describes a health problem; usually consists of a category label plus the etiology or contributing factors. It may also describe manifestations.

**Diaphragm** A contraceptive device consisting of a latex dome that covers the cervix and prevents entrance of sperm; must be used with spermicide to be effective.

**Diastasis recti** Separation of the longitudinal muscles of the abdomen (rectus abdominis) during pregnancy.

**Dilation and curettage (D&C)** Stretching of the cervical os to permit suctioning or scraping of the walls of the uterus. The procedure is performed in abortion, to obtain samples of uterine lining tissue for laboratory examination, and during the postpartum period to remove retained fragments of placenta.

**Dilation and evacuation (D&E)** Wide cervical dilation followed by mechanical destruction and removal of fetal parts from the uterus. Following complete removal of the fetus, a vacuum curet is used to remove the placenta and remaining products of conception.

**Diploid** Having a pair of chromosomes (46 in humans) that represents one copy of every chromosome from each parent; the number of chromosomes normally present in body cells other than **gametes.**

**Disturbance in body image** Negative feelings about characteristics, functions, or limits of one's body.

**Duration** Period from the beginning of a uterine contraction to the end of the same contraction.

**Dysmenorrhea** Painful menstruation.

**Dyspareunia** Difficult or painful coitus in women.

**Dysplasia** Abnormal development of tissue.

**Dystocia** Difficult or prolonged labor; often associated with abnormal uterine activity and **cephalopelvic disproportion.**

**Dysuria** Painful urination, often associated with urinary tract infection.

**Early deceleration** Slowing of the fetal heart rate that occurs during the uterine contraction.

**Eclampsia** Convulsive form of pregnancy-induced hypertension.

**Ectopic pregnancy** Implantation of a fertilized ovum in any area other than the uterus; the most common site is in the fallopian tube.

**EDD** Abbreviation for estimated date of delivery; this date may also be abbreviated **EDB** (estimated date of birth).

**Effleurage** Massage of the abdomen or other body part performed during labor contractions.

**Egocentrism** Interest centered on the self rather than on the needs of others.

**Ejaculation** Expulsion of **semen** from the penis.

**Embolus** A clot, usually part or all of a **thrombus,** brought by the blood from another vessel and forced into a smaller one, thus obstructing circulation.

**Embryo** The developing baby from the beginning of the third week through the eighth week after conception.

**Endometrial hyperplasia** Excessive proliferation of normal cells of the uterine lining; may be due to administration of estrogen during the postmenopausal period.

**Endometriosis** Presence of tissue resembling endometrium outside the uterine cavity.

**Endometrium** Lining of the uterus.

**Endorphins** Morphine-like substances that occur naturally in the central nervous system and modify pain sensations.

**En face** Position that allows eye-to-eye contact between the newborn and a parent; optimal distance is 20 to 22 cm (8 to 9 inches).

**Engagement** Descent of the widest diameter of the fetal presenting part to at least a zero **station** (the level of the ischial spines in the maternal pelvis).

**Engorgement** Swelling of the breasts resulting from feedings that are delayed, too short, or not frequent enough.

**Engrossment** Intense fascination and close face-to-face observation between father and newborn.

**Enteral feeding** Nutrients supplied to the gastrointestinal tract orally or by feeding tube.

**Entrainment** Newborn movement in rhythm to adult speech, particularly high-pitched tones, which are more easily heard.

**Epidural space** The area outside the dura, between the dura mater and the vertebral canal.
**Episiotomy** Surgical incision of the perineum to enlarge the vaginal opening.
**Epispadias** Abnormal placement of the urinary meatus on the dorsal side of the penis.
**Erythema toxicum** Benign rash of unknown cause in newborns with blotchy red areas that may have white or yellow papules in the center.
**Erythroblastosis fetalis** Agglutination and hemolysis of fetal erythrocytes due to incompatibility between maternal and fetal blood. In most cases, the fetus is Rh-positive and the mother is Rh-negative.
**Esophageal atresia** Condition in which the esophagus is separated from the stomach and ends in a blind pouch.
**Essential amino acids** Amino acids that cannot be synthesized by the body and must be obtained from foods.
**Ethical dilemma** A situation in which no solution seems completely satisfactory.
**Ethics** Rules or principles that govern right conduct and distinctions between right and wrong.
**Ethnic** Pertaining to religious, racial, national, or cultural group characteristics, especially speech patterns, social customs, and physical characteristics.
**Ethnicity** Condition of belonging to a particular **ethnic** group; also refers to ethnic pride.
**Ethnocentrism** Opinion that the beliefs and customs of one's own ethnic group are superior.
**Euglycemia** Normal blood glucose level.
**Extrusion reflex** Automatic nervous system response that causes an infant to push anything solid out of the mouth.
**Familial** Presence of a trait or condition in a family more often than would be expected by chance alone.
**Fantasy** Mental images formed to prepare for the birth of a child.
**Ferning** (or **fern test**) Microscopic appearance of amniotic fluid that resembles fern leaves when the fluid is allowed to dry on a microscope slide. Used to determine whether the woman's membranes have ruptured. Also describes the microscopic fern-like appearance of dried cervical mucus that is most apparent at the time of ovulation.
**Fertilization age** Prenatal age of the developing baby calculated from the date of conception. Also called **postconceptional age.**
**Fetal alcohol syndrome** A group of physical and mental disorders of the offspring associated with maternal use of alcohol during pregnancy.
**Fetal lung fluid** Fluid that fills the fetal lungs, expanding the alveoli and promoting lung development.
**Fetus** The developing baby from 9 weeks after conception until birth. In everyday practice, this term is often used to describe a developing baby during pregnancy, regardless of age.
**FHR** Abbreviation for fetal heart rate.
**Finger-tipping** First tactile (touch) experience between mother and newborn; the mother explores the infant's body with her fingertips only.
**First period of reactivity** Period beginning at birth in which newborns are active and alert. It ends when the infant first falls asleep.
**Fontanelle** Space at the intersection of sutures connecting fetal or infant skull bones.
**Foremilk** First breast milk received in a feeding.
**Fornix** (pl. **fornices**) An arch or pouch-like structure at the upper end of the vagina. Also called a **cul-de-sac.**
**Fourth trimester** First 12 weeks following birth; a time of transition for parents and siblings.
**Frequency** Period from the beginning of one uterine contraction until the beginning of the next.
**Fundus** Part of the uterus that is farthest from the cervix, above the openings of the fallopian tubes.
**Gamete** Reproductive cell; in the female an **ovum,** and in the male a **spermatozoon.**
**Gametogenesis** Development and maturation of the **sperm** and **ova.**
**Gastroschisis** Protrusion of the intestines through a defect in the abdominal wall. Intestines are not covered by a peritoneal sac or skin.
**General anesthesia** Systemic loss of sensation with loss of consciousness.
**Genetic** Pertaining to the genes or the chromosomes.
**Genetic sex** Sex determined at conception by union of two X chromosomes (female) or an X and a Y chromosome (male). Also called **chromosomal sex.**
**Genogram** See **Pedigree.**
**Genotype** Genetic makeup of an individual.
**Gestational age** Prenatal age of the developing baby (measured in weeks) calculated from the first day of the woman's last menstrual period. Also called **menstrual age.** About 2 weeks longer than the **fertilization age.**
**Gestational diabetes** Impaired glucose tolerance that is induced by pregnancy and diagnosed during pregnancy. Usually disappears after childbirth.
**Gestational surrogate** A woman who carries the embryo of an infertile couple and relinquishes the child after birth.
**Gestational trophoblastic disease** A spectrum of diseases that includes benign hydatidiform mole and gestational trophoblastic tumors, such as invasive moles and choriocarcinoma.
**Gluconeogenesis** Formation of glycogen by the liver from noncarbohydrate sources, such as amino or fatty acids.
**Gonad** Reproductive (sex) gland that produces gametes and sex hormones. The female gonads are *ovaries*; the male gonads are *testes.*
**Gonadotropic hormones** Secretions of the anterior pituitary gland that stimulate the gonads, specifically follicle-stimulating hormone and luteinizing hormone. Chorionic gonadotropin is secreted by the placenta during pregnancy.
**Goodell's sign** Softening of the cervix, uterus, and vagina during pregnancy.
**Graafian follicle** A small sac within the ovary that contains the maturing ovum.
**Gravida** A pregnant woman. Also refers to a woman's total number of pregnancies, including the one in progress, if applicable.
**Gynecologic age** The number of years since menarche (first menstrual period).
**Habituation** Decreased response to a repeated stimulus.
**Haploid** Having one copy of a chromosome from each pair (23 in humans, or half the diploid number). **Gametes** normally have a haploid number of chromosomes.
**Hematoma** Localized collection of blood in a space or tissue.
**Heme iron** Iron obtained from meat, poultry, or fish sources; the form most usable by the body.
**Heterozygous** Having two different **alleles** for a genetic trait.
**Hindmilk** Breast milk received nearer the end of a feeding; contains higher fat content than **foremilk.**
**Homozygous** Having two identical **alleles** for a genetic trait.

**Hormone implant** Small capsules of progestin inserted subcutaneously to provide contraception.
**Human immunodeficiency virus (HIV)** A retrovirus that results in the development of AIDS (see **Acquired immunodeficiency syndrome**).
**Hydatidiform mole** Abnormal pregnancy resulting from proliferation of chorionic villi that give rise to multiple cysts and rapid growth of the uterus.
**Hydramnios** Excess volume of amniotic fluid (more than 2000 ml at term). Also called **polyhydramnios.**
**Hydrops fetalis** Heart failure and generalized edema in the fetus secondary to severe anemia resulting from destruction of erythrocytes.
**Hyperbilirubinemia** Excessive amount of bilirubin in the blood.
**Hypercapnia** Excess carbon dioxide in the blood, evidenced by an elevated $Pco_2$.
**Hyperemia** Excess of blood in a part of the body.
**Hyperglycemia** An abnormally high blood glucose level.
**Hypertonic contractions** Uterine contractions that are too long or too frequent, have too short a resting interval, or have an inadequate relaxation period to allow optimal uteroplacental exchange.
**Hypertonic labor dysfunction** Ineffective labor characterized by erratic and poorly coordinated contractions. **Uterine resting tone** is higher than normal.
**Hypoglycemia** An abnormally low blood glucose level.
**Hypospadias** Abnormal placement of the urinary meatus on the ventral side of the penis.
**Hypotonic labor dysfunction** Ineffective labor characterized by weak, infrequent, and brief but coordinated uterine contractions. **Uterine resting tone** is normal.
**Hypovolemia** Abnormally decreased volume of circulating fluid in the body.
**Hypovolemic shock** Acute peripheral circulatory failure due to loss of circulating blood volume.
**Hypoxemia** Reduced oxygenation of the blood, evidenced by a low $Po_2$.
**Hypoxia** Reduced availability of oxygen to the body tissues.
**Iatrogenic** An adverse condition resulting from treatment.
**Impotence** Inability of a man to achieve or maintain an erection of the penis that is sufficiently rigid to permit successful sexual intercourse.
**Incompetent cervix** Inability of the cervix to remain closed long enough during pregnancy for the fetus to survive.
**Incomplete protein food** Food that does not contain all the essential amino acids.
**Increment** Period of increasing strength of a uterine contraction.
**Independent nursing interventions** Nurse-prescribed actions used in both nursing diagnoses and collaborative problems. See also **Delegated nursing interventions.**
**Induction of labor** Artificial initiation of labor.
**Infant mortality rate** Number of deaths per 1000 live births that occurs within the first 12 months of life.
**Inference** The act of drawing a conclusion or making a deduction.
**Infertility** Inability of a couple to conceive after 1 year of regular intercourse (two to three times weekly) without using contraception; also, the involuntary inability to conceive and produce viable offspring when the couple chooses. **Primary infertility** occurs in a couple who has never conceived; **secondary infertility** occurs in a couple who has conceived at least once before.
**Intensity** Strength of a uterine contraction.
**Intermittent monitoring** A variation of electronic fetal monitoring in which an initial strip is obtained on admission. If patterns are reassuring, the woman is remonitored for 15 minutes at regular intervals (about every 30 to 60 minutes).
**Interval** Period between the end of one uterine contraction and the beginning of the next.
**Intrapartum** Term describing the time of labor and childbirth.
**Intrauterine device (IUD)** A mechanical device inserted into the uterus to prevent pregnancy.
**Intrauterine growth restriction (IUGR)** Failure of a fetus to grow as expected for gestational age. May also be called *intrauterine growth retardation*.
**Intraventricular hemorrhage (IVH)** Bleeding into the ventricles of the brain.
**Introversion** Inward concentration on oneself and one's body.
**Involution** Retrogressive changes that return the reproductive organs, particularly the uterus, to their pre-pregnancy size and condition.
**Jaundice** Yellow discoloration of the skin and sclera caused by excessive bilirubin in the blood.
**Judgment** An opinion.
**Karyotype** A photomicrograph of a cell's chromosomes, arranged from largest to smallest pairs.
**Kegel exercises** Alternate contracting and relaxing of the pelvic muscles; these movements strengthen the pubococcygeal muscle, which surrounds the urinary meatus and vagina.
**Kernicterus** Staining of brain tissue caused by accumulation of unconjugated bilirubin in the brain.
**Ketosis** Accumulation of ketone bodies (metabolic products) in the blood; frequently associated with acidosis.
**Kilocalorie** A unit of heat; used to show the energy value in foods; commonly called **calorie.**
**Lactation** Secretion of milk from the breasts; also describes the time when a child is breastfed.
**Lacto-ovovegetarian** A **vegetarian** whose diet includes milk products and eggs.
**Lactose intolerance** Inability to digest most dairy products because of a lack of the enzyme lactase.
**Lactovegetarian** A **vegetarian** whose diet includes milk products.
**Laminaria** Slender cones of prepared seaweed or a similar substance inserted into the cervix to dilate it as they absorb water.
**Lanugo** Fine, soft hair covering the fetus.
**Laparoscopy** Insertion of an illuminated tube into the abdominal cavity to visualize contents, locate bleeding, and perform surgical procedures.
**Laparotomy** Incision through the abdominal wall to examine the abdominal or pelvic organs.
**Large-for-gestational age (LGA) infant** An infant whose size is above the 90th percentile for gestational age.
**Latch-on** Attachment of the infant to the breast.
**Late deceleration** Slowing of the fetal heart rate after the onset of a uterine contraction and persisting after the contraction ends.
**Lecithin/sphingomyelin ratio (L/S ratio)** Ratio of two phospholipids in amniotic fluid that is used to determine fetal lung maturity; an L/S ratio greater than 2:1 usually indicates fetal lung maturity.
**Let-down reflex** See **Milk-ejection reflex.**
**Letting-go** A phase of maternal adaptation that involves relinquishment of previous roles and assumption of a new role as a parent.
**Libido** Sexual desire.

**Lie** Relationship of the long axis of the fetus to the long axis of the mother.
**Lightening** Descent of the fetus toward the pelvic inlet before labor.
**Linear salpingostomy** Incision along the length of a fallopian tube to remove an ectopic pregnancy and preserve the tube.
**Lipogenic** Substance, such as insulin, that stimulates the production of fat.
**Lochia** Vaginal drainage after birth.
**Lochia alba** Whitish or clear vaginal discharge that follows **lochia serosa;** occurs when the amount of blood is decreased and the number of leukocytes is increased.
**Lochia rubra** Reddish vaginal discharge that occurs immediately after childbirth; composed mostly of blood.
**Lochia serosa** Pinkish or brown-tinged vaginal discharge that follows **lochia rubra** and precedes **lochia alba;** composed largely of serous exudate, blood, and leukocytes.
**Low-birth-weight (LBW) infant** An infant weighing less than 2500 g at birth.
**Maceration** Discoloration and softening of tissues and eventual disintegration of a fetus that is retained in the uterus after its death.
**Macrosomia** Unusually large fetal size; infant birth weight more than 4000 g.
**Malpractice** Negligence by a professional person.
**Mammogram** Study of breast tissue using very-low-dose x-ray; primary tool in the discovery of breast tumors.
**Marfan's syndrome** A hereditary condition that involves weakness in connective tissue, bones, and muscles; the vascular system is affected, particularly the aorta.
**Mastitis** Inflammation of the breast, usually caused by stasis of milk in the ducts or by infection.
**Maternal mortality rate** Number of maternal deaths from births and complications of pregnancy, childbirth, and puerperium (the first 42 days after termination of the pregnancy) per 100,000 live births.
**Mature milk** Breast milk that appears after the first 2 weeks of lactation.
**Meconium aspiration syndrome** Obstruction and air trapping due to meconium in the infant's lungs, which may cause severe respiratory distress.
**Meiosis** Reduction cell division in **gametes** that halves the number of chromosomes in each cell.
**Menarche** Onset of menstruation; average age is 13 years.
**Meningocele** Protrusion of the meninges through a defect in the verterbrae; a form of **neural tube defect.**
**Menometrorrhagia** Uterine bleeding that is irregular in frequency and also excessive in amount.
**Menopause** Permanent cessation of menstruation during the **climacteric.**
**Menorrhagia** Excessive bleeding at the time of menstruation in number of days' duration, amount of blood lost, or both.
**Menstrual age** See **Gestational age.**
**Methadone** A synthetic compound with opiate properties. Used as an oral substitute for heroin and morphine in the opiate-addicted person.
**Metrorrhagia** Bleeding from the uterus at any time other than during the menstrual period.
**Milia** White cysts, 1 to 2 mm in size, from distended sebaceous glands.
**Miliaria (prickly heat)** Rash caused by heat.
**Milk-ejection reflex** Release of milk from the alveoli into the ducts; also known as the **let-down reflex.**
**Mimicry** Copying the behaviors of other pregnant women or mothers as a method of "trying on" the role of advanced pregnancy or motherhood.
**Miscarriage** See **Abortion.**
**Mitosis** Cell division in body cells other than the **gametes.**
**Mittelschmerz** Low abdominal pain that occurs at **ovulation.**
**Molding** Shaping of the fetal head during movement through the birth canal.
**Mongolian spots** Bruise-like marks that occur mostly in newborns with dark skin tones.
**Monosomy** Presence of only one of a chromosome pair in every body cell.
**Motor block** Loss of voluntary movement caused by **regional anesthesia.**
**Multifetal pregnancy** A pregnancy in which the woman is carrying two or more fetuses. Also called **multiple gestation.**
**Multipara** A woman who has given birth after two or more pregnancies of at least 20 weeks of gestation. Also informally used to describe a pregnant woman before the birth of her second child.
**Multiple gestation** See **Multifetal pregnancy.**
**Mutation** Variation in a gene that affects its function.
**Myelomeningocele** Protrusion of the meninges and spinal cord through a defect in the vertebrae; a form of **neural tube defect.**
**Myometrium** Uterine muscle.
**Narcissism** Undue preoccupation with oneself.
**Natural family planning** Method of predicting **ovulation** based on normal changes in a woman's body.
**Necrotizing enterocolitis (NEC)** A condition of injury, invasion by bacteria, and possible necrosis of the intestines.
**Negligence** Failure to act in the way a reasonable, prudent person of similar background would act in similar circumstances.
**Neonatal abstinence syndrome** A cluster of physical signs exhibited by the newborn who was exposed in utero to maternal use of substances such as cocaine or heroin. See also **Abstinence syndrome.**
**Neonatal mortality rate** Number of deaths per 1000 live births occurring at birth or within the first 28 days of life.
**Neonatologist** A physician who specializes in the care of newborn infants (from birth until the 29th day of life).
**Neural tube defect** A congenital defect in closure of the bony encasement of the spinal cord or of the skull. Neural tube defects include **anencephaly, spina bifida, meningocele, myelomeningocele,** and others.
**Neutral thermal environment** Environment in which body temperature is maintained without an increase in metabolic rate or oxygen use.
**Nevus flammeus** Permanent purple birthmark. Also called *port wine stain.*
**Nevus vasculosus** Rough red collection of capillaries with a raised surface that disappears with time.
**Nidation.** Implantation of the fertilized ovum **(zygote)** in the uterine endometrium.
**Nitrazine paper** Paper used to determine pH; helps to determine whether the amniotic sac has ruptured.
**Noncompliance** Resistance of the lungs and thorax to distention with air during respirations. Also, failure of the client to adhere to a therapeutic plan.
**Non-heme iron** Iron obtained from plant sources.
**Non-nutritive sucking** Sucking during which no milk flow is obtained.
**Nonshivering thermogenesis** Process of heat production, without shivering, by oxidation of **brown fat.**

**Nonstress test** A method for evaluating fetal status during the antepartum period by observing the response of the fetal heart rate to fetal movement.
**Nuchal cord** Umbilical cord around the fetal neck.
**Nullipara** A woman who has not completed a pregnancy to at least 20 weeks' gestation.
**Nurse-anesthetist** A registered nurse who has advanced education and certification in administration of anesthetics. Also *certified registered nurse anesthetist* (CRNA).
**Nurse-midwife** See **Certified nurse-midwife.**
**Nurse practice acts** Laws that determine the scope of nursing practice in each state.
**Nutrient density** The quality of protein, vitamins, and minerals per 100 calories in foods.
**Nutritive suckling or sucking** Steady rhythmic suckling at the breast or sucking at a bottle to obtain milk.
**Occult prolapse** See **Prolapsed cord.**
**Oligohydramnios** Abnormally small quantity of amniotic fluid (less than 500 ml at term).
**Oligospermia** A decreased number of sperm in semen, usually considered to be under 20 million per milliliter.
**Omphalocele** Protrusion of the intestines into the base of the umbilical cord. Intestines are covered by a peritoneal sac. May be associated with other anomalies.
**Oogenesis** Formation of **gametes (ova)** in the female.
**Opiate** Any narcotic containing opium or a derivative of opium.
**Oral contraceptive** Drug that inhibits ovulation; contains progestins alone or in combination with estrogen.
**Osmotic diuresis** Secretion and passage of large amounts of urine as a result of increased osmotic pressure that can result from **hyperglycemia.**
**Osteoporosis** Increased spaces (porosity) in bone; process greatly accelerates following menopause.
**Ovovegetarian** A vegetarian whose diet includes eggs.
**Ovulation** Release of the mature **ovum** from the ovary.
**Ovum** (pl. **ova**) Female **gamete,** or sex cell.
**Oxytocin** Hormone produced by the posterior pituitary gland that stimulates uterine contractions and the **milk-ejection reflex;** also prepared synthetically.
**Paced breathing** Learned breathing technique used during labor contractions to promote relaxation and increase pain tolerance.
**Pain threshold** (or **pain perception**) The lowest level of stimulus one perceives as painful. Pain threshold is relatively constant under different conditions.
**Pain tolerance** Maximum pain one is willing to endure. Pain tolerance may increase or decrease under different conditions.
**Para** A woman who has given birth after a pregnancy of at least 20 weeks' gestation. Also designates the number of a woman's pregnancies that have ended after at least 20 weeks of gestation. (A multifetal gestation, such as twins, is considered one birth when calculating parity.)
**Parenteral nutrition** Intravenous infusion of all nutrients needed for metabolism and growth.
**Peau d'orange** Dimpled skin condition that resembles an orange; associated with lymphatic edema and often seen over the area of breast cancer.
**Pedigree** A graphic representation of a family's medical and hereditary history and the relationships among the family members. May be called a **genogram.**
**Percutaneous umbilical blood sampling (PUBS** or **cordocentesis)** Procedure for obtaining fetal blood through ultrasound-guided puncture of an umbilical cord vessel to detect fetal problems such as inherited blood disorders, acidosis, or infection.
**Perinatologist** A physician who specializes in the care of the mother, the fetus, and the infant during the perinatal period (from the 20th week of pregnancy to 4 weeks after childbirth).
**Periodic breathing** Cessation of breathing lasting no more than 10 seconds without changes in color or heart rate.
**Periventricular-intraventricular hemorrhage (PIVH)** Bleeding into and around the ventricles of the brain.
**Persistent fetal circulation** Failure of the pulmonary vessels to dilate and the ductus arteriosus to close; caused by low blood oxygen levels.
**Persistent pulmonary hypertension** Vasoconstriction of the infant's pulmonary vessels after birth; may result in right-to-left shunting of blood flow through the ductus arteriosus, the foramen ovale, or both.
**Phenotype** The outward expression of one's genetic makeup.
**Phosphatidylglycerol (PG)** A major phospholipid of **surfactant;** its presence in amniotic fluid indicates fetal lung maturity.
**Phosphatidylinositol (PI)** A phospholipid of **surfactant;** produced and secreted in increasing amounts as the fetal lungs mature. Its presence in amniotic fluid indicates fetal lung maturity.
**Physiologic anemia of pregnancy** Decrease in hematocrit values caused by dilution of erythrocytes by expanded plasma volume rather than by an actual decrease in erythrocytes or hemoglobin.
**Pica** Ingestion of a nonfood substance, such as laundry starch, dirt, or ice.
**Placenta** Fetal structure that provides nourishment and removes waste from the developing baby and secretes hormones necessary for the pregnancy to continue.
**Placenta accreta** A placenta that is abnormally adherent to the uterine muscle. If the condition is more advanced, it is called **placenta increta** (the placenta extends into the uterine muscle) or **placenta percreta** (the placenta extends through the uterine muscle).
**Placenta previa** Abnormal implantation of the placenta in the lower uterus.
**Point of maximum impulse (PMI)** Area of the chest in which the heart sounds are loudest when auscultated.
**Polycythemia** Abnormally high number of erythrocytes.
**Polydactyly** More than 10 digits on the hands or feet.
**Polydipsia** Excessive thirst.
**Polyhydramnios** See **Hydramnios.**
**Polymorphism** Common variation in a gene that does not affect its function or the individual's health negatively.
**Polyphagia** Excessive ingestion of food.
**Polyploidy** Having additional full sets of chromosomes.
**Polyuria** Excessive excretion of urine.
**Position** Relation of a fixed reference point on the fetus to the quadrants of the maternal pelvis.
**Postconceptional age** See **Fertilization age.**
**Postmaturity syndrome** Condition in which a **postterm infant** shows characteristics indicative of poor placental functioning before birth.
**Postneonatal mortality rate** Number of deaths between 28 days and 1 year of life per 1000 live births.
**Postpartum** Term describing the first 6 weeks following childbirth.
**Postpartum blues** Temporary, self-limiting period of weepiness experienced by many new mothers within the first few days following childbirth.
**Postterm birth** A birth that occurs later than 42 weeks of gestation.
**Postterm infant** An infant born after 42 weeks of gestation.

**Precipitate birth** A birth that occurs without a trained attendant present.

**Precipitate labor** An intense, unusually short labor (less than 3 hours).

**Pre-eclampsia** A hypertensive disorder induced by pregnancy that usually includes a triad of signs and symptoms: hypertension, edema, and proteinuria.

**Premature infant** See **Preterm infant.**

**Premature rupture of the membranes** Spontaneous rupture of the membranes before the onset of labor. The gestation may be term, preterm, or postterm.

**Presentation** Fetal part that enters the pelvic inlet. Also, the **presenting part.**

**Presenting part** See **Presentation.**

**Preterm birth** A birth that occurs after the 20th week and before the 38th week of gestation.

**Preterm infant** An infant born before the beginning of the 38th week of gestation. Also called **premature infant.**

**Preterm labor** Onset of labor after 20 weeks and before the beginning of the 38th week of gestation.

**Primary infertility** See **Infertility.**

**Primigravida** A woman who is pregnant for the first time.

**Primipara** A woman who has given birth after a pregnancy of at least 20 weeks of gestation. Also used informally to describe a pregnant woman before the birth of her first child.

**Progestin** Any natural or synthetic form of progesterone.

**Prolactin** Anterior pituitary hormone that promotes growth of breast tissue and stimulates production of milk.

**Prolapsed cord** Displacement of the umbilical cord in front of or beside the fetal presenting part. An **occult prolapse** is one that is suspected on the basis of fetal heart rate patterns; the umbilical cord cannot be palpated or seen.

**Prune-belly syndrome** An absence of abdominal muscles that results in a flabby, distended, and creased abdomen that may occur in the infant exposed to cocaine in utero.

**Pseudomenstruation** Vaginal bleeding in the newborn, resulting from withdrawal of placental hormones.

**Psychoprophylaxis** Method of prepared childbirth that emphasizes mental concentration and relaxation to increase **pain tolerance.**

**Psychosis** Mental state in which a person's ability to recognize reality, communicate, and relate to others is impaired.

**Puberty** Period of sexual maturation accompanied by the development of secondary sex characteristics and the capacity to reproduce.

**Puerperium** Period from the end of childbirth until **involution** of the uterus is complete; approximately 6 weeks.

**Pulse oximetry** Method of determining the level of blood oxygen saturation using sensors attached to the skin.

**Reciprocal bonding behaviors** Repertoire of infant behaviors that promote attachment between parent and newborn.

**Recommended dietary allowances (RDA)** Levels of nutrient intake considered to meet the needs of healthy individuals.

**Rectocele** Herniation (protrusion) of the rectum through the posterior vaginal wall.

**REEDA** Acronym for redness, ecchymosis, edema, discharge, and approximation; useful for assessing wound healing or the presence of inflammation or infection.

**Reflection** Meditation, attentive consideration.

**Reflux** A condition in which stomach contents enter the esophagus and may be aspirated into the lungs.

**Regional anesthesia** Anesthesia that blocks pain impulses in a localized area without loss of consciousness.

**Respiratory distress syndrome (RDS)** Condition caused by insufficient production of **surfactant** in the lungs; results in atelectasis (collapse of the lung alveoli), **hypoxemia,** and **hypercapnia.**

**Resting tone** See **Uterine resting tone.**

**Retinopathy of prematurity (ROP)** Condition in which interference with blood supply to the retina may cause decreased vision or blindness.

**Retrograde ejaculation** Discharge of **semen** into the bladder rather than from the end of the penis.

**Role transition** Changing from one pattern of behavior and one image of self to another.

**Ruga** (pl. **rugae)** Ridge or fold of tissue, as on the male's scrotum and in the female's vagina.

**Salpingectomy** Surgical removal of a fallopian tube.

**Seborrheic dermatitis (cradle cap)** Yellowish, crusty area of the scalp.

**Second period of reactivity** Period of 4 to 6 hours after the first sleep following birth when the newborn may have an elevated pulse and respiratory rate and excessive mucus.

**Secondary infertility** See **Infertility.**

**Secondary sex characteristics** Physical differences between mature males and females that are not directly related to reproduction.

**Semen** **Spermatozoa** with their nourishing and protective fluid; discharged at **ejaculation.**

**Sensory block** Loss of sensation caused by **regional anesthesia.**

**Seroconversion** Change in a blood test result from negative to positive, indicating the development of antibodies in response to infection or immunization.

**Sex chromosome** The X or Y **chromosome.** Females have two X chromosomes; males have one X and one Y chromosome.

**Sexually transmissible** (or **transmitted) disease (STD)** A disease that is passed to others primarily through sexual contact.

**Shoulder dystocia** Delayed or difficult birth of the fetal shoulders after the head is born.

**Sibling rivalry** Feelings of jealousy and fear of replacement when a young child must share the attention of the parents with a newborn infant.

**Skepticism** Doubt in the absence of conclusive evidence.

**Small-for-gestational age (SGA) infant** An infant whose size is below the 10th percentile for gestational age.

**Somatic cells** Body cells other than the **gametes,** or germ cells.

**Somatic sex** Gender assignment as male or female on the basis of form and structure of the external genitalia.

**Sperm** See **Spermatozoon.**

**Spermatogenesis** Formation of male **gametes (sperm)** in the testes.

**Spermatozoon** (pl. **spermatozoa** or **sperm)** Male **gamete,** or sex cell.

**Spermicide** A chemical, such as nonoxynol 9, that kills **sperm.**

**Spina bifida** Defective closure of the bony spine that encloses the spinal cord; a type of **neural tube defect.**

**Spinnbarkeit** Clear, slippery, stretchy quality of cervical mucus during ovulation.

**Standard of care** Level of care that can be expected of a professional. This level is determined by laws, professional organizations, and health care agencies.

**Standardized procedures** Procedures determined by nurses, physicians, and administrators that allow nurses to perform duties usually part of the medical practice.

**Station** Measurement of fetal descent in relation to the ischial spines of the maternal pelvis. See also **Engagement.**

**Sterility** Total inability to conceive.

**Stork bites** See **Telangiectatic nevi.**

**Strabismus** A turning inward ("crossing") or outward of the eyes due to poor muscle tone.

**Striae gravidarum** Irregular reddish streaks resulting from tears in connective tissue; during pregnancy, these streaks generally appear on the woman's abdomen, breasts, or thighs.

**Subarachnoid space** Space between the arachnoid mater and the pia mater containing **cerebrospinal fluid.**

**Suckling** Giving or taking nourishment from the breast. Sometimes used interchangeably with sucking, which refers only to drawing into the mouth with a partial vacuum, as with a bottle or pacifier.

**Sudden infant death syndrome (SIDS)** Sudden death of an infant that is unexplained by autopsy, examination of the scene of death, or history.

**Surfactant** Combination of lipoproteins produced by the lungs of the mature fetus to reduce surface tension in the alveoli, thus promoting lung expansion after birth.

**Surrogate mother** A fertile woman who is inseminated with the purpose of conceiving and relinquishing a child to an infertile couple.

**Suspend** To delay or to bring to a stop temporarily.

**Sutures** Narrow areas of flexible tissue that connect fetal skull bones, permitting slight movement during labor.

**Syndactyly** Webbing between fingers or toes.

**Tachypnea** Respiratory rate above 60 breaths per minute in the newborn after the first hour of life.

**Taking-hold** Second phase of maternal adaptation during which the mother assumes control of her own care and initiates care of the infant.

**Taking-in** First phase of maternal adaptation during which the mother passively accepts care, comfort, and details of the newborn.

**Telangiectatic nevi (stork bites, nevus simplex)** Flat pink areas on the nape of the neck and over the eyelids resulting from dilation of the capillaries.

**Telemetry** Transmission of electronic fetal monitoring data to the bedside monitor unit with radio signals.

**Teratogen** An agent that can cause defects in a developing baby during pregnancy.

**Term** A birth that occurs between the 38th and 42nd week of gestation.

**Thermogenesis** Heat production.

**Thermoregulation** Maintenance of body temperature.

**Thrombus** Collection of blood factors, primarily platelets and fibrin, that may cause vascular obstruction at the point of formation.

**Tocolytic** A drug that inhibits uterine contractions.

**Total parenteral nutrition (TPN)** Intravenous infusion of all nutrients needed for metabolism and growth.

**Toxemia** An old term occasionally used to denote pregnancy-induced hypertension, **pre-eclampsia,** and **eclampsia.**

**Toxic shock syndrome** Rare, potentially fatal disorder caused by toxin produced by *Staphylococcus aureus*; has been associated with improper use of tampons.

**Tracheoesophageal fistula** Abnormal connection between the esophagus and the trachea.

**Transcutaneous oxygen/carbon dioxide monitoring** Method of continuous noninvasive measurement of oxygen and carbon dioxide levels in the blood by transducers attached to the skin.

**Transducer** A device that translates one physical quantity to another, such as fetal heart motion to an electrical signal for rate calculation or generation of sound or of a written record.

**Transient tachypnea of the newborn** Condition of rapid respirations due to inadequate absorption of **fetal lung fluid.**

**Transitional milk** Breast milk that appears between secretion of **colostrum** and **mature milk.**

**Translocation** Attachment of all or part of a **chromosome** to another chromosome.

**Trimester** A division of pregnancy into three equal parts of 13 weeks each.

**Triple-marker screening** Analysis of maternal serum for abnormal levels of **alpha-fetoprotein,** human chorionic gonadotropin, and estriols that may predict chromosomal abnormalities of the fetus.

**Trisomy** Presence of three copies of a **chromosome** in each body cell.

**Tubal ligation** Occluding of the fallopian tubes to prevent passage of **ova** or **sperm,** thus preventing pregnancy.

**Ultrasonography** Technique for visualizing deep structures of the body by recording the reflections (echoes) of sound waves directed into the tissue.

**Uterine inversion** Turning of the uterus inside out after birth of the fetus.

**Uterine resting tone** Degree of uterine muscle tension when the woman is not in labor or during the interval between labor contractions.

**Uterine rupture** A tear in the wall of the uterus.

**Uteroplacental insufficiency (UPI)** Inability of the placenta to exchange oxygen, carbon dioxide, nutrients, and waste products properly between the maternal and fetal circulations.

**Utilitarian theory** Ethical theory stating that the right course of action is the one that produces the greatest good.

**Vacuum curettage (vacuum aspiration)** Removal of the uterine contents by application of a vacuum through a hollow curet or cannula introduced into the uterus.

**Validate** To make certain that the information collected during assessment is accurate.

**Valsalva's maneuver** Increasing pressure within the abdomen and thorax by holding the breath and pushing against a closed glottis.

**Variable deceleration** Slowing of the fetal heart rate having an inconsistent relationship to uterine contractions.

**Varicocele** Abnormal dilation or varicosity of veins in the spermatic cord.

**Vasectomy** Occluding the vas deferens to prevent passage of **sperm,** thus preventing pregnancy.

**Vasoconstriction** Narrowing of the lumen of blood vessels.

**VBAC** Acronym for vaginal birth after cesarean.

**Vegan** A complete **vegetarian** who does not eat any animal products.

**Vegetarian** An individual whose diet consists wholly or mostly of plant foods and who avoids animal food sources.

**Vernix caseosa** Thick white substance that protects the skin of the fetus.
**Version** Turning the fetus from one presentation to another before birth, usually from breech to cephalic.
**Very-low-birth-weight (VLBW) infant** An infant weighing 1500 g or less at birth.
**Vibroacoustic stimulation test** Use of sound stimulation to elicit fetal movement and acceleration (speeding up) of the fetal heart rate.
**Withdrawal syndrome** See **Abstinence syndrome.**
**Zygote** The developing baby from conception through the first week of prenatal life.

# Appendix A

# Infection Control in Maternity and Women's Health Care

Pathogens such as human immunodeficiency virus (HIV) and hepatitis B virus (HBV) have resulted in significant changes in infection control. Early infection control practices were based on segregation of infected persons, or on disease-specific categories of isolation such as respiratory, wound and skin, or blood precautions. The major shortcoming of these systems is that they were applied after the infection status of the person was known. They also involved use of warning signs on the doors to the person's room, which compromised his or her privacy.

Increases in HIV and HBV infections required a new approach because these pathogens could be transmitted long before the infected person had signs and symptoms. To prevent transmission of blood-borne pathogens to caregivers, the infection control practice of *universal precautions* was established. Universal precautions stressed that all clients are presumed infectious for HIV and other blood-borne pathogens. Universal precautions required use of protective equipment if contact with certain fluids, or articles contaminated with these fluids, was likely. A major advantage of universal precautions was that they could protect the worker from blood-borne pathogens even if the client's infection status was unknown. A shortcoming of universal precautions was that the guidelines did not address sources of infection other than blood-borne. However, universal precautions did specify use of general infection control practices, such as hand washing.

Because *all* body substances may contain pathogens, the more comprehensive guidelines of body substance isolation were adopted by many hospitals in the late 1980s. These guidelines specified use of barriers, primarily gloves, for contact with all moist body substances, mucous membranes, and nonintact skin. They also included signs on the doors to check with the nurse before entering the rooms of clients who might have infections transmitted by the airborne route. The advantages of using body substance isolation guidelines were that they protected the client's privacy better and that they protected workers from more pathogens than did universal precautions.

## New Infection Control Guidelines

The newest guidelines for infection control have two levels of protection. The first level, *standard precautions*, combines features from universal precautions and body substance isolation and applies to all clients. Standard precautions specify the use of personal protective equipment for potential contact with

- Blood
- All body fluids, secretions, and excretions except sweat
- Nonintact skin
- Mucous membranes

Hand washing before and after care is essential. Immediate, thorough hand washing should follow unexpected contact with body substances.

The second level of protection, *transmission-based precautions*, is used for care of specific clients. Transmission-based precautions are designed to limit spread of pathogens that may not be confined by use of standard precautions. These pathogens can be spread by air, droplet, or contact with dry skin or contaminated surfaces. Transmission-based precautions are used in addition to standard precautions.

Gloves are a major component of personal protective equipment, but gloves do not prevent injuries from needles or sharp instruments. Caregivers should not recap needles, purposely bend or break them by hand, remove them from disposable syringes, or otherwise manipulate used needles and other sharp instruments by hand. After use, disposable syringes and needles, scalpel blades, and other sharp items are placed in puncture-resistant containers for disposal.

## Sources of Infection in Maternal, Newborn, and Women's Health Care

Maternal, newborn, and women's health care nursing includes many situations in which the nurse must expect exposure to pathogens, both blood-borne and other infectious agents:

- Handling tissue specimens or specimens of body secretions
- Surgical procedures, including circumcision of the neonate (scrub personnel near the operative site need more protective equipment than circulating personnel)
- Contact with nonintact skin, including surgical incisions
- Contact with mucous membranes, such as vaginal examinations or assessment of the infant's mouth
- Parenteral procedures, such as venipunctures, injections, finger sticks, and heel sticks
- Application of medication to nonintact skin or mucous membranes, such as rectal or vaginal suppositories, topical analgesic preparations, infant eye prophylaxis, and care of the umbilical cord
- Preoperative shaving, perineal care, enemas
- Handling linens, gowns, underpads, perineal pads, and dressings, especially during the intrapartum and postpartum periods, when these items are likely to be contaminated with amniotic fluid, blood, or both
- Handling the infant before the first bath
- Changing diapers and cleaning the infant's diaper area
- Assessing breasts or contact with colostrum or breast milk
- Suture or staple removal

# Appendix B

# Laboratory Values in Pregnant and Non-Pregnant Women and in the Newborn

## Laboratory Values in Pregnant and Non-Pregnant Women

| Value | Non-pregnancy | Pregnancy |
|---|---|---|
| Blood volume, total (ml/kg) | 60–80 | Increases 45% |
| Plasma volume (ml/kg) | 40–50 (average 4700 ml) | Increases 45% by 32 weeks (average 5200 ml) |
| Red blood cell mass (ml/kg) | 20–30 | Increases 20–30% (average increase of 250–450 ml) |
| Red blood cell count (million/mm³) | 3.8–5.1 | Increases 20–30%, 4.5–6.5 |
| Hemoglobin (g/dl) | 12–16 | 11–12 (<11 g/dl during late pregnancy suggests anemia) |
| Hematocrit, packed cell volume (%) | 36–48 | 33–46 |
| White blood cell count | 5000–10,000/mm³ | 5000–12,000/mm³ Rises during labor and post partum up to 25,000/mm³ |
| Platelets | 150,000–400,000/mm³ | Slight decrease (values <100,000/mm³ are considered abnormal); marked increase 3–5 days after birth |
| Prothrombin time (sec) | 11–15 | Slight decrease |
| Activated partial thromboplastin time (sec) | 21–35 | Slight decrease |
| Glucose, serum | | |
| Fasting (mg/dl) | 65–110 | Decreases approximately 11 mg/dl |
| Postprandial (mg/dl) | 1 hr: 120–170<br>2 hr: 70–120 | Screening glucose challenge test: <140 mg/dl<br>1 hr: <190 mg/dl<br>2 hr: <165 mg/dl |
| Creatine, serum (mg/dl) | 0.8 average | End of first trimester: 0.7<br>Late pregnancy: 0.5–0.6 |
| Creatinine clearance, urine (ml/min) | 85–120 | 150–200 |
| Fibrinogen (mg/dl) | 200–400 | 300–600 |

Data from Creasy, R.K., and Resnik, R. (1994). *Maternal-fetal medicine: Principles and practice* (3rd ed.). Philadelphia: W.B. Saunders; Cunningham, F.G., MacDonald, P.C., Gant, N.F., Leveno, K.J., Gilstrap, L.C., Hankins, G.D.V., et al. (1997). *Williams obstetrics* (20th ed.). Norwalk, Conn.: Appleton & Lange; Fischbach, F. (1996). *A manual of laboratory and diagnostic tests* (5th ed.). Philadelphia: J.B. Lippincott; and Tietz, N.W. (1995). *Clinical guide to laboratory tests* (3rd ed.). Philadelphia: W.B. Saunders.

# Laboratory Values in the Newborn

| Test, Specimen, and Unit of Measurement | Age | Normal Ranges (Conventional Units) |
|---|---|---|
| Red blood cell count, whole blood (million/$mm^3$) | Cord | 3.9–5.5 |
| | 1–3 days | 4.0–6.6 |
| | 1 wk | 3.9–6.3 |
| | 1 month | 3.0–5.4 |
| Hemoglobin, whole blood (g/dl) | 1–3 days (cap) | 14.5–22.5 |
| | 2 months | 9.0–14.0 |
| Hematocrit, whole blood (%) | 1 day (cap) | 48–69 |
| | 2 days | 48–75 |
| | 3 days | 44–72 |
| | 2 months | 28–42 |
| White blood cell count, whole blood (thousand/$mm^3$) | Birth | 9.0–30.0 |
| | 24 hr | 9.4–34.0 |
| | 1 month | 5.0–19.5 |
| White blood cell differential count, whole blood | | |
| Myelocytes (%) | | 0 |
| Neutrophils ("bands") (%) | | 3–5 |
| Neutrophils ("segs") (%) | | 54–62 |
| Lymphocytes (%) | | 25–33 |
| Monocytes (%) | | 3–7 |
| Eosinophils (%) | | 1–3 |
| Basophils (%) | | 0–0.75 |
| Platelet count, whole blood (thousand/$mm^3$) | Newborn | 84–478 |
| | >1 wk | 150–400 |
| Glucose, serum (mg/dl) | Cord | 45–96 |
| | Newborn, 1 day | 40–60 |
| | Newborn, >1 day | 50–90 |

| Test, Specimen, and Unit of Measurement | Age | PRETERM | FULL-TERM |
|---|---|---|---|
| Bilirubin, total serum (mg/dl) | Cord | <2.0 | 2.0 |
| | 0–1 day | <8.0 | <6.0 |
| | 1–2 days | <12.0 | <8.0 |
| | 2–5 days | <16.0 | <12.0 |
| | >5 days | <2.0 | 0.2–1.0 |
| Bilirubin, direct (conjugated) serum (mg/dl) | | 0–0.2 | |

Adapted from Behrman, R.E. (1996). *Nelson textbook of pediatrics* (15th ed.). Philadelphia: W.B. Saunders.

# Appendix C

# Effects of Drug Use During Pregnancy and Breastfeeding

## FDA Pregnancy Risk Categories

The U.S. Food and Drug Administration (FDA) has assigned pregnancy risk categories to many drugs on the basis of their known relative safety or danger to the fetus and on whether safer alternative drugs exist. For many drugs, little is known about the fetal risk. The categories are as follows:

A: No evidence of risk to the fetus.
B: Animal reproduction studies have not demonstrated a risk to the fetus. No adequate and well-controlled studies have been done in pregnant women.
C: Animal reproduction studies have shown an adverse effect on the fetus but no adequate, well-controlled studies have been done in humans. Potential benefits may warrant use of the drug in pregnant women despite fetal risks.
D: There is positive evidence of human fetal risk based on adverse reaction data, but potential benefits may warrant use of the drug in pregnant women despite fetal risks. Essentially, no safer alternatives to the drug are available.
X: There is positive evidence of human fetal risk based on animal or human studies and/or adverse reaction data. The risks of using the drug in pregnant women clearly outweigh potential benefits. Safer alternatives to these drugs may be available.

## Drug Use During Lactation

The effects of many drugs, when used during lactation, have not been studied. In general, if a drug is safe for use in infants, it is probably safe for the lactating woman to take. Other drugs are known not to be excreted in breast milk or to be excreted in an inactive form or in very low concentrations. Modifying the time of maternal ingestion may reduce transfer of the drug to the infant. Other drugs are undesirable because they suppress lactation.

The American Academy of Pediatrics (AAP) has established classifications for safety of some drugs during lactation. The categories are as follows:

AAP compatible: Usually compatible with breastfeeding
AAP contraindicated: Contraindicated for use in breastfeeding mothers
AAP reason for concern: Reports of infant side effects cause concern about use in breastfeeding mothers

Social and illicit drugs, such as alcohol and cocaine, are discussed in Chapters 22 and 24.

| Drug | Use During Pregnancy | Use During Breastfeeding |
|---|---|---|
| **ANALGESICS** | | |
| Aspirin | Risk category D. May prolong pregnancy because of its antiprostaglandin effects. May cause bleeding disorders in mother or newborn if used during late pregnancy. | AAP reason for concern. Toxicity unlikely in normal doses, but higher doses could cause bleeding in infant. |
| Acetaminophen | Risk category B. Problems have not been documented, but drug does cross placenta. Use with caution. | AAP compatible. Very small amounts secreted into breast milk. |
| Narcotic analgesics (butorphanol, hydrocodone, meperidine, morphine, nalbuphine, propoxyphene) | Most are risk category C. Neonatal respiratory depression is the most significant adverse effect when narcotic analgesics are used during labor. Neonatal withdrawal may occur if the woman is addicted to the narcotic. | Most narcotics given briefly and in therapeutic doses are compatible with breastfeeding. Infant lethargy and poor feeding may be noted with large doses. Prolonged use may result in infant drug dependence and subsequent withdrawal when the mother no longer takes the drug. |
| Nonsteroidal anti-inflammatory drugs (NSAIDs) (fenoprofen, flurbiprofen, ibuprofen, indomethacin, ketoprofen, naproxen) | Risk category B. Not recommended after 34 weeks. May prolong pregnancy or labor because of antiprostaglandin effects. Associated with premature closure of ductus arteriosus in newborn. | Ibuprofen and indomethacin are AAP compatible. All should be used cautiously owing to potential for infant bleeding. Ketoprofen and naproxen have long half-lives and may remain in mother's blood a long time. |
| **ANTIALLERGIC AND ANTIASTHMATIC DRUGS (See also *Hormones, Corticosteroids*)** | | |
| Antihistamines | Risk category B: brompheniramine, chlorpheniramine, clemastine, cyproheptadine, diphenhydramine, loratadine, meclizine, triprolidine.<br>Risk category C: astemizole, phenylephrine, phenylpropanolamine, terfenadine | All should be used with caution. Most are safe, but may cause infant drowsiness. If these adverse effects occur, a different drug may be tried. Clemastine is rated as AAP reason for concern and is contraindicated. |
| Cromolyn | Risk category B | Minimal oral absorption, so it is unlikely to adversely affect infant. |
| Epinephrine | Risk category C | Unlikely to be absorbed in infant's gastrointestinal tract after early newborn period, or if preterm. |
| Metaproterenol (Alupent) | Risk category C | Unknown if secreted in milk; use cautiously. |
| **ANTICOAGULANTS** | | |
| Heparin | Risk category C. Does not cross placenta; anticoagulant of choice during pregnancy | AAP compatible. Not excreted in breast milk |
| Warfarin (Coumadin) | Risk category D. Associated with facial abnormalities and neurologic deficit. Traumatic intracranial hemorrhage may occur in neonate if ingested near term. If used, it is typically avoided between 6 and 12 weeks' gestation and for 2 to 3 weeks before term. | AAP compatible, but should be used with caution. Very small amounts secreted in milk. No reported bleeding abnormalities in infant, but observe for bruising or petechiae. |
| **ANTICONVULSANTS** | | |
| Carbamazepine (Tegretol) | Risk category C. Associated with craniofacial abnormalities, underdeveloped fingernails, neural tube defects, and developmental delay | AAP compatible. Small amounts secreted in breast milk; accumulation does not seem to occur. Observe infant for sedation. |
| Magnesium sulfate | Risk category A. Infants exposed to magnesium sulfate shortly before birth may exhibit respiratory depression, hypotonic muscle tone, depressed reflexes, hypocalcemia, or cardiac dysrhythmias. | AAP compatible. Moderate amounts secreted in milk, but most remains in infant's gastrointestinal tract. Milk levels return to normal about 24 hr after drug is stopped. |

| Drug | Use During Pregnancy | Use During Breastfeeding |
|---|---|---|
| **ANTICONVULSANTS** | | |
| Phenobarbital | Risk category D. Fetal addiction with subsequent withdrawal is possible but rare at dose levels used for seizure control. Abnormalities similar to those seen in infants exposed to carbamazepine, phenytoin, and valproic acid have been reported. | AAP reason for concern. Significant amounts accumulate in infant's plasma. Psychomotor delay and sedation possible. Use cautiously. |
| Phenytoin (Dilantin) | Risk category D. The fetal hydantoin syndrome includes prenatal-onset growth deficiency, small head, mental retardation, craniofacial and other anomalies, underdeveloped nails or distal phalanges. | AAP compatible. Minimal effects if maternal dose is low. Observe for sedation and decreased sucking. |
| Trimethadione (Tridione) | Risk category D. Fetal risk for malformations is greater than with other anticonvulsants. Associated with developmental delay, craniofacial abnormalities, cardiovascular and other internal abnormalities. | Enters breast milk. Use cautiously. |
| Valproic acid (Depakene) | Risk category D. Associated with neural tube defects, craniofacial abnormalities. | AAP compatible. Secreted in small amounts. May cause drowsiness. Used for infant seizures. |
| **ANTIDIABETIC AGENTS** | | |
| Insulin | Risk category B. Insulin is only appropriate drug to control diabetes during pregnancy because it does not cross placenta. | AAP compatible. Any insulin secreted would be destroyed in infant's gastrointestinal tract. |
| Oral hypoglycemic agents | Contraindicated; cross placenta. Insulin controls blood glucose levels without crossing placenta. May cause prolonged neonatal hypoglycemia. | Safety not established for most. Observe for infant hypoglycemia. |
| **ANTIHYPERTENSIVES See also *Diuretics* because these drugs are often used to treat hypertension.** | | |
| ACE inhibitors (benazepril, captopril, enalapril, fosinopril, ramipril) | Risk categories C and D. Suspected teratogenic effects. May reduce uteroplacental perfusion and cause fetal hypotension. Renal malformations with anuria, leading to oligohydramnios, lung hypoplasia, and cranial and facial deformities. | Use with caution. Captopril and enalapril are AAP compatible. Small amounts are transferred to infant. Observe for infant hypotension. |
| Beta-adrenergic blockers (acebutolol, atenolol, betaxolol, labetalol, metoprolol, nadolol, penbutolol, pindolol, propranolol, timolol) | Risk category C, except acebutolol, atenolol, and pindolol, which are risk category B. Possible fetal or neonatal effects include transient bradycardia, respiratory depression, and hypoglycemia. | AAP compatible, but potentially hazardous: acebutolol, labetalol, nadolol, timolol. Observe infant for pharmacologic effects if mother is taking a beta-adrenergic blocker: hypotension, bradycardia, sedation, fatigue. |
| Calcium channel blockers (amlodipine, diltiazem, nicardipine, nifedipine, nimodipine, verapamil) | Risk category C. Hypotensive effects may reduce uteroplacental perfusion and may lead to fetal heart failure and atrioventricular block. Nifedipine has been used on an investigational basis to inhibit preterm labor. | Drugs excreted in breast milk. AAP compatible: diltiazem, nifedipine, and verapamil. Use with extreme caution; overdoses in young children are very dangerous. Observe for hypotension and bradycardia. Delaying nursing for 3–4 hr after the *non–sustained-release* form may reduce transfer to infant. |
| Centrally acting sympatholytics (clonidine, guanabenz, guanfacine, methyldopa) | Risk category C, except for guanfacine (risk category B). | Methyldopa is AAP compatible. Others should be used cautiously, as safety is not established. Observe for hypotension and sedation. |
| Vasodilators (hydralazine, minoxidil) | Risk category C. No adverse fetal effects associated with long-term use. Excessive hair has been reported. | Listed drugs are AAP compatible. |

*Table continued on following page*

| Drug | Use During Pregnancy | Use During Breastfeeding |
|---|---|---|
| **ANTIMICROBIALS** | | |
| Aminoglycosides (gentamicin, kanamycin, neomycin, streptomycin) | Risk categories C and D. Associated with hearing loss and renal toxicity. | AAP compatible: kanamycin and streptomycin. Most drugs in this class are poorly absorbed orally. |
| Azithromycin (Zithromax) | Risk category B. Chemically related to erythromycin. | Only small amounts are likely to be ingested by infant. |
| Cephalosporins | Most are risk category B. | Secretion into milk is generally poor. Observe for diarrhea. |
| Chloramphenicol | Risk category C. Not recommended for use at term because it is associated with neonatal "gray baby syndrome" (rapid respiration, ashen and pale color, poor feeding, abdominal distention, vasomotor collapse, death). | AAP reason for concern. Generally contraindicated in breastfeeding mothers. May cause infant sensitivity. |
| Erythromycins | Risk category C. Little transfer to fetus across placenta, which limits the drugs' usefulness for treating syphilis. | AAP compatible. May cause alteration in gastrointestinal flora, allergies, interference with infant's cultures for infection. |
| Fluoroquinolones (includes ciprofloxacin, norfloxacin, ofloxacin) | Risk category C. Animal studies have shown joint abnormalities. | Contraindicated. Possible association with cartilage damage and colitis. |
| Metronidazole (Flagyl) | Risk category B. However, not recommended to treat *Trichomonas* infections during first trimester. | AAP reason for concern (primarily for oral form). Breastfeeding may be discontinued for 12–24 hr to allow mother to excrete last dose, then restarted. |
| Nitrofurantoin (Macrodantin) | Risk category B. Use should be avoided near term because it may cause hemolytic anemia in newborn. | AAP compatible for older infants. Should avoid if infant is younger than 1 month. Risk for hemolytic anemia if infant has an enzyme (G-6-PD) deficiency. |
| Penicillins (includes amoxicillin, ampicillin, penicillin G) | Risk category B. No reported adverse fetal effects. Penicillins combined with beta-lactamase inhibitors (Augmentin, Timentin, and Unasyn) have not been adequately studied, although fetal effects are unlikely. | Penicillins are AAP compatible. Observe for infant diarrhea or development of sensitivity. |
| Sulfonamides | Risk category B (D near term). May result in neonatal hyperbilirubinemia. | Potentially hazardous. Sulfisoxazole is considered compatible, but all should be used with great caution. Associated with jaundice, diarrhea, rash. |
| Tetracyclines | Risk category D. Can interfere with tooth enamel formation and cause discolored teeth. Prenatal exposure does not affect permanent teeth. | AAP compatible for short periods. Tooth discoloration, slowed bone growth, and altered bowel flora are possible. |
| **ANTINEOPLASTICS** | | |
| Few cases have been studied because of the relative rarity with which these drugs are used in women of childbearing age. Therefore, their relative safety or danger cannot be accurately determined. Additionally, reported congenital defects may be more related to the mother's serious disease than to the drug itself. | | |
| Alkylating agents | Probable association with fetal anomalies. Risk category D | Contraindicated |
| Antimetabolites | Risk category D. Methotrexate is contraindicated for treatment of psoriasis or rheumatoid arthritis during pregnancy (risk category X). | Contraindicated |
| Tamoxifen (Nolvadex) | Risk category D | Contraindicated |
| **ANTITUBERCULOSIS AGENTS (see also *Antimicrobials*)** | | |
| Ethambutol | Risk category B. No evidence of increased abnormalities. Fetal effects of combinations of ethambutol with other antituberculosis drugs are unknown. | AAP compatible. Concentration in breast milk is similar to that in maternal serum, so caution is indicated. |

| Drug | Use During Pregnancy | Use During Breastfeeding |
|---|---|---|
| **ANTITUBERCULOSIS AGENTS (see also *Antimicrobials*)** | | |
| Isoniazid | Risk category C | AAP compatible, but infant should be observed for liver toxicity and neuritis. |
| Pyrazinamide | Risk category C. Safety is not established; try to avoid use. | Use cautiously. |
| Rifampin | Risk category C | AAP compatible. No reported adverse effects |
| **ANTITUSSIVES AND EXPECTORANTS** | | |
| Dextromethorphan | Risk category C | Safety not established |
| Guaifenesin | Risk category C | Unlikely to cause side effects |
| **ANTIVIRAL AGENTS** | | |
| Acyclovir | Risk category C | AAP compatible. Few reported toxicities. If topical drug is used on nipples, wash thoroughly before nursing. |
| Ribavirin (Virazole) | Risk category X. Administered by aerosol. Women who are pregnant or may become pregnant should avoid exposure. | Not known if drug is excreted in milk. |
| Zidovudine (formerly called AZT) | Risk category C. Given to HIV-seropositive women to reduce risk for perinatal transmission of the virus. | Contraindicated |
| **BRONCHODILATORS** | | |
| Albuterol | Risk category C | Small amounts likely to be secreted. Observe infant for tremors and excitement. |
| Terbutaline (Brethine) | Risk category B. Also used in treatment of preterm labor | AAP compatible. Observe infant for tremors and nervousness. |
| Theophylline | Risk category C | AAP compatible. Excreted in milk. May result in infant irritability, insomnia, and fretfulness. |
| **CARDIAC GLYCOSIDES** | | |
| Digoxin | Risk category C | AAP compatible |
| **DECONGESTANTS** | | |
| Ephedrine, epinephrine, oxymetazoline, phenylephrine | Risk category C. Should not be used during third trimester. | Use with caution. May cause irritability in infant. |
| Pseudoephedrine | Risk category C. Avoid during third trimester. | AAP compatible. Minimal amounts secreted in milk. |
| **DIURETICS** | | |
| Furosemide (Lasix) | Risk category C | Effects unknown but probably minimal. May reduce milk production. |
| Thiazides | Risk categories B and C. Decreased intravascular volume may reduce uteroplacental perfusion. Metabolic disturbances and thrombocytopenia may occur in mother and fetus. | Probably safe. May reduce milk production. |
| **HORMONES** | | |
| Corticosteroids | Risk category C. Prednisone is agent of choice for asthmatic woman who needs steroids. Betamethasone and dexamethasone are used to accelerate maturation of fetal lungs if preterm delivery is likely. | Potentially hazardous in high doses or with long-term use. Delay nursing 4 hr after dose to reduce transfer to infant. Do not apply topically to nipples. |
| Estrogens | Risk category X. Diethylstilbestrol (DES) is associated with development of vaginal cancer in female offspring during adolescence or adulthood. | Reduces milk volume and protein content. Try to delay drug until breastfeeding is firmly established. DES should not be used. |

*Table continued on following page*

| Drug | Use During Pregnancy | Use During Breastfeeding |
|---|---|---|
| **HORMONES** | | |
| Oral contraceptives (estrogen-progestin combinations) | Risk category X. Doses much higher than those used in oral contraceptives are associated with masculinization of the female fetus' genitalia. | Should not be used until lactation is well established, or drugs may decrease milk quantity and quality. |
| Clomiphene citrate (Clomid) | Risk category X. Questionable association with neural tube defects. Drug is discontinued after pregnancy is achieved. | May suppress lactation. Unlikely to be prescribed during lactation because it is given for infertility. |
| **PSYCHOACTIVE DRUGS** | | |
| Benzodiazepines | Most are risk category D. The following benzodiazepines are risk category X and contraindicated during pregnancy: estazolam, quazepam, temazepam, and triazolam. Some reports of mild facial abnormalities and developmental delay, but no conclusive studies. | Potentially hazardous. Preferred drugs in this class are lorazepam or oxazepam. |
| Lithium | Risk category D. Slightly increased risk for cardiac abnormalities. | AAP contraindicated |
| Meprobamate | Contraindicated. Associated with a significant increase in malformations. Equagesic contains meprobamate. | Concentrations in milk are higher than in maternal serum. May cause sedation in infant. |
| Phenothiazines (chlorpromazine, perphenazine, prochlorperazine, thioridazine, trifluoperazine) | Risk category C. Risk of malformations is uncertain. Continued use during pregnancy should be carefully evaluated. | AAP reason for concern; some sources say these drugs are probably safe in usual doses. Observe infant for sedation or jerking movements. |
| Tricyclic antidepressants | Risk category C | Use with caution. Probably safe in usual doses. Desipramine and nortriptyline are preferred. Some sources consider these drugs contraindicated for breastfeeding mothers. |
| **THYROID DRUGS** | | |
| Antithyroids (methimazole, propylthiouracil [PTU]) | Risk category D. May result in neonatal goiter or hypothyroidism, although uncommon at usual therapeutic doses. Methimazole has possible association with scalp defects. | AAP compatible. Propylthiouracil is preferred drug. |
| Iodine, iodides | Risk category C. Long-term exposure may produce fetal thyroid enlargement. | Use caution. May cause rash or suppress infant's thyroid function. Large quantities of iodides are contraindicated. |
| Thyroid replacement hormones (levothyroxine, liothyronine, liotrix) | Risk category A. Crosses placenta only to limited extent. | Small amounts secreted in milk. Observe infant for nervousness and agitation. Infant should have periodic thyroid studies. |
| **VITAMINS AND RETINOIDS** | | |
| Retinoids (etretinate [Tegison], isotretinoin [Accutane]) | Risk category X. Related to vitamin A. Associated with severe fetal malformations (microcephaly, ear abnormalities, cardiac defects, central nervous system abnormalities). Etretinate has a long half-life and may have fetal effects up to 18 months after drug is stopped. | AAP contraindicated |
| Vitamin A | Risk category A (X at high doses). Excess intake may lead to abnormalities noted for etretinate and isotretinoin. | Breast milk usually supplies sufficient vitamin A to infant. Mother should not take more than 6000 units per day. |

| Drug | Use During Pregnancy | Use During Breastfeeding |
|---|---|---|
| **VITAMINS AND RETINOIDS** | | |
| Vitamin $B_6$ (pyridoxine) | Risk category A. Large doses could produce pyridoxine deficiency in infant. | AAP compatible, but a maximum of 10 mg/day should be prescribed, and only to women having deficiencies. |
| Vitamin D | Risk category C (D at high doses). Excess intake associated with malformations, including aortic stenosis, facial abnormalities, and mental retardation. | AAP compatible. Should be supplemented with caution. High doses could cause high infant calcium levels. |
| **MISCELLANEOUS DRUGS** | | |
| Nicotine gum; nicotine transdermal | Risk category X | AAP contraindicated. Nicotine levels from drug may be less than those from smoking, *if* the mother does not smoke at all. Smoking plus use of nicotine-containing drugs could lead to high levels in infant. Observe for infant shock, vomiting, diarrhea, tachycardia, and restlessness. |

### *References*


American Academy of Pediatrics Committee on Drugs (1994). Transfer of drugs and other chemicals into human milk. *Pediatrics*, 93(1), 137–150.

Caldwell, J. (1996). Hyperthyroidism during pregnancy: Nursing care issues. *Journal of Obstetric, Gynecologic and Neonatal Nursing*, 25(5), 395–400.

Conover, E. (1994). Hazardous exposures during pregnancy. *Journal of Obstetric, Gynecologic and Neonatal Nursing*, 23(6), 524–532.

Corbett, J.V., & Kenney, C. (1995a). Anticoagulants during pregnancy. *MCN: American Journal of Maternal-Child Nursing*, 20(1), 56.

Corbett, J.V., & Kenney, C. (1995b). Zidovudine in pregnancy. *MCN: American Journal of Maternal-Child Nursing*, 20(2), 122.

Cunningham, F.G., MacDonald, P.C., Gant, N.F., Leveno, K.J., Gilstrap, L.C., Hankins, G.D.V., et al. (1997). *Williams obstetrics* (20th ed.). Norwalk, Conn.: Appleton & Lange.

Deglin, J.H., & Vallerand, A.H. (1997). *Davis's drug guide for nurses* (5th ed.). Philadelphia: F.A. Davis.

Gilstrap, L.C., & Little, B.B. (1994). Medication during pregnancy: Maternal and embryofetal considerations. In D.K. James, P.J. Steer, C.P. Weiner, & B. Gonik (Eds.), *High risk pregnancy: Management options* (pp. 239–251). Philadelphia: W.B. Saunders.

Hale, T. (1996). *Medications and mothers' milk* (4th ed.). Amarillo, Tex.: Pharmasoft Medical Publishing.

Hodgson, B., Kizior, R., & Kingdon, R. (1996). *Nurse's drug handbook*. Philadelphia: W.B. Saunders.

Jones, K.L. (1994). Effects of therapeutic, diagnostic, and environmental agents. In R.K. Creasy & R. Resnik (Eds.), *Maternal-fetal medicine: Principles and practice* (3rd ed., pp. 171–181). Philadelphia: W.B. Saunders.

Karch, A.M. (1996). *Lippincott's nursing drug guide*. Philadelphia: J.B. Lippincott.

Kliegman, R.M. (1996). Parent-infant bonding. In R.E. Behrman, R.M. Kliegman, A.M. Arvin, & W.E. Nelson, *Nelson textbook of pediatrics* (15th ed., pp. 439–440). Philadelphia: W.B. Saunders.

Lindberg, C.E. (1995). Perinatal transmission of HIV: How to counsel women. *MCN: American Journal of Maternal-Child Nursing*, 20(4), 207–212.

Mastrobattista, J.M., (1997). Angiotensin converting enzyme inhibitors in pregnancy. *Seminars in Perinatology*, 21(2), 124–134.

Rebar, R.W. (1994). The breast and the physiology of lactation. In R.K. Creasy & R. Resnik (Eds.), *Maternal-fetal medicine: Principles and practice* (3rd ed., pp. 144–161). Philadelphia: W.B. Saunders.

Simpkins, S.M., Hench, C.P., & Ghatia, G. (1996). Management of the obstetric patient with tuberculosis. *Journal of Obstetric, Gynecologic and Neonatal Nursing*, 25(4), 305–312.

# Appendix D

# Keys to Clinical Practice: Components of Daily Care

## Intrapartum Care

### Text to Prepare You for Clinical Practice

Chapter 11: Breathing techniques
Figure 12–4: Pelvic divisions and measurements
Table 13–1: Intrapartum assessment guide
Table 13–2: Assessment and documentation of fetal heart rate
Figure 13–1: Vaginal examination during labor
Figure 13–6: Sequence for delivery
Figure 13–7: Vaginal birth
Table 13–4: Apgar score

### New Terms

Amniotomy
Bloody show
Crowning
EDD
Gravida
Lochia
Multipara
Nullipara
Para
Presentation
Station
VBAC

### Equipment and Supplies

Sterile and nonsterile gloves
Lubricant
Urine specimen containers
Amniotic membrane perforator
Emesis basin
Bedpan
Disposable underpads
Extra linens
Fetal monitoring equipment and related supplies
Electronic fetal monitor and supplies
Doppler transducer
Intravenous fluids, tubing, venipuncture supplies, intravenous pumps
Urinary catheters (indwelling and straight)
Oxygen equipment, including water, tubing, and face mask
Emergency cart
"Precip tray" (for emergency birth)

### Normal Assessments

**Fetus**

*Gestation.* 38 to 42 weeks.

*Fetal Heart Rate* (FHR). Lower limit of 110–120 beats/minute and upper limit of 150–160 beats/minute at term. The rate may slow during contractions but should return to its original level by the end of the contraction.

*Amniotic Fluid.* Clear (may have particles of white vernix); no foul odor.

**Woman**

*Temperature.* Lower than 38°C (100.4°F).

*Blood Pressure.* Near baseline levels established during pregnancy. (Report elevations of 140/90.)

*Pulse.* 60 to 100 beats/minute.

*Respirations.* 12 to 20 breaths/minute.

*Contractions.* No more than 90 seconds in duration, with at least 60 seconds of uterine relaxation between the end of one contraction and the beginning of the next.

*Bloody Show.* Dark blood mixed with mucus (has a distinct mucous component). The amount varies but increases as full dilation nears.

*Lochia (Fourth Stage).* No more than one saturated pad in 1 hour. (Perineal pads with cold packs in them absorb less and are saturated sooner than standard pads.)

*Fundus (Fourth Stage).* Firm, between the symphysis and the umbilicus, midline.

## Nursing Care

Clinical experiences in the intrapartum setting are primarily observational. The beginning nurse works with an experienced nurse and takes limited responsibility for the woman's care. Primary responsibilities of the novice are to promote family attachment, provide comfort and support to the woman and her family, and report maternal or fetal assessments that are not expected.

*Personal protective equipment, such as gloves and water-repellent gowns or aprons, must be worn whenever the possibility of contact with body fluids (amniotic fluid, blood, lochia, colostrum, breast milk, urine, or stool) exists to conform with standard precautions. Protective eyewear also must be worn if splash or spray contamination of the eyes is a possibility.*

## Assessments

Unless directed otherwise by the experienced nurse, assess the woman and fetus who do not have complications using the following guidelines:

1. FHR with continuous electronic fetal monitoring or intermittent auscultation: every hour during the latent phase; every 30 minutes during the active phase; every 15 minutes during the second stage.
2. The woman's temperature every 4 hours unless her membranes have ruptured, then every 2 hours.
3. The woman's blood pressure, pulse, and respirations every hour.
4. Contractions: Assess at same time as FHR.
5. If the woman's membranes rupture, assess FHR for at least 1 minute, and observe the color, odor, and amount of fluid. Notify an experienced nurse that the woman's membranes have ruptured.
6. After birth, during the recovery phase, assess the mother's uterine fundus, lochia, blood pressure, pulse, and respirations every 15 minutes for the first hour.

## Interventions

1. Assess the woman and the fetus using the guidelines above or according to the facility's policy. Document all assessments, and *report any findings that do not fall within the expected limits.*
2. If there is no contraindication, give the woman ice chips, and encourage her to change position as much as she desires. Ask an experienced nurse to be sure.
3. The woman can usually walk to the bathroom if she is not in advanced labor and has not had analgesia or anesthesia that impairs mobility. Record each time she voids or has a bowel movement.
4. Help the woman cope with labor:
   a. A cool, damp washcloth often feels good on her face, arms, and abdomen.
   b. If her back hurts, offer to rub it, or apply firm pressure in the sacral area. Ask her where and how firmly to press. Encourage her to try alternate positions.
   c. Give generous praise and encouragement for her efforts to give birth. Praise the partner's efforts as a coach.
5. Offer a snack to the woman's partner, or encourage him or her to take a break and have a meal.
6. Look at the woman's perineum if she says that the baby is coming or begins making grunting sounds or bearing down. Summon the experienced nurse with the call bell immediately, but *do not leave the woman.*
7. When the infant is born, focus on the respiratory efforts and maintain warmth. Use a bulb syringe (see p. 560) to suction excess secretions. Keep the infant under a radiant warmer or wrap in warmed blankets. Be sure not to get between the radiant heat source and the infant.
8. Observe parent-infant attachment behaviors, such as making eye contact, talking in soft, high-pitched tones, and making remarks about the infant.
9. In many facilities, the infant remains with the parents during the recovery period, and the same nurse cares for both the mother and the newborn. If so, continue to observe the infant's respiratory effort and maintain the temperature.

# Postpartum Care: Physiologic Aspects

## Text to Prepare You for Clinical Practice

Procedure 17–1: Assessing the uterine fundus
Procedure 17–2: Assessing the perineum
Figure 17–2: Estimating volume of lochia
Figure 17–7: Clinical Pathway for Vaginal Birth
Figure 17–8: Assessing Homans' sign
Table 17–1: Characteristics of lochia
Table 17–4: Observations of the fundus requiring nursing actions
Critical to Remember: Signs of a distended bladder

## New Terms

Afterpains
Atony
Colostrum

Engorgement
Episiotomy
Fundus
Lochia rubra, serosa, alba
Puerperium
REEDA (redness, edema, ecchymosis, drainage, approximation)

## Equipment and Supplies

Thermometer
Blood pressure equipment
Watch
Stethoscope
Flashlight
Nonsterile gloves
Peripads
Clean linen
Disposable underpads or linen liners

## Normal Assessments

### *Vital Signs*

*Temperature.* Lower than 38°C (100.4°F).

*Blood Pressure.* Near the baseline levels established during pregnancy.

*Pulse.* 50 to 60 beats/minute is not unusual. Bradycardia reflects increased amount of blood returning to the central circulation.

*Respirations.* 16 to 20 breaths/minute. Should be unchanged from preconception levels; the lungs should be free of adventitious breath sounds.

### *Breasts*

a. First 24 hours. Soft.
b. Days 2 to 3. Firm to very firm, as milk comes in.

*Nipples.* Free of redness, abraded areas, or fissures.

### *Gastrointestinal System*

1. Mother hungry and thirsty.
2. Abdomen soft; temporary constipation may occur because of dehydration and decreased intake during labor.
3. Bowel sounds usually present within 24 to 36 hours after cesarean birth.
4. Hemorrhoids may be obvious, particularly during first 24 hours.

### *Genitourinary System*

1. Fundus should be firm, midline, and located at the umbilicus (± 1 cm).
2. Lochia rubra should be scant to moderate with fleshy, earthy odor.
3. Episiotomy edges should be approximated and without redness or edema.
4. Perineum, labia, or both may be slightly bruised or swollen
5. Abdominal dressing for cesarean birth should be dry and intact. When dressing is removed, edges of surgical incision should be approximated and without signs of infection.
6. Diuresis normal for first 2 to 3 days; mother often unaware of need to urinate.
7. After voiding, bladder should not be palpable; fundus should remain firm and at the level of the umbilicus.

## Nursing Care

Preparation before approaching the new mother helps the beginning nurse to recognize unusual or abnormal data and to initiate the necessary nursing interventions. Moreover, it builds self-confidence that, in turn, inspires confidence in the new mother and sets the stage for individualized nursing care.

*Nonsterile gloves must be worn whenever the possibility of contact with body fluids (blood, lochia, colostrum, breast milk, urine, or stool) exists.*

The sequence in which postpartum assessments are performed is important because they should progress from areas that are least likely to be contaminated, such as the breasts, to areas that are associated with pathogenic organisms, such as the perineum and anal areas. The following sequence is recommended.

## Assessments

1. Explain the purpose of the assessments: "I know we do these assessments several times a day, but it is necessary to be sure that everything is progressing as it should. It is also a good time for you to ask any questions you might have."
2. Assess vital signs, usually every 2 to 8 hours, depending on facility protocols and the condition of the mother.
3. Observe and report edema of the face or hands, which may suggest pregnancy-induced hypertension.
4. Auscultate breath sounds and ability to deep breathe and cough if the woman had a cesarean birth, if she smokes, or if she has a history of respiratory disorders.
5. Ask the mother to unfasten her bra or to lower the bra flaps to assess the nipples for redness, fissures, or blisters that may occur with breastfeeding. Note nipple size and shape that may make breastfeeding more difficult (flat, retracted, inverted). Palpate the breasts; this is a good time to ask how well breastfeeding is progressing and if she has any questions.
6. Lower the top of the bed, and ask the mother to flex her knees for comfort; palpate the ab-

domen (soft or distended?). If the woman had a cesarean birth, auscultate the abdomen for bowel sounds and ask if she is passing flatus.

7. Observe the dressing covering the incision for intactness and discharge; if the dressing has been removed, observe the cesarean incision for REEDA and note if staples, Steri-Strips, or skin clips remain in place.
8. Assess for bladder distention: time and amount of last voiding (can be validated from the chart before beginning the assessment), observable or palpable bulge above symphysis pubis. If an indwelling catheter is in place, note the color and amount of urine.
9. Palpate the lower extremities for the presence and extent of edema; press the thumb on the pretibial area and the feet to determine if pitting edema is present; note how long it takes for the pit to disappear.
10. Observe and palpate the lower extremities for signs of thrombophlebitis (areas of redness, tenderness, swelling). Sharply dorsiflex the foot to elicit Homans' sign.
11. Lower the perineal pad(s) and observe flow of lochia while palpating the fundus for firmness and location.
12. Observe the perineal pad(s) for color and amount of lochia; ask how long since the peripad(s) was changed to determine the amount of flow; note unpleasant or foul odor.
13. Ask the mother to turn to her side to assess the perineum for REEDA. Note the number and size of hemorrhoids.
14. Evaluate the mother's ability to ambulate, and elicit information about dizziness, weakness, or lightheadedness during ambulation. Observe gait for steadiness and balance.
15. Ask the mother about particular problems and concerns. How is her appetite? How much rest is she getting? Does she have discomfort (where, when)? Does she require medication?

## Interventions

1. Changes in vital signs may be within expected limits or they may indicate the beginning of serious problems. Tachycardia or lower-than-expected blood pressure may indicate excessive bleeding and should be reported. Blood pressure that is higher than expected may indicate pregnancy-induced hypertension. The blood pressure should be reassessed in both arms with the woman in a left lateral recumbent position. *Temperature above 38°C (100.4°F) suggests infection rather than dehydration and should be reassessed and reported to the primary nurse. Diminished or abnormal breath sounds (wheezes or crackles), as well as difficulty breathing or coughing, should be reported at once.*
2. Nipple trauma provides a portal for entry of pathogenic organisms and creates discomfort during breastfeeding. The new mother often needs information, guidance, and encouragement with breastfeeding.
3. *Report at once if you are unable to locate the fundus, if the fundus feels soft (boggy), or if it is above the umbilicus or displaced from the midline.* Be prepared to assist the mother to void or to catheterize her if she is unable to empty her bladder. Use uterine massage to contract a boggy uterus.
4. Report positive Homans' sign as well as areas of redness, edema, or tenderness of the legs. Assist woman to ambulate if her gait is unsteady or she experiences lightheadedness when she ambulates.
5. If necessary, teach self-care measures, such as perineal care and sitz bath, to reduce perineal discomfort and to prevent infection.
6. Provide medication for afterpains or perineal discomfort according to the physician's orders; reassure the mother that very little of the medication administered for discomfort crosses into the breast milk and that the infant should not be affected.

# Postpartum Care: Psychosocial Aspects

## Text to Prepare You for Clinical Practice

Table 18–1: Assessing maternal adaptation
Table 18–2: Assessing family adaptation
Critical to Remember: Reciprocal attachment behaviors

## New Terms

Attachment
Bonding
En *face*
Engrossment
Entrainment
Finger-tipping
Letting-go
Reciprocal bonding behaviors
Taking-hold
Taking-in

### Normal Assessments

***Maternal Touch.*** During the first 24 hours, the mother progresses from the discovery phase, when she "finger-tips" the infant, to enfolding the infant and demonstrating a range of consoling behaviors.

***Verbal Expressions.*** The mother progresses from referring to the infant as "it" to "he" or "she" and finally to calling the infant by a given name.

***Taking-in Phase.*** Mothers are concerned with their own physical needs and the need to recount details of their labor and delivery.

***Taking-hold Phase.*** Mothers become more independent and focus on learning how to care for themselves and the infant.

***Fathers.*** Fathers demonstrate intense fascination with the infant and are often observed to respond gently to infant signals, such as fussing and crying.

***Family.*** Family support is obvious when the grandparents visit, offer to assist the mother, and demonstrate interest in the newborn.

## Nursing Care

Although a psychological assessment is never as precise as a physical assessment, it is nevertheless essential, and a fairly systematic method can be developed. In order to sharpen observational skills, students should review expected maternal behaviors, progression of maternal touch, and verbal interactions before beginning a psychosocial assessment.

Pertinent observations may escape those who are unprepared and who make a casual, uninformed assessment. However, with preparation and careful practice, observational skills increase rapidly.

### Assessments

1. Collect data from the woman's chart (age, gravida, para, time and type of delivery, sex and weight of infant, unusual characteristics or anomalies of infant, time mother was last medicated for discomfort) to identify factors that might affect adjustment.
2. Be prepared to begin a psychosocial assessment during the physical assessment, and continue to make observations throughout the day.
3. Observe maternal mood, general energy level, and activity.
4. Ask about the mother's comfort, how she slept, and whether she has special concerns.
5. Note the focus of the mother's attention—is it on her own needs or on care of the infant? Does she require assistance with hygiene and self-care measures? How much does she talk of the birth experience?
6. Observe the mother's interaction with the infant and her readiness to participate in infant care. Note voice tone and verbal interaction.
7. Watch how the mother touches the infant and how she responds to infant cues, such as crying and fussing.
8. Note the father's participation in infant care and his comfort handling the infant.
9. Notice infant behavior (awake, response to parents' voices, gazing); watch closely how the infant responds to the parents and whether the parents are successful in consoling the infant.
10. Observe visitors, particularly the grandparents and family, who may provide assistance to the parents during the early weeks at home.

### Interventions

1. Anticipate needs and provide physical care and comfort measures that are particularly important in the early hours following childbirth.
2. Allow time to listen; this is very important in establishing rapport and assisting the mother to integrate the birth experience into her reality system.
3. Promote bonding and attachment by providing long periods of uninterrupted contact between the parents and the infant and by modeling behaviors, such as gentle response when the infant cries and talking to the infant in a high-pitched voice. Point out positive characteristics of the infant to the parents.
4. Prepare to teach basic infant care by observing videos and staff demonstrations. Clarify questions of care with instructor or primary nurse.
5. Answer questions or demonstrate care as the mother indicates a readiness to learn.

# The Newborn: Initial Assessments and Care

### Text to Prepare You for Clinical Practice

Procedure 20–1: Weighing and measuring the newborn
Procedure 20–2: Assessing vital signs in the newborn
Procedure 20–3: Assessing blood glucose in the newborn
Procedure 21–1: Administering intramuscular injections to newborns
Procedure 21–2: Using a bulb syringe
Table 20–1: Summary of newborn assessment

### New Terms

Acrocyanosis
Caput succedaneum
Cephalhematoma
Hyperbilirubinemia
Lanugo

Milia
Molding
Mongolian spots
Vernix caseosa

## Equipment and Supplies

Scale
Radiant warmer
Nonsterile gloves
Stethoscope
Thermometer
Tape measure
Vitamin K, syringe, filter needle, alcohol wipes
Eye medication
Bulb syringe

## Normal Assessments

**Vital Signs**
*Temperature*
a. Axillary—36.5 to 37.5°C (97.7 to 99.5°F)
b. Rectal—36.5 to 37.6°C (97.7 to 99.7°F)

*Heart Rate.* 120 to 160 beats/minute
*Respirations.* 30 to 60 breaths/minute. Average 30 to 40 breaths/minute
**Blood Glucose.** Above 45 mg/dl by screening tests or above 40 mg/dl by laboratory analysis

**Measurements**
*Weight.* 2500 to 4000 g (5 pounds, 8 ounces to 8 pounds, 13 ounces)
*Length.* 48 to 53 cm (19 to 21 inches)
*Head Circumference.* 33 to 35.5 cm (13 to 14 inches)
*Chest Circumference.* 30.5 to 33 cm (12 to 13 inches)

## Nursing Care

A typical order in which assessments and care are done in the labor, delivery, recovery unit or the admission nursery is given here. The elements actually included and the order in which they are performed depend on the facility's routine and the circumstances.

*Adhere to standard precautions at all times. Wear nonsterile gloves at all times when handling the infant until the bath is given and all blood is removed from the skin. After the bath, wear gloves when soiling with body fluids may occur.*

Include family members who are present. They are often very interested in explanations of the assessments and care being given. Promote bonding by encouraging them to touch and talk to the infant.

## Assessments

Begin with a quick overall assessment of the infant's general condition. Attend to major problems, such as severe respiratory distress, before continuing the more detailed assessment and care. Observe for signs of distress or abnormality in the early hours after birth, as this is the time when they are most likely to appear. Report and take action, as necessary, for any abnormal findings.

1. Perform a quick general assessment to identify gross abnormalities. *Be constantly alert for signs of respiratory distress.*
2. Assess vital signs. *Report and follow up on abnormalities immediately.*
3. Weigh infant and measure length and head and chest circumferences.
4. Assess blood glucose according to signs of hypoglycemia and agency policy.
5. Perform in-depth assessment (see Table 20–2).
6. Continue monitoring vital signs every 30 minutes until infant has been stable for 2 hours. Assess more often if necessary. Once the infant is stable, vital signs should be checked every 8 hours, or more frequently if abnormal.

## Interventions

1. Position the infant with the head lower than the body for a short time to drain airways. Suction as necessary. Return the infant to flat position as soon as drainage of airways is completed.
2. Take footprints, if not done previously.
3. Administer antibiotic to the eyes, and administer vitamin K injection. *Note:* Do not give vitamin K until after the bath if the mother is hepatitis B or HIV positive.
4. Allow the infant to rest quietly under a radiant warmer between assessments and care. Keep positioned on side with a rolled blanket to promote drainage of secretions. When initial assessment and procedures are completed, wrap the infant in two blankets, place a hat on the head, and give the infant to the parents to hold.
5. Bathe the infant under a radiant warmer when the temperature is stable or according to agency policy to remove blood and excess vernix. Keep the infant warm by drying as quickly as possible and removing wet linens. Dry the hair thoroughly to prevent heat loss.
6. Assist the mother with the initial feeding. If the infant is formula fed, give no more than 1 ounce. Burp the infant halfway through feeding.
7. Watch continuously for circumoral or central cyanosis, indicating that the infant is not breathing when sucking. Stop feeding, suction with a bulb syringe, and stimulate the infant by rubbing his or her back. Continue feeding

when the infant has regained color. Place the infant on his or her right side with a rolled diaper behind the back after feeding, or elevate head of bed slightly.
8. Complete gestational age assessment.
9. Prepare for transfer from radiant warmer to crib. Place clothing and blankets under the warmer to heat. Take last set of vital signs, dress, apply hat, wrap in two warmed blankets. Complete charting.
10. Give report if another nurse is taking over care of the infant. Include gravida, para, length of labor, medications/anesthesia used in labor and delivery, time of rupture of membranes, any complications during birth, any problems in early hours, feeding, voids and stools, and any other pertinent information.

## The Newborn: Continued Care

### Text to Prepare You for Clinical Practice

Procedure 21–3: Identifying infants
Parents Want to Know: Caring for the uncircumcised penis
Parents Want to Know: How to care for the circumcision site

### New Terms

Erythema toxicum
Hypoglycemia
Nonshivering thermogenesis

### Equipment and Supplies

Stethoscope
Thermometer
Alcohol wipes

### Normal Assessments

**Vital Signs**

*Temperature*

a. Axillary—36.5 to 37.5°C (97.7 to 99.5°F)
b. Rectal—36.5 to 37.6°C (97.7 to 99.7°F)

*Heart Rate.* 120 to 160 beats/minute

*Respirations.* 30 to 60 breaths/minute. 30 to 40 breaths/minute average

***Blood Glucose.*** Above 45 mg/dl by screening tests or above 40 mg/dl by laboratory analysis

### Nursing Care

Assess and care for infants using the following list as a guide. Keep in mind that the role of the nurse is to continue to observe for abnormalities and complications, as well as to assess progress of mother-infant bonding and the mother's ability to care for the infant.

### Assessments

1. *Vital signs.* Assess vital signs once every 8 hours and more often if there are any abnormalities. Begin with respirations and pulse before disturbing the infant, if asleep. Temperature should be stable after the first day, and action is needed if it is not. Continue to listen for abnormal heart sounds. Murmurs heard earlier may disappear after the first day as transition to neonatal circulation becomes complete. Note acrocyanosis or central cyanosis. Listen to breath sounds, which should be clear.
2. *Weight.* Weigh infants daily at the same time of day according to agency routine.
3. *Neurologic.* Note state of alertness (six stages), movement of extremities, and reflexes (especially Moro, rooting, suck). Observe the eyes for signs of inflammation (redness, drainage); may be due to reaction to eye medication or infection. Cleanse drainage with sterile water from inner to outer canthus, being certain no drainage from one eye contaminates the other. Watch for signs of hypoglycemia ("jitteriness," tremors). Check fontanelle with the infant in an upright position. It should be soft and flat. *Report fullness, bulging, depression.*
4. *Skin.* Assess all skin areas to observe for new marks or changes in existing ones. Compare with previous assessments. Expect skin to be dry and peeling. Look for redness, scratches (keep hands covered), rashes, signs of skin breakdown, or infection. Erythema toxicum may become more apparent. Caput succedaneum may resolve as early as 12 hours or may take several days. Cephalhematoma resolves in several weeks. Physiologic jaundice may begin to develop after the first 24 hours. Blanch skin over nose and bony prominences, and note color. Check cord and base of cord for redness, foul odor, and serosanguinous or purulent drainage. Note how well cord is drying. Remove clamp when end of cord is dry and crisp (about 24 hours).
5. *Musculoskeletal.* Note movement of extremities and muscle tone. The infant should resist when extremities are extended. Note stiffness, arching of the infant's back, or molding of the infant to the caregiver's body.
6. *Gastrointestinal.* Abdomen should be soft and bowel sounds present. Observe part of feeding if the mother is doing all feedings. Assess for suck and swallow coordination, choking, length

of time feeding lasts, amount taken, and any regurgitation. Ask the mother how she feels the feedings are going. Note type and number of stools. Know whether the infant has had stool on present shift and when last stool occurred. (First stool is generally within 24 hours of birth, usually sooner.)

7. *Genitourinary.* Note number of voidings, color of urine on diaper. Know whether the infant has voided on present shift and when last voiding occurred. Teach parents to expect the infant to have at least two to six wet diapers per day during the first 2 days of life and six to 10 wet diapers per day thereafter. (First voiding should occur within 24 hours, usually sooner.) Observe circumcision site for drainage (purulent, serous, sanguinous—frank bleeding or oozing). Determine if the infant is voiding after circumcision is performed.
8. *Bonding.* Observe bonding behaviors in the mother and infant. Note how the mother holds the infant, whether she talks to the infant, calls the infant by name, and the like. Note response of the infant to the mother's care.
9. *Teaching.* Assess in which areas the mother (or the parents) need teaching.

### Interventions

The following care of the infant is typical for every shift. In addition, make rounds frequently (at least every hour) to monitor the progress of the mother in infant care and to determine the need for further interventions.

1. *Cord care.* Apply alcohol to the cord once or more each shift, according to agency routine. Use an alcohol wipe or an applicator dipped in alcohol. Cleanse all parts of the cord and the crevices of the umbilicus. Do not apply alcohol to the skin around the cord because this is drying to the skin. Some units use "triple dye" or other bactericidal agents once daily.
2. *Care of circumcision site.* Assess the parent's knowledge of care of the circumcision site, and teach as necessary. If a Plastibell was used, no special care is necessary other than observation for complications. If a Gomco clamp was used, instruct parents to squeeze petroleum jelly liberally over the circumcision site (and apply gauze if part of agency routine) at each diaper change for the first 24 hours. Assess incision throughout the shift for redness, edema, purulent or sanguinous drainage, and odor.
3. *Identification.* If the mother and infant are separated at any time, use the proper identification process each time the infant is reunited with the mother.
4. *Protection.* Maintain vigilance against kidnappers at all times. Follow methods to provide for infant security.
5. *Feedings.* Determine if the infant is taking feedings adequately (every 2 to 3 hours if breastfed, every 4 hours if formula fed). Record each feeding with type, amount (or how long the infant nursed at each breast), how feedings are taken, and any regurgitation. Teach the parents as necessary.
6. *Elimination.* Record each wet diaper and stool. Note color, amount, consistency.
7. *Continue observation.* Observe for problems throughout the shift.
8. *Continue teaching.* Teach parents as needed along with the "scheduled" teaching that is part of the plan made at the beginning of the shift.

## Assisting the Inexperienced Breastfeeding Mother

### Text to Prepare You for Clinical Practice

Figure 22–3: Cradle hold
Figure 22–4: Football hold
Figure 22–5: Side-lying position
Figure 22–6: C position of hand on breast
Mothers Want to Know: Is my baby getting enough milk?
Mothers Want to Know: Solutions to common breastfeeding problems
Mothers Want to Know: Breastfeeding after the birth of more than one infant
Mothers Want to Know: How to wean from breastfeeding
Table 22–3: The LATCH Scoring Tool

### New Terms

Latch-on
Non-nutritive suckling or sucking
Nutritive suckling or sucking

### Normal Assessments

1. The infant is positioned facing the breast, and the infant's body is well supported.
2. The mother is comfortable and holds her breast so that the infant can take it into the mouth without interference.
3. The infant's mouth covers the nipple and as much of the areola as possible.
4. Suckling includes audible swallowing.

## Nursing Care

This is a summary of information that nurses can use to help the inexperienced mother, especially during the first breastfeeding sessions.

### Assessments

1. Assess the mother's knowledge about breastfeeding techniques.
2. Assess the mother's breasts to identify engorgement, flat or inverted nipples, or nipple trauma.
3. Assess the infant's behavior state, sucking reflex, and coordination of sucking and swallowing.

### Interventions

1. Plan with the mother when the infant will be fed, and note any questions or concerns that she has about breastfeeding. Be sure that she is comfortable (e.g., pain relief needs met) and not in the middle of other care (A.M. care, meals). However, if the infant must eat immediately because of concerns about hypoglycemia, meet the mother's needs quickly or postpone care.
2. Explain that breastfeeding is a learned skill for both the mother and the infant and that practice is required to perfect the skill.
3. Begin the feeding when the infant is awake and showing signs of hunger. Do not wait until the infant is ravenously hungry and upset.
4. Assist the mother to position herself and the infant. Use pillows or blankets for comfort, to protect an abdominal incision, and to raise the infant to nipple level.
   a. Sitting. Place the bed in a high Fowler's position. Position a pillow behind the mother's back and under her elbow to support her arm.
   b. Cradle hold. Place the infant in the mother's arms, with the head at the antecubital space (or at nipple level) and the mother's arm extending along the infant's body. The mother's other hand positions the breast. The infant should be totally on the side facing the breast so that no turning of the head is necessary.
   c. Football hold. Place the infant's head in the mother's hand, with the body along her side.
   d. Side-lying. Place pillows behind the mother's back and between her legs. Her lower arm may go under her head or around the infant, while her upper hand positions the breast. Place the infant on the side facing the breast, using pillows to pad siderails and to maintain position.
5. Demonstrate proper hand position, with the hand cupped around the breast, thumb on top, and fingers supporting the breast below. Keep the fingers and thumb behind the areola.
6. Elicit latch-on. Brush the nipple against the center of the infant's lower lip until the infant opens the mouth wide. Bring the infant toward the breast while inserting the nipple and as much of the areola as possible into the infant's mouth.
7. Assess the mouth position. The infant's lips should be 1 to 1 1/2 inches from the base of the nipple with the lips flared. Remove the infant from the breast and start over if dimpling of cheeks, clicking, or smacking sounds occur.
8. Assess the infant's suck. Nutritive suckling is smooth and continuous with occasional pauses. A swallow follows every one to three sucks and has a "ka" or "ah" sound. Non-nutritive suckling is choppy with no swallowing. When swallowing stops, remove the infant from the breast and burp, change sides, awaken, or let sleep if feeding is finished. Do not jiggle the breast in the infant's mouth to stimulate suckling or the infant may lose the grip and chew on the nipple.
9. Demonstrate removal from the breast. Have the mother insert a finger into the corner of the infant's mouth between the gums to release suction. Remove the infant immediately.
10. Instruct the mother to nurse an average of at least 15 minutes per feeding to begin, increasing as the infant shows interest. Burp the infant between breasts. Instruct her to nurse every 2 to 3 hours during the day and at least every 4 hours throughout the night to build the milk supply.
11. Observe the mother at intervals after the feeding begins. Help her switch sides to observe for difficulty. Then observe the mother at other feedings to give reinforcement and correct technique as needed. Offer praise generously because feeding the infant may affect the mother's view of her mothering abilities.

# Appendix E

# Answers to Check Your Reading

## Chapter 1

1. Federal involvement and consumer demands created change in maternity care in the last 4 decades.
2. Family-centered maternity care provides safe, quality care that adapts to both the physical and the psychological needs of the entire family during reproduction and greatly increases the responsibilities of nurses providing care.
3. Birthing centers provide professional care during pregnancy and childbirth in a home-like environment for women with low-risk pregnancies. They are associated with a nearby hospital, to which the woman can be moved in case of unexpected complications. The home setting, although providing comfort and closeness, may not have adequate equipment to handle unexpected developments.
4. Cost-containment strategies have shortened the length of stay in the birth facility of mothers and their infants. This has created concern for nurses, who must provide information for parents in a very short time.
5. Clinical pathways are guidelines that define expected outcomes for clients, including the length of stay and the time and sequence of interventions that will accomplish the outcomes.
6. A variety of standards guide home care. These include agency and organizational standards that spell out the preparation and responsibilities of nurses. Legal standards define the scope of practice, and other regulatory bodies, such as OSHA, CDC, and FDA, provide guidelines. Accrediting agencies, such as JCAHO and CHAP, give their stamp of approval when standards reach a certain level.
7. Traditional families are headed by a man and a woman, usually married, who view parenting as the major priority in their lives and whose energies are not depleted by poverty, illness, or substance abuse. Nontraditional families are defined by their unique structure and include single-parent families, blended families, extended families, homosexual families, and adoptive families.
8. Families may be identified as "high risk" if they are below the poverty level; headed by a single teenaged parent; have a preterm, ill, or disabled infant; or have lifestyle problems, such as substance abuse or family violence.
9. A healthy family can adapt, without undue stress, to the changes precipitated by childbirth. Members communicate openly, volunteer assistance, and agree on basic principles of child care.
10. Factors that interfere with family functioning are lack of family resources, absence of adequate family support, birth of an infant who requires specialized care, unhealthy habits (smoking, substance abuse), and the inability to make mature decisions.
11. Nurses should examine their own cultural values and beliefs to determine ways that their beliefs may generate conflict with those who hold different cultural beliefs.
12. Differences in language create the greatest difficulty; however, differences in style add to potential conflicts.
13. Culture is difficult to understand because, like an iceberg, only the tip (behavior) shows. Reasons for the behavior (e.g., religious beliefs, moral values) are hidden like the submerged part of an iceberg and require serious study.
14. The infant mortality rate is lower today than at the beginning of the 20th century because of improved health of the population, application of basic principles of sanitation, increase in medical knowledge, widespread availability of antibiotics, and improved prenatal care.
15. The higher incidence of poverty among African-American families is associated with inadequate prenatal care and the birth of low-birth-weight infants who are less likely to survive than white children.
16. The infant mortality rate in the United States

ranks 21st in the world. Japan, Switzerland, and Canada all have lower infant mortality rates.

## Chapter 2

1. Therapeutic communication is purposeful, goal-directed, and focused.
2. Major communication techniques include clarifying, paraphrasing, reflecting, silence, structuring, pinpointing, questioning, directing, and summarizing.
3. Major blocks to communication are conveying a lack of interest or haste, closed posture, interrupting, providing false reassurance, inappropriate self-disclosure, giving advice, and failure to acknowledge comments or feelings.
4. Major principles of teaching and learning include readiness to learn, participation, repetition, positive feedback, and acknowledgment of frustration. Effective methods include role modeling, presenting simple tasks before more complex material, and using a variety of teaching methods.
5. Factors that affect learning include developmental level, language, culture, previous experience, environment, and the skill of the instructor.
6. The purpose of critical thinking is to identify and overcome habits or impulses that result in poor decisions or inappropriate actions and to make the best clinical judgments.
7. Steps that may be helpful in learning critical thinking include a recognition of assumptions, an examination of personal biases, an analysis of pressure one feels for closure, an examination of how one collects and analyzes data, and an evaluation of how emotions may interfere with ability to think critically.
8. Reflective skepticism means to suspend judgment to avoid making decisions in haste or with insufficient data.
9. The data base assessment gathers information about all aspects of the woman's health. A focus assessment gathers information about an actual health problem.
10. Actual nursing diagnoses reflect health problems that can be validated by the presence of defining characteristics. At-risk nursing diagnoses indicate that risk factors are present that make the client vulnerable to the development of a particular problem.
11. Goals and outcomes should be stated in terms of the client, they should be observable and measurable, they must have a time frame, and they should be realistic.
12. Nursing interventions that are not specific and do not spell out clearly exactly what is to be done are difficult to implement. Clearly written interventions that provide detailed instructions correct the problem.
13. Nursing diagnoses describe health problems that nurses can treat independently and for which they are legally responsible. Collaborative problems are potential complications that require physician-prescribed as well as nursing-prescribed interventions.
14. Client-centered goals are inappropriate for collaborative problems because client-centered goals imply accountability for problems that nurses cannot manage independently.

## Chapter 3

1. Ethics examines conduct and distinctions between right and wrong. Bioethics applies only to the ethics of health care.
2. Deontologic ethical theory applies ethical principles to determine what is right. It does not vary the solution according to individual situations. Utilitarian theory analyzes the benefits and burdens to determine a course of action that provides the greatest amount of good in a given situation.
3. Ethical principles may conflict when applying one principle may violate another.
4. *Assessment* is used to gather data from all concerned persons. Ethical theories and principles are *analyzed* to determine if an ethical dilemma exists. *Planning* involves identifying as many options as possible and choosing a solution. *Interventions* must be identified to implement the chosen solution, and the results are *evaluated*.
5. The Supreme Court decision in *Roe v. Wade* declared that abortion was legal anywhere in the United States and that existing state laws prohibiting abortion were unconstitutional because they interfered with a woman's right to privacy.
6. The belief that abortion is a private choice conflicts with the belief that abortion is taking a life.
7. States cannot give a husband veto power over his spouse's decision to have an abortion; states do not have an obligation to pay for abortions; physicians are given broad discretion to determine fetal viability; states may restrict abortions of viable fetuses. In addition, states may require parental consent for minors to obtain abortion as long as an alternative (judge's approval) is available; states may require a woman to wait 24 hours before seeking

and obtaining an abortion; states may not require a married woman to inform her husband before obtaining an abortion.

8. At the time they are hired, nurses must disclose their feelings about caring for women having an abortion.
9. Punitive approaches are against the principle of autonomy, bodily integrity, and personal freedom. The resulting fear may jeopardize the health care of pregnant women who may avoid seeking prenatal care.
10. Problems involved in the use of advanced reproductive techniques include high cost, low success rate, limitation to the affluent, control of unused embryos, and problem pregnancy outcomes.
11. Poverty is the underlying factor that causes many other problems, such as inadequate access to health care. The lack of access to health care is a major reason for the large number of low-birth-weight infants and the high infant mortality rate.
12. The focus has been on treatment and cure of illness, often with expensive technology. However, prevention is less expensive and provides care for greater numbers.
13. Standards of care and agency policies influence judgment about malpractice because they describe the level of care that can be expected from practitioners.
14. Negligence is failure to perform the way a reasonable and prudent person of similar background would act in a like situation. Malpractice is negligence by professionals (including nurses) in the performance of their duties.
15. Nurses can help to prevent malpractice claims by following guidelines for informed consent, refusal of care, and documentation; by acting as client advocates; and by maintaining their level of expertise.
16. Concerns about the use of unlicensed assistive personnel include whether this use compromises the quality of care and the nurse's ability to supervise unlicensed personnel adequately with increased workloads.
17. Early discharge leads to concerns about the woman's ability to care for herself and her infant, complications that may develop that new parents may not identify, and the fact that parents will not have had time to take in the teaching needed.

## Chapter 4

1. Development of the breasts is the first sign of puberty in girls. In boys, growth of the testes is the first sign, followed by growth of the penis about a year later.
2. Usually, Asians and Native Americans have less and finer body hair than either whites or African-Americans. African-Americans usually have body hair that is coarser and curlier than Asians, Native Americans, or whites.
3. The female pelvis has a wide, rounded basin shape that favors efficient passage of the fetus during birth. The male pelvis is heavier, narrower, and structurally suited for tasks requiring load bearing.
4. Males generally attain a greater adult height than females because they begin their growth spurt about 1 year later than girls and continue growing for a longer period of time.
5. The female's secondary sex characteristics include round hips and breasts and growth of pubic hair, finer skin texture, and a higher-pitched voice. Male secondary sex characteristics include the presence of facial and pubic hair, a deeper voice, broader shoulders, and a greater muscle mass.
6. The female external reproductive organs are collectively called the vulva. The labia majora extend from the mons pubis to the perineum. The labia minora are within and parallel to the labia majora. The clitoris is at the anterior junction of the labia minora. The urinary meatus and vaginal introitus are found within the vestibule (the area enclosed by the labia minora). The hymen partly closes the vaginal opening. The perineum extends from the fourchette (posterior rim of the vaginal opening) to the anus.
7. The three divisions of the uterus are the corpus (body), isthmus, and cervix (neck). The fundus is the part of the corpus that lies above the entry points of the fallopian tubes.
8. Myometrium is the middle layer of thick uterine muscle, between the perimetrium and the endometrium. The myometrium has three types of muscle fibers within it: (1) longitudinal fibers, mostly in the fundus, to expel the fetus during birth; (2) interlacing figure-8 fibers to compress bleeding blood vessels after birth; and (3) circular fibers to provide constrictions near the fallopian tubes and the internal cervical os, enabling the proper implantation of the fertilized ovum and preventing the reflux of menstrual blood into the tubes.
9. The fallopian tubes are lined with cells that have cilia that beat rhythmically toward the uterine cavity to propel the ovum through the fallopian tube. The fertilized ovum undergoes its early cell divisions in the fallopian tube so that implantation is most likely to occur in the uterine fundus.

10. The two functions of the ovaries are to produce hormones (primarily estrogen and progesterone) and to mature on ovum for release during each reproductive cycle.
11. The pelvis is located at the lower end of the spine. The true pelvis is the part that is located below the linea terminalis. The true pelvis is the most relevant during birth.
12. Pelvic muscles and ligaments enclose the lower pelvis and support internal reproductive, urinary, and bowel structures.
13. The ripening follicle secretes estrogen. After ovulation, the follicle (now called the corpus luteum) secretes large amounts of estrogen and progesterone.
14. Three ovarian phases of the female reproductive cycle are the follicular (maturation of an ovum), ovulatory (release of the mature ovum), and luteal (secretion of estrogen and progesterone by the corpus luteum). There is greater variation among women in the length of the follicular phase than of the other two phases.
15. The three phases are the proliferative, the secretory, and the menstrual. The proliferative phase occurs during the first half of the cycle and is when the endometrium becomes thicker in preparation for a fertilized ovum. The secretory phase occurs during the last half of the cycle and is characterized by continued growth of the endometrium, growth of blood vessels and glands, and secretion of substances to nourish a fertilized ovum. If pregnancy does not occur, the endometrium becomes ischemic and necrotic as secretion of estrogen and progesterone from the corpus luteum falls. The old endometrium is shed in the menstrual phase.
16. The cervical mucus becomes thin, clear, and elastic during ovulation to facilitate entrance of sperm from the vagina into the uterus and fallopian tube, thus enhancing the chances for conception.
17. Montgomery's tubercles secrete a substance during pregnancy and lactation that keeps the nipples soft.
18. A woman's breast size is not related to the amount of milk she can produce. It is influenced by the amount of fatty tissue in the breast.
19. Milk secretion does not occur during pregnancy because estrogen and progesterone produced by the placenta inhibit its production.
20. As a urinary organ, the penis transports urine from the bladder to outside the body during urination. As an organ of reproduction, it carries and deposits the semen into the vagina during coitus.
21. The two types of erectile tissue in the penis are the corpus spongiosum that surrounds the urethra and the two columns of corpus cavernosum tissue on each side of the penis. The function of erectile tissue is to facilitate entry of the penis into the female's vagina.
22. The scrotum holds the testes away from the body to keep them cooler than the core body temperature, thus facilitating sperm production.
23. The testes function as endocrine glands, producing testosterone, and produce the male gametes (spermatozoa).

## Chapter 5

1. DNA is the building block of genes. A varying number of genes, in turn, make up each chromosome.
2. Genes are too small to be seen under a microscope. They can be studied by analyzing the products they instruct cells to produce, by direct study of the DNA, or by their close association with another gene that can be studied more easily.
3. Chromosomes can be seen under a microscope when living nucleated cells are dividing. They may be photographed under the microscope and the resulting picture of chromosomes arranged in a karyotype. Fluorescent in situ hybridization (FISH) is a newer technique that uses DNA probes to identify numerical chromosomal abnormalities.
4. 46,XY is an abbreviation that describes the chromosome makeup of a normal human male. 46,XX describes the chromosomes of a normal human female.
5. The child of a parent who has an autosomal dominant disorder has a 50 percent chance of having the same disorder.
6. Blood relationship (consanguinity) of parents increases the likelihood that both share some of the same harmful autosomal recessive genes, increasing the chance that their offspring will be affected with a disorder.
7. If both parents carry an abnormal gene for an autosomal recessive disorder, each of their children has a 25 percent chance of receiving both copies of the defective gene and having the disorder. Each child also has a 50 percent chance of receiving only one copy of the defective gene, thus being a carrier like the parents. Each child also has a 25 percent chance of receiving the normal gene from each parent, thus being neither a carrier nor affected.
8. Males are more likely to have X-linked recessive disorders because they do not have a

compensating X chromosome that has a normal gene. Each son of a female carrier has a 50 percent chance of having the trait and a 50 percent chance of being unaffected. Each daughter of the female carrier has a 50 percent chance of being a carrier and a 50 percent chance of being unaffected.

9. A trisomy exists when each body cell contains an extra copy of one chromosome. Down syndrome is the most common trisomy and involves three copies of chromosome 21 for a total of 47 chromosomes in each cell.
10. A monosomy exists when each body cell is missing a chromosome. Turner's syndrome (a female with a single X chromosome) is the only monosomy compatible with postnatal life.
11. Genetic material can be lost or duplicated when a chromosome has a structural abnormality. Also, the position of genes on the chromosome may be altered, preventing them from functioning normally.
12. A parent with a balanced chromosomal translocation may have a child with completely normal chromosomes, or the child may have a balanced chromosomal translocation similar to that of the parent. The offspring may also receive an unbalanced amount of chromosomal material (too much or too little), which often results in spontaneous abortion or birth defects.
13. Multifactorial disorders are typically present and detectable at birth. They are usually isolated defects rather than being present with other unrelated defects. However, sometimes the primary multifactorial defect alters further development and results in other related defects.
14. Factors that may affect the likelihood that a multifactorial disorder will occur or recur include the following:
    a. The number of affected close relatives.
    b. The severity of the defect in those affected.
    c. The sex of the affected person.
    d. Geographic location.
    e. Seasonal variations.
15. The woman may be able to avoid exposing her fetus to teratogens by immunization against infections such as rubella, eliminating the use of nontherapeutic drugs such as alcohol or illicit drugs, changing therapeutic drugs to those having a lower risk to the fetus, and avoiding x-rays at a time when she may be pregnant.
16. A pregnant woman who has phenylketonuria (PKU) should return to her low-phenylalanine diet when she is pregnant to avoid buildup of toxic products that would damage her developing baby.

## Chapter 6

1. Meiosis is a type of cell division that halves the number of chromosomes so that only one of each chromosomal pair goes into each gamete. Meiosis also promotes genetic variation by the process of crossing over, or exchange of chromosomal material between each member of the pair of chromosomes. The union of male and female gametes at conception restores the number of chromosomes to 46 in the offspring.
2. One mature ovum results from two meiotic divisions of the oogonium. The first meiotic division begins in fetal life and is not completed until shortly before that ovum is ovulated. The second meiotic division begins at ovulation but is not completed unless fertilization occurs.
3. Each spermatogonium undergoes two meiotic divisions to result in four mature spermatozoa. Meiosis begins at puberty and both meiotic divisions are completed before the sperm mature and are ejaculated.
4. Fertilization usually occurs in the distal one third of the fallopian tube, near the ovary.
5. Seminal fluid nourishes and protects the sperm from the acidic environment of the woman's vagina.
6. As sperm approach the ovum, they secrete hyaluronidase to digest a pathway through the corona radiata and zona pellucida. When one spermatozoon finally penetrates the ovum, changes in the zona pellucida prevent other spermatozoa from entering. The ovum also completes its second meiotic division.
7. Fertilization is complete when the nuclei of the ovum and spermatozoon unite.
8. Implantation begins 6 days after conception and is complete by the 10th day.
9. The fundus, or upper uterus, is the ideal location for implantation for three reasons. It has a rich blood supply for fetal gas exchange and nutrition. The thick uterine lining prevents the placenta from attaching too deeply. The strong interlacing muscle fibers in the fundus contract to limit blood loss after birth.
10. Nutritive fluids produced in the thick decidua pass to the conceptus by diffusion before a placental circulation is established. Primary chorionic villi (which will form the fetal side of the placenta) extend from the conceptus into the decidua basalis (which will become the maternal side of the placenta) to tap these nutrients.
11. During the first 8 weeks after conception, all major organ systems develop. The woman may be unaware that she is pregnant and may ex-

pose the embryo to harmful substances inadvertently.

12. At 4 weeks, the trachea develops as a bud of the upper digestive tract and branches into the two bronchi. The main bronchi branch to form the three lobes of the right lung and the two lobes of the left. Branching continues until terminal air sacs develop.
13. The intestines are contained mostly within the umbilical cord until 10 weeks because they grow more rapidly than the abdominal cavity and because the liver and kidneys are relatively large. By 10 weeks, the abdominal cavity has caught up with the growth of its contents and can accommodate them.
14. Vernix caseosa protects fetal skin from constant exposure to amniotic fluid. Lanugo helps vernix adhere to the skin. Brown fat helps the infant maintain temperature stability in the cooler external environment. Surfactant keeps the lung alveoli from collapsing with each expiration, thus making breathing easier after birth.
15. The fetus usually assumes a head-down position because this position fits the egg shape of the uterus best. Also, the head is heavier and tends to go downward with gravity in the pool of amniotic fluid.
16. Gestational age is calculated from the woman's last menstrual period and is about 2 weeks longer than fertilization age. Gestational age is most commonly used because the menstrual period provides a specific marker.
17. The placenta gradually takes over the function of the corpus luteum and secretes estrogen and progesterone.
18. Exchange of oxygen, nutrients, and waste products between the woman and the fetus takes place in the intervillous spaces of the placenta.
19. Maternal and fetal blood may be of incompatible blood types and thus should not mix.
20. The fetus can thrive in a relatively low-oxygen environment because of the following:
    a. Fetal hemoglobin carries more oxygen than adult hemoglobin.
    b. The fetus has a higher hemoglobin and hematocrit level than does the newborn or adult.
    c. Rapid diffusion of carbon dioxide into the maternal blood causes her to give up oxygen more readily and causes oxygen to combine with fetal blood more readily.
21. Human chorionic gonadotropin (hCG) causes the corpus luteum of the ovary to persist and secrete estrogens and progesterones, which are essential to maintain the uterine lining for implantation. It also facilitates fetal testosterone secretion in the male fetus. Human placental lactogen promotes normal fetal nutrition and growth and maternal breast development. Estrogens cause enlargement of the woman's uterus and genitalia and enlargement and development of the breasts. Progesterone changes the endometrium into the decidua to nourish the conceptus and reduces uterine contractions to prevent spontaneous abortion. Progesterone also facilitates growth and development of the mother's breasts and the cells that will secrete milk.
22. The fetal membranes contain the amniotic fluid, which cushions the fetus, maintains a stable temperature, and promotes normal prenatal structural development.
23. Oxygenated blood enters the fetus through the umbilical vein. Half the blood goes to the liver, and the rest passes through the ductus venosus to the inferior vena cava. Blood enters the right atrium, where a small amount goes to the right ventricle and the rest goes through the foramen ovale to the left atrium and then to the left ventricle. Some blood from the right ventricle goes to the lungs, and the rest goes through the ductus arteriosus, where it joins blood ejected from the left ventricle. After circulation through the body, deoxygenated blood returns to the placenta through the two umbilical arteries.
24. Monozygotic twins occur when one spermatozoon fertilizes one ovum and the resulting conceptus later divides into two inner cell masses that will become two fetuses.
25. The placentas and chorions may fuse before birth, making it difficult to determine if the twins are monozygotic or dizygotic.
26. Dizygotic twins develop from two ova that are each fertilized by a spermatozoon and are like other siblings in a family.

## Chapter 7

1. Uterine growth has generally reached the level of the umbilicus by 20 weeks' gestation; at 36 weeks, the uterus extends to the xiphoid process, the highest level of uterine growth.
2. In early pregnancy, most of the blood flow to the uterus is to the endometrium and myometrium. As pregnancy progresses, there is an increase in blood flow into intervillous spaces of the placenta, where oxygen and nutrients are transferred through the chorionic villi and carried to the fetus.
3. The major purpose of progesterone in early pregnancy is to maintain the pregnancy.

4. The cervical mucus plug blocks ascent of bacteria from the vagina into the uterus, thereby protecting the membranes and fetus from infection.
5. During pregnancy the breasts enlarge and become more vascular; the areola increases in size and becomes more pigmented; the nipples increase in size and become more erect.
6. Physiologic anemia of pregnancy is caused by a greater increase in plasma volume than in red blood cells, resulting in a dilution but not inadequate hemoglobin concentration. Iron deficiency anemia is due to inadequate hemoglobin concentration.
7. During pregnancy increased circulation through the kidneys is needed to remove metabolic wastes generated by the mother and fetus; increased circulation through the skin is necessary to dissipate heat that is generated by accelerated metabolism.
8. In a supine position, the weight of the gravid uterus on the vena cava and descending aorta impedes blood flow to and from the lower extremities, resulting in decreased cardiac output and a supine hypotensive syndrome.
9. It is important to standardize techniques for taking blood pressure because blood pressure in the pregnant woman is affected by position. It is lowest in a lateral recumbent position and highest when standing. Moreover, there is an increase when the arm is in a dependent position.
10. During pregnancy the ribs flare, the substernal angle widens, and the circumference of the chest increases.
11. Progesterone stimulates the minute volume by raising the sensitivity of the respiratory center to carbon dioxide and breathing becomes thoracic as the uterus lifts the diaphragm.
12. Estrogen causes hyperemia of the gums that may lead to bleeding or gingivitis. Excessive salivation (ptyalism) is a problem for some. Progesterone relaxes smooth muscle in the gastrointestinal tract, allowing additional time for nutrients to be absorbed but also resulting in some of the discomforts of pregnancy, such as heartburn and constipation.
13. Expectant mothers are at increased risk for urinary tract infection because of compression of the ureters between the uterus and the pelvic bones, resulting in dilation of the ureters and consequent stasis of urine, which allows prolonged time for bacterial growth.
14. Softening of pelvic ligaments and joints due to relaxin, a maternal hormone, creates instability and results in a wide stance and "waddling" gait. As the uterus increases in size, the woman must lean backward to maintain balance, which creates a progressive lordosis.
15. Progesterone maintains the uterine lining, prevents uterine contractions during pregnancy, and helps prepare the breasts for lactation.
16. Maternal hormones (human placental lactogen, estrogen, and progesterone) create increasing resistance of maternal tissues to insulin during the second and third trimesters. Moreover, insulinase speeds up the breakdown of insulin.
17. Presumptive signs are subjective, probable signs are objective; both can be caused by conditions other than pregnancy.
18. Many things such as gas, peristalsis, or pseudocyesis (false pregnancy) can be mistaken by the woman for fetal movement.
19. The most common causes of false-negative pregnancy tests are pregnancy tests performed too soon, or with other than the first urine of the day, urine that is too dilute, or urine that is allowed to stand for too long; impending spontaneous abortion; and tubal pregnancy.
20. A medical-surgical history as well as an obstetric history is necessary to identify chronic conditions or past trauma that can affect the outcome of the pregnancy.
21. Blood pressure should be obtained while the woman is sitting with the arm supported in a horizontal position at heart level. Documentation should include position as well as pressures obtained to maintain consistency.
22. There is a gradual, predictable increase in uterine size as gestation advances; from approximately 22 weeks until term, fundal height in centimeters is nearly equal to gestational age in weeks.
23. Major risk factors during pregnancy are age under 18 years, low socioeconomic status, preexisting medical disorders or infections, and use of substances such as alcohol, tobacco, or illicit drugs.
24. Antepartum visits should begin in first trimester, every 4 weeks until 28 weeks; every 2 to 3 weeks from 29 to 36 weeks, and weekly from 37 weeks to birth.
25. Maternal adaptation differs in multifetal pregnancies because increased blood volume results in additional work for the heart. The greatly increased size of the uterus intensifies mechanical effects, such as greater elevation of the diaphragm, and compression of the ureters and bowel.
26. Increased levels of placental hormones, such as estrogen, and hCG plus periodic hypoglycemia are believed to be responsible for "morning sickness."
27. Correct posture and body mechanics, plus ex-

ercises such as pelvic rocking can alleviate backache during pregnancy.

28. "Cultural negotiation" means acknowledging that the family may hold different views, being sensitive to special concerns, and providing information in an acceptable manner.

## Chapter 8

1. The fetus seems vague and unreal during the first trimester. Gradually, physical changes (uterine growth, weight gain, "quickening") confirm that a fetus is developing, and the expectant mother begins to perceive the fetus as a separate, though dependent being.
2. Sexual responses vary widely and depend on how the mother-to-be feels, her body image, and response of the expectant father to the physical changes of pregnancy.
3. The pregnant woman explores the role of mother to develop a sense of herself in the role and selects behaviors that confirm her sense of how she wants to fulfill the role.
4. The pregnant woman often experiences a temporary sense of sadness when she realizes that she must give up certain aspects of her previous self when she moves into the role of mother.
5. The pregnant woman seeks safe passage for herself and the baby when she seeks the care of a physician or nurse-midwife and follows recommendations about diet, vitamins, rest, and subsequent prenatal care.
6. Experiences that make the child more real are "reality boosters"; the most frequently mentioned are hearing the fetal heart tones, feeling the fetus move, and seeing the fetus via ultrasound.
7. Nurses can help men in their struggle for recognition as parents by viewing the mother/father/fetus as their clients and focusing on the father as well as the mother by encouraging the father's questions and including him in the plan of care.
8. Information about infant behaviors and care is more relevant and therefore more useful after the infant is born.
9. A number of factors shape the way grandparents respond to a grandchild, including their own ages, the number and spacing of other grandchildren, and how they perceive their role as grandparents.
10. Toddlers may feel threatened and abandoned when attention must be shared with an infant. They may revert to infantile behaviors to gain the attention of their parents. Preschoolers may like to be involved and to help prepare for the birth. Adolescents may be embarrassed by confirmation of their parents continued sexuality.
11. Parents can make any changes in sleeping arrangements several weeks before the infant is born so that the toddler does not feel displaced by the newborn. They can encourage family and friends to give as much time and attention to the child as they give to the infant, and they can reassure the child of their love and acceptance.
12. Priorities of the poor often focus on present needs, such as food and shelter, and less on preventive activities, such as prenatal care.
13. Many health care workers are unsympathetic to the plights of poor families, who experience long delays at health care facilities, hurried examinations, and rudeness from members of the health care team.
14. Cultural differences that cause conflict between health care workers and families during pregnancy occur most often in the areas of health care beliefs, communication, and time orientation.

## Chapter 9

1. Weight gain helps determine fetal growth. Too little may be associated with low birth weight, and too much with large infants.
2. The average woman should gain 25 to 35 pounds. Underweight women and those carrying more than one fetus should gain more, and overweight women should gain less.
3. The average woman should gain approximately 3 to 4 pounds the first trimester and 1 pound a week in the second and third trimesters.
4. A woman should eat 300 kcal more each day during pregnancy.
5. Sixty g of protein per day, an increase of 10 to 16 g above pre-pregnancy needs, is recommended during pregnancy.
6. Vitamins $B_6$, D, E, and folic acid are likely to be low in the diets of pregnant women.
7. Fat-soluble vitamins (A, D, E, and K) are stored in the fat and are available for longer periods than the water-soluble vitamins ($B_6$, $B_{12}$, folic acid, thiamin, riboflavin, niacin, and C), which must be replenished daily. Excessive intake of fat-soluble vitamins may cause toxicity.
8. Iron, calcium, zinc, and magnesium are often below the recommended amounts in the diets of pregnant women.
9. Excessive intake of vitamins and minerals may

result in toxicity and may interfere with use of other vitamins and minerals.

10. During pregnancy, a woman should drink eight to ten 8-ounce glasses daily, mostly water.
11. During pregnancy, the following servings from the food pyramid are recommended: whole grains: seven or more; fruits and vegetables: five or more (with one serving of vitamin A and one serving of vitamin C source); dairy products: three or more; protein: servings to equal 7 ounces; unsaturated fats: 3 teaspoons.
12. The nurse should consider traditional foods from the woman's culture, the degree to which she follows the traditional diet, and nontraditional foods she includes.
13. Both Southeast Asian and Latina women balance yin and yang or cold and hot food during pregnancy and may be low in calcium, iron, and vitamin D.
14. The nurse should assess for the woman's financial resources for food purchase, need for financial assistance, and education about nutrition.
15. The adolescent may skip meals, eat snacks and fast foods of low nutrient value, and experience peer pressure.
16. The vegan can include nonanimal sources of iron, calcium, and vitamin $B_{12}$ and combine incomplete protein foods to ensure intake of all essential amino acids.
17. Lactose-intolerant women can choose calcium-containing foods like leafy green vegetables, broccoli, corn tortillas, tofu, sunflower seeds, nuts, salmon, and sardines.
18. Other conditions that present nutritional risk factors during pregnancy are excessive nausea and vomiting, anemia, abnormal pre-pregnancy weight, eating disorders, pica, grand multiparity, substance abuse, closely spaced pregnancies, and multiple pregnancy.
19. The lactating woman needs more of most nutrients than the woman who is not pregnant. She needs 200 more calories and a little more protein and vitamin C than the pregnant woman.
20. The breastfeeding woman should avoid alcohol, caffeine, and foods that seem to cause distress in the infant.
21. The woman who is not breastfeeding should decrease calories by 300 daily, continue to eat a well-balanced diet, and plan to lose extra weight slowly.

## Chapter 10

1. Major reasons for ultrasonography during the first trimester are to confirm pregnancy, locate the fetus, determine multifetal pregnancy, confirm fetal viability, and locate the best area for chorionic villus sampling (CVS). Indications during the second and third trimesters are to confirm gestational maturity, locate the placenta, determine fetal presentation, perform biophysical profile, guide needle placement for amniocentesis and cordocentesis, and evaluate fetal anatomy and physiology.
2. Transvaginal ultrasonography is most often performed during the first trimester when the uterus lies within the pelvis. A transabdominal procedure is more common during the second and third trimesters when the uterus is above the pelvic brim and the contents are clearly visible.
3. Major advantages of ultrasonography are that it allows clear visualization of the fetus and surrounding structures; it is safe, noninvasive, and relatively comfortable; and the results are available immediately. The major disadvantage is the cost.
4. Maternal serum alpha-fetoprotein (MSAFP) must be viewed as the first step in a series of diagnostic procedures that are offered if abnormal concentrations are found.
5. Elevated AFP indicates open neural tube defects, esophageal obstruction, abdominal wall defects, or undetected fetal demise. Additional causes include multiple gestation, inaccurate fetal age, and threatened abortion.
6. Low levels of AFP suggest chromosomal abnormalities or inaccurate gestational age.
7. Triple marker screening determines maternal serum levels of AFP, human chorionic gonadotropin, and unconjugated estriols. Low levels of all three more accurately predict chromosomal abnormalities than level of AFP alone.
8. Chorionic villus sampling is performed in the first trimester, and results are available in 24 to 48 hours. Obtaining information about fetal anomalies this early in the pregnancy allows the woman to make a decision about pregnancy termination before the second trimester.
9. Pregnancy loss is slightly higher following CVS than following amniocentesis. Additional risks for CVS before 12 weeks include limb reduction defect.
10. Amniocentesis is most often performed to detect chromosomal abnormalities. Additional indications include investigating abnormal levels of MSAFP, determining fetal lung maturity, and testing for fetal hemolytic disease.
11. Fetal lung maturity is confirmed by a 2:1 ratio of lecithin/sphingomyelin and by the presence of other lipoproteins, such as phosphatidylglyc-

erol (PG), and phosphatidylinositol (PI), which make up pulmonary surfactant.

12. Bilirubin is a waste product of red blood cell destruction and thus indicates the degree of compromise in an Rh-positive fetus whose mother is Rh-sensitized.
13. Early amniocentesis has the same advantages as CVS; information is available early in the pregnancy, which allows parents to make decisions about the pregnancy as early as possible.
14. A nonstress test measures acceleration, or lack of acceleration, of the fetal heart in response to fetal movement. Acceleration provides reassurance of fetal health. It is so named because the fetus is not challenged or stressed to obtain data.
15. In a vibroacoustic stimulation test, a false larynx is used to stimulate fetal movement. Otherwise, the procedure and interpretation are the same as those in a nonstress test.
16. A contraction stress test (CST) indicates how the fetus responds to periodic hypoxia that occurs as a result of uterine contractions. Contractions are initiated by intravenous administration of oxytocin. As contractions compress the placental arterioles that supply oxygen to the fetus, there is a recurrent decrease in fetal oxygen levels.
17. Late decelerations in a CST indicate fetal oxygen reserves are inadequate to tolerate contractions and fetal acidosis or myocardial depression or both may result.
18. Loss of fetal tone in a biophysical profile indicates advanced hypoxia and fetal acidosis.
19. Decreased amniotic fluid volume is associated with chronic fetal hypoxia, when blood is shunted away from the fetal lungs and kidneys, which produce amniotic fluid, and toward vital organs, such as the fetal heart and brain.

## Chapter 11

1. The goals of perinatal education are to help women and their support persons become knowledgeable consumers and active participants in pregnancy and childbirth.
2. Women must choose a health care professional, birth setting, support persons and techniques for labor, and type of education for preparation (if any).
3. Early pregnancy classes emphasize adapting to pregnancy, coping with common discomforts, and learning what to expect in later pregnancy. Later classes discuss preparation for childbirth, the postpartum period, breastfeeding, and parenting concerns.
4. The chance that a couple may experience cesarean birth is more than 20 percent. Therefore, all women need to know about cesarean birth.
5. Classes for family members help ease family transition by providing information and opportunity for discussing common feelings.
6. Education, relaxation, and conditioning reduce pain and increase coping ability for childbirth by helping to decrease muscle and mental tension.
7. Cutaneous stimulation and imagery help reduce pain by sending other messages to the brain so that pain messages are not recognized as strongly and perception of pain is reduced.
8. Breathing techniques are used to enhance relaxation during labor.
9. A support person during labor increases a woman's satisfaction by helping her deal with stress, focus on her learned techniques, and feel that her experience is being shared.
10. Support roles include active assistance with coaching techniques, verbal encouragement, minimal physical assistance, or being present without active involvement.
11. Specific techniques used by support persons during labor include assisting with relaxation, breathing, encouragement, sacral pressure, massage, and comfort measures.

## Chapter 12

1. Effacement and dilation of the cervix occur because contractions pull the cervix upward over the fetus and amniotic sac and, at the same time, push the fetus and amniotic sac downward against the cervix. The muscle fibers of the upper uterus become shorter to maintain these forces between contractions. In addition, the uterus changes shape, becoming more elongated and narrow, to maintain pressure of the fetus and amniotic sac against the cervix.
2. The cervix of the nullipara effaces more before it dilates. The multipara's cervix is usually thicker than a nullipara's during all of labor.
3. Maternal changes that occur during labor include the following:
   a. Cardiovascular system: Slight increase in blood pressure and decrease in pulse rate as each contraction temporarily stops blood flow to her uterus. Supine hypotension may occur if she lies on her back because the heavy uterus compresses her inferior vena cava and reduces blood flow to her heart.

b. Respiratory system: Increased depth and rate of respirations.
c. Gastrointestinal system: Although a controversial belief, many authorities think that peristalsis slows during labor.
d. Renal system: Reduced sensation of a full bladder.
e. Hematopoietic system: Leukocytes as high as 25,000 to 30,000. Elevated clotting factors.

4. Uterine contractions temporarily stop blood flow to the placenta. If the contractions were sustained, the fetus could not receive freshly oxygenated blood or nutrients, or dispose of waste products through the placenta.
5. Labor and vaginal birth benefit the newborn by increasing absorption of fetal lung fluid and compressing the upper airways, causing some lung fluid to be expelled. These effects reduce the amount of lung fluid remaining in the newborn's respiratory tract when breathing begins. Labor also stimulates the fetus to secrete catecholamines, which help speed clearance of the lung fluid after birth, stimulate cardiac contraction and breathing, and aid in temperature regulation.
6. The power of labor during the first stage of labor involves uterine contractions. The powers during the second stage are uterine contractions, augmented by the woman's voluntary pushing efforts.
7. The three divisions of the true pelvis are the inlet, the midpelvis, and the outlet.
8. The vertex presentation, with the fetal head fully flexed forward, allows the smallest diameter of the fetal head to enter the pelvis. It also more effectively dilates the cervix.
9. ROP: The fetal landmark is the occiput, indicating a vertex presentation. It is located in the mother's right posterior pelvic quadrant. OA: The fetal landmark is the occiput, which is located in the mother's anterior pelvis and is not directed toward her left or her right. RSA: The fetal landmark is the sacrum, indicating that the fetus is in a breech presentation. It is located in the mother's right anterior pelvis. LMA: The fetal landmark is the mentum, or chin, indicating that the fetus is in a face presentation. The chin is in the mother's left anterior pelvis.
10. If the fetus is in a face presentation, the occiput is not accessible to the examiner's fingers during vaginal examination. For this reason, the fetal chin (mentum) is used to describe position (e.g., RMA or right mentum anterior).
11. The woman may note any of several changes as labor approaches: increased strength and frequency of Braxton Hicks contractions, lightening, increased vaginal mucus, bloody show, an energy spurt, or a small weight loss.
12. False labor tends to differ from true labor in three major ways. True labor is characterized by contractions that become progressively more frequent, of longer duration, and of greater intensity. The discomfort of true labor begins in the lower back and sweeps to the lower abdomen. The key difference between true and false labor is that in true labor, progressive effacement and dilation of the cervix occur.
13. The transverse diameter of the pelvic inlet is slightly larger than the inlet's anteroposterior diameter. The anteroposterior diameter of the fetal head (in line with the sagittal suture) is slightly larger than the transverse diameter. Therefore, the fetal head best fits the pelvis if the sagittal suture is aligned with the pelvic transverse diameter.
14. Because the woman's pelvic outlet is usually slightly larger in its anteroposterior diameter than its transverse, the fetal head turns in the mechanism of internal rotation so that the sagittal suture aligns with the anteroposterior diameter.
15. During the first stage, latent phase, the expectant mother is often sociable, excited, and somewhat anxious. During the first stage, active phase, the woman becomes less sociable and is inwardly focused. During the first stage, transition phase, the woman may become irritable and temporarily lose control. During the second stage, the woman usually concentrates her energy toward pushing her baby out, interacting little with others. She often regains a feeling of being in control and being an active participant in the birth.
16. Contractions vary among women, but there is a general pattern of increasing frequency, duration, and intensity throughout labor. In the first stage, latent phase, contractions gradually increase until they are about 5 minutes apart, lasting for 30 to 40 seconds with mild to moderate intensity. In the first stage, active phase, contractions increase to about 2 to 5 minutes apart, with a duration of about 40 to 60 seconds and a moderate to strong intensity. In the first stage, transition phase, contractions are strong, with a frequency of 1½ to 2 minutes and a duration of 60 to 90 seconds. In the second stage, contractions are about 2 to 3 minutes apart, strong, and have a duration of about 40 to 60 seconds.
17. Signs that the placenta may have separated include a spheric uterine shape; the rising of the uterus upward in the abdomen; protrusion

of the umbilical cord farther out from the vagina; and a gush of blood.

18. Hemorrhage may occur if the uterus does not remain contracted after birth of the placenta, because open blood vessels at the site will not be compressed by the interlacing muscle fibers of the uterus.

## Chapter 13

1. The nurse should show warmth, concern, and friendliness when the woman and her family enter the hospital or birth center. In addition, a nonjudgmental attitude facilitates communication and shows respect to the woman as an individual.
2. The nurse should try to identify and incorporate beneficial or neutral cultural practices into care during labor and birth. For example, ask if there are specific practices that are important during birth and facilitate communication by obtaining a fluent interpreter.
3. The nurse should promptly evaluate the maternal and fetal conditions and the nearness of birth when a woman comes to the hospital or birth center. Prompt assessments should include checking the maternal vital signs, fetal heart rate and patterns, and progress of labor.
4. The average fetal heart rate (FHR) at term has a lower limit of 110–120 BPM and an upper limit of 150–160 BPM, with variability in the rate. Accelerations in the rate and absence of decelerations after contractions are also reassuring.
5. Impending birth should be suspected if the woman is grunting, bearing down, sitting on one buttock, or urgently signifying that her baby is about to be born. In that case, the nurse should abbreviate the initial assessment and collect other information after the birth.
6. Two tests assist the nurse, nurse-midwife, or physician to determine whether a woman's membranes have ruptured: the nitrazine test and examination of the amniotic fluid under a microscope for ferning.
7. Hypertonic contractions (too frequent, too long, or an inadequate rest period) reduce blood flow to and from the placenta. This interferes with fetal oxygenation and waste disposal.
8. Routine FHR assessments in uncomplicated labor are done every hour during latent (early) labor, every 30 minutes during active labor, and every 15 minutes during the second stage. The FHR should be assessed after the membranes rupture to detect whether the fetal umbilical cord was displaced with the gush of fluid and is being compressed between the fetal presenting part and the maternal pelvis.
9. Greenish amniotic fluid contains meconium, which may have been passed by the fetus in response to transient hypoxia. Cloudy, yellowish, or foul-smelling fluid suggests infection in the amniotic sac.
10. Frequent vaginal examinations may cause infection because microorganisms from the perineal area can be introduced into the uterus.
11. The woman may express ineffectiveness of nonpharmacologic measures, show muscle tension during and between contractions, have a tense facial expression, express an inability to tolerate the pain, or specifically request other pain management measures, including medication.
12. Hypotension reduces blood flow to the placenta (and therefore reduces fetal oxygenation) because it diverts blood away from the uterus to better supply the mother's brain, heart, and kidneys. Hypertension may result in vasospasm that can reduce exchange of oxygen, nutrients, and waste products in the placenta. Fetal hypoxia and acidosis can be the ultimate result of maternal hypotension or hypertension.
13. The supine position allows the heavy uterus to compress her vena cava, reducing blood flow to her heart and reducing placental blood supply. A small wedge under her side is effective to relieve vena cava compression.
14. General physical comfort measures during labor include soft, dim lighting; a comfortable temperature; maintaining cleanliness; mouth care; observations for a full bladder; positioning for comfort; and a warm bath or shower. Caring for the support person includes respect for the couple's wishes about partner involvement in birth. The nurse should provide support that the partner cannot and should consider his or her physical needs for food and rest.
15. Shortly before birth, the woman's perineum bulges and the fetal head may become visible during contractions. At this time, birth can occur suddenly.
16. Perineal massage or heat applications relax the perineal tissues, facilitating birth of the head. An episiotomy or perineal lacerations may thus be avoided.

## Chapter 14

1. Fetal oxygenation depends on normal maternal blood flow and volume; normal oxygen satura-

tion of the maternal blood; adequate oxygen-carbon dioxide exchange in the placenta; patent umbilical cord vessels; and normal fetal circulatory and oxygen-carrying function.

2. When the umbilical cord is compressed, the umbilical vein is compressed first, resulting in a slight fetal hypotension and acceleration of the fetal heart rate. Continued compression obstructs the umbilical arteries, resulting in fetal hypertension and slowing of the fetal heart rate. As compression is relieved, these changes are reversed.
3. The fetus increases cardiac output, and therefore oxygenation, primarily by increasing the heart rate. Rates lower than 50 BPM may reduce fetal oxygenation. Rates higher than 200 BPM also may reduce fetal oxygenation because the ventricles do not have time to refill with oxygenated blood.
4. Fetal monitoring should be done more frequently if there are risk factors present. These may include antepartum factors in the woman's history or course of pregnancy. They may also include problems in the woman or fetus that develop intrapartally. Although there are no absolute indications for continuous electronic fetal monitoring, most hospitals use it in both low- and high-risk intrapartum care.
5. Intermittent auscultation promotes the laboring woman's mobility and creates a more natural atmosphere. However, it can assess the fetus for only a small part of labor, may be distracting for some women, and may require more staff. Continuous electronic fetal monitoring provides more data, is often expected by parents, and can assist the nurse to better observe more than one laboring woman. It allows the nurse to devote more time to coaching the woman and her partner through labor. Its primary drawback is reduced maternal mobility, adjustments to the equipment, and the technical atmosphere it lends to the birth process.
6. The upper grid on the paper strip of the electronic fetal monitor records the constant changes in the fetal heart rate. The lower grid records contractions as a series of bell-shaped curves.
7. The Doppler ultrasound transducer senses fetal heart motion and translates the motion into a heart rate.
8. Four factors may affect the accuracy of the external uterine activity monitor: fetal size, abdominal fat thickness, maternal position, and where the transducer is located.
9. The two types of internal uterine activity catheters are the solid and the fluid-filled catheter. The solid catheter tends to record higher intrauterine pressures because it senses fluid pressure above its sensor inside the uterus. The fluid-filled catheter can be affected by its height in relation to the mother's transducer.
10. Fetal heart rate accelerations are a reassuring sign of fetal responsiveness and nonacidosis.
11. In early decelerations, the fetal heart rate slows after the contraction begins and returns to the baseline rate by the end of the contraction. They are caused by fetal head compression and are reassuring. Late decelerations are characterized by slowing of the fetal heart rate late in the contraction cycle, often after the peak. They do not return to the baseline until after the contraction has ended. Late decelerations are associated with decreased uteroplacental perfusion and are nonreassuring.
12. Variable decelerations show a fetal heart rate that rises and falls abruptly. They are not consistent in appearance and may not occur at similar times in relation to the contractions. They are caused by compression of the umbilical cord.
13. Fetal scalp stimulation or vibroacoustic stimulation may be done to clarify fetal heart rate patterns as reassuring or nonreassuring when they are vague. The reassuring response to stimulation is an increase in the fetal heart rate of 15 BPM for at least 15 seconds. This suggests that the fetus has a normal oxygen and acid-base balance.
14. Cord blood gas and pH analysis assesses the newborn's oxygen and acid-base status immediately after birth and identifies if the fetus was adjusting to the stresses of labor.
15. Basic nursing actions for nonreassuring fetal heart rate patterns vary according to the pattern. They include identifying the cause of a nonreassuring pattern by vaginal examination, taking vital signs, reviewing medications, or applying internal monitoring; increasing placental perfusion by reducing excess uterine activity and positioning the woman on her side; giving the mother oxygen; and reducing cord compression by position changes and amnioinfusion.
16. A tocolytic drug reduces the intensity and frequency of uterine contractions, thus allowing more time for the placenta to be supplied with oxygen-rich maternal blood.
17. Amnioinfusion may be used to replace the fluid cushion around the umbilical cord, reducing compression. It may also be used to dilute thick meconium, which might otherwise cause respiratory distress in the newborn.

## Chapter 15

1. Childbirth pain differs from other painful experiences because it is part of a normal process, the woman has time to prepare for it, it is self-limited and intermittent, and it ends with the birth of her baby.
2. Excessive, unrelieved labor pain may result in a stress response (diverting blood flow from the uterus and compromising fetal oxygenation), maternal acid-base imbalance, and fetal acidosis. It may increase the length of labor. Poor pain relief can lessen the joy of childbirth for the woman and her partner and may have lasting psychological effects.
3. Physical and psychological factors interact to alter the ability to tolerate pain. For example, relaxation and working with the forces of labor enhance the chance that the woman who has a large baby and a small pelvis will give birth vaginally.
4. Four sources of pain present in most labor are cervical dilation, uterine ischemia, pressure and pulling on pelvic structures, and distention of the vagina and perineum.
5. Physical factors that influence pain include the following:
   a. A short, intense labor may be more painful because dilation, effacement, and fetal descent occur rapidly.
   b. A cervix that does not efface or dilate easily is likely to be associated with a longer and more uncomfortable labor.
   c. An abnormal fetal position may cause a longer labor as the woman's body maneuvers it into a better position. Back pain is especially noticeable if the fetus is in an occiput posterior position.
   d. Variations in the mother's pelvic size or shape may result in abnormal fetal presentations or positions and in a longer labor because the fetus does not fit through the pelvis easily.
   e. Fatigue reduces the woman's pain tolerance and ability to use coping skills.
6. Psychosocial factors that influence labor pain include culture, anxiety and fear, previous experiences, preparation for childbirth, and the mother's support system.
7. Relaxation (a) promotes uterine blood flow, (b) promotes efficient uterine contractions, and (c) reduces maternal tension that increases pain perception, decreases pain tolerance, and inhibits fetal descent.
8. Nursing actions to promote relaxation include arranging for environmental comfort, maintaining the woman's personal comfort, reducing factors that cause anxiety and fear, and using specific directed relaxation techniques such as helping the woman focus on relaxing specific tense muscles.
9. Accurate information and a focus on the normal aspects of childbirth help reduce anxiety and fear. Avoid referring to the woman as a "patient," because this word is associated with illness. Empowerment of the birthing partners helps them see themselves as competent to give birth successfully.
10. Touch techniques include effleurage, firm palm or sole pressure, back rubs, and warm or cool applications. Firm pressure to the sacral area may help manage back pain during labor.
11. Drugs taken by the mother can affect the fetus directly, such as decreased fetal heart rate variability, or indirectly, such as hypotension that reduces placental blood flow and fetal oxygen supply.
12. (a) Aortocaval compression should be offset by placing a wedge under the woman's hip if a supine position is required. (b) The woman is more sensitive to general anesthesia and may have a greater fall in oxygenation when general anesthesia is induced. (c) The reduced peristalsis and tone of the sphincter at the junction of the esophagus and stomach can lead to regurgitation and aspiration of gastric contents, primarily with general anesthesia. (d) Lower doses of anesthetic agents will be needed for epidural or subarachnoid blocks.
13. Higher endorphin levels provide a natural analgesia and reduce the woman's requirements for pharmacologic analgesia.
14. Drugs (prescribed, over-the-counter, or illicit) may interact with one another. These interactions may be harmful to the woman, the fetus, or both. Knowledge of exactly what drugs she uses allows the safest choices in pharmacologic pain relief methods.
15. Neonatal respiratory depression is the primary drawback to the use of opioid analgesia. This effect can be reduced by timing the dose to reduce the amount transferred to the fetus (which varies according to the drug) and by giving the narcotic in small, frequent, intravenous doses at the beginning of the contraction. Naloxone (Narcan) is the drug commonly given to reverse narcotic respiratory depression.
16. Because naloxone's effects are shorter than those of the narcotic, the nurse must observe for a recurrence of respiratory depression.
17. The correct dose of naloxone for a 3178-g (7-pound) infant is 0.3 mg.
18. The two major advantages of regional pain

management are that the woman can have pain relief and remain alert.

19. Epidural and subarachnoid blocks can cause maternal hypotension. The fall in blood pressure may result in reduced placental blood flow, compromising fetal oxygen supply. Giving the woman intravenous fluids before the block reduces this effect. Other less serious adverse effects are bladder distention, prolonged second stage of labor (epidural), and postspinal headache (subarachnoid block).
20. Epidural or intrathecal opioid analgesics may cause nausea, vomiting, itching, or a combination of these. They may also result in delayed respiratory depression (up to 24 hours), depending on the drug used. Management includes promethazine for nausea and vomiting; diphenhydramine, Naloxone, or Naltrexone for itching; and pulse oximetry and monitoring of respirations while the opioid is given and up to 24 hours after administration ends, depending on the drug.
21. Maternal regurgitation with aspiration of acidic gastric contents is the major potential adverse effect of general anesthesia. The risk may be reduced by limiting intake to clear fluids, giving drugs to raise the gastric pH, giving drugs to reduce gastric secretions or speed emptying of the stomach, and using cricoid pressure (Sellick's maneuver) to block the esophagus while the endotracheal tube is being inserted. Respiratory depression, primarily in the infant, is minimized by delaying general anesthesia until the surgery team is prepared and by keeping the anesthesia level as light as possible until the umbilical cord is cut.

## Chapter 16

1. Three major risks of amniotomy are prolapsed umbilical cord, infection, and abruptio placentae.
2. The fetal heart rate is assessed before the membranes rupture to identify whether the fetus has a normal rate and pattern and to establish a baseline. It is checked after the membranes rupture to identify patterns that suggest umbilical cord compression or other problems.
3. Green amniotic fluid contains meconium, passed from the fetal intestines. It may be seen in postterm gestation or placental insufficiency.
4. Signs of chorioamnionitis include fetal tachycardia (often the first sign), elevated maternal temperature, and amniotic fluid that has a foul or strong odor or a cloudy or yellowish appearance.
5. Five precautions that promote safe oxytocin induction or augmentation of labor include the following:
   a. Dilution of the oxytocin in a physiologic electrolyte solution
   b. Piggybacking the oxytocin solution into the port nearest the venipuncture site
   c. Starting the oxytocin infusion slowly
   d. Increasing its rate gradually
   e. Monitoring uterine contractions and fetal heart rate
6. Labor may be augmented if it stops or if contractions become ineffective. The woman whose labor is augmented with oxytocin usually needs less of the drug than the woman whose labor is being induced because her uterus is more sensitive to its effects.
7. The fetus may have an adverse reaction to oxytocin, manifested by nonreassuring fetal heart rate patterns, such as bradycardia, tachycardia, late decelerations, and decreased fetal heart rate variability.
8. Signs of hypertonic uterine activity include incomplete relaxation of the uterus between contractions or a rest period shorter than 60 seconds, which may result in inadequate placental blood flow and a fall in fetal oxygenation.
9. Administration of oxytocin for a prolonged time may lead to postpartum hemorrhage because the fatigued uterus cannot contract properly to compress bleeding vessels at the placenta site (uterine atony).
10. The fetal heart rate should be monitored before external version to identify nonreassuring patterns. It should be monitored (by Doppler or real-time ultrasound) as much as possible during, and for a short while after, to detect cord compression that can occur if the umbilical cord becomes entangled during change of the fetal presentation.
11. Uterine activity should be observed after external version for possible onset of labor because this procedure may cause uterine irritability or possible abruptio placentae and is done near term.
12. Both forceps and vacuum extractor are used to provide traction to assist the mother in rotation or expulsion of the fetal head, or both. Special forceps (Piper) can be used to deliver the aftercoming head of the fetus in a breech presentation, but vacuum extractor can be used only for the fetus in a cephalic presentation. Forceps may cause fetal injury such as facial bruising or nerve injury. The vacuum extractor may create an artificial caput called a chignon.

13. Catheterization before forceps are used eliminates a full bladder, which would reduce available room in the pelvis. Emptying the bladder also reduces the risk of bladder injury.
14. Use of cold immediately (for the first 12 hours) following episiotomy reduces pain, edema, and formation of hematomas. The nurse should also observe for continuous bright red bleeding that suggests a vaginal wall laceration. Warmth after 12 hours promotes resolution of the edema and hematoma.
15. The infant with an asymmetric facial appearance when crying may have facial nerve injury, usually a temporary condition that sometimes occurs when forceps are used to assist birth.
16. The low transverse uterine incision is less likely to rupture during another pregnancy than are either of the two vertical incisions. There are, however, valid reasons for the use of vertical incisions.
17. The woman expecting a cesarean birth should be taught the following about the operating room and recovery area:
    a. Preoperative procedures, such as the skin preparation and indwelling catheter.
    b. Personnel who will be present and their functions.
    c. The narrow table, safety strap, and positioning measures.
    d. When her partner or support person can come in.
    e. If a regional anesthetic is planned, explain that she will be awake and will feel pulling and pressure sensations but should not expect pain. If a general anesthetic is planned, explain that all preparations will be made before she is put to sleep, but that the surgery will not begin before she is asleep and that she will not awaken during it.
    f. In the recovery area, oxygen, pulse oximeter, and automatic blood pressure cuff will be in use. Her fundus, incision, lochia, and pain relief needs will be checked regularly.
18. The woman who has cesarean birth needs care similar to the woman who delivers vaginally in terms of vital signs and fundus and lochia assessments. Additional care includes assessment of oxygen saturation and respiratory status, observation of urine output from the indwelling catheter, pain needs, and respiratory care (turning, coughing, deep breathing). Anesthesia-related care includes level of consciousness (primarily if general anesthesia was used) and return of movement and sensation (primarily if epidural or subarachnoid block was used).

## Chapter 17

1. The three processes involved in involution are contraction of muscle fibers, catabolism, and regeneration of uterine epithelium.
2. The fundus is expected to descend 1 centimeter (approximately 1 fingerbreadth) per day so that, by the 10th postpartum day, it cannot be palpated.
3. A multipara is expected to experience afterpains because repeated stretching of the uterus makes uterine contraction more difficult. Afterpains are treated by analgesics, which should be taken at least one-half hour before breastfeeding. Lying in a prone position with a small pillow under the abdomen also provides relief. The birth of twins or a large infant also results in overdistention of the uterus. Breastfeeding aggravates afterpains.
4. Lochia rubra lasts for 3 days following childbirth and consists mostly of blood and is therefore red. Lochia serosa is pinkish and usually lasts from the fourth to the 10th day. Lochia alba is clear or colorless and may last from 3 to 6 weeks.
5. The mother is at risk for urinary retention because there is diminished sensitivity to fluid pressure and the mother may not have the urge to void even when her bladder is distended. Trauma of childbirth may also make it difficult to void. Urinary tract infection is more likely because stasis of urine allows time for bacteria to multiply. Postpartum hemorrhage may occur because a full bladder displaces the uterus, resulting in inability of uterine muscles to contract.
6. Hyperpigmentation decreases because the melanocytes-stimulating hormone decreases rapidly following childbirth.
7. Breastfeeding delays the return of both ovulation and menstruation.
8. The best method for suppressing lactation is to prevent breast distention by wearing a snug bra and preventing nipple stimulation. Ice is sometimes used for discomfort.
9. Uterine massage is necessary when the uterus is not firmly contracted. The nurse places the nondominant hand above the woman's symphysis pubis to anchor and support the uterus during massage.
10. A cervical or vaginal laceration may cause excessive bleeding even when the uterus is firmly contracted.
11. When tachycardia is noted, temperature, blood pressure, location and firmness of the uterus,

amount of lochia, estimated blood loss at delivery, hemoglobin, and hematocrit values are necessary. Excitement, fatigue, dehydration, infection, or hypovolemia may cause tachycardia.

12. Orthostatic hypotension, a drop in blood pressure when the mother goes from a supine to standing position quickly, produces symptoms of dizziness, lightheadedness, or feeling faint.
13. Frequent respiratory assessments, auscultation of breath sounds, auscultation of bowel sounds, and inspection of the surgical dressing and wound are necessary for the postcesarean mother.
14. Hypostatic pneumonia can be prevented by frequent turning, coughing, and breathing deeply, as well as early and frequent ambulation.
15. Early ambulation, pelvic lifts, and restriction of carbonated beverages and straws for drinking prevent or minimize abdominal distention.
16. Providing adequate information in a very short time is a major problem associated with early discharge. Clinical pathways list guidelines for goals and a specific time frame for interventions that will help the new mother achieve the stated outcomes.
17. For early discharge, maternal vital signs must be stable; estimated blood loss during delivery should not exceed 250 to 300 ml; the fundus must be firm; lochia rubra should be scant and without offensive odor or clots; the mother must be able to ambulate and empty her bladder; and the perineum should be free of signs of infection. For early discharge, the infant should weigh more than 2500 g (5.5 pounds) and have a robust cry and normal reflexes. In addition, the infant must have voided, and the umbilical cord and circumcision must be free of signs of bleeding or infection.
18. Information lines can help meet educational needs by answering questions and providing reassurance. The disadvantage of information lines is that nurses must rely on the family to initiate contact and they usually deal only with the concern that precipitated the call.

Telephone interviews allow a nurse to assess new families and to provide information. They are relatively inexpensive. The major disadvantage is that nurses cannot confirm the data but must rely on observations made by the family.

Home visits allow physical examination of the mother, infant, and environment. Teaching and counseling can be reinforced. The disadvantage is that home visits are expensive because they require the time of a well-prepared nurse.

Outpatient clinics are less expensive and can be used to replace home visits. Transportation is a problem for some families, and not all families will take advantage of clinics.

## Chapter 18

1. Bonding describes the initial attraction felt by the parents for the infant. Attachment is the development of an enduring, loving relationship between parents and child. It is progressive and requires response from the infant.
2. Maternal touch may progress from finger-tipping in the discovery phase to enfolding the infant and a full range of consoling behaviors.
3. Parents progress from referring to the newborn as "it" to he or she and then to using the given name.
4. The mother is focused primarily on her own needs during the taking-in phase; she is often passive and dependent and repeatedly recounts her birth experience. In the taking-hold phase she becomes more independent and shifts her attention to the infant and exhibits a heightened readiness to learn.
5. In the letting-go phase, mothers (and fathers) relinquish previous lifestyle patterns to assume the parenting role.
6. The anticipatory stage begins during pregnancy as mothers prepare for the birth of the child. The formal stage begins with birth when parents become acquainted with their child. During the informal stage parents respond to the unique cues of their child rather than following textbook or health professionals. The personal stage is attained when the parents feel comfortable with their roles as parents.
7. Postpartum blues is believed to be related to wide hormonal fluctuations that occur during and following childbirth. It is helpful if nurses focus on how the mother is feeling and reassure her that what she is feeling is normal and self-limited.
8. Fathers who are sometimes ignored and not included in infant care may feel left out and unneeded.
9. Siblings may feel jealousy and fear that they will be replaced by the newborn in the affection of the parents.
10. Time must be allowed for the parents to form attachment with each newborn individually.

## Chapter 19

1. Hypoxia causes decreased $Po_2$ and pH and increased $Pco_2$ to affect chemoreceptors that stimulate the respiratory center in the brain. Cool air and handling at birth cause skin sensors to stimulate the respiratory center. Mechanical factors include pressure against the chest that is released and helps air to enter the lungs. These factors all contribute to the initiation of respirations at birth.
2. Surfactant reduces surface tension in the alveoli and allows them to remain partially open on expiration.
3. Fetal lung fluid begins to move into the interstitial spaces shortly before birth owing to changes in the sodium levels. A very small part of the fluid is squeezed out during birth. The rest is absorbed by the lymphatic and vascular systems.
4. The ductus arteriosus closes as a result of increases in blood oxygen levels and decreased prostaglandin $E_2$ from the placenta. The foramen ovale closes when pressure in the left atrium exceeds that in the right atrium. The ductus venosus closes when the vessels of the cord become occluded.
5. At birth, increasing levels of oxygen cause the pulmonary blood vessels to dilate. In addition, movement of fetal lung fluid into the interstitial tissues allows more room for expansion of the pulmonary blood vessels.
6. Newborns have thinner skin with less subcutaneous fat, blood vessels close to the surface, and a larger skin surface area. These all contribute to greater loss of heat than in older children or adults.
7. Newborns respond to low temperatures by increased metabolism, vasoconstriction, and nonshivering thermogenesis. This increases oxygen and glucose consumption and may cause respiratory distress, hypoglycemia, acidosis, and jaundice.
8. Newborns have higher levels of erythrocytes, hemoglobin, and hematocrit than adults because during fetal life, the available oxygen is lower than after birth, causing a need for increased red blood cells.
9. Stools progress from thick, greenish-black meconium, to loose greenish-brown transitional stools to milk stools that are frequent, soft, seedy, and mustard-colored if the infant is breastfed, and pale yellow or light brown, firmer, and less frequent if formula fed.
10. Hypoglycemia is a problem for the newborn because the brain requires a constant supply of glucose and may be damaged without an adequate supply.
11. Physiologic jaundice occurs in normal newborns after the first 24 hours of life as a result of hemolysis of red blood cells and immaturity of the liver. Pathologic jaundice begins within the first 24 hours and may necessitate phototherapy. Breast milk jaundice begins later than physiologic jaundice and is thought to be due to enzymes in the milk.
12. The newborn's body is composed of a greater percentage of water, with more located in the extracellular compartment, than that in adults.
13. Newborns receive passive immunity to infections when IgG crosses the placenta in utero. After birth, infants produce IgM and IgA to protect against infection. IgA lines the gastrointestinal and respiratory tracts to prevent infection and is present in breast milk.
14. During both periods of reactivity, newborns are active and alert, may be interested in feeding, have elevated pulse and respiratory rates, and may have transient signs of respiratory distress.
15. In the quiet sleep state, the infant is in a deep sleep with regular respirations and little response to outside stimuli. In active sleep, infants move about and may have irregular respirations. The drowsy state is the time between sleep and waking. In the quiet alert state the infant is awake and interested in stimuli. The active alert state is a fussy period that may lead to the crying state if the infant's needs are not met.

## Chapter 20

1. Molding of the head is change in shape due to normal temporary overriding of bones during birth. Caput succedaneum is localized swelling from pressure against the cervix. Cephalhematoma is bleeding between the periosteum and the bone that never crosses suture lines. Molding and caput disappear within a few days, whereas cephalhematoma may last for several weeks.
2. The quick initial assessment of the infant immediately after birth helps detect serious abnormalities and anomalies that may need immediate attention. It is followed by a more complete assessment.
3. Measurements of the infant help determine if in utero growth was adequate and if complications are present.
4. The cardiovascular assessment includes history, airway, color, heart sounds, pulses, and blood pressure.

5. Taking a rectal temperature is dangerous because it risks perforation of the rectum, which turns sharply after about 1 inch.
6. Some signs of hypoglycemia are jitteriness, poor muscle tone, respiratory distress, diaphoresis, low temperature, and poor suck.
7. Using an incorrect site for heel punctures risks damage to the bone, nerves, or blood vessels of the heel.
8. Newborn reflexes provide information about the status of the neonate's central nervous system.
9. The first feeding allows the nurse to assess for signs of a connection between the trachea and the esophagus and to evaluate the newborn's ability to suck, swallow, and breathe in coordination.
10. Newborns usually pass the first stool within 24 hours of birth. Feeding and taking a rectal temperature may stimulate stool passage.
11. Infants should void within 24 to 48 hours. Infants void two to six times during the first 2 days and five to 25 times daily thereafter.
12. The nurse documents location, size, color, elevation, and texture, explains marks to parents; and offers emotional support as needed.
13. The gestational age provides an estimate of the infant's age since conception and alerts the nurse to possible complications related to age and development.
14. The periods of reactivity are important because the infant may need nursing intervention for low temperature, elevated pulse and respirations, and excessive respiratory secretions. During the sleep period, the infant will sleep deeply, have relaxed muscle tone, and no interest in feeding.

## Chapter 21

1. All newborns receive vitamin K to prevent hemorrhagic disease of the newborn. The eyes are treated with an antibiotic to prevent ophthalmia neonatorum.
2. Nurses can prevent heat loss in newborns by keeping them dry and covered and away from cold objects or surfaces, drafts, and outside windows and walls.
3. When infants show signs of hypoglycemia, the nurse should check the blood glucose level and temperature, feed the infant, and watch for signs of other complications.
4. Interventions for preventing jaundice include ensuring that the infant is feeding well by working with mothers and infants having difficulty with the process and teaching parents about jaundice and what observations to make.
5. Parents choose circumcision because of the decreased incidence of urinary tract infections and inflammation of the glans, prepuce, or meatus; religious dictates; parent preference; and lack of knowledge about care of the foreskin. Parents decide against circumcision because of the risk of hemorrhage, infection, overremoval, urethral stenosis or fistula, adhesions and damage to the glans, pain, and questions about the need for surgery.
6. Do not retract the foreskin on an uncircumcised penis until it becomes separated from the glans later in childhood. Teach the child to retract it to clean after separation occurs. Teach parents of circumcised infants to watch for bleeding and infection and to apply petroleum jelly for 24 to 48 hours unless a Plastibell was used.
7. Nurses can prevent a parent from getting the wrong baby by always checking the identification band of the infant against that of the mother or support person.
8. Parents and nurses can prevent infant abductions by always being alert for suspicious behavior and stopping any person that might be taking a baby. Parents must know how to identify hospital staff and should never allow anyone without proper identification to remove their infant from them.
9. Scrupulous hand washing by staff and all who come in contact with newborns is the most important way to prevent newborn infections.
10. Important considerations in planning parent teaching include determining who will teach which subjects, setting priorities based on parents' needs, using a variety of teaching techniques, modeling behavior, including other family members, and considering culture.
11. The first hepatitis B vaccine is often given to infants at the birth facility because it is a widespread disease and some infants are exposed during birth if their mothers are infected.
12. Newborn screening tests should be performed as close to discharge as possible as the tests are more sensitive after the first 24 hours of life. If infants are discharged earlier, they should be retested so that any disorders can be diagnosed early.

## Chapter 22

1. Some infants lose weight after birth because of insufficient intake and normal loss of extracellular fluid.

2. Colostrum is rich in protein, vitamins, minerals, and immunoglobulins. Transitional milk has less protein and immunoglobulin but more lactose, fat, and calories than colostrum. Mature milk appears less rich than colostrum and transitional milk but supplies all nutrients needed.
3. Breast milk nutrients are in an easily digested form and in proportions required by the newborn. Commercial formulas contain cow's milk adapted to simulate human milk. Infants may develop allergies to modified cow's milk and may need other types of formula, but they are not allergic to human milk.
4. Breast milk contains bifidus factor, leukocytes, lysozymes, and immunoglobulins.
5. Commercial formulas include modified cow's milk formula, soy-based or protein hydrolysate formulas, and special formulas for preterm infants or those with special needs.
6. Cultural influences, employment demands, support from family and friends, knowledge about each method, age, and education may influence a woman's choice of feeding method.
7. Suckling causes release of oxytocin from the posterior pituitary, which produces the let-down reflex. It also causes the anterior pituitary to release prolactin to increase milk production.
8. The more frequently the infant breastfeeds, the more prolactin is produced. This increases the milk supply. The opposite is also true: infrequent feedings decrease prolactin output and milk production.
9. During pregnancy, identification of flat and inverted nipples and possible use of breast shells may help correct them.
10. The nurse can help the mother establish breastfeeding during the initial feeding session by initiating early feeding, helping to position the infant at the breast, and showing the mother how to position her hands. The nurse also can help the infant latch on to the breast, assess the position of the mouth on the breast, check for swallowing, and remove the infant from the breast.
11. The mother should feed the infant every 2 to 3 hours (8 to 12 times each day) for about 10 to 15 minutes at the first breast and until the infant is satisfied at the second breast. Length of feedings may vary but should average at least 15 minutes.
12. (See Mothers Want to Know: Solutions for Common Problems.) To wake up a sleepy infant, unwrapping the infant's blankets, talk to the infant, change the diaper, rub the infant's back, and express colostrum onto the breast.
13. Sucking from a bottle requires pushing the tongue against the nipple to slow the flow of milk. Suckling from the breast requires drawing the nipple far into the mouth so that the gums compress the areola as the tongue moves over the milk sinus in a wave-like motion.
14. To help the mother who has engorged breasts, the nurse can encourage frequent nursing, applying heat and cold, massaging, and expressing milk to soften the areola.
15. The nurse should advise the mother with sore nipples to ensure proper positioning of the infant at the breast, vary the position of the infant, apply colostrum or warm water compresses to the nipples, and expose the nipples to air.
16. Care available after discharge for the breastfeeding mother includes home visits by nurses, outpatient clinics where nurses assess breastfeeding, and telephone access to nurses.
17. The mother who plans to work and breastfeed should be taught use of a breast pump, proper storage of milk, and ways to maintain her milk supply.
18. A mother might ask about the types of formula available, how to prepare it correctly, and feeding techniques.

## Chapter 23

1. Parents obtain information about infant care from friends, family, nurses, child care classes, books, and magazines.
2. Nurses may offer follow-up phone calls, home visits, and classes about parenting.
3. All equipment should be checked for safety, and parts should be inspected to see that they are in good condition and functioning properly.
4. Car seats must be chosen according to the size of the infant and must be used correctly to maintain safety.
5. Infants are not "spoiled" by prompt attention to their needs.
6. Nurses can assist parents of crying infants to determine the cause and appropriate techniques for dealing with a crying infant. Nurses can also use therapeutic communication techniques to help parents deal with negative feelings.
7. Signs of teething include drooling, irritability, decreased appetite and sleep, rash, loose stools, and red, swollen gums.
8. Diaper rash can be prevented by keeping the area clean and dry and avoiding plastic pants or products to which the infant seems sensitive. If rash occurs, parents should expose the area to air and apply creams sparingly.

9. The amount infants eat during the early weeks will vary but will average about 1 ounce per feeding at first and 5 to 6 ounces per feeding at 12 weeks.
10. Solid foods cannot be digested completely until age 4 to 6 months and may cause allergies, gastric upsets, and decreased intake of needed nutrients from milk.
11. Understanding the infant's changing capabilities helps parents assess situations to prevent accidents.
12. Well baby checkups provide for assessment of growth and development, guidance, and immunizations.
13. Immunizations safeguard infants and communities from spread of communicable diseases.
14. Immediate help should be obtained if infants have difficulty breathing, show cyanosis, or are hard to arouse from sleep.
15. The cause of sudden infant death syndrome remains unknown, but the risk may be increased with maternal smoking, maternal drug abuse, or prone sleep position.

## Chapter 24

1. Pregnancy interrupts developmental tasks such as the achievement of a stable identity, development of a personal value system, completion of educational goals, and achievement of independence from parents.
2. Teenagers experience greater risk for pregnancy-induced hypertension, anemia, nutritional deficiencies, and sexually transmissible diseases. There is also increased risk for infants to be born prematurely and to be under 2500 g. Both infant and maternal mortality rates are higher during the teenage years.
3. Adolescent parents may have unrealistic expectations of infants; they demonstrate less empathy, tend to be less sensitive to infant signals, and provide less infant stimulation than older parents.
4. Teenagers may not benefit from printed materials to the same degree as older clients. A variety of teaching methods, such as visual aids, videos, group classes, and one-to-one counseling, may be effective.
5. Infants develop a sense of trust, which is necessary for future development, when their needs are met promptly and gently; crying indicates a need and does not mean the infant is "spoiled"; physical growth and development proceed slowly from the head downward.
6. Mature primigravidas often have maturity and problem-solving skills as well as emotional and financial resources that are still unavailable to younger women.
7. Women older than 35 years are at increased risk for chromosomal anomalies that may be detected by prenatal screening.
8. The nurse's role in genetic counseling is to be informed and to reinforce or clarify information provided by genetic counselors or physicians.
9. The older mother may have less energy than younger mothers, and it is important to conserve her energy for care of self and infant.
10. The effects of smoking on the fetus include low birth weight, prematurity, and increased perinatal loss. Long-term effects on the child include delayed neurologic and intellectual development, including hyperactivity, shorter attention span, and lower reading and spelling scores during the primary grades.
11. Fetal alcohol syndrome is characterized by slow growth, central nervous system disorders, and cranial and facial anomalies. Fetal alcohol effect describes mild or partial manifestations of fetal alcohol syndrome.
12. The long-term effects of maternal cocaine use on the child include learning difficulties, slower intellectual development, delayed language and motor development, and limited interaction with people and objects in the environment.
13. Caregivers may be frustrated by the infant's hypertonicity and continuous crying and by their inability to console the infant during the abstinence syndrome.
14. Prenatal behaviors that indicate substance abuse include seeking prenatal care late in pregnancy, failing to keep appointments, inconsistent follow-through with recommended regimens, poor grooming, inadequate weight gain, needle punctures, thrombosed veins, or signs of cellulitis.
15. Signs and symptoms of recent cocaine use include profuse sweating, high blood pressure, irregular respirations, dilated pupils, increased body temperature, sudden onset of severely painful uterine contractions, fetal tachycardia, and excessive fetal activity. Emotional signs include anger, caustic or abusive reactions to the caregiver, emotional lability, and paranoia.
16. Interventions are focused on preventing maternal or fetal injury and may require setting limits in a firm, nonjudgmental manner with a woman who may be abusive and in great pain.
17. To promote positive parenting, nurses should provide anticipatory guidance about the growth and development of infants, measures that prevent a frantic cry state, instructions in how to feed the infant with uncoordinated suck and

swallow reflexes, and instructions in how to mobilize a support system that is knowledgeable and reliable.

18. Parents experience less anxiety when they are gently told the condition of the infant and allowed to hold their newborn as soon as possible.
19. Facial and genital defects are believed to affect parenting most.
20. The reaction of parents can be described in terms of a grief response. Initial reactions include shock and disbelief.
21. Nurses can promote bonding and attachment by handling the infant gently, emphasizing normal traits, helping parents hold and cuddle the infant, using communication skills to help parents come to terms with their feelings.
22. Discharge planning for the family of an infant with congenital anomalies should include special feeding, holding, and positioning techniques that the infant may require.
23. How the stillborn infant is presented creates memories that the parents will retain. If necessary, the infant should be washed; lotion or powder may be applied. If possible, the infant should be presented while still warm and soft, wrapped in a soft, warm blanket.
24. The "rights of the baby" are to be recognized as a person who was born and died; to be named; to be seen, touched, and held by the family; to have life-ending acknowledged; and to be put to rest with dignity.
25. Most parents treasure a memory packet that includes a photograph, footprints, a birth bracelet, and crib card, and if possible a lock of hair.
26. Mothers see adoption as an act of sacrifice and love when they give up the child to those who can provide a better life.
27. Adoptive parents must be taught how to care for an infant and what to expect in terms of growth and development.
28. Battering may start or become worse during pregnancy; the abdomen may replace the face and breasts as the target for battery.
29. Nurses can examine their own biases to determine whether they accept a common myth that blames the victim. In addition, nurses can consciously practice in ways that empower women and make it clear that the woman owns her body and that no one deserves to be beaten.
30. The battered woman often appears hesitant, embarrassed, or evasive; she may avoid eye contact and appear ashamed, guilty, or frightened. There may be signs of present and past injury, such as bruising, swelling, lacerations, scars, and old fractures, as well as genital injuries.
31. Nurses can help establish short-term goals:
    a. Acknowledge the abuse.
    b. Develop a specific plan of action to implement to protect the safety of the woman and her children.
    c. Identify community resources that provide protection.

## Chapter 25

1. Bleeding is the most common sign of threatened abortion. It may be accompanied by rhythmic cramping, backache, or feelings of pelvic pressure. When there is gross rupture of membranes followed by uterine contractions and bleeding, the abortion becomes inevitable.
2. Disseminated intravascular coagulation is a life-threatening disorder in which procoagulation and anticoagulation factors are activated simultaneously, resulting in profuse bleeding from any vulnerable area.
3. Recurrent spontaneous abortions most often occur as a result of genetic or chromosomal abnormalities of the embryo or anomalies of the maternal reproductive tract. Additional causes are believed to be hormonal and immunologic factors, as well as systemic diseases or infections.
4. Nurses can facilitate the grief response by being aware that although many couples grieve over an early pregnancy loss, they often feel a lack of support from family, friends, and health care personnel. When nurses demonstrate empathy and unconditional acceptance of the feelings expressed, they facilitate the grief response. Providing information about the grieving and referrals to additional support groups may also be helpful.
5. Ectopic pregnancy remains the leading cause of maternal death due to hemorrhage, and it sharply reduces the woman's chance of subsequent pregnancies because of damage to a fallopian tube.
6. The increase in incidence of ectopic pregnancy may occur as a result of pelvic inflammatory disease that may complicate untreated sexually transmissible diseases. Scarring of the fallopian tubes that may result may make it difficult for the fertilized ovum to pass through the obstructed tube. Treatment may be medical (chemotherapeutic agent) or surgical (salpingostomy or salpingectomy).
7. Hydatidiform mole is a form of gestational trophoblastic neoplasia that involves abnormal

development of the placenta as the fetal part of the pregnancy fails to develop. The first phase of treatment is evacuation of the molar pregnancy from the uterus. The second phase is follow-up to detect malignant changes in remaining trophoblastic tissue.

8. Painless bleeding from the vagina in the latter half of pregnancy is the classic sign of placenta previa. Strict bedrest, no sexual intercourse, an adult caregiver present at all times, and availability of immediate transportation to the hospital are essential for home care. The woman must also be taught to monitor fetal movement and to report a decrease in movement or vaginal bleeding.
9. The four classic signs of abruptio placentae are vaginal bleeding, abdominal pain, uterine hyperactivity, and uterine tenderness.
10. Hemorrhagic shock is the major danger of placental abruption for the mother; anoxia, excessive blood loss, or delivery before maturity are the major dangers for the fetus.
11. Both morning sickness and hyperemesis gravidarum begin in the first trimester. Morning sickness is self-limiting and causes no serious complications. Hyperemesis is persistent, uncontrollable vomiting that can result in dehydration, and electrolyte or acid-base imbalance.
12. Goals of management are to maintain hydration, replace electrolytes and vitamins, maintain nutrition, and provide emotional support.
13. Nurses must use critical thinking to examine biases that may result in lack of comfort and support for women with hyperemesis.
14. Persistent vasospasm of uterine arterioles may result in fetal hypoxemia, intrauterine growth restriction, or even fetal death.
15. Signs and symptoms of pre-eclampsia include hypertension, proteinuria, and may include generalized edema. Headache, hyperreflexia, visual disturbances, and epigastric pain indicate the disease is worsening. Bedrest in a lateral position increases cardiac return and circulatory volume, thus improving perfusion of vital organs. Increased renal perfusion decreases angiotensin II levels, thus lowering blood pressure.
16. Vasospasms cause cerebral edema and small cerebral hemorrhages.
17. Magnesium sulfate prevents convulsions by reducing central nervous system irritability and decreasing vasoconstriction. The primary adverse effect is central nervous system depression, which includes depression of the respiratory center.
18. Pulmonary edema, circulatory or renal failure, and cerebral hemorrhage are complications of eclampsia.
19. Assessments for the woman with pre-eclampsia include daily weights, location and degree of edema, vital signs, hourly urinary output, urine for protein, deep tendon reflexes, and subjective signs such as headache, visual disturbances, and epigastric pain. Fetal heart rate and fetal movement should be assessed. Respiratory rate, level of consciousness, and laboratory data such as creatinine, liver enzymes, and magnesium level should be evaluated. Psychosocial assessment should include the reaction of the woman's family and support system. Nursing assessment is the only way to determine whether the condition is responding to medical management or the disease is worsening.
20. To prevent convulsions, maintain a quiet environment, reduce environmental stimuli, and maintain a therapeutic level of magnesium. Nurses must remain with the woman and call for help if a convulsion occurs. If there is time, attempt to turn the woman on her side. Note the sequence and time of the convulsion. Insert an airway following the convulsion and suction the woman's nose and mouth, administer oxygen, administer medications, and prepare for additional medical interventions.
21. To prevent seizure-related injury, the side rails should be padded and raised. The bed should be in the lowest position with the wheels locked. Oxygen and suction should be readily available. Necessary equipment and medications should be kept in the room.
22. Signs of magnesium toxicity include respiratory rate below 12 breaths per minute, hyporeflexia, sweating or flushing, altered sensorium (lethargy, drowsiness, disorientation), and serum magnesium level beyond the therapeutic range. If toxicity occurs, discontinue magnesium and notify the physician so the dose can be altered. Calcium gluconate is the antidote for magnesium toxicity.
23. H = hemolysis; EL = elevated liver enzymes; LP = low platelets. Major symptoms are pain and tenderness in the right upper quadrant. Additional signs and symptoms may include nausea, vomiting, and severe edema. Laboratory data include irregular, damaged red blood cells, progressive anemia, thrombocytopenia, and elevated liver enzymes.

    Palpating the liver could cause trauma, including rupture of a subcapsular hematoma.
24. Pre-eclampsia occurs only during pregnancy and the early postpartum period; chronic hypertension is present before pregnancy

and persists following the postpartum period. Treatment may be similar during pregnancy; however, chronic hypertension is often treated with antihypertensive medications before and during pregnancy.

25. Administration of RhoGAM prevents development of maternal Rh antibodies and is recommended following any procedure that includes the possibility of maternal exposure to Rh-positive fetal blood.
26. Maternal antibodies cross the placental barrier and cause destruction of fetal red blood cells. The fetus becomes anemic, bilirubin increases, and severe neurologic disease can result.
27. Many women with blood type O have anti-A or anti-B antibodies before they become pregnant so the first pregnancy can be affected. The effects of ABO incompatibility are milder than Rh sensitization because fewer antibodies cross into fetal blood.

## Chapter 26

1. The hormones of pregnancy cause resistance of maternal cells to insulin, which increases the availability of glucose for the fetus.
2. The mother is at risk to develop pregnancy-induced hypertension, urinary tract infections, ketoacidosis, and preterm labor. Possible fetal and neonatal effects include congenital malformations, variations in fetal size, fetal hypoxemia, and polycythemia. Neonatal effects include hypoglycemia, hypocalcemia, hyperbilirubinemia, and respiratory distress syndrome.
3. Glycosylated hemoglobin gives an accurate evaluation of blood glucose for the past 4 to 8 weeks and is not affected by recent intake of food.
4. Insulin needs decrease during the first trimester and increase sharply during the second and third trimesters (when placental hormones initiate insulin resistance). During labor, insulin needs vary and must be determined by frequent checks of blood glucose. In the postpartum period insulin needs decrease as placental hormones decline.
5. Gestational diabetes mellitus is first diagnosed during pregnancy. It is most often managed by diet and exercise, although insulin may be needed.
6. A glucose challenge test is a screening procedure only and requires no preparation. A glucose tolerance test is diagnostic for diabetes mellitus; it requires preparation and 3 hours of testing.
7. Maternal effects of gestational diabetes mellitus include increased incidence of urinary tract infections, hydramnios (excessive amniotic fluid), premature rupture of membranes, and development of pregnancy-induced hypertension. Fetal effects may include macrosomia that can result in shoulder dystocia or cesarean birth. The newborn is at risk for hypoglycemia.
8. Increased vascular volume and increased cardiac output (particularly stroke volume) impose an added burden on the woman who has a cardiac defect.
9. Rheumatic and congenital heart disease are the two major categories of heart disease. Functional classification depends on the person's ability to tolerate activity. Class I indicates no limitation on activity. Class II indicates slight restriction if necessary. In Class III there is marked limitation, and Class IV indicates inability to perform any physical activity.
10. Goals of treatment are to prevent anemia so there is an adequate supply of red blood cells to transport oxygen and thus reduce the demands on the heart, limit physical activity so cardiac demand does not exceed the capacity of the heart, and limit weight gain, which places further demands on the heart.
11. With every contraction, blood is shifted from the uterus and placenta into central circulation; this can lead to fluid overload if fluids are administered rapidly.
12. Five hundred ml of blood are added to the central circulation with delivery of the placenta. This increases cardiac output and can lead to further compromise of the heart.
13. Most women do not have adequate iron stores to meet the demands of pregnancy, and it is difficult to meet needs by diet alone.
14. The fetus usually receives adequate iron, even at a cost to the mother. Therefore, neonatal effects of moderate maternal anemia are rare.
15. The fetal and neonatal effects of folic acid deficiency are increased risk of spontaneous abortion, abruption of the placenta, and fetal anomalies (particularly neural tube defects).
16. Pregnancy exacerbates sickle cell anemia, and the risk of "sickle cell crisis" is increased.
17. Frequent evaluations of hemoglobin, blood count, serum iron, and iron-binding capacity as well as folate are necessary to determine the degree of anemia. Frequent fetal surveillance and monitoring for signs of sickle cell crisis are also necessary.
18. Thalassemia is associated with increased iron absorption and storage, making women with this disorder susceptible to iron overload.
19. The maternal and fetal effects of systemic lu-

pus erythematosus are increased incidence of abortion, preterm delivery, and fetal death. Pregnancy can exacerbate the disease and renal complications pose a special risk.

20. There is often marked improvement of rheumatoid arthritis during pregnancy; however, relapse often occurs soon after childbirth.
21. Some anticonvulsant drugs are teratogenic.
22. The recommended supportive care for women with Bell's palsy includes eye patching, applying ointment or drops to prevent trauma to the cornea, facial massage, and psychological support.
23. Two percent of all live neonates are infected with cytomegalovirus; 90 percent of these are asymptomatic and appear normal. The most serious complications of those affected are deafness, mental retardation, seizures, blindness, and dental abnormalities.
24. The first trimester is the time of organogenesis, when damage can be done to all developing organ systems.
25. A vaccine is available to prevent rubella; however, it cannot be given during pregnancy.
26. Immunization with varicella-zoster immune globulin is recommended. Mothers and infants must be isolated from those who are not immune.
27. Vertical transmission of herpesvirus occurs when organisms ascend following rupture of membranes and during birth when the fetus comes into contact with infectious tissue and secretions.
28. The fetal and neonatal effects of parvovirus 19 infection are failure of red blood cell production, severe fetal anemia, hydrops, and heart failure.
29. Hepatitis B virus is transmitted by contact with infected blood, saliva, vaginal secretions, semen, or breast milk. A newborn whose mother is known to carry the hepatitis B surface antigen should receive hepatitis B immune globulin soon after birth, followed by hepatitis B vaccine.
30. Avoid sexual transmission by abstinence, avoiding intercourse with infected persons, or using recommended barrier methods. Intravenous drug users who refuse rehabilitation must avoid transmission that occurs when needles are shared with those who are infected.
31. A variety of antiviral medications may be administered to delay replication of the virus. Medications are also available to prevent *Pneumocystis carinii* pneumonia. Opportunistic diseases are treated.
32. Toxoplasmosis can be prevented by cooking meat thoroughly, not touching mucous membranes while handling raw meat, washing kitchen surfaces and hands thoroughly after handling raw meat, avoiding uncooked eggs and unpasteurized milk, washing vegetables and fruit before consumption, and avoiding contact with materials that may be contaminated with cat feces.
33. Preterm labor, premature rupture of the mother's membranes, prolonged rupture of membranes, a sibling affected by symptomatic group B streptococcal infection, or maternal fever during labor are risk factors for colonization of the newborn with group B streptococcus. Intravenous antibacterial therapy is used to prevent colonization.
34. Isoniazid plus rifampin and pyridoxine are used to treat tuberculosis in the mother. Ethambutol may be added if drug resistance is suspected. Treatment must continue over several months. The infant is skin tested at birth and may be started on INH therapy until the skin test, which will be repeated, remains negative.

## Chapter 27

1. Hypotonic labor dysfunction usually occurs during the active phase of first-stage labor (4 cm cervical dilation or more), whereas hypertonic dysfunction usually occurs during the latent phase (within the first 3 cm of cervical dilation). Uterine contractions become weaker, shorter, and less frequent in hypotonic dysfunction; in hypertonic dysfunction, they are painful but inefficient and the uterine resting tone is high. Hypotonic dysfunction is not painful because the contractions decrease, although the woman may become tired; hypertonic dysfunction is characterized by a cramping type of pain. Management of both depends on the identified cause. Hypotonic dysfunction is often managed by ensuring adequate intake of fluids and electrolytes, position changes, amniotomy, and oxytocin augmentation. Hypertonic dysfunction may be managed by mild sedation or tocolytic drugs to reduce excess uterine activity.
2. Maternal position changes encourage the fetus to rotate from an occiput transverse or occiput posterior position to an occiput anterior position, similar to nesting two spoons together. The convex surface of the rounded fetal back rotates toward the convex surface of the anterior uterus. The squatting position also increases pelvic diameters and straightens the pelvic curve to facilitate both fetal rotation and descent.

3. Other complications are associated with a fetus in a breech presentation that may cause problems, regardless of the method of birth. These include low birth weight, fetal anomalies, and associated pregnancy or labor complications.
4. The staff must be prepared for care of multiple infants. Duplicate staff and equipment should be ready for every infant expected.
5. Bladder distention during labor can consume available room in the woman's pelvis, thus impeding labor progress and fetal descent. In addition, it is a potential source of discomfort.
6. Psychological support helps reduce excess stress that can otherwise consume energy that the uterus needs, inhibit uterine contractions, reduce placental blood supply, impair the woman's pushing efforts, and increase the woman's pain experience.
7. The average nullipara's cervix dilates about 1.2 cm per hour; minimum fetal descent is 1.0 cm per hour. The average parous woman's cervix dilates about 1.5 cm per hour, with minimum descent of 2 cm per hour.
8. Nursing care for the woman who has prolonged labor is similar to that for dysfunctional labor. Promoting comfort, energy conservation, position changes, and assessments for related complications, such as infection, should be done.
9. Trauma is the primary maternal risk of a precipitate labor and may include uterine rupture, cervical lacerations, and hematomas. Fetal risks may include trauma, such as intracranial hemorrhage or nerve damage, and hypoxia.
10. Premature rupture of the membranes occurs before true labor any time during pregnancy. Preterm premature rupture of the membranes (PPROM) occurs before 37 weeks of gestation are completed and may or may not be accompanied by contractions; PPROM is more likely to be associated with preterm labor and birth.
11. Infection may be both a cause of and a result of premature rupture of the membranes.
12. Labor is usually induced if a woman with ruptured membranes is near term and has a favorable cervix and if labor does not spontaneously begin within about 4 to 6 hours after rupture. If her cervix is not favorable for induction, the procedure may be delayed for 24 hours or more, as long as infection is not present.
13. The physician will balance the risks of prematurity against the risk for infection when deciding the best management of PPROM.
14. Symptoms of preterm labor are often vague. They include uterine contractions that may often be painless, the fetus "balling up," menstrual-like cramps, backache, pelvic pressure, change or increased vaginal discharge, abdominal cramps, thigh pain, or a sense of "feeling bad."
15. Early identification of preterm labor enables management that may delay birth and allow further maturation of the fetus or permit transfer to a facility equipped to care for an immature infant.
16. $\beta$-Adrenergics, such as ritodrine or terbutaline, magnesium sulfate, prostaglandin synthesis inhibitors (indomethacin), or calcium channel blockers (nifedipine) may be used to stop preterm labor.
17. Corticosteroids are given to the woman who expects to deliver prematurely to accelerate maturation of the fetal lungs. These drugs may also reduce the incidence of intraventricular hemorrhage and necrotizing enterocolitis. The greatest benefits occur if steroids are in the mother's system at least 24 hours.
18. The three potential fetal or newborn risks are reduced placental function and umbilical cord compression before birth and meconium aspiration after birth.
19. The priority of care if umbilical cord prolapse occurs is to reduce compression of the cord and restore normal blood flow through it. At the same time, the nurse should summon help to expedite delivery.
20. Oxytocin-stimulated contractions are potentially more powerful than natural ones and may cause the pressure in the uterus to exceed the uterine wall's ability to withstand that pressure.
21. Shock and hemorrhage are rapidly developing complications of uterine inversion. They are managed by rapid intravenous fluid and blood replacement, often using two intravenous lines. A drug that relaxes the uterus is often needed to allow uterine replacement; oxytocin is given *after* the uterus is replaced in the proper position.
22. The risk for amniotic fluid embolism is greater if the woman has a very strong labor with ruptured membranes because the amniotic fluid can be forced into her blood vessels.
23. Care focuses initially on treatment of any life-threatening maternal injuries to stabilize her condition.
24. Maternal death is the most common cause of fetal death when trauma occurs. The fetus may also suffer direct blunt or penetrating trauma.
25. For intrapartum emergencies, nursing considerations include the following; *Prolapsed umbilical cord*: Relieve pressure on the cord to restore adequate blood flow through it. *Uterine rupture*: Attempt to prevent by cautious intrapartum use of oxytocin and close monitoring of uterine

contractions. *Uterine inversion*: Avoid pressure on the poorly contracted fundus after birth; assess for and correct shock. *Amniotic fluid embolism*: Respiratory support; observe for coagulation deficits. *Trauma*: Stabilize the mother's condition, and treat any life-threatening injuries; place wedge under right hip to improve hemodynamic stability.

## Chapter 28

1. The nurse examines a woman's prenatal record as well as her labor and delivery record to determine whether there are factors that predispose her to have postpartum hemorrhage.
2. Overdistention of uterine muscles makes their contraction more difficult and predisposes to excessive bleeding.
3. The nurse cannot be certain that bleeding is controlled because concealed bleeding can occur in soft tissue and produce a hematoma.
4. Initial management of uterine atony focuses on measures to contract the uterus, such as massaging, expressing clots, and emptying the bladder. Pharmacologic measures include administration of dilute oxytocin, methylergonovine, or both, as well as fluid replacement.
5. Large hematomas may require incision and evacuation of clots, as well as ligation of the bleeding vessel.
6. It is sometimes difficult to recognize that the woman is becoming hypovolemic because of compensatory mechanisms, such as carotid and aortic baroreceptors that are stimulated to constrict peripheral blood vessels. This shunts blood to central circulation and maintains blood pressure. Moreover, catecholamines promote constriction in nonessential organs, increasing the heart rate and raising blood pressure.
7. The major signs of subinvolution are prolonged lochial discharge, irregular or excessive uterine bleeding, pelvic pain, feelings of pelvic heaviness, backache, fatigue, and persistent malaise.
8. Nurses must teach the mother how to locate and palpate the fundus and how to estimate fundal height in relation to the umbilicus. They also teach the mother to report any deviation from the expected pattern or duration of lochia, a foul odor, or pelvic pain.
9. There is increased venous stasis during pregnancy because of compression of the large vessels by the enlarging uterus. Venous stasis may also occur if the woman spends a prolonged period of time in stirrups during labor and birth. Pregnancy and the postpartum are also characterized by changes in the coagulation and fibrinolytic systems that elevate the factors that favor coagulation and decrease the factors that favor lysis of clots.
10. Superficial venous thrombosis occurs most often in the calf area with signs and symptoms that include swelling, tenderness, warmth, and redness.
11. Heparin remains the long-term treatment of the pregnant woman with deep venous thrombosis because warfarin (Coumadin), which crosses the placental barrier, may be teratogenic and it predisposes the fetus to hemorrhage. If the woman is in the postpartum period, heparin is changed to warfarin after several days of treatment.
12. Strict bedrest is prescribed for the woman with deep vein thrombosis to decrease interstitial swelling and to promote venous return from that leg.
13. When the mother is receiving anticoagulation medicine, additional nursing assessments include visual inspection of the mother for bruising, petechiae, or bleeding from the nose, bladder, gums, or increased vaginal bleeding. Signs of hemorrhage, such as tachycardia, falling blood pressure, or other signs of shock should also be noted.
14. The home care nurse should assess family structure and function that will need to change as a result of prolonged treatment for the mother. The nurse should evaluate mother-infant interaction and determine what support system may be available to provide assistance.
15. Cesarean birth, the use of forceps, or vacuum extraction may result in trauma that provides a portal for infectious organisms.
16. Every part of the reproductive tract is connected to every other part, and organisms can move from the vagina through the cervix, uterus, fallopian tubes, and out into the peritoneal cavity. Moreover, alkalinity of the vagina during labor encourages bacterial growth. In addition, necrosis of the endometrium and the presence of lochia provide an excellent medium for bacterial growth.
17. Metritis is more likely to develop in a woman who had prolonged labor because organisms have time and opportunity to ascend from the vagina into the uterus during prolonged labor. Also she may have more vaginal examinations and ruptured membranes for a longer time. It is likely to develop in a mother who gave birth by cesarean because of surgical trauma, an incision that provides an entrance for bacteria, the possibility of contamination during surgery,

and the presence of foreign bodies such as sutures.

18. Fever, chills, lethargy, malaise, anorexia, abdominal pain and cramping, uterine tenderness, and purulent foul-smelling lochia are the major symptoms of metritis. Additional symptoms include tachycardia and subinvolution. Metritis is usually treated by intravenous administration of antibiotics. Antipyretics are used to control fever, and oxytocin is often administered to promote involution.
19. Wound infection most often occurs in sites of episiotomies and lacerations. Surgical incisions performed for cesarean birth are also common sites.
20. Incisions and lacerations should be inspected for redness, tenderness, edema, and approximation of the edges of the wound, which may pull apart with infection.
21. To prevent urinary tract infection, the woman should be advised to drink at least 2000 ml of fluid each day. She should empty her bladder every 2 to 3 hours during the day and should practice meticulous hygiene. Cystitis is treated with oral antibiotics on an outpatient basis. Pyelonephritis requires readmittance to the hospital and intravenous administration of antibiotics.
22. Measures to prevent mastitis include correct positioning of the infant, frequent emptying of the breasts, and avoiding nipple trauma and supplemental feedings. In addition the woman should avoid continuous pressure on the breasts caused by tight bras or infant carriers. Treatment includes antibiotic therapy with continued decompression of the breast. Analgesics and supportive therapy, such as warm, moist compresses, may also be helpful.
23. Septic pelvic thrombophlebitis spreads along the venous system, often from a wound infection.
24. The symptoms of postpartum depression differ from those of postpartum "blues" by the number, intensity, and persistence of symptoms, which are intensely and persistently present for at least 2 weeks. These symptoms include a loss of interest in one's surroundings and a loss of a woman's usual emotional response to her family. The woman may also have feelings of unworthiness, guilt, and shame.
25. Nurses can demonstrate care, provide anticipatory guidance, help the mother verbalize her feelings, and make appropriate referrals.
26. Postpartum psychosis usually requires hospitalization, psychotherapy, and appropriate medication.

## Chapter 29

1. Poor women are at risk for preterm birth because they may have impaired general health and may receive little or no prenatal care.
2. Preterm infants appear frail and weak and are small, with limp extremities, poor muscle tone, red skin, and immature ears, nipples, areola, and genitals.
3. Factors that increase respiratory problems in preterm infants include lack of surfactant, poor cough reflex, small air passages, and weak muscles.
4. Nursing responsibilities for preterm infants with respiratory problems include working with respiratory therapists to manage equipment, monitoring the infant's changing oxygen needs, positioning infants to promote drainage, and suctioning.
5. Nurses wean infants to the open crib by making gradual changes in the environmental temperature, dressing the infant, and using blankets and a hat when the infant is out of the incubator.
6. To measure intake and output for infants, all fluids, intravenous and oral, including medications, are measured. Diapers are weighed to calculate urine output.
7. Preterm infants' kidneys do not concentrate or dilute urine well, and they have large insensible water losses. They lack passive antibodies from the mother and have an immature immune system. Pain causes physiologic responses such as vital signs changes and decreases in oxygenation.
8. The nurse can diminish overstimulation by organizing care to provide for rest periods, reduce environmental stimuli, minimize pain, and discuss the plan of care with others.
9. Feeding tolerance is assessed by checking gastric residual before gavage feedings, measuring abdominal girth, testing stools for reducing substances and blood, and observing for regurgitation. During nipple feedings, the nurse watches for signs of respiratory difficulty, decreased oxygenation, and fatigue.
10. The nurse can help breastfeeding mothers of preterm infants by teaching them how to pump and store milk and breastfeeding techniques adapted to the preterm's needs and by providing support and encouragement.
11. The nurse can help parents feel comfortable with preterm infants by providing warm support, realistic encouragement, and information about the neonatal intensive care unit environ-

ment, the infant's condition and characteristics, and the equipment and care.

12. Helping parents take on partial responsibility for care, beginning early in hospitalization, and gradually increasing their responsibility will help them prepare for discharge of their infant.
13. Postmature infants may be thin, have loose skin folds, cracked and peeling skin, minimal vernix or lanugo, and meconium staining. They look hyperalert and worried.
14. Postmature infants may have polycythemia, meconium aspiration, hypoglycemia, and poor temperature regulation.
15. In symmetric growth restriction, all body parts are proportionately small. In asymmetric growth restriction, the head is normal in size but seems large for the small body.
16. Large-for-gestational age infants may have birth injuries, such as fractures, nerve damage, cephalhematoma, hypoglycemia, or polycythemia.

## Chapter 30

1. Asphyxia before or during birth may cause meconium aspiration, apnea, acidosis, failure of the ductus arteriosus and foramen ovale to close, brain damage, and death.
2. The nurse's role in asphyxia is to begin resuscitation promptly, assist the team, and provide follow-up and parental support.
3. Transient tachypnea of the newborn is caused by failure of fetal lung fluid to be absorbed completely in full-term or preterm infants. Respiratory distress syndrome occurs in preterm infants as a result of inadequate surfactant.
4. Meconium in amniotic fluid enters the lungs before birth or is drawn in during the first breaths after birth, causing obstruction, air trapping, and inflammation.
5. When meconium-stained amniotic fluid is seen during labor, the nurse must notify the physician, prepare equipment, assist with intubation, and observe for infection or other problems.
6. Jaundice is considered pathologic when it occurs in the first 24 hours of life or continues beyond the second week of life, when total bilirubin is above 12 mg/dl in full term infants or 10–14 mg/dl in preterm infants, or it rises more than 5 mg/dl in 24 hours.
7. In caring for infants receiving phototherapy, the nurse must prevent cold stress, hypoglycemia, inadequate intake, and injury due to improper use of lights. Monitoring for complications is also important.
8. Vertical infection is transmitted from the mother to the infant during pregnancy or birth. Horizontal infection is transmitted from other people to the infant after birth.
9. The role of the nurse in sepsis is to identify early signs, notify the physician, coordinate treatment, observe for change, and support the family.
10. Problems of infants of diabetic mothers include congenital anomalies, macrosomia or intrauterine growth restriction, respiratory distress syndrome, hypoglycemia, hypocalcemia, and polycythemia.
11. Care of the infant of a diabetic mother includes identifying complications, performing glucose screenings, providing early feedings, and supporting parents.
12. Infants who are exposed to drugs in utero are subject to congenital defects, neonatal abstinence syndrome, behavior and feeding problems, failure to gain weight, and abnormal social interaction.
13. Infants with neonatal abstinence syndrome need decreased environmental stimuli and assistance with feeding. Their mothers need help with bonding and learning to care for them.
14. Cyanotic heart defects allow unoxygenated blood flow into the systemic circulation, producing cyanosis. Acyanotic heart defects cause impairment of blood flow or circulation of oxygenated blood into the pulmonary system, usually without cyanosis. Other categories are by blood flow in which there is increased or decreased pulmonary blood flow, obstruction to blood flow, or mixing of venous and oxygenated blood.

## Chapter 31

1. Almost all contraceptive methods are used by women, and failure will affect them most.
2. The nurse's role in helping women with contraception is to provide information so that women can choose appropriately and use contraceptives correctly.
3. Important considerations in choosing contraceptive techniques include safety, protection from sexually transmissible diseases, effectiveness, convenience, education needed, side effects, interference with spontaneity, availability, expense, preference of the woman and her partner, and culture.
4. Sterilization, hormonal contraceptives, and intrauterine devices require signed informed consents.
5. Incorrect beliefs adolescents may have are that

they cannot conceive during first intercourse, without orgasm, or without having menstruated a certain length of time or that douching will prevent pregnancy.

6. Adolescents may not seek contraception because they may fear lack of acceptance, loss of sexual privacy, pelvic examination, or that contraception will affect their health adversely.
7. The nurse can increase teaching effectiveness with adolescents by showing sensitivity to their feelings, being accepting, and providing extensive teaching without hurry, using understandable terms and audiovisual materials.
8. Women can conceive until menstruation has ceased for 2 years, but pregnancy is rare after age 50. Perimenopausal women who do not smoke and have no other contraindications can use any method of contraception.
9. Important factors to consider when choosing a method of sterilization include time involved, cost, need for hospitalization, and feelings of each partner about a permanent end to having more children.
10. Hormonal contraceptives alter normal hormone changes, preventing ovulation, altering the endometrium, and making the cervical mucus unfavorable to sperm.
11. Education for women choosing intrauterine devices includes information about side effects, when and how to check the strings, and when to seek medical treatment.
12. Barrier methods kill sperm and prevent them from entering the cervix.
13. Natural family planning methods avoid drugs, chemicals, and devices; are inexpensive; and are acceptable to most religions. However, couples need extensive education and high motivation, and they risk pregnancy if they make an error.

## Chapter 32

1. Infertility is strictly defined as the inability to conceive after 1 year of unprotected regular intercourse. Primary infertility is that which occurs in couples who have never conceived; secondary infertility occurs in those who have conceived before and are not able to conceive again.
2. The normal average number of sperm released at ejaculation is 400 million. Twenty million per ml is probably the minimum required for unassisted fertility. At least half of the sperm must be normal, have normal forward movement, and be living. The seminal fluid should liquefy within 30 minutes and should have few white blood cells.
3. Erection problems exist if the man cannot initiate and maintain a penile erection that is sufficient to deposit seminal fluid, with its sperm, near the woman's cervix. Ejaculation abnormalities may result from retrograde ejaculation, hypospadias, or abnormal ejaculation response (premature, slow, or absent).
4. Abnormalities of the sperm, ejaculation, or the seminal fluid can result from many factors, such as systemic illness, infections or abnormalities of the reproductive tract, exposure to toxins, excessive alcohol consumption, illicit drug use, elevated scrotal temperature, obstruction, and immunologic factors.
5. Abnormal ovulation can occur because of hormone disruptions caused by cranial tumors, stress, obesity, anorexia, systemic disease, and abnormalities in the ovaries or other endocrine glands.
6. Ovulation disorders are often associated with abnormal menstrual periods because hormone abnormalities associated with the ovulation problem interfere with normal buildup and decline of the endometrium. Menstrual periods may be absent, scant, or very heavy.
7. Fallopian tube obstruction may be caused by scarring or adhesions secondary to infections, endometriosis, or pelvic surgery. Congenital anomalies of the reproductive structures can also cause mechanical interference with successful pregnancy.
8. Abnormal cervical mucus can trap sperm and prevent them from entering the uterus and fallopian tube or prevent their preparation (capacitation) for fertilization.
9. Anatomic abnormalities of the woman's reproductive tract may prevent normal implantation or prevent normal placental or fetal growth.
10. Endocrine abnormalities associated with repeated pregnancy loss include inadequate progesterone secretion, inadequate endometrial response to progesterone, hypothyroidism and hyperthyroidism, and maternal diabetes.
11. Immunologic causes of repeated pregnancy loss include an intolerance of the conceptus' foreign tissue and lupus erythematosus.
12. Elements included in the history and physical examination include a reproductive history, past medical history, examination for undiagnosed endocrine disturbances, tumors, chronic disease, and abnormalities of the reproductive organs. Chromosome analysis is sometimes done.
13. Medications used to induce ovulation include clomiphene citrate, chorionic gonadotropin, go-

nadotropic-releasing hormone, menotropins, and urofollitropin. Clomiphene is a common drug for this purpose.

14. Screening tests related to donor sperm use include those for blood type and Rh factor, possible genetic defects, and infection. In addition, the man's history, physical examination, and lifestyle are reviewed for possible problems that might not be revealed by standard tests. Donor sperm is frozen for 6 months to allow identification of infections or other problems that may not have been evident at the time of collection.
15. In vitro fertilization mixes the male and female gametes outside the body and places embryos back into the uterus. Gamete intrafallopian transfer places the ova and sperm into the fallopian tubes, where fertilization takes place. Tubal embryo transfer mixes male and female gametes and places the fertilized ova into the fallopian tubes.
16. Factors couples consider when seeking infertility help include their age, the length of their attempt to conceive, their desire for a biologic child, and their feelings about adoption or a child-free life. Financial constraints are often another consideration.
17. When deciding about infertility evaluations and treatments, the couple considers their social, cultural, and religious values; how difficult treatment may be; the probability of success with treatment; and financial concerns.
18. Psychological reactions to infertility include guilt, isolation, depression, and stress on the relationship.
19. Parenthood after infertility may be marked by anxiety about the pregnancy, loss of support from infertile couples, and unrealistic expectations about their parenting abilities.
20. Couples considering adoption must confront their personal preferences, limitations, and prejudices.
21. Couples who lose a pregnancy after a period of infertility often experience grief, but sometimes the grief is mixed with optimism because they were able to achieve pregnancy.

## Chapter 33

1. Family history is an important part of a health history to assess risk factors for conditions such as heart disease, breast and colon cancer, and osteoporosis.
2. When taking a sexual history, the nurse should ask about sexual activity, number of partners, age when sexual activity began, method of contraception, and knowledge and practice of measures to protect self from sexually transmissible diseases (STDs).
3. Three screening procedures for cancer of the breast are breast self-examination, professional breast examination, and mammography.
4. Vulvar self-examination is recommended to detect signs of precancerous conditions or infections.
5. A Pap test is a smear of the superficial layers of the cervix and endocervix to detect precancerous and cancerous cells of the cervix.
6. Fecal occult blood testing is important to detect colon or rectal cancer.
7. Additional screening tests include tests for STDs, rubella antibodies, cholesterol, thyroid function test, transvaginal ultrasonography and CA 125, and a sigmoidoscopy or colonoscopy. These tests are recommended for women with increased risk for a specific condition.
8. Medical treatment of fibrocystic breast changes is rare because side effects of the drugs may be more distressing than the breast discomfort. If drugs are used, they may include progesterone, tamoxifen, or bromocriptine.
9. Ultrasound examination, needle aspiration biopsy, or surgical biopsy is used to determine whether a breast disorder is benign or malignant.
10. The major risk factors for breast cancer are gender (female), age (increases with age), and prior history of breast cancer.
11. Staging of breast cancer is important to determine the extent of the breast cancer and to plan appropriate therapy.
12. Adjuvant therapy is supportive or additional therapy recommended following surgery to improve the chance of long-term survival.
13. Breasts may be reconstructed during the initial surgery or later. Two major methods are the tissue expansion method and autogenous grafts.
14. Preoperative teaching should include a description of the pressure dressing, portable suction apparatus, the wound, and any special exercises that may be recommended.
15. Discharge planning should emphasize the need for follow-up care, side effects of adjuvant therapy, and signs and symptoms that should be reported to the physician. Referral to local groups may also be helpful.
16. Primary amenorrhea describes menstruation that fails to occur by the age of 14 to 16 years; causes include hormonal imbalances, congenital anomalies, chromosomal defects, and systemic diseases as well as rigorous dieting and

exercise; treatment is aimed at identifying and treating the underlying cause.

Secondary amenorrhea describes cessation of menstruation for a period of at least 6 months in a woman who has an established pattern of menstruation; additional causes include use of drugs such as oral contraceptives, phenothiazines, and antihypertensives; once pregnancy is ruled out, treatment may include hormonal replacement therapy and ovulation stimulation.

17. Possible causes of abnormal uterine bleeding include systemic diseases, uterine myomas, cervical polyps, genital infections, or cancer of the cervix or uterus, which must be investigated before diagnosis and treatment can be initiated.
18. Primary dysmenorrhea is caused by excessive endometrial prostaglandin that diffuses into endometrial tissue, causing abnormal uterine contractions, uterine ischemia, and tissue hypoxia. Effective treatment includes rest, application of warmth, oral contraceptives, and prostaglandin inhibitors.
19. Endometriosis lesions grow and proliferate during the follicular and luteal phases of the menstrual cycle and then slough during menstruation. The menstruation from endometriosis lesions occurs in a closed cavity, which causes pressure and pain on adjacent tissue. Endometriosis is often treated by interrupting the menstrual cycle and thus preventing bleeding into the pelvic cavity.
20. Side effects of danazol include headache, dizziness, irritability, decreased libido, and masculinizing effects. Most common side effects of GnRH are hot flashes, vaginal dryness, decreased libido, and loss of bone mineral density.
21. Symptoms of premenstrual syndrome (PMS) must be cyclic and recur in the luteal phase of the menstrual cycle; the woman should be symptom free during the follicular phase, and there must be at least 7 symptom-free days during the cycle; symptoms must be severe enough to alter the lifestyle of the woman.
22. Edema, weight gain, and bloating are the most common physical symptoms of PMS. Anxiety, depression, and irritability are the most common behavioral symptoms.
23. Lifestyle changes to reduce the symptoms of PMS include decreased consumption of caffeine, simple sugars, and salty foods; drinking at least 2000 ml of water per day; avoiding alcohol; eating six small meals per day to prevent hypoglycemia; increasing exercise; and using stress management techniques.
24. Menopause is called the "change of life" because physical changes are accompanied by psychological and social changes, and the woman must come to terms with aging.
25. Without estrogen the reproductive organs begin to atrophy; the vagina and labia are thinner and more fragile.
26. Depression, mood swings, and irritability are the most common psychological symptoms of menopause.
27. Hormonal replacement controls hot flashes, alleviates genital atrophy, and protects against coronary heart disease and osteoporosis.
28. Osteoporosis is called the "silent thief" because there are no signs or symptoms until fractures occur.
29. Osteoporosis can be prevented by hormonal replacement therapy, calcium supplementation, and weight-bearing exercise.
30. Nurses can help women with osteoporosis prevent falls by making their environment as safe as possible.
31. With a cystocele, the weakened upper anterior wall of the vagina cannot support the weight of urine, and the bladder protrudes downward into the vagina, resulting in incomplete emptying of the bladder and consequent cystitis and stress incontinence. With a rectocele, the rectum protrudes into the vagina as the upper posterior wall of the vagina becomes weakened, which may result in difficulty emptying the rectum.
32. Uterine prolapse is caused when the cardinal ligaments are unduly stretched during pregnancy and do not return to normal. This condition generally is treated surgically according to severity.
33. Pelvic exercises and bladder training may alleviate symptoms of pelvic floor relaxation and urinary incontinence. Additional measures include teaching about the need to maintain hydration, restrict alcohol and caffeine, and use of commercial products to protect the skin and prevent odor.
34. Symptoms of leiomyomas are increased uterine size and excessive vaginal bleeding. Treatment depends on size and symptoms and may include removal of the fibroid or hysterectomy.
35. Ultrasound is used to distinguish a fluid-filled ovarian cyst from a solid tumor, which necessitates additional evaluation.
36. Signs and symptoms that suggest cancer of the reproductive organs are irregular vaginal bleeding, unexplained postmenopausal bleeding, unusual vaginal discharge, dyspareunia, persistent vaginal itching, elevated or discolored le-

sions of the vulva, abdominal bloating, persistent constipation, anorexia, and nausea.

37. Cancer of the cervix can be treated by cryosurgery, destruction of tissue by laser, loop electrodiathermy excision, or surgical conization.
38. Pregnancy, diabetes mellitus, oral contraceptive use, and antibiotic therapy may result in vaginitis.
39. Candidiasis causes a thick, white ("cottage cheese") discharge, whereas trichomoniasis causes a thin, malodorous, greenish-yellow discharge.
40. Barrier methods of contraception (particularly condoms) prevent potentially infected ejaculate from entering the genital tract.
41. The major symptom of primary syphilis is a painless chancre that disappears in about 6 weeks; the disease is highly infectious at this time. Symptoms of secondary syphilis are enlargement of the liver and spleen, headache, anorexia, and skin rash. Condylomata lata that contain numerous spirochetes and are highly contagious may develop.
42. Condylomata acuminata (genital warts) are caused by human papillomavirus (HPV), which is increasingly associated with cervical intraepithelial neoplasia (CIN).
43. *Staphylococcus aureus* causes toxic shock syndrome.
44. The risk of toxic shock syndrome can be reduced by changing tampons every 1 to 4 hours, avoiding use of superabsorbent tampons, using pads rather than tampons during hours of sleep, and careful hand washing before as well as after inserting tampons or changing perineal pads.

# Index

Note: Page numbers followed by f refer to illustrations; page numbers followed by t refer to tables, and those followed by d refer to displayed material.

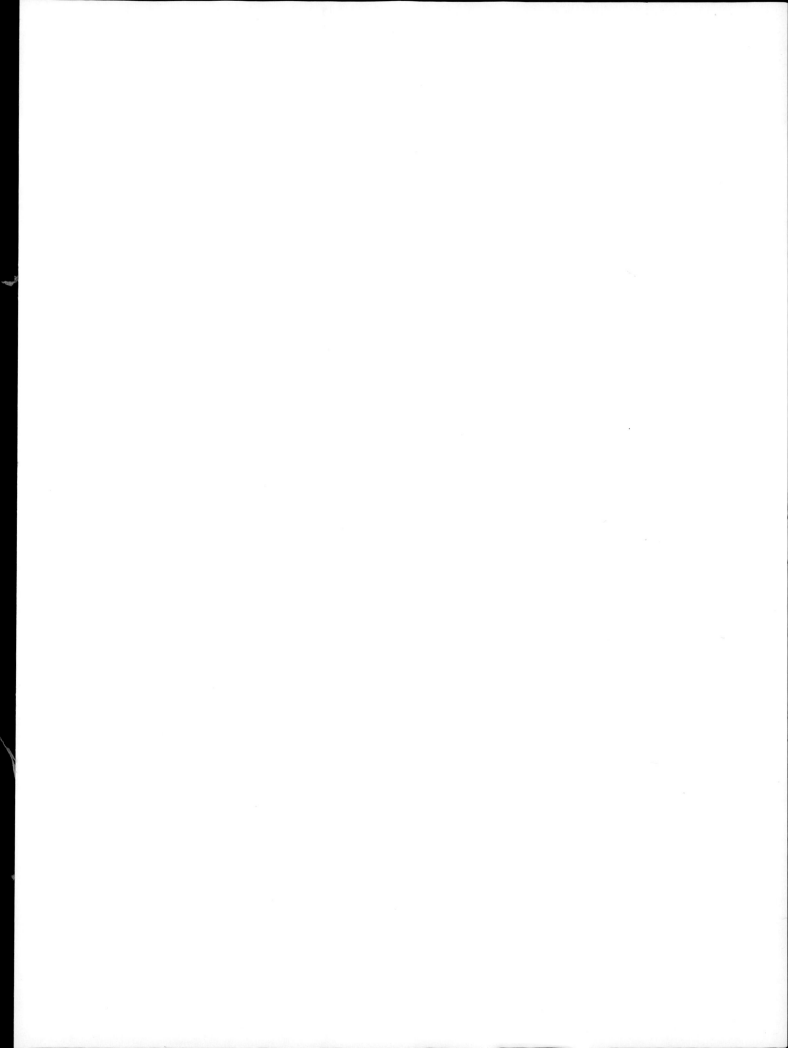